T3-AKE-751

Textbook of

DIAGNOSTIC IMAGING

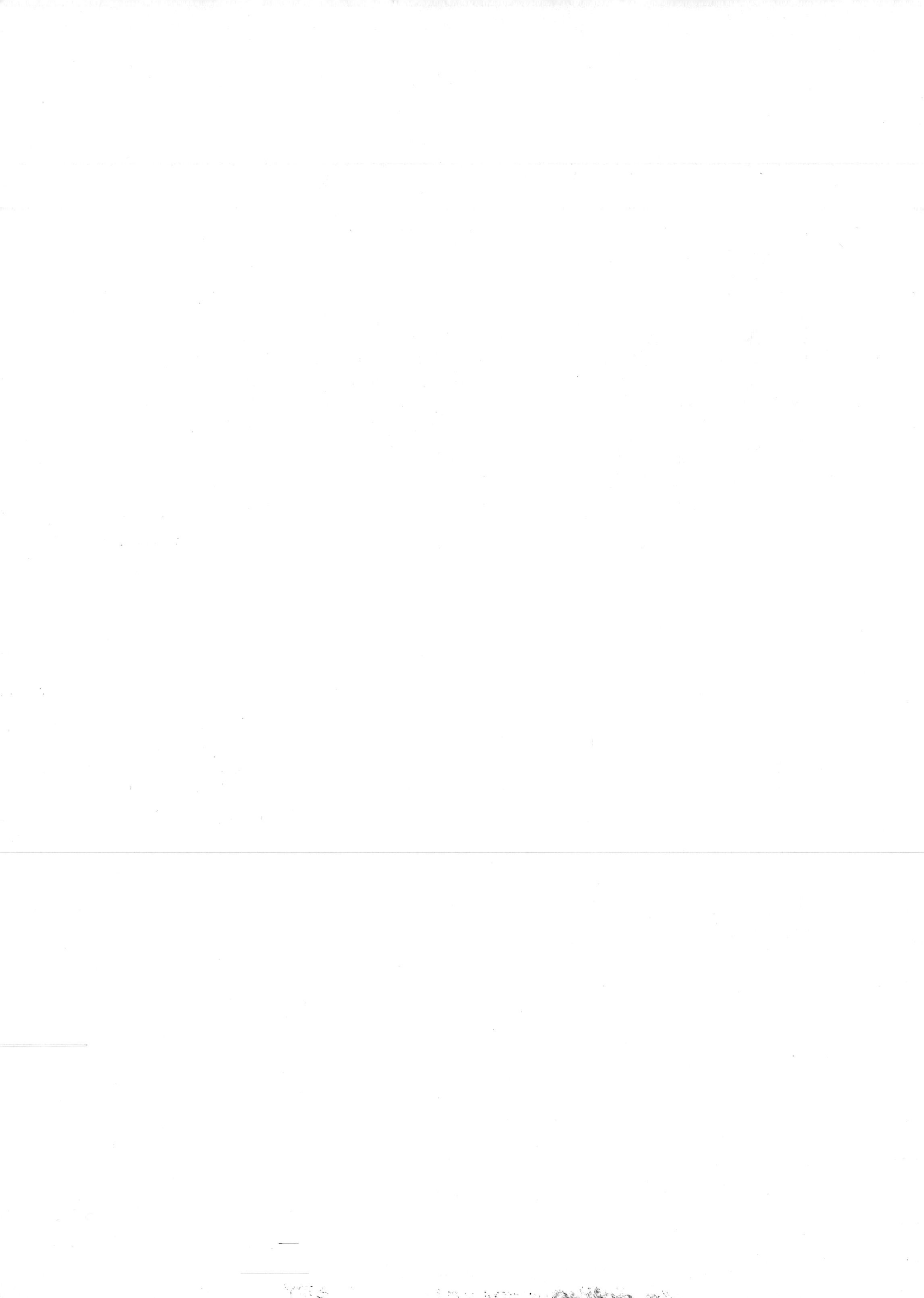

Textbook of DIAGNOSTIC IMAGING

SECOND EDITION

Volume 2

CHARLES E. PUTMAN, M.D.
Executive Vice President for Duke University
James B. Duke Professor of Radiology
and Professor of Medicine
Vice Provost for Research and Development
Duke University Medical Center
Durham, North Carolina

CARL E. RAVIN, M.D.
Professor and Chairman
Department of Radiology
Duke University Medical Center
Durham, North Carolina

W.B. SAUNDERS COMPANY
A Division of Harcourt Brace & Company
Philadelphia London Toronto Montreal Sydney Tokyo

W.B. SAUNDERS COMPANY
A Division of
Harcourt Brace & Company

The Curtis Center
Independence Square West
Philadelphia, Pennsylvania 19106

Library of Congress Cataloging-in-Publication Data

Textbook of diagnostic imaging / [edited by] Charles E. Putman, Carl E. Ravin.—2nd ed.

p. cm.

Includes bibliographical references and index.

ISBN 0–7216–3697–7 (set)

1. Diagnostic imaging. I. Putman, Charles E. (Charles Edgar). II. Ravin, Carl E.

[DNLM: 1. Diagnostic Imaging. WN 100 T3545 1994]

RC78.7.D53T49 1994

616.07′54—dc20

DNLM/DLC
for Library of Congress 94–4061
CIP

TEXTBOOK OF DIAGNOSTIC IMAGING 2/E

Volume 1 ISBN 0–7216–3698–5
Volume 2 ISBN 0–7216–3699–3
Two Volume Set ISBN 0–7216–3697–7

Printed in the United States of America.

Last digit is the print number: 9 8 7 6 5 4 3 2 1

To our Residents, Medical Students, and Fellows,
whose enthusiasm, energy, and eagerness to learn
provided the inspiration for this book;
and to our wives, Mary and Alison,
and our children, Cammie, Shannon, Garrett, David, Adam, and Todd,
without whose patience, understanding, and continued support
this project could not have been completed

EDITORS

James D. Bowie, M.D.
Professor of Radiology, Director of Radiology Education, Duke University Medical Center, Durham, North Carolina
IMAGING THE FEMALE PATIENT

N. Reed Dunnick, M.D.
Professor and Chair, Department of Radiology, University of Michigan, Ann Arbor, Michigan
GENITOURINARY SYSTEM

William R. Hendee, Ph.D.
Senior Associate Dean for Research and Vice President for Technology, Medical College of Wisconsin, Milwaukee, Wisconsin
FUNDAMENTALS OF DIAGNOSTIC IMAGING

Michael J. Kelley, M.D.
Clinical Associate Professor of Radiology, Department of Radiology, Duke University Medical Center, Durham, North Carolina; Staff Radiologist, Department of Radiology, Carolinas Medical Center, Charlotte, North Carolina
CARDIOVASCULAR SYSTEM

Thomas L. Lawson, M.D.
Professor and Chairman, Department of Radiology, Loyola University Chicago, Stritch School of Medicine; Loyola University Medical Center and Foster McGaw Hospital, Loyola University Chicago, Maywood, Illinois
GASTROINTESTINAL SYSTEM

B. J. Manaster, M.D., Ph.D.
Professor of Radiology, University of Utah School of Medicine; Radiologist–Staff Physician, University of Utah Medical Center and Salt Lake City Veterans Administration Medical Center, Salt Lake City, Utah
MUSCULOSKELETAL SYSTEM

Charles E. Putman, M.D.
Executive Vice President for Duke University, James B. Duke Professor of Radiology and Professor of Medicine, Vice Provost for Research and Development, Duke University Medical Center, Durham, North Carolina
PULMONARY SYSTEM

Carl E. Ravin, M.D.
Professor and Chairman, Department of Radiology, Duke University Medical Center, Durham, North Carolina
PULMONARY SYSTEM

Charles M. Strother, M.D.
Professor, University of Wisconsin Medical School; Professor of Radiology, Neurology and Neurosurgery, University of Wisconsin Hospital and Clinics, Madison, Wisconsin
CENTRAL NERVOUS SYSTEM

Daniel C. Sullivan, M.D.
Associate Professor of Radiology, Department of Radiology, Duke University Medical Center, Durham, North Carolina
THE BREAST

CONTRIBUTORS

Amjad Ali, M.D.
Associate Professor, Rush Medical College; Associate Attending, Rush-Presbyterian-St. Luke's Medical Center, Chicago, Illinois
Radiology of Renal Transplantation

E. Stephen Amis, Jr., M.D.
Professor of Radiology, The Albert Einstein College of Medicine; Chairman, Department of Radiology, Albert Einstein College of Medicine and Montefiore Medical Center, Bronx, New York
The Prostate

Carol L. Andrews, M.D.
Department of Radiology, University of Utah; Housestaff, University of Utah Medical Center, Salt Lake City, Utah
Imaging Modalities; Tumor and Tumor-Like Conditions: Musculoskeletal Tumor Imaging; Tumor-Like Lesions

Yong Ho Auh, M.D.
Professor and Chairman of Radiology, Department of Radiology, Asan Medical Center–Ulsan University, Seoul, Korea
Normal Computed Tomographic Anatomy of the Pelvis with Ultrasound and MRI Correlations

Mark E. Baker, M.D.
Associate Professor of Radiology, Duke University Medical Center; Chief, Section of Abdominal Imaging, Duke University Medical Center, Durham, North Carolina
Postpartum Sonography

Dennis M. Balfe, M.D.
Professor of Radiology, Washington University School of Medicine; Chief of Gastrointestinal Radiology, Barnes Hospital, St. Louis, Missouri
The Pharynx; The Esophagus

Marc P. Banner, M.D.
Professor of Radiology, University of Pennsylvania School of Medicine; Director of Uroradiology, University of Pennsylvania Medical Center, Philadelphia, Pennsylvania
Urolithiasis and Nephrocalcinosis

Claire E. Bender, M.D.
Assistant Professor of Diagnostic Radiology, Mayo Medical School; Consultant, Diagnostic Radiology, Mayo Clinic Rochester, Rochester, Minnesota
The Gallbladder

Michael E. Bernardino, M.D.
Professor of University Radiology, Emory University School of Medicine; Director, Abdominal Division and Magnetic Resonance Imaging, Emory Hospital, Atlanta, Georgia
The Liver and Spleen

Kenneth Bird, M.D.
Associate Clinical Professor of Diagnostic Radiology, Yale University School of Medicine, New Haven, Connecticut; Senior Attending Radiologist, Middlesex Memorial Hospital, Middletown, Connecticut
Scrotal Imaging

Morton A. Bosniak, M.D.
Professor of Radiology and Urology, Chief, Uroradiology Section, New York University School of Medicine, New York, New York
Nonfunctioning Adrenal Masses; Benign Renal Tumors; Renal Lymphoma and Metastatic Disease to the Kidneys

Richard A. Bowerman, M.D.
Associate Professor of Radiology, University of Michigan School of Medicine; University of Michigan Hospitals, Ann Arbor, Michigan
Ultrasound Imaging of Normal Fetal Anatomy

James D. Bowie, M.D.
Professor of Radiology, Director of Radiology Education, Duke University Medical Center, Durham, North Carolina
IMAGING THE FEMALE PATIENT
Miscellaneous Fetal Abnormalities; General Obstetric Sonography

Jeffrey C. Brandon, M.D.
Assistant Professor in Residence, University of California Irvine, Irvine, California
The Duodenum

Michael N. Brant Zawadzki, M.D.
Clinical Professor, Department of Radiology, School of Medicine, Stanford University, Stanford, California; Chairman, Department of Radiology, Director of MRI, Hoag Memorial Hospital, Newport Beach, California
Imaging of Spine Trauma

Ethan M. Braunstein, M.D.
Professor of Radiology and Adjunct Professor of Anthropology, Indiana University Hospital, Indianapolis, Indiana
Arthropathies: The Spondyloarthropathies

Patricia E. Burrows, M.D., F.R.C.P.(C.)
Associate Professor, Harvard Medical School; Staff Radiologist, Chief, Section of Vascular/Interventional Radiology, Children's Hospital, Boston, Massachusetts
Congenital Cardiovascular Disease

William J. Burtis, M.D.
Associate Professor of Medicine, Yale University School of Medicine, New Haven, Connecticut; Acting Chief of Metabolism, West Haven Veterans Administration Hospital, West Haven, Connecticut; Staff Physician, Yale–New Haven Hospital, New Haven, Connecticut
Basic Principles (Musculoskeletal System): Bone Metabolism; Metabolic Disorders: Osteoporosis

William H. Bush, Jr., M.D., F.A.C.R.
Professor, Department of Radiology, University of Washington School of Medicine; Director of Genitourinary Radiology, University of Washington Medical Center, Seattle, Washington
Stone Therapy: Extracorporeal Lithotripsy and Percutaneous Techniques

Alan V. Cadkin, M.D.
Director of Ultrasound, Division of Reproductive Endocrinology, Department of Obstetrics and Gynecology, Illinois Masonic Medical Center, Chicago, Illinois
Normal First Trimester

Peter W. Callen, M.D.
Professor of Radiology, Obstetrics-Gynecology, University of California San Francisco, San Francisco, California
Fetal Skeletal Abnormalities

Frank E. Carroll, Jr., M.D., F.A.C.R.
Associate Professor of Radiology and Radiologic Sciences, Vanderbilt University School of Medicine; Chief, Chest Radiology, Vanderbilt University Medical Center, Nashville, Tennessee
Chest Wall and Hemidiaphragm

Robert J. Cassling, M.D.
Assistant Clinical Professor of Radiological Sciences, University of California, Los Angeles, UCLA School of Medicine; Attending Physician, UCLA Medical Center, Los Angeles, California
Conventional and Digital Angiography of the Peripheral Vascular System; Diseases of the Peripheral Vascular System

James T. T. Chen, M.D.
Professor of Radiology, Duke University School of Medicine; Senior Staff, Department of Radiology, Duke University Medical Center, Durham, North Carolina
Chest Radiography and Cardiac Fluoroscopy; Cardiac Pacemakers and Prosthetic Valves

Caroline Chiles, M.D.
Associate Professor of Radiology, Bowman Gray School of Medicine–Wake Forest University, Winston-Salem, North Carolina
Alveolar Disease in the Adult

Michael R. Clair, M.D.
Co-Director of Cross Sectional Imaging and Director of Ultrasound, Fox Chase Cancer Center and Jeanes Hospital, Philadelphia, Pennsylvania
Benign Ovarian Disease

Richard L. Clark, M.D.
Professor of Radiology and Vice-Chair for Research, Department of Radiology, University of North Carolina School of Medicine; Attending Radiologist, University of North Carolina Hospitals, Chapel Hill, North Carolina; Consultant, Dorothea Dix Hospital, Raleigh, North Carolina
Vascular Diseases of the Kidney; Bladder Cancer

R. Edward Coleman, M.D.
Professor of Radiology and Director of Nuclear Medicine, Duke University Medical Center, Durham, North Carolina
Radionuclide Cardiac Imaging; Coronary Artery Disease: Radionuclide Evaluation

Robert O. Cone, M.D.
Clinical Assistant Professor, Department of Radiology, University of Texas; Staff

Physician, St. Luke's Hospital and South Texas Methodist Hospital, San Antonio, Texas
Arhthropathies: Degenerative Joint Disease

Cirrelda Cooper, M.D.
Assistant Professor, Georgetown University Hospital, Washington, DC
Malignant Ovarian Masses

Daniel L. Crosby, M.D.
Assistant Professor of Radiology, The University of Iowa; Faculty Neuroradiologist, The University of Iowa Hospital and Clinics, Iowa City, Iowa
Imaging of Spine Trauma

Nancy S. Curry, M.D.
Associate Professor (Director, Genitourinary Section), Department of Radiology, Medical University of South Carolina; Medical University Hospital, Ralph H. Johnson VA Medical Center, and Charleston Memorial Hospital, Charleston, South Carolina
Interventional Techniques

Anne McB. Curtis, M.D.
Professor, Diagnostic Radiology, Chief, Chest Radiology, Yale University School of Medicine; Chief, Chest Radiology, Yale–New Haven Hospital, New Haven, Connecticut
Adult Respiratory Distress Syndrome; Drug-Induced Lung Disease

Murray K. Dalinka, M.D.
Professor of Radiology, University of Pennsylvania; Staff Radiologist, University of Pennsylvania Hospital, Philadelphia, Pennsylvania
Infectious Diseases

David L. Daniels, M.D.
Professor of Radiology, Section of Neuroradiology, Medical College of Wisconsin; Radiologist, Milwaukee County Medical Complex, Froedtert Memorial Lutheran Hospital; Consultant in Radiology, VA Medical Center, Milwaukee, Wisconsin
Normal Anatomy of the Brain; Spinal Anatomy; Normal Anatomy of the Orbits

Lane A. Deyoe, M.D.
Instructor in Radiology, Washington University School of Medicine, Mallinckrodt Institute of Radiology; Fellow in Radiology, Barnes Hospital, St. Louis, Missouri
The Pharynx; The Esophagus

Anthony J. Doyle, B.Sc., M.B., Ch.B.
Assistant Professor, Radiology, University of Utah, Salt Lake City, Utah
Musculoskeletal Trauma

N. Reed Dunnick, M.D.
Professor and Chair, Department of Radiology, University of Michigan, Ann Arbor, Michigan
GENITOURINARY SYSTEM
Functional Lesions of the Adrenal Cortex; Primary Renal Carcinoma; The Prostate

F. Marc Edwards, Ph.D.
Clinical Professor of Radiology, University of Missouri–Kansas City; Radiological Physicist, St. Luke's Hospital of Kansas City, Kansas City, Missouri
Risks of Medical Imaging

Eric L. Effman, M.D.
Professor, University of Washington; Director, Department of Radiology, Children's Hospital and Medical Center, Seattle, Washington
Pediatric Chest Diseases

Dieter R. Enzmann, M.D.
Professor of Radiology, Stanford University Medical Center, Stanford, California
Central Nervous System Infections

Charles J. Fagan, M.D.
Professor of Radiology, Director of Body CT and Ultrasound, University of Texas Medical Branch; John Sealy Hospital and University of Texas Medical Branch Hospitals, Galveston, Texas
Hysterosalpingography

Michael P. Federle, M.D.
Professor of Radiology, University of Pittsburgh Medical Center, Pittsburgh, Pennsylvania
The Peritoneal Cavity

Arthur C. Fleischer, M.D.
Professor, Departments of Radiology and Obstetrics/Gynecology, Vanderbilt University Medical Center, Nashville, Tennessee
Gynecologic Sonography

Olof Flodmark, M.D., Ph.D., F.R.C.P.(C.)
Associate Professor, Department of Neuroradiology, Karolinska Institute; Director, Department of Neuroradiology, Karolinska Hospital, Stockholm, Sweden
Hydrocephalus

D. M. Forrester, M.D.
Associate Professor of Radiology, Medicine and Orthopedics, University of Southern California; Los Angeles County–USC Medical Center, Harbor-UCLA, Los Angeles, California
Arthropathies: General Approach to Joint Disease

Patrick C. Freeny, M.D.
Professor, University of Washington School of Medicine; Professor and Director, Abdominal Imaging, CT/MR, University of Washington School of Medicine, Department of Radiology, Seattle, Washington
The Pancreas

Gary D. Fullerton, Ph.D.
Professor of Radiology, University of Texas Health Science Center at San Antonio; Staff Physicist, Medical Center Hospital, San Antonio, Texas
Transmission Imaging: Computed Tomography

R. Kristina Gedgaudas-McClees, M.D.
Clinical Professor of Radiology, Emory University School of Medicine; Staff Radiologist, St. Joseph's Hospital, Atlanta, Georgia
The Liver and Spleen

Robert A. Gelfand, M.D.
Associate Clinical Professor of Medicine, Yale University School of Medicine; Attending Physician, Yale–New Haven Hospital, New Haven, Connecticut
Endocrine Disorders: Pituitary; Adrenal; Thyroid

Nancy B. Genieser, M.D.
Professor of Radiology, New York University School of Medicine; Attending Radiologist, New York University Medical Center, Bellevue Hospital Center; Consultant Pediatric Radiologist, Manhattan Veterans Administration Medical Center, New York, New York
Diseases of the Airways

Lindell R. Gentry, M.D.
Associate Professor of Radiology, University of Wisconsin Hospital and Clinics, Madison, Wisconsin
Normal Facial Anatomy; Facial Trauma

Seth N. Glick, M.D.
Professor of Radiology, Hahnemann Hospital, Philadelphia, Pennsylvania
The Duodenum

J. David Godwin, M.D.
Professor of Radiology, University of Washington, Seattle, Washington
Pleural Disease

Stanford M. Goldman, M.D.
Chairman and Professor of Radiology, University of Texas Medical School at Houston; Chief of Radiology, Hermann Hospital, Houston, Texas
Renal Infection

Antoinette S. Gomes, M.D.
Associate Professor, Radiological Sciences and Medicine, University of California, Los Angeles, UCLA School of Medicine; Chief, Cardiovascular Radiology, UCLA Medical Center, Los Angeles, California
Conventional and Digital Angiography of the Peripheral Vascular System; Diseases of the Peripheral Vascular System

Lawrence R. Goodman, M.D.
Professor of Radiology, Head of Thoracic Radiology, Medical College of Wisconsin, Milwaukee, Wisconsin
Chest Trauma

Lawrence P. Gordon, M.D.
Associate Professor of Pathology, State University of New York Health Science Center at Syracuse; Staff Pathologist, Crouse Irving Memorial Hospital, Syracuse, New York
Ultrasound of the Placenta

Michael T. Gorey, M.D.
Assistant Professor of Clinical Radiology, Northwestern University Medical School, Chicago, Illinois; Associate Attending, Evanston Hospital, Evanston, Illinois
Congenital Anomalies of the Spine and Spinal Cord

Katsuya Goto, M.D., D.M.Sc.
Director of The Institute of Central Nervous Diseases, Chief of Interventional Neuroradiology, Iizuka Hospital, Fukuoka, Japan
Arteriovenous Malformations and Fistulas

Douglas A. Graeb, M.D., F.R.C.P.C.
Associate Professor, Department of Radiology, Faculty of Medicine, University of British Columbia; Active Staff, Department of Radiology, Vancouver General Hospital; Consulting Staff, BC Children's Hospital, BC Cancer Agency, University Hospital, Vancouver, British Columbia, Canada
Intracranial Trauma

Curtis E. Green, M.D.
Professor of Radiology and Medicine, Georgetown University; Director of Cardiac Radiology, Georgetown University Hospital, Washington, DC
Interventional Techniques for Coronary Artery Disease; Coronary Artery Disease: Radiographic Evaluation

Giampaolo Grisolia, M.D.
Universita deli Studi Bologna, Cattedra di Fisiopatologia Prenatale, Clinica Obstetrica e Ginecologica, University of Bologna, Bologna, Italy
Prenatal Diagnosis of Anomalies of the Central Nervous System

Julius H. Grollman, Jr., M.D., F.A.C.R.
Clinical Professor of Radiological Sciences, Department of Radiological Sciences, UCLA School of Medicine; Chief, Cardiovascular and Interventional Radiology, Department of Radiology, Little Company of Mary Hospital, Torrance, California; Department of Radiology, Memorial Hospital Long Beach, Long Beach, California
Conventional and Digital Angiography of the Heart; Conventional and Digital Angiography of the Peripheral Vascular System; Diseases of the Peripheral Vascular System

Frank P. Hadlock, M.D.
Professor of Radiology, Baylor College of Medicine, Department of Radiology; Chief of Radiology, The Woman's Hospital of Texas, Houston, Texas
The Role of Fetal Biometry in Obstetric Sonography

Lynwood Hammers, D.O.
Clinical Director of Ultrasound, Associate Professor of Diagnostic Radiology, Department of Diagnostic Radiology, Yale University School of Medicine, New Haven, Connecticut
Scrotal Imaging

Michael W. Hanson, M.D.
Assistant Professor of Radiology (Nuclear Medicine), Associate in Internal Medicine (Cardiology), Duke University Medical Center; Chief of Nuclear Cardiology, Duke University Medical Center, Durham, North Carolina
Radionuclide Cardiac Imaging; Coronary Artery Disease: Radionuclide Evaluation

Robert R. Hattery, M.D.
Professor of Radiology, Mayo Graduate School of Medicine; Consultant, Mayo Clinic, Saint Marys Hospital, and Rochester Methodist Hospital, Rochester, Minnesota
Adrenal Medulla

Victor M. Haughton, M.D.
Professor of Radiology, Medical College of Wisconsin; Director of MRI Research, Medical College of Wisconsin; Radiologist, Froedtert Memorial Lutheran Hospital, Milwaukee County Medical Complex; Consultant in Radiology, VA Medical Center, Milwaukee, Wisconsin
Normal Anatomy of the Brain; Spinal Anatomy; Normal Anatomy of the Orbits

William R. Hendee, Ph.D.
Senior Associate Dean for Research and Vice President for Technology, Medical College of Wisconsin, Milwaukee, Wisconsin
FUNDAMENTALS OF DIAGNOSTIC IMAGING
The Imaging Process; Characteristics of the Radiologic Image; Image Analysis and Perception; Introduction to Imaging Techniques; Transmission Imaging: Roentgenography, Transillumination; Reflection Imaging (Ultrasound); Emission Imaging: Magnetic Resonance

R. Edward Hendrick, Ph.D.
Associate Professor and Chief, Division of Radiological Sciences, Department of Radiology, University of Colorado Health Sciences Center, Denver, Colorado
Emission Imaging: Magnetic Resonance

Barbara S. Hertzberg, M.D.
Associate Professor, Duke University Medical Center; Associate Professor of Radiology, Assistant Professor of Obstetrics/Gynecology, Duke University Medical Center, Durham, North Carolina
Ultrasound Evaluation for Intrauterine Growth Retardation

John R. Hesselink, M.D.
Professor of Radiology and Neurosciences, UCSD School of Medicine; Chief of Neuroradiology, Chief of Magnetic Resonance, UCSD Medical Center, San Diego, California
Infections of the Sinuses and Face; Neoplasms of the Sinuses and Adjacent Structures

Grant B. Hieshima, M.D.
Professor in Residence, Department of Radiology and Neurological Surgery, U.C.S.F. Medical Center, San Francisco, California
Arteriovenous Malformations and Fistulas

James F. Holman, M.D.
Assistant Clinical Professor, Department of Obstetrics and Gynecology, Duke University School of Medicine; Attending Gynecologist, Durham County General Hospital, Durham, North Carolina
Clinical Considerations in Imaging the Nonpregnant Female Patient

Marc J. Homer, M.D.
Professor of Radiology, Tufts University School of Medicine; Chief, Mammography Section, New England Medical Center, Boston, Massachusetts
Benign Diseases of the Breast

C. Carl Jaffe, M.D.
Professor of Diagnostic Radiology and Medicine (Cardiology), Yale University School of Medicine; Attending Radiologist, Yale–New Haven Hospital, New Haven, Connecticut
Echocardiography

R. Brooke Jeffrey, Jr., M.D.
Professor of Radiology, Chief of Abdominal Imaging, Stanford University School of Medicine; Stanford University Medical Center, Stanford, California
The Peritoneal Cavity

Pamela S. Jensen, M.D.
Chief, Radiology Service, Veterans Administration Hospital, Tobus, Maine
Infectious Diseases: Conditions of Undetermined Etiology; Arthropathies: Rheumatoid Arthritis; Hematologic Disorders: Bleeding Disorders, Multicentric Reticulohistiocytosis; Endocrine Disorders: Pituitary, Adrenal, Parathyroid; Metabolic Disorders: Osteomalacia and Rickets; Neurologic and Vascular Disorders

Lee D. Katz, M.D.
Associate Professor of Diagnostic Radiology and Internal Medicine, Yale University School of Medicine; Yale–New Haven Hospital, New Haven, Connecticut; VA Medical Center, Norwalk, Connecticut
Metabolic Disorders: Hypervitaminoses and Hypovitaminoses; Heavy Metal and Chemical Exposures; Drug-Induced Disorders

Richard W. Katzberg, M.D.
Professor, University of California Davis Medical Center in Sacramento, Sacramento, California
Intravascular Contrast Media

Elias Kazam, M.D.
Professor of Radiology, Head of the Division of Ultrasound and Computed Body Tomography, New York Hospital–Cornell Medical Center (Cornell Medical College); Attending Radiologist, New York Hospital, New York, New York
Normal Computed Tomographic Anatomy of the Pelvis with Ultrasound and MRI Correlations

Marc S. Keller, M.D.
Professor of Diagnostic Radiology and Pediatrics, Yale University School of Medicine; Director, Pediatric Diagnostic Imaging, Children's Hospital at Yale–New Haven, New Haven, Connecticut
The Duodenum

Michael J. Kelley, M.D.
Clinical Associate Professor of Radiology, Department of Radiology, Duke University Medical Center, Durham, North Carolina; Staff Radiologist, Department of Radiology, Carolinas Medical Center, Charlotte, North Carolina
CARDIOVASCULAR SYSTEM
Cardiovascular Anatomy and Function; Vascular Interventional Techniques in the Abdominal Aorta and Its Pelvic and Peripheral Branches; Acquired Valvular Heart Disease; Diseases of the Myocardium; Diseases of the Pericardium

Frederick M. Kelvin, M.D.
Clinical Professor of Radiology, Indiana University School of Medicine; Staff Radiologist, Methodist Hospital of Indiana, Indianapolis, Indiana
The Large Bowel and Appendix

Bernard F. King, M.D.
Assistant Professor of Radiology, Mayo Medical School; St. Marys Hospital and Rochester Methodist Hospital, Rochester, Minnesota
Impotence

Faye C. Laing, M.D.
Associate Professor of Radiology, Harvard University; Co-Director, Radiology Residency Program, Brigham and Women's Hospital, Boston, Massachusetts
Complications of Early Pregnancy; The Diagnosis of Ectopic Pregnancy

Robert Lang, M.D.
Endocrinologist, Yale–New Haven Hospital, New Haven, Connecticut
Basic Principles (Musculoskeletal System): Bone Metabolism; Metabolic Disorders: Osteoporosis

John C. Lappas, M.D.
Professor of Radiology, Indiana University School of Medicine; Wishard Memorial Hospital, Indiana University Medical Center, Indianapolis, Indiana
The Small Bowel

Jack P. Lawson, M.B., Ch.B., F.R.C.R.
Professor of Radiology and Orthopedic Surgery, Yale University School of Medicine; Attending Radiologist, Yale–New Haven Hospital, New Haven, Connecticut
Hematologic Disorders: Hemoglobinopathies

Thomas L. Lawson, M.D.
Professor and Chairman, Department of Radiology, Loyola University Chicago, Stritch School of Medicine; Loyola University Medical Center and Foster McGaw Hospital, Loyola University Chicago, Maywood, Illinois
GASTROINTESTINAL SYSTEM
The Biliary Ductal System; The Pancreas

Fred T. Lee, Jr., M.D.
Assistant Professor of Radiology, University of Wisconsin Clinical Science Center, Madison, Wisconsin
The Ureter

Mark H. LeQuire, M.D.
Staff Radiologist, Department of Radiology, Carolinas Medical Center, Charlotte, North Carolina
Vascular Interventional Techniques in the Abdominal Aorta and Its Pelvic and Peripheral Branches

Elsie Levin, M.D.
Assistant Professor (Clinical), Boston University Medical School; Staff Radiologist, Faulkner Hospital, Boston, Massachusetts
Radiologic Diagnosis of Breast Cancer

Errol Levine, M.D., Ph.D., F.A.C.R., F.R.C.R.(Eng.)
Professor of Diagnostic Radiology and Surgery (Urology), The University of Kansas Medical Center; Head, Sections of Body Computed Tomography and Uroradiology, The University of Kansas Medical Center, Kansas City, Kansas
The Retroperitoneum

Robert A. Levine, M.D.
Endocrinologist and Vice-Chairman of Medicine, Nashua Memorial Hospital, Nashua, New Hampshire
Endocrine Disorders: Pituitary; Adrenal

David Ling, M.D.
Assistant Professor, Mallinckrodt Institute of Radiology, Washington University School of Medicine, St. Louis, Missouri; Active Staff, Wake Medical Center, Raleigh, North Carolina
The Pharynx; The Esophagus

Kerry M. Link, M.D.
Associate Professor of Radiology, Bowman Gray School of Medicine, Wake Forest University; Director of MRI, Bowman Gray School of Medicine, North Carolina Baptist Hospital, Winston-Salem, North Carolina
Cardiac MRI

Stephen P. Loehr, B.A.
Medical Student, Bowman Gray School of Medicine, Winston-Salem, North Carolina
Cardiac MRI

Beatrice L. Madrazo, M.D.
Clinical Associate Professor of Radiology, University of Michigan Medical School, Ann Arbor, Michigan; Head, Division of Diagnostic Ultrasound, Department of Diagnostic Radiology and Medical Imaging, Henry Ford Hospital, Detroit, Michigan
Postpartum Sonography

Dean D. T. Maglinte, M.D.
Clinical Professor of Radiology, Indiana University School of Medicine; Methodist Hospital of Indiana, Indianapolis, Indiana
The Small Bowel

Barry S. Mahony, M.D.
Director, Division of Ultrasound, Swedish Hospital Medical Center, Seattle, Washington
Fetal Urinary Tract Abnormalities; Fetal Skeletal Abnormalities

B. J. Manaster, M.D., Ph.D.
Professor of Radiology, University of Utah School of Medicine; Radiologist–Staff Physician, University of Utah Medical Center and Salt Lake City Veterans Administration Medical Center, Salt Lake City, Utah
MUSCULOSKELETAL SYSTEM
Tumor and Tumor-Like Conditions: Musculoskeletal Tumor Imaging; Musculoskeletal Trauma

John A. Markisz, M.D., Ph.D.
Associate Professor of Radiology, Director of Division of MRI; Associate Attending

Radiologist, The New York Hospital, New York, New York
Normal Computed Tomographic Anatomy of the Pelvis with Ultrasound and MRI Correlations

Eric M. Martin, Ph.D.
Medical Student, Bowman Gray School of Medicine, Winston-Salem, North Carolina
Cardiac MRI

Terence A. S. Matalon, M.D.
Associate Professor, Rush Medical College; Associate Attending, Rush-Presbyterian-St. Luke's Medical Center, Chicago, Illinois
Radiology of Renal Transplantation

Gerald R. May, M.D.
Assistant Professor of Diagnostic Radiology, Mayo Medical School; Consultant, Diagnostic Radiology, Mayo Clinic Radiology, Jacksonville, Florida
The Gallbladder

Ronald W. McCallum, M.B., F.R.C.P.(C), F.A.C.R.
Professor of Radiology, University of Toronto; Chief of Radiology, St. Michael's Hospital, Toronto, Ontario, Canada
The Urethra and Seminal Vesicles

Kevin E. McCarthy, M.D.
Assistant Professor of Radiology, Louisiana State University; Staff Radiologist, Louisiana State University Medical Center, New Orleans, Louisiana
Infectious Diseases

Bruce L. McClennan, M.D.
Professor of Radiology, Washington University School of Medicine; Barnes Hospital, Jewish Hospital, and St. Louis Children's Hospital, St. Louis, Missouri
Urography—Anatomy and Technique

Charles M. McCurdy, Jr., M.D.
Assistant Professor, University of Arizona, Tucson, Arizona
Amniotic Fluid Volume Abnormalities: Ultrasonic Evaluation

David G. McLone, M.D., Ph.D.
Professor of Surgery (Neurosurgery), Northwestern University Medical School; Division Head, Pediatric Neurosurgery, Children's Memorial Hospital, Chicago, Illinois
Congenital Anomalies of the Spine and Spinal Cord

Theresa C. McLoud, M.D.
Associate Professor of Radiology, Harvard Medical School; Chief of Thoracic Radiology, Massachusetts General Hospital, Boston, Massachusetts
Diseases of Altered Immunologic Activity

Christopher R. B. Merritt, M.D.
Chairman, Department of Radiology, Ochsner Clinic and Alton Ochsner Medical Foundation, New Orleans, Louisiana
Breast Imaging Techniques

Harold A. Mitty, M.D.
Professor of Radiology, The Mount Sinai School of Medicine of the City University of New York; Attending Radiologist and Director of Interventional Radiology, The Mount Sinai Hospital, New York, New York
Anatomy and Techniques of Examination of the Adrenal Gland

C. A. F. Moes, M.D.
Professor Emeritus, Department of Diagnostic Imaging, Faculty of Medicine, University of Toronto; Professor Emeritus, Diagnostic Imaging, Hospital for Sick Children, Toronto, Ontario, Canada
Congenital Cardiovascular Disease

Deborah L. Morton-Turski, M.D.
Associate Clinical Professor of Pathology, University of Wisconsin Medical School; Chair, Department of Pathology, St. Mary's Hospital, Madison, Wisconsin
Magnetic Resonance Imaging of the Pituitary Gland and Juxtasellar Regions

Paul H. Murphy, Ph.D.
Associate Professor, Nuclear Medicine Section, Department of Radiology, Baylor College of Medicine; Assistant Chief, Nuclear Medicine Service, St. Luke's Episcopal Hospital, Houston, Texas
Emission Imaging: Nuclear Medicine

David P. Naidich, M.D.
Professor of Radiology, New York University Medical Center; Attending Physician, Tisch Hospital and Bellevue Hospital, New York, New York
Diseases of the Airways

Thomas P. Naidich, M.D.
Professor of Radiology, Northwestern University Medical School; Director of Neuroimaging, The Children's Memorial Hospital, Chicago, Illinois
Congenital Anomalies of the Spine and Spinal Cord

Lewis H. Nelson, III, M.D.
Professor, Obstetrics and Gynecology, Associate Dean, Medical School Admissions, Bowman Gray School of Medicine, Wake Forest University; North Carolina Baptist Hospital and Forsyth Memorial Hospital, Winston-Salem, North Carolina
Fetal Anomalies of the Abdomen and Abdominal Wall

John D. Newell, Jr., M.D., F.C.C.P.
Professor of Radiology and Co-Director of Thoracic Radiology, Department of Radiology, University of Colorado Health Sciences Center; Staff Radiologist, University Hospital (University of Colorado HSC); Director of Radiology, National Jewish Center for Immunology and Respiratory Medicine, Denver, Colorado
Acquired Valvular Heart Disease

Gary S. Novick, M.D.
Clinical Assistant Professor, Yale University School of Medicine; Staff Physician, Yale–New Haven Hospital and Temple Radiology Group, New Haven, Connecticut
Imaging Modalities

David A. Nyberg, M.D.
Co-Director of Obstetrics-Gynecology Ultrasound, Swedish Hospital Medical Center; Associate Clinical Professor of Radiology and Obstetrics-Gynecology, University of Washington Medical Center, Seattle, Washington
Complications of Early Pregnancy

John A. Ogden, M.D.
Professor of Orthopaedic Surgery, University of South Florida College of Medicine; Staff Physician, Tampa General Hospital; Chief of Staff, Shriner's Hospital, Tampa, Florida
Basic Principles (Musculoskeletal System): Skeletal Growth and Development

William W. Olmsted, M.D.
Professor of Radiology, The George Washington University; The George Washington University Medical Center, Washington, DC
Congenital Dysplasias Primarily Involving the Skull; Primary and Secondary Neoplasms of the Skull

Randolph S. Pallas, M.D.
Assistant Professor of Medicine, Georgetown University School of Medicine, Washington, DC
Acquired Valvular Heart Disease

Suresh K. Patel, M.D.
Professor, Rush Medical College; Senior Attending, Rush-Presbyterian-St. Luke's Medical Center, Chicago, Illinois
Radiology of Renal Transplantation

Richard R. Pelker, M.D., Ph.D.
Professor, Department of Orthopaedics and Rehabilitation, Yale University School of Medicine; Attending, Yale–New Haven Hospital, New Haven, Connecticut
Arthropathies: Surgical Treatment of Joint Disease

Antonella Perolo, M.D.
Universita deli Studi Bologna, Cattedra di Fisiopatologia Prenatale, Clinica Obstetrica e Ginecologica, University of Bologna, Bologna, Italy
Prenatal Diagnosis of Anomalies of the Central Nervous System

Val Michael Phillips, M.D.
Clinical Assistant Professor at Emory University School of Medicine, Atlanta, Georgia; Staff Radiologist at Gwinnett Medical Center, Lawrenceville, Georgia
The Liver and Spleen

Gianluigi Pilu, M.D.
Clinical Attending Physician, Prenatal Pathophysiology Unit and Department of Obstetrics and Gynecology, University of Bologna, Bologna, Italy
Prenatal Diagnosis of Anomalies of the Central Nervous System

C. F. Pope, M.D.
Instructor, Magnetic Resonance Imaging, Department of Diagnostic Radiology, Yale University School of Medicine; Instructor, Section of Magnetic Resonance Imaging, Yale–New Haven Hospital, New Haven, Connecticut
Venous Thromboembolic Disease

Thomas Lee Pope, Jr., M.D.
Professor of Radiology, Bowman Gray School of Medicine, North Carolina Baptist Hospital, Wake Forest University, Winston-Salem, North Carolina
Normal Roentgen Anatomy of the Breast

Janet L. Potter, Ph.D., M.D.
Associate Professor, University of Texas Health Science Center at San Antonio; Bexar County Hospital District, Audie Murphy Memorial Veterans Hospital, San Antonio, Texas
Transmission Imaging; Computed Tomography

Andrew K. Poznanski, M.D.
Professor of Radiology, Northwestern University; Radiologist-in-Chief, Children's Memorial Hospital, Chicago, Illinois
Congenital and Developmental Anomalies

Robert Pugatch, M.D.
Associate Professor of Radiology, Harvard Medical School; Co-Director, Division of Thoracic Imaging, Brigham and Women's Hospital, Boston, Massachusetts
Thoracic Neoplasms

Charles E. Putman, M.D.
Executive Vice President for Duke University, James B. Duke Professor of Radiology and Professor of Medicine, Vice Provost for Research and Development, Duke University Medical Center, Durham, North Carolina
PULMONARY SYSTEM
Infectious Pneumonias—Including Aspiration States

Elizabeth Ramirez de Arellano, M.D.
Assistant Professor of Radiology, New York Hospital–Cornell Medical Center (Cornell Medical College); Assistant Attending Radiologist, New York Hospital–Cornell Medical Center, New York, New York
Normal Computed Tomographic Anatomy of the Pelvis with Ultrasound and MRI Correlations

Carl E. Ravin, M.D.
Professor and Chairman, Department of Radiology, Duke University Medical Center, Durham, North Carolina
PULMONARY SYSTEM
Introduction to Chest Radiography

Helen C. Redman, M.D.
Professor of Radiology, University of Texas Southwestern Medical School; Attending, Parkland Memorial Hospital, Zale-Lipshy Hospital, and Dallas VA Hospital, Dallas, Texas
Radiologic Imaging in Renal Trauma

Kathryn L. Reed, M.D.
Professor, Obstetrics/Gynecology, University of Arizona College of Medicine, Department of Obstetrics and Gynecology, Tucson, Arizona
Ultrasound Studies of Fetal Cardiac Anatomy

Donald L. Resnick, M.D.
Professor of Radiology, University of California, San Diego; Chief, Osteoradiology, VA Medical Center, San Diego, California
Arthropathies: Degenerative Joint Disease; Crystal-Induced and Related Arthropathies

Charles S. Resnik, M.D.
Associate Professor of Radiology, University of Maryland Medical Center, Baltimore, Maryland
Arthropathies: Crystal-Induced and Related Arthropathies

Christopher M. Rigsby, M.D.
Attending Radiologist, The Fairfax Hospital, New Haven, Connecticut
Drug-Induced Lung Disease

E. Russell Ritenour, Ph.D.
Director of Graduate Studies, Biophysical Sciences Graduate Program, University of Minnesota School of Medicine; Director of Physics for Radiology, University of Minnesota Hospital and Clinics, Minneapolis, Minnesota
Emission Imaging: Magnetic Resonance

William D. Robertson, M.D.
Professor of Radiology, University of Washington; Department of Radiology, Washington Medical Center; Department of Radiology, Harborview Medical Center, Seattle, Washington
Neoplasms of the Brain, Cranial Nerves, and Meninges

Neil M. Rofsky, M.D.
Assistant Professor of Radiology, New York University School of Medicine, New York, New York
Benign Renal Tumors

Roberto Romero, M.D.
Associate Professor of Obstetrics and Gynecology and Director of Perinatal Research, Yale University School of Medicine, New Haven, Connecticut
Prenatal Diagnosis of Anomalies of the Central Nervous System

Arthur T. Rosenfield, M.D.
Professor of Diagnostic Radiology, Yale University School of Medicine; Attending Physician and Head, Section of Computed Tomography, Yale–New Haven Hospital, New Haven, Connecticut
Scrotal Imaging

Nancy S. Rosenfield, M.D.
Associate Professor of Radiology, Cornell University Medical College; Associate

Radiologist, Memorial Sloan-Kettering Cancer Center, New York, New York
Hematologic Disorders: Myeloproliferative Disorders

Stuart A. Royal, M.S., M.D.
Associate Clinical Professor of Radiology and Pediatrics, The University of Alabama at Birmingham; Radiologist-in-Chief, The Children's Hospital of Alabama, Birmingham, Alabama
Congenital Abnormalities of the Urinary Tract

William A. Rubenstein, M.D.
Associate Professor of Clinical Radiology, Cornell University Medical College (New York Hospital–Cornell Medical Center); Associate Attending Radiologist, New York Hospital, New York, New York
Normal Computed Tomographic Anatomy of the Pelvis with Ultrasound and MRI Correlations

William M. Rumancik, M.D.
Associate Professor of Clinical Radiology, State University of New York Health Sciences Center at Brooklyn; Attending Radiologist, The Long Island College Hospital, Brooklyn, New York
Nonfunctioning Adrenal Masses

Rudy E. Sabbagha, M.D.
Professor, Obstetrics and Gynecology, Northwestern University Medical School; Director, Diagnostic Ultrasound Center in Obstetrics and Gynecology Practice, Women's Pavilion of Northwestern Memorial Hospital, Chicago, Illinois
Ultrasonic Imaging in Obstetrics

Joseph F. Sackett, M.D.
Professor and Chairman, Department of Radiology, University of Wisconsin Hospital and Clinics, Madison, Wisconsin
Degenerative Change of Spinal Column Causing Neurologic Deficit

Norman L. Sadowsky, M.D.
Professor of Radiology (Clinical), Tufts University School of Medicine; Instructor of Radiology, Harvard Medical School; Chief, Department of Radiology, Faulkner Hospital; Director, Faulkner-Sagoff Centre for Breast Health Care, Boston, Massachusetts
Radiologic Diagnosis of Breast Cancer

Carl M. Sandler, M.D.
Professor of Radiology and Surgery (Urology), University of Texas Medical School at Houston; Chief of Radiology Service, Lyndon B. Johnson General Hospital, Houston, Texas
The Bladder; The Urethra and Seminal Vesicles

Michael A. Sandler, M.D.
Clinical Professor of Radiology, University of Michigan, Ann Arbor, Michigan; Department of Diagnostic Radiology, Henry Ford Hospital, Detroit, Michigan
Endometriosis and Pelvic Inflammatory Disease

Lowell F. Satler, M.D.
Clinical Assistant Professor of Medicine, Georgetown University; Interventional Cardiologist, Washington Hospital Center, Washington, DC
Interventional Techniques for Coronary Artery Disease; Coronary Artery Disease: Radiographic Evaluation

Francis J. Scholz, M.D.
Clinical Assistant Professor, Tufts University School of Medicine; Clinical Instructor, Harvard Medical School, Boston, Massachusetts; Radiologist, Lahey Clinic Medical Center, Burlington, Massachusetts
The Stomach

John W. Seeds, M.D.
Professor, Department of Obstetrics and Gynecology, University of Arizona; Professor and Director of Maternal-Fetal Medicine, Department of Obstetrics and Gynecology, University of Arizona, Tucson, Arizona
Amniotic Fluid Volume Abnormalities: Ultrasonic Evaluation

Joachim F. Seeger, M.D.
Professor of Radiology, University of Arizona College of Medicine; Head of Neuroradiology, University Hospital and Veterans Administration Medical Center, Tucson, Arizona
Extracranial Vascular Disease

Arthur J. Segal, M.D.
Clinical Professor of Radiology and Urology, University of Rochester School of Medicine and Dentistry; Associate Chairman, Department of Radiology, Rochester General Hospital, Rochester, New York
Renal Cystic Disease

Katherine A. Shaffer, M.D.
Professor of Clinical Radiology, Medical College of Wisconsin; Staff Radiologist,

Milwaukee County Medical Complex, Froedtert Memorial Lutheran Hospital, Milwaukee, Wisconsin
Normal Temporal Bone and Temporal Bone Trauma

Douglas R. Shearer, Ph.D.
Associate Professor, Brown University; Director of Medical Physics, Rhode Island Hospital, Providence, Rhode Island
Transmission Imaging: Roentgenography

Patrick F. Sheedy II, M.D.
Professor of Radiology, Mayo Graduate School of Medicine; Consultant, Mayo Clinic, Saint Marys Hospital, and Rochester Methodist Hospital, Rochester, Minnesota
Adrenal Medulla

Marilyn J. Siegel, M.D.
Professor of Radiology, Mallinckrodt Institute of Radiology, Washington University School of Medicine; Associate Radiologist, Barnes Hospital and St. Louis Children's Hospital, St. Louis, Missouri
The Pharynx; The Esophagus

Jeffrey F. Smallhorn, M.B.B.S., F.R.A.C.P., F.R.C.P.(C.)
Associate Professor, University of Toronto Faculty of Medicine; Staff Paediatric Cardiologist, The Hospital for Sick Children, Toronto, Ontario, Canada
Congenital Cardiovascular Disease

James G. Smirniotopoulos, M.D.
Associate Professor, Department of Radiology and Nuclear Medicine, Uniformed Services University of the Health Sciences, Bethesda, Maryland; Associate Professor (Clinical), Georgetown University; Associate Professor (Clinical), George Washington University, Washington, DC
Congenital Dysplasias Primarily Involving the Skull; Primary and Secondary Neoplasms of the Skull

Stephen W. Smith, Ph.D.
Adjunct Associate Professor, Department of Radiology, Duke University School of Medicine, Durham, North Carolina; Senior Scientist, Center for Devices and Radiological Health, Rockville, Maryland
The Use of Diagnostic Ultrasound Imaging in Pregnancy

Suzanne J. Smith, M.D.
Associate Professor of Clinical Radiology, Columbia University College of Physicians and Surgeons; Director of Breast Imaging, Columbia-Presbyterian Medical Center, New York, New York
Renal Lymphoma and Metastatic Disease to the Kidneys

Wendy R. K. Smoker, M.D.
Professor of Radiology, Director of Neuroradiology and Head and Neck Radiology, Medical College of Virginia, Richmond, Virginia
Intracranial Aneurysms

Stephen H. Smyth, M.D.
Assistant Professor of Clinical Radiology, University of Arizona College of Medicine; University Health Sciences Center and Department of Veterans Affairs Medical Center, Tucson, Arizona
Renovascular Hypertension: Etiologic, Diagnostic, and Therapeutic Considerations

H. Dirk Sostman, M.D.
Professor of Radiology and Attending Radiologist, Duke University Medical Center, Durham, North Carolina
Venous Thromboembolic Disease

Robert F. Spataro, M.D.
Clinical Associate Professor of Radiology, University of Rochester School of Medicine and Dentistry; Department of Radiology, The Genesee Hospital, Rochester, New York
The Ureter

Beverly A. Spirt, M.D., F.A.C.R.
Professor of Radiology, Chief of Ultrasound, State University of New York Health Science Center at Syracuse, Syracuse, New York
Ultrasound of the Placenta

Paul Stark, M.D.
Associate Professor of Radiology, Harvard Medical School; Co-Director, Section of Thoracic Radiology, Brigham and Women's Hospital, Boston, Massachusetts
Radiology of Pneumoconioses

Charles M. Strother, M.D.
Professor, University of Wisconsin Medical School; Professor of Radiology, Neurology and Neurosurgery, University of Wisconsin Hospital and Clinics, Madison, Wisconsin
CENTRAL NERVOUS SYSTEM
Technique for Examination of the Skull; Traumatic Abnormalities of the Skull; Techniques for Evaluation of the Brain; Techniques for Evaluation of the Spine and Spinal Contents; The Abnormal Intervertebral Disc; Techniques for Examination of the Eye, Orbit, and Sinuses

Steven K. Teplick, M.D.
Professor of Radiology, University of Arkansas for Medical Sciences; University Hospital, J. L. McClellan VA Hospital, Arkansas Children's Hospital, Little Rock, Arkansas
The Duodenum

John R. Thornbury, M.D.
Professor of Radiology, University of Wisconsin Clinical Science Center, Madison, Wisconsin
The Ureter

Robert D. Tien, M.D., M.P.H.
Associate Professor of Radiology, Department of Radiology, Duke University Medical Center, Durham, North Carolina
Neurodegenerative Diseases, Metabolic Diseases, White Matter Diseases, and the Neurocutaneous Syndromes

Ina L. D. Tonkin, M.D.
Professor of Radiology and Pediatrics, University of Tennessee, Memphis, The Health Science Center; Director of Cardiovascular/Interventional Radiology, Le Bonheur Children's Medical Center and St. Jude Children's Research Hospital; Attending Radiologist, The Regional Medical Center at Memphis, Memphis, Tennessee
Diseases of the Thoracic Aorta

Patrick A. Turski, M.D.
Professor of Radiology, Neurology and Neurosurgery, University of Wisconsin Medical School; Chief, Section of Neuroradiology, University of Wisconsin Hospital and Clinic, Madison, Wisconsin
Magnetic Resonance Imaging of the Pituitary Gland and Juxtasellar Regions

Arl Van Moore, M.D.
Clinical Assistant Professor of Radiology, Department of Radiology, Duke University Medical Center, Durham, North Carolina; Staff Radiologist, Department of Radiology, Carolinas Medical Center, Charlotte, North Carolina
Vascular Interventional Techniques in the Abdominal Aorta and Its Pelvic and Peripheral Branches

Michael G. Velchik, M.D.
Staff Physician, Nuclear Medicine, Fairfax Hospital (Virginia)
Infectious Diseases

Miriam E. Vincent, M.D.
Professor of Radiology, Tufts University School of Medicine; Associate Chief and Head, Gastrointestinal Section, Radiology Service, Veterans Administration Medical Center, Boston, Massachusetts
The Stomach

James W. Walsh, M.D.
Professor of Radiology, Director, Body Computed Tomography, Department of Radiology, University of Minnesota Hospital and Clinic, Minneapolis, Minnesota
Imaging of Uterine Masses and Tumors

W. Richard Webb, M.D.
Professor of Radiology, Co-Director of Thoracic Imaging, University of California, San Francisco, San Francisco, California
Diseases of the Mediastinum

Alfred L. Weber, M.D.
Professor of Radiology, Harvard Medical School; Chief of Radiology, Massachusetts Eye and Ear Infirmary; Radiologist, Massachusetts General Hospital, Boston, Massachusetts
Infections of the Sinuses and Face; Neoplasms of the Sinuses and Adjacent Structures

Barbara N. Weissman, M.D.
Associate Professor, Radiology, Harvard Medical School; Radiologist, Brigham and Women's Hospital, Boston, Massachusetts
Arthropathies: Juvenile Rheumatoid Arthritis; Systemic Lupus Erythematosus; Progressive Systemic Sclerosis; Mixed Connective Tissue Disease

Timothy J. Welch, M.D.
Assistant Professor, Mayo Graduate School of Medicine; Consultant, Mayo Clinic, Saint Marys Hospital, and Rochester Methodist Hospital, Rochester, Minnesota
Adrenal Medulla

Jeffrey D. Wicks, M.D., F.A.C.R.
Clinical Professor of Radiology, University of Colorado Health Sciences Center; Chairman, Department of Radiology, St. Anthony Hospitals, Denver, Colorado
Imaging of Gestational Trophoblastic Disease

Margaret E. Williford, M.D.
Assistant Clinical Professor, Department of Radiology, Duke University Medical Center, Durham, North Carolina
The Large Bowel and Appendix

Peter J. Yang, M.D.
Assistant Professor of Radiology, University of Arizona College of Medicine, Tucson, Arizona
Extracranial Vascular Disease

Bradford A. Yeager, M.D.
Staff Radiologist, Lehigh Valley Regional Hospital, Allentown, Pennsylvania
Infectious Diseases

Ronald J. Zagoria, M.D.
Associate Professor of Radiology at Wake Forest University, Bowman Gray School of Medicine; Director, Division of Uroradiology, North Carolina Baptist Hospital, Winston-Salem, North Carolina
Ureteral Obstruction and Dilatation

Kenneth Zirinsky, M.D.
Adjunct Assistant Professor of Radiology, New York Hospital–Cornell Medical Center, New York, New York; Attending Physician, Tacoma Specialty Center, Department of Radiology, Tacoma, Washington
Normal Computed Tomographic Anatomy of the Pelvis with Ultrasound and MRI Correlations

PREFACE

The second edition of the *Textbook of Diagnostic Imaging* has been extensively revised to provide a comprehensive state-of-the-art text emphasizing the role of imaging in the diagnostic and therapeutic management of patients. Following the positive reviews and constructive criticisms of the first edition, the following principles of writing and editing were applied to the second edition:

1. Provision of current clinical and scientific data to promote an improved understanding of the pathophysiologic events occuring within each clinical entity.
2. More strenuous emphasis on the utility and efficacy of complementary but often competing technologies.
3. A pragmatic approach to each clinical problem, rather than overemphasizing the role of any particular imaging modality.
4. Formulation of the content of each chapter on proven clinical assessments, and embracing a common style of presentation throughout the volume.

We, again, are grateful for the enthusiastic efforts and cooperation of each of our previous Associate Editors: James D. Bowie, M.D.; N. Reed Dunnick, M.D.; William R. Hendee, Ph.D.; Michael J. Kelley, M.D.; Thomas L. Lawson, M.D.; and Charles M. Strother, M.D.

We are also delighted to welcome to the second edition two new Associate Editors: Dr. B. J. Manaster, who has assumed responsibility for the section on musculoskeletal imaging; and Dr. Daniel C. Sullivan, who has developed the section on breast imaging.

Each chapter author has been selected on the basis of documented contribution to the better understanding of a disease entity and the knowledge of multiple imaging modalities. We are most grateful for their patience, perseverance, and dedication to this effort.

W. B. Saunders Company deserves our special recognition and appreciation for their continued confidence and support of the *Textbook of Diagnostic Imaging*. We would like to particularly recognize the efforts of Dolores Meloni, Developmental Editor, and Lisette Bralow, Vice President and Editor-in-Chief, Medical Books, in the assembly and production of this book.

The second edition of the *Textbook of Diagnostic Imaging* is intended to strengthen the understanding of clinical diagnostic imaging for students, residents, and practitioners. We hope that those individuals utilizing the special skills and services of radiologists will find the clinical emphasis throughout the textbook to have practical implications for their daily practice. At a time when health care costs and the provision of health care to all citizens of this country are receiving appropriate review and recognition, it is timely that a textbook encompassing objective criteria for the selection of various imaging systems be made available. We hope you will find that this edition meets your professional needs and fosters the improved care of patients referred for imaging studies.

CHARLES E. PUTMAN
CARL E. RAVIN

CONTENTS

Volume 1

Volume 2

Textbook of
DIAGNOSTIC IMAGING

GENITOURINARY SYSTEM

The past 15 years have seen a dramatic change in the practice of uroradiology. Modalities such as computed tomography and ultrasonography have developed into primary imaging methods. Technical advances such as digital angiography and low-osmolality contrast agents have improved the safety of many procedures and have contributed to their widespread use. Magnetic resonance is an entirely new imaging modality that promises to expand even further on the inroads developed by computed tomography. Finally, a host of interventional techniques has allowed radiologists to play a more active role in treating patients.

Although each of these procedures has something to contribute in almost every aspect of uroradiology, some have proven so valuable that they have altered our approach to certain clinical problems. Ultrasonography is routinely used to detect hydronephrosis, to determine if a mass is solid or cystic, and to evaluate the female pelvis. Furthermore, it is a particularly useful modality for patients who may be at increased risk for ionizing irradiation, such as children and pregnant women. Computed tomography has become the primary imaging modality for suspected adrenal pathology and is the most sensitive method of detecting renal masses. Since it is not operator-dependent and precisely delineates the size and extent of many tumors, it has become an essential modality for oncologic imaging.

Radionuclide imaging has long been valued for its reflection of physiology. These techniques continue to prove useful in determining renal function. The most recent addition to physiologic imaging, metaiodobenzylguanidine (MIBG), is an analog of guanethidine that is concentrated in adrenergic tissue. MIBG may become the most reliable method of detecting pheochromocytomas and may preclude the tedious search sometimes required to locate ectopic tumors.

Digital subtraction is yet another benefit derived from modern high-speed computers. This method of data manipulation provides better contrast resolution than conventional film screen combinations and has reopened the field of intravenous arteriography. These same techniques can be used with arterial contrast injections to save time and film and reduce the contrast burden to the patient.

A major breakthrough in contrast material has been the development of non-ionic and other low-osmolality agents. Early clinical experience suggests that these agents provide equivalent radiographic images with a greater margin of patient comfort and safety.

Continued improvements in angiographic catheters, guidewires, and needles have expanded the role of the interventional radiologist to virtually every body cavity. This is especially true in the urinary tract, where the percutaneous nephrostomy has become an essential tool for the preservation of function of hydronephrotic kidneys and provides access for a variety of endourologic procedures. Percutaneous angioplasty can be used to dilate ureteral strictures as well as cure renovascular hypertension. Vascular occlusion techniques are often employed as adjunctive therapy for renal malignancies or their complications.

Radiologists must understand not only the uses but also the limitations and potential pitfalls of these modalities. This is an especially difficult task, as the modalities continue to evolve with technical advances. Furthermore, the use of the new techniques must be integrated with conventional methods to provide the safest and most efficient assessment of the patient. It is our responsibility to assist our clinical colleagues and care for our patients not only by performing these examinations but also by designing the most effective plan for evaluation and treatment.

N. Reed Dunnick

63 Adrenal Gland

Anatomy and Techniques of Examination of the Adrenal Gland

Harold A. Mitty

ANATOMY

The adrenals are only 3 to 6 mm in thickness, but the area containing the bulk of the medulla is thicker. Since normal glands range from 4 to 6 cm in length and 2 to 3 cm in width, this variability may explain in part why some hyperfunctioning glands measure within the normal range. The weight of the normal gland in individuals who die suddenly is 4 to 5 g. Illness may be associated with hypertrophy; autopsy specimens would then be heavier—6 g or more. Adrenal volume determination in normal nonstressed adult volunteers was performed by Rubin and Phillips. Mean right and left volumes were slightly greater by computed tomography (CT). The left adrenal volume was larger than the right by both CT and magnetic resonance imaging (MRI). Body surface area was highly correlated with volume on both sides. CT, by an average of 42 per cent, and MRI, by 20 per cent, overestimated known volumes in a set of phantoms. This was thought to be due to partial volume averaging.

Since CT and MRI have become the backbone of adrenal imaging, an understanding of the cross-sectional anatomy of this area is vital (Fig. 63–1). The images obtained by these modalities realistically represent the orientation and shape of the glands in the body.

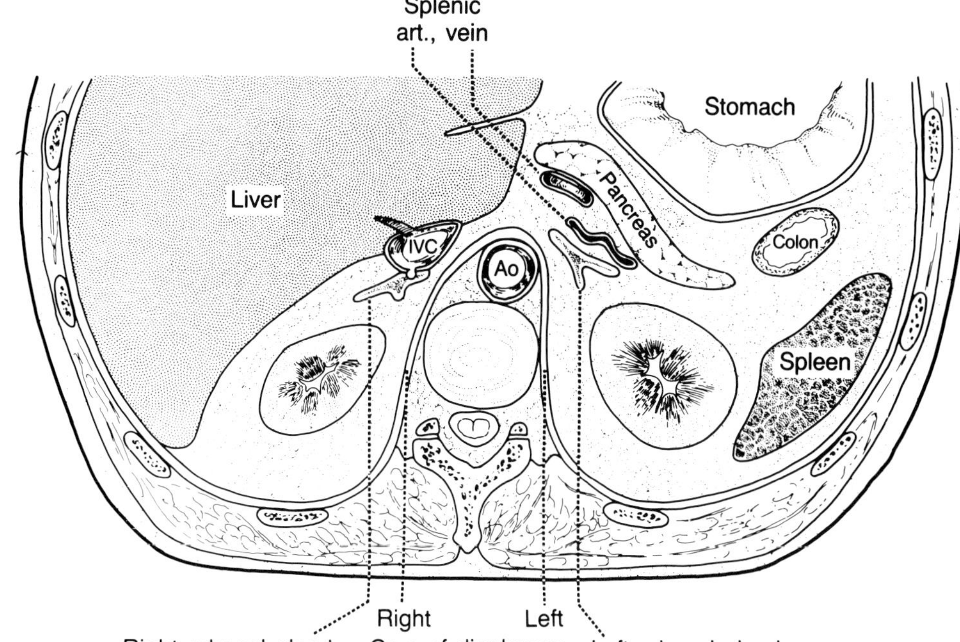

Figure 63–1. Cross-sectional anatomy of adrenal glands and adjacent structures.

The adrenals are thin structures folded to form an anteromedial ridge and two posterior or posterolateral wings. These wings (limbs) are close together in the superior aspect of the gland but become widely open inferiorly so that each gland appears to straddle the medial anterior aspect of the upper portion of the kidney. The angles between the wings at the base of the gland may exceed 120 degrees.

The features shown on cross-sectional images of the gland depend on the level of the section. At the superior level, the gland often assumes a linear appearance in an anteroposterior orientation. Often this linear appearance slants in a lateral direction. In the middle portion of the gland, the cross-sectional image is that of an inverted Y-shaped structure. In the more inferior section, the inverted Y assumes the wide angle of the two wings. When the anteromedial ridge is small or not developed, an inverted V shape is produced.

The adrenal glands are situated at the superoposterior extreme of the retroperitoneal space lateral to the vertebrae at the level of the eleventh or twelfth rib. The left gland extends as low as L1. The glands are fixed to the inner surfaces of the superoanteromedial aspect of the perirenal fascia. The glands are surrounded by fibrofatty areolar tissue that separates them from surrounding structures including the kidneys, aorta, and liver. On the right this areolar tissue is practically nonexistent between the gland and the inferior vena cava. Since the kidney is not fixed to the perirenal fascia, the upright position or deep inspiration often causes increased separation of kidney and adrenal gland.

The inferior portion of the right gland is anteromedial to the upper pole of the right kidney, and the superior portion is above the kidney. On the left, the gland is lower and is actually anteromedial to the kidney and frequently extends to the renal hilum. Often, only small portions of the left gland project above the kidney. Thus, the use of the term "suprarenal" is misleading.

The anteromedial portion of the right adrenal gland is nonperitonealized and is immediately behind the inferior vena cava. The anterolateral portion is posterior to the liver. Its superior aspect is behind the bare area of the liver. Its inferior aspect is beneath the peritoneal reflection. In some individuals, the duodenal loop is anterior to this area of the right gland.

The left gland is usually lateral or posterolateral to the aorta. Its upper two thirds are covered by the peritoneum of the lesser sac, which is behind the stomach. The lower third of the left gland is nonperitonealized and lies posterior to the body of the pancreas and the splenic vessels.

The arterial supply to the adrenal glands is through 50 to 60 thread-like arteries (arteriae comitantes) that enter the superior, medial, and inferior aspects of the gland. These arterial branches can be divided into three groups according to their vessel of origin: (1) the superior group from the inferior phrenic artery, (2) the medial group of the aorta, and (3) the inferior group from the renal artery. Branches have also been described arising from the intercostal arteries and left gonadal vessels.

The venous drainage of each gland is mainly through a single central vein. These veins exit the adrenal hilum without a corresponding major artery. On the right, the hilum is at the anteromedial aspect of the gland and the vein enters the vena cava directly. Rarely, the right adrenal vein may join an accessory hepatic vein before entering the vena cava on its posterior or posterolateral wall at the level of the twelfth rib.

The hilum of the left gland is located inferomedially. The left adrenal vein exits the gland and joins with the inferior phrenic vein before draining into the superior aspect of the left renal vein.

The right adrenal vein is smaller and shorter than the left, which in part accounts for the difficulty in finding and catheterizing this vessel. Its average length is 12 mm (range, 0.5 to 15 mm), and its average diameter is 4 mm (range, 2 to 7 mm). The left adrenal vein is larger and longer than the right. Its length averages 18 mm (range, 4 to 41 mm), while its diameter averages 5 mm (range, 3 to 8 mm).

The central adrenal vein and its intraglandular branches are connected to a pericapsular venous system by emissary veins. These emissary veins may also connect to other retroperitoneal veins such as the gonadal veins. The capsular veins may also communicate with the inferior phrenic vein, renal vein, or splenic vein. These communications provide collateral drainage for the adrenal gland. In addition, the adrenal venous system may act as a collateral drainage path for these adjacent structures. For example, the connection to the portal system via splenic vein–adrenal emissary communication may enlarge in portal hypertension to become a spontaneous splenoadrenal-renal shunt.

TECHNIQUES

Urography

The plain film is important in the demonstration and localization of calcifications. Adrenal cysts calcify in approximately 15 per cent of cases. The pattern is usually curvilinear and peripheral in location. Other common causes of adrenal calcification include prior neonatal adrenal hemorrhage and neuroblastoma. Tumor is also a common cause of adrenal calcification, occurring in 10 to 14 per cent of cases. The pattern of calcification varies from punctate to peripheral "eggshell" type. Rarer causes of adrenal calcification include myelolipoma, Wolman's disease, and hemangioma.

Following the plain film, we generally perform 10-degree zonography at 3 to 5 minutes after the administration of the contrast agent. For better detail, we may increase the arc of the tomogram to 30 to 40 degrees so that the glands are studied by thinner sections. In order to get optimal total body opacification effect, one should use 1 ml of water-soluble contrast material per pound of body weight. This may be done using the bolus technique or the infusion method. It is important to rule out cardiac, renal, or other relative contraindications to larger doses of contrast material. Eighty per cent of adrenal cortical tumors and pheochromocytomas can be demonstrated by nephrotomography. The rate of tumor detection decreases for the aldosteronoma, since these lesions are often quite small.

Some normal structures may be confused with adrenal masses. These include the spleen and fundus of the stomach on the left. The spleen is usually quite lateral in position. In questionable cases, the fundus of the stomach can be identified by turning the patient into the prone position so that gas collects in that area.

Adrenal masses on the left tend to rotate the upper pole of the kidney laterally while displacing the kidney inferiorly. This is not surprising, since the gland occupies an anteromedial position relative to the kidney.

On the right the gland tends to be more suprarenal in location, so that indentation of the upper pole of the kidney as well as inferior displacement is common. It is important to emphasize that large right-sided adrenal tumors may compress and thin the liver as they extend anteriorly. Such large adrenal masses may be thought to be of hepatic origin. This differentiation is usually resolved by CT or sonography. In questionable cases, the blood supply may have to be identified to define the organ of origin.

Computed Tomography

CT is the most widely used imaging modality for evaluating the patient with suspected adrenal disease. Modern scanners are capable of producing images in 2 to 5 seconds. Slice thickness of 2 to 4 mm is readily available.

The optimal use of CT requires proper patient preparation. We routinely administer orally a solution of dilute barium so that bowel loops are opacified, precluding their misidentification as adrenal masses. One may examine the adrenals without the use of intravenous contrast enhancement, since the perirenal fat provides natural contrast to the water-density adrenal glands. Nevertheless, we have found it useful to know exactly where the upper pole of the kidney ends, particularly in patients with suspected adrenal masses. Adjacent vessels may be erroneously interpreted as adrenal tumors. Contrast enhancement will usually correctly identify these pseudotumors. For this reason, we generally use intravenous contrast material in the evaluation of the patient with suspected adrenal pathology. If there is a relative contraindication to the use of intravenous contrast material, we perform an unenhanced scan before resorting to the use of contrast agents. We use either a bolus technique, injecting 50 to 150 ml of 50 per cent diatrizoate; or an infusion technique, using 300 ml of 30 per cent diatrizoate.

It is most important to include the entire adrenal gland in the scans. We have made it a practice to scan from the superiormost aspect of the right gland at least to the level of the left renal hilum using an initial slice thickness of 10 mm. If a small tumor or nodule is suspected, 5-mm scans are performed.

This technique should lead to demonstration of the adrenals in almost every case. Rarely, patients with diminished retroperitoneal fat due to long-standing disease may prove to be poor candidates for adrenal evaluation by CT. These rare patients can be evaluated by ultrasound and/or venography.

The anteromedial ridge and part of the lateral wing of the right adrenal are situated posterior to the inferior vena cava without interposed fat. It is at this point that the right gland and vena cava may appear as a single confluent structure (Fig. 63–2*A*). This problem does not exist on the left, where the gland is surrounded completely by perirenal fat. The appearance of the right gland varies as sequential scans are obtained from apex to base. Most superior sections disclose a linear structure between the liver laterally and the crus of the diaphragm medially (Fig. 63–2*B*). More inferior sections reveal the gland to have a V or inverted Y configuration (Fig. 63–2*C*). The apex of the V corresponds to the anteromedial ridge and part of the lateral wing. The limbs of the gland that form the base of the V or inverted Y are directed posteriorly. The lateral limb extends in the direction of the adjacent liver, while the medial limb parallels the crus of the diaphragm. This limb is longer and extends more posteriorly. The right adrenal extends above the kidney in normal individuals. The base of the V or inverted Y widens as one progresses more inferiorly. In addition, the upper pole of the kidney is often visualized posterolateral to the base of the gland. Thus, the adrenal is more anteromedial to the kidney than it is suprarenal. Separation between the limbs of the adrenals is accentuated in obese patients.

The left adrenal is truly anteromedial to the kidney. In fact, the left gland extends above the upper pole of the kidney in less than half of the cases. The left gland extends in the direction of the renal hilum where the adrenal vein enters the superior aspect of the renal vein.

The left gland is also identifiable as an inverted Y or V shape on the cross-sectional images obtained on CT scan (Fig. 63–3). The anteromedial ridge (apex of V or stem of inverted Y) is larger than that of the right side, while the wings that form the base of the gland are smaller. These posterolateral and posteromedial wings or limbs widen as one progresses in a caudal direction. Anterolateral to the gland is the splenic vein and body or tail of the pancreas. Medial to the left gland is the crus of the diaphragm.

The actual size of the adrenal glands has been studied by a variety of modalities. In clinical practice, one "eyeballs" the glands to determine enlargement. Normal size may not indicate absence of disease. For example, patients with Cushing's syndrome due to hyperfunction have normal size glands in 50 per cent of cases. Normal length of the adrenals has been described as 2.5 to 4 cm. In our experience, the left gland tends to be slightly larger than the right. This correlates well with postmortem studies.

The thickness of the limbs of the gland are of more significance than the overall length of the gland or its individual limbs. Karstaedt et al (1978) described a mean of 5.1 mm (SD, 1.1 mm) for the right and 6.7 mm (SD, 1.7 mm) for the left. In general, a gland with limbs that are greater than 1.0 cm in thickness must be considered abnormal. A presumptive diagnosis of hyperplasia should be made if this thickening involves most of the gland. If these areas of thickening are localized, the possibility of nodular hyperplasia should be considered.

Ultrasonography

Since the glands are situated deep in the upper abdomen and surrounded by ribs, demonstration may present quite a challenge. These anatomic and technical problems explain why CT and MRI are currently the methods of choice for imaging these glands.

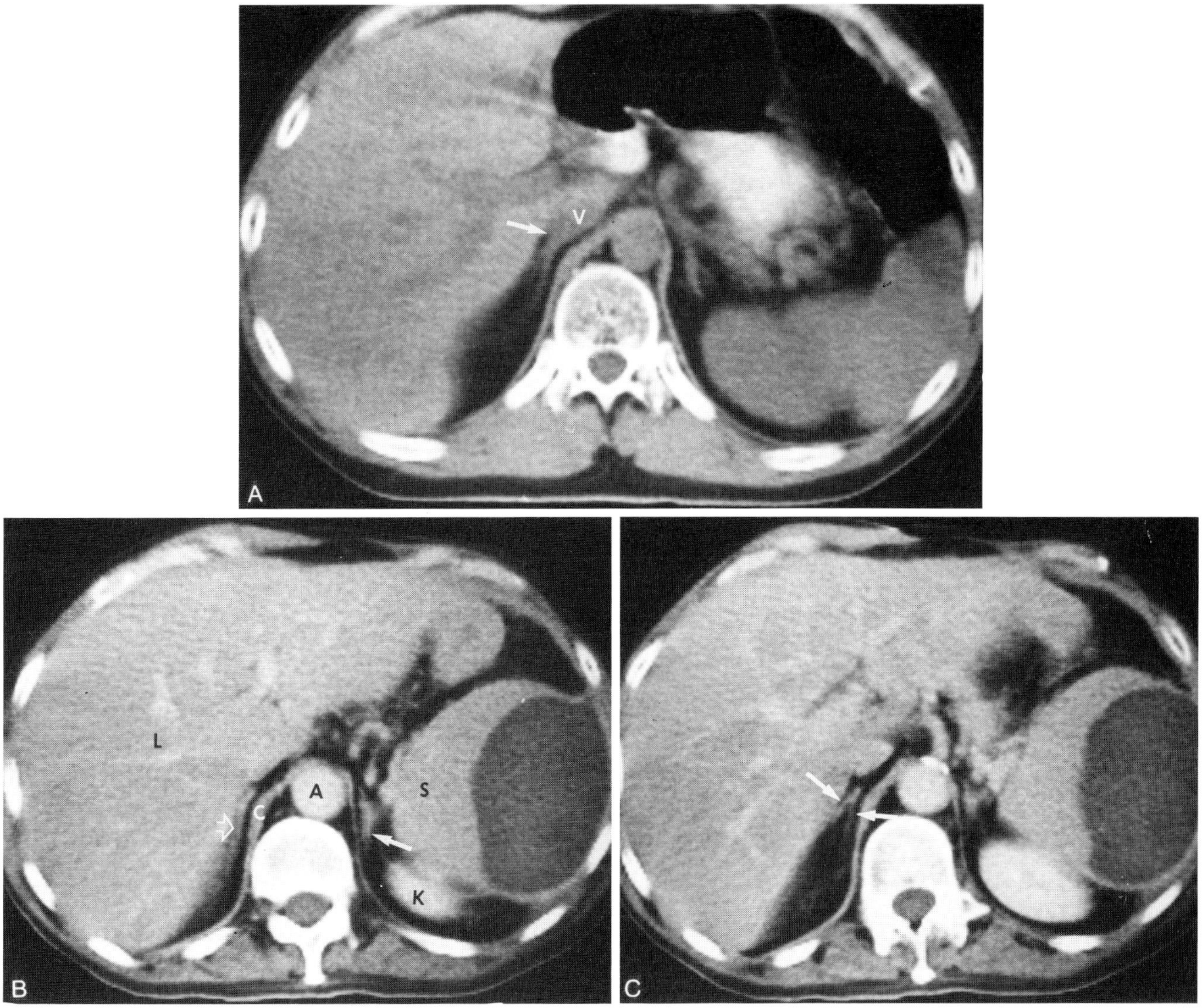

Figure 63–2. CT scans. *A,* Anteromedial ridge of right gland *(arrow)* appears as a single confluent structure with vena cava (V) due to lack of interposed fat. *B,* CT scan demonstrates the superior portion of right gland as a linear structure *(open arrow)* between the liver laterally and the crus of the diaphragm medially. Note that the left medial wing *(arrow)* is seen as a linear structure extending posterior from a short anteromedial ridge. The lateral wing is just visible in this cephalad section. (L = liver; S = spleen, with organized hematoma; A = aorta; K = kidney; C = crus of diaphragm.) *C,* Same patient as in *B* but at a more caudal level revealing inverted V configuration of the right gland *(arrows).*

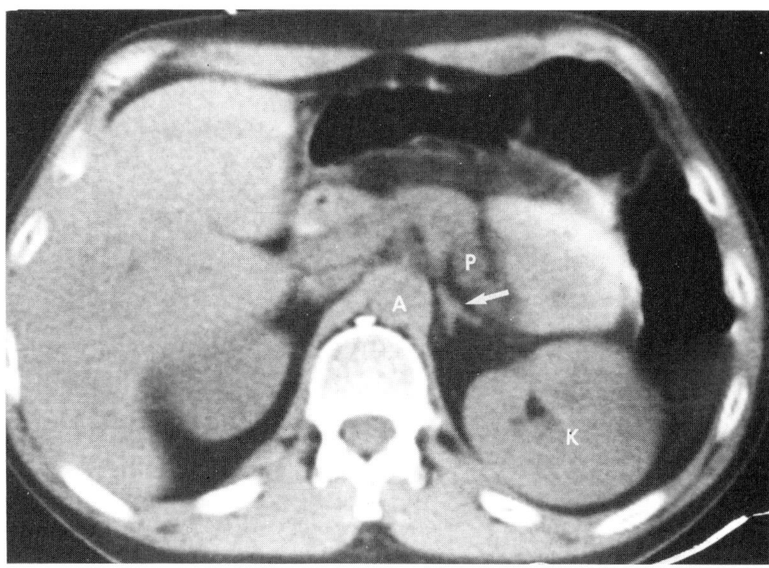

Figure 63–3. CT scans. Left adrenal. The anteromedial ridge as well as the medial and lateral wings are clearly demonstrated, giving the typical inverted Y appearance *(arrow).* Note that the gland is lateral to the aorta (A), anteromedial to the kidney (K), and posteromedial to the tail of the pancreas (P).

One should use a high-quality sector real-time scanner to study these patients and obtain satisfactory sonographic images. Generally, a 3.5-mHz transducer is used, although a 2.25-mHz transducer may also suffice. In the case of obese patients, a 1.7- to 2.25-mHz transducer is used for better penetration. A 5-mHz transducer may improve resolution in small children or babies. A smaller transducer surface is preferred in small children so that the intercostal spaces can be scanned more effectively.

Overlying ribs and transverse processes usually preclude posterior scanning of the adrenal glands. The anterior transverse scan usually provides the most information. The patient is scanned in the supine position using a series of sector scans from an intercostal space somewhat posterior to the anterior axillary line. These scans extend from the level of the renal hilum cephalad until reverberation echoes appear from the costophrenic sulcus. This anterior transverse series visualizes the adrenal area, the upper half of the kidneys, the lateral border of the spine, the crus of the diaphragm, the liver or spleen, and part of the aorta or inferior vena cava. This is easier on the right than on the left, where gastric or bowel gas often presents a problem. One can improve this situation on the left by elevating the patient's left side slightly and scanning from a more posterior location. Often, the spleen provides a good sonographic window to the left side (Fig. 63–4). In the average hospital population the right adrenal can be defined in one or more scans in 78.5 per cent of cases, the left in 44 per cent, and both glands in 31.5 per cent.

The anterior longitudinal scan can also be quite useful in demonstrating the normal right gland as well as right adrenal masses. A series of scans at close intervals is done from a point medial to the inferior vena cava and extending laterally until the gland is seen. The right gland will usually appear as a horizontal V- or Y-shaped structure immediately posterior to the vena cava. At times, it is difficult to separate the normal right adrenal from the upper pole of the kidney. This can usually be accomplished by having the patient take a deep breath just before the scan. The kidney usually moves inferiorly, while the adrenal remains relatively fixed.

Small masses are best demonstrated on the anterior transverse scan. Masses as small as 1.2 cm have been demonstrated with this approach. Moderate size masses are easily shown in any projection. When masses are greater than 6 cm in diameter, the posterior longitudinal approach becomes useful because the relationship to the kidney is important and well-defined in this view.

Right adrenal masses may compress the posterior aspect of the inferior vena cava. As right adrenal masses increase in size, they tend to extend lateral to the vena cava and make contact with the posterior aspect of the liver. Very large right adrenal tumors may compress and thin the right lobe of the liver. On occasion, the hepatic or adrenal origin of such a mass may be in doubt. Angiography may be useful in such cases by defining the vessel providing supply to the mass.

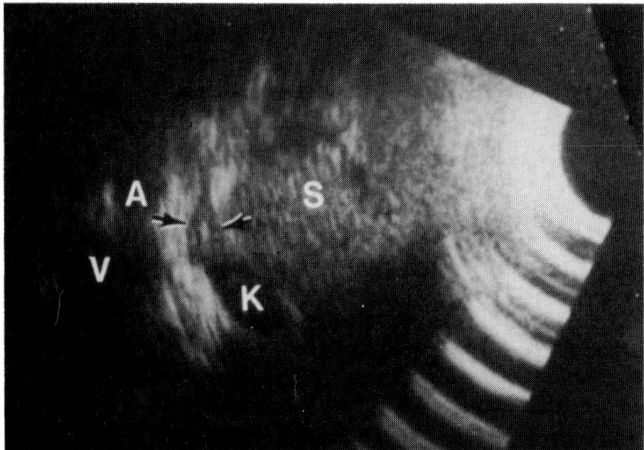

Figure 63–4. Sonogram of normal left adrenal gland. This sector scan was made from the left upper flank. The gland appears as an inverted Y *(arrows)* lateral to the aorta (A) and medial to the spleen (S). (K = upper pole of kidney; V = vertebral body.) (Courtesy of Dr. H-C Yeh.)

Abrams and coworkers undertook a prospective study of the usefulness of CT and ultrasound in a study of the adrenal gland in 110 patients. CT had a sensitivity of 83 per cent, a specificity of 98 per cent, and an accuracy of 90 per cent. Sonography had a sensitivity of 76 per cent, a specificity of 57 per cent, and an accuracy of 68 per cent. This study supports the concept that CT is preferred over sonography in the evaluation of adrenal disease.

Arteriography

The arteriographic study of the adrenal is rarely indicated. Those patients who come to arteriography usually have large adrenal masses. The blood supply to such lesions may be of importance to the surgeon for preoperative planning. In some patients, the origin of large masses may be in doubt, and demonstration of the major blood supply may indicate the nature of the lesion.

The three groups of arteries that supply the adrenal are superior adrenals from the inferior phrenic, middle adrenals from the aorta, and inferior adrenals from the renal. In fact, there is frequent variation in blood supply. Some patients lack major branches and have one or two vessels that are dominant. The important thing to remember is that one must account for all adrenal parenchyma regardless of the site of origin of the supplying vessels. Selective injection of all major adrenal arteries can be a tedious and time-consuming endeavor, but this is rarely necessary in the CT era.

Venography

The venous approach to the adrenal has two advantages: (1) each gland is drained by a single vein, making catheterization less tedious; and (2) blood samples can be obtained for assay in order to localize functioning lesions.

Opacification of the adrenals by retrograde injection requires careful hand injections, so that rupture of the veins does not occur. This is the most common complication of adrenal venography and occurs in approximately 5 per cent of patients. Although usually self-limited, adrenal insufficiency may occur.

Extravasation following rupture of the adrenal veins is usually accompanied by severe back pain that may radiate to the shoulder. This pain is often quite persistent and may require narcotics for several days. If the extravasation occurs on the side of subsequent surgery, the local hematoma and inflammatory reaction can make the surgeon's job significantly more difficult. Since adrenal insufficiency can occur as a complication of contrast material extravasation, it is not surprising that this procedure has been employed for adrenal ablation. Purposeful extravasation of contrast material has been used in patients with metastatic breast carcinoma to effect a nonsurgical adrenalectomy.

RIGHT ADRENAL VENOGRAPHY

A variety of catheters has been employed for right adrenal venography. We have found the "cobra" shape quite adequate for this purpose. The right adrenal vein is usually found at a level between the eleventh and twelfth ribs. It is important to remember that the vein enters the posterior aspect of the vena cava at this level. The most common error in attempting right adrenal vein catheterization is to orient the tip of the catheter to the right. In most cases, this will result in entrance into one of the accessory hepatic veins at this level. Injection of an hepatic vein results in the characteristic hepatic parenchymal blush.

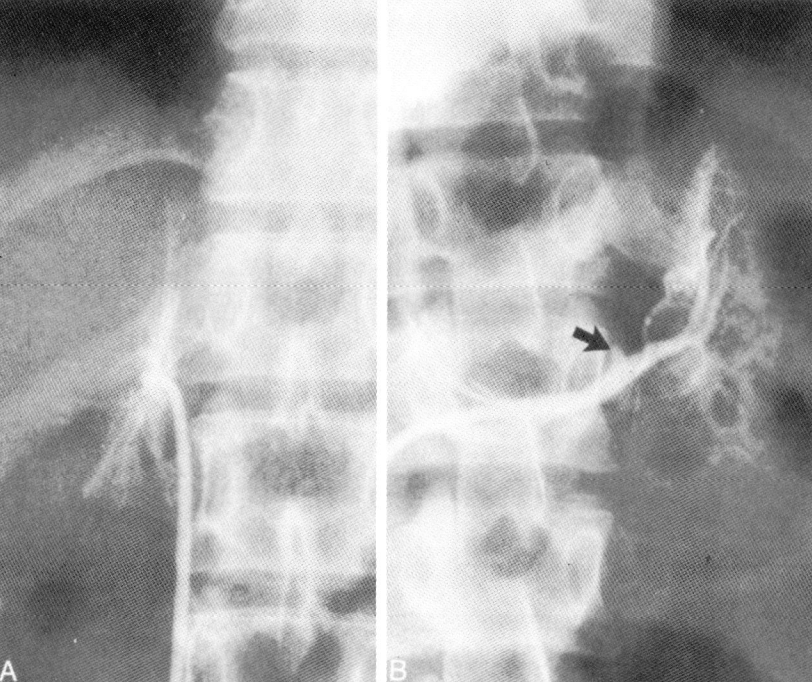

Figure 63–5. Normal adrenal venograms. *A*, Right. A normally triangular structure is demonstrated. Note that the catheter tip is oriented almost directly posterior. *B*, Left. Note the tendency to convex contours of the normal left gland. The point of entrance of the inferior phrenic vein is also demonstrated *(arrow)*.

The normal right adrenal venogram demonstrates a more or less triangular gland (Fig. 63–5*A*). Injection studies by McLachlan and Roberts have demonstrated a medial convex border in 80 per cent of cases and a superior convex border in 40 per cent. One third of normal right adrenals have more than one convex border. The frontal radiographic appearance is more frequently that of a concave lateral-inferior border. The medial border may be flat or concave. The intraglandular configuration on venography is an orderly branching pattern. There are small communicating veins (venae comitantes) that drain through the capsule of the gland to join adjacent retroperitoneal branches including the inferior phrenic, renal capsule, and lumbars. For this reason, one may inject the main adrenal vein and see filling of these adjacent veins. Similarly, one can inject these adjacent veins and see communication with the adrenal venous system. On two occasions in 220 adrenal venograms, we have encountered a situation in which the right adrenal vein joins with an accessory hepatic vein before entering the inferior vena cava.

LEFT ADRENAL VENOGRAPHY

Since the left adrenal vein joins the renal vein in a rather constant position, it is catheterized more easily than the right. In general, the point of junction is over the left pedicle of the T12-L1 vertebrae. In addition, the left adrenal vein is larger where it joins the inferior phrenic vein.

Several manufacturers produce catheters with a double-curve configuration designed to enter the left adrenal vein. The proximal curve matches the renal vein, and the distal curve is angulated cephalad to facilitate entrance into the adrenal vein. Once this preformed catheter has entered the renal vein it is usually a simple matter to engage the tip into the adrenal vein. However, one must be sure that the catheter tip does not enter the inferior phrenic vein. This will result in poor adrenal vein filling and erroneous adrenal blood samples.

The normal left adrenal venogram demonstrates a structure with borders that are almost always convex (Fig. 63–5*B*). The left gland is somewhat larger than the right but has a similar regular internal branching pattern. The central adrenal vein is usually larger than the right. Here, too, venae comitantes are seen to anastomose with adjacent veins. Some of these communications can be quite prominent and may overlie the gland, making interpretation more difficult. One communication on the left that deserves special mention is that with the portal system via small branches. We have opacified the splenic vein in otherwise normal patients during left-sided adrenal venography in 2 to 3 per cent of cases. These communications may enlarge in patients with portal hypertension to produce a spontaneous splenoadrenal-renal shunt. We have encountered several instances in which such enlarged veins have produced an image resembling an adrenal mass on CT. In the presence of portal hypertension, a patient with a suspected left adrenal mass should have an enhanced CT scan to be sure that such a mass is not an enlarged vein. In questionable cases, venography or MRI may be performed to establish the nature of such a "mass."

Venous Sampling

Obtaining blood from the right adrenal vein can be tedious and time-consuming. One cannot aspirate blood with a syringe, because it may result in collapse of the small veins under the negative pressure or possibly suction of the intima against the catheter tip. The best method for obtaining a sample on the right is to keep the catheter hub in a dependent position and simply allow the blood to drip into the test tube. Collecting a sample on the left is usually not a problem, since the preformed catheter tip is oriented along the long axis of the vessel. On the right, it is often helpful to rotate the catheter slightly while the tip remains in the orifice until maximum flow is obtained. A catheter sidehole cannot be used for sampling. Since the right vein is so short, one may actually be sampling vena cava via the sidehole while the tip is occluded by intima. On occasion, we have cut a notch in the inferior aspect of the end of a right adrenal vein catheter to facilitate sampling.

Adrenal sampling should always be performed prior to venography. In this way, a valid sample can be used for diagnosis even if extravasation occurs as a complication of the venography.

Other Sampling

There is good evidence that simultaneous bilateral petrosal sinus sampling is an effective means of localizing the source of adrenocorticotropic hormone (ACTH) in patients with adrenal hyperfunction. This is particularly important because trans-sphenoidal hypophysectomy is the preferred method of treating patients with Cushing's disease due to a basophilic microadenoma. Confirmation that the pituitary rather than an ectopic location is the source of increased ACTH production is good practice before pituitary surgery is performed in these patients.

The procedure is performed by passing catheters from both femoral veins into the petrosal sinuses. Contrast material is injected to confirm correct catheter position. Simultaneous samples are obtained. One may augment the gradients between right and left by injecting corticotropin-releasing hormone before sampling.

Radioisotope Scanning

Iodine-131 19-iodocholesterol is administered intravenously in a dose of 2 mCi. Thyroid accumulation is minimized by giving the patient Lugol's solution before the tracer and continuing this blocking agent for two weeks. Scans are performed at 2 to 14 days after administration of the isotope. This delay, which is an inherent disadvantage of this method, is necessary because the isotopic agent must be incorporated into adrenal steroid synthesis. The patient will require an average of three visits for scanning in order to identify the optimal time for obtaining the best image.

Right adrenal visualization may be impaired by the radioactivity in the liver and gallbladder. Similarly, GI tract accumulation of the isotopic agent may obscure the left adrenal. These problems are easily overcome by fatty meals and/or enemas, depending on the site of extra-adrenal localization of the isotope. Further definition of the adrenals can be accomplished by means of computer enhancement or by subtracting hepatic accumulation.

Radioisotope scanning has been employed with success in patients with adrenal hyperfunction causing Cushing's syndrome (Fig. 63–6). In these patients, one sees bilateral uptake of the agent. This method is particularly useful in the patient who has had bilateral adrenalectomy but continues to have Cushing's syndrome. The isotopic agent will localize in the causative adrenal remnant, which may be in a distorted postsurgical area.

In the case of a functioning adrenocortical adenoma, one obtains intense uptake in the mass while the suppressed normal gland will not visualize. Adrenocortical carcinomas usually have poor uptake of the isotope per gram of excised tissue. At the same time, the normal gland is also suppressed. For this reason, the isotopic scan usually shows little uptake on either side in the patient with adrenocortical carcinoma and Cushing's syndrome.

Hyperaldosteronism due to an adenoma does not suppress the contralateral gland's ability to take up and metabolize the isotope. In order to define the side of the lesion, dexamethasone suppression is usually employed. In this way, uptake by normal adrenal tissue is prevented so that the tumor of Conn's syndrome can be localized. The dexamethasone-suppressed scan is also useful in differentiating aldosteronism of Conn's tumor from that due to nodular hyperplasia. The suppression occurs in patients with hyperfunction, but the Conn tumor will continue to take up the isotope. Using this method, the correct differential diagnosis can be made in 80 to 90 per cent of cases.

Reports have emphasized the usefulness of ^{131}I-metaiodobenzylguanidine (^{131}I-MIBG) for the localization of pheochromocytomas. This agent localizes in adrenergic tissues in both the adrenal medulla and extra-adrenal sites. The normal adrenal medulla and extra-adrenal chromaffin tissues are too small to be visualized by this agent. Pheochromocytomas, which are usually several centimeters in size, contain many adrenergic storage vesicles and as a result are imaged by ^{131}I-MIBG. This agent also localizes in neuroblastomas.

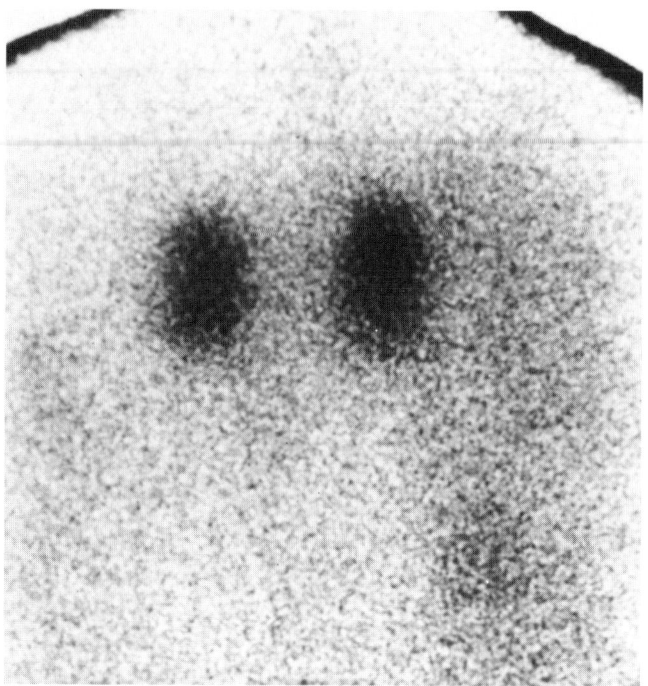

Figure 63–6. Posterior scintiscan of a patient with adrenal hyperfunction due to Cushing's syndrome with relatively normal size glands using ^{131}I-NP-59.

The dose of this radiopharmaceutical is 0.5 mCi, or 0.5 mCi/1.7 m^2 of body surface area if that is a smaller amount. A saturated solution of one drop of potassium iodide orally is administered twice a day for one day before giving the isotope, and for one week thereafter to protect the thyroid gland. Most pheochromocytomas will be visualized optimally two to three days after giving the isotope. Sisson et al reported that they were able to localize tumors in 76 of 84 patients with pheochromocytoma, including 12 that were extra-adrenal in location. The reason for not localizing all pheochromocytomas by this method is not clear but may be related to low storage capacity in these particular lesions or other metabolic aberration. This method has its greatest usefulness in localizing lesions in extra-adrenal areas, particularly in patients with multiple lesions and as a confirmatory study to CT and MRI.

Van Gils et al reported on the results of MRI and MIBG scanning in 33 patients and found that MIBG scintigraphy was more specific but MRI was more sensitive. As a result, they recommended MRI as the initial technique for evaluating these patients.

Magnetic Resonance Imaging (MRI)

Modern MRI has become a valuable imaging modality for the study of the adrenal gland. As early as 1983, Moon et al reported their results in the evaluation of 42 patients. Both CT and MRI demonstrated the pathology in the six abnormal cases. The spatial resolution was superior with CT, while soft-tissue contrast was better with MRI.

MRI has the advantage of allowing reconstruction in sagittal and coronal planes as well as the standard axial projection (Fig. 63–7). One inherent advantage of MRI is its non-ionizing nature. MRI also allows tissue characterization. Thus, pheochromocytomas are shown as very bright lesions on T_2-weighted images. At 1.5 T, there is evidence that MRI is useful for distinguishing adenomas from non-

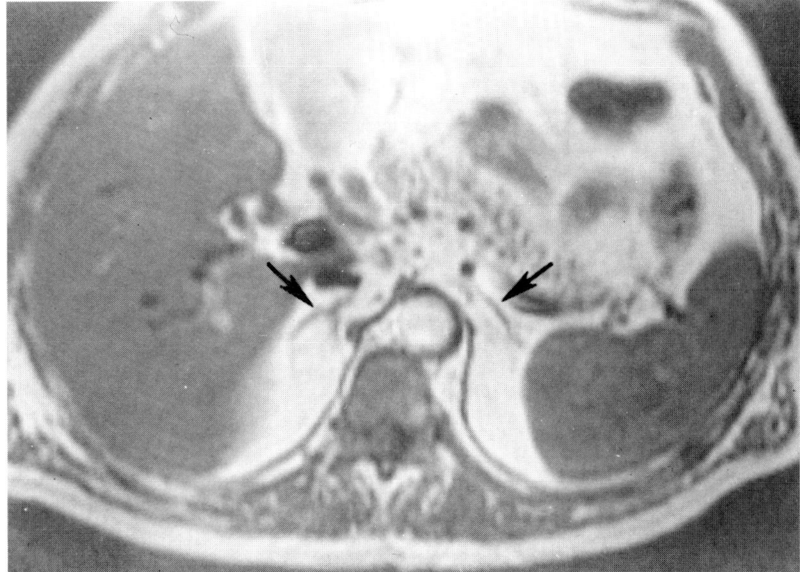

Figure 63–7. Magnetic resonance image. Portions of both adrenal glands *(arrows)* are well-visualized.

adenomas. These differences may be enhanced by administering Gd-DTPA before the study. MR spectroscopy has also been employed in vivo as an additional method to help differentiate benign from malignant adrenal lesions.

Bibliography

Abrams HL, Siegelman SS, Adams DF, et al: Computed tomography versus ultrasound of the adrenal gland: A prospective study. Radiology 143:121, 1982.

Anson BJ, Caudwell EW, Pick JW, Beaton LE: The anatomy of the pararenal system of veins, with comments on the renal arteries. J Urol 60:714, 1948.

Baker ME, Blinder R, Spritzer C, et al: MR evaluation of adrenal masses at 1.5 T. AJR 153:307, 1989.

Bayliss RIS, Edwards OM, Starer F: Complications of adrenal venography. Br J Radiol 43:531, 1970.

Cho KJ: Current role of angiography in the evaluation of adrenal disease causing hypertension. Urol Radiol 3:249, 1982.

Doppman JL, Oldfield E, Krudy AG, et al: Petrosal sinus sampling for Cushing syndrome: Anatomical and technical considerations. Radiology 150:99, 1984.

Dunnick NR, Doppman JL, Gill JR, et al: Localization of functional adrenal tumors by computed tomography and venous sampling. Radiology 142:429, 1982.

Dunnick NR, Korobkin M: Computed tomography of the adrenal gland in hypertension. Urol Radiol 3:245, 1982.

Francis IR, Glazer GM, Shapiro B, et al: Complementary roles of CT and ^{131}I-MIBG scintigraphy in diagnosing pheochromocytoma. AJR 141:719, 1983.

Gross MD, Thompson NW, Beierwaltes WH: Scintigraphic approach to the localization of adrenal lesions causing hypertension. Urol Radiol 3:241, 1982.

Hattner RS, Huberty JP, Engelstad BL, et al: Localization of M-Iodo (^{131}I) benzylguanidine in neuroblastoma. AJR 143:373, 1984.

Holmes RO, Moon HD, Rinehart JE: A morphologic study of the adrenal gland with correlations of body size and heart size. Am J Pathol 27:724, 1951.

Huebener KH, Treugut H: Adrenal cortex dysfunction: CT finding. Radiology 150:195, 1984.

Karstaedt N, Sagel SS, Stanley RJ, et al: Computed tomography of the adrenal gland. Radiology 129:723, 1978.

Kier R, McCarthy S: MR characterization of adrenal masses. Radiology 171:671, 1989.

Krestin GP, Steinbrich W, Friedmann G: Adrenal masses: Evaluation with fast gradient echo MR imaging and Gd-DPTA–enhanced dynamic studies. Radiology 171:675, 1989.

Leroy-Willig A, Bittoun J, Lujon JP, et al: In vivo MR spectroscopic imaging of the adrenal glands. AJR 153:771, 1989.

McLachlan MSF, Roberts EE: Demonstration of normal adrenal gland by venography and gas insufflation. Br J Radiol 44:664, 1971.

Mitty HA, Nicolis GL, Gabrilove JL: Adrenal venography: Clinical-roentgenographic correlation in 80 patients. AJR 119:564, 1977.

Mitty HA, Shapira H: Total body opacification in the adult. AJR 115:630, 1972.

Moon KL, Hricak H, Crooks LE, et al: Nuclear magnetic resonance imaging of the adrenal gland: A preliminary report. Radiology 147:155, 1983.

Oldfield EH, Doppman JL, Nieman LK, et al: Petrosal sinus sampling with and without corticotrophin releasing hormone for the differential diagnosis of Cushing's syndrome. N Engl J Med 325:877, 1991.

Raisanen J, Shapiro B, Glazer GM, et al: Plasma catecholamines in pheochromocytoma: Effect of urographic contrast media. AJR 142:43, 1984.

Rubin RT, Phillips JJ: Adrenal gland volume determination by computed tomography and magnetic resonance imaging in normal subjects. Invest Radiol 26:465, 1991.

Sisson JC, Shapiro B, Beierwaltes WH, Copp JE: Locating pheochromocytomas by scintigraphy using I^{131} metaiodobenzylguanidine. CA 34:86, 1984.

van Gils APG, Falke THM, van Erkel AR, et al: MR imaging and MIBG scintigraphy of pheochromocytomas and extraadrenal functioning paragangliomas. Radiographics 11:37, 1991.

Yeh HC: Sonography of the adrenal glands: Normal glands and small masses. AJR 135:1167, 1980.

64 Functional Lesions of the Adrenal Cortex

N. Reed Dunnick

Although small, the adrenal glands are active endocrine organs. Patients with diseases of the adrenal glands often present as a result of either excess or inadequate hormone secretion. In the adrenal cortex, these endocrine syndromes include hypersecretion of cortisol, aldosterone, androgens, and estrogens. In addition, adrenal insufficiency may develop as a result of destruction of adrenal tissue by a variety of processes.

CUSHING'S SYNDROME

Cushing's syndrome is the result of excess glucocorticoid and can be either iatrogenic or spontaneous. The clinical manifestations of truncal obesity, hirsutism, abdominal striae, muscle atrophy, and hypertension are accompanied by osteoporosis and glucose intolerance. The diagnosis of Cushing's syndrome can be confirmed by finding elevated plasma or urinary 17-hydroxycorticosteroids that are not suppressed with dexamethasone. Hypersecretion of cortisol may result from an adrenal tumor, either adenoma or carcinoma, or from adrenal hyperplasia. Although biochemical tests help to differentiate among these entities, there is overlap and the radiologist is often asked to help in this distinction.

Adrenal hyperplasia is a bilateral process that results from stimulation of the cortex by excess adrenocorticotropic hormone (ACTH). Adrenal hyperplasia is the most common cause of Cushing's syndrome and typically occurs in women in the third or fourth decade of life. This hormone's oversecretion is usually due to a pituitary adenoma (Cushing's disease), but other tumors may also elaborate ACTH. Oat cell carcinoma and bronchial adenomas are the most common ACTH-producing tumors, although a variety of other sources, including tumors of the thymus, pancreas, ovary, and medullary carcinoma of the thyroid, have been reported. Although Cushing's syndrome is more common in women, there is a male preponderance among cases due to ACTH production by a nonpituitary tumor.

The adrenal glands enlarge in response to ACTH stimulation, and this generalized enlargement can usually be detected by computed tomography (CT). Both adrenal glands enlarge symmetrically, such that they maintain the normal adrenal configuration (Fig. 64–1). However, the appearance of hyperplasia overlaps with that of the normal gland, so that one cannot always predict upon the basis of size alone whether or not there is adrenal hyperfunction. Excess cortisol secretion, however, is easily confirmed biochemically, so that the distinction between normal and hyperplastic glands is not usually a clinical problem. The role of CT is to identify and localize a focal adrenal mass that would indicate a cortisol-secreting adrenal tumor.

Nodular cortical hyperplasia may represent a transition from ACTH-dependent hyperplasia to an autonomous adenoma. These cortical nodules vary from small microscopic whirls to a single large nodule that dominates the gland. Functionally, nodular hyperplasia responds the same as hyperplasia to ACTH or metyrapone tests. If a dominant nodule is present, it may be impossible to distinguish from an autonomous adenoma by CT, as both will be seen as a focal adrenal mass. Nodular hyperplasia is more common in children than in adults.

Adrenal adenomas are the most common adrenal tumor causing Cushing's syndrome. These tumors average about 4 cm in diameter and are readily detected by CT (Fig. 64–2). Furthermore, the abundant retroperitoneal fat present in these patients displays the adrenal glands and aids in tumor detection. Adrenal adenomas are homogeneous, rounded masses that seldom calcify. The density is variable, from near water to the soft tissue density of muscle.

Although less common, a significant number of cases of Cushing's syndrome are due to primary adrenal carcinoma. Approximately three-fourths of primary adrenal malignancies produce recognizable hormones, and cortisol is the hormone most commonly overproduced. It is likely that virtually all adrenal carcinomas are functional, but the steroids produced are incomplete and not recognized clinically.

It is often possible to predict that an adrenal tumor will be malignant based on the radiographic characteristics. Primary adrenal carcinomas are almost always very large by the time they are clinically detected. In one series, the smallest primary adrenal carcinoma was 8 cm in diameter, with the largest measuring 25 cm. This large size and the general hypovascular nature of adrenal cortical tumors contribute to the central necrosis and dystrophic calcification often seen.

Adrenal carcinoma is readily identified on CT examination, which can also be used to define the extent of the tumor. Involvement or displacement of adjacent organs, as well as extension of tumor through the adrenal vein to the left renal vein or inferior vena cava, can usually be shown (Fig. 64–3). Due to their large size, these tumors often abut and may invade adjacent organs, such as the kidney, liver, or spleen.

The presence or absence of tumor invasion into an adjacent organ may be critical in determining resectability. The abundant retro-

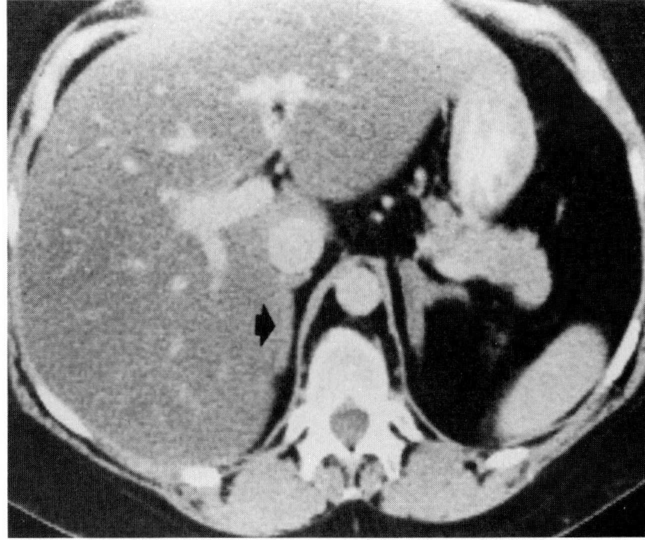

Figure 64–1. Bilateral adrenal hyperplasia. This 41-year-old female presented with Cushing's syndrome. Both adrenal glands are symmetrically enlarged. The low-density, fatty infiltration of the liver helps to identify the right adrenal gland *(arrow).*

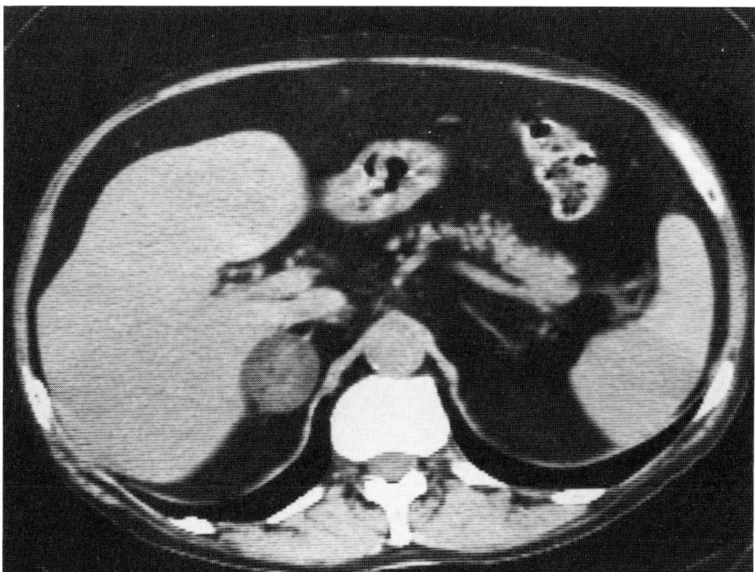

Figure 64–2. Adrenal adenoma. A 3.5-cm right adenoma is clearly seen in this patient with Cushing's syndrome.

peritoneal fat helps to define the local extent of these tumors. The presence of a fat plane indicates the limit of tumor extension. The absence of a fat plane, however, does not necessarily mean the tumor is invading the adjacent organ.

Magnetic resonance imaging (MRI) may also help to identify an adrenal carcinoma by the high signal intensity on T_2-weighted sequences (Fig. 64–4). With the improved spatial resolution of current systems, MRI can also be applied to small adenomas. However, the differences in signal intensity are not great enough to distinguish between functional and nonfunctional adenomas.

The primary value of MRI is in the detection and delineation of venous extension of adrenal carcinomas. Limited flip angle techniques are readily acquired and clearly demonstrate flowing blood to show vessel patency. This technique does not distinguish tumor thrombus from bland thrombus.

Arteriography is seldom needed but may be required in three specific settings: (1) to help identify the tissue of origin of a large upper quadrant mass, (2) to detect invasion of adjacent organs, and (3) to define the arterial supply to the tumor prior to surgery. Many times a large mass in the upper abdomen displaces and distorts adjacent organs to such an extent that it is unclear from which organ the tumor arose. Arteriography is used to identify the primary vascular supply to the tumor and thus provide further support for the tissue of origin (Fig. 64–5). Local invasion of adjacent organs may result in parasitization of arterial supply, but the predominant feeding vessels can usually still be recognized. Identification of tumor supply by other organ vessels, such as hepatic arteries, indicates direct invasion of the tumor into the liver. If surgery is anticipated, precise delineation of the feeding vessels and the identification of any vascular anomalies may be particularly valuable.

The accuracy of CT in detecting tumors causing Cushing's syndrome is excellent. Adenomas range from approximately 2 to 5 cm in diameter, and carcinomas are usually greater than 5 cm in diameter. The CT examination is also aided by the abundance of retroperitoneal fat resulting from the excess cortisol secretion. Although the symmetrically enlarged glands of adrenal hyperplasia are often easily recognized, there is significant overlap with the size of normal glands and this distinction is unreliable.

CONN'S SYNDROME

The syndrome of primary aldosteronism was described by Conn in 1955 and consists of hypertension, hypokalemia, and hyporeninemia as well as elevated serum and urine levels of aldosterone. In the adult the most common etiology is an adrenal adenoma, while bilateral adrenal hyperplasia is more common among children with this syndrome. Although several cases of primary adrenal carcinoma have been reported, it is a rare cause of primary aldosteronism.

Hyperaldosteronism results in excessive sodium retention, an increase in plasma volume, and hypertension. Hypokalemia is a result of the sodium retention as potassium is exchanged for sodium in the distal tubule. Patients with primary aldosteronism have a low serum renin concentration, which distinguishes them from patients with secondary aldosteronism, in which the serum renin activity is elevated. The definitive diagnosis of primary aldosteronism depends upon nonsuppressible plasma aldosterone levels and low plasma renin activity.

Although biochemical tests, such as the level of 18-hydroxycorticosterone and the change in serum aldosterone after upright posture, tend to distinguish hyperplasia from an adenoma, they are not absolute. Furthermore, if an adenoma is present, it must be lateralized and radiologic methods are needed.

The initial radiographic examination for patients with Conn's syndrome is CT. Aldosterone-secreting adenomas often have a homogeneous low density (Fig. 64–6). Since aldosterone-secreting adenomas tend to be small, averaging less than 2 cm in diameter, contiguous, narrowly collimated scans must be obtained. Intravenous contrast material is unlikely to be helpful, as the glands are usually well-defined by the surrounding fat, and the tumors are not hypervascular (Fig. 64–7). Even when carefully examined, some adenomas will be missed by CT due to their small size. The sensitivity of CT for the detection of aldosteronomas is approximately 85%.

Adrenal venous sampling may be employed when the CT examination fails to reveal a suspected adenoma or to evaluate equivocal cases. Since the syndrome is a function of hormone oversecretion rather than tumor mass, it is logical to selectively measure hormone levels to determine the location of the adenoma. By placing a catheter in the adrenal vein, blood samples may be obtained that reflect the hormone secretion. The technical difficulty of selectively catheterizing the right adrenal vein has prevented this technique from gaining widespread acceptance. It is, however, extremely accurate when adequate adrenal vein samples can be obtained. Furthermore, the use of anticoagulation during the procedure has markedly reduced the most troublesome complication of the procedure—venous thrombosis.

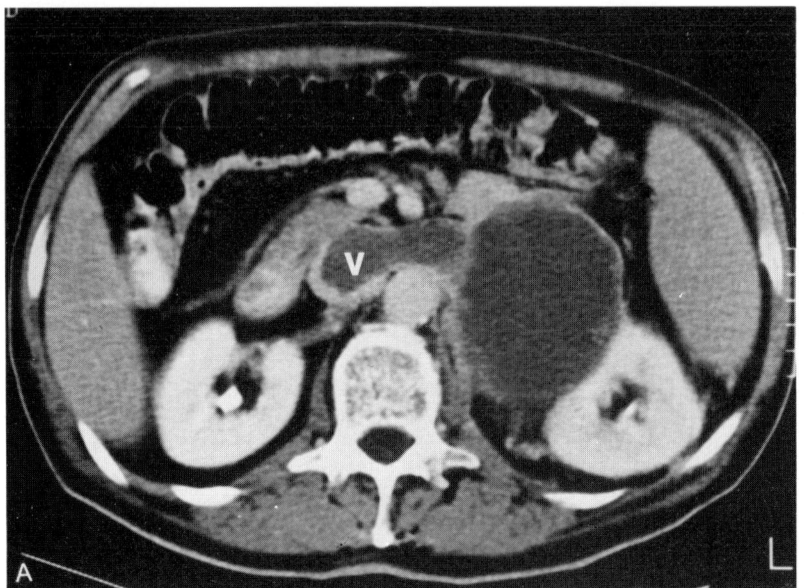

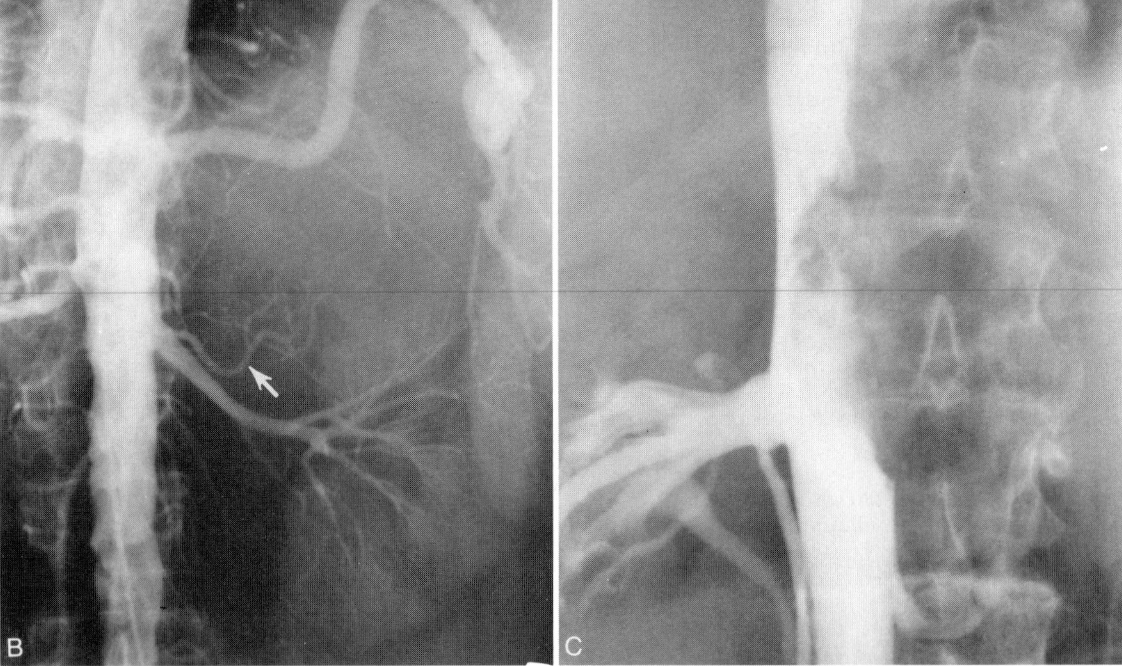

Figure 64–3. Adrenal carcinoma. *A,* A large left adrenal mass is causing lateral displacement of the left kidney. The low-density center of the adrenal mass indicates central necrosis. The tumor can be seen extending down into the renal vein and across to the inferior vena cava (V). *B,* Arteriography confirms the displacement of the kidney and demonstrates the supply to the tumor by the inferior adrenal artery *(arrow)* arising from the renal artery. *C,* An inferior venacavogram confirms the extent of the tumor into, but not occluding, the vena cava.

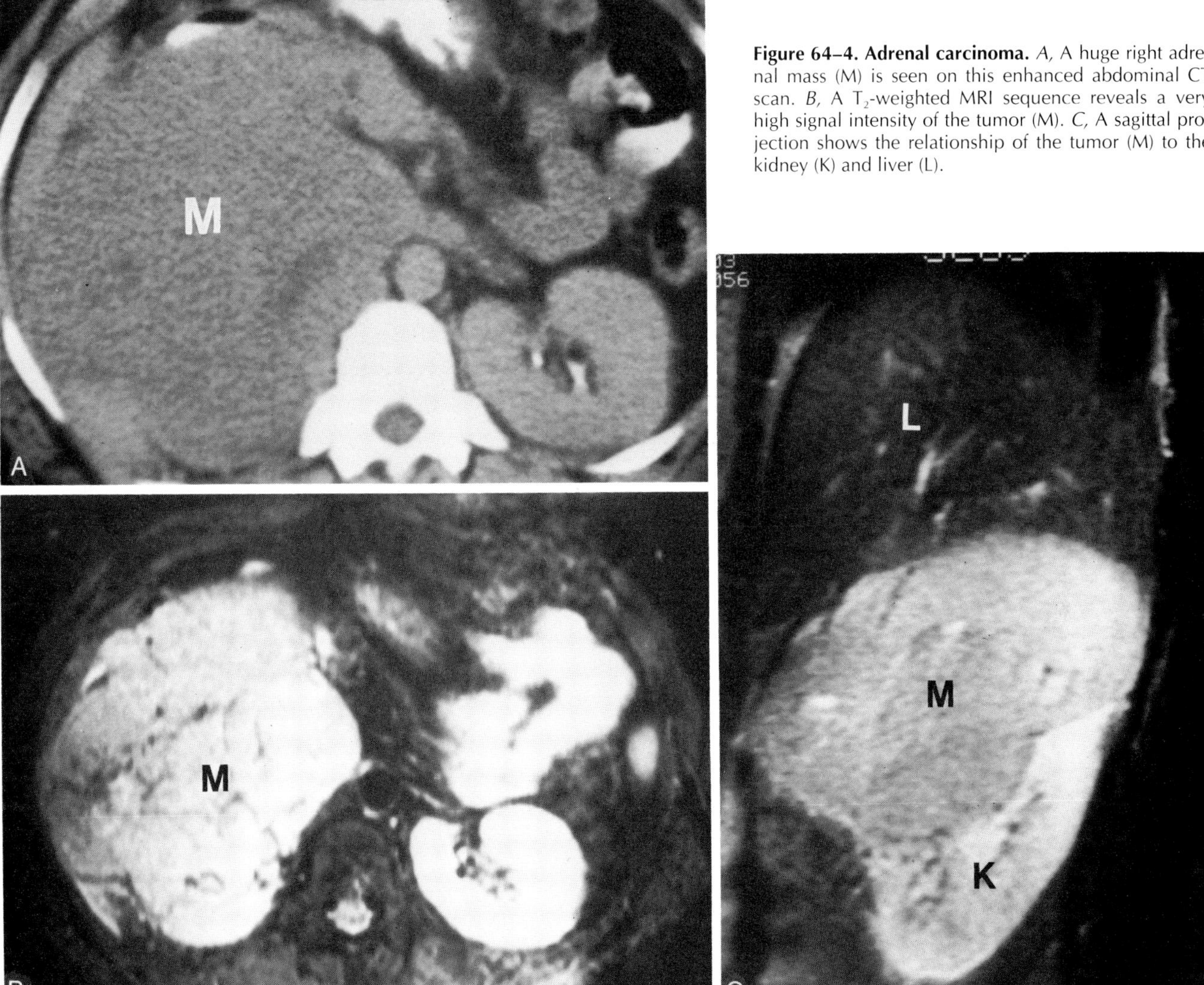

Figure 64–4. Adrenal carcinoma. *A,* A huge right adrenal mass (M) is seen on this enhanced abdominal CT scan. *B,* A T_2-weighted MRI sequence reveals a very high signal intensity of the tumor (M). *C,* A sagittal projection shows the relationship of the tumor (M) to the kidney (K) and liver (L).

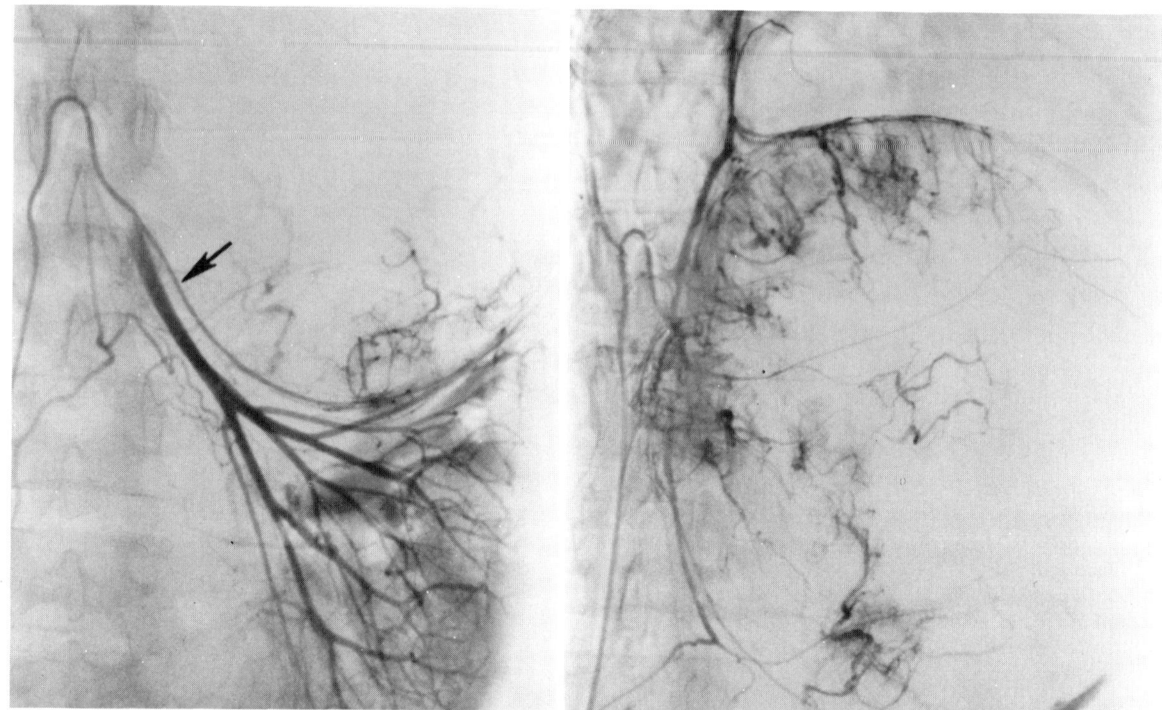

Figure 64–5. Adrenal carcinoma. *A,* Conventional arteriography was used to help determine the tissue of origin. Tumor vascularity is seen arising from the inferior adrenal artery *(arrow). B,* The largest supply to the tumor is coming from the superior adrenal artery.

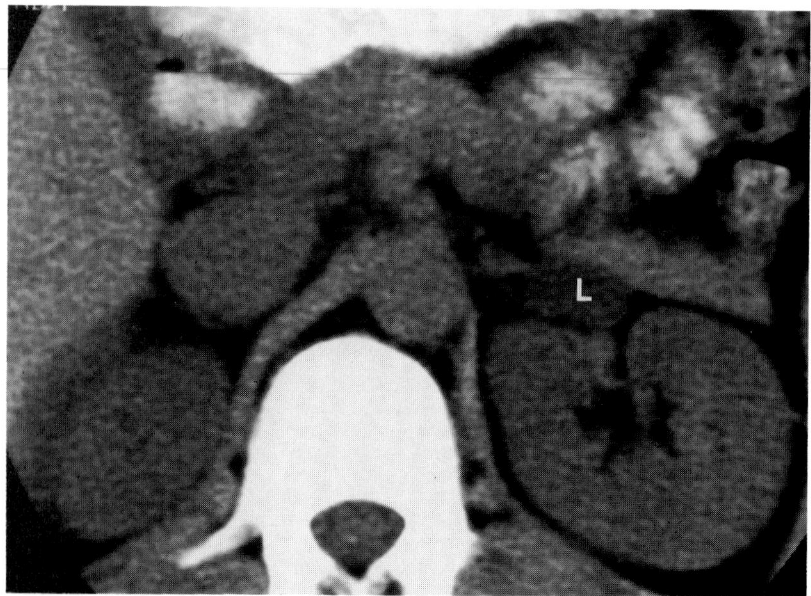

Figure 64–6. Adrenal adenoma. The low-density (L) adrenal mass seen on this unenhanced CT examination was proven to be an aldosterone-secreting adenoma.

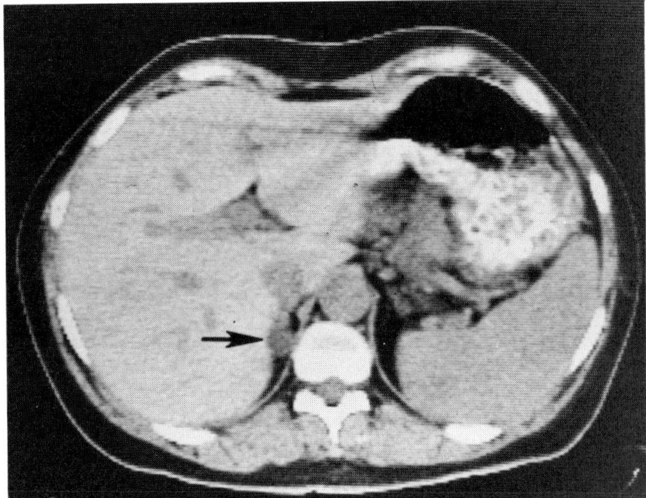

Figure 64–7. Adrenal adenoma. A 1.5-cm right adrenal adenoma *(arrow)* is clearly identified in this patient with Conn's syndrome.

Since the adrenal vein sample may be diluted with blood from the inferior phrenic vein or renal vein on the left or the caval blood on the right, some correction must be made to determine the actual aldosterone concentration. This may be done by measuring a second hormone, such as cortisol, which is unaffected by the hyperaldosteronism. A ratio of the aldosterone to cortisol levels then provides a relative aldosterone concentration corrected for dilution. A hyperfunctioning adrenal tumor will be demonstrated by a marked increase over both the sample from the contralateral adrenal vein and the vena cava (Fig. 64–8 and Table 64–1). The aldosterone level is elevated in both adrenal veins, as compared with the vena cava, when adrenal hyperplasia is present.

The treatment of an adrenal adenoma causing Conn's syndrome is surgical removal. However, bilateral adrenal hyperplasia is treated medically. Thus, the distinction between an adenoma and hyperplasia is essential. Furthermore, with accurate radiographic localization, a simple adrenalectomy can be performed via a posterior or flank approach. This avoids the transperitoneal route required to examine both adrenal glands before surgical removal. This more direct surgical approach has contributed to improved morbidity and mortality but depends upon accurate tumor localization.

ADRENOGENITAL SYNDROMES

Congenital adrenal hyperplasia results from an error in the adrenal enzyme system that impairs or blocks the synthesis of cortisol or aldosterone. Low serum levels of cortisol result in increased ACTH secretion by the pituitary, while inadequate levels of aldosterone lead to compensatory increases in renin and angiotensin. At least six different enzyme deficiencies are recognized, each resulting in a different variety of congenital adrenal hyperplasia. The clinical manifestations are determined by the deficiency of cortisol or aldosterone and the biologic properties of those biochemical intermediates that are secreted in excess.

The most common forms of congenital adrenal hyperplasia are a deficiency of either 21-hydroxylase or 11β-hydroxylase. When a deficiency of 21-hydroxylase exists, production of both cortisol and aldosterone is impaired. If the deficiency is severe, signs of adrenal insufficiency will present in the first few weeks of life.

Adrenal androgens do not require 21-hydroxylase for their synthesis, and they are overproduced in response to high levels of ACTH. The precise clinical manifestation—virilization—depends

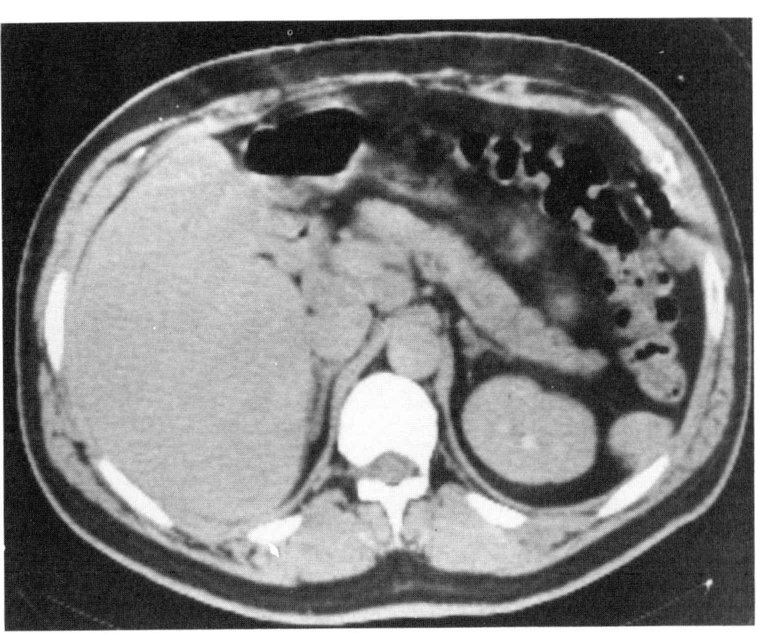

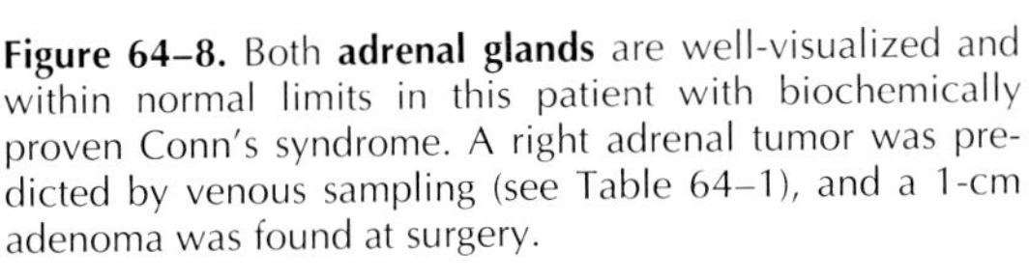

Figure 64–8. Both **adrenal glands** are well-visualized and within normal limits in this patient with biochemically proven Conn's syndrome. A right adrenal tumor was predicted by venous sampling (see Table 64–1), and a 1-cm adenoma was found at surgery.

TABLE 64–1. ADRENAL VENOUS SAMPLING

	RIGHT	LEFT
Aldosterone	800	500
Cortisol	36.6	400
Aldosterone/cortisol ratio	21.9	1.3

upon the sex of the patient and the age at which the androgen excess occurs. A deficiency of 11β-hydroxylase results in impaired cortisol secretion and thus an increase in ACTH. The precursor, 11-deoxycortisol, which is secreted in excess, is a mineralocorticoid that induces hypertension. Virilization also results in this syndrome, as adrenal androgens do not require 11β-hydroxylation.

The radiographic manifestation of these patients is adrenal hyperplasia, which is most readily detected by CT. The symmetrical enlargement of both adrenal glands is typical. The glands maintain a normal configuration and do not have a focal mass (Fig. 64–9).

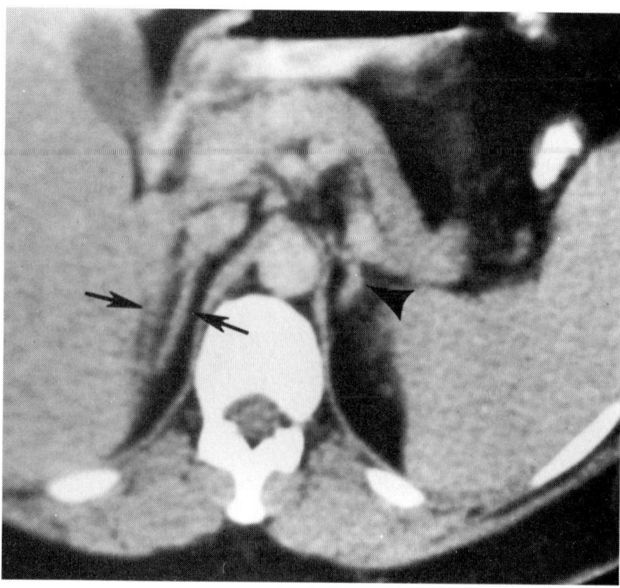

Figure 64–9. Adrenal hyperplasia causing virilization. The adrenal glands are enlarged, but no focal mass is present. Both limbs of the right adrenal gland *(arrows)* are demonstrated, but only a portion of the left gland *(arrowhead)* is seen in this section.

VIRILIZING AND FEMINIZING TUMORS

Although rare, virilizing tumors may be either benign or malignant and may occur at any age. The clinical syndrome of virilization is limited to women and children, where it may be seen in either boys or girls.

These patients must be differentiated from those with congenital adrenal hyperplasia, which can usually be done by the later onset of manifestations. Hirsutism, amenorrhea, enlargement of the clitoris, and deepening of the voice are the most common clinical features. There is no difference in clinical presentation between benign and malignant tumors.

Since testosterone levels are frequently elevated in adrenal tumors, a high testosterone concentration cannot be used to distinguish a gonadal from an adrenal tumor. The adrenal tumors are usually sufficiently large to be readily detected by CT. Adrenal venous sampling has also been used successfully to localize virilizing adrenal tumors.

Feminizing adrenal tumors, presenting as gynecomastia, are exceedingly rare. They are more common in males but have been reported in prepubertal girls and most menopausal women. Gynecomastia is the predominant clinical manifestation. Both benign and malignant tumors have been reported and are usually large enough to be detected by CT.

ADRENAL INSUFFICIENCY

Primary adrenal insufficiency (Addison's disease) does not usually occur until approximately 90 per cent of the adrenal cortex has been destroyed. Worldwide, the most common etiologies are granulomatous diseases (especially tuberculosis) and disseminated fungal infections. Idiopathic atrophy, which may be an autoimmune

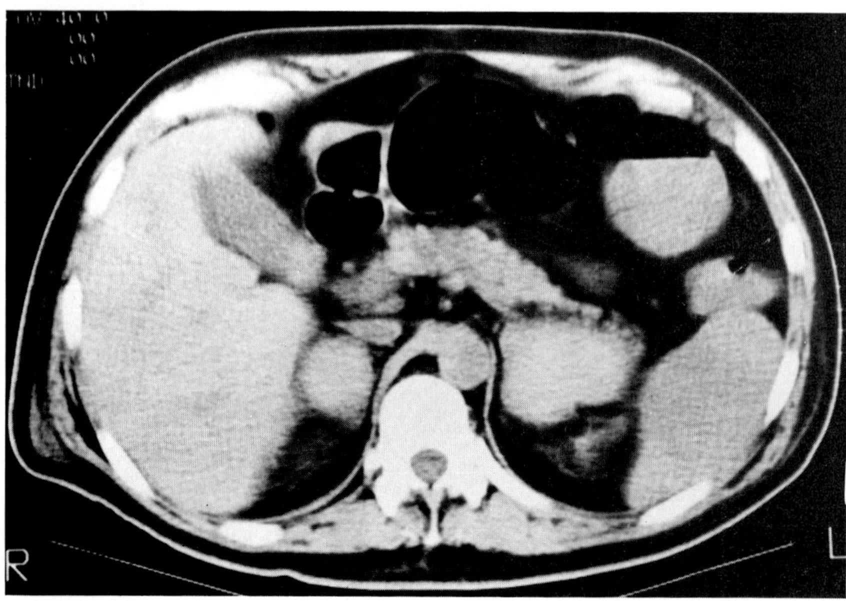

Figure 64–10. Adrenal hemorrhage. Bilateral adrenal masses are easily seen in a patient with adrenal insufficiency. The increased density indicates recent hemorrhage.

disorder, is the most common etiology in the United States. However, a variety of causes have been reported, including hemorrhage, amyloidosis, and metastatic tumor.

The clinical manifestations are hypotension, anorexia, weight loss, weakness, and increased skin pigmentation. In such patients, the clinical suspicion of adrenal insufficiency can be confirmed biochemically and treatment begun with replacement corticosteroids. In patients hospitalized with complex medical problems, however, the diagnosis may not be obvious. The first suggestion of Addison's disease may be made after the demonstration of bilateral adrenal masses on a CT scan obtained to examine other areas of the abdomen.

When adrenal insufficiency is due to involvement by granulomatous disease, normal glandular tissue is usually not present. The gland may be replaced with dense calcification, or if active disease is present, there may be bilateral adrenal masses.

Although the adrenal glands are a common site of metastases, adrenal insufficiency is unusual. The metastatic deposit that destroys only a portion of the gland does not significantly affect adrenal function. Both glands must be extensively involved before the patient will become addisonian.

Although uncommon, spontaneous bilateral adrenal hemorrhage may also result in adrenal insufficiency. This may be seen in association with severe stress but may also be a complication of a bleeding diathesis. Bilateral adrenal masses are readily identified on CT (Fig. 64–10). Hyperdense areas help to confirm recent hemorrhage. Follow-up CT examinations show a diminution in size and density as the hematomas resolve.

Bibliography

Conn JW: Primary aldosteronism: A new clinical syndrome. J Lab Clin Med 45:3, 1955.

Doppman JL, Gill JR, Nienhuis AW, et al: CT findings in Addison's disease. J Comput Assist Tomogr 6:757–761, 1982.

Dunnick NR, Doppman JL, Gill JR, Jr, et al: Localization of functional adrenal tumors by computed tomography and venous sampling. Radiology 142:429–433, 1982.

Dunnick NR, Doppman JL, Mills SR, et al: Preoperative diagnosis and localization of aldosteronomas by measurement of corticosteroids in adrenal venous blood. Radiology 133:331, 1979.

Dunnick NR, Heaston D, Halvorsen R, et al: CT appearance of adrenal cortical carcinoma. J Comput Assist Tomogr 6:978–982, 1982.

Dunnick NR, McCallum RW, Sandler CM: A Textbook of Uroradiology. Baltimore, Williams & Wilkins, 1991.

Guerin CK, Wahner HW, Gorman CA, et al: Computed tomographic scanning versus radioisotope imaging in adrenocortical diagnosis. Am J Med 75:653–657, 1983.

Mitty HA, Yeh H-C: Radiology of the Adrenals. Philadelphia, WB Saunders Company, 1982, pp 80–186.

Schaner EG, Dunnick NR, Doppman JL, et al: Adrenal cortical tumors with low attenuation coefficients: A pitfall in computed tomography diagnosis. J Comput Assist Tomogr 2:11–15, 1978.

65 Adrenal Medulla

Timothy J. Welch, Robert R. Hattery, and Patrick F. Sheedy II

Tumors of the adrenal medulla are relatively uncommon. Pheochromocytoma and neuroblastoma account for the vast majority of the medullary neoplasms. Their interesting and often unusual presentations are the stimulus for the clinical and diagnostic interest generated in these tumors. The role that diagnostic imaging plays in the successful diagnosis and treatment of these tumors has rapidly grown in recent years.

PHEOCHROMOCYTOMA

Clinical, Laboratory, and Pathologic Findings

Pheochromocytomas are rare, occurring in less than 1 per cent of patients with systemic hypertension, and in 1 in 200,000 patients in the general population. The characteristic signs and symptoms of pheochromocytomas are related to the excessive release of catecholamines. All or part of the release may be episodic in nature. The systemic effects bear no relationship to the size, location, or histologic character of the tumor.

Hypertension is the most common finding in patients with pheochromocytoma and was present in 91 per cent of patients in one review. About half of the patients have paroxysmal hypertension. These paroxysms are usually short-lived, lasting minutes to hours in duration. Certain clinical observations help differentiate essential hypertension from hypertension secondary to pheochromocytomas. Patients with pheochromocytoma more commonly have (1) labile blood pressure, (2) paroxysms of hypertension, (3) accelerated hypertension, and (4) pressure response to the induction of anesthesia.

Symptomatic episodes are the result of a sudden excessive release of catecholamines and consist of palpitations, pallor, perspiration, hypertension, and headache. These spells occur in approximately one half of patients with pheochromocytoma. Other clinical findings, such as tachyarrhythmias, myocardiopathy, and myocardial infarction, are also due to excessive circulating catecholamines. Cholelithiasis of unknown etiology is seen in 23 per cent of patients. Intra-adrenal and ectopic pheochromocytomas may also cause renovascular hypertension secondary to renal artery compression. Several other interesting presentations of pheochromocytoma have been reported, including primary lung tumor, intra-adrenal tumor secreting ACTH, and bladder tumor causing spells with micturition.

Patients with certain syndromes have an increased incidence of pheochromocytoma. The most important of these is multiple endocrine neoplasia (MEN) 2. There are two subtypes of MEN 2: (1) MEN 2A—medullary carcinoma of thyroid, pheochromocytoma, and parathyroid hyperplasia; and (2) MEN 2B—orofacial neuromas, medullary carcinoma of thyroid, and pheochromocytoma. These syndromes are of autosomal dominant inheritance. In one series, 15 per cent of patients with pheochromocytoma had MEN 2, which was also present in 7 per cent of patients with a negative family history of pheochromocytoma.

Other syndromes associated with an increased incidence of pheochromocytoma include von Hippel–Lindau disease and neurofibromatosis. There are also well-documented cases of familial inheritance of pheochromocytoma. More recently, an association between renal cell carcinoma and pheochromocytoma has been reported.

Pathologically, pheochromocytomas are tumors of chromaffin cells that occur in the adrenal medulla in 90 per cent of cases. They are extra-adrenal in 10 per cent, multicentric in 10 per cent, bilateral intra-adrenal in 5 per cent, and malignant in 13 per cent. Of intra-adrenal tumors, 60 per cent occur in the right gland. Extra-adrenal pheochromocytomas (paragangliomas) can occur from the base of the brain to the epididymis. However, they usually occur along the sympathetic chain. There is an increased incidence of multicentric, bilateral, and malignant pheochromocytomas in MEN 2 patients. The gross and microscopic pathology of the adrenal medulla in MEN 2 patients is different from that in cases of sporadic occurrence. In sporadic cases, the tumor is well-encased within a normal background of adrenal medulla. However, in MEN 2 patients, the background adrenal medulla is usually hyperplastic and the tumor is often multicentric and not well-encased. These pathologic differences are useful to alert the clinician to the possible presence of MEN 2.

The diagnosis of pheochromocytoma is often difficult despite characteristic symptomatology. It is estimated that only 24 per cent of these tumors are correctly diagnosed before death. The basis of the correct diagnosis is the demonstration of elevated plasma and urine levels of certain catecholamines and their metabolites. The tests most commonly used are urinary metanephrines and vanillylmandelic acid (VMA). Both are measured in 24-hour urine collections. Urinary metanephrines are elevated in 95 per cent of cases, while urinary VMA levels are elevated in 89 per cent. The false-negative rates of these tests are 2 per cent and 5 per cent, respectively. It is important to note that methylglucamine, a common component of many contrast agents, may cause urinary metanephrine values to be falsely normal for 72 hours. The addition of plasma and urinary catecholamine levels (norepinephrine, epinephrine, and dopamine) obtained by high-pressure liquid chromatography has added to the accuracy of the diagnostic work-up of patients with pheochromocytoma. Falsely high catecholamine levels may be encountered in patients on medications such as methyldopa and methenamine mandelate (Mandelamine). It is important to stress the need for at least two separate determinations of urinary and/or plasma catecholamine or their metabolites in patients suspected of harboring a pheochromocytoma. Many factors, such as drug ingestion, poor specimen collection, and noncompliance, can lead to misdiagnosis if these laboratory determinations are not verified.

The role of provocative tests using glucagon or histamine in the diagnosis of pheochromocytoma has been largely abandoned. These tests offer no advantage in the diagnosis of pheochromocytoma owing to the excellent imaging studies available.

The surgical management of patients with pheochromocytoma is often complex, yet with proper technique, cure rates of 90 per cent can be achieved. The cornerstone of proper surgical treatment is preoperative localization of the tumor. Another key factor in the management of these patients is the presurgical treatment with alpha-blocking agent (propranolol) to control the effect of excessive catecholamine release. The intraoperative management consists of central venous monitoring, arterial lines, and the use of nitroprusside to control hypertension. These overall advances in preoperative and perioperative treatment have decreased surgical mortality to less than 4 per cent.

The surgical approach used in most patients is a transabdominal incision with resection of the involved gland. Patients with MEN 2 are treated with bilateral total adrenalectomy to decrease the incidence of local recurrence and metastatic disease. The approach to ectopic and metastatic tumors is tailored to the individual patient's overall medical condition and the site of the tumor.

The medical management of inoperable cases of pheochromocytoma is limited to radiation therapy and high-dose, ^{131}I-labeled meta-iodobenzylguanidine (MIBG). Experience with both is limited, but they appear effective in limiting tumor growth. No chemotherapeutic agents have proved to be successful in the therapy of pheochromocytoma.

The follow-up of surgically treated patients reveals that about 10 per cent recur. Therefore, urinary metanephrines and VMA should be measured annually for at least five years. In patients surgically cured of disease, hypertension will persist in 33 per cent of cases, while paroxysms of hypertension will persist in 5 per cent. The five-year survival rate for a malignant tumor is 44 per cent, with pulmonary metastases being a poor prognostic sign.

Diagnostic Imaging

The basis of successful treatment of pheochromocytoma lies in the accurate preoperative localization of these tumors. The task is often complex, sometimes requiring multiple imaging modalities. The diagnostic approach depends on the site of the tumor, whether it is primary or recurrent, and whether it is benign or malignant. In the past 15 years, there has been a profound change in the diagnostic imaging work-up of patients with suspected pheochromocytoma. This change has occurred largely because of advances in computed tomography (CT) and nuclear medicine.

The majority (90 per cent) of pheochromocytomas are unilateral intra-adrenal tumors. CT has supplanted other forms of imaging as the primary method of tumor localization. CT has an accuracy near 100 per cent.

On CT scans, intra-adrenal pheochromocytomas are discrete round or oval masses whose density is homogeneous and often only slightly less than that of the adjacent liver or pancreas (Fig. 65–1). Areas of central decreased density secondary to tumor necrosis or cystic changes occur in 23 per cent of cases, especially after the administration of contrast material (Figs. 65–2 and 65–3). Calcification occurs in 7 per cent of these tumors. Intra-adrenal pheochromocytomas vary in size from 2 cm, weighing a few hundred grams, to 20 cm with a weight of 3600 g. Bilateral intra-adrenal tumors are usually smaller in size than solitary intra-adrenal tumors, but they have the same CT appearance as solitary tumors (Fig. 65–4). The degree of contrast enhancement in intra-adrenal tumors varies, with approximately 33 per cent showing enhancement greater than that of the surrounding organs.

MIBG, an adrenergic localizing radiopharmaceutical labeled with ^{131}I, has been used with success in the localization of pheochromocytomas. This radiopharmaceutical is given intravenously with

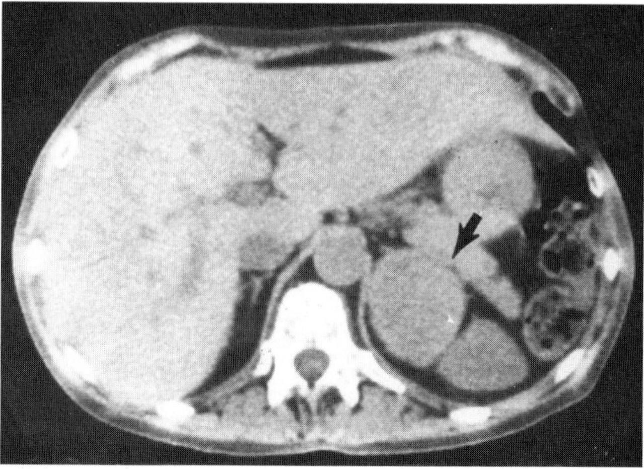

Figure 65–1. Solid left intra-adrenal pheochromocytoma *(arrow).* No intravenous or oral contrast given. Normal right adrenal.

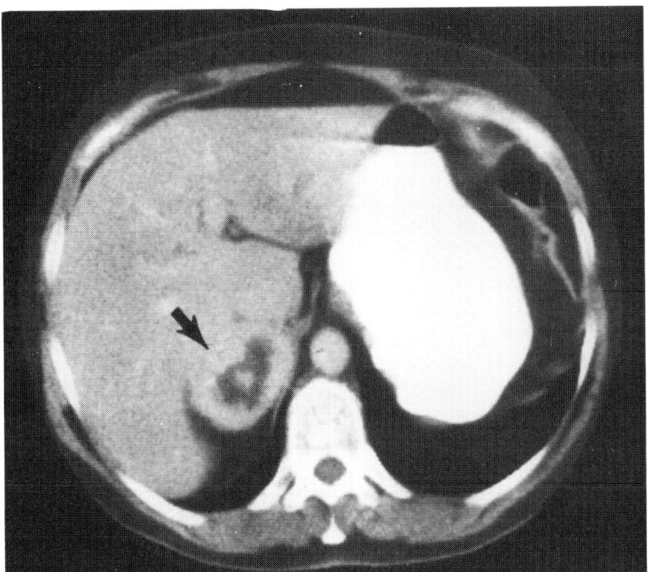

Figure 65–2. Right intra-adrenal pheochromocytoma *(arrow).* Scan made during IV contrast infusion. Note inhomogeneous CT density with enhancing periphery and central area surrounded by an irregular area of decreased density.

scanning performed at 24, 48, and 72 hours. Radiation dose is 0.11 rad total body and 17.5 rad to the normal adrenal medulla. Tumors appear as circumscribed collections of increased activity. The bladder, liver, spleen, and salivary gland are the only normal organs that demonstrate faint accumulation of the tracer. The role of MIBG in intra-adrenal pheochromocytomas is primarily in those patients with positive clinical and laboratory findings and a negative CT scan. CT should be employed as the first diagnostic imaging procedure for suspected pheochromocytoma, as it is faster, cheaper, more widely available, and at least as accurate as MIBG.

Pheochromocytomas occur in extra-adrenal locations in 10 per cent of cases. These locations are primarily in the abdominal cavity, but they may occur in a variety of other locations. Reports of tumors occurring in the bladder, cardiac intra-atrial septum, lung, posterior mediastinum, and the cervical region are well-documented. However, the most common ectopic sites are the organ of Zuckerkandl, the abdominal para-aortic region, and the retroperitoneum. On CT scans, ectopic tumors appear as soft-tissue masses that may be solid or partially necrotic (Fig. 65–5). Ectopic tumors vary in size from several centimeters to as large as 8 cm. If the initial CT scan of the adrenals and abdomen through the aortic bifurcation is negative, the next step should be an MIBG scan, if available. MIBG scans are effective in localizing ectopic tumors, especially those outside the abdomen. The combination of abdominal CT and an MIBG localized the great majority of ectopic pheochromocytomas.

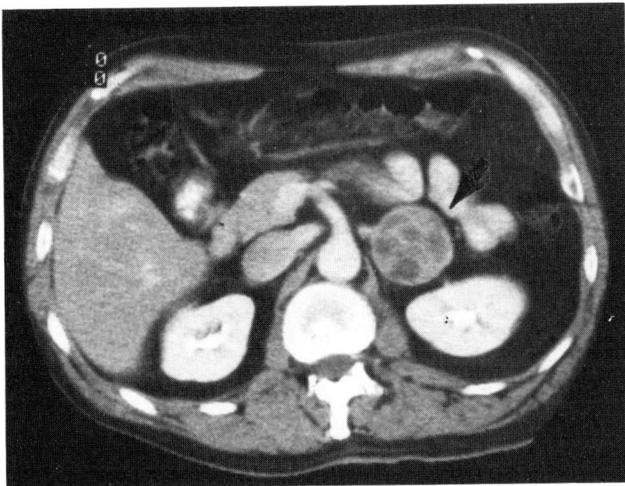

Figure 65–3. Left intra-adrenal pheochromocytoma *(arrow).* Irregular cystic decreased density in tumor seen on scan made during infusion of contrast media.

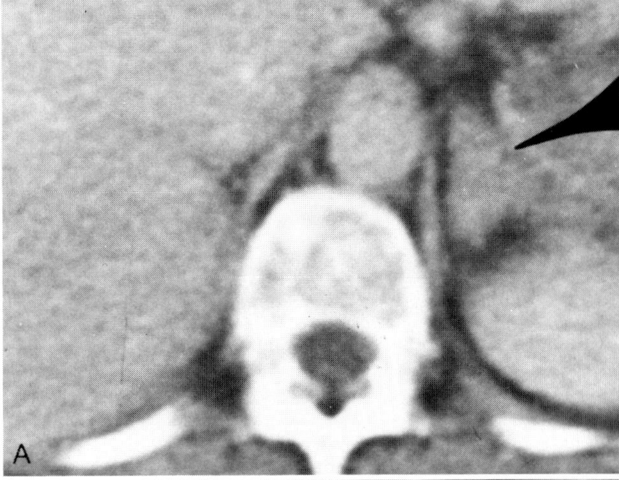

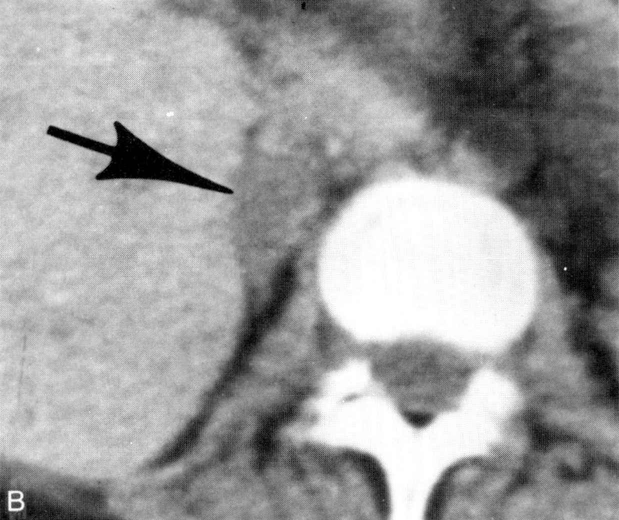

Figure 65–4. *A* and *B,* **Solid bilateral intra-adrenal pheochromocytoma** *(arrows)* in a patient with MEN 2A syndrome.

Pheochromocytomas recur in approximately 10 per cent of cases. These recurrent tumors may present anywhere from six months to five years after the removal of the initial tumor. Sites of recurrence include the contralateral adrenal gland, the bed of a resected adrenal gland, and other sites in the retroperitoneum. The remaining sites of recurrence are primarily thoracic and sometimes pelvic. A unique feature of these tumors is multiple recurrences in the same patient separated by months or years.

There is an increased incidence of recurrent tumors in MEN 2 patients. On CT, the recurrent tumor may appear as a solid soft-tissue mass or multiple small nodules in the area of a previous resection. The initial imaging procedure in suspected recurrent tumors should be an MIBG scan. While CT is accurate in localizing over 70 per cent of recurrent tumors, MIBG scans have the advantage of imaging tumors regardless of previous surgery in the area, and avoid the need for a total-body CT search.

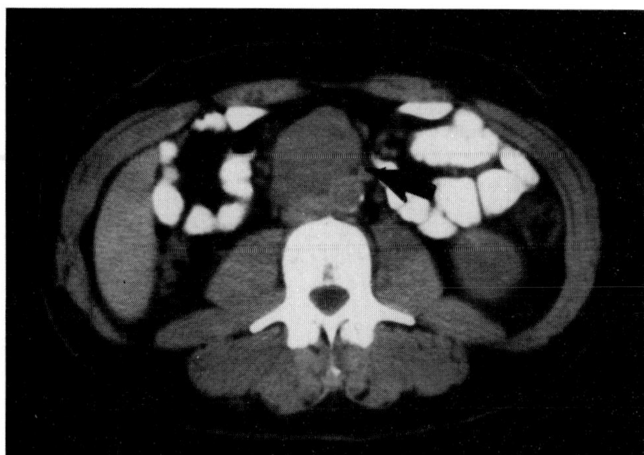

Figure 65–5. Ectopic pheochromocytoma arising in the organ of Zuckerkandl and extending superiorly *(arrow)*.

The incidence of malignancy in pheochromocytoma ranges from 3 to 13 per cent (Fig. 65–6). Malignancy poses a difficult problem because of the multicentric origin and the absence of specific histologic, biochemical, or electron microscopic criteria of malignancy. Therefore, the diagnosis of malignancy can be made only by the identification of tumor where chromaffin tissue is not normally found. Common sites of metastatic involvement include lung, bone, and liver. MIBG plays the primary role in the localization of these metastatic tumors. It has the advantages of localizing multiple metastatic deposits with one scan, of visualizing tumors in locations not normally imaged by CT, and of not being affected by previous surgical interventions. The role of CT in these patients is to provide a better anatomic definition of a suspected metastatic deposit when surgery or radiation therapy is planned. The appearance of malignant pheochromocytomas on CT and MIBG scans is indistinguishable from that of nonmalignant tumors in the vast majority of cases. However, in some cases, secondary evidence of malignancy is identifiable such as liver metastases or bone destruction.

In the recent past, multiple other imaging modalities have played a role in the work-up of suspected pheochromocytoma. These tests have largely been supplanted by CT and MIBG scans. Excretory urography and bolus nephrotomography were once the mainstay of the evaluation of patients with suspected pheochromocytoma. These studies were 70 to 90 per cent accurate in localizing intra-adrenal or perirenal tumors. Tumors were identified as solid, partially cystic or necrotic, or calcified suprarenal masses. Angiography with or without venous sampling was also widely used in the diagnosis of pheochromocytoma. It was highly accurate in localizing intra-abdominal tumors. Findings at angiography included cystic changes, dense stain, and central necrosis with peripheral enhancement ("ring sign"). However, excretory urography, bolus nephrotomography, and angiography were all poor at localizing ectopic or recurrent tumors. Angiography had the additional handicap of being an invasive procedure, and is also prone to cause a hypertensive crisis, particularly with selective injections. Ultrasound is not often used in the evaluation of pheochromocytomas, owing to the limitation of imaging the normal adrenals, especially the left adrenal gland. Ultrasound is also limited in evaluating the common ectopic locations of these tumors. Magnetic resonance imaging (MRI) has shown the ability to accurately delineate adrenal masses in various patient populations. The strengths of MRI of suspected pheochromocytomas is the ability to image in multiple planes, superior contrast delineation, and the lack of exposure to ionizing radiation or iodinated contrast material. The real hope for MRI in adrenal tumors is the use of a unique signal signature to differentiate various adrenal tumors. Pheochromocytomas consistently have high signal intensity on T_2-weighted images. This can be used to separate them from other adrenal masses. Unfortunately, there is a significant overlap of the various signal characteristics of adrenal tumors and therefore, MRI does not appear to be superior to MIBG scintigraphy in respect to specificity. The other disadvantages of MRI include expense of the examination and a small but significant patient non-compliance secondary to claustrophobia with scanning (Figs. 65–7 and 65–8).

The localization of pheochromocytomas can be a diagnostic challenge that may require several studies for diagnostic success. The outcome of therapy is ultimately dependent on accurate localization;

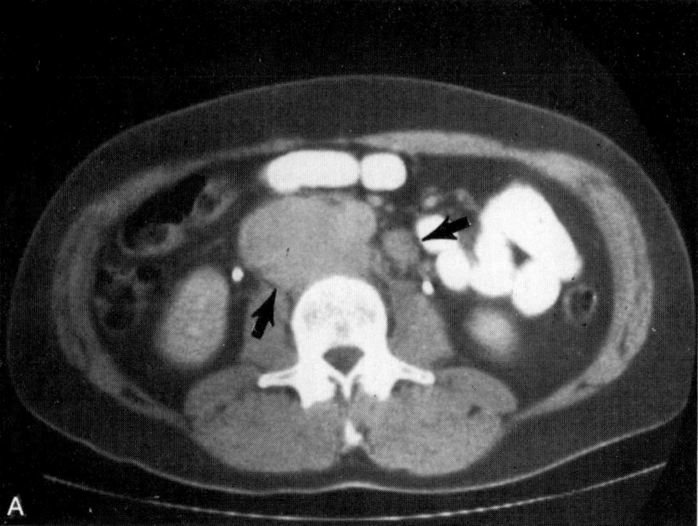

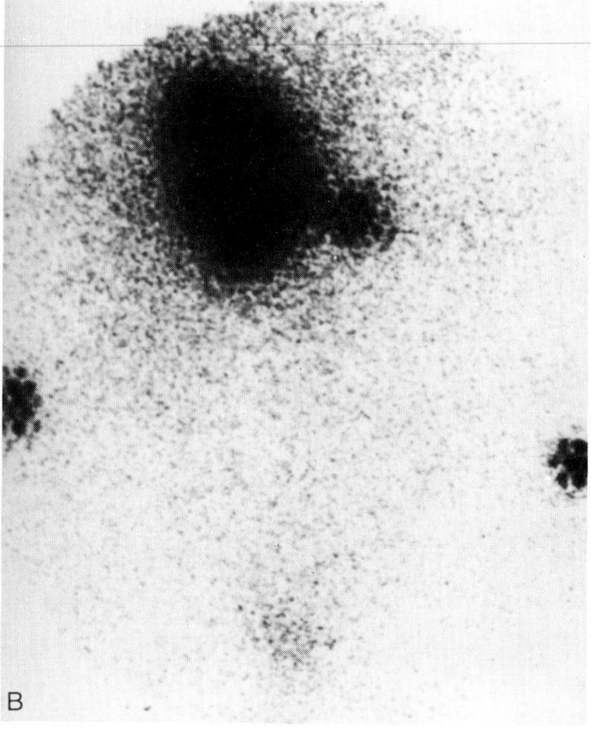

Figure 65–6. *A,* **Solid multicentric malignant pheochromocytoma** in the periaortic region *(arrows)*. Oral and IV contrast given. *B,* ^{131}I-MIBG scan clearly demonstrating the multicentric nature of this tumor.

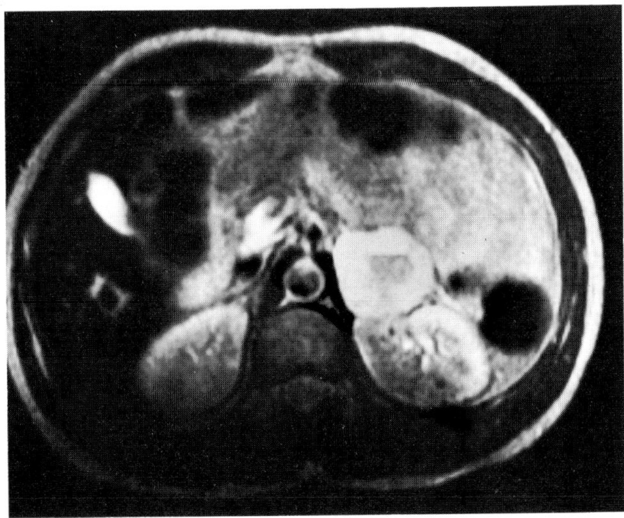

Figure 65–7. T_2-weighted MRIs demonstrate a high-signal intensity mass in the left adrenal gland compatible with an **intra-adrenal pheochromocytoma**.

therefore, every effort must be made to fully define the location and extent of each tumor. Abdominal CT through the aortic bifurcation should be the initial study in most patients suspected of harboring a pheochromocytoma. For patients with recurrent or metastatic tumors, and for patients with a negative CT scan, the MIBG scan is the procedure of choice. MRI with further development of signal characteristics and contrast agents may play a greater role in the evaluation of adrenal tumors. However, currently this role is relegated to a complementary nature to CT scanning and MIBG scintigraphy.

NEUROBLASTOMA

Clinical, Laboratory, and Pathologic Findings

Neuroblastoma represents the most common solid malignant tumor of children excluding intracranial malignancies. It is estimated that the incidence is between one and three cases per 100,000 children per year. Neuroblastoma is a highly aggressive tumor with an overall survival rate ranging from 30 to 40 per cent. The age range of neuroblastoma patients is from a few months to nine years. The site of neuroblastoma is generally in the adrenal gland or abdomen. However, 29 per cent occur in the pelvis, thorax, or unknown locations. Neuroblastomas tend to metastasize early in the course of the disease. Common sites of metastases include bone, liver, and bone marrow. Neuroblastoma is also characterized by the highest rate of spontaneous remission and dedifferentiation into benign histology of any malignant tumor.

The common presenting findings in neuroblastoma include a palpable abdominal mass, weight loss, abdominal pain, and bone pain. However, these tumors may present in a variety of less common ways, including ataxia, chorea, pyrexia, intestinal obstruction, and excessive sweating. There is prognostic importance to the age at presentation, site of primary tumor, and stage and histology of these tumors. Younger patients with extra-abdominal tumors appear to have the better prognosis.

Pathologically, neuroblastomas are primitive tumors derived from neural crest ectoderm. Therefore, they can occur at any location where such cells exist. They are often biochemically active, secreting catecholamines and their metabolites. Elevated VMA, the most common metabolic abnormality seen in these patients, occurs in 76 per cent of cases. As with pheochromocytomas, there is no correlation between tumor size and levels of urinary metabolites.

Staging of neuroblastomas has both prognostic and therapeutic significance. The current staging protocol is outlined in Table 65–1. Stages I and II of the disease are treated with surgery alone with a 60 to 90 per cent cure rate. Stages III, IV, and IV S are best treated with initial radiation therapy and/or chemotherapy, then possibly followed by surgery. Cure rates for these stages range from 5 to 20 per cent.

Diagnostic Imaging

The importance of proper diagnosis and staging in patients with neuroblastoma is critical to prognostic and therapeutic decisions. The diagnostic work-up of suspected neuroblastoma patients centers on the use of CT scanning in the initial evaluation. This is especially true in the older age group. In the neonate, abdominal masses are frequently evaluated using ultrasonography. If there is question of intraspinal extension, MRI is the most accurate way of detecting intraspinal involvement. MIBG scintigraphy is primarily used in the follow-up of known tumors to judge the activity within treated tumors.

Neuroblastomas appear as solid soft-tissue masses on CT scans (Fig. 65–9). They may have cystic or necrotic areas located within

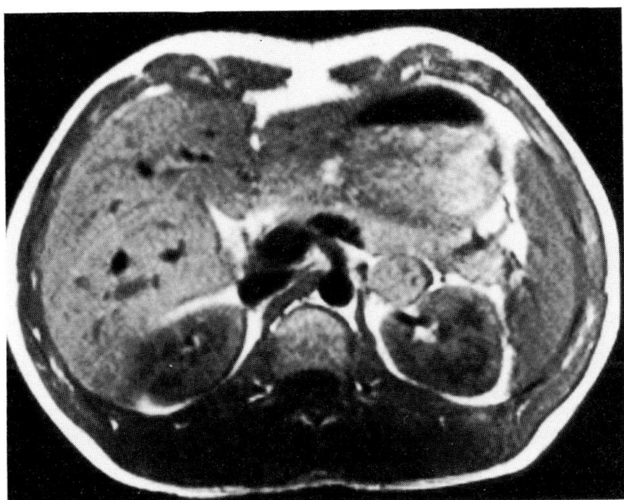

Figure 65–8. "Snapshot" MRI illustrating a **left intra-adrenal pheochromocytoma.**

TABLE 65–1. STAGING FOR NEUROBLASTOMA

STAGE	FINDING
I	Tumor confined to organ of origin and completely excised.
II	Tumor extending in continuity beyond the organ or structure of origin, but not crossing the midline. Regional lymph nodes on the homolateral side may be involved.
III	Tumor extending in continuity beyond the midline. Regional nodes bilaterally may be involved.
IV	Remote disease involving the skeleton, parenchymatous organs, soft tissues, or distant lymph nodes.
IV S	Disease that would otherwise be Stage I or Stage II, but is remote and confined only to one or more of the following sites: liver, skin, or bone marrow.

Modified from Evans AE, d'Angio GJ, Randolph J: A proposed staging for children with neuroblastoma. Cancer 27:374–378, 1971.

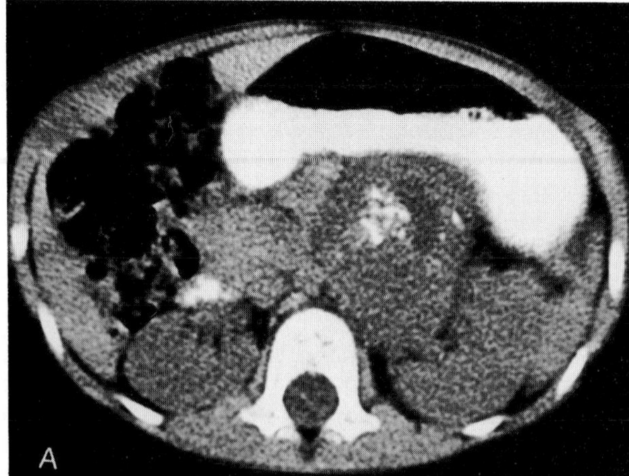

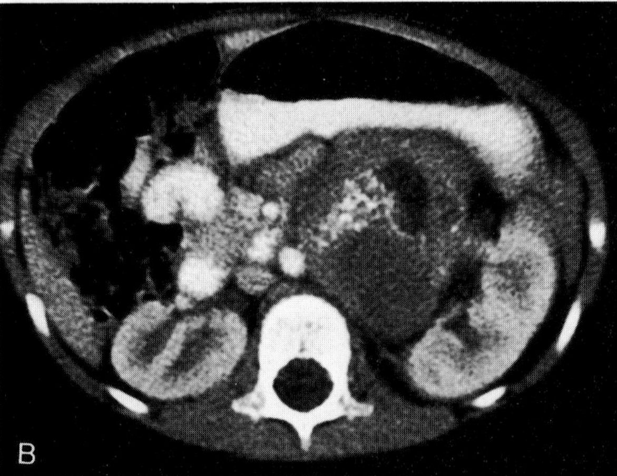

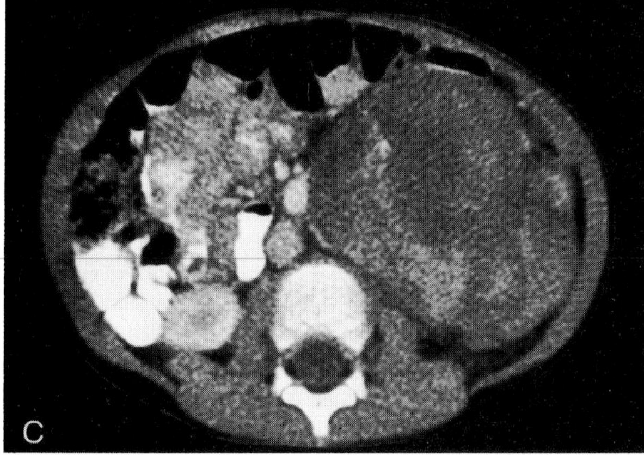

Figure 65–9. Four-year-old male with abdominal mass. *A* to *C,* Fast CT performed without and with intravenous contrast material demonstrates a partially calcified, mixed density **left paraspinal neuroblastoma.**

the tumor. Calcification has long been an important factor in differentiating neuroblastomas from Wilms' tumor. CT is more accurate in detecting calcifications in neuroblastomas than either plain radiography or bone scintigraphy. Calcification may take a variety of forms, including ring, multiple dotted, or dense mottled patterns. The last form is the most common, but ring calcifications in neuroblastomas are not as rare as previously thought.

Certain other imaging tests can play an important role in the evaluation of patients with suspected neuroblastoma. Ultrasound is accurate in the evaluation of intra abdominal and pelvic neuroblastoma; however, it is severely limited in extra-abdominal and extrapelvic tumors. Ultrasound is also an excellent method for delineation of tumor involvement of vascular structures such as the inferior vena cava or aorta. Bone and liver scintigraphy may also be helpful in evaluating suspected metastatic disease in neuroblastomas. Fifty-nine per cent of all neuroblastomas have uptake of bone scanning agents in the primary tumor. MIBG scintigraphy is primarily used in neuroblastoma patients to follow known or metastatic lesions. There are, however, reports of using ^{125}I-labeled MIBG instead of ^{131}I-labeled MIBG in the treatment of neuroblastoma patients.

Another area of active research that may be valuable in the future imaging of ^{131}I-neuroblastoma patients is the use of monoclonal antibodies for diagnostic imaging. This work is under preliminary investigation and shows promising results.

The diagnostic imaging approach to suspected neuroblastoma patients is based on the use of ultrasound and CT to evaluate suspected cases. Bone scintigraphy plays an important role to detect skeletal metastases, which occur in a high number of patients with neuroblastoma. The combination of CT scanning, bone scintigraphy, and bone marrow aspiration accurately stages over 90 per cent of neuroblastoma patients (see Fig. 67–9). MRI is reserved to evaluate for intraspinal extension of patients with known neuroblastoma. MIBG scintigraphy is useful in the follow-up of known tumors and to judge their activity level following treatment.

Bibliography

Alcock MK, Morris LL, LeQuesne GW, Savage JP: Imaging in neuroblastoma: A 12-year experience. Australas Radiol 1986;30:38–45.

Bousvaros A, Kirks DR, Grossman H: Imaging of neuroblastoma: An overview. Pediatr Radiol 16:89–106, 1986.

Dietrich RB, Kangarloo H, Lenarsky C, Feig SA: Neuroblastoma: The role of MR imaging. AJR 148:937–942, 1987.

Figueroa RE, El Gammal T, Brooks BS, et al: MR findings on primitive neuroectodermal tumors. J Comput Assist Tomogr 13 (5), 1989.

Jacobs A, Delree M, Desprechins B, et al: Consolidating the role of I-MIBG-scintigraphy in childhood neuroblastoma: Five years of clinical experience. Pediatr Radiol 20:157–159, 1990.

Quint LE, Glazer GM, Francis IR, et al: Pheochromocytoma and paraganglioma: Comparison of MR imaging with CT and I-131 MIBG scintigraphy. Radiology 165:89–93, 1987.

Reinig JW, Doppman JL, Dwyer AJ, et al: Adrenal masses differentiated by MR. Radiology 158:81–84, 1986.

Sheps SG: Pheochromocytoma. In Spittel JA (ed): Clinical Medicine. Philadelphia, Harper and Row, 1981.

Sheps SG, Van Heerden JA, Sheedy PF: Current approach to the diagnosis of pheochromocytoma. In Blaufox MD, Branchi D (eds): Secondary Forms of Hypertension: Current Diagnosis and Management. New York, Grune and Stratton, 1981, pp 11–18.

Sisson JC, Hutchinson RJ, Shapiro B, et al: Iodine-125-MIBG to treat neuroblastoma: Preliminary report. J Nucl Med 31:1479–1485, 1990.

Van Heerden JA, Sheps SG, Hamberger B, et al: Pheochromocytoma: Current status and changing trends. Surgery 91:367–373, 1982.

Velchik MG, Alavi A, Kressel HY, Engelman K: Localization of pheochromocytoma: MIBG, CT, and MRI correlation. J Nucl Med 30:328–336, 1989.

Webb TA, Sheps SG, Carney JA: Differences between sporadic pheochromocytoma and pheochromocytoma in multiple endocrine neoplasia, type 2. Am J Surg Pathol 4:121–126, 1980.

Welch TJ, Sheedy PF II, Van Heerden JA, et al: Pheochromocytoma: Value of computed tomography. Radiology 148:501–503, 1983.

66 Nonfunctioning Adrenal Masses

Morton A. Bosniak and William M. Rumancik

Adrenal lesions that do not elaborate a recognizable hormone in excess are considered nonfunctioning or nonhyperfunctioning. In some cases they are detected as an incidental finding during examination of the upper abdomen whereas in other cases they are discovered during the staging of neoplastic disease. Clues to their etiology lie in their radiographic appearance and clinical presentation.

These nonfunctional (in some cases, nonhyperfunctional) lesions have a wide variety of etiologies that may be categorized as neoplastic, either benign or malignant, or non-neoplastic lesions. Primary adrenal carcinoma, which also may be nonfunctional, is discussed separately in Chapter 64.

ADRENAL METASTASES

After lungs, liver, and bones, the adrenal gland is the fourth most common site for metastatic disease from all tumors. The most common primary malignancies to metastasize to the adrenal glands are lung, breast, kidney, and melanoma; however, any tumor may metastasize to the adrenals. In one autopsy series, 27 per cent of 1000 patients with malignant epithelial neoplasms had adrenal metastases.

Adrenal metastases from lung cancer occur in 35 to 38 per cent of patients in autopsy series. When computed tomography (CT) was used to evaluate the adrenal glands in patients with non-small cell bronchogenic carcinoma, solid adrenal masses were discovered in 12 to 21 per cent of patients. For this reason, the adrenals should be carefully evaluated in all patients undergoing preoperative staging for non-small cell bronchogenic carcinoma (Fig. 66–1).

Various autopsy reports note adrenal metastases from renal cell carcinoma in 18 to 25 per cent of patients. Metastases are usually ipsilateral; however, metastases to the contralateral adrenal gland can occur. Angiographically, these metastases are vascular and similar in appearance to the primary renal lesion. Without histologic evaluation, it may be impossible to distinguish between a metastasis from a primary renal carcinoma and a benign adrenal adenoma.

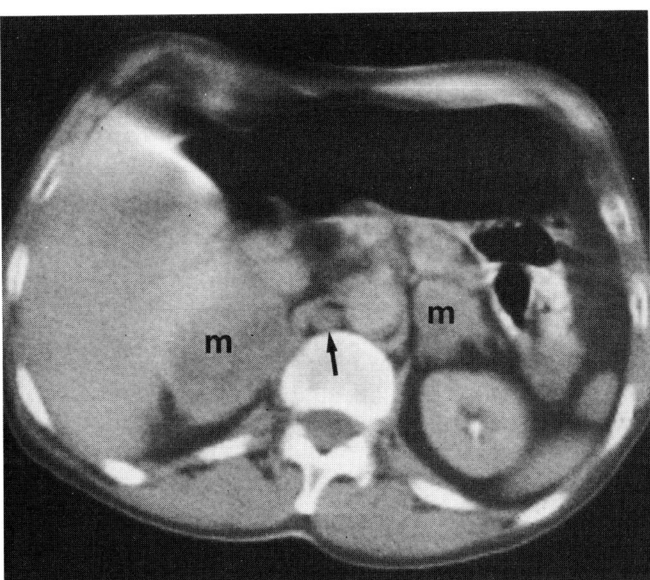

Figure 66–1. Bilateral adrenal metastases. Both adrenal glands contain large, heterogeneous masses (m) consistent with metastatic disease. Note the right retrocrural node *(arrow)*.

Malignant melanoma is discovered in autopsy series to metastasize to the adrenal gland with an incidence of 50 per cent. Lesions are usually bilateral and other areas in the body are often involved. Solitary, unilateral metastatic lesions are unusual. Although primary melanoma of the adrenal has been reported, malignant melanoma of the adrenal gland almost always represents metastatic disease.

Direct contiguous extension of malignancy into the adrenal may occur. This has been described in carcinomas of the pancreas, stomach, liver, and kidney, in sarcomas of the retroperitoneum and diaphragm, and in lymphoma.

Metastasis to the adrenals may undergo necrosis or hemorrhage. Although most patients with adrenal metastasis are asymptomatic, adrenal insufficiency may result from bilateral metastases that totally infiltrate the glands.

It is important not only to detect adrenal metastases but also to differentiate an adrenal metastasis from other adrenal masses (e.g., adrenal adenoma). In a patient with known primary malignancy, an adrenal mass must be considered a metastatic deposit until proved otherwise. However, reports indicate that more than 50 per cent of adrenal masses in oncologic patients depicted by CT represent benign nonhyperfunctioning adenomas. Because clinical staging and therapy are dependent on knowing whether an adrenal metastasis is present, imaging studies often are necessary to detect these lesions and distinguish them from benign adrenal adenomas or other conditions.

Metastases to the adrenals can be visualized by most imaging techniques. Larger lesions can be seen on urography, particularly with tomography. Sonography can visualize adrenal metastases, and their appearance will vary depending on the size of the mass and whether necrosis is associated. Usually, a hypoechoic pattern is seen. CT remains the technique of choice for staging neoplastic disease and can visualize the adrenals and adrenal metastases readily. The CT appearance of adrenal metastases, however, is not specific. The lesions can be large or small, unilateral or bilateral. When small (< 3 cm) they appear as solid, homogeneous masses. As they enlarge, areas of decreased attenuation often appear within them representing hemorrhage and/or necrosis. Margins are usually irregular as well, but smooth margination can occur. Thus, an adrenal metastasis cannot be distinguished clearly from a benign lesion of the adrenal on the basis of CT findings alone. In a patient with an adrenal mass who also has obvious widespread metastatic disease to other organs and structures, evaluation of the etiology of the adrenal mass becomes relatively less important because the patient's management is not dependent on this information. However, in those cases when the adrenal lesion is the only evidence of possible metastatic disease (particularly in a patient with a known primary tumor of the lung), a definite diagnosis of the adrenal lesion as to whether it represents a metastasis or some other condition becomes critically important because it may very well change the treatment approach. Magnetic resonance imaging (MRI) can be helpful in making this distinction but at this time it has not proven to be accurate enough, so that needle aspiration biopsy is the only definitive way of determining whether an adrenal lesion represents metastatic neoplasm or a benign lesion (usually adenoma) (Fig. 66–2).

MRI is helpful in identifying the nature of an adrenal mass because it is capable of providing tissue characterization not possible with CT or ultrasound. Adrenal metastases characteristically

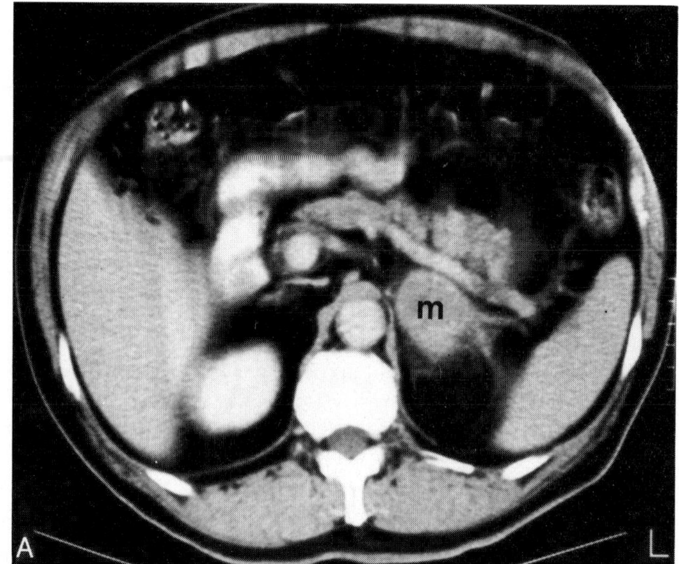

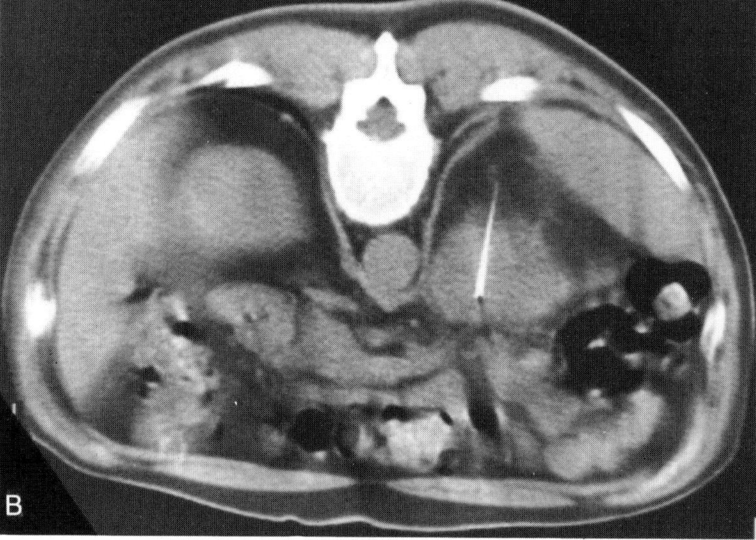

Figure 66–2. Adrenal metastasis with percutaneous biopsy. A 63-year-old man with non-small cell lung carcinoma. The patient had no other evidence of metastases. *A,* A left adrenal mass (m) is present. The right adrenal gland is normal. *B,* CT scan with the patient in the prone position demonstrates the percutaneous biopsy needle within the left adrenal mass. The needle was angled superiorly to avoid the pleural space at the left lung base. Pathology of the biopsy specimen showed the lesion to be a metastasis.

display high signal intensity on long TR and long TE pulse sequence (T_2-weighted) images; they display low signal intensity similar to that of liver or muscle on short TR and short TE pulse sequence (T_1-weighted) images (Fig. 66–3). (The metastatic lesion usually has similar MRI characteristics to the primary tumor). On the other hand, the characteristic signal intensity and behavior of nonhyperfunctioning adrenal adenomas (the most common lesion from which metastatic neoplasm must be distinguished) are parallel to those of the liver and remain relatively low on T_2-weighted images. However, in some instances, it may be difficult to accurately separate adrenal metastases from nonhyperfunctioning adenomas based solely on the MRI appearance of the adrenal lesion since an overlap in signal behavior may occur. Some adenomas demonstrate more signal than usual on T_2-weighted images and some metastases less signal than expected, often depending on the signal characteristics of the primary tumor. Approximately 21 to 31 per cent of adrenal metastases evaluated in various reported series behaved similarly to some benign nonfunctioning adenomas and could not be differentiated reliably. Some studies using calculated T_1 values to distinguish benign from malignant adrenal masses have shown a similar overlap. Most of the early studies that used MRI to distinguish metastatic neoplasm from benign adenoma were performed with low field strength (0.35–0.5 T) units. Later studies using higher strength units (1.5 T) have shown some improvement in accuracy but considerable overlap is still present. MRI spectroscopy might be able to provide additional information to help distinguish metastatic lesions from benign adenomas. In one report the lipid content was found to be lower in carcinomas than adenomas when measured by proton spectroscopy. However, this difference in lipid content between adenoma and carcinoma may well become the basis for differentiating these lesions by imaging techniques (see later under Adrenal Adenoma).

Aspiration biopsy is the most definite method of confirming the existence of metastatic neoplasm in an adrenal mass and is necessary when treatment depends on this information. A positive biopsy result is close to 100 per cent accurate and definitive. A negative biopsy result, however, is not as definitive because sampling error or an inadequate specimen may preclude a confident diagnosis. Aspirations with negative results can be repeated to increase the confidence that the lesion is benign. Overall accuracy rates reported for adrenal biopsy in these cases are between 80 and 100 per cent.

ADRENAL LYMPHOMA

Adrenal involvement in lymphoma is a relatively common occurrence. In autopsy series, the adrenals were involved in 25 per cent

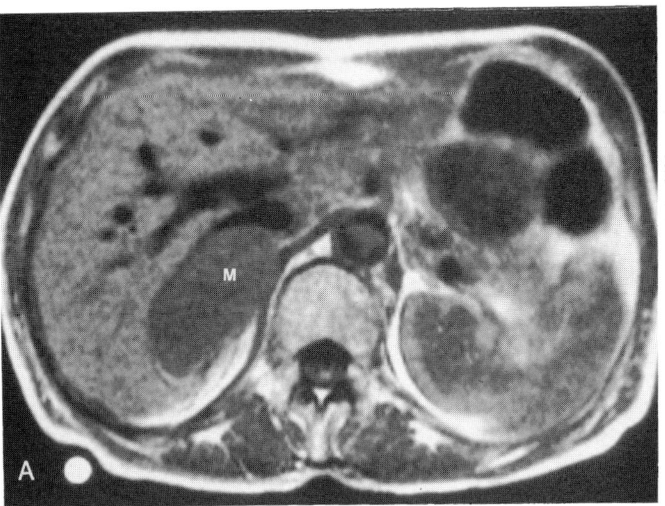

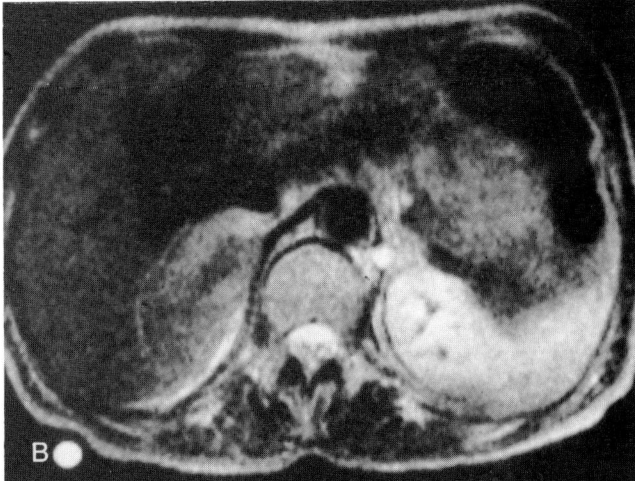

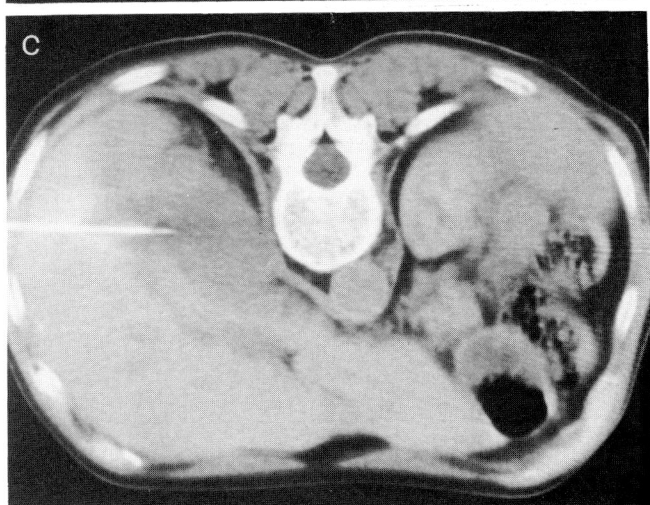

Figure 66–3. Metastatic carcinoma to the right adrenal from adenocarcinoma of the lung. In a 63-year-old woman with carcinoma of the lung, a CT scan revealed a mass in the right adrenal gland (M). *A,* Spin-echo T_1-weighted MRI image (TR 550, TE 30 msec). A large mass is demonstrated in the right adrenal gland (M). Note that the mass has a signal less than that of the liver. *B,* T_2-weighted MRI image (TR 1968, TE 100 msec). Most of the mass has an increased signal compared with the liver, which indicates that it is likely to be a metastatic neoplasm. *C,* CT-guided biopsy of the right adrenal mass. The needle is placed in the adrenal mass via a percutaneous transhepatic approach. Specimen obtained indicated metastatic adenocarcinoma.
(*Comment:* In this case percutaneous needle biopsy was performed to be certain of the diagnosis. The transhepatic biopsy approach demonstrated here is a route used to obtain tissue from the right adrenal.) (*A* to *C* courtesy of Peter Schlossberg, M.D.)

of patients with lymphoma. This was due mainly to contiguous spread of retroperitoneal lymphoma to the adrenal glands. However, the adrenals may contain heterotopic lymphoid elements that may be involved intrinsically by lymphoma. This may result in discrete adrenal masses similar in appearance to metastases, adenomas, or other adrenal neoplasms. It is estimated that discrete adrenal involvement occurs in 4 per cent of patients with non-Hodgkin's lymphoma at some time during the course of their disease. Adrenal insufficiency is rare but may occur if both adrenal glands are affected.

Adrenal involvement is usually associated with retroperitoneal nodal disease, but may occasionally represent the sole site of detectable disease in a patient. The adrenals have also been described as an isolated site of recurrent lymphomatous disease after therapy.

Although adrenal involvement in Hodgkin's lymphoma has been described, non-Hodgkin's lymphoma overwhelmingly represents the most common type of histology. Lymphomas of diffuse cell type occur more frequently than the nodular type.

The imaging characteristics of adrenal lymphoma are much like those seen in lymphoma in other portions of the body. On sonography the characteristic sonolucent (hypoechoic) pattern is seen. On CT, lymphomatous tissue has a very homogeneous appearance. The attenuation values vary between 30 and 50 HU on non-contrast scans and show a relatively low degree of enhancement with intravenous contrast (depending on amount and speed of contrast injection) (Fig. 66–4). Necrosis is uncommon but can be seen following treatment and occasionally with extremely rapid growth. Occasionally, very large adrenal masses will be seen (Fig. 66–5). On MRI, lesions behave similarly to other metastatic neoplasms with relatively higher signal on T_2-weighted sequences. Thus, the imaging characteristics of adrenal lymphoma can be quite similar to those seen in hypovascular metastatic malignancy to the adrenals. Therefore, in a patient not known to have systemic lymphoma, the diagnosis of adrenal lymphoma may require needle aspiration biopsy.

The therapeutic response of adrenal lymphomatous lesions is similar to that of coincidental nonadrenal masses in these patients. If an adrenal mass fails to respond to therapy as do other sites of disease, percutaneous biopsy of the adrenal lesion may be necessary to exclude other adrenal gland pathology.

ADRENAL ADENOMAS

Nonhyperfunctioning adenomas are the most common benign tumor of the adrenal cortex, occurring in 2 to 8 per cent of the population at autopsy. The incidence of adenoma is greater with increasing age and has been reported to be higher in patients with renal, urinary bladder, and endometrial neoplasms. An unexplained increased frequency of occurrence has also been described in patients with hypertension, hyperthyroidism, and diabetes mellitus.

Nonhyperfunctioning adrenal adenomas are small tumors, usually 2 to 3 cm in diameter. Larger adenomas of up to 12 cm in diameter

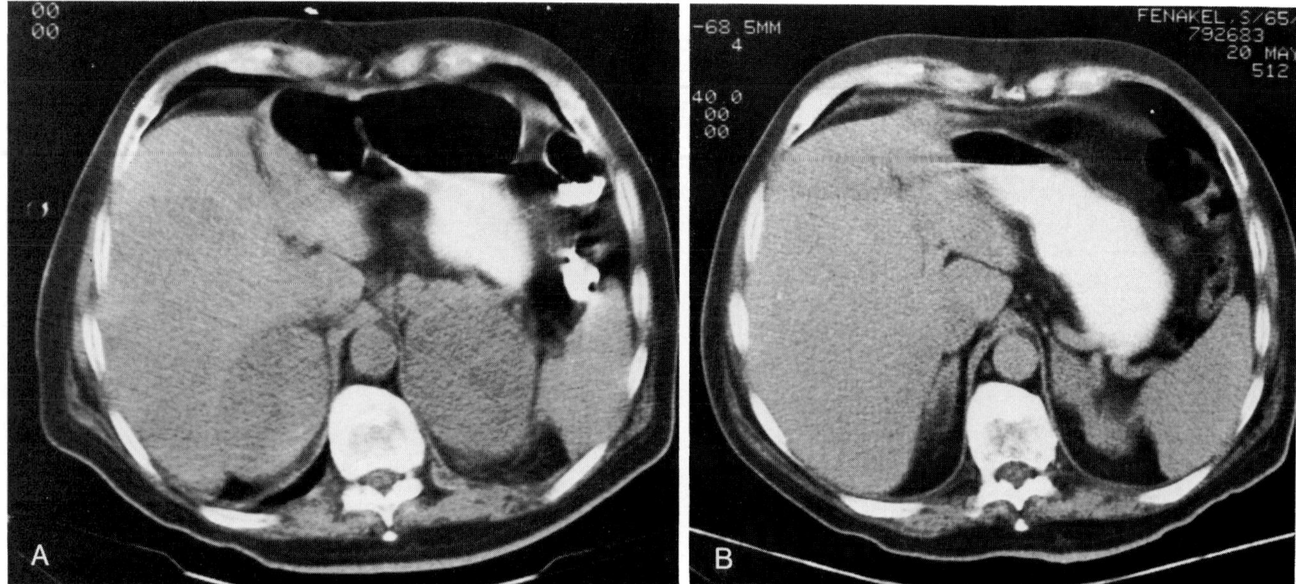

Figure 66–4. Bilateral adrenal lymphoma. A 65-year-old male entered the hospital with symptoms of malaise, weakness, and fever. *A,* CT scan reveals bilateral large adrenal masses that are relatively smooth and homogeneous. Because of the large size of these masses, the CT appearance is most consistent with lymphoma and metastatic carcinoma (most commonly from oat cell carcinoma of the lung). Percutaneous needle biopsy revealed non-Hodgkin's lymphoma, and chemotherapy was instituted. *B,* CT scan performed 6 months later reveals that the large adrenal masses are dramatically smaller. The adrenal glands are still slightly enlarged, particularly on the left, but have resumed their normal configuration. The patient had marked clinical improvement. (*A* and *B* from Bosniak MA, Rumancik WM: Metastatic neoplasm of the adrenal gland and adrenal lymphoma. In Pollack HM (ed): Clinical Urography. Philadelphia, WB Saunders Company, 1990.)

have been reported but are unusual. Unless there is hemorrhage into the adenoma, patients are asymptomatic.

Most adenomas are single and encapsulated. Small adenomas often project from one of the limbs of the adrenal, with a normal-appearing gland seen otherwise. Larger adenomas often distort the contour of the entire gland. Microscopically, encapsulated adenomas usually can be distinguished from the nonencapsulated nodules of adrenal nodular hyperplasia. However, when adenomas are smaller than 1.0 cm, radiologic differentiation between adenoma and nodular hyperplasia may be impossible.

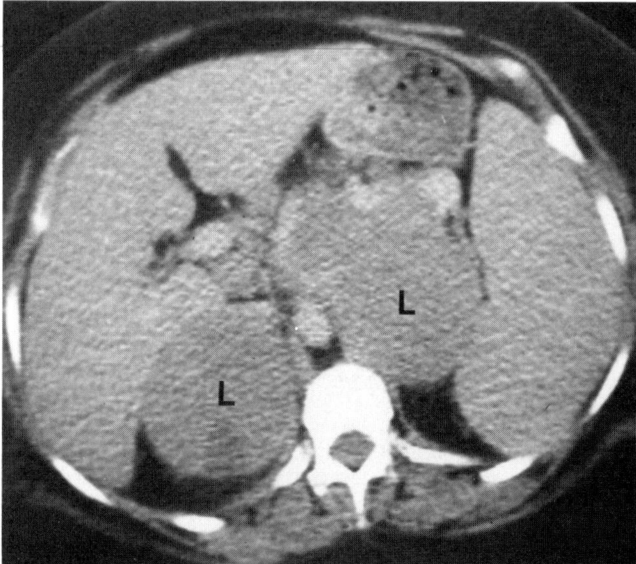

Figure 66–5. Adrenal lymphoma. Large, bilateral hypodense adrenal masses are present (L). Note also splenomegaly. No other evidence of lymphoma was present in this patient. Percutaneous biopsy revealed lymphoma of the adrenal glands.

With CT, several criteria are typical of benign adenomas: (1) The contour of the lesion is smooth and either rounded or oval; minimal smooth bulging can be noted occasionally. (2) The tumor margin is well delineated and clearly separate from adjacent structures. (3) The lesion measures less than 4 cm. (4) No growth is detected on serial CT studies (Fig. 66–6). Attenuation values may vary from water to soft-tissue density on non-enhanced CT scans, with values lower than 0 HU frequently seen. This is believed to be related to different proportions of lipid content within the adenoma. Punctate calcifications may infrequently be present within or on the edge of an adenoma. Areas of diminished attenuation within the lesion may represent hyalinization or necrosis. No CT differentiation can be made between functioning and nonfunctioning adenomas. No distinct pattern of intravenous contrast enhancement is observed or useful in distinguishing benign from malignant lesions.

On angiography, adenomas are characteristically vascular with a homogeneous capillary blush. The adrenal artery may enlarge to supply the adenoma.

MRI may be useful in distinguishing benign nonhyperfunctioning adenomas from adrenal metastases. On T_2-weighted images metastases have shown a high signal intensity (greater than liver) whereas nonhyperfunctioning adenomas have a signal intensity equal to or lower than liver (Fig 66–7). But, as discussed previously, there is an overlap in these findings so that although MRI can suggest that a lesion is probably a benign adenoma rather than a metastatic lesion, needle aspiration biopsy is usually needed for definitive diagnosis when this information is necessary for a proper treatment approach.

However, it has become apparent that the difference in the fat content of adrenal adenomas and metastatic neoplasm may lead to a reliable imaging differentiation between adenoma and malignancy. Since adenomas have a high intracellular fat content due to lipid-laden adrenocortical cells, some of these lesions have enough intracellular fat to have an attenuation of -5 to -15 HU on *non-enhanced* CT scans. This high fat content may allow the differentia-

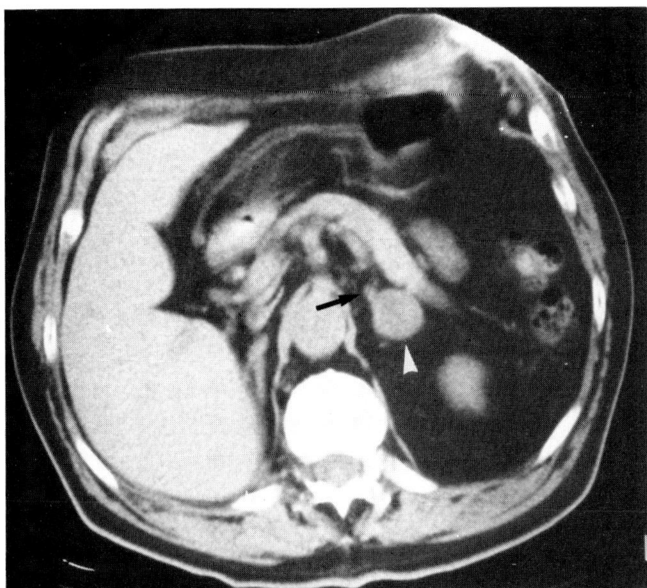

Figure 66–6. Adrenal adenoma. CT scan shows a round, 2.8-cm mass in the posterior limb of the left adrenal gland *(arrowhead)*. The lesion is smooth, and a normal anterior adrenal limb is present *(arrow)*. The right adrenal gland is normal. Follow-up CT studies at three and six months showed no change in this adenoma.

tion of adrenal adenoma from metastatic neoplasm because metastases to the adrenal apparently do not contain a high lipid content and therefore will not demonstrate negative attenuation numbers on CT. MRI may even be more sensitive in detecting the fat content of adrenal masses. The presence of fat within an adenoma can be clearly established when a dramatic decrease in signal intensity is noted on opposed-phase T_1-weighted gradient echo sequences. Since, as yet, this level of lipid has not been seen in metastatic neoplasm to the adrenals or in adrenal carcinoma, the use of this finding may well enable differentiation between adenoma and malignancy. (It should be emphasized that the intracellular fat content of adenomas should not be confused with the fatty tissue seen in myelolipomas, and this difference in the amount and type of fatty tissue should clearly be able to differentiate myelolipoma from adenoma based on imaging characteristics.)

There is little evidence for malignant transformation of adrenal adenomas. Adrenal carcinoma is generally considered to arise *de novo* rather than in adenomas. Pathologically, distinction between benign and malignant tumors can be difficult. Differentiation is usually based on the pattern of growth, not on the histology. Indications of malignancy include invasion of the capsule and/or adrenal vein and distant metastases. Radiologically, malignant lesions are usually large (greater than 5 cm), have an irregular contour, invade adjacent structures (kidney, pancreas, diaphragm), and are often associated with metastases to distant organs such as the liver and lung. Furthermore, malignant lesions exhibit a rapid growth pattern and would be expected to change in character and/or size on serial CT studies.

Because the prevalence of adrenal adenoma is far greater than that of biochemically silent adrenocortical carcinoma (less than 1 per 250,000), it is important to accurately diagnose an adrenal mass and avoid unnecessary surgical intervention. Therefore, in a patient with no known history of malignancy, a nonhyperfunctioning adrenal mass can be considered a benign adenoma if (1) the diameter of the lesion is less than 4 cm, (2) it has a smooth contour with well-defined margins, and (3) there is no change in size of the lesion on follow-up CT examination, which could be performed at a 6- to 12-month interval. Detection of the intracellular fat content, as noted above, also could be used to diagnose benign adrenal adenoma.

MYELOLIPOMA

Myelolipomas are rare benign tumors of the adrenal glands composed of mature fat and cells like those of bone marrow. Autopsy incidence ranges from 0.08 to 0.2 per cent. A questionable association between myelolipoma, obesity, and various chronic illnesses such as hypertension and cardiovascular disease has been noted. However, these tumors are almost always incidental findings often at CT or ultrasonography and generally not considered to be associated with any clinical findings or conditions. Rarely, if they grow to a large size, they may be associated with symptoms related to their bulk.

Pathologically, these tumors arise in the adrenal cortex. A myelolipoma contains mature fat cells with large vacuoles, interspersed

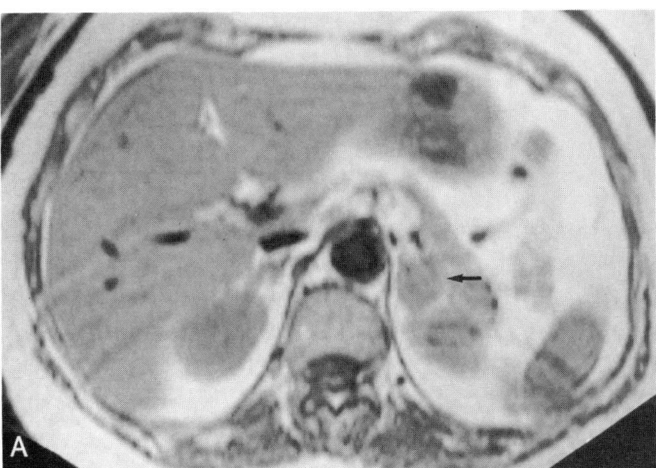

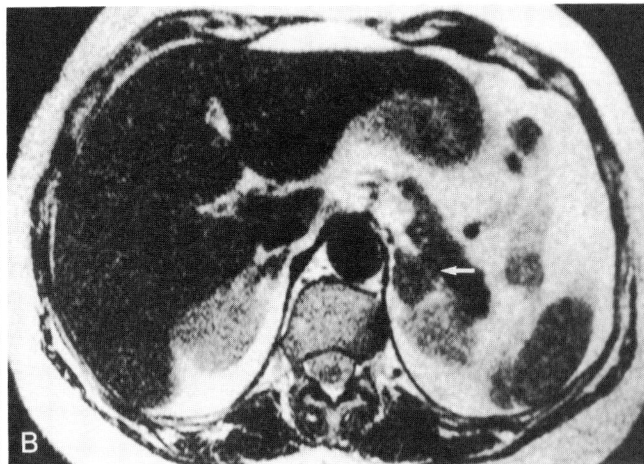

Figure 66–7. Benign nonhyperfunctioning adenoma of the left adrenal gland in a 68-year-old female. *A,* spin-echo T_1-weighted MRI image (TR 70, TE 6 msec). Note that the left adrenal gland mass has a relatively low signal similar to that of liver *(arrow)*. *B,* T_2-weighted image (TR 2000, TE 100 msec) reveals that the mass has a low signal similar to that of liver *(arrow)*. These findings are highly indicative of benign nonhyperfunctioning adenoma.

with cells resembling bone marrow myelocytes, megakaryocytes, lymphocytes, and erythrocytes. Hemorrhage, calcification, or ossification may also be present. Tumors range in size from microscopic to 30 cm in diameter.

Myelolipomas have no known malignant potential and are nonfunctioning. The etiology is not clear. It is possible that these lesions represent an embryonal rest of primitive mesenchyme or a metaplasia of reticuloendothelial system cells. Myelolipomas do not represent extramedullary hematopoiesis, nor are they associated with any known cause of it.

On ultrasonography, a mass containing high-amplitude echoes in the region of the adrenal gland should suggest the diagnosis of a myelolipoma (Fig. 66–8*A*). On CT, myelolipomas are usually well-defined, discrete masses that may have a pseudocapsule. Attenuation values vary with the proportion of fat and myeloid elements present. In the majority of lesions, attenuation values corresponding to fat can be readily found within the lesions (Figs. 66–8*B* and 66–9*A*). MRI can also readily diagnose the lesion by detecting fat in the tumor (Fig. 66–9*B*). In some lesions the amount of fat present is minimal and must be searched for carefully to be able to make the diagnosis. Particularly, in these cases, a large amount of punctate calcification or clumps of calcium may be present (Fig. 66–10). In those rare cases in which fat tissue can not be recognized, the lesion cannot be distinguished from other adrenal tumors by imaging techniques.

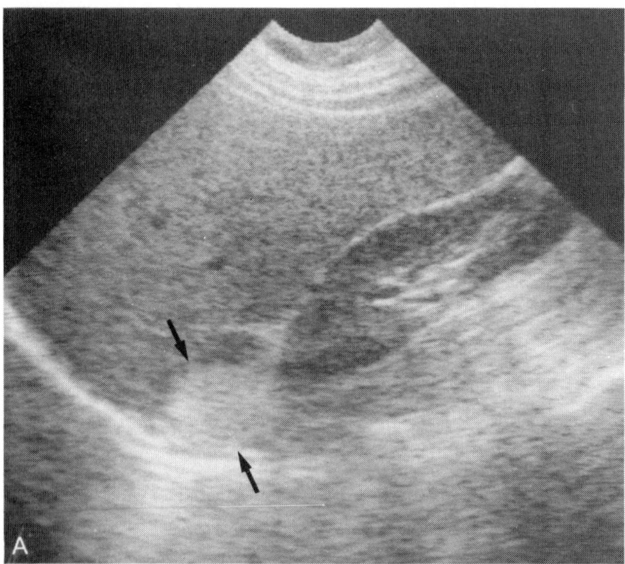

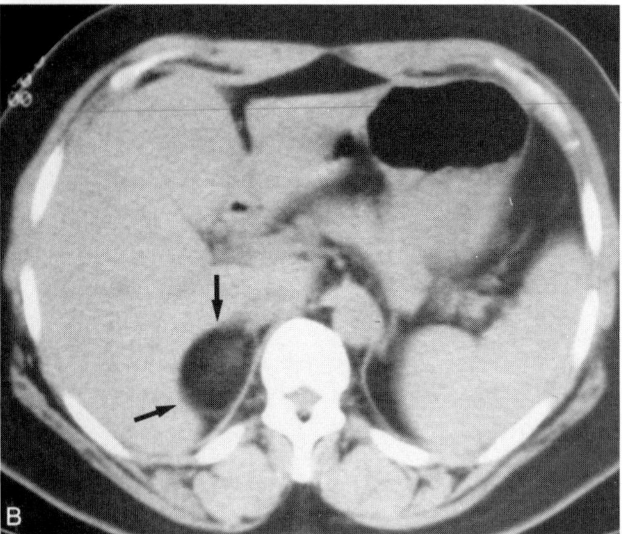

Figure 66–8. Adrenal myelolipoma. *A,* Longitudinal sonogram shows a 3-cm echogenic mass in the right suprarenal region *(arrows)*. *B,* CT scan identifies an encapsulated, fat-containing right adrenal lesion *(arrows)*. Note some areas of increased attenuation within the lesion representing myeloid elements. The left adrenal gland is normal. Follow-up CT studies of this patient show no change.

Angiographically, these lesions are hypovascular and indistinguishable from other hypovascular adrenal lesions. Most myelolipomas can be accurately diagnosed by imaging criteria, especially when the lesions can be shown to be clearly originating in the adrenal. However, when myelolipomas are large, radiologic differentiation between liposarcoma originating in the adjacent retroperitoneum and myelolipoma may be impossible, because the site of origin of the tumor may be difficult to determine. Angiography may be helpful in differentiation, but percutaneous biopsy may be required to establish the diagnosis. The presence of mature fat cells and myeloid elements in a biopsy specimen is characteristic for myelolipoma. Needle aspiration biopsy is required if there is a suspicion that a metastatic lesion is associated with the myelolipoma.

ADRENAL HEMANGIOMA

Hemangiomas of the adrenal gland are rare. Their pathologic and radiologic appearance can resemble that of analogous hemangiomas of the liver, brain, and peripheral soft tissues. The presence of phleboliths is a characteristic finding. Degenerative changes such as thrombosis, necrosis, hemorrhage, and calcification are commonly present. Interestingly, what are thought to be hemorrhagic adrenal cysts may actually be hemangiomas that have undergone episodes of internal hemorrhage with subsequent complete destruction of the original architecture. For this reason, the true incidence of hemangiomas may be higher than the actual small number of reported cases.

Histologically, the diagnosis is made on the basis of dilated, endothelium-lined, blood-filled channels. Tumors may be large, weighing up to 5000 g. There is no endocrine abnormality associated with these lesions, although a case of adrenal insufficiency in a patient with bilateral hemangiomas has been reported.

Most tumors are incidental findings. Patients are asymptomatic but may present with pain due to hemorrhage or to the mechanical mass effect of the tumor on associated structures. Phleboliths may be observed within a suprarenal mass, strongly suggesting the diagnosis of adrenal hemangioma.

Angiographic findings include sparse tumor vascularity, pooling of contrast material within areas of the tumor, and abnormally prolonged venous filling. On CT, these tumors are smoothly marginated and heterogeneous. Attenuation coefficients are relatively low (15 to 20 HU on non–contrast-enhanced scans). Contrast-enhanced scans may show only minimal enhancement or mixed areas of enhancement because the lesion may be filled with dilated venous lakes or areas of thrombosis might be present within the lesion. Calcifications representing phleboliths may be seen (Fig. 66–11). Internal irregular stellate calcific deposits or crescentic peripheral calcifications may also be present and most likely represent residua from previous hemorrhage. MRI might be helpful in diagnosis as it is in hemangiomas of the liver. However, little imaging experience using MRI with this tumor in the adrenal is available.

Surgical removal is almost always encouraged. This is to avoid the possibility of future hemorrhagic complications and/or to relieve the mass effect produced by large lesions. Furthermore, the rare presence of a hemangiosarcoma cannot be excluded radiographically.

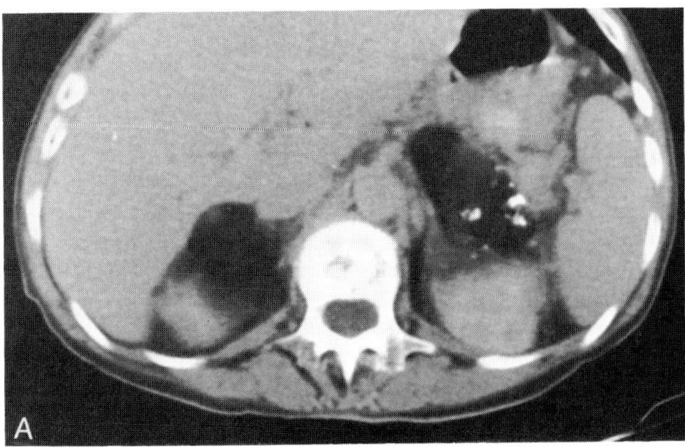

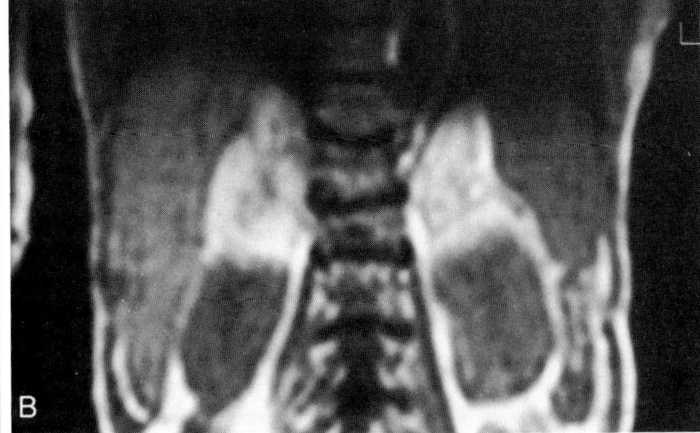

Figure 66–9. Bilateral adrenal myelolipomas, incidentally discovered in an 82-year-old woman being studied for pelvic malignancy. *A,* Contrast-enhanced CT scan reveals fatty masses in the suprarenal areas bilaterally. Attenuation of these masses measured −35 to −50 HU. Note punctate calcifications in the left-sided tumor. *B,* T_1-weighted coronal MRI scan (TR 700, TE 20 msec) of the abdomen reveals bilateral adrenal masses with a signal consistent with fatty tissue. The masses are less intense than the surrounding perinephric fat, however, probably because of the presence of myeloid and stromal elements. (*A* and *B* from Rumancik WM, Bosniak MA: Miscellaneous conditions of the adrenals and adrenal pseudotumors. In Pollack HM (ed): Clinical Urography. Philadelphia, WB Saunders Company, 1990.)

MISCELLANEOUS NEOPLASMS OF THE ADRENAL

Rare and unusual tumors have been described occurring in the adrenal glands. These may have nonspecific appearances, and the diagnosis is usually made histologically. These include teratoma, leiomyosarcoma, neurofibroma, osteoma, ganglioneuroma, fibroma, and myoma. Lipoma of the adrenal can be suggested by its fat content, although differentiation from a myelolipoma might be difficult.

ADRENAL CYSTS

Adrenal cysts are rare lesions with an incidence at autopsy of about 0.06 per cent. The vast majority are of minute size and are found only incidentally at autopsy. Larger cysts are rare and seldom exceed 10 cm in diameter. Those found clinically usually measure 3 to 4 cm in diameter. There is no lateral predominance. Females are affected more commonly than males, with a ratio of about 3:1. Adrenal cysts may occur at any age but are most frequently observed in the fifth and sixth decades.

Cysts of the adrenal have multiple origins. A classification of adrenal cysts includes:

1. *Parasitic* (7 per cent)—These are most commonly echinococcal in origin. Disseminated echinococcal disease is frequently associated with adrenal involvement.
2. *Epithelial* (9 per cent)—These may represent rare glandular or retention cysts, cystic transformation of embryonal remnants, or unusual cystic adenomas.
3. *Endothelial* (45 per cent)—These can be further subdivided into lymphangiectatic cysts, angiomatous cysts, and hamartomas. Some observers believe that obstructed adrenal lymph vessels may result in the formation of endothelium-lined, multiloculated cystic

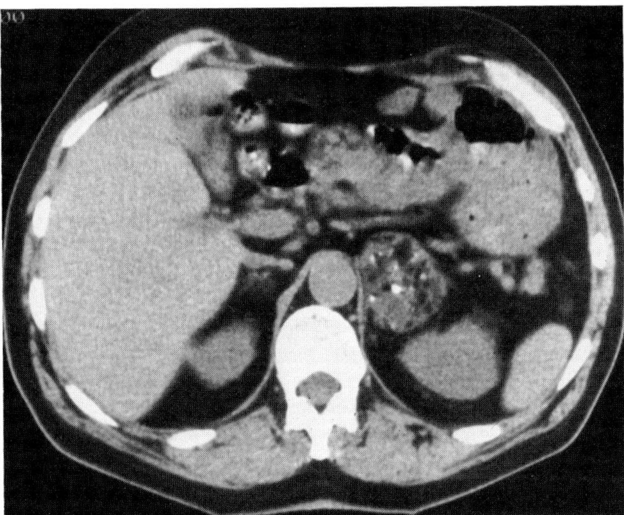

Figure 66–10. Myelolipoma of left adrenal gland. A left adrenal mass measuring 4.0 cm in diameter is seen that contains multiple punctate areas of calcification and areas of low attenuation tissue measuring −53 HU.

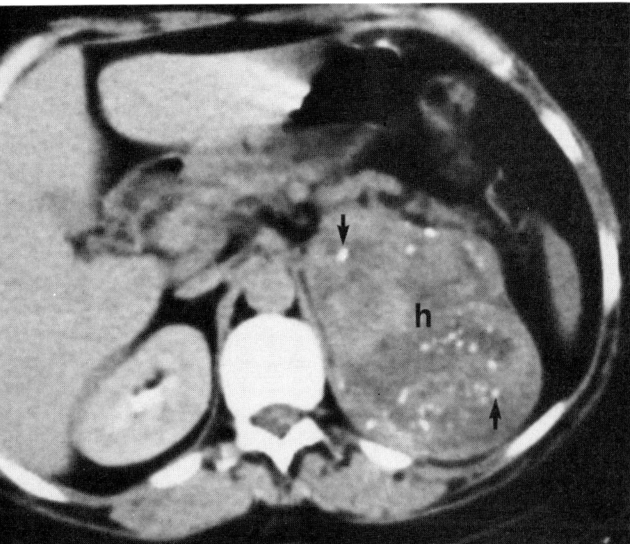

Figure 66–11. Adrenal hemangioma. CT scan after intravenous contrast administration shows a large heterogeneous mass (h) in the region of the left adrenal gland containing phleboliths *(arrows).* This adrenal hemangioma was removed surgically.

cavities. These may also represent the end result of repeated hemorrhage into an adrenal hemangioma, with destruction of the original architecture.

4. *Pseudocysts* (39 per cent)—These are the result of hemorrhage into a normal gland or are secondary to degenerative necrosis and hemorrhage into an adrenal tumor (particularly adenoma).

Calcification occurs in the wall in about 15 per cent of cases. This is especially true of echinococcal cysts but can be seen in cysts of all origins, particularly pseudocysts due to hemorrhage in adrenal tumors (Fig. 66–12).

On urography with tomography a well-marginated radiolucent mass will be seen. Angiography reveals a well-marginated, avascular mass often with vessels stretched over its surface. In uncomplicated cysts, ultrasonography may show a typical fluid-filled lesion with sharp margination and good through transmission (similar to renal cysts), but internal debris or calcification is often present, especially in those lesions containing hemorrhagic components. CT shows well-demarcated lesions that do not enhance with IV contrast. The fluid in the cyst measures water density or much higher depending on the amount of hemorrhagic debris and protein in the fluid. On MRI, uncomplicated adrenal cysts are low in signal intensity on T_1-weighted images and high on T_2-weighted images. Complicated or hemorrhagic adrenal cysts will, however, be high on both T_1- and T_2-weighted images and may be difficult to differentiate from fat-containing adrenal lesions. When the cysts are large, it may be impossible to determine their adrenal origin. Here again, coronal or sagittal plane MRI may be quite helpful. Percutaneous aspiration of the cyst with analysis of its fluid for adrenal hormones or cholesterol may help confirm its origin as adrenal.

Because adrenal cysts are benign, small lesions that meet the criteria for a cyst can usually be monitored with serial imaging studies. However, surgery may be needed in large lesions in which the diagnosis is in doubt or when lesion size produces symptoms.

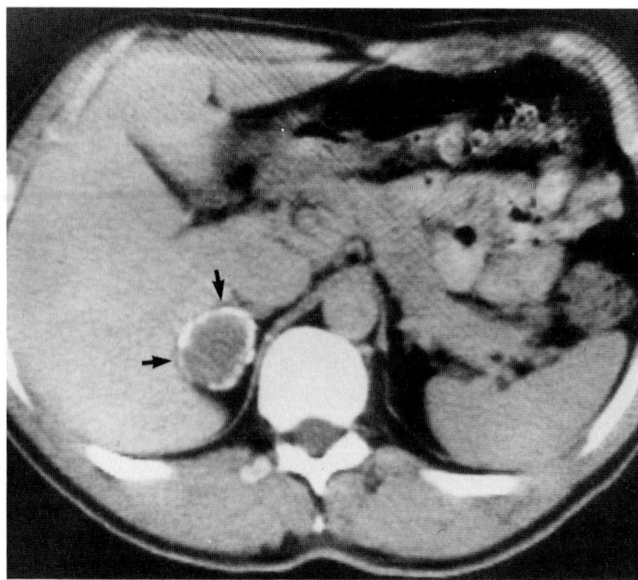

Figure 66–12. Adrenal cyst. A right adrenal mass with a densely calcified wall is present *(arrows)*. There was no change in this lesion on follow-up CT studies. This represents a benign hemorrhagic adrenal cyst.

ADRENAL HEMORRHAGE

Adrenal hemorrhage can be seen in the neonate or adult. The clinical presentations and prognostic implications differ greatly in these two groups of patients.

Neonatal Adrenal Hemorrhage

Adrenal hemorrhage in the neonate is not rare. It occurs most frequently between the second and seventh days of life. The presenting symptoms vary with the amount of hemorrhage. Classically, patients present with prolonged neonatal jaundice and hyperbilirubinemia. An abdominal mass may be palpated, and patients may have a mild anemia. Hemorrhage into the right adrenal gland occurs in 70 per cent of cases. Bilateral involvement is seen in only 5 to 10 per cent of cases. Adrenal insufficiency is rare, if ever present.

The pathogenesis of adrenal hemorrhage of the newborn is unknown. Associated factors include stress and trauma at birth, anoxia, septicemia, hemorrhagic disorders, hypoprothrombinemia, and congenital syphilis. Stress and trauma appear to be the most common factors.

The unusual susceptibility of the right adrenal gland for hemorrhage is unknown. The right adrenal vein usually drains directly into the inferior vena cava. This may make the right adrenal more prone to changes in central venous pressure and subsequent rupture of the medullary sinusoids.

In the past, diagnosis of adrenal hemorrhage was made with intravenous urography (IVU), which revealed a smooth, homogeneous mass displacing the kidney inferiorly. The mass was avascular and relatively lucent during the phase of total body opacification. Sonography is now the primary imaging study in the diagnosis of neonatal adrenal hemorrhage and shows a hypoechoic suprarenal mass that may contain some degree of solid component representing blood elements. Most lesions exhibit mixed echogenicity early and then progress to a echo-free center as the hematoma undergoes lysis and coalesces (Fig. 66–13).

On follow-up, shrinkage of the hemorrhagic lesions is apparent. By six to eight weeks, the kidney usually returns to a normal axis and position. Follow-up sonograms show liquefaction and progressive decrease in the size of the hemorrhage. Dense calcification in the region of the hemorrhagic adrenal usually develops by two years of age.

Adult Adrenal Hemorrhage

Adrenal hemorrhage is an uncommon condition in the adult. It is usually associated with severe stress, surgery, septicemia, hypotension, burns, or trauma. Other causes include anticoagulant therapy, thrombocytopenia, or disseminated intravascular coagulation. Most anticoagulant-associated adrenal hemorrhage occurs during the initial three weeks of treatment. It is apparently not due to excessive anticoagulation because hemorrhage into other organs or the rest of the retroperitoneum does not usually occur. Increased stimulation of the adrenal glands by endogenous ACTH produced during periods of stress may predispose the gland to increased activity and hemorrhage.

Post-traumatic adrenal hemorrhage can be bilateral or unilateral. If unilateral, it is more common on the right. This is possibly due to compression of the gland between the liver and the spine or perhaps due to increased pressure in the right gland due to increased central venous pressure readily transmitted to the gland via the short adrenal vein entering directly into the inferior vena cava. Metastatic neoplasm to the adrenal is also associated with adrenal hemorrhage, which can become massive. Carcinoma of the lung and metastatic melanoma are the most common primary neoplasms.

Subsequent adrenal insufficiency is a recognized complication of bilateral adrenal hemorrhage. The clinical manifestations of adrenal insufficiency are nonspecific. They may occur days to weeks after

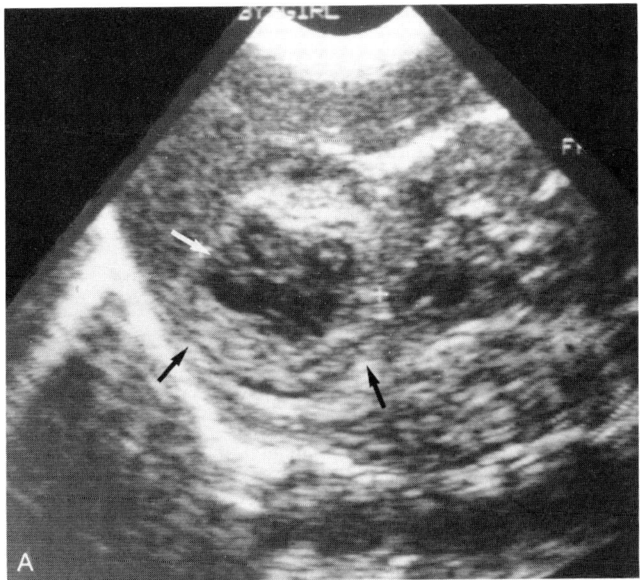

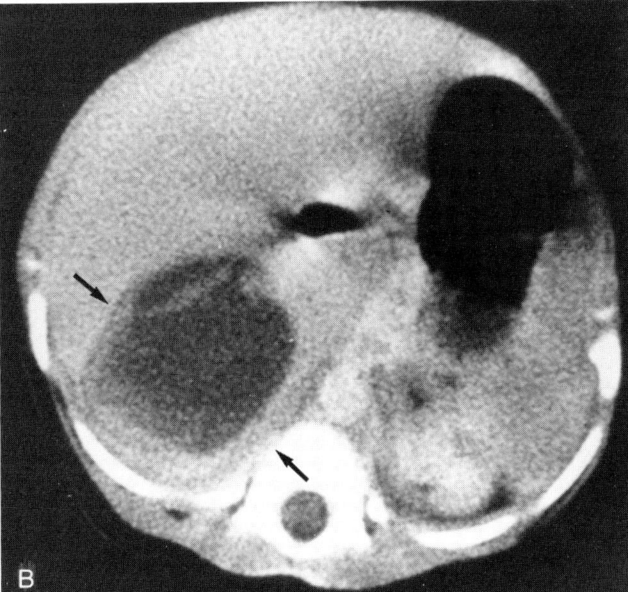

Figure 66–13. Adrenal hematoma in an infant. *A,* Longitudinal sonogram shows a heterogeneous mass in the right suprarenal region *(arrows). B,* Contrast-enhanced CT scan shows a large, low-attenuation mass in the region of the right adrenal gland representing a hematoma *(arrows).* Follow-up studies showed progressive resolution and calcification of the lesion.

the hemorrhagic episode and are easily confused with those of the patient's underlying condition.

On CT, an adrenal mass may be identified that appears similar to an adenoma or metastasis (Fig. 66–14). However, if the CT scan is performed within a week of the hemorrhage, the characteristic increased attenuation (50 to 60 HU) of fresh blood will be present. If the scan is performed without intravenous contrast, the presence of an adrenal mass measuring 60 HU will be diagnostic of an adrenal hematoma (Fig. 66–15). If the scan was performed with intravenous contrast, differentiation from metastatic neoplasm based on attenuation can be difficult. However, repeat CT scan before and after intravenous contrast to show that the lesion does not enhance would be diagnostic because hematomas do not enhance and other adrenal lesions that might be considered will.

Follow-up CT usually shows diminution or disappearance of the areas of hemorrhage and progressive diminution of attenuation values, consistent with resolving hematomas (Fig. 66–14). As the hematoma resolves, calcification within the gland often occurs.

Ultrasound findings in adrenal hematoma may show a moderately echogenic mass. MRI will demonstrate a high–signal intensity mass on the T_1-weighted pulse sequence. Differentiation from the high signal intensity of fat can be achieved by fat suppression techniques.

ADRENAL INFECTIONS

Most infections of the adrenals are granulomatous in origin and most commonly are due to tuberculosis. Pyogenic adrenal infections can be observed in infants and children, usually as a result of superinfection in an adrenal hemorrhage.

The most common radiologic appearance of adrenal tuberculosis is bilateral adrenal calcifications (Fig. 66–16). This is usually irregular, dense, and chunky. Calcification is often visible on plain radiographs. The main differential diagnosis is posthemorrhagic

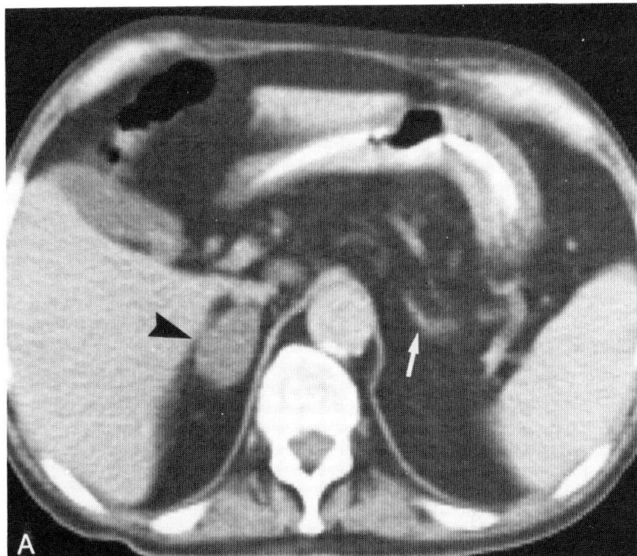

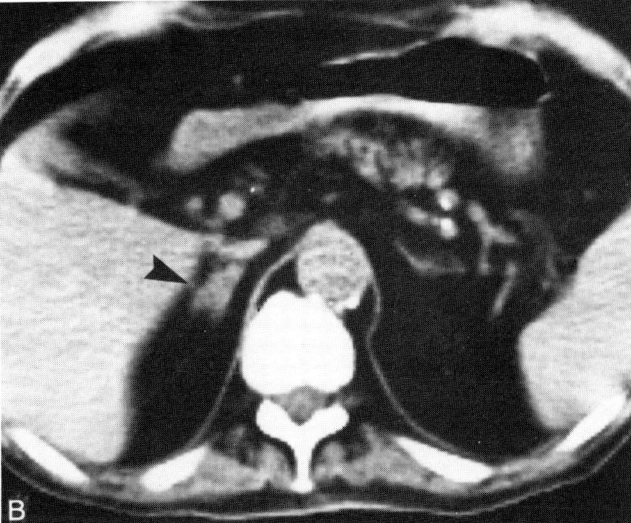

Figure 66–14. Adrenal hematoma in an adult. *A,* A homogeneous mass is present in the right adrenal gland *(arrowhead).* The left adrenal *(arrow)* is normal. *B,* Scan obtained two months later shows almost complete resolution of the right adrenal hematoma *(arrowhead).*

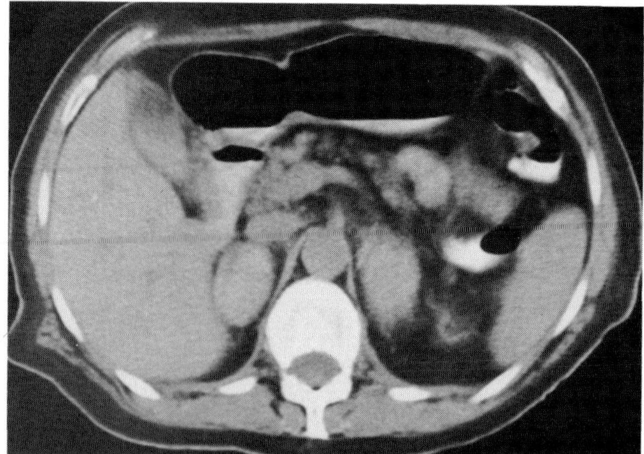

Figure 66–15. Acute bilateral adrenal hemorrhage in a 74-year-old female with gram-negative sepsis and shock followed by weakness. CT scan reveals bilateral adrenal masses. The adrenals have increased attenuation consistent with recent hemorrhage. A previous CT scan performed 3 weeks earlier revealed normal adrenal glands. (From Rumancik WM, Bosniak MA: Miscellaneous conditions of the adrenals and adrenal pseudotumors. In Pollack HM (ed): Clinical Urography. Philadelphia, WB Saunders Company, 1990.)

calcification, but calcification can occur in carcinoma, other infections, neuroblastoma, cysts, hemangioma, myelolipoma, or adenoma.

Caseous adrenal tuberculosis can be seen as a much rarer form of adrenal tuberculosis. CT shows a low-attenuation adrenal mass with a thick, irregular wall having dense peripheral enhancement after intravenous contrast administration. Adrenal tuberculosis is the most common granulomatous infection causing Addison's disease.

Histoplasmosis of the adrenal is uncommon except in endemic areas. CT findings include unilateral but more commonly bilateral enlargement of the gland with focal low-attenuation areas within. Adrenal gland shape may be preserved but round masses of low attenuation in the adrenals are commonly seen. A characteristic peripheral contrast enhancement is often seen. Flecks of calcification may be present but usually in the healing phase. Adrenal insufficiency is frequently associated. CT-guided aspiration biopsy can be diagnostic, but special stains of the aspirate may be necessary.

Other granulomatous infections such as cryptococcosis and blastomycosis have been reported. Although adrenal gland morphology is grossly normal, a necrotizing adrenalitis due to cytomegalovirus is commonly seen in patients with acquired immune deficiency syndrome.

WOLMAN DISEASE

Wolman disease was originally described as a generalized xanthomatosis associated with adrenal calcifications. This acid lipase deficiency presents as an autosomal recessive error of lipid metabolism that results in marked accumulation of cholesteryl esters and triglycerides in many tissues of the body. The cells involved include those active in cholesterol synthesis. The tissues most affected include liver, spleen, intestinal mucosa, lymph nodes, aorta, bone marrow, neurons, skin fibroblasts, and adrenals.

Wolman disease becomes clinically evident in the first few weeks of life and is usually fatal by the age of six months. It is characterized by abdominal distention, steatorrhea, failure to thrive, hepatosplenomegaly, lymphadenopathy, and retarded motor development. There is symmetrical enlargement of both adrenal glands associated with punctate or diffuse calcifications.

In patients with Wolman disease, CT shows an enlarged liver of diminished density and enlarged adrenals with cortical calcifications (Fig. 66–17).

PSEUDOTUMORS

Adrenal pseudotumors comprise those conditions that can mimic an adrenal tumor but in reality are not a true adrenal mass. Most of these conditions are due to normal anatomic structures or variations and to certain pathologic conditions in adjacent organs or structures that project into the region of the adrenal. Adrenal pseudotumors were occasionally a diagnostic problem in the pre-CT era on plain

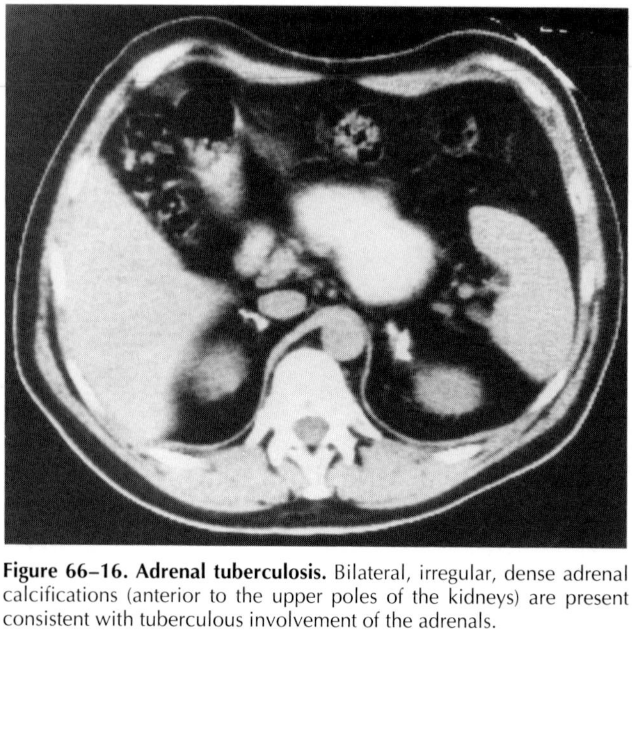

Figure 66–16. Adrenal tuberculosis. Bilateral, irregular, dense adrenal calcifications (anterior to the upper poles of the kidneys) are present consistent with tuberculous involvement of the adrenals.

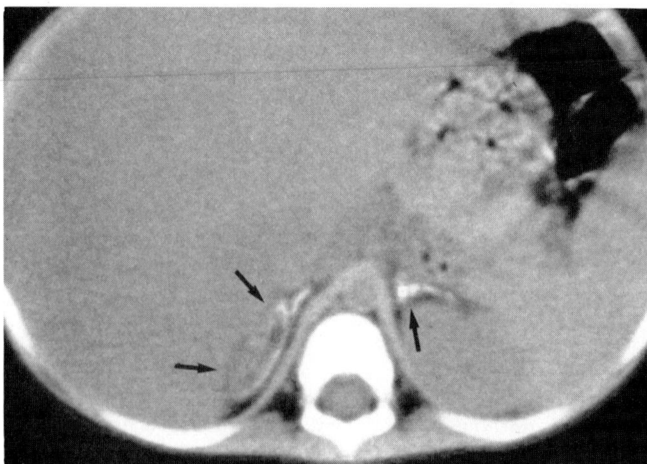

Figure 66–17. Wolman disease. A 28-month-old child with a diagnosis of Wolman disease. Dense cortical calcification is present within both adrenal glands *(arrows)*. The enlargement of the right adrenal gland can be appreciated. Also note the enlarged liver typical of this disease. (Reprinted with permission from Hill SC, Hoeg JM, Dwyer AJ, et al: CT findings in acid lipase deficiency. Wolman disease and cholesteryl ester storage disease. J Comput Assist Tomogr 7:815–818, 1983.)

films of the abdomen and even in the early CT era, when first- and second-generation scanners were used. However, with the use of modern CT equipment, the difficulty in differentiating an extra-adrenal from an adrenal mass should not occur if one is aware of this potential pitfall. Thin-section CT scans can be obtained and the normal adrenal gland identified in almost all cases. Occasionally selective angiography is necessary to determine whether a large mass projecting into the adrenal bed is adrenal in origin or is due to a tumor in an adjacent organ. By noting the major feeding vessel to the tumor, one can usually make this differentiation. MRI, particularly with the use of coronal and sagittal sections, frequently can determine the likely origin of large masses in the adrenal bed.

Adrenal pseudotumors include the following:

1. Fluid-Filled Gastric Fundus. On plain abdominal films or routine linear tomography of the kidney, a soft-tissue mass may be seen in the left suprarenal region, representing gastric fundus. On CT, the fluid-filled gastric fundus, which has not been opacified by orally administered contrast material, may produce a mass-like density in the expected region of the left adrenal gland (Fig. 66–18). Similarly, a focal gastric diverticulum projecting from the juxtacardial region of the stomach may mimic an adrenal tumor.

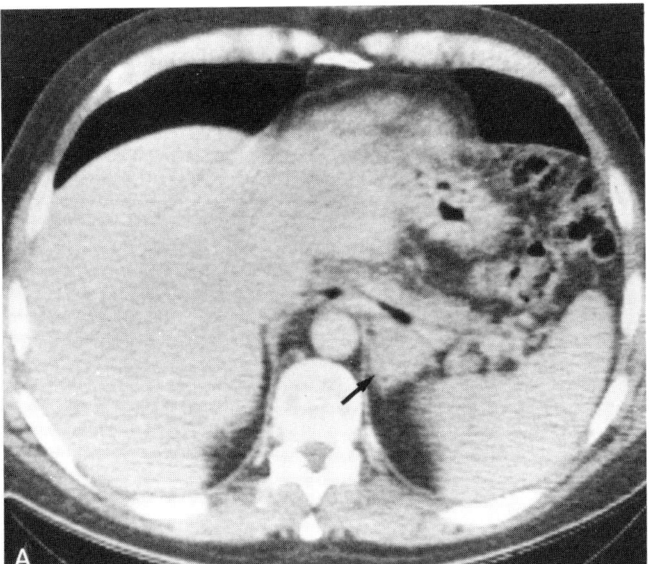

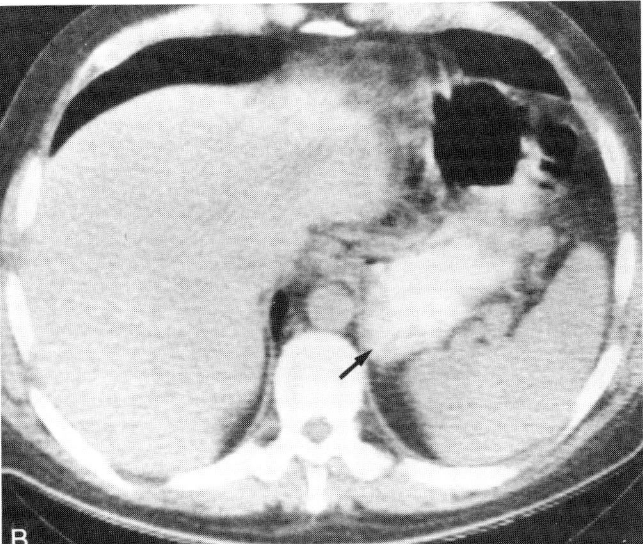

Figure 66–18. Adrenal pseudotumor: fluid-filled gastric fundus. *A,* CT scan with no oral contrast shows a mass-like lesion in the region of the left adrenal *(arrow). B,* CT scan after oral contrast shows the oral contrast to fill the presumed lesion seen in *A (arrow),* demonstrating that it was only a fluid-filled gastric fundus and not an actual adrenal lesion. (*A* and *B* from Berliner L, Bosniak MA, Megibow AJ: Adrenal pseudotumors on computed tomography. J Comput Assist Tomogr 6:281–285, 1982.)

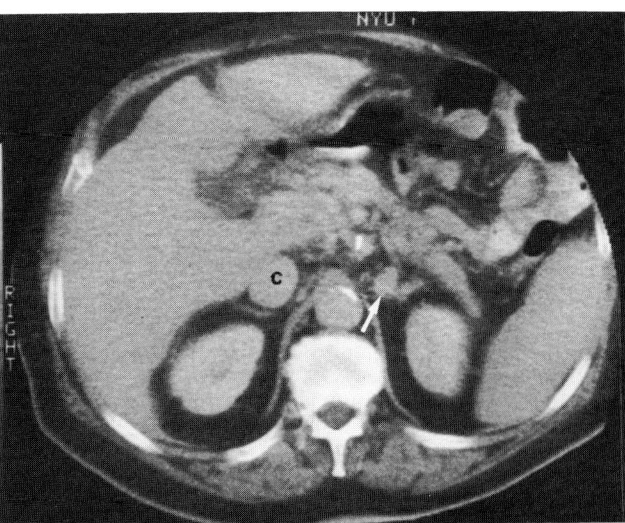

Figure 66–19. Pseudotumor of the left adrenal due to dilated adrenal vein in a patient with portal hypertension. CT scan reveals a small "mass" in the region of the left adrenal gland *(arrow).* Note that the "mass" has a high attenuation similar to that seen in other vessels such as the inferior vena cava (c). Evidence of upper abdominal varices in the peripancreatic area is also noted.

2. Prominent Splenic Lobulation or Accessory Spleen.

3. Upper Pole Renal Tumor or Cyst. Coronal or longitudinal ultrasound scans may be helpful in showing the mass to be contiguous with the kidney. Routine transaxial CT scans may be inadequate to exclude an adrenal lesion in these cases. MRI, ultrasonography, or in some cases angiography may be necessary for differentiation.

4. Tortuous Splenic and Retroperitoneal Vessels. Intravenous contrast administration in CT scanning is necessary to show opacification of vessels in the region of the adrenal gland to exclude an intrinsic adrenal lesion. This is particularly true when dilated retroperitoneal veins associated with portal hypertension and cirrhosis occur (Fig. 66–19). An enlarged adrenal vein draining into the left renal vein (splenorenal anastomosis) can simulate an adrenal tumor. MRI with its ability to image vessels can readily evaluate this and similar entities.

5. Pancreatic Mass. Neoplastic, inflammatory, and/or cystic masses arising in the tail of the pancreas may extend to the region of the left adrenal gland. Normal variations in the position of the pancreatic tail may also simulate a left adrenal mass.

6. Nodules or Variations of the Diaphragmatic Crura.

7. Hepatic Tumor. Because of the close association of the right adrenal to the liver, liver lesions particularly in the caudate lobe can project into the area of the right adrenal gland, causing an adrenal pseudotumor. If the adrenal gland cannot be identified, the differentiation on CT may not be possible. In such cases, MRI or angiography is usually able to make the distinction.

8. Colon. Interposition of a fluid-filled colon into the right adrenal bed can also appear as a cystic adrenal lesion. With careful technique a normal adrenal gland should be identified; however, if this cannot be done, air or contrast can be instilled into the colon to establish the diagnosis.

Acknowledgments

The authors would like to thank Dr. John L. Doppman, Bethesda, MD, for the use of Figure 66–17; Dr. Barry Held, New York, NY, for the use of Figure 66–13; Dr. Leon Love, Maywood, IL, for the use of Figure 66–11; and Angela Oleske and Esther Roman for manuscript preparation.

Bibliography

Abrams HL, Spiro R, Goldstein N: Metastases in carcinoma: Analysis of 1000 autopsied cases. Cancer 3:74–85, 1950.

Baker ME, Blinder R, Spritzer C, et al: MR evaluation of adrenal masses at 1.5 T. AJR 153:307–312, 1989.

Berliner L, Bosniak MA, Megibow AJ: Adrenal pseudotumors on computed tomography. J Comput Assist Tomogr 6(2):281–285, 1982.

Bernardino ME: Management of the asymptomatic patient with a unilateral adrenal mass. Radiology 166:121–123, 1988.

Bernadino ME, Walther MM, Phillips VM, et al: CT-guided adrenal biospy: Accuracy, safety and indications. AJR 144:67–69, 1985.

Bosniak MA, Siegelman SS, Evans JA: The Adrenal, Retroperitoneum, and Lower Urinary Tract. Chicago, Year Book Medical Publishers, 1976, pp 14–17, 29–53, 72–103, 192–229.

Brady TM, Gross BH, Glazer GM, Williams DM: Adrenal pseudomasses due to varices: Angiographic–CT–MRI pathologic correlations. AJR 145:301–304, 1985.

Cheema P, Cartagena R, Staubitz W: Adrenal cysts. Diagnosis and treatment. J Urology 126:396–399, 1981.

Cohen EK, Daveman A, Stringer DA, et al: Focal adrenal hemorrhage. A new US appearance. Radiology 161:631–633, 1986.

Derchi LE, Rapaccini GL, Banderali A, et al: Ultrasound and CT findings in two cases of hemangioma of the adrenal gland. J Comput Assist Tomogr 13:659–661, 1989.

Dunnick NR. Adrenal imaging: Current status. AJR 154:927–936, 1990.

Falke THM, te Strake L, Shaff MI, et al: MR imaging of the adrenals. Correlation with computed tomography. J Comput Assist Tomogr 10:242–253, 1986.

Feldberg MAM, Hendriks MJ, Klinkhamer AC: Massive bilateral non-Hodgkin's lymphomas of the adrenals. Urol Radiol 8:85–88, 1986.

Glazer GM, Woolsley EJ, Borello J, et al: Adrenal tissue characterization using MR imaging. Radiology 158:73–79, 1986.

Glazer HS, Lee JKT, Balfe DM, et al: Non-Hodgkin lymphoma. Computed tomographic demonstration of unusual extranodal involvement. Radiology 149:211–217, 1983.

Hill SC, Hoeg JM, Dwyer AJ, et al: CT findings in acid lipase deficiency. Wolman disease and cholesteryl ester storage disease. J Comput Assist Tomogr 7:815–818, 1983.

Itoh K, Yamashita K, Satoh Y, Sawada H: MR imaging of bilateral adrenal hemorrhage. J Comput Assist Tomogr 12:1054–1056, 1988.

Jafri SZH, Francis IR, Glazer GM, et al: CT detection of adrenal lymphoma. J Comput Assist Tomogr 7(2):254–256, 1983.

Khuri FJ, Alton DJ, Hardy BE, et al: Adrenal hemorrhage in neonates. Report of 5 cases and review of the literature. J Urology 124:684–687, 1980.

Kier R, McCarthy S: MR characterization of adrenal masses: Field strength and pulse sequence considerations. Radiology 171:671–674, 1989.

Lee MJ, Hahn PF, Papanicolaou N, et al: Benign and malignant adrenal masses: CT distinction with attenuation coefficients, size and observer analysis. Radiology 179:415–418, 1991.

Lee WJ, Weinreb J, Kumari S, et al: Adrenal hemangioma. J Comput Assist Tomogr 6(2):392–394, 1982.

Leroy-Willig A, Bittoun J, Luton JP, et al: In vivo MR spectroscopic imaging of the adrenal glands: Distinction between adenomas and carcinomas larger than 15 mm based on lipid content. AJR 153:771–773, 1989.

Levine E: CT evaluation of active adrenal histoplasmosis. Urol Radiol 13:103–106, 1991.

Ling D, Korobkin M, Silverman PM, Dunnick NR: CT demonstration of bilateral adrenal hemorrhage. AJR 141:307–308, 1983.

Mitchell DG, Crovello M, Matteucci T, et al. Benign adrenocortical masses: Diagnosis with chemical shift MR imaging. Radiology 185:345–351, 1992.

Mitnick JS, Bosniak MA, Megibow AJ, Naidich DP: Non-functioning adrenal adenomas discovered incidentally on computed tomography. Radiology 148(2):495–499, 1983.

Mitty JA, Cohen BA, Sprayregen S, Schwartz K: Adrenal pseudotumors on CT due to dilated portosystemic veins. AJR 141:727–730, 1983.

Miyake H, Maeda H, Tashiro M, et al: CT of adrenal tumors: Frequency and clinical significance of low attenuation lesions. AJR 152:1005–1007, 1989.

Murphy BJ, Casillas J, Yrizarry JM: Traumatic adrenal hemorrhage: Radiologic findings. Radiology 169:701–703, 1988.

Musante F, Derchi LE, Bazzocchi M, et al: MR imaging of adrenal myelolipomas. J Comput Assist Tomogr 15:111–114, 1991.

Musante F, Derchi LE, Zappasodi F, et al: Myelolipoma of the adrenal gland: Sonography and CT features. AJR 151:961–964, 1988.

Oliver TW Jr, Bernardino ME, Miller JI, et al: Isolated adrenal masses in non-small-cell bronchogenic carcinoma. Radiology 153:217–218, 1984.

Pagani JJ: Non-small cell lung carcinoma adrenal metastases. Computed tomography and percutaneous needle biopsy in their diagnosis. Cancer 53:1058–1060, 1984.

Paling MR, Williamson BRJ: Adrenal involvement in non-Hodgkin's lymphoma. AJR 141:303–305, 1983.

Pastakia B, Miller I, Wolfman M, et al: MR imaging of a large adrenal cyst. J Comput Assist Tomogr 10:710–711, 1986.

Reinig JW, Doppman JL, Dwyer AJ, et al: Adrenal masses differentiated by MR. Radiology 158:81–84, 1986.

Reinig JW, Doppman JL, Dwyer AJ, et al: Distinction between adrenal adenomas and metastases using MR imaging. J Comput Assist Tomogr 9:898–901, 1985.

Remer EM, Weinfeld RM, Glazer GM, et al: Hyperfunctioning and nonhyperfunctioning benign adrenal cortical lesions: Characterization and comparison with MR imaging. Radiology 171:681–685, 1989.

Rofsky NM, Bosniak MA, Megibow AJ, Schlossberg P: Adrenal myelolipoma: CT appearance with tiny amounts of fat and punctate calcification. Urol Radiol 11:148–152, 1989.

Sandler MA, Pearlberg JL, Madrazo BL, et al: Computed tomographic evaluation of the adrenal gland in the preoperative assessment of bronchogenic carcinoma. Radiology 145:733–736, 1982.

Schwartz JM, Bosniak MA, Megibow AJ, Hulnick DH: Right adrenal pseudotumor caused by colon: CT demonstration. J Comput Assist Tomogr 12:153, 1988.

Shah HR, Love L, Williamson MR, et al: Hemorrhagic adrenal metastases: CT findings. J Comput Assist Tomogr 13:77–81, 1989.

Siekavizza JL, Bernardino ME, Samaan NA: Suprarenal mass and its differential diagnosis. Urology 18(6):625–632, 1981.

Silverman PM: Gastric diverticulum mimicking adrenal mass: CT demonstration. J Comput Assist Tomogr 10:709–711, 1986.

Tung GA, Pfister RC, Papanicolaou N, Yoder IC: Adrenal cysts: Imaging and percutaneous aspiration. Radiology 173:107–110, 1989.

Vick CW, Zeman RK, Mannes E, et al: Adrenal myelolipoma. CT and ultrasound findings. Urol Radiol 6:7–13, 1984.

Vicks BS, Perusek M, Johnson J, Tio F: Primary adrenal lymphoma. CT and sonography appearances. JCU 15:135, 1987.

Welch K, Finkbeiner W, Alpers CE, et al: Autopsy findings in the acquired immune deficiency syndrome. JAMA 252(9):1152–1159, 1984.

Wilms G, Marchal G, Baert A, et al: CT and ultrasound features of post-traumatic adrenal hemorrhage. J Comput Assist Tomogr 11:112–115, 1987.

Wilms GE, Baert AL, Kint EJ, et al: Computed tomographic findings in bilateral adrenal tuberculosis. Radiology 146:729–730, 1983.

Wilson DA, Muchmore HG, Tisdale RG, et al: Histoplasmosis of the adrenal glands studied by CT. Radiology 150:779–783, 1984.

Wolverson MK, Kannegiesser H: CT of bilateral adrenal hemorrhage with acute adrenal insufficiency in the adult. AJR 142:311–314, 1984.

67 Kidney
Urography—Anatomy and Technique

Bruce L. McClennan

The intravenous urogram (IVU) can accurately demonstrate the anatomy and pathology of the urinary tract, and, despite the wide variety of alternative imaging tests, has remained the cornerstone of uroradiologic diagnosis. The indications for intravenous urography have undergone considerable change in the modern imaging era. Although there may not be any absolute contraindications to the performance of intravenous urography, circumstances such as previous severe life-threatening contrast reaction, congestive heart failure, pulmonary edema, pregnancy, and severe azotemia are cause for prudent clinical correlation and risk assessment. The availability of alternative imaging procedures such as ultrasonography (US), computed tomography (CT), and magnetic resonance imaging (MRI), which may provide equal or more comprehensive information, is one reason for the decline in the overall number of urograms performed today. Additionally, the knowledge that the use of urography may have little or no effect on patient outcome (treatment) in certain, low-yield circumstances—for example, males with benign prostatic hypertrophy and females with lower urinary tract infection or incontinence—has further contributed to a decline in the volume of urograms. Finally, better understanding of the risks attendant to the administration of contrast material in the azotemic patient has virtually eliminated the use of urography for evaluation of the patient in renal failure. Awareness of the need for cost containment exerts further pressure on the radiologist to be selective in his or her choice of contrast media as well as the choice and sequence of imaging tests.

RENAL ANATOMY

The kidneys lie in the retroperitoneum surrounded by perirenal fat that is enveloped by the perinephric (Gerota's) fascia. The normal position of the kidney in the retroperitoneum varies considerably (Fig. 67–1). The upper posterior surface of both kidneys usually lies in contact with the diaphragm, but lower positions are common, especially on the right, and ectopia exists when the kidney fails to ascend out of the true bony pelvis. The right kidney is usually situated more caudad than the left but may be situated more cephalad than the left kidney in 10 to 15 per cent of cases. The long axis of the kidney usually runs parallel to the psoas muscle, but the lower poles of both kidneys tend to move more laterally with age and increase in the amount and deposition of perinephric fat. The right kidney is much more mobile than the left, varying 1 to 4 cm in position with deep respiration. The kidneys are about equal in overall size, but the left kidney tends to be 0.5 cm longer than the right. Average renal length ranges from 11 to 15 cm or greater depending upon body habitus. The length of most kidneys is about the length of 3 to 4 lumbar vertebral bodies in the average adult. Renal mass tends to decrease with age, and fibrofatty replacement may expand the renal sinus. Anomalous (fused or duplex) kidneys may be much larger, and congenital solitary kidneys will be large, nearing the overall mass of two normal-sized kidneys. Compensatory renal hypertrophy may occur after loss of the contralateral kidney. It is most marked when kidney loss occurs early in life and is rare after the fifth decade.

The normal renal shape seen at urography often reflects the lobular architecture of the kidney (Fig. 67–2). The kidney is made up of, on the average, 14 lobes, each lobe having its own medulla and cap of cortex. The normal septum or partition of cortical tissue that extends between the papillae, when enlarged, can mimic a neoplasm. The enlarged or prominent septum has been called a column of Bertin after its original description by Bertin in 1744. During growth, fusion between lobes, particularly at the renal poles, occurs. Therefore the renal parenchyma is thickest in the polar regions. The lobular renal contour occasionally seen during the early nephrogram phase of the urogram may represent persistent lobulation (fetal) and usually is manifest as a slight notching in the cortical outline occurring between the calyces, rather than directly over them. The distance between a line drawn connecting the papillary tips (interpapillary line of Hodson) and the cortical edge tends to be uniform and

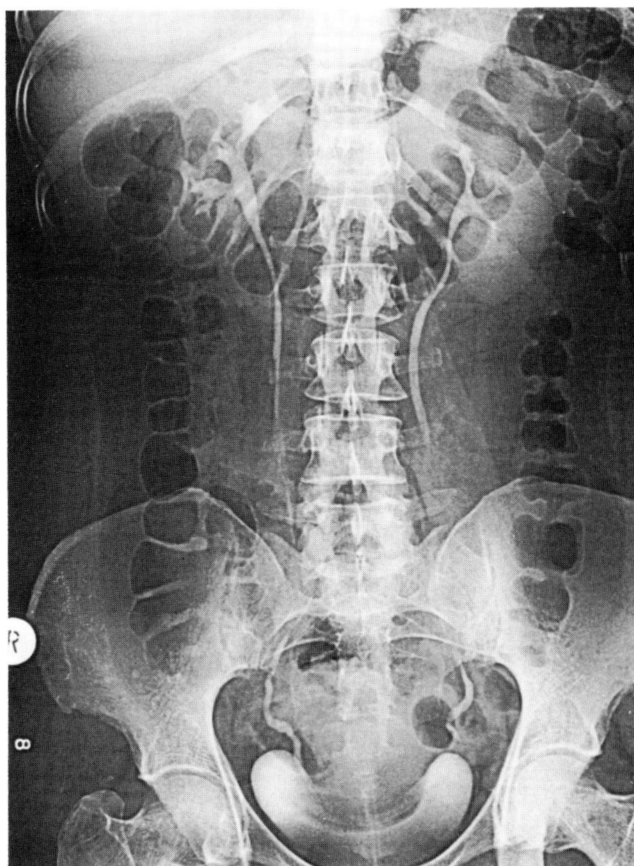

Figure 67–1. Intravenous urogram depicts **normal urinary tract** (kidneys, ureters, bladder). Prominent uterus indents dome of bladder.

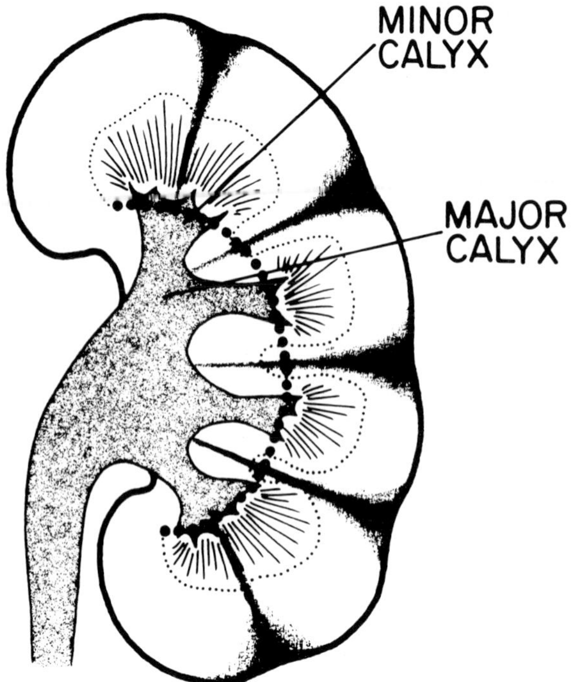

Figure 67–2. Diagram of **normal renal lobular architecture.** Lobular fusion in polar regions leads to compound calyces at both poles. Two or three *major* calyces drain numerous minor calyces. The interpapillary line (dotted line) links the tip of the pyramids. Shaded areas denote septa of cortical tissue that extend toward the renal hilum. Indentations in the cortical margin between calyces represent persistent fetal lobulation.

symmetrical, side to side (Fig. 67–2). Even when so-called dromedary humps or parenchymal bulges are present due to splenic or hepatic compression, this rule holds true. Correct urographic diagnosis of parenchymal loss depends upon the knowledge of the interpapillary line and its relationship to the cortical margin.

COLLECTING SYSTEM

The normal pelvicalyceal system consists of calyces, pelvis, and ureter. The pelvis is a triangular or funnel-shaped structure that may be entirely intrarenal but usually is partially extrarenal as it tapers to join the ureter at the ureteral-pelvic junction. The pelvis drains the collecting system, typically composed of major and minor calyces. While there is wide variation in size, shape, and branching pattern of the collecting system, the major calyces (n = 2 to 4) in turn drain the minor calyces (n = 4 to 12), which may receive one or more papillae; this accounts for the greater variation in minor calyceal appearance on the urogram. Although the collecting system patterns tend to be symmetrical side to side, minor anatomic variations and vascular impressions, particularly on the right, create minor differences in the urographic appearance. A more common variation is the propensity for polar calyces to be fused (compound) especially in the upper poles. The minor calyces are usually arranged in two rows, an anterior and a posterior one. Hodson has noted that the calyces rarely overlap directly on a frontal radiograph. In the interpolar region, the anterior calyces are usually profiled and seen to lie lateral to the posterior calyces, which are typically seen en face (Fig. 67–3). The infundibulum (isthmus) is the portion of the pelvicalyceal system connecting the minor and the major calyces.

The normal adult ureter is close to 30 cm in length but varies with body habitus. It begins at the ureteral-pelvic junction and descends on the ventral surface of the psoas muscle to the bladder (ureteral vesicle junction), passing over the transverse processes of the lower lumbar vertebrae en route. Ureters rarely extend medial to the pedicle of the lumbar vertebral body. The widest portion of the ureter is usually its proximal half, and it is unusual to see the entire ureter on a single urogram film because of peristaltic activity. Three areas of relative ureteral narrowing are typically present on urography: (1) at the ureteral-pelvic junction, (2) at the ureteral-vesicle junction, and (3) at the pelvic brim where the ureter crosses over the iliac vessels before descending somewhat posterior to the dorsal ventral body plane to enter the bladder. Transient kinks or concentric constrictions are common findings in the proximal ureter. The ureters usually follow the curvature of the true bony pelvis as they course to the bladder. However, obstruction, malrotation, ectopia, ptosis, diuresis, bladder diverticula, and skeletal deformity may all affect ureteral size, configuration, and course.

CONTRAST MATERIAL FOR UROGRAPHY

Currently, available sodium and/or meglumine ionic salts of iothalamic or diatrizoic acid are in use for intravenous urography. Newer, low osmolality, nonionic contrst media offer improved safety and efficacy for urography. Concentrations range from 32 to 66.8 per cent (weight/volume) for those agents used for urography. The mechanisms for excretion of contrast by the kidney are well described. Water-soluble contrast agents are pure glomerular filtrates—osmotic diuretics that freely dissociate in solution (if ionic) and are essentially not protein-bound. Normally, an extremely small amount of contrast material is excreted by the liver and small intestine. In the presence of azotemia and/or renal obstruction, this amount may increase and cause gallbladder or small bowel visualization on a radiograph.

Urographic quality depends on numerous technical factors, but two features related to the renal handling of contrast material are

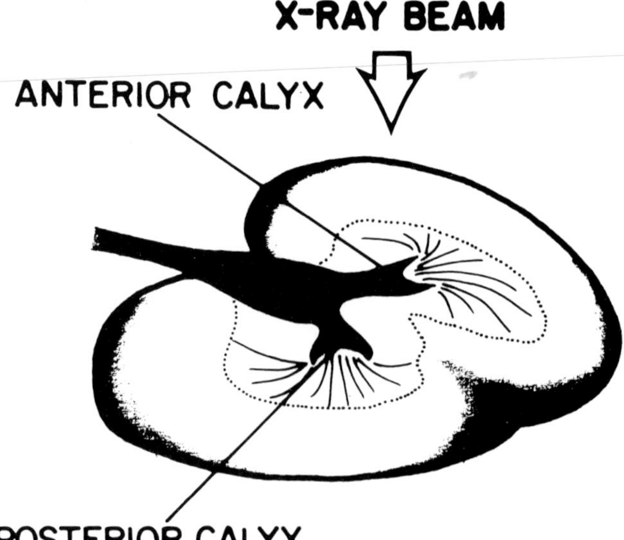

Figure 67–3. Diagram in **transaxial plane through the kidney** relates anterior and posterior calyceal groups to a frontal x-ray beam. On frontal urograms, posterior calyces would be viewed en face and anterior calyces in profile. Based on this principle, oblique radiographs provide optimal calyceal diagnosis in two planes.

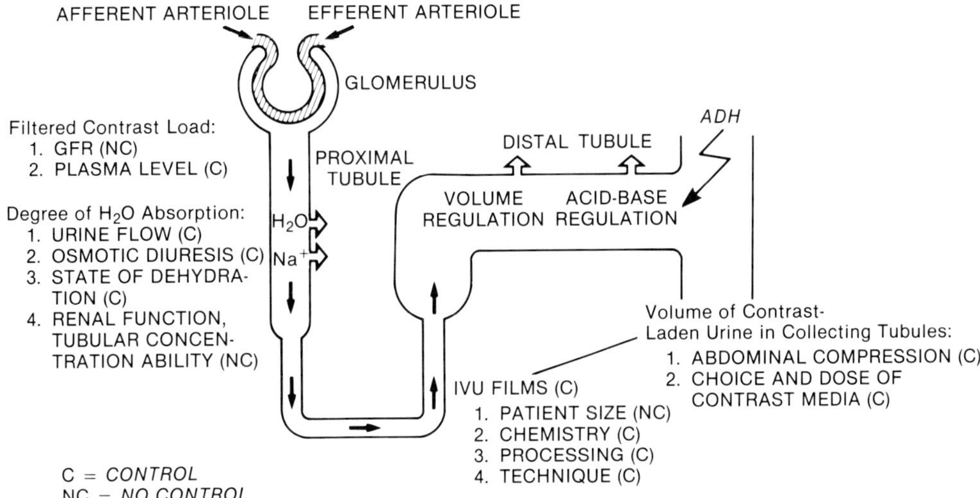

Figure 67–4. Schematic diagram of a nephron illustrating the **control that the radiologist has over the performance and quality of an intravenous urogram.** An increase in the dose of contrast medium will increase the amount of iodine in the filtered load that is delivered to the proximal tubule. Salt and water resorption from the proximal tubular lumen concentrates the contrast media, providing nephrographic opacification on the urogram. Volume and acid-base regulatory functions performed at the distal tubular level have little effect on overall urographic quality. Film quality and the choice of various contrast materials are under direct control of the radiologist.

critical to the performance of optimal urography. They are (1) adequate concentration of the contrast media within the collecting system, and (2) adequate distention (diuresis) of the pelvicalyceal systems. Most attempts to improve urographic quality are aimed at these two factors. Successful achievement of both results in excellent quality diagnostic urograms. The end result of these physiologic processes is production of enough urine containing an adequate amount of radiopaque contrast material for diagnostic radiographs. It is the amount of contrast material excreted per unit volume of urine that is critical. This is one aspect of the urogram over which the urographer has considerable control (Fig. 67–4).

NEPHROGRAM-PYELOGRAM

The fundamental building blocks of the urogram, the nephrogram and the pyelogram, depend on understanding and application of the previously described principles. The nephrogram directly depends upon the amount of contrast material (plasma level) delivered to the glomerulus and the time of delivery (injection). In other words, the filtered load in the proximal tubule depends on the plasma level of contrast material × the glomerular filtration rate (GFR). The GFR is fixed in most patients, but the radiologist controls the plasma level of contrast material. The nephrographic phase of the urogram is then both a vascular and a proximal tubular event. The pyelogram, on the other hand, depends on the "3 D's": density, distention, and diuresis. The time of delivery of the contrast material is less critical in terms of the character of the pyelogram, but the state of hydration and the amount of diuresis may affect pyelographic quality.

CHOICE OF CONTRAST MATERIAL

Numerous studies have examined the subjective and objective differences in urograms performed with sodium or meglumine salts of ionic high osmolality contrast material. Higher urinary concentrations have been measured with the sodium agents. Greater osmotic diuresis occurs with pure meglumine salts. Sodium salts tend to be less viscous, making injection through smaller needles much easier. However, for all practical purposes, for standard adult urography, there are no significant differences among the various formulations of sodium and meglumine salts of ionic contrast material. There are no substantial differences in urographic quality among currently available nonionic monomers. Ultimately, factors such as cost, availability, packaging, service, and safety must determine the choice of contrast medium used for adult urography.

DOSE

Considerable confusion still exists concerning an optimal dose of contrast material for urography in the average adult. Simply stated, it is the amount of iodine delivered to the kidney, not its volume or concentration, that is the determining factor. This author reviewed the literature in 1971 and found a consensus recommendation of 1 ml/kg (0.5 ml/lb) body weight of a 60 per cent solution of sodium or meglumine salt. We then concluded, based on further investigations of our own, that a dose of 0.5 to 0.75 ml/lb body weight was optimal for adult urography if approximately 20 g of iodine were administered in that volume. Rather than be concerned with volume per unit body weight or milligrams of iodine per unit body weight or total volumes, one should focus on the amount of iodine delivered with any conventional contrast agent or new, low-osmolality nonionic agent. Dosages of iodine above the 20-g level may necessitate larger volumes and will cause greater osmotic diuresis. Such diuresis may diminish urogram quality. The amount of diuresis is less with nonionic compounds, and 16 to 20 g of iodine will provide an optimal urogram. With attention to the technical details of urography such as abdominal compression and tomography, a high-quality urogram can be obtained in most adult patients with 16 to 20 g of iodine. Advanced age, obesity, hydrated states, trauma, urinary diversion, or even azotemia may require increased dose levels of 30 to 40 g of iodine or more for adequate urographic evaluation.

INJECTION TECHNIQUE

Most contrast material for urography today is administered by bolus injection using a syringe and a scalp vein needle apparatus. Drip infusion methods were shown by Cattell et al in 1967 to be of no advantage over conventional bolus techniques for equivalent doses of iodine. Since it is the amount of contrast material that makes a difference in the diagnostic quality of the urogram, not the method of delivery, routine infusions have been largely abandoned. There is an advantage to the rapid bolus technique for achieving maximal nephrographic density during urography. The highest peak plasma concentration of contrast material is achieved immediately after the rapid bolus injection of contrast material. Therefore, films such as tomograms to evaluate the nephrogram are best taken early in the study to take advantage of this circumstance. The maximal plasma concentration of contrast material after a bolus injection exceeds that achieved with infusion. Bolus injection of 50 to 75 ml of a 50 to 60 per cent solution of contrast material can be administered intravenously in less than 30 seconds in many, but slower injections should be used in older patients with cardiovascular disease. Unlike the nephrogram, the pyelographic quality is not affected by the time of injection of contrast material. Because the pyelogram depends on diuresis, it may be delayed in time when using low-osmolality contrast materials that have a less effective osmotic diuretic effect.

PATIENT PREPARATION

Fluid Restriction

For the majority of adult patients, fluid restriction prior to urography has little effect on the quality of the urogram. Overnight abstinence from food or liquids, the ''NPO after midnight'' regimen, does little to change the effective urine osmolality of most adult patients. Longer periods (up to 20 hours) are required before urine osmolality or specific gravity increase sufficiently to make visible differences on the urogram. Individual patients will vary their early morning urine osmolality, day to day, with similar overnight fluid deprivation. The benefit to the patient and radiologist of overnight pre-urography food and fluid deprivation is that the patient's stomach will be empty should emesis occur after injection of contrast material. Additionally, inadvertent overhydration with resultant increased urine flow rates will not occur. Most importantly, however, attempted dehydration through fluid restriction or vigorous bowel preparation may be dangerous to certain groups of patients. Patients with abnormal or fixed urinary concentrating mechanisms, i.e., renal failure, multiple myeloma, elderly, debilitated, diabetic patients, or young infants and children may be harmed by dehydration. Patients with tenuous electrolyte balance may be adversely affected, or develop contrast-induced renal failure. Overnight fluid deprivation in most patients represents neither undue hardship nor risk of serious harm.

Bowel Preparation

Vigorous bowel preparation for urography, like fluid restriction, is not routinely necessary, nor is it uniformly successful even when ordered. Preliminary cathartics and enemas have been met with poor patient compliance and are often uncomfortable and ineffective. All too often, the bowel gas is increased and/or rearranged and potentially obscuring feces are merely shifted to the distal gastrointestinal tract. Extensive bowel preparation may in fact take longer than one day to be successful. Such efforts are only necessary in isolated situations or for renal or ureteral calculi evaluation or when tomography is not available. Routine tomography with multiple sections (n = 3) now obviates vigorous bowel preparation. Mild, oral cathartics such as milk of magnesia or citrate of magnesia the evening before and/or a rectal suppository the morning of the examination is usually all that is required.

RADIOGRAPHIC TECHNIQUE

kVp and mAs

Pertinent pathologic findings must be observed on a urogram before they will be diagnosed. Use of proper radiographic technique factors will assure optimal urographic conspicuity. The best achievable subject contrast on the film should be the ideal goal. Equipment and generators that allow 60 to 70 kVp coupled with 500 to 1000 mA, three-phase circuitry are optimal. This is particularly important for high-quality nephrotomography, thus allowing shorter exposure times. Computed radiography (digital) systems require similar exposure factors but usually shorter times.

Films and Screens

A number of workable combinations of film and intensifying screens in light-weight cassettes are available today. High-contrast film with par or high-speed screens can allow sufficient use to be made of available radiographic equipment. Exposure dose should be kept as low as possible while obtaining high-contrast, high-quality urograms. New rare-earth film/screen combinations significantly lower radiation dose and decrease motion artifacts. Excellent quality diagnostic urograms can be obtained with these faster film/screen systems, especially in very large patients. However, attention to radiographic technique, especially when phototiming is not available, is important. Computed radiography utilizing photostimulable phosphor plates provides wide dynamic range and exposure latitude. Both adults and pediatric patients benefit from such systems. Exposure dose, repeat films, and possibly dose of contrast media are reduced using such systems.

PROCESSING AND CHEMISTRY

Film processing must carefully match the film/screen system used for intravenous urography. Control through a quality assurance program that monitors chemistry and processing factors, e.g., time and temperature, should be routine. The radiologist has complete control over this aspect of urographic quality. This control is very important because he or she has no control over the size of the object being examined—the patient. Laser readers, printers, and processors matched to corresponding computed radiography systems require the same monitoring programs.

FILM SEQUENCE

The film sequence for adult urography must get maximal utilization of the contrast material as it passes from the glomerulus to the bladder. Allowance must be made for the degree and adequacy of supervision of the study. Any scheme must be flexible to allow adaptation to individual patient variables, and utilitarian to suit varied clinical problems and patient populations. It should, however, be geared to the physiology of contrast material excretion outlined previously. The routine urogram detailed herein takes ad-

TABLE 67–1. CONTRAINDICATIONS TO ABDOMINAL COMPRESSION

1. Aortic aneurysm
2. Abdominal pain
3. Recent surgery
4. Extreme obesity
5. Ascites
6. Urinary diversion (loops)
7. Ureteral obstruction (calculi)

vantage of a rapid bolus injection of contrast material. It is designed to be neither a short, limited film study nor a less discriminate long series of sequential radiographs.

There are two fundamental principles for the performance of an optimal urogram—abdominal compression and routine tomography. In 1937, Berger stressed the importance of "accurately located and maintained abdominal pressure" for the production of diagnostic urograms. Abdominal compression is best performed using a device that attaches directly to the patient. Such inflatable devices are readily available, comfortable, and economical. Patient mobility is not compromised, and even prone or erect filming is possible with such devices. Alternatives to routine abdominal compression have proved less than satisfactory. Prone films are rarely as effective as adequately placed abdominal compression devices. Devices that attach directly to the table (table binders) limit patient mobility and tend to compress the abdomen over an unnecessarily large area. Increased amounts of contrast may improve calyceal and ureteric filling but at a greater monetary expense. All adult patients should have abdominal compression during urography unless contraindicated (Table 67–1).

Tomography should be an integral part of the modern urogram. Linear tomography is sufficient and equipment is readily available, including attachable tomogram arms for most pre-existing units. Although the timing of tomography during the urogram may still be somewhat controversial, it is well documented that significant pathology, particularly renal masses, will go undetected without tomography. Older et al retrospectively analyzed 24 urograms in patients with proven renal adenocarcinomas and found that 19 per cent of the lesions would have been missed without the tomograms. Signs and symptoms of significant renal disease must always be considered prior to urography, but frequently renal neoplasia is discovered in asymptomatic patients. Cost-benefit analysis for routine tomography is a positive one because tomography decreases the need for repeat studies and increases diagnostic confidence. Nondiagnostic studies may be salvaged and faster film review is possible. Improved visualization of the renal margins and parenchyma is obtained with routine tomography, particularly in patients with marginally compromised renal function.

The most efficacious time for routine tomography during a urogram is when nephrographic density is greatest, that is, immediately after the rapid bolus injection of contrast. The main purpose of the tomogram is to assess renal parenchymal contours. Nontomographic, frontal and oblique films are for analysis of the pelvicalyceal system. Delayed tomograms are less useful because parenchymal opacification fades rapidly as calyceal opacification occurs.

Linear tomography, performed with a long arc (40 to 50 degrees), provides thin (1 to 2 mm) section images with satisfactory blurring of the overlying tissues (Fig. 67–5). Thicker sections (20- to 30-degree arc) or zonograms give more tissue in the plane of focus with shorter exposure times. Thin-section, longer arc tomograms, at three levels between 7 and 10 cm from the table top, provide adequate screening of the kidney contours.

Ideally, all urograms should be carefully monitored by a radiologist who will take a problem-oriented approach to the study. Preliminary scout or survey films of the abdomen and kidneys must be obtained prior to injection. These films should be appropriately exposed and coned to the areas of interest. A standard 14 × 17 inch radiograph of the abdomen often suffices, but frequently a coned down (10 × 12 inch) radiograph of the bony pelvis to include the prostate gland or a radiograph coned to the region of the kidneys is necessary. Additional plain radiographs in oblique projections may be necessary for evaluation of suspected renal calculi. A preliminary scout tomogram of the kidneys is usually taken to assess technique and positioning. Digital images obtained with phosphor plates are printed on smaller format films. Early tomograms taken with a 40-degree arc at three predetermined levels (1 cm apart) through the kidneys should be obtained immediately after the injection of contrast material (Fig. 67–5*A*). Renal margins can be seen during the parenchymal opacification phase. If circumstances mandate that urography be performed without tomography, an immediate postinjection film coned to the kidneys should be obtained (Fig. 67–5*B*). Next a 4- or 5-minute film coned to both kidneys allows pyelographic analysis prior to the application of abdominal compression (Fig. 67–6*A*). An 8- or 10-minute film in

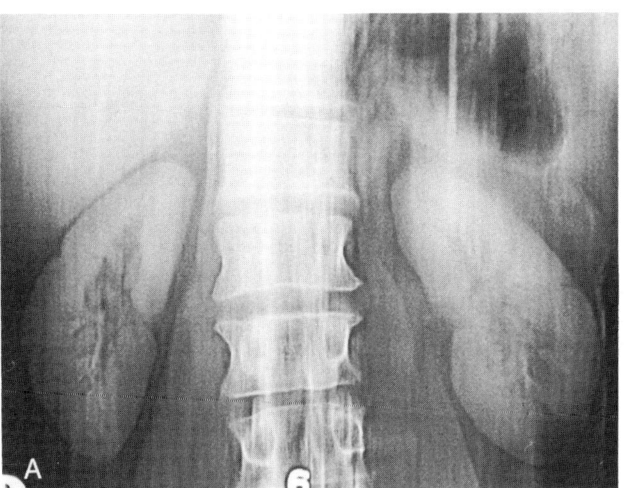

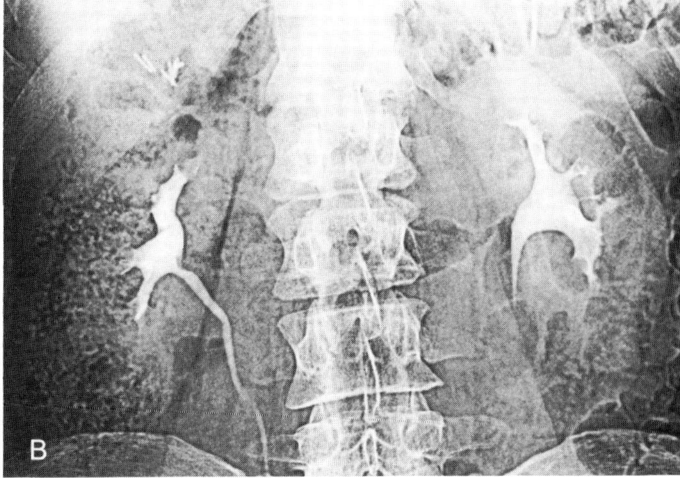

Figure 67–5. *A,* Initial postinjection tomogram (nephrogram phase) shows excellent parenchymal opacification and clearly displays the renal margins. Renal sinus fat and calyces appear as "negative" (black) stellate areas within the center of the kidneys. *B,* Calyces and pelves are well filled on the 8-minute film but renal margins are obscured by overlying bowel contents especially on the right.

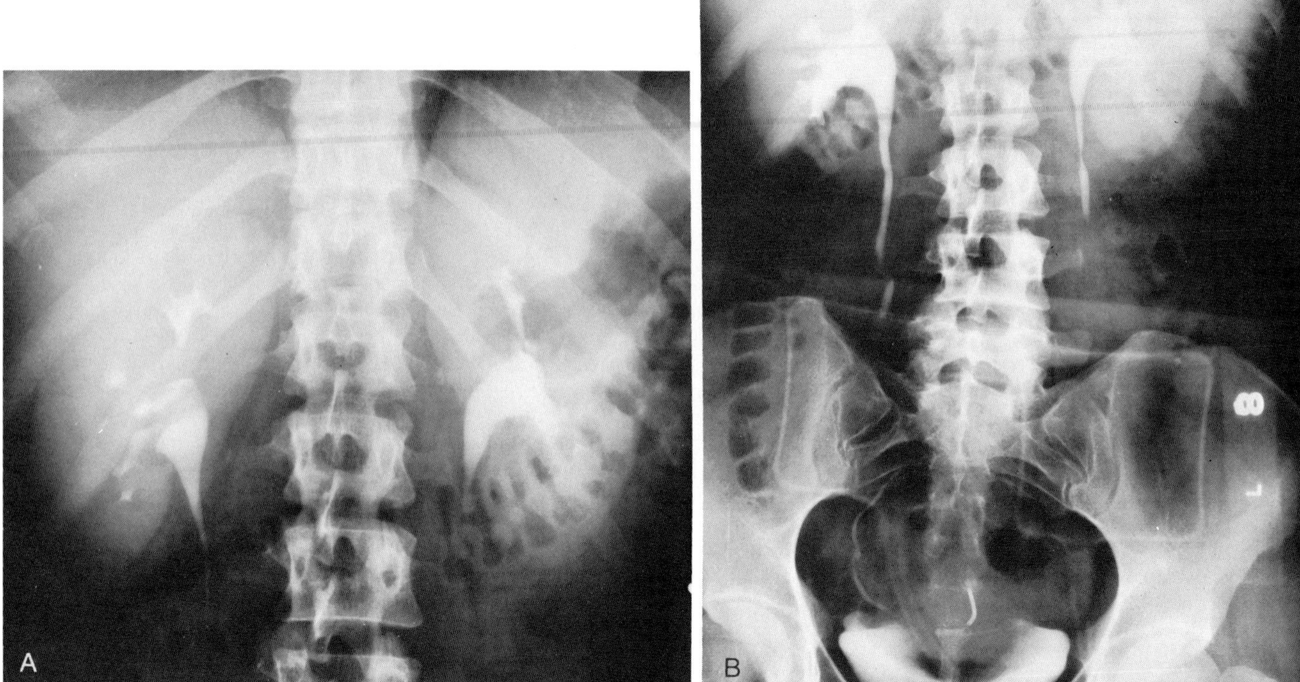

Figure 67–6. *A,* A 4-minute film coned to kidneys after a bolus injection of 50 cc of Conray 400. Calyces appear sharp. Pelves and proximal ureters are filled. Impression on right renal pelvis is due to crossing vessels. *B,* An 8-minute film after abdominal compression was applied shows the collecting systems well distended. Extrinsic compression defects on right renal pelvis are obliterated by the effect of abdominal compression.

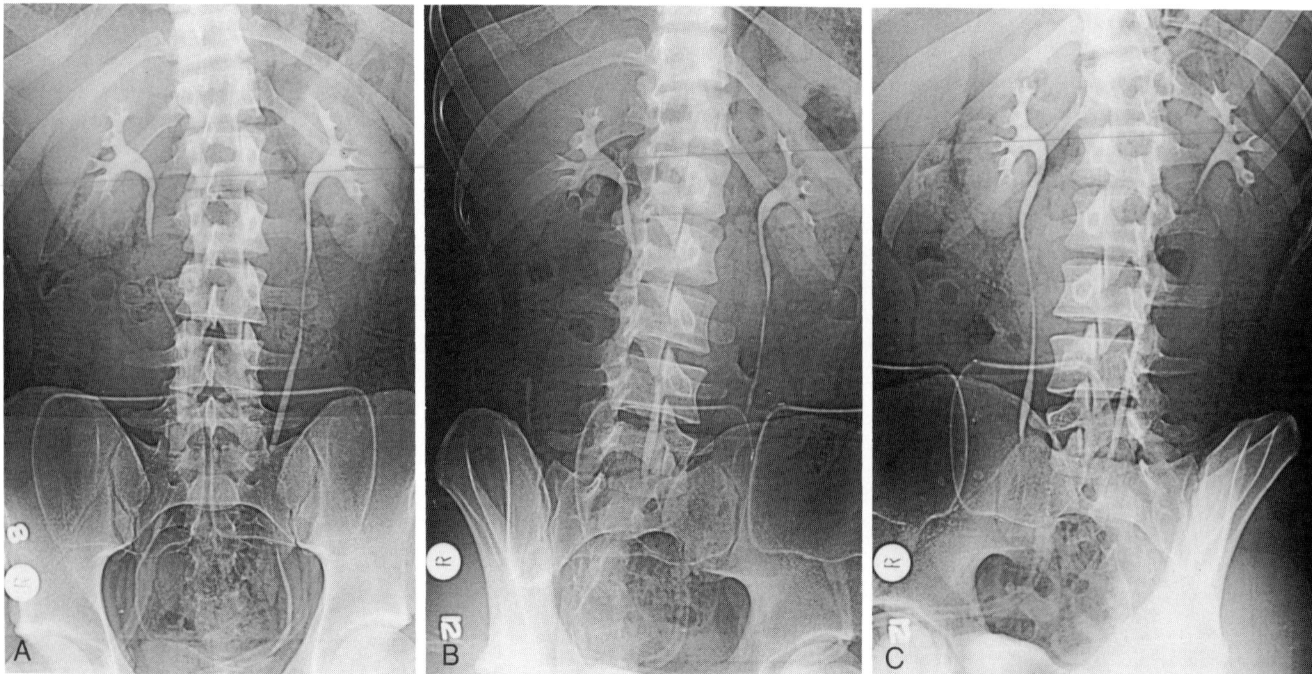

Figure 67–7. *A,* An 8-minute view of both kidneys taken after application of the abdominal compression band. *B,* A left posterior oblique view and *(C)* right posterior oblique view allow optimal visualization of the collecting system of both kidneys in two planes. Calyces are seen both en face and in profile. Infundibulae are best displayed on oblique views. (R = right.)

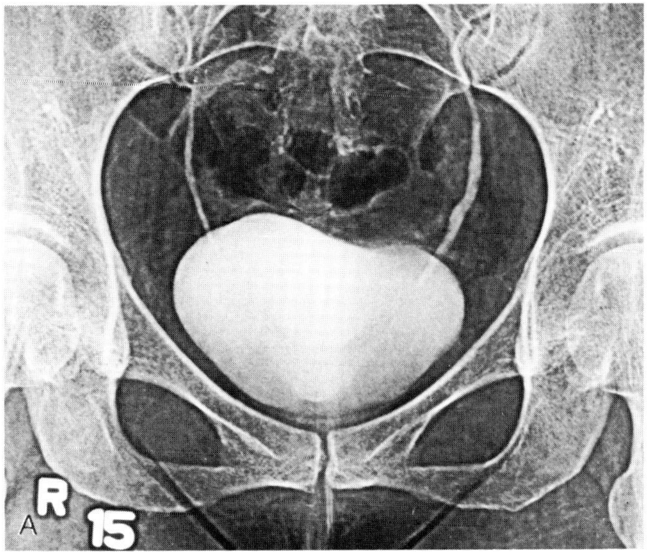

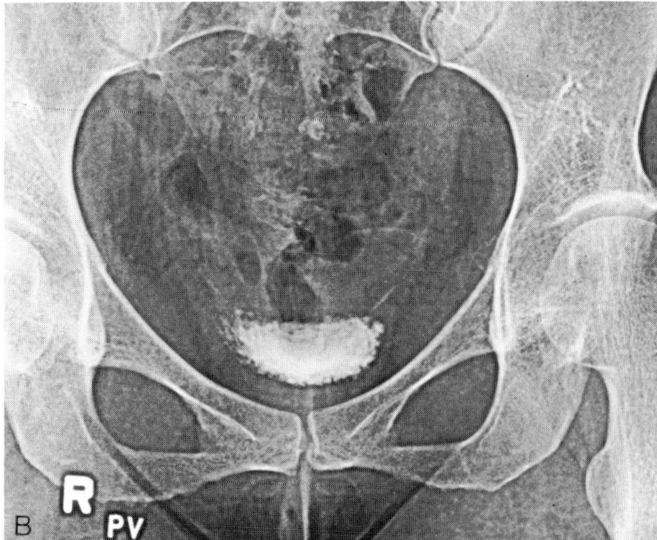

Figure 67–8. *A,* A coned view of the bladder at 15 minutes taken after the release of the abdominal compression device. *B,* A post-void film shows a normal bladder mucosal pattern and no significant residual urine.

the frontal projection with abdominal compression in place will demonstrate the pelvocalyceal system in a distended state (Fig. 67–6*B*). Both oblique views with a compression device still in place may then be obtained at 10 to 15 minutes after injection (Fig. 67–7). These may be coned to the kidneys or at best are full abdominal films to include the ureters. Oblique views are most helpful for calyceal assessment because if only frontal views are obtained, the anterior calyceal system will be only seen in profile and the posterior calyces en face (Fig. 67–7*B* and *C*). A postcompression release view of the bladder often allows evaluation of the distal ureters (Fig. 67–8). Oblique views of the filled bladder may be necessary in males older than 40 years of age for evaluation of prostatic enlargement. The post-void film may also be routine for older males and often is the best film for detecting bladder abnormalities.

As a minimum routine urographic examination, this film sequence will allow diagnostic radiographic evaluation of the urinary tract. Additional ancillary views may be required such as lateral, inspiration-expiration, prone, erect, or fluoroscopic spot films. Repeat injection of additional contrast media is rarely required but may be useful for evaluation of collecting system abnormalities. Computed tomography has largely obviated inspiration-expiration or lateral views, but the prone and erect films still have important uses. The prone position facilitates pelvic or ureteric filling when obstruction is present. Appropriate use of the prone film when evaluating obstruction may save time and an excessive number of delayed films. Erect filming can also be useful for diagnosing ureteric obstruction, and fluoroscopic spot films in the upright position may expedite the diagnostic process, also saving extra delayed films.

Suggestions for a reduced or shortened urogram in terms of the number of films have not proven efficacious in clinical practice. A routine conventional multifilm urogram remains one of the best screening tests available for detection of urinary tract disease. Definition of pathology (for example, renal masses) depends heavily today on ultrasonography, computed tomography, and magnetic resonance imaging. Limited or shortened urograms do not provide an acceptable level of diagnostic confidence and neglect the duty of the radiologist to declare the urinary tract normal whenever possible. Although there may be a saving in cost and radiation dose with a limited film urogram, significant pathology will be missed. Attention to sound uroradiographic principles will allow the urogram to continue to provide a high level of diagnostic accuracy.

Bibliography

Berger RA: Increasing the value of intravenous urography by improvements in technique. AJR 38:156, 1937.

Bertin R: Memoire pour servir à l'histoire des reins. Histoire de L'Academie Royale des Sciences 79:108–159, 1744.

Bosniak MA: Nephrotomography: A relatively unappreciated but extremely valuable diagnostic tool. Radiology 113:313, 1974.

Cantwell KG, Press HC: Evaluation of the renal outline by excretory urography. Radiology 137:223, 1980.

Cattell WR, et al: Excretion urography. I. Factors determining the excretion of Hypaque. Br J Radiol 40:561–571, 1967.

Davison AJ (ed): Radiologic Diagnosis of Renal Parenchymal Disease. Philadelphia, WB Saunders Company, 1985.

Dobrin R, Kricheff I, Fite W, Weathers R: The effect of the variability of automatic film processing systems on the quality of radiographs. Radiology 113:545, 1974.

Dure-Smith P: Fluid restriction before excretory urography. Radiology 118:487, 1976.

Dure-Smith P, McArdle GH: Tomography during excretory urography. Technical aspects. Br J Radiol 45:896, 1972.

Ekberg O, Bondestam S, Wehlin L: Screening for urinary tract abnormalities with single-film urography after phlebography and angiography. Radiology 138:325, 1981.

Elkin M: Radiology of the urinary tract: Some physiological considerations. Radiology 116:259, 1975.

Fajardo LL, Hillman BJ, Hunter TB, et al: Excretory urography using computed radiography. Radiology 162:345, 1987.

Green WM, Pressman BD, McClennan BL, Casarella WJ: Column of Bertin: Diagnosis by nephrotomography. AJR 116:714, 1972.

Hamilton G: The vascular nephrogram phase of excretory urography and its implications. Radiology 102:37, 1972.

Hardt VH, Rohrl C: Inadequate demonstration of the calyces—A disadvantage of infusion urography. Fortschr Röntgen 119:588, 1973.

Hattery RR, Williamson B, Hartman GW: Urinary tract tomography. Radiol Clin North Am 14:23, 1976.

Hattery RR, Williamson B, Hartman GW, et al: Intravenous urographic technique. Radiology 167:593, 1988.

Hillman BJ, Silvert M, Cook G, et al: Recognition of bladder tumors by excretory urography. Radiology 138:319, 1981.

Hodson CJ: The lobar structure of the kidney. Br J Urol 44:246, 1972.

Lloyd LK, Witten DM, Bueschen AJ, Daniel WW: Enhanced detection of asymptomatic renal masses with routine tomography during excretory urography. Urology 2:523–528, 1978.

McClennan BL: Optimal evaluation at intravenous urography. CRC Crit Rev Radiol Sci 577, 1971.

McClennan BL, Becker JA: Excretory urography: Choice of contrast material—clinical. Radiology 100:591, 1971.

McClennan BL, Becker JA, Berdon WE: Excretory urography: Choice of contrast material—experimental. Radiology 100:585, 1971.

Mellins HZ, McNeil BJ, Abrams HL, et al: The selection of patients for excretory urography. Radiology 130:293, 1979.

Murphey MD, Huang HKB, Siegel EL, et al: Clinical experience in the use of photostimulable phosphor radiographic systems. Invest Radiol 26:590, 1991.

Newberg AH, Mindell HJ: Predicting tomographic levels for urography. Radiology 118:460, 1976.
Older RA, McLelland R, Cleeve DM, et al: Importance of routine vascular nephrotomography in excretory urography. Urology 15:312, 1980.
Strautman PR, Fajardo LL, Hillman BJ, et al: Evaluation of contrast dose reduction for excretory urography using computed radiography. Eur J Radiol 9:60, 1989.
Thomsen HS, Vestergaard A, Dorph S: Quality of urography and renal clearance of ionic and nonionic contrast media. Invest Radiol 27:41, 1992.

68 Intravascular Contrast Media

Richard W. Katzberg

Intravascular contrast media are administered to more than six million patients in the United States on a yearly basis. The indications have continued to increase: Examinations requiring contrast media include excretory urography, angiography, head and body computed tomography, and digital subtraction angiography. There has been a trend toward higher doses and higher concentrations of rapidly injected media and toward the increasing utilization of low osmolar media.

Contrast media are necessary for imaging because small density differences in soft tissues of the body do not allow optimal radiographic evaluation without enhancement. These agents should ideally be inert in every respect; however, significant toxicity related mainly to hyperosmolality does exist. Newer, low-osmolality intravascular agents are a further, significant step toward decreased toxicity.

This chapter discusses the basic properties of contrast media, their pharmacologic and physiologic actions within the human body, general and specific organ injury, and a comparison with new agents.

CHARACTERISTICS OF CONTRAST MEDIA

Contrast agents available for intravascular use depend upon iodine for their radiopacity and are unlike any other intravascular drugs. Therapeutic agents are given in very small quantities at regularly spaced intervals. Contrast media are administered in quantities as large as 100 g and are most often administered as a bolus lasting only one or two minutes. Therapeutic drugs are given to effect biological or chemical change, whereas contrast media are used for organ or tissue enhancement. Most intravascular drugs are nearly isotonic, yet some contrast media have osmolalities even up to seven times that of plasma.

Even with the increasing utilization of low osmolar agents, commonly used angiographic and urographic contrast agents are water-soluble, fully saturated, tri-iodinated benzoic acid derivatives that are manufactured either as a sodium or a meglumine salt of either diatrizoic or iothalamic acid (Fig. 68–1). The theoretical ratio of iodine atoms to dissolved particles in solution for these agents is 1.5:1 because they are ionic and dissociate into two particles in solution, with the anion containing three iodine atoms and with a cation of sodium or methylglucamine (meglumine) containing no iodine atoms. Osmolalities range from 1200 to over 2000 mOsm/kg H_2O.

The ionic monomers are small molecules at high concentrations in solution which are not metabolized and which are excreted by pure glomerular filtration. While some patients will react adversely to small quantities of these agents, many investigators believe that most of the toxic effects are mediated by the large osmotic load. Thus, the nonionic monomers (ratio 3:1) and nonionic dimers (ratio 6:1) have been developed. These agents, however, are also not metabolized and are also excreted by pure glomerular filtration.

Contrast agents come labeled as per cent concentration of the weight of the solute to the volume of solution (g/100 ml). Thus, a 76 per cent sodium/meglumine diatrizoate solution represents 76 g of solute per 100 ml of solvent. A more meaningful comparison of agents is, however, based upon an expression of iodine concentration (mg I) per milliliter (ml) of solution. For monomeric or single tri-iodinated benzene ring media, per cent concentrations can be converted to *iodine concentrations* using the following relationship:

$$\text{Iodine concentration (mg I/ml)} = \frac{381}{\text{M}} \times 1000\text{P}$$

where M is the molecular weight of the medium and 381 is three times the atomic weight of iodine (the resulting fraction gives the proportion of iodine in the molecule); P is the per cent concentration expressed as a decimal (i.e., 76 per cent = 0.76); and 1000 converts to mg/ml. Iodine concentrations can then be used to calculate the approximate *osmolality* of the various agents. Thus, for monomeric agents:

$$\text{Osmolality (mOsm/kg)} = \frac{\text{mg I/ml}}{381} \times \text{KG}$$

where K is the number of particles in solution (2 for ionic and 1 for nonionic media); G is the osmotic coefficient, which varies with concentration and with specific media (for most ionic media, G is between 0.85 and 1.0); and dividing by 381 gives the molar concentration of the agent. Thus the newer, nonionic media have lower tonicity for a given concentration of iodine because K is one half as large. Their generally lower osmotic coefficients (G) give them a further osmotic advantage.

Ion composition is another important characteristic of the water-soluble contrast media. Transitory changes in the ionic composition of extracellular fluids can affect membrane potentials in any excitable tissue. Thus, coronary arteriography, which involves the direct injection of contrast media into the coronary vasculature, can result in arrhythmias, including ventricular fibrillation. Changes in calcium flux and ionic gradients can lead to contraction abnormalities of the cardiac musculature, and these have, indeed, been observed during rapid contrast medium injections.

A third characteristic of contrast media is increased *viscosity*. The viscosity effect of contrast media can cause a transient reduction in

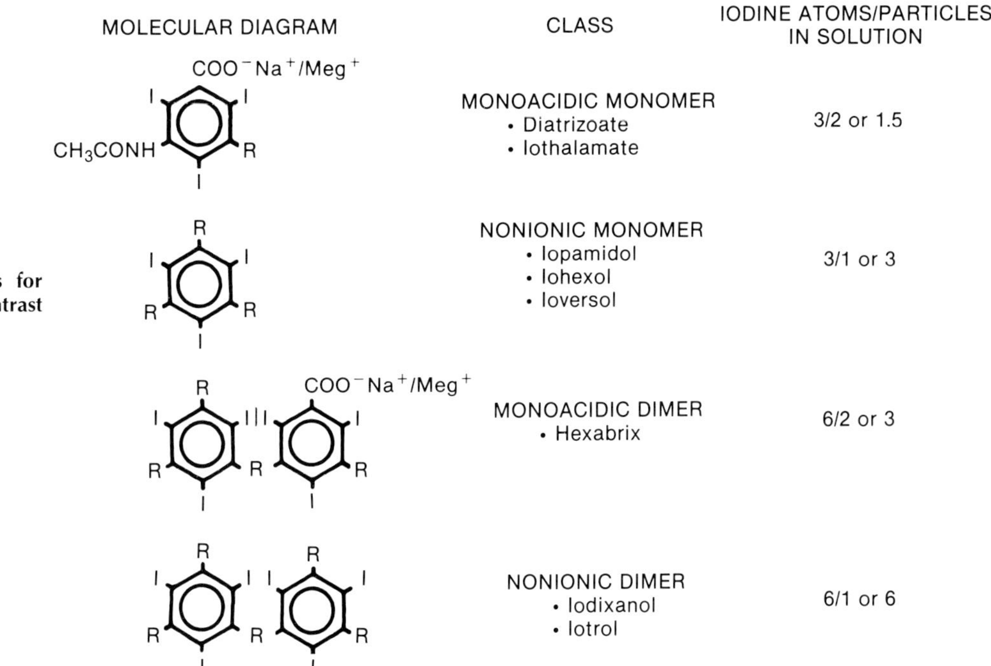

Figure 68–1. Structural formulas for ionic, nonionic, and dimeric contrast media with iodine ratios.

flow as the relatively viscous material passes through the resistance vasculature. This effect is superimposed upon and is thus often masked by the marked vasodilatation associated with hypertonicity. The newer contrast agents are generally higher in viscosity, and these effects may become more noticeable but do not appear to be a significant risk. Warming the contrast material prior to administration reduces this effect by decreasing the viscosity.

Recent developments have aimed at reducing high osmolality by changing the substituted side groups. This results in nonionic monomers in which the ratio of iodine atoms to dissolved particles in solutions is increased to 3:1 and the osmolality is more than halved (see Fig. 68–1). Nonionic monomers thus developed include Iopamidol and Iohexol. A monoacidic dimer, ioxaglate (Hexabrix) is a ratio-3 contrast medium that has an ionized anion in solution with an osmolality of about 600 mOsm/kg H_2O at 320 mg I/ml. Nonionic dimer ratio-6 contrast media, Iotrol and Iodixanol, were developed later and reduce the osmolality to approximately 300 mOsm/kg H_2O at 300 mg I/mg, which is isotonic with blood (see Fig. 68–1).

PHYSIOLOGIC ACTIONS OF CONTRAST MEDIA

Hyperosmolality, *hypertonicity*, and *viscosity* are the major characteristics of water-soluble contrast media that are responsible for the hemodynamic, cardiac, and subjective effects. Hyperosmolality is the single most important factor in the renal handling and thus elimination of contrast media from the human body.

When injected rapidly, intravenous contrast media quickly equilibrate across capillary membranes (except an intact blood-brain barrier) (Fig. 68–2). In the first phase of distribution, the marked

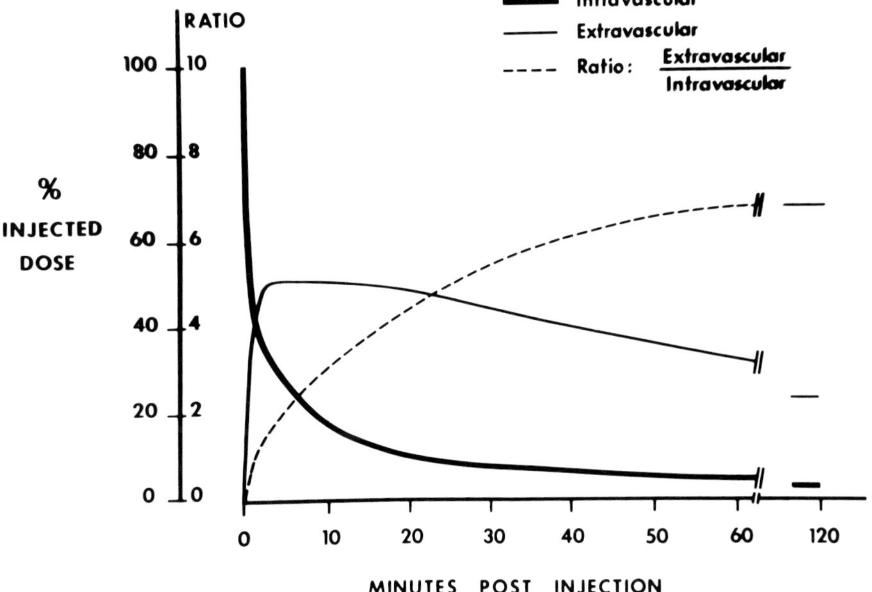

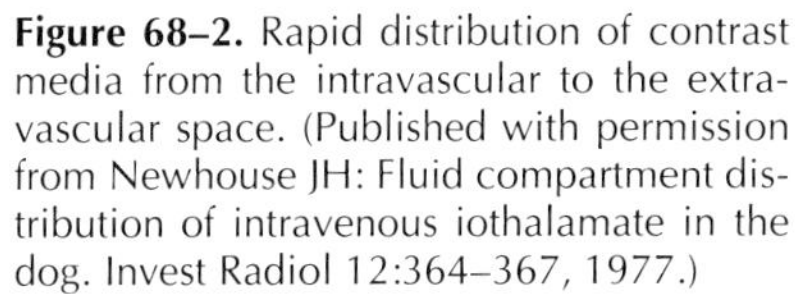
Figure 68–2. Rapid distribution of contrast media from the intravascular to the extravascular space. (Published with permission from Newhouse JH: Fluid compartment distribution of intravenous iothalamate in the dog. Invest Radiol 12:364–367, 1977.)

increase in intravascular osmolality causes a rapid fluid shift across capillary membranes toward the hypertonic (intravascular) compartment. Because the agents cannot cross normal cell membranes, cellular desiccation, particularly of red blood cells, is one possible effect of this shift. The net loss of intracellular water can influence cell membrane potential. This may be one mechanism responsible for the generalized stimulation of peripheral receptors that results in the sensation of heat, pain, and involuntary movement patients so often experience.

After the intravenous injection of large quantities of hypertonic ionic contrast media there is a significant increase in serum osmolality. This leads to a rapid influx of water from the interstitial space into the vascular compartment that causes a rapid increase in blood volume of up to 16 per cent, a decrease in hematocrit, an increase in cardiac output, and a decrease in peripheral vascular resistance. A clinical study that employed an automated heart rate/blood pressure monitor in 97 patients undergoing routine excretory urography demonstrated that in over half the patients the most common systemic response was a decrease in blood pressure. Indeed, a significant number of patients (6 per cent) showed a decrease in mean blood pressure below 60 mm Hg yet exhibited no overt clinical manifestations of hypotension. This study underscores the important physiologic activity of hypertonic contrast media when they are administered in customary doses via the venous route.

The osmotic gradient across the red blood cell (RBC) membrane results in shrinkage, making the cells more rigid with loss of the normal deformability. These microcirculatory changes are associated with crenation and aggregation of RBCs, adherence of leukocytes to the vessel wall, and palisading of leukocytes. There is also a sudden decrease in blood coagulation that has its maximum activity after about five minutes. The depression, however, is transient and returns to normal within four hours. A transient decrease in platelet aggregation from contrast medium has also been observed.

Contrast media can cause damage to the vascular endothelium, leading to increased permeability of the vessel wall and to the induction of thrombus formation. Clinically, thrombosis has been observed as a complication after intravenous injections of hypertonic contrast media for phlebography and urography. For this reason, the American College of Radiology has recommended that 60 per cent solutions of ionic contrast media be diluted to 45 per cent when used for phlebography, a practice that may, however, result in the degradation of image quality. Lower osmolality agents should be an advantage because they deliver at least twice the concentration of iodine in a given osmotic load.

Intracoronary injections of contrast media cause a decrease in heart rate, a decrease in peak left ventricular (LV) volume, a decrease in the maximum rate of increase in LV pressure, an increase in LV end-diastolic pressure, an increase in LV end-diastolic diameter, a decrease in systemic arterial pressure, and a biphasic decrease then increase in coronary blood flow. Injection of contrast material into the coronary artery causes a direct inhibitory effect on the sinoatrial node. A similar inhibitory effect has been observed in conduction through the bundle of His and Purkinje fibers. To a lesser extent, the decline in heart rate during coronary arteriography is cholinergically mediated. The major direct actions of hypertonic contrast media on the myocardium are mechanical and electrophysiologic alterations.

Intra-aortic and intra-arterial injections of hyperosmolar contrast media cause a decrease in systemic arterial pressure, an increase in pulmonary arterial pressure, tachycardia, and peripheral vasodilatation with a decrease in peripheral vascular resistance and an increase in blood flow. The major direct action on the peripheral circulation is vasodilation. The indirect effects, for the most part, are reflexly mediated and tend to offset the direct effects.

The central nervous system (CNS) is separated from many of the substances circulating in the blood by means of the blood-brain barrier (BBB). The endothelial cells of the CNS capillary have a continuous basement membrane and are connected to each other by a tight junction. There are, however, certain areas within the CNS that lack this barrier: the median eminence, pineal gland, area postrema, subfornical organ, neurohypophysis, supraoptic crest, and choroid plexus. In these particular areas, certain low–molecular weight substances in the blood will diffuse freely into the interstitial tissue. The common symptoms of nausea and vomiting following injection of contrast media may thus be due to the contrast medium entering the area postrema of the medulla, where it is devoid of a BBB.

Diseases that affect the integrity of the BBB may place the patient at increased risk from contrast administration. Brain metastases, for example, have capillaries characteristic of the originating tumor and these do not have such a barrier. Under certain circumstances contrast media can more readily enter the brain in these regions and may cause seizures. Seizures after intravenous contrast medium administration are rare in the general population, about 0.01 per cent, but have been reported to be as high as 6 to 19 per cent in patients with brain metastasis. The risk for seizure development, especially in cases of brain metastasis, may be reduced by an intravenous injection of 5 mg of diazepam prior to the injection of contrast medium. Should seizures develop, most are also controlled with diazepam.

Injections of hypertonic contrast media into the carotid arteries can cause a decrease in the pulse rate, periods of asystole, and lowering of the arterial blood pressure. It has been shown that the meglumine salts of contrast media have fewer cardiovascular effects with these procedures.

The circulatory effects from rapid injections of hypertonic contrast media in the vicinity of the right atrium, as may occur with digital subtraction angiography, can be summarized as follows: (1) increase in pulmonary artery pressure (PAP), (2) increase in left atrial pressure, (3) increase in the end-diastolic pressure of the left ventricle, and (4) decrease in systemic arterial pressure.

In toxicity studies, animals given a lethal dose of contrast medium develop pulmonary edema as well as evidence of CNS damage prior to death. Intravenous injections of contrast media also result in an increase in PAP along with subclinical bronchospasm, as measured by pulmonary function tests. The effects on PAP have been related to the osmotic effects of the solution for the most part, and, less significantly, to the viscosity. Acute pulmonary edema of noncardiogenic etiology is seen, but rarely in healthy patients after the intravascular administration of contrast media. In infants, pulmonary edema may be seen after urography owing to the hypertonicity of the contrast material, particularly because of the small volumes involved. The exact frequency of pulmonary edema occurring in clinical studies is difficult to ascertain inasmuch as it is known that interstitial edema may be present without symptoms. Possible causes of contrast medium-induced pulmonary edema include: (1) increase in pulmonary microvascular pressure from rapid injection of contrast material in the vicinity of the right atrium, (2) decrease in protein concentration of plasma as a result of dilution, (3) binding of plasma proteins to certain contrast media, and (4) increase in capillary permeability of fluid and proteins as a result of endothelial damage by toxic effects of contrast media. In these animal studies, the severity of pulmonary edema formation seems related to dose.

Intravascular injections of contrast media produce transient systemic hypocalcemia. This is likely due to the chelating effect of disodium edetate and sodium citrate, which are present as stabilizing agents; the high ionic strength of contrast media; hemodilution; and a small amount of direct binding by the contrast agent per se. Hypocalcemia may have potentially serious effects because this ion is important to cardiac function and rhythm.

Complement activation and coagulopathy secondary to hypertonic contrast media have been described and are believed to be important factors in the development of adverse reactions. Contact activators are known to be present in subendothelial areas that would be subject to release by contrast media-endothelium interactions. Platelet activation also activates the contact system, leading to production of kallikrein and bradykinin. These substances may play a major role in reactions by producing (1) hypotension, (2) smooth muscle spasm, (3) increased capillary permeability, and (4) potentiation of arachidonic acid production favoring the release of vasoactive prostaglandins and SRSA (leukotrienes).

Increased prekallikrein transformation rates and increased endogenous heparin levels may be additional pieces of the puzzle in the etiology of adverse reactions to contrast media. Histamine release induced by hypertonic contrast media has been described as a possible contributing factor. However, histamine release is not consistent and may be a nonspecific response to the hypertonic medium itself. Biochemical events in patients with true hypersensitivities and in patients with contrast media and other nonimmunologic reactions may, in whole or in part, follow common metabolic pathways. The effects of hyperosmolality and chemical toxicity of contrast materials and the induction of complement activation, histamine release, and coagulopathies continue under intense investigation.

RENAL HANDLING OF CONTRAST MEDIA

Water-soluble contrast agents are excreted almost exclusively by the kidney; less than 1 per cent is excreted by extrarenal routes that include liver, bile, small and large bowel, sweat, tears, and saliva. The plasma level of contrast media is totally dose-dependent, and the filtered load is proportional to the glomerular filtration rate times the plasma level.

The average adult dose routinely used for conventional urography with high osmolar contrast agents is 20 g of iodine, which would be in the range of 1 to 1.5 ml/kg body weight for most adults, although larger doses up to 40 to 80 g of iodine have been advocated. On the other hand, due to the high costs of the low osmolar agents but the higher densities achieved, some advocate somewhat lower dose ranges for these agents. The peak time for excretion of contrast media is about three minutes following the intravenous injection. Peak urine iodine concentrations occur approximately 60 minutes after administration. Urine flow rates are increased with the meglumine salts when compared with the sodium salts. The excretion of the nonopaque cation meglumine in the tubule accounts for the finding of higher urinary iodine concentrations with sodium salts. Thus, some investigators have noted that the sodium salts of diatrizoate or iothalamate give higher urinary concentrations than do comparable doses of the meglumine salt.

The administration of hypertonic contrast media either intravenously or directly into the renal arterial circulation induces a unique biphasic alteration in renal blood flow (RBF). There is an initial increase in flow followed by a decline; the latter is more marked following the intra-arterial route than with the intravenous route of administration. Interest in the nephrotoxic effects of contrast media has stimulated a number of investigations into the nature of the decrease in blood flow. Attempts to identify mediators such as serotonin, norepinephrine, angiotensin, and the prostaglandins using blocking agents have failed to implicate the most likely candidates. It has been shown that the decrease in RBF is directly related to the osmolality of the contrast agent and that similar changes can be induced by other hypertonic solutions, including mannitol. Studies comparing the effects on RBF with low osmolar agents confirm a marked lessening of hemodynamic changes consistent with and directly related to the lessened osmolality. Thus, the qualitative effects are identical, whereas the quantitative effects reflect the osmolality differences. The osmotic influence of the initial contrast medium bolus within the renal vascular bed attracts water and electrolytes from interstitial space, and possibly from the renal tubules, and this water leaves the kidney with the renal venous effluent. This fluid shift can explain the initial decrease in renal size and intrarenal pressure for the time of the initial increase in RBF.

Micropuncture studies have defined the Starling forces that are important in determining the GFR. Briefly, hydrostatic pressure in the glomerular capillary loop minus the pressure in Bowman's capsule in the proximal tubule acts in favor of filtration but is opposed by the osmotic pressure exerted by the plasma proteins. Hydraulic permeability of the filtering membrane of the glomerulus, surface area available for filtration, and plasma flow rate within capillary loops are also factors. Endogenous vasoconstrictors have been shown to reduce GFR, predominantly by their influence on the plasma flow rate through glomerular capillary loops. This is thought to be modulated by changes in resistance in the afferent and efferent arterioles. It has been assumed that these agents decrease GFR less than renal blood flow because of a predominant influence on efferent arterioles. The contrast medium-induced reductions in both filtration fraction and GFR coincide with the decrease in renal perfusion. This is in marked contrast to the response known to occur with renal vasoconstrictors, such as norepinephrine and angiotensin II, which produce a relatively smaller decrease in GFR than in renal blood flow and thus a net increase in filtration fraction.

The marked initial rise in renal blood flow following injection of contrast material delivers a large osmotic load into the renal tubules. Because molecules of contrast material, like those of mannitol, are not reabsorbed, they continue to exert an osmotic effect, markedly reducing reabsorption of water from the tubules. This increases pressure in Bowman's capsule and in the proximal tubules and reduces GFR in two ways: (1) by decreasing the effective hydrostatic pressure gradient across the interfaces between the glomerular capillaries and Bowman's capsule, and (2) by compressing the glomerular capillary loops, thereby reducing the available surface area of the filtering membrane. Thus, it is likely that the contrast-induced reductions in glomerular filtration rate, filtration fraction, and renal perfusion are explainable on the basis of intratubular (and hence intracapsular) pressure changes caused by the hypertonic solution. These effects are markedly attenuated using the low osmolality agents.

Osmotic diuretics are low–molecular weight substances that are freely filtered by the glomeruli and remain in the tubular lumen in a high concentration because of a limitation on their reabsorption. By virtue of their relatively small size and high concentration, they contribute notably to the osmolality of the filtrate, and this osmotic property is an important factor responsible for the diuretic effect. The hypertonic water-soluble contrast media are potent osmotic diuretics that are qualitatively indistinguishable from mannitol.

Within minutes after an intravascular osmotic diuretic is injected, water and sodium excretion increases markedly (Fig. 68–3). Much of the diuretic action can be accounted for on the basis of inhibition of sodium and water reabsorption in the proximal tubule, along with inhibition of sodium and water transport in the loop of Henle. During brisk osmotic diuresis, the distal tubule and collecting duct fail to recapture any notable portion of the increased sodium and water load delivered into the early distal tubule. Increases in the rate of perfusion of the distal portion of the loop of Henle lead to a decrease in whole kidney GFR, which is a function of the glomerulotubular feedback mechanism. This is, in part, related to the marked increase in proximal tubular pressure with increased flow rates within the nephron associated with a relative increase in resistance to tubular flow at the level of the collecting duct (Fig. 68–3). The increase in urine flow induced by the osmotic diuresis is associated with an increase in excretion of a wide variety of substances other than water and sodium, and these include potassium, calcium, phosphorus, magnesium, uric acid, urea, and oxalate. Patients with persistent osmotic diuresis are typically volume contracted and hyperosmolar.

Early clinical investigators focused on ways to improve the concentration of contrast media in the urine, including the use of larger

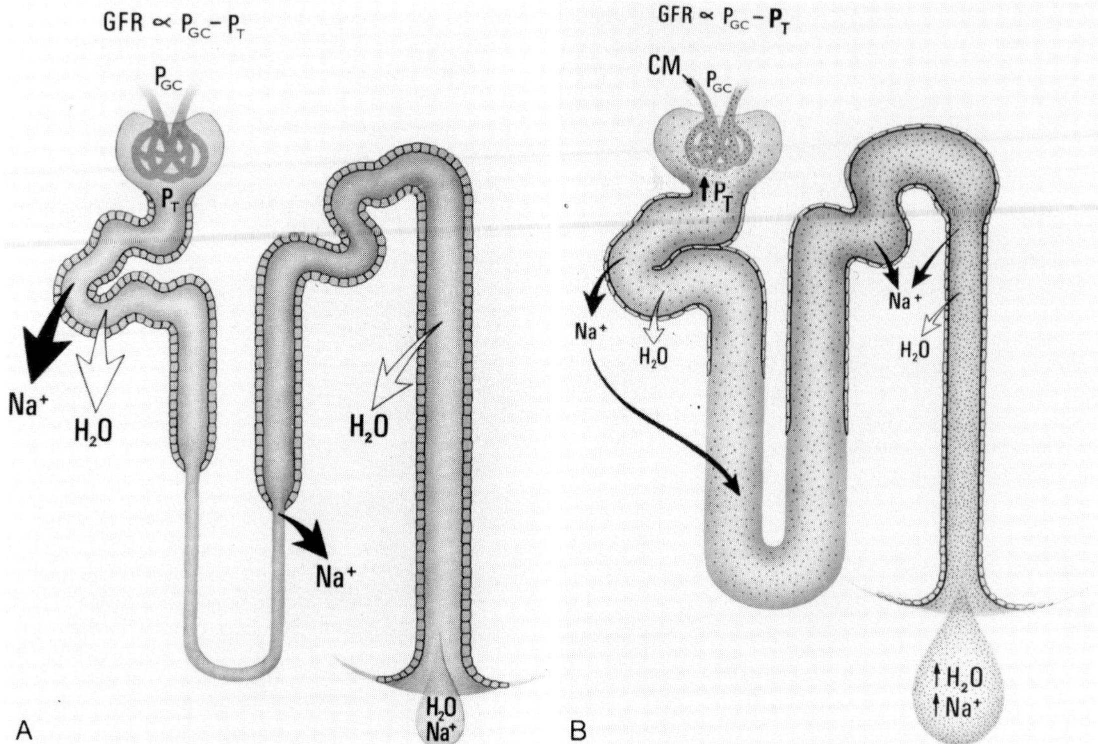

Figure 68–3. Diagrammatic representation of the osmotic effects in the nephron. *A,* Antidiuretic state shows nondistended nephron and nephron with sodium and water reabsorption. The GFR is proportional to glomerular capillary pressure, P_{GC} minus proximal tubular pressure, P_T. *B,* With hypertonic contrast media the nephron distends because of the large osmotic gradient, leading to a decrease in water and sodium reabsorption. An increase in P_T leads to a decrease in GFR because there is a resultant decrease in the hydrostatic gradient for filtration.

doses and prior dehydration. It was subsequently realized that the total quantity of contrast media excreted was more important for image quality than concentration; thus, a ureter that is distended with less concentrated contrast medium that actually contains more iodine will produce more information on intravenous urography than one incompletely filled with more highly concentrated contrast medium. Dehydration does produce a more concentrated urine but leads to a significantly reduced glomerular filtration rate. Hence, the current trend toward the use of larger doses and away from dehydration is logical. Harvey and Caldicott have also shown that glomerular functional responses to contrast media are, however, dose related: the magnitude and duration of the reductions in filtration fraction are increased by logarithmic increments in the injected dose. These findings suggest that further attempts at improving the excretion of contrast media by injecting larger doses meet with diminishing returns.

REACTIONS TO INTRAVASCULAR CONTRAST MEDIA

The majority of patients receiving intravascular contrast media do not experience adverse reactions, but such responses do occur and may be life-threatening. Adverse reactions may be classified into three types based upon the severity of the response: (1) *minor reactions* include nausea, a feeling of heat, pain, and limited urticaria; (2) *intermediate reactions* include faintness, severe vomiting, dyspnea, chest pain, and seizures, and these usually require some form of treatment; and (3) *severe reactions* include shock, anaphylactoid effects, pulmonary edema, cardiac arrest, myocardial infarction, and death (Fig. 68–4). The minor and intermediate reactions are the most often seen but are not life-threatening. This discussion will emphasize the various aspects of severe and fatal reactions.

Severe and fatal contrast reactions are uncommon, accompanying approximately 0.022 per cent and 0.0025 per cent, respectively, of 158,500 urograms reported by Ansell et al. They noted an apparent increased incidence of severe and fatal reactions that appear to be related to increased dose. An iodine content of 5 to 19 g in 59,462 adult excretory urograms led to nine severe and fatal reactions (0.015 per cent), whereas an iodine content greater than or equal to 20 g in 71,344 adult excretory urograms resulted in 27 such reactions (0.038 per cent), suggesting that a chemotoxic effect of contrast material may be important. The following observations were emphasized: severe reactions show a slight predominance in the older age groups; patients with a history of allergy have approximately a four-fold increased risk of a severe reaction; patients with a history of asthma have a five-fold increased risk of a severe reaction; there is an eleven-fold increased risk of a severe reaction in those patients with a previous history of a reaction to contrast media; and patients with a history of cardiac disease have a 4.5 times increased risk for severe reactions. The lower osmolar contrast agents cause fewer adverse systemic reactions and fewer severe and potentially life-threatening reactions than the high osmolar agents. The reaction rate with these newer nonionic agents is about one fifth that of conventional standard ionic contrast agents. Katayama et al reported the largest comparative series of the 340,000 patients, half of whom received the low osmolar contrast agents and half received the high osmolar contrast agents. Serious reactions were reduced significantly in the low osmolar group, but only a single fatal reaction occurred in each group. These two fatal reactions may not have been related to the contrast media, per se, however. Use of these newer low osmolar agents, has, unfortunately, not completely eliminated serious reactions, and fatal reactions with each class of contrast agents continue to occur.

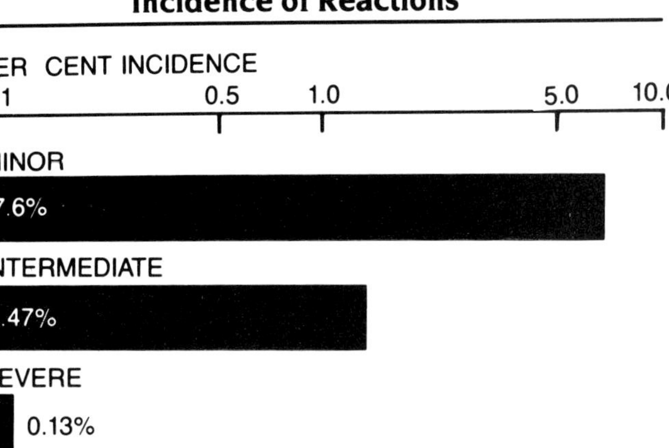

Figure 68–4. Incidence of contrast media reactions. (Adapted from Ansell G, Tweedie MCK, West CR, et al: The current status of reactions to intravenous contrast media. Invest Radiol 15:532–539, 1980.)

Various mechanisms have been implicated in the pathogenesis of severe and fatal responses to intravascular contrast materials. Recent literature suggests mediation by the cardiovascular and central nervous systems, complement or allergic activation. More recent investigations have also identified dehydration as a significant major risk factor for severe hypotension and shock during excretory urography and contrast-enhanced CT scanning. Hyperviscosity states, such as those found in macroglobulinemia or multiple myeloma, have also been identified as risk factors. *Chemotoxicity* may be particularly important in patients with dehydration, with ventricular arrhythmogenic areas of the myocardium that could trigger fibrillation, or with compromised blood-brain barriers. *Antigen-antibody reactions* may be involved, but it is usually not possible to demonstrate antibodies in patients who have experienced severe reactions. Lasser has proposed an *anaphylactoid* mechanism involving a cascade of the complement, coagulation, kinin, and fibrinolytic system subsequent to osmotic injury to the vascular endothelium. Others have suggested that *psychogenic* factors complicated by blood-brain barrier leakage are responsible. It is also possible that there are combinations of responses that must occur in synergism to lead to the severe and fatal responses.

Some investigators have proposed prophylactic premedication in those patients at high risk for contrast media reactions whose condition requires the clinical investigation. One commonly used regimen includes 50 mg predisone PO q6h × 3 and 50 mg diphenhydramine IM. Another regimen that has been suggested recommends the administration of prednisone, 50 mg PO on the two nights and the morning before the contrast examination. This 36-hour pretreatment is thought to be more effective than steroid regimens of shorter duration. Other investigators have advocated careful attention to the state of hydration and have suggested the use of intravenous fluids prior to study. Withholding fluids prior to intravenous urography is no longer recommended now that larger dose regimens have been advocated and are general clinical practice. There is no evidence that pretesting for sensitivity to contrast media is of value.

Specific treatment regimens for severe contrast media reactions are controversial. Primary attention should be given to maintaining circulation and respiration along with rapid volume expansion with intravenous fluids. Epinephrine may be indicated if auscultation of the lung fields indicates the wheezing of laryngospasm or bronchospasm. On the other hand, a poor pulse or irregular rhythm may indicate the presence of myocardial infarction or arrhythmia; in this case epinephrine is contraindicated. A well-trained resuscitation team that is quickly available is the most effective regimen.

NEPHROTOXICITY

Acute renal failure that is the direct result of contrast administration is a matter of continued concern. Although recent surveys suggest an overall incidence of approximately 0.15 per cent of clinical procedures, they actually approach 12 per cent in certain clinical settings. Predisposing factors include dehydration, diabetes mellitus, multiple myeloma, advanced age, cardiac disease, use of diuretics, renal insufficiency, hyperuricemia, and undergoing several contrast examinations within 24 hours. Clinically, contrast-induced acute renal failure is defined as a rise in serum creatinine of at least 1.0 mg/dl occurring within 48 hours after the contrast medium administration. Oliguria (urine volume of less than 400 ml/day) is observed in approximately 75 per cent. Non-oliguric renal failure also occurs. (It has been re-emphasized that the most important predisposing factors to contrast medium–induced renal injury are pre-existing renal insufficiency together with diabetes mellitus. The advantages of low osmolar contrast agents, if any, have not been clearly established. Indeed, recent investigations show little benefit with the newer agents. The importance of prerenal factors, including hypotension and hypovolemia with dehydration, have not been adequately examined but appear highly important.)

A significant but transient proteinuria develops after renal angiography in animals and in man with the use of the hypertonic agents and with the nonionic agent metrizamide. Abnormal enzymuria has also been reported after both the intra-arterial and intravenous injections of contrast materials.

Hypertonic contrast agents induce vacuolization in the cytoplasm of the renal proximal tubular cells. This had been termed "osmotic" nephrosis and is seen most commonly in patients with pre-existing renal insufficiency after the administration of contrast materials. However, similar changes have been found after urography with metrizamide, and in a small number of patients studied, osmotic nephrosis was seen in some patients after urography with Hexabrix and Iopamidol. Because these are low-osmolality agents, chemotoxicity rather than osmolality may be a factor. These changes have not been shown to have a direct relationship to significant renal toxicity and are clearly nonspecific.

Most examples of contrast medium-induced nephrotoxicity are self-limited without serious sequelae. However, attention to risk factors and adequate patient hydration provide the best means for prevention.

NEWER CONTRAST AGENTS

Research has been aimed at the development of new contrast media that reduce toxicity, unpleasant side effects, and adverse reactions while improving diagnostic quality. The new contrast materials are of three basic types: (1) nonionic monomers, (2) monoacidic dimers, and (3) nonionic dimers. These agents have one major characteristic in common: a markedly lower osmolality. Clinical usage in Europe, Australia, and Japan has shown fewer side effects, less toxicity, and equivalent or better diagnostic opacification than the current agents. The newer agents are ratio-3 to ratio-6, with less than half the osmolality of the current agents. They include Iodixanol, Iohexol, Iopamidol, Iotrol, Ioversol and Ioxagtate. Acute toxicity (LD_{50}) in mice for new agents shows an LD_{50} of 13 to 25 g I/kg vs 7 to 10 g I/kg with the current ionic monomers. Low-osmolality media produce significantly higher urinary iodine concentrations, less urine volume (less diuretic effect), and similar total iodine excretion rates compared with the currently available urographic contrast materials. Clinical investigations comparing subjective responses and radiographic quality in the United States demonstrate a significant decrease in subjective patient complaints of warmth, heat, or other unpleasant sensations after intravenous injections of low-osmolality agents, in comparison with more hypertonic solutions. Radiographs are consistently better for caliceal opacification, and voided urine specimens show a significantly higher iodine concentration and lower urine volume with the newer agents. Thus, new low-osmolality contrast media represent a significant advantage.

Bibliography

Ansell G, Tweedie MCK, West CR, et al: The current status of reactions to intravenous contrast media. Invest Radiol (Suppl) 15:S32–S39, 1980.

Benness GT: Urographic contrast agents: A comparison of sodium and methylglucamine salts. Clin Radiol 21:150, 1970.

Berger RE, Comez LS, Mallette LE: Acute hypocalcemic effects of clinical contrast media injections. AJR 138:283–288, 1982.

Berkseth RO, Kjellstrand CM: Radiologic contrast-induced nephrotoxicity. Med Clin North Am 68:351–370, 1984.

Bettman MA, Salzman EW, Rosenthal D, et al: Reduction of venous thrombosis complicating phlebography. AJR 134:1169–1172, 1980.

Brasch RC: Allergic reactions to contrast media: Accumulated evidence. AJR 134:797–801, 1980.

Committee on Drugs of the Commission on Public Health and Radiation Protection, American College of Radiology: Prevention and Management of Adverse Reactions to Intravenous Contrast Media, 1977.

Deutsch AL, Gerber KH, Haigler FH, et al: Effects of low osmolality contrast materials on coronary hemodynamics, myocardial function and coronary sinus osmolality in normal and ischemic states. Invest Radiol 17:284–291, 1982.

Düre-Smith P: The dose of contrast medium in intravenous urography: A physiologic assessment. AJR 108:691–697, 1970.

Ekholm SE: Adverse reactions to intravascular and intrathecal contrast media. Iatrogenic diseases. Crit Rev Diagnostic Imag 5:115–136, 1986.

Fischer HW, Doust VL: An evaluation of pretesting in the problem of serious and fatal reactions to excretory urography. Radiology 102:497, 1972.

Fischer HW, Katzberg RW, Morris TW, Spataro RF: Systemic response to excretory urography. Radiology 151:31–33, 1984.

Fischer HW, Kido DK, Morris TW: Understanding contrast media: The promise of nonionic agents. New York, Winthrop-Breon Consult Series, 1985.

Harvey LA, Caldicott WJH: The influence of contrast medium dose on filtration fraction in the rabbit kidney. Invest Radiol 18:441–444, 1983.

Higgins CB, Gerber KH, Mattrey RF, et al: Evaluation of the hemodynamic effects of intravenous administration of ionic and nonionic contrast materials. Radiology 142:681–686, 1982.

Higgins CB, Sovak M, Schmidt WS, et al: Direct myocardial effects of intracoronary administration of new contrast materials with low osmolality. Invest Radiol 15:39–46, 1980.

Katayama H, Yamaguchi K, Kozuka T, et al: Adverse reactions to ionic and nonionic contrast media: A report from the Japanese Committee on the Safety of Contrast Media. Radiology 175:621–628, 1990.

Katzberg RW (ed): The Contrast Media Manual. Baltimore, Williams and Wilkins, 1992.

Katzberg RW, Morris TW, Schulman G, et al: Intravenous contrast media. Part I: Severe and fatal reactions in a canine dehydration model. Radiology 147:327–330, 1983.

Katzberg RW, Morris TW, Schulman G, et al: Reaction to intravenous contrast media. Part II: Acute renal response in euvolemic and dehydrated dogs. Radiology 147:331–334, 1983.

Katzberg RW, Schulman G, Meggs LG, et al: Mechanism of the renal response to contrast medium in dogs: Decrease in renal function due to hypertonicity. Invest Radiol 18:74–80, 1983.

Kelley JF, Patterson R, Lieberman P, et al: Radiographic contrast media studies in high-risk patients. J Allergy Clin Immunol 62:181–184, 1978.

Lalli AF, Greenstreet R: Reactions to contrast media: Testing the CNS hypothesis. Radiology 138:47–49, 1981.

Lasser EC: Mechanisms of contrast media reactions. Implications for avoidance and treatment based on hypothesis of causation. In Katckey RW (ed): The Contrast Media Manual, Part III. Baltimore, Williams and Wilkins, 1992, pp 171–179.

Moreau J-F, Droz D, Noel L-H, et al: Tubular nephrotoxicity of water soluble iodinated contrast media. Invest Radiol (Suppl) 15:S54–S60, 1980.

Palmer FJ: The R.A.C.R. survey of intravenous contrast media reactions: A preliminary report. Australas Radiol 32:8–11, 1988.

Parfrey PS, Griffiths SM, Barrett BJ, et al: Contrast-media induced renal failure in patients with diabetes mellitus, renal insufficiency, or both. A prospective controlled study. N Engl J Med 320:149–153, 1989.

Schwab SJ, Hlatky MA, Pieper KS, et al: Contrast nephrotoxicity: A randomized controlled trial of a nonionic and an ionic radiographic contrast agent. N Engl J Med 320:149–153, 1989.

Spataro RF, Fischer HW, Boylan L: Urography with low-osmolality contrast media: Comparative urinary excretion of Iopamidol, Hexabrix, and Diatrizoate. Invest Radiol 17:494–500, 1982.

69 Congenital Abnormalities of the Urinary Tract

Stuart A. Royal

UPPER URINARY TRACT ANOMALIES

Renal Agenesis, Ectopia, and Fusion

The ureteral bud first arises from the mesonephric duct in the fourth week of gestation and begins to induce the metanephrogenic blastema from the nephrogenic ridge by the fifth week. The kidneys then migrate cranially either by differential growth or by forceful extrusion from the pelvis. Finally, the renal pelvis rotates medially to end in its normal position by eight weeks. A variety of insults may occur at different stages, leading to a multitude of upper urinary tract anomalies, occurring in 1 in 500 children.

RENAL AGENESIS

Bilateral renal agenesis occurs once in 4800 births. It can be secondary to absence of the metanephrogenic blastema and nephrogenic ridge or to failure of the mesonephric duct or ureteral bud to develop. It is invariably fatal, with the children having "Potter

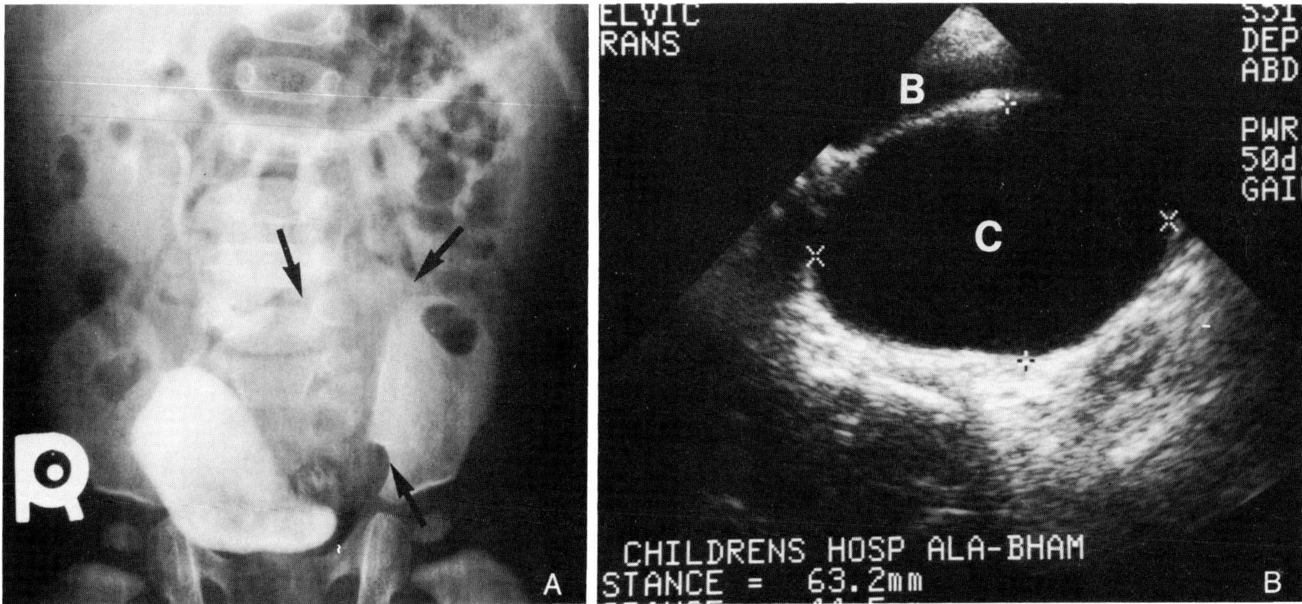

Figure 69–1. Unilateral renal agenesis with ipsilateral seminal vesicle cyst. *A,* Intravenous urogram in this 9-month-old male reveals compensatory hypertrophy of the right kidney with absent visualization of the left kidney. A large mass in the left pelvis *(arrows)* is seen displacing the urinary bladder to the right. *B,* Transverse pelvic ultrasonogram demonstrates the urinary bladder (B) displaced anteriorly by the large retrovesical cystic mass (C).

facies'' (flattened face, low-set large floppy ears, hypertelorism, micrognathia, and prominent skin folds at the inner canthus) and frequently dying of pulmonary hypoplasia, most likely from lack of urine production and resultant oligohydramnios and uterine compression of the fetal thorax.

Ultrasound and nuclear medicine are sufficient to demonstrate the condition postnatally, although ultrasound promises to provide accurate in utero detection. However, one must be careful not to mistake the normal adrenal gland in utero for the kidney and therefore miss the diagnosis. Persistent failure to image the fetal urinary bladder after furosemide infusion confirms fetal anuria and establishes fetal nonviability.

Unilateral renal agenesis is more common (1 in 1100 births) than bilateral renal agenesis and may be detected on a screening examination or suspected because of an associated anomaly of the external or internal genitalia. Genital anomalies occur in 25 to 50 per cent of females with this condition, with unicornuate or bicornuate uterus being most common. An occasional pubertal woman will present with painful menstruation, enlarging pelvic mass, and unilateral renal agenesis with ipsilateral obstructed duplicate vagina and hematocolpos. Genital anomalies occur in 10 to 15 per cent of males, with ipsilateral seminal vesicle cyst most commonly reported (Fig. 69–1). Ipsilateral adrenal agenesis occurs in 10 per cent of cases. Cardiac (30 per cent), gastrointestinal (25 per cent), and musculoskeletal (14 per cent) anomalies are also associated findings.

At birth, the single kidney in a patient with unilateral renal agenesis will be normal in size because maternal renal function prevents compensatory hypertrophy. After birth, it takes approximately 18 months for complete contralateral compensatory renal hypertrophy to occur, although the majority occurs in the first 6 to 12 months of life. Ultrasonography and nuclear medicine complement one another in making the diagnosis of unilateral renal agenesis, demonstrating normal function in a single kidney. However, ultrasonography can also demonstrate the associated genital anomaly. Occasionally, medial deployment of the splenic or hepatic flexure of the colon or displacement of small bowel, duodenum, spleen, and tail of pancreas may suggest renal agenesis (Fig. 69–2). A

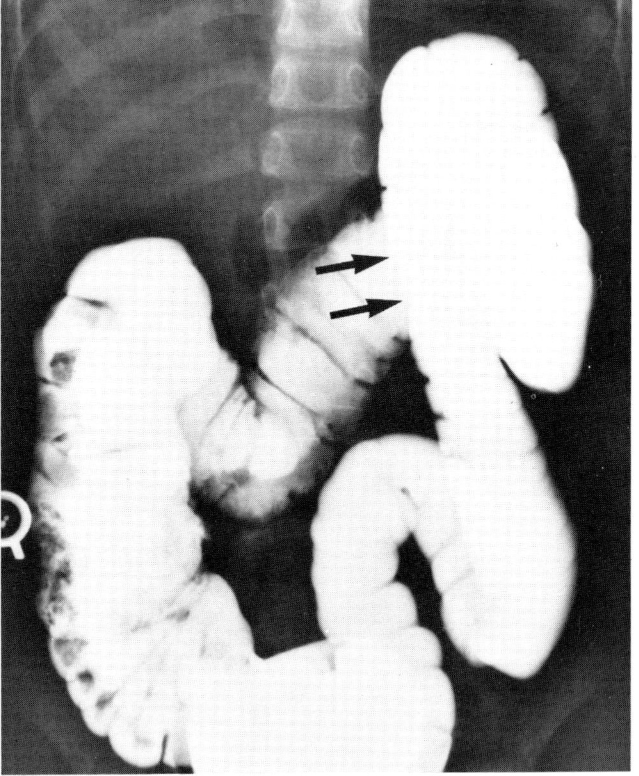

Figure 69–2. Renal agenesis. Unilateral left renal agenesis with the anatomic splenic flexure of the colon in the left renal fossa. Barium enema demonstrates the anatomic splenic flexure of the colon in the left renal fossa *(arrows).* This can be seen in anterior transperitoneal nephrectomies in which the ligamentous attachments of the kidney are freed, allowing the colon to fall into the renal fossa. This is not seen in retroperitoneal nephrectomies.

comprehensive review of all organ systems should be undertaken to discover other associated anomalies.

RENAL ECTOPIA

Ectopic kidneys may occur anywhere below or even above the normal path of ascent of the kidney. Ectopic kidneys may also cross to the opposite side and may be unilateral or bilateral. Embryologic abnormalities of ureteral bud formation, defective metanephric tissue, genetic abnormalities, and teratogenic influences have all been implicated as etiologic factors. Various names have been given to these kidneys depending on their location and gross appearance (pelvic, lumbar, pancake, disc, lump, etc.). The kidneys frequently appear dysmorphic, with a nonreniform shape, anteriorly located pelvis, tilted axis, and bizarre calyces that should not be mistaken for intrinsic pathology.

Crossed ectopia is a unique type of renal ectopia in which the ectopic kidney is located on the opposite side of the retroperitoneum, usually adjacent to the lower pole of the contralateral kidney, with its ureter emptying into the bladder on the ipsilateral side. A deep anteroposterior notch between the two kidneys is felt to be characteristic of this entity. Ninety per cent of crossed ectopic kidneys are fused to the contralateral kidney. Solitary or bilateral crossed ectopia is exceedingly rare. The embryologic basis for crossed ectopia is uncertain. As in all types of ectopia, the kidney usually appears dysmorphic and has an increased risk for hydronephrosis (perhaps from aberrant vessels), infection (with reflux), multicystic dysplasia, trauma, and stones (Fig. 69–3).

HORSESHOE KIDNEY

Horseshoe kidney (1 in 400 population) is probably the most common of all renal fusion anomalies. It is usually formed by

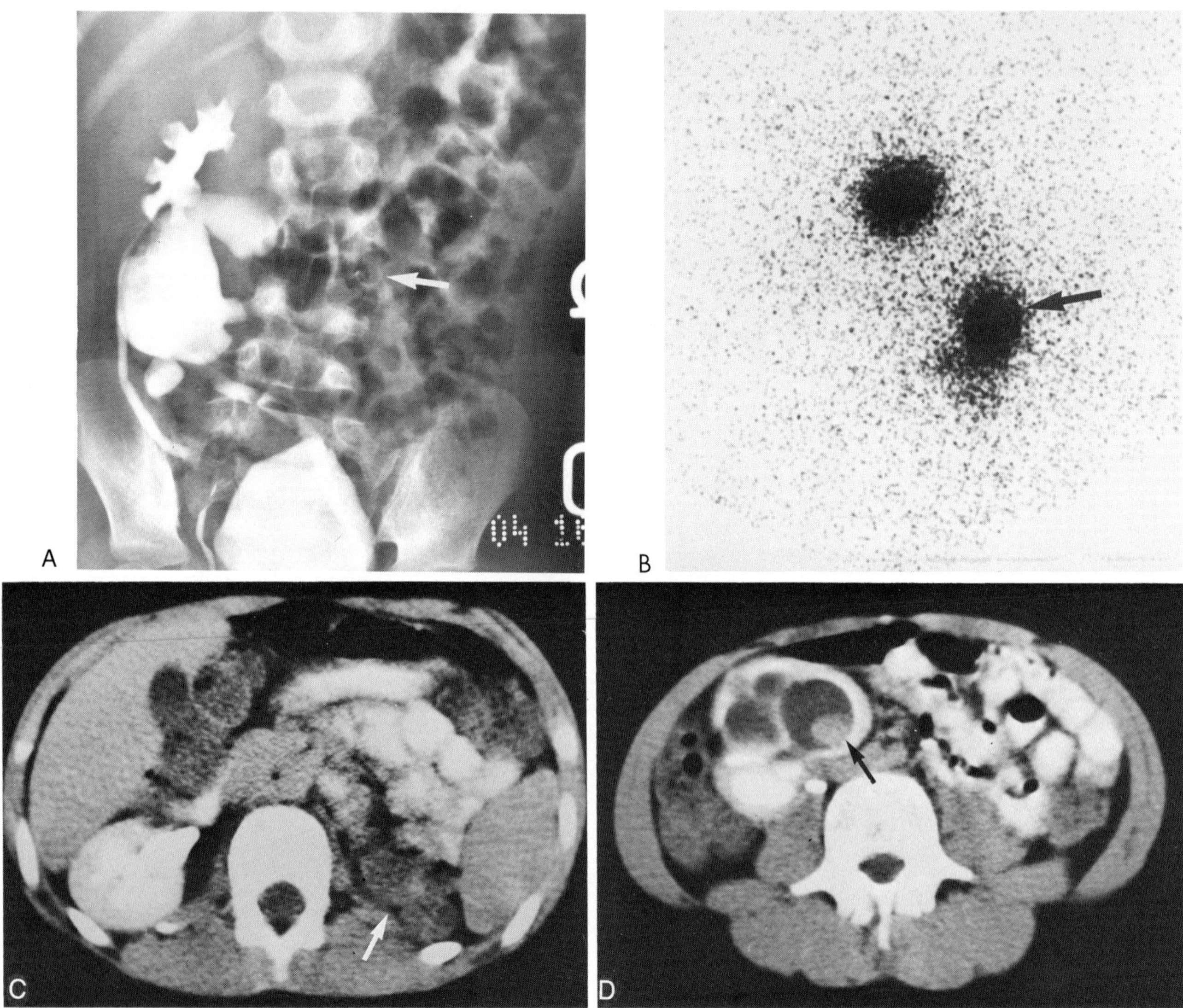

Figure 69–3. Crossed fused renal ectopia with ureteropelvic junction obstruction of the ectopic kidney. *A,* Intravenous urography reveals the left kidney adjacent to the lower pole of the normally positioned right kidney, with both ureters emptying into their normal positions in the bladder. A urographic appearance of ureteropelvic junction obstruction of the lower moiety is present. Note the hemivertebra at L3-L4 *(arrow)* typically seen in the VATER association. *B,* A technetium-99m DTPA scan reveals left crossed renal ectopia with retention of radionuclide in the renal pelvis of the crossed ectopic kidney *(arrow),* typical of ureteropelvic junction obstruction. *C* and *D,* An 11-year-old male with hematuria after minor trauma. CT scan reveals no kidney in left renal fossa *(arrow),* with the ectopic left kidney in right abdomen, with hydronephrosis from ureteropelvic junction obstruction. A blood clot *(arrow)* is seen in a dilated calyx.

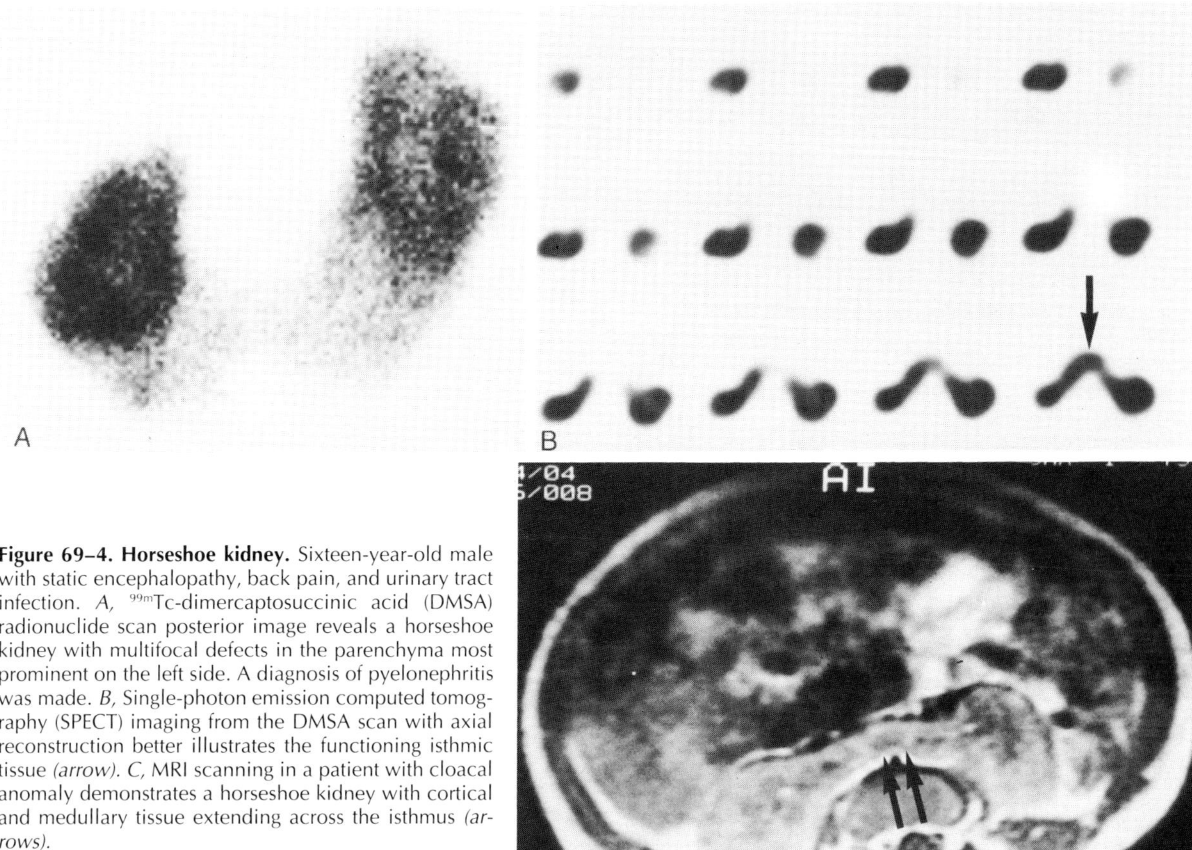

Figure 69–4. Horseshoe kidney. Sixteen-year-old male with static encephalopathy, back pain, and urinary tract infection. *A,* ^{99m}Tc-dimercaptosuccinic acid (DMSA) radionuclide scan posterior image reveals a horseshoe kidney with multifocal defects in the parenchyma most prominent on the left side. A diagnosis of pyelonephritis was made. *B,* Single-photon emission computed tomography (SPECT) imaging from the DMSA scan with axial reconstruction better illustrates the functioning isthmic tissue *(arrow). C,* MRI scanning in a patient with cloacal anomaly demonstrates a horseshoe kidney with cortical and medullary tissue extending across the isthmus *(arrows).*

fusion of the lower poles of the kidneys between the fourth and sixth weeks of gestation after the ureteral bud has entered the metanephrogenic blastema. The anomaly consists of two distinct renal masses that lie vertically, low on either side of the midline, and are connected by a parenchymatous or fibrous isthmus that is usually anterior to the aorta and inferior vena cava, and crosses the midline just below the junction of the inferior mesenteric artery and the aorta. The pelves are frequently extrarenal and are usually anteriorly placed with the ureters crossing ventral to the isthmus. The arterial supply is quite variable with multiple, unpredictable accessory vessels arising from the abdominal aorta or even the iliac arteries. As is usual for ectopic kidneys, the collecting system appears dysmorphic. Associated anomalies are only mildly increased in frequency, with horseshoe kidney being the most common anomaly in Turner's syndrome.

On urography, the vertical or reversed axis of the calyces is easily seen. Ultrasonography may directly demonstrate the isthmus. CT, MRI, and nuclear medicine (Fig. 69–4) aid in distinguishing the fibrous from the parenchymatous isthmus, which is helpful preoperatively because the isthmus frequently must be divided during surgical procedures. Urography, ultrasonography, nuclear medicine, and computed tomography may all be necessary in evaluating the two thirds of patients with horseshoe kidney who develop complications such as hydronephrosis, infection, calculus formation, trauma, or the occasional renal cell carcinoma or Wilms' tumor.

Screening for Anomalies

Renal agenesis, ectopia, and fusion anomalies are more common among patients with certain extraurinary anomalies or syndromes, and these patients should be screened for underlying renal anomalies (Table 69–1). However, it is unclear whether patients with congenital heart disease, simple hypospadias, or cryptorchidism should have such a screening evaluation. Patients with isolated single umbilical artery, meatal stenosis, or anomalies only of the ear are not at risk for urinary anomalies and need not be screened for renal anomalies. Because such defects are rarely life-threatening, these patients should be screened on an elective basis. In the neonatal period, this is best accomplished by ultrasonography or radionuclide imaging because urography may not satisfactorily image the kidneys in the first week of life. A voiding cystourethrogram may be necessary to evaluate for vesicoureteral reflux in patients with the VATER association (see Table 69–1).

Renal Dysplasia

Renal dysplasia is a type of parenchymal maldevelopment resulting in a microscopic picture of abnormal nephrons with primitive glomeruli, tubules, and ducts in embryonic mesenchymal connective tissue; disordered parenchyma with cystic transformation of collecting ducts; and rests of metaplastic cartilage. The changes may affect the entire kidney or only segments thereof. Congenital anomalies of the ureter or lower urinary tract are associated findings in 90 per cent of the cases. Although primarily a histologic diagnosis, renal dysplasia may be inferred from imaging studies when evaluating diseases associated with renal dysplasia.

The etiology of renal dysplasia is unclear, although contributions from congenital obstruction (with or without vesicoureteral reflux), ureteral bud anomalies, and maldevelopment associated with a va-

TABLE 69–1. VATER ASSOCIATION

*V*ertebral segmentation defects
*V*ascular anomalies
*A*norectal anomalies
*T*racheoesophageal fistula
*E*sophageal atresia
*R*adial ray aplasia
*R*enal anomalies

riety of syndromes appear to be important. Renal dysplasia is most commonly associated with urinary obstruction. The most common congenital obstructions associated with renal dysplasia are multicystic dysplastic kidney (MCDK) and posterior urethral valves with reflux. Prune belly may also be included, although congenital obstruction has not been proven to be the etiology of this disorder. Generally, the more severe the obstruction, the more severe the dysplasia.

Renal dysplasia can also be explained by an ectopic origin of the ureteral bud off the mesonephric duct, producing faulty induction of the metanephrogenic blastema. The further from the trigone the ureteral orifice is located, the more dysplastic the renal unit. The best-studied example of this is the segmental dysplasia of the upper pole of a complete duplex collecting system with or without ectopic ureterocele. However, the dysplasia occasionally seen in primary vesicoureteral reflux and in posterior urethral valves with reflux may also be explained by ectopic ureteral bud origination. Cystic renal dysplasia can also be seen independent of obstruction or ureteral ectopia in syndromes such as Meckel syndrome (encephalocele, polydactyly), Beckwith-Wiedemann syndrome (macroglossia, omphalocele, visceromegaly), Jeune syndrome (asphyxiating thoracic dystrophy), Zellweger syndrome (cerebrohepatorenal syndrome), trisomy 13, and trisomy 18.

When classic MCDK is encountered by imaging procedures, the diagnosis of renal dysplasia is assured. In patients with posterior urethral valves, finding parenchymal cysts by ultrasound (in utero or ex utero), increased parenchymal echogenicity, or reflux into parenchymal cysts on voiding cystourethrography is highly predictive of renal dysplasia. Similarly, one can speculate about renal dysplasia in a patient with posterior urethral valves and reflux if the kidney functions poorly or in a poorly functioning upper pole moiety of a complete duplex collecting system. However, in the absence of renal cysts, histologic confirmation of renal dysplasia will be necessary for diagnosis. Patients having syndromes known to be associated with renal dysplasia can be diagnosed by ultrasonography and clinical correlation, with biopsy necessary only for absolute confirmation.

MULTICYSTIC DYSPLASTIC KIDNEY

Multicystic dysplastic kidney (MCDK) is an expression of collecting system atresia occurring early in gestation. MCDK and ureteropelvic junction (UPJ) obstruction are the two most common etiologies of neonatal abdominal masses and are believed to be entities along the same pathologic spectrum. The classic MCDK (pelvoinfundibular atresia, type II cystic diseases of Potter) results from complete ureteral, pelvic, and infundibular atresia before eight to ten weeks' gestation during the metanephric stage of development. The collecting tubules enlarge to form a variable number of macroscopic cysts that do not intercommunicate and are interspersed with glomeruli, fibrovascular tissue, and primitive mesenchyma in a nonreniform shape. However, if obstruction occurs between the tenth and thirty-sixth weeks of gestation, the pelves may be dilated, the cysts may or may not intercommunicate, and variable amounts of dysplastic parenchyma will persist, forming the hydronephrotic form of MCDK. After 36 weeks of gestation, hydronephrosis without dysplasia will result from obstruction.

MCDK is usually discovered as a neonatal abdominal mass (80 per cent detected in first two years), with hypertension being a rare complication seen in untreated adults. In classic MCDK (Fig. 69–5*A*), ultrasonography demonstrates multiple cysts of varying size randomly distributed throughout the mass, with septations separating the cysts, no parenchymal rim, non-medial deployment of the largest cyst, and an echogenic central core representing the obliterated renal pelvis. Radionuclide imaging (Fig. 69–5*B*) and urography will demonstrate no function, although one may appreciate septations between the cysts on urography. Occasional cyst-wall calcifi-

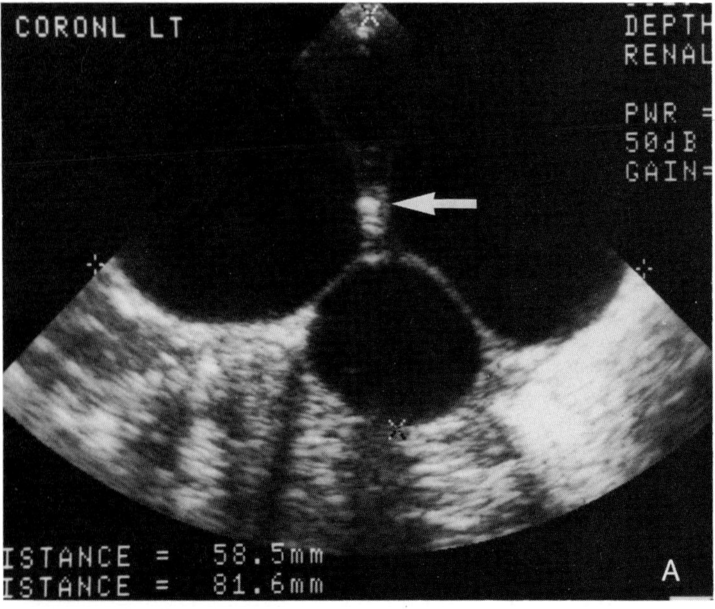

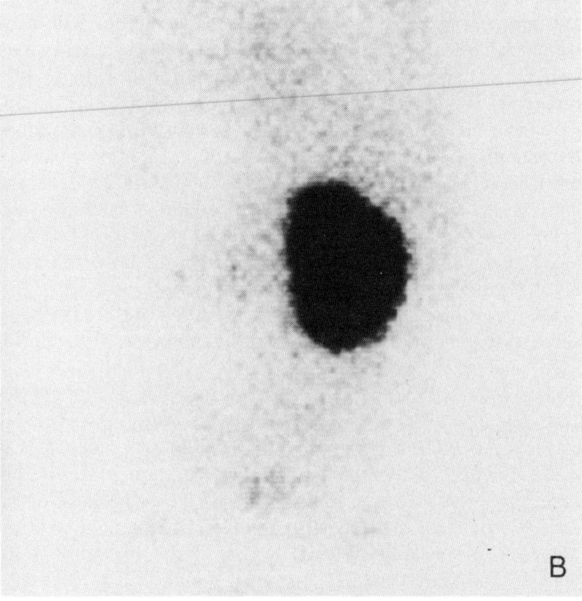

Figure 69–5. Multicystic dysplastic kidney. This newborn presented with a left abdominal mass. *A,* Coronal ultrasonogram of the left renal fossa reveals the left kidney replaced by multiple cysts of varying size with the obliterated renal pelvis represented by an echogenic core *(arrow).* Careful real-time ultrasonography will demonstrate septations separating the noncommunicating cysts with nonmedial deployment of the largest cyst. *B,* ^{99m}Tc-DMSA radionuclide scan demonstrates nonfunction of the left multicystic dysplastic kidney.

cation is seen in adults. Occasionally, a cystogram will reveal reflux into a bulbous, blind-ending ureter in its mid to upper segment. As the pathology approaches the hydronephrotic form of MCDK, the largest cyst becomes medially deployed, the peripheral smaller cysts become radially arranged around the largest cyst, parenchyma becomes visible, and the radionuclide renogram begins to demonstrate function. In up to 41 per cent of cases, abnormalities will be present on the contralateral side, with the most common being UPJ obstruction.

The differential diagnosis of MCDK largely involves distinguishing it from hydronephrosis. In utero, this can be difficult and may require serial studies that may demonstrate enlargement, reduction in size, or even complete disappearance of the entire dysplastic kidney. After birth, in classic MCDK and hydronephrosis, ultrasonography, and, if necessary, radionuclide imaging will provide all the diagnostic information necessary. In intermediate forms, cyst puncture with antegrade pyelography may be necessary for accurate diagnosis. Although still controversial, nonoperative management of MCDK in infancy has gained favor. Ultrasonography in follow-up will demonstrate no change or decrease in size in 85 to 90 per cent of MCDK, with the remainder showing an increase in size frequently requiring nephrectomy.

Renal Hypoplasia

Congenital renal hypoplasia denotes a deficiency in the total number of nephrons per unit volume of parenchyma. In *simple global hypoplasia,* the kidney is small with a reduced number of reniculi and a corresponding decrease in the number of calyces. If bilateral, the child will present in the first months of life with progressive renal failure. It is difficult to distinguish primary renal hypoplasia from acquired vascular or pyelonephritic insults to the kidney or from some types of dysplasia (dysplasia and hypoplasia may coexist) (Fig. 69–6*A* and *B*). However, in bilateral *oligomeganephrotic hypoplasia* (Fig. 69–6*C* and *D*), the kidneys are characteristically unipapillary or bipapillary, and therefore are recognizable radiographically as a form of renal hypoplasia. These patients usually present later in childhood with polyuria, proteinuria, and progressive renal failure, and therefore must be distinguished from patients with familial juvenile nephronophthisis and bilateral generalized dysplasia.

Segmental hypoplasia, when used to describe unilateral focal or multifocal renal parenchymal loss overlying calyceal dilatation in association with hypertension, has been designated the *Ask-Upmark kidney.* In most cases, it is not possible radiographically or pathologically to distinguish these findings from chronic pyelonephritis or vascular disease, and many authors doubt that they are separate entities.

LOWER URETERAL ANOMALIES

Single Ectopic Ureter

Single ectopic ureters (10 to 20 per cent of all ectopic ureters) occur when a single ureteral bud arises more cephalic off the mesonephric duct than normal, with its orifice being anywhere from near normal to extravesical in location. The location of the ectopic ureteral orifice corresponds to the location of ultimate mesonephric duct tissue. In the male, this is always suprasphincteric, and the ureter enters the prostatic urethra, ejaculatory duct, seminal vesicle, or vas deferens. This explains why males with single ectopic ureters do not present with wetting problems but rather with epididymo-orchitis or seminal vesicle mass.

In the female, the ectopic orifice may be either supra- or infrasphincteric, with entry into the urethra, vestibule, or vagina being most common. Therefore, females with single ectopic ureters frequently present with urinary dribbling. If the ureter empties through the sphincter, the ureter will be obstructed during bladder filling and will reflux during voiding. Therefore, the sphincteric ectopic ureter may present with urinary tract infection. Since ectopic ureters frequently drain ectopic dysplastic renal units, the ipsilateral kidney will frequently show diminished or no function by urography, although occasionally the ectopic ureter will be directly visualized, especially if tomography is utilized. Ultrasonography, nuclear medicine, or computed tomography may demonstrate the hydronephrotic system with a retrovesicle dilated ureter. Voiding cystourethrography, especially with multiple voiding sequences at the same setting, may demonstrate reflux into the urethral ectopic ureter (which in the male may also fill the seminal vesicle and vas deferens) or demonstrate a ureterocele. Vaginography, endoscopy, or retrograde injections may be necessary for complete evaluation. Nephroureterectomy is required in most unilateral cases, although reimplantation can be performed if preservation of function is important. Rare bilateral single ectopic ureters may be associated with underdevelopment of the trigone and bladder incontinence.

Duplication of the Collecting System

Duplication (1.7 to 2.4 per cent of autopsy and urographic series) is the most common anomaly of the upper urinary tract and may vary from a bifid pelvis to a complete duplex collecting system. Although usually a normal variant, complications occur in a wide variety of forms and can be detected in utero.

A duplex collecting system arises when two ureteral buds arise from the mesonephric duct. The ureter draining the upper renal segment is carried caudally to open in a variably ectopic position caudad to the ureter draining the lower renal segment. This ureteral arrangement is predicted by the *Weigert-Meyer rule.* Because the ureter draining the lower pole moiety is frequently lateral and superior to its normal location in the trigone, it lacks a submucosal tunnel and may reflux. If vesicoureteral reflux into the lower pole moiety is significant, the patient may present with urinary tract infection and demonstrate chronic pyelonephritis selectively involving the lower pole moiety (Fig. 69–7). Occasionally, UPJ junction obstruction of the lower pole moiety occurs. The ureter draining the upper pole moiety may have a ureterocele and therefore will have obstructed hydronephrosis. Other complications of the upper pole moiety are similar to those seen with a single ectopic ureter—wetting in the female (Fig. 69–8), epididymo-orchitis or seminal vesicle mass in the male, infection with sphincteric ureters, and renal dysplasia. Rarely, the diagnosis of a duplex collecting system can be difficult if the upper pole moiety functions poorly and is nondilated. Computed tomography and surgical exploration with direct injection of the ectopic upper pole ureter may be necessary in exceptional cases.

Ureterocele

A ureterocele is attributed to obstruction of the developing ureter during embryogenesis, because of either failure of disintegration of Chwalle's membrane where the mesonephric duct joins the primitive urogenital sinus or failure of expansion of the ureteral orifice. This results in a submucosal mass in the bladder or urethra that on urography will be a filling defect if it drains a nonfunctioning renal unit, or a "cobra-head" appearance if it fills with contrast from a functioning renal unit.

SIMPLE URETEROCELE

An orthotopic or simple ureterocele is usually associated with a single ureter that has its orifice in normal position in the trigone.

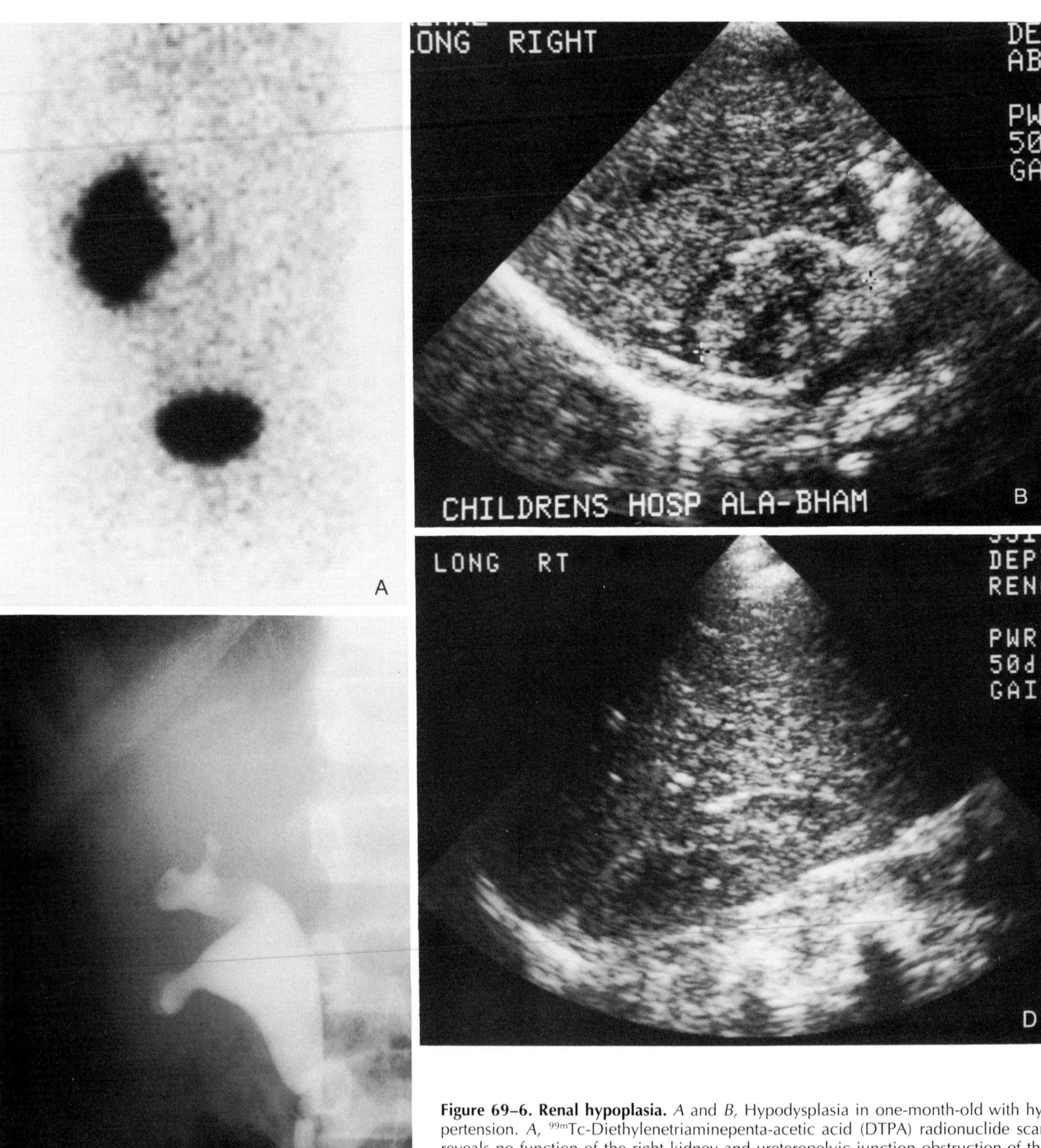

Figure 69–6. Renal hypoplasia. *A* and *B,* Hypodysplasia in one-month-old with hypertension. *A,* ^{99m}Tc-Diethylenetriaminepenta-acetic acid (DTPA) radionuclide scan reveals no function of the right kidney and ureteropelvic junction obstruction of the left kidney. *B,* Longitudinal right renal ultrasonogram reveals a small echogenic kidney with poor corticomedullary distinction. Surgical resection of this kidney revealed multifocal renal dysplasia. *C* and *D,* Oligomeganephronic renal hypoplasia. *C,* Radiograph of the right kidney with vesicoureteral reflux during voiding cystourethrography demonstrates three calyces with few papillary impressions. *D,* Longitudinal right renal ultrasound scan demonstrates lack of corticomedullary distinction of this mildly small kidney.

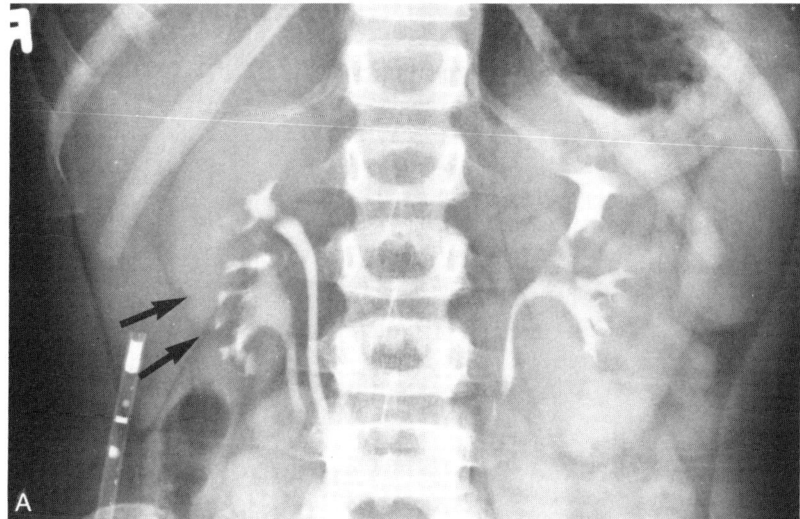

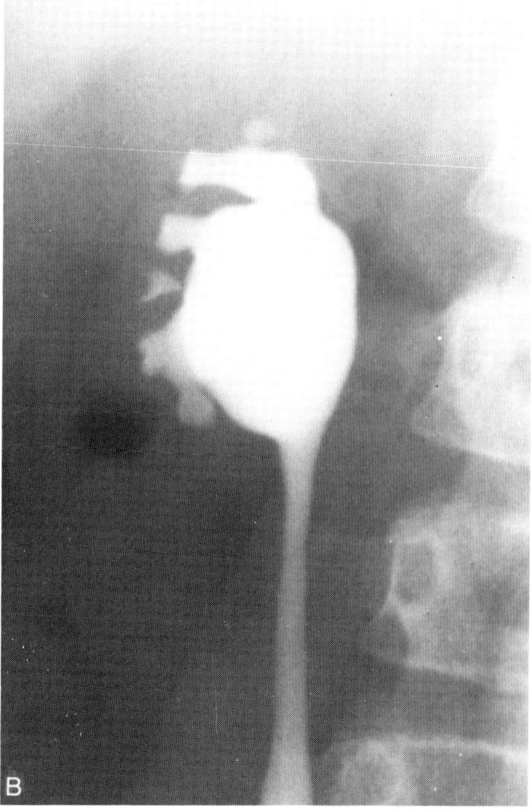

Figure 69–7. Complete duplex collecting system with lower pole reflux nephropathy. *A,* Intravenous urogram demonstrates multifocal renal parenchymal scarring and calyceal clubbing *(arrows)* isolated to the lower pole of the right duplex collecting system, the "nubbin sign." *B,* Voiding cystourethrogram reveals vesicoureteral reflux into the lower pole of the right renal collecting system, permitting lower pole reflux nephropathy. This proves complete duplication of the right collecting system because reflux would occur into both upper and lower poles with incomplete duplication.

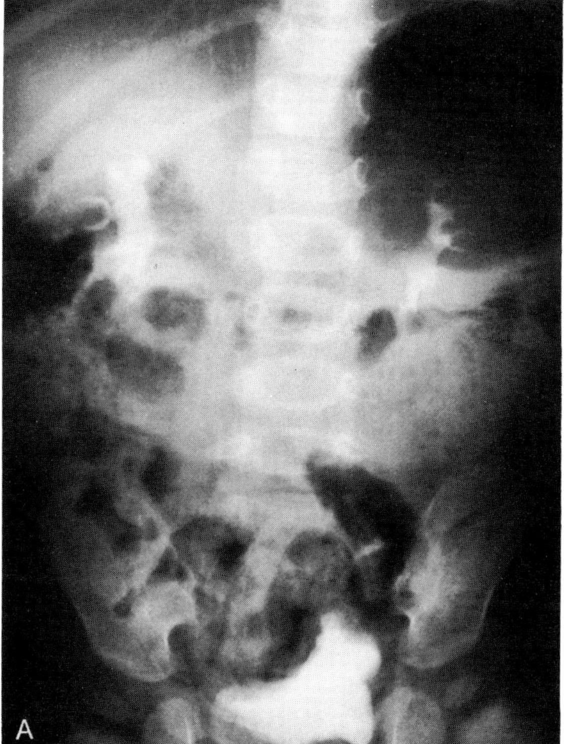

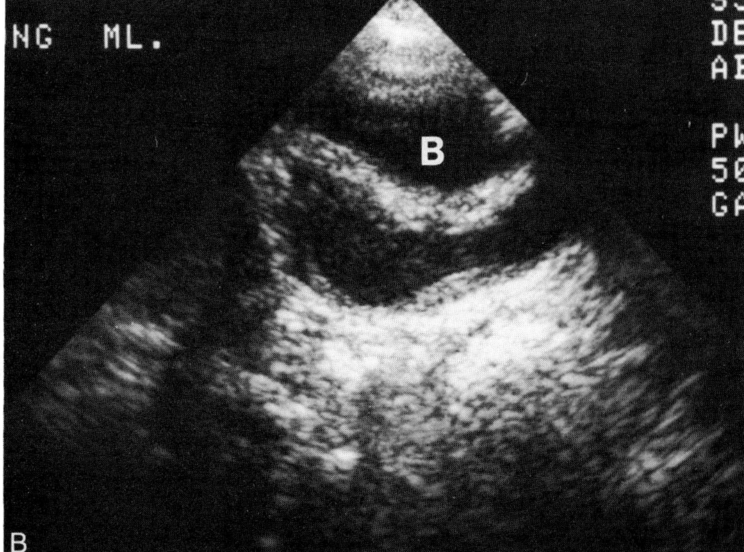

Figure 69–8. Vaginal ectopic ureter. Six-month-old female with vaginal discharge. *A,* Intravenous urogram reveals subtle lateral displacement of the upper pole of the right kidney. *B,* Longitudinal pelvic ultrasonogram demonstrates the dilated, thick-walled retrovesical ectopic ureter extending below the bladder (B) with echogenic luminal debris *(small arrows).*

Simple ureteroceles are more commonly discovered in adults than in children and in adults are usually small with little or no obstruction. However, in children they more frequently lead to severe hydroureteronephrosis and require reimplantation or nephroureterectomy.

ECTOPIC URETEROCELE

Ectopic ureteroceles are more common in children than simple ureteroceles (4:1), almost invariably involve the upper pole of a complete duplex collecting system, and are located distal to the trigone with the orifice at the bladder neck or urethra. It is the most common cause of severe lower urinary tract obstruction in girls and is bilateral in 10 per cent. The main types are stenotic (40 per cent), sphincteric (40 per cent), and sphincterostenotic (5 per cent), with other types rarely encountered (cecoureterocele, blind ectopic ureterocele, and nonobstructive ectopic ureterocele). Patients usually present in the first year of life with urinary tract infection; however, failure to thrive, an abdominal mass, or prolapse of the ureterocele through the urethra may occur.

In the typical ectopic ureterocele (Fig. 69–9), the upper pole of the complete duplex collecting system functions poorly because of either severe obstruction or associated dysplasia. Ultrasonography, CT, or MRI (Fig. 69–9*D*) can demonstrate the hydronephrotic upper pole with a dilated ureter, and usually shows the ureterocele in the bladder (Fig. 69–9*C*). The diagnosis of ectopic ureterocele may be

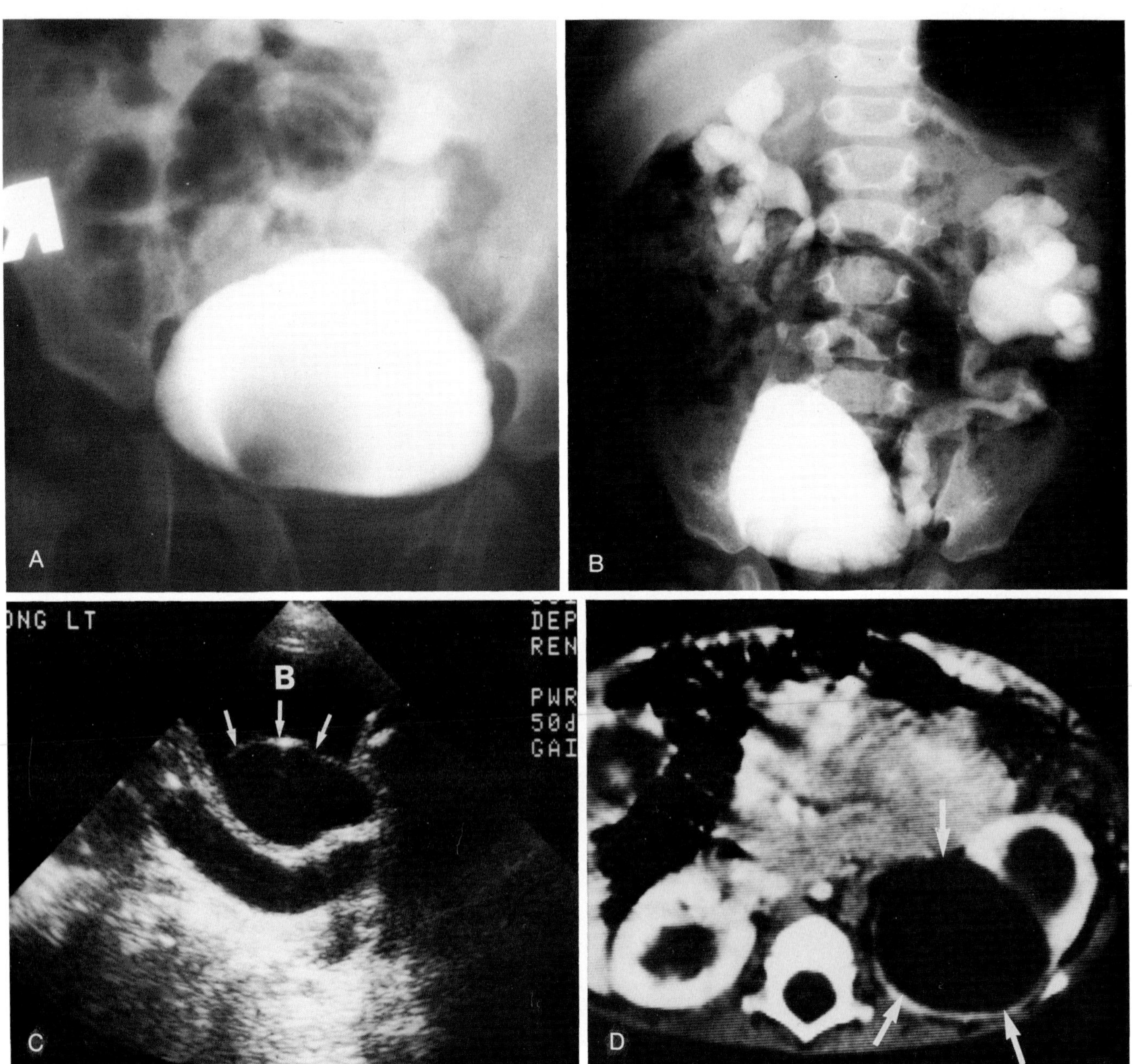

Figure 69–9. Ectopic ureterocele. Seven-month-old female with urinary tract infection. *A,* Cystogram reveals a radiolucent filling defect in the bladder. There was reflux into the left lower pole of this complete duplex collecting system. *B,* Intravenous urogram reveals lateral and inferior displacement of the visualized lower pole of the left kidney. There is a tortuous lower pole left ureter that is winding around the nonopacified upper pole ureter. The ureterocele is not visualized because contrast is not opacifying the posterior aspect of the bladder on this prone film. *C,* Longitudinal ultrasonogram of the pelvis reveals the dilated left upper pole ureter ending in the ureterocele *(arrows),* which projects into the bladder lumen (B). *D,* CT scan demonstrates direct visualization of the medially deployed dilated left upper pole collecting system *(arrows).*

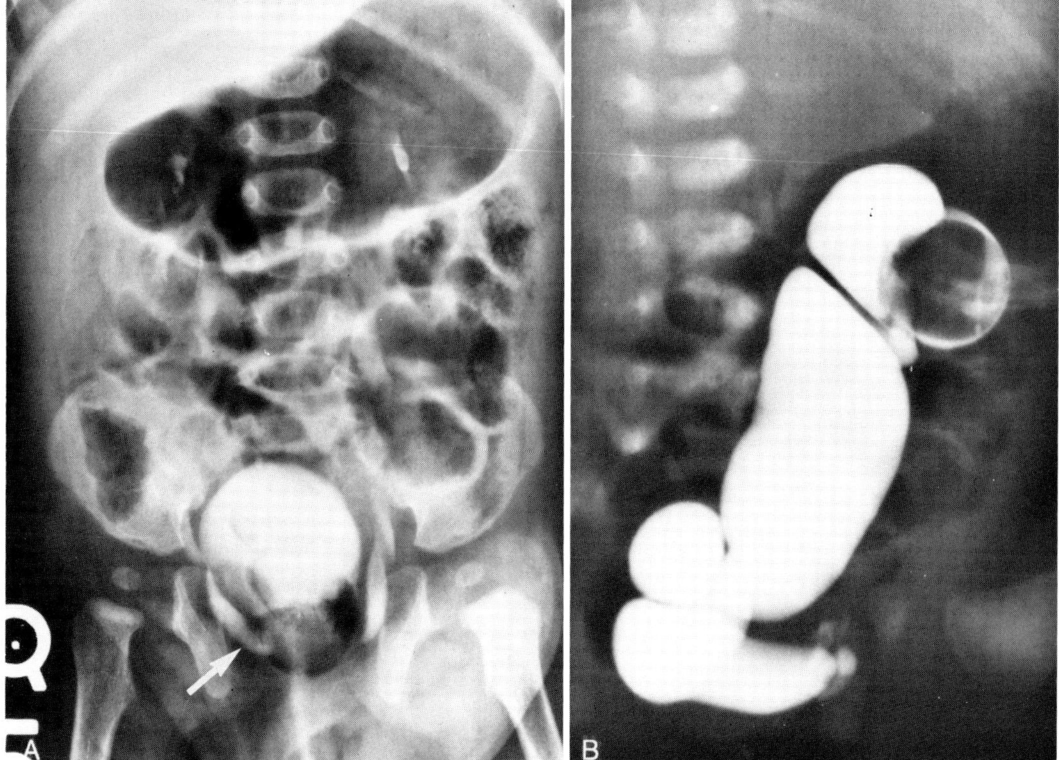

Figure 69–10. Typical bladder exstrophy reveals widening of the pubic symphysis and the "hockey stick" appearance of the distal ureters *(arrow)*. The upper urinary tracts are normal. The bladder has been turned in, allowing visualization of the bladder lumen. *B*, Antegrade pyelogram in **cloacal exstrophy** reveals a dysmorphic left kidney with no visualized calyces and a markedly hydronephrotic, tortuous ureter emptying through a stenotic orifice on the perineum. This anomalous appearance is to be contrasted with bladder exstrophy, in which the upper urinary tracts are normal.

difficult if the upper pole ureter is not dilated, if massive dilatation obscures the lower pole parenchyma, or if the ureterocele is not recognized owing to bladder distention. However, several signs aid in the urographic diagnosis:

1. Contralateral duplication (30 to 50 per cent).
2. Displacement of the lower pole parenchyma and ureter laterally by the hydronephrotic upper pole collecting system ("drooping lily" appearance).
3. Decreased number of calyces in the lower pole, with a notch at the junction of the upper and lower pole parenchyma.
4. Characteristic corkscrew appearance of the lower pole ureter owing to its close association with the dilated and tortuous obstructed upper ureter (Fig. 69–9*B*).
5. Radiolucent filling defect of the ectopic ureterocele in the bladder on a supine film of the partially filled bladder (Fig. 69–9*A*).

Voiding cystourethrography will demonstrate the ureterocele if a small amount of contrast is infused into the bladder so as not to obscure the ureterocele. The ureterocele may evert or intussuscept into its own ureter if the intraluminal bladder pressure exceeds that of the ureterocele or may prolapse into the urethra to cause bladder outlet obstruction and bilateral hydronephrosis. Reflux into the lower pole ureter frequently occurs (50 per cent) as in other complete duplex collecting systems. This may be caused by lack of muscular support in the bladder or by the mass effect of the ureterocele.

The surgical approach to ectopic ureteroceles depends on the functional status of the obstructed upper pole (which can be determined by radionuclide scanning) and the degree of reflux. If no salvageable upper pole function is present, upper pole heminephroureterectomy with decompression of the ureterocele from above is performed. With salvageable function, a pyelopyelostomy or common sheath reimplantation can be performed depending on the status of the lower pole reflux. Reflux will frequently resolve with heminephroureterectomy and ureterocele decompression. Occasionally, ureterocele incision may be used as a temporary procedure to relieve obstruction or to drain an infected, obstructed system. Total nephroureterectomy may be necessary if both upper and lower poles do not have salvageable function.

LOWER URINARY TRACT ANOMALIES

Exstrophy-Epispadias Complex

Exstrophy of the bladder (1 in 30,000 births) is due to failure of fusion of the midline mesodermal elements of the infraumbilical anterior abdominal wall. Defects involving only the urethra and sphincter produce *epispadias*, whereas a more extreme form is *exstrophy of the cloaca.*

Clinically, exstrophy and epispadias are obvious in the male, in whom either the bladder lies everted on the lower abdominal wall with the ureteral orifices visible or the mucosal surface of the urethra is exposed. Female epispadias is more occult clinically and can present as an undiagnosed cause of wetting. In bladder exstrophy (Fig. 69–10*A*), diastasis of the pubic symphysis and outward rotation of the innominate and iliac bones are obvious on a plain radiograph. In epispadias, there is mild widening of the symphysis pubis (greater than 10 mm). The upper urinary tracts are normal at birth in bladder exstrophy and epispadias, but the lower ureters typically have a "hockey stick" appearance.

Surgical correction of bladder exstrophy is a staged procedure. Closure of the abdominal wall can be accomplished in the neonatal period by manual compression of the iliac bones or assisted by iliac osteotomies, converting bladder exstrophy to the anatomy of epispadias. This can be accomplished only if the bladder is adequate in size. Otherwise, cystectomy is necessary to prevent later bladder malignancy. Surgery to correct vesicoureteral reflux (which is universal), create continence, reconstruct the urethra, and augment the bladder is accomplished in early childhood. Some patients still require upper tract diversion if the above procedures fail. Serial imaging studies are necessary to detect postoperative complications such as hydronephrosis, reflux, pyelonephritis, stones, small bladder capacity, or bladder malignancy (4 to 7.5 per cent of turned-in bladders).

Cloacal exstrophy is even rarer (Fig. 69–10*B*) and differs from bladder exstrophy in the local manifestations (terminal ileum and atretic colon prolapse in addition to bifid exstrophied bladder), associated anomalies (lipomyelomeningocele, genital anomalies, omphalocele, imperforate anus, vertebral segmentation anomalies), and upper urinary tract anomalies (60 per cent). Hydronephrosis, ectopia, and agenesis are common.

Bladder Diverticula

Bladder diverticula consist of herniation of bladder mucosa through congenital defects in the muscle and fascia of the bladder wall. Most bladder diverticula are therefore primary in nature, although bladder outlet obstruction (posterior urethral valves, neurogenic dysfunction) may worsen a pre-existing congenital diverticulum. The majority of diverticula are located at the ureterovesical junction, where they are called Hutch diverticula. Those at the dome of the bladder are called urachal diverticula. A ureterocele may evert and cause a diverticulum. Secondary causes of bladder diverticula include ureteral reimplantation, suprapubic tube placement, and enlargement of remnants of rectovesical fistulae in patients with imperforate anus. Diverticula can be seen in syndromes such as prune belly, Menke's kinky hair, Williams, Ehlers-Danlos, and cutis laxa.

Most bladder diverticula in children are incidental but are of clinical importance if they (1) cause urine stasis with the potential development of infection, bleeding, or stones; (2) have the same orifice as the ureter, which leads to vesicoureteral reflux that will be unlikely to resolve; or (3) become so large that they obstruct the ureter or bladder outlet. The rare neonatal bladder diverticulum can be a difficult diagnosis because of anatomic distortion and poor renal function and leads to significant morbidity.

In any clinical situation in which bladder diverticula may present (urinary tract infection, hematuria, voiding difficulties, unexplained ureteral dilatation down to the bladder) a fluoroscopically controlled voiding cystourethrography will best exclude bladder diverticula as the cause. Most large bladder diverticula should be removed. However, if a paraureteral diverticulum is associated with vesicoureteral reflux, cystoscopy may be necessary to determine the relation of the diverticulum to the ureteral orifice. If the ureter enters into the diverticulum, reflux will likely continue and may require reimplantation with diverticulectomy, whereas if the ureter enters beside the diverticulum, reflux will frequently disappear spontaneously.

Urachal Disorders

The urachus is the normal embryologic remnant of the connection between the allantois and the bladder and persists as a narrow cord between the umbilicus and bladder dome. Congenital urachal disorders are manifestations of arrested developmental regression of the urachus and may present in four forms. *Patent urachus* usually presents in the newborn with discharge of urine from the umbilicus and represents an open communication from the bladder to the umbilicus. This condition may be associated with urethral obstruction or prune belly syndrome but can be seen in normal infants. Voiding cystourethrography or direct injection will demonstrate the connection. *Urachal cyst* (Fig. 69–11) is an encapsulation of fluid within a urachus that has closed at both bladder and umbilical ends and frequently presents infected. The patient presents with a palpable mass, abdominal pain, fever, and urinary tract infection. The diagnosis can be made with ultrasonography and computed tomography, although cystography is necessary to evaluate the entire urachus. *Urachal sinus* exists when only the urachal apex persists and presents with umbilical discharge. The patient should be evaluated with cystography as well as direct injection of the urachal sinus. In *urachal diverticulum,* only the vesical end of the urachus remains open and is nicely demonstrated with voiding cystourethrography. A wide-mouthed urachal diverticulum is seen typically in prune belly syndrome or urethral obstruction and may be calcified at birth.

Posterior Urethral Valves

Posterior urethral valves (PUV) represent the most common obstructive anomaly of the male urethra. Young, in 1919, originally described three types of posterior urethral valves, but the existence of type II and III valves is controversial and only type I valves will be considered here. Type I valves attach to the urethral wall along the distal portion of the verumontanum, and their margins fuse centrally from dorsal to ventral to form a variable-sized aperture along the ventral aspect of the urethra. Embryologically, PUV are felt to represent remnants of the mesonephric duct fusion with the urogenital sinus.

PUV range from nonobstructive to highly obstructive. This accounts for the variable pathology and clinical presentation of this disease. Approximately half of the patients with significant urethral obstruction present in the neonatal period. Typically, bilateral flank masses with a distended bladder and urinary dribbling will be present. Ultrasonography will demonstrate bilateral hydroureteronephrosis with parenchymal thinning and a thick-walled bladder, either in utero or ex utero. Voiding cystourethrography is diagnostic, demonstrating bladder trabeculations and diverticula, dilatation of the posterior urethra, ballooning of the valve membranes distally, an eccentric caliber change in the urethral stream ventrally, and a post-voiding residue (Fig. 69–12*A*). Forty to 60 per cent will have vesicoureteral reflux that predisposes to cystic renal dysplasia (type IV cystic disease of Potter). This can be suspected if ultrasonography shows parenchymal cysts or increased echogenicity, or if the kidney functions poorly after successful treatment of the valves. Other complications include urosepsis, urinary ascites, perirenal urinoma (Fig. 69–12*B*), and electrolyte problems with renal tubular acidosis, salt-losing nephropathy, and nephrogenic diabetes insipidus. Initial management includes antibiotics, fluid and electrolyte therapy, and decompression of the urinary tract. Bladder catheters may be sufficient for decompression, although percutaneous nephrostomy, cutaneous ureterostomy, or vesicostomy may be necessary for deteriorating renal function or persistent infection.

With lesser degrees of obstruction, the patient may present later in childhood with urinary tract infection, voiding dysfunction, or chronic retention with failure to thrive. In this situation, or eventually in the sick neonate, the valves are fulgurated for treatment. Reflux will resolve in approximately 50 per cent of those with successful valve treatment. Complications after valve fulguration include urethral stricture (8–50 per cent), post-obstructive diuresis, incontinence, and secondary ureterovesical junction obstruction.

Patients must be imaged postoperatively in a serial fashion, frequently employing urography, voiding cystourethrography, ultrasonography, and nuclear imaging. Prognosis relates to the initial degree of renal damage, presence of renal dysplasia, correction of obstruction, and avoidance of infection. Reconstruction of the urinary tract, including diversion, reimplantation of the ureters, and nephroureterectomy for renal dysplasia, may be necessary. Of those

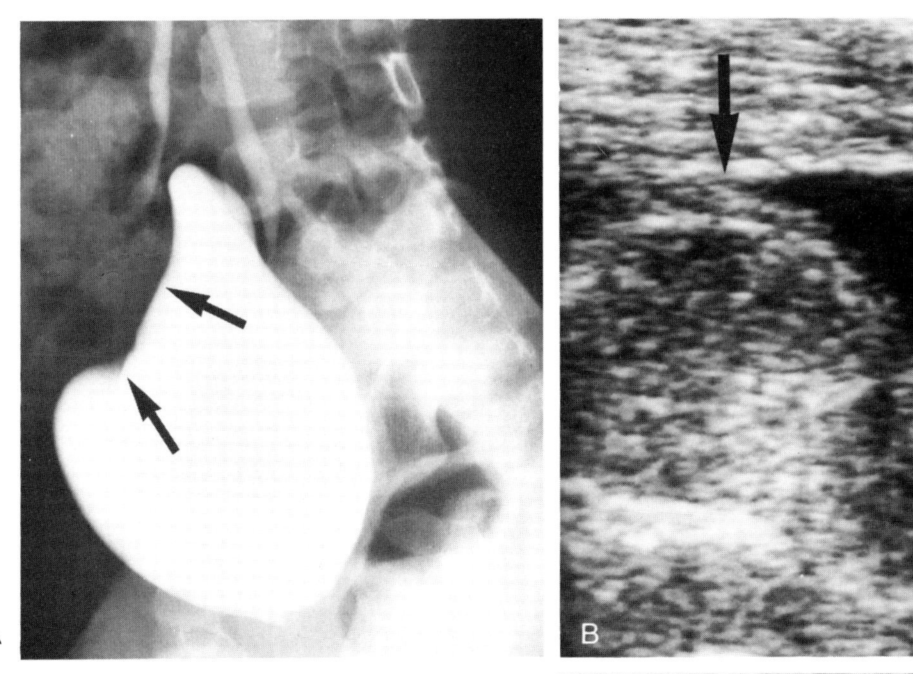

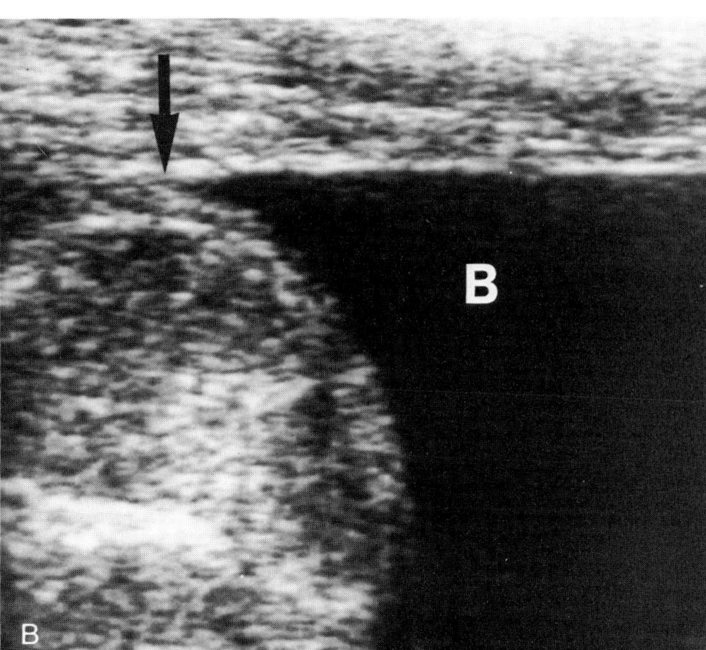

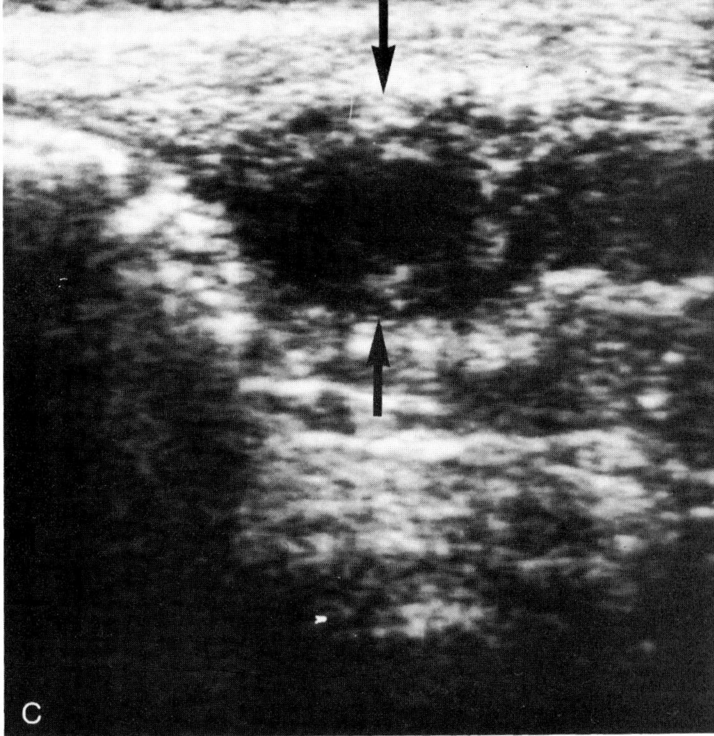

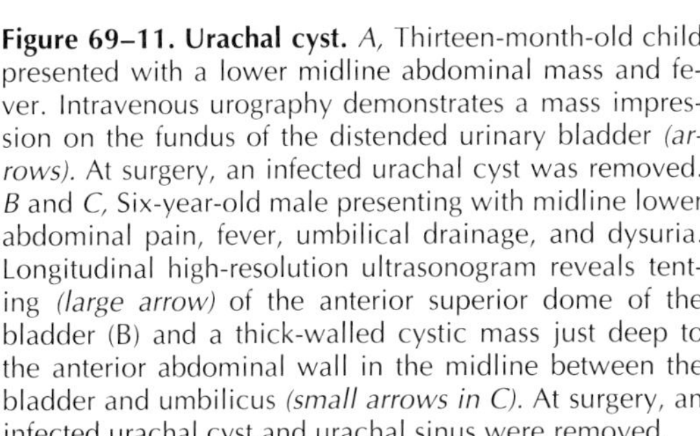

Figure 69–11. Urachal cyst. *A,* Thirteen-month-old child presented with a lower midline abdominal mass and fever. Intravenous urography demonstrates a mass impression on the fundus of the distended urinary bladder *(arrows).* At surgery, an infected urachal cyst was removed. *B* and *C,* Six-year-old male presenting with midline lower abdominal pain, fever, umbilical drainage, and dysuria. Longitudinal high-resolution ultrasonogram reveals tenting *(large arrow)* of the anterior superior dome of the bladder (B) and a thick-walled cystic mass just deep to the anterior abdominal wall in the midline between the bladder and umbilicus *(small arrows in C).* At surgery, an infected urachal cyst and urachal sinus were removed.

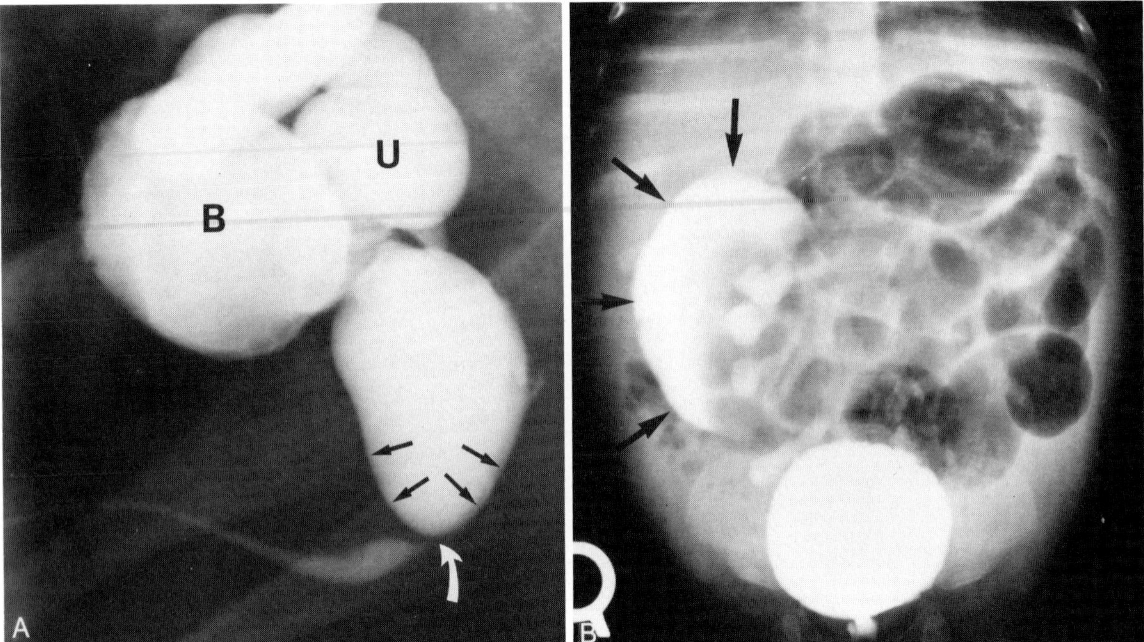

Figure 69–12. Posterior urethral valves. *A,* Voiding cystourethrography (VCUG) reveals dilatation of the posterior urethra with valves ballooning distally *(arrows)* and a ventrally eccentric opening in the valves *(curved arrow).* Vesicoureteral reflux and reflux into prostatic ducts are seen (U = ureter; B = bladder). *B,* Post-void film following the VCUG demonstrates subcapsular extravasation around the right kidney *(arrows),* probably from a ruptured calyceal fornix. This may progress to perirenal urinoma or urinary ascites. This kidney functioned poorly in follow-up after successful valve fulguration, probably from underlying renal dysplasia.

with hydroureteronephrosis, approximately 60 per cent will eventually show normal renal function.

MISCELLANEOUS DISORDERS

Hydrometrocolpos

Hydrometrocolpos, the third most common abdominal mass in the neonate, is dilatation of the uterus and/or vagina from congenital obstruction of the vagina and accumulation of cervical secretions. *Imperforate hymen* is a common cause of this condition and will present as an abdominopelvic mass either in the neonatal period or during adolescence when menses begin. Other than hydronephrosis from ureteral compression, there are no associated abnormalities with imperforate hymen, and incision of the obstructing membrane is curative.

A more serious etiology of hydrometrocolpos is *vaginal atresia* in the middle to upper third of the vagina with or without urogenital sinus or cloacal abnormalities. Obviously, the surgical reconstruction of the perineum is challenging and requires precise delineation of the pelvic organs and orifices by radiographic contrast injections. However, there is a high incidence of other anomalies such as renal hypoplasia and agenesis, bicornuate uterus, ectopic ureter, imperforate anus, and congenital heart disease. These associated anomalies must be delineated because they cause increased morbidity and mortality in these patients. Delay in diagnosis may result in infection, with pyometrocolpos. Rarely, fluid from the hydrometrocolpos refluxes into the peritoneal cavity via the fallopian tubes and causes adhesive, plastic peritonitis.

Ultrasonography or MRI scanning can provide a confident diagnosis by demonstrating a vagina and/or uterus distended with cystic or echogenic material representing urine and uterovaginal secretions and will also show the associated hydronephrosis and upper urinary tract anomalies. Combined contrast examinations of the rectum, vagina, and bladder are necessary when urogenital sinus or cloacal abnormalities are associated findings.

Prune Belly Syndrome

Prune belly syndrome classically occurs in males with a triad of abdominal wall muscular deficiency, cryptorchidism, and urinary tract abnormalities. Pathologically, the kidneys in this uncommon disorder show hypoplasia and dysplasia with the ureters and bladder showing dilatation with patchy absence of smooth muscle and replacement by fibrous connective tissue. One proposed etiology explaining the concordant absent abdominal wall and urinary tract musculature is a disorder of mesodermal development. Alternatively, it has been suggested that the abdominal wall musculature deficiency is secondary to in utero abdominal distention with subsequent muscular atrophy, and that the primary abnormality is in utero urethral obstruction with secondary hydronephrosis and secondary musculature atrophy.

The pathologic spectrum of urinary tract involvement in prune belly syndrome is quite broad, ranging from absent or mild to severe hydronephrosis. The kidneys range from normal size with mild dysmorphism to gross distortion of form, poor function, or even multicystic dysplasia (Fig. 69–13*A*). The ureters are extremely tortuous and usually quite dilated with poor peristalsis. Vesicoureteral reflux is present in many but not all cases. The bladder is of large capacity, although it functions surprisingly well. The bladder outline is undulating, frequently demonstrating a urachal or other diverticulum (Fig. 69–13*B*). The posterior urethra usually has a tapering dilatation down to the membranous urethra, where a variable constriction or even atresia occurs (Fig. 69–13*C*). Posterior urethral valves are not a common occurrence. Occasionally, a megalourethra is present, resulting from deficiency of the corpus spongiosum or coexisting deficiency of the corpora cavernosa. Associated anomalies are important, including microcephaly, imperforate anus, malrotation, congenital heart disease, congenital hip dislocation, scoliosis, and club feet.

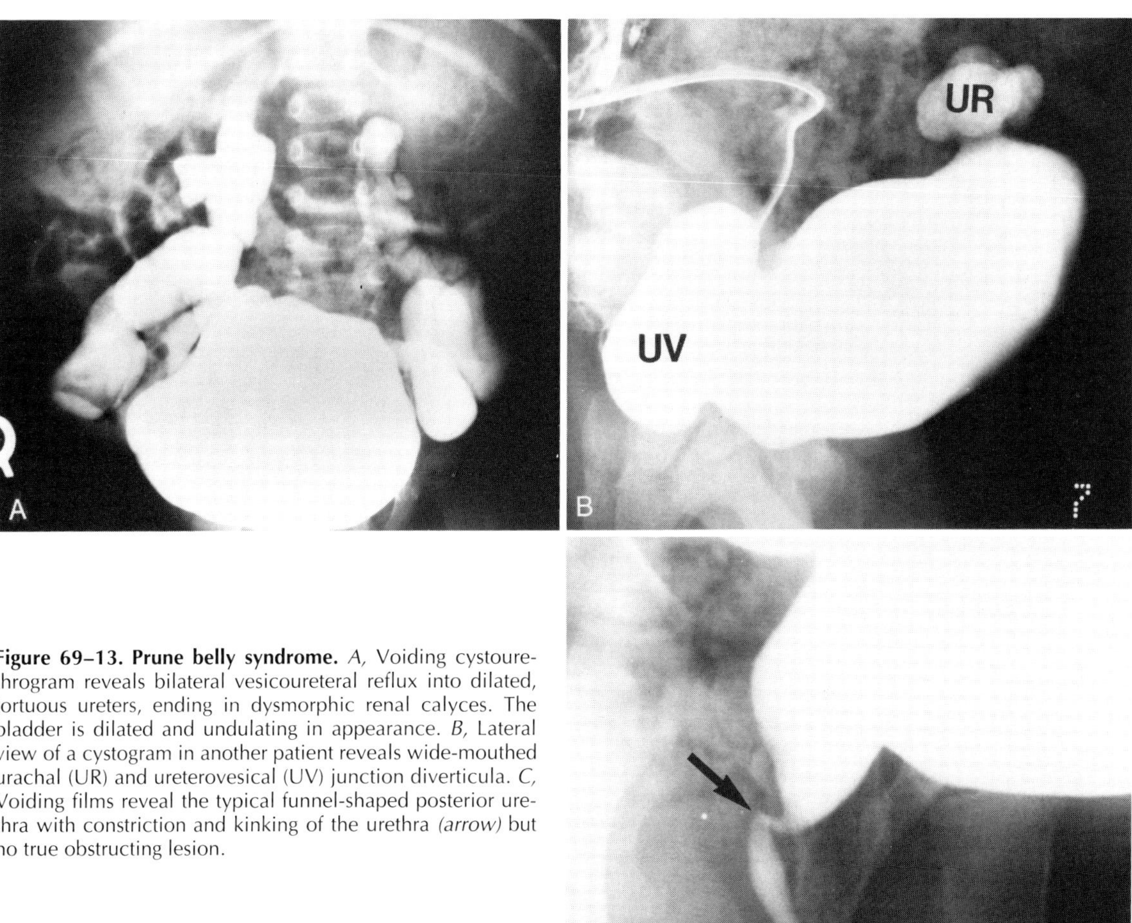

Figure 69–13. Prune belly syndrome. *A,* Voiding cystourethrogram reveals bilateral vesicoureteral reflux into dilated, tortuous ureters, ending in dysmorphic renal calyces. The bladder is dilated and undulating in appearance. *B,* Lateral view of a cystogram in another patient reveals wide-mouthed urachal (UR) and ureterovesical (UV) junction diverticula. *C,* Voiding films reveal the typical funnel-shaped posterior urethra with constriction and kinking of the urethra *(arrow)* but no true obstructing lesion.

Clinically, the severity of the urinary tract anomalies determines the prognosis. With extreme disease, the patients have pulmonary hypoplasia typical of Potter's syndrome and die of respiratory failure with pneumothorax and pneumomediastinum soon after birth. Patients with lesser degrees of disease may develop early renal failure, with superimposed infection having disastrous consequences. However, the majority of neonates with this disease survive infancy, although frequent atelectasis and pneumonia occur. Close urologic follow-up is mandatory. Various surgical procedures may be necessary with time, including urethrotomy, reduction cystoplasty, ureteral reimplantation, nephroureterectomy, urinary diversion, orchiopexy, and plication of the abdominal wall.

Intersex

The evaluation of the newborn with ambiguous genitalia is one of the most complicated challenges in medicine. Genetic sex, gonadal sex, and phenotypic sex may be abnormal and quite confused in these patients. Several basic embryologic and hormonal aspects of normal genital development are important in understanding these disorders: (1) sex chromosomes are important in gonadal differentiation, (2) internal and external genitalia tend to follow a female pattern in the absence of gonads, and (3) the testes have a dual role in masculinizing the external genitalia and in promoting ipsilateral involution of the müllerian ducts.

The goals in evaluating a newborn with ambiguous genitalia are to define the underlying diagnosis, determine the precise anatomy of the internal genitalia, assign the sex of rearing (with major consideration being achievement of functional genitalia), and, when necessary, determine the gonadal histology by biopsy. Appropriate investigation includes a carefully performed history and physical examination, chromosomal evaluation, hormonal evaluation, gonadal biopsy when indicated, and evaluation of the urogenital sinus and internal genitalia by genitography and ultrasonography. Ultrasonography has largely replaced clinical examination under anesthesia in evaluating the internal genitalia. With this information, the four most common disorders producing ambiguous genitalia in the newborn can be diagnosed: (1) female pseudohermaphroditism, (2) male pseudohermaphroditism, (3) true hermaphroditism, and (4) mixed gonadal dysgenesis.

Female pseudohermaphroditism is a disorder of phenotypic sexual differentiation in which 46XX individuals with ovaries differentiate partially as phenotypic males. It usually results from virilization of a female embryo with congenital adrenal hyperplasia and is the most common cause of ambiguous genitalia in the newborn. At birth, there is usually clitoral hypertrophy with variable fusion of the labioscrotal folds and differing degrees of virilization of the urethra. Diagnosis must be expedited to avoid consequences of hydrocortisone or mineralocorticoid deficiency. Most patients are reared in the gender of chromosomal and gonadal sex.

Male pseudohermaphroditism is a disorder in which genetic males with bilateral testes differentiate partially or completely as phenotypic females. It can result from defects in either androgen synthesis, androgen action, or müllerian duct regression. The expression of this subset of disorders of sexual differentiation is quite variable and requires detailed biochemical evaluation. Testicular feminization syndrome, a common form of male pseudohermaphroditism, is caused by target tissue androgen resistance, and is a common cause of primary amenorrhea (after gonadal dysgenesis and congenital absence of the vagina). Although the external genitalia are those of a normal female, the vagina is a vestigial blind pouch with no uterus or cervix. The testes may be intra-abdominal or located anywhere along the anatomic pathway of normal descent. In the neonatal period, these patients usually present as phenotypic females with testes and inguinal hernias.

True hermaphroditism is a rare condition in which both an ovary and a testis are present, or a gonad with histologic features of both (ovotestis) is present. Most patients are masculinized to some degree, with 60 to 75 per cent being reared as males although the majority have XX chromosomes. Almost all patients have a urogenital sinus, and in most cases a uterus is present (the internal ducts usually correspond to the adjacent gonad). In males, menstruation may present as cyclic hematuria. Gonadal biopsy is necessary for final diagnosis.

In *mixed gonadal dysgenesis,* a phenotypic male or female has a testis on one side and a streak gonad on the other. It is the second most common cause of ambiguous genitalia in the newborn. It usually presents with an enlarged phallus and a urogenital sinus. The majority have 45,XO/46,XY mosaic chromosomes, all have a uterus and vagina, and most are reared as females. One third have somatic stigmata of Turner's syndrome. Gonadal tumors develop in approximately 25 per cent of patients (seminomas, gonadoblastomas, dysgerminomas, and embryonal carcinomas), so that prophylactic gonadectomy is usually advised.

The precise delineation of the genital anatomy by imaging studies in patients with ambiguous genitalia is important for determining the underlying diagnosis, sex assignment, and preoperative evaluation. Genitography is accomplished by retrograde injection of water-soluble contrast material through the perineal orifice with a closed system present. Either a blunt-ended syringe or a No. 8 French catheter placed through a nipple feeder can be an effective system to employ. Important features to delineate are the length of the urogenital sinus, the length of the urethra and presence of a verumontanum, and the size of the vagina and the presence of a cervical impression on the vagina (which provides incontrovertible evidence for the presence of a uterus) (Fig. 69–14*B*). Voiding cystourethrography is sometimes of supplemental value. Ultrasonography is quite valuable in demonstrating the presence of the uterus (Fig. 69–14*A*), with the gonads being somewhat more difficult to identify.

The most common appearance on genitography and ultrasonography is that seen in a female pseudohermaphrodite with congenital adrenal hyperplasia. There is a long urogenital sinus, a short urethra, and a normal-appearing vagina and cervical impression (occasionally reflux into the uterus and fallopian tubes is seen). Ultrasonography will demonstrate a uterus (which is normally prominent in newborns due to maternal estrogen stimulation), vagina, and ovaries. With progressive masculinization, the urogenital sinus gets longer, a verumontanum begins to be evident, the vagina gets smaller, and the uterus gets smaller. Finally, variable degrees of hypospadias exist, with the urethral orifice located somewhere between the shaft of the penis and the perineum, and a prominent utriculus masculinus (a remnant of the müllerian structures representing the proximal two thirds of the vagina) is present. The findings on genitography and ultrasonography are not specific for the individual disorders of sexual differentiation; however, the precise internal anatomy is quite important in gender assignment and preoperative evaluation.

Congenital Absence of the Vagina (Mayer-Rokitansky-Kuster-Hauser Syndrome)

The combination of congenital absence of the vagina with some form of abnormal or absent uterus is second only to gonadal dysgenesis as a cause of primary amenorrhea. The external genitalia and remainder of the phenotype are normal female, but on exami-

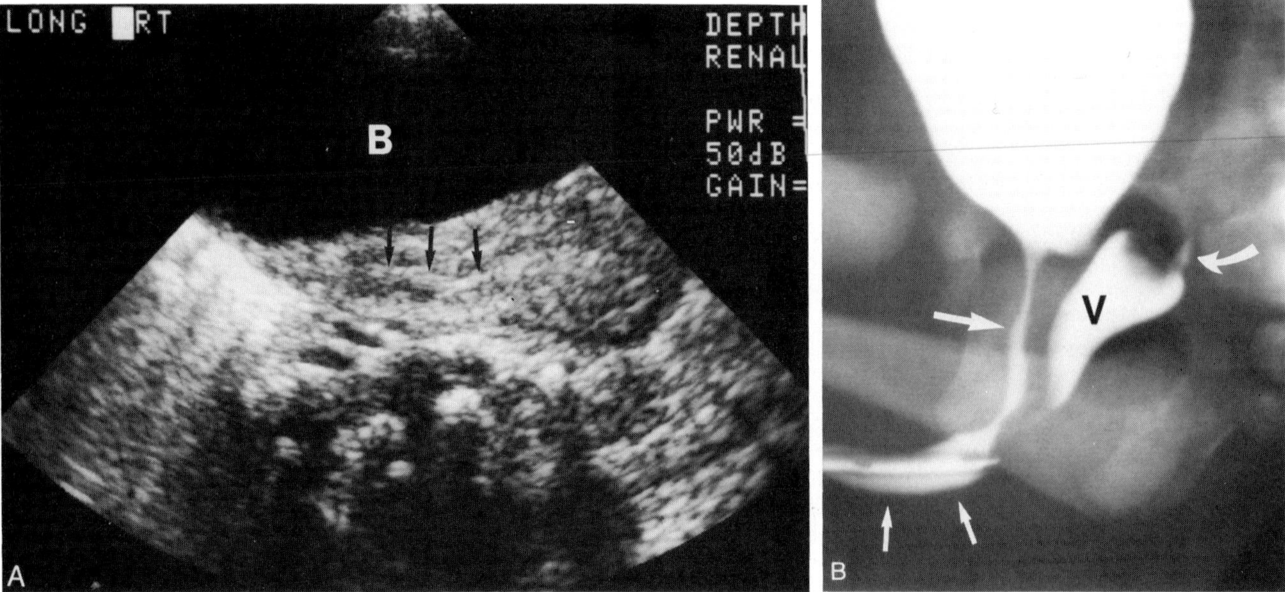

Figure 69–14. Female pseudohermaphrodite with congenital adrenal hyperplasia. The patient presented as a newborn with phallic enlargement and a single perineal orifice. *A,* Longitudinal midline pelvic ultrasonogram reveals a normal infantile uterus behind the bladder (B). Note the endocervical and endometrial canals *(arrows).* The cervical portion of the uterus is larger than the body and fundus, an expected appearance at this age. *B,* Genitography by retrograde injection reveals the urogenital sinus *(arrows),* vagina (V), and urethra *(long arrow).* Possible reflux into the uterine canal was seen *(curved arrow).*

nation only a rudimentary distal vaginal pouch is present. The ovaries and fallopian tubes are present, and ovarian function is generally normal. Approximately one third of patients have renal anomalies, with renal agenesis and ectopia being most common. Skeletal anomalies occur in 12 per cent, with vertebral segmentation anomalies or even Klippel-Feil syndrome being present.

The exact pathogenesis of this disorder is not clear. The origin of the müllerian duct, which is the anlage of the uterus, fallopian tubes, and upper two thirds of the vagina, has two components. The cephalic portion gives rise to the fallopian tubes, and the caudal end, which is derived from the mesonephric duct, gives rise to the uterus and upper two thirds of the vagina. Failure of development of the caudal end of the müllerian duct can account for the genital abnormalities in this syndrome. It is believed that a mesodermal defect could account for the vertebral segmentation anomalies and interference with the mesonephric duct, the latter leading to renal anomalies and the absent uterus and proximal two thirds of the vagina. Chromosomal analysis may be necessary to exclude the testicular feminization syndrome, which can have a similar presentation. Ultrasonography or MRI scanning will demonstrate the absent uterus, presence of the ovaries, and absence of hydrocolpos, confirming the diagnosis.

Bibliography

Blask ARN, Sanders RC, Gearhart JP: Obstructed uterovaginal anomalies: Demonstration with sonography. Part I. Neonates and infants. Radiology 179:79, 1991.

Blask ARN, Sanders RC, Rock JA: Obstructed uterovaginal anomalies: Demonstration with sonography. Part II. Teenagers. Radiology 179:84, 1991.

Blyth B, Duckett JW: Gonadal differentiation: A review of the physiological process and influencing factors based on recent experimental evidence. J Urol 145:689, 1991.

Boechat MI, Lebowitz RL: Diverticula of the bladder in children. Pediatr Radiol 7:22, 1978.

Burbige KA, Amodio J, Berdon WE, et al: Prune belly syndrome: 35 years of experience. J Urol 137:86, 1987.

Curtis JA, Pollack HM: Renal duplication with a diminutive lower pole: The nubbin sign. Radiology 131:327, 1979.

Chaim W, Kammehl P, Kopernik G, Meizner I: Uterus didelphis with unilateral imperforate vagina and ipsilateral renal agenesis: The challenge of noninvasive diagnosis. J Clin Ultrasound 19:583, 1991.

DiSantis DJ, Siegel MJ, Katz ME: Simplified approach to umbilical remnant abnormalities. Radiographics 11:59, 1991.

Kleiner B, Filly RA, Mack L, Callen PW: Multicystic dysplastic kidney: Observations of contralateral disease in the fetal population. Radiology 161:27, 1986.

Laufer I, Griscom NT: Compensatory renal hypertrophy: Absence in utero and development in early life. AJR 113:464, 1971.

Louie A, Arger PH: Fetal genitourinary tract. Seminars in Roentgenology 25:342, 1990.

Lubat E, Hernanz-Schulman M, Genieser NB, et al: Sonography of the simple and complicated ipsilateral fused kidney. J Ultrasound Med 8:109, 1989.

MacPherson RI, Leithiser RE, Gordon L, Turner WR: Posterior urethral valves: An update and review. Radiographics 6:753, 1986.

Meglin AJ, Balotin RJ, Jelinek JS, et al: Cloacal exstrophy: Radiologic findings in 13 patients. AJR 155:1267, 1990.

Merguerian PA, McLorie GA, McMullin ND, et al: Continence in bladder exstrophy: Determinants of success. J Urol 145:350, 1991.

Nakayama DK, Harrison MR, Chinn DH, DeLorimier AA: The pathogenesis of prune belly. Am J Dis Child 138:843, 1984.

Nussbaum AR, Dorst JP, Jeffs RD, et al: Ectopic ureter and ureterocele: Their varied sonographic manifestations. Radiology 159:227, 1986.

Prewitt LH, Lebowitz RL: The single ectopic ureter. AJR 127:941, 1976.

Sanders RC, Hartman DS: The sonographic distinction between neonatal multicystic kidney and hydronephrosis. Radiology 151:621, 1984.

Sanders RC, Nussbaum AR, Solez K: Renal dysplasia: Sonographic findings. Radiology 167:623, 1988.

Shane JC, Lebowitz RL: The unsuspected double collecting system on imaging studies and at cystoscopy. AJR 155:561, 1990.

Smith SJ, Cass AS, Aliabadi H, et al: Unipapillary kidney: A case report and literature review. Urol Radiol 6:43, 1984.

Steffens J, Mast GJ, Braedel HU, et al: Segmental renal hypoplasia of vascular origin causing renal hypertension in a 3-year-old-girl. J Urol 146:826, 1991.

Stephens FD: The Mayer-Rokitansky Syndrome. J Urol 135:106, 1986.

Uehling PT, Gilbert E, Chesney R: Urologic implications of the Vater association. J Urol 129:352, 1983.

White D, Lebowitz RL: Exstrophy of the bladder. Radiol Clin North Am 15:93, 1977.

Wyly JB, Lebowitz RL: Refluxing urethral ectopic ureters: Recognition by the cyclic voiding cystourethrogram. AJR 142:1263, 1984.

70 Renal Infection

Stanford M. Goldman

With the advent of the newer imaging modalities, the dynamism of renal infection is just being appreciated. These new techniques allow for rapid, early diagnosis and have had a significant impact on management. There is a great deal of confusion in the terminology used for both acute and chronic infectious pyelonephritis. Many terms have no pathologic corollaries and are used differently by radiologists. There is a growing sentiment to abandon these terms and merely describe the degree of involvement (unifocal, multifocal, or diffuse) and its evolution. However, because this approach is not uniformly accepted, we have elected to use the current classification of these terms along with their evolution so that the reader will be better able to appreciate the meanings of these terms as they are currently used in the literature.

ACUTE INFECTIOUS PYELONEPHRITIS

Prior to the development of present-day antibiotics, hematogenous spread of gram-positive organisms such as *Staphylococcus* and *Streptococcus* was a major route for the development of renal infection. Although bacterial seeding of the kidney does occur in cases of septicemia, adequate treatment directed toward the infecting organism will usually leave the kidney without major sequelae. At present, ascending involvement of the kidney with a gram-negative organism, usually originating in colonic flora (*Escherichia coli, Proteus, Pseudomonas,* etc.), is believed to represent the major route of renal involvement. AIDS patients are also susceptible to these infections.

Anovulvar or anoscrotal flora obtain entrance to the urinary tract via the urethra. Because of the shortness of the urethra, urinary tract infections (UTI) are encountered far more frequently in females. Once bacteria are within the bladder, attempts at colonization are partially prevented by the constant flow of urine. On the other hand, many of the gram-negative bacteria have fimbria that attach to the mucosa and prevent their dislodgement.

Access to the kidney is secondary to pre-existent ureterovesical reflux. The theory that the reflux is secondary to the infection has been largely abandoned. Once bacteria are within the ureter, they enter the renal parenchyma predominantly through the upper or lower pole of the kidney. Anatomically, compound calyces are present more often in these locations and more readily permit bacteria to enter retrograde into the collecting tubules. Finally, infecting organisms may excrete an endotoxin that causes paralysis of the ureter and ureteral stasis, thus permitting further bacterial colonization.

Radiographically, acute pyelonephritis presents as a swollen kidney with poor filling of the calyceal system. This is secondary to the intrarenal outpouring of fluid and polymorphonuclear leukocytes as a result of the infection (Fig. 70–1*A*). Linear striations under the mucosa in the pelvis and ureter may be seen secondary to submucosal edema. A striated nephrogram also has been reported.

In some patients, the ureter will be poorly filled secondary to decreased renal excretion from an edematous kidney. In others, the ureter is noted to be dilated secondary to endotoxin-induced aperistalsis.

It should be noted that in many patients with acute pyelonephritis the urogram will be normal, and in uncomplicated cases urography is unnecessary in the acute stage. In boys, a work-up should be performed after the first infection abates (i.e., two to four weeks later). In girls, radiographic evaluation is sometimes delayed to the second documented episode of pyelonephritis.

In the past, an excretory urogram and a voiding cystourethrogram were performed in the initial work-up. Currently, ultrasound and/or nuclear medicine studies are recommended, especially in the pediatric population, in order to limit the patient's radiation exposure. A voiding cystourethrogram should also be included in the initial work-up.

On ultrasound, one most often demonstrates a swollen kidney with diminished echogenicity secondary to the edema. Rarely increased echogenicity is noted if hemorrhage occurs or if focal clumps of leukocytes are present. The renal pelvis is not dilated, thus excluding hydronephrosis. A ^{99m}Tc glucoheptonate or ^{99m}Tc MAG scan will show decreased or delayed isotope accumulation in the affected kidney while there is an increased uptake with indium-labeled white blood cells or gallium. On CT, a swollen kidney with poor uptake of contrast or a striated nephrogram is seen (Fig. 70–1*B*). These linear streaks represent a few overlapping contrast-filled tubules separated by other unopacified tubules. In many cases, alternating wedge-shaped areas (i.e., in a lobar distribution) of normal uptake are seen separated by similarly shaped areas of low attenuation. The latter are probably secondary to vasospasm, tubular obstruction, and/or interstitial edema. These areas may be shown to pick up contrast on delayed CT images. On occasion, perinephric extension with thickening of the perinephric septa and focal thickening of Gerota's fascia are noted. MRI is not of clinical value but may show an enlarged kidney with loss of corticomedullary junction definition.

As compared with the diffuse form described above, focal involvement is recognized as well, usually localized to the upper or lower pole of the involved kidney where the compound calyces are usually situated. The affected, wedge-shaped area is varyingly described as hypoechoic on ultrasound, hypodense on CT, or showing poor or no uptake of ^{99m}Tc diethylenetriaminepenta-acetic acid (DTPA), dimercaptosuccinic acid (DMSA), or mercaptoacetylglycl glyclglycene (MAG3). The latter two techniques are more sensitive than ultrasound. We prefer using the pathologic term, *acute focal infectious pyelonephritis,* for these cases, although other radiologists use *focal lobar nephronia* to describe this same entity to emphasize its lobar distribution. Still others use *focal bacterial nephritis* to describe the same localized pyelonephritis. Please note that the term *focal lobar nephronia* is also used by some uroradiologists to describe another stage of renal infection, also termed the *preabscess state,* described below.

ACUTE BACTERIAL NEPHRITIS (ABN)

ABN is a term popularized among radiologists by Talner and Davidson. However, it is not recognized as a separate pathologic entity by many uropathologists. In its original usage, ABN represented a severe acute or suppurative pyelonephritis. Today, the term *ABN* is most often used synonymously with an diffuse infectious pyelonephritis. However, as originally described, ABN was found in extremely ill, diabetic females, immunosuppressed individuals, and patients on steroids with absent or extremely poor function noted. On angiography, no flow is recognized in the renal cortex owing to the swelling, but instead there is shunting of flow into the medulla (the so-called Trueta phenomenon). The severe inflammatory cortical reaction of fluid and polymorphonuclear leukocytes will disappear if aggressive antibiotic therapy is instituted. A nephrectomy is contraindicated. The sequela is renal papillary necro-

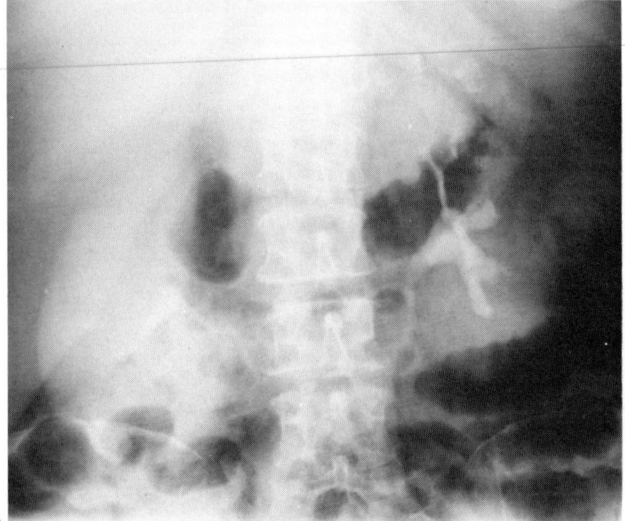

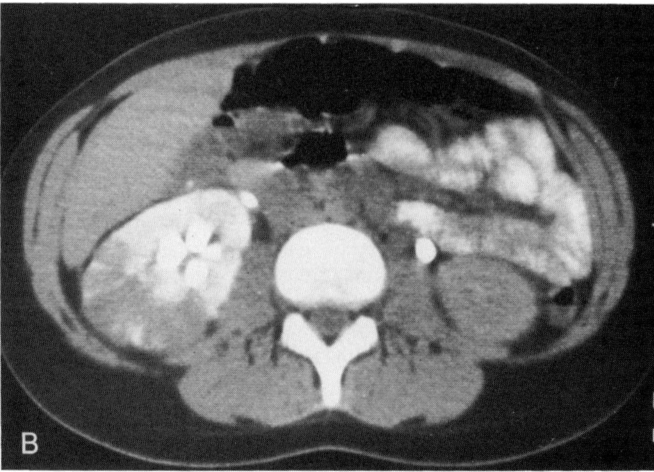

Figure 70–1. Acute pyelonephritis. *A,* Intravenous pyelogram shows right kidney to be swollen with a dense nephrogram. The normal calyceal system precludes obstruction as the cause. *B,* CT in another case showing multiple wedge-shaped areas of low attenuation characteristic of multifocal pyelonephritis.

sis, but the kidney is usually still functional. To our knowledge, the CT corollary of acute suppurative pyelonephritis has not been described.

THE PREABSCESS STATE (FOCAL LOBAR NEPHRONIA, FOCAL BACTERIAL NEPHRITIS)

Occasionally, a focal acute pyelonephritis fails to resolve and becomes indolent. In the radiologic literature, the term *preabscess state, acute focal bacterial nephritis,* or *focal lobar nephronia* (FLN) has been applied to such situations if a frank abscess has not occurred in the affected area. We consider FLN to be midway in the spectrum between an acute pyelonephritis and actual abscess formation. Percutaneous aspiration will yield positive cultures but little in the way of fluid.

Although intravenous pyelography (IVP) may be normal, more often a focal, ill-defined mass is seen that is of lower density than the surrounding parenchyma. This may be more obvious on nephrotomography. This area will be hypoechoic on ultrasound without the good through transmission characteristic of an abscess. However, the differentiation between FLN and a frank abscess may be extremely difficult by this technique. On CT, a nonenhancing elliptic or rounded defect with CT numbers slightly above water is identified (Fig. 70–2). We consider a few small areas of necrosis to be compatible with a diagnosis of FLN. Technetium-99m glucoheptonate or ^{99m}Tc MAG3 will not accumulate in areas of FLN, but indium-tagged white blood cells and gallium citrate will.

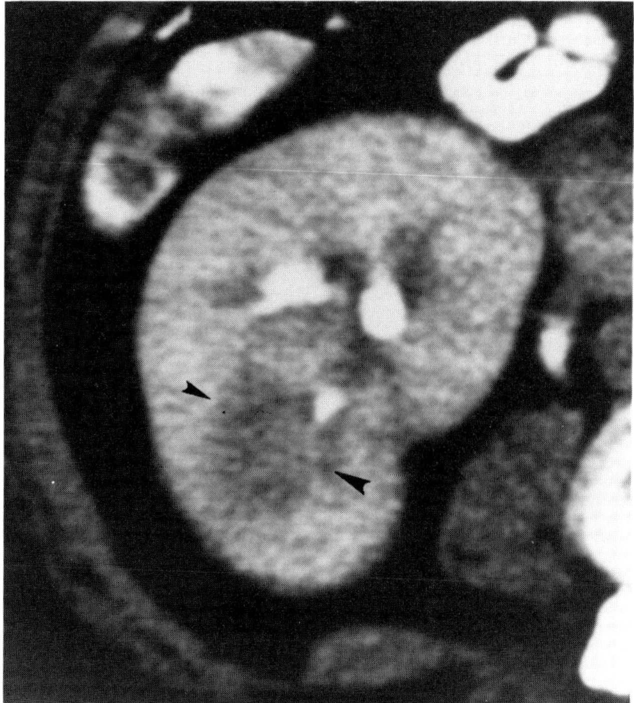

Figure 70–2. Preabscess state (focal lobar nephronia, focal bacterial nephritis). CT shows area of low density *(arrowheads)* with irregular, somewhat ill-defined borders and CT density slightly greater than water. Pathologically, such an area consists of white blood cells, debris, interstitial edema, and both normal and destroyed parenchyma. Percutaneous aspiration would yield organisms but no drainable fluid.

INTRARENAL ABSCESS

Intrarenal abscesses can be considered the opposite end of the spectrum from acute pyelonephritis, preabscess state being viewed as an intermediate. We reserve the term abscess for a cavity filled with fluid, frank pus, and debris. There should be no recognizable functioning parenchyma within the involved areas. In many cases, the abscess has a thickened capsule. These lesions are often difficult to diagnose because the fever may be low grade and symptoms are nonspecific and few. Drug abuse is a common source for abscess in young individuals. AIDS patients are also affected.

On urography, a nonenhancing mass is identified that may or may not have irregular walls. The lesion can superficially resemble a benign simple cyst, but an abscess will usually have a thickened wall. Ultrasonically, the abscess is predominantly anechoic, but one can usually recognize a few internal echoes. If the study is performed in a decubitus position, these echoes will be found in the dependent portion of the abscess and represent intracavitary debris. Ultrasound is less sensitive than CT and we advocate the latter if an abscess is suspected or the clinical picture is unclear. The CT picture is that of a low-density, fluid-filled mass sometimes containing some evidence of debris (Fig. 70–3). Angiograms need not be performed in patients suspected of abscesses and, if anything, they may be confusing. The interlobar arteries are stretched with loss of corticomedullary definition. There is no evidence of central contrast enhancement during the nephrographic phase. Usually the angiogram is obtained because a tumor is suspected clinically. Unfortunately, inflammatory and neoplastic neovascularity are indistinguishable, and neither responds to epinephrine. Nuclear scintigrams using gallium-67 or indium-labeled white blood cells will be positive, but one cannot distinguish focal infection or even tumor from an abscess by isotopic techniques. Treatment formerly required surgical intervention. By means of percutaneous techniques and/or intravenous antibiotics, most abscesses can now be successfully treated without surgical intervention.

PERIRENAL AND PARARENAL ABSCESSES

Perirenal infection is most often secondary to a primary intrarenal process. On occasion, extrarenal sources such as pancreatitis and

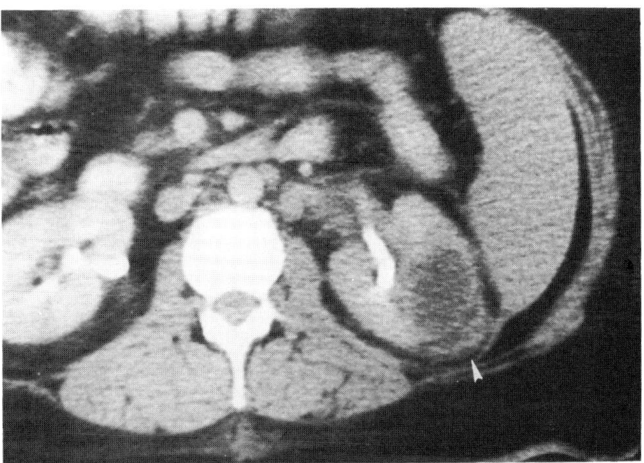

Figure 70–3. Renal abscess in a 32-year-old female with fever and leukocytosis. CT shows the rounded low-density intrarenal mass with extension posteriorly into the perinephric space *(arrowhead).*

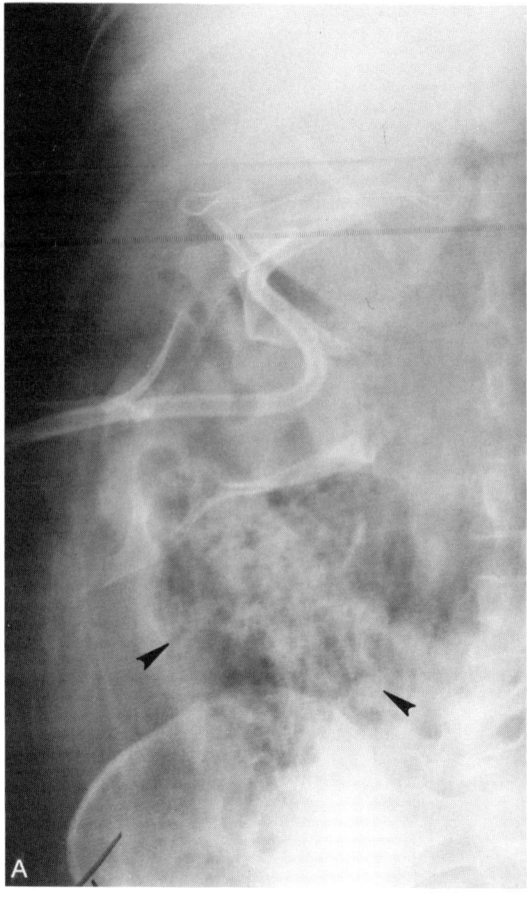

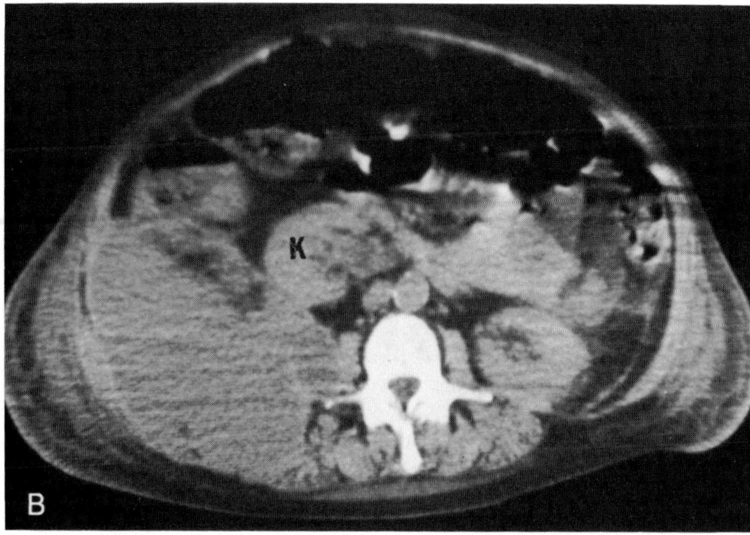

Figure 70–4. Perirenal and pararenal abscess. *A,* Typical perirenal abscess *(arrowheads)* with gas bubbles confined to the cone-shaped Gerota's fascia. Care should be taken not to confuse this with air and feces in the cecum and ascending colon. *B,* CT of a posterior pararenal abscess extending into the back muscles in a 61-year-old female with cervical cancer. Note the right kidney (K) and the fat in the perirenal space to be displaced anteriorly.

diverticulitis also affect this area. On plain film, perirenal gas may be mistaken for air in the ascending colon (Fig. 70–4*A*). Care should be taken to differentiate these two entities on all abdominal films. On urography, Gerota's fascia may be bulging and the kidney displaced. On inspiratory and expiratory double-exposure films, the involved kidney may show absence of movement. Although ultrasound can demonstrate perirenal disease, CT is the study of choice because of the ease of defining the extent and location of the abscess. The abscess itself will not enhance and is of low CT attenuation. Gerota's fascia can usually be delineated, thus differentiating perirenal from pararenal disease.

The pararenal spaces are more often affected by extrarenal and even extra-abdominal sources; however, intrarenal spread to perirenal and subsequently to pararenal spaces does occur (Fig. 70–6*B*).

EMPHYSEMATOUS PYELONEPHRITIS; EMPHYSEMATOUS PYELITIS, PERINEPHRIC EMPHYSEMA

The recognition of intrarenal gas requires aggressive management. Although surgical intervention had been considered mandatory, conservative management may be appropriate in certain select situations. Although most often secondary to the presence of a gas-forming organism, emphysematous pyelonephritis must be differentiated from air refluxing from the bladder or an ileal conduit and from air entering through a percutaneous stent. Another important cause of intrarenal air is a fistula from bowel, bronchus, or skin.

The diagnosis of intrarenal air should be made on plain films but can be difficult because of overlying bowel gas (Fig. 70–5*A*). Similarly, normal bowel loops or renal calculi cause multifocal shadowing on ultrasound that can be confused with a similar pattern that has been described in emphysematous pyelonephritis. CT is an ideal method for demonstrating and localizing intrarenal air. CT will clearly differentiate air confined to the collecting system (emphysematous pyelitis) and/or air confined to the perinephric space (perinephric emphysema) from true emphysematous pyelonephritis (air within the parenchyma and collecting system). However, small amounts of intrarenal air seen on CT may not have the same grave consequences as the increased volume of gas necessary for plain film recognition (Fig. 70–5*B*).

CHRONIC PYELONEPHRITIS

In some patients, acute pyelonephritis leads to renal scarring (i.e., chronic pyelonephritis). Although chronic pyelonephritis is most often the result of recurrent acute infection or persistent low-grade inflammation, there are individuals who apparently develop renal scars after only a single acute insult. Interestingly, screening studies have documented patients with renal scars and no history of urinary tract infections (UTI). On the other hand, other studies have identified individuals with untreated asymptomatic urinary infections and no evidence of scarring. Unfortunately, the issue is complicated and unresolved.

Radiographically, the sine qua non for diagnosing chronic pyelonephritis is a renal scar overlying a blunt renal calyx (Fig. 70–6*A*), often involving a compound calyx. This is due to the inflammatory retraction that occurs secondary to scarring. In severe cases, the opposite kidney or uninvolved portions of the affected kidney may undergo compensatory hypertrophy. This hypertrophy may be focal

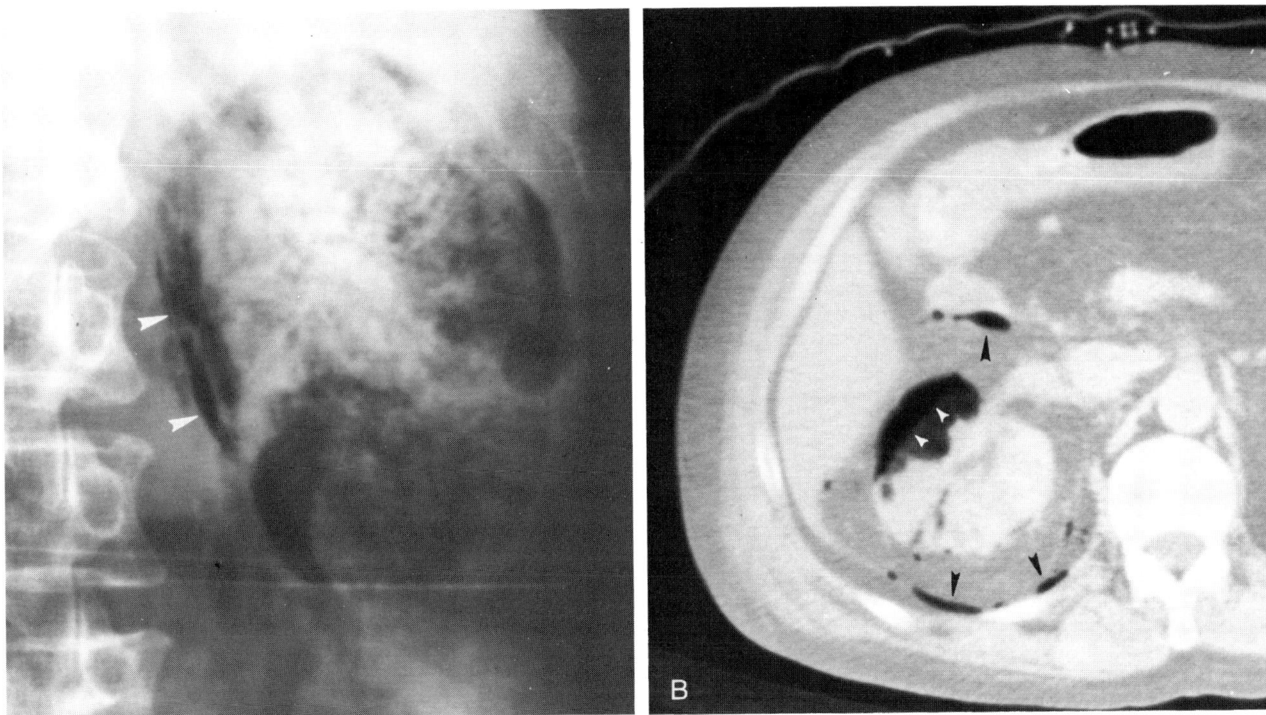

Figure 70–5. Emphysematous pyelonephritis. *A,* Classic plain film diagnosis. Note air in perirenal space *(arrowheads)* as well as radiating spokes of air in the kidney itself. (*A* courtesy of Sanford Minkin, M.D., Pikesville, MD.) *B,* CT in a 52-year-old female. Note the multiple small intraparenchymal air, subcapsular air *(white arrowhead),* and linear air streaks just beneath Gerota's fascia (perinephric emphysema) *(black arrowhead).*

in nature on the involved side and may simulate a mass (Fig. 70–6*A*). Occasionally, chronic pyelonephritis will be identified on other radiographic studies being performed for entirely different reasons. On ultrasound, a highly echogenic focal scar will be denoted, often in a small kidney. On CT, the renal outline is irregular with evidence of renal shrinkage, cortical loss, and blunt calyces (Fig. 70–6*B*). Angiographic studies may, if anything, be confusing, because inflammatory and neoplastic vasculature can be indistinguishable. In the final stages, the renal artery is small except at its origin; the interlobar arteries are widened proximally and tortuous peripherally, with a "gnarled tree" appearance. In the cortex there may be pseudoencasement and crowding of vessels, neovascularity, and a mottled nephrogram. It is believed that radioisotopic studies are the most sensitive for demonstrating renal scarring. The use of the

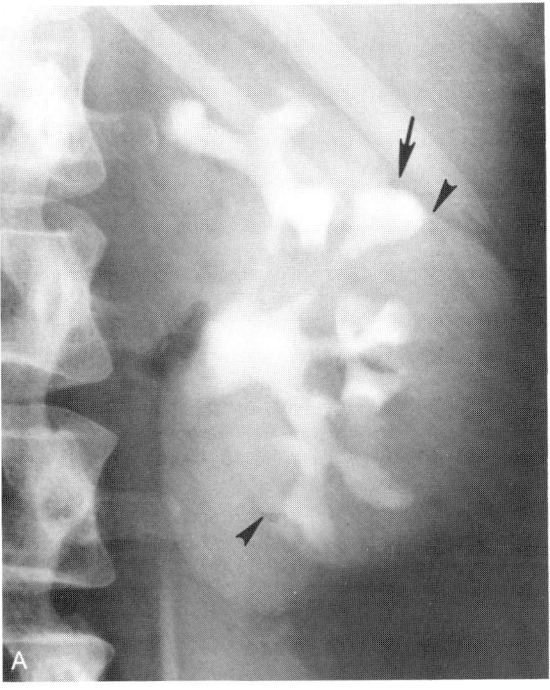

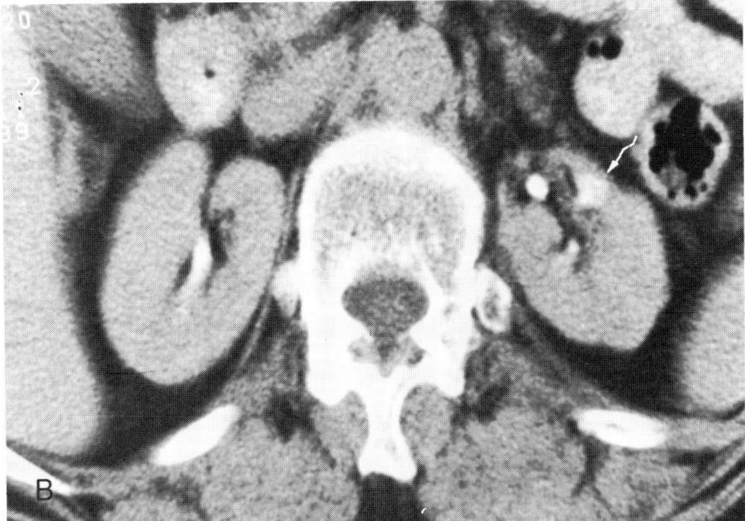

Figure 70–6. Chronic pyelonephritis. *A,* Hallmark of chronic pyelonephritis is a blunt calyx and overlying scar *(arrow). Arrowheads* point to a pseudotumor representing focal compensatory hypertrophy. *B,* CT in a 70-year-old black female with recurrent urinary tract infections. Note the blunt dilated calyx and the overlying scar *(arrow).*

radioisotopic renogram is often important in those patients in whom surgery is being contemplated in order to determine differential renal function.

It is important to monitor children regularly once the diagnosis of pyelonephritis has been made. For those with demonstrable reflux on initial work-up, isotopic voiding cystourethrograms should be performed. Renal ultrasonograms, with MAG3 radioisotopic studies, possibly with a single initial urogram, seem appropriate to further minimize the radiation exposure. Yearly renal growth should be documented. As a guide, the width of renal cortex in the upper pole and lower pole on one side should be approximately the same. Similarly, the width of cortex laterally from side to side should be equal. Otherwise, the possibility of renal damage must be seriously considered.

ATROPHIC PYELONEPHRITIS, REFLUX NEPHROPATHY

As originally demonstrated by Hodson in pigs, vesicoureteral reflux can cause chronic renal changes that are often indistinguishable from chronic pyelonephritis in humans. He also reported a few individuals in whom there was renal scarring but no documented infection. The appellation *chronic atrophic pyelonephritis* or *reflux nephropathy* was applied to these cases. In all probability, reflux alone rarely, if ever, causes renal damage in humans. Reflux, however, is a primary prerequisite for bacteria to enter the renal parenchyma via the ascending route.

ACUTE AND CHRONIC PYONEPHROSIS

An infected dilated renal collecting system is termed pyonephrosis. The infection may itself have caused the obstruction or may have secondarily involved an initially sterile obstructed hydronephrosis. The abdominal film may reveal either a large or a small kidney. The urogram with nephrotomography will reveal a hydronephrotic pattern with dilated calyces, pelvis, and/or ureter, and a thinned cortex. Function may or may not be present. A retrograde pyelogram, if performed, will demonstrate a site of obstruction. The ultrasonogram will also demonstrate an obstructive, hydronephrotic pattern. Internal echoes representing debris may possibly be noted within the calyces; the echoes may layer if ultrasonography is performed in the decubitus position. With CT as well, dilated calyces and pelvis, possibly with thickening of the wall of the collecting system, will be noted and, with careful technique, the site of obstruction can be identified. The density within the collecting system may be that of water or slightly above, reflecting infected and/or hemorrhagic urine. In our experience, MRI usually does not distinguish between simple hydronephrosis and pyonephrosis and its expense precludes its use. Debris also can occasionally be identified by CT as well. On many occasions, however, the differentiation between a hydronephrosis and pyonephrosis may be impossible. Percutaneous drainage and antibiotics can be a successful mode of therapy.

RENAL FISTULA

Primary inflammatory fistula may arise from the kidney and connect to the bowel, skin, or bronchus. Trauma, neoplasms, and surgery are other causes of fistulae. A fistulogram may localize the tract, but CT will identify the extent of the accompanying inflammation, which is vital information in planning the surgical approach.

TUBERCULOSIS

Tuberculosis is the most common granulomatous disease involving the kidney. Just as in the lung, these patients are unable to annihilate the invading bacillus using their primary defense mechanisms. Instead, using histiocytes, macrophages, and fibroblasts, a granuloma is formed with a fibrotic outer rim laid down in an effort to avert spread. Cavitation can ensue and, pathologically, a process similar to pulmonary tuberculosis develops. It is by hematogenous spread from the lung that almost all present-day cases of renal tuberculosis occur. Although renal tuberculosis is said to develop in as many as 3 to 5 per cent of pulmonary cases, reliance should not be placed on finding active tuberculosis on chest x-ray. In one series, only 14 of 200 cases of renal tuberculosis had demonstrable active pulmonary tuberculosis. The tubercle bacillus enters the kidney parenchyma through the glomerular or cortical arteries. Focal necrosis allows the bacteria to enter into tubules. This permits further advancement to the loop of Henle, where a destructive papillitis ensues. A reactive fibrosis usually leads to narrowing at the infundibulum or ureteropelvic or ureterovesicle junction. Occasionally, a small end-stage autonephrectomized kidney will result.

Occasionally, if seen during acute infection, an enlarged kidney with decreased function will be noted on the urogram that is indistinguishable from that seen in any acute pyelonephritis. More often, the earliest recognizable radiographic finding on IVP is that of a necrotizing papillitis leading to an irregular fuzzy calyx (Fig. 70–7*A*). The next development is an infundibular stricture secondary to the reactive fibrosis described above (Fig. 70–7*B*). This is followed by nonvisualization of the involved papilla secondary either to the infundibular obstruction or to renal papillary necrosis. Cavities, which are often filled with caseous material, can usually be appreciated in the cortex. Strictures that develop at the ureteropelvic junction will cause a pyonephrotic pattern. With stricture formation, the kidney may undergo an ''autonephrectomy'' with amorphous calcification (Fig. 70–7*C*). Subsequent seeding from the kidney causes a reactive fibrosis, leading to a pipestem or ''string of beads'' appearance to the ureter. The bladder also can become contracted as a result of fibrosis of the wall, and there is often unilateral reflux secondary to a reactive fibrosis occurring at the ureterovesical angle. On retrograde pyelography, the renal pelvis and/or calyx is either completely obstructed or demonstrates a fibrosed renal pelvis with the pelvis and calyces lined by multiple rounded wall lesions representing granulomatous masses. Although some believe that retrograde pyelography is contraindicated because of fear of infection, urine cultures can be obtained by this method.

Both ultrasonography and CT can be confusing. In the former, a pyonephrotic pattern, often with dependent debris, may be noted. In cases with an infiltrative pattern, there is a degree of increased echogenicity throughout the kidney. On CT, one may also note a variable pattern from a focal process with a few obstructed calyces possibly containing debris, amorphous calcification (Fig. 70–7*D*), and stones to a nonfunctioning small fibrosed renal pelvis and a thinned cortex draped over a pyonephrotic kidney. The kidney is usually small in the late stages of the disease, unlike in xanthogranulomatous pyelonephritis. With obstruction, the kidney may atrophy and calcify, with a typical ground-glass appearance seen on plain film. CT has also significant value in demonstrating perirenal, pararenal, and/or psoas involvement (i.e., the cold abscess). In spite of all the above, tuberculosis still remains a ''great imitator,'' with radiographic patterns indistinguishable from acute or chronic pyelonephritis, papillary necrosis, obstructive pyonephrosis, xanthogranulomatous pyelonephritis (XGP), tumors, and tumor-like lesions.

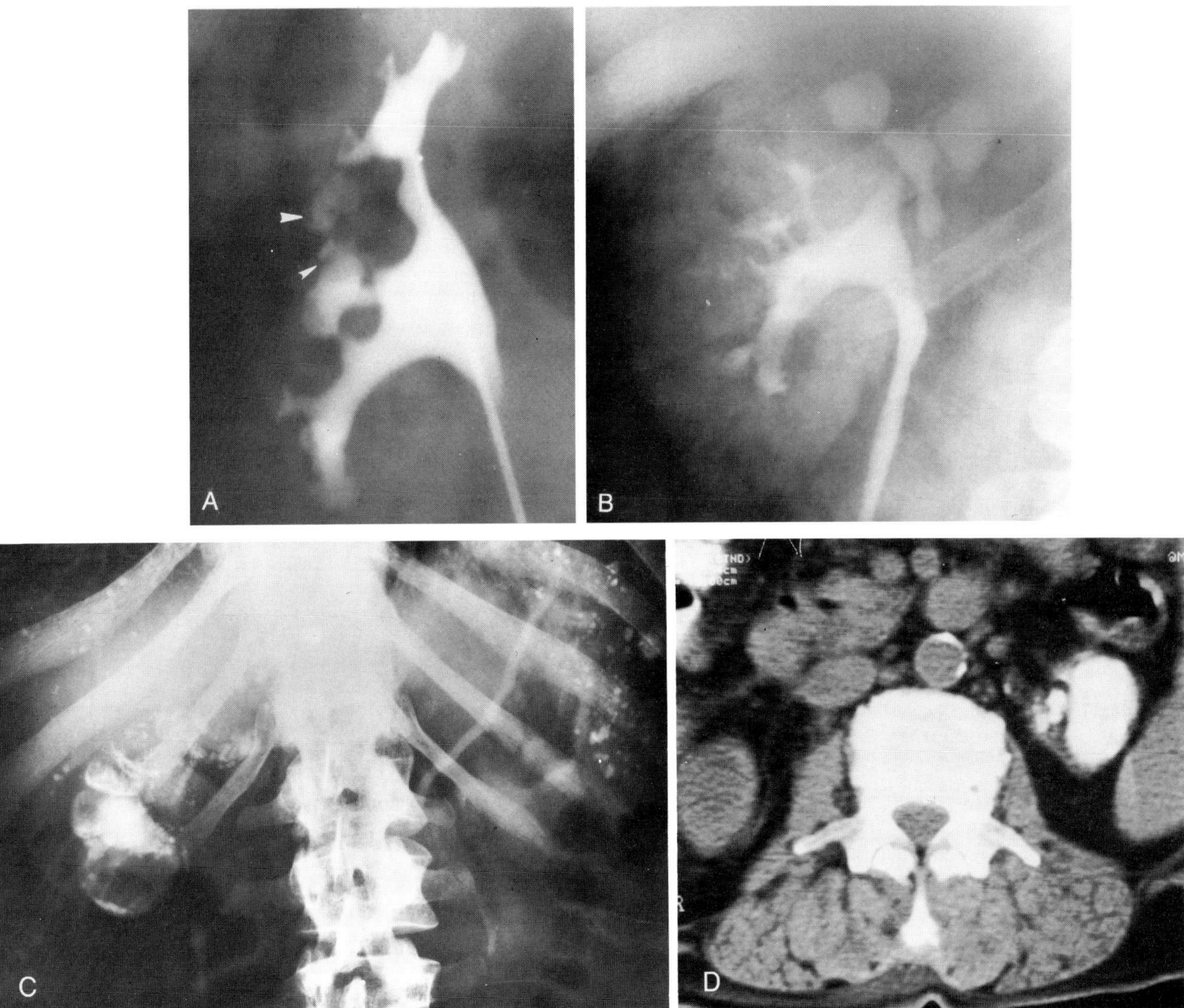

Figure 70–7. Tuberculosis. *A,* Early lesion of middle group of calyces *(lower arrowhead).* A medullary abscess *(upper arrowhead)* connects with calyx. *B,* More advanced lesion. Minor and major infundibular stenosis (i.e., fibrosis) in upper pole calyx. The blunt calyces may be secondary to obstruction, renal papillary necrosis, or both. *C,* End-stage nonfunctioning calcified right kidney. Note splenic calcified granuloma. *D,* CT scan of another end-stage calcified right kidney in a new Russian immigrant.

XANTHOGRANULOMATOUS PYELONEPHRITIS (XGP)

The hallmark of XGP is the presence of the xanthoma cell (a lipid-laden macrophage) in response to subchronic renal infection. Just as in tuberculosis, the development of the xanthoma cell, the fibrotic reaction, and the granuloma formation are all part of the host's defense mechanisms invoked against the causative gram-negative organisms. XGP usually starts in the obstructed pelvis or calyx with the xanthoma cells creeping along the calyceal wall, causing destruction, cavitation, and/or abscess formation first in the medulla and then in the cortex. Usually a staghorn calculus is present, with the involved calyces filled with yellowish-orange tissue and fluid. It can be seen at any age, but it is usually found in middle-aged females who are often diabetic. They usually present with malaise, low-grade fever, weight loss, nonspecific pain, and/or dysuria. There are two forms of XGP: diffuse XGP, in which the whole kidney is involved, and focal, in which one or two calyces or a portion of the kidney is affected.

In about three quarters of patients, an obstructing pelvic or calyceal stone is present. Often, a mass representing the enlarged kidney is recognized. If, in addition, there is absence of function, XGP is a very likely diagnosis (Fig. 70–8). However, in 10 to 30 per cent, function is present, usually in the focal variety. More difficult to diagnose is the focal variety that may mimic a neoplasm or an abscess. Retrograde studies will demonstrate either a small constricted pelvis or calyces lined with irregular, granulomatous tissue, or total occlusion.

In the diffuse form, the angiograms will usually reveal an enlarged kidney with stretched interlobar vessels in a pattern initially indistinguishable from the radiographic pattern of hydronephrosis. However, variable amounts of inflammatory neovasculature can usually be identified, which should help differentiate between the two entities. With focal XGP, a hypo- to hypervascular lesion may be seen that resembles a tumor and an abscess. Ultrasonically the

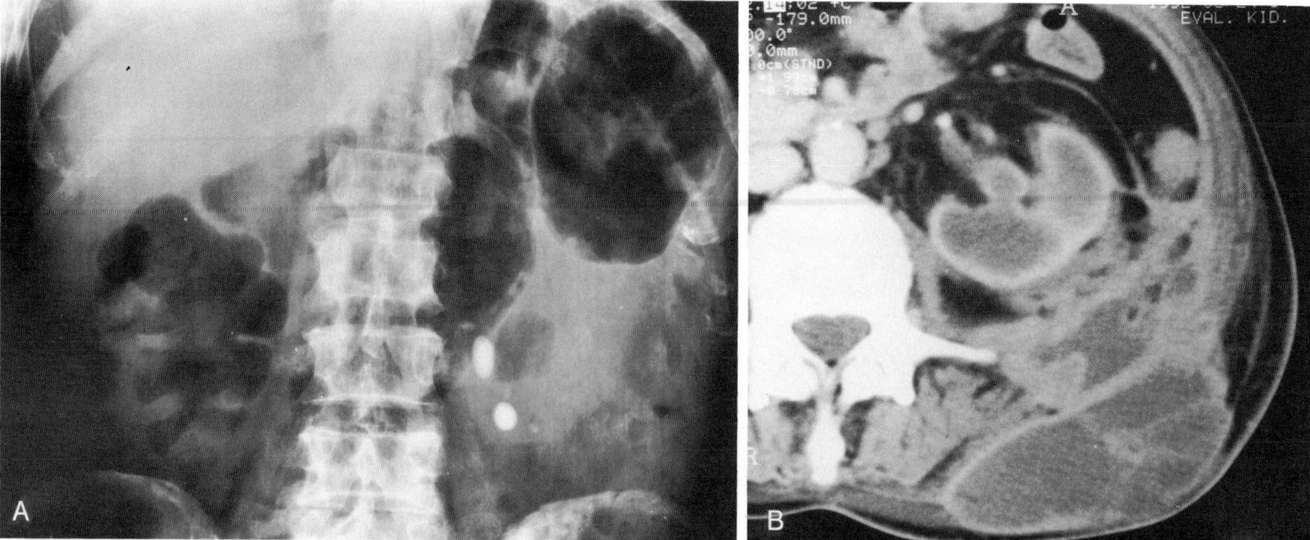

Figure 70–8. Xanthogranulomatous pyelonephritis with extension into the posterior pararenal space and back muscles. Sixty-eight-year-old female seen with large flank mass. *A,* Plain film shows left-sided stones. *B,* CT scan shows low-density dilated calyces with a small contracted renal pelvis. Abscess extension into the posterior pararenal space and back muscles is readily apparent.

enlarged kidney is replaced with multiple fluid-filled masses representing dilated calyces or parenchymal abscesses with a small contracted pelvis. A few layered internal echoes can occasionally be recognized representing debris. Shadowing from a staghorn calculus may or may not be present. On CT, they are multiple, rounded, predominantly cortical or medullary low-density areas, representing the dilated calyces, with a small renal pelvis. These CT numbers are never in the range of fat. Scattered calcifications and stones are noted within the parenchyma and the calyces. A staghorn pelvic calculus is often present. With contrast injection, the residual cortical rim enhances, making the nonenhancing calyces and abscesses stand out. In the focal form, one or two dilated calyces, with an obstruction often secondary to a calyceal stone, are seen. Not infrequently, marked posterior pararenal and psoas involvement is noted with only minimal perirenal infection. Extrarenal involvement can occur in both focal and diffuse XGP.

MALAKOPLAKIA

Malakoplakia is another granulomatous disease in which histiocytes are involved, but these contain Michaelis-Gutmann inclusion bodies (which are basophilic) instead of the fat found in XGP. Apparently, the bacteria are incorporated within the lysosome of the histiocyte but cannot be completely destroyed. Usually seen in diabetic females or in immunosuppressed individuals, malakoplakia most frequently involves the bladder.

In the multifocal form, either the cortex or the medulla is involved and there is usually absence of function. If the cortex is involved, multiple individual masses may be seen on nephrotomography. These masses are hypoechoic on ultrasonography and hypovascular on angiography. In the medullary form, an obstructive hydro- or pyonephrosis is identified using these same modalities. If unifocal, a hypovascular mass that may mimic a tumor may be recognized. There may even be renal vein and vena cava thrombosis. In the presence of simultaneous bladder and kidney lesions in a female with recurrent UTI, malakoplakia can be reasonably suggested in the differential diagnosis.

SCHISTOSOMIASIS

Schistosoma hematobium, endemic in the Near East and Africa, will affect the kidney if there is ureterovesical reflux. Usually, but not always, heavy calcification of the bladder and/or lower ureters will be present to suggest the diagnosis. In the kidney, a staghorn calculus, nephrocalcinosis, or a mass may be present on the plain film, and ureteral obstruction may be noted on urography. A secondary squamous cell carcinoma may develop in the urinary tract infested with schistosomiasis.

CANDIDIASIS

Involvement of the kidney may be secondary to reflux from the bladder or part of a fulminant systemic process. It occurs in patients with altered defense mechanisms secondary to chronic debilitating diseases, steroid or antibiotic therapy, or diabetes. On plain film, air may be noted in the bladder surrounding the rope-like mycelia. Several different patterns can be seen on urography. These include acute pyelonephritis, a swollen kidney with multiple renal abscesses, renal failure, chronic pyelonephritis, hydronephrosis, or renal papillary necrosis. In those kidneys involved secondarily from the bladder, fungus balls will be identified within the calyces, bladder, and/or renal pelvis. These irregular, usually mobile mycetomas should be recognizable but can be confused with blood clot. On ultrasonography, the fungus ball is demonstrated to be echogenic but without shadowing. This excludes a renal calculus. On CT, patterns consistent with chronic or acute pyelonephritis, unifocal or multifocal abscesses, or hydronephrosis will be noted. The presence of the mycetoma within the collecting system is an important clue to the diagnosis.

ECHINOCOCCOSIS

Most often involved by hematogenous spread, direct spread occasionally occurs from nearby organs. Although classically divided

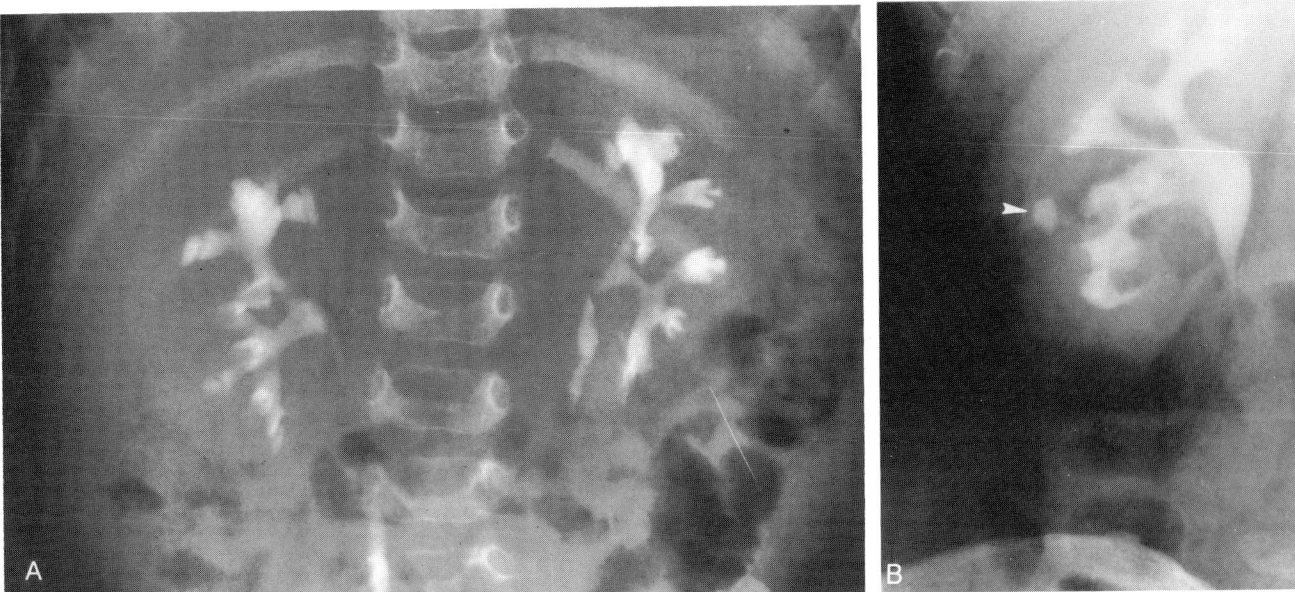

Figure 70–9. Renal papillary necrosis. *A,* Medullary type. Note small contrast-filled areas involving almost all the calyces in a 2-month-old child. *B,* Papillary form. Note blunt calyx *(arrowhead)* where a sloughed papilla had been. Follow-up studies showed slough of other papillae.

into "closed," "exposed," and "open" cysts, radiographically this is of little importance in relationship to the kidney. The kidney is almost always involved subcortically.

On plain films, rim-like wall calcification may be noted. There may be one or more cysts that may be mistaken for either a renal tumor or polycystic kidneys. CT and nephrotomography will usually reveal the cyst walls to be thickened but not always calcified. The cysts may be filled with debris or may be septated, mimicking a multilocular cyst. A mass effect on the calyces may be present, and air-fluid levels can sometimes be found. The cysts are usually angiographically avascular. No attempts at cyst puncture should be made if echinococcal infection is suspected, except by experienced individuals because seeding and spillage are serious complications.

PYELITIS CYSTICA

This is the focal form of ureteritis cystica and, as such, is related to a chronic mucosal and submucosal inflammatory process, usually infectious in nature. Others relate this to a cystic change in von Bruin's glands. Typically, multiple small filling defects are seen on IVP or retrograde pyelography.

RENAL PAPILLARY NECROSIS

Renal papillary necrosis (RPN) is an ischemic necrosis of one or more pyramids secondary either to damage to the vessels supplying the medulla (i.e., the vasa recta) or to red blood cell sludging. There are multiple etiologies, including pyelonephritis, obstruction, sickle cell anemia, tuberculosis, cirrhosis, analgesic abuse, renal vein thrombosis, diabetes mellitus, and renal transplantation. Of these, analgesic abuse is most important and can be discovered only after careful investigation. The disease is classically divided into two types: medullary and papillary. In the former, irregular linear cavities filled with contrast are seen in one or more pyramids on IVP. Usually only one or two such streaks are identified per pyramid, in contradistinction to medullary sponge kidney, in which multiple linear streaks representing dilated tubules are recognized (Fig. 70–9). In the papillary form, fistulae develop from adjacent fornices, with ultimate slough of the entire papilla. These fistulae will fill with contrast on urography. In time, the contrast will connect one fornix to an adjacent one, and the papilla will then be identified freely floating in the calyx surrounded by a ring of contrast. In the rare situation where the necrotic papillary form does not slough, RPN in situ is present and may eventually calcify. This papilla may calcify or may pass down the ureter, giving symptoms of ureteral colic. After passage, the involved calyx mimics a hydrocalyx secondary to past obstruction, reflux, or infection. On CT and ultrasonography, the sloughed papilla can be seen within the calyx, and, if calcified, the sloughed papilla will shadow on ultrasonography. It should be noted that there is no known relationship between the type of RPN (i.e., medullary or cortical) and the etiology.

Bibliography

Al-Ghorab MM: Radiological manifestation of genitourinary bilharziasis. Clin Radiol 19:100–111, 1968.

Ben Amni T: The sonographic evaluation of urinary tract infections in children. Semin Ultrasound CT & MR 5:19–33, 1984.

Bohlman ME, Sweren BS, Khazan R, et al: Emphysematous pyelitis and emphysematous pyelonephritis. South Med J 84:1438–1443, 1991.

Caberwal D, Katz J, Reid R, et al: A case of nephrobronchial and colonobronchial fistula presenting as lung abscess. J Urol 117:371–373, 1977.

Claes H, Vereeken R, Oyen R, et al: Xanthogranulomatous pyelonephritis with emphasis on computerized tomographic scan. Urology 29:389–393, 1987.

Conrad MR, Sanders RC, Mascardo AD: Perinephric abscess aspiration using ultrasound guidance. AJR 128:459–466, 1977.

Davidson AJ, Talner LB: Urographic and angiographic abnormalities in adult-onset acute bacterial nephritis. Radiology 106:249–256, 1973.

Davidson AJ, Talner LB: Late sequelae of adult-onset acute bacterial nephritis. Radiology 127:367–371, 1978.

Ellis LR, Kenny GM, Nellans RE: Urogenital aspects of actinomycosis. J Urol 122:132–133, 1979.

Friedland GW: Long term effects of urinary tract infections. Radiology 124:263–264, 1977.

Gerle RD: Roentgenographic features of primary renal candidiasis. AJR 119:731–738, 1973.

Gold RP, McClennan BL, Rottenberg RR: CT appearance of acute inflammatory disease of the renal interstitium. AJR 141:343–349, 1983.

Goldman SM, Fishman EK: Upper urinary tract infection: The current role of CT, ultrasound, and MRI. Semin Ultrasound, CT, MRI 12:335–360, 1991.
Goldman SM, Fishman EK, Hartman DS, et al: Computed tomography of renal tuberculosis and its pathological correlates. J Comput Assist Tomogr 9:771–776, 1985.
Goldman SM, Fishman EK, Soulen MC: CT/MRI of inflammatory disease of the kidney. In Goldman SM, Gatewood OMB (eds): CT and MRI of the Genitourinary Tract. Contemporary Issues in Computed Tomography. New York, Churchill Livingstone, 1990, pp 59–96.
Goldman SM, Hartman DS, Fishman EK, et al: CT of xanthogranulomatous pyelonephritis: Radiologic-pathologic correlation. AJR 143:963–969, 1984.
Goldman SM, Minkin SD, Naraval DC, et al: Renal carbuncle: The use of ultrasound in its diagnosis and treatment. J Urol 118:525–528, 1977.
Goodman M, Curry T, Russel T: Xanthogranulomatous pyelonephritis: A local disease with systemic manifestations. Medicine 58:171–181, 1979.
Gross GW, Lebowitz RL: Infection does not cause reflux. AJR 137:929–932, 1981.
Haines JG, Mayo ME, Allan NA, Ansell JS: Echinococcal cyst of the kidney. J Urol 117:788–789, 1977.
Hall JRW, Choa RG, Wells JP: Percutaneous drainage in emphysematous pyelonephritis: An alternative to major surgery. Clin Radiol 39:622–624, 1988.
Hare WSC, Poynter JD: The radiology of renal papillary necrosis as seen in analgesic nephropathy. Clin Radiol 25:423–443, 1974.
Hartman DS, Davis CJ Jr, Lichtenstein JE, Goldman SM: Renal parenchymal malakoplakia. Radiology 136:33–42, 1980.
Hartman DS, Sanders RS, Davis CJ Jr, et al: Xanthogranulomatous pyelonephritis: Sonographic-pathologic correlation of 16 cases. J Clin Ultrasound Med. 3:481–488, 1984.
Ishikawa I, Saito Y, Onouchi Z, et al: Delayed contrast enhancement in acute focal bacterial nephritis: CT features. J Comput Assist Tomogr 9:894–897, 1985.
Kalalis PP, Greene LF, Weed LA: Brucellosis of the urogenital tract: A mimic of tuberculosis. J Urol 88:347–353, 1962.
Kay CJ, Rosenfield AT, Taylor KJW, Rosenberg MA: Ultrasonic characteristics of chronic atrophic pyelonephritis. AJR 132:47–49, 1979.
Kim DS, Woesner ME, Howard TF, Olson LK: Emphysematous pyelonephritis demonstrated by computed tomography. AJR 132:287–288, 1979.
Kollins SA, Hartman GW, Carr DT, et al: Roentgenologic findings in urinary tract tuberculosis: A 10 year investigation. AJR 121:487–500, 1974.
Lalli AF: Renal papillary necrosis. AJR 114:741–745, 1972.
Lapides J: Mechanism of urinary tract infection. Urology 14:217–225, 1978.
Malek RS, Elder JS: Xanthogranulomatous pyelonephritis: A critical analysis of 26 cases and the literature. J Urol 119:589–593, 1978.
Margolian HN: Fungal infections of the urinary tract. Semin Roentgenol 6:323–330, 1971.
Mellins HZ: Chronic pyelonephritis and medullary necrosis. Semin Roentgenol 6:292–308, 1971.
Mendez G Jr, Isikoff MP, Morillo G: The role of computed tomography in the diagnosis of renal and perirenal abscesses. J Urol 122:582–586, 1979.
Mogle JM, Perlberg S, Heiman S, Caine M: Emphysematous pyelonephritis. J Urol 131:203–208, 1984.
Morehouse HT, Weiner SN, Hoffman JC: Imaging in inflammatory disease of the kidney. AJR 143:135–141, 1984.
Morgan WR, Nyberg LM Jr: Perinephric and intrarenal abscess: A review article. Urology 26:529–536, 1985.
Mulopulos GP, Patel SK, Pessis D: MR imaging of xanthogranulomatous pyelonephritis. J Comput Assist Tomogr 10:154–156, 1986.
Piccirillo M, Rigsby CM, Rosenfield AT: Sonography of renal inflammatory disease. Urol Radiol 9:66–78, 1987.
Premkumar A, Lattimer J, Newhouse JH: CT and sonography of advanced urinary tract tuberculosis. AJR 148:65–69, 1987.
Rigsby CM, Rosenfield AT, Glickman MG, et al: Hemorrhagic focal bacterial nephritis findings on gray-scale sonography and CT. AJR 146:1173–1177, 1986.
Roberts JA: Pathogenesis of pyelonephritis. J Urol 129:1102–1106, 1983.
Rosenfield AT, Glickman MG, Taylor KJW, et al: Acute focal bacterial nephritis (acute lobar nephronia). Radiology 132:553–561, 1979.
Silver TM, Kass EJ, Thornbury JR: The radiological spectrum of acute pyelonephritis in adults and adolescents. Radiology 118:65–71, 1976.
Stanton MJ, Maxted W: Malacoplakia: A study of the literature and current concepts of pathogenesis, diagnosis and treatment. J Urol 125:139–146, 1981.
Subramanyam BR, Raghavendra BN, Bosniak MA, et al: Sonography of pyonephrosis: A prospective study. AJR 140:991–993, 1983.
Wills JS, Pollack HM, Curtis JA: Cholesteatoma of the upper urinary tract. AJR 136:941–944, 1981.
Yoder IC, Lindfors KK, Pfister RC: Diagnosis and treatment of pyonephrosis. Radiol Clin North Am 22:407–414, 1984.

71 Renal Cystic Disease

Arthur J. Segal

SIMPLE RENAL CYST

Simple renal cysts are filled with clear, straw-colored fluid. Their sizes and volumes vary from a few millimeters to liters. They are uncommon under 30 years of age but are present in approximately 50 per cent of patients over 50 years of age. Sex distribution is equal and there is no evidence of inheritance. Simple cysts are located in both cortex and medulla. The wall is yellowish-white and semitransparent. The inner surface of the cyst is usually smooth but may have septa that are usually incomplete. Microscopically, they are lined by flattened epithelium, and occasionally, this lining may have papillary projections. There is no confirmed etiology, but they may be the result of obstruction occurring in the setting of ischemia.

Although cysts are usually asymptomatic, they have been associated with hematuria, hypertension, and polycythemia. They may compress and obstruct or occasionally may communicate with the collecting system. Rarely, pedunculated cysts have been associated with torsion.

With good quality nephrotomography, cortical cysts may present with the following findings: (a) relative lucency, (b) very fine (1 mm) peripheral margin, (c) sharp demarcation from adjacent renal parenchyma, and (d) undermining of the adjacent parenchyma, producing a "claw" or "beak" (Fig. 71–1). Medullary and cortical cysts that are small and totally within the renal parenchyma may demonstrate only criteria (a) and (c). Urography cannot distinguish these from other hypovascular lesions of the kidney. When all criteria (a to d) are present, the accuracy of diagnosis is in the range of 95 to 97 per cent.

On ultrasonography (US), renal cysts have (a) a smooth spherical or ovoid contour, (b) no internal echoes, (c) sharp demarcation of the far wall, and (d) accentuation of sound transmission distal to the cyst (Fig. 71–2). When performed by an experienced ultrasonographer, accuracy of up to 98 per cent has been reported.

CT criteria for diagnosis of a simple cyst include (a) sharp demarcation from adjacent renal parenchyma, (b) attenuation value near water density, (c) complete homogeneity, (d) no enhancement with intravenous contrast, and (e) an imperceptible peripheral margin (Fig. 71–3). There may be a pseudo-thick peripheral margin that can occur if the axial section occurs at the level of a "beak" or "claw." When strict CT criteria are applied, accuracy is near 100 per cent.

Using CT as a standard, Warshauer et al defined the sensitivity of excretory urography with nephrotomography in detecting renal masses as follows: 10 per cent when less than 1 cm; 21 per cent

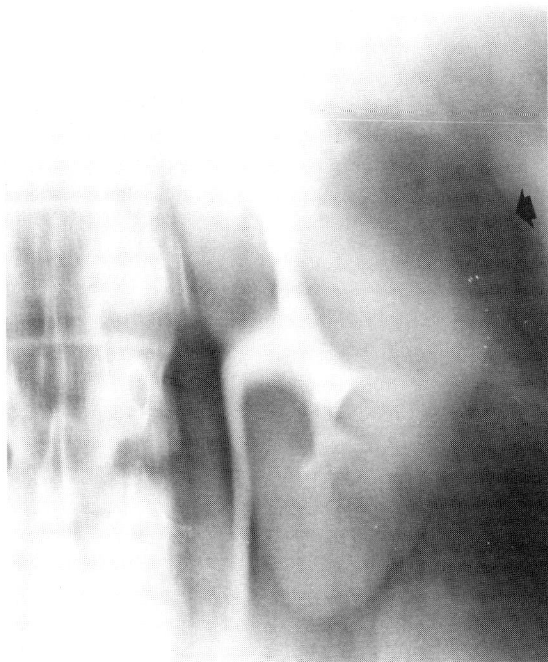

Figure 71–1. Simple renal cyst (nephrotomogram). There is a 6-cm mass with relative lucency, sharp demarcation ("claw" or "beak") at the superior and inferior margins, and a very fine peripheral margin *(arrow)* at the lateral aspect of the left kidney.

between 1 and 2 cm; 52 per cent between 2 and 3 cm; and 85 per cent greater than 3 cm. They also determined the sensitivity of ultrasonography as follows: 26 per cent—less than 1 cm; 60 per cent between 1 and 2 cm; 82 per cent between 2 and 3 cm; and 85 per cent when greater than 3 cm.

Diagnosis by magnetic resonance imaging (MRI) requires the same sharp demarcation and homogeneity characteristics necessary

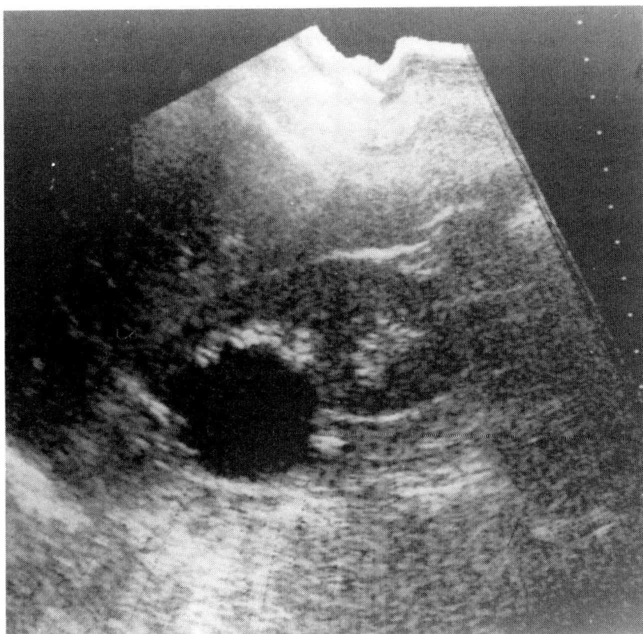

Figure 71–2. Simple renal cyst (ultrasonogram). There is a mass in the upper pole of the right kidney with no internal echoes, a sharply demarcated far wall, and accentuation of sound transmission.

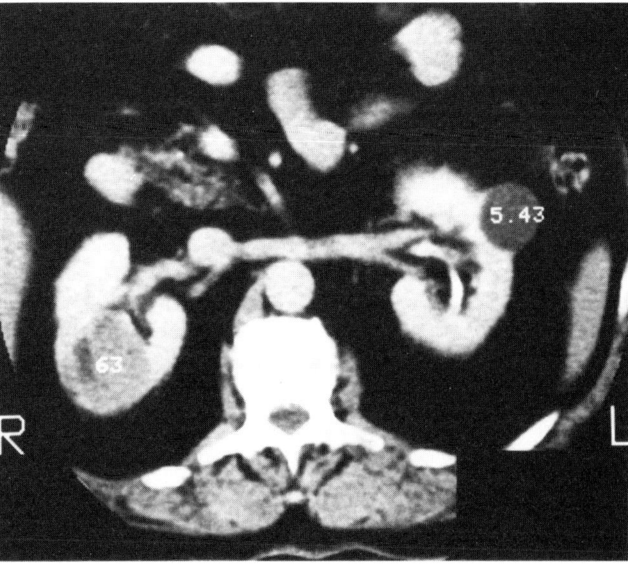

Figure 71–3. Simple renal cyst (CT). A simple cyst of the left kidney is contrasted with a hypernephroma of the right kidney. Note the homogeneous water density (5.43 HU), the sharp demarcation from adjacent renal parenchyma, and the imperceptible peripheral margin of the left renal cyst.

for US or CT diagnosis. Additionally, a renal cyst is represented as a low-intensity lesion with relaxation parameters characteristic of water (spin-echo technique). There are long T_1 and T_2 values.

In selected cases, percutaneous aspiration may be performed to further characterize a cystic mass. Clear fluid without malignant cells may be aspirated. After contrast is instilled into the cyst cavity, the entire mass is opacified. When septations are present, they are thin (1 mm or less), usually incomplete, and the inner walls are otherwise smooth.

BILATERAL MULTIPLE SIMPLE RENAL CYSTS

It is common to see multiple cysts in one or both kidneys. Each is assessed individually by the previously mentioned criteria. There is no associated deterioration of renal function. These cysts are countable with normal intervening parenchyma that enhances (nephrogram) following intravenous contrast administration (Fig. 71–4). This normal renal parenchyma helps to distinguish this benign process from autosomal dominant polycystic kidney disease.

PARAPELVIC CYSTS

A parapelvic cyst is a cyst within the renal sinus, often compressing the renal pelvis. It occurs in the same age population as simple cysts. Its etiology is controversial. Lymphatic, wolffian body, or other embryonic rest theories of origin have been postulated. It may represent a noncommunicating duplication, a diverticulum, or a cyst arising from the adjacent renal parenchyma.

Most are asymptomatic and incidental. Occasionally, there is focal compression on the collecting system or adjacent vasculature and, as a result, there may be hydronephrosis or, rarely, hypertension. Its importance rests in the differential diagnosis from more ominous mass lesions in the region of the renal hilum.

The urogram demonstrates a mass effect on the renal pelvis and

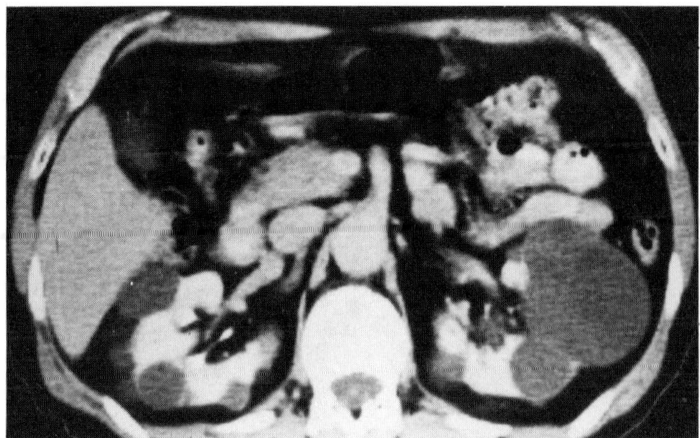

Figure 71–4. Bilateral multiple simple renal cyst (CT). This 74-year-old woman had no evidence of decreased renal function. The cysts are multiple and countable and there is normal intervening renal parenchyma. The liver is free of cysts.

occasionally calyceal infundibula. Ultrasonographic criteria are those of a simple cyst. The mass should be anechoic and have a well-demarcated wall. Problems may occur as a result of echoes from adjacent vessels or the renal sinus. The CT criteria are the same as those for simple cysts. However, the cyst wall may project into the renal sinus and appear thicker secondary to the adjacent hilar vessels, collecting system, or renal parenchyma (Fig. 71–5). Intravenous contrast should be used to distinguish it from a dilated renal pelvis and to confirm the lack of enhancement.

The differential diagnosis varies with the detecting modality. On urography the primary diagnostic considerations include a simple renal cyst, renal sinus lipomatosis, or other tumor. Occasionally, aneurysm or vascular malformation is possible. If the abnormality is detected on ultrasonography, hydronephrosis and occasionally renal sinus lipomatosis must be considered.

COMPLEX CYSTS

The classic simple cyst has been classified by Bosniak as a category I lesion. Complex cysts are simple cysts that become secondarily affected by hemorrhage or infection "Benign, minimally complicated" cysts have been classified as category II lesions. As these processes resolve, some calcify. Peripherally located calcification ("eggshell") has been seen in approximately 3 per cent of cysts. It has been suggested that a calcified cyst is benign (category II) when the calcium is thin and within a wall or septum, there is no associated soft-tissue mass, the central portion of the mass measures water density, and no portion of the mass enhances. There are reports of carcinoma arising in the wall of a simple cyst. Additionally, it is estimated that approximately one third of all hemorrhagic cysts are malignant and probably started as carcinomas.

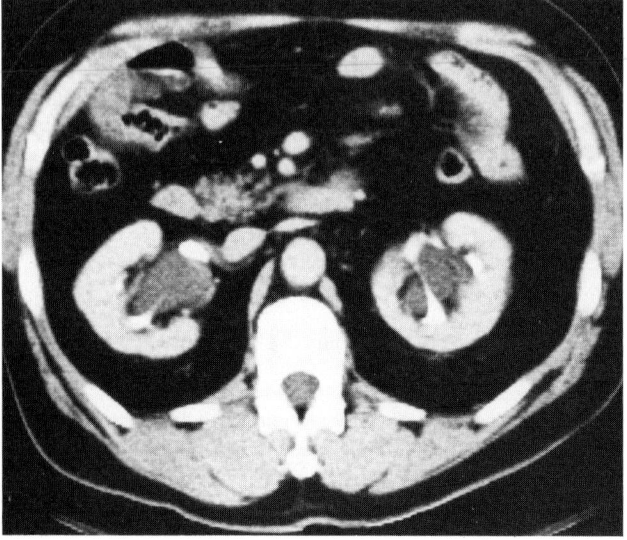

Figure 71–5. Parapelvic cyst (CT). This is a 60-year-old man with bilateral parapelvic cysts (8 HU). Calyceal infundibula are displaced and the peripheral margins are not sharply demarcated where they appose the adjacent renal parenchyma.

There may be a thickened peripheral margin. If calcification is present and peripheral, there is an 80 per cent chance that it is the result of hemorrhage or infection complicating a simple cyst. However, 20 per cent of masses with such calcifications are malignant. If the mass contains central calcification, the chance of carcinoma rises dramatically. Ultrasonography may demonstrate a thickened wall, internal echoes, poor acoustic enhancement, and acoustic shadowing (if mural calcification is present).

Complex cysts show CT attenuation values greater than that of water and as high as 60 HU. The wall can be thickened and the contour irregular. There may be discernible calcification, and the cross-sectional images provide better definition of its location (peripheral or central). Hyperdense renal cysts have been identified (greater than 60 HU) but must be detected on an unenhanced scan. Most are the result of hemorrhage into a benign cyst. Other causes include intravenous or retrograde contrast entering a simple cyst, high protein content of the fluid, or "paste-like calcification" filling the cyst.

To maximize the likelihood of benignity of these hyperdense cysts, it has been suggested that the lesion should be 3.0 cm or smaller; at least 25 per cent of its circumference should extend outside the renal margin; its shape should be round and borders sharply circumscribed; and there should be no enhancement following intravenous contrast.

When examined with MRI, hemorrhagic cysts show a high intensity on spin-echo and inversion recovery images. The T_1 and T_2 values are shorter than those of simple cysts. Note should be made that MRI cannot detect calcification, a deficiency of this modality. However, with the addition of plain films, this is not a major drawback.

Since the advent of CT or ultrasonography combined with needle aspiration, angiography has been of little value in confirming the diagnosis of a benign complex cyst. Renal mass puncture may be helpful if the nature of the fluid is in doubt and cytology and/or culture are required.

AUTOSOMAL RECESSIVE POLYCYSTIC DISEASE

This is a rare disease characterized by cystic dilatation of renal tubules and hepatic periportal fibrosis. It is inherited as an autosomal recessive trait. Although its pathogenesis is unknown, Osathanondh and Potter have attributed this abnormality to "hyperplasia of the interstitial portions of the collecting tubules." Grossly, the kidneys are symmetrically enlarged with smooth contours, despite the fact that the cortices are studded with tiny cysts. Microscopically, there is diffuse distribution of radially oriented collecting tubules that are lined by cuboidal or low columnar epithelium. Histology of the liver reveals "bizarre infolding, proliferation, and dilation of well-differentiated portal bile ducts and ductules, associated with a variable degree of periportal fibrosis."

Intravenous contrast may opacify long, radially oriented, and dilated collecting tubules. This produces opaque streaks, sometimes

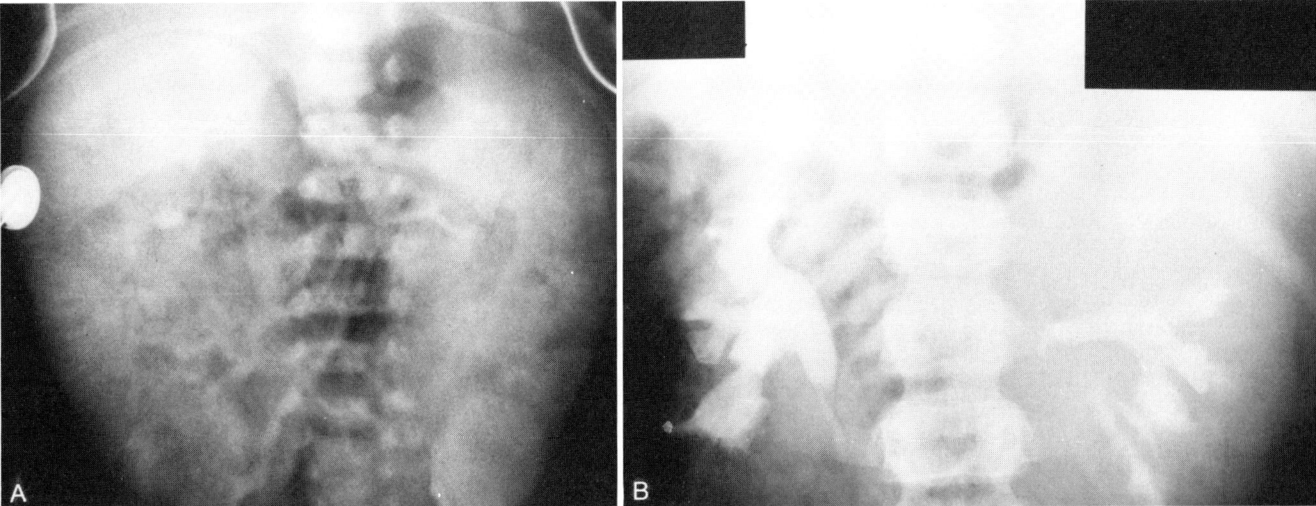

Figure 71–6. Autosomal recessive polycystic disease (urography). *A,* Perinatal form. This is a 24-hour film of a one-day-old male infant with massively enlarged kidneys. Note the radially oriented streaks of contrast in dilated tubules extending to the periphery of both kidneys. *B,* Infantile form. There is moderate enlargement of both kidneys and splenomegaly in this eight-year-old girl. Note opacification of dilated renal tubules extending to the periphery.

extending to the periphery of the kidney. These may be better seen on delayed films up to 24 to 48 hours (Fig. 71–6*A*). Pelvocalyceal systems and ureters are not opacified in the severe form of the disease. With increased age, there is more likely to be liver and spleen enlargement (Fig. 71–6*B*). Renal enlargement and opacification of dilated ducts become less likely. With mild renal involvement, there may be dilated distal collecting tubules only, similar in appearance to those of medullary sponge kidney.

Increased echogenicity is seen throughout both cortex and medulla. There is poor definition of the renal sinus and renal contours. In one study investigators were able to confirm the presence of this entity in utero between the seventeenth and twenty-sixth week of gestation in five of six cases. As children mature, the likelihood of discrete macroscopic cysts increases. Hepatic abnormalities are more variable. With increased periportal fibrosis, there is diffuse increase in echogenicity that varies from subtle to obvious.

Blyth and Ockenden suggested clinicopathologic features of four distinct subgroups. Perinatal is the most severe form, with maximum renal tubular involvement (greater than 90 per cent) and minimal hepatic periportal fibrosis. There may be diminished urine production in utero, oligohydramnios with associated pulmonary hypoplasia, and possibly Potter's facies. If they are not stillborn, they may develop respiratory failure and pneumothorax, uremia, hypertension, or cardiac failure. Most die within the first day or two of life, although some may live as long as six weeks. The juvenile subgroup has the longest survival. They have less than 10 per cent dilated renal tubules and the greatest degree of periportal fibrosis. Intermediate between perinatal and juvenile are the neonatal group (60 per cent dilated renal tubules and mild periportal fibrosis) and the infantile group (25 per cent dilated renal tubules and moderate periportal fibrosis). Neonatal polycystic kidney disease is diagnosed between one day and one month of age and is associated with a life expectancy of 6 to 12 months; those with infantile type disease are diagnosed between three and six months of age and usually die before the age of 10; diagnosis of the juvenile type occurs between six months and five years of age, although they may live to late childhood, adolescence, or even young adulthood. As longevity progresses, hepatic fibrosis with associated portal hypertension dominates the clinical picture and enlarged kidneys may get smaller.

In perinatal polycystic disease, there is massive enlargement of both kidneys, often with bulging flanks and elevation of the diaphragm.

In the neonate with bilateral flank masses and renal failure, the rare bilateral total renal dysplasia may be considered in the differential diagnosis. In the older child with minimum renal involvement, medullary sponge kidney has been considered. The above-mentioned diagnostic criteria, especially periportal fibrosis, are distinguishing features of childhood polycystic disease.

AUTOSOMAL DOMINANT POLYCYSTIC KIDNEY DISEASE

Autosomal dominant polycystic kidney disease is associated with progressive enlargement of cysts that are diffusely distributed throughout both kidneys. It is an autosomal dominant trait with high penetrance. The frequency at autopsy is between 1:222 and 1:1019. There is no sex predilection. Although its pathogenesis is unknown, there are two popular theories. Hildebrand has suggested that there is a "failure of union of branches of the ureteric bud with the metanephric anlage, which, deprived of an organizing influence, forms cysts." Kampmeier postulates that "cysts result from the failure of involution and eventual cyst formation by the first generation of nephrons to differentiate in the metanephros." Grossly, both kidneys are asymmetrically enlarged. Cysts are present in both cortex and medulla and deform adjacent collecting structures as well as the renal contours. They may contain clear, straw-colored fluid. If there has been previous hemorrhage, the fluid may be reddish-brown and inspissated. Microscopically, many cysts contain glomerular tufts and probably arise from dilatation of Bowman's capsule. However, there are others that arise from proximal and distal tubules.

Many pathologic series show hepatic cysts in only 33 per cent of patients. However, more recent studies utilizing CT indicate an overall incidence of 74 per cent and, in patients over 30 years of age, 89 per cent. Ten per cent of patients have pancreatic cysts and 5 per cent have splenic cysts. Other organs with associated cysts include seminal vesicles, epididymis, thyroid, endometrium, ovary, and lung. Berry aneurysms have been reported in as many as 15 per cent of this polycystic population. Subarachnoid hemorrhage, whether from ruptured aneurysm or hemorrhagic infarction unassociated with aneurysm, may be seen in approximately 10 per cent of patients. Periportal fibrosis or other significant hepatic disease is absent.

Although the disease is congenital, it is frequently not apparent until the third to fifth decades. However, there are well-documented reports of autosomal dominant polycystic kidneys occurring in infancy and childhood and as late as the ninth decade. The patient may present with hypertension, renal colic (secondary to calculus disease or spontaneous hemorrhage into a cyst), hematuria, proteinuria, and/or bilateral flank masses. Associated polycythemia has been reported. Renal calculi are present in 20 per cent of patients, and there may be associated infection or obstruction. Rarely, subarachnoid hemorrhage may be a presenting symptom. Mean survival has increased from 50 to 57 years because of dialysis and renal transplantation. Causes of death include uremia (50 per cent), myocardial infarction (10 per cent), cerebral hemorrhage (not always associated with aneurysms—10 per cent), congestive heart failure (10 per cent), and unrelated disease (10 per cent).

The early urographic findings may be unassociated with renal enlargement and include multiple, round, relative radiolucencies causing an inhomogeneous nephrogram (best seen with nephrotomography). As the disease progresses and the cysts enlarge, there is commensurate increase in renal size and poorly defined margins due to a multitude of cysts studding the cortical surface (Fig. 71–7*A*). The pelvocalyceal system may be stretched and distorted, and there may be segmental obstruction due to calculus, blood clot, or deforming cyst. Hepatic cysts can be identified at the time of nephrotomography.

Ultrasonography is excellent for screening families of polycystic patients and may be helpful in genetic counseling. It is also used to document progression of disease. CT provides excellent anatomic resolution. Diagnosis of diffuse cystic disease at early stages of renal and hepatic involvement is possible (Fig. 71–7*B*). Evidence of recent hemorrhage or hyperdense cysts from previous hemorrhage may be defined.

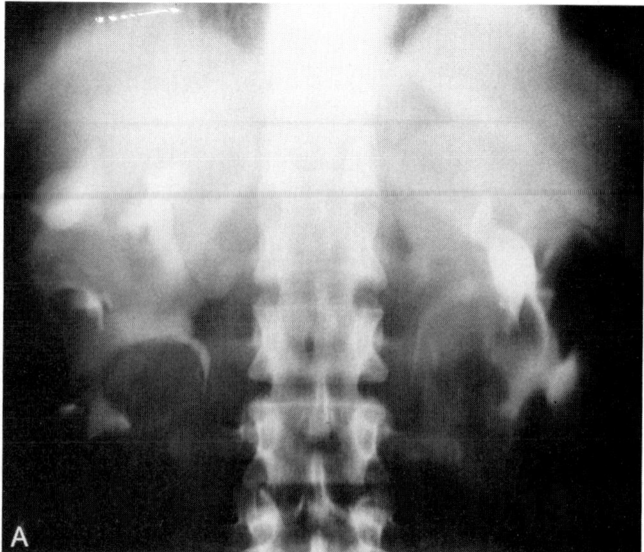

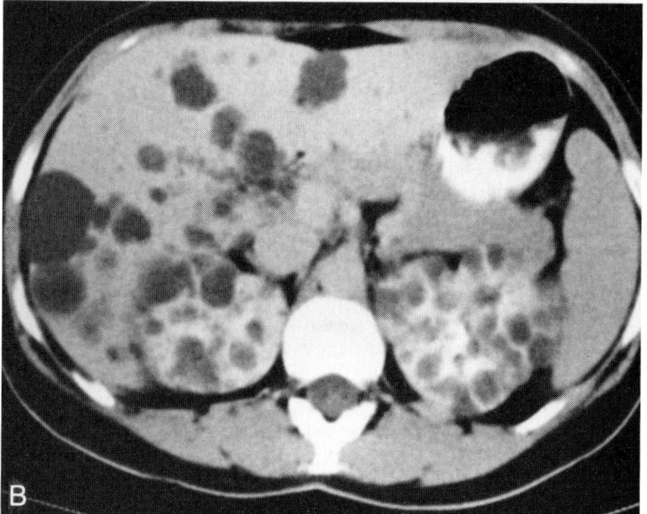

Figure 71–7. Autosomal dominant polycystic kidney disease. *A,* Nephrotomogram. There are asymmetrically enlarged kidneys with poor definition of most borders and compression of the pelvocalyceal structures. *B,* CT scan (different patient than in *A*). The kidneys are massively enlarged, with diffuse cystic disease and no normal intervening renal parenchyma. There are multiple hepatic cysts.

Differential Diagnosis

The main differential diagnosis at the time of urography is bilateral multiple simple cysts and diffuse, multiple angiomyolipomas. Bilateral multiple simple cysts have normal intervening renal parenchyma and no extrarenal cystic disease. Angiomyolipomas have been characterized by both US and CT. The ultrasonogram can detect one or more very echogenic intrarenal masses. Although this finding is suggestive of angiomyolipoma, it is not diagnostic. On CT, fat density may be measured and frequently ranges from −40 to −90 HU. Associated hemorrhage may also be defined. Angiomatous components enhance with intravenous contrast. Diffuse multiple renal cysts, independent of angiomyolipomas, may mimic polycystic kidney disease in those rare cases in which they are associated with tuberous sclerosis. Differentiation is made by detection of angiomyolipomas, skin lesions, and/or the presence of convulsions. This entity may present in infancy.

MEDULLARY SPONGE KIDNEY (RENAL TUBULAR ECTASIA)

Medullary sponge kidney (MSK) consists of multiple cystic dilatations of the papillary collecting tubules. This abnormality was first described by Lenarduzzi in 1939. It is felt to be developmental, although a few familial cases have been described. Sex distribution favors males, 2.5 to 1. Palubinskas reported an incidence of 0.5 per cent on excretory urography. Most patients are between the ages of 30 and 60 at the time of diagnosis. The abnormality is bilateral in 75 per cent of patients. Associated somatic asymmetry and hemihypertrophy have been reported.

Most of the papillae contain cysts, although sometimes several or only one may be abnormal. The cysts are usually less than 5 mm in diameter and may contain calculi. They are lined by columnar or flattened cuboidal epithelium, although rarely transitional or squamous epithelium has been found.

Patients are usually asymptomatic until they form calculi, which is presumably the result of stasis in dilated collecting tubules. Patients may present with hematuria. Other complications include infection and obstruction, which, if not properly treated, can result in significant renal damage.

It is estimated that 40 to 50 per cent of patients with MSK have calculi that are demonstrable on an abdominal radiograph. The calculi are frequently tiny, particularly when confined to the dilated distal tubules. They are composed primarily of mixed calcium phosphates or carbonates. When they pass into the pelvocalyceal system, they can grow larger or even provide the nidus for staghorn calculus formation.

Early in the disease, there is opacification of discrete linear densities (''brush'' or ''fan'' appearance) in the papillae with or with-

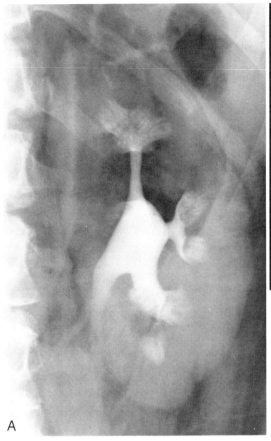

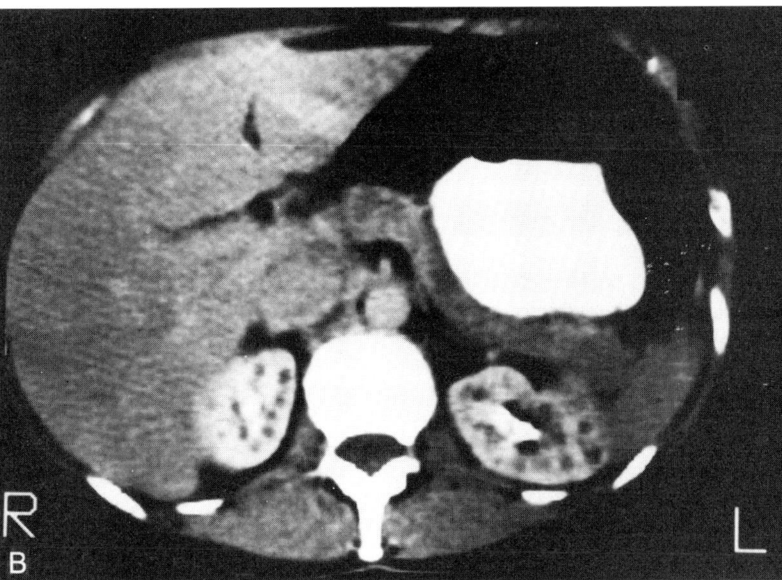

Figure 71–8. Medullary sponge kidney. *A,* Urogram. Note diffusely dilated and contrast-filled papillary ducts in this 54-year-old woman. *B,* CT scan (different patient than in *A*). This 53-year-old woman has multiple medullary cysts that have not filled with contrast on the enhanced scan.

A

out associated tiny calcifications. As the disease progresses, clusters of calculi may be detected in the papillary regions. There is opacification of cystically dilated tubules, some of which contain calculi (Fig. 71–8). As dilatation increases, the papillae may broaden with associated flattening of the calyceal cup.

MSK must be distinguished from other causes of medullary nephrocalcinosis, particularly hyperparathyroidism and renal tubular acidosis. The latter two have abnormalities with distinguishing metabolic features. They are not associated with dilated collecting ducts or medullary cysts. Medullary necrosis produces a single cavity in the renal papillae and therefore is distinct from the multiple ectatic tubules of MSK. Renal tuberculosis results in cavities and calcifications. But these are rarely limited to the papillae alone. They are not usually clustered. There are frequently other stigmata of TB such as cicatrization of the pelvocalyceal structures, ureter, and bladder. A calyceal diverticulum is usually larger than the cystic cavities of MSK. Diverticulae tend to be singular and to extend from the fornix of the calyx rather than the papillary region.

UREMIC MEDULLARY CYSTIC DISEASE/JUVENILE NEPHRONOPHTHISIS

Both of these entities are thought to represent the same disease. They occur in children and young adults and are characterized by medullar cysts and progressive renal failure. The most prevalent subset of this group (juvenile) is associated with autosomal recessive inheritance and usually presents in the first decade of life. A less common (adult) subset is characterized by autosomal dominant inheritance and frequently appears in the latter portion of the second decade, the third decade, or, less commonly, even later. X-linked inheritance has been suggested in some patients. Approximately 25 per cent of cases of this disease are nonfamilial (sporadic). There is no sex predilection. It is estimated that this disease accounts for 10 to 20 per cent of renal failure in childhood.

Grossly, the kidneys are smaller than normal and are typically granular. Corticomedullary cysts, which are variable in size but do not usually exceed 1 to 2 cm, are the characteristic finding. Microscopic features include interstitial cortical fibrosis, glomerular sclerosis, tubular atrophy, and hyaline thickening of the tubular basement membranes.

There is progressive azotemia and anemia, decreased urine specific gravity, salt wasting, polyuria, and polydipsia. There is typically no proteinuria and no urinary sediment abnormalities. Hypertension may develop late in the disease.

Urography is usually not helpful because there is poor concentration of the contrast medium owing to renal failure. Occasionally, small cysts can be identified as radiolucencies in the nephrogram. In early disease, an "inhomogeneous, streaky nephrogram confined to the medulla" has been reported. In those cases in which the collecting system is opacified, there is mild calyceal blunting and occasional distortion from medullary cysts.

Small medullary cysts, loss of corticomedullary differentiation, and increased parenchymal echogenicity are seen with ultrasonography.

ACQUIRED RENAL CYSTIC DISEASE

This is a complication of chronic renal failure and hemodialysis. During the dialysis period, there is an increased incidence of cyst and tumor formation. Ishikawa et al studied this group of patients with computed tomography. An incidence of 43.5 per cent cystic disease was noted in those patients undergoing dialysis for less than three years. When dialysis exceeded three years, the incidence increased to 79.3 per cent.

The kidneys are typically small and usually weigh less than 300 g. Cysts vary in number and are usually less than 2 cm in diameter; however, mean renal volume tends to increase over time as the cysts enlarge. They may be cortical or medullary. When present in the medulla, the appearance is similar to that of uremic medullary cystic disease. Histologically, cysts are lined by flattened cuboidal epithelium. There is usually disorganization of the renal architecture, glomeruli are few, tubules are atrophic, and there is interstitial fibrosis. Extensive arterial disease is present. Oxalate crystals are present in the collecting tubules, and associated obstruction has been suggested as a possible etiology for cyst formation.

The main complications of this disease include hemorrhage and the development of tumors. Estimates of the frequency of renal cell carcinoma complicating acquired renal cystic disease have been between 4 and 7 per cent. Patients present with pain and/or hematuria. The pain may be the result of hemorrhage into a cyst or tumor but is sometimes associated with perirenal hemorrhage. The frequency of this complication has been explained by the fact that sclerotic blood vessels are unsupported because of loss of renal architecture in the diseased kidneys. Minor trauma to these vessels, particularly in the uremic patient with frequently diminished coagulability, has been suggested to explain the ease of hemorrhage. Polyamines, which may be present in greater quantities in the uremic patient, may explain epithelial proliferation and tumor development.

With sonography, bilaterally small kidneys with multiple cysts and one or more echogenic masses may be seen. The latter finding may be associated with hemorrhage or primary neoplasm. CT can confirm the presence of hemorrhage by demonstrating high density before contrast administration. The demonstration of a primary tumor is often difficult in these small kidneys with multiple cystic lesions. Nevertheless, dynamic contrast-enhanced CT with supplemental use of ultrasonography, in problematic cases, has been recommended as the best way to define these complications.

RENAL DYSPLASIA

Renal dysplasia has been called renal dysgenesis, unilateral polycystic disease, renal aplasia, polycystic disease with abundant stroma, multicystic renal dysplasia, and multicystic kidney. It is a sporadic abnormality of embryogenesis resulting in a cluster of varying-sized cysts and no normal renal tissue. It is not inherited. It is the result of early (less than 8 to 10 weeks gestation) obstruction in the developing kidney. Its gross appearance is variable depending upon the number and size of the cysts, and it may be smaller or larger than a normal kidney. There is absence or atresia of the upper third of the ureter. No renal pelvis or infundibulum is present. Microscopically, there may be focally dilated collecting ducts, primitive mesenchyma, and cartilage. Cyst walls are fibrous with a cuboidal or flattened epithelial lining.

Total renal dysplasia is the most common abdominal cystic mass and the second most common abdominal mass in the neonate (hydronephrosis being slightly more common). It is almost always unilateral but may rarely occur bilaterally. The bilateral form is associated with Potter's facies, hypoplastic lungs, and pneumothoraces and is not compatible with life. Some series indicate no sex predominance, although others suggest that it is twice as common in males.

The more common unilateral total renal dysplasia is associated with anomalies in the contralateral kidney (30 per cent) and extrarenal anomalies as frequent as 45 per cent. The prognosis is excellent if anomalies are not present or not serious.

Segmental renal dysplasia is always associated with duplication of the renal pelvis and ureter. Atresia or stenosis affects one of the two collecting systems usually in the pelvoinfundibular region or proximal ureter. The ureter associated with the dysplastic segment frequently has an ectopic distal orifice and usually drains the upper pole of the kidney.

In infancy, there may be an observable mass. If the diagnosis is delayed until adulthood, the plain film may show multiple areas of ring-like calcification in the cyst walls. Most commonly there is nonfunction of the involved kidney or segment. Occasionally, opacification of septations and/or delayed puddling of contrast in cysts has been demonstrated during urography. Abnormalities of the contralateral kidney (e.g., ureteropelvic junction obstruction, malrotation) may be shown.

Cysts that vary in size and shape can be demonstrated with ultrasonography in the classic case of renal dysplasia. The largest cyst is not medially situated and there is absence of an identifiable renal sinus or surrounding renal parenchyma. There is no demonstrable communication between adjacent cysts. There are echogenic areas (due to multiple tiny cysts) that may be in an eccentric location (Fig. 71–9).

In the pediatric population, it has been shown that the kidney may be large with multiple large or moderate-sized cysts when the obstruction is at the ureteropelvic junction; distal ureteral obstruction is associated with a smaller kidney with few variably sized cysts; urethral obstruction can result in small kidneys with few or no cysts; small echogenic kidneys can be seen in those few cases without obstruction. "In one recent study utilizing prenatal ultrasound, 10/14 cases were accurately detected in the second trimester and 7/14 cases had abnormalities in the contralateral kidney, 5 of which were lethal."

Retrograde pyelography is usually not necessary. There may be a small, blind lower ureteral segment indicating atresia of the upper

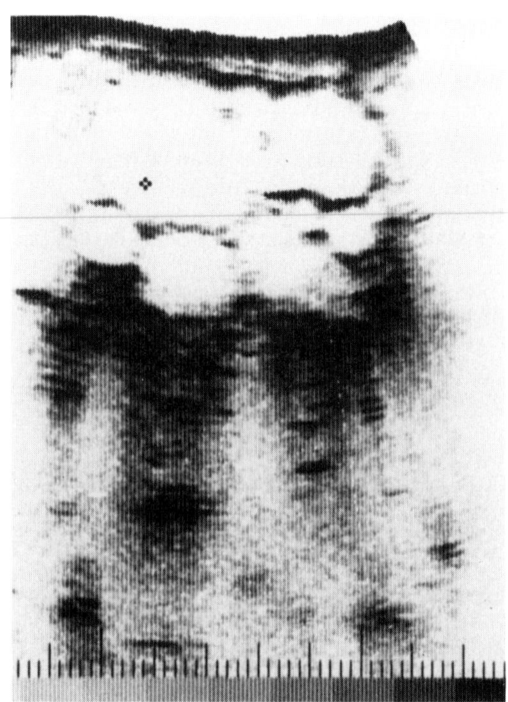

Figure 71–9. Total renal dysplasia (ultrasonogram). Note multiple cysts of varying size and shape. No identifiable renal sinus is present, and there is no surrounding renal parenchyma.

ureter. There may be no hemitrigone and ureter. If there is segmental disease, an ectopic distal ureteral orifice may be identified.

The most important differential diagnosis is hydronephrosis. Usually, this can be distinguished by ultrasonography, but occasionally other modalities such as urography or retrograde pyelography may be helpful.

CALYCEAL DIVERTICULUM/PYELOGENIC CYST

This is a cyst-like structure that usually extends from the fornix of a minor calyx via a narrow infundibulum and is located in the medullary region at the periphery of the renal pyramid. They are usually 2 to 5 mm in size, but can exceed 1 cm. They are most frequently unifocal and unilateral but may be multifocal and bilateral. The etiology is not clear, but formation has been attributed to either a congenital anomaly or rupture of a small cyst or abscess into a calyx.

Clinically they are usually asymptomatic; however, many do not drain well and are associated with stasis of urine that may become secondarily infected. Additional complications include calculus formation, renal colic, and hematuria. Occasionally, milk of calcium may be present.

A calyceal diverticulum may be suspected on the plain film if a cluster of calculi is noted in a spherical configuration in the region of minor calyces.

Delayed filling of a calyceal diverticulum relative to the pelvocalyceal system is seen at urography. The isthmus is not always defined but enters the fornix of the calyx. Intraluminal calculi may be noted (Fig. 71–10).

If no calculi are present, ultrasonography may demonstrate a small cystic structure (sometimes confused with a renal cyst) extending from the region of the minor calyces. If calculi are present, shadowing may obscure detail.

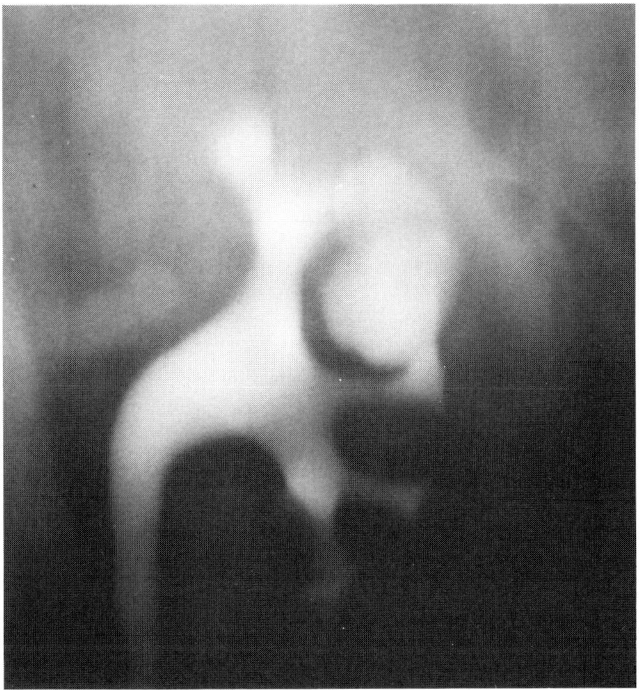

Figure 71–10. Calyceal diverticulum (nephrotomogram). There is a bilobed calyceal diverticulum between the upper and middle calyces. The isthmus is not defined. There is a 3-mm calculus that is not seen but was detected on the plain film.

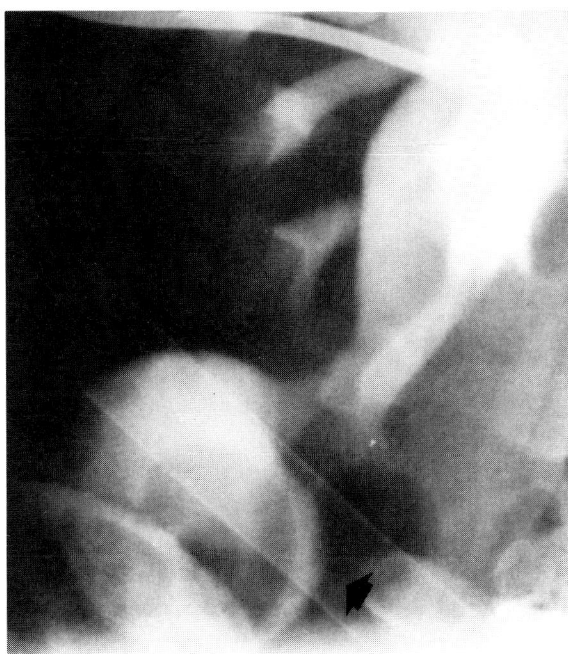

Figure 71–11. Perinephric pseudocyst (urinoma) (nephrostogram). There is opacification of a well-defined urinoma *(arrow)* extending from the ureteropelvic junction following pyeloplasty. It resolved with nephrostomy drainage.

A calyceal diverticulum must be differentiated from medullary necrosis. The cavity of medullary necrosis is in the center of a papilla and different in location from a diverticulum. Both medullary necrosis and microcalyces opacify at the same time as the remainder of the collecting structures, while a calyceal diverticulum opacifies after the calyx fills with contrast. A hydrocalyx can be diagnosed because of its typical position relative to the renal pelvis and other minor calyces.

PERINEPHRIC PSEUDOCYST (URINOMA)

This abnormality has also been called uriniferous perirenal pseudocyst, pararenal pseudocyst, traumatic perinephric cyst, pseudohydronephrosis, hydrocele renalis, perirenal cyst, and perinephric cyst. Blunt trauma or iatrogenic injury can lead to encapsulation of extravasated urine. It is usually secondary to laceration of the collecting system. Occasionally, it is the result of obstruction with spontaneous extravasation. If ureteral obstruction persists and the pelvocalyceal system does not heal or seal, urine will continue to leak into adjacent perirenal adipose tissue with subsequent development of a fibrous capsule (produced experimentally in animals in 12 to 40 days). There is no epithelial lining.

Patients present most frequently between two weeks and two months following injury with extravasation. They may experience pain and there may be a palpable flank mass.

With urography, there is an elliptical soft-tissue mass inferomedially with resultant superolateral displacement of the kidney's lower pole and medial displacement of the ureter. Hydronephrosis may occur or there may be extravasation of contrast into the mass.

Ultrasonography and CT can demonstrate the cystic mass but retrograde and/or antegrade pyelography may be necessary to define the anatomy and the point of communication (Fig. 71–11).

Bibliography

Amis ES Jr, Hartman DS: Renal ultrasonography 1984: A practical overview. Radiol Clin North Am 22:315–332, 1984.

Aronson D, Frazier HA, Baluch JD, et al: Cystic renal masses: Usefulness of the Bosniak classification. Urol Radiol 13:83–90, 1991.

Becker JA, Schneider M: Simple cyst of the kidney. Semin Roentgenol 10:103–111, 1975.

Blyth H, Ockenden BG: Polycystic disease of kidneys and liver presenting in childhood. J Med Genet 8:257–284, 1971.

Boal DK, Teele RL: Sonography of infantile polycystic kidney disease. AJR 135:575–580, 1980.

Bosniak MA: Difficulties in classifying cystic lesions of the kidney. Urol Radiol 13:91–93, 1991.

Dungan JS, Fernandez MT, Abbitt PL, et al: Multicystic dysplastic kidney: Natural history of prenatally detected cases. Prenat Diagn 10:175–182, 1990.

Dunnick NR, Korobkin M: Computed tomography of the kidney. Radiol Clin North Am 22:297–313, 1984.

Feiner HD, Katz LA, Gallo GR: Acquired cystic disease of kidney in chronic dialysis patients. Urology 17:260–264, 1981.

Griscom NT, Vawter GF, Fellers FX: Pelvoinfundibular atresia: The usual form of multicystic kidney: 44 unilateral and two bilateral cases. Semin Roentgenol 10:125–131, 1975.

Grossman H, Rosenberg ER, Bowie JD, et al: Sonographic diagnosis of renal cystic diseases. AJR 140:81–85, 1983.

Hartman DS, Aronson S, Frazier H: Current status of imaging indeterminate renal masses. Radiol Clin North Am 29:475–496, 1991.

Hidalgo H, Dunnick ND, Rosenberg ER, et al: Parapelvic cysts: Appearance on CT and sonography. AJR 138:667–671, 1982.

Hricak H, Newhouse JH: MR imaging of the kidney. Radiol Clin North Am 22:287–296, 1984.

Ishikawa I, Saito Y, Onouchi Z, et al: Development of acquired cystic disease and adenocarcinoma of the kidney in glomerulonephritic chronic hemodialysis patients. Clin Nephrol 14:1–6, 1980.

Kissane JM: Congenital malformations. In Heptinstall's Pathology of the Kidney. Boston, Little, Brown and Company, 1983, pp 83–140.

Lebowitz RL, Griscom NT: Neonatal hydronephrosis: 146 cases. Radiol Clin North Am 15:49–59, 1977.

Levine E, Slusher SL, Grantham JJ, Wetzel LH: Natural history of acquired renal cystic disease in dialysis patients: A prospective longitudinal CT study. AJR 156:502–506, 1991.

Madewell JE, Hartman DS, Lichtenstein JE: Radiologic-pathologic correlations in cystic disease of the kidney. Radiol Clin North Am 17:261–279, 1979.

Osathanondh V, Potter EL: Pathogenesis of polycystic kidneys: Historical survey. Arch Pathol 77:459–473, 1964.

Palubinskas AJ: Medullary sponge kidney. Radiology 76:911–918, 1961.

Reuss A, Wladimiroff JW, Stewart PA, Niermeijer MF: Prenatal diagnosis by ultrasound in pregnancies at risk for autosomal recessive polycystic kidney disease. Ultrasound Med Biol 16:355–359, 1990.

Sanders RC, Hartman DS: The sonographic distinction between neonatal multicystic kidney and hydronephrosis. Radiology 151:621–625, 1984.

Sanders RC, Nussbaum AR, Solez K: Renal dysplasia: Sonographic findings. Radiology 167:623–626, 1988.

Scanlon MH, Karasick SR: Acquired renal cystic disease and neoplasia: Complications of chronic hemodialysis. Radiology 147:837–838, 1983.

Segal AJ, Spataro RF, Barbaric ZL: Computed tomography of adult polycystic disease. J Comput Assist Tomogr 6:777–780, 1982.

Stuck KJ, Koff SA, Silver TM: Ultrasonic features of multicystic dysplastic kidney: Expanded diagnostic criteria. Radiology 143:217–221, 1982.

Taylor AJ, Cohen EP, Erickson SJ, et al: Renal imaging in long-term dialysis patients: A comparison of CT and sonography. AJR 153:765–767, 1989.

Warshauer DM, McCarthy SM, Street L, et al: Detection of renal masses: Sensitivities and specificities of excretory urography/linear tomography, US, and CT. Radiology 169:363–365, 1988.

72 Benign Renal Tumors

Neil M. Rofsky and Morton A. Bosniak

Benign tumors of the kidney may arise from the renal parenchyma or the capsule. Many of the benign tumors are very small in size, asymptomatic, often found incidentally at autopsy, and of no clinical significance. However, some benign tumors become clinically significant. Although the nature of these lesions cannot always be established with imaging studies, some, such as angiomyolipomas, display imaging features that can distinguish them from malignant tumors. Every effort should be made to accurately characterize these lesions to direct the proper management of these patients. This chapter deals with the radiologic features of these benign renal tumors with emphasis on imaging studies in detection, diagnosis, and management.

The following benign tumors of the kidney will be discussed: (1) renal adenoma, (2) renal oncocytoma, (3) angiomyolipoma (hamartoma), (4) multilocular cystic nephroma, and (5) mesenchymal tumors including leiomyoma, lipoma, hemangioma, reninoma (juxtaglomerular tumor), and miscellaneous tumors.

RENAL ADENOMA

Renal adenomas are one of the most common benign tumors of the renal parenchyma. The great majority of these are small adenomas (less than 2 cm) that are generally subcapsular in location and discovered incidentally at autopsy. Rarely, large adenomas may be detected serendipitously or during evaluation for symptoms caused by their large size.

The relationship between renal adenomas and well-differentiated renal cell carcinomas has been debated for many years and is still not universally agreed upon. Most pathologists believe that renal adenomas are "premalignant" lesions, or "potentially" malignant or are precursors of renal cell carcinoma. As Willis has written, "Adenomas show a structure indistinguishable from that of carcinoma, and it is purely a matter of opinion whether we regard such tumors as atypical adenomas or as young carcinomas that happen to have been discovered before they have metastasized. Many an 'adenoma' found incidentally at necropsy differs not one whit from some of those small symptomless carcinomas which have produced precocious metastases." The criterion of size that was used for many years that small renal cortical tumors (less than 3.0 cm) were adenomas and those over 3.0 cm were carcinomas has been completely abandoned.

Many aspects are common to renal adenomas and renal cell carcinomas: (1) both occur in the same age group, (2) both occur more often in tobacco users and in men, (3) both have their origin from the proximal convoluted tubules, (4) the same kidney can harbor both an adenoma and a carcinoma, and (5) histology and electron microscopy may not differentiate an adenoma from a carcinoma of the same cell type.

Microscopically, the cellular arrangement of renal adenomas includes tubular, papillary, and alveolar, and the cell types are basophilic, eosinophilic, and clear-cell. (One type of tubular adenoma is distinctive and will be discussed in the next section on oncocytoma.) The tubular and papillary adenomas are the most common, the next being mixed adenomas, and the alveolar type is the least common.

The imaging features of renal adenomas are nonspecific and are similar to those seen with renal cell carcinomas. It should be emphasized that the differentiation between an adenoma and a carcinoma is not possible radiologically.

RENAL ONCOCYTOMA

Although renal oncocytomas were initially described during the 1960s, there has been increased interest in the tumor ever since Klein and Valenci reported 13 cases in 1976. Renal oncocytomas are also known as proximal tubular adenomas with so-called oncocytic features and also as oxyphilic adenomas. They are benign neoplasms, believed to have their origin from the proximal tubular epithelium, and composed exclusively of oncocytes. These tumors generally occur in the fifth and sixth decade with a mean age of 52 years, and a male to female ratio of about 1.7 to 1. They can be multicentric and bilateral and can be associated with renal cell carcinoma. Oncocytomas can occur in the adrenal, thyroid, parathyroid, and salivary glands as well as in the kidney.

Oncocytomas vary in size from about 1 to 2 cm to very large bulky lesions. In contrast to renal cell carcinomas, which are yellow or orange on cut section, the oncocytomas have a typical tan to brown color similar to that of normal renal tissue. Tumor necrosis or hemorrhage, which is common in renal cell carcinomas, is uncommon in oncocytomas. A central fibrotic scar may be seen in larger oncocytomas (Figs. 72–1 and 72–2).

There is some difference of opinion about the significance and pathologic diagnosis of oncocytomas. Most pathologists believe that these tumors are distinct benign adenomas of the kidney that can be clearly differentiated from other adenomas or renal cell carcinomas. Some pathologists have divided oncocytomas into grades I, II, and III. The grade I tumors are benign, proximal tubular adenomas made up of pure, well-differentiated eosinophilic granular cells that are nonaggressive tumors and have a highly favorable prognosis. Grade II and III oncocytomas are less well differentiated and show features such as capsule and venous invasion with prominent nuclear and nucleolar characteristics. Most pathologists consider these tumors as renal cell carcinoma with oncocytic features. For the remainder of this section, the term *oncocytoma* will refer to these clearly benign grade I lesions.

Oncocytomas are composed entirely of oncocytes that contain finely granular eosinophilic cytoplasm and an increased cytoplasmic volume. Ultrastructurally, the hallmark of these tumors is the presence of abundant mitochondria, scanty organelles, and the absence of fat vacuoles.

The conspicuous cellular pleomorphism and anaplasia with high mitotic rates seen in granular cell carcinomas are typically absent in oncocytomas. To establish a conclusive pathologic diagnosis of renal oncocytoma, it is important that a large sample of tumor tissue (in most instances the entire tumor) be obtained so that necrosis, hemorrhage, and cellular heterogeneity seen with renal cell carcinoma can be excluded in all portions of the tumor.

It is reported in one series that the majority of oncocytomas are asymptomatic and discovered incidentally. The larger tumors may present as palpable masses (28 per cent), gross hematuria (9 per cent), and microscopic hematuria (40 per cent).

Radiologic Diagnosis

Renal oncocytomas have a nonspecific appearance on excretory urography and are seen as well-demarcated renal masses. Calcification within the tumor is extremely rare, but has been reported. Nuclear medicine scans have proven not to be helpful because these tumors display a defect on the renal scan indistinguishable from other renal masses.

The gross pathologic features of oncocytomas determine their sonographic appearance. The smaller neoplasms are generally well-circumscribed and homogeneously solid masses due to lack of hemorrhage or tumor necrosis. The tumors are of medium amplitude echogenicity, closely resembling the echogenicity of normal renal parenchyma. The larger tumors could be either poorly or well-demarcated and appear homogeneously solid or heterogeneously solid when associated with internal hemorrhage or necrosis. The presence of a central echogenic or echo-poor area corresponding to the central cleft or scar is sometimes seen (see Fig. 72–2).

Oncocytomas appear on CT as discrete, well-marginated masses. They are generally homogeneous on non-contrast and contrast scans (see Figs. 72–1 and 72–2). On non-contrast scans, the attenuation of these neoplasms and adjacent renal parenchyma is similar, and hence small tumors confined to the renal margins may not be visible. Oncocytomas are generally quite vascular and show homogeneous enhancement after an intravenous bolus injection of contrast. During the early vascular phase, they may be hypervascular compared with renal tissue, but during the nephrogram phase the degree of enhancement is generally less than that of normal renal parenchyma. In the presence of intratumoral hemorrhage and/or necrosis the tumors will appear heterogeneous, in which case a diagnosis of oncocytoma cannot be suggested by CT criteria. In a significant proportion of oncocytomas, generally in larger lesions, a characteristic central low attenuation cleft can be demonstrated (see Figs. 72–1 and 72–2); however, this finding is not pathognomonic as a similar central scar (or area of decreased attenuation) can be seen with some renal cell carcinomas. The invasive features seen with renal cell carcinomas are absent with oncocytomas.

Angiographically, a typical oncocytoma is a vascular mass and shows ''spoke-wheel'' configuration of the feeding vessels, homogeneous dense nephrogram, sharp margination, and a smooth rim (see Figs. 72–1 and 72–2). All these features are present in 23 to 57 per cent of renal oncocytomas. The remainder of the tumors may show one or more of these angiographic features. Some oncocytomas may be hypovascular or avascular. Large, irregular, clearly malignant vessels are not seen in oncocytomas, nor is arteriovenous (AV) shunting with early venous filling. However, the angiographic findings can be occasionally mimicked by well-differentiated, well-encapsulated renal cell carcinoma.

The MRI appearance of oncocytomas is variable and nonspecific. Some of these lesions may demonstrate a central scar. When present, the scar can be seen as a dark stellate area on T_1-weighted images and may brighten considerably on T_2-weighted images. However, because this finding can be seen with renal cell carcinoma, it cannot be used to definitively establish the diagnosis of oncocytoma.

Percutaneous needle aspiration for diagnosis of oncocytoma has been performed. However, because only a small sample of tumor tissue is obtained by needle aspiration, there is a potential for confusing an oncocytoma with a renal cell carcinoma that contains areas with oncocytic features. However, in cases in which renal surgery must be avoided because of poor operative risk, this approach might be used.

Since oncocytomas are benign tumors, achieving a preoperative radiographic diagnosis would have an important effect on patient management. However, because the radiologic features of oncocytomas and some malignant renal tumors overlap, this is not possible.

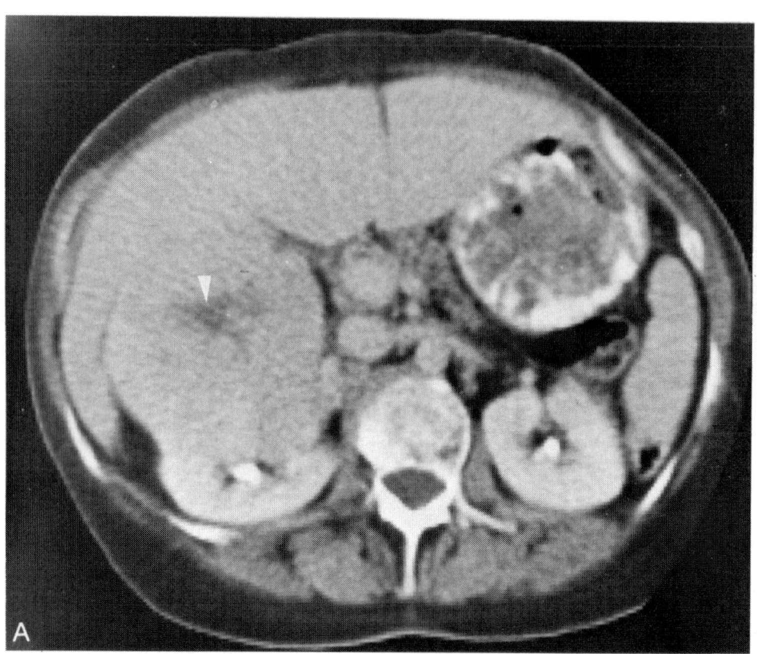

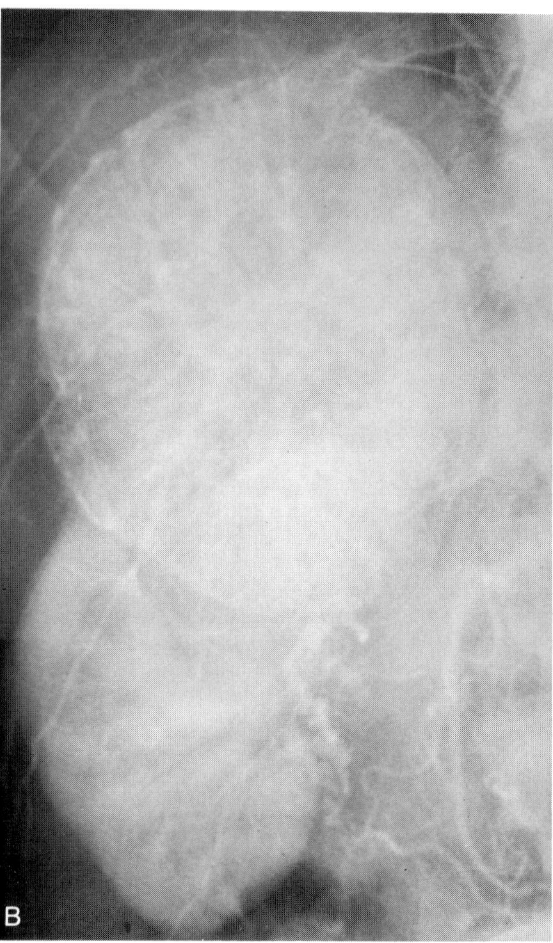

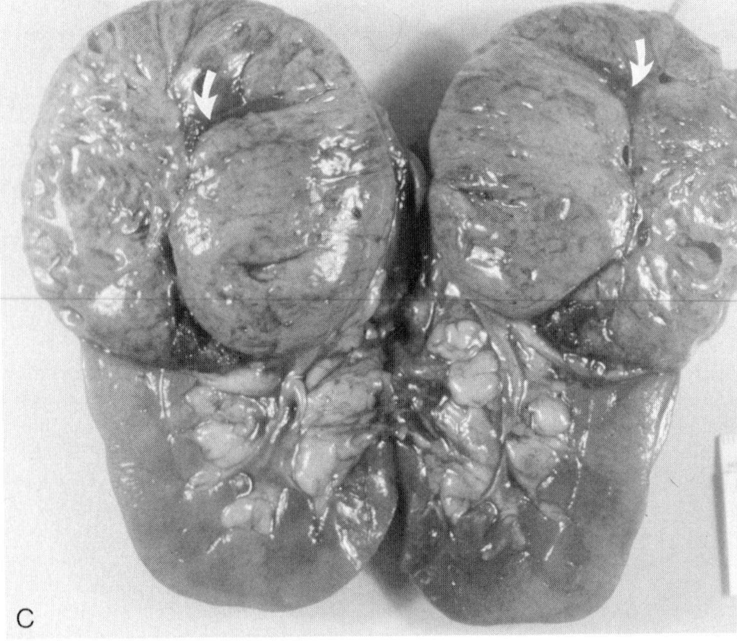

Figure 72–1. Characteristic findings in renal oncocytoma. *A,* Contrast-enhanced CT scan shows a well-circumscribed, homogeneously solid mass with a central low attenuation cleft *(arrowhead)*—features considered typical of an oncocytoma. *B,* Angiography reveals a sharply marginated vascular mass with "spoke-wheel" configuration, typical of an oncocytoma. *C,* Gross pathology of an oncocytoma that is homogeneous and contains a "stellate" scar *(arrows)*. The brown color of the tumor is very similar to that of the normal renal parenchyma. (*B* courtesy of Richard Gordon, M.D. *C* reprinted with permission from Ambos MA, Bosniak MA, Valensi QJ, et al: Angiographic patterns in renal oncocytomas. Radiology 129:615–622, 1978.)

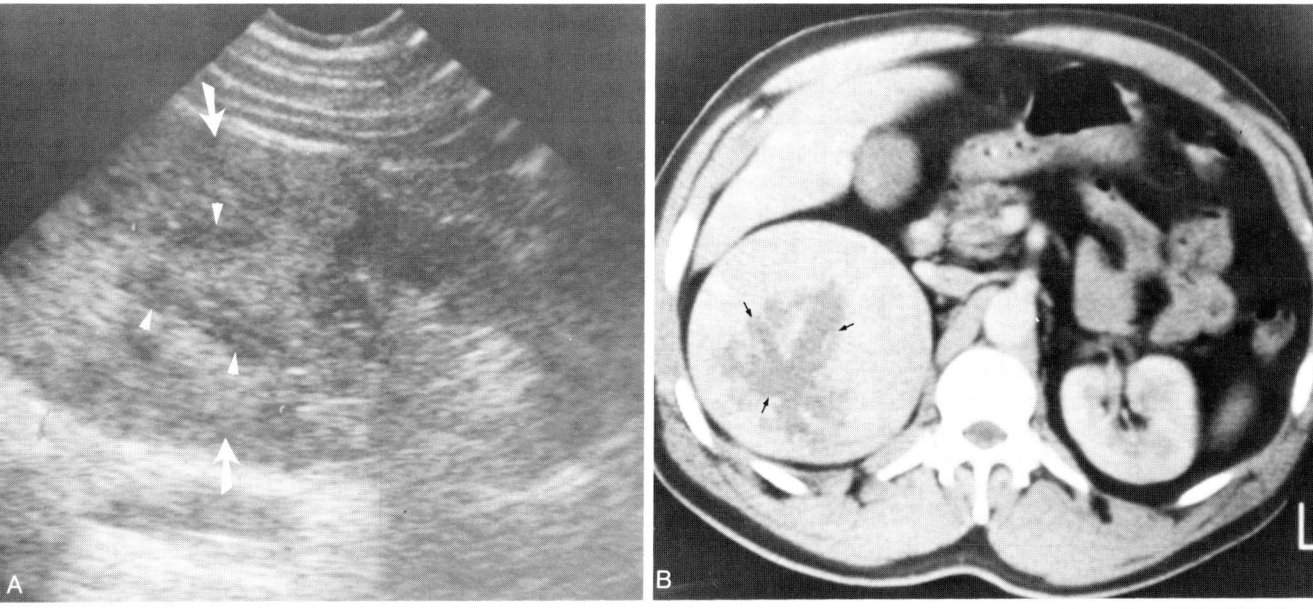

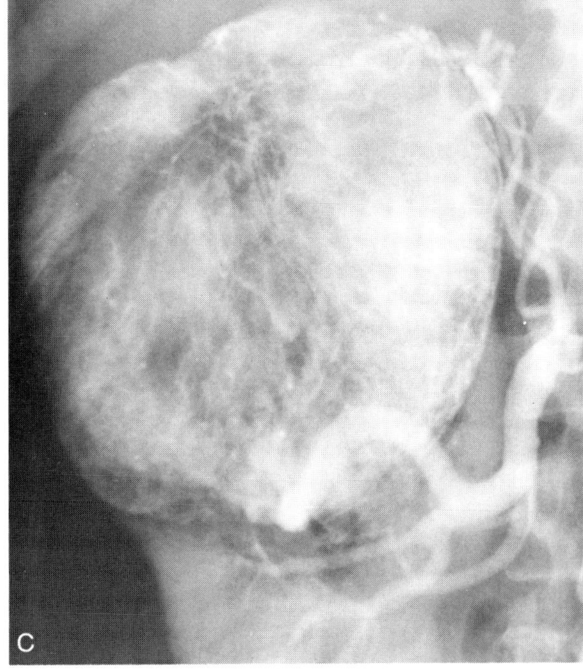

Figure 72–2. Oncocytoma in a 42-year-old man with history of trauma. *A,* Sonogram. Longitudinal scan reveals normal lower half of the right kidney and a large, heterogeneously solid mass *(arrows)* involving the upper half. Note the echo-poor areas *(arrowheads)* within the mass, representing the central scan often seen in oncocytomas. *B,* Contrast-enhanced CT scan shows a well-marginated mass with homogeneous contrast enhancement with a very prominent "stellate" scar *(arrows). C,* Selective renal angiogram reveals a well-marginated hypervascular mass with "spoke-wheel" configuration of vessels. (*C* courtesy of Richard S. Lefleur, M.D.)

Although well-circumscribed, homogeneously solid masses with a central scar on sonography and/or CT and a typical angiographic appearance of spoke-wheel configuration and sharp margination are strongly suggestive of oncocytomas, this diagnosis cannot be made with 100 per cent confidence. For this reason, it is difficult to justify an alternative approach to nephrectomy for these renal tumors. In certain clinical settings an alternative approach might be justified. In those cases in which the radiologic features strongly suggest oncocytoma, partial nephrectomy could be considered an alternative to total nephrectomy if the lesion is small and located in a polar position. In those cases in which there is a need to preserve renal tissue because of chronic renal disease, a single kidney, or bilateral tumors, a partial nephrectomy or tumorectomy could be justified. Because of the vastly greater incidence of renal cell carcinoma as compared with oncocytoma and the inability to reach a firm radiologic diagnosis of oncocytoma, the current surgical approach to these lesions is the same as for other renal parenchymal malignancies.

MESENCHYMAL TUMORS

Benign mesenchymal tumors are generally found incidentally at autopsy with a frequency of 8 to 11 per cent. Most of these tumors are not detected in life because they are small (often measuring several millimeters in size) and asymptomatic, although some larger tumors may manifest clinically. The tumors discussed in this group of lesions include angiomyolipoma, leiomyoma, lipoma, hemangiomas, reninomas and other rare miscellaneous tumors.

ANGIOMYOLIPOMA (HAMARTOMA)

Renal angiomyolipomas are not true neoplasms, but hamartomatous tissue rests. They occur in about 80 per cent of patients with tuberous sclerosis, whereas less than 40 per cent of patients with angiomyolipomas show one or more features of the tuberous sclerosis complex. An occasional manifestation of tuberous sclerosis is renal cystic disease resembling autosomal dominant polycystic disease. However, pathologically in tuberous sclerosis, the renal cyst may have a hyperplastic eosinophilic epithelial lining, a finding not seen in polycystic renal disease. The combination of renal involvement by cystic disease and angiomyolipomas is felt to be virtually pathognomonic for tuberous sclerosis. Angiomyolipomas may also be seen in patients with pulmonary lymphangiomyomatosis (Fig. 72–3). Angiomyolipomas could be very small in size (1 cm or less) or may attain very large size. At autopsy, it is not uncommon (7 to 10 per cent) to find in the renal parenchyma very small nodules containing adipose tissue and smooth muscle. These are frequently unilateral and found in women. In addition to smooth muscle and fat (myolipomas), they may contain angiomatous tissue, and these are indistinguishable from angiomyolipomas seen in patients with tuberous sclerosis. In patients with tuberous sclerosis, the angiomyolipomas are usually small, multiple (13 to 30 per cent), bilateral (15 per cent) (Fig. 72–4), and generally asymptomatic; however, it is not unusual for the tumors to be quite large and cause significant symptoms, particularly due to bleeding. The great majority of angiomyolipomas found in patients without tuberous sclerosis are asymptomatic, relatively small lesions (measuring 1 to 3 cm in size) and are incidental findings at sonography or CT. In symptomatic patients without tuberous sclerosis, the tumors are usually large, solitary lesions occurring in women between the ages of 30 and 60 years, with a female to male ratio of 2.6 to 1.

Angiomyolipomas are round or oval tumors that arise in both the cortex and medulla and elevate the renal capsule. They grow by expansion and local invasion. In about 25 per cent, the tumors extend into the perirenal space. Involvement of regional lymph nodes is usually due to separate hamartomatous foci (see Fig. 72–3). Vascular extension is extremely rare but has been reported.

Typically, angiomyolipomas contain three tissue elements: adipose tissue, smooth muscle, and angiomatous tissue. The proportion of these tissue elements is variable from patient to patient and within different segments of the tumor in the same patient. According to the proportion and distribution of the tissue elements, the tumors on cut surface are yellow to gray in color and frequently consist of masses of fat. The tumors are often associated with areas of hemorrhage within the tumor and in a subcapsular location. Old hemorrhage is seen as areas of necrosis and calcification.

The microscopic features of angiomyolipomas typically consist of a variable combination of mature adipose tissue, sheets of smooth muscle, and a cluster of thick-walled blood vessels lacking normal

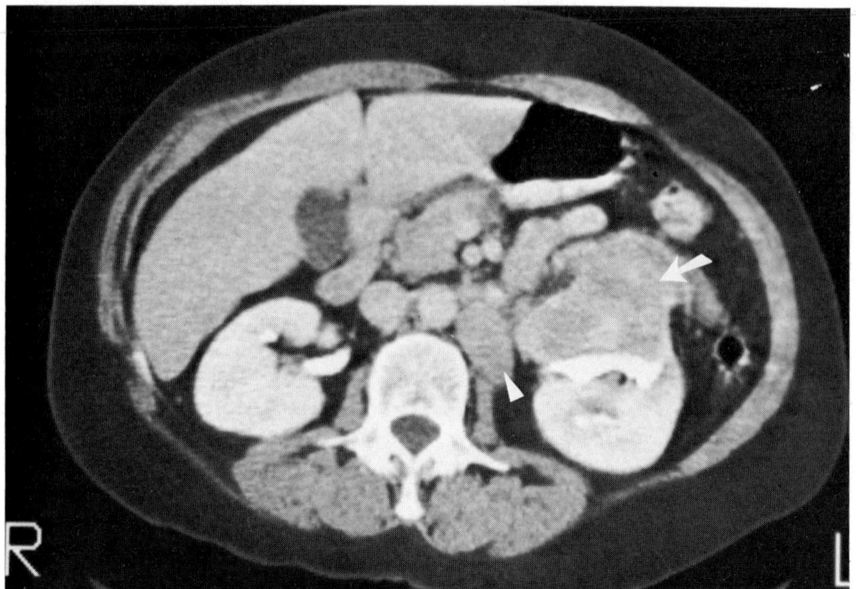

Figure 72–3. Hamartoma in a 52-year-old female with pulmonary lymphangiomyomatosis. Contrast-enhanced CT scan reveals a left renal mass *(arrow)* representing an angiomyoma without discernible fatty tissue. The para-aortic mass *(arrowhead)* represents a hamartoma in a pararenal lymph node. A subsequent angiogram revealed the characteristic angiomatous vessels seen in these tumors. (Reprinted with permission from Rumancik WM, Bosniak MA, Rosen RJ, et al: Atypical renal and pararenal hamartomas associated with lymphangiomyomatosis. AJR 142:971–972, 1984. © 1984, American Roentgen Ray Society.)

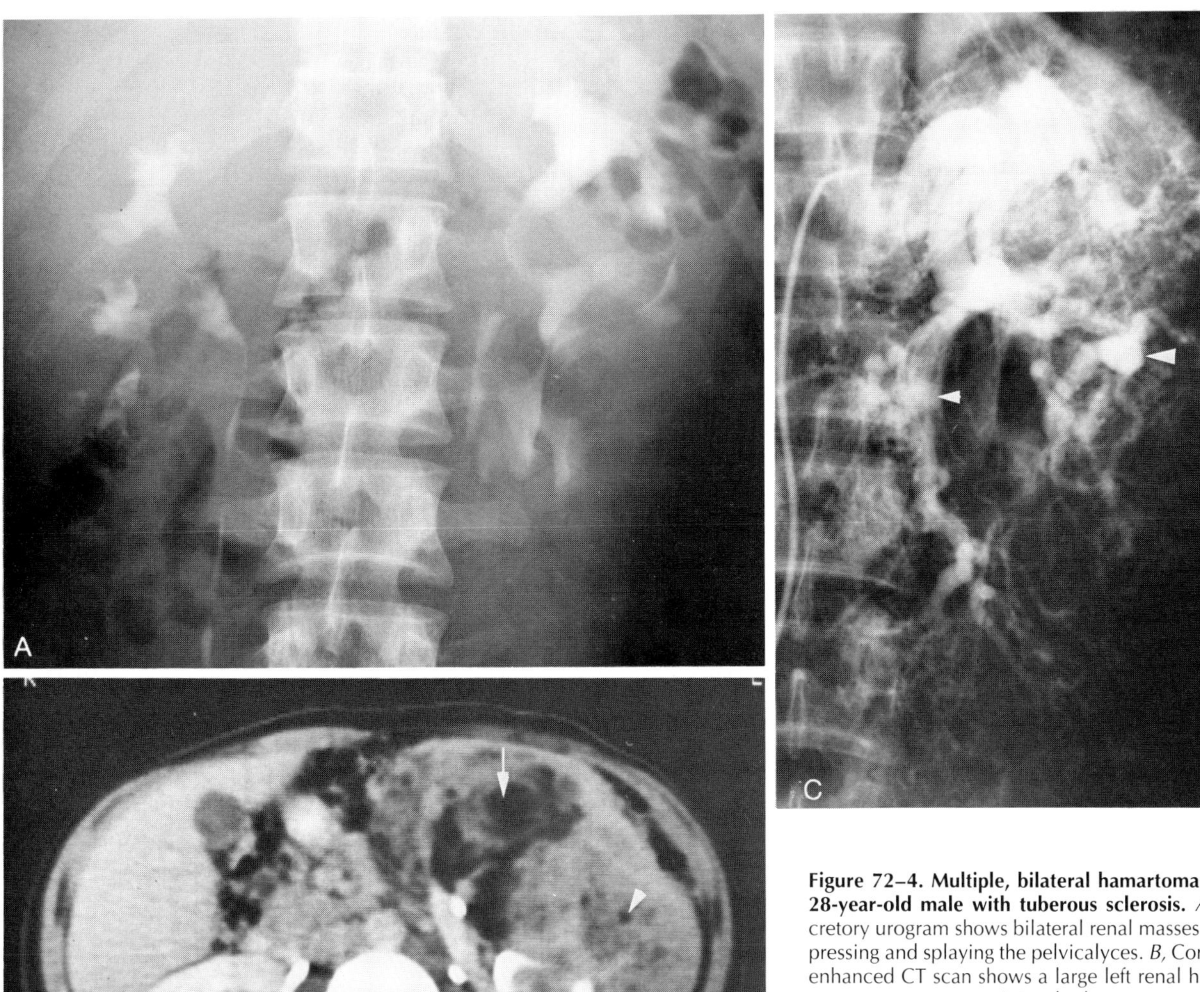

Figure 72–4. Multiple, bilateral hamartomas in a 28-year-old male with tuberous sclerosis. *A,* Excretory urogram shows bilateral renal masses compressing and splaying the pelvicalyces. *B,* Contrast-enhanced CT scan shows a large left renal hamartomatous mass containing both myomatous elements and fatty portions *(straight arrow).* Note numerous small foci of fat within the tumor and in the remainder of the kidney *(arrowheads).* The right kidney shows a soft-tissue mass *(curved arrow)* without fatty areas and represents an angiomyoma. *C,* Selective left renal angiogram shows a vascular mass supplied by hypertrophiedrenal arterial branches. Note the presence of multiple aneurysms *(arrowheads),* characteristic of an angiomatous tumor. (*A* to *C* reprinted with permission from Rosen RJ, Schlossberg P, Roven SJ, et al: Management of symptomatic renal angiomyolipomas by embolization. Urol Radiol 6:196–200, 1984.)

elastic membranes that contribute to the tortuosity and aneurysmal dilatation of the blood vessels. The vessels in general are poorly formed and show varying thickness, subintimal fibrosis, hyalinization of the media, and eccentrically placed lumina. Based on the proportion and distribution of the tissue elements within the tumor, the microscopic features will differ, but generally all three components will be present.

Diagnostic Imaging

On plain film of the abdomen angiomyolipomas can be detected if they are relatively large in size with a significant amount of fat. Because of the widespread use of sonography and CT in the diagnosis of abdominal disease, increased serendipitous detection of these tumors has occurred. More importantly, the ability to accurately diagnose many angiomyolipomas has resulted which has had important implications in patient management with particular emphasis on preservation of renal tissue.

ULTRASONOGRAPHY

There is a spectrum of sonographic features in renal angiomyolipomas that is attributed to variable pathology of each angiomyolipoma and within different parts of the same tumor. Sonographic detection of angiomyolipomas will depend on the proportion of fat to smooth muscle and angiomatous tissue within the tumors. In addition, the presence or absence of intratumoral hemorrhage further alters the sonographic appearance. The interaction between ultrasound beam and fatty tissue and tumors is somewhat variable. However, the great majority of renal angiomyolipomas have a predictable sonographic appearance, that of a highly echogenic mass due to the usual high fat content or the multiple tissue interfaces of these tumors (Figs. 72–5 and 72–6). Occasionally, a renal cell carcinoma or an area of renal infarct may appear highly echogenic; hence, it is essential to recognize that "high echogenicity" of a renal mass although highly suggestive does not always equate to the diagnosis of angiomyolipoma. This lack of specificity mandates the need for unequivocal identification of fat within the tumor by CT.

As mentioned above, the overwhelming majority of angiomyolipomas contain abundant fatty tissue and will be highly echogenic on ultrasonography, which allows detection of very small lesions (see Fig. 72–5). Angiomyolipomas, which contain a greater proportion of smooth muscle, or tumors with internal hemorrhage will appear as heterogeneous solid masses. The highly echogenic areas represent fatty parts of the tumor, whereas the low or medium echogenic segments correspond to areas of smooth muscle or hemorrhage and/or necrosis. The least common sonographic appearance is that of a medium-amplitude solid mass without obvious areas of high echogenicity. Such tumors have been shown to be angiomyolipomas containing primarily smooth muscle and very little fat, or angiomyomas containing only smooth muscle and angiomatous tissue. The sonographic appearance of such tumors will be indistinguishable from that of other solid neoplasms. Sonography can detect perinephric hemorrhage due to an angiomyolipoma. A large perinephric hematoma can obscure an underlying small angiomyolipoma, and hence meticulous scanning, follow-up study, and the use of CT and angiography may be necessary for diagnosis.

COMPUTED TOMOGRAPHY

The pathologic features of angiomyolipomas discussed earlier determine their appearance on CT. CT is extremely accurate in the positive identification of fat, and a preoperative diagnosis of angiomyolipoma can therefore be made in almost all cases. The CT diagnosis of angiomyolipoma depends on obtaining negative attenuation values from fatty tissue within the tumor.

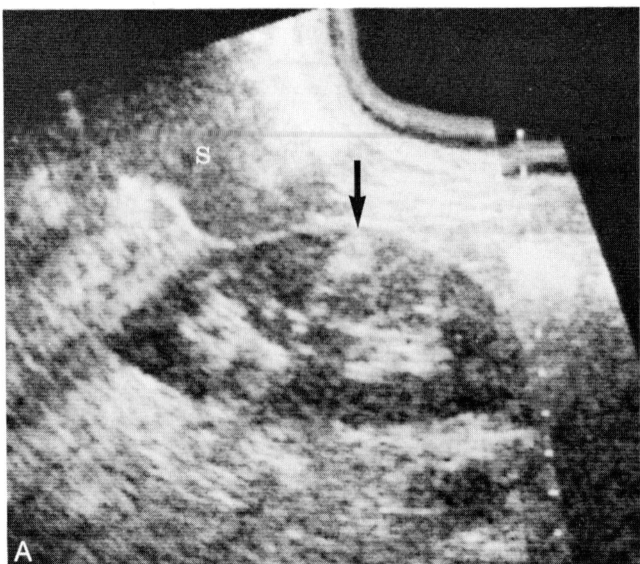

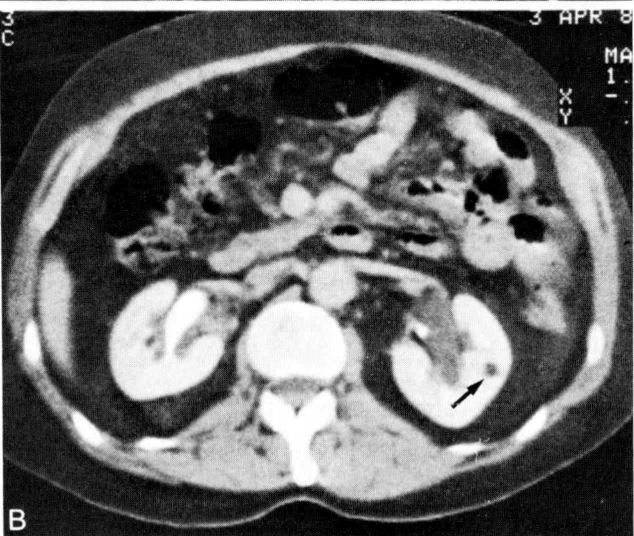

Figure 72–5. Incidental angiomyolipoma in a 56-year-old male. *A,* Sonogram: Longitudinal scan through the kidney reveals a 1-cm highly echogenic mass *(arrow)* characteristic of an angiomyolipoma. The adjacent spleen (S) is seen. *B,* Contrast-enhanced CT scan shows the left renal mass *(arrow)* to contain fat (−50 HU) diagnostic of an angiomyolipoma.

Most angiomyolipomas contain abundant adipose tissue, and the CT diagnosis is usually straightforward (Fig. 72–7; see Figs. 72–4 and 72–6). Even small tumors (less than 1 cm) can be accurately diagnosed by unequivocal identification of fat (see Fig. 72–5). Although partial-volume phenomenon could be a potential problem in obtaining negative values, it has been possible to identify fat even within tumors that have extremely small amounts of fat by meticulous scanning using thin sections (5 mm) if necessary. If uncertainty exists as to whether fat is present in a lesion, thin sections (as small as 3 mm) should be obtained without the use of intravenous contrast to further facilitate the detection of negative attenuation values, characteristic of fat. It must be remembered that the only imaging finding that will distinguish between a renal cell carcinoma (which requires surgery) and a benign angiomyolipoma (which often does not) is proving the existence of fat within the lesion. The radiologist should be suspicious of the possibility of fat in a lesion that shows areas of low attenuation within it and then make every effort to facilitate its detection to prove the diagnosis (Fig. 72–8). It has to

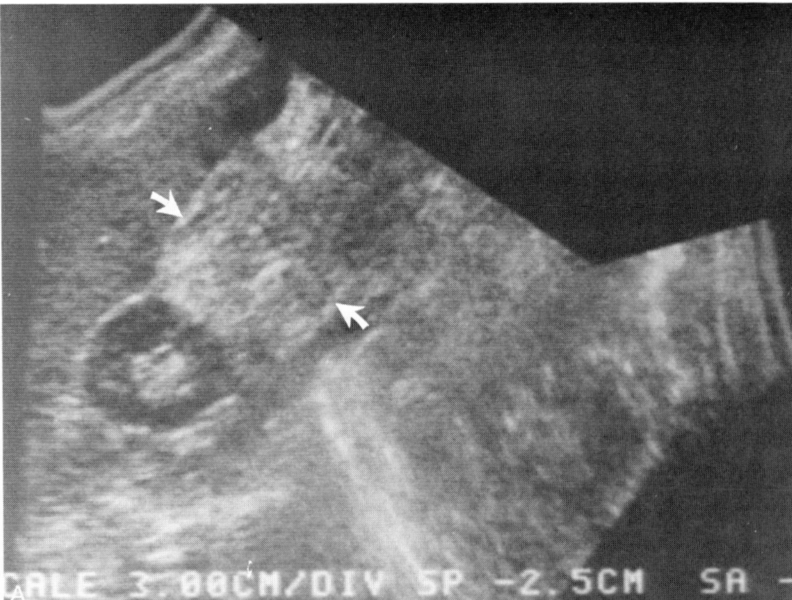

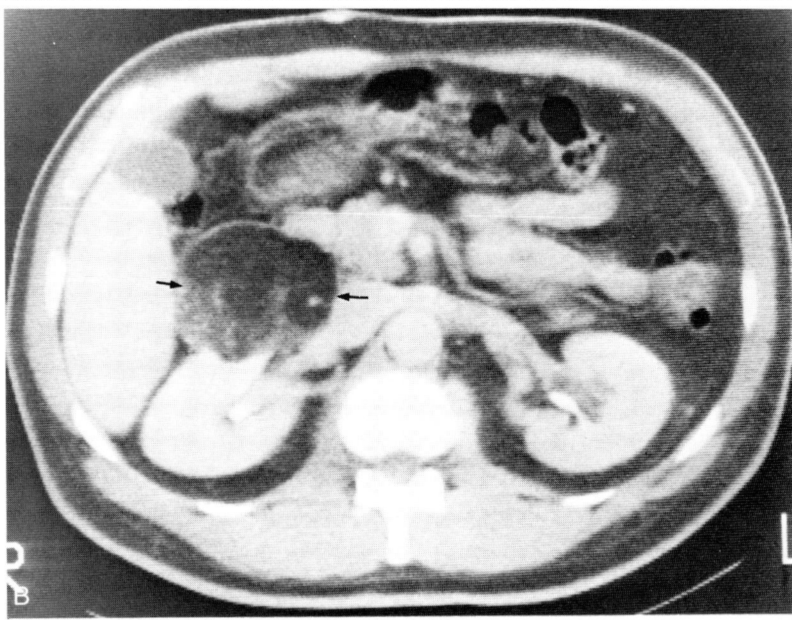

Figure 72–6. Incidental angiomyolipoma in a 53-year-old female referred for sonography for gall-bladder disease. *A,* Transverse sonogram reveals a highly echogenic mass *(arrows)* arising from the right kidney. *B,* Contrast-enhanced CT scan confirms an angiomyolipoma by detecting fat (−95 HU) within the mass *(arrows).*

be noted that very small tumors located adjacent to the renal sinus or at the periphery of the renal cortex may escape detection because the fat within the tumor may merge with the renal sinus or perinephric fat and therefore not be able to be clearly identified as a separate mass of tissue. Also it must be certain that the fat detected in a lesion is truly an intrinsic component of the lesion and not normal fat (renal sinus or perirenal) that has been engulfed by the lesion (see Fig. 72–7). Angiomyolipomas containing increased smooth muscle or complicated by internal hemorrhage and/or necrosis will show a mixed appearance on CT. In addition to fat within the tumor, CT may show areas of soft-tissue density corresponding to smooth muscle components of the tumor or hemorrhagic areas. Despite the presence of marked hemorrhage within the tumor, CT can usually readily identify at least some fatty component to the tumor. This is particularly important in patients who present with spontaneous subcapsular or perirenal hematomas because approximately one third of cases of spontaneous perirenal hemorrhage are due to bleeding angiomyolipomas. Patient management will be significantly guided if the existence of a fat-containing tumor as the etiology of the bleed can be firmly established. Finally, hamartomas without fatty tissue (angiomyomas) are rare and will be unable to be diagnosed by CT because they will appear similar to other solid renal neoplasms (see Figs. 72–3 and 72–4).

Recently, two cases of renal cell carcinoma containing fat have been reported. However, in both instances, the lesions also contained significant amounts of calcification. Intratumoral calcification is rare in angiomyolipoma and strongly suggestive of malignancy. Therefore, a diagnosis of angiomyolipoma cannot be made when a fat-containing renal tumor also contains calcification and renal cell carcinoma must be strongly considered.

MRI

The characteristic MRI signal intensities of fat can be used to help diagnose angiomyolipomas. When fatty elements predominate, the tumor will display hyperintense signal compared with other tissues on T_1-weighted images. The signal characteristics of subcutaneous and retroperitoneal fat demonstrated on T_1- and T_2-weighted

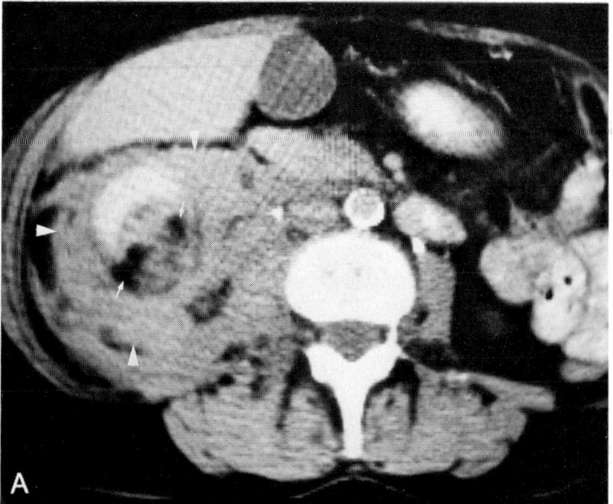

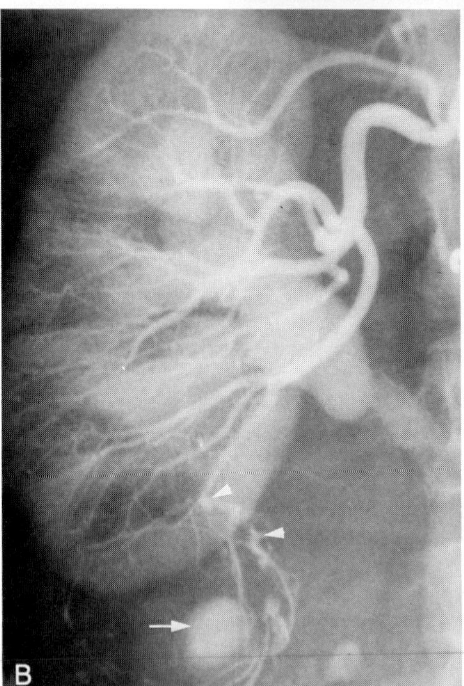

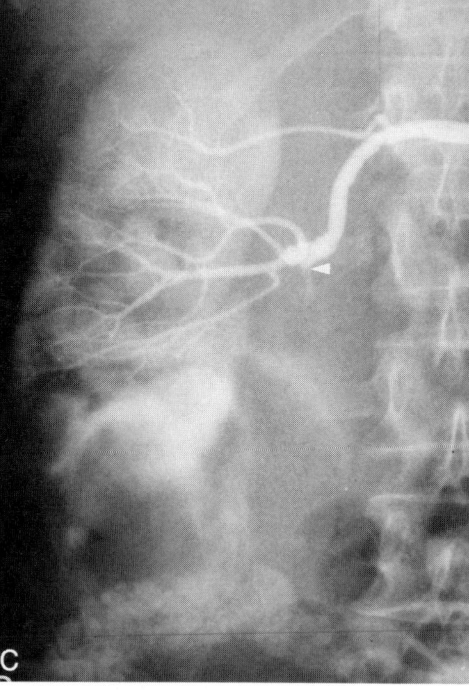

Figure 72–7. Perinephric hematoma due to an angiomyolipoma in a 68-year-old female with right flank pain. *A,* Contrast-enhanced CT scan reveals a large perinephric hamartoma *(arrowheads)* due to a renal neoplasm at the lower pole of the right kidney. Note the fatty areas *(arrows)* within the tumor, which are diagnostic of an angiomyolipoma. *B,* Selective right renal angiogram shows a vascular tumor at the lower pole with small aneurysms *(arrowheads).* A large collection of contrast medium is seen *(arrow)* that represents either a ruptured macroaneurysm or localized extravasation of contrast medium. *C,* Angiogram performed after embolization of the tumor with Ivalon particles shows complete obliteration of the branch *(arrowhead)* feeding the lesion. Note contrast accumulation at the lower pole of the kidney from previous extravasation. CT scan performed 14 months later showed a shrunken, fat-containing calcified mass without contrast enhancement, and the patient has remained asymptomatic. (*A* to *C* reprinted with permission from Zerhouni, EA, Schellhammer P, Schaefer JC, et al: Management of bleeding renal angiomyolipomas by transcatheter embolization following CT diagnosis. Urol Radiol 6:205–209, 1984.)

images can be used for comparison to positively identify fat within a tumor. Additionally any of a variety of selective fat suppression techniques can be employed to establish the presence of fat. These techniques may be of particular value in distinguishing fat from hemorrhage, which can be confused at times owing to similar MRI signal characteristics.

The relative amounts of the tissues composing the tumor will influence the signal characteristics with MRI. When large amounts of smooth muscle are present a definitive diagnosis may be precluded and the tumor may be indistinguishable from other tumors, including adenocarcinoma.

ANGIOGRAPHY

The noninvasive and accurate diagnosis of angiomyolipomas by sonography and CT has limited the use of angiography. However, angiography still has an important role in selected situations and remains unique in detailed depiction of renal arterial anatomy in treatment planning.

The angiographic appearance of angiomyolipomas is governed primarily by the proportion of angiomatous tissue. In about a third of cases, a characteristic vascular pattern is seen related to the angiomatous elements. This includes tortuous and aneurysmally dilated vessels, localized berry-like aneurysms, and stagnation of contrast in these vessels (see Figs. 72–4 and 72–7). A frequent finding in larger tumors is the presence of a single prominent hypertrophied intrarenal artery feeding the tumor. Of the remaining two thirds of angiomyolipomas, approximately a third will show vascular tumors indistinguishable from renal cell carcinoma, and the rest will be hypovascular because of lack or sparseness of angiomatous tissue. Although angiography cannot reliably differentiate renal cell carcinoma and angiomyolipoma, it should be noted that arteriovenous shunting, not uncommon in renal cell carcinoma, is reported not to occur in angiomyolipoma.

Renal angiomyolipomas, which may be amenable to renal-sparing surgery such as tumorectomy or partial nephrectomy, require preoperative angiography. In patients with perinephric hemorrhage due to angiomyolipomas that are bilateral or occurring in a solitary kidney, a nonsurgical approach of embolization of the bleeding tumor can be achieved to preserve functioning renal tissue.

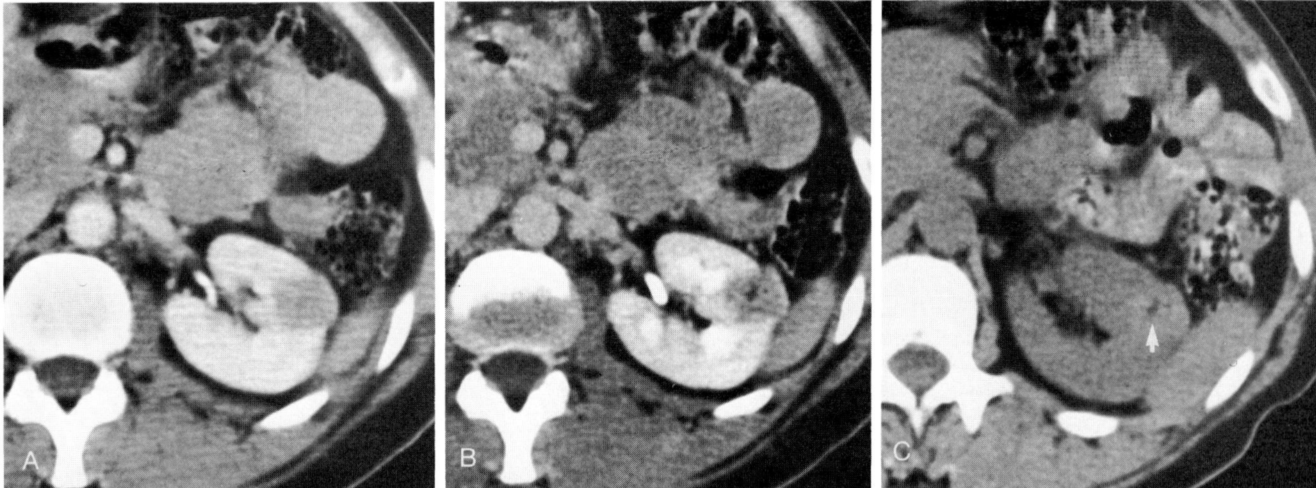

Figure 72–8. Angiomyolipoma with minimal amount of fat in a 43-year-old female. *A,* IV contrast–enhanced CT scan (10-mm section) reveals a well-marginated enhancing mass. *B,* IV contrast–enhanced CT scan (5-mm section) shows a tiny area of decreased attenuation in the center of lesion. However, negative attenuation values in this area could not be obtained. *C,* Nonenhanced CT scan (5-mm section) again shows tiny area of decreased attenuation in center of lesion *(arrow)* that demonstrates negative attenuation values indicative of fat. Tumorectomy revealed a hamartoma with mostly myomatous tissue with a small focus of fat in lesion center. (*A* to *C* reprinted with permission from Bosniak MA, Megibow AJ, Hulnick DH, et al: CT diagnosis of renal angiomyolipoma: The importance of detecting small amounts of fat. AJR 151:497–501, 1988.)

Management

Sonography and CT have made great contributions in the detection, diagnosis, and evaluation of complications of angiomyolipomas. Because of the accuracy in diagnosis of this benign condition, a change in the management of these lesions has occurred. Most small (<4.0 cm), asymptomatic lesions are managed by follow-up studies rather than surgical resection. If surgery is indicated because of repeated bleeding episodes or other severe symptomatology, tumorectomy or partial nephrectomy should be performed if surgically possible, guided by the angiographic findings. The use of arteriography with embolization to stop gross bleeding has been added to the management of some of these lesions in the appropriate setting (see Fig. 72–7) and has become an important part of the overall management of these cases.

LEIOMYOMA

Leiomyomas can either be very small in size or may attain a larger size. They are believed to arise from the muscle fibers of the capsule, renal pelvis, calyces, or blood vessels. They are usually well-encapsulated, pearly gray nodules and may contain calcification or cystic degeneration. Microscopically, they are composed of typical smooth muscle cells.

The findings on excretory urography are those of an intrarenal or a subcapsular mass. Sonographically, they are solid masses of variable echogenicity, similar to renal cell carcinomas. The features on CT are nonspecific and appear as soft-tissue masses with variable enhancement on contrast scans. On angiography, the tumors show variable vascularity—they may be hypervascular, moderately vascular, or hypovascular. These features are indistinguishable from renal cell carcinomas. In contrast to the intrarenal leiomyomas, the capsular leiomyomas may show some features on angiography that may be helpful in suggesting the diagnosis and assisting in surgical planning. Capsular leiomyomas are generally hypovascular, may displace the renal cortex inward, have a distinct interface with the parenchyma, and are characteristically supplied by renal capsular arteries.

LIPOMA

Renal lipomas, although frequently small in size, may attain larger proportions. They may be located in the renal parenchyma or arise from the capsule but are rarely seen in clinical practice. On cut section, lipomas are generally multiloculated and reddish or yellowish gray in color due to fatty tissue interspersed with fibrous trabeculae. Microscopically, they consist of adult fat cells with vacuolated cytoplasm and peripherally displaced deep staining nuclei. Vascularized loose connective tissue and various degrees of mucoid degeneration are present.

Plain radiographs may show increased lucency corresponding to fat in the tumor. Sonography will show a highly echogenic mass similar to renal angiomyolipoma. Similarly, CT and MRI will readily demonstrate a fat-containing mass, and the differentiation from an angiomyolipoma may not be possible. However, the treatment approach to a renal lipoma would be similar to that of an angiomyolipoma. The very small, clinically silent, fat-containing renal tumors, whether they be pure lipomas, myolipomas, or angiomyolipomas, can often be detected serendipitously by cross-sectional imaging techniques. These ''tiny'' lesions are managed best by conservative nonsurgical approach, since they have not shown any growth on follow-up studies.

HEMANGIOMA

Renal hemangiomas are uncommon lesions that generally manifest beyond the third decade of life. They are frequently small in size, measuring only a few millimeters, but can be larger. They can occur anywhere in the renal parenchyma but are generally located between the cortex and medulla and can occasionally project into the renal pelvis. The clinical manifestation is hematuria in a majority of patients, and flank pain can occur from obstruction by blood clots. Capillary hemangiomas consist of capillary-size vessels and clusters of endothelial cells, and cavernous hemangiomas contain larger, dilated vessels.

Renal hemangiomas, because of their small size, are not generally

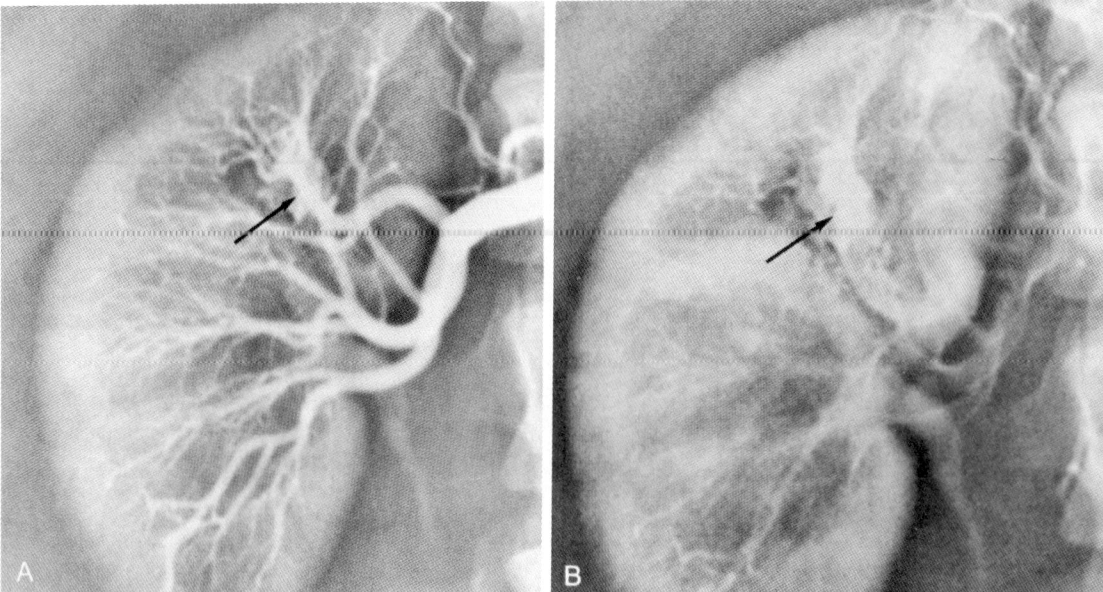

Figure 72–9. Hemangioma in a 40-year-old female with gross hematuria. *A,* Selective right renal angiogram reveals a small vascular lesion *(arrow)* in the arterial phase. *B,* The lesion *(arrow)* is more evident during the capillary phase. (*A* and *B* reprinted with permission from Evans JA, Bosniak MA: The Kidney. An Atlas of Tumor Radiology. Chicago, Year Book Medical Publishers, 1971.)

evident on excretory urography, sonography, or CT. The larger lesions may produce displacement of the infundibulum or pelvis or filling defect in the pelvocalyces. Renal angiography is best suited for diagnosis of hemangiomas, and even very small lesions can be detected with the aid of magnification technique and pharmacoangiography (Fig. 72–9). Typically, the hemangiomas are fed by irregular and tortuous arteries. Arteriovenous shunting is often present within the hemangioma, and there may be decreased perfusion distal to the shunt with resultant ischemia and hypertension. Occasionally a larger hemangioma may be confused with a vascular renal cell carcinoma. Most hemangiomas are diagnosed by angiography in the search for the source of unexplained hematuria.

RENINOMA (JUXTAGLOMERULAR TUMOR)

Reninomas (juxtaglomerular cell tumors) are benign tumors and, as their name indicates, originate from the juxtaglomerular cells and actively produce and secrete excessive amounts of renin into the blood stream and cause hypertension. Reninomas cause primary reninism, which is defined as a clinical syndrome comprising hypertension, hyper-reninemia, and secondary aldosteronism. These tumors are uncommon but constitute a distinct syndrome that is completely reversible by removal of the tumor. They represent a definite cause of surgically curable hypertension.

Reninomas are most common in young people and women but can also occur in older age groups. The clinical presentation includes headache due to hypertension, muscular weakness related to hypokalemia, and polyuria. Clinically, there is moderate to severe hypertension and elevated peripheral renin activity, which generally shows no change with sodium restriction but may show an increase with upright position.

The tumors are generally small in size (2 to 3 cm) but may occasionally attain a larger size or may even be very small, measuring only a few millimeters. They are usually located beneath the renal capsule and are sharply marginated. On cut section, they are tan or gray in color and may show foci of hemorrhage. There has been no evidence of invasive or metastatic behavior.

Microscopically, the tumors are composed of small, fairly uniform cells with little pleomorphism or mitotic activity. Reninomas contain many deeply staining cytoplasmic granules, and cytoplasmic glycogen or lipid is absent. The presence of renin in the cytoplasmic granules can be shown by immunofluorescence. The ultrastructural characteristics of the cytoplasmic granules are identical to those of the epithelial cells of the normal human juxtaglomerular complex. The electron microscopic demonstration of tumor cells containing polyhedral, polygonal, or elongated protogranules is diagnostic of juxtaglomerular tumors.

Radiologic Features

Reninomas, being generally small in size, may not be detected on excretory urograms. The larger tumors will be seen as nonspecific renal masses.

The reports on the sonographic features of reninomas are limited. In one report, all seven patients with reninomas measuring from 3.0 to 6.5 cm were detected by sonography. However, the sonographic appearance is nonspecific because the tumors show variable echogenicity as compared with the normal renal parenchyma.

The features on CT are nonspecific, and the tumors are seen as isodense masses on noncontrast scans; hence intravenous contrast should be used. On contrast scans, the tumors may show some enhancement, but they are less dense than normal renal parenchyma.

The indications for angiography include detection of reninomas, assessment of the vascularity of these tumors seen on sonography or CT, depiction of the detailed vascular anatomy for possible local resection of the tumor or heminephrectomy, and exclusion of renal artery stenosis as the cause of secondary reninism. Although reninomas contain numerous microscopic vascular spaces, they are hypovascular masses. They may show displacement of vessels and mild neovascularity, but tumor blush is absent. In the context of normal ultrasonography, CT, and angiography, sampling for renin from the main renal veins and segmental branches is advocated.

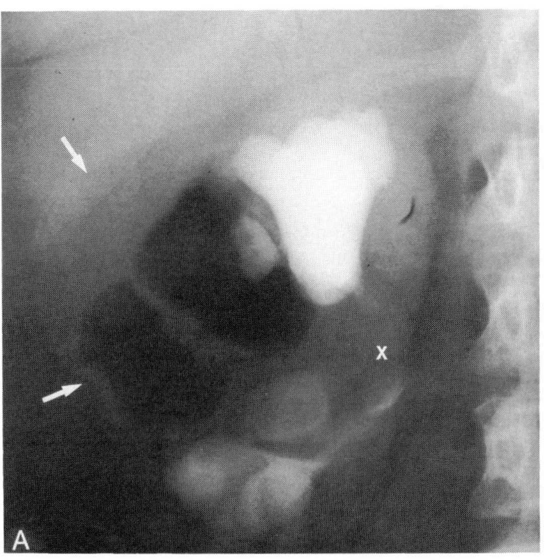

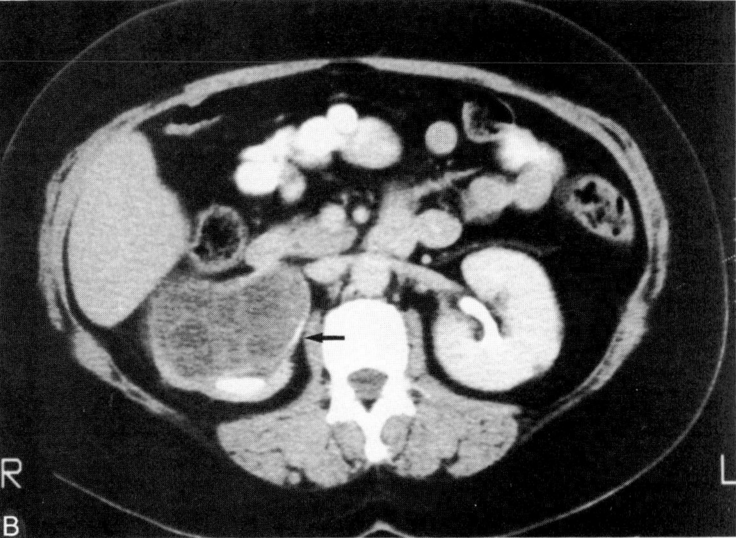

Figure 72–10. A multilocular cystic nephroma in a 53-year-old female found to have a renal mass. *A,* Intravenous urogram. A large defect fills the renal pelvis of the right kidney (x). The full extent of this mass is outlined *(arrows)*. The mass obstructs the upper pole calyces causing hydrocalycosis. Similar but less marked changes are seen at the lower pole. This herniation of the tumor mass into renal pelvis is a characteristic but not specific finding in this tumor. *B,* Contrast-enhanced CT scan. The large cystic tumor in the midportion of the right kidney is outlined. The multiloculated cystic tumor has some faintly seen septa running throughout the lesion. Note, again, that the tumor mass is seen to protrude into the renal pelvis filling it. Note thin line of contrast in renal pelvis medially *(arrow)* corresponding to urogram seen in *A.* A benign multiloculated cystic nephroma was removed at nephrectomy. (*A* and *B* courtesy of Edward H. Smith, M.D., Worcester, MA.)

MULTILOCULAR CYSTIC NEPHROMA (MLCN)

MLCN is an uncommon cystic renal lesion that has an unique age distribution, affecting predominantly males in the first two years of life whereas in adulthood, a 2:1 female predominance is observed. This renal mass consists of multiple noncommunicating cysts surrounded by a thick, fibrous capsule. The masses are located within the renal parenchyma and do not communicate with the renal pelvis, although cysts may herniate into the renal pelvis. The content of the cysts usually is clear fluid but occasionally myxomatous, proteinaceous, or hemorrhagic material will be present.

Theories of pathogenesis have included dysplasia, hamartoma, and neoplasm. The confusion surrounding the nature of this mass has led to the application of many terms including multicystic nephroma, multilocular cyst, cystic nephroblastoma, cystic Wilms' tumor, cystic hamartoma, and segmental polycystic disease, to name a few.

Microscopically, individual locules lined by epithelium are separated by septa of spindle cells. No differentiated renal elements are present although the septa may contain tissue resembling renal blastema. The lesions are usually benign but cases with microscopic foci of nephroblastoma or sarcoma have been reported.

In children this lesion is usually discovered as an incidental mass. In adults MLCN is more likely to be symptomatic, and abdominal pain, hematuria, hypertension, or urinary tract infection can be presenting features.

Plain radiographs of the abdomen are nonspecific and usually indicate the presence of a mass with displacement of adjacent bowel loops. Calcifications, which usually arise from the capsule or septa, may be present. Excretory urography typically demonstrates a well-defined intrarenal mass with compression, dilatation, and displacement of the collecting system. Herniation of a portion of the lesion into the renal pelvis can occur, resulting in a focal filling defect (Fig. 72–10). This finding is highly suggestive of MLCN. If there is obstruction, pyelocaliectasis or delayed or absent excretion of contrast material will occur. Tomograms can reveal the septated nature of this lesion.

The appearance of MLCN with sonography is related to the size and content of the cysts and the amount of stroma. Multiple sonolucent lesions with through transmission separated by highly echogenic septations is the characteristic appearance, but when the cysts are small or are not composed of simple fluid, internal echoes may be present.

CT demonstrates a well-defined intrarenal mass with cystic spaces of varying size separated by septa (Figs. 72–10, 72–11, and 72–12). Following intravenous contrast administration, it is common for the septations to demonstrate enhancement. The size and

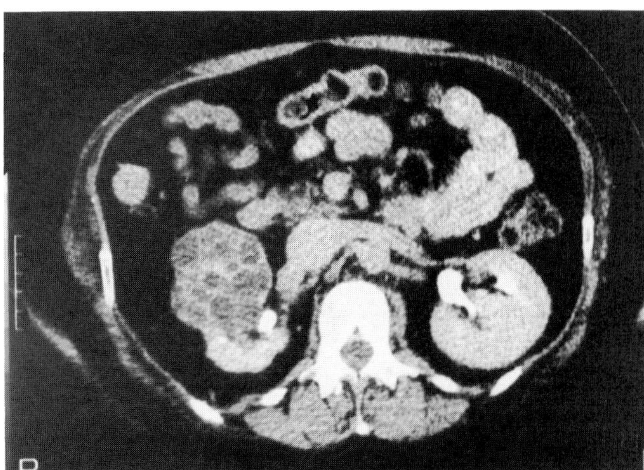

Figure 72–11. A multilocular cystic nephroma in a 47-year-old female with right flank pain. Contrast-enhanced CT scan reveals a 6.5-cm multiloculated cystic mass in the right kidney. Septa are thick and enhance with contrast media although no significant solid areas are present. Lesion extends into renal sinus. A right nephrectomy revealed a multiloculated cystic nephroma without any malignant portions.

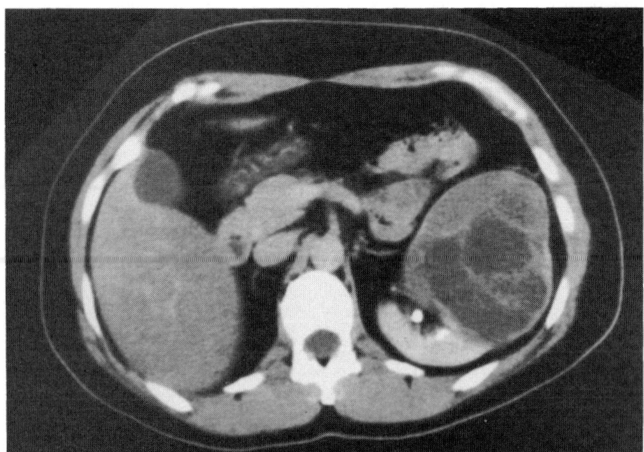

Figure 72–12. A multilocular cystic nephroma in a 46-year-old female who was discovered to have an abdominal mass. Contrast-enhanced CT scan reveals a 9.5-cm multiloculated cystic mass in the left kidney. The mass has an enhancing thick wall and multiple enhancing septa. The fluid in some of the compartments is of higher attenuation than in others, demonstrating that these locules do not communicate. Some contain degenerated bloody fluid; others contain clear fluid but some with increased amounts of protein. A left nephrectomy was performed, and a benign multilocular cystic nephroma was present.

content of the cysts influence their appearance. When the cysts are very small or when proteinaceous, myxomatous, or hemorrhagic material is present, these masses may be very difficult to distinguish from renal cell carcinoma. Even when characteristic findings are present, cystic renal cell carcinoma and Wilms' tumor still need to be considered. It is important to realize that this lesion consists of cystic spaces confined within a single lesion. This is in contrast to the appearance of benign localized cystic disease of the kidneys, in which multiple, distinct cystic lesions are diffusely scattered throughout the kidney.

Similarly, the size and content of the component cysts influences the appearance with MRI. Locules containing simple fluid will demonstrate the characteristic signal intensities of prolonged T_1 and T_2 values (decreased intensity on T_1-weighted images and increased intensity on T_2-weighted images, compared with skeletal muscle). The presence of proteinaceous or hemorrhagic material may shorten T_1 and result in lesions with increased signal intensity on T_1-weighted images. In some cases cysts may be too small to be resolved and mimic the appearance of a solid mass. The tumor capsule is typically hypointense on all sequences but the signal intensity of the septa may be variable. Hypo- and hyper-intense septa have been reported on T_2-weighted images, likely related to the degree of cellularity within this collagenous tissue.

The ability of cross-sectional imaging techniques to demonstrate the morphologic characteristics of MLCN allows for a highly suggestive diagnosis when characteristic features are demonstrated. However, cystic renal cell carcinoma and Wilms' tumor are diagnoses that cannot be completely excluded and therefore, these lesions are treated surgically. Lesions that are located in either renal pole can be removed by partial nephrectomy, and this approach seems reasonable in cases demonstrating classic findings.

MISCELLANEOUS TUMORS

Renal medullary fibromas are benign tumors that arise from the interstitial cells of the renal medulla. These are most commonly discovered as an incidental finding at autopsy and rarely present clinically. Imaging findings with urography, CT, and angiography are nonspecific, simulating malignant tumors. However, the MRI appearance of medullary fibroma, low signal intensity on both T_1- and T_2-weighted images, is highly suggestive. These signal characteristics are expected in densely collagenous, hypocellular tissue. Unfortunately, similar findings have been reported in renal carcinoma, thereby precluding a definitive MRI diagnosis.

Lymphangiomas are extremely rare, generally occur in children, and may be associated with similar lesions in the chest. Dermoid cyst of the kidney is rare but can occur. Neurogenic tumors, rhabdomyoma, myxoma, and cholesteatoma complete the list of extremely rare benign renal tumors.

Acknowledgments

The authors would like to acknowledge the contributions of Bala R. Subramanyan who was a coauthor from the first edition.

Bibliography

Ambos MA, Bosniak MA, Valensi QJ, et al.: Angiographic patterns in renal oncocytomas. Radiology 129:615–622, 1978.

Ball DS, Friedman AC, Hartman DS, et al: Scar signal of renal oncocytoma: Magnetic resonance imaging appearance and lack of specificity. Urol Radiol 8:46–48, 1986.

Bell ET: Renal Disease, 2nd ed. Philadelphia, Lea and Febiger, 1950, p 435.

Bennington JL: Renal adenoma. World J Urol 5:66–70, 1987.

Bennington JL, Beckwith JB: Tumors of the kidney, renal pelvis and ureter. In Atlas of Tumor Pathology, 2nd Series, Fascicle 12. Washington, DC, Armed Forces Institute of Pathology, 1975, pp 201–212.

Bosniak MA: Angiomyolipoma (hamartoma) of the kidney: A preoperative diagnosis is possible in virtually every case. Urol Radiol 3:135–142, 1981.

Bosniak MA: Spontaneous subcapsular and perirenal hematomas. Radiology 172:601–602, 1989.

Bosniak MA: The small (≤ 3.0 cm) renal parenchymal tumor: Detection, diagnosis and controversies. Radiology 179:307–317, 1991.

Bosniak MA, Megibow AJ, Hulnick DH, et al: CT diagnosis of renal angiomyolipoma: The importance of detecting small amounts of fat. AJR 151:497–501, 1988.

Bruneton N, Ballanger P, Ballanger R, et al: Renal adenomas. Clin Radiol 30:343–352, 1979.

Camunez F, Lafuente J, Robledo R, et al: CT demonstration of extension of renal angiomyolipoma into the inferior vena cava in a patient with tuberous sclerosis. Urol Radiol 9:152–154, 1987.

Chonko AM, Weiss JM, Stein JH, et al: Renal involvement in tuberous sclerosis. Am J Med 56:124–132, 1974.

Cohan RH, Dunnick NR, Degysys GE, et al: Computed tomography of renal oncocytoma. J Comput Assist Tomogr 8:284–287, 1984.

Cormier P, Patel SK, Turner DA, Hoeksema J: MR imaging findings in renal medullary fibroma. AJR 153:83–84, 1989.

Defossez SM, Yoder IC, Papanicolaou N, et al: Nonspecific magnetic resonance appearance of renal oncocytomas: Report of 3 cases and review of the literature. J Urol 145:552–554, 1991.

Dikengil A, Benson M, Sanders L, Newhouse JH: MRI of multilocular cystic nephroma. Urol Radiol 10:95–99, 1988.

Dunnick NR, Hartman DS, Ford KK, et al: The radiology of juxtaglomerular tumors. Radiology 147:321–326, 1983.

Ekelund L, Gothlin J: Renal hemangiomas: An analysis of 13 cases diagnosed by angiography. AJR 125:788–794, 1975.

Erwin BC, Carroll BA, Walter JF, et al: Renal infarction appearing as an echogenic mass. AJR 138:759–761, 1982.

Evans JA, Bosniak MA: The Kidney. An Atlas of Tumor Radiology. Chicago, Year Book Medical Publishers, 1971.

Forman HP, Middleton WD, et al: Hyperechoic renal cell carcinomas: Increase in detection at US. Radiology 188:431–434, 1992.

Goldman, SF: Benign renal tumors: Diagnosis and treatment. Urol Radiol 11:203–209, 1989.

Helenon O, Chrestien Y, Paraf F, et al: Renal cell carcinoma containing fat: Demonstration with CT. Radiology 188:429–430, 1993.

Klein MJ, Valensi GJ: Proximal tubular adenomas of the kidney with so-called oncocytic features: A clinicopathologic study of 13 cases of a rarely reported neoplasm. Cancer 38:906–914, 1976.

Lieber MM, Tomera KM, Farrow GM: Renal oncocytoma. J Urol 125:481–485, 1981.

Madewell JE, Goldman SM, Davis CJ, et al: Multilocular cystic nephroma: A radiologic pathologic correlation of 58 patients. Radiology 146:309–321, 1983.

Mitnick JS, Bosniak MA, Hilton S, et al: Cystic renal disease in tuberous sclerosis. Radiology 147:85–87, 1983.

Oesterling JE, Fishman EK, Goldman SE, Marshall FF: Management of angiomyolipoma. J Urol 135:1121–1124, 1986.

Quinn MJ, Hartman DS, Friedman AC, et al: Renal oncocytoma: New observations. Radiology 153:49–53, 1984.

Raghavendra BN, Bosniak MA, Megibow AJ: Small angiomyolipoma of the kidney: Sonographic-CT evaluation. AJR 141:575–578, 1983.

Reese AJM, Winstanley DP: The small tumor-like lesions of the kidney. Br J Cancer 12:507–516, 1958.

Rodriguez CA, Buskop A, Johnson J, et al: Renal oncocytoma: Preoperative diagnosis by aspiration biopsy. Acta Cytol 24:355–359, 1980.

Rosen RJ, Schlossberg P, Roven SJ, et al: Management of symptomatic renal angiomyolipomas by embolization. Urol Radiol 6:196–200, 1984.

Rumancik WM, Bosniak MA, Rosen RJ, et al: Atypical renal and pararenal hamartomas associated with lymphangiomyomatosis. AJR 142:971–972, 1984.

Strotzer M, Lehner KB, Becker K: Detection of fat in a renal cell carcinoma mimicking angiomyolipoma. Radiology 188:427–428, 1993.

Uhlenbrock D, Fischer C, Beyer HK: Angiomyolipoma of the kidney. Comparison between magnetic resonance imaging, computed tomography, and ultrasonography for diagnosis. Acta Radiologica 29:523–526, 1988.

Willis RA: Pathology of Tumours, 4th ed. London, Butterworth, 1967, p 459.

Zerhouni EA, Schellhammer P, Schaefer JC, et al: Management of bleeding renal angiomyolipoma by transcatheter embolization following CT diagnosis. Urol Radiol 6:205–209, 1984.

73 Primary Renal Carcinoma

N. Reed Dunnick

Renal adenocarcinoma is the most common primary malignant tumor of the adult kidney, accounting for approximately 3 per cent of all malignancies. It arises from proximal convoluted tubular epithelial cells and is most common in males in the fifth and sixth decades. Although a primary renal cancer can grow from any tissue, malignant tumors arising in muscular, adipose, vascular, or fibrous elements within the kidney are rare.

The most common presenting signs and symptoms of renal carcinoma include hematuria, flank pain, fever, hypertension, proteinuria, an abdominal mass, and weight loss. However, the classic clinical triad of hematuria, flank pain, and an abdominal mass is present in only 15 to 20 per cent of cases. In some patients, the diagnosis of renal carcinoma is made after identification of anemia, polycythemia, leukemoid reaction, peripheral neuropathy, or hypercalcemia, or after detection of a metastasis such as a pulmonary nodule or pathologic bone fracture.

The traditional screening examination has been excretory urography (ECU). If there is strong clinical suspicion of a renal lesion despite a negative ECU, additional studies, such as CT, ultrasound, or magnetic resonance imaging (MRI), may be used. It must be recognized that urography is not nearly as sensitive as either CT or MRI in detecting renal masses.

Once a renal mass is detected, it must be further characterized in an effort to arrive at a diagnosis. On urography, a benign renal cyst is seen as a rounded renal mass that has an imperceptibly thin wall and a sharp interface with normal renal parenchyma, and does not enhance with intravenous contrast injection. When all of these criteria are met, the diagnosis of a benign renal cyst can be made with confidence (Fig. 73–1). However, in most cases the lesion cannot be so clearly defined on ECU, and an additional study is needed. When a benign cyst is likely, ultrasound is indicated, as it is the most efficient means of confirmation.

However, if the urogram indicates a complex or solid mass, ultrasound can be bypassed, as it will likely confirm the presence of a renal lesion that needs further evaluation. In this case, CT is recommended. The axial image plane and excellent density differentiation of CT allow further characterization of renal masses. Renal cysts are readily detected and identified by the same principles used in urography. However, CT provides additional information, such as the attenuation coefficient of the cyst fluid and a precise assessment of any contrast enhancement.

Solid mass lesions may also be more clearly defined by CT than ultrasound, and occasionally a benign diagnosis can be made or strongly suggested. However, a histologic diagnosis cannot be made radiographically in most solid renal masses, and such lesions must be considered renal adenocarcinoma until proven otherwise. In many patients, a surgical nephrectomy is planned and a staging evaluation is required. If evidence of metastatic disease is present to further support the diagnosis of malignancy, a percutaneous biopsy may be all that is needed prior to therapy.

Percutaneous biopsy of a renal mass provides valuable information as to the nature of the lesion. The accuracy of the aspiration biopsy depends upon the needle placement, the quality of the cellular aspirate, and the experience of the cytopathologist. When adequately cellular biopsy specimens are obtained, the sensitivity is very high and false-positive diagnoses are rare.

The complications of percutaneous renal mass biopsy are similar to those of any soft-tissue biopsy. Hemorrhage is the most likely complication, but this is rarely clinically significant when an aspi-

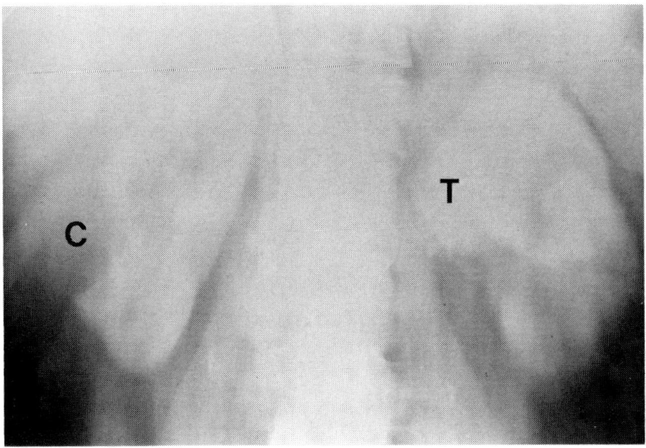

Figure 73–1. Cyst versus carcinoma. The mass in the right kidney (C) is a well-defined, rounded, peripheral lesion that does not enhance. These are the features of a benign cortical cyst. The mass in the left kidney (T) is approximately the same size but is a solid lesion that merges with the normal renal parenchyma and enhances with contrast injection. At surgery it was found to be a renal adenocarcinoma.

TABLE 73–1. STAGING RENAL CARCINOMA

Stage I	Confined by renal capsule
Stage II	Confined by Gerota's fascia
Stage III A	Main renal vein and/or IVC
Stage III B	Regional lymph nodes
Stage IV	Adjacent organs, or distant metastases

rating, rather than a cutting needle, is used. Tumor seeding of the needle tract has been reported, but it is rare and should not deter the use of percutaneous biopsy when clinically helpful information can be obtained.

For most patients, CT can accurately stage the extent of disease. The perirenal fat and Gerota's fascia can usually be identified, and the local extent of tumor delineated. Tumors confined to the kidney are Stage I, while those contained by Gerota's fascia are Stage II (Table 73–1). Since the adrenal gland lies within the perirenal space, ipsilateral adrenal involvement is still Stage II. CT is also useful for delineating tumor extension into the main renal vein and inferior vena cava (Stage III A) or involvement of regional lymph nodes (Stage III B). Extension through Gerota's fascia, into adjacent organs, or the presence of distant metastases indicates Stage IV disease.

The spatial resolution of MRI has improved and is now approximately equal to that of CT. The use of gadolinium as a contrast agent has made MRI as sensitive as CT for the detection of renal masses. For most patients, however, CT should be used to detect and characterize a renal mass. MRI is recommended when CT cannot clearly define the venous extension of a renal carcinoma or provide clarification of possible local invasion through Gerota's fascia into the liver.

Renal adenocarcinoma is usually a solid renal mass, although cystic tumors do exist. On urography, the tumor is poorly delineated from normal renal parenchyma (see Fig. 73–1). The plain film is helpful for the detection of calcification. Although simple cysts may show calcification in the wall, the presence of any calcification, but especially central calcification, increases the likelihood of the mass being carcinoma.

The primary use of ultrasound is often the distinction between solid and cystic masses. In situations in which CT is not readily available, however, ultrasound may also provide useful additional information about the character of the tumor. The highly echogenic fat of an angiomyolipoma or multiple septations of a multilocular cystic nephroma may be characteristic. In most cases, a solid mass lesion that may contain areas of hemorrhage or cystic degeneration is seen. Involvement of the renal vein or inferior vena cava may also be identified with sonography but is more reliably detected by CT or MRI.

In all but the most obese patients, a technically satisfactory ultrasound examination can be performed. The right kidney is often easier to study than the left kidney, as the liver can provide a "window" to examine the kidney. Often the most difficult area to image is the upper pole of the left kidney. A variety of positions, including prone, supine, and decubitus, may be required for a complete examination.

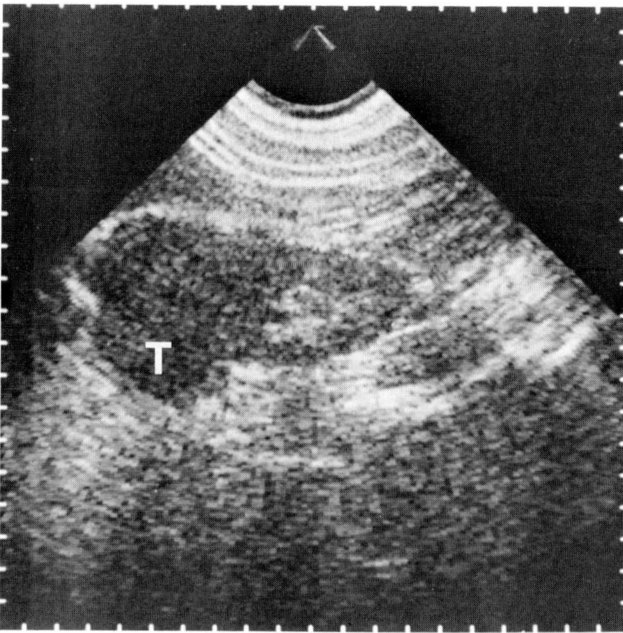

Figure 73–2. Renal adenocarcinoma. The right kidney is well-seen in this longitudinal sonogram. The collecting system in the upper pole is displaced by a large solid tumor (T) that is causing a contour deformity in the posterior wall of the kidney.

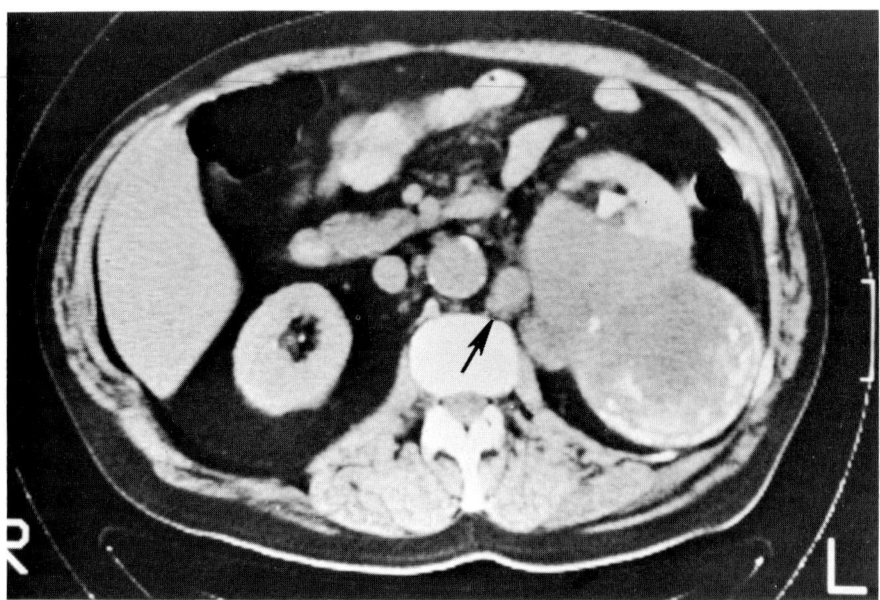

Figure 73–3. Renal adenocarcinoma. The large mass growing out of the posterior half of the left kidney has a calcified rim, as well as some central calcifications. A regional lymph node metastasis *(arrow)* is also noted.

The sonographic appearance of renal adenocarcinoma is an echogenic mass (Fig. 73–2). The character of the internal echo texture is quite variable. Cystic areas may represent areas of hemorrhage or tumor necrosis. Calcification within the tumor is characteristically highly echogenic and may cause acoustic shadowing. In general, highly vascular tumors tend to be more echogenic than hypovascular masses.

The characteristic features of renal adenocarcinoma on CT include a poorly defined mass of mottled density that shows inhomogeneous enhancement with intravenous contrast injection (Fig. 73–3). Occasionally, however, the tumor will be homogeneous and well-defined, suggesting a benign tumor or lymphoma. Cystic renal carcinomas may mimic an abscess or complicated renal cyst but can occasionally be differentiated by a thickened wall and the presence of a tumor nodule. Occasionally, a renal carcinoma may arise in the wall of an otherwise benign cyst, but this is rare.

Renal adenocarcinomas have a variable signal intensity on both T_1- and T_2-weighted MRI. On T_1 sequences, the tumor has a signal intensity intermediate between that of the cortex and the medulla. On T_2-weighted sequences, the signal intensity is often higher than the parenchyma but is quite variable due to areas of necrosis and hemorrhage. Since the kidney has an intrinsically high signal intensity, MRI has not been sensitive for the detection of renal masses. However, gadolinium contrast agents are proving to be valuable in the examination of the kidney and the sensitivity of MRI is now approximately equal to that of CT for the detection of renal masses.

Arteriography has been used for many years to diagnose renal adenocarcinoma, but the accuracy of cross-sectional imaging techniques has markedly reduced the number of angiograms performed. A "vascular roadmap" can be provided with a midstream aortogram. Selective renal angiography provides clearer images to define neovascularity. Renal carcinoma is typically hypervascular, although approximately 15 to 20 per cent of tumors will be hypovascular, as compared with the normal renal parenchyma. Tumor vascularity is disordered and irregular with areas of vascular encasement, venous laking or puddling, and often early draining veins (Fig. 73–4). Arteriovenous fistulas and microaneurysms may also be present.

Surgical resection requires precise delineation of the venous extension so that vascular control can be gained quickly during the operation. CT relies upon enlargement of the renal vein (Fig. 73–5*A*) or inferior vena cava, and on greater enhancement of the blood within the renal vein than the tumor thrombus.

Renal adenocarcinoma is readily detected by magnetic resonance, but MRI is more expensive and less readily available than CT. Thus, CT is sufficient for most patients. However, MRI is indicated if the CT findings are equivocal or if intravascular contrast material is contraindicated. MRI is useful in evaluating the renal vein and inferior vena cava, as it does not rely upon contrast material to identify flowing blood. Limited flip angle techniques are used to identify venous invasion by the tumor and precisely delineate its extent (Fig. 73–5*B*).

Extension of the renal tumor through Gerota's fascia is often apparent on CT. Invasion of the liver, psoas muscle, spine, or posterior abdominal wall indicates Stage IV disease. However, involvement may not be easy to predict if there is a paucity of retroperitoneal fat making the normal tissue planes difficult to distinguish. Furthermore, the determination of hepatic involvement is frequently difficult by CT due to the curved adjacent surfaces (Fig. 73–6). Arteriography may be useful in this setting. If tumor vessels are identified after selective opacification of hepatic arteries, liver invasion may be diagnosed. Ultrasound may also be helpful in this setting. If the renal mass and liver move separately, hepatic invasion is unlikely. However, neither of these techniques are completely satisfactory and MRI is often applied when the CT findings are uncertain. In addition to greater tissue differentiation, MRI can be acquired in the sagittal plane, which makes the interface with the liver easier to assess.

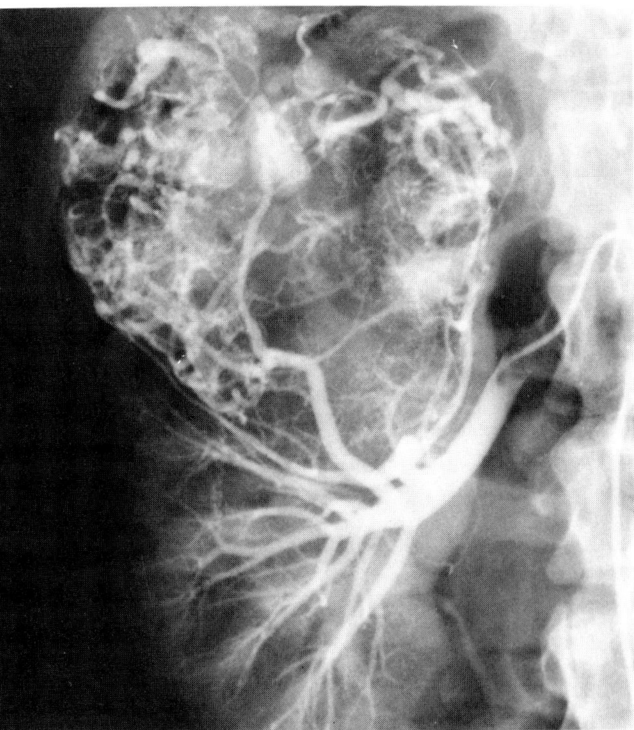

Figure 73–4. Renal adenocarcinoma. A selective right renal arteriogram demonstrates the disordered vascular supply to the tumor. Vascular encasement and venous laking and puddling indicate its malignant etiology.

It is important to include evaluation of the contralateral kidney in the presurgical examination of a patient suspected of having a renal adenocarcinoma. The incidence of bilateral renal adenocarcinomas is less than 2 per cent. These may be either synchronous primary tumors or a metastasis to the contralateral kidney. However, the contralateral kidney may be affected by other disease processes, and an assessment of its functional status must be made during the presurgical evaluation.

PAPILLARY NEOPLASMS

Papillary adenocarcinoma is a subgroup of renal carcinoma in which vascularized connective tissue stalks are lined by neoplastic cells. They are present in less than 10 per cent of adenocarcinomas but are characterized by slower growth and a better prognosis than nonpapillary renal adenocarcinomas.

The radiographic features of papillary tumors reflect their pathologic appearance. They tend to be smaller than nonpapillary types and are more likely to be calcified. The classic hypervascularity seen in many renal carcinomas is uncommon in the papillary type. This diminished vascularity can often be appreciated on contrast-enhanced CT scans (Fig. 73–7).

TUMORS IN ACQUIRED CYSTIC KIDNEY DISEASE

Acquired cystic kidney disease is seen in patients who are treated with either hemodialysis or peritoneal dialysis. Cystic changes are usually detected after three years of dialysis and, if followed long enough, will be seen in almost all patients.

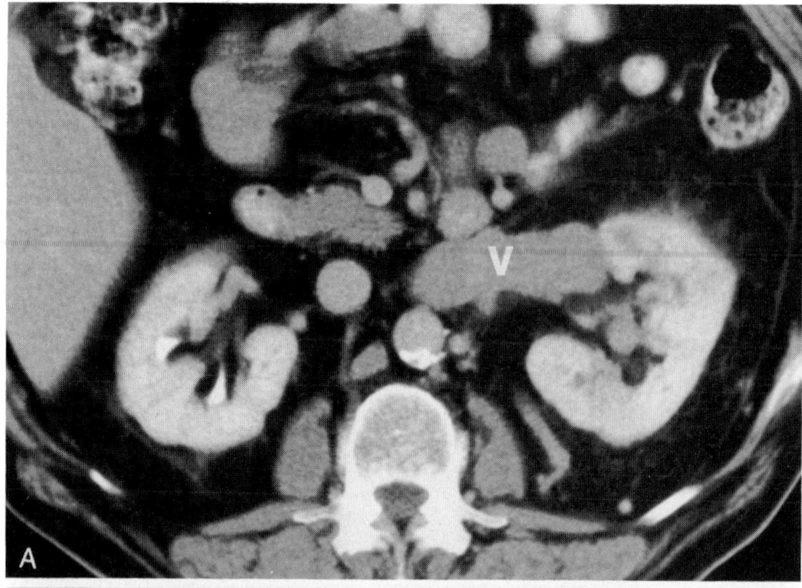

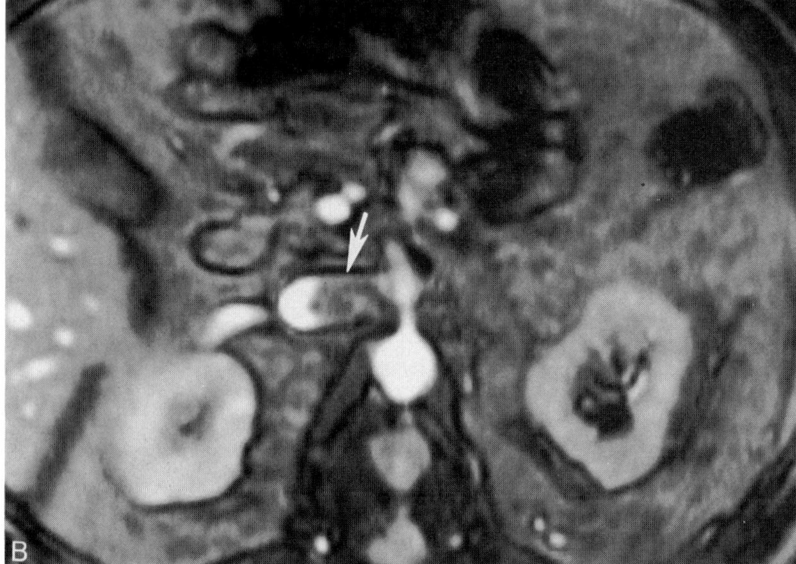

Figure 73–5. Renal adenocarcinoma. *A,* On CT, the left renal vein (V) is enlarged and does not enhance as brightly as other venous structures, indicating tumor thrombus. *B,* Venous extension is confirmed on this MRI performed with gadolinium enhancement and a limited flip angle technique. Tumor thrombus *(arrow)* can be seen entering the inferior vena cava.

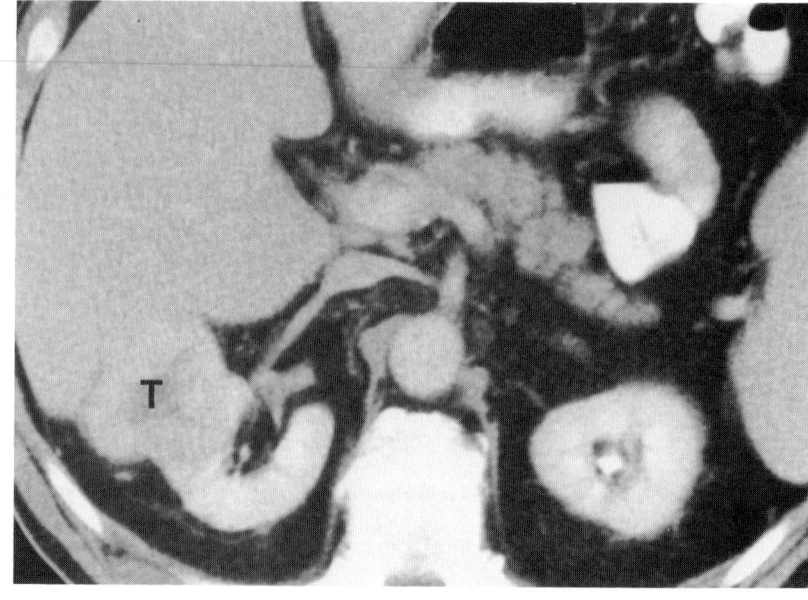

Figure 73–6. Renal adenocarcinoma invading liver. The absence of a fat plane between the renal tumor (T) and the liver suggests hepatic invasion.

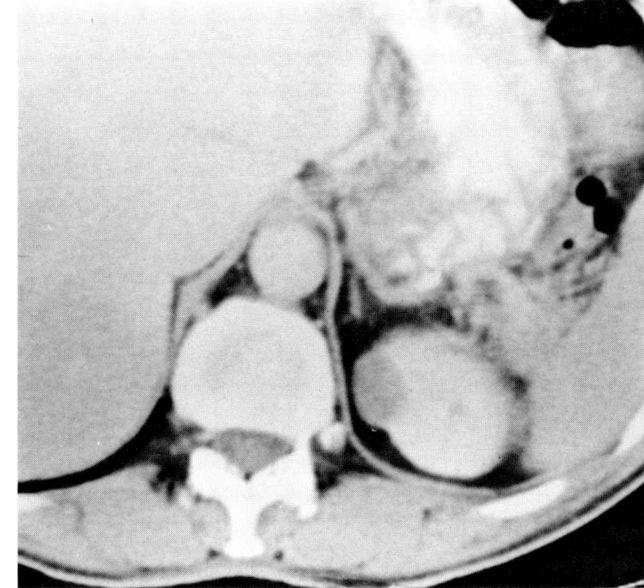

Figure 73–7. Papillary adenocarcinoma. The hypovascular nature of this small tumor is seen by its relatively lucent appearance on the contrast-enhanced CT examination.

The native kidneys of patients in chronic renal failure are small but enlarge with the development of multiple cysts. Dystrophic calcification and hemorrhage are common. As many as 7 per cent of patients develop solid renal neoplasms, approximately half of which are malignant.

The changes of acquired cystic kidney disease may be detected by ultrasound, CT, or MRI. CT is more sensitive than sonography and has become the primary imaging modality. However, the malignant neoplasms are difficult to identify, as the tumors are small and the kidneys are distorted by numerous cysts and do not concentrate intravenous contrast material (Fig. 73–8).

RARE RENAL MALIGNANCIES

Primary renal sarcomas comprise only about 1 per cent of all malignant renal tumors. The age range and clinical presentation are similar to those of patients with renal adenocarcinoma. Leiomyosarcoma is the most common renal sarcoma, but other primary tumors, including liposarcoma, osteosarcoma and chondrosarcoma, have been reported. Although experience with these rare tumors is limited, most should be detectable with CT. The tumors are often disseminated when detected, and the prognosis is poor.

RENAL CAPSULAR TUMORS

The tissues comprising and blending with the renal capsule include fat, smooth muscle, fibrous tissue, nerves, and blood vessels. Although rare, tumors may arise from any of these components and may be benign or malignant. The malignant capsular neoplasms are often large by the time they are detected and frequently invade the renal parenchyma.

The radiographic appearance is of a mass that is usually hypovas-

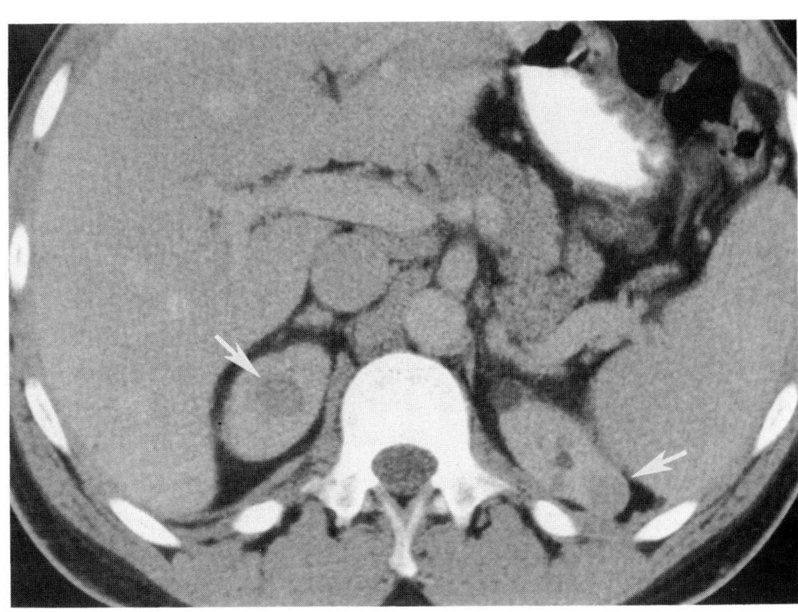

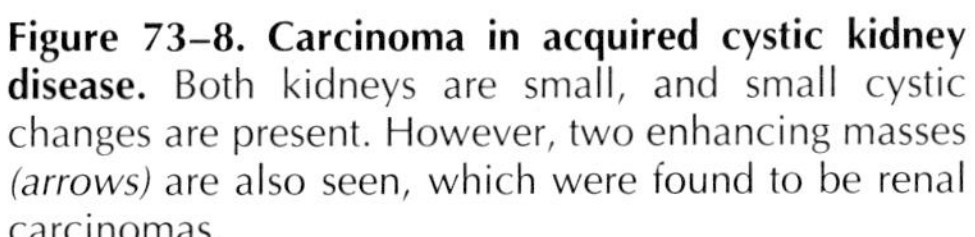

Figure 73–8. Carcinoma in acquired cystic kidney disease. Both kidneys are small, and small cystic changes are present. However, two enhancing masses *(arrows)* are also seen, which were found to be renal carcinomas.

cular. The kidney is compressed or flattened by the extrarenal mass, but the collecting system is not splayed. Arteriography is useful in demonstrating the prominent vascular supply from the capsular rather than the parenchymal renal vessels.

CARCINOMA OF THE RENAL PELVIS

Transitional cell carcinoma (TCC) of the renal pelvis constitutes approximately 5 per cent of primary renal malignancies. Similar to renal adenocarcinoma, it has a peak incidence in the fifth and sixth decades and occurs more commonly in men than in women.

Several chemical agents have been recognized as contributing to the development of TCC. Aniline dye workers in the textile, printing, or plastics industries have an increased incidence of TCC. Abuse of phenacetin, which is an aniline derivative whose major metabolite is excreted in the urine, is also associated with invasive TCC. Urine stasis prolongs contact of these carcinogens with the urothelium and may increase the incidence of malignant transformation.

Most patients present with hematuria, and an ECU is the screening examination for detection. Calcification is uncommon. A filling defect in the collecting system is the typical urographic manifestation. Since these tumors grow with a frond-like pattern, contrast material can frequently be seen within the interstices of the tumor. This results in a sharply defined but irregular filling defect. TCCs are also frequently multifocal, so multiple filling defects may be appreciated (Fig. 73–9).

The differential diagnosis for a filling defect in the collecting system also includes a renal stone or blood clot. Most renal stones are sufficiently radiopaque that they can be detected on plain radiographs. However, a significant number of renal stones will be "lucent"—that is, not dense enough to be seen on an abdominal radiograph. Since CT has superior density differentiation, even these "lucent" stones are readily detected. Thus, a CT scan through the filling defect will identify a renal stone.

The appearance of a filling defect due to blood clot is usually smooth and conforms to the collecting system. Since it is constantly undergoing changes of clot lysis and new clot formation due to continued bleeding, the appearance of a filling defect due to blood clot will change from day to day. Follow-up excretory urography or retrograde pyelography should be sufficient to demonstrate this evolution.

The CT appearance of TCC is a soft-tissue mass within the collecting system (Fig. 73–9). Mild dilatation of the portion of the collecting system containing the tumor and compression of the renal sinus fat may be seen. These tumors are usually small, but occasionally large infiltrating lesions are seen. Angiography is rarely needed for these patients but, when performed, demonstrates a hypovascular mass.

WILMS' TUMOR

Wilms' tumor, or nephroblastoma, is the most common primary renal tumor in children. It arises from metanephric blastema, which may be persistent after birth. The peak incidence ages are three to four years, and presentation after age seven is rare.

The most common presentation is a palpable abdominal mass that may be detected by parents or during routine physical examination. Other manifestations include pain, hematuria, fever, and anorexia. In addition to the abdominal mass, physical examination often reveals hypertension, which may be due to production of renin by the tumor or secondary to renin release by the kidney in response to decreased renal blood flow from pressure by the tumor mass.

Wilms' tumor is associated with congenital anomalies in approximately 15 per cent of cases, particularly in the urinary tract. Children with aniridia or hemihypertrophy also have an increased inci-

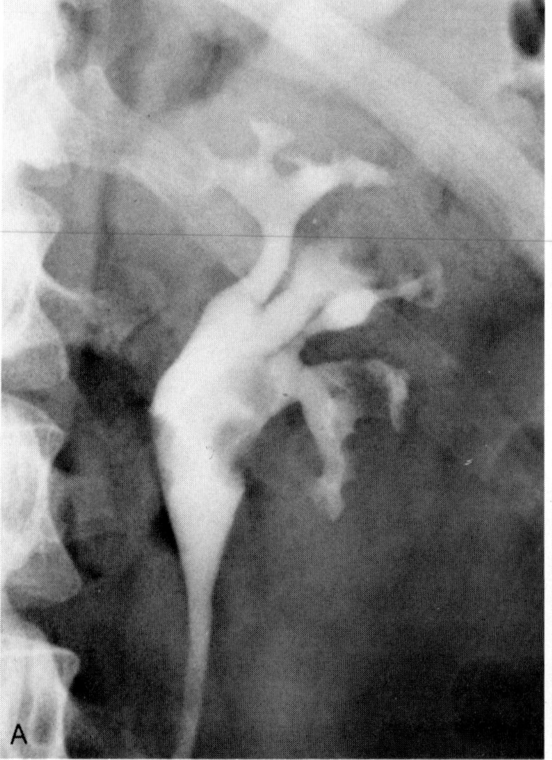

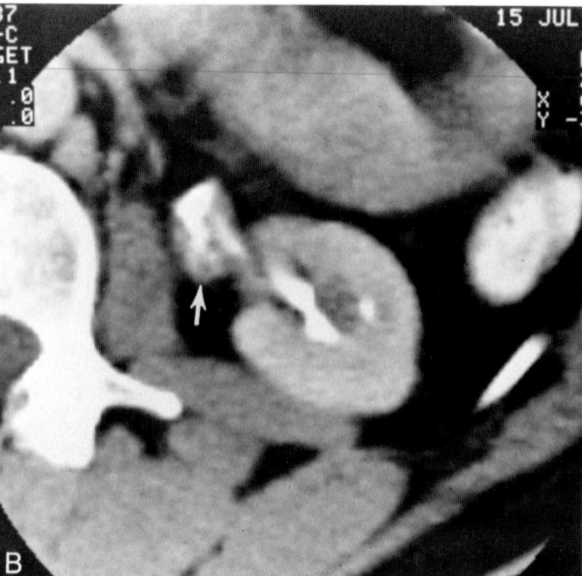

Figure 73–9. Transitional cell carcinoma. *A,* Multiple filling defects in the renal pelvis and lower pole calyces represent a multifocal transitional cell carcinoma. *B,* These irregular soft-tissue masses *(arrow)* can be seen on this contrast-enhanced CT scan.

TABLE 73–2. WILMS' TUMOR STAGING

Stage I	Limited to kidney, and completely resected
Stage II	Extension beyond kidney, but completely resected
Stage III	Residual nonhematogenous tumor confined to abdomen
Stage IV	Hematogenous metastases
Stage V	Bilateral renal involvement

dence of Wilms' tumor. Wilms' tumor is also associated with several chromosomal abnormalities; the best known is deletion of the short arm of chromosome 2.

The radiographic evaluation of patients suspected of having Wilms' tumor has traditionally begun with ECU. However, cross-sectional imaging techniques, especially sonography, have largely replaced the urogram. The plain radiograph demonstrates curvilinear or amorphous calcification in 5 to 10 per cent of these tumors. If the mass is large, it may be detectable by the obliteration of the ipsilateral psoas margin and displacement of bowel.

Since Wilms' tumors are often large, there may be confusion as to the tissue of origin. Most Wilms' tumors arise in the upper pole of the kidney, which adds to the possible confusion with neuroblastoma or a nonmalignant upper pole mass, such as an obstructed duplication. Distortion of the intrarenal collecting system is the primary clue to the renal origin, as extrarenal masses tend to displace the kidney, leaving the intrarenal structures intact.

Sonography demonstrates an echogenic intrarenal mass. Hypoechoic areas within the tumor represent areas of hemorrhage or central necrosis. Tumor extension into the renal vein or inferior vena cava may also be detected by demonstrating an echogenic mass within the vein. If this examination is unsatisfactory, MRI is recommended for complete evaluation.

CT has been limited by the relative lack of retroperitoneal fat in children, which results in an image that is often inferior to that which can be obtained with ultrasound. However, CT helps to confirm the presence of an intrarenal mass and is particularly valuable in tumor staging (Table 73–2). A large rounded mass that splays the intrarenal collecting system is readily seen with CT (Fig. 73–10). Diminished density and poor contrast enhancement of the central portions of the tumor reflect tumor necrosis. As with renal adenocarcinoma in the adult, it is most important to evaluate the contralateral kidney.

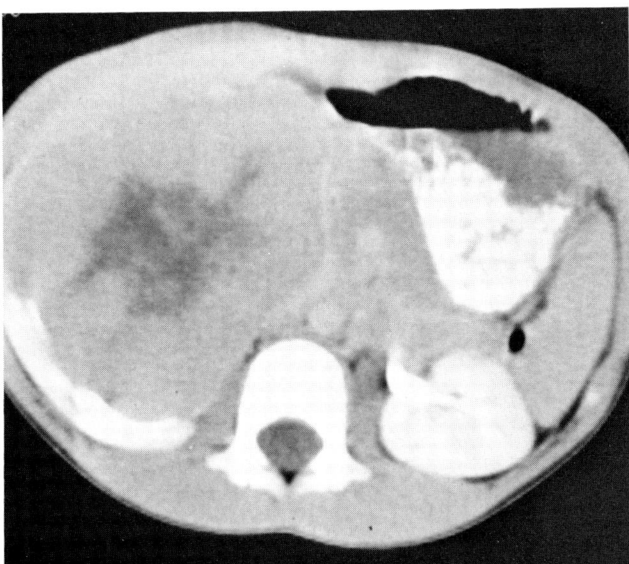

Figure 73–10. Wilms' tumor. A huge tumor is arising from the right kidney, splaying the intrarenal collecting system.

MRI is being increasingly used to study patients with Wilms' tumor. It provides much the same information as CT in terms of delineation of the tumor mass and detection of local invasion or regional lymph node involvement. The tumor has an increased signal on both T_1- and T_2-weighted sequences. The limited flip angle techniques are especially useful for evaluating the venous structures for tumor extension.

Conventional arteriography is seldom needed in children with Wilms' tumor. It can be valuable, however, if the tissue of origin of the tumor is in doubt. Demonstration of primary vascular supply from renal arteries supports a primary renal neoplasm. Venography, particularly inferior venacavography, may be required to confirm patency of the inferior vena cava prior to surgery.

Bibliography

Bisset GS III, Strife JL, Kirks DR: Tumors. In Kirks DR (ed), Practical Pediatric Imaging, 2nd ed. Boston, Little, Brown, 1991, pp 994–1032.

Bosniak MA: The small (≤3.0 cm) renal parenchymal tumor: Detection, diagnosis, and controversies. Radiology 179:307–317, 1991.

Bush WH Jr, Burnett LL, Gibbons RP: Needle tract seeding of renal cell carcinoma. AJR, 129:725–727, 1977.

Castellino RA: The non-Hodgkin's lymphomas: Practical concepts for the diagnostic radiologist. Radiology 178:315–321, 1991.

Charbit L, Gendreau MC, Mee S, Cukier J: Tumors of the upper urinary tract: Ten years of experience. J Urol 146:1243–1246, 1991.

Choyke PL, Filling-Katz MR, Shawker TH, et al: Von Hippel–Lindau disease: Radiologic screening for visceral manifestations. Radiology 174:815–820, 1990.

Cohan RH, Dunnick NR, Leder RA, Baker ME: Computed tomography of renal lymphoma. J Comput Assist Tomogr 14(6):933–938, 1990.

Dalla-Palma L, Pozzi-Mucelli F, di Donna A, Pozzi-Mucelli RS: Cystic renal tumors: US and CT findings. Urol Radiol 12:67–73, 1990.

Dunnick NR, McCallum RW, Sandler CM: A Textbook of Uroradiology. Baltimore, Williams and Wilkins, 1991.

Hartman DS, Davis CJ Jr, Madewell JE, Friedman AC: Primary malignant renal tumors in the second decade of life: Wilms' tumor versus renal cell carcinoma. J Urol 127:888–891, 1982.

Jafri SZH, Freeman JL, Rosenberg BF, et al: Clinical and imaging features of rhabdoid tumor of the kidney. Urol Radiol 13:94–97, 1991.

Johnson CD, Dunnick NR, Cohan RH, Illescas FF: Renal adenocarcinoma: CT staging of 100 tumors. AJR 148:59–63, 1987.

Kass DA, Hricak H, Davidson AJ: Renal malignancies with normal excretory urograms. AJR 141:731–734, 1983.

Kollias G, Giannopoulos T: Primary malignant fibrous histiocytoma of the kidney: Report of a case. J Urol 138:400–401, 1987.

Leder RA, Dunnick NR: Transitional cell carcinoma of the pelvicalices and ureter. AJR 155:713–722, 1990.

Levine E, Slusher SL, Grantham JJ, Wetzel LH: Natural history of acquired renal cystic disease in dialysis patients: A prospective longitudinal CT study. AJR 156:501–506, 1991.

Narumi Y, Sato T, Hori S, et al: Squamous cell carcinoma of the uroepithelium: CT evaluation. Radiology 173:853–856, 1989.

Parienty RA, Pradel J, Parienty I: Cystic renal cancers: CT characteristics. Radiology 157:741–744, 1985.

Press GA, McClennan BL, Melson GL, et al: Papillary renal cell carcinoma: CT and sonographic evaluation. AJR 143:1005–1009, 1984.

Roubidoux MR, Dunnick NR, Sostman HD, Leder RA: Detection of venous extension of renal carcinoma by magnetic resonance imaging with gradient recalled echo sequences. Radiology 182:269–272, 1992.

Srinivas V, Sogani PC, Hajdu SI, Whitmore WF Jr: Sarcoma of the kidney. Radiology 132:13–16, 1984.

Steiner M, Quinlan D, Goldman SM, et al: Leiomyoma of the kidney: Presentation of four new cases and the role of the computerized tomography. J Urol 143:994–998, 1990.

Taylor AJ, Cohen EP, Erickson SJ, et al: Renal imaging in long-term dialysis patients: A comparison of CT and sonography. AJR 153:765–767, 1989.

Warshauer DM, McCarthy SM, Street L, et al: Detection of renal masses: Sensitivities and specificities of excretory urography/linear tomography, US, and CT. Radiology 169:363–365, 1989.

Yousem DM, Gatewood OMB, Goldman SM, Marshall FF: Synchronous and metachronous transitional cell carcinoma of the urinary tract: Prevalence, incidence, and radiographic detection. Radiology 167:613–618, 1988.

74 Renal Lymphoma and Metastatic Disease to the Kidneys

Morton A. Bosniak and Suzanne J. Smith

RENAL LYMPHOMA

Lymphomatous involvement of the kidneys is present in 33.5 per cent of patients dying of widespread lymphoma of all histologic types and is more common in non-Hodgkin's lymphoma than in Hodgkin's disease. Excluding the hematopoietic and reticuloendothelial systems, the kidney is the most common site of this malignancy. However, there is a marked discrepancy between the incidence of disease found at autopsy and that recognized clinically, probably due to the lack of clinical symptoms in many patients with lymphomatous infiltration of the kidneys and to the fact that the presentation of renal lymphoma was below the sensitivity of radiologic techniques before the advent of ultrasound and computed tomography (CT). Because lesions had to grow to critical size to be detected, there was an early misconception that renal involvement was only a late manifestation of the disease. However, since the more widespread use of CT for tumor staging, renal involvement has been found in 2.7 to 8.3 per cent of cases of lymphoma even though half of these patients have no clinical signs of the disease. Occasionally, renal involvement may be the initial presentation of lymphoma (although it is rarely the sole site of lymphoma), or it may occur anytime during the course of the disease, from weeks to years after the initial diagnosis.

In recent years, because of the increased incidence of AIDS cases, an increased number of cases of renal lymphoma have been seen. The incidence of lymphoma is 60 times more common in patients with AIDS than in the general population. Extranodal lymphoma with organ involvement is common in AIDS-related lymphoma patients, so that lymphomatous involvement of the kidney has been seen with greater frequency.

Pathology

In an autopsy series of 696 patients, Richmond et al found histologic renal involvement in 35 per cent of non-Hodgkin's lymphoma and 13 per cent of Hodgkin's disease. However, the pathologic pattern of renal involvement appears to be similar. There are three general patterns of renal involvement: primary tumor, hematogenous metastasis, and direct invasion. Primary renal lymphoma, where the kidney is the only site of lymphoma, is rare, since the kidney is devoid of lymphoid tissue. Most renal lesions are the result of hematogenous metastases to the kidneys from lymphoma elsewhere in the body, and in most of these cases there is lymphomatous involvement of the retroperitoneum as well, although it is not contiguous. Hematogenous dissemination results in metastastic deposits in the renal cortex. These usually present as nodular lesions and are more frequently multiple than single, and bilateral than unilateral (3:1). This type of renal involvement is more common in lymphoma in AIDS patients, in which blood-borne dissemination of disease occurs more frequently, leading to an extranodal distribution of disease with increased organ involvement (Fig. 74–1). Less common forms of metastatic deposits are discrete single or focal masses, and diffuse infiltration. Renal involvement by direct invasion from a contiguous retroperitoneal mass is a commonly observed manifestation of the disease. Retroperitoneal lymphoma may extend through the renal capsule into the cortex or ascend along the ureteral wall and renal pelvis into the renal sinus and parenchyma. Rarely a retroperitoneal mass will surround and displace but not invade the kidney.

Radiology

Radiologic findings depend on the type and extent of renal involvement and whether there is focal involvement by nodules or masses, diffuse infiltration, or extension from retroperitoneal tumor.

EXCRETORY UROGRAPHY

Urography is rarely performed in patients with lymphoma, as its role has almost entirely been taken over by sonography and CT. Urography is a fairly insensitive technique in the evaluation of renal lymphoma and is limited to the detection of large lesions of the kidney and retroperitoneum. Retroperitoneal extrarenal disease can lead to displacement of the kidneys or ureters, with extrinsic compression on the ureters by lymphomatous nodes, sometimes leading to ureteral obstruction and hydronephrosis. Obstructive uropathy can also be due to uric acid stones. Occasionally a perirenal mass will be apparent.

Visualization of the involved kidney can be normal, decreased, or absent. The kidneys may be diffusely enlarged, or discrete masses may be demonstrated in enlarged or normal-sized kidneys. Occasionally renal lymphoma will present as a single large renal mass not unlike carcinoma. When diffuse infiltration has occurred, urography may demonstrate poor visualization, renal enlargement, and distortion of the collecting system with splaying, attenuation, and compression of the collecting system. Penetration into the ureter with a filling defect is very uncommon, although perinephric extension is often seen.

ULTRASONOGRAPHY

In general, lymphomatous tissue is homogeneous without tissue interfaces. Sonography displays homogeneous hypoechoic masses with little or no augmented through transmission and lack of a sharply defined wall (Fig. 74–2*B*). Fine internal echoes may be present if the tumor has undergone necrosis or infiltrating tumor has traversed several tissue interfaces. Rarely, lymphomatous masses can present as anechoic lesions with smooth, well-defined margins; they are distinguishable from renal cysts by the degree of through transmission but can be difficult to distinguish from thickened, homogeneous fluid collections such as pus. In diffuse renal infiltration, the kidneys are enlarged with a diffuse hypoechoic appearance. Hydronephrosis can be present with obstructing masses in or near the renal hilum or with enlarged lymph nodes causing ureteral obstruction. Differential diagnosis of renal lymphoma by ultrasonography includes polycystic kidneys; cystic or necrotic tumors; abscess; intra- or perirenal collections of blood, urine, pus, or lymph; and hydronephrosis.

COMPUTED TOMOGRAPHY

Computed tomography is the procedure of choice for the detection and follow-up of renal lymphoma, since it can demonstrate

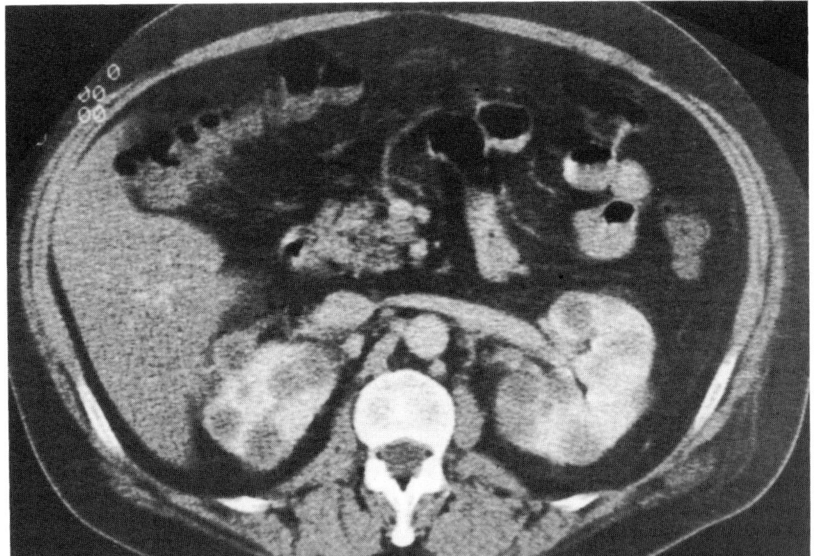

Figure 74–1. A 48-year-old male with **AIDS and lymphoma**. Contrast-enhanced CT scan reveals multiple round areas of decreased attenuation (31 HU) scattered throughout both kidneys. Some of the nodules of tumor extend outside the contour of the kidney. Masses of lymphoma were seen in the liver, spleen, and right adrenal as well. Some slightly enlarged lymph nodes were also present in the retroperitoneum.

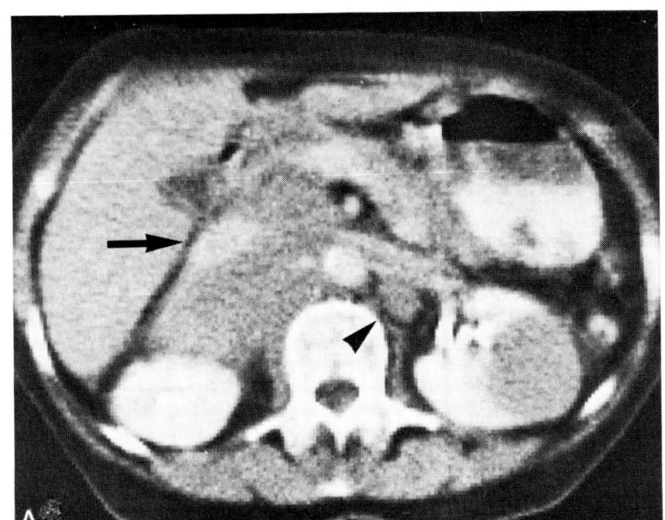

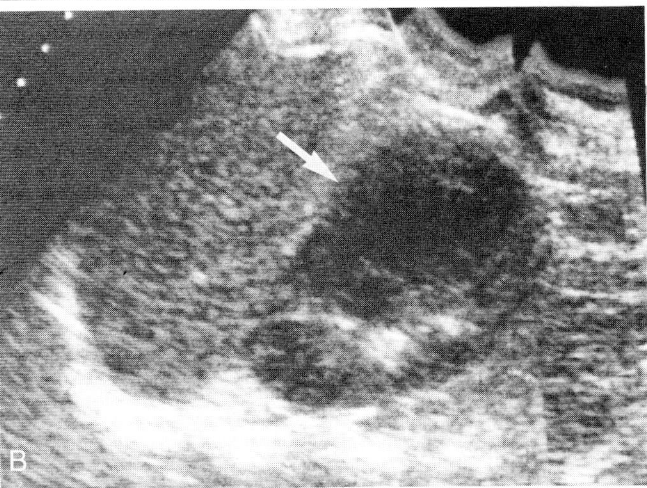

Figure 74–2. A 56-year-old woman with **diffuse histiocytic lymphoma.** *A,* A contrast-enhanced CT scan at the level of the upper pole right kidney demonstrates a low-attenuation right retroperitoneal mass that displaces the IVC anteriorly *(arrow).* A left renal mass of similar attenuation is seen laterally in the midportion of the left kidney. The *arrowhead* points to an enlarged retroperitoneal lymph node. *B,* Coronal sonogram through the spleen and left kidney shows a mass projecting from the lateral aspect of the kidney *(arrow),* corresponding to the mass seen on CT scan. Although the mass is hypoechoic, it does not demonstrate the augmented transmission expected with a fluid-filled mass of similar size. (Reprinted with permission from Horii SC, Bosniak MA, Megibow AJ, et al: Correlation of CT and ultrasound in evaluation of renal lymphoma. Urol Radiol 5:69–76, 1983.)

both renal involvement and extrarenal disease (Fig. 74–2). CT optimally demonstrates the extent of retroperitoneal disease and its contiguous spread to the kidneys as well as showing lymphadenopathy in the region of the renal hilum and para-aortic and paralumbar regions. The majority of patients with renal lymphoma demonstrate retroperitoneal adenopathy as well as the renal lesion.

When lymphoma presents as intraparenchymal nodules, these lesions are usually multiple and bilateral (Fig. 74–3). Nodules as small as 3 to 5 mm in diameter have been demonstrated by CT, although they usually range in size from 1 to 4.5 cm. They are located predominantly in the renal cortex. On unenhanced scans, lymphomatous nodules are usually isodense or hypodense in comparison with normal renal parenchyma and may be difficult to appreciate. Occasionally, lymphoma is hyperdense compared with renal parenchyma. Following contrast administration, the masses demonstrate enhancement of approximately 10 to 50 HU (depending on the amount of contrast used and the speed of injection), considerably less than the enhancement seen in normal renal tissue. Enhancement is usually uniform (see Fig. 74–2). In fact, it is characteristic for lymphomatous tissue to be homogeneous. Rarely, areas of decreased attenuation within the lymphomatous mass indicating necrosis may be present. This is usually seen in cases of very aggressive disease or after chemotherapy.

In cases of infiltrative involvement of the kidneys, CT appearance can vary depending on whether the lymphoma is focal or diffuse. Focal infiltration usually results from predominantly extrarenal lymphoma that has extended into the kidneys (Fig. 74–4). Diffuse infiltration may be due to a hematogenous metastasis with continuing extensive infiltration and growth or, more commonly, to extension of contiguous retroperitoneal disease. With diffuse infiltration, the entire kidney is enlarged and replaced by tumor but may retain its reniform shape (Fig. 74–5). There is dilatation, distortion, and elongation of the collecting system due to compression by the infiltrative tumor. Occasionally, complete disruption of renal architecture with tumor growing across and obliterating tissue planes can be seen (Fig. 74–6*A*). Lymphoma not infrequently extends into the kidney via the renal hilus with extension into the renal sinus and then into the renal parenchyma (Fig. 74–4).

CT is able to demonstrate perirenal changes due to tumor infiltration. There may be extension of a focal renal mass into the perirenal space or, more often, extension of a lymphomatous process around the kidney directly into the renal parenchyma (Fig. 74–7). These extrarenal changes secondary to tumor infiltration were seen in 19 of 35 affected kidneys in one CT series.

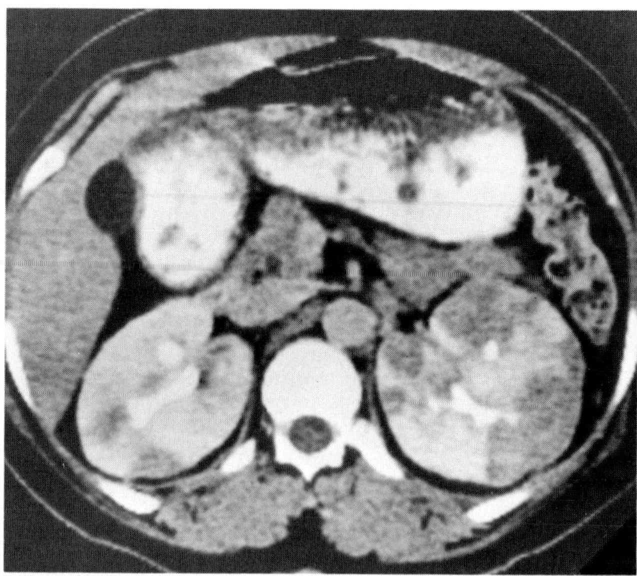

Figure 74–3. A 46-year-old woman with **CNS lymphoma** diagnosed one year previously presented with abdominal discomfort. Contrast-enhanced CT reveals both kidneys to be involved by multiple 1 to 2 cm nodules of lymphomatous tissue. The left kidney shows coalescence of these multiple nodules. Note that they are predominantly cortical and that the kidney margins maintain a smooth contour. Following chemotherapy, there was regression of the lymphomatous masses with focal scars in the areas of tumor involvement.

In two series of cases of renal lymphoma studied by CT reported by Cohan et al and Reznek et al, multiple renal masses were the most common manifestation of renal lymphoma. Invasion of the kidney by contiguous retroperitoneal masses was the next most common presentation, with perinephric masses, solitary renal mass, and diffuse renal infiltration less commonly seen.

CT can also demonstrate the mechanical effects of extrarenal tumor on the kidney. When retroperitoneal disease causes secondary ureteral obstruction, the resultant hydronephrosis is well seen by CT and the level and nature of the obstruction can be clearly assessed.

CT is the most effective means of following the results of therapy for renal and retroperitoneal lymphoma. CT can clearly show de-

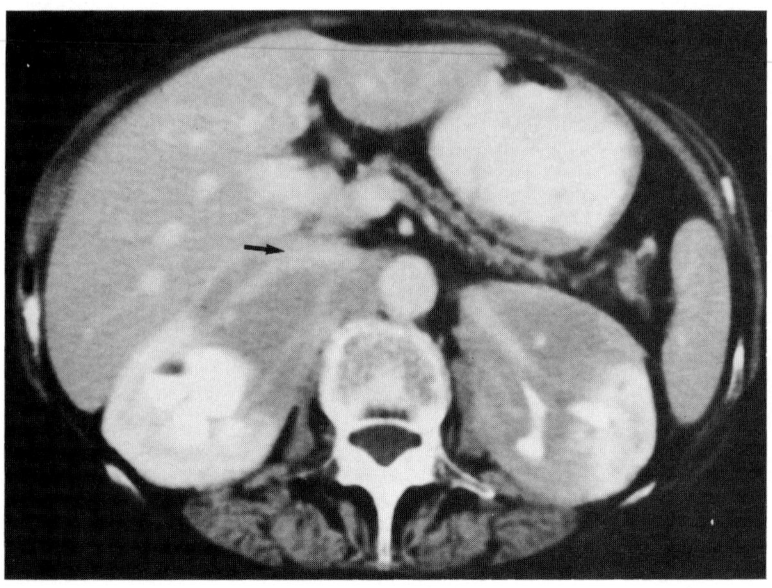

Figure 74–4. A 67-year-old female with **generalized non-Hodgkin's lymphoma**. A contrast-enhanced CT scan reveals a characteristic picture of lymphoma extending into the hilar portions of both kidneys. Dilation of the collecting systems of both kidneys has resulted. Note that the renal vessels can be seen coursing through the lymphomatous mass, which is relatively homogeneous in appearance. The inferior vena cava can be seen elevated anteriorly *(arrow)*.

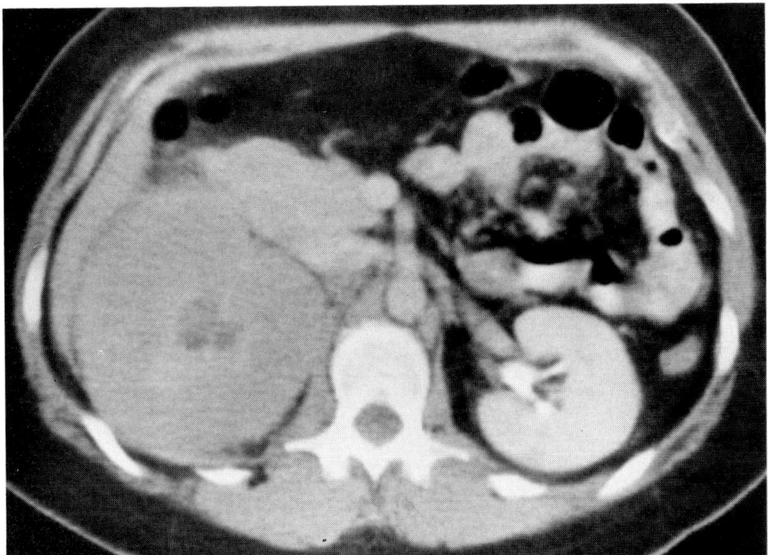

Figure 74–5. A 24-year-old woman with **lymphoma** had a staging CT examination. Contrast-enhanced CT of the abdomen taken through the midportion of the kidneys reveals diffuse infiltration of the right kidney by lymphoma. The infiltrated kidney is greatly enlarged and demonstrates no contrast in the collecting system. Note that there is symmetrical enlargement of the kidney, which maintains its reniform shape.

creased size or disappearance of nodules or shrinkage of retroperitoneal lymphomatous masses. Rarely, nodular masses are replaced by renal scars, and diffusely infiltrated kidneys may become atrophic following therapy.

Differential diagnosis for the CT appearance of renal lymphoma depends on the type of renal involvement. When lymphoma presents as multiple renal masses, other types of blood-borne disease in the kidney could give a similar picture, such as metastatic tumor to the kidney, infarction, infection, and leukemia. A single renal lymphomatous mass could be difficult to differentiate from renal cell carcinoma, and in some cases of diffuse lymphomatous infiltration, invasive transitional cell carcinoma might give a similar picture. The latter could be differentiated by evaluation of the collecting system, which would show a filling defect or destruction in transitional cell carcinoma but would only be compressed and distorted by lymphoma. The presence of retroperitoneal adenopathy and often splenomegaly and especially a history of lymphoma can assist in this differential diagnosis. Correlation with sonography can be helpful. Decreased size of the renal mass following chemotherapy suggests renal lymphoma.

ANGIOGRAPHY

Angiography is rarely performed in patients with renal lymphoma, and this section is included only for historical interest. In the days prior to CT and percutaneous biopsy, angiography had a role in differentiating renal lymphoma from renal cell carcinoma and other tumors. Renal lymphoma is usually relatively hypovascular (see Fig. 76–6*B*), with stretched and pruned vessels often with encasement and amputation. This appearance was somewhat helpful

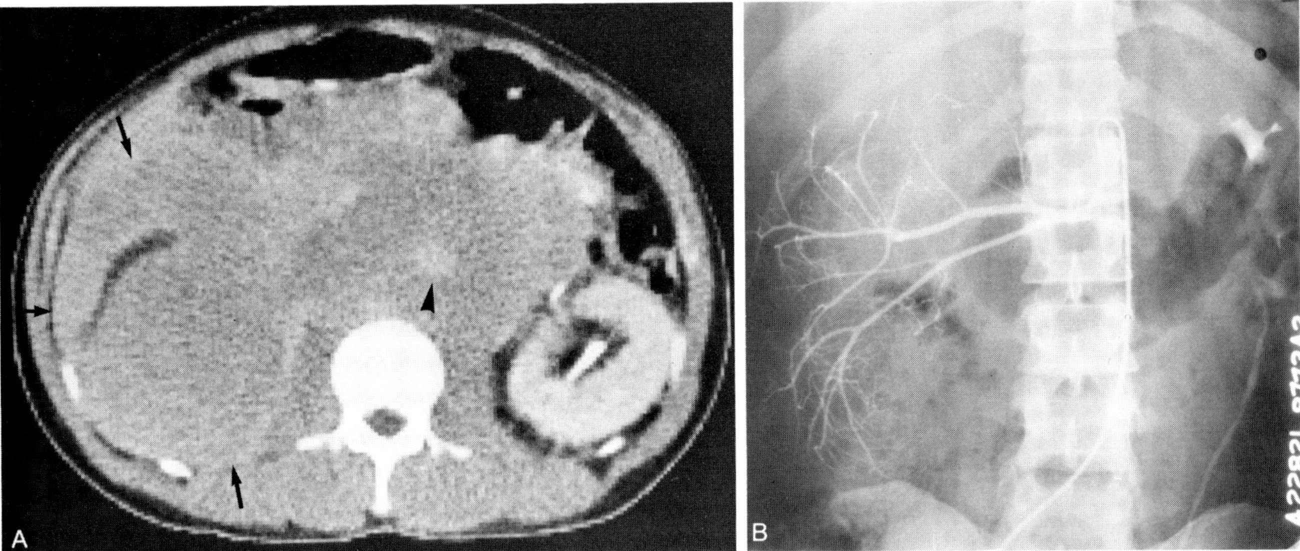

Figure 74–6. A 34-year-old man with **mixed-cell lymphoma**. *A*, A contrast-enhanced CT scan at the level of the mid–left kidney shows a huge retroperitoneal mass that extends into the right renal fossa and the mesentery, obliterating all tissue planes. Slight opacification of the aorta is seen *(arrowhead)*. The right kidney is infiltrated and completely replaced by the lymphomatous mass *(arrows)*. *B*, Selective right renal arteriogram reveals stretching and attenuation of intrarenal arteries as well as apparent amputation of peripheral vessels and loss of side branches, findings that are characteristic of infiltrating renal masses such as lymphoma. (Reprinted with permission from Horii SC, Bosniak MA, Megibow AJ, et al: Correlation of CT and ultrasound in evaluation of renal lymphoma. Urol Radiol 5:69–76, 1983.)

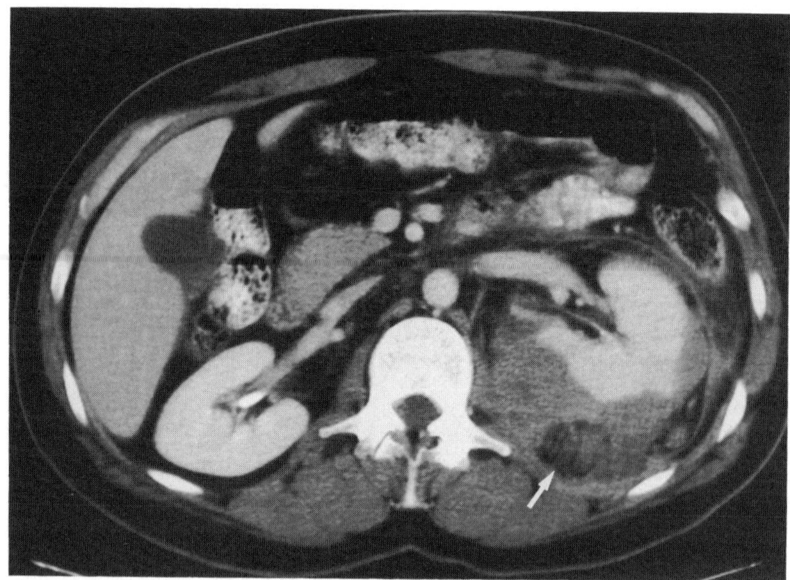

Figure 74–7. A 33-year-old male with **non-Hodgkin's lymphoma.** A contrast-enhanced CT scan reveals a large lymphomatous mass surrounding the kidney. Note actual invasion of the renal parenchyma by the tumor. The tumor is homogeneous, but some areas of decreased attenuation are seen posteriorly *(arrow)*, which represent perirenal fat being caught up in the neoplasm (which can be appreciated by reviewing scan sections above and below this section).

in differentiating lymphoma from other malignancies. However, at this time there is no role for angiography in the diagnosis and management of renal lymphoma.

MAGNETIC RESONANCE IMAGING

Lymphomatous tissue is relatively homogenenous and tends to be hypointense to fat and slightly hyperintense to muscle on T_1-weighted images and isointense to fat and hyperintense to muscle on T_2-weighted images. These characteristics are similar to other malignant tissues in the kidney. Perirenal tissue involvement and nodal involvement is well seen with MRI but intrarenal involvement is probably less well seen, as differentiation from normal kidney is not as clear in MRI as in contrast-enhanced CT.

RADIOISOTOPES

The role of the gallium scan in lymphoma has been well-established. Gallium-67 may demonstrate areas of increased uptake within the kidneys corresponding to the location of lesions demonstrated on ultrasonography and CT. However, due to normal bowel excretion of gallium, and even with extensive bowel cleaning with laxatives and enemas, evaluation of abnormal gallium uptakes in the abdomen has been difficult. However, with the use of single photon emission computed tomography (SPECT) scanning and using a relatively larger dose and more frequent follow-up images, the value of the technique seems to have increased. Since a similar uptake of gallium can be seen in other renal neoplasms, inflammatory conditions, acute tubular necrosis, renal vasculitis, and severe liver impairment, use of gallium in the diagnosis and differentiation of a renal lesion as representing lymphoma is significantly limited.

PERCUTANEOUS NEEDLE BIOPSY

The diagnosis of renal lymphoma can often be suggested by radiologic findings, distribution of disease, and clinical history. However, occasionally percutaneous or open renal biopsy is required for histologic diagnosis. For instance, in a patient with lymphoma in whom a renal mass is discovered, which is not radiologically characteristic of lymphoma or does not appear to be resolving under treatment, particularly if other areas of disease are responding to treatment, renal biopsy may be necessary to rule out a renal cell carcinoma.

LEUKEMIA

In general, the radiologic findings in leukemia of the kidneys closely resemble those of lymphoma. However, in contradistinction to the lymphomas, which are thought to begin as a local disease that may spread to become systemic, leukemia is a systemic disease from the onset. The kidney is the most frequently involved organ in all forms of leukemia. Renal involvement at autopsy in patients with leukemia varies from 31 to 80 per cent, being highest in chronic lymphocytic leukemia. There is a greater tendency toward bilateral and diffuse renal involvement with leukemia than with lymphoma. Leukemia causes a diffuse nodular infiltration of the cortex with little involvement of the medulla. Renal infiltration may produce moderate to marked bilateral symmetrical renal enlargement. A focal renal mass is much less common and represents a local aggregate of leukemic cells or hemorrhage. Nonvisualization of the kidneys results most commonly from uric acid nephropathy, especially after therapy, and rarely from complete leukemic infiltration of both kidneys.

METASTATIC NEOPLASMS TO THE KIDNEY

Secondary neoplasms to the kidneys may arise either from direct extension or, more commonly, by hematogenous metastasis. Direct extension may occur by invasion of a contiguous neoplasm growing into the kidney or via lymphatics or renal veins. Hematogenous metastases arise from tumor emboli carried to the kidneys via the renal arteries, and this section deals primarily with blood-borne metastatic disease.

The kidney is the fifth most common site of metastases in the body, with metastases more common to liver, lung, bone, and adrenals in decreasing order of frequency. Blood-borne metastases to the kidneys occur in 7.6 to 12.6 per cent of patients dying of malignant disease. Metastasis to the kidney may be present when the primary tumor is initially diagnosed or may occur anytime during the course of the disease, even years later. Any primary neoplasm can metastasize to the kidneys, although carcinoma of the lung is the primary site in about half of these cases. Less commonly, melanoma or malignancies in the breast, stomach, colon, opposite kidney, or pancreas are the source of metastases.

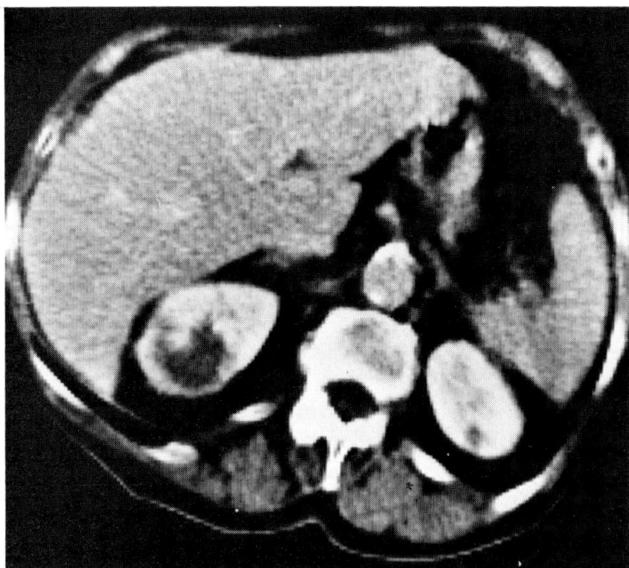

Figure 74–8. An 86-year-old woman presented with back pain. A chest film demonstrated a large mass in the lung, which was biopsied and revealed **adenocarcinoma**. CT of the abdomen performed as part of her staging showed defects in both kidneys and in the liver. A contrast-enhanced CT scan through the upper abdomen reveals an irregular area of diminished attenuation in the upper pole of the right kidney and a small similar defect in the left kidney. These lesions measured 70 HU. These metastatic lesions are completely intrarenal and do not distort the renal contours. (Reprinted with permission from Mitnick JS, Bosniak MA, Rothberg M, et al: Metastatic neoplasm to the kidney studied by computed tomography and sonography. J Comput Assist Tomogr 9:43–49, 1985.)

Because of the vascularity of the glomeruli, the cortex is frequently the area for entrapment and proliferation of tumor emboli, and indeed tumor emboli trapped in the glomerular capillary tuft have been demonstrated. Metastatic lesions are usually multiple and bilateral. Their location is cortical, frequently subcapsular. Most renal metastases are microscopic to millimeters in size and only rarely form masses large enough to be roentgenologically detectable.

In contrast to the relative frequency of autopsy findings, clinical suspicion and antemortem detection of secondary neoplasms of the kidney have been comparatively rare. Excretory urography may show solitary or multiple masses in the kidney when there is sufficient tumor volume, although in most cases of metastasis the lesion will be below critical size for detection. However, with the more widespread use of CT for tumor diagnosis and staging, renal metastases—even in asymptomatic patients—have been more commonly discovered. The majority of these lesions will be detected between 1 and 12 months following the diagnosis of the primary tumor, although some will be found at the time of tumor staging for the primary neoplasm. It is unusual for the metastasis to the kidney to be found prior to the diagnosis of the primary neoplasm.

CT generally shows multiple, bilateral, small parenchymal nodules (Fig. 74–8). They range in size from 1 to 11 cm in diameter, with a mean of 3.8 cm. In the majority of cases the lesions are entirely confined to the renal contour, with only the very large lesions projecting beyond the renal outline. The appearance will vary depending on the primary site. Lung and melanoma metastases in general are small and multifocal and even occur in perinephric locations, while colon metastases tend to be large and exophytic (Figs. 74–9 and 74–10*A*). On the unenhanced scans, the attenuation of the metastases is similar to that of normal renal parenchyma. With contrast, lesion enhancement is variable depending on dose and speed of IV contrast infusion and vascularity of the metastatic tissue but usually considerably less than normal renal parenchyma. There is usually evidence of metastatic disease elsewhere besides the kidney, and in one series, 89 per cent of cases demonstrated metastases in other areas (Fig. 74–11).

Ultrasonography demonstrates hypoechoic areas with few echoes and no through transmission in the majority of cases. Some lesions may have a mixed pattern of hypoechoic and echoic areas, or the echogenicity may be similar to that of normal renal parenchyma.

While angiography has little role currently in the diagnosis of

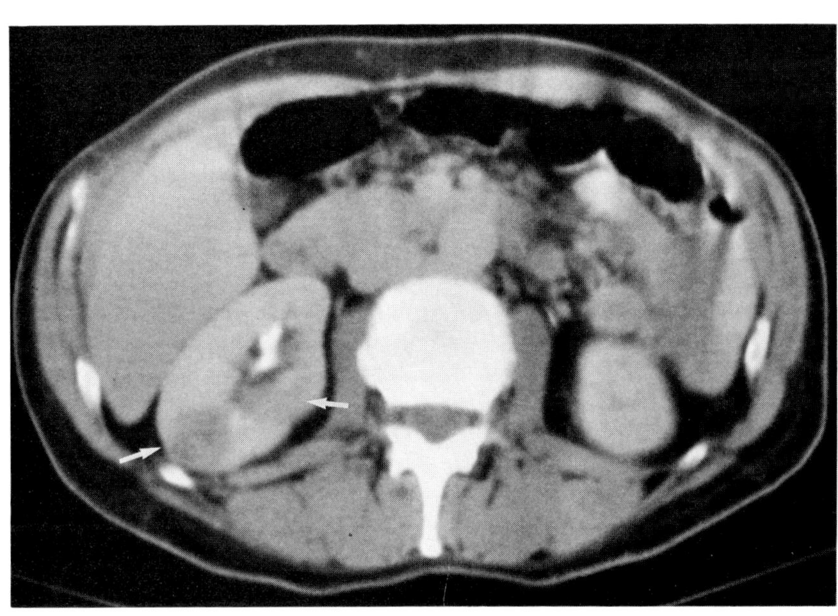

Figure 74–9. A 42-year-old man who had resection of the rectum for **squamous cell carcinoma of the anus** one year earlier and experienced current weight loss. A contrast-enhanced CT scan of the abdomen taken near the lower poles of the kidney demonstrates two small distinct nodules in the right kidney *(arrows)*. They could not be distinguished from renal parenchyma on the non-enhanced scan and increased in attenuation by 20 HU following contrast. At other levels, retroperitoneal adenopathy was seen, and multiple nodules were seen in the lungs. Percutaneous needle biopsy of the posteriorly placed renal lesion was performed, and squamous cell carcinoma identical to the previous tumor was obtained.

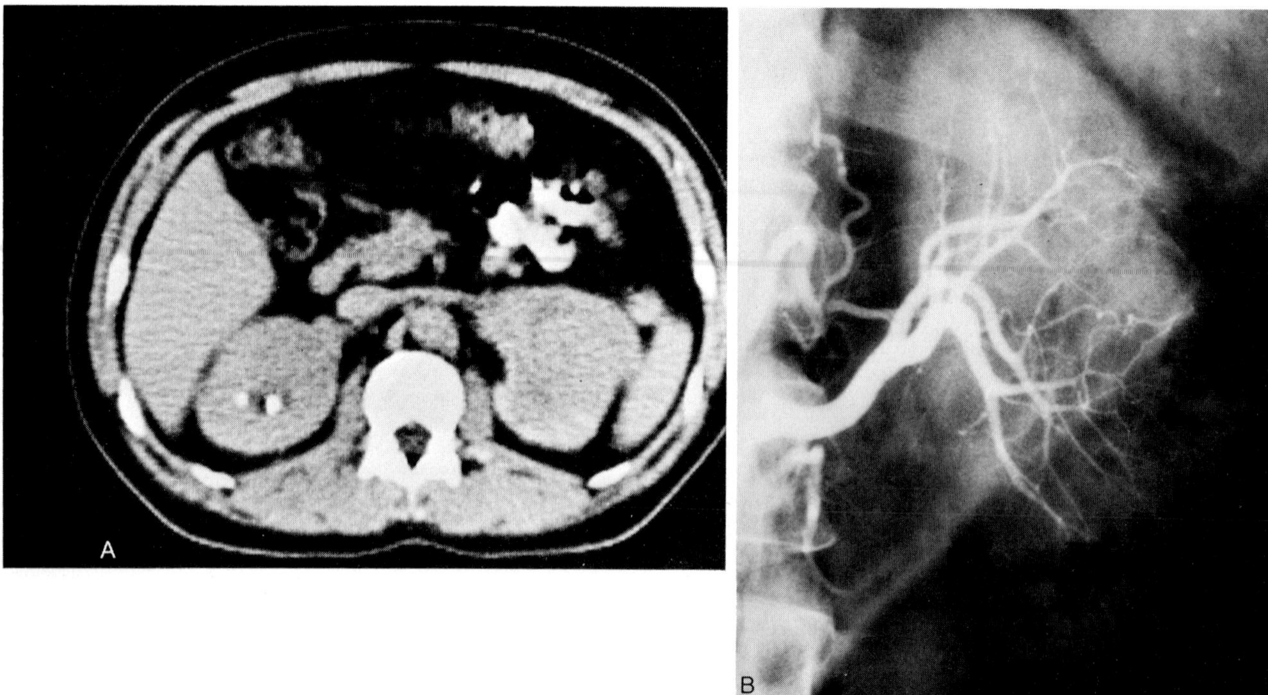

Figure 74–10. A 53-year-old man with **squamous cell carcinoma of the larynx and metastasis to cervical lymph nodes**. The patient was treated with radiotherapy and chemotherapy. Five months later he developed back pain, a soft-tissue mass in the thigh, and elevated blood urea nitrogen levels. *A*, Low-dose contrast-enhanced CT scan reveals a large, irregularly shaped mass of the midportion of the left kidney extending along the renal vein, which appears collapsed. A smaller similarly located mass is present in the right kidney. *B*, Selective left renal arteriogram demonstrates a hypovascular mass with encasement and amputation of peripheral vessels and a diminished nephrogram. These findings are characteristic of an infiltrating renal mass and are consistent with squamous cell carcinoma metastatic to the kidney. Subsequent needle biopsy of the thigh mass confirmed metastatic squamous cell carcinoma. (Reprinted with permission from Mitnick JS, Bosniak MA, Rothberg M, et al: Metastatic neoplasm to the kidney studied by computed tomography and sonography. J Comput Assist Tomogr 9:43–49, 1985.)

renal metastases, information that was accumulated in previous years with this technique helps explain the variable vascularity of these lesions on CT. Metastatic lesions show a variable angiographic appearance depending upon the histology of the primary neoplasm. The degree of vascularity and the presence of tumor encasement are in part related to the nature of the primary neoplasm. Avascular primaries give avascular metastases, and vascular primaries give vascular ones. Squamous cell carcinoma of the lung is the most frequent metastatic tumor to the kidney, and this metastasis demonstrates an infiltrating pattern, with irregularity, amputation, and encasement of smaller branch vessels and uneven distribution of flow (see Fig. 74–10*B*). Most lesions are avascular or hypovascular, although metastases from vascular primaries may show profuse neovascularity.

In patients with a known primary tumor, the presence of multiple bilateral solid renal masses strongly favors metastases, and histo-

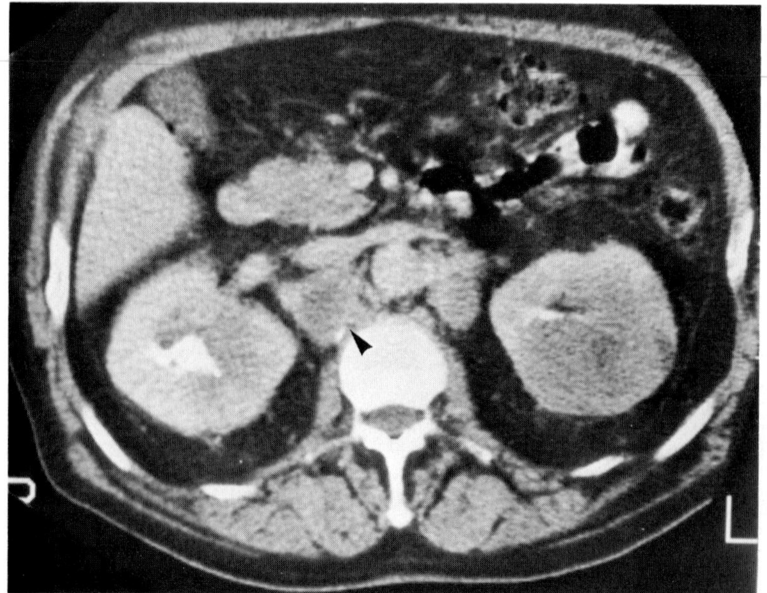

Figure 74–11. A 71-year-old man with **squamous cell carcinoma of the lung** had hematuria. Urography revealed bilateral renal masses. A contrast-enhanced CT scan demonstrates large hypovascular masses in both kidneys. The lesions are completely intrarenal and do not distort the renal contour. Multiple necrotic retroperitoneal lymph nodes were noted in the para-aortic area *(arrowhead)* on this and sequential slices. (Reprinted with permission from Mitnick JS, Bosniak MA, Rothberg M, et al: Metastatic neoplasm to the kidney studied by computed tomography and sonography. J Comput Assist Tomogr 9:43–49, 1985.)

logic diagnosis can be proven by percutaneous aspiration biopsy if necessary. About 11 per cent of patients demonstrate a solitary renal metastasis without evidence of metastasis elsewhere. When a solitary renal lesion is discovered in a patient with a known tumor, the possibility of a second primary must be considered and percutaneous needle biopsy is indicated to make the differentiation. Although renal metastases are twice as common as primary renal carcinoma at autopsy, many of these lesions are below the threshold of CT detection. It was noted in one small series of oncologic patients that the occurrence of a second primary in the kidney was 4.5 times more common than detection of metastasis to the kidney. On the other hand, a more recent larger series of cases reported by Choyke et al demonstrated that renal metastases outnumbered a second renal primary tumor by approximately 4 to 1. In the case of a solitary renal lesion, differentiation of metastasis from primary cell carcinoma can be difficult. In most instances, neither angiography nor CT will be able to differentiate these two possibilities, and needle biopsy will be required for diagnosis.

When metastatic disease to the kidney presents with multiple lesions, the differential diagnosis includes lymphoma, bilateral renal cell carcinomas, multiple renal infarcts, and multiple areas of renal inflammation. Clinical history as well as CT pattern is usually able to make the differentiation. In difficult cases, aspiration biopsy may be necessary.

Acknowledgment

The authors would like to thank Esther Roman and Angela Oleske for manuscript preparation.

Bibliography

Abrams HL, Spiro R, Goldstein N: Metastases in carcinoma. Analysis of 1,000 autopsied cases. Cancer 3:74–85, 1950.

Ambos MA, Bosniak MA, Madayag MA, Lefleur RS: Infiltrating neoplasms of the kidney. AJR 129:859–864, 1977.

Beral V, Peterman T, Berkelman R, Jaffe H: AIDS-associated non-Hodgkin's lymphoma. Lancet 337:805–809, 1991.

Bhatt GM, Bernardino ME, Graham SD Jr: CT diagnosis of renal metastases. J Comput Assist Tomogr 7:1032–1034, 1983.

Burgener FA, Hamlin DJ: Histiocytic lymphoma of the abdomen: Radiographic spectrum. AJR 137:337–342, 1981.

Choyke PL, White EM, Zeman RK, et al: Renal metastases: Clinicopathologic and radiologic correlation. Radiology 162:359–363, 1987.

Cohan RH, Dunnick NR, Leder RA, Baker ME: Computed tomography of renal lymphoma. J Comput Assist Tomogr 14:933–938, 1990.

Dunnick NR, Leder RA, Roubidoux MA: Percutaneous biopsy of the kidney and adrenal glands. Urol Radiol 12:125–129, 1990.

Heiken JP, Gold RP, Schnur MJ, et al: Computed tomography of renal lymphoma with ultrasound correlation. J Comput Assist Tomogr 7:245–250, 1983.

Horii SC, Bosniak MA, Megibow AJ, et al: Correlation of CT and ultrasound in the evaluation of renal lymphoma. Urol Radiol 5:69–76, 1983.

Jafri SZH, Amendola MA, Brady TM, et al: Angiographic patterns of involvement in renal and perirenal lymphoma. Urol Radiol 6:14–19, 1984.

Kuhlman JE, Browne D, Shermak M, et al: Retroperitoneal and pelvic CT of patients with AIDS: Primary and secondary involvement of the genitourinary tract. Radio Graphics 11:473–483, 1991.

Mitnick JS, Bosniak MA, Rothberg M, et al: Metastatic neoplasm to the kidney studied by computed tomography and sonography. J Comput Assist Tomogr 9:43–49, 1985.

Negendank WG, Al-katib AM, Karanes C, Smith MR: Lymphomas. MR imaging contrast characteristics with clinical-pathologic correlations. Radiology 177:209–216, 1990.

Nyberg DA, Jeffrey RB, Federle MP, et al: AIDS related lymphoma: Evaluation by abdominal CT. Radiology 159:59–63, 1986.

Pagani JJ: Solid renal mass in the cancer patient. Second primary renal cell carcinoma versus renal metastasis. J Comput Assist Tomogr 7:444–448, 1983.

Reznek RH, Mootosamy I, Webb JAW, Richards MA: CT in renal and perirenal lymphoma: A further look. Clin Radiol 42:233–238, 1990.

Richmond J, Sherman RS, Diamond HS, Craver LF: Renal lesions associated with malignant lymphomas. Am J Med 32:184–207, 1962.

Shapiro JH, Ramsay CG, Jacobson GH, et al: Renal involvement in lymphomas and leukemias in adults. AJR 88:928–941, 1962.

Shimkin PM, Buchignani JS, Soloway MS: Blood borne metastases to the kidney. Angiographic investigation of three vascular tumors. Acta Radiol Diagn 12:387–395, 1972.

Shirkhoda A, Staab EV, Mittelstaedt CA: Renal lymphoma imaged by ultrasound and gallium-67. Radiology 137:175–180, 1980.

Townsend RR, Laing FC, Jeffrey RB, Bottles K: Abdominal lymphoma in AIDS. Evaluation with US. Radiology 171:719–724, 1989.

Viadana E, Bross IDJ, Pickren JW: An autopsy study of the metastatic patterns of human leukemia. Oncology 35:87–96, 1978.

75 Vascular Diseases of the Kidney

Richard L. Clark

Our increased understanding of renal vascular disease has paralleled the technical advances of renal angiography over the past 30 years. From its infancy in Scandinavia, following the development of the Seldinger technique of percutaneous catheterization, to the modern era of magnification and digital subtraction techniques, renal angiography has often provided diagnostic information that has been critical to the management of patients with renal vascular disease. Coupled with the increased use of magnification techniques and the resulting improvement in resolution has been a continued interest in in vitro microangiographic studies that has helped bridge the gap between the viewbox (or CRT) and the histologic slide. Knowledge of renal microvascular anatomy and pathology does indeed permit more rational interpretation of clinical studies, even though structures such as glomeruli, peritubular capillaries, and cortical lymphatics are too small to be seen in vivo. Because a detailed discussion of any of the subjects covered in the following sections is beyond the scope of a general text, the interested reader is referred to the list of additional sources at the end of this chapter.

VASCULAR ANATOMY

Arterial Anatomy

Usually, a single renal artery arises from each side of the abdominal aorta at about the level of L1 to L2. However, in about 40 per cent of normal individuals (Fig. 75–1), one or both kidneys will be found to be supplied by more than one vessel. Looking at it another way, about one fourth of all human kidneys will have two or more renal arteries identified. Accessory vessels are more likely to be seen on the left side and usually arise from the aorta distal to the origin of the main renal artery. Rarely, the kidney may receive accessory, usually polar, vascular supply from the hepatic, celiac, superior mesenteric, iliac, or contralateral renal arteries. The renal arteries lie posterior to the renal veins, and because of the left-of-midline position of the abdominal aorta, the right renal artery has a slightly longer course than the left as it passes behind the inferior vena cava.

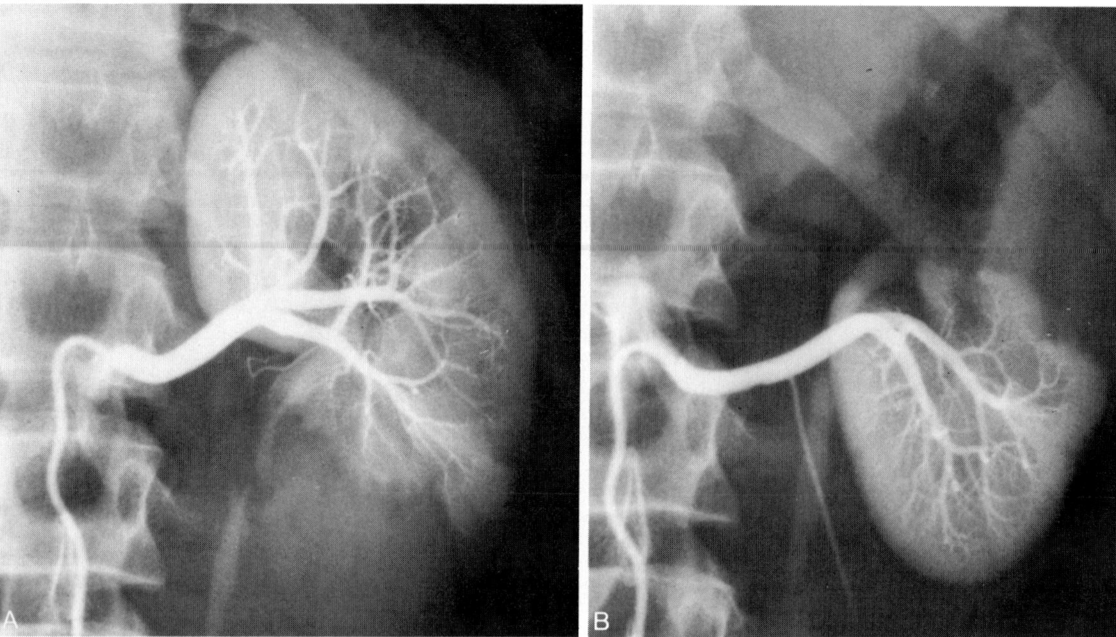

Figure 75–1. *A* and *B*, Dual blood supply in an otherwise normal kidney.

The renal arteries together carry 20 per cent of the normal cardiac output, making the kidneys second only to the thyroid gland in rate of organ perfusion (600 ml/minute/kidney). Normally, the renal cortex receives 70 per cent of this blood flow and the medulla 30 per cent. However, in certain renal parenchymal diseases, during systemic hypotension, or with aging, this distribution can be altered considerably.

The proximal main renal artery gives off the inferior adrenal artery and branches to the renal capsule, renal pelvis, and ureter. Occasionally the inferior phrenic, gonadal, and middle and superior adrenal arteries arise from the main renal artery.

As the renal artery nears the kidney, it divides into anterior (ventral) and posterior (dorsal) rami that pass in front of and behind the renal pelvis. Although many variations occur, the normally larger anterior division usually supplies the anterior and inferior (caudal) aspects of the kidney, while the posterior division supplies the posterior and superior (cephalad) aspects.

First-order branches of these dorsal and ventral rami are called segmental arteries as they traverse the proximal pericalyceal extensions of the renal sinus. Second-order branches (called interlobar arteries) follow along the sides of the septa of Bertin and usually divide again as they pass between medullary pyramids and supply the multiple (average 14) renal lobes. These vessels then penetrate the renal parenchymal substance, becoming arcuate arteries that partially encircle the base of each medullary pyramid and define the corticomedullary junction. Thus, each renal lobe is usually supplied by at least two interlobar arteries, and each interlobar artery via its terminal arcuate branches may supply two or more renal lobes. Arcuate arteries, contrary to their name, do not form continuous arcades between lobes but taper rapidly as they terminate in interlobular arteries (Fig. 75–2).

Microvascular Anatomy

Conventional angiographic studies are usually unable to resolve interlobular arteries (70 to 200 μm in diameter) that are the candelabrum-like arborizations of arcuate arteries. These vessels, after an initial zig-zag course between bundles of tubules and collecting ducts (medullary rays) during which they may divide again, run perpendicular to the corticomedullary junction and supply the cortex, each giving off approximately 20 afferent arterioles that in turn supply one or more glomeruli. Occasionally, an interlobular artery will supply the renal capsule, permitting some potential extrarenal collateral supply to the outer cortex in instances of more proximal renal arterial obstruction.

There are approximately 1.5 million glomeruli in each young adult human kidney. Each structure is about 300 μm in diameter and consists primarily of capillary loops. It therefore has a large vascular capacitance that is expressed angiographically as the dense cortical nephrogram normally seen during the first few seconds following injection. Once blood has passed through glomerular capillaries, it then, depending on whether it is in an outer or inner cortical glomerulus, will flow through efferent arterioles to either the peritubular capillary plexus of the cortex or to the arteriolae rectae spuriae that ramify as the medullary capillary plexus. The kidney thus has a portal circulation with two sequential capillary beds (glomerular capillaries and cortical peritubular or medullary capillaries) linked by efferent arterioles.

As a result of normal aging, glomerular capillary sclerosis occurs and about one fourth of the glomeruli present at birth degenerate. This phenomenon, which may be accelerated by hypertension and various renal parenchymal diseases, permits some blood to reach the cortical peritubular plexus or the medullary capillaries directly. These lower-resistance pathways (not true shunts), particularly to the medulla, have been the source of much controversy among renal physiologists over the years.

The urothelial and renal sinus blood supply is derived from small aglomerular branches of segmental or interlobar vessels. Blood supply to the renal capsule and perirenal fat is from vessels that originate from the main renal artery and from inferior adrenal, gonadal, and perforating interlobular arteries.

Venous Anatomy

Except for four important points, the intrarenal venous structures parallel the arterial circulation in both anatomic detail and nomenclature. First, retro- or circumaortic left renal veins are occasionally seen. Second, the main renal vein and its major segmental tributar-

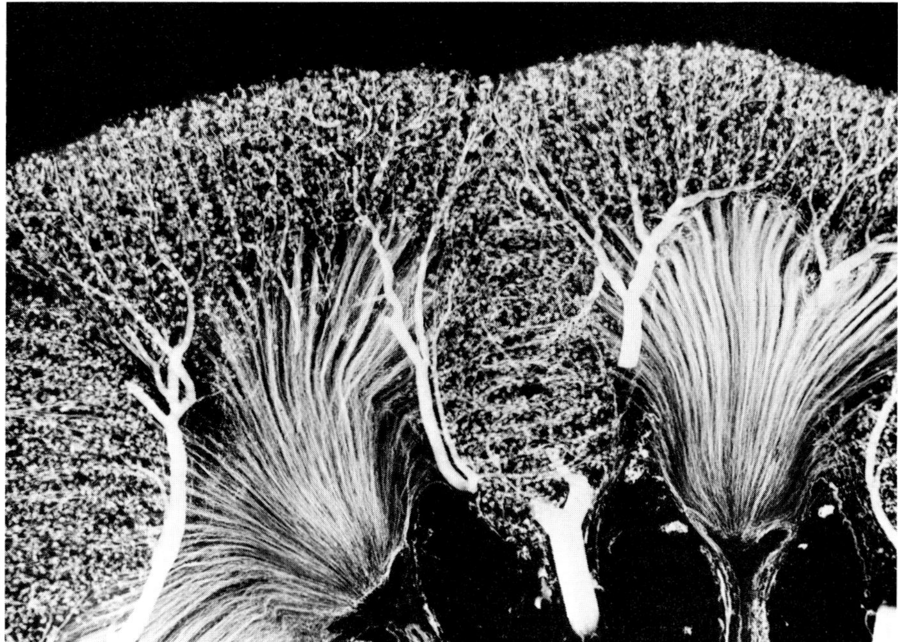

Figure 75–2. Normal renal microangiogram (×7). The typical appearance of two adjacent renal lobes can be seen with an intervening cortical septum. The striking difference between the microvascular pattern of the cortex with interlobular arteries, afferent arterioles, and glomeruli and the medulla containing vasa recta is emphasized by this illustration. Several interlobar arteries, which taper to arcuate vessels, can also be seen. (From Bookstein JJ, Clark RL: Renal Microvascular Disease: Angiographic-Microangiographic Correlates. Boston, Little, Brown and Company, 1980, p 22.)

ies occasionally contain valves. Third, despite classic anatomic teaching, the arcuate veins do not communicate directly with one another at the corticomedullary junction (Fig. 75–3). However, frequent anastomoses do occur between segmental and interlobar veins. Fourth, although not as well-developed in humans as in lower animals, a subcapsular stellate venous plexus exists that drains the outer cortex and then communicates with interlobular and capsular veins.

The main renal vein is less frequently duplicated than the renal artery. Accessory veins are present only 16 per cent of the time on the right and 3 per cent on the left. The left renal vein receives the inferior phrenic, adrenal, capsular, ureteral, and gonadal veins and anastomoses with the left ascending lumbar vein. The right renal vein receives the capsular and ureteral vein and anastomoses with the right ascending lumbar vein. Therefore, a rich potential collateral network exists and is clinically important during renal vein thrombosis. Any obstruction downstream from these numerous venous tributaries will permit these collateral paths of drainage to occur.

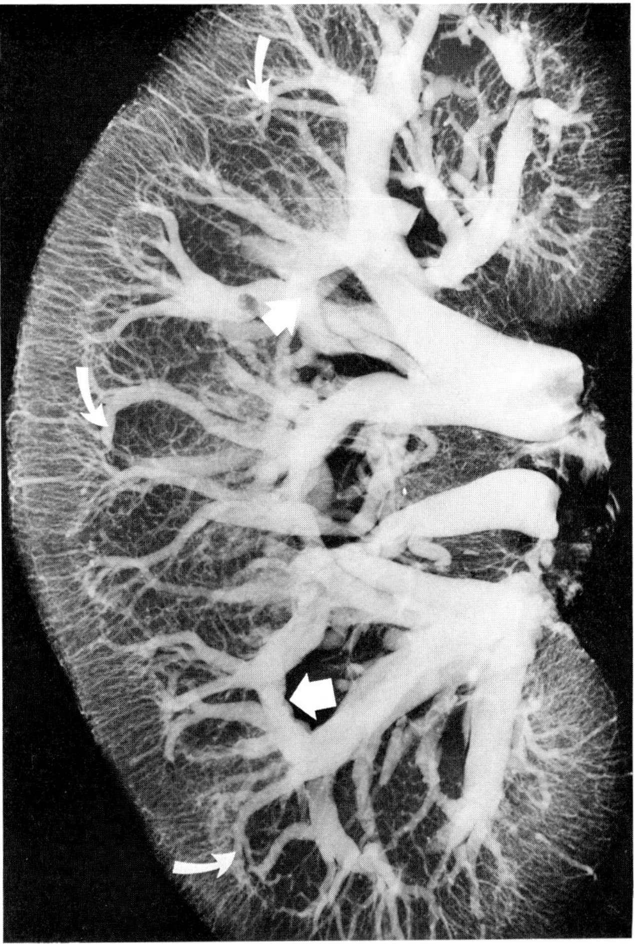

Figure 75–3. Venous microangiogram (×2) of a central 1-cm section of a normal kidney. Note the presence of communications between segmental veins *(straight arrows)* but absence of arcuate venous arcades *(curved arrows)*. (From Clark RL, Klein S: Renal arcuate veins: New microangiographic observations. AJR 141:755–759, 1983.)

Renal Lymphatics

Although the lymphatic circulation of the kidney is not easily visualized with conventional radiographic techniques, this alternative vascular system is extremely important because it provides an accessory route for renal drainage during altered physiologic states.

Normal renal lymphatic flow in humans is about 4 ml/minute or more than 2500 ml/day. This rather large volume of fluid gains access to the parenchymal microlymphatics as they arise in the periglomerular and medullary interstitium. In the renal cortex, these small and histologically inconspicuous vessels course around interlobular arteries like vines around tree trunks on their way to form a plexus in the periarcuate region. Subsequent drainage via larger valve-containing trunks to the renal hilum occurs. About one fourth of renal lymph flow leaves the kidney via small lymphatic channels that permeate the renal capsule and communicate with perirenal lymphatics in Gerota's space. Medullary lymphatics, although not as conspicuous as cortical lymphatics, do exist and may play an important role in maintaining the osmotic gradients necessary for countercurrent mechanisms to work.

Large perihilar lymphatics are occasionally visualized as a form of back-flow during retrograde pyelography or following contrast media extravasation secondary to acute ureteral obstruction (Fig. 75–4). CT has also allowed us to indirectly assess renal lymphatic flow by demonstrating changes in the appearance of the perirenal fat and Gerota's fascia during hydronephrosis, intrarenal inflammation, and renal vein occlusion.

The ability of the kidney to recover from an episode of obstruction or renal vein thrombosis is in part related to the success with which the renal lymphatics drain off excess interstitial fluid. Thus, if this accessory microcirculation is damaged or obliterated by chronic infection, irreversible hydronephrotic damage will occur more rapidly.

Normal Aging

Progressive glomerulosclerosis is a normal phenomenon of aging. As many as half a million glomeruli will degenerate during a normal lifetime. With the accompanying loss of nephrons, benign glomerulosclerosis accounts for the normal renal atrophy that occurs with age. Together with this loss in renal parenchymal volume (as much as 20 per cent), changes are noted in the renal vessels. Increased tortuosity of all intrarenal vessels is seen, and more abrupt tapering of distal interlobar and arcuate arteries is noted. In addition, the dense and sharply demarcated cortical nephrogram will be less clearly defined. It should be emphasized, however, that the vascular changes due to aging are subtle and not unlike the effects of mild essential hypertension (benign arterial and arteriolonephrosclerosis).

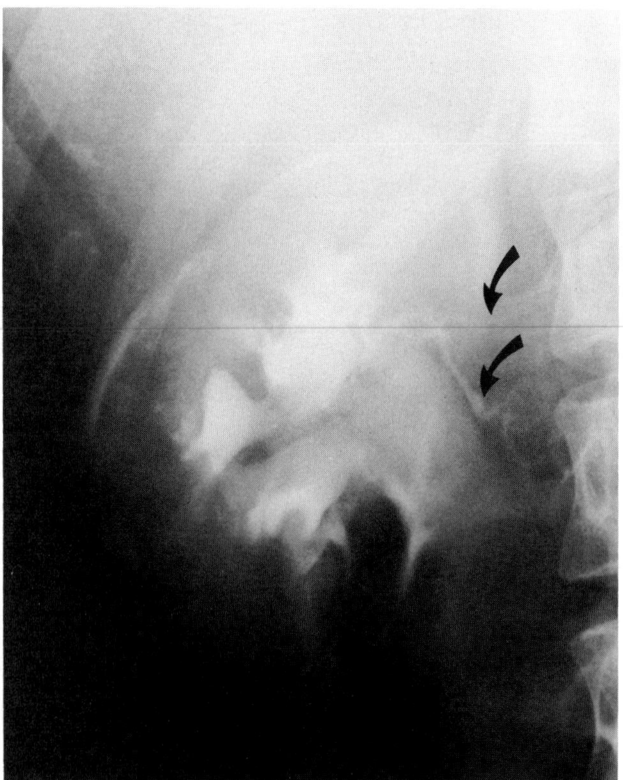

Figure 75–4. Perihilar lymphatics *(arrows)* visualized during IVU for acute obstruction. Note also subcapsular and pericalyceal extravasation.

DISEASES OF THE RENAL VASCULATURE

Pathologic conditions affecting the main renal arteries and their proximal branches such as atherosclerosis and fibromuscular disease frequently may produce arterial stenosis and renovascular hypertension. These lesions are potentially correctable with either surgical or interventional radiologic techniques and are discussed in detail elsewhere. What remains to be discussed, however, is the large number of ''medical'' vascular diseases that, although frequently associated with (or due to) hypertension, can only be treated with pharmacologic agents that either lower the blood pressure or reduce the microvascular inflammatory changes that may underlie these complex and often immunologically mediated conditions.

The renal vasculature, when affected directly or indirectly by diverse widespread parenchymal processes, responds in only a limited fashion. It is therefore convenient to divide the diffuse renal microvascular diseases into two groups: (1) conditions that primarily affect the preglomerular vascular tree (arcuate and interlobular arteries and afferent arterioles), and (2) conditions primarily affecting the glomeruli. Pathologic entities that focally and secondarily alter the circulation, such as emboli and aneurysms, will be treated separately. Renal vein thrombosis will also receive special attention later in this chapter.

Conditions Primarily Affecting Preglomerular Vessels

There are few distinctive characteristics of the intravenous urogram or of renal computed tomography (CT) in patients with diseases that affect primarily the preglomerular vessels. The kidneys are usually smaller than normal, and there may be fine irregularity of the renal outline because of cortical microinfarcts. Function may be considerably diminished, but the pelvicalyceal system is invariably normal. Plain films may demonstrate atherosclerotic calcification of the larger renal vessels (main renal artery, segmental branches, and proximal interlobar vessels), particularly if there is underlying diabetes mellitus. As will be described subsequently, angiographic findings in this group of ''medical'' diseases are fairly characteristic, but there is little variation in the vascular manifestations exhibited by individual diseases in this section.

NEPHROSCLEROSIS

Nephrosclerosis is a widely used but often poorly defined term that refers to the broad spectrum of degenerative and obstructive vascular changes associated with normal aging and to all forms of hypertension from the mild essential type to the malignant variety. As mentioned earlier in the section on aging, it is usually impossible to distinguish histologically, microangiographically, and angiographically between the benign nephrosclerosis of aging and early hypertensive changes. Intimal fibrosis, and elastosis of interlobular arteries and afferent arterioles seen histologically, are coupled with microvascular irregularity, tortuosity, and occasional occlusions. Larger vessels will show abrupt tapering and increased tortuosity (Fig. 75–5). As the condition becomes more severe in reaction to increasingly higher blood pressure, microvascular and larger vessel occlusions predominate with the development of numerous small cortical scars that result in a finely irregular renal outline. Fibrinoid necrosis and small hemorrhages are seen, and glomerular ischemic changes are to be expected.

Advanced nephrosclerosis will evoke a collateral response by the kidney. Frequent new corticomedullary junction vessels are seen that bypass obstructed interlobular and arcuate arteries. Prominent penetrating capsular vessels can often be demonstrated to supply the outer rim of ischemic cortex.

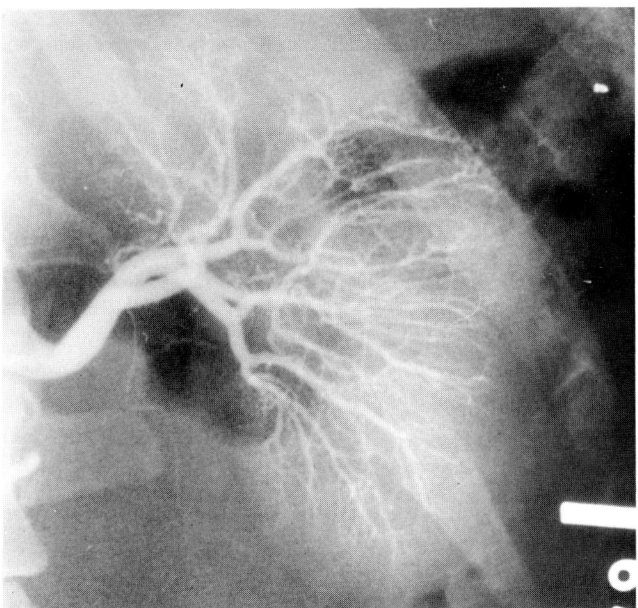

Figure 75–5. Nephrosclerosis in a 26-year-old black male with long-standing hypertension. Note the small renal size and abrupt tapering and increased tortuosity of intrarenal vessels. The nephrogram phase demonstrated very poor corticomedullary differentiation.

It is likely that in malignant nephrosclerosis the kidneys are no longer just passive recipients of hypertensive damage, but are in fact contributing to their own destruction by the production of renin from ischemic areas, which continues to augment a vicious circle of ever-increasing blood pressure, renal damage, and renin release.

SCLERODERMA

Progressive systemic sclerosis, or scleroderma, is a multisystem disease of unknown cause characterized by widespread vascular and connective tissue fibrosis. The kidneys are involved in up to 80 per cent of patients, and death due to renal failure and hypertension is common. Intimal thickening and thrombosis of interlobular arteries are present but because inflammatory changes are rare, the microaneurysms characteristic of necrotizing arteritis (see below) are not seen. The angiographic findings are similar to those of advanced nephrosclerosis (Fig. 75–5) with interlobular obliteration, cortical infarcts, and collaterals being the predominant findings.

THE ARTERITIDES

Several systemic "autoimmune" diseases affect primarily the walls of small arteries, resulting in inflammatory degeneration and subsequent microaneurysm formation, microvascular occlusions, and microinfarcts. Periarteritis nodosa (PAN) is the best-known of these necrotizing vasculitides, but identical lesions can be seen in drug abuse-related syndrome (usually methamphetamine) and less commonly in Wegener's granulomatosis, systemic lupus erythematosus, serum sickness, and following insect bites. PAN is a systemic disease, with liver, lung, spleen, mesentery, muscle, and brain often showing the characteristic microaneurysms of vessel wall degeneration. However, the kidney in most angiographic series has been the most common organ involved (80 to 100 per cent of cases). These vascular lesions, which appear to have a preference for bifurcation points, have been found to heal occasionally but most often result in arterial thrombosis and small cortical infarcts (Fig. 75–6). Vessel wall or aneurysm rupture may also occur with resultant intrarenal or subcapsular hemorrhage. Occasionally, the larger vessels of the kidney may be involved with variants of Takayasu's aortitis and arteritis, but usually this involvement is of little clinical significance compared with the effects this condition has on the central nervous system because of neck vessel involvement.

INTRAVASCULAR COAGULATION

Several different clinical entities with similar microvascular findings are characterized as disorders of intravascular coagulation. These conditions include hemolytic-uremic syndrome, microangiopathic hemolytic anemia, thrombotic thrombocytopenic purpura, postpartum renal failure, and to some extent acute allograft rejection. No definite unifying concept has been able to link all of these diseases because it is thought that the intravascular coagulation is precipitated by a number of different factors such as immune mechanisms, viral or bacterial inflammation, trauma, and amniotic fluid emboli. Hemolytic anemia and, to a lesser extent, thrombocytopenia have been attributed to mechanical damage to red cells and platelets passing through narrow and roughened vessels.

Angiographic findings are similar to other conditions that affect the preglomerular microcirculation such as malignant nephrosclerosis, scleroderma, and the arteritides (without microaneurysms). More frequently, however, the acute nature of these syndromes results in frank cortical necrosis (see below).

RADIATION NEPHRITIS

Any discussion of renal microvascular diseases that involve primarily the preglomerular microcirculation should also include radiation nephritis. Levels of radiation greater than 2500 rad in five weeks will produce small vessel changes. An initial increase in vascular wall permeability or fragility that results in edema will eventually lead to wall thickening, irregularity, and luminal occlusion. Glomeruli seem to be less affected primarily, although ische-

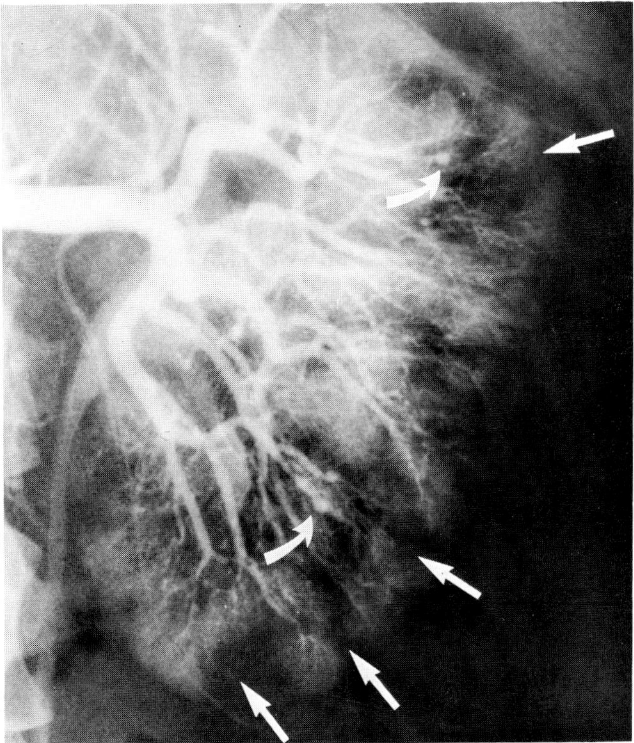

Figure 75–6. Periarteritis nodosa in a 21-year-old female with malignant hypertension. Note the small cortical infarcts *(straight arrows)* and microaneurysms *(curved arrows).* (Case courtesy of Paul F. Jaques, M.D.)

mic changes are seen later on. Angiographic findings again may be nonspecific and resemble benign or malignant nephrosclerosis (see Fig. 75–5) and the necrotizing arteritides. Focal hypertrophy of adjacent irradiated renal parenchyma should also be expected.

Conditions Primarily Affecting Glomeruli

Several different diseases have as their commonality the acute but usually transient reduction of glomerular perfusion with resultant renal failure. The two most frequently encountered conditions with this characteristic are acute tubular necrosis (ATN) and acute rapidly progressive glomerulonephritis (ARPG). Imaging studies in patients with these conditions are usually aimed at ruling out surgically correctable causes of acute renal failure such as bilateral obstruction. Since contrast media may exacerbate the acute renal failure, ultrasound is the initial procedure of choice. Renal nuclear medicine studies are valuable in assessing functional damage and in predicting or documenting recovery.

In addition to those conditions resulting in temporary loss of glomerular function, there are a large number of diseases that cause primary or secondary chronic and permanent glomerular damage. Imaging studies in patients with chronic renal failure usually are designed to evaluate the native kidneys (e.g., CT or ultrasound to rule out neoplasia or follow acquired cystic disease), complications of dialysis (catheter or shunt occlusions), or renal transplantation (Doppler ultrasound or nuclear medicine studies to rule out rejection).

ACUTE TUBULAR NECROSIS

ATN is usually the result of either a transient episode of renal ischemia or a renal toxin such as mercury, certain antibiotics, or iodinated contrast media. Various mechanisms have been postulated to account for the renal failure. These include (1) direct tubular damage with resultant tubular obstruction, (2) vasoconstriction of afferent arterioles and subsequent decrease in glomerular perfusion, (3) leakage of glomerular filtrate from damaged tubules into the interstitium, and (4) diminished glomerular filtration secondary to basement membrane changes that affect glomerular permeability. Although a large and often controversial literature appears to support a multifactorial etiology of ATN, the radiographic findings reflect the common denominator of diminished glomerular perfusion. Angiography, although rarely indicated, will show somewhat enlarged kidneys with markedly reduced blood flow. The intense cortical blush will be absent, and the images of overlapping interlobular arteries will be seen without overlying glomerular granularity. A persistent, albeit somewhat diminished, tubular nephrogram is frequently seen as contrast that is filtered, persists, and may be concentrated in obstructed tubules. We have been impressed with the frequency with which abdominal plain films, following vascular or contrast-enhanced CT procedures in patients at high risk for ATN (dehydration, myeloma, diabetes, congestive heart failure, and sepsis), will suggest the developing renal failure by documenting a persistent nephrogram and renal enlargement. In these cases, it is not easy to ignore the possible deleterious effects of contrast media on the already marginal renal function that these patients may possess. Although there are theoretical reasons to use non-ionic or other lower-osmolarity contrast agents in patients with deteriorating renal function, accumulated empirical evidence to date does not suggest that these newer agents are significantly safer in these difficult to manage patients.

ACUTE RAPIDLY PROGRESSIVE GLOMERULONEPHRITIS

It is not surprising that ARPG is also associated with diminished glomerular perfusion. This disease is usually easy to differentiate from ATN on clinical grounds (history of upper respiratory tract infections, increased ASO titers, hypertension, and urine sediment analysis). The kidneys are often markedly swollen, and histologic studies demonstrate glomerular inflammation with capillary obliteration and proliferation of cells in Bowman's capsule. Again, as in ATN, contrast studies are usually contraindicated, but if obtained, will show renal enlargement, a markedly diminished nephrographic intensity, loss of glomerular granularity, and increase in the interlobular pattern.

Two other causes of acute glomerular obliteration include eclampsia, in which intravascular coagulation is thought to account for glomerular capillary occlusion, and Henoch-Schönlein purpura, which is an angiitis with a predilection for glomerular microvasculature.

CHRONIC GLOMERULAR OBLITERATION

It is not surprising that a number of pathologic entities such as chronic glomerulonephritis, diabetes mellitus, and systemic lupus erythematosus, all of which are characterized by diffuse glomerular degeneration, have a similar constellation of radiologic findings. The renal outlines on tomography are smooth, and the renal size is markedly diminished. A relatively lucent cortex compared with the medullary regions is seen at angiography (Fig. 75–7) because of the absence of glomerular capillary perfusion and capacitance. Secondary hypertensive changes, or nephrosclerosis, may be present, such as arterial tortuosity and obstruction. Vessel wall irregularity may also be evident. Unlike the shrunken kidneys of chronic pyelonephritis, in which residual function is usually present and areas of focal compensatory hypertrophy may be seen, the kidney with chronic diffuse glomerular disease is usually nonfunctioning and may even exhibit diffuse cortical calcification. In the modern dialysis and transplantation era, more patients are surviving with their nonfunctioning kidneys in situ, and there has been an increasing awareness of the potential for these kidneys to develop cysts and neoplasms.

Renal Infarction and Ischemia

Renal infarction and ischemia often are associated with radiologic findings that are usually quite prominent and characteristic. In addition, cortical necrosis will be discussed because it also is a manifestation of renal infarction but is due to diffuse intrarenal microvascular insufficiency.

RENAL EMBOLISM

Segmental or lobar renal infarction is usually due to large emboli that have their origin in a diseased heart. Ventricular mural thrombi secondary to myocardial infarction and atrial thrombi secondary to rheumatic heart disease with atrial enlargement and atrial fibrillation are common causes. Smaller emboli may come from the valvular vegetations of subacute bacterial endocarditis or from the cholesterol plaques of a severely atherosclerotic abdominal aorta. Unlike progressive intrarenal vascular narrowing due to hypertension or atherosclerosis, which often is asymptomatic and may evoke a collateral response (Fig. 75–8), emboli produce acute focal infarcts that may cause a variety of clinical symptoms. Flank pain, hematuria, fever, transient increase in blood pressure, and leukocytosis are all frequently seen, and angiography will often demonstrate the focal vascular obstruction(s) and characteristic wedge-shaped and sharply demarcated nephrographic defects. If clot lysis occurs, the findings may revert to normal, but subsequent parenchymal scarring (classically between normal calyces) should be looked for at urography. CT, besides demonstrating sharply demarcated nephrographic defects, will often show outer cortical rim enhancement due to capsular collaterals (Fig. 75–9).

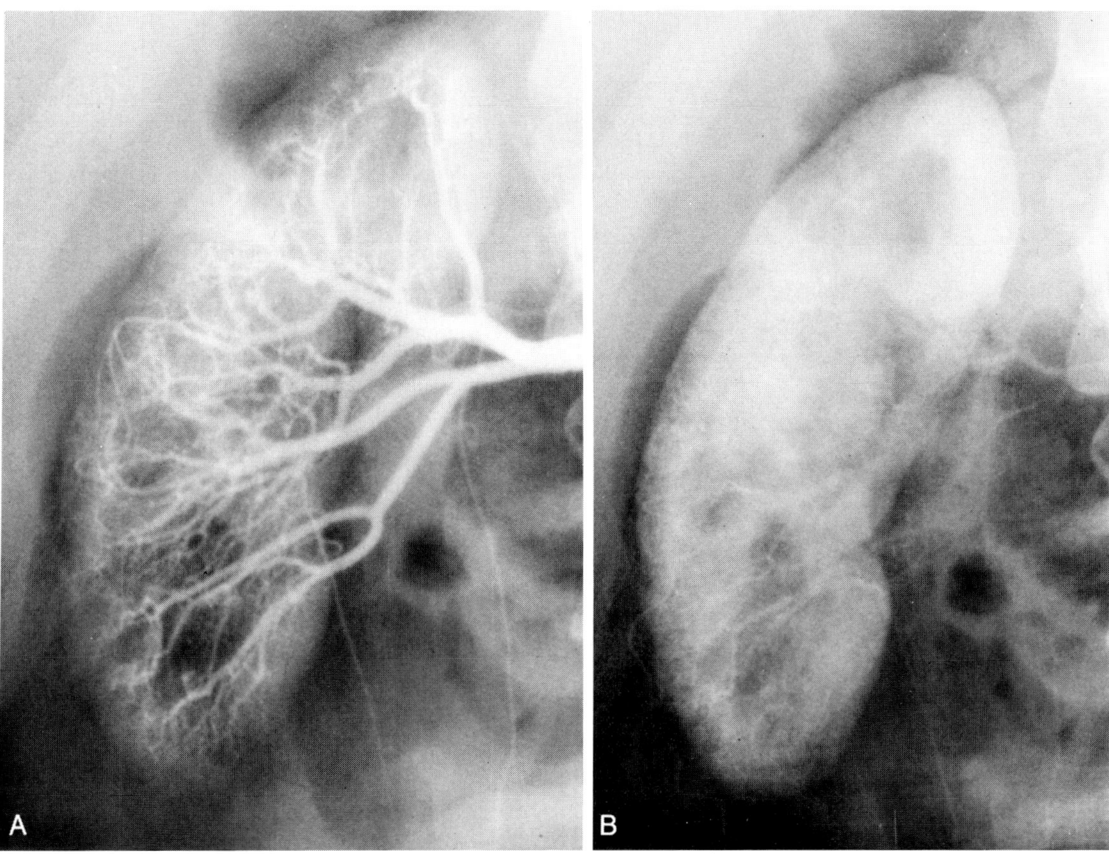

Figure 75–7. Chronic glomerulonephritis with nephrosclerosis in a 26-year-old male with progressively deteriorating renal function and hypertension. Note the poor cortical nephrogram *(B)* due to the lack of glomeruli. Marked vascular tortuosity and obliteration of smaller intrarenal branches can also be seen *(A)*.

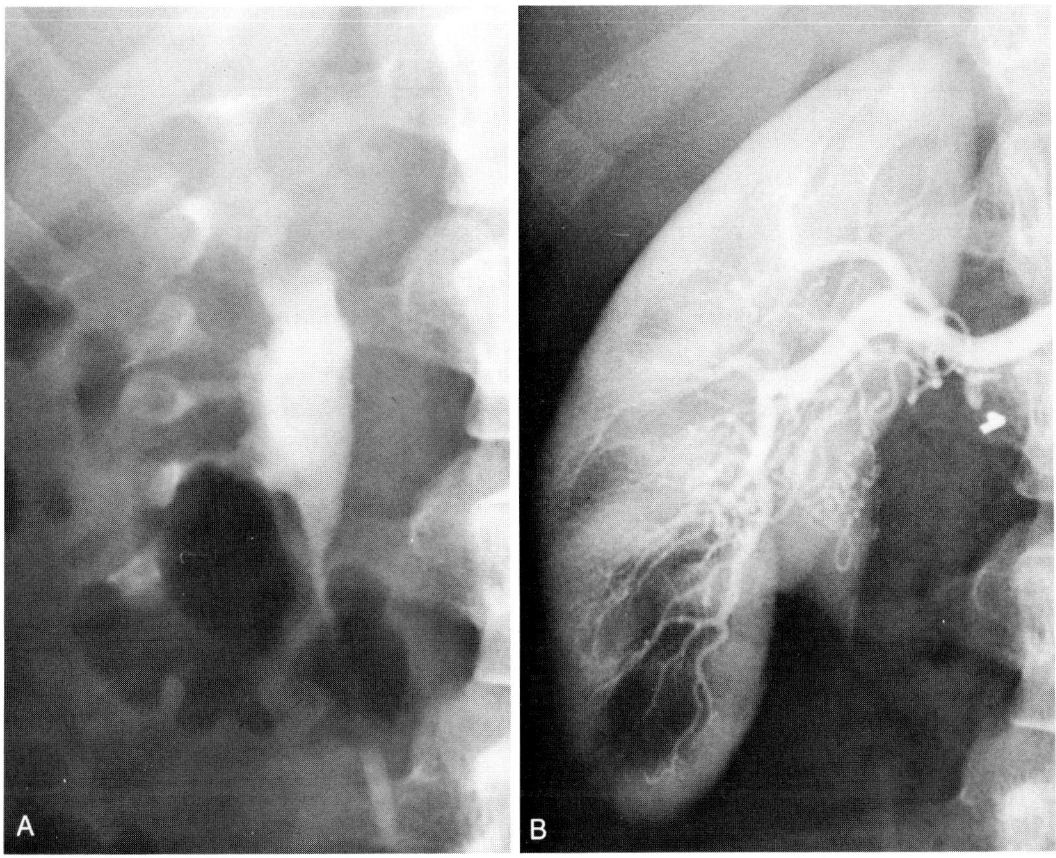

Figure 75–8. Irregularity of the renal pelvic mucosa *(A)* because of arterial collaterals *(B)* that developed following occlusion of a major branch of the renal artery.

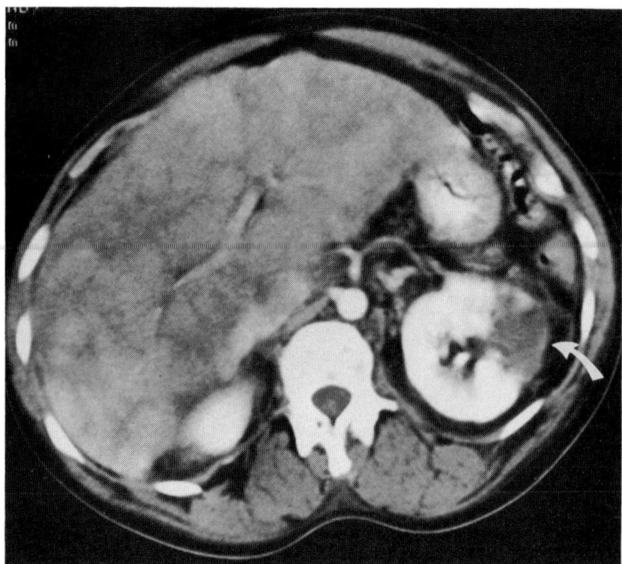

Figure 75–9. Renal infarct following embolus from a left ventricular thrombus. Note segmental nephrographic defect and slight outer cortical rim enhancement *(arrow)* from collateral flow. Massive hepatic congestion is also present.

RENAL VEIN THROMBOSIS

Renal vein thrombosis (RVT), because of its many ways of pathologically affecting the kidney, may present a broad spectrum of clinical and radiologic manifestations. This condition, if unilateral and gradual in its development, may be asymptomatic. In contrast are those situations in which onset is acute and involvement is bilateral. In patients with this more fulminant course, symptoms are severe and survival may be in jeopardy.

RVT is more frequently recognized in infants and children, in whom it is usually associated with dehydration due to gastroenteritis or other systemic infection. In adults with RVT, there may be a recent history of trauma or evidence of underlying tumor, amyloidosis, polycythemia, diabetes mellitus, systemic lupus erythematosus, pyelonephritis or, most commonly, membranous glomerulonephritis. Many of these conditions are associated with a marked reduction in renal blood flow as well as the presence of a coagulopathy. Because of these factors, it is believed that thrombi first develop in the small intrarenal veins and propagate centrally with time. It is also now generally accepted that the nephrotic syndrome, frequently seen in patients with renal RVT, is, despite some experimental evidence to the contrary, usually a consequence of the underlying renal parenchymal disease rather than being caused by the venous obstruction per se.

In the acute stage, patients will present with flank pain, hematuria, fever, leukocytosis, and varying amounts of proteinuria. Pulmonary emboli are a frequent associated finding that may clinically overshadow the acute renal disease.

Urography will demonstrate enlarged, very poorly functioning kidneys that are, on gross pathologic examination, markedly congested and cyanotic. Rupture may occasionally occur. Hemorrhagic infarction will ensue if treatment with anticoagulants or surgical intervention is not forthcoming.

More commonly, particularly in adults, onset is insidious and alternate venous and lymphatic drainage pathways (see Venous Anatomy) can be established. This is particularly true on the left side, where there is a greater potential for collateral development. Urography at this time, besides showing a delayed but persistent nephrogram and normal to slightly increased renal size with calyceal attenuation, will frequently demonstrate evidence of peripelvic or periureteric collaterals such as ureteral notching or pelvic urothelial irregularity (Fig. 75–10).

Ultrasound may also suggest the diagnosis of RVT, particularly in infants and small children, by the demonstration of bilateral or unilateral renal enlargement and increased medullary sonolucency corresponding to congestion of the renal pyramids. Recent application of color Doppler techniques has also proven useful in detecting absent flow in the main renal vein.

CT can confirm the correct diagnosis by revealing clot in a dilated renal vein as well as collateral vessels. Because of its noninvasive character, CT has begun to replace renal venography in making the definitive diagnosis.

Renal venography, and to a lesser extent inferior venacavography, although certainly specific, is not without risk (Fig. 75–11).

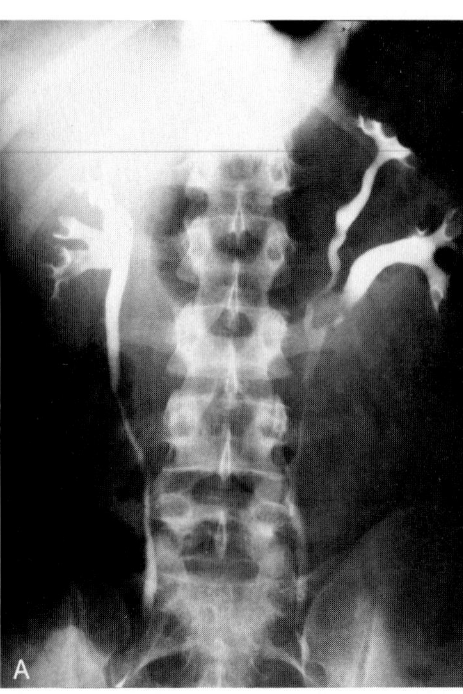

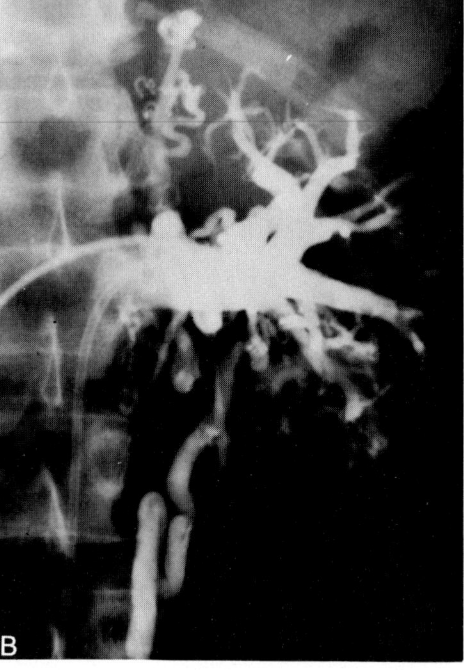

Figure 75–10. Segmental posttraumatic renal vein thrombosis with large collateral peripelvic and periureteric veins *(B)* producing irregularity of the left upper collecting system *(A)* in a 19-year-old male. (Case courtesy of Paul F. Jaques, M.D.)

There is always the rare but real chance that the catheter will dislodge potentially fatal clots from the inferior vena cava or renal vein. Of course, potential contrast media toxicity may be heightened by the possible marginal renal function.

Renal angiography is a less specific invasive procedure but potentially less dangerous. It may suggest a diagnosis because of the demonstration of a striated nephrogram that is due to interstitial edema, lymphatic engorgement, and dilated interlobular veins separating medullary rays that are the bundles of tubules and collecting ducts extending from the cortex to the medulla.

Magnetic resonance imaging (MRI), with its developing potential for the noninvasive assessment of larger vessels, may eventually become the modality of choice in the diagnosis of renal thrombosis.

CORTICAL NECROSIS

Unlike the focal cortical infarcts produced by emboli from an extrarenal source, cortical necrosis is a more diffuse process caused by acute intrarenal microvascular obstruction or severe systemic hypotension. Whereas in ATN there is damage to, or death of, tubular epithelium, and the potential for some regeneration, the histologic hallmark of acute cortical necrosis (ACN) is irreversible glomerular injury and permanent loss of function. Many causes have been described, including sepsis, dehydration, burns, hemorrhage, allograft rejection, and a variety of toxins such as diethylene glycol and carbon tetrachloride. Complications of pregnancy such as abruptio placentae and other intravascular coagulopathies are frequently associated with ACN. The radiologic work-up of the acute renal failure associated with ACN should be designed to exclude urinary obstruction and assess functional loss. Studies utilizing iodinated contrast agents are rarely indicated. If patient survival is prolonged by dialysis, cortical calcification is to be expected.

SHOCK

If systemic hypotension occurs during intravenous contrast administration owing either to a systemically mediated allergic reaction to the contrast medium or to some other factor such as hemorrhage, a persistent nephrogram (Fig. 75–12) will be observed. This phenomenon is caused by stasis of contrast in renal tubules due to reduced glomerular perfusion and filtration. Some enhancement of nephrographic density may be seen with the passage of time, as tubular water may continue to be reabsorbed. When the blood pressure is returned to normal, usually by a combination of fluid replacement and cardiac stimulants, the contrast is flushed from the nephrons. Transient renal shrinkage may also be documented during episodes of hypotension due to diminished perfusion of this extemely vascular organ.

Renal Aneurysms

Although not as common as aneurysms of the splanchnic circulation, renal artery aneurysms are of importance because of their fairly frequent association with renal ischemia and hypertension. They also may be the source of emboli that may produce renal infarcts, and of course there is always the danger, although remote, of rupture. Most aneurysms are acquired and may be post-stenotic in location and secondary to atherosclerosis or, more commonly, fibromuscular dysplasia. They seem to have a predilection for bifurcations of segmental branches. Aneurysms may also occur following penetrating trauma (false aneurysms), and occasionally they may be seen in patients with neurofibromatosis. Dissecting aneurysms are seen as extensions of aortic dissections or they may result from catheterization mishaps or percutaneous transluminal angioplasty. Congenital lesions do occur and are one of the causes of hypertension in the pediatric age group. Calcification is often present on plain films, and bruits are frequently heard (Fig. 75–13).

Renal Arteriovenous Malformations and Fistulas

True arteriovenous malformations are rare congenital vascular lesions that vary in size from a few millimeters to several centimeters in diameter (Figs. 75–14 and 75–15). They may also be known as angiodysplasias, angiomas, or telangiectases. Usually, hematuria is the presenting complaint, but because of the inconspicuous nature of many of these lesions, magnification angiography may not demonstrate abnormality. In most series of patients with hematuria, arteriovenous malformations account for less than 1 per cent of

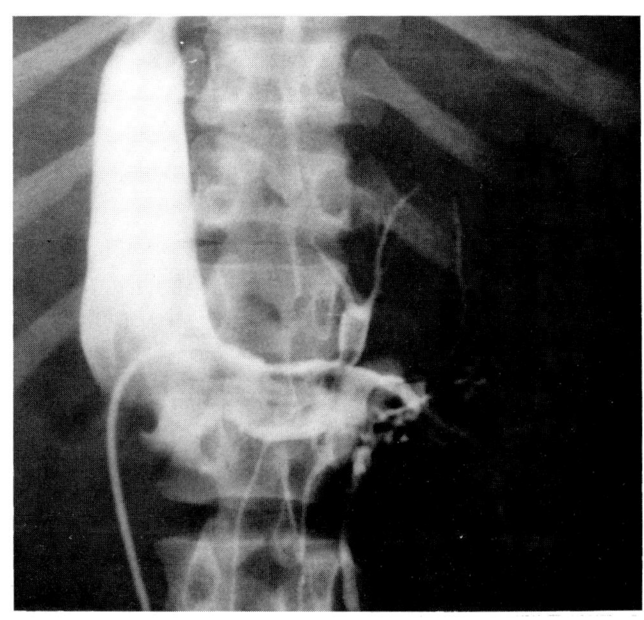

Figure 75–11. Left renal venogram in a 33-year-old female with systemic lupus erythematosus and bilateral renal vein thrombosis with extension of clot into the IVC. Pulmonary emboli were also suspected clinically.

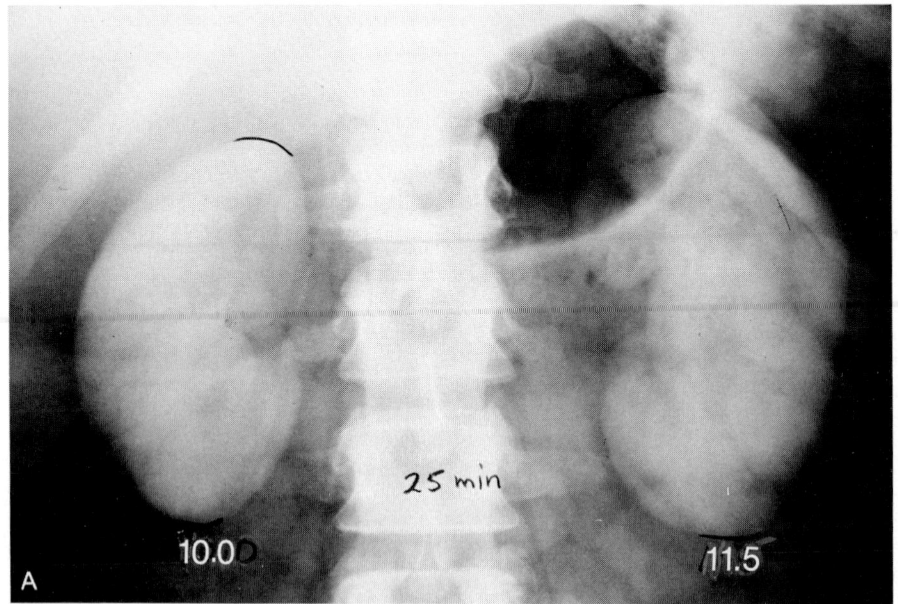

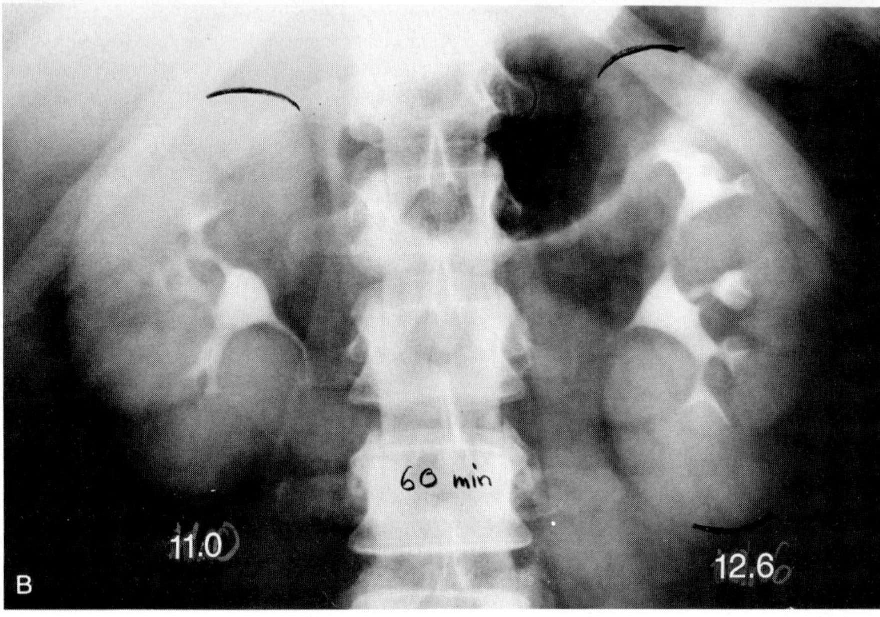

Figure 75–12. Shock following intravenous urography in a 55-year-old female, resulting in a dense, persistent nephrogram *(A)*. Following restoration of normal blood pressure and renal perfusion, the nephrogram fades, a pyelogram develops, and the kidneys increase 1 cm in length *(B)*. (Case courtesy of John T. Cuttino Jr, M.D.)

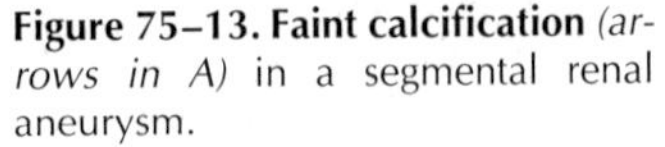

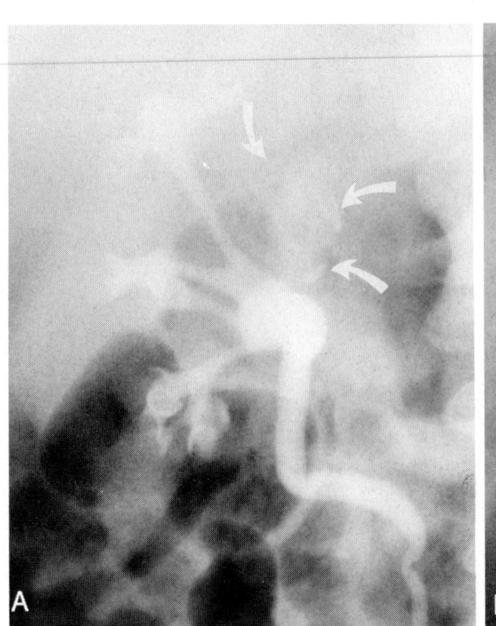

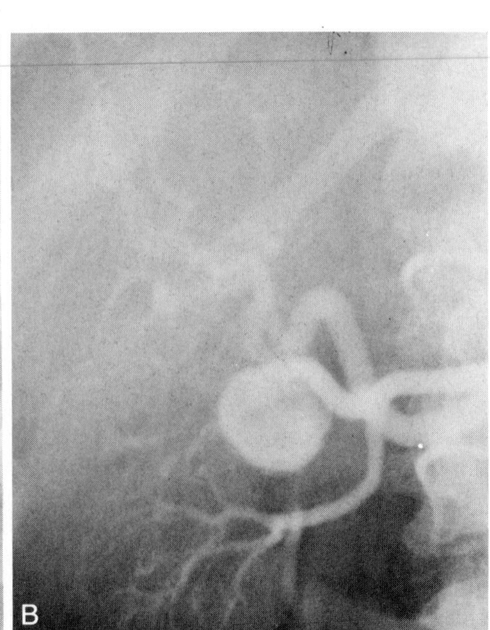

Figure 75–13. Faint calcification *(arrows in A)* in a segmental renal aneurysm.

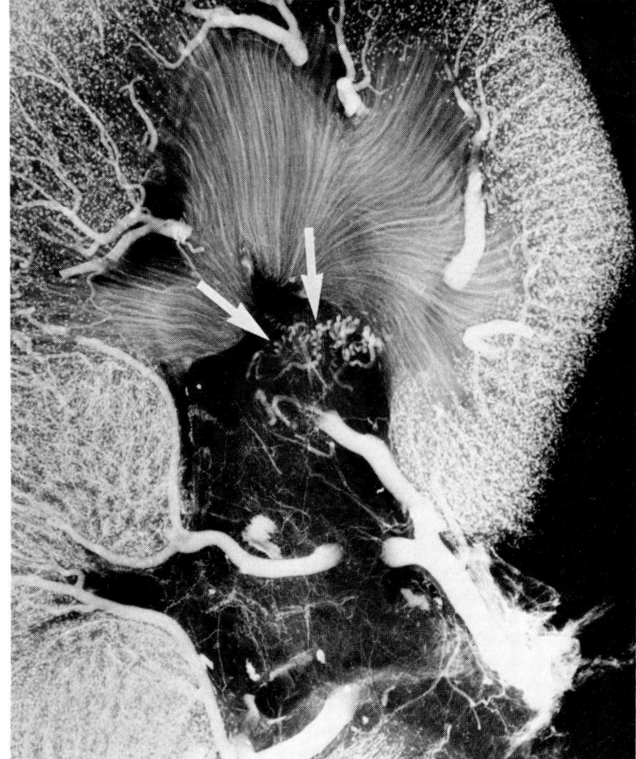

Figure 75–14. A pericalyceal angiodysplasia *(arrows)* that caused intractable bleeding, necessitating nephrectomy in a 34-year-old male. The lesion was not seen at angiography, but specimen contrast perfusion and microangiography (×4) easily demonstrated the vascular abnormality.

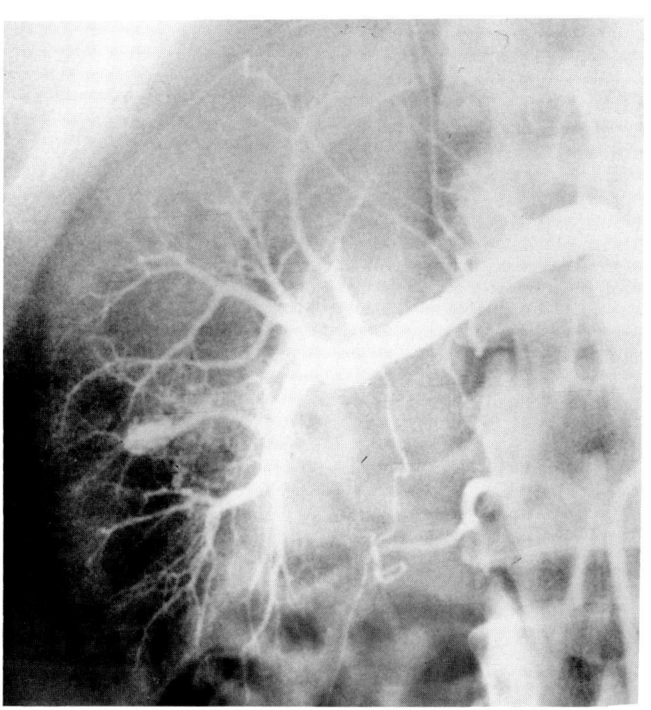

Figure 75–15. A congenital arteriovenous malformation causing recurrent hematuria in a 29-year-old female. (Case courtesy of Paul F. Jaques, M.D.)

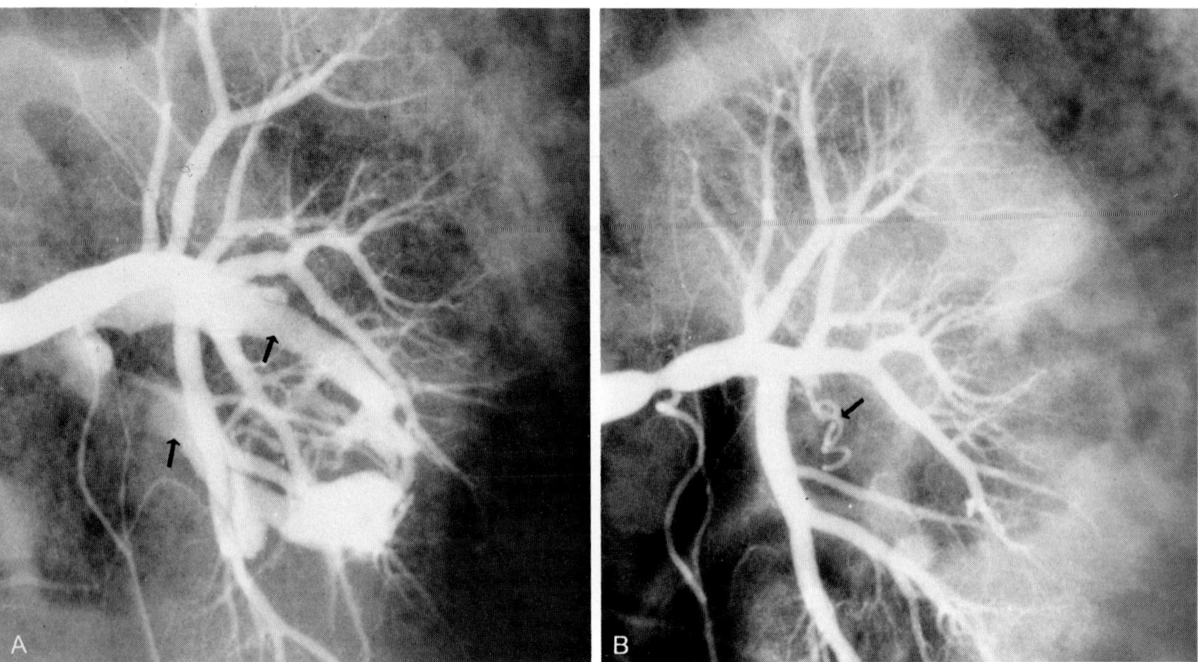

Figure 75–16. A large arteriovenous fistula developed following renal biopsy in this young male. Note the early opacification of segmental renal veins *(arrows in A)*. Following subselective catheterization of the feeding segmental artery, a Gianturco coil was used to occlude the vessel *(arrow in B)*. Focal spasm of the main renal artery due to catheter manipulation is incidently seen. (Case courtesy of Paul F. Jaques, M.D.)

cases. However, these lesions can be treated with therapeutic embolization, particularly if there is uncontrolled hypertension and/or gross hematuria. If nephrectomy must be performed, the importance of specimen angiography to assist the pathologist in locating and characterizing these rare and difficult to diagnose lesions cannot be overemphasized (see Fig. 75–14).

Arteriovenous fistulas, in comparison to arteriovenous malformations, are usually acquired abnormal vascular communications that are seen following penetrating trauma, abdominal surgery, percutaneous nephrostomy, or, most commonly, renal biopsy (Fig. 75–16). Although angiographic studies following renal biopsy have shown a fairly high frequency of arteriovenous fistulas (10 per cent), fortunately most of these close spontaneously. As with other vascular lesions of the kidney, arteriovenous fistulas may cause hypertension (''steal'' phenomenon) and hematuria.

Bibliography

Baker SB: The blood supply of the renal papilla. Br J Urol 31:53, 1959.

Barger AC, Herd JA: The renal circulation. N Engl J Med 284:482, 1971.

Beeuwkes R, Bonventre J (with graphics by Lavey KH): Tubular organization and vascular-tubular relations in the dog kidney. Am J Physiol 229:695, 1976.

Boijsen E: Angiographic studies of the anatomy of single and multiple renal arteries. Acta Radiol 183 (Suppl), 1959.

Bookstein JJ, Clark RL: Renal Microvascular Disease: Angiographic-Microangiographic Correlates. Boston, Little, Brown, 1980.

Clark RL, Cuttino JT Jr: Microradiographic studies of renal lymphatics. Radiology 124:307, 1977.

Davidson AJ, Talner LB: Lack of specificity of renal angiography in the diagnosis of renal parenchymal disease: A point of view. Invest Radiol 8:90, 1973.

Elkin M: Radiology of the Urinary System. Boston, Little, Brown, 1980.

Foley WD: Color Doppler Flow Imaging. Reading, MA, Andover Medical Publishers, 1991.

Fourman J, Moffat DB: The Blood Vessels of the Kidney. Oxford, Blackwell Scientific Publications, 1971.

Friedland GW, et al (ed): Uroradiology: An Integrated Approach. New York, Churchill Livingstone, 1983.

Graves FT: The Arterial Anatomy of the Kidney. Baltimore, Williams and Wilkins, 1971.

Hartman DS: Renal Cystic Disease. AFIP Atlas of Radiologic-Pathologic Correlations. Fascicle 1. Philadelphia, WB Saunders Company, 1989, Chapter 3: Renal Cystic Diseases Associated with Renal Neoplasms.

Heptinstall RH: Pathology of the Kidney, 4th ed. Boston, Little, Brown, 1992.

Hillman BJ: Imaging and Hypertension. Philadelphia, WB Saunders Company, 1983.

Hodson CJ: The Renal Parenchyma and Its Blood Supply. Current Problems in Diagnostic Radiology. Chicago, Year Book Medical Publishers, 1978.

Ljungqvist A: The intrarenal arterial pattern in essential hypertension: A micro-angiographic and histological study. J Pathol Bacteriol 84:313, 1962.

Pollack HM (ed): Clinical Urography. Philadelphia, WB Saunders Company, 1990, Chapters 15, 65, 69, 71, 80, 81.

Schrier RW, Gottschalk CW (eds): Diseases of the Kidney, 4th ed. Boston, Little, Brown, 1988.

76 Renovascular Hypertension: Etiologic, Diagnostic, and Therapeutic Considerations

Stephen H. Smyth

Renovascular hypertension is defined as systemic hypertension caused by narrowing of the major renal arteries. It represents one of the several etiologies of secondary hypertension (Table 76–1). The significance of secondary hypertension and, in particular, renovascular hypertension is the potential for therapeutic intervention and cure. In the United States, the estimated prevalence of systemic hypertension is 60 million individuals, representing the important risk factor of morbidity and mortality for cardiovascular disease, stroke, and renal insufficiency. The prevalence estimate for renovascular hypertension has been cited as high as 32 per cent, but most sources quote a prevalence of 1 to 5 per cent. More likely accurate are estimates of less than 1 per cent of systemic hypertension in the adult population, which is the most common etiology of secondary hypertension.

Although occlusive disease of the major renal arteries can cause systemic hypertension, it can be found in normotensive individuals, as a coincidental finding with essential hypertension, or in conjunction with other causes of hypertension. Only with treatment of renal artery stenosis and resolution or improvement of blood pressure can an individual be said to have had renovascular hypertension. Surgical and percutaneous interventional, rather than medical, treatment of renovascular hypertension reduces end-organ damage and better maintains patients' life spans, which, along with safer and less expensive means of diagnosis and treatment, has resulted in a more aggressive approach to this entity.

RENO-OCCLUSIVE DISEASE: ETIOLOGIES

Angiographic demonstration of renal artery disease has been seen in 32 per cent of normotensive patients and has been demonstrated at autopsy in 49 per cent of patients who were normotensive in life. In hypertensive patients of the Cooperative Study on Renovascular Hypertension, lesions of the renal arteries were found in 36 per cent, with approximately two thirds of the lesions caused by atherosclerosis, approximately one third by fibrodysplasia, and 5 per cent by other causes.

Atherosclerosis

Arteriosclerotic disease (hardening of the arteries) accounts for approximately 50 per cent of all deaths in the United States. The three morphologic types of arteriosclerotic disease are atherosclerosis, Monckeberg's medial calcific sclerosis, and arteriolosclerosis.

Atherosclerosis is the most common etiology of renal artery stenoses in both normotensive and hypertensive patients, representing approximately two thirds of cases. Bilateral involvement can be seen in 33 to 43 per cent of cases. Fibrofatty eccentric intimal plaques occur in large and medium-sized muscular arteries. Progressive development of ulceration, thrombus, hemorrhage, calcification, aneurysm, and dissection can occur, but may take 20 to 40 years before symptoms occur. Usually the patient is over 50 years old before symptoms of the disease are evident.

The proximal third and ostium of the renal artery are most frequently involved, with the lesions usually eccentric and in 40 to 45 per cent of cases progressive. Although branch vessels may be involved with atherosclerotic lesions, they are unusual in isolation. Irregularity of the luminal margin is usually seen, and poststenotic dilatation may be present. The osteal lesions result from extensions of aortic disease with encroachment of the orifice, an important factor when angioplasty of these stenoses is considered. Atherosclerotic disease of the renal arteries is almost always associated with involvement of the abdominal aorta (Fig. 76–1). The appearance of this involvement may be stenotic, occlusive, or aneurysmal (Fig. 76–2). Aortic aneurysm can compress the renal artery and result in stenosis.

Fibrodysplasia

Fibrodysplasia is of unknown pathogenesis and may affect the intima, media, or adventitia of the artery. Fibrous, muscular, or fibromuscular hyperplasia occurs. Although its most common manifestation is in the renal arteries, it has been described in carotid and iliac arteries. It occurs in approximately one third of renal artery stenoses and is seen more frequently in younger individuals. Females are affected more often than males. There is a predilection

TABLE 76–1. CAUSES OF SECONDARY HYPERTENSION

Coarctation
Cushing's syndrome
Drugs and hormones
- Amphetamines
- Estrogens
- Oral contraceptives
- Steroid or thyroid
- Hormone excess

Increased intracranial pressure
Pheochromocytoma
Primary aldosteronism
- Conn's syndrome
- Idiopathic hyperaldosteronism

Renal parenchymal disease
- Chronic pyelonephritis
- Congenital renal disease
- Diabetic nephropathy
- Glomerulonephritis
- Interstitial nephropathy
- Obstructive uropathy
- Polycystic disease
- Renin-secreting tumors
- Vasculitis

Renovascular hypertension

McCarron DA, Haber E, Slater EE: High Blood Pressure. Scientific American Medicine, Section 1, Subsection VII.

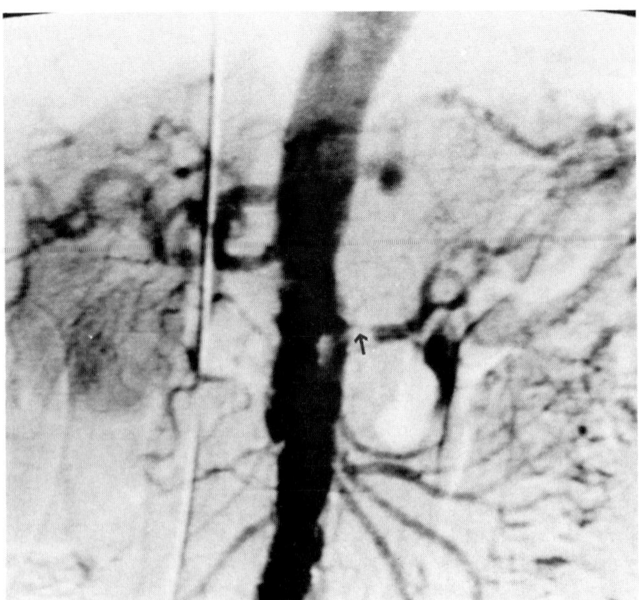

Figure 76–1. Intravenous digital subtraction angiogram (IV-DSA) examination performed on a middle-aged man with hypertension. There is **diffuse aortic atherosclerosis.** A post-orificial stenosis *(arrow)* is seen to involve the left renal artery.

for unilateral involvement of the right renal artery, with bilateral disease occurring in two thirds of patients. It is the most frequent cause of renovascular hypertension in children. Progression appears to occur in both asymptomatic and hypertensive individuals with the disease.

A classification of the fibrodysplasia subtypes separates the lesions into intimal, medial, and adventitial locations. One of the subtypes primarily involves the intima and another the adventitia; four subtypes affect the media. Distinguishing between atherosclerotic and fibrodysplasia lesions by arteriography has been shown to be 82 per cent accurate, but arteriography is not effective at distinguishing among the histologic types. If renal artery stenosis is found in the setting of aortic disease, there is a 76 per cent likelihood that the etiology is atherosclerotic disease. Without aortic disease, there is a 94 per cent likelihood that fibrodysplasia is the etiology.

Intimal fibroplasia is characterized by circumferential accumulation of a loose and moderately cellular fibrous tissue in the intima with no lipid or inflammatory component. It represents 1 to 2 per cent of fibrodysplasia lesions. Most commonly affected are children and young adults; intimal fibrodysplasia is the most frequent type of fibrodysplasia causing renal artery stenosis in children. Involvement is typically of the middle and distal renal artery or major segmental branches. Arteriographically, there are smooth tubular or funnel-shaped focal stenoses. A predisposition to dissection with irregularity or thrombosis may result.

Medial fibroplasia is characterized by alternating areas of medial thinning with occurrence of mural aneurysms and regions of fibromuscular ridges that result in stenoses (Fig. 76–3). It is the most common subtype and represents 60 to 70 per cent of the fibrodysplasia lesions. Most commonly affected are females from early adulthood to middle age. Involvement is typically of the distal two thirds of either the main or the branch arteries. Carotid and iliac arteries may also be involved. The pathognomonic arteriographic appearance of these lesions is a "string of beads," with alternating stenotic and aneurysmal regions.

Medial hyperplasia is characterized by smooth muscle hyperplasia of the media with neither disruption of the media nor mural aneurysms. It represents 5 to 15 per cent of fibrodysplasia lesions. Main and branch renal arteries are most commonly affected. It occurs most frequently in teenagers and middle-aged males. The arteriographic appearance is of focal or tubular smooth narrowing. With dissection and thrombosis, a more irregular appearance is seen with these stenoses.

Perimedial fibroplasia is characterized by focal or multifocal nonuniform fibroplasia of the outer one half to two thirds of the media. It represents 15 to 25 per cent of fibrodysplasia lesions, affecting main or branch arteries. It occurs most commonly in young females.

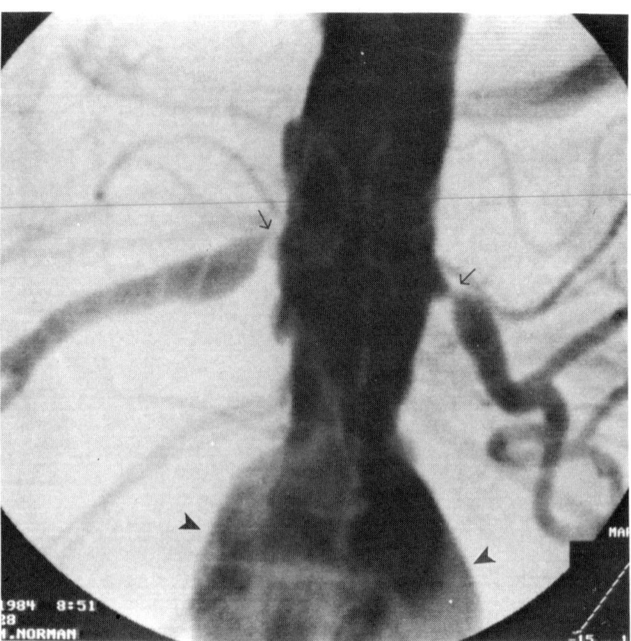

Figure 76–2. Intra-arterial digital subtraction angiogram (IA-DSA) depicting **bilateral renal artery stenoses** *(small arrows)* in a man with hypertension. The infrarenal aorta is irregular with atherosclerotic plaques and there is a large aneurysm *(arrowheads).*

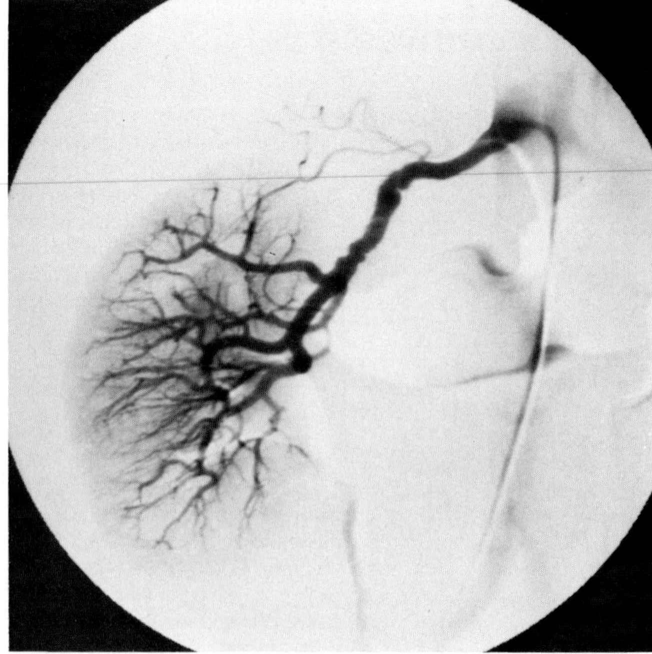

Figure 76–3. Medial fibroplasia of right kidney. IA-DSA of the right renal artery in a young woman demonstrates serial stenoses and aneurysms in the distal two thirds of the artery.

Arteriographically, irregular stenoses and beading without aneurysms are identified, although mural or saccular aneurysm can rarely occur.

Medial dissection is characterized by regions of fibroplasia in the outer one third of the media, with dissections. Main or branch arteries are affected. It represents 5 to 10 per cent of fibrodysplasia lesions. Arteriographically, false channels and aneurysms may be seen.

Adventitial fibroplasia is the least common of the fibrodysplasia lesions, representing less than 1 per cent of cases. It is characterized by adventitial and periarterial proliferation, affecting main or branch arteries. Arteriographically, the stenoses are focal or tubular.

Trauma

Blunt trauma, usually decelerations from motor vehicle accidents, can result in shearing injuries to the renal arteries with consequent hematoma, dissection, or disruption. These injuries can result in stenoses or occlusions of the renal arteries. Subcapsular hematoma with resultant Page kidney (Fig. 76–4), aneurysm, arteriovenous fistula (Fig. 76–5), arterial occlusion or stenosis, dissection, and pseudoaneurysm can occur from penetrating injury (stab wound) or iatrogenic injury. These lesions have been seen after percutaneous needle biopsy, nephrostolithotomy, nephrostomy drain placement, and arteriography. Arteriographic findings include occlusion, intimal disruption, an intimal flap, a false channel, an arteriovenous fistula, and an aneurysm or perirenal hematoma.

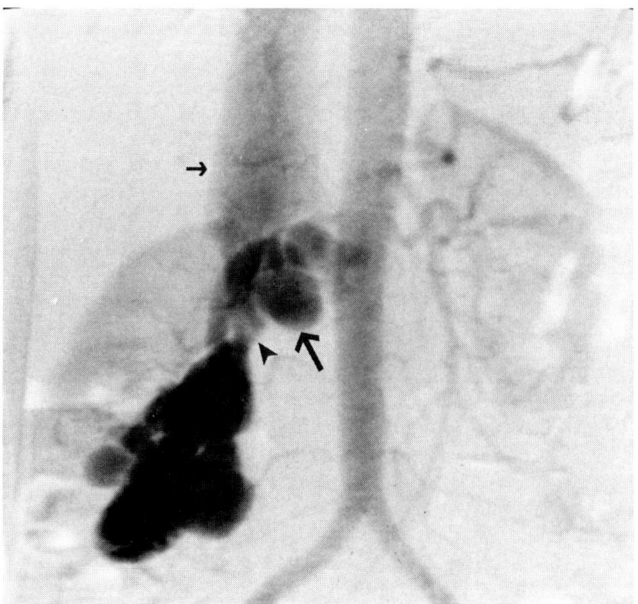

Figure 76–5. IV-DSA of a **traumatic arteriovenous fistula.** There is simultaneous opacification of the dilated, **tortuous renal artery** *(large arrow)*, renal vein *(arrowhead)*, and vena cava *(small arrow)*.

Dissection

Renal artery dissection without concomitant aortic dissection is rare and usually occurs in the setting of fibromuscular disease of the renal arteries. Most commonly, dissection of the renal artery occurs in the setting of atherosclerotic aortic dissection and is most frequent in elderly males. Aortic dissection may extend into the renal artery, causing narrowing, or it may occlude the main renal artery at its origin. The left renal artery is more frequently involved by extension of the dissection than is the right. A retrospective review of 63 patients with aortic dissection (86 per cent with hypertension), found 10 patients (16 per cent) with antecedent hypertension and hemodynamically significant renal artery stenosis. Five of these patients had atherosclerotic lesions, and five fibromuscular disease. This suggests a need to exclude synchronous aortic dissection and renal artery stenosis occurring from causes other than the dissection. Blunt abdominal trauma and arterial catheterization can also result in dissection. Arteriography may show an intimal flap extending into the renal artery lumen, an irregular and widened lumen from opacification of the false lumen, or occlusion from thrombosis.

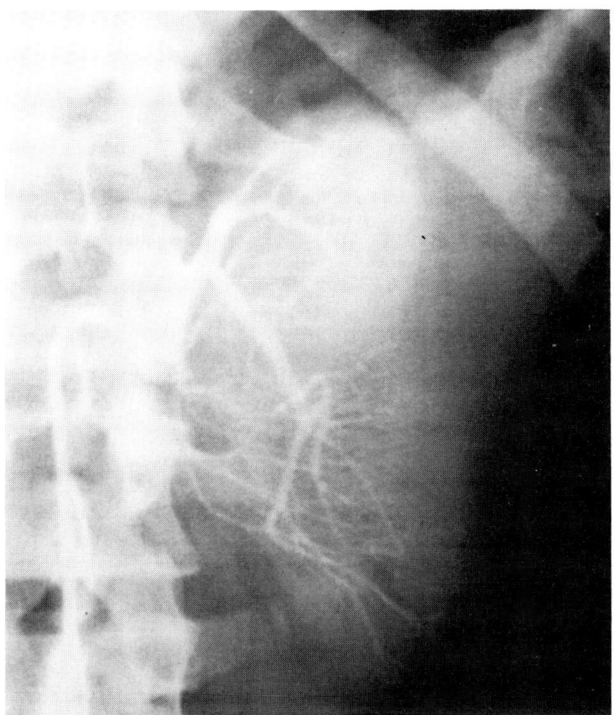

Figure 76–4. Page kidney with hypertension following renal trauma. Left selective renal arteriogram shows gross lateral parenchymal deformity due to fibrotic residual hematoma; surgery relieved the hypertension. (Courtesy of K. J. Cho, M.D.)

Other Etiologies of Renal Artery Stenosis

Renal artery stenosis has been seen in association with pheochromocytoma. Most commonly, it is believed to be a consequence of mechanical compression of the renal artery from extra-adrenal tumors arising in the sympathetic ganglia at the renal hilum. Other cases have been seen without mechanical compression, perhaps due to arterial spasm caused by high concentrations of catecholamine secretion by the tumor, which initially may be reversible but can result in irreversible myointimal proliferation. Arteriographically depicted stenoses are smooth and circumferential and are seen in conjunction with the extrinsic vascular tumor.

Congenital encasement of the renal artery with stenosis caused by muscular fibers of the diaphragmatic crus has been described in association with hypertension. Most of these cases have involved the right crus. Arteriographically, there is sharp angulation of the renal artery with poor opacification. The stenosis may mimic a focal atherosclerotic plaque.

Extrinsic compression of the renal artery from a syphilitic aortic aneurysm has been reported. Intimal thickening of the renal artery with stenosis has also been reported in a patient with syphilis.

Stenosis and occlusion of renal arteries have been reported in patients with thromboangiitis obliterans. The lesion, in acute stages, has polymorphonuclear infiltration of all layers of the vessel wall with mural or occlusive thrombosis. Microabscesses in the thrombus occur. There is organization over time, and fibrosing granulomas develop. Arteriographic findings are multiple segmental occlusions, thready recanalized vessels, collateral vessels, and arterial spasm.

Two patients with moyamoya disease and renal artery stenosis have been reported. The association of moyamoya disease with other vascular processes (saccular aneurysms of the carotid siphon and occlusive peripheral vascular disease) suggests a process of multiple vessels. Arteriographic findings are focal stenoses of the renal arteries. Extrinsic compression by renal masses (hydatid cyst, leiomyosarcoma, papillary carcinoma of the renal pelvis, and bronchial carcinoma metastasis) has been reported to cause renal artery stenosis in addition to hypertension. Arteriography demonstrates extrinsic compression of the renal arteries, resulting in smooth, tapered stenoses.

Takayasu's arteritis is characterized by nonspecific inflammation of the aorta, great vessels of the arch, and pulmonary arteries. It also affects the abdominal aorta and its branches. Renal artery stenoses usually occur near their origins and tend to be progressive. Severe focal or long stenoses are seen. Aneurysms can be seen involving the aorta in 9 per cent of patients and can be associated with hypertension both with and without renal artery lesions.

Stenosis of renal artery origin has also been identified in neurofibromatosis. The arterial stenoses are caused by disorganized intimal and medial proliferation and can result in aneurysms. Neurofibromata may surround vessels and cause stenoses, which tend to progress over time. Abdominal aortic coarctation is seen with and without renal artery stenosis. If the coarctation occurs superior to the renal arteries, reduced blood flow may cause hypertension. Stenoses of neurofibromatosis are smooth or nodular with saccular aneurysms. This is an appearance similar to fibrodysplasia, except that lesions of neurofibromatosis are usually at the orifice or proximal artery.

PATHOPHYSIOLOGY OF RENOVASCULAR HYPERTENSION

The kidney regulates blood pressure through three control mechanisms located at the juxtaglomerular apparatus. The first is a baroreceptor believed to be located in the afferent arteriole. The second is the macula densa, which senses the flow of filtrate and sodium excretion in the distal convoluted tubule. The third is the postganglionic renal sympathetic nerves that end in the juxtaglomerular apparatus, providing central nervous system control. In response to a significant renal artery stenosis, these mechanisms interact to release an increased amount of renin, which, through the renin-angiotensin system, results in blood pressure elevation. The increased renin secretion cleaves circulating angiotensinogen, forming a decapeptide, angiotensin I. Upon passing through the lungs, it is converted to angiotensin II. Although mild vasoactive properties are present in angiotensin I, the major vasoactive factor is angiotensin II. It stimulates the central nervous system to increase vessel tone, in addition to having a direct vasoconstrictive effect on blood vessels, and increases adrenal secretion of aldosterone, resulting in retention of salt and water. As hypertension accelerates, the initially reversible changes in the renal resistance circulation become fixed, and a decrease in renal function occurs.

CLINICAL EVALUATION

The Cooperative Study on Renovascular Hypertension concluded that no single clinical finding is capable of consistently diagnosing renovascular hypertension. Age younger than 30 years or older than 50 years, absence of family history of hypertension, and accelerated target organ damage were all found to be poor discriminators of renovascular hypertension. The only physical finding of use was the presence of an abdominal or flank bruit, which is present in 50 per cent of patients with renovascular hypertension and in 10 per cent of patients without the disease. Of patients with severe hypertension (diastolic pressure $\geqslant$ 125 mm Hg) and grade III or IV retinopathy on funduscopic examination, renovascular hypertension was found only in 31 per cent.

Attempts to identify patients with renovascular hypertension using blood tests have high false-negative rates. Provocative tests that look for alterations of peripheral serum renin and blood pressures by use of an angiotensin-II antagonist or angiotensin-converting enzyme inhibitor have been inadequate for screening.

The lack of signs, symptoms, clinical history, laboratory studies, and provocative tests that adequately discriminate between patients with and without renovascular hypertension has prevented the development of a reasonable clinical screening protocol.

DIAGNOSTIC IMAGING

Excretory Urography

When described in 1964, the hypertensive urogram reflected radiologically the physiologic events and consequences of renovascular disease. The current version of the study consists of bolus intravenous contrast administration followed by renal tomograms at one, two, and three minutes after injection. An abdominal image at five minutes is followed by routine completion of the examination. Significant findings that may indicate ischemia are a right kidney 1.0 cm or a left kidney 1.5 cm smaller than the contralateral kidney; asymmetric time of first appearance of excreted contrast media (Fig. 76–6); or hyperconcentration of contrast in the renal collecting system of the affected kidney on delayed films, which suggests prolonged tubular transit time and increased water absorption.

If the most reliable sign is used (late asymmetric opacity of contrast material in the collecting systems), a true-positive rate of 59 per cent and a false-positive rate of 2 per cent are found. With a greater severity of stenosis, the true-positive rate increases. The sensitivities of this test for detection of renovascular hypertension have ranged from 71 to 94 per cent. Because the examination only implies disease, has poor accuracy, and is a poor prediction of the likelihood of cure, it is seldom used as a screening test for renovascular hypertension.

Radionuclide Studies

Iodine-131 hippuran renography with blood-flow imaging using either ^{99m}Tc-diethylenetriaminepenta-acetic acid or glucoheptonate has been evaluated as a screening test for renovascular hypertension. Signs of a positive study are asymmetry in the rates of rise in activity, the time to peak activity, and rates of decline in activity. Reported sensitivities and specificities are 76 to 100 per cent and 75 to 90 per cent, respectively. Patients with renovascular hypertension and some patients with nonvascular abnormalities may have similar findings on radionuclide studies. When performed in conjunction with excretory urography, increased sensitivity is seen, although the specificity remains low. Positive results for either test correctly predict renovascular hypertension in only 12% of cases.

Use of renal scintigraphy with administration of an angiotensin converting enzyme (ACE) inhibitor has recently shown promise as a screening diagnostic test with reportedly high sensitivity and specificity for renovascular hypertension. The hallmark of significant renal artery stenosis is deterioration of the renogram after ACE

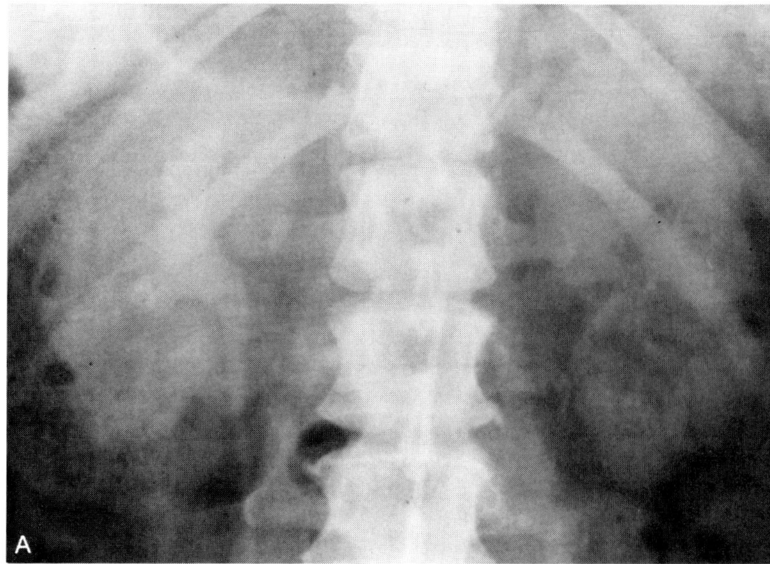

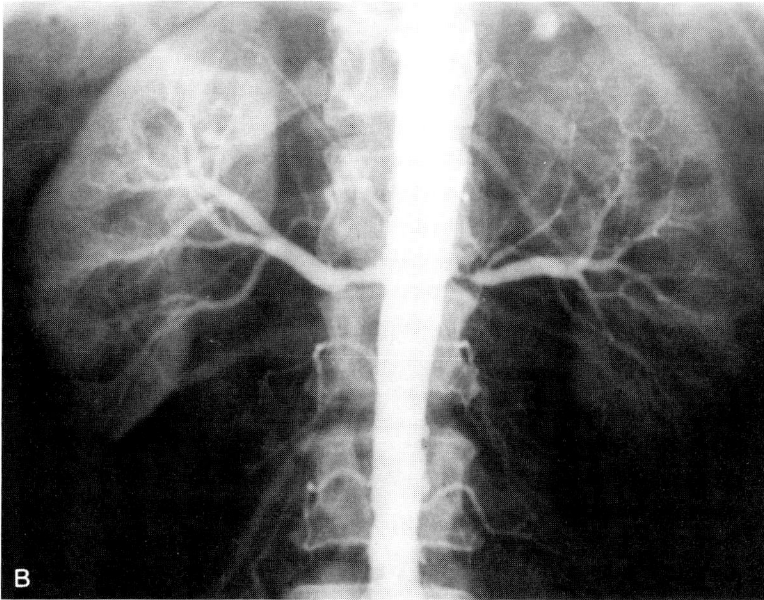

Figure 76–6. Renal artery stenosis. *A,* Positive hypertensive urogram with smaller left kidney and delayed appearance time. *B,* Aortogram showing tight atherosclerotic stenosis of proximal left renal artery and minimally stenotic atherosclerotic lesion of proximal right renal artery. Left lesion was successfully treated by transluminal angioplasty.

inhibitor administration, which removes the vasoconstrictive effect of angiotensin II on the efferent arteriole, resulting in a fall in glomerular filtration. In the study by Sfakianakis et al., false-negative results were noted to occur with stenoses less than 60 per cent but not in more severe stenoses, suggesting that this test may be a means for detection of significant hemodynamic lesions. Two more recent studies of 155 patients have reported sensitivities of 91 & 92 per cent and specificities of 93 & 97 per cent. Although these results are encouraging, larger studies with a more typical screening population are necessary to evaluate the efficacy of these examinations.

Renal Artery Ultrasound and Doppler

With the development of duplex sonography, a number of studies have suggested its use to identify renal artery stenosis. In addition to broadening of the Doppler shift and increased amplitude of the systolic peak, the following have also been reported: acceleration time, acceleration indices, and acceleration time ratio; renal-to-aortic peak velocity ratio; pulsatility flow index and end-diastolic-to-peak systolic frequency ratio; and peak systolic velocity. In comparisons with arteriography, color Doppler-flow imaging has been found inadequate as a screening examination. In addition, these examinations have been found to be time and technician intensive. However, one area in which renal artery ultrasound, duplex Doppler, and color Doppler imaging may be useful is in the detection of vascular complications of renal transplants. The proximity to the skin and the lack of interfering soft tissues and bowel enhance its ability to evaluate the transplanted kidneys.

Renal Vein Renin

In an attempt to detect renovascular hypertension and predict which patients may respond to revascularization, sampling of the renal veins and inferior vena cava for renin activity has been performed. A comparison of renin activity of the involved and contralateral kidney using a ratio method has been used to suggest renovascular hypertension. A ratio greater than or equal to 1.5:1 represents a positive study. More complex measurements and indices have been described to obtain higher sensitivities and specificities. Major problems with this study are difficulties in patient preparation, technical expertise, and handling and measurements of samples, which result in inconsistent replication of results. False-negative rates between 30 and 50 per cent have been reported. Contrast administration for catheter localization and single catheter serial sampling versus bilateral simultaneous sampling with two catheters have not been shown to have an impact on the examination.

An attempt at improving the results of renal vein renin sampling by administering the ACE inhibitor captopril 30 to 60 minutes before sampling has demonstrated a false-positive rate of 47.8 per cent, a positive predictive value of 18.6 per cent, and a negative predictive value of 89.3 per cent. So far this test has been poor at accomplishing the task of excluding nonrenovascular patients with hypertension and predicting which patients will respond to therapy. In a recent study of captopril-stimulated renal vein renin sampling before and after mannitol administration in seven patients with renal artery stenosis, renal vein renin levels were found to be suppressed by more than 32 per cent on the involved side and less than 32 per cent on the uninvolved side. Although it has been suggested that the degree of suppression might serve as a tool for diagnosing significant stenotic lesions, there was no discussion of the response to angioplasty in the four treated patients. Further study including long-term follow-up is required to evaluate this as a potential test of renal artery stenosis significance and possible response to revascularization.

Digital Intravenous Angiography

In the late 1970s and early 1980s, intravenous digital subtraction angiography (Fig. 76–7) was used to evaluate renal arteries of hypertensive patients for possible renovascular disease. This technique was an advance over hypertensive urography because it actually depicted artery stenoses, allowing detection of bilateral stenosis and stenoses in solitary kidneys. The initial enthusiasm has diminished, however, as variation in the quality of digital equipment and in technique has been recognized and problems with patient bowel, respiratory, and vascular motion and function as well as the missing or poor depiction of lesions because of less resolution than with conventional arteriography have been reported.

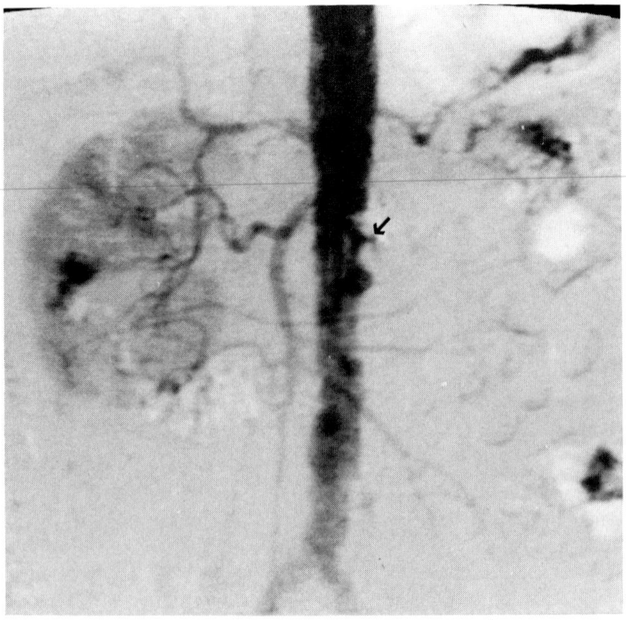

Figure 76–7. This IV-DSA demonstrates **occlusion of the left renal artery.** There is present diffuse infrarenal atherosclerosis. A small "nipple" *(arrow)* protrudes from the left aortic margin, which may represent the occluded left renal artery.

Conventional and Digital Arteriography

With well-performed technique, conventional film screen arteriography is an excellent examination for the detection of renal artery stenoses. The accuracy of detecting major arterial lesions using intra-arterial digital subtraction arteriography is comparable to that using conventional film screen arteriography. Because of the speed with which it can be performed (film does not need to be processed immediately), the smaller volumes and concentrations of contrast media and smaller catheters (decreased complication risk) used, and accrued cost savings, intra-arterial digital subtraction arteriography has increasingly become an outpatient procedure.

Magnetic Resonance Angiography

Methods for producing images using magnetic resonance imaging have included a subtraction technique in which images created by suppression of signal from blood are subtracted from images with preserved or enhanced signal from blood, as well as three-dimensional image sets from gradient-recalled echoes with static tissues having partially saturated steady states and inflowing blood with unsaturated spins. Prolonged data acquisition time, resulting in degradation of images from patient motion, was the primary disadvantage of these techniques. To increase the speed of data acquisition, serial breath-hold, gradient-echo imaging, requiring eight seconds per section and less than 30 minutes per study, and high-speed imaging requiring two to five minutes per study have been developed. A few studies in which magnetic resonance imaging has been tested as a means of evaluating the main renal artery suggest that it may develop as a reliable noninvasive test for stenosis. Although promising, this technique is still its early stages of development and requires further evaluation.

TREATMENT OF RENOVASCULAR HYPERTENSION

Percutaneous Treatment

The first description of transluminal angioplasty was made in 1964 by Dotter and Judkins. Their technique involved serial passage of Teflon dilators, first over a guidewire, then over other dilators. They suggested that this technique could be applied to open arterial stenoses of the coronary, renal, carotid, and vertebral arteries. With development of the angioplasty balloon in 1974, transluminal angioplasty for coronary and renal angioplasty rapidly followed. Percutaneous transluminal balloon angioplasty is now extensively used in the arterial system, including the renal arteries. Although bilateral renal artery stenoses or stenosis in a solitary kidney has been viewed as a relative contraindication to angioplasty, patients with these lesions are commonly treated with success.

Because none of the diagnostic imaging modalities are currently satisfactory as screen for physiologically significant stenosis, severe stenosis (>75 per cent) or pressure gradients measured at the time of arteriography are often used to initiate treatment.

PATHOPHYSIOLOGY OF DILATATION

Cadaveric and in vivo studies have discounted the previously held belief that angioplasty worked by compressing or molding atheromata. These studies showed longitudinal splitting of the atheromata with intimal disruption, separation from the media, and injury to medial muscle fibers. With this splitting and separation of the plaque, subintimal dissections may be seen in the dilated segment. Deposition of platelets and fibrin begins the healing process, and approximately three days after the procedure, arteriographic evidence of moderately smooth intimal walls of the dilated segment can be seen.

TECHNIQUES

Preparation for renal angioplasty includes review of the diagnostic images, patient history, physical findings, and laboratory testing to confirm the need for angioplasty. Backup by a vascular surgeon should also be available, because performing renal angioplasty without prompt surgical backup places the patient at needless risk. In the angiography suite, the patient should have a route of venous access established for medication administration, continuous or frequent electrocardiography, and vital sign monitoring. Oxygenation monitoring should be considered.

Although the usual choice for vascular access is the right common femoral artery, the decision for the route should consider the presence of occlusive or stenotic disease of the femoral, iliac, and aortic vessels. Although an axillary approach may be more advantageous for engagement of the inferiorly oriented renal arteries, the femoral artery approach can be used most times. In addition, the axillary approach carries a higher risk of hematoma and nerve and vascular injury, especially with the need for anticoagulation.

Access to and crossing of the renal artery stenosis can be accomplished by a number of catheters, including cobra configuration, Simmons, multipurpose, and guiding catheters. The stenosis is first crossed with a guidewire (Bentson, tapered attenuated-diameter, hydrophilic-coated, or interventional injectable wire), followed by the catheter. Although each combination has its proponents, the more important factors are the operator's familiarity and comfort with the system and the care taken in traversing the stenosis. After the stenosis is crossed, contrast assessment for location and possible complication (dissection/occlusion) is performed. Once the location is determined, the catheter is exchanged for the balloon catheter for the angioplasty. Balloon catheters are available in straight, cobra, or Simmons configurations, with a number of balloon shapes, maximum inflation pressures, and catheter shaft sizes available. Although there may be advantages of one catheter over another, a straight configuration balloon catheter on a small diameter shaft (5 Fr) is satisfactory for most angioplasties. By creating a gentle curve in the catheter using steam, the operator can easily pass the catheter over the guidewire at the origin of the renal artery without having to eject the guidewire from the renal artery. Introduction of a sheath into the common femoral artery at the beginning of the procedure is often advisable, because there catheter exchange is usually frequent during the diagnostic and therapeutic portions of the procedure. This is particularly important in patients with tortuous iliac arteries.

The size of the balloon to use for dilation of the stenosis is determined from the normal nondilated portion of the renal artery. Measuring the diameter from the arteriogram overestimates the size because of magnification effects. However, most angiographers favor overdilation by 25 per cent or 1 mm larger than the measured diameter. If the measurements from the arteriogram are used, there will usually be enough magnification for sufficient overdilation of the stenosis.

The guidewire should be left across the stenosis when the balloon is inflated to protect the arterial wall from injury should the catheter straighten its curve and to maintain access. Typically, a waist deformity is seen as the balloon is inflated. If it is seen during deflation, reinflation is usually performed. If it persists, consideration of a larger balloon is appropriate. As the stenosis is dilated, the patient will usually complain of some moderate back or possibly abdominal pain. It should resolve after deflation of the balloon. Persistent pain suggests either rupture or occlusion of the artery and requires prompt investigation of the artery with contrast injection through the catheter. Low-pressure balloon catheters (6 to 8 atm) are usually adequate for successful dilation, although high-pressure balloons are occasionally required. Thirty to sixty seconds is usually a sufficient duration for balloon inflation.

A number of medications are used during the angioplasty procedure to diminish the risk of complications and to treat complications should they arise. Vasospasm can occur in the renal artery upon selective catheterization and traversal of the stenosis. Nifedipine (a calcium channel blocker), given 20 minutes before the procedure in a dose of 10 to 20 mg, is effective in preventing vasospasm. The duration of effect is two to four hours. If vasospasm occurs despite pretreatment, intra-arterial administration of 100 μg of nitroglycerin may reverse the process (Fig. 76–8). Anticoagulation is performed to decrease the risk of thrombosis from decreased flow through the stenosis once the stenosis is crossed by the catheter and from the intimomedial injury of angioplasty. An adult-dose aspirin (325 mg) should be given for its antiplatelet effect before the procedure, and aspirin should be continued as life-long self-medication with 80 mg (one baby aspirin) per day. Once the stenosis is successfully crossed, 3000 to 5000 units of heparin should be administered intravenously. Heparinization is not reversed at the close of the procedure and is not continued beyond the initial dose in uncomplicated procedures.

RESULTS

The success of renal artery angioplasty for atheromatous disease varies with the location of the disease. For osteal lesions, reported success is low (approximately 25 per cent), whereas for nonosteal lesions (Fig. 76–9) a 75 to 80 per cent success rate has been reported. For fibromuscular disease (Fig. 76–10), an initial success rate of approximately 87 to 90 per cent is reported, with 90 per cent of these patients showing blood pressure benefit (60 per cent cured and 30 per cent improved). Blood pressure benefit was found in 85 per cent of patients with aortoarteritis (Takayasu's arteritis) who received angioplasty, as opposed to 60 per cent of patients with aortoarteritis who received surgical revascularization.

Delayed response to angioplasty has been described with fibrodysplasia, Takayasu's arteritis, and neurofibromatosis. In these cases there initially was incomplete dilation of the stenosis, but on follow-up dilation was found to be complete.

For occluded vessels, technical success (crossing the occlusion and dilating the stenosis) is achievable in 50 per cent of patients. If the occlusion is due to acute thrombosis, thrombolytic agents may be given before dilatation.

Restenosis rates are reported to be 15 to 20 per cent, but this rate is difficult to assess because of the difficulty in obtaining follow-up arteriograms and because in some studies patients with atheromatous and fibromuscular disease were combined. One study reports a patency rate at 5 years of 80 per cent in patients with atherosclerosis, 89 per cent in those with fibrodysplasia, and 74 per cent in an indeterminate group and an overall mortality rate of less than 1 per cent.

No randomized clinical trials exist comparing percutaneous treatment with surgical treatment of renal artery stenosis. Results of a series of studies in which the renal artery stenosis could be crossed and dilated are comparable to surgical results.

COMPLICATIONS

A recent review of the literature reports an overall complication rate of 14 per cent for percutaneous transluminal renal angioplasty. Puncture site trauma requiring surgery or transfusion was seen in 1.2 per cent of patients. Injury to the renal artery required surgery in 2.5 per cent did not require surgery in 1.6 per cent and resulted

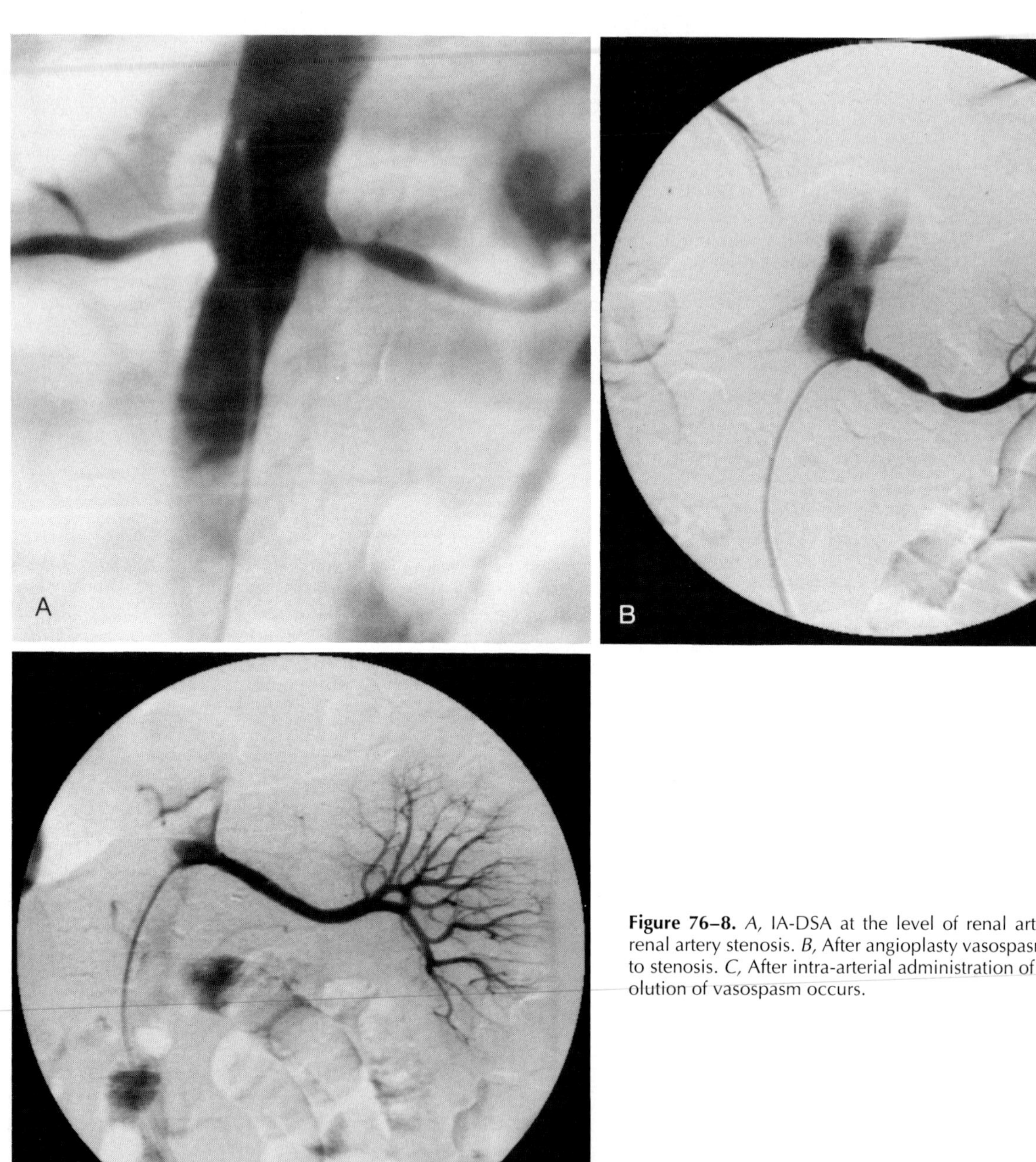

Figure 76–8. *A,* IA-DSA at the level of renal arteries shows a left renal artery stenosis. *B,* After angioplasty vasospasm is present, distal to stenosis. *C,* After intra-arterial administration of nitroglycerin, resolution of vasospasm occurs.

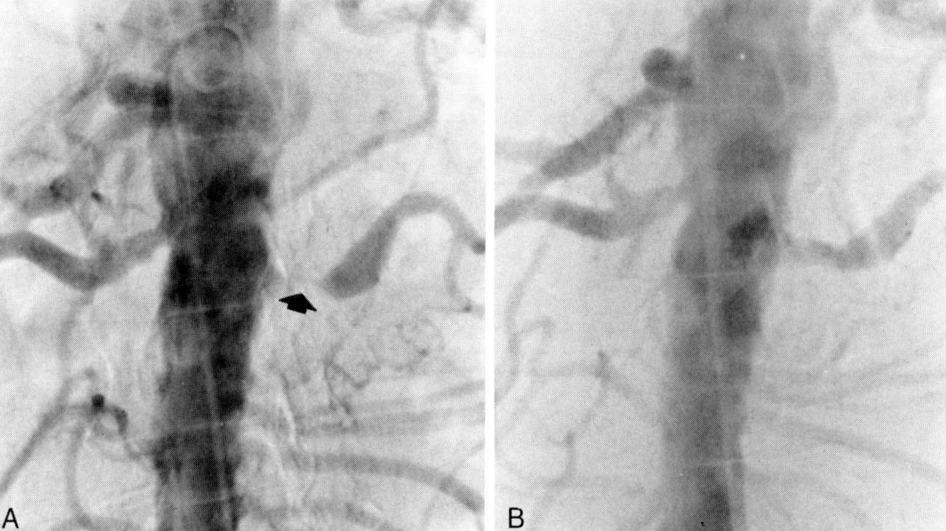

Figure 76–9. *A,* IA-DSA demonstrates a **high grade stenosis** *(arrow)* **of the proximal left renal artery.** *B,* Percutaneous angioplasty has resulted in effective dilation of the narrowed segment and relief of the patient's hypertension.

in renal artery rupture in 0.6 per cent. Acute renal failure was seen in 1.5 per cent of cases and worsening of chronic renal failure in 2.3 per cent. Symptomatic embolization occurred in 1.1 per cent of patients. Death has been reported in up to 1 per cent of angioplasties. Other complications have been reported, but they are less frequent.

Surgical Revascularization

In a nonrandomized study in 1974, comparison of medical treatment with surgical therapy of renal vascular hypertension showed that after 7 to 14 years of follow-up, only 60 per cent of patients treated medically were alive, compared with 84 per cent of patients treated with definitive surgery. Control of hypertension was seen in a cooperative study reported in 1975 but with a complication rate of 13 per cent and an overall mortality rate of 5.9 per cent. More recent reports show lower mortality rates (approximately 2 per cent) and cures approaching 90 per cent. Surgical revascularization does not appear to be compromised by prior attempted percutaneous transluminal renal angioplasty.

Several operative therapies are used to treat renal artery stenoses. When the obstruction of the renal arteries is due to atherosclerosis and involves the renal artery ostia, endarterectomy can be performed, with reported benefit in 82 per cent. Aortorenal bypass grafts using autogenous saphenous vein or artery and synthetic materials are commonly performed with satisfactory results. Other origins of grafts to the renal arteries are the iliac, hepatic, and splenic arteries. Autotransplantation has also been used as a mean of treating renal artery stenosis with significant success.

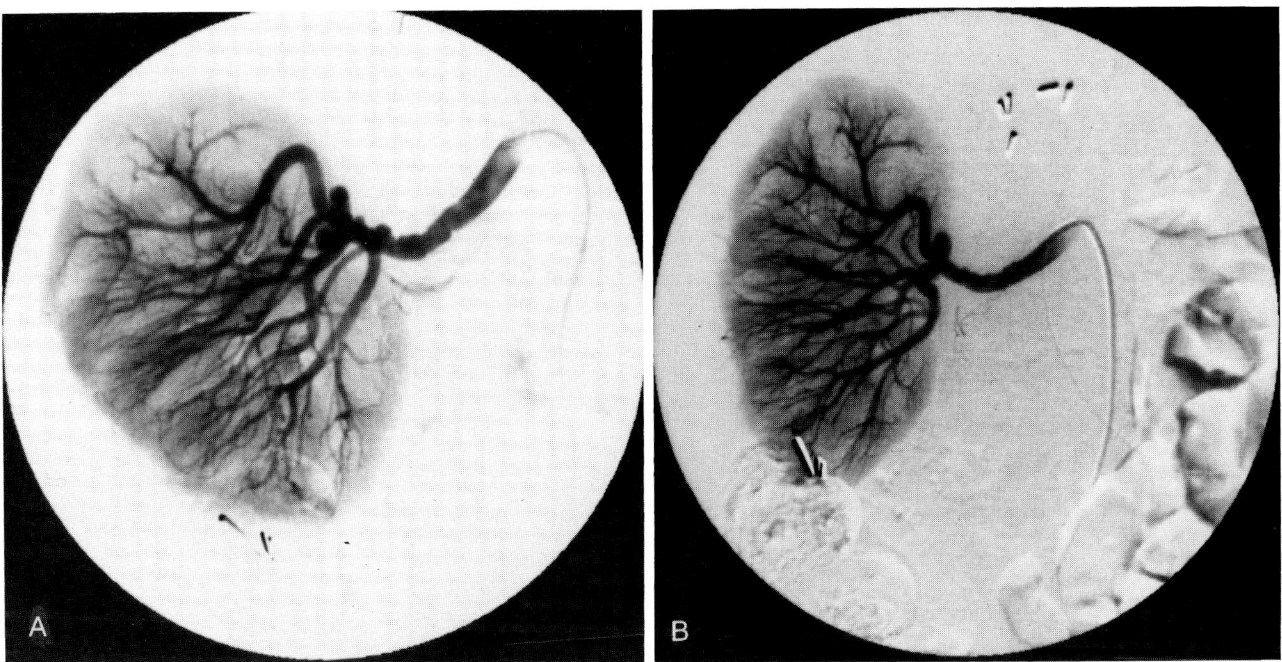

Figure 76–10. *A,* IA-DSA of right kidney demonstrates stenoses of medial fibroplasia. *B,* Image obtained after successful balloon angioplasty with resolution of the stenoses.

Bibliography

Abel BJ, Kennedy JH: Severe hypertension following traumatic renal infarction. Br J Urol 50:54, 1978.

Abeshouse BS, Tankin LH, Lerman S, et al: Dissecting aneurysm of the aorta: Report of case with anuria and prolongation of life by peritoneal lavage. Urol Cutan Rev 52:196, 1948.

Abrams HL: Dissecting aortic aneurysm. In Abrams HL (ed): Abrams Angiography, 3rd ed. Boston, Little, Brown, 1983, pp 441–466.

Adams TS Jr, Roub LW: Outpatient angiography and interventional radiology: Safety and cost benefits. Radiology 151:81, 1984.

Ahlmen J, Bergentz S-E, Ohlsson L, Hood B, Two causes of hypertension in a subject with generalized neurofibromatosis. Scand J Urol Nephrol 6:94, 1972.

Allan TN, Davies ER: Neurofibromatosis of the renal artery. Br J Radiol 43:906, 1970.

Andersson I: Renal artery lesions after pyelolithotomy. A potential cause of renovascular hypertension. Acta Radiol (Diagn) (Stockh) 17:685, 1976.

Andersson I, Boijsen E, Hellsten S, Linell F. Lesions of the dorsal renal artery in surgery for renal pelvic calculus. A potential cause of renovascular hypertension. Eur Urol 5:343, 1979.

Athanasoulis CA: Percutaneous transluminal angioplasty. General principles. AJR 135:893, 1980.

Avasthi PS, Voyles WF, Greene ER: Noninvasive diagnosis of renal artery stenosis by echo-Doppler velocimetry. Kidney Int 25:824, 1984.

Baxi R, Epstein HY, Abitbol C: Percutaneous transluminal renal artery angioplasty in hypertension associated with neurofibromatosis. Radiology 139:583, 1981.

Becker GJ, Katzen BT, Dake MD: Noncoronary angioplasty. Radiology 170:921, 1989.

Benz RL, Teehan BP, Sigler MH, et al: Suppression of renal vein renin profiles by Mannitol prophylaxis: Implications in the evaluation of renovascular hypertension. Am J Kidney Dis 18:649, 1991.

Berbner H: Dissecting aortic aneurysm of the aorta with renal complications. Br Med J 1:394, 1951.

Bergqvist D, Jonsson K, Weibull H: Complications after percutaneous transluminal angioplasty of peripheral and renal arteries. Acta Radiol 28(I):3, 1987.

Berland LL, Koslin DB, Routh WD, Keller FS: Renal artery stenosis: Prospective evaluation of diagnosis with color duplex US compared with angiography. Radiology 174:421, 1990.

Block PC, Myler R, Sterzer S: Morphology after transluminal angioplasty in human beings. N Engl J Med 305:382, 1981.

Bookstein JJ, Abrams HL, Buenger RE, et al: Radiologic aspects of renovascular hypertension. Part II: The role of urography in unilateral renovascular disease. JAMA 220:1225, 1972.

Bookstein JJ, Abrams HL, Buenger RE, et al: Radiologic aspects of renovascular hypertension. Part III. Appraisal of arteriography. JAMA 221:368, 1972.

Bookstein JJ, Maxwell MH, Abrams HL, et al: Cooperative study of radiologic aspects of renovascular hypertension. JAMA 237:1706, 1977.

Bookstein JJ, Walter JF: The role of abdominal radiography in hypertension secondary to renal or adrenal disease. Med Clin North Am 59:169, 1975.

Borlin I: Renal artery changes in hypertension. Acta Radiol Diagn 6:401, 1967.

Brown DG, Riederer SJ, Jack CR, et al: MR angiography with oblique gradient-recalled echo technique. Radiology 176:461, 1990.

Buda JA, Baer L, Parra-Carrillo JZ, et al: Predictability of surgical response in renovascular hypertension. Arch Surg 111:1243, 1976.

Bunker SR, Cutaia FI, Fritz AL, et al: Femoral intraarterial digital angiography: An outpatient procedure. AJR 141:593, 1983.

Buonocore E, Meaney TF, Borkowski GP, et al: Digital subtraction angiography of the aorta and renal arteries. Radiology 139:281, 1981.

Burns AB, Tesluk H, Palmer JM: Hypertension associated with vascular lesions of neurofibromatosis. J Urol 108:676, 1972.

Busch HP, Strass LG, Hoevels J, et al: Fibromuscular dysplasia, a pitfall in intravenous digital subtraction angiography. Eur J Radiol 4:42, 1984.

Campbell DR, Masson WF, Flemming BK, et al: Digital subtraction arteriography in the diagnosis of renovascular hypertension. J Can Assoc Radiol 34:261, 1983.

Carini M, Selli C, Trippitelli A, et al: Surgical treatment of renovascular hypertension secondary to renal trauma. J Urol 126:101, 1981.

Case DB, Laragh JH: Reactive hyperreninemia in renovascular hypertension after angiotensin blockade with Saralasin or converting enzyme inhibitor. Ann Intern Med 91:153, 1979.

Castaneda-Zuniga WR, Formanek A, Tadavarthy M, et al: The mechanism of balloon angioplasty. Radiology 135:565, 1980.

Chen CC, Hoffer PB, Vahjen G, et al: Patients at high risk for renal artery stenosis: A simple method of renal scintigraphic analysis with Tc-99m DTPA and captopril. Radiology 176:365, 1990.

Chrispin AR, Scatlif JH: Systemic hypertension in childhood. Pediatr Radiol 1:75, 1973.

Clark RA, Alexander ES: Digital subtraction angiography of the renal arteries prospective comparison with conventional arteriography. Invest Radiol 18:6, 1983.

Clayman AS, Bookstein JJ: The role of renal arteriography in pediatric hypertension. Radiology 108:107, 1973.

Cohn DJ, Sos TA, Saddekni S, et al: Transluminal angioplasty for atherosclerotic renal artery stenosis. Semin Intervent Radiol 1:279, 1984.

Collins HA, Jacobs JK: Acute arterial injuries due to blunt trauma. J Bone Joint Surg 43A:193, 1961.

Cope C, Zeit RM: Pseudoaneurysms after nephrostomy. AJR 139:255, 1982.

Cotran RS, Kumar V, Robbins SL: Robbins Pathologic Basis of Disease, 4th ed. Philadelphia, WB Saunders Company, 1989.

Cragg AH, Smith TP, Thompson BH, et al: Incidental fibromuscular dysplasia in potential renal donors: Long-term clinical follow-up. Radiology 172:145, 1989.

Crummy AB, Stieghorst MF, Turski PA, et al: Digital subtraction angiography: Current status and use of intra-arterial injection. Radiology 145:303, 1982.

D'Abreu F, Strickland B: Developmental renal artery stenosis. Lancet 2:517, 1962.

Davis BA, Crook JE, Vestal RE, et al: Prevalence of renovascular hypertension in patients with grade III or IV hypertensive retinopathy. N Engl J Med 301:1273, 1979.

Davis TC, Hoffman JC: Work in progress. Intraarterial digital subtraction angiography. Evaluation in 150 patients. Radiology 148:9, 1983.

Davson AJ: Malignant hypertension associated with hydatid disease of the kidney. J Pathol 53:207, 1941.

Dean RH, Kieffer RW, Smith BM, et al: Renovascular hypertension: Anatomic and renal function changes during drug therapy. Arch Surg 116:1408, 1981.

Depner TA, Sullivan MJ, Ryan KG, et al: Post-traumatic renal artery stenosis. Arch Surg 110:1150, 1975.

Desberg AL, Paushter DM, Lammert GK, et al: Renal artery stenosis: Evaluation with color Doppler flow imaging. Radiology 177:749, 1990.

Dondi M, Franchi R, Levorato M, et al: Evaluation of hypertensive patients by means of captopril enhanced renal scintigraphy with technetium-99m DTPA. J Nucl Med 30:615, 1989.

Dong Z, Li S, Lu X: Percutaneous transluminal angioplasty for renovascular hypertension in arteritis: Experience in China. Radiology 162:477, 1987.

Dotter CT, Judkins MP: Transluminal treatment of arteriosclerotic obstruction: Description of a new technique and a preliminary report of its applications. Circulation 30:654, 1964.

Dubbins PA: Renal artery stenosis: Duplex Doppler evaluation. Br J Radiol 59:225, 1986.

Dunnick NR, Ford KK, Johnson A, et al: Digital intravenous subtraction angiography for investigating renovascular hypertension: Comparison with hypertensive urography. South Med J 78:690, 1985.

Dunnick NR, Svetky LP, Cohan RH, et al: Intravenous digital subtraction renal angiography: Use in screening for renovascular hypertension. Radiology 171:219, 1989.

Dustan HP, Humphries AW, De Wolfe VG, et al: Normal arterial pressure in patients with renal arterial stenosis. JAMA 187:138, 1964.

Ekelund L, Gerlock J, Molin J, Smith C: Roentgenologic appearance of fibromuscular dysplasia. Acta Radiol (Diagn) (Stockh) 19:433, 1978.

Ellison PH, Largent JA, Popp AJ: Moya-moya disease associated with renal artery stenosis. Arch Neurol 38:467, 1981.

Eyler WR, Clark MD, Garman JE, et al: Angiography of the renal areas including a comparative study of renal artery stenosis in patients with and without hypertension. Radiology 78:879, 1962.

Foster JH, Maxwell MD, Franklin SS, et al: Renovascular occlusive disease. Results of operative treatment. JAMA 231:1043, 1975.

Franklin SS, Young JD, Maxwell MH, et al: Operative morbidity and mortality in renovascular disease. JAMA 231:1148, 1975.

Freiha FS, Kavaney PB, Cunningham JJ, et al: Extra-adrenal pheochromocytoma causing renal artery stenosis. Relationship to hypertension and renin levels. Urology 2:303, 1973.

Gardiner GA Jr, Freedman AM, Shlansky-Goldberg R: Percutaneous transluminal angioplasty: Delayed response in neurofibromatosis. Radiology 169:79, 1988.

Gardiner GA Jr, Meyerovitz MF, Stokes KR, et al: Complications of transluminal angioplasty. Radiology 159:201, 1986.

Gavant ML, Gold RE, Church JC: Delayed rupture of renal pseudoaneurysms: Complications of percutaneous nephrostomy. AJR 138:948, 1982.

Gewertz BL, Stanley JC, Fry WR: Renal artery dissections. Arch Surg 112:409, 1977.

Geyskes GG, Oei HY, Puylaert C, Ulees EJ: Renovascular hypertension identified by captopril-induced changes in the renogram. Hypertension 9:451, 1987.

Geyskes GG, Puylaert CBA, Dei HY, et al: Follow-up study of 70 patients with renal artery stenosis treated by percutaneous transluminal dilatation. BR Med J 287:333, 1983.

Gifford RW Jr: Epidemiology and clinical manifestations of renovascular hypertension. In Stanley JC, Ernst CB, Fry WJ (eds): Renovascular Hypertension. Philadelphia, WB Saunders Company, 1984, pp 77–104.

Gill WE, Cole AT, Wong RJ: Renovascular hypertension developing as a complication of selective renal arteriography. J Urol 107:922, 1972.

Gill WM, Meaney TF: Medial fibroplasia of the renal artery. Radiology 92:861, 1969.

Godin M, Helias A, Tadie M, et al: Moya-moya syndrome and renal artery stenosis. Kidney Int 15:450, 1978.

Goncherenko V, Gerlock AJ Jr, Shaff MI, Holifield JW: Progression of renal artery fibromuscular dysplasia in 42 patients as seen on angiography. Radiology 139:45, 1981.

Greene ER, Avasthi PS, Hodges JW: Noninvasive Doppler assessment of renal artery stenosis and hemodynamics. J Clin Ultrasound 15:653, 1987.

Greene ER, Venters MD, Avasthi PS, et al: Noninvasive characterization of renal artery blood flow. Kidney Int 20:523, 1981.

Grenier N, Douws C, Morel D, et al: Detection of vascular complications in renal allografts with color Doppler flow imaging. Radiology 178:217, 1991.

Grim CE, Luff FC, Yune HY: Percutaneous transluminal dilatation in the treatment of renal vascular hypertension. Ann Intern Med 95:439, 1981.

Gruntzig A, Hopff H: Perkutane rekanalisation chronischer arterieller verschlusse mit einem neuen dilatationskatheter. Modifikation der Dotter-Technik. Dtsch Med Wochenschr 99:2502, 1974.

Gruntzig A, Kuhlmann U, Vetter W, et al: Treatment of renovascular hypertension with percutaneous transluminal dilatation of a renal-artery stenosis. Lancet 1:801, 1979.

Gruntzig A, Turina MI, Schneider JA: Experimental percutaneous dilatation of coronary artery stenosis. Circulation 54:81, 1976.

Gullberg GT, Wehrli FW, Shimakawa A, Simons MA. MR vascular imaging with a fast gradient refocusing pulse sequence and reformatted imaged from transaxial sections. Radiology 165:241, 1987.

Hachiya J: Current concepts of Takayasu's arteritis. Semin Roentgenol 5:245, 1970.

Handa N, Fukunaga R, Etani H, et al: Efficacy of echo-Doppler examination for the evaluation of renovascular disease. Ultrasound Med Biol 14:1, 1988.

Hare WSC, Kincaid-Smith PK: Dissecting aneurysm of the renal artery. Radiology 97:255, 1970.

Harrington DP, Whelton PK, Mackenzie EJ, et al: Renal venous renin sampling: Prospective study of techniques and methods. Radiology 138:571, 1981.

Harrison EG Jr, Hunt JC, Bernatz PE: Morphology of fibromuscular dysplasia of the renal artery in renovascular hypertension. Am J Med 43:97, 1967.

Harrison EG Jr, McCormack LJ: Pathologic classification of renal arterial disease in renovascular hypertension. Mayo Clin Proc 46:161, 1971.

Hillman BJ: Digital radiology of the kidney. Radiol Clin North Am 23:211, 1985.

Hillman BJ, Ovitt TW, Capp MP, et al: Digital video subtraction angiography of renal vascular abnormalities. Radiology 139:277, 1981.

Hillman BJ, Ovitt TW, Capp MP, et al: Renal digital subtraction angiography: 100 cases. Radiology 145:643, 1982.

Hirst AE Jr, Johns VJ Jr, Kime SW Jr, et al: Dissecting aneurysm of the aorta: A review of 505 cases. Medicine 37:217, 1938.

Hoffman BJ: Renal ischemia produced by aneurysm of abdominal aorta. JAMA 120:1028, 1942.

Holley KE, Hunt JC, Brown AL Jr, et al: Renal artery stenosis: A clinical pathologic study in normotensive and hypertensive patients. Am J Med 37:14, 1964.

Hunt JC, Sheps SG, Harrison EG Jr, et al: Renal and renovascular hypertension. Arch Intern Med 133:988, 1974.

Hunt JC, Sheps SG, Harrison EG Jr, et al: Renal and renovascular hypertension. A reasoned approach to diagnosis and management. Arch Int Med 133:988, 1974.

Hunt JC, Strong CG: Renovascular hypertension: Mechanisms, natural history, and treatment. Am J Cardiol 32:562, 1973.

Illescas FF, Braun SC, Cohan RH, et al: Fibromuscular dysplasia of renal arteries: Comparison of intravenous digital subtraction angiography with conventional angiography. J Can Assoc Radiol 39:167, 1988.

Jenni R, Vieli A, Luscher ThF, et al: Combined two-dimensional ultrasound Doppler technique: New possibilities for the screening of renovascular hypertension and parenchymatous hypertension? Nephron 44 (Suppl 1):2, 1986.

Jensen SR, Novelline RA, Brewster DC, Bonventre JV: Transient renal artery stenosis produced by a pheochromocytoma. Radiology 144:767, 1982.

Juncos LI, Strong CG, Hunt JC: Prediction of results of surgery for renal artery renovascular hypertension. Arch Intern Med 134:655, 1974.

Kadir S: Diagnostic Angiography. Philadelphia, WB Saunders Company, 1986.

Kadir S, Athanasoulis CA: Angiographic diagnosis and control of postoperative bleeding. CRC Crit Rev Diagn Imaging 12:1 35, 1979.

Kannel WB: Role of blood pressure in cardiovascular morbidity and mortality. Prog Cardiovasc Dis 17:15, 1974.

Kannel WB, Dawber TR, Sorlie P, Wolf PA: Components of blood pressure and risk of atherothrombotic brain infraction: The Framingham study. Stroke 7:327, 1976.

Kaplan NM: Renin profiles. The unfulfilled promises. JAMA 238:611, 1977.

Kaufman JJ: Renovascular hypertension: The UCLA experience. J Urol 121:139, 1979.

Kaufman SL, Chang R, Kadir S, et al: Intraarterial digital subtraction angiography in diagnostic arteriography. Radiology 151:323, 1984.

Keller PJ, Drayer BP, Fram EK, et al: MR angiography with two-dimensional acquisition and three-dimensional display: Work in progress. Radiology 173:527, 1989.

Kent KC, Edelman RR, Kim D, et al: Magnetic resonance imaging: A reliable test for the evaluation of proximal atherosclerotic renal arterial stenosis (abstract). Radiology 181:293, 1991.

Kerlan RK Jr, Pogany AC, Burke DR, et al: Recognition and management of renovascular hypertension. AJR 145:119, 1985.

Kim D, Edelman RR, Kent KC, et al: Abdominal aorta and renal artery stenosis: Evaluation with MR angiography. Radiology 174:727, 1990.

Kim PK, Spriggs DW, Rutecki GW, et al: Transluminal angioplasty in patients with bilateral renal artery stenosis or renal artery stenosis in a solitary functioning kidney. AJR 153:1305, 1989.

Klatte EC, Worrell JA, Forster JH, et al: Diagnostic criteria of bilateral renovascular hypertension. Radiology 101:301, 1971.

Klecker RL, Roth JB: Visceral neurofibromatosis and hypertension childhood. Pediatrics 53:417, 1974.

Klinge J, Mali WPTM, Puijlaert CBAJ, et al: Percutaneous transluminal renal angioplasty: Initial and long term results. Radiology 171:501, 1989.

Kohler TR, Zierler RE, Martin RL, et al: Noninvasive diagnosis of renal artery stenosis by ultrasonic duplex scanning. J Vasc Surg 4:450, 1986.

Korobkin M, Pick RA, Merten DF, et al: Etiologic radiographic findings in children and adolescents with non-uremic hypertension. Radiology 110:615, 1974.

Krakoff LR, Ribeiro AB, Gorkin JU, et al: Saralasin infusion in screening patients for renovascular hypertension. Am J Cardiol 45:609, 1980.

Lande A: Takayasu's arteritis and congenital coarctation of the descending thoracic and abdominal aorta: A critical review. AJR 127:227, 1976.

Lawrie GM, Morris GC Jr, Glaeser DH, et al: Renovascular reconstruction: Factors affecting long-term prognosis in 919 patients followed up to 31 years (abstract). Radiology 174:294, 1990.

Lepke RA, Pagani JJ: Renal artery compression by an aortic aneurysm: An unusual cause of hypertension. AJR 139:812, 1982.

Lewin A, Blaufox D, Castle H, et al: Apparent prevalence of curable hypertension in the hypertension detection and follow-up program. Arch Intern Med 145:424, 1985.

Lewin JS, Laub G, Hausmann R: Three-dimensional time-of-flight MR angiography: Applications in the abdomen and thorax. Radiology 179:261, 1991.

Liu YQ: Radiology of aorto-arteritis. Radiol Clin North Am 23:671, 1985.

Ludgate CM, Watson GS: Unilateral renal hypertension following major trauma. Br J Urol 48:362, 1976.

Manashil GD, Thunstrom BS, Thorpe CD, Lipson SR: Outpatient transluminal angioplasty. Radiology 147:7, 1983.

Marks LH, Lupo AN, Cahill PJ, et al: Predictive value of renin determinations in renal artery stenosis. JAMA 238:2617, 1978.

Martin LG: Angioplasty of renal artery stenosis. In Kadir S (ed): Current Practice of Intervention Radiology. Philadelphia, BC Decker, 1991, pp 605–611.

Martin LG, Casarella WJ, Alspaugh JP, et al: Renal artery angioplasty: Increased technical success and decreased complications in the second 100 patients. Radiology 159:631, 1986.

Martin ED, Mattern RF, Baer L: Renal angioplasty for hypertension: Predictive factors for long-term success. AJR 128:951, 1981.

Masaryk TJ, Modic MT, Ruggieri PM, et al: Three-dimensional (volume) gradient-echo imaging of the carotid bifurcation: Preliminary clinical experience. Radiology 171:801, 1989.

Maxwell MH, Gonick HC, Wiita R, Jaufman JJ: Use of the rapid-sequence intravenous pyelogram in the diagnosis of renovascular hypertension. N Engl J Med 270:213, 1964.

Maxwell MH, Varady P, Zawada ET, et al: Maximal discrimination of renovascular hypertension by the Saralasin test. Clin Sci Mol Med 55:297S, 1978.

McCann RL, Bollinger R, Newman GE: Surgical renal artery reconstruction after percutaneous transluminal angioplasty. J Vasc Surg 8:389, 1988.

McCormack LJ, Dusten HP, Meaney TF: Selected pathology of the renal artery. Semin Roentgenol 2:126, 1967.

Miller GA, Ford KK, Braun SD, et al: Percutaneous transluminal angioplasty vs. surgery for renovascular hypertension. AJR 144:447, 1985.

Nally JV, Chen C, Fine E, et al: Diagnostic criteria of renovascular hypertension with captopril renography. Am J Hypertension 4:748S, 1991.

Nishimura DG, Macovski A, Pauly JM: Magnetic resonance angiography. IEEE Trans Med Imaging 5:140, 1986.

Norman D, Ulloa N, Brant-Zawadzki M, Coould RG: Intraarterial digital subtraction imaging cost considerations. Radiology 156:33, 1985.

Norris CS, Pfeiffer JS, Rittgers SE, Barnes RW: Noninvasive evaluation of renal artery stenosis and renovascular resistance. J Vasc Surg 1:192, 1984.

Novick AC: Surgical management of renovascular hypertension. In Kaplan NM, Brenner BM, Laragh JH (eds): The Kidney in Hypertension. New York, Raven Press, 1987, pp 225–237.

Oei HY, Geyskes GG, Mees EJ, Puylaert CB: The significance of captopril renography in renovascular hypertension. Contrib Nephrol 56:95, 1987.

Oparil S, Haber E: Renin in differential diagnosis of hypertension. Am Heart J 82:568, 1971.

Pickering TG, Sos TA, Laragh JH: Role of balloon dilatation in the treatment of renovascular hypertension. Am J Med 77:61, 1984.

Pickering TG, Sos TA, Vaughan ED Jr, et al: Predictive value and changes of renin secretion in hypertensive patients with unilateral renovascular disease undergoing successful renal angioplasty. Am J Med 76:398, 1984.

Pohl MA, Novick AC: Natural history of atherosclerotic and fibrous renal artery disease: Clinical implications. Am J Kidney Dis 5:A120, 1985.

Powers TA, Lorenz CH, Holburn GE, et al: Renal artery stenosis: In vivo perfusion MR imaging. Radiology 178:543, 1991.

Price RK, Skelton R: Hypertension due to syphilitic occlusion of the main renal arteries. Br Heart J 10:29, 1948.

Quinones JD, Varma V, Macal O: Radionuclide and pyelographic tests in screening for renovascular hypertension. Arch Intern Med 129:570, 1972.

Rackson ME, Lossef SV, Sos TA: Renal artery stenosis in patients with aortic dissection: Increased prevalence. Radiology 177:555, 1990.

Raghaviah NV, Singh SM: Extra-adrenal pheochromocytoma producing renal artery stenosis. J Urol 116:243, 1976.

Rao CN, Blaivas JG: Primary renal artery dissecting aneurysms: A review. J Urol 118:716, 1977.

Riemenschneider A, Emmanouilides GC, Hirose F, Linde LM: Coarctation of the abdominal aorta in children: Report of three cases and review of the literature. Pediatrics 44:716, 1969.

Robertson R, Murphy A, Dubbins PA: Renal artery stenosis: The use of duplex ultrasound as a screening technique. Br J Radiol 61:196, 1988.

Ross R Jr, Ackerman E, Pierce JM Jr: Traumatic subintimal hemorrhage of the renal artery. J Urol 104:11, 1970.

Roubidoux MA, Dunnick NR, Klotman PE, et al: Renal vein renins: Inability to predict response to revascularization in patients with hypertension. Radiology 178:819, 1991.

Saint-Georges G, Aube M: Safety of outpatient angiography. A prospective study. AJR 144:235, 1985.
Schwarten DE, Yune HY, Klatte EC, et al: Clinical experience with percutaneous transluminal angioplasty (PTA) of stenotic renal arteries. Radiology 135:601, 1980.
Scott JA, Rabe FE, Becker GJ, et al: Angiographic assessment of renal artery pathology. AJR 141:1299, 1983.
Segura JW, Patterson DE, LeRoy AJ, et al: Percutaneous removal of kidney stones: Review of 1,000 cases. J Urol 134:1077, 1985.
Sfakianakis GN, Bourgoignie JJ, Jaffe D, et al: Single dose captopril scintigraphy in the diagnosis of renovascular hypertension. J Nucl Med 28:1383, 1987.
Sharma S, Rajani M, Kamalakar T, et al: Association between aneurysm formation and systemic hypertension in Takayasu's arteritis. Clin Radiol 42:182, 1990.
Silver D, Clements JB: Renovascular hypertension from renal artery compression by congenital bands. Ann Surg 183:161, 1976.
Simon N, Franklin SS, Bleifer KH, et al: Cooperative study of renovascular hypertension. Clinical characteristics of renovascular hypertension. JAMA 220:1209, 1972.
Sniderman KW, Sos TA: Percutaneous transluminal recanalization and dilatation of totally occluded renal arteries. Radiology 142:607, 1982.
Sos TA, Pickering TG, Phil D, et al: Percutaneous transluminal renal angioplasty in renovascular hypertension due to atheroma or fibromuscular dysplasia. N Engl J Med 309:274, 1983.
Spies JB, LeQuire MH, Robison JG, et al: Renovascular hypertension caused by compression of the renal artery by the diaphragmatic crus. AJR 149:1195, 1987.
Srur MF, Sos TA, Saddekni S, et al: Intimal fibromuscular dysplasia and Takayasu arteritis: Delayed response to percutaneous transluminal renal angioplasty. Radiology 157:657, 1985.
Stables DP, Fouche RF, van Niekerk JPDV, et al: Traumatic renal artery occlusion: 21 cases. J Urol 115:229, 1976.
Stanley JC, Fry WJ: Pediatric renal artery occlusive disease and renovascular hypertension. Arch Surg 116:669, 1981.
Stanley JC, Fry WJ: Renovascular hypertension secondary to arterial fibroplasia in adults. Arch Surg 110:922, 1975.
Stewart BH, DeWeese MS, Conway J, Correa RJ: Renal hypertension: An appraisal of diagnostic studies and of direct operative treatment. Arch Surg 85:617, 1962.
Stewart BH, Dustan HP, Kiser WS, et al: Correlation of angiography and natural history in evaluation of patients with renovascular hypertension. J Urol 104:231, 1970.
Stockigt JR, Collins RD, Noakes CA, et al: Renal vein renin in various forms of renal hypertension. Lancet 1:1194, 1972.
Streeten DH, Freiberg JM, Anderson GH, Dalakos TG: Identification of angiotensinogenic hypertension in man using 1-sar-8-ala-a-angiotensin II (Saralasin, P-113). Circ Res 36(Suppl 1):125, 1975.
Stringer DA, O'Halpin D, Daneman A, et al: Duplex Doppler sonography for renal artery stenosis in the post-transplant pediatric patient. Pediatr Radiol 19:187, 1989.
Subcommittee on Definition and Prevalence of the 1984 Joint National Committee: Hypertension prevalence and the status of awareness, treatment, and control in the United States (final report). Hypertension 7:457, 1985.
Sutton D: Arteriography in the diagnosis of dissecting aneurysm. Clin Radiol 11:85, 1960.
Talner LB: Renal complications of angiography. In Ansell G (ed): Complications in Diagnostic Radiology. Oxford, England, Blackwell Scientific Publications, 1976, pp 111–133.
Taylor DC, Kettler MD, Moneta GL, et al: Duplex ultrasound scanning in the diagnosis of renal artery stenosis: A prospective evaluation. J Vasc Surg 7:363, 1988.
Tegtmeyer CG, Dyer R, Teates CD: Percutaneous transluminal dilatation of renal arteries. Radiology 135:589, 1980.
Tegtmeyer CG, Dyer R, Teates CD: Percutaneous transluminal angioplasty: The treatment of choice for renovascular hypertension due to fibromuscular dysplasia. Radiology 143:631, 1982.
Tegtmeyer CG, Dyer R, Teates CD, et al: Percutaneous transluminal dilatation of the renal arteries: Techniques and results. Radiology 135:589, 1980.
Tegtmeyer CG, Kellum CD, Ayers A: Percutaneous transluminal angioplasty of renal arteries: Results and long-term follow-up. Radiology 153:77, 1984.
Thorstad BL, Russell CD, Dubovsky EV, et al: Abnormal captopril renogram with a technetium-99m-labeled hippuran analog. J Nucl Med 29:1730, 1988.
Tilford DL, Kelsch RC: Renal artery stenosis in childhood neurofibromatosis. Am J Dis Child 126:665, 1983.
Vander AJ: Renin-angiotensin system. In Stanley JC, Ernst CB, Fry WJ (eds): Renovascular Hypertension. Philadelphia, WB Saunders Company, 1984, pp 20–45.
Veterans Administration Cooperative Study Group on Antihypertensive Agents: Effects of treatment of morbidity in hypertension: Results in patients with diastolic blood pressures averaging 115 through 129 mm Hg. JAMA 202:1028, 1967.
Wang Y: Regional renogram. A screening test for renal hypertension evaluation. Arch Intern Med 134:463, 1974.
Webb JA, Talner LB: The role of intravenous urography in hypertension. Radiol Clin North Am 17:187, 1979.
Wedeen VJ, Meuli RA, Edelman RR, et al: Projective imaging of pulsatile flow with magnetic resonance. Science 230:946, 1985.
Weidmann P, Siegenthaler W, Ziegler WH, et al: Hypertension associated with tumors adjacent to renal arteries. Am J Med 47:528, 1969.
Weiss ER, Blahd WH, Winston MA, et al: The scintillation camera in the dynamic evaluation of renal disorders. Radiology 98:165, 1971.
Wilms GE, Baert AL, Staessen JA, et al: Renal artery stenosis: Evaluation with intravenous digital subtraction angiography. Radiology 160:713, 1986.
Winter CC: Renogram and other radioisotope tests in the diagnosis of renal hypertension. Am J Surg 107:43, 1964.
Wise KL, McCann RL, Dunnick NR, Paulson DF: Renovascular hypertension. J Urol 140:911, 1988.
Working Group on Renovascular Hypertension: Final report of the Working Group on Renovascular Hypertension. Arch Intern Med 147:820, 1987.
Yamato M, Lecky JW, Hiramatsu K, Khoda E: Takayasu's arteritis: Radiographic and angiographic findings in 59 patients. Radiology 161:329, 1986.
Youngberg SP, Sheps SG, Strong CG: Fibromuscular disease of the renal arteries. Med Clin North Am 61:623, 1977.

77 Urolithiasis and Nephrocalcinosis

Marc P. Banner

The evaluation and management of patients with urinary tract stone disease (urolithiasis) and nephrocalcinosis are very much dependent upon radiologic imaging. Because approximately 90 per cent of all urinary tract calculi are radiopaque, the plain film of the abdomen (KUB) is the keystone of radiographic diagnosis. The KUB is usually supplemented with an intravenous urogram (IVU) or ultrasonogram. These studies answer most of the questions that affect patient management, including the number, size, and location of calculi; the presence or absence of underlying uropathology predisposing to stone formation and of urinary tract damage produced by the stone (primarily obstruction); and the status of the remainder of the urinary tract. Serial KUBs or IVUs show whether a stone has enlarged over time (metabolic activity). One other important factor in patient management is the composition or etiology of a stone, a determination that usually requires integrating urinary tract morphologic changes as displayed on the urogram and the roentgenographic characteristics of the calculus with clinical and biochemical information regarding the patient.

RADIOGRAPHIC CHARACTERISTICS OF URINARY CALCULI

Urinary calculi are composed of a mucoprotein matrix and a crystalline aggregate of varying chemical composition. The most commonly encountered calculi are composed of calcium oxalate, calcium phosphate, magnesium ammonium phosphate, and uric acid. Less frequent are calcium carbonate, cystine, xanthine, matrix, and fibrin calculi. Although each of these constituents has a fairly characteristic radiographic appearance when pure, crystalline admixtures occur frequently and produce varied radiographic images. Nonetheless, analysis of the size, shape, and appearance of a calculus often suggests its pathogenesis.

Calcium oxalate calculi may be smooth or mammillated and round or oval, and are densely opaque. The mammillations impart a characteristic stippled appearance to the calculus radiographically (Fig. 77–1). Large calcium oxalate stones may exhibit a jagged or stellate shape, resembling a jackstone.

Calcium phosphate (apatite) rarely forms a pure calculus but commonly combines with either calcium oxalate or magnesium ammonium phosphate, imparting a concentrically laminated appearance to such mixed stones. Apatite is an important constituent of calculi present in infected, alkaline urine. A pure apatite calculus is opaque and may be difficult to distinguish radiographically from a smooth calcium oxalate stone.

Magnesium ammonium phosphate (struvite) calculi are associated with an alkaline urine and almost always are accompanied by, and are the result of, a urea-splitting bacillary urinary tract infection, usually with *Proteus mirabilis* and occasionally with *Staphyloccus aureus* and *Klebsiella, Serratia,* and *Pseudomonas* species. Pure struvite or infection stones are rare and of relatively low radiopacity, but they are often laminated with more dense calcium salts, usually calcium phosphate, resulting in a magnesium-ammonium-calcium phosphate, or triple phosphate stone. These laminations suggest that recurrent infections with changes in urinary pH have favored different rates of crystallization for various calculus constituents. Struvite-apatite is the most common constituent of a staghorn calculus. A triple phosphate calculus is more dense than a pure struvite stone but less dense than a calcium oxalate calculus of the same volume (Fig. 77–2).

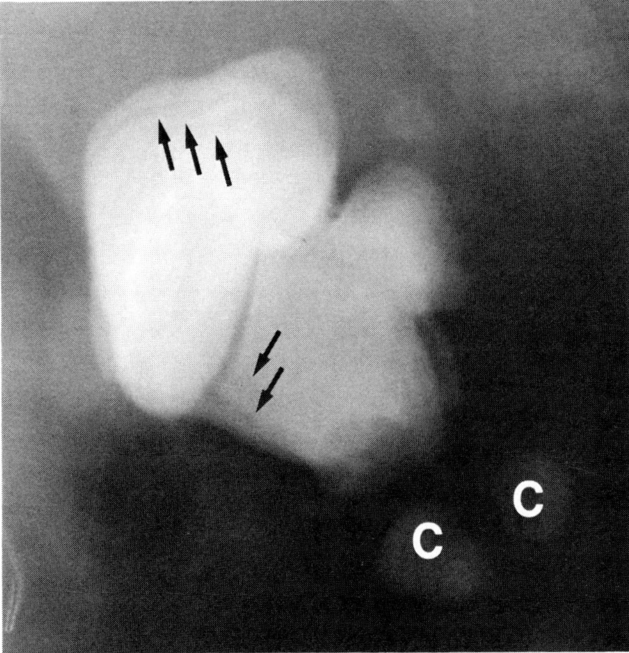

Figure 77–2. Magnesium-ammonium-calcium (triple) phosphate branched calculus. A plain film of the abdomen (KUB) demonstrates an inhomogeneously opaque calculus conforming to the contour of the left renal pelvis. *Arrows* point to some of the alternately opaque and lucent laminations that are characteristic of a triple phosphate calculus. The stone extends into the major infundibula, thereby qualifying as a branched, dendritic, or staghorn calculus. Two round stones (C) located in lower pole calyces are of lesser radiographic density than the major portion of the calculus and are probably predominantly composed of magnesium ammonium phosphate (struvite), with relatively little calcium phosphate (apatite). Pure struvite is only faintly opaque. When laminated with apatite (from multiple urinary infections), the opacity of the stone increases.

Uric acid calculi account for approximately 5 to 10 per cent of stones in the United States. When pure, they are radiolucent. However, over half of such calculi are adventitiously covered with calcium oxalate or, less commonly, calcium phosphate, imparting varying degrees of radiopacity and facilitating radiographic identification. Factors favoring formation of uric acid calculi are hyperuricosuria and an acid, concentrated urine. When pure, uric acid stones tend to be relatively small and smooth and are often disc shaped. Large uric acid calculi can attain a staghorn configuration and are usually of mixed composition, i.e., uric acid layered with calcium salts.

Cystine stones comprise 1 to 4 per cent of urinary calculi. They usually occur in a pure state and exhibit a homogeneous appearance.

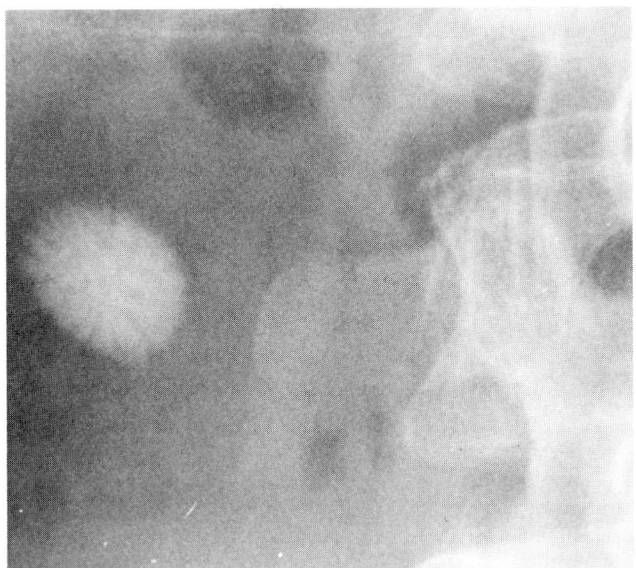

Figure 77–1. A 15 × 20 mm **densely opaque ovoid right renal pelvic calculus** exhibits peripheral spiculations or mammillations, which when viewed en face impart an inhomogeneous stippled appearance to the calculus. This appearance is characteristic of a stone composed entirely, or at least peripherally, of calcium oxalate.

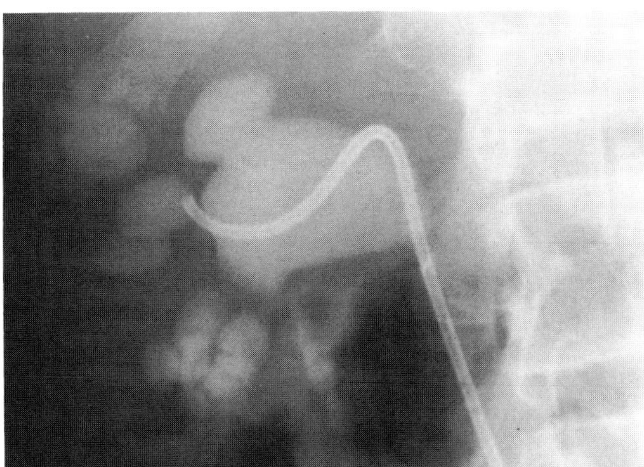

Figure 77–3. KUB shows a moderately opaque **staghorn calculus in the right kidney.** Most of the calyceal components of this large calculus are not attached to the renal pelvic stone. All portions of the stone appear very homogeneous and smoothly outlined. This appearance is characteristic of a cystine calculus. A ureteral stent has been inserted to relieve renal obstruction.

Their opacity, less than that of calcium-containing calculi, is related to the sulfur atoms within the cystine. Cystine calculi may be single, multiple, or of the staghorn variety. Cystine staghorn calculi usually exhibit multiple small unattached satellite stones (Fig. 77–3).

Xanthine stones are extremely rare and are essentially nonopaque. *Matrix, mucopus,* and *fibrin* constitute other varieties of nonopaque "calculi." Each may become secondarily calcified, especially matrix.

NEPHROCALCINOSIS

Nephrolithiasis refers to calcification within the pyelocalyceal lumina, while intraparenchymal calcification is termed *nephrocalcinosis.* A limited group of diseases may produce calcification confined to or predominantly located in the renal cortex—cortical nephrocalcinosis. Other conditions spare the cortex and deposit calcium salts in the medullary interstitium or lumina of the nephrons—medullary nephrocalcinosis. Table 77–1 lists the numerous causes of nephrocalcinosis.

Cortical Nephrocalcinosis

The two most common causes of cortical nephrocalcinosis are acute cortical necrosis and chronic glomerulonephritis, although radiographically evident calcification is rare in both conditions. In cortical necrosis, calcification most commonly appears as a single thin peripheral band with extensions radiating centrally into the necrotic septa of Bertin. The uninvolved medullary pyramids remain of soft-tissue density. Another pattern of involvement is that of two thin parallel tracks, or "tramlines," at the interfaces of the necrotic cortex and viable subcapsular cortex and corticomedullary junction on either side. Less frequently, a diffuse distribution of punctate calcific densities is seen, representing necrotic calcified cortical tubules as seen both in profile and en face. By the time calcification becomes radiographically evident, both renal size and cortical thickness have often decreased.

TABLE 77–1. CAUSES OF NEPHROCALCINOSIS

CORTICAL NEPHROCALCINOSIS	MEDULLARY NEPHROCALCINOSIS
Acquired immune deficiency syndrome (AIDS)	Acetazolamide administration
Acute cortical necrosis	AIDS (infection with *Pneumocystis carinii* or *Mycobacterium avium–intracellulare*)
Alport's syndrome	Bone metastases
Chronic glomerulonephritis	Chronic pyelonephritis
Chronic hypercalcemic states	Cushing's syndrome (endogenous, exogenous)
Ethylene glycol poisoning	Hyperparathyroidism
Excessive oxalate ingestion	Hyperthyroidism
Methoxyflurane toxicity	Hypophosphatasia
Oxalosis	Hypothyroidism
Pyridoxine deficiency	Idiopathic hypercalcemia
Rejected renal transplants	Malignancy
Sickle cell disease	Medullary sponge kidney disease
	Milk-alkali syndrome
	Nephrotoxic drugs (amphotericin B, outdated tetracycline)
	Ochronosis
	Primary hyperoxaluria
	Renal papillary necrosis, especially analgesic nephropathy
	Renal tuberculosis
	Sarcoidosis
	Sickle cell disease
	Triamterene administration
	Vitamin D intoxication
	Wilson's disease

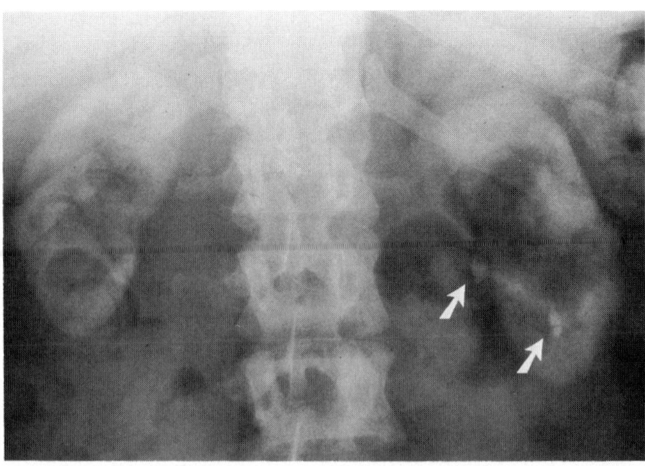

Figure 77–4. A diffuse increase in renal density on this KUB is indicative of **cortical nephrocalcinosis.** The patient, a 28-year-old male with congenital (primary) hyperoxaluria, has oxalate crystal deposition in multiple peripheral joints as well as his kidneys (oxalosis). He also has two oxalate calculi in a left lower pole calyx and one in the left renal pelvis *(arrows).* (From Banner MP: Calculous disease of the urinary tract. In Pollack HM (ed): Clinical Urography. Philadelphia, WB Saunders Company, 1990.)

These patterns of calcification may also occur in chronic glomerulonephritis, rejected renal transplants, and Alport's syndrome (hereditary nephropathy with deafness). Infants or children with a severe form of primary hyperoxaluria known as oxalosis may deposit calcium oxalate crystals in many solid organs, including the kidneys. These intratubular deposits impart a diffuse stippled opacity to the kidneys (Fig. 77–4). A similar intranephronic deposition of oxalate crystals with resultant diffuse nephrocalcinosis may follow methoxyflurane (penthrane) anesthesia and ethylene glycol (antifreeze) poisoning.

A punctate pattern of cortical nephrocalcinosis can occur in patients with acquired immune deficiency syndrome (AIDS), usually the result of prior infection with *Pneumocystis carinii* (Fig. 77–5). Similar calcifications often occur in other solid abdominal viscera, including the liver, spleen, adrenal glands, and lymph nodes. Nonhomogeneous cortical and patchy medullary calcifications in patients with AIDS have also been attributed to infection with *Mycobacterium avium-intracellulare.*

Medullary Nephrocalcinosis

Medullary nephrocalcinosis is usually associated with hypercalciuria and often with hypercalcemia. The typical radiographic picture is bilateral, diffuse fan-shaped clusters of stippled calcifications corresponding in distribution to the pyramids (Fig. 77–6). Approximately 40 per cent of cases of medullary nephrocalcinosis are attributable to primary hyperparathyroidism, another 20 per cent to renal tubular acidosis, and the remaining 40 per cent divided among many other causes, some of which are discussed below. Because most of the conditions that cause medullary nephrocalcinosis can also result in nephrolithiasis, these two groups of disorders are considered together. Their coexistence helps establish the etiology of the calculi and may significantly affect patient management.

Both ultrasonography and computed tomography (CT) can detect nephrocalcinosis at an earlier stage than can film radiography. CT readily depicts the exact location of the calcification. With ultrasonography, cortical echogenicity is increased and may produce

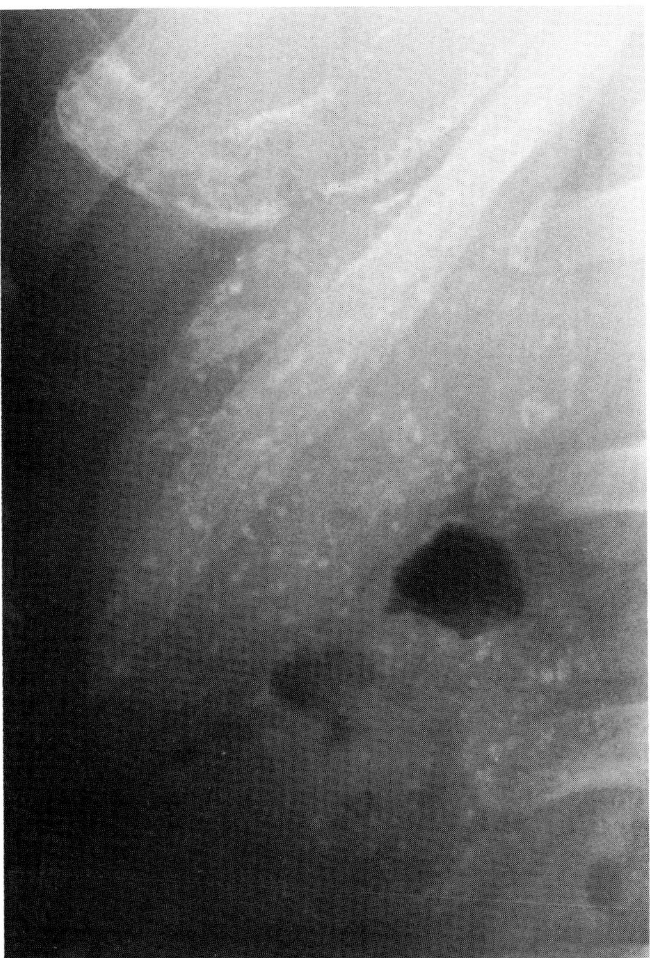

Figure 77–5. Multiple punctate calcifications scattered throughout the renal parenchyma is one of the patterns of **cortical nephrocalcinosis,** in this case attributable to systemic *Pneumocystis carinii* infection in a patient with acquired immune deficiency syndrome. Similar findings were present in the other kidney.

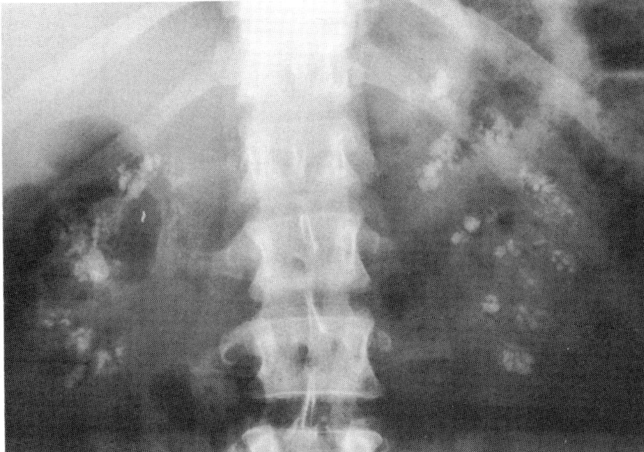

Figure 77–6. KUB shows multiple round clustered calcifications corresponding to each medullary pyramid, an appearance pathognomonic of **medullary nephrocalcinosis.** The diffuse and symmetrical pattern of calcification is more in keeping with renal tubular acidosis (which this patient had) than with other causes of medullary nephrocalcinosis.

acoustic shadowing in cases of cortical nephrocalcinosis (Fig. 77–7). In the medullary variety, there is a reversal of the normal differential corticomedullary echogenicity. The medullary pyramids increase in echogenicity and often become more echogenic than the adjacent cortex, although acoustic shadowing may not be demonstrable.

CAUSES OF UPPER URINARY TRACT CALCULI AND MEDULLARY NEPHROCALCINOSIS

Table 77–2 lists many of the causes of urolithiasis.

Structural Abnormalities

Any urinary tract structural abnormality that produces stasis of urine predisposes to urolithiasis, especially in the presence of urinary tract infection. These abnormalities include both obstructive and nonobstructive dilatation of the pyelocalyceal system, ureter, and urinary bladder. They may be generalized or localized. An example of the latter is a calyceal diverticulum containing multiple small clustered seed calculi or "milk-of-calcium," a colloidal suspension of minute calcific granules that appears as a finely granular opaque cloud on a KUB. These granules of calcium phosphate and/or carbonate layer in dependent fashion and are diagnosable on horizontal beam radiographs, ultrasonography, or CT (Fig. 77–8). Milk-of-calcium has also been observed in hydronephrotic kidneys

TABLE 77–2. COMMON CAUSES OF UROLITHIASIS

Urinary tract structural abnormalities	Hyperoxaluria
Pyelocalyceal diverticulum	Primary hyperoxaluria
Ureteropelvic junction obstruction	Secondary hyperoxaluria
Megacalyces/hydrocalyces	Excessive ingestion of oxalate or a precursor
Horseshoe kidney	Ileal disease
Renal ectopy	Pyridoxine deficiency
Polycystic kidney disease	Ethylene glycol poisoning
Medullary sponge kidney disease	Methoxyflurane toxicity
Megaureter	Hypercystinuria
Ureterocele	Xanthinuria
Bladder diverticulum	Hyperuricosuria
Urethral diverticulum	Gout
Bladder outflow obstruction	Myeloproliferative disorders, especially if treated
Hypercalciuria	Uricosuric agents
Hyperparathyroidism	Intestinal disease
Renal tubular acidosis	Lesch-Nyhan syndrome (juvenile gout)
Immobilization	Idiopathic
Milk-alkali syndrome	Urinary tract infection
Vitamin D intoxication	Miscellaneous
Sarcoidosis	Ingested substances (silica, sulfonamides, phenacetin, triamterene)
Idiopathic hypercalciuria	Ochronosis
Cushing's syndrome (endogenous, exogenous)	Long bone fractures (urostealithiasis)
Hyperthyroidism	Ureteral diversion to bowel segments
Hypothyroidism	Foreign bodies
Bone metastases	Dietary deficiencies
Multiple myeloma	
Paget's disease	
Acetazolamide therapy	
Furosemide therapy	
Wilson's disease	
Hyperalimentation	
Hyperpituitarism (acromegaly)	

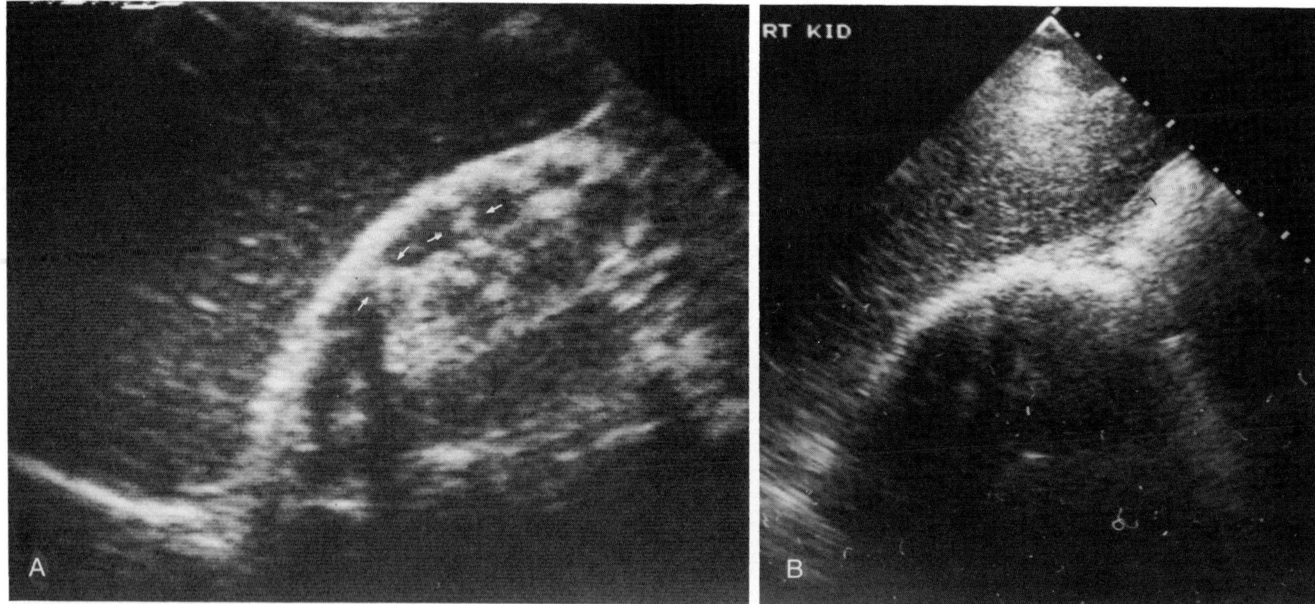

Figure 77–7. Sonographic demonstration of **cortical nephrocalcinosis.** *A,* Sagittal view of the right kidney shows the cortex to be even more echogenic than the renal sinus fat. Calcification in septal cortex *(arrows)* is also evident. The renal pyramids, which are unaffected, stand out in bold relief from the calcified cortex. The patient has Alport's syndrome. (*A* from Banner MP: Calculous disease of the urinary tract. In Pollack HM (ed): Clinical Urography. Philadelphia, WB Saunders Company, 1990.) *B,* More extensive cortical nephrocalcinosis in a patient with oxalosis. Sagittal view of the right kidney demonstrates highly echogenic renal margins with virtually complete absorption of sound, producing an acoustic shadow equal in size to the kidney itself. At this normal gain setting, the liver is imaged, but renal architecture cannot be evaluated. The ultrasonic appearance could also be due to a large amount of gas in the perinephric or subcapsular spaces.

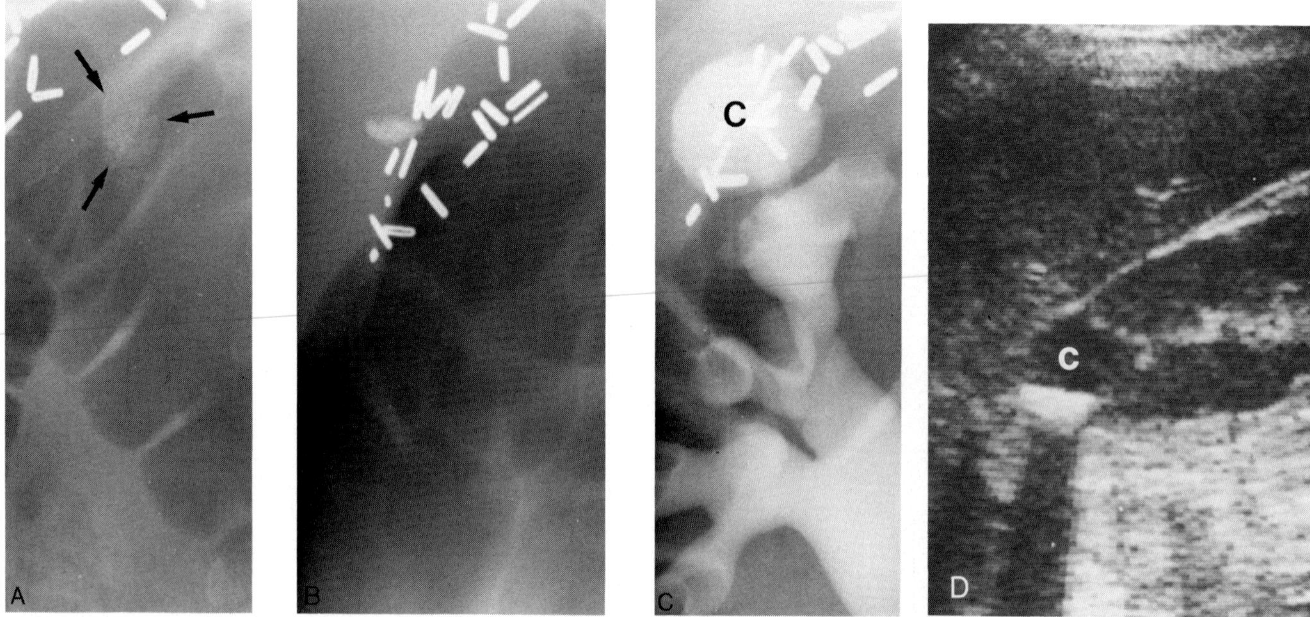

Figure 77–8. *A,* A coarsely granular, moderately opaque **right-upper–pole renal calculus** *(arrows)* is seen on a supine KUB. Despite its stippled en face appearance, the periphery of the stone is smooth rather than mammillated, as might be expected with a calcium oxalate stone. Metallic clips were placed at the time of cholecystectomy. *B,* On an erect radiograph the configuration of the calculus has changed, and the stone has apparently become more dense. This behavior and appearance are characteristic of both seed calculi and, as in this case, milk-of-calcium. The calcareous material gravitates to the most dependent portion of the enclosed space in which it is located, here a calyceal diverticulum (C) originating from the upper pole calyx as shown in *C* on an intravenous urogram (IVU). The milk-of-calcium is obscured by the contrast material that has passively opacified the diverticulum by way of its adjacent calyx. *D,* On this sagittal ultrasonogram of the right kidney, the milk-of-calcium layers in dependent fashion within the fluid-filled calyceal diverticulum (C) and casts a distinct acoustic shadow.

resulting from ureteropelvic junction (UPJ) obstruction and in chronically dilated ureters.

Tubular ectasia, or medullary sponge kidney, is a disease in which the terminal nephrons and ducts of Bellini are dilated. Calculi form in about half of cases owing to stasis of urine in these dilated ducts. These medullary nephrocalcific deposits not infrequently pass into the pyelocalyceal lumina. On urography, the concretions are engulfed by excreted contrast material and may appear to enlarge after contrast administration if the ectatic duct is larger than the calcification it contains (Fig. 77–9).

Calculi may complicate a simple ureterocele, the stones having arisen in the kidney. Their passage into the bladder is arrested by the narrowed ureteral orifice. Because of the chronic urinary stasis in ureteroceles, calculi can grow to rather large size and assume unusual shapes by conforming to the ureterocele (Fig. 77–10).

Hypercalciuria

Hypercalciuria may be due to dissolution of bone, excessive ingestion or absorption of calcium from the gastrointestinal tract, or faulty renal reabsorption of calcium, and can result in medullary nephrocalcinosis and renal calculi, usually of the calcium oxalate or phosphate type. The numerous hypercalciuric conditions associated with nephrolithiasis are listed in Table 77–2.

Nephrolithiasis occurs in 50 to 80 per cent of patients with primary *hyperparathyroidism,* and nephrocalcinosis in about 5 per cent. Both are seen less commonly in secondary hyperparathyroidism. The radiographic appearance of hyperparathyroid-induced nephrocalcinosis and lithiasis superficially resembles that of medullary sponge kidney disease. In the former, however, the medullary calcific deposits are not confined to the lumina of the nephron but also occur in the medullary interstitium. Thus, on urography, the interstitial nephrocalcific deposits will not be engulfed by excreted contrast medium, whereas the tubular concretions will be, as in sponge kidney. Contrast-filled ectatic tubules devoid of calculi, the diagnostic sine qua non of sponge kidney disease, will not be evident in hyperparathyroid-related nephrocalcinosis.

Renal tubular acidosis (RTA) is characterized by abnormal renal tubular function that results in chronic systemic acidosis and a persistently alkaline urine. Patients with proximal renal tubular abnormalities (type II RTA), in which there is a greater than normal urinary loss of bicarbonate, do not form metabolic renal calculi. Distal tubular dysfunction (type I RTA) interferes with hydrogen ion transfer into the urine and may result in stone formation, usually apatite in nature. Medullary nephrocalcinosis and lithiasis occur in

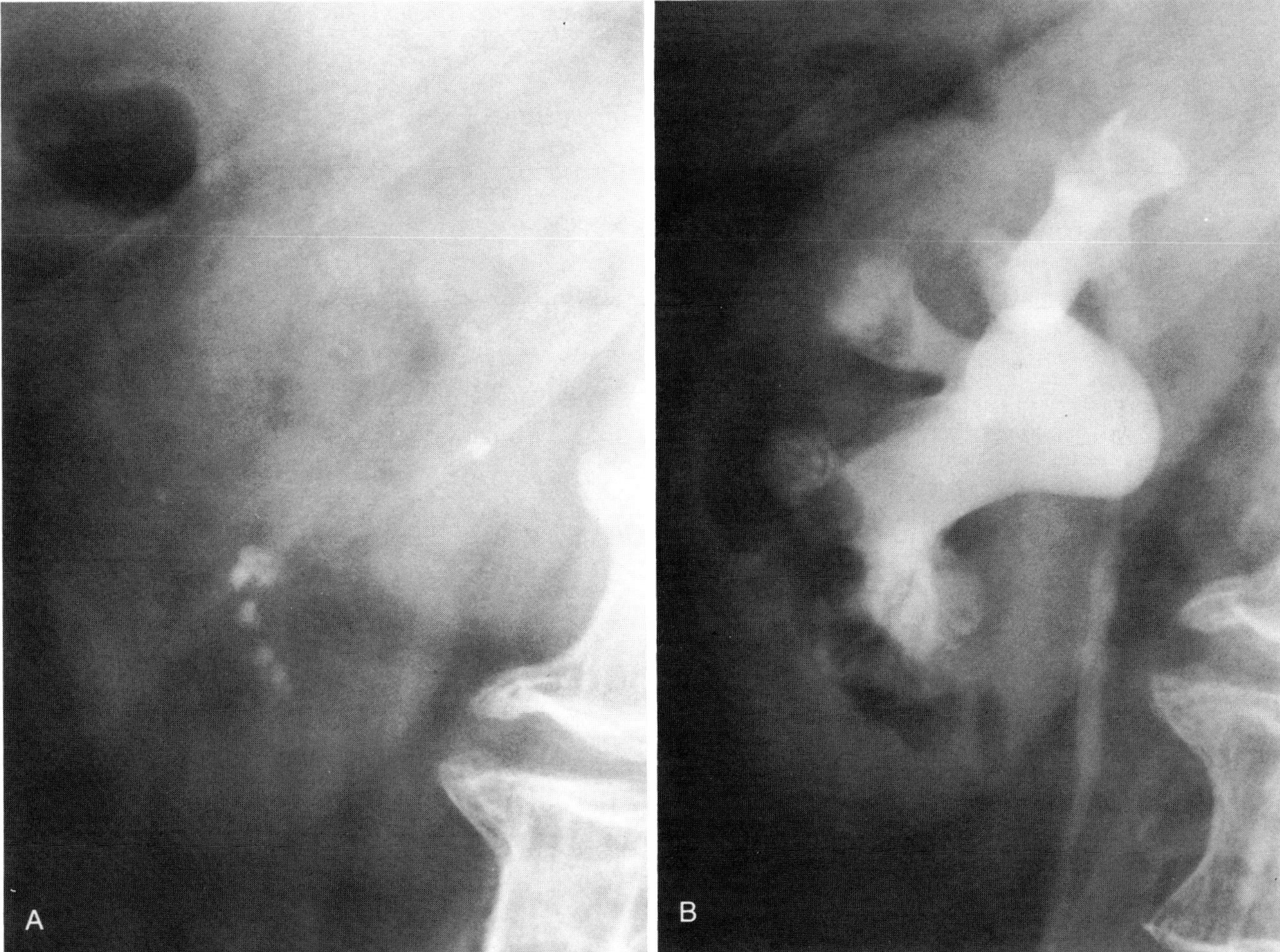

Figure 77–9. *A,* Multiple densely opaque **calcifications** are scattered throughout the right kidney, predominantly in the lower pole. *B,* On excretory urography, most of the calcifications lie in the distribution of the medullary pyramids and therefore represent **medullary nephrocalcinosis.** Also evident are multiple dilated, contrast-filled collecting tubules, most evident in the interpolar and lower polar kidney, not all of which contain calculi. This is the diagnostic sine qua non of medullary sponge kidney disease. The most medially situated calcification lies in the renal pelvis and therefore represents nephrolithiasis.

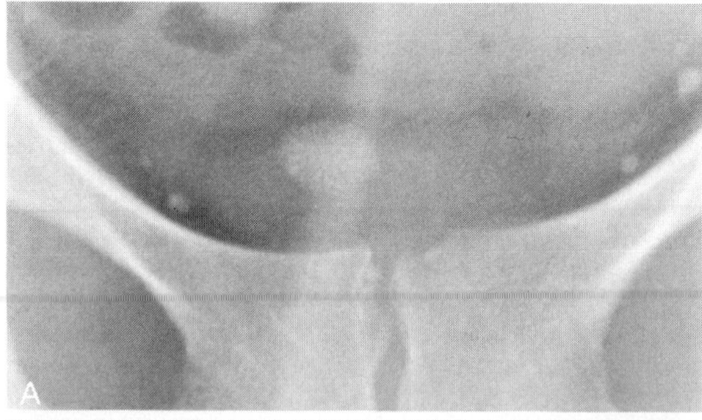

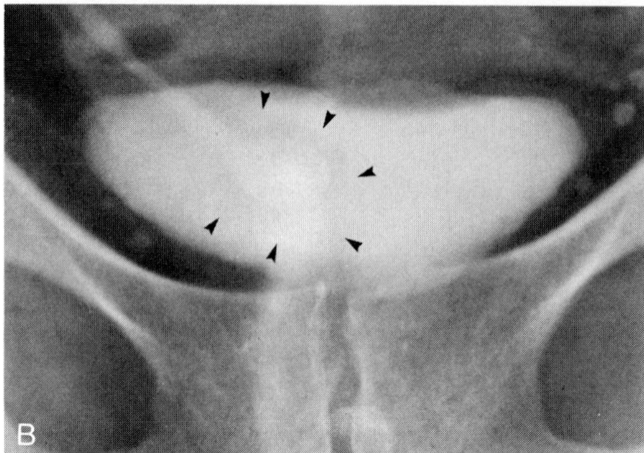

Figure 77–10. *A,* **An ovoid stippled calculus,** characteristic of calcium oxalate, appears to be located in the urinary bladder on a KUB, but is shown on urography *(B)* to reside in a ureterocele, too large to spontaneously pass into the bladder. Both the smooth, regular radiolucent collar surrounding the stone *(arrowheads)* and the absence of significant ureteral dilatation proximal to the calculus bespeak a simple or orthotopic ureterocele with secondary stone formation and militate against a primary intramural ureteral calculus producing a pseudoureterocele.

approximately 30 per cent of infants with primary or idiopathic RTA and in 73 per cent of adults. The nephrocalcinosis may be spotty in distribution, but more often it is diffuse and uniform, involving all medullary pyramids similarly (see Fig. 77–6). Delayed skeletal maturation and osteomalacia may also be seen. Other diseases can damage renal tubules, interfere with distal tubular hydrogen ion excretion, and produce a secondary RTA with nephrocalcinosis and lithiasis. These include Wilson's disease, Fanconi's syndrome, hyperglobulinemias, nephrotoxic drugs (out-dated tetracycline, amphotericin B), and acetazolamide administration.

Medullary nephrocalcinosis and urolithiasis may occur in a variety of other conditions, including immobilization, especially when accompanied by urinary infection; the milk-alkali syndrome, in which patients ingest large amounts of calcium and absorbable alkali, usually for treatment of peptic ulcer disease; hypervitaminosis D with excessive calcium absorption from the gastrointestinal tract; sarcoidosis, wherein hypercalciuria, with or without hypercalcemia, is not infrequently present, probably owing to hypersensitivity to vitamin D with increased intestinal absorption of calcium; idiopathic hypercalciuria, a condition that characteristically affects white males over the age of 20 years; diseases that cause bone destruction or dissolution with resultant hypercalcemia and hypercalciuria, including multiple myeloma, bone metastases, Paget's disease, Cushing's syndrome (both endogenous and exogenous from steroid administration), and hyperthyroidism; and in preterm infants treated for long periods of time with furosemide for either congestive heart failure secondary to a patent ductus arteriosus or pulmonary disease (hyaline membrane disease or bronchopulmonary dysplasia). Calcium stones can develop in the collecting system or medullary interstitium.

Hyperoxaluria

Hyperoxaluria can result in either nephrocalcinosis or calcium oxalate calculi. In primary hyperoxaluria, an autosomal recessive inborn error of metabolism, there is excessive production and urinary excretion of oxalate. Affected patients usually present with calcium oxalate lithiasis in early childhood. The disease often causes progressive renal failure and death in adolescence. In its advanced stage, known as oxalosis, calcium oxalate crystal deposition occurs in multiple organs. Radiographically, diffuse mottled calcification occurs throughout the renal parenchyma (see Fig. 77–4).

Secondary hyperoxaluria can also cause nephrolithiasis or nephrocalcinosis, usually of the cortical variety. It can result from increased ingestion of oxalate or one of its precursors, ileal disease, pyridoxine deficiency, ethylene glycol poisoning, and methoxyflurane anesthesia. The most common cause of secondary hyperoxaluria with calcium oxalate stones is increased intestinal absorption of dietary oxalate secondary to small bowel disease (Crohn's disease, ileal resection, or bypass).

Hypercystinuria

Only the most severely affected of these patients with an autosomal recessive defect of renal tubular transport of cystine and related amino acids suffer from urinary calculi, the majority of which are pure cystine.

Xanthinuria

Calculi develop in less than half the patients with this uncommon inborn error of metabolism and also develop rarely in patients taking allopurinol.

Hyperuricosuria

Myeloproliferative disorders, especially after cytolytic therapy, account for about 40 per cent of uric acid calculi and gout for another 25 per cent. Other calculogenic factors are uricosuric agents and an acid, concentrated urine. Uric acid stones also occur in patients with intestinal disease, although not as frequently as calcium oxalate lithiasis. Such patients, typified by those with ileostomies, lose large amounts of alkaline intestinal fluid by way of chronic diarrhea. Their kidneys respond by secreting an acidic, highly concentrated urine, so setting the stage for uric acid stone formation.

In the Lesch-Nyhan syndrome (juvenile gout), enzymatic overproduction of purine and consequently of uric acid occurs. Affected children exhibit growth and mental retardation, a tendency to self-mutilation often manifested by amputation of the fingertips and phalanges, and multiple radiolucent uric acid calculi.

Miscellaneous Causes

Infection stones may form after ureteroenteric diversion, whether by an isolated bowel conduit or by ureterosigmoidostomy. The stones are seen most commonly 5 to 10 years after surgery and are related to hyperchloremic acidosis, reflux of bowel contents, and infection. Such calculi are almost always composed of mixtures of struvite, apatite, and calcium oxalate.

Calcification can accompany papillary necrosis, especially when related to analgesic abuse, diabetes mellitus, or renal tuberculosis. The small necrotic foci within the center of the papilla, characteristic of analgesic-induced papillary necrosis, may contain calcific debris, or the papilla itself may undergo ischemic necrosis and calcification. These calcific foci can detach from the papilla, or a completely necrotic papilla may slough from its base and, free in the pyelocalyceal system, calcify secondarily.

RADIOLOGIC EVALUATION OF UPPER URINARY TRACT CALCULI

Plain Film of the Abdomen

Because most urinary calculi are opaque, the plain film of the abdomen, or KUB, is invaluable in diagnosis. Stones are customarily described as densely opaque, moderately opaque, faintly opaque, and nonopaque (Fig. 77–11). Opaque calculi can be obscured or easily overlooked when they overlie bony structures such as the sacrum or a vertebral transverse process. Numerous extraurinary calcific shadows (e.g., calcified costal cartilages, gallstones, and vascular calcifications) may overlie the urinary tract and be confused with nephroliths. Prior to contrast injection, one must ascertain whether these calcifications lie within the kidneys. This can be accomplished with oblique films, plain film renal tomograms, or sequential films exposed in inspiration and expiration. Ureteral calculi can be confused with bone islands in the sacrum and with phleboliths. To reliably distinguish the latter from distal ureteral calculi, one can opacify the ureter by urography or pyelography, demonstrate that a calcification touches an opaque catheter in the ureter in two projections (i.e., anteroposterior and oblique), or demonstrate a calculus in the disal ureter on cross-sectional imaging (ultrasonography, CT, or magnetic resonance imaging [MRI]).

Excretory Urography

The excretory urogram or the IVU can specifically locate a calculus within the kidney or ureter as well as evaluate the degree of obstruction it is producing. Stones may be either partially or completely obscured by excreted contrast, or they may appear as a filling defect.

Aside from the growth characteristics of various stones discussed above, the anatomy of the renal pelvis and the presence or absence of urinary infection help determine calculus shape and whether or not a given calculus will be obstructive to the collecting system. Box-shaped pelves may restrict stone passage and, by allowing mobility, help shape a round calculus. On the other hand, a rapidly growing infection stone is often molded by contact with the pelvic and infundibular walls, promoting growth in a branched or dendritic fashion (staghorn calculus). Noninfection stones (calcium oxalate and cystine) usually become obstructive before excessive branching occurs, while the mucous coating of an infected branched struvite stone encourages predominant appositional growth at the terminal portions of the staghorn within the calyces. The site of maximal obstruction is therefore usually calyceal for infection stones and renal pelvic or infundibular for noninfection stones.

Urography is the traditional (and most consistently reliable) method of establishing the diagnosis of a ureteral calculus, whether or not a suspicious density is seen on the KUB. As ureteral calculi usually arise in the kidney, their composition is the same as that of renal calculi. The shape of a ureteral calculus recently expelled from the kidney is usually round or oval; one that resides in the ureter for some time may grow in length. Important considerations in the management of patients with ureterolithiasis include stone size and location and the presence or absence of obstructive uropathy. Stones greater than 1 cm in largest diameter have only a small likelihood of spontaneous passage, whereas those measuring less than 5 mm usually will do so. The management of those in between is individualized on the basis of both clinical and radiologic features. Stones tend to come to rest at the narrowest sites in the ureter, i.e., where the ureter crosses the iliac vessels; in the intramural ureter; and, in some patients, in areas of ureteral stricture from prior ureteral surgery or secondary to fibrosis.

Many of the urographic signs of an obstructing ureteral calculus are discussed in the section on ureteral obstruction; however, a few observations specific to ureteral calculi deserve emphasis.

The diagnosis of a ureteral calculus is established by demonstrating ureteral dilatation that ends abruptly at a density in the ureter and that is seen on at least two films, supine and prone, supine and oblique, or recumbent and erect. Multiple projections are also often necessary with calculi overlying the sacrum and in the pelvis when phleboliths are present in the vicinity of a ureteral obstruction.

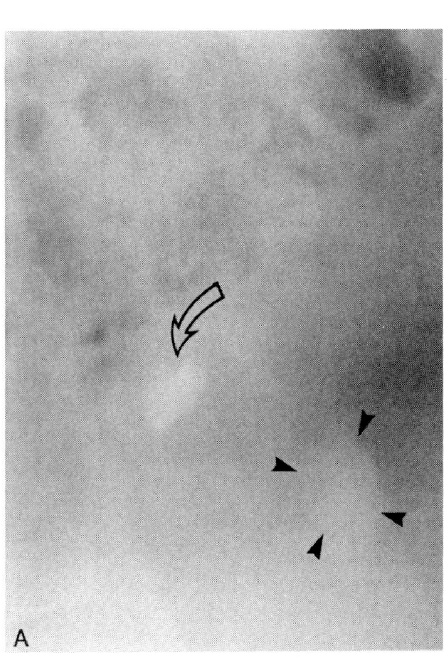

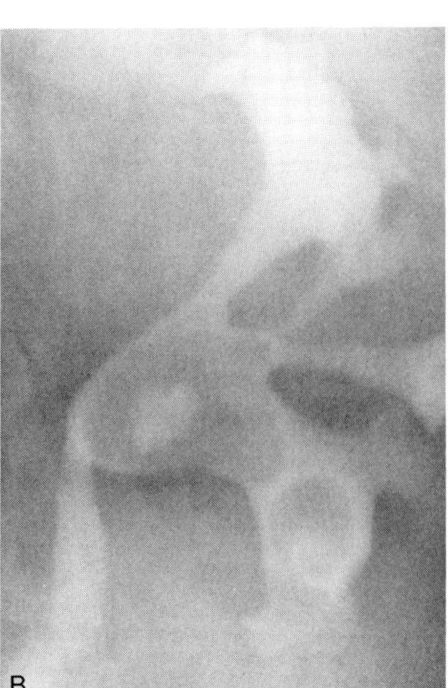

Figure 77–11. *A,* KUB shows a 10 × 12 mm **densely opaque pyramid-shaped calculus** in the region of the left renal pelvis. The overall shape of the stone as well as the small depression in its base *(arrow)* suggests that it may have formed in a calyx attached to the base of a medullary pyramid and subsequently passed into the renal pelvis where it enlarged. A 12 × 14 mm faintly opaque density *(arrowheads)* inferolateral to the calculus could easily be mistaken for bowel contents but actually represents a second stone. *B,* On excretory urography, the faintly opaque stone is shown to be located in the lower pole major infundibulum, where it appears as a filling defect. Were it totally nonopaque, it could also represent a blood clot and could not be differentiated by urography alone. The densely opaque calculus is seen to represent only the center of a much larger stone that occupies the entire renal pelvis and is growing in dendritic fashion into multiple infundibula—the beginnings of a staghorn calculus. On chemical analysis, the larger stone was composed of a calcium oxalate center and a uric acid (nonopaque) periphery; the smaller stone was uric acid adventitiously covered with a small amount of calcium oxalate, thereby accounting for its faint radiopacity.

Demonstrating that even part of an opaque density in the pelvis lies outside the opacified ureteral lumen proves that the density is not a ureteral calculus, a rare exception being a stone that has eroded through the ureteral wall.

The degree of obstructive uropathy often bears no relation to the size of a ureteral calculus. If the distal migration of a rather small calculus is suddenly halted in the ureter, severe colic and urographic changes of an acute high-grade obstruction may result (progressively dense nephrogram, marked delay in contrast excretion, contrast extravasation from the collecting system, etc.).

The most consistent urographic finding with a ureteral calculus is the presence of a continuous column of opacified ureter extending from the renal pelvis to the site of a stone, indicating that the obstructing calculus has diminished or abolished ureteral peristalsis. Some degree of ureterectasis is also usually present if ureteral obstruction has been present for more than a few hours (Fig. 77–12). If a calculus is incompletely obstructing the ureter, contrast will flow by it. The ureteral lumen just distal to a stone often appears narrowed because of inflammation and mucosal edema. This narrowing may give the false impression of a ureteral stricture that has prevented further distal migration of the stone. Calculi in the intramural ureter often provoke severe focal edema, suggesting a ureterocele or even bladder neoplasm. The combination of focal distal ureterectasis and vesical edema is referred to as a ''pseudoureterocele'' and usually can be differentiated from a true orthotopic ureterocele by the somewhat irregular and asymmetric radiolucency surrounding the dilated intramural ureter (see Fig. 77–10).

Lesser degrees of ureteral obstruction may be apparent only on erect radiographs that show impaired drainage of opacified urine from the affected ureter above the site of obstruction. Rarely, a relatively small ureteral calculus may not produce any urographic abnormality. Patients harboring such nonobstructive calculi are usually asymptomatic.

Ultrasonography

The ultrasonic diagnosis of a calculus is based on the demonstration of an echogenic focus that casts a discrete posterior acoustic shadow. Stones as small as 1.5 mm can be reliably detected in this manner. This technique assumes greatest importance when faced with a nonopaque filling defect in the kidney on urography (Fig. 77–13). Tumors and blood clots are less echogenic than stones, do not absorb sound as fully as do stones, and therefore lack a distal acoustic shadow.

Transabdominal ultrasonography is not able to evaluate the ureter except for its most proximal and distal portions, and then only when it is dilated. To differentiate nonopaque calculi from tumors or clots in the ureter, pyelography or CT is usually necessary unless acoustic shadowing can be demonstrated in association with a ureteral lesion. Ultrasonographic evaluation of the distal ureter (transabdominal, transrectal, or transvaginal) may be helpful (and possibly even more sensitive than excretory urography) for evaluating distal ureteral obstruction of uncertain cause. The sonographic criteria for a distal ureteral calculus (opaque or nonopaque) include demonstration of a highly echogenic reflector with a distinct acoustic shadow in the expected location of the distal ureter and a history of renal colic and/or a dilated ureter proximal to the shadowing reflector.

This technique can be of help in patients in whom urography should be avoided (e.g., pregnant women and patients with contrast media sensitivity), when a distal ureteral calculus is suspected on an IVU but cannot be identified on the KUB because of confusing or obscuring shadows, or in differentiating edema of the intramural ureter secondary to recent passage of a ureteral calculus (which has not been recovered) from continued calculous obstruction (Fig. 77–14).

In the patient with acute flank pain whose urographic findings are unclear, ultrasonography can usually differentiate obstructive pye-

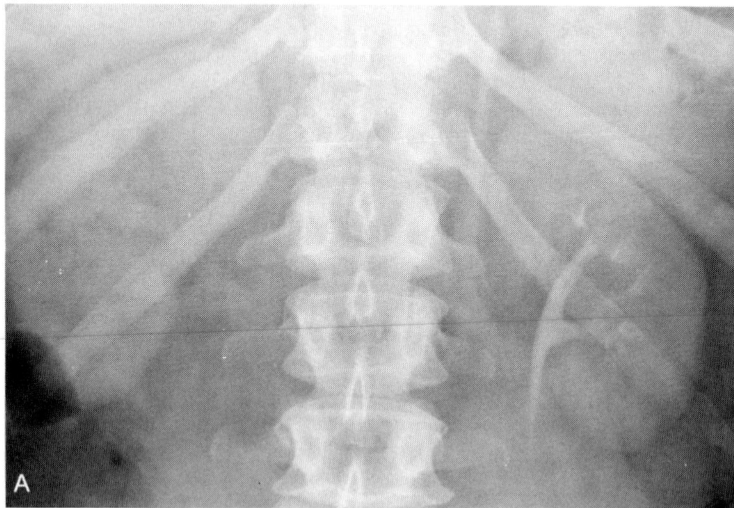

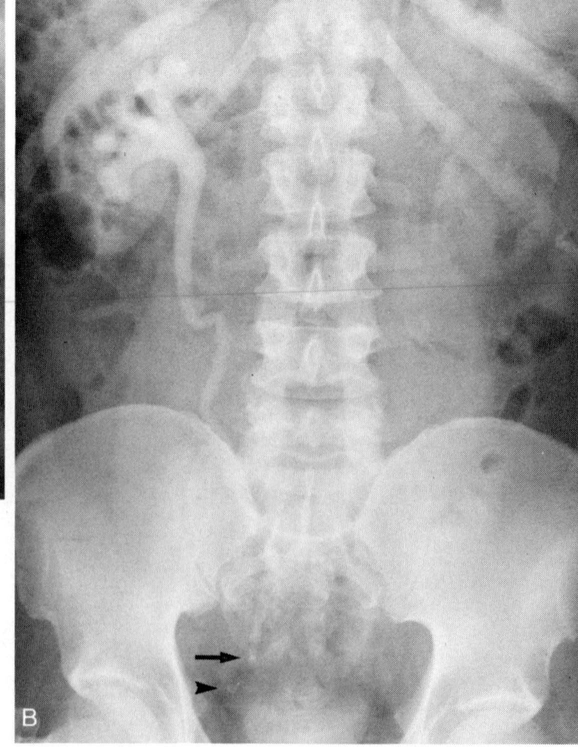

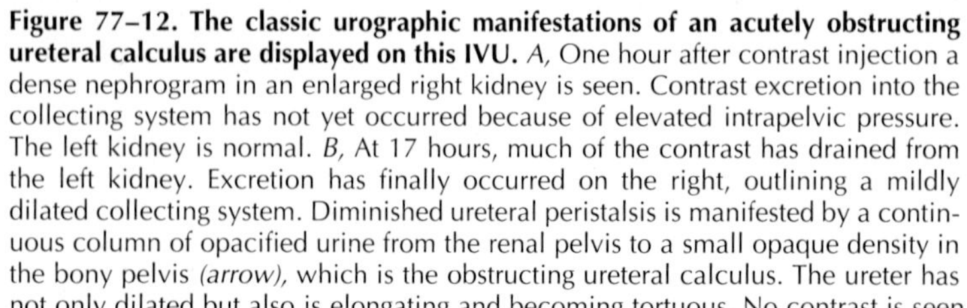
Figure 77–12. The classic urographic manifestations of an acutely obstructing ureteral calculus are displayed on this IVU. *A,* One hour after contrast injection a dense nephrogram in an enlarged right kidney is seen. Contrast excretion into the collecting system has not yet occurred because of elevated intrapelvic pressure. The left kidney is normal. *B,* At 17 hours, much of the contrast has drained from the left kidney. Excretion has finally occurred on the right, outlining a mildly dilated collecting system. Diminished ureteral peristalsis is manifested by a continuous column of opacified urine from the renal pelvis to a small opaque density in the bony pelvis *(arrow),* which is the obstructing ureteral calculus. The ureter has not only dilated but also is elongating and becoming tortuous. No contrast is seen in the ureter distal to the stone. The bladder has been filled from the left kidney. A phlebolith is present *(arrowhead)* just distal to the ureteral calculus. Note its characteristic radiolucent center and opaque periphery.

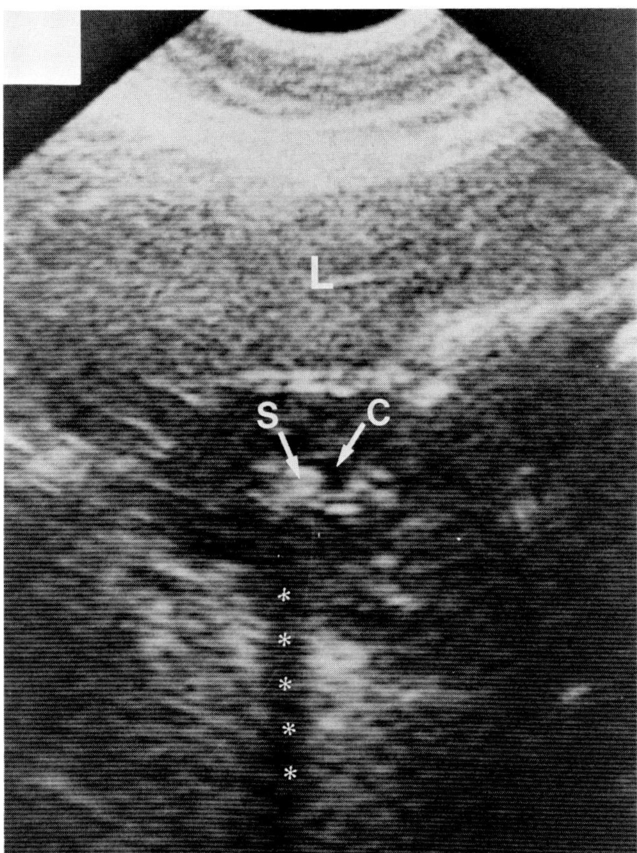

Figure 77–13. Sagittal ultrasonogram of the right kidney imaged through the liver (L) in a patient with hematuria and a nonopaque filling defect in a dilated lower pole calyx on urography. The filling defect appears as an echogenic focus (S) within a mildly dilated calyx (C). The former is impeding sound transmission, as evidenced by the acoustic shadow it is casting *(asterisks)*. This combination of ultrasonic findings identifies the filling defect as a nonopaque renal calculus, in this case composed of uric acid.

localyceal dilatation from renal infarction, pyelonephritis, spontaneous renal bleeding, or acute renal vein thrombosis.

Ultrasonography has been proposed as an alternative to IVU for evaluating patients with suspected calculous obstruction. Although it is quite sensitive in detecting hydronephrosis, gray scale ultrasound cannot depict the early physiologic changes that occur within hours of acute calculous obstruction (e.g., delayed contrast excretion) and precede the development of hydronephrosis. In addition, ultrasonography is not as sensitive as urography in detecting fornix rupture and contrast extravasation.

It has recently been shown that an elevated resistive index on pulsed Doppler ultrasound often accompanies acute urinary obstruction, and it has been suggested that this determination may be helpful in evaluating patients with flank pain and suspected calculous obstruction. However, pulsed or duplex Doppler is associated with too many false positives and false negatives to be as yet a reliable discriminator of obstructive uropathy.

Another area of investigation is the potential use of color Doppler ultrasound in the evaluation of distal ureteral peristalsis and intravesicle ureteral jets in patients with calculous ureteral obstruction. Until the technique of the examination is standardized and its statistical validity evaluated, its use should be adjunctive but certainly helpful, especially in those patients in whom urography should be avoided if possible.

Computed Tomography

Nonopaque calculi, although invisible on a KUB, are clearly depicted by CT since they are much denser than urine or any soft tissue. CT attenuation values for all stones are greater than those of renal parenchyma, transitional cell neoplasms and fresh blood clots (Fig. 77–15). Unfortunately, attempts to characterize the chemical composition of calculi based on their CT numbers have met with limited success. The diagnostic accuracy of CT is no greater than that of plain film analysis.

CT assumes great importance in differentiating nonopaque calculi from other causes of nonopaque filling defects in the renal collecting system; in depicting nonopaque ureteral calculi in cases of ureteral obstruction of uncertain cause; and in evaluating many of the complications of upper urinary tract calculus disease, as discussed later in this chapter.

Retrograde Ureterography

The insertion of an opaque ureteral catheter without contrast injection can confirm that a density lying in the expected course of the ureter or UPJ is a urinary calculus. More commonly, retrograde ureterography is used to substantiate a diagnosis of a nonopaque ureteral calculus when urographic opacification of the ureter sufficient for diagnosis is not forthcoming. The fluoroscopically controlled injection of contrast through a cystoscopically placed ureteral catheter can usually differentiate ureteral calculi from other

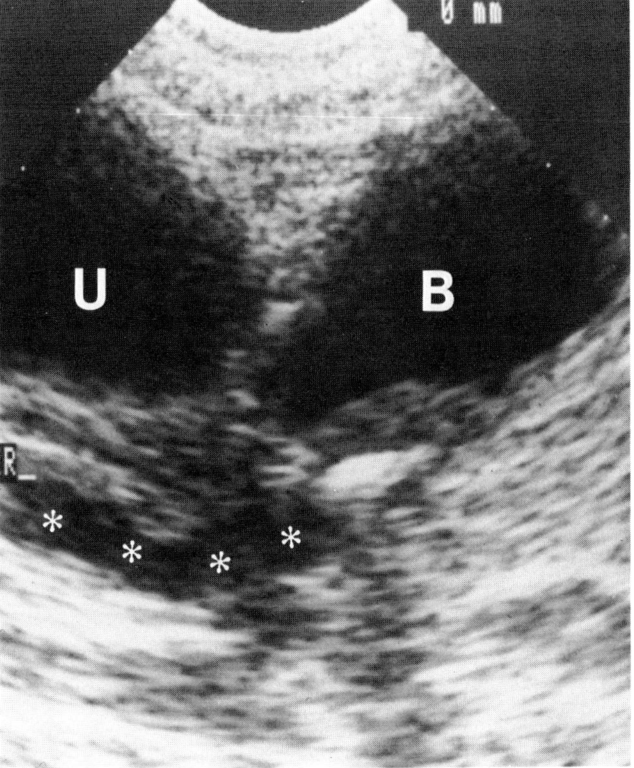

Figure 77–14. Longitudinal pelvic ultrasonogram in a patient 32 weeks pregnant shows a highly echogenic **calculus** with an acoustic shadow in the juxtavesical portion of a dilated and obstructed right ureter (asterisks). The patient presented with five days of right pyelonephritis that was unresponsive to medical therapy. The ultrasonogram obviated the need to perform radiographic studies. (B = bladder; U = lower uterine segment.)

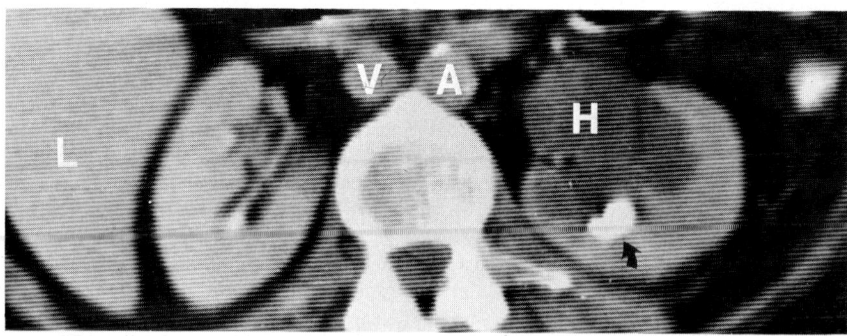

Figure 77–15. Computed tomographic scan following intravenous contrast administration in a patient with left proximal ureteral obstruction but no opaque calculi on an IVU. A highly attenuating uric acid calculus *(arrow)* is seen in one of the posterior calyces, unchanged in appearance from precontrast scans. There is also marked hydronephrosis (H = hydronephrotic renal pelvis). Contrast has not yet been excreted into the left collecting system but is present in a normal-appearing right kidney. Other sections showed the hydronephrosis to be due to a similar appearing obstructing proximal ureteral uric acid calculus. (L = liver; V = inferior vena cava; A = partially calcified abdominal aorta.)

nonopaque filling defects. A calculus usually exhibits a smooth convex lower margin as opposed to the more irregular margin of most ureteral tumors, benign ureteral polyps being an unusual but notable exception. In addition, owing to edema, there may be narrowing of the contrast-filled ureter just distal to a stone. In the absence of significant edema, the ureter may simply be collapsed beyond the stone. On the other hand, ureteral tumors grow slowly and tend to be accompanied by ureteral widening for a centimeter or so just distal to their lowest margin (Bergman's sign) because of the continued effect of ureteral peristalsis on the growing intraluminal neoplasm.

If the ureter distal to a calculus has not been well seen on urography, a retrograde ureterogram in the operating room just before endourologic manipulation is desirable to exclude previously unsuspected additional calculi as well as coexistent ureteral disease (such as stricture or retroperitoneal fibrosis) that might complicate management, even if direct visualization of the ureter via ureteroscopy is contemplated.

The occasional symptomatic calculus in a ureteral stump requires retrograde ureterography, CT, or ureteroscopy for diagnosis.

Antegrade Pyeloureterography and Loopography

Antegrade pyeloureterography via a needle percutaneously inserted into the renal collecting system may be preferable to retrograde ureterography if long-term renal drainage is anticipated, in infants and small children, if a nephrostomy catheter is present, and if the ureter cannot be catheterized cystoscopically. Ureters that have been diverted to an ileal conduit can easily be opacified by instilling contrast medium into the conduit and fluoroscopically positioning the patient for optimal demonstration of filling defects in the pyelocalyceal system and ureter by way of ureteral reflux.

Perioperative Radiography and Intraoperative Imaging

A KUB should be obtained just before open surgical or endourologic intervention for ureteral calculi to ascertain exact stone location, because ureteral calculi can occasionally exhibit great mobility. Although this is usually caudal (toward the bladder), cranial migration can occur, especially if the ureter is dilated.

Intraoperative ultrasonography and occasionally radiography may facilitate the identification of small stones or stone fragments during surgical lithotomy. Ultrasonic contact scanning with a high-frequency transducer can detect and localize stones as small as 2 to 3 mm in diameter at depths of up to 3.0 to 3.5 cm from the kidney surface. Stones that may not have been apparent on a KUB may be disclosed by these techniques.

Renal Arteriography

As noninvasive imaging modalities replace arteriography to evaluate renal integrity and nonoperative techniques replace surgical lithotomy, renal arteriography is infrequently performed to assist stone management. Renal arteriography may be helpful when a partial nephrectomy is contemplated for localized stone disease or if surgical lithotomy is contemplated in cases of congenital abnormalities of renal parenchymal development, such as horseshoe kidney, where renal arterial anomalies are often present.

Nuclear Radiology

Although radionuclide renal imaging is superior to urography for assessing renal function, it is inferior to the other imaging modalities discussed above for depicting anatomic detail. Urography and radionuclide imaging therefore complement each other and may be used together to assess the anatomic changes and functional derangements associated with urolithiasis, especially in patients with bilateral stone disease and associated parenchymal damage. The noninvasive, isotopic split renal functional analysis may influence not only which renal unit merits initial consideration (the one contributing the majority of total renal function) but also the type of intervention most appropriate (nephrectomy, segmental resection, lithotomy, or nephrostomy).

In the patient with unilateral obstruction secondary to a renal or ureteral calculus, the quantitative contribution of such a kidney to overall renal function may be small at the time of obstruction, yet that kidney may possess significant recuperative capability if treated in conservative fashion. This cannot always be predicted accurately by radionuclide techniques. The length of the obstruction and the presence of urinary infection may alter the initial nuclide assessment to give a rather low estimation of renal function. Temporary relief of the obstruction prior to deciding on definitive therapy (nephrectomy versus lithotomy) often significantly improves the kidney's functional status and contribution to overall renal function to make appropriate management options more apparent than at the time of initial evaluation.

Magnetic Resonance Imaging

Although MRI is not used primarily to image urinary calculi, it can differentiate stones from other nonopaque filling defects in the kidney, bladder, and elsewhere. On T_2-weighted images, stones

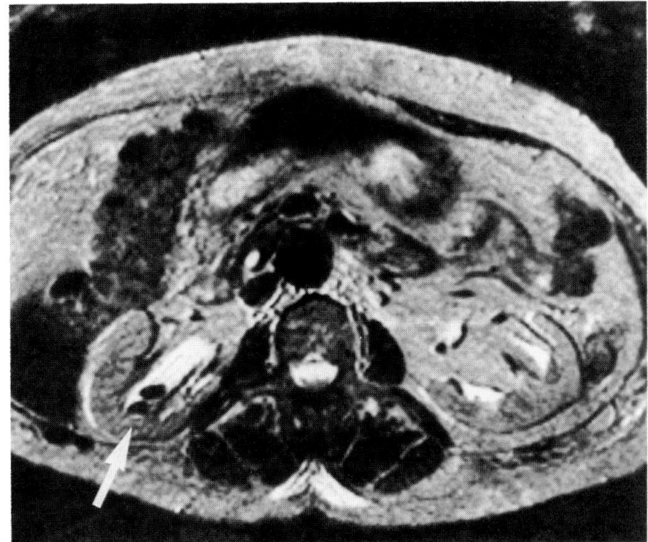

Figure 77–16. Two right-sided **nonobstructing calyceal calculi** are depicted as rounded areas of signal void *(arrow)* within the fluid-filled collecting system on this proton density axial image. Various combinations of magnetic resonance pulse sequences can be used to elucidate the nature of radiographically nonopaque urinary tract filling defects.

appear as foci of signal void within fluid (urine or contrast material)-filled structures (Fig. 77–16).

COMPLICATIONS OF UPPER URINARY TRACT UROLITHIASIS

An acutely obstructing upper urinary tract calculus rarely gives rise to significant complications, since its dramatic clinical presentation usually leads to prompt medical attention. On the other hand, the chronically stone-bearing kidney or ureter, especially if infected, may be the seat of not inconsequential complications.

While spontaneous urinary extravasation from forniceal rupture during acute obstruction is of little clinical consequence, chronic obstruction may perpetuate extravasation and produce retroperitoneal fibrosis, UPJ obstruction, or a urinoma.

Chronic calculous pyelonephritis may lead to pyonephrosis or perinephric abscess. The latter may spread widely in the retroperitoneum if untreated, and may even rupture into adjacent viscera. In such cases, renal calculi may migrate into these viscera or lie within an infected retroperitoneal urinoma. Another complication of chronic calculous pyelonephritis is xanthogranulomatous pyelonephritis. This is often accompanied by a perinephric abscess.

Long-standing urothelial irritation from infection or calculus disease can cause squamous metaplasia or leukoplakia. This keratinized squamous epithelium can desquamate to form a mass of keratin in the collecting system known as a cholesteatoma. Cellular atypia of the lower squamous epithelial layers may develop, and is a premalignant condition for squamous cell carcinoma. Renal or ureteral calculi are present in 25 to 50 per cent of cases of leukoplakia.

Although not as clinically or radiographically dramatic as these complications, a chronically obstructing renal pelvic or ureteral calculus can produce sufficient obstructive atrophy as to render the affected kidney functionless.

LOWER URINARY TRACT UROLITHIASIS

Vesical Calculi

There are relatively few causes of lower tract calculi. The majority of these stones are found in the urinary bladder. Ureteral calculi that pass into the bladder are referred to as migrant calculi. The remainder are endemic calculi, stasis calculi, or foreign body nidus calculi.

Endemic or primary calculi form in patients in whom obstruction, infection, or other calculogenic factors are not present. They are especially prevalent in young boys of low socioeconomic class in Middle and Far Eastern countries, probably related to dietary protein deficiencies. These stones are usually ammonium hydrogen urate (nonopaque), but they may be admixed with calcium salts (poorly opaque). Radiologic discovery of endemic bladder or urethral calculi occurs when evaluating such children for lower tract irritative symptoms or intermittent involuntary interruption of the urinary stream.

Most secondary calculi occur in adults (although they can occur in children) and are related to urinary stasis, as may occur with bladder outflow obstruction in males with residual urine, vesical diverticula, and/or lower urinary tract infection (Fig. 77–17); females with large cystoceles; and patients with neurogenic bladder dysfunction and residual urine, especially if infected. These calculi may be single or multiple, small or large, smooth or faceted, and of almost any composition.

Bladder calculi composed of struvite, oxalate, apatite, or mixtures thereof vary in size, shape, and radiodensity. They may attain considerable size before causing symptoms. As in the kidney, struvite and apatite calculi are usually associated with alkaline urine and urinary infection and often appear opaquely laminated (Fig. 77–18).

Stones may form in a bladder diverticulum, related in part to the stasis of urine it causes and in part to the urinary infection it may promote. A large calculus may block its neck and prevent intravesical contrast material from entering the diverticulum. The radiographic appearance is so characteristic, however, as to allow almost a definitive diagnosis of a stone-bearing diverticulum without the benefit of contrast material. Diverticular stones are usually accompanied by concretions of similar composition and appearance in the bladder itself. On occasion a dumb-bell-shaped stone may develop with one end lodged in a diverticulum and the other projecting into the bladder (Fig. 77–19).

Adenomucosa in the urinary tract probably plays a role in lithogenesis as well. It is assumed that the mucus produced provides a nidus for the formation of calculi. This occurs (a) when the bladder is augmented with intestine, (b) when bowel is used to bridge a ureteral gap (e.g., during "undiversion"), and (c) when there is exstrophy of the urinary bladder and the bladder itself contains rests of bowel mucosa.

Another major cause of vesical calculi is phosphatic encrustation

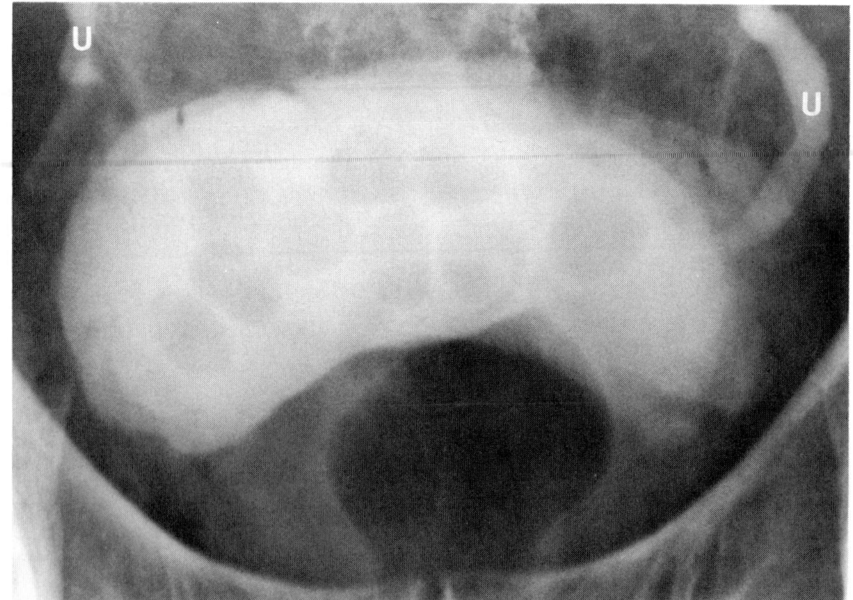

Figure 77–17. Multiple uric acid vesical calculi are imaged as nine nonopaque filling defects in the partially opacified urinary bladder of an elderly male with bladder outflow obstruction secondary to benign prostatic hyperplasia. Also note a prostatic impression on the bladder base, luminal irregularity attributable to trabeculation, and mild bilateral distal ureteral stasis due to the thickened bladder wall that the ureters traverse. (U = ureters.)

Figure 77–18. *A,* **Pelvic radiograph** obtained before an IVU in a 62-year-old male with urinary frequency and urgency shows a large laminated densely opaque bladder calculus (C), multiple small prostatic calculi overlying the superior pubic rami and, at the bottom of the film, an ovoid density *(arrowheads),* which was subsequently shown on *B,* a voiding cystourethrogram, to represent a proximal bulbar urethral calculus *(arrowheads).* The latter had not passed because of urethral stricture disease, most marked in the midbulbar urethra *(arrows).* The prostatic calculi are also well seen on this voiding study surrounding the most proximal urethra and represent a normal finding. The bladder calculus formed as a result of outflow obstruction secondary to benign prostatic hyperplasia complicated by bladder infections. (B = bladder filled with excreted contrast material from the IVU.)

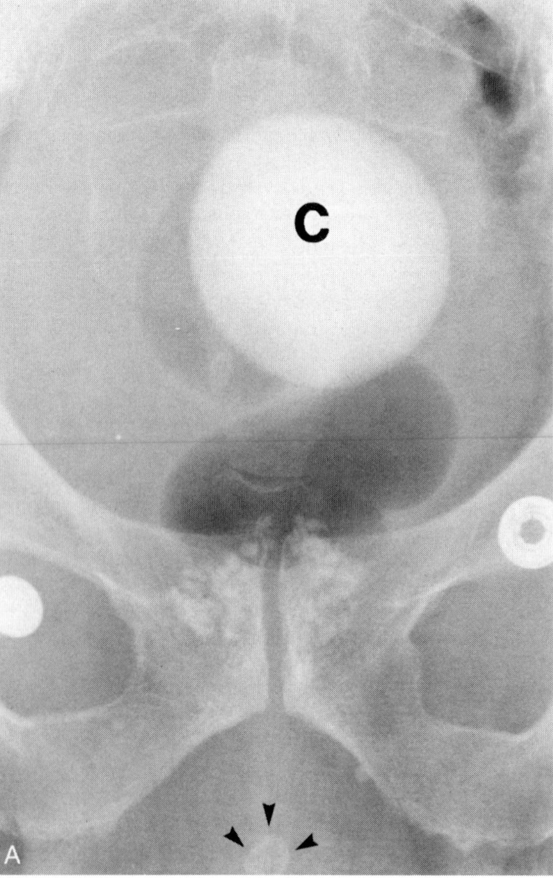

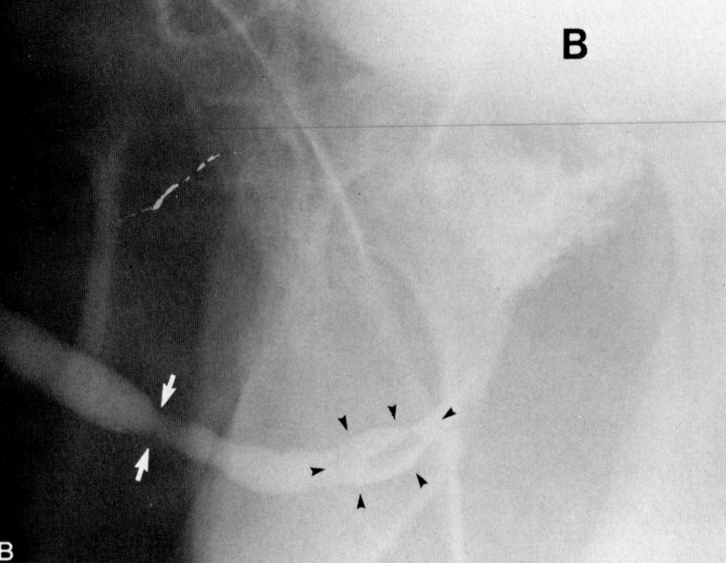

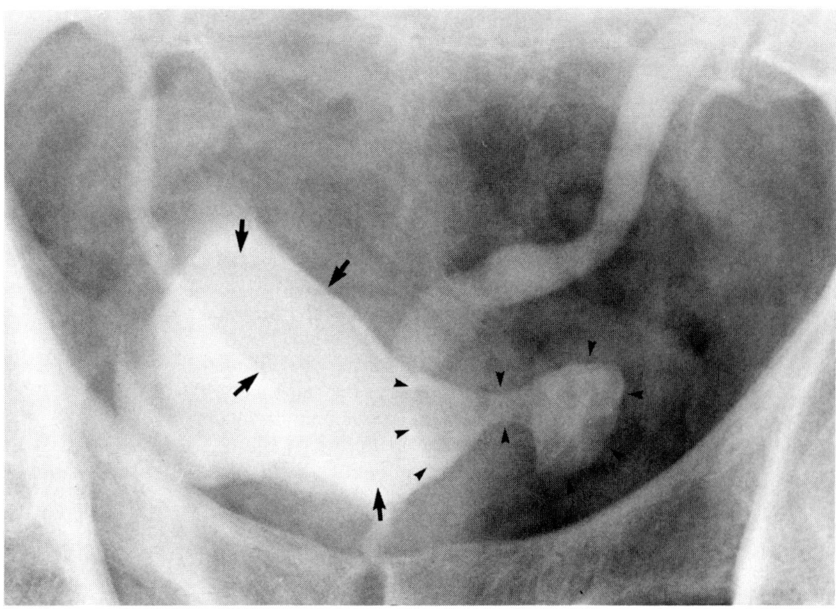

Figure 77–19. Two triple phosphate vesical calculi in an elderly male with bladder outflow obstruction and recurrent urinary bladder infections. The larger ovoid calculus *(arrows)* appears as a filling defect in the opacified bladder. Laminations in this calculus are faintly seen but were more evident on a KUB. A second dumb-bell–shaped stone is outlined by *arrowheads*. The medial portion of this stone resides in the bladder proper and the lateral half in a bladder diverticulum that has not filled with contrast material owing to calculous obstruction of its neck. The hourglass appearance of this stone should allow a diagnosis of a bladder diverticulum to be made on the KUB alone. The medial deviation of the left pelvic ureter is further evidence of a large bladder diverticulum. The ureter is dilated because of irritation and edema of the left ureteral orifice by the adjacent calculi.

on a foreign body. These calculi may be seen in both sexes and in patients of any age. Common nidi include a variety of objects self-introduced transurethrally, bone fragments from prior pelvic fractures that penetrated the bladder wall, nonabsorbable suture material used during prior pelvic surgery, prostatic chips, and Foley catheter balloon fragments. Stones may form on surgical staples that are inadvertently left exposed to urine in the pouch during the creation of a continent urinary reservoir.

The radiographic diagnosis of vesical calculus is not always straightforward, because of either poor stone opacity or mistaken identity as a phlebolith. Definitive roentgen diagnosis usually requires cystography, either an excretory cystogram as part of an IVU or a retrograde cystogram with very dilute contrast material instilled through a urethral catheter. Faintly opaque bladder calculi can be easily obscured on a KUB by fecal material in the rectosigmoid colon. On contrast studies, nonopaque calculi occasionally mimic blood clots, bladder tumors, or even intravesical growth of a hypertrophied prostate. Demonstration of the mobility of such filling defects can exclude tumor. Although the need infrequently arises to differentiate nonopaque vesical calculi from clots or tumors radiologically, these stones also exhibit acoustic shadowing on ultrasonography and may be readily identified thereby. Bladder stones are also readily apparent on CT or MRI.

Aside from phleboliths, other densities in the pelvis may simulate vesical calculi on a KUB. These include scybalous masses; baroliths; opaque suppositories or foreign bodies in the rectum; calcified rectal tumors; calcification in the cul-de-sac; stones or foreign bodies in the vagina; calcification elsewhere in the female genital tract; unusual prostatic calcifications; and a variety of bladder abnormalities, including calcified bladder tumors, inflammatory vesical calcification, calcification in areas of vesical or urachal necrosis (prune belly syndrome), or phosphatic encrustation on an intact Foley catheter balloon.

Prostatic Calculi

Most prostatic calculi result from deposition of inorganic salts (calcium phosphate and carbonate) on the corpora amylacea normally found within the prostate. These calculi, which originate in the glandular acini and ducts of the prostate, are usually multiple and relatively small, ranging from 1 to 10 mm in diameter. They are rare in boys but frequent in men, especially after the age of 40 years, and are usually of no clinical significance. Two radiographic patterns may be observed—a diffuse pattern and a horseshoe one. In the former, encountered more commonly, the small calcific densities are scattered throughout the gland (see Fig. 77–18). Depending on the size of the gland, they may be seen above, over, or even beneath the symphysis pubis. In some hyperplastic glands the calculi may be projected a considerable distance above the symphysis and mimic bladder stones. In the horseshoe or ring arrangement, the calculi are located in both sides of the gland but are absent anterior to the urethra, as evidenced by a calculus-free space that represents the opening of the horseshoe. These concretions are referred to as native prostatic calculi.

Secondary calculi form in conjunction with obstruction, stasis, or infection. Single or multiple calculi larger than those usually noted incidentally on a KUB or IVU should suggest pathologic dilatation of prostatic ducts (cavitary prostatitis) or excavation of glandular substance, as in an old abscess cavity. Such calculi are most often seen in conjunction with urethral stricture disease or other forms of urethral obstruction. Because their appearance may be mimicked by tuberculous excavation of the prostate with secondary dystrophic calcification, a careful radiographic search for other evidence of genital tuberculosis (calcified seminal vesicles or vasa or epididymides) should be made.

Occasionally, calculi form in the prostatic fossa following open prostatectomy. Persistent postoperative urinary infection and bladder neck contracture are the usual clinical findings. These calculi are usually hourglass in shape, with the upper portion of the calculus lodged in the bladder neck and the lower portion in the excavated prostatic urethra.

Urethral Calculi

Stones that form as a primary event within the urethra are known as native calculi; migrant calculi originate in the bladder or kidney and secondarily descend into the urethra. Both are seen infrequently in the United States. Most native calculi form in association with chronic stasis and infection, either within a urethral diverticulum or proximal to urethral obstruction. They are generally composed of struvite, apatite, or calcium carbonate and are usually solitary, although a large diverticulum may harbor several small stones. Migrant calculi are noted more often than native calculi, probably because they call attention to their presence by suddenly passing from the bladder into the urethral lumen, often impacting proximal to a urethral stricture or in the fossa navicularis. Urethral calculi are more common in males, in whom they are usually located in the posterior urethra, than in females, in whom virtually all reside in a urethral diverticulum. The occasional anterior urethral diverticulum in the male, if large enough to accumulate urine, may contain stones.

Even though some urethral calculi may be suspected on an IVU, radiographic diagnosis requires urethrography, performed in either retrograde or antegrade (voiding) manner. These studies localize the density in question to the urethral lumen as well as disclose associated urethral pathology (stricture, diverticulum) that may require surgical or endoscopic correction when removing the calculus (see Fig. 77–18). Urethrography can also differentiate urethral calculi from the calcific corporal and fascial plaques of Peyronie's disease, which they might mimic when seen en face on a pelvic radiograph.

Both ultrasonography and magnetic resonance imaging can be helpful in evaluating women with suspected stone-bearing urethral diverticula, especially when a diverticulum does not fill on urethrography.

Miscellaneous Lower Tract Calculi

Rarely, calculi may occur in the seminal vesicles, in an enlarged prostatic utricle or müllerian duct cyst, in a patent urachus or urachal diverticulum, in Cowper's ducts or glands, within the testicle or tunica vaginalis, or under the foreskin in association with marked phimosis (preputial calculi).

Bibliography

Banner MP: Urinary tract calculi and calcifications. In Pollack HM (ed): Clinical Urography—An Atlas and Textbook of Urological Imaging. Philadelphia, WB Saunders Company, 1989, pp 1758–1761.

Bergman H, Friedenberg RM, Sayagh V: New roentgenologic signs of carcinoma of the ureter. AJR 86:707, 1961.

Bertle M, Resnick MI: Intraoperative imaging in renal calculus surgery. Urol Radiol 6:144, 1984.

Besemann EF: Renal leukoplakia. Radiology 88:872, 1967.

Burge HJ, Middleton WD, McClennan BL, Hildebolt CF: Ureteral jets in healthy subjects and in patients with unilateral ureteral calculi: Comparison with color Doppler US. Radiology 180:437, 1991.

Courey WR, Pfister RC: The radiographic findings in renal tubular acidosis: Analysis of 21 cases. Radiology 105:497, 1972.

Douenias R, Rich M, Badalani G, et al: Predisposing factors in bladder calculi: Review of 100 cases. Urology 37:240, 1991.

Dretler SP: The pathogenesis of urinary tract calculi occurring after ileal conduit diversion: I. Clinical study. II. Conduit study. III. Prevention. J Urol 109:204, 1973.

Ezzedeen F, Adelman RD, Ahlfors CE: Renal calcification in preterm infants: Pathophysiology and long-term sequelae. J Pediatr 113:532, 1988.

Falkoff GE, Rigsby CM, Rosenfield AT: Partial, combined cortical, and medullary nephrocalcinosis: US and CT patterns in AIDS-associated MAI infection. Radiology 162:343, 1987.

Gilsanz V, Fernal LW, Reid BS, et al: Nephrolithiasis in premature infants. Radiology 154:107, 1985.

Hill MC, Rich JI, Mardiat JG, Finder CA: Sonography vs. excretory urography in acute flank pain. AJR 144:1235, 1985.

Hillman BJ, Drach GW, Tracey P, Gaines JA: Computed tomographic analysis of renal calculi. AJR 142:549, 1984.

Hinman F Jr: Directional growth of renal calculi. J Urol 121:700, 1979.

Hinman F Jr: Peripelvic extravasation during intravenous urography. Evidence for an additional route for backflow after ureteral obstruction. J Urol 85:385, 1961.

Kirks DR: Lithiasis due to interruption of enterohepatic circulation of bile salts. AJR 133:383, 1979.

Laing FC, Jeffrey RB, Wing VW: Ultrasound versus excretory urography in evaluating acute flank pain. Radiology 154:613, 1985.

Lebowitz RL, Vargas B: Stones in the urinary bladder in children and young adults. AJR 148:491, 1987.

Lesch M, Nyhan WL: A familial disorder of uric acid metabolism and central nervous system function. Am J Med 36:561, 1964.

Malek RS: Urolithiasis. In Kelalis PP, King LR, Belman AB (eds): Clinical Pediatric Urology. Philadelphia, WB Saunders Company, 1976, p 866.

Middleton WD, Dodds WJ, Lawson TL, Foley WD: Renal calculi: Sensitivity for detection with US. Radiology 167:239, 1988.

Murray RL: Milk-of-calcium in the kidney. Diagnostic features on vertical beam roentgenograms. AJR 113:455, 1971.

Newhouse JH, Prien AL, Amis ES, et al: Computed tomographic analysis of urinary calculi. AJR 142:545, 1984.

Platt JF: Duplex Doppler evaluation of native kidney dysfunction: Obstructive and nonobstructive disease. AJR 158:1035, 1992.

Pollack HM, Arger PH, Banner MP, et al: Computed tomography of renal pelvic filling defects. Radiology 138:645, 1981.

Pyrah LN, Hodgkinson A, Anderson CK: Primary hyperparathyroidism. Br J Surg 53:245, 1966.

Radin DR, Baker EL, Klatt EC, et al: Visceral and nodal calcification in patients with AIDS-related *Pneumocystis carinii* infection. AJR 154:27, 1990.

Smith LH: Medical evaluation of urolithiasis: Etiologic aspects and diagnostic evaluation. Urol Clin North Am 1:241, 1971.

Spouge AR, Wilson SR, Gopinath N, et al: Extrapulmonary *Pneumocystis carinii* in a patient with AIDS: Sonographic findings. AJR 155:76, 1990.

Thornbury JR, Silver TM, Vinson RK: Ureteroceles *vs* pseudoureteroceles in adults: Urographic diagnosis. Radiology 122:81, 1977.

Uln A, Kawamura T, Ogawa A, et al: Relation of spontaneous passage of ureteral calculi to size. Urology 10:544, 1977.

Weber AL: Primary hyperoxaluria: Roentgenographic, clinical and pathologic findings. AJR 100:155, 1967.

Whelan JG Jr, Ling JT, Davis LA: Antemortem roentgen manifestations of bilateral renal cortical necrosis. Radiology 89:682, 1967.

Williams HE: Nephrolithiasis. N Engl J Med 290:33, 1974.

Wolfman MG, Thornbury JR, Braunstein EM: Nonobstructing radiopaque ureteral calculi. Urol Radiol 1:97, 1979.

78 Stone Therapy: Extracorporeal Lithotripsy and Percutaneous Techniques

William H. Bush, Jr.

Nonsurgical removal of kidney stones has become the method of choice for most patients with symptomatic calculi. The majority of these patients can be treated by extracorporeal lithotripsy. Larger stones and staghorn calculi are treated best with initial percutaneous lithotripsy, often combined with extracorporeal lithotripsy for remaining fragments. Upper ureteral calculi are treated with extracorporeal lithotripsy. Some lower ureteral calculi can be similarly treated; others require ureteroscopy for fragmentation and removal.

INITIAL EVALUATION

The extent of calculous disease must be assessed accurately. Plain film renal tomography without contrast will suffice for all calculi except for the "nonopaque" uric acid stones. For these, computed tomography (CT) without intravenous contrast is used, since they are always opaque on CT.

Anatomy of the upper collecting system also must be defined; this is best accomplished by excretory urography. Retrograde ureteropyelography is occasionally necessary and is best done in a fluoroscopic suite following cystoscopic ureteral catheter placement; the patient can be positioned to determine the exact relationship of the calculus to the collecting system.

Renal function (serum creatinine) and hematologic status (prothrombin time) should be determined. Additional studies are indicated if clinical evaluation reveals potential problems. Infected urine dictates preoperative antibiotic therapy. If an obstructing calculus is causing pyonephrosis or sepsis, the obstruction should first be relieved by retrograde ureteral catheter placement or by a percutaneous nephrostomy, and the infection should be treated appropriately.

Metabolic evaluation of the patient should proceed concurrent with determination of therapeutic approaches. Correction of a causative metabolic disorder (which can be identified in nearly 75 per cent of patients with urolithiasis) usually arrests growth of existing stones and prevents formation of new ones. Analysis of the chemical composition of removed stones is also helpful in subsequent clinical management.

EXTRACORPOREAL LITHOTRIPSY

The term "lithotripsy" describes various nonoperative techniques and is derived from the Greek *lithos* (stone) and *tribo* (to grind down, wear away). The brittleness of kidney stones makes them vulnerable to treatment by shock waves. Cavitation in fluid adjacent to the calculus creates shock wave forces that develop tensile stresses in the calculus, leading to the formation of cracks and ultimately disintegration of the calculus into particles; these, in turn, are fragmented into granules (Fig. 78–1). Compared with ultrasonic waves, the impulses produced by shock waves in the propagation medium are of high amplitude but short duration.

Soft tissues are also affected by shock wave passage and these same cavitation effects, evidenced by skin bruising after treatment with the high-energy Dornier HM-3 extracorporeal shock wave lithotripsy (ESWL) unit; similar organ tissue changes are demonstrated by CT and by magnetic resonance imaging (MRI). Contusions have been demonstrated in the kidneys, bowel, and pancreas. Lung tissue, because of its many air-water interfaces, is highly susceptible to shock wave trauma. Conversely, living bone is relatively unaffected by shock wave energy because of its resiliency, although bone does constitute acoustic interfaces and prevents passage of the shock waves.

Differing substantially in technical components, all lithotripters share basic features of an energy source, a focusing method, a coupling medium, and an imaging/stone localization system. The Dornier HM-3 ESWL unit uses electrohydraulic shock waves generated by a spark gap in a water medium or water bath that are focused by an ellipsoidal reflector (Fig. 78–2). The shock waves are of such high energy that stones are usually fragmented adequately in one treatment; however, epidural anesthesia is necessary. A newer model with a larger ellipsoid permits a broader entrance pathway that is much less painful. These patients are treated with only intravenous sedation and analgesia. The piezoelectric lithotripter generates shock waves by the sudden expansion of ceramic elements excited by a high-voltage pulse.

With the ultrasonic devices, waves from the large curved source are propagated through either a water bag (EDAP and Diasonics) or a water basin (Wolf); the broad zone of entry eliminates the need for anesthesia. However, the lower peak pressures generated at the treatment focus of these lower-energy units usually necessitate repeated treatments of the calculus for adequate stone fragmentation. In the electromagnetic unit (Siemens), shocks are formed when an electrical impulse moves a metallic membrane in a water-filled conduction tube.

Stone imaging or localization is achieved with fluoroscopy (Dornier HM-3), ultrasonography (Dornier MPL-9000, EDAP, Wolf), or a combination of fluoroscopy and ultrasonography (Siemens). Fluoroscopic localization has advantages in that it is an imaging technique familiar to urologists and can be used to locate and target calculi in the ureter. However, contrast material is necessary to localize radiolucent calculi. Ultrasonography is the calculus localization method on most newer lithotripsy machines, although quality of the ultrasonic image varies with the unit. Although computer-coordinated, articulated, locating ultrasonic heads are of high quality, in-line units provide poorer quality images, particularly with larger patients. Separation of large fragments from a collection of small fragments can become quite difficult with the in-line units.

Clinical Results with Extracorporeal Lithotripsy

The stone location, size, number, and composition, as well as the anatomy of the renal collecting system, all affect the success of treatment by extracorporeal lithotripsy and, therefore, the selection

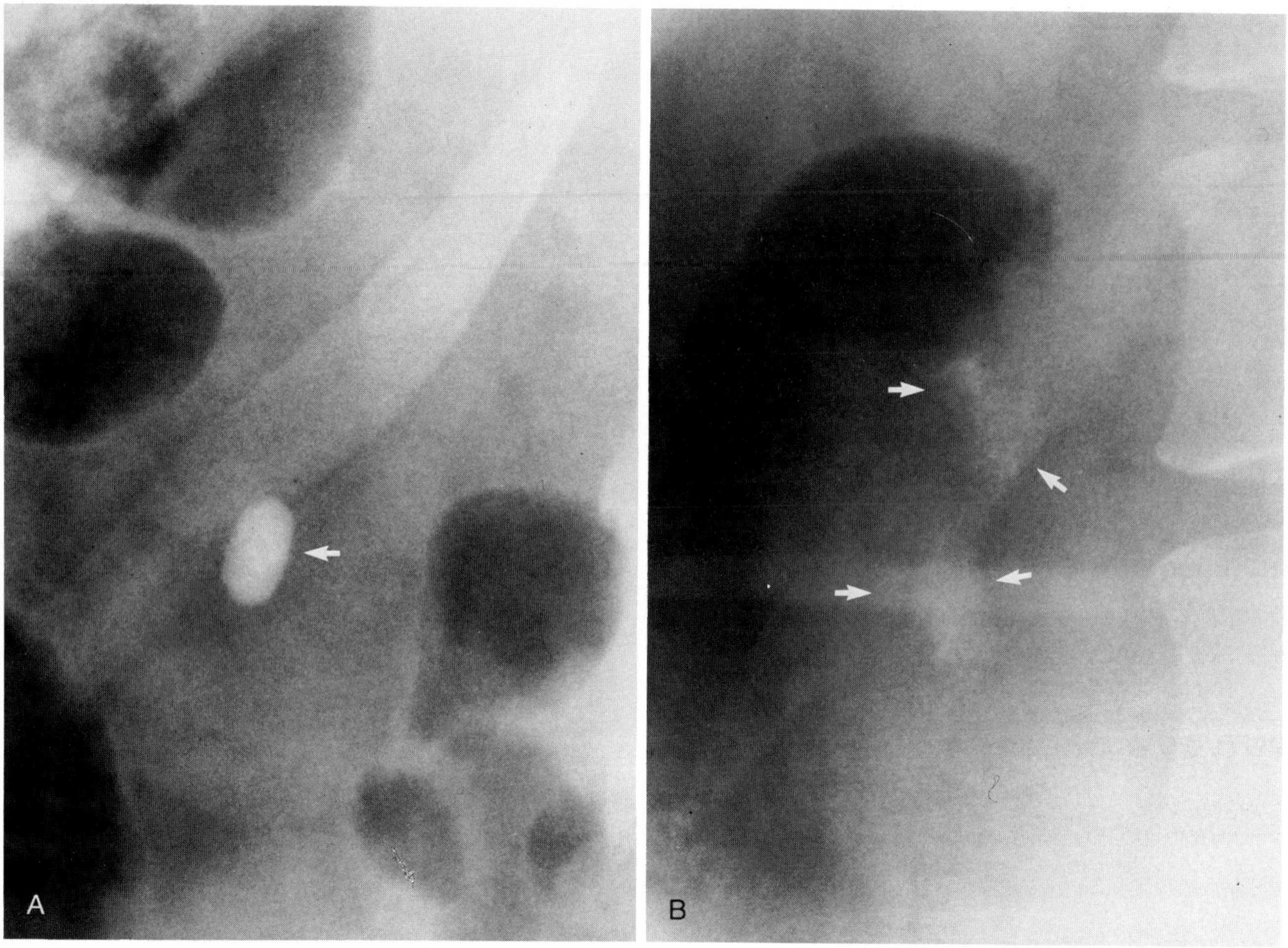

Figure 78–1. Example of stone fragmentation by extracorporeal shock wave lithotripsy (ESWL). *A,* Two-cm calculus in the lower infundibulum of the right kidney *(arrow). B,* Following 600 shocks, the stone has been totally fragmented, and the small particles and granules fill the lower infundibulum and calices *(arrows).*

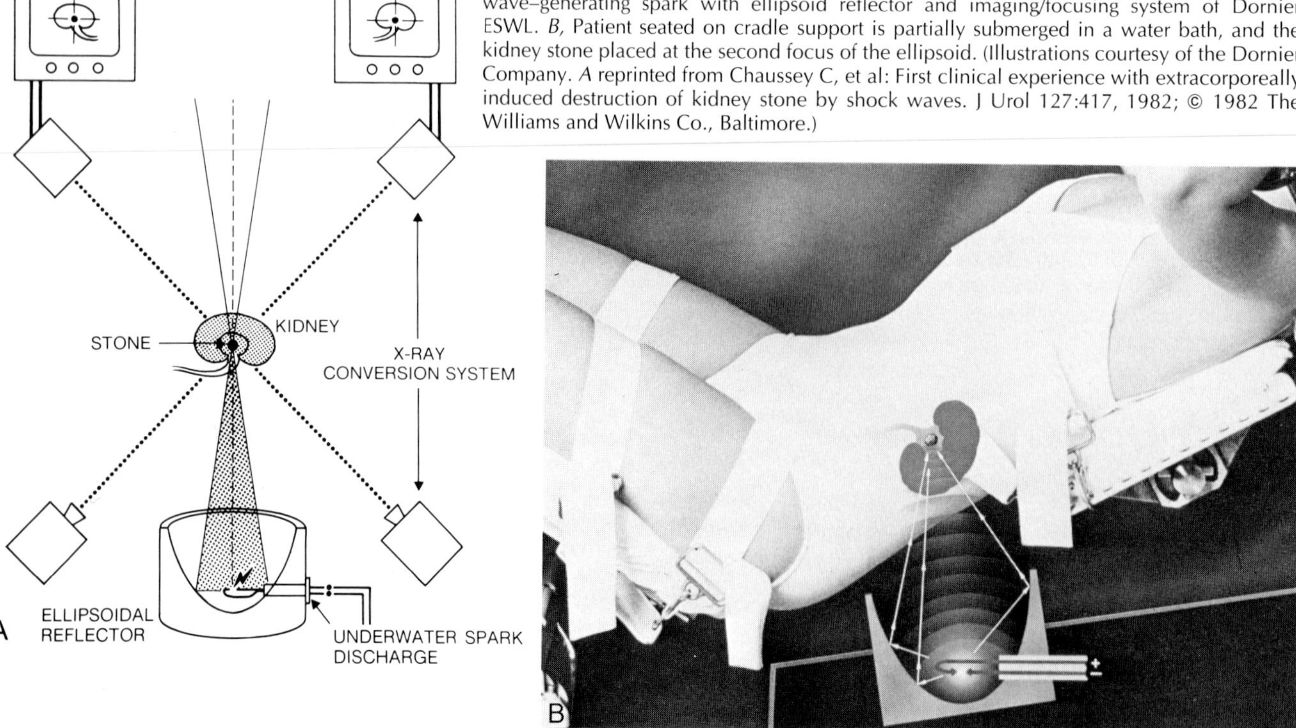

Figure 78–2. Extracorporeal shock wave lithotripsy (ESWL). *A,* Diagram of shock wave–generating spark with ellipsoid reflector and imaging/focusing system of Dornier ESWL. *B,* Patient seated on cradle support is partially submerged in a water bath, and the kidney stone placed at the second focus of the ellipsoid. (Illustrations courtesy of the Dornier Company. *A* reprinted from Chaussey C, et al: First clinical experience with extracorporeally induced destruction of kidney stone by shock waves. J Urol 127:417, 1982; © 1982 The Williams and Wilkins Co., Baltimore.)

of this modality as the primary treatment method. Obstruction of the collecting system distal to the calculus, whether it be due to a stenotic infundibulum, congenital ureteropelvic junction narrowing, or stricturing in the ureter, is a primary contraindication to extracorporeal lithotripsy. Usually, patients with such an obstruction can be treated by combining the techniques of percutaneous nephrostolithotomy and extracorporeal lithotripsy. The stenotic infundibulum or ureteropelvic junction area is treated with incision, dilation, and stenting, and at the same session, the calculus is removed percutaneously; any residual fragments are treated by extracorporeal lithotripsy.

Calculi in a horseshoe kidney are more effectively treated by percutaneous nephrostolithotomy than by ESWL. With extracorporeal lithotripsy, only about 50 per cent of patients will achieve freedom from their calculi, whereas nearly all of patients treated with percutaneous techniques can be rendered stone-free. Access to a horseshoe kidney is best achieved by a posterior approach through an upper calyx, which provides optimal access to the collecting system.

Stone size determines significantly the effectiveness of extracorporeal lithotripsy. Of patients with a calculus less than 1 cm in diameter, over 95 per cent will be stone-free at three months following lithotripsy with a high-power unit. However, if the stone is 2 to 3 cm in diameter, only about 50 per cent of patients are stone-free at three months after treatment. Extracorporeal lithotripsy of a staghorn calculus inevitably requires multiple sessions with long intervals between sessions to permit passage of the fragments. Even so, a high incidence of remaining particles is still observed at three months. By combining initial percutaneous nephrostolithotomy for debulking, with subsequent extracorporeal lithotripsy of the remaining portions of the calculus (particularly those in the calyces), 80 to 90 per cent of patients with a staghorn calculus can be rendered stone-free at three months.

A calculus in a calyceal diverticulum can be fragmented easily with extracorporeal lithotripsy, though the patient is rendered stone-free in only 20 to 30 per cent of cases; the fragments remain trapped in the diverticulum. Interestingly, twice that number will have improvement or resolution of their symptoms. Milk-of-calcium stones, however, because of their nature, do not fragment with extracorporeal lithotripsy. If they are symptomatic, percutaneous nephrostolithotomy of the calyceal calculi and dilatation and stenting of the diverticular neck are recommended.

Composition determines the hardness or brittleness of the calculus and the effectiveness of the treatment method. Harder stones, such as calcium oxalate monohydrate and cystine, require more shocks at higher intensity to achieve adequate fragmentation.

The various combinations of collecting system anatomy, stone location, and composition result in the following recommendations:

1. For calculi less than or equal to 2 cm in diameter, extracorporeal lithotripsy is recommended unless the stone is composed of cystine, or the calculus is located in a calyceal diverticulum or a dilated dependent calyx; in these latter situations, percutaneous nephrostolithotomy is recommended.
2. For calculi 2 to 3 cm in diameter, extracorporeal lithotripsy is recommended for suspected calcium oxalate dihydrate. Percutaneous nephrostolithotomy is recommended for the larger, harder calculi of calcium oxalate monohydrate, brushite, or cystine, or for stones associated with chronic bacteriuria and/or dilation of the collecting system.
3. Most larger calculi—that is, over 3 cm in diameter—are better treated with percutaneous nephrostolithotomy followed by extracorporeal lithotripsy; the exception is a soft stone in a system that will provide adequate drainage.

Success of treatment by any modality depends on how one defines success and the sensitivity of the imaging techniques to identify residual fragments. One definition of a successful treatment is a patient who is stone-free or has residual fragments smaller than 3 mm, determined by ultrasonography and abdominal radiographs, or when at least 90 per cent of the stone mass has passed and the remaining fragments are smaller than 3 mm at the last follow-up. Plain film radiography has been the imaging modality used to determine the success of lithotripsy treatments; this use certainly can be challenged. Based on evaluation by flexible nephroscopy, plain radiographs and renal tomograms overestimate stone-free rates by 35 per cent and 17 per cent, respectively. Renal tomography is superior to a plain film radiograph alone, and it is the rare patient who will have a negative tomogram yet a positive radiograph. Conversely, when the abdominal plain film is "negative," tomography will often find small or mildly opaque calculus fragments up to 6 to 7 mm in diameter. The significance of residual fragments is controversial but relates to stone regrowth and persistent "infection" (struvite) stones.

Most institutions and groups are no longer using ureteral stents routinely for extracorporeal lithotripsy. Although many urologists believed initially that stents decreased morbidity following treatment of larger stones and assisted fragment passage, subsequent studies have shown that ureteral stents do not reduce post-lithotripsy complications, do not markedly improve stone passage from the kidney, and are clearly associated with their own irritative-type morbidity. About 15 per cent of patients treated with extracorporeal lithotripsy will develop a steinstrasse ("street of stones") in the ureter as fragments pass (Fig. 78–3), and this occurs as frequently with stents as without them.

Ureteral Calculi

For calculi in the upper and distal ureteral segments, in situ extracorporeal lithotripsy is the treatment of choice. Success rates of over 80 per cent and over 75 per cent, respectively, can be expected. Mid-ureteral calculi treated in situ with the Dornier HM-3 lithotripter will be successfully fragmented in over 80 per cent of patients.

Patients with ureteral stones may be managed expectantly, or treated with a variety of invasive and noninvasive techniques depending on stone composition, size, location, anatomy, and expectations of the patient. As shown by Morse and Resnik at the Cleveland Clinic, of ureteral calculi 5 mm in diameter or smaller in the middle or lower ureter, approximately 50 per cent will pass spontaneously. The percentage of stone passage will increase with a decrease in stone size. Passage rate for similar size stones in the upper ureter is substantially less, likely reflecting the availability and efficacy of in situ ESWL for the stone, combined with an unwillingness of the patient to tolerate the discomfort of stone passage. For stones in the mid and lower ureter, it is important, in this era of high technology, to not lose sight of the fact that the majority of small stones will pass spontaneously.

Complications of Extracorporeal Lithotripsy

Although renal contusion after ESWL is demonstrated readily with MRI, clinically significant subcapsular hematomas occur uncommonly, or about 0.5 per cent of the time. Risk factors include hypertension and aspirin. Patients who have taken aspirin have altered platelet function; since platelet half-life is 5 to 7 days, discontinuance of aspirin 14 days before the procedure is recommended.

Trauma by extracorporeal shock waves to organs in the region of

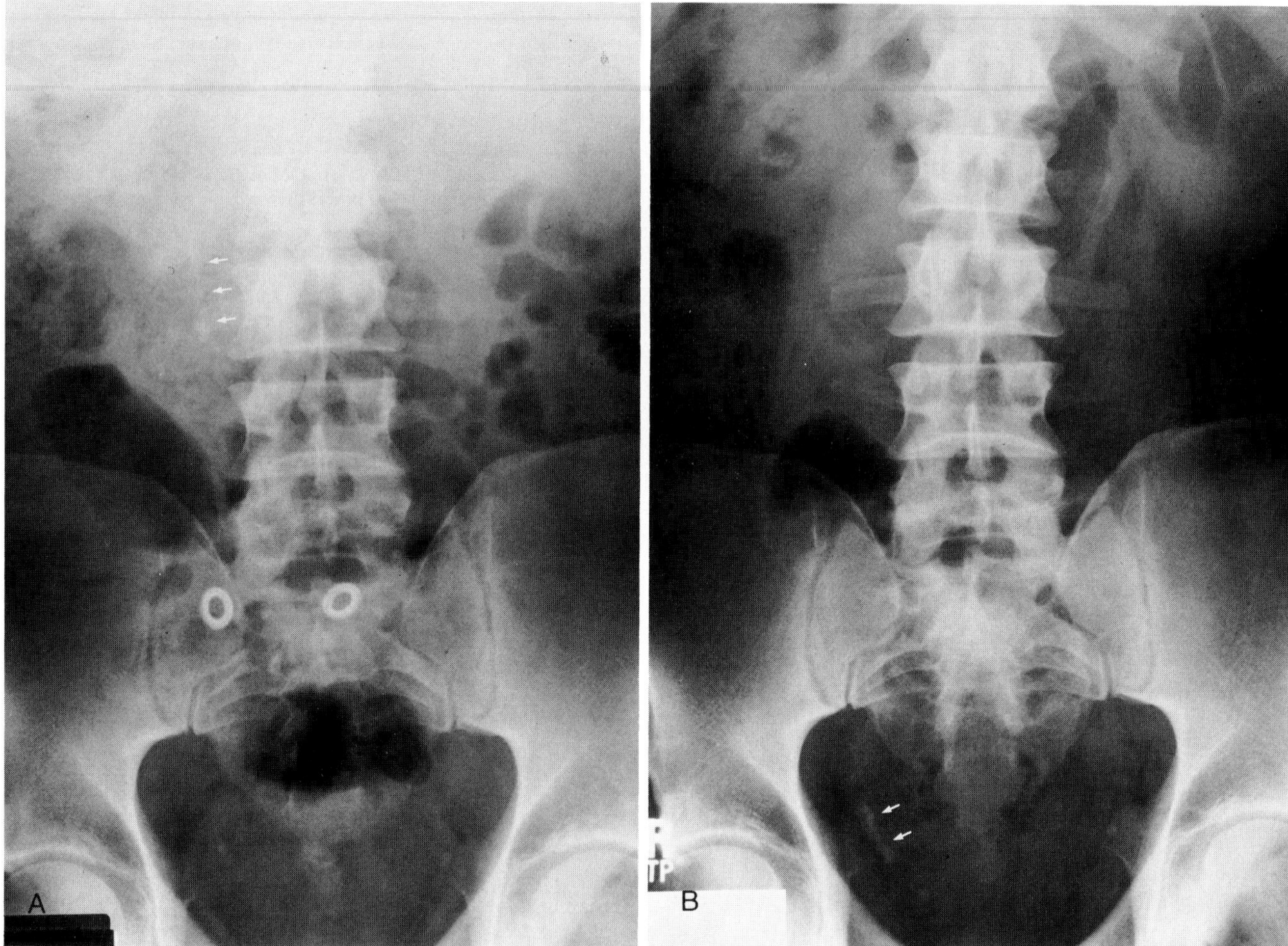

Figure 78–3. Illustration of stone granule passing down the ureter after fragmentation of a renal pelvic caculus by ESWL. *A,* The column of granules and stone fragments ("steinstrasse") is seen in the upper ureter *(arrows)* four days after ESWL. *B,* Further passage of the steinstrasse through the ureter. One day later, the column of granules and fragments is seen in the lower ureter *(arrows)*. The ureter was completely clear of fragments two weeks later.

the kidneys or in the shock wave path present as a clinical problem only uncommonly. A case of shock wave–induced pancreatic trauma has been reported. Similarly, in our own patients we have encountered one who developed a hematoma of the hepatic flexure of the right colon after receiving ESWL for gallstones.

In a clinical study of patients undergoing ESWL, 14.3 per cent developed bacteremia during treatment. In three of these seven patients, the urine culture was sterile. As similarly shown in a study of nephrostomy tube placement, culture of voided urine is an unreliable indicator of the kidneys being a potential source of bacteremia.

Hypertension was reported as a sequela of ESWL, but initial data were conflicting. Lingeman et al reported initially an alarmingly high incidence (8.2 per cent) of new-onset hypertension in their patients treated by ESWL. In a larger and more controlled study, these authors have now found that the annualized incidence of hypertension (2.4 per cent) in patients who received ESWL did not differ significantly from controls (4.0 per cent). Although a rise in diastolic pressure after treatment was noted in the study, the effect was more pronounced in patients who had treatment of stones in the ureter. In conclusion, the authors find no evidence that ESWL patients have a higher incidence of hypertension over an average two-year follow-up.

PERCUTANEOUS STONE REMOVAL: ACHIEVING ACCESS

Single-Stage or Staged Procedure

Percutaneous stone removal may be completed in one or more stages. For the single-stage procedure, both percutaneous access and calculus removal are accomplished in one session in the operating room, usually under general anesthesia. For the staged procedure, percutaneous access is obtained at an initial session, usually with local anesthesia; calculus removal is done later under general anesthesia. With either method, a radiologist-urologist team approach is advocated. Extending fluoroscopic and angiographic skills to this application, the radiologist establishes the percutaneous access route and dilates the tract for the instruments. Applying cystoscopic and clinical skills, the urologist utilizes the nephroscope to inspect the kidney and identify and remove the calculus. Fluoroscopic assistance by the radiologist during the removal process is often helpful. Undoubtedly, one person can learn to do all components of the procedure; however, patient care is usually optimized if the procedure is done as a joint radiologist-urologist effort.

COLLECTING SYSTEM OPACIFICATION

Having an opacified, distended collecting system facilitates percutaneous access. Intravenous contrast injection, augmented by a diuretic, may achieve this in some cases. Renal pelvis puncture with a 22-gauge needle (Chiba type) may also be used for contrast injection, although adequate distention of a nonobstructed collecting system may not be possible by this means. Cystoscopic placement of a retrograde ureteral catheter for injection of dilute (e.g., 20 per cent) contrast optimizes collecting system distention and opacification. If the calculus is first identified fluoroscopically and contrast injection is monitored fluoroscopically, the exact position of the calculus relative to the collecting system can be defined. Since a posterior calyx in a prone patient may not fill adequately with contrast owing to residual urine, gas or air can be injected through the retrograde catheter to outline the collecting system and calculus.

PUNCTURE FOR ACCESS

Antegrade percutaneous entrance can be done with a variety of needles (22-gauge coaxial, 21-gauge coaxial, 18-gauge). A dual or parallel-needle approach with single-needle puncture has some advantages; the 22-gauge allows directional assessment with minimal trauma to tissue, whereas the 18-gauge is stiff enough to permit exact calyx or proximal infundibular puncture.

A point on the skin of the posterolateral torso below the twelfth rib is selected for needle insertion. This point is near the posterior axillary line in obese patients, and two to three fingerbreadths lateral to the margin of the erector spinae muscles in thinner patients. This point of entrance varies considerably with body build. Also, it is important to realize that the colon can be located far posteriorly, particularly in thin, older females. The relationships of the calculus and kidney to other organs, particularly the diaphragm, spleen, and colon, should be determined if placement of the main percutaneous tract to an upper calyx or through an intercostal approach is being considered. Abdominal CT scanning will be necessary in the more complex cases.

Initially a 22-gauge "localization" needle is inserted toward the calculus and down to the renal capsule. This defines direction for the "puncture" needle. An 18-gauge, 15-cm-long, stylet-tipped or blunted cannula needle is then inserted gradually in a parallel course, and its position appropriately adjusted (Fig. 78–4). With the fluoroscopic beam parallel to the needle, the mediolateral location of the needle is defined. With the fluoroscopic beam perpendicular to the needle, the depth of insertion is defined, as well as cephalocaudad location. The 18-gauge needle is inserted incrementally

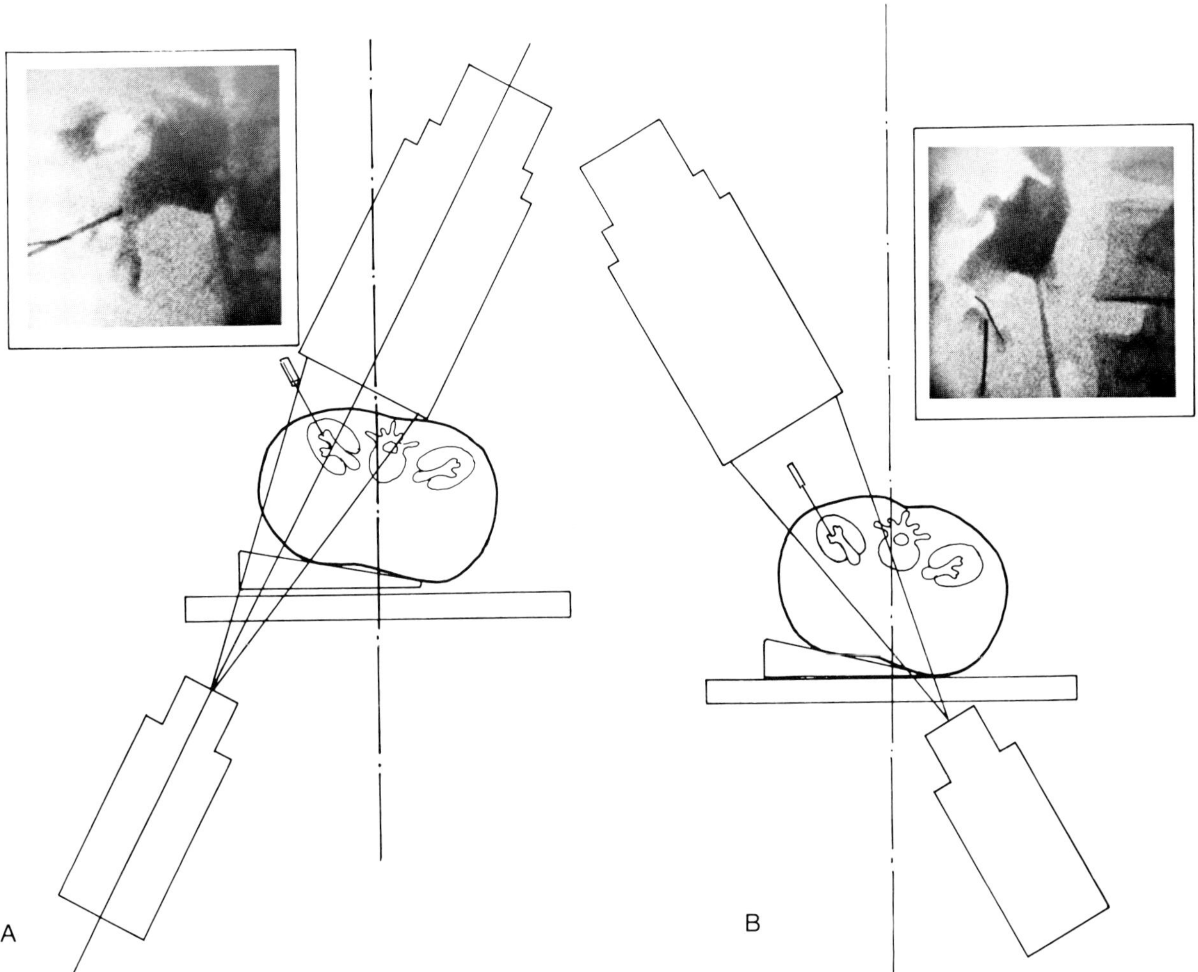

Figure 78–4. Multidirectional C-arm fluoroscopy and radiographic images obtained during percutaneous access for calculus removal. *A,* C-arm fluoroscope rotated so that x-ray beam is perpendicular to needles. Cephalocaudad direction and depth of needles are defined. *B,* C-arm fluoroscope rotated so that x-ray beam is parallel to the needle. Mediolateral orientation of the needles is defined. (Reprinted from Bush WH, et al: Access techniques for successful percutaneus nephrostolithotomy. Appl Radiol 14:86–92, 1985, with permission of the publisher.)

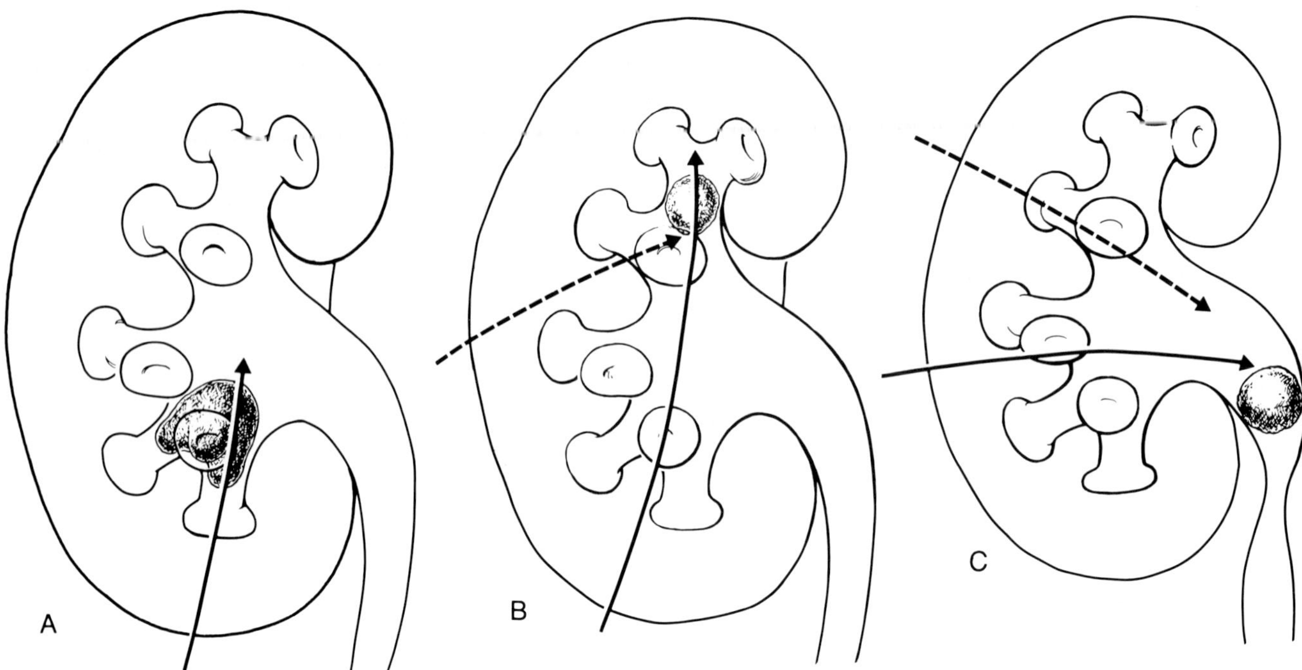

Figure 78–5. Location of stone determines entrance site for percutaneous nephrostolithotomy. *A,* Calculus in the lower calyceal area is approached directly with nephroscope inserted into the calculus-containing calyx. *B,* An upper calyx calculus is approached through an inferior calyx and subcostal insertion *(solid arrow),* or may be approached directly through an intercostal insertion *(dotted arrow). C,* Calculus in the ureteropelvic junction is approached through a lateral calyx; an upper ureter calculus is approached either through a lateral calyx *(solid arrow)* or, if necessary, intercostally through an upper calyx, intercostal approach *(dotted arrow).* (Reprinted from Bush WH, et al: Access techniques for successful percutaneous nephrostolithotomy. Appl Radiol 14:86–92, 1985, with permission of the publisher.)

(e.g., at 2-cm intervals) as the fluoroscope is rotated frequently between the parallel and perpendicular positions. The combination of multidirectional imaging and a stiff needle permits placement of the needle tip in the specific calyx desired. Successful removal of more difficult calculi depends on this precise placement.

The point of cutaneous entry and the calyx chosen for renal entrance are determined by the location of the calculus to be removed (Fig. 78–5). A calculus in a lateral, posterior, or inferior calyx is approached directly. A calculus in an upper-pole calyx may be approached through subcostal insertion by way of a lower calyx, or it may be approached directly through a posterior intercostal insertion. A calculus at the ureteropelvic junction or in the upper ureter is approached subcostally by way of a lateral calyx or intercostally through an upper calyx. Preferably, the major nephrostomy tract is created below the twelfth rib to allow best mobility of instruments; to minimize trauma to the lung, spleen, and pleura; and to minimize periosteal pain. For lower anterior calyx calculi, and for some upper lateral calyx calculi, it may be necessary to place the major tract between the eleventh and twelfth ribs. With a supra-twelfth access route, complications of hydro- and/or pneumothorax occur in 6 per cent of these patients and are substantially more frequent when the approach is above the eleventh rib. A major nephrostomy route above the eleventh rib should be avoided if at all possible.

The entrance point into the collecting system should also be peripherally in a calyx. This approach leaves more room in the collecting system to maneuver the instruments and provides better fixation for the postoperative nephrostomy tube. It also minimizes injury to vessels during the access procedure, although inadvertent damage to smaller interlobar arteries cannot be avoided completely. Major vessels cross the renal pelvis and are closely applied to the infundibular regions, particularly around the upper infundibulum (Fig. 78–6). Posterolateral access into the kidney is also in the region of Brödel's "avascular" zone, which should also decrease the risk of vessel injury.

DILATATION OF TRACT

With appropriate access established, the tract must be dilated to accept a working sheath (24 to 30 Fr) or the 24 Fr nephroscope. Initially, however, a safety guidewire is placed down the ureter. This essential step should not be skipped, as it provides a secure route for access back into the kidney if the nephroscope becomes dislodged during the calculus removal process.

A variety of dilator systems are available. The Amplatz system uses a series of polyethylene fascial dilators (12 to 30 Fr) inserted over an 8 Fr Teflon catheter and a guidewire. Fascial dilator systems that pass directly over a guidewire have a more tapered tip and are more flexible in a curved tract. Rigidity of the system can be improved by using a stiff wire such as the Lunderquist exchange wire. High-pressure balloon catheters facilitate a rapid, smooth dilation, and they are particularly helpful with curved tracts or an angulated entrance at the kidney.

A Teflon working sheath can be inserted after dilation, and through this, extraction instruments, such as a basket or grasper, can be directly inserted and monitored fluoroscopically. The nephroscope can be inserted through the working sheath or directly through the tract into the kidney without a working sheath. If the ureteropelvic region is patulous, an occlusion balloon should be placed to prevent migration of the calculus or fragments into the upper ureter.

PERCUTANEOUS REMOVAL TECHNIQUES

Irrigation

Saline irrigation or flushing through a working sheath is only occasionally helpful. However, for calculi composed of struvite,

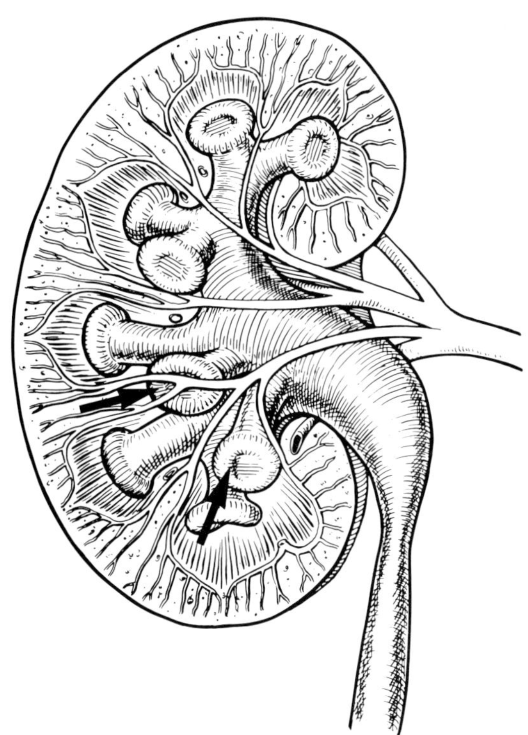

Figure 78–6. Diagram of **renal vascularity,** showing how major vessel injury can be avoided by peripheral nephrostomy insertion *(arrows).* (After Melloni BJ: Melloni's Illustrated Medical Dictionary. Baltimore, Williams and Wilkins Company, 1979.)

cystine, or uric acid, chemolysis can be effective. It is important that the stone be directly bathed with the solution and that there be a second catheter for drainage. The ureter itself is usually not adequate for drainage, since it may become obstructed, and continued irrigation into a "closed" system can quickly endanger the patient.

Grasp Removal

Direct removal of calculi less than 1 cm in diameter with grasping instruments avoids the problem of residual fragments. A variety of instruments are available for use through the nephroscope. The Mazzariello-Caprini forcep is used directly through the tract and is most effective through a matured tract (e.g., one week after a nephrostomy creation). This forcep has the advantage of a "twisting" shaft rather than a "scissors" action and requires minimal tract diameter for complete opening.

Fragmentation

Some method of fragmentation must be employed for calculi greater than 1 cm. The electrohydraulic lithotripter fragments stones by shock waves in water produced by a discharging spark. However, the electrohydraulic instruments lack adequate suction for fragment removal, and the shock wave discharge can cause mucosal damage. For routine use, ultrasonic lithotripters have supplanted the electrohydraulic instruments.

Percutaneous Ultrasonic Lithotripsy (PUL)

Current equipment for PUL consists of a rigid hollow probe that is inserted through a 24 Fr nephroscope (Fig. 78–7). The probe visually is placed in contact with the calculus, and ultrasonic energy up to 23 mHz is conducted to the stone, causing it to fragment. The combination of suction through the hollow probe and infusion of saline irrigant around the probe removes the fragments as they are created. Complete calculus removal will be achieved at the initial session in 80 per cent of patients; residual calyceal fragments are treated with extracorporeal lithotripsy. PUL offers the ability to fragment and remove large or multiple calculi.

Problem Calculi and Special Techniques

Staghorn Calculi. A large staghorn calculus can fill the collecting system. Special attention is required in selecting the point of access, which must be a calyx or infundibulum with adequate space to allow initial access for the nephroscope. A safety back-up wire should be maintained. Although this can be coiled in a large dilated part of the collecting system, preferably the wire should be placed down the ureter.

Calyceal Diverticulum. Treatment of calculi in a calyceal diverticulum or calyx with stenotic infundibulum requires treatment not only of the calculus but also of the narrowed drainage lumen. A tract entering the specific calyx or one giving a direct line approach to an anterior or upper calyx simplifies removal and greatly increases the likelihood of success. The stenotic infundibulum or neck of the calyceal diverticulum is treated by overdilation and stenting with a modified pigtail catheter that includes not only holes in the renal pelvis pigtail loop but also additional holes along the stent segment traversing the infundibular and calyceal areas. Duration of stenting has varied from two to six weeks. Lack of parenchyma over the diverticulum or dilated calyx can adversely affect healing of the percutaneous tract, although with adequate treatment of the stenotic infundibulum, this has not been a problem in our experience.

The Medi-Tech steerable catheter combined with a snare made from guidewires is an effective flexible instrument for calculus retrieval from large and small calyces. The blunt tip of the guidewire loop snare avoids the problem of parenchymal penetration encountered with using stone baskets to retrieve calculi from small calyces. The "steerable loop snare system" can be used intraoperatively through a working sheath or later through a mature tract. A double-loop snare of 0.071 cm (0.028 inch) wires is used through a 13 Fr catheter, and a double-loop snare of 0.053 cm (0.021 inch) wires through a 10 Fr catheter.

Ureteral Calculi. Ureteral calculi pose special problems in management. Natural passage depends on size, and most calculi less than 4 mm in diameter will pass spontaneously. Urologic techniques are available for removing symptomatic calculi from the lower ureter.

Symptomatic calculi in the upper ureter that fail to pass spontaneously or cannot be treated by ESWL require interventional procedures. Ureteroscopy and fragmentation of the calculus with electrohydraulic lithotripsy or laser lithotripsy are very effective for larger stones in the mid and upper ureter. Selection of the best method for removing ureteral calculi depends on many factors, including body habitus, previous surgery in the region, collecting system anatomy, and composition of the stone.

Extraction by percutaneous nephrostomy is an effective alternate method for upper ureteral calculi. Following cystoscopic placement of a retrograde ureteral catheter, some calculi can be flushed into the renal pelvis or displaced upward with the catheter. Through the percutaneous nephrostomy, these are then removed by grasping or ultrasonic lithotripsy. For those calculi that remain in the upper ureter, the retrograde catheter is advanced past the stone. Retrieval with a stone basket is then tried; the Burhenne or other basket that can be removed from its sheath is used for the "basket-sheath exchange maneuver." If basket extraction fails, a steerable catheter loop-snare system similar to that used for calyceal calculi is tried.

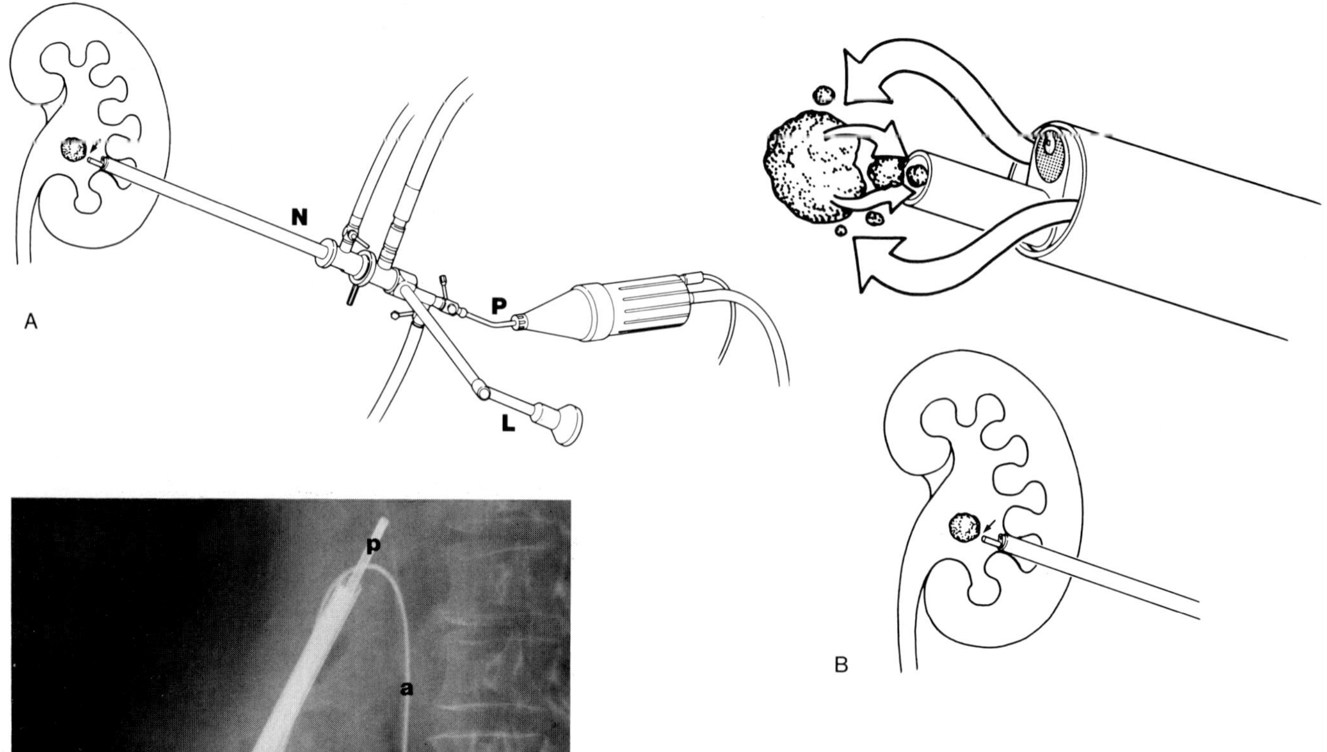

Figure 78–7. Diagram of **percutaneous ultrasonic lithotriptor.** *A,* Nephroscope (N) with side-viewing lens (L) is inserted into kidney. Ultrasonic probe (P) is passed through nephroscope to contact calculus *(arrow). B,* Percutaneous ultrasonic fragmentation of calculus. Hollow probe is visually placed in contact with the stone *(arrow).* During saline irrigation about the probe, stone fragmentation is initiated and sand-like granules are aspirated through the hollow probe. *C,* Radiograph of nephroscope (N) and ultrasonic probe (p) during PUL. (a = Antegrade safety ureteral catheter.)

If a stone can be brought up into the renal pelvis but not out of the kidney, an occlusion balloon should be inserted to block the ureteropelvic junction and avoid progression of the stone back down the ureter during the final nephroscopic removal process.

Postoperative or Conclusion Studies

Patients are given intravenous antibiotics during the stone removal procedure and for one to two days thereafter. A large-bore nephrostomy tube (22 to 24 Fr) drains the kidney, and for the first 12 to 24 hours the ureteral safety guidewire or catheter is left in place. One or two days following the procedure, tomograms of the kidney are obtained to ensure that all stones and fragments have been removed (Fig. 78–8*A*). CT is used for those stones that are composed primarily of uric acid. If no fragments remain, the ureteral wire is removed and a nephrostogram is done to check nephrostomy tube position and to evaluate the integrity of the collecting system (Fig. 78–8*B*). The nephrostomy tube can then be clamped. The tube is removed after it has been clamped for 6 to 12 hours without causing symptoms. Usually the tube can be removed before the patient is discharged from the hospital, although some patients require longer outpatient nephrostomy drainage because of edema in the ureter or ureteropelvic junction.

Radiation Exposure to Patient and Personnel During Stone Removal

Fluoroscopy is an integral part of percutaneous stone removal; C-arm or multidirectional fluoroscopy facilitates greatly the entrance procedure and guidance of non-nephroscopic instruments. Therefore, the patient and uroradiologic personnel receive measurable radiation exposure. Surface radiation dose to the gonad area of the patient has been in the range of 600 mrem (6 mSv) for women, and 150 mrem (1.5 mSv) for men. These levels are similar to exposures from a seven-view excretory urogram. Radiation dose to personnel performing the procedure has been at levels similar to those from other interventional procedures, about 10 mrem (0.10 mSv) per case.

Minimizing radiation exposure is important and can be achieved by proper shielding (radiation-resistant glasses with side shields, thyroid shield, 0.5-mm lead-equivalent apron, radiation-resistant surgical gloves), and by judicious use of fluoroscopy. The incorporation of a single-frame video disc recording unit can often greatly decrease fluoroscopy time.

Radiation dose to the patient during ESWL with the Dornier HM-3 lithotripter is less than doses from percutaneous procedures and is similar to that incurred during an upper gastrointestinal barium study. Radiation to personnel in the lithotripter suite is minimal.

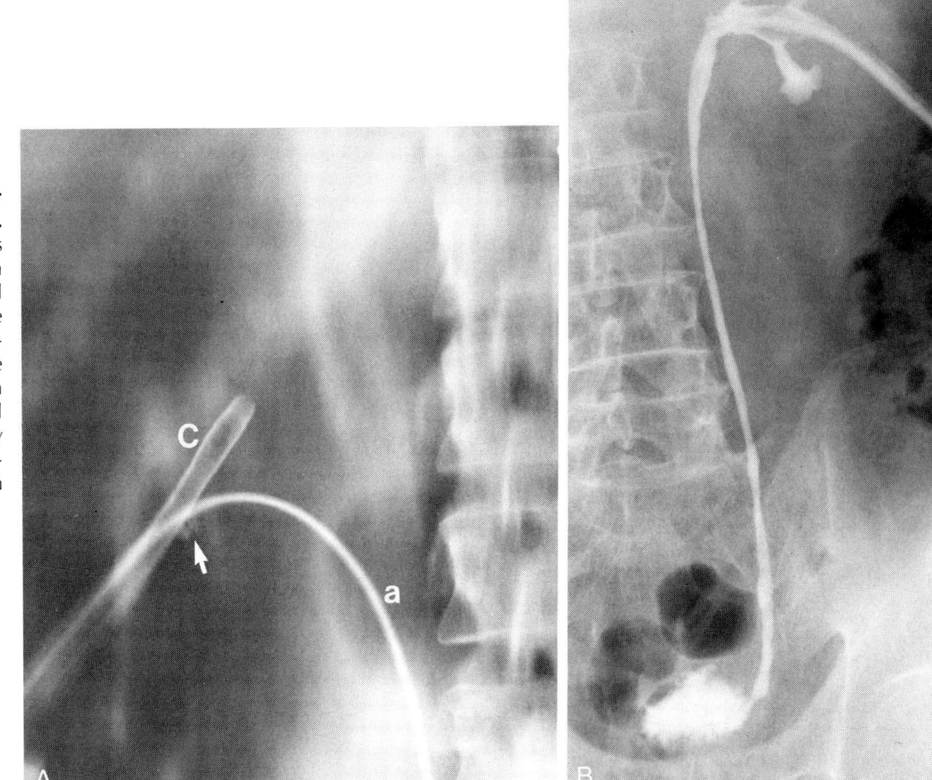

Figure 78–8. Conclusion studies after percutaneous stone removal procedures. *A,* Linear tomography after percutaneous nephrostolithotomy shows two 3-mm fragments *(arrow)* adjacent to the Councill nephrostomy catheter (C). a = Antegrade ureteral catheter and guidewire. The fragments were easily extracted with a stone basket. *B,* Nephrostogram obtained on postprocedure day one following removal of antegrade guidewire. The nephrostomy tube is in good position, there is no extravasation, and there is free flow down the ureter to the bladder.

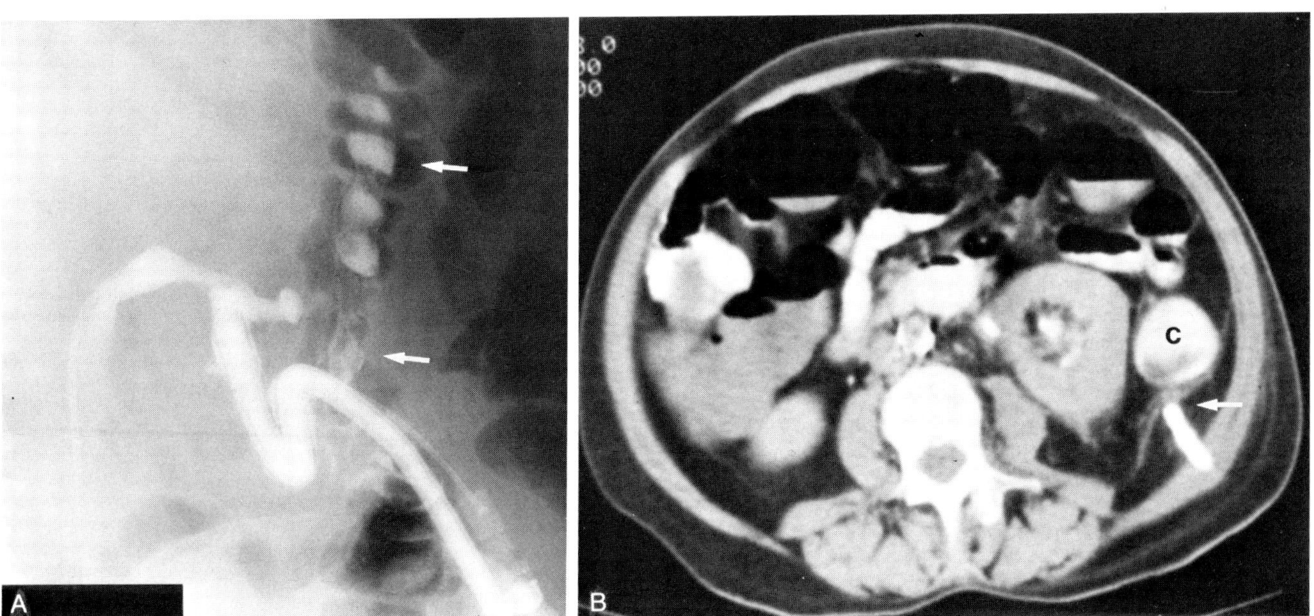

Figure 78–9. Colon perforation during percutaneous nephrostomy for stone removal. *A,* Nephrostogram obtained on postprocedure day one shows nephrostomy tube in the renal collecting system, but contrast along the nephrostomy tract enters the descending colon *(arrows)*. A retrograde ureteral stent was placed to ensure kidney drainage; the nephrostomy tube was withdrawn so that the tip was out of the kidney and adjacent to the colon perforation so it could act as a drain. *B,* Transverse abdominal CT scan (oral and intravenous contrast) at kidney level shows nephrostomy tube tip *(arrow)* at site of colon (C) perforation. The tube was left in place as a drain for three days and then gradually removed over two days; the fistula closed, and the patient recovered without complication.

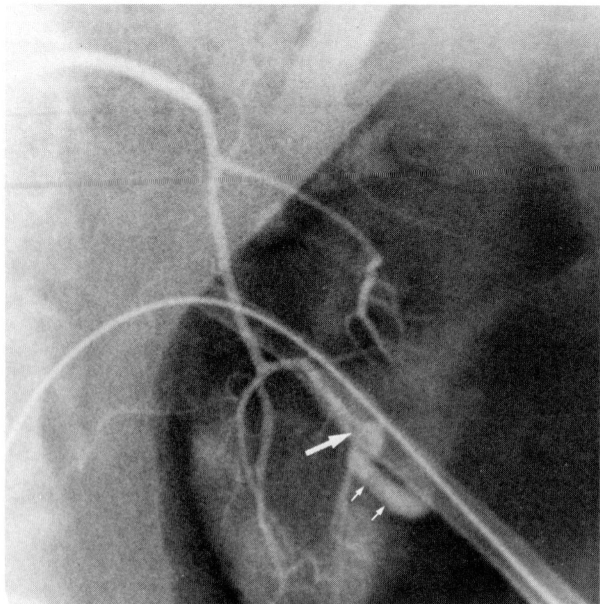

Figure 78–10. Bleeding pseudoaneurysm at nephrostomy site following percutaneous stone removal. A 93-year-old woman had uncomplicated percutaneous ultrasonic lithotripsy of a 2-cm left renal pelvic calculus. Persistent heavy bleeding through the nephrostomy led to angiography, which showed extravasation *(small arrows)* from the interlobar artery. The interlobar artery at the nephrostomy *(large arrow)* was embolized with Gelfoam and minicoils. (Reprinted from Brannen GE, et al: Kidney stone removal: Percutaneous versus surgical lithotomy. J Urol 133:6–12, 1985; © 1985 The Williams and Wilkins Co., Baltimore.)

COMPLICATIONS OF PERCUTANEOUS STONE THERAPY

Small rents or tears in the uroepithelium are common (31 per cent) but heal rapidly and are usually not apparent on the next day's nephrostogram. Even large tears will heal quickly if the tissue can approximate and there is good drainage of urine by way of a nephrostomy. A large tear in the upper ureter should be stented internally. Loss of small stone fragments through a rent occurs occasionally. Extruded fragments of a noninfected calculus are left in the retroperitoneum, as continued attempts at retrieval can cause serious complications of excessive extravasation of irrigation fluid or major vessel damage. Extruded noninfected fragments left in the pararenal areas have not affected recovery adversely.

Major complications are infrequent with percutaneous techniques. Extravasation and/or absorption of large amounts of irrigation fluid can occur surprisingly quickly and pose a serious threat to the patient; therefore, inflow and fluid return must be monitored closely.

A nephrostomy tract placed above the twelfth rib and into an upper calyx not infrequently traverses the lower pleural sulcus; a small pleural effusion frequently develops, but pneumothorax is uncommon. Injury to the spleen or liver also is a potential problem with high nephrostomy placement. A relatively lateral nephrostomy placement can enter or damage the colon (Fig. 78–9). This colon fistula often can be treated conservatively by providing separate drainage for the kidney (either a new separate small nephrostomy tract or, preferably, a retrograde ureteral stent) and partially withdrawing the major nephrostomy tube to act as a colocutaneous drain for three to five days.

Persistent or recurrent bleeding is the most common serious complication associated with percutaneous stone removal. It usually originates at the nephrostomy site from trauma to an interlobar artery of the posterior division. It can arise from larger vessel injury if the nephrostomy location is more centrally positioned (see Fig. 78–6). If bleeding does not cease with tamponade from a large nephrostomy tube, or if bleeding and clots with obstruction occur persistently after the procedure, angiography is necessary. A pseudoaneurysm with or without an arteriovenous fistula usually will be found (Fig. 78–10). The incidence varies from 0.6 to 1.2 per cent. Nephrectomy can usually be avoided by treating these with angiographic embolization of the small feeding artery using substances such as Gelfoam particles and minicoils. Selective embolotherapy will help preserve renal function, although the patients still need to be followed clinically for possible development of hypertension.

FOLLOW-UP OF PATIENTS WITH CALCULI

Calculus removal alone is not adequate for patients with renal calculus disease. In addition to careful chemical analysis of the retrieved stone fragments, medical management to prevent stone recurrence is essential. A causative metabolic disorder can usually be identified; correction of this metabolic disorder usually prevents formation of new calculi. Follow-up clinical management includes appropriate adjustment in patient diet and fluid intake and oral medication appropriate for the composition of the stone.

Bibliography

Brannen GE, Bush WH, Correa RJ, et al: Kidney stone removal: Percutaneous versus surgical lithotomy. J Urol 133:6–12, 1985.

Bush WH, Brannen GE, Burnett LL, Wales LR: Ultrasonic renal lithotripsy: Single-stage percutaneous technique and adjuvant radiological procedures. Radiology 152:387–389, 1984.

Bush WH, Brannen GE, Gibbons RP, et al: Radiation exposure to patient and urologist during percutaneous nephrostolithotomy. J Urol 132:1148–1152, 1984.

Bush WH, Brannen GE, Lewis GP, Burnett LL: Upper ureteral calculi: Antegrade extraction via percutaneous nephrostomy. AJR 144:795–799, 1985.

Bush WH, Crane RS, Brannen GE: Steerable loop snare for percutaneous retrieval of renal calix calculi. AJR 142:367–368, 1984.

Castaneda-Zuniga WR, Clayman R, Smith A, et al: Nephrostolithotomy: Percutaneous techniques for urinary calculus removal. AJR 139:721–726, 1982.

Chaussy C, Schmiedt E, Jocham D, et al: Extracorporeal shock-wave lithotripsy (ESWL) for treatment of urolithiasis. Urology 23:59–66, 1984.

Coleman CC, Castaneda-Zuniga WR, Kimura Y, et al: A systematic approach to puncture-site selection for percutaneous urinary tract stone removal. Semin Intervent Radiol 1:42–49, 1984.

Denstedt JD, Clayman RV, Picus DD: Comparison of endoscopic and radiological residual fragment rate following percutaneous nephrolithotripsy. J Urol 145:703–705, 1991.

Dunnick NR, Carson CC, Braun SD, et al: Complications of percutaneous nephrostomy. Radiology 157:51–55, 1985.

Dunnick NR, Carson CC, Moore AV, et al: Percutaneous approach to nephrolithiasis. AJR 144:451–455, 1984.

Fuchs EF, Forsyth MJ: Supracostal approach for percutaneous ultrasonic lithotripsy. Urol Clin North Am 17:99–102, 1990.

Krysiewicz S: Complications of renal extracorporeal shock wave lithotripsy reviewed. Urol Radiol 13:139–145, 1992.

LeRoy AJ, May GR, Bender CE, et al: Percutaneous nephrostomy for stone removal. Radiology 151:607–612, 1984.

LeRoy AJ, Segura JW: Percutaneous ultrasonic lithotripsy. AJR 143:785–788, 1984.

Lingeman JE, Woods JR, Toth PD: Blood pressure changes following extracorporeal shock wave lithotripsy and other forms of treatment of nephrolithiasis. JAMA 263:1789–1794, 1990.

Narasimham DL, Jacobsson B, Vijayan P, et al: Percutaneous nephrolithotomy through an intercostal approach. Acta Radiol 32:162–165, 1991.

Pollack HM, Banner MD: Percutaneous extraction of upper urinary tract calculi. Urol Radiol 6:124–137, 1984.

Wilson WT, Preminger GM: Extracorporeal shock wave lithotripsy. An update. Urol Clin North Am 17:231–242, 1990.

79 Interventional Techniques

Nancy S. Curry

INTERVENTIONAL URORADIOLOGY

Percutaneous Nephrostomy

Percutaneous nephrostomy was first accomplished in 1954 by large-bore needle puncture of the hydronephrotic kidney, with insertion of polyethylene tubing through the needle serving as a temporary drainage catheter. Although guided by radiographs made before and during the puncture, the procedure was essentially "blind" and generated little enthusiasm until advances in radiographic equipment made fluoroscopically controlled catheter placement safe and practical.

Indications. The indications for percutaneous nephrostomy include temporary relief of obstruction and assessment of renal function; pyohydronephrosis drainage; calculus dissolution, extraction, or disintegration; and creation of access for ureteral stenting, dilation, ablation, or foreign body retrieval.

A common clinical setting requiring percutaneous nephrostomy is obstruction with infection or renal failure in patients who are often critically ill. Ureteral obstruction may occur from a multitude of causes, most commonly calculi, postsurgical complications, congenital causes, and malignancy. Whatever the etiology, an infected, obstructed urinary tract can rapidly lead to sepsis, hypotension, and death. When obstruction is bilateral, usually owing to neoplasm, the patient becomes uremic, eventually developing severe metabolic acidosis and electrolyte disturbances. Attempts to relieve obstruction by retrograde cystoscopic ureteral stenting may fail, and surgical decompression is fraught with high morbidity and mortality rates. The alternative is the placement of catheters percutaneously for temporary or long-term drainage.

Patient Preparation. Preliminary preparations include informed consent, blood coagulation screen, and antibiotic coverage. When there is no history of clinical infection, prophylactic coverage utilizing a cephalosporin is appropriate. When infection is likely but a specific organism has not yet been identified, an aminoglycoside and ampicillin will cover the usual infective organisms. A well-established intravenous line is essential.

Intravenous sedation and analgesia with midazolam (Versed, Roach Laboratories, Nutley, NJ) and fentanyl (Sublimaze, Janssen Pharmaceutica, Titusville, NJ) during the procedure yield better results than premedication. Although respiratory depression does not usually occur with these agents unless high doses are given, monitoring pulse oximetry is advisable.

Technique. Most interventional radiologists utilize fluoroscopy to perform percutaneous nephrostomy, although some advocate the use of ultrasound or CT. A combined approach of ultrasound and fluoroscopy is probably the most useful when renal function is too poor to visualize the collecting structures, when the patient's anatomy is distorted as in severe scoliosis, or when the system is not very distended. The preferred needle path, depth, and angulation can be easily planned with ultrasound and the remainder of the procedure conducted under fluoroscopy.

The collecting system is visualized by administration of an intravenous contrast agent or a preliminary antegrade pyelogram is performed by a direct 22-gauge "skinny" needle puncture of the renal pelvis guided by ultrasound.

The patient may be positioned prone oblique, prone, or supine oblique. Occasionally the supine oblique position is necessary because complicating factors such as flexion contractures of the extremities, endotracheal intubation and ventilation, or recent abdominal surgery prevent the usual prone or prone oblique approach. The angled needle path required by the prone position is facilitated by C-arm fluoroscopy, if available. With only single-plane imaging, the prone oblique position is used.

The location of needle puncture is below the twelfth rib approximately two fingerbreadths lateral to the lateralmost extent of paraspinal muscles. The angulated needle path will allow entry parallel to the larger renal arterial branches along the junction of the anterior and posterior division of the renal blood supply. The renal parenchyma traversed will serve to tamponade bleeding and provide resistance to catheter removal. The longer path also will keep the needle farther away from large hilar vessels. Finally, the patient is likely to tolerate the catheter better because it exits the skin obliquely and therefore will have less of a tendency to kink and obstruct on recumbency.

There are two main techniques of percutaneous nephrostomy placement. The most commonly used is the Seldinger or angiographic approach, in which a guidewire is placed through the puncturing needle cannula or sheath and fascial dilators are used to enlarge the tract until a final catheter is placed. Others advocate use of a trocar system, in which a hollow metal trocar with a pencil-point tip and a single sidehole fits inside a Teflon cannula. After the puncture, the trocar is removed and a silicone catheter is placed through the peel-away cannula. This system is more direct but has fewer advocates because of the fear of hemorrhagic complications from the large-bore needle.

With a background in angiography, most radiologists feel comfortable with the angiographic method, which is more complex and time-consuming than the trocar method. It is better suited for the mildly dilated collecting system, which is a more challenging target. Initial puncture may be made with a 21-gauge skinny needle or an 18-gauge sheathed needle. A variety of fine-needle, single-puncture sets are available, which consist of pediatric-size exchange wires and introducer catheters (Fig. 79–1) or coaxially loaded large needles introduced over the puncture needle. These systems are most useful in minimally dilated to nondilated collecting systems. Trocar puncture techniques are more suited to very dilated systems. After a working guidewire is established in the collecting system, fascial dilators are used to dilate the tract to 8 or 10 Fr with subsequent placement of the nephrostomy catheter.

To prevent accidental dislodgement, self-retaining catheters are preferred. A Cope loop catheter* has an internal suture attached to its end, which, when pulled at the hub, causes the distal end of the catheter to circle on itself to form a fixed loop. The advantage of this catheter is that it is very resistant to accidental removal; unfortunately, crystalline deposits on the fixation thread may make removal very difficult. Forward pressure exerted by a Teflon sheath while pulling back on the catheter will break the suture and allow removal. A Foley balloon catheter can be made into a satisfactory nephrostomy drainage system by creating an endhole and advancing the catheter piggybacked over a straight 8 Fr Teflon catheter. Problems with this system include balloon leakage and decompression. Another self-retaining catheter is the Malecot catheter,* which has expanding flanges (Fig. 79–2). An introducer inserted inside the catheter straightens the flanges for placement into the nephrostomy tract over a guidewire. When the introducer is removed, the flanges re-expand to prevent dislodgement. Regardless of the system used, the catheters should be exchanged every two to three months.

---

*Cook Inc., 925 South Curry Pike, Bloomington, IN 47402.

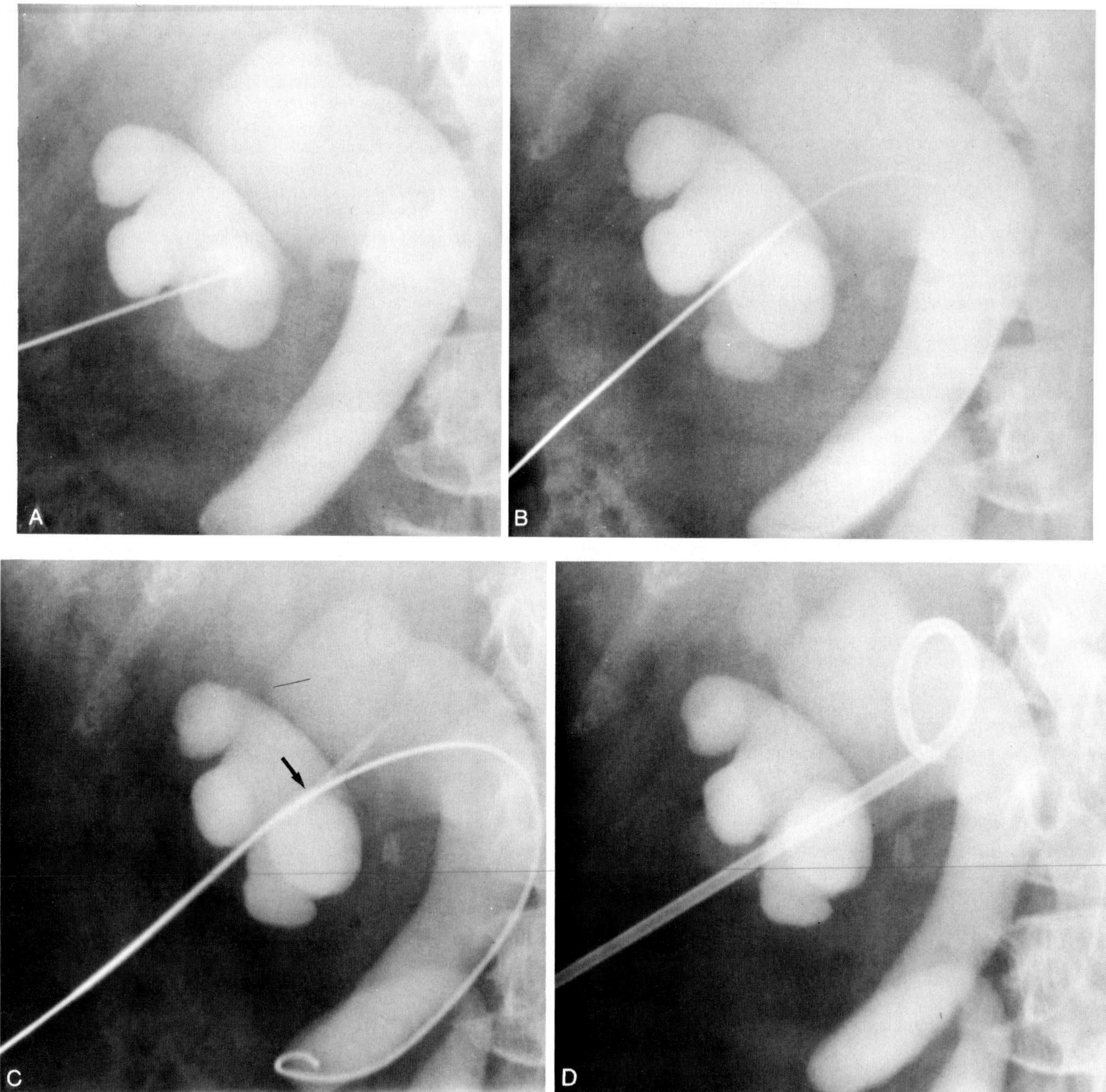

Figure 79–1. Percutaneous nephrostomy. *A,* Initial puncture with a 21-gauge needle into a lower pole calyx. *B,* An 0.018-inch guidewire is introduced through the needle. *C,* The needle has been replaced by a 6.3 Fr catheter tapered to fit the 0.018-inch guidewire. The fine guide has been removed, and a standard 0.038-inch tight J guidewire exits through the catheter sidehole *(arrow). D,* An 8.3 Fr pigtail nephrostomy catheter is placed over the 0.038-inch wire after dilatation with appropriate dilators.

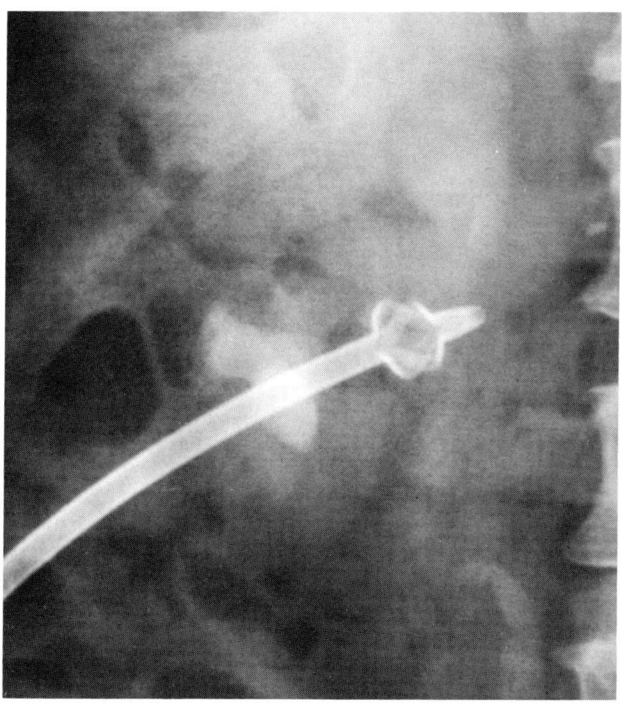

Figure 79–2. Malecot self-retaining nephrostomy catheter. Expanded wings are flattened on introduction and open by removing the internal introducer.

COMPLICATIONS. The overall major complication rate for percutaneous nephrostomy ranges from 0.7 to 4 per cent, with infection being the most common complication, followed by hemorrhage and urinary leakage. A mortality rate of 0.2 per cent is markedly better than the surgical nephrostomy mortality rate of 6 to 12 per cent, which may rise even higher when nephrectomy is performed for pyohydronephrosis.

The infective complications of percutaneous nephrostomy are the result of superinfection of an obstructed system or exacerbation of an existing infection. Careful attention to sterile technique and routine use of antibiotics will decrease the incidence of these complications. Overinjection of contrast causing pyelointerstitial and pyelovenous contamination with infected material must be avoided. The amount of contrast injected should be no more than the amount of fluid evacuated from the collecting system. Also, it is advisable to defer diagnostic antegrade pyelography until drainage is well-established and infection under control.

Virtually all patients will have hematuria, often gross, as a consequence of the percutaneous nephrostomy, and this is therefore not regarded as a complication. Hematuria should clear within 24 hours. Persistent hematuria and a falling hematocrit should be cause for concern; in some cases it may be a result of slight withdrawal of the catheter, allowing sideholes to lie within the renal parenchyma. Readjustment of the catheter may remedy the situation. In many serious cases of bleeding, there has been an underlying hemorrhagic diathesis. Clotting factors should always be checked and anticoagulant therapy stopped or reversed.

A less frequent complication is urinary leakage that may occur with perforation of the collecting system or when catheter sideholes extend outside the kidney. Pneumothorax and puncture of other organs (duodenum, colon, and bile ducts) have been reported consequent to attempted percutaneous nephrostomy. CT evaluation of kidneys several years after uncomplicated percutaneous nephrostomy, however, shows no evidence of any significant late effects on renal morphology or function.

The safety and ease with which percutaneous nephrostomy catheters can be placed has led to their use in pediatric patients and even the fetus in utero. The procedure has also been useful in the renal transplant, in which it is simpler because of the superficial position of the transplanted kidney and painless because of renal denervation (Fig. 79–3). Complications must be scrupulously avoided because the procedure involves a solitary kidney in an immunocompromised patient.

Catheter dislodgement and obstruction are potential problems after successful placement. An obstructed catheter may be filled with debris that can be dislodged by firm back-and-forth motion with a stiff guidewire. If this fails, the hub of the catheter is cut off and a sheath passed over it to maintain access to the collecting system. The obstructed catheter is removed through the sheath and a new nephrostomy catheter placed through it. A recently placed catheter that has become dislodged demands immediate attention, as the nephrostomy tract may close within hours, necessitating repuncture. A tract that has matured over several weeks or months will stay patent longer. In either case, the tract can be opacified by attaching a Christmas tree adaptor to a contrast-filled syringe and injecting with the adaptor snugly fitted into the tract. The tract may then be renegotiated by small, soft catheters aided by a floppy-tipped guidewire.

Ureteral Intervention

Once a percutaneous nephrostomy catheter is in place, access to the ureter may provide treatment for ureteral fistulas, strictures, calculi, foreign bodies, or neoplasms. The traditional approach to such ureteral lesions is via retrograde cystoscopic manipulations or surgery. The patient may not be a good surgical candidate, however, because of debilitation or extensive malignancy, and retrograde intervention may fail. Because percutaneous ureteral intervention is fluoroscopically guided and general anesthesia is avoided, the procedure is safe and often successful.

Ureteral stenting for strictures or leaks is common urologic practice. The stent serves to maintain the ureteral lumen and allow healing while providing a route for urinary drainage. Extrinsic ureteral obstruction by malignancy or retroperitoneal fibrosis may be

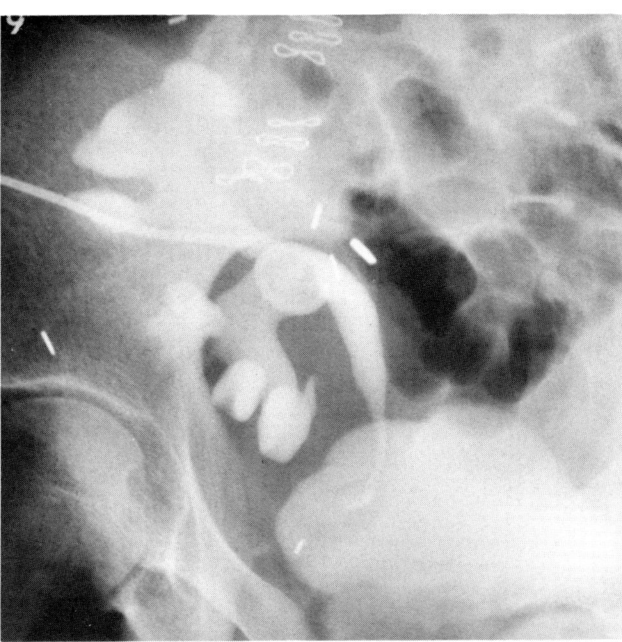

Figure 79–3. Pigtail nephrostomy catheter in a renal transplant. Intermittent obstruction occurred with ureteral kinking by a distended bladder.

similarly treated. When retrograde stenting attempts have failed and the flank approach is required, a percutaneous nephrostomy is established as discussed previously. The only difference is that the puncture should be made into a mid- or upper-pole calyx rather than lower-pole calyx to facilitate stent passage. The nephrostomy tract should have matured for at least several days before the procedure is attempted.

The ureteropelvic junction is negotiated by a Cobra angiographic catheter. A straight, floppy-tipped guidewire placed through the catheter will negotiate ureteral kinks and bends. When a stricture or marked tortuosity causes difficulty, a "glidewire" (Meditech, Inc., Watertown, MA) is usually successful in achieving passage. The catheter is then advanced into the bladder, and the soft guidewire is replaced by an Amplatz superstiff wire. Once the guidewire has reached the bladder, further maneuvers depend on whether a permanent indwelling or temporary external type stent is desired. For external stenting, a non-Teflon angiographic pigtail catheter is introduced after sideholes are placed along the shaft to the level of the pelvis. External stenting is usually performed in the patient with a benign process such as a leak that can be expected to heal within a short period of time. External stents are easily flushed and exchanged but have the disadvantage of increasing the likelihood of infection.

Internal stents used for long-term drainage must resist encrustation, fracturing, and migration. Soft, biocompatible copolymer ureteral stent catheters (Percuflex, Meditech, Inc., Watertown, MA) are now available, which can be expected to maintain patency for at least six months. A double-pigtail 8 Fr catheter of sufficient length to extend from renal pelvis to mid-bladder is selected. A stent that is too long will irritate the bladder, and one that is too short will not drain properly. The exact length required can be determined by placing the guidewire tip within the middle of the bladder and making a kink in the wire where it exits the skin. The guidewire is then pulled back until its tip is at the renal pelvis, and another kink is made at the skin site. The length of guidewire between the bends is the appropriate length of the stent. Once the appropriate length is established, the stent is advanced over the stiff wire by a pusher while placement is monitored fluoroscopically. When the wire is retracted, the stent assumes a pigtail configuration proximally and distally. A nephrostomy catheter may be reintroduced into the pelvis for 24 hours to ensure adequate drainage (Fig. 79–4).

Before a stent is passed, dilatation of a ureteral stricture may be necessary. Sequentially larger angiographic catheters, tapered Teflon dilating (van Andel) catheters, and angioplasty balloon catheters have all been successfully used to dilate strictures. The angioplasty balloon method allows local dilatation without having to enlarge the nephrostomy tract. Recent postoperative strictures and inflammatory strictures of the ureter due to Crohn's disease and tuberculosis have been successfully dilated. Ischemic or densely fibrotic strictures may not respond to dilatation.

Percutaneous ureteral stenting can be performed with greater than 90 per cent success in experienced hands. Apparent complete obstruction on antegrade pyelography does not mean that a given lesion is impassable. Wedging a straight catheter in the obstructed segment and pushing a straight guidewire through the stricture have been successful in recannulating the ureteral lumen.

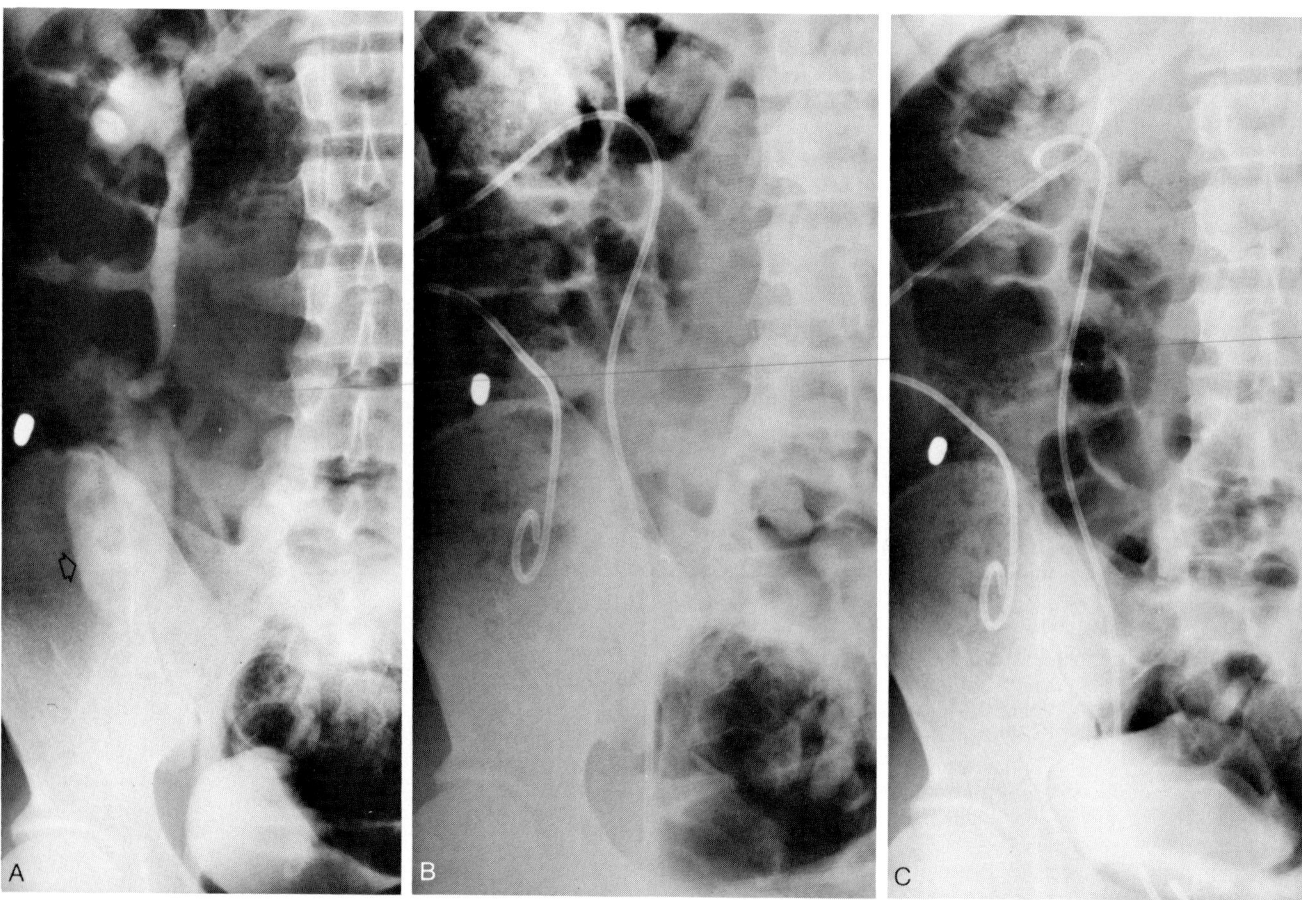

Figure 79–4. *A,* **An excretory urogram** obtained after gunshot trauma to the mid-ureter demonstrates a urinoma *(arrow). B,* The urinoma was drained by a pigtail catheter, and a percutaneous catheter was successfully manipulated across the partially disrupted ureter. *C,* An internal double-pigtail stent in place. A temporary percutaneous nephrostomy catheter was removed the following day.

Ureteral fistulas to skin, bowel, vagina, or other sites can be successfully treated by percutaneous stenting when the retrograde method fails or is unsuitable. Despite nearly complete ureteral disruption or multiple fistulas, it is often possible to advance a guidewire along existing tissue bridges. A stent is then placed, taking care to ensure that no sideholes are located at the fistula site. With the stent in place, healing can occur without the need for surgical intervention, although a stricture may later develop at the fistula site. Large, inoperable urinary fistulas may not heal despite stenting in the patient with advanced malignancy, and in some cases continence can be achieved by transcatheter occlusion of the ureter with tissue adhesives.

Patients with ureteroileal urinary diversion may develop leaks or strictures at the ureteroileal anastomosis. These conditions are also amenable to stenting. The procedure is the same as in an intact urinary system except that the guidewire may easily be retrieved from the loop to facilitate the stenting process.

Another use of ureteral catheters placed percutaneously is to aid the surgeon in localization of the ureter when it lies in an abnormal position or is surrounded by intense fibrosis or tumor. A large-caliber ureteral catheter can be palpated during surgical dissection or reconstruction. If such a catheter cannot be placed in the usual retrograde fashion, the antegrade approach is appropriate.

Percutaneous Retroperitoneal Biopsy

A common difficult clinical problem is the patient who develops ureteral obstruction after surgery or radiation therapy for a pelvic neoplasm. Whether the patient has postsurgical fibrosis, radiation fibrosis, or recurrent neoplasm influences future therapy. Because imaging procedures cannot distinguish among these possibilities, tissue sampling is necessary, and until the late 1970s, this required laparotomy. The development of thin-needle aspiration biopsy, with its negligible morbidity, provided a safe, quick, inexpensive alternative.

The procedure may be performed on an outpatient basis. Imaging is via either biplane fluoroscopy or CT, with ureteral opacification by intravenous contrast. If the patient has a nephrostomy catheter or external ureteral stent, the catheter may be injected to localize the stricture site. While multiple biopsies increase the chances of obtaining a positive diagnosis, interpretation by an experienced cytopathologist is essential. A positive result will obviate the need for exploratory surgery, but a negative biopsy result is inconclusive because false-negatives and true-negatives are indistinguishable. The same biopsy techniques may be used to determine whether lymph node abnormalities seen on lymphangiography are secondary to inflammatory changes or metastases.

Renal Transplant Intervention

Percutaneous nephrostomy is occasionally useful in the diagnosis and localization of ureteral obstruction, while providing temporary therapeutic diversion in a transplant kidney. Obstruction may be due to the development of a large fluid collection around the kidney, representing either hematoma, urinoma, abscess, or lymphocele. Such collections may cause obstruction because of their size and contribute to a decline in renal function. Aspiration, usually under ultrasound control, can establish the source and nature of the fluid and provide temporary therapy. Lymphoceles tend to recur, requiring a second drainage procedure in a significant number of patients. Sclerosing agents such as providone-iodine and tetracycline have been used with success to prevent recurrence.

Cyst Puncture/Mass Biopsy

Ultrasound and CT have gained acceptance in establishing whether a renal lesion is cystic or solid, thus severely reducing the need for renal cyst puncture. A lesion deemed indeterminate by imaging studies may be aspirated, but since benign lesions may contain bloody fluid and malignant lesions may contain clear fluid, only unequivocally positive cytology from the fluid is clinically useful. Truly indeterminate masses are therefore surgical lesions. Needle aspiration is appropriate, however, when the patient is febrile and might have an infected renal cyst or abscess.

Solid renal lesions rarely require puncture because most are renal cell carcinomas, which are managed surgically. Biopsy is indicated, however, when there is suspicion that the renal lesion might represent a single metastasis from a known non-renal primary tumor, lymphoma, or Wilms' tumor in an adult.

Fluoroscopy, ultrasound, and CT may all be utilized to localize the mass to be punctured. The choice depends on multiple factors: the patient's renal function; body habitus; size and location of the lesion; equipment availability; cost and time considerations; and physician preference. Localization by ultrasound is independent of renal function and avoids exposure to contrast material and irradiation. Continuous monitoring of the lesion and needle tip is possible with a real-time transducer. Unfortunately, obesity, small lesion size, or sound transmission interference by overlying ribs may make a puncture under ultrasound technically impossible. Large lesions can be safely aspirated utilizing fluoroscopy with or without primary depth localization by ultrasound (Fig. 79–5). Puncture under CT is time-consuming and expensive but occasionally necessary in small lesions (Fig. 79–6).

A variety of sizes and types of aspiration biopsy needles are available. Fine-gauge "skinny" needles (22 or 23 gauge) are relatively atraumatic but tend to deflect from the target with deep lesions. Less flexible 18 to 20 gauge needles are easier to direct to the lesion and provide better tissue samples. Spring-loaded biopsy guns are now available, which provide excellent core specimens.

The lesion is punctured from a posterior approach, which avoids the peritoneum and bowel. The measured depth to the center of the lesion may be marked on the needle by wrapping it with a small strip of sterile tape. No matter what the imaging modality used, care must be taken in upper pole masses to avoid transgression of the

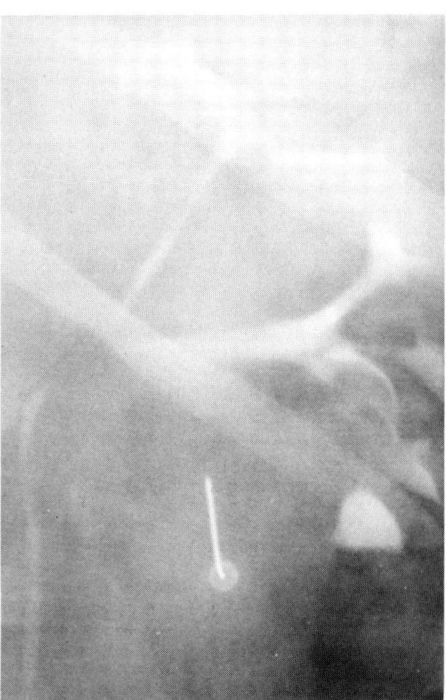

Figure 79–5. A parapelvic mass in the left kidney was equivocal on CT evaluation. Percutaneous puncture by fluoroscopic guidance yielded no fluid. A renal cell carcinoma was found at operation.

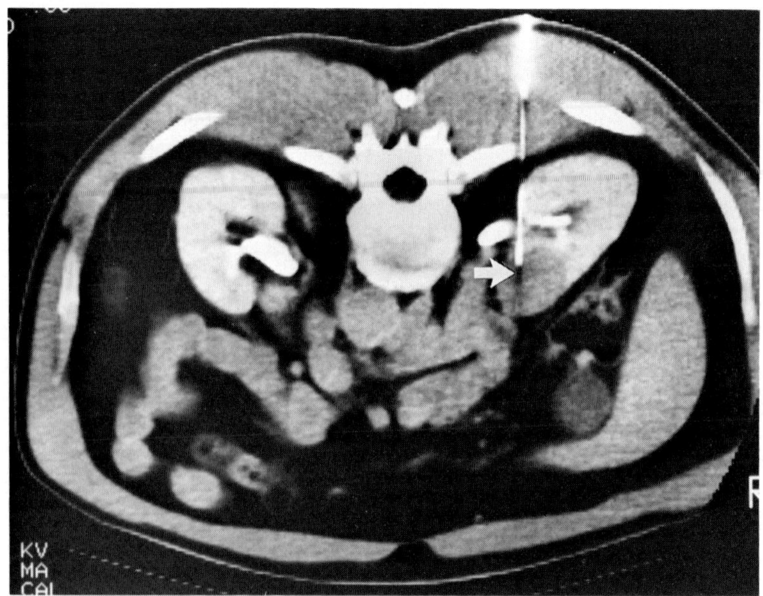

Figure 79–6. Prone CT scan demonstrates **skinny needle within a renal cell carcinoma** proven by aspiration biopsy. The patient had a primary squamous cell carcinoma of the esophagus. Note low-density artifact created by the needle tip *(arrow)*.

posterior pleural space, which will cause pneumothorax. A directly perpendicular orientation of the needle to the table is preferred when vertical-beam fluoroscopy alone is used. To avoid causing a pneumothorax in aspirating an upper pole lesion, however, cephalad needle angulation from a more caudal entry site is often necessary. Needle angulation is also possible when CT or ultrasound is used.

A sudden loss of resistance is usually felt when the needle punctures a cystic lesion. The inner stylet of the needle is then removed, and fluid usually wells up and drips spontaneously from the hub. Microbiologic stains and cultures should be obtained. Contrast and air can be injected into the cyst and horizontal beam radiographs obtained to study the wall of the structure, but this is rarely necessary. The injection of contrast can identify, however, communication with the intrarenal collecting structures (Fig. 79–7).

A clear aspirate with negative cytology and normal lactate dehydrogenase is considered diagnostic for a benign renal cyst. The presence of turbid or hemorrhagic fluid in a nontraumatic puncture suggests the possibility of malignancy. A lesion that yields no fluid is usually a neoplasm that will require surgery for definitive diagnosis. Biopsy may be performed when a metastasis from a known primary of other than adenocarcinoma cell type or lymphoma is suspected. The small number of cells obtained from an aspiration biopsy will not allow the cytopathologist to distinguish a benign renal adenoma from a well-differentiated adenocarcinoma, nor is it possible to distinguish renal carcinoma from adenocarcinoma metastatic from another organ.

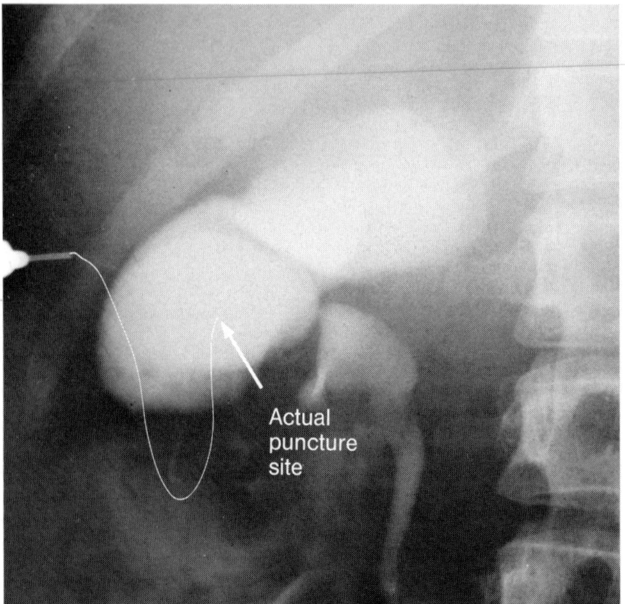

Figure 79–7. Sheathed needle puncture of **obstructed upper pole collecting system** due to tuberculous stricture.

The vast majority of renal mass lesions are cysts, and these are nearly always asymptomatic. In rare cases, however, large cysts may be responsible for hydronephrosis, pain, or hypertension. Ablation of a symptomatic renal cyst can be accomplished percutaneously by puncture and injection of a sclerosing agent. Hypertonic glucose, quinacrine, phenol, alcohol, and iophendylate have all been used with variable success in shrinking cysts and preventing their recurrence. After the cyst fluid is evacuated by catheter drainage, one quarter of the volume is replaced by 95 per cent ethanol. The inner surface of the cyst is exposed to the alcohol by rotating the patient. The ethanol is reaspirated after five minutes, and the catheter is removed.

The incidence of major complications associated with cyst puncture is 1.4 per cent, including perirenal hemorrhage, pneumothorax, infection, arteriovenous fistulas, urinoma formation, bile peritonitis, and massive hematuria. Obstruction can occur following aspiration from renal rotation, fibrosis from the injection of sclerosing agents, or obstructive migration of renal calculi. Care must be taken not to overinject a cyst, as contrast material extravasation, pain, fever, and perirenal fibrosis may result. The potential for massive bleeding exists if the mass punctured is not a cyst but a hypervascular neoplasm or a large arteriovenous malformation or aneurysm. The theoretical risk of seeding malignant tumor cells along the needle tract has not proved to be of significance in the use of "skinny" needles in the kidney.

Perinephric and Renal Abscess

Traditionally, a patient with a renal abscess underwent surgical drainage. This conventional therapy has been challenged in recent years by the success of medical therapy combined with percutaneous drainage.

In the era before antibiotics were available, most abscesses of the

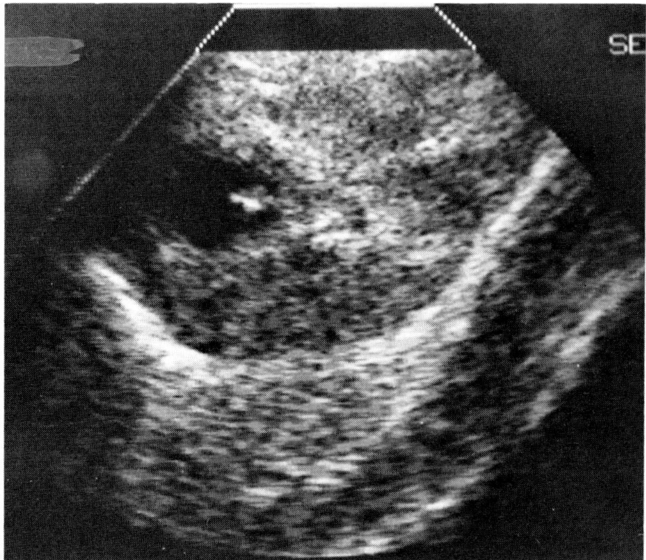

Figure 79–8. Renal transplant with a cortical abscess. The aspirating needle tip can be seen as a bright echo within the abscess.

kidney developed from a blood-borne staphylococcal infection. At the present time, most cases arise from infection by a gram-negative coliform microorganism superimposed on a pre-existing abnormality of the GU tract such as obstruction or calculi. A simple cyst may become infected and then is virtually indistinguishable from a cortical abscess unless there is a baseline study confirming the pre-existence of a cyst. In most cases a perinephric abscess arises from rupture of an intrarenal abscess into the perinephric space.

CT, ultrasound, and fluoroscopy all may be utilized in the diagnosis and treatment of renal and perirenal abscesses.

On CT a renal abscess usually appears as a low-density mass that is either well-defined or irregular, depending on the stage of development and whether the abscess developed from a pre-existing cyst or a primary renal infection. An enhancing rim representing inflammatory hypervascularity of the abscess wall may be present. Extension into the perinephric space will result in localized obliteration of normal perirenal tissue planes with mass effect and thickening of the renal fascia. Occasionally, gas bubbles can be seen in the affected tissues. On ultrasound examination, a renal abscess may have the characteristics of a simple cyst, although internal debris may produce internal echoes and layer out as a fluid-fluid level.

CT best demonstrates the extent of the inflammatory mass and its relationship to contiguous structures and allows planning of the entry site for percutaneous drainage. Avoidance of other organs and major vessels is essential, and an extraperitoneal posterior or posterolateral approach is mandatory. Angulation and depth to the most safely accessible portions of the lesion can easily be determined. While the initial localization may be best accomplished by CT or ultrasound, fluoroscopy is essential to the safe manipulation of catheters and guidewires.

Various approaches to the percutaneous treatment of renal abscesses have been advocated: intravenous antibiotics and simple aspiration, aspiration combined with antibiotic instillation, or saline irrigation. While a single aspiration may be curative (Fig. 79–8), catheter drainage may be necessary when there is thick pus (Fig. 79–9). It is essential that appropriate antibiotics be administered prior to the drainage procedure to prevent the complication of sepsis.

The two techniques for abscess catheterization are the modified Seldinger or angiographic method and the trocar method. When an abscess is large and easily accessible, the trocar technique is used: a large catheter is introduced in one step over a pencil-point stylet. Alternatively, catheter placement can be accomplished by initial entry with a 21-gauge needle or 18-gauge sheathed needle requiring subsequent guidewire exchanges and tract dilatation. The trocar method is faster and less complicated, but the size of the puncturing apparatus increases the potential for harm when misdirected.

The catheter ultimately placed should be soft, opaque, biologically inert, and resistant to clogging. Biocompatible polymer materials have been developed to satisfy these requirements. A curved or pigtail configuration will prevent erosion of the tip through the abscess wall. The sideholes should be along the inner aspect of the curve to prevent surrounding tissues from obstructing the catheter. Additional sideholes can be created to enhance drainage, but care must be taken to ensure that none extends into normal tissue. The catheter size should be at least 8 Fr to promote adequate drainage, and multiple catheters may be necessary in loculated abscesses. Once the abscess cavity has been entered, the collection should be

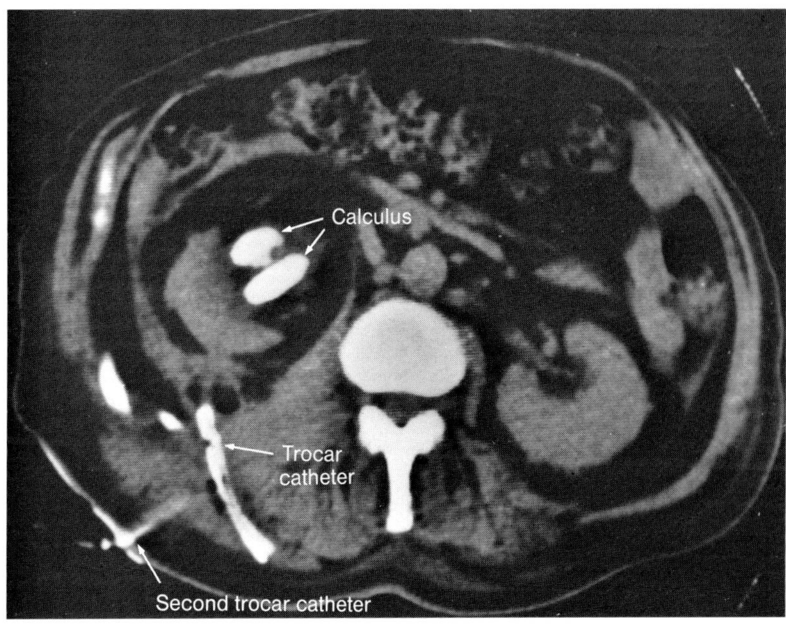

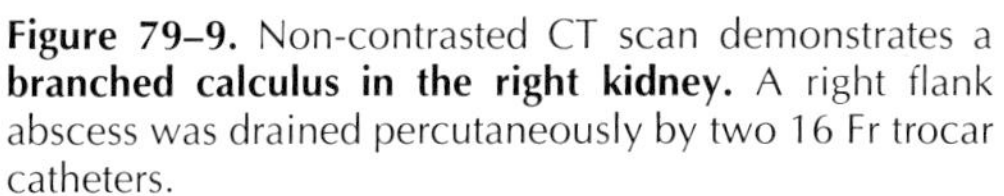

Figure 79–9. Non-contrasted CT scan demonstrates a **branched calculus in the right kidney.** A right flank abscess was drained percutaneously by two 16 Fr trocar catheters.

completely drained and the contents sent for appropriate microbiologic stains and cultures. Fluoroscopy and cautious contrast injection may then be employed to check catheter position, size of cavity, and relative position of the sideholes. Special care must be taken to avoid overinjection because of the possibility of intravasation and sepsis.

The complications of abscess drainage are the same as those for other renal mass punctures, although the risk of sepsis is higher. A close watch on vital signs is mandatory following the procedure. Possible contraindications to the procedure are a bleeding diathesis, lack of patient cooperation, and the suspicion of hydatid disease.

Bibliography

Barbaric ZL, MacIntosh PK: Periureteral thin-needle aspiration biopsy. Urol Radiol 2:181–185, 1981.

Baron RL, Lee JKT, McClennan BL, Melson GL: Percutaneous nephrostomy using real-time sonographic guidance. AJR 136:1018–1019, 1981.

Bean WJ: Renal cysts: Treatment with alcohol. Radiology 138:329–331, 1981.

Beckmann CF, Roth RA, Bihrle W III: Dilatation of benign ureteral strictures. Radiology 172:437–441, 1989.

Bettmann MA, Murray PD, Perlmutt LM, et al: Ureteroileal anastomotic leaks: Percutaneous treatment. Radiology 148:95–100, 1983.

Boren SR, Dotter CT, McKinney M, Rosch J: Percutaneous removal of ureteral stents. Radiology 152:230–231, 1984.

Cope C: Improved anchoring of nephrostomy catheters: Loop technique. AJR 135:402–403, 1980.

Curry NS, Cochran S, Barbaric ZL, et al: Interventional radiologic procedures in the renal transplant. Radiology 152:647–653, 1984.

Cragg RF, Smith TP, Berbaum KS, Nakagawa N: Randomized double-blind trial of midazolam/placebo and midazolam/fentanyl for sedation and analgesia in lower extremity angiography. AJR 157:173–176, 1991.

Cronan JJ, Amis ES Jr, Dorfman GS: Percutaneous drainage of renal abscesses. AJR 142:351–354, 1984.

Dunnick NR, Illescas FF, Mitchell S, et al: Interventional uroradiology. Invest Radiol 24:831–841, 1989.

Hruby W, Marberger M: Late sequelae of percutaneous nephrostomy. Radiology 152:383–385, 1984.

Lang EK, Glorioso LW: Antegrade transluminal dilatation of benign ureteral strictures: Long-term results. AJR 150:131–134, 1988.

Lang EK, Price ET: Redefinitions of indications for percutaneous nephrostomy. Radiology 147:419–426, 1983.

Lang EK: Renal, perirenal and pararenal abscesses: Percutaneous drainage. Radiology 174:109–113, 1990.

Matalon TS, Silver B: US guidance of interventional procedures. Radiology 174:43–47, 1990.

Meranze SG, Pollack HM, Banner MP: The use of grasping forceps in the upper urinary tract: Technique and radiologic implications. Radiology 144:171–173, 1982.

Mitty HA, Rackson ME, Dan SJ, Train JS: Experience with a new ureteral stent made of a biocompatible copolymer. Radiology 168:557–559, 1988.

Mitty HA, Train JS, Dan SJ: Antegrade stenting in the management of fistulas, strictures and calculi. Radiology 149:433–438, 1983.

Newhouse J, Pfister RC: Percutaneous catheterization of the kidney and perinephric space: Trocar technique. Urol Radiol 2:157–164, 1981.

Rezneck RH, Talner LB: Percutaneous nephrostomy and related pyeloureteral manipulative techniques. Urol Radiol 2:147–157, 1981.

Spies JB, Rosen RJ, Lebowitz AS: Antibiotic prophylaxis in vascular and interventional radiology: A rational approach. Radiology 166:381–387, 1988.

Stables DP: Percutaneous nephrostomy: Techniques, indications and results. Urol Clin North Am 9:15–29, 1982.

Stanley P, Bear JW, Reid BS: Percutaneous nephrostomy in infants and children. AJR 141:473–477, 1983.

van Waes PFGM, Feldberg MAM, Mali WPTHM, et al: Management of loculated abscesses that are difficult to drain: A new approach. Radiology 147:57, 1983.

Wein AJ, Ring EJ, Freiman DB, et al: Applications of thin needle aspiration biopsy in urology. J Urol 121:626–629, 1979.

80 Radiology of Renal Transplantation

Suresh K. Patel, Terence A. S. Matalon, and Amjad Ali

Renal transplantation and long-term dialysis have both proved to be successful modes of therapy for treatment of chronic renal failure or end-stage renal disease (ESRD). Renal transplantation is the optimal treatment for many patients with ESRD, leading to recovery of normal renal function, cure of the uremic syndrome, and full rehabilitation from renal disease. Over 10,210 renal transplants were performed in the United States in 1992. Approximately 25,185 patients currently on dialysis are on waiting lists to receive renal transplants.

DONORS AND RECIPIENTS

Transplantation from living related donors offers ideal therapy for chronic renal failure. Superior long-term results are obtained by using parental or sibling donors, and the ideal donor is an identical twin.

Careful evaluation of a potential live donor is carried out to exclude medical or psychologic conditions that may impair the future health of the donor. Radiologic evaluation of a live donor begins with excretory urography to determine the number of renal units, size, position, and presence of any parenchymal or collecting system abnormality. If excretory urography is normal, arteriography is then performed to exclude unsuspected renal arterial or parenchymal diseases and to determine the number and position of the renal arteries. The incidence of multiple renal arteries in the general population is approximately 25 per cent, and most surgeons will not transplant a kidney supplied by multiple renal arteries. Aortographic evaluation of potential donors is supplemented by selective studies when necessary. Digital subtraction angiography is an attractive alternative but has limitations of less spatial resolution, smaller field size, and artifacts from patient motion.

Cadaver kidneys are being increasingly utilized in renal transplantation, because of the difficulty in obtaining suitable live donors. This form of transplantation represents 60 to 70 per cent of all renal transplants performed in the United States. Cadaver kidneys are obtained under nearly normal physiologic circumstances from patients in whom brain death has been ascertained.

Retrospective studies have shown that recipients between the ages of 16 and 45 years with primary renal disease have the lowest risk for morbidity and mortality. Older patients with evidence of cardiovascular disease are considered for a transplant on an individual basis. Administration of a blood transfusion to the recipient prior to transplantation increases the survival rate of transplanted cadaver kidneys. Patients with renal failure secondary to chronic reflux pyelonephritis or analgesic nephropathy are prime transplant candidates. Uroradiologic work-up of the recipient includes voiding cystourethrography to rule out vesicoureteral reflux and urethral stricture and to ascertain the residual capacity of the urinary bladder.

SURGICAL TECHNIQUE

Prior to transplantation, the recipient's own kidneys are removed if they may represent a persistent source of recurrent pyelonephritis, or if they are very large owing to polycystic kidney disease and may interfere with transplant placement. Pretransplantation splenectomy or partial splenic embolization has largely been supplanted by the effectiveness of newer immunotherapeutic agents.

At present, renal transplantation is performed in the contralateral iliac fossa of the recipient. The left kidney has the advantage of a longer renal vein that is easier to anastomose. Typically, end-to-end anastomosis is carried out between the internal iliac artery and transplant renal artery, and end-to-side anastomosis between the common or external iliac vein and transplant renal vein. There are many variations in the surgical technique of vascular anastomosis, depending on the number of renal arteries and the experience and eagerness of the surgeon. Urine drainage is established by a ureteroneocystostomy of the donor ureter. Even though most renal transplants are placed extraperitoneally in the iliac fossa, some surgeons place them intraperitoneally in the pelvis.

PATIENT AND GRAFT SURVIVAL

First-year patient and graft survivals for living, related transplant recipients are now approximately 95 and 85 per cent, respectively, and for cadaveric transplant recipients, 90 and 65 per cent. Both mortality and graft loss are greater in the first year than in subsequent years; after the first two years the annual risks of death and graft loss are lower and nearly constant. Subsequent yearly patient and graft survival are from 95 to 99 per cent for living related transplant recipients and from 90 to 95 per cent for cadaveric transplant recipients.

COMPLICATIONS OF RENAL TRANSPLANTATION

Impairment of renal function in the post-transplant period can be secondary to two broad categories of complications: (1) parenchymal failure due to acute tubular necrosis, rejection, infection, etc.; and (2) surgical complications that include vascular problems, ureteral and bladder leaks, and ureteral obstruction from a variety of causes. Depending upon clinical findings and suspicion, appropriate diagnostic studies are promptly carried out. In cases in which mechanical causes of transplant failure have been ruled out, renal biopsy remains the definitive way to diagnose rejection.

Acute Tubular Necrosis

Acute tubular necrosis (also known as acute vasomotor nephropathy) occurs in 5 to 75 per cent of renal transplants. It is a direct result of renal ischemia, usually self-limited, with renal function returning to normal within a few days to a few weeks. It is most commonly seen in patients with cadaver transplants, in which the tubules may have suffered ischemic damage if the donor was hypotensive for a prolonged period before the kidneys were removed. A prolonged ischemic interval between perfusing and cooling the kidneys will have a similar effect. A kidney with a warm ischemic time of 20 minutes will inevitably suffer some degree of acute tubular necrosis.

Rejection

Allograft rejection represents the most common cause of transplant dysfunction, with the incidence of rejection episodes being as high as 93 per cent with cadaveric transplants. Rejection is the cause of up to 80 per cent of graft losses within the first year. In clinical transplantation, rejection is best described in terms of its pathologic effect on the graft and the extent to which it alters renal function. Clinically, there are three distinct types of rejection: hyperacute, acute, and chronic.

HYPERACUTE REJECTION

Hyperacute rejection usually occurs within hours to one or two days after transplantation. It is observed in patients who have developed circulating cytotoxic antibodies to one or more of the donor lymphocyte antigens as a result of previous blood transfusions, previous pregnancies, or a previous allograft. The circulating humoral lymphotoxic antibody is solely responsible for this type of rejection. It is characterized by the presence of fibrin thrombi in small arteries and arterioles with extensive cortical necrosis.

Clinically, hyperacute rejection manifests itself as failure of the kidney to perfuse properly on release of the vascular clamps; typically, the graft initially becomes firm and then rapidly becomes blue and flabby. Renal biopsy confirms the diagnosis by demonstrating the presence of polymorphonuclear leukocytes in the glomeruli and peritubular capillaries. In this situation, the kidney should be removed. Hyperacute rejection within the first 48 hours manifests itself with severe systemic symptoms, high fever, rigors, and thrombocytopenia on peripheral blood smear. Attempts to treat hyperacute rejection have been unsuccessful, and graft removal is the usual treatment. Fortunately, hyperacute rejection is becoming rare owing to advances in the histocompatibility testing procedures, particularly for detecting circulating antibodies to donor lymphocyte antigens.

ACUTE REJECTION

This type of rejection is experienced by most transplant patients during the first three to four months. The term *acute* refers to a group of morphologic changes that include a large, swollen, and edematous kidney with tense capsule, and patchy areas of cortical necrosis on cut section. Microscopic examination demonstrates a marked interstitial and perivascular infiltrate of mononuclear cells, fibrinoid necrosis of small arteries, arterioles, and glomerular capillaries, marked interstitial edema, tubular necrosis, cortical necrosis, and patchy hemorrhagic infarcts. The signs of rejection are fever, decreased urine output, and increased serum creatinine. There is often associated renal enlargement and tenderness. Acute rejection is the result of activation of the recipient's immune system to the graft, owing to a proliferation of sensitized T-lymphocytes. The changes of acute rejection often involve the donor portion of the ureter and can result in ureteral necrosis and urinary leakage.

Accelerated acute rejection is a particularly severe form of acute rejection seen during the first week after transplantation. It is characterized by sudden onset of oliguria or even anuria after satisfactory initial urine production. It is accompanied by fever and graft tenderness. The presence of interstitial hemorrhage on renal biopsy specimen is an ominous sign with no hope of graft survival in spite of treatment.

The goal of immunosuppressive therapy is the prevention and reversal of these immunologic events without impairment of host defenses. Current immunosuppressive therapies begin shortly before or at the time of transplantation; additional therapy is used to reverse acute rejection.

CHRONIC REJECTION

The term *chronic rejection* signifies a group of morphologic changes that include an irregular outer surface, corresponding to areas of old infarcts, and, on microscopic examination, obliterative arteritis secondary to marked subintimal fibroplasia with severe narrowing of the lumen of medium and small arteries. Other morphologic changes of chronic rejection are membranous thickening of glomeruli, interstitial fibrosis, tubular atrophy, and patchy interstitial lymphocytic infiltrate.

Clinically, chronic rejection manifests itself as slow deterioration in renal function over a period of weeks or months with rising serum creatinine and development of proteinuria and hypertension. Chronic rejection does not respond to increased immunosuppressive therapy. Clinical judgment usually indicates when to remove the graft and return the patient to dialysis.

Surgical Complications of Renal Transplantation

Surgical complications following renal transplantation occur more frequently than after general surgical procedures. Impaired clotting mechanisms, uremia, metabolic disorders, anemia, hypertension, and postoperative treatment with immunosuppressive drugs are all factors that contribute to the high complication rates. The incidence of surgical complications varies widely. However, gentle graft handling, careful ureteral implantation, and the use of low-dose immunosuppressive therapy will lower the complication rate to below 10 per cent. Once the complications are detected, they demand prompt and aggressive management to prevent loss of the transplanted kidney or death of the patient.

Surgical complications of renal transplantation can be classified as follows:

1. Vascular complications
   a. Arterial
   b. Venous
   c. Arteriovenous fistula
2. Peritransplant fluid collections
   a. Hematoma
   b. Abscess
   c. Urinoma
   d. Lymphocele
3. Urinary extravasation (leak)
4. Ureteral obstruction
5. Miscellaneous unusual complications: papillary necrosis, calculus formation, cortical necrosis, renal neoplasms, etc.

VASCULAR COMPLICATIONS

Vascular complications may occur in either the early or the late postoperative period. The incidence of such complications in reported series has been between 6.5 and 12.5 per cent. Vascular complications include renal artery thrombosis, renal artery stenosis, arterial dehiscence with anastomotic leak, pseudoaneurysm, renal vein thrombosis, and renal arteriovenous fistula.

Arterial Complications

RENAL ARTERY THROMBOSIS. Renal artery thrombosis is a rare complication that occurs in 1 to 2 per cent of renal transplants and results in loss of the graft. The causes of arterial thrombosis are hyperacute or acute rejection, improper vascular anastomosis resulting in an intimal flap, torsion or kinking of the renal artery, and intimal elevation as a result of perfusion. Renal artery thrombosis should be suspected in any patient who suddenly becomes anuric after transplantation. Prompt nephrectomy is the treatment of choice.

RENAL ARTERY STENOSIS. Renal artery stenosis is a well-recognized complication occurring in 3 to 12 per cent of renal transplants. It should be suspected in patients with severe or uncontrolled hypertension, with or without deterioration of renal function, or with recent onset of an arterial bruit. Stenosis either occurs at the anastomotic site or involves the donor renal artery. Anastomotic stenosis is more common after end-to-end arterial anastomosis and is probably due to faulty surgical technique. Stenosis of the donor renal artery occurs distal to the anastomosis and is characterized by gross intimal thickening. It may be the result of rejection involving the renal artery, excessive length or angulation of the renal artery causing turbulent flow, or intimal damage caused at the time of organ perfusion. This type of stenosis is more commonly seen in patients with end-to-side anastomosis. Duplex Doppler sonography typically demonstrates increased peak frequency shift (>7.5 kHz with 3-mHz scanning or velocity >3 m/second) at the stenotic site with turbulence of the signal distal to the stenosis. Color flow imaging facilitates identification of flow velocity at the stenotic site. Selective renin determinations are very helpful in confirming hemodynamic significance of stenotic lesions. Percutaneous transluminal angioplasty is the preferred mode of therapy, with surgical correction reserved for patients with unsuccessful angioplasty.

ANASTOMOTIC LEAK. Early anastomotic leaks are due to technical problems with resultant dehiscence. Immediate re-exploration is indicated for salvage of the transplant and the patient. Delayed leaks are seen in patients with wound infection extending to the vascular suture line. Emergency nephrectomy and wound drainage are the preferred mode of therapy.

PSEUDOANEURYSM. This is an uncommon complication, usually of mycotic origin. Hypertension may be a presenting symptom because of compression of the renal artery by the aneurysm. Rupture of the aneurysm has been reported. Intrarenal pseudoaneurysms are secondary to needle biopsy. On duplex Doppler sonography, pseudoaneurysms demonstrate highly turbulent pulsatile flow in their central lumen with classic ''machine-like'' to-and-fro flow at their neck. Intrarenal pseudoaneurysms are treated by selective embolization.

Venous Complications

RENAL VEIN STENOSIS. Renal vein stenosis is a rare complication of transplantation. Early recognition and treatment by angioplasty can reverse graft dysfunction.

RENAL VEIN THROMBOSIS. Renal vein thrombosis usually occurs in the early postoperative period. The incidence of renal vein thrombosis is 0.5 to 4 per cent. It may be secondary to twisting or kinking of the renal vein at the time of surgery, or it may be a secondary complication of thrombosis of iliac veins. External compression of the renal vein by lymphocele, abscess, or urinoma is also possible. Renal vein thrombosis is more common in transplants placed in the left iliac fossa. This has been attributed to compression of the left common iliac vein against the sacral promontory by the overlying right common iliac artery or the bifurcation of aorta.

Graft swelling, oliguria, and proteinuria suggest renal vein thrombosis. Since these symptoms are also seen in acute rejection, a high index of suspicion is necessary. Duplex Doppler sonography demonstrates absence of renal vein blood flow, and the arterial waveform may show high resistance and reversed diastolic flow. Diagnosis is established by renal venography. Surgical exploration with thrombectomy is indicated. Anticoagulation is advisable in patients with thrombophlebitis of iliac veins.

Renal Arteriovenous Fistula

Arteriovenous fistula complicating renal transplantation occurs most commonly after percutaneous needle biopsy of the transplant kidney. Rupture of a mycotic aneurysm may also result in an arteriovenous fistula. Injury to the major transplant vessels during surgery may also be responsible. Clinically patients may present with hematuria, hypertension, and bruit. Duplex Doppler sonography demonstrates turbulence with increased flow in the supplying artery and arterialization of the waveform from the draining vein. Color flow imaging demonstrates increased flow in the area of the fistula. Angiography will be necessary for definitive diagnosis. Treatment depends upon the size and location of the fistula. Most small fistulas following renal biopsy close spontaneously. Large central fistulas may require embolization or nephrectomy. Conservative surgery is carried out in selected cases.

PERITRANSPLANT FLUID COLLECTIONS

Peritransplant fluid collections occur in a high percentage of patients. Increased detection of such fluid collections is attributed to improved resolution of ultrasound equipment and routine serial examinations following the transplantation procedure. Early detection and close monitoring of peritransplant fluid collections are important to avoid and/or effectively deal with resultant clinical problems.

In the early postoperative period, the fluid collection is hematoma, abscess, or urinoma. Lymphocele generally occurs later. Ultrasonically guided percutaneous aspiration can provide definitive diagnosis.

Hematoma. Small, clinically insignificant hematomas are frequent in the early postoperative period. A large hematoma may develop secondary to graft rupture or injury to the vascular pedicle of the transplanted kidney. The most common clinical signs and symptoms are hypotension, decreased urinary output, hematuria, and acute pain over the transplant site. Hematoma may be a complication of percutaneous renal biopsy.

Abscess. Most patients with an abscess have fever, leukocytosis, and decreased renal function. Abscess can be seen in the early as well as the late postoperative period. Gallium scanning as well as percutaneous aspiration is helpful in definitive diagnosis.

Urinoma. Peritransplant fluid collection associated with free intraperitoneal fluid raises the possibility of urinoma. Decreased renal function is associated with decreased urine output, anuria, or urine drainage from the surgical incision. Uroradiographic examinations are necessary to delineate the exact site of urine leak.

Lymphocele. Lymphocele is the most common peritransplant fluid collection and is seen in 1 to 15 per cent of patients. It is generally seen in the late post-transplant period. Lymphocele is a localized accumulation of lymph in the extraperitoneal space that occurs as a result of interruption of the recipient's pelvic lymphatics or secondary to lymph seepage from the surface of the transplanted kidney. It is usually asymptomatic and manifests itself as fluctuant swelling around the kidney. Large lymphoceles can cause iliac vein compression and obstruction of the ureter. On sonography, lymphocele appears as a cystic fluid collection with internal septations in a high percentage of cases. There may be secondary hydronephrosis. Percutaneous aspiration of a lymphocele is usually inadequate treatment and results in infection, recurrence, or leak. Drainage is therefore required either to the surface or by marsupialization through a very large hole into the peritoneum.

UROLOGIC COMPLICATIONS

Urologic complications continue to be a frequent and significant problem in renal transplant recipients. The incidence of such complications is approximately 13 per cent. Even though the complication rate has remained constant during the last 30 years, the rate of death caused by such complications has decreased significantly during the last 10 years. This is attributed to early recognition of such complications by routine ultrasonography and radionuclide studies of transplant recipients. The majority of urologic complications occur in the first month after transplantation. Contributing factors include technical problems, ischemia, and perhaps rejection phenomenon.

Urinary Extravasation (Leak)

Elevated serum creatinine in post-transplant patients may be related to urinary leakage with reabsorption of creatinine from the retroperitoneal space. The reported incidence of urinary extravasation varies between 0.5 and 17 per cent. The most common causes of urinary extravasation in renal transplant recipients are defects at the ureteropelvic, ureteroureteric, or ureterovesical anastomoses. Extravasation can also occur from the bladder where it has been opened for ureteroneocystostomy. Most urinary extravasations occur in the early postoperative period and are manifested by a decrease in urine output from the bladder and an increase in wound drainage or urinary ascites, if the extravasation is intraperitoneal. Chronic urinary extravasation leads to urinoma formation. Urinary extravasation may be the result of ureteral necrosis secondary to compromised blood supply or ureteral graft rejection.

Radionuclide studies are very useful to detect urinary leaks. Cystography, excretory urography, or retrograde or antegrade pyelography will demonstrate the exact site of extravasation. Ureteral extravasation is best managed by percutaneous nephrostomy and ureteral stenting. Extravasation from the bladder may be managed by catheter drainage.

A calyceal-cutaneous fistula is an uncommon complication, particularly seen in donor kidneys with multiple renal arteries. Polar arteries inadvertently cut during nephrectomy or occluded during the post-transplant period may lead to segmental infarction with fistula formation.

Urinary Obstruction

Ureteral obstruction occurs in 2 to 7.5 per cent of renal transplants. It is a late complication, as opposed to urinary extravasation, which occurs in the early post-transplant period. Urinary obstruction in the immediate postoperative period is a normal phenomenon and is due to either edema at the ureterovesical junction or lack of peristalsis in the transplanted ureter. The causes of obstruction include stricture at the ureterovesical junction, extrinsic compression from lymphocele or abscess, ureteral necrosis, torsion of the transplanted kidney with concomitant ureteral obstruction, ureteral calculus, and blood clots. Ureteropelvic fibrosis with obstruction has been described in a few cases. Ureteral stricture may occur as a manifestation of the rejection phenomenon. Fungus ball and necrotic papillae are rare causes of obstruction of the ureter. Ultrasonography is the most useful screening test. Radionuclide studies will also discover this problem. However, the exact level and cause of obstruction are best identified by excretory urography, retrograde pyelography, or percutaneous antegrade pyelography. Percutaneous nephrostomy allows easy decompression of the dilated collecting system and rapid improvement of renal function prior to balloon dilatation and subsequent ureteral stenting or surgical repair.

MISCELLANEOUS COMPLICATIONS

Papillary necrosis, cortical necrosis, and renal neoplasms are unusual complications that have been reported in the literature. Urinary tract infection is also seen in renal transplants, with diabetic patients being particularly susceptible.

Calculus formation in the renal transplant patient is an unusual and late complication occurring two months to seven years after transplantation. Hyperparathyroidism, obstruction, and recurrent urinary tract infections are contributing factors.

IMAGING TECHNIQUES IN RENAL TRANSPLANTATION

Impaired renal allograft function during the post-transplant period warrants an immediate and thorough evaluation to distinguish between the parenchymal and surgical complications discussed earlier. The goal of pelvic imaging in such cases is to expeditiously obtain the most information in the least invasive manner possible so that appropriate therapy may be promptly instituted. Plain radiography, excretory urography, ultrasonography, radionuclide scintigraphy, computed tomography, angiography, cystography, and retrograde pyelography are established imaging techniques in transplant recipients. Digital subtraction angiography and magnetic resonance imaging are promising new techniques. Ultrasonography facilitates percutaneous renal biopsy, antegrade pyelography, and aspiration and drainage of fluid collections. Ureteral stenting, ureteral stricture dilatation, and percutaneous transluminal angioplasty serve as useful therapeutic adjuncts.

Plain Radiographs of the Transplant Kidney

Prior to the days of ultrasonography, transplant surgeons routinely attached silver clips around the kidney and plain radiographs of the transplant kidney were very helpful to evaluate kidney enlargement. However, this practice has now been abandoned. Plain radiographs are useful in demonstrating radiopaque calculi and gas in the renal parenchyma and collecting system in rare cases of emphysematous pyelonephritis.

Excretory Urography

Prior to routine use of radionuclide scanning and ultrasonography, excretory urography was frequently carried out to identify surgically treatable causes of transplant failure. Excretory urography remains a useful study when ureteral obstruction (Fig. 80–1) or extravasation is suspected in a transplant recipient with adequate renal function. Contrary to popular belief, the use of contrast medium carries little risk to transplants with normal renal function and does not significantly increase the risk of allograft dysfunction or likelihood of rejection. Adequate dose of contrast medium is necessary to opacify the collecting system, as the patient is generally well-hydrated. Oblique projections as well as tomography are necessary to provide good anatomic detail.

Cystography

Cystography is indicated in patients with suspected urinary extravasation from the bladder. Oblique views and post-voiding films are necessary to demonstrate small bladder leaks. Extrinsic compression of the bladder will be seen in patients with large, loculated fluid collections in the pelvis. In patients with persistent or recurrent urinary tract infection, cystography is indicated to rule out vesicoureteral reflux.

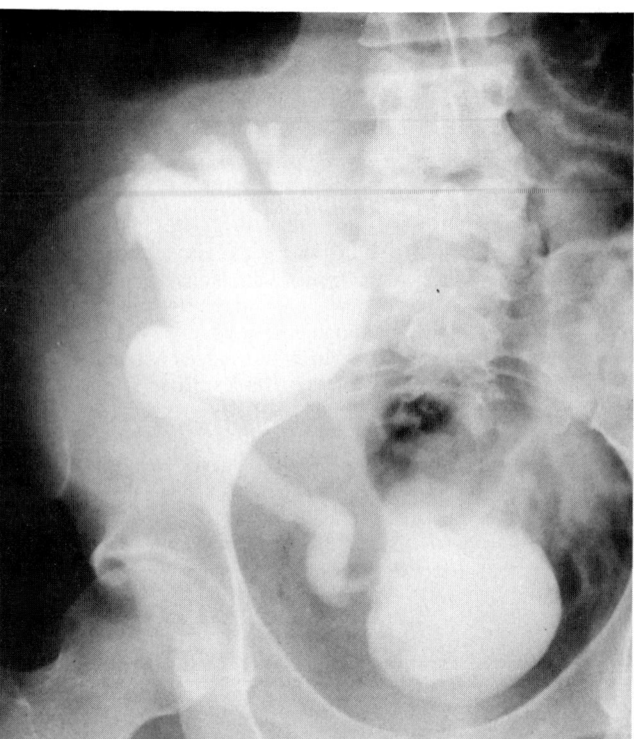

Figure 80–1. Excretory urogram in a 20-year-old transplant recipient demonstrates **distal ureteral stricture with proximal dilatation.**

Retrograde Pyelography

In patients with impaired renal function, retrograde pyelography is sometimes indicated to localize the exact site of obstruction or extravasation. However, it may be technically difficult to perform because of ureteroneocystostomy.

Ultrasonography

Because of the relatively superficial position of the transplant kidney in the iliac fossa and no intervening bowel gas or bony structures, renal transplants are particularly well-suited for ultrasonic study. Routine use of a 3.5- or 5-mHz transducer provides excellent detail. Real-time studies facilitate prompt and accurate assessment of post-transplantation problems.

High-frequency transducers (5 mHz or higher) provide excellent detail of the transplant because of its superficial location. Real-time ultrasonography, combined with duplex Doppler or color flow imaging techniques (Fig. 80–2*C*), is the most frequently used examination to evaluate worsening renal function in the post-transplantation period and provides prompt and accurate assessment of post-transplantation problems. Resistive index (RI) was initially thought to separate rejection from other causes of worsening renal function. However, recent studies suggest that the increased RI may be due to a variety of causes other than rejection. The RI should be used to alert the examiner that there may be problems that may necessitate arteriography or other investigations.

ULTRASOUND FINDINGS

Normal

The normal renal configuration is preserved, with a smooth renal outline. There is a distinct corticomedullary interface, with the cortex being echogenic when compared with echo-poor pyramids. Centrally, the pelvocalyceal echo complex is seen as a highly echogenic ellipsoid or stellate area of varying thickness depending upon the amount of fat in the renal sinus (Fig. 80–2*A*). The arcuate artery and vein and surrounding fatty envelope produce short, curvilinear, high-amplitude echoes in the corticomedullary region. Real-time ultrasonography usually demonstrates strong vascular pulsations in the allograft.

Rejection

During the course of acute tubular necrosis, the renal anatomy remains sonographically unaltered. During the course of acute rejec-

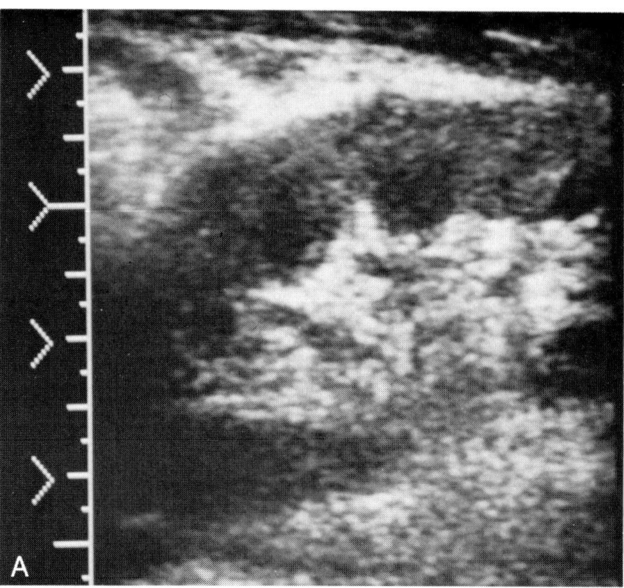

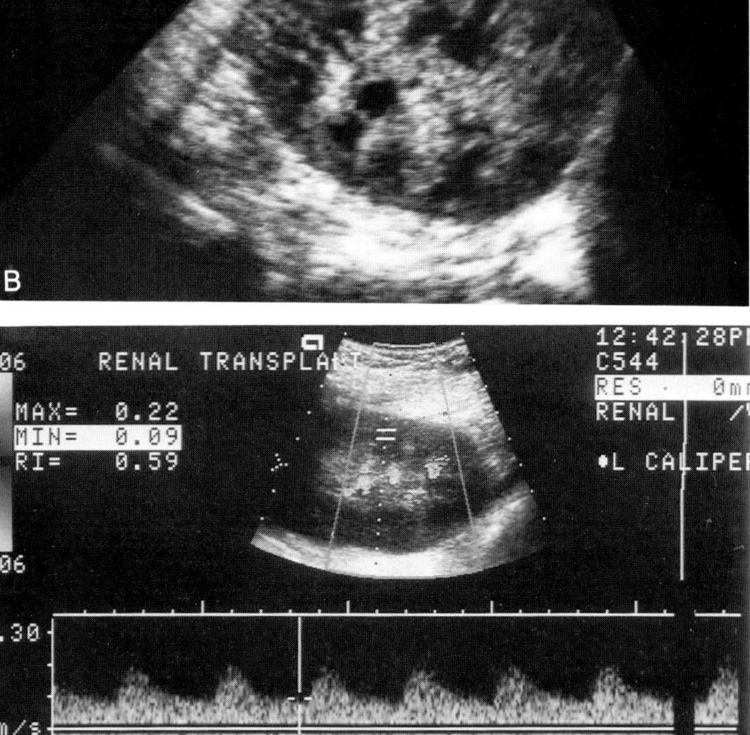

Figure 80–2. *A,* **Normal transplant ultrasound** demonstrates excellent corticomedullary differentiation with normal-sized hypoechoic pyramids and a central echogenic renal sinus. *B,* **Longitudinal ultrasonic examination** demonstrates multiple enlarged sonolucent medullary zones extending to the periphery of the kidney. In addition, there is poor differentiation between parenchyma and renal sinus secondary to decreased amplitude of the renal sinus in this biopsy-proven **acute rejection.** *C,* Doppler examination with color flow imaging defines location of arcuate arteries and demonstrates normal spectral waveform obtained at this level.

tion, however, there is a spectrum of sonographic findings that depend upon the stage that the rejection process has reached. The sonographic findings include increased renal volume, decreased amplitude of the renal sinus echoes (Fig. 80–2*B*), enlarged medullary pyramids, indistinct corticomedullary boundary, increased echogenicity of the renal cortex, focal sonolucent areas in the renal parenchyma, decreased echogenicity of the renal parenchyma, sparse cortical echoes, perirenal fluid collections, localized bulging of the renal outline, and submucosal edema of the collecting system. To suggest a diagnosis of acute rejection sonographically, at least two of the above-described findings should be present. In chronic rejection, parenchymal atrophy with consequent fibrosis and shrinkage results in an irregular parenchymal echo pattern.

Ureteral Obstruction

Minimal dilatation of the collecting system is acceptable in the immediate post-transplantation period and is usually due to edema at the ureteroneocystostomy site. Hydronephrosis in the presence of a distended urinary bladder should be interpreted with caution, and a repeat study after emptying the bladder should be carried out. Hydronephrosis may be secondary to ureteral stricture or peritransplant fluid collections such as urinoma or lymphocele.

Peritransplant Fluid Collections

Fluid collections near or around the kidney include hematoma, abscess, urinoma, and lymphocele. Hematomas and abscesses may have low-level echoes due to cellular debris. Lymphoceles are typically multilocular and free of internal echoes. Urinomas are generally echo-free collections near the bladder. Repeat scans after voiding are necessary to determine which fluid-filled structure is bladder. While ultrasonography is sensitive for detection of fluid collections, it is not specific for fluid type, and aspiration of fluid collection with ultrasonic guidance is extremely helpful in management of the transplant recipient.

Radionuclide Scintigraphy

Radionuclide scintigraphy of the renal transplant has assumed an important role in the diagnosis and management of post-transplant complications. The radionuclide studies can provide useful information about renal perfusion, renal morphology, tubular function, and the status of the collecting system (Fig. 80–3*A*). The commonly used radiopharmaceuticals are technetium-99m diethylenetriamine-penta-acetic acid (DTPA), technetium-99m glucoheptonate, and ^{131}I- or ^{123}I-labeled orthoiodohippurate.

Technetium-99m DTPA and technetium-99m glucoheptonate are commonly employed to study renal perfusion. The patient is positioned under a large-field gamma camera so that the abdominal aorta, renal transplant, and urinary bladder are in the field of view. Serial dynamic images are obtained at one-, two-, or three-second intervals when the injected radioactivity starts appearing in the abdominal aorta. Normally the vascular flush in the transplant kidney appears almost simultaneously with that of the external iliac artery. It reaches a peak within the next four to six seconds, and the successive images show uniform activity within the kidney, which falls rapidly to lower levels in the next few frames. Following the radionuclide angiogram, serial static images of the kidney at two- or three-minute intervals are obtained for 10 to 20 minutes. These images provide information concerning renal morphology and excretory function. Since technetium-99m DTPA is excreted only by glomerular filtration, its rate of clearance from the blood indirectly reflects the glomerular filtration rate.

The most commonly used radiopharmaceutical for evaluation of renal tubular function is ^{131}I- or ^{123}I-labeled orthoiodohippurate (Hippuran). About 80 per cent of the intravenously administered dose is extracted from renal blood by renal tubular cells and actively excreted into the urine. The remaining 15 to 20 per cent is filtered at the glomerular level. Sequential two- or three-minute static images are obtained after administration of 100 to 250 microcuries of ^{131}I Hippuran on a standard or large-field gamma camera fitted with a high-energy collimator. Normally there is rapid uptake of Hippuran within the renal cortex and maximal cortical concentration is reached in two to six minutes. There is prompt excretion into the collecting system. The urinary bladder is normally visualized within six minutes after radiopharmaceutical injection. Most of the radiopharmaceutical is cleared from the renal parenchyma by 20 minutes after injection.

It is generally agreed that a baseline renal study using technetium-99m DTPA and ^{131}I Hippuran should be performed at 24 hours after surgery. Thereafter, based on the results of the baseline study and clinical situation, serial renal studies are obtained at such intervals as considered appropriate to determine any changes in functional status of the renal transplant. It is the change in renal function on serial studies that is considered useful in diagnosis and management of any renal complication. Complete knowledge of the patient's clinical condition is also necessary to interpret the significance of change in graft function on radionuclide studies.

Acute tubular necrosis (ATN) and acute and chronic rejection are some of the important and common complications of renal transplantation. Renal perfusion study with a technetium complex in a typical case of ATN would demonstrate a mild to moderate reduction in renal blood flow and glomerular filtration rate. Delayed static images will show poor uptake in the graft owing to impaired GFR. I-131 Hippuran study will show relatively good concentration in the graft because localization of Hippuran in the kidneys is primarily related to renal blood flow (Fig. 80–3*B*). However, there is slow or no excretion of radiopharmaceutical in the urinary bladder because of dysfunction of the tubular cells. On serial studies there is a gradual improvement in renal function, provided that rejection or any other complication does not hinder the recovery.

In acute rejection, the technetium DTPA study shows considerable decrease in renal perfusion, usually more severe than seen in patients with ATN. There is marked delay and considerably diminished uptake of ^{131}I Hippuran in the renal cortex and extremely slow excretion into the collecting system and urinary bladder (Fig. 80–3*C*). Subtle changes of early rejection can best be diagnosed on serial renal studies. However, it is apparent from the above discussion that both ATN and acute rejection are manifest by a decrease in renal perfusion and function on technetium DTPA and ^{131}I Hippuran studies, which makes it extremely difficult to accurately differentiate between these two complications. The differentiation between ATN and acute rejection is made primarily on clinical grounds. The radionuclide studies reveal the severity and extent of the deterioration in renal function, which can be used as a guide in daily management of these complications. The diagnosis of acute rejection should be suspected in patients who initially show evidence of ATN and if there is continuing deterioration of renal function on serial examinations over a period of several days.

Hyperacute rejection usually occurs within 48 hours of renal transplantation. The renal perfusion study would demonstrate lack of blood flow to the transplanted kidney, and there is no concentration of ^{131}I Hippuran in the transplant kidney. However, similar findings are also noted in patients who develop complete occlusion of the renal artery or thrombosis of the renal vein, and it is impossible to differentiate between these conditions on radionuclide studies. Kirchner and Rosenthal have shown the importance of renal perfusion studies in these conditions. If a technetium DTPA study reveals a "photopenic zone" at the expected position of the renal transplant on dynamic and delayed static images, it indicates total lack of renal perfusion and generally warrants surgical removal of the kidney. If there is just nonvisualization of the renal transplant without any "photopenic zone," some degree of functional recovery is still possible, since renal perfusion is at least as much as the surrounding soft tissues.

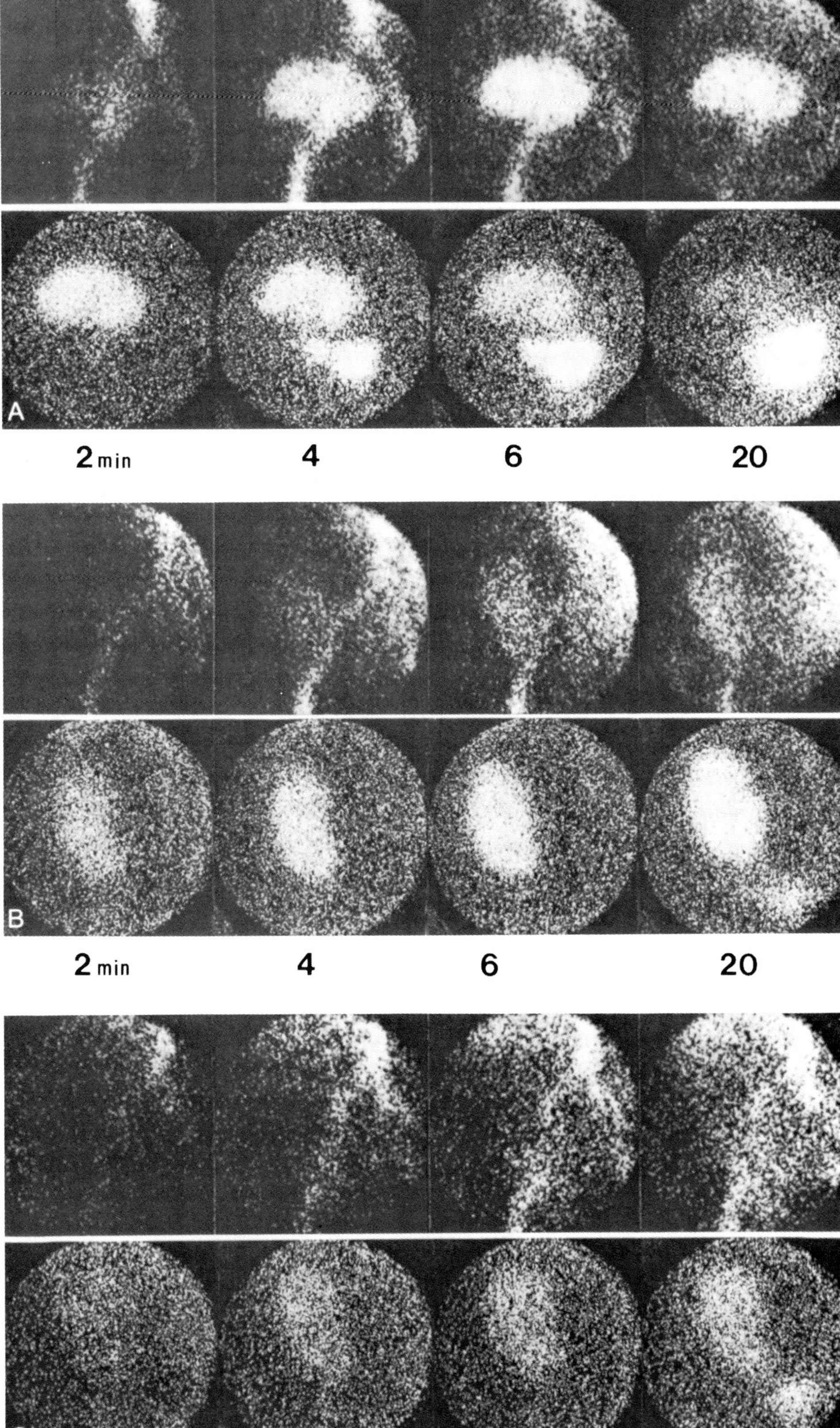

Figure 80–3. *A,* Selected frames from a ^{99m}Tc DTPA dynamic study *(top row)* and a ^{131}I Hippuran study *(bottom row)* demonstrate **normal perfusion and function of a transplant kidney**. *B,* Radionuclide studies demonstrate relatively intact renal perfusion *(top row)* but delayed transit of ^{131}I Hippuran *(bottom row)* in a patient with **acute tubular necrosis.** *C,* Radionuclide studies demonstrate decreased renal perfusion *(top row)* and poor concentration and excretion of ^{131}I Hippuran *(bottom row)* in a patient with **acute rejection.**

Urinary obstruction in a renal transplant may result from several causes. The renal collecting system is visualized very well with technetium-99m complexes, especially technetium-99m DTPA. Usually the appearance of radioactivity in the collecting system with absent or markedly delayed visualization of the urinary bladder suggests the diagnosis of urinary obstruction. A diuretic renogram may be needed to differentiate a dilated collecting system from an obstructed one. In some situations, delayed images of the kidney may be needed at one or two hours to detect urinary obstruction. Reliable detection of urinary extravasation is also aided by delayed images that would demonstrate increasing accumulation of radiopharmaceutical in an extraurinary location. A post-void image will demonstrate persistent activity at the site of urinary extravasation.

Formation of a lymphocele or hematoma adjacent to the renal transplant usually produces a relatively photopenic area that does not change in intensity on delayed images. These lesions can be detected only if they are larger than 2 cm in size. Infarcts of the transplant kidney are recognized on early static images as irregular or wedge-shaped defects in the renal cortex.

Angiography

Angiography of renal transplants can be very helpful in making a relatively precise diagnosis in post-transplantation dysfunction. However, because of its invasive nature, it plays a limited role in the work-up of most patients with renal impairment in the early post-transplant period. Indications for arteriography of renal transplants are (1) acute anuria, (2) hypertension not responding to medication and usually associated with a bruit in the area of the transplanted kidney, and (3) functional deterioration of the allograft in which confirmatory evidence of rejection or renal artery stenosis is necessary in order to proceed with definitive surgery. Selective injections and magnification studies, as well as oblique views, are very helpful in arriving at a proper diagnosis.

In patients with acute anuria, when radionuclide studies fail to visualize the allograft, arteriography is useful in differentiating arterial thrombosis from hyperacute rejection. Delayed clearance of contrast medium, a pruned tree appearance, and an absent nephrogram suggest hyperacute rejection.

In acute rejection, there is tapering, attenuation, constriction, or occlusion of intrarenal branches. There is a pruned tree appearance secondary to loss of second- and third-order branches, with prolongation of arterial clearance time and diminished or absent nephrogram. In contrast, the arteriogram is essentially normal in patients with acute tubular necrosis.

In chronic rejection, arteriography demonstrates small graft size with irregularity, attenuation, and occlusion of interlobular arteries, and a patchy nephrogram secondary to areas of cortical infarction. Renal artery aneurysms have also been described as a manifestation of chronic rejection.

Hypertension that does not respond to medical therapy and that is associated with a bruit over the transplanted kidney is an indication for angiography (Fig. 80–4*A* and *B*). Digital subtraction angiography is the preferred screening test in the evaluation of these patients. If it is technically unsuccessful, selective arteriography is necessary to demonstrate the degree of renal artery stenosis. Percutaneous transluminal angioplasty is an attractive alternative to surgical correction for the relief of arterial stenosis.

Renal venography is indicated in those rare cases in which there is strong clinical suspicion of renal vein thrombosis.

Computed Tomography

Computed tomography (CT) is an accurate, noninvasive technique that can be easily performed for the diagnosis of complications after renal transplant surgery. It is less operator-dependent than ultrasound, and the examination can be performed in spite of drains, tubes, open wounds, and surgical dressings. It helps to dif-

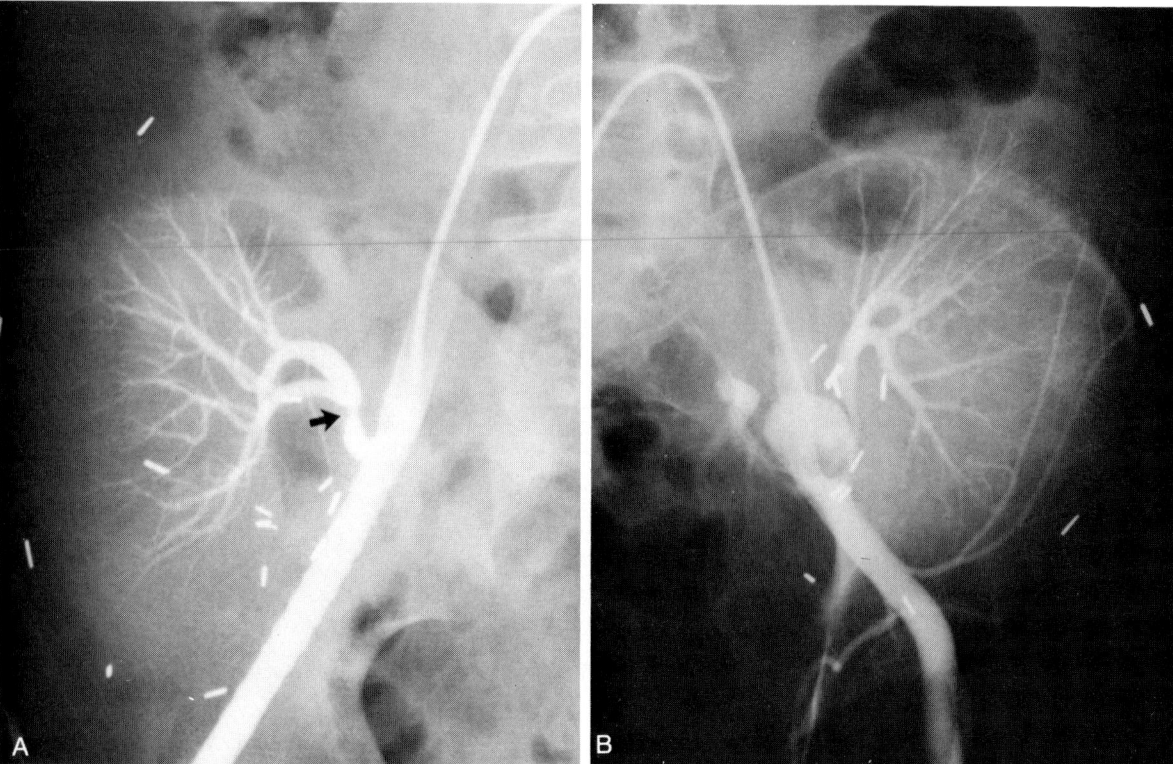

Figure 80–4. *A,* Selective right iliac arteriogram demonstrates **short focal stenosis** *(arrow)* **of the renal artery.** *B,* Left external iliac arteriogram in a patient with bruit and hypertension demonstrates **anastomotic pseudoaneurysm** causing compression of the renal artery.

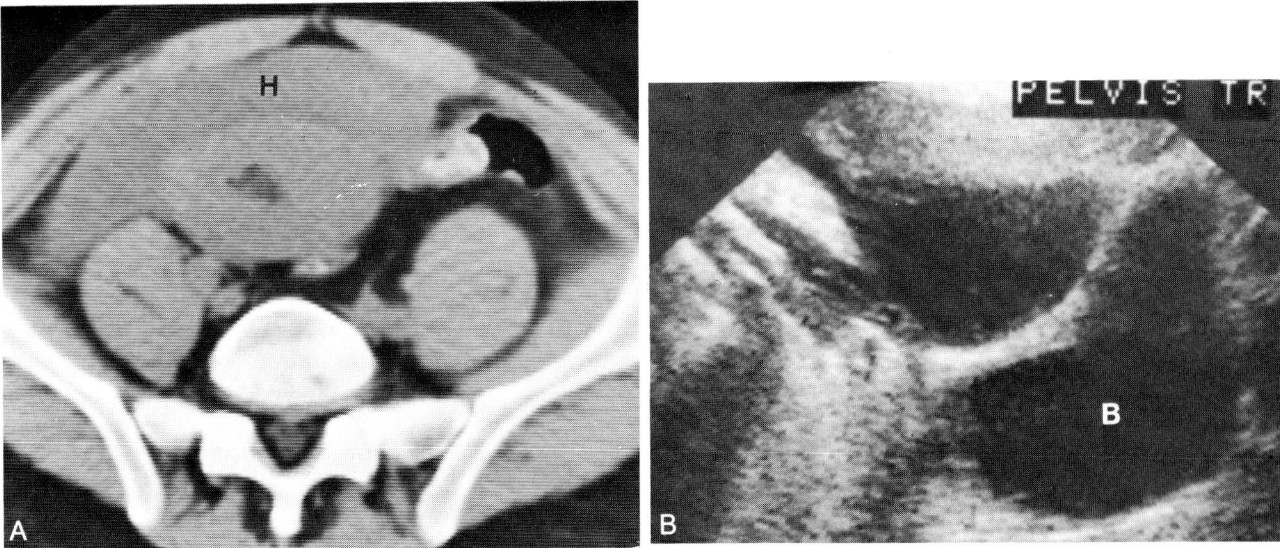

Figure 80–5. *A,* **Computed tomographic evaluation** of patient three weeks following transplantation. Biopsy was complicated by an anterior peritransplant hematoma (H). *B,* Transverse ultrasonic examination of the pelvis demonstrates a loculated fluid collection anterior and to the right of the bladder (B).

ferentiate acute rejection from obstructive uropathy, urinary fistula, or significant perinephric fluid collections (Fig. 80–5*A*).

In acute rejection, CT reveals normal anatomy of the allograft—ureter, bladder, and adjacent structures—with no evidence of hydronephrosis or perinephric fluid collection. Dynamic CT has been used in the evaluation of physiologic status of renal transplants with corticoarterial junction time as an index of renal blood flow and corticomedullary junction time as an index of renal function.

CT can define the position of the graft and the extent of peritransplant fluid collections. Absorption coefficient values expressed as Hounsfield units (HU) are helpful in distinguishing the nature of fluid collections. Fresh blood in the form of hematoma has the highest value, frequently in the range of 55 to 65 HU. The attenuation values of lymphoceles are between 10 and 20 HU (Fig. 80–5*B*), whereas attenuation values of abscesses are often between 20 and 30 HU.

CT after infusion of contrast medium will readily demonstrate urinary leaks and urinomas. CT and ultrasound both provide useful guidance in performing percutaneous biopsy, aspiration of fluid collections, or percutaneous nephrostomy in selected cases.

Magnetic Resonance Imaging

The role of magnetic resonance imaging (MRI) in post-transplant dysfunction is still evolving. However, MRI is of limited value in the differentiation of ATN from acute rejection because loss of corticomedullary differentiation is a nonspecific finding. ^{31}P MRI spectroscopy may be useful for evaluating renal metabolism during episodes of transplant dysfunction. Preliminary work to determine the clinical potential of MRI for evaluation of renal transplants appears promising.

T_1-weighted images appear to provide the best differentiation between the cortical and medullary portions of the transplanted kidney (Fig. 80–6). T_2-weighted images demonstrate fluid collec-

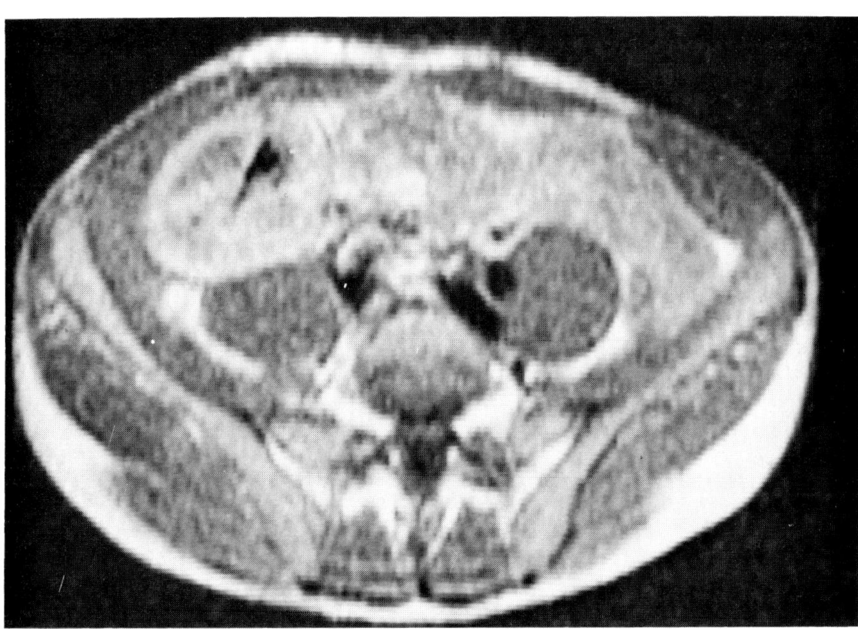

Figure 80–6. T_1-weighted magnetic resonance image demonstrates excellent corticomedullary differentiation in this **normal transplant.**

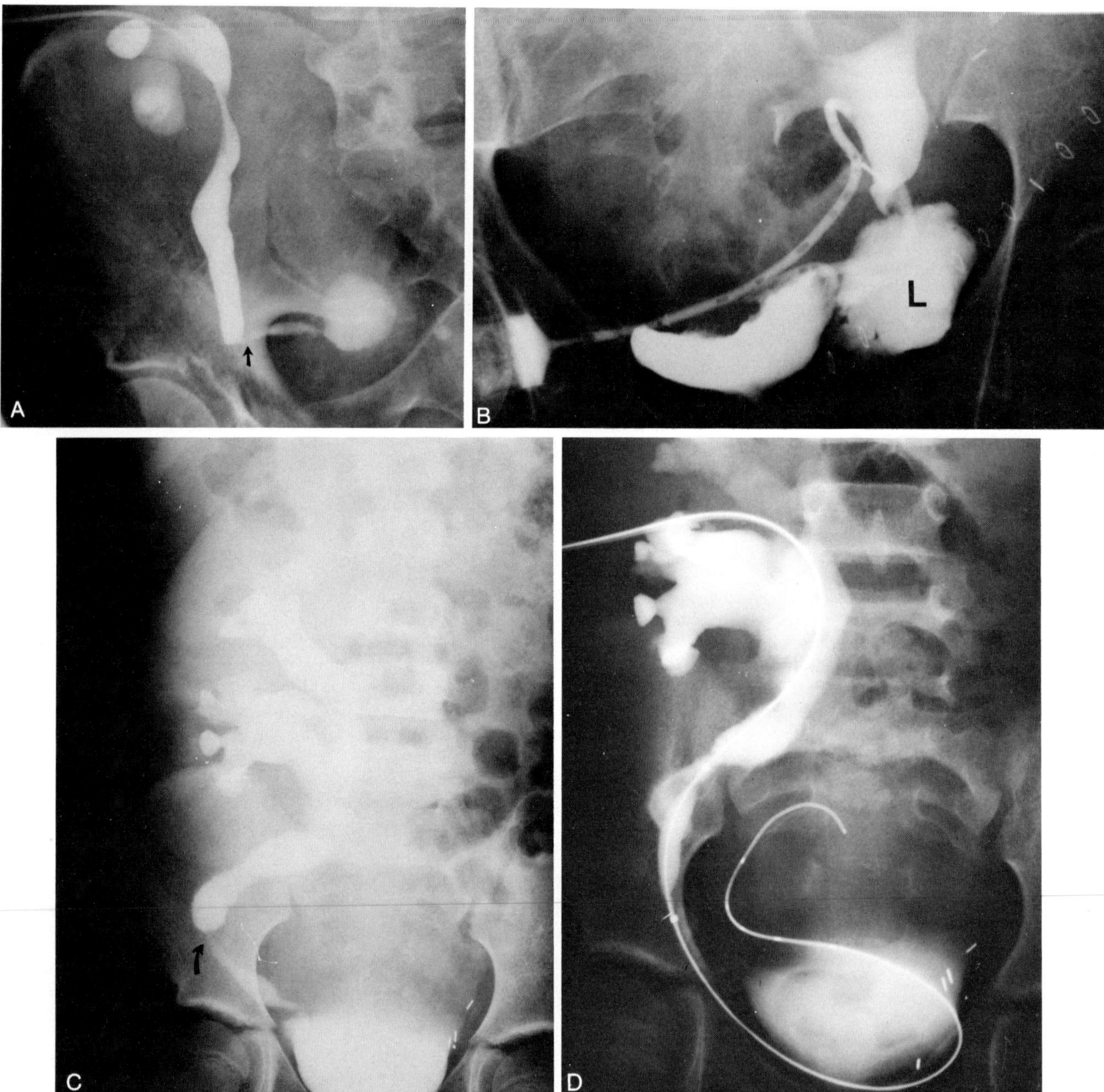

Figure 80–7. *A,* Antegrade pyelography in a patient with deteriorating renal function and ultrasonic demonstration of hydronephrosis demonstrates **stricture of the distal ureter** *(arrow). B,* A 35-year-old male was noted to have ascites and urine leakage (L) from the mid-ureter. Follow-up study three weeks after internal-external ureter stenting demonstrated no further extravasation, and the stent was removed. *C,* Excretory urography demonstrates stricture of the mid-ureteral stenting *(arrow)* with resultant ureteropyelocaliectasis. *D* demonstrates balloon catheter in place dilating the stricture.

tions either within or around the kidney to best advantage. Lymphoceles can be readily distinguished from hematomas because of inherent differences in relaxation times, with lymphoceles having low signal intensity on the T_1-weighted images and high signal intensity on T_2-weighted images, in contrast to hematomas, which have high signal intensity on both T_1- and T_2-weighted images.

MRI readily demonstrates the size, shape, and position of the transplanted kidney. In acute rejection, there is a decrease in corticomedullary differentiation and a decrease in overall signal intensity on T_1-weighted images, reflecting a prolongation of T_1 relaxation time. In chronic rejection, there is complete loss of corticomedullary differentiation.

PERCUTANEOUS TECHNIQUES IN THE MANAGEMENT OF UROLOGIC COMPLICATIONS IN RENAL TRANSPLANT PATIENTS

Antegrade pyelography by fine-needle puncture of the transplant kidney is a remarkably safe procedure with no clinically significant complications. It provides superior anatomic detail of the transplant ureter. It is the most accurate and informative examination for demonstration of ureteral stricture (Fig. 80–7*A*) as well as the site of ureteral leak.

Indications for placement of a nephrostomy drainage catheter are urine leak (Fig. 80–7*B*) and ureteral obstruction that have resulted in renal impairment, symptoms (pain, fever, oliguria, or anuria), or urinary tract infection.

Following improvement in the patient's clinical status, ureteral strictures can be dilated percutaneously by using angioplasty catheters and indwelling ureteral stents left in place (Fig. 80–7*C* and *D*).

Renal stone extraction through a percutaneous nephrostomy in a renal transplant patient has also been successfully accomplished.

Bibliography

Baxter GM, Morley P, Dall B: Acute renal vein thrombosis in renal allografts: New Doppler ultrasonic findings. Clin Radiol 43:125–127, 1991.

Coyne SS, et al: Surgically correctable renal transplant complications: An integrated clinical and radiologic approach. AJR 163:113–119, 1981.

Deodhar SD, Benjamin SP: Pathology of human renal allograft rejections. Surg Clin North Am 51:1141–1159, 1971.

DeSouza NM, Reidy JF, Koffman CG: Arteriovenous fistulas complicating biopsy of renal allografts: Treatment of bleeding with superselective embolization. AJR 156:507–510, 1991.

Dodd GD, Tublin ME, Shah A, Zajko A: Imaging of vascular complications associated with renal transplants. AJR 157:449–459, 1991.

Geisinger MA, et al: Magnetic resonance imaging of renal transplants. AJR 143:1229–1234, 1984.

Hunter DW, et al: Percutaneous techniques in the management of urological complications in renal transplant patients. Radiology 148:407–412, 1983.

Kirchner PT, Rosenthal L: Renal transplant evaluation. Semin Nucl Med 12:370–378, 1982.

Kumar R, Wilson DD, Santa-Cruz FR: Postoperative urological complications of renal transplantation. Radiographics 4:531–547, 1984.

Levey AS: The improving prognosis after kidney transplantation. New strategies to overcome immunologic rejection. Arch Intern Med 144:2382–2387, 1984.

Matalon TAS, Thompson MJ, Patel SK, et al: Percutaneous transluminal angioplasty for transplant renal artery stenosis. JVIR 3:55–58, 1992.

Middleton WD, Kellman GM, Melson LG, Madrazo BL: Post-biopsy renal transplant arteriovenous fistulas: Color Doppler US characteristics. Radiology 171:253–257, 1989.

Needleman L, Kurtz A: Doppler evaluation of the renal transplantation. J Clin Ultrasound 15:661–673, 1987.

Novick AC, et al: The role of computerized tomography in renal transplant patients. J Urol 125:15–18, 1981.

Pozniak, MA, Kelcz F, Dodd GD: Renal transplant ultrasound: Imaging and Doppler. Semin US, CT, MR 12(4):319–334, 1991.

Rijksen JFWB, et al: Vascular complications in 400 consecutive renal allotransplants. J Cardiovasc Surg 23:91–98, 1982.

Smith RB, Ehrlich RM: The surgical complications of renal transplantation. Urol Clin North Am 3:621–646, 1976.

Snider JF, Hunter DW, Moradian GP, et al: Transplant renal artery stenosis: Evaluation with duplex sonography. Radiology 172:1027–1030, 1989.

Streem SB, Novick AC: Pelvic imaging techniques in renal transplantation. Urol Clin North Am 10:301, 1983.

Surratt JT, Seigel MJ, Middleton WD: Sonography of complications in pediatric renal allografts. RadioGraphics 10:687–699, 1990.

81 Radiologic Imaging in Renal Trauma

Helen C. Redman

The surgical approach to acute renal trauma is conservative. Most patients with acute renal trauma are observed, as surgery is usually reserved for those patients with a serious vascular injury, a significant leakage of urine, or uncontrollable renal hemorrhage. Radiographic studies are used to help define which patients can be observed and which require surgical intervention.

Computed tomography (CT) is the most comprehensive radiologic technique for the evaluation of renal trauma. Other radiologic procedures that may be useful in specific patients include abdominal radiographs, excretory urography, ultrasound, and angiography. When the integrity of the collecting system is in doubt, either antegrade or retrograde pyelography may demonstrate a leak from the renal pelvis or ureter. Chronic or delayed sequelae of trauma often require a more extensive radiologic evaluation.

CLINICAL FEATURES

Blunt injuries are most frequently due to motor vehicle accidents, falls, or assaults. Although hematuria commonly occurs after blunt abdominal injury, significant injury to the kidney is infrequent. Furthermore, there is poor correlation between the amount of hematuria and the degree of renal injury. Thus, the amount of hematuria that should trigger a radiologic evaluation after blunt trauma remains controversial. Patients with gross hematuria and patients with a combination of microscopic hematuria and clinical indications of significant injury such as shock generally undergo radiologic evaluation of the urinary tract.

Penetrating injuries are most commonly due to gunshot or stab wounds. Penetrating trauma is either high- or low-velocity in nature. These injuries may be extensive or quite localized in their effect. Hematuria after penetrating injury is usually a sign of renal damage.

CLASSIFICATION

Since there is no universally accepted classification of renal injuries, it is important to clearly communicate the results of the radiographic evaluation to the referring physician. A functional classification by which injuries are grouped by severity is useful because of the therapeutic implications.

Minor injuries are often treated by observation and rarely require surgical intervention. They are the most common renal injury and are usually small. They include intrarenal hematomas, lacerations, subcapsular or perinephric hematomas, and subsegmental infarcts.

Intermediate injuries are often managed conservatively but may require surgical intervention, especially if there is clinical deterioration. Intermediate injuries include major renal lacerations and hematomas. If the laceration extends through the kidney such that a portion is distracted, it may be termed a renal fracture. If the collecting system is involved, there will be extravasation of urine and excreted contrast material. A perirenal hematoma is usually present.

Major renal injuries account for only approximately 5 per cent of all renal injuries but usually require surgical exploration. If the patient is hemodynamically unstable, immediate surgical exploration is necessary and often results in nephrectomy. Major renal injuries include damage to the renal pedicle, avulsion of the ureteropelvic junction, and multiple large renal lacerations.

RADIOLOGIC FINDINGS

Abdominal films provide only nonspecific information in renal trauma. Posterior fractures of the lower three ribs indicate forceful trauma to the flank in the region of the kidney. Obscuration of the renal contour or a kidney enlarging over several hours raises the question of perinephric bleeding or leakage of urine. These observations are vague and need confirmation.

Excretory urography is a reasonable screening technique for renal trauma but is not needed if an abdominal CT examination is to be obtained. When a urogram is performed to exclude traumatic injury, a one-minute film should be included. The nephrograms should be equal and symmetrical bilaterally, ensuring patency of the renal arteries and excluding most renal lacerations. Unilateral absence of renal opacification and contrast excretion suggest injury to the renal pedicle, usually traumatic occlusion of the renal artery. If the kidney is to be saved, emergent surgery is required. Thus, immediate arteriography is often requested to confirm the vascular lesion and define the arterial anatomy.

Normal calyces, infundibula, and pelvis on a 10-minute film make serious renal injury unlikely. Delayed function or spidery collecting systems raise the question of diffuse renal swelling or subcapsular hematoma. Filling defects within the collecting system are most likely due to blood clots and suggest hemorrhage. Contrast extravasation usually occurs in major renal injury but may be seen in less severe injury. In the setting of trauma, these findings assume significance, but the radiologist must always remember that preexisting disease and congenital abnormalities may have identical urographic findings.

Ultrasound is an excellent procedure to identify fluid collections in and around the kidney. It can also demonstrate parenchymal swelling and disruption. While some patients with rib fractures or abdominal wall tenderness are difficult to study because of pain caused by the transducer, the primary drawback is the inability to reliably demonstrate renal arterial injury. Renal function is also not evaluated. Therefore, ultrasound is most satisfactorily used to follow patients who are treated conservatively after CT has demonstrated the nature and extent of the renal injury. Percutaneous needle biopsies provide an exception to this rule. Percutaneous needle biopsies cause low-velocity penetrating injuries that may lead to pseudoaneurysms, frank hemorrhage, or arteriovenous fistulas. Ultrasound is a reasonable survey technique in these patients since fluid collections are easily seen and abdominal tenderness does not interfere with the examination.

In a patient suspected of having renal injury, CT is preferably performed after the administration of intravenous contrast material, though scans performed both before and after intravenous contrast media is given can be useful (Fig. 81–1). The kidneys can be evaluated without intravenous contrast material, but patency of the main renal arteries and their branches cannot be determined on unenhanced scans. Oral contrast material is not necessary in the evaluation of renal injury per se, but it is also usually given since the remainder of the abdomen is generally surveyed in the evaluation of any abdominal trauma. Contiguous 10-mm collimation is routinely employed. Since these scans generally include the entire abdomen, a common scanning sequence includes contiguous 10-mm sections from the dome of the diaphragm through the lower poles of the kidneys followed by 10-mm sections at 15- or 20-mm intervals to the symphysis pubis. The ureters and the bladder are evaluated on these lower sections.

The CT findings of renal injury include an absent or incomplete nephrogram caused by arterial occlusion, an abnormal contour (Fig. 81–2), abnormal position (Fig. 81–3), hemorrhage in the renal parenchyma, delayed or absent function, hemorrhage or fluid in the tissues around the kidney (Fig. 81–4), and frank extravasation of contrast material. Lacerations are generally linear or stellate parenchymal defects that are often accompanied by hemorrhage. Subcapsular hematomas may be crescentic or biconvex and generally distort the adjacent renal parenchyma. Arterial injuries severe enough to occlude a renal artery cause absence of the nephrogram in the portion of the kidney served by that artery. The entire kidney may be devascularized, or segmental defects may be seen. Pseudoaneurysms and arteriovenous fistulas can sometimes be detected with dynamic scanning.

Figure 81–1. Acute hematuria with massive clot retention occurred one week after a minor fall and two months after severe injury in a motor vehicle accident in this 31-year-old woman. *A,* A retrograde pyelogram was performed during placement of a ureteral stent. A filling defect extends from the hydronephrotic kidney to the distal ureter. At cystoscopy, the bladder was filled with clot. The bladder and ureter were irrigated and a double pigtail stent was placed. Because of continued hematuria and clot retention, a CT scan was ordered. *B,* A section through the mid-kidney taken before the administration of intravenous contrast material demonstrates blood in the renal pelvis and parenchyma *(arrows)*. *C,* A section at the same level as in *B* after intravenous contrast material has been administered demonstrates an irregular, somewhat poorly defined filling defect where the increased density was seen in *B*. This defect includes blood both in the collecting system and in a renal parenchymal laceration. *D,* Selective angiography of the more cephalad of two renal arteries using digital subtraction technique demonstrates frank extravasation. *E,* The injured artery was embolized with gelatin sponge. A nubbin of the branch artery is seen *(arrow)*, and other branches are narrowed by spasm caused by the instrumentation.

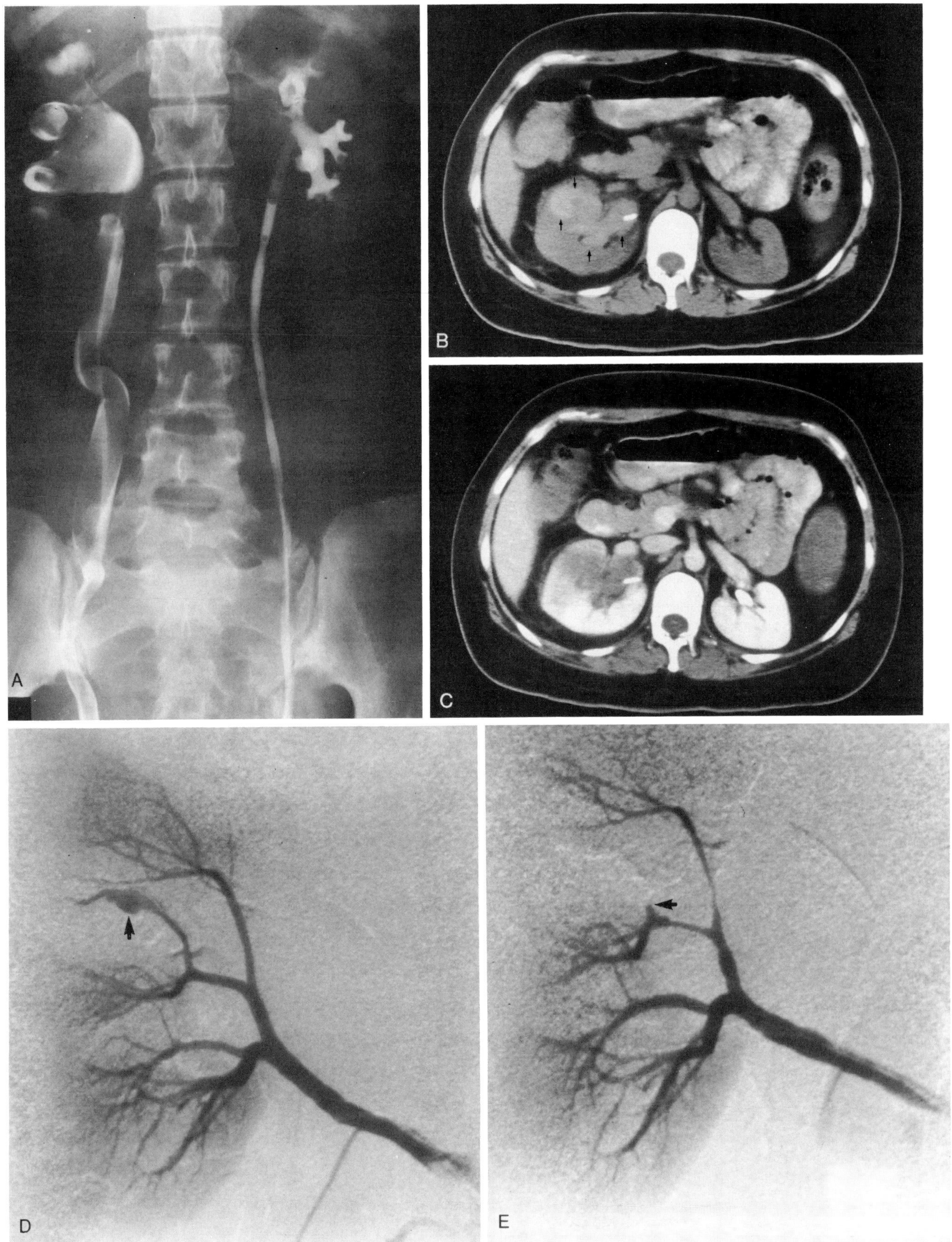

Figure 81–1. *See legend on opposite page*

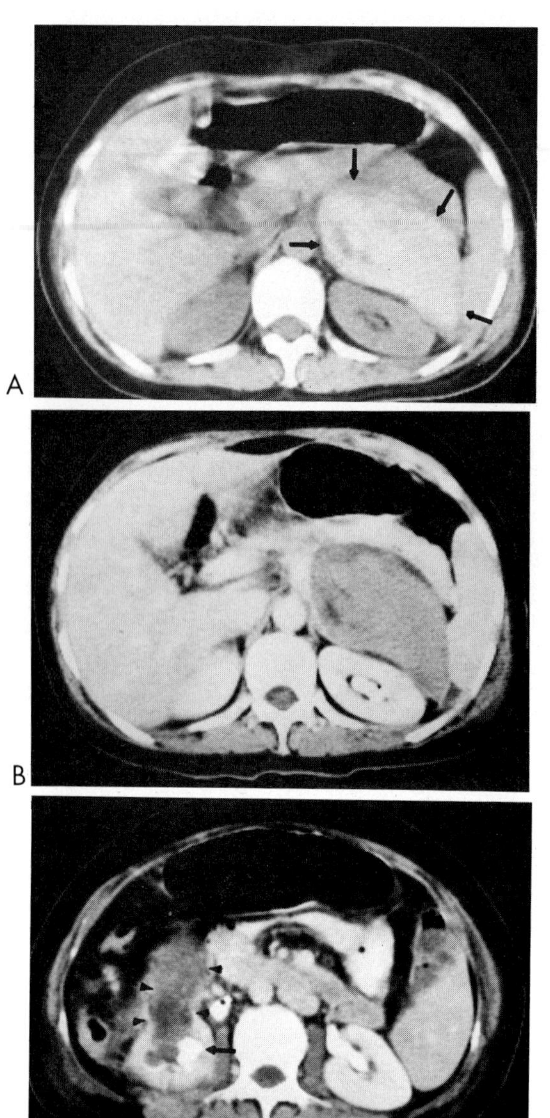

Figure 81–2. Renal injury occurred during electrohydraulic lithotripsy for renal stones in this 48-year-old woman. Three days after placement of a 26 Fr catheter into her renal pelvis, the patient hemorrhaged through the nephrostomy tube. CT was requested because angiography suggested renal compression by a subcapsular or perinephric hematoma. *A*, A section through the left upper pole before administration of contrast material demonstrates a large high-density mass *(arrows)* compressing the left kidney. The mass is in the anterior perirenal space. *B*, A similar section after intravenous contrast material has been given shows that the kidney is now of higher attenuation than the mass, a finding typical of recent hemorrhage. *C*, A section through the lower pole demonstrates residual calculus *(arrows)*. The ventral parenchyma is markedly disrupted, and the calyces communicate directly with the anterior perirenal hematoma *(arrowheads)*.

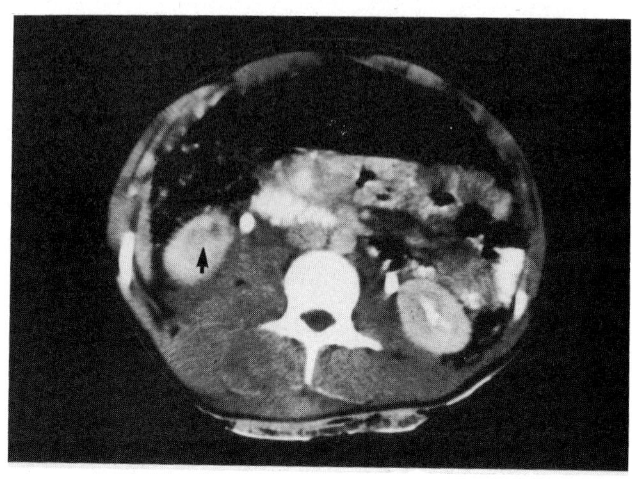

Figure 81–3. Stab wound to the right kidney has caused **a parenchymal laceration** *(arrow)*. In addition, the kidney is displaced anteriorly by a large perirenal and psoas hematoma.

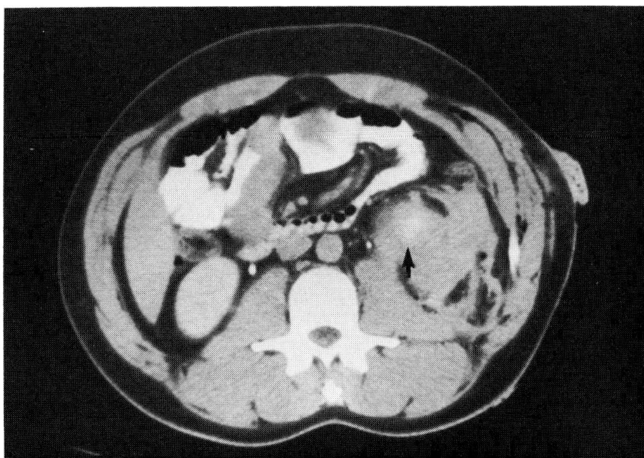

Figure 81–4. The lower pole of the left kidney is displaced ventrally *(arrow).* It is surrounded by an irregular abnormal fluid collection. The injury was caused by a gunshot wound to the flank.

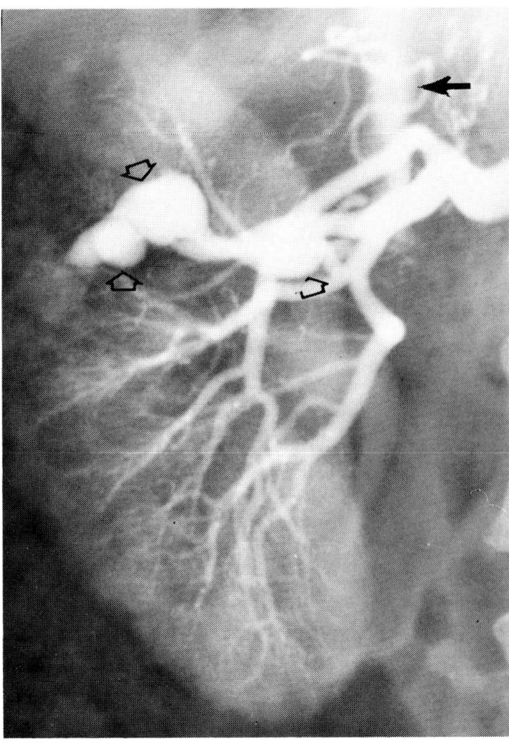

Figure 81–6. Traumatic arteriovenous fistula. Selective right renal angiogram in a 49-year-old man who had been stabbed in the flank six weeks earlier. The angiogram was requested because of persistent microscopic hematuria with episodes of gross hematuria. One second into the injection, contrast medium is seen in the inferior vena cava *(arrow).* There has been very rapid filling of a vein that has become dilated *(open arrows).* The remainder of the kidney is normal.

Although most traumatic arteriovenous fistulas close spontaneously, this one has not done so. It can be treated radiographically by embolization of the feeding artery or by partial nephrectomy.

Angiography has both diagnostic and therapeutic applications in renal trauma. Arterial injury is most fully evaluated angiographically. Main or branch renal artery occlusions (Fig. 81–5), intimal injuries, pseudoaneurysms, arteriovenous fistulas (Fig. 81–6), and frank extravasation are all well-demonstrated. Selective embolization of bleeding arteries, pseudoaneurysms (see Fig. 81–1), and some arteriovenous fistulas may obviate the need for surgical intervention in many of these patients.

The site of persistent urine leakage following either blunt or penetrating injury is often difficult to locate. These patients sometimes require a carefully performed retrograde or antegrade pyelogram to identify the site of leakage. In some patients, a percutaneous nephrostomy will allow closure of the tear, and in others percutaneous placement of a ureteric stent is indicated.

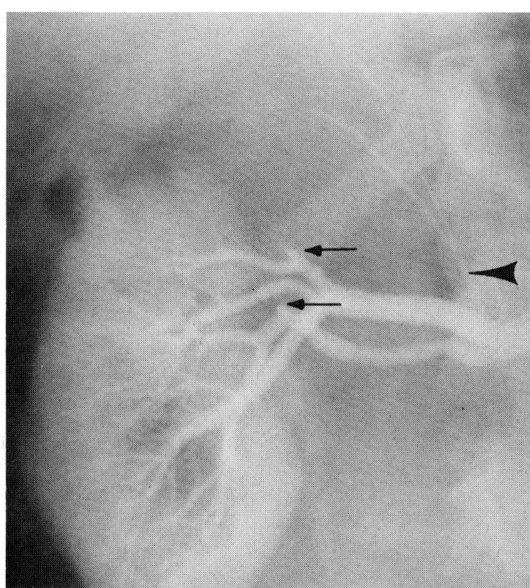

Figure 81–5. Selective right renal angiogram in a 25-year-old man with **hematuria** after a motorcycle accident. A lumbar aortogram had demonstrated a normal main renal artery, but the right upper pole was poorly defined. Two right renal artery branches *(arrows)* are occluded. The capsular artery *(arrowhead)* is stretched, suggesting a hematoma. The patient was treated conservatively and experienced no known sequelae. Renin-mediated hypertension is a possibility if collaterals develop into the ischemic upper pole.

RADIOLOGIC APPROACH TO RENAL TRAUMA

No two patients with suspected renal injury are identical. Therefore, no rigid protocol for diagnosis of renal injury can or should be established. Clinical concern for renal injury usually is caused by hematuria in the presence of an appropriate trauma history. Some institutions evaluate patients with as few as two to four red blood cells per high-power field; others have more detailed guidelines. The decision to evaluate a patient radiographically is generally quite simple; deciding on the correct radiologic course is more complex.

At present, a contrast-enhanced CT examination is the preferred survey technique for renal trauma since it rapidly evaluates the entire abdomen in addition to the kidneys and their surrounding tissues. The additional information that can be gained from an unenhanced examination seldom justifies the added time, and most trauma centers proceed immediately to an enhanced study.

Isolated renal injury, such as might be caused by percutaneous renal biopsy, can be evaluated by ultrasound, but angiography is more suited to demonstrate arterial injury and can be used therapeutically to occlude the bleeding site. If injury to the renal pelvis or ureter is of concern, an excretory urogram may demonstrate the site and nature of the injury, but antegrade or retrograde pyelography is often required. Both CT and ultrasound demonstrate the location and extent of any resultant fluid collections. Both can be used to guide placement of a drainage catheter, though CT is preferable in most patients.

The radiologic evaluation of each patient with suspected renal injury must be tailored to that individual. CT is the most comprehensive survey technique, but even it should not be performed in all patients. It is important to avoid unnecessary procedures in these patients so that the appropriate therapy can be instituted without undue delay.

Bibliography

Bernath AS, Schutte H, Fernandez RRD, et al: Stab wounds of the kidney: Conservative management in flank penetration. J Urol 129:468, 1983.

Bergqvist D, Grenabo L, Hedelin H, et al: Long-time follow-up of patients with conservatively treated blunt renal injuries. Acta Chir Scand 146:291, 1980.

Carroll PR, McAninch JW: Operative indications in penetrating renal trauma. J Trauma 25:587, 1985.

Carroll PR, McAninch JW: Staging of renal trauma. Urol Clin North Am 16:193–201, 1989.

Kisa E, Schenk WG III: Indications for emergency intravenous pyelography (IVP) in blunt abdominal trauma: A reappraisal. J Trauma 26:1086, 1986.

Lang EK, Sullivan J, Frentz G: Renal trauma: Radiological studies. Comparison of urography, computed tomography, angiography, and radionuclide studies. Radiology 154:1, 1985.

Mee SL, McAninch JW: Indications for radiographic assessment in suspected renal trauma. Urol Clin North Am 16:187–192, 1989.

Oakland CDH, Britton JM, Charlton CAC: Renal trauma and the intravenous urogram. J Royal Soc Med 80:21, 1987.

Pollack HM, Wein AJ: Imaging in renal trauma. Radiology 172:297, 1989.

Rhyner P, Federle MP, Jeffrey RB: CT of trauma to the abnormal kidney. AJR 142:747, 1984.

Retroperitoneum and Ureter

82 The Retroperitoneum

Errol Levine

Accurate radiologic evaluation of the nature and location of retroperitoneal disease processes is dependent on an understanding of the complex anatomy of the retroperitoneum. Excellent delineation of this anatomy is obtained by computed tomography (CT), which is currently the preferred imaging method for evaluating the retroperitoneum. Magnetic resonance imaging (MRI) may provide additional information about retroperitoneal abnormalities because it produces sagittal and coronal images, in addition to axial images. In this chapter, the anatomy of the retroperitoneum and the role of CT and other imaging techniques in the assessment of retroperitoneal diseases are discussed.

ANATOMY AND PATHOLOGY OF THE RETROPERITONEAL COMPARTMENTS

The retroperitoneal space is bounded anteriorly by the posterior parietal peritoneum and posteriorly by the transversalis fascia, within the confines of which the space is further subdivided by the renal fascia (Figs. 82–1 and 82–2). The renal fascia is a dense connective tissue sheath that envelops the kidney and perinephric fat. One layer covers the kidney anteriorly and is called the anterior renal fascia (Gerota's fascia). A second layer covers the kidney posteriorly and is called the posterior renal fascia (Zuckerkandl's fascia) (Fig. 82–2). For simplification, *Gerota's fascia* is currently often used as a general term describing both layers. Lateral to the kidney the two layers fuse to form the lateroconal fascia. This continues laterally behind the ascending or descending colon and ends by blending with the connective tissue layer just deep to the peritoneum. The renal fascial layers divide the retroperitoneal space into three compartments extending from the diaphragm to the pelvic brim—namely, the anterior pararenal, perinephric, and posterior pararenal spaces. The psoas muscle and fascia may be considered an additional retroperitoneal compartment. Because of its ability to differentiate between fat and fascial tissue, CT shows the renal fascia and major extraperitoneal compartments in most patients (Fig. 82–3).

Anterior Pararenal Space

NORMAL ANATOMY

The anterior pararenal space lies between the posterior parietal peritoneum and the anterior renal fascia. It contains the pancreas, duodenal loop, ascending and descending colon, and a modest amount of fat. The presence of the pancreas provides continuity across the midline between the right and left anterior pararenal spaces. The space is bounded laterally by the lateroconal fascia and extends longitudinally from the posterior-superior bare area of the liver to the iliac fossa, where it has a potential communication with the posterior pararenal space (see Fig. 82–1).

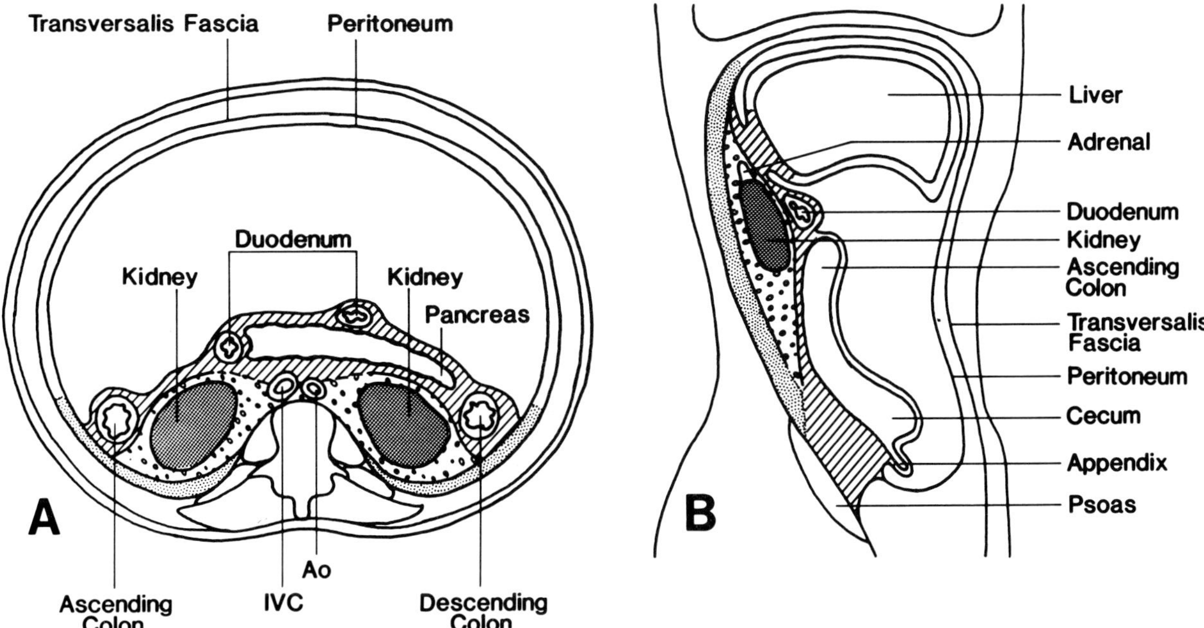

Figure 82–1. Transverse *(A)* and parasagittal *(B)* sections of the three retroperitoneal compartments. The striped area indicates the anterior pararenal space, the area with small circles indicates the perinephric space, and the stippled area indicates the posterior pararenal space. (IVC = inferior vena cava; Ao = aorta.) (Modified from Meyers MA: Dynamic Radiology of the Abdomen. Normal and Pathologic Anatomy, 3rd ed. New York, Springer-Verlag, 1988, p. 184, with permission.)

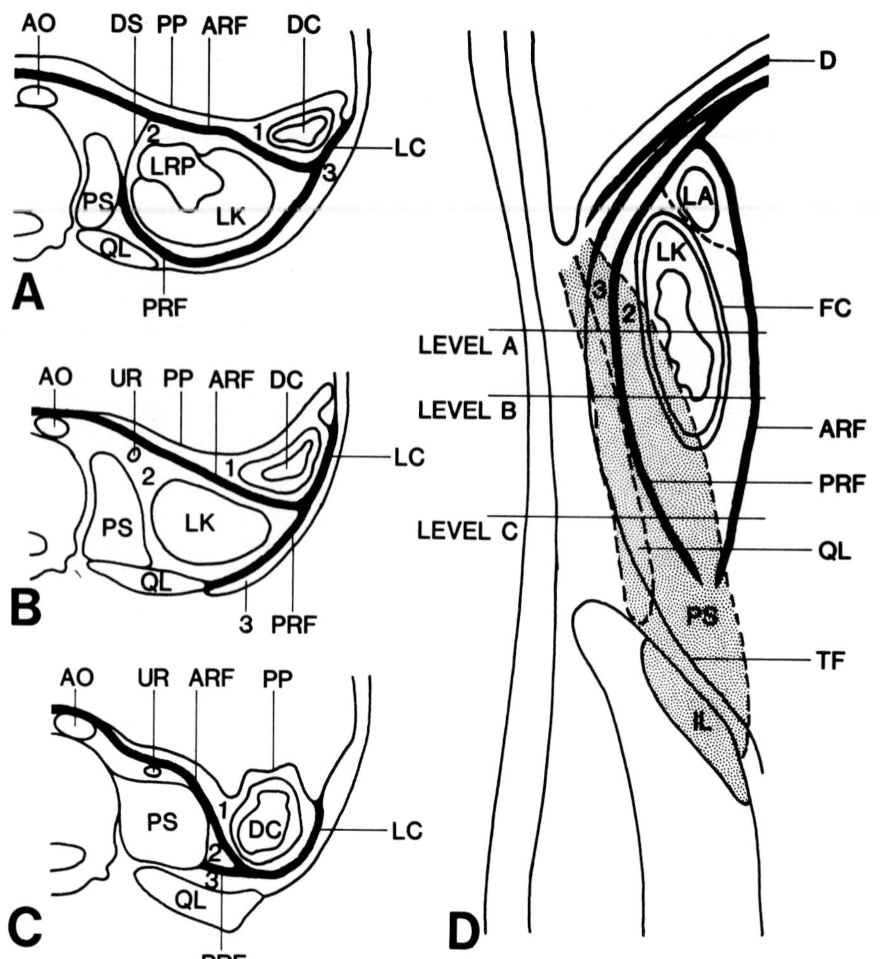

Figure 82–2. Transverse *(A to C)* and parasagittal *(D)* sections of the left flank. Sections *A* to *C* show the cross-sectional anatomy at the three levels indicated in *D*—the level of the renal hilus *(A)*, lower renal pole *(B)*, and above the iliac crest *(C)*. In *D*, the approximate positions of the psoas and quadratus lumborum muscles *(stippled areas)* are indicated by dashed lines. (AO = aorta; PS = psoas muscle; QL = quadratus lumborum muscle; LK = left kidney; LRP = left renal pelvis; UR = ureter; PP = parietal peritoneum; ARF = anterior renal fascia; PRF = posterior renal fascia; LC = lateroconal fascia; DS = deeper stratum of renal fascia; DC = descending colon; 1 = anterior pararenal space; 2 = perinephric space; 3 = posterior pararenal space; D = diaphragm; LA = left adrenal; FC = fibrous capsule of kidney; TF = transversalis fascia; IL = iliacus muscle.) (Modified from Feldberg MAM, Koehler PR, van Waes PFGM: Psoas compartment disease studied by computed tomography. Analysis of 50 cases and subject review. Radiology 148:505, 1983, with permission.)

PATHOLOGIC CONDITIONS

The anterior pararenal space is a common site of extraperitoneal infection and fluid collections. Pancreatitis is the most frequent cause of fluid collections in this space. These are most common in the left anterior pararenal space, but they may also occur on the right. Retrorenal fluid collections may also occur in patients with pancreatitis (Fig. 82–4). The mechanism for this has been described. The posterior renal fascia is usually composed of two laminae. The thinner anterior lamina becomes continuous with the anterior renal

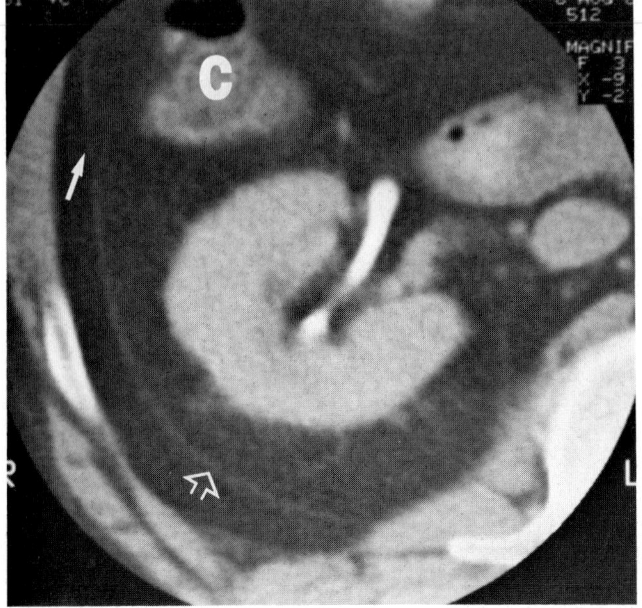

Figure 82–3. Normal CT anatomy. The posterior renal fascia *(open arrow)* is well-shown and separates the perinephric and posterior pararenal spaces. The anterior renal fascia is only faintly shown. The lateroconal fascia *(arrow)* extends lateral to the ascending colon (C).

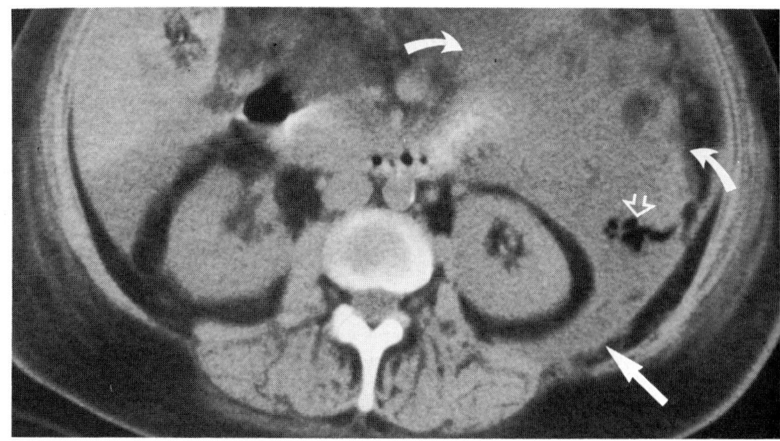

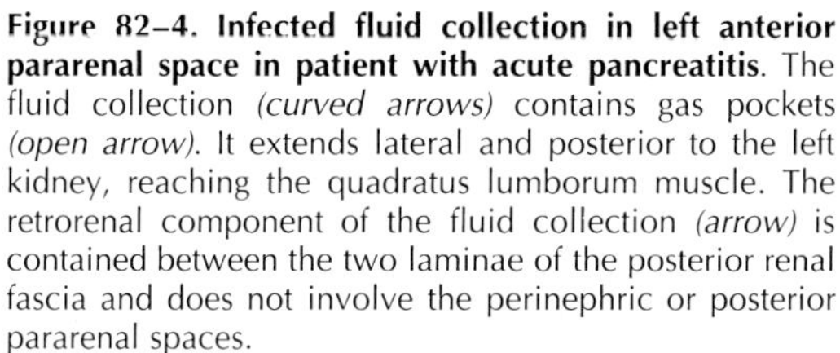

Figure 82–4. Infected fluid collection in left anterior pararenal space in patient with acute pancreatitis. The fluid collection *(curved arrows)* contains gas pockets *(open arrow)*. It extends lateral and posterior to the left kidney, reaching the quadratus lumborum muscle. The retrorenal component of the fluid collection *(arrow)* is contained between the two laminae of the posterior renal fascia and does not involve the perinephric or posterior pararenal spaces.

fascia, while the thicker posterior lamina becomes the lateroconal fascia. A potential space between the two laminae is thus anatomically continuous with the anterior pararenal space. However, normally, septa connect the lateroconal and anterior renal fasciae and serve as a barrier between the anterior pararenal space and the potential space in the posterior renal fascia. In acute pancreatitis, proteolytic enzymes dissolve these septa, thus allowing fluid in the anterior pararenal space to extend between the laminae of the posterior renal fascia in a retrorenal location, sparing the posterior pararenal and perinephric spaces (Fig. 82–4).

Anterior pararenal fluid collections may also result from extraperitoneal perforations of the colon, duodenum, or appendix due to inflammatory conditions, perforating malignancies, penetrating ulcers, and trauma (Fig. 82–5). Other causes of anterior pararenal masses include invasive pancreatic and colonic neoplasms and hemorrhage after rupture of hepatic, peripancreatic, and splenic artery aneurysms or pseudoaneurysms. Anterior pararenal masses or fluid collections do not cause loss of the renal or psoas contours or of the flank stripe on plain films or CT. Thickening of the anterior renal fascia commonly occurs. Anterior pararenal fluid collections may cause anterior displacement of the ascending or descending colon, duodenum, or pancreas.

Perinephric Space

NORMAL ANATOMY

The perinephric space is the largest of the retroperitoneal compartments and is bounded by the anterior and posterior layers of the renal fascia and is demarcated by their sites of fusion (see Figs. 82–1 and 82–2). Above the adrenal glands, the two renal fascial layers fuse and adhere firmly to the underside of the diaphragmatic fascia, while laterally they fuse to form the lateroconal fascia. Medially, the anterior fascial layer blends into the connective tissue near the midline around the renal pedicle and behind the pancreas and duodenum. However, at or just below the level of the renal hila, the right and left anterior renal fasciae sometimes fuse for a variable distance, producing a potential site of communication of the two perinephric spaces across the midline anterior to the lower aorta and inferior vena cava.

Medially, the posterior renal fascia fuses with the psoas fascia above the level of the renal hilus. Below this level, the posterior renal fascia often does not extend to the psoas muscle but fuses with the fascia near the lateral margin of the psoas or even with that of the quadratus lumborum muscle (see Fig. 82–2). Accordingly, the lower part of the kidney is not separated from the psoas muscle by the posterior renal fascia but is merely surrounded by fat that is in direct contact with the psoas fascia (see Fig. 82–2). The caudal insertion of the posterior renal fascia courses medially to rejoin the psoas fascia. As the anterior and posterior renal fasciae course inferiorly below the kidney, they converge and weakly blend with the iliac fascia. Laterally, below the kidney, the fusion line of the two layers to form the lateroconal fascia courses medially. This results in an inverted cone of fascia extending inferiorly to the kidney and medially towards the lower part of the psoas muscle. The compartment enclosed by the cone is an inferior extension of the main perinephric space (see Figs. 82–1 and 82–2) and contains the ureters and gonadal vessels. The caudal apex of the compart-

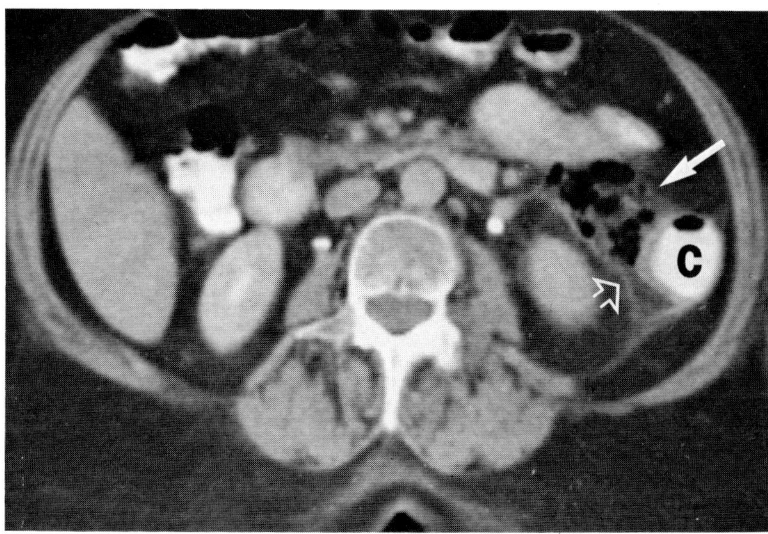

Figure 82–5. Anterior pararenal space abscess. There is a gas-containing abscess *(arrow)* in the left anterior pararenal space. This resulted from perforation of the descending colon in a patient with nonspecific colitis. The medial wall of the descending colon (C) and the renal fascia *(open arrow)* are thickened, but the perinephric and posterior pararenal spaces are normal.

ment remains open towards the iliac fossa, and effusions may escape from the perinephric space at this site.

The perinephric space is divided into multiple compartments by fibrous lamellae, the bridging septa. Some of these structures arise from the renal capsule and extend to the anterior and posterior renal fascia. Others are attached only to the renal capsule and are arranged nearly parallel to the renal surface. One of the more constant of these is the posterior renorenal bridging septum. It arises from the renal capsule at its posteromedial aspect and runs nearly parallel to the posterior surface of the kidney, inserting into the posterolateral aspect of the renal capsule. Still other bridging septa connect the anterior to the posterior leaves of the renal fascia.

The perinephric space contains the kidney, adrenal gland, inferior vena cava, lower aorta, renal pelvis, ureter, renal vessels, renal capsular vessels, and perinephric fat, which is most abundant behind and lateral to the lower pole of the kidney.

PATHOLOGIC CONDITIONS

Abscesses, hematomas, urinomas, and neoplasms may all cause perinephric masses. Most perinephric abscesses result from renal infection with capsule perforation, and they sometimes contain gas (Fig. 82–6). Perinephric hematomas may be due to renal trauma or may occur spontaneously with renal neoplasms (renal cell carcinoma and angiomyolipoma), segmental renal infarction, polyarteritis nodosa, arteriovenous malformations, bleeding diatheses and renal cystic disease (Fig. 82–7). Renal cell carcinomas, which are often small, are the most common cause of spontaneous perinephric hemorrhage and are usually well-shown by CT. When abdominal aortic aneurysms rupture, bleeding occurs primarily into the perinephric space. Perinephric urinomas develop as a result of perforation of the renal collecting system in patients who have obstructive uropathy or who have had abdominal trauma, renal surgery, or urinary tract instrumentation. The nature of a urinoma may be confirmed by contrast-enhanced CT that shows layering of contrast medium in the dependent part of the fluid collection (Fig. 82–8). Renal cell carcinomas often penetrate the renal capsule and invade the perinephric space. Sarcomas may arise primarily in the perinephric space.

The bridging septa described above play an important role in determining the distribution of blood, pus, or urine collections in the perinephric space. When such a collection is confined by the posterior renorenal bridging septum, it may compress and indent the renal surface and, because it is separated from the renal fascia, it may be misdiagnosed as a subcapsular collection. However, while subcapsular hematomas are confined to the kidney, perinephric hematomas usually extend caudally below the kidney into the cone of renal fascia (see Fig. 82–7). The bridging septa that connect the renal capsule to the renal fascia may form compartments that separate a fluid collection into several locules (Fig. 82–8).

Perinephric fluid collections generally collect posteriorly and often displace the kidney anteriorly (see Figs. 82–6 to 82–8). Anterior displacement of the inferior vena cava may occur. Perinephric fluid collections that are adjacent to the kidney usually cause loss of the renal outline. The psoas contour may be obliterated if there is an adjacent fluid collection, but it may be preserved if the bridging septa separate the fluid collection from the muscle. The flank stripe is preserved. Thickening of the renal fascia may be shown on plain films and CT.

Posterior Pararenal Space

NORMAL ANATOMY

The posterior pararenal space extends from the posterior renal fascia to the transversalis fascia. Medially, it is bounded by the line of fusion of the posterior renal fascia with the psoas or quadratus lumborum fascia (see Figs. 82–1 and 82–2). Laterally, it continues external to the lateroconal fascia and communicates with the space between the peritoneum and transversalis fascia that contains the properitoneal fat. The latter is visualized radiologically as the "flank stripe." Caudally, the posterior pararenal space communicates with the anterior pararenal space in the region of the tip of the renal fascial cone. The posterior pararenal space contains no organs and is occupied only by a thin layer of fat.

PATHOLOGIC CONDITIONS

The posterior pararenal space is the most common site of spontaneous retroperitoneal hemorrhage in conditions such as bleeding diathesis and excessive anticoagulation (Fig. 82–9). Trauma, including stab wounds, percutaneous renal biopsy, and rib fractures, may also cause posterior pararenal hematomas. Infection limited solely to this compartment is rare. Infections originating in the lower abdomen or pelvis below the tip of the renal fascia cone may extend cephalad in the posterior pararenal space. Consequently, perforation of a sigmoid diverticulum or of an inflamed pelvic appendix may cause posterior pararenal space abscesses.

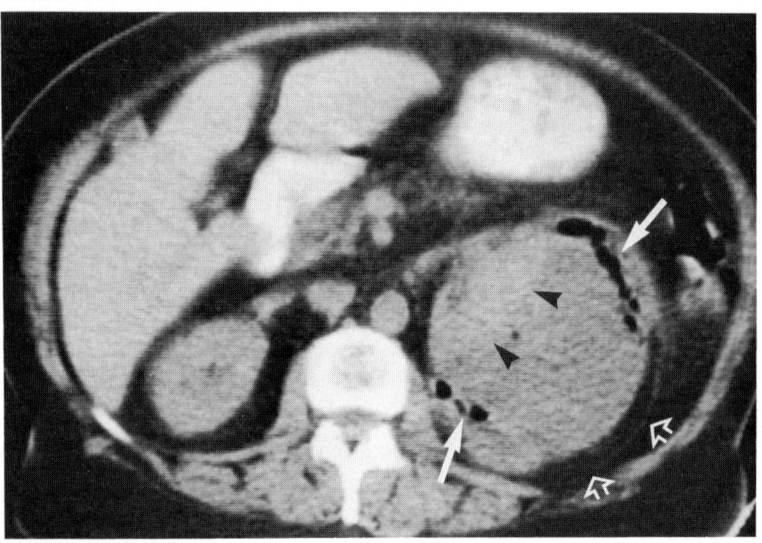

Figure 82–6. Perinephric abscess complicating acute pyelonephritis in a diabetic patient. Note gas collections *(solid arrows)* in the abscess and anteromedial displacement of the left kidney *(arrowheads)*. The abscess is contained posteriorly by the posterior renorenal bridging septum and does not extend to the posterior renal fascia *(open arrows)*.

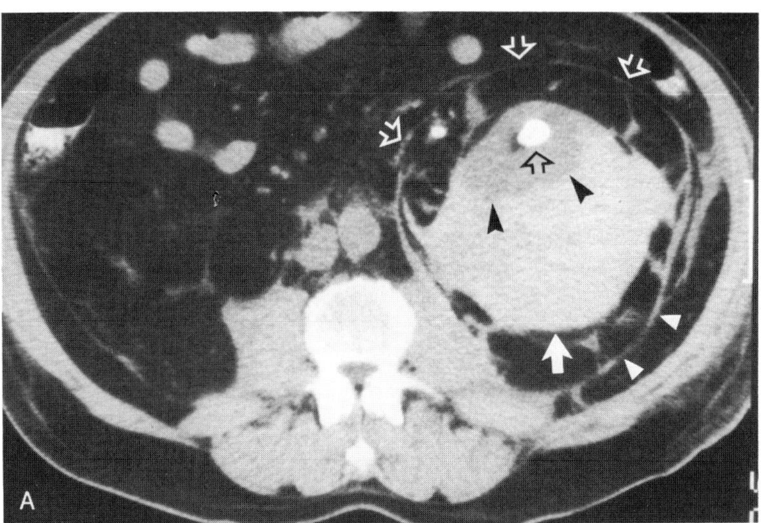

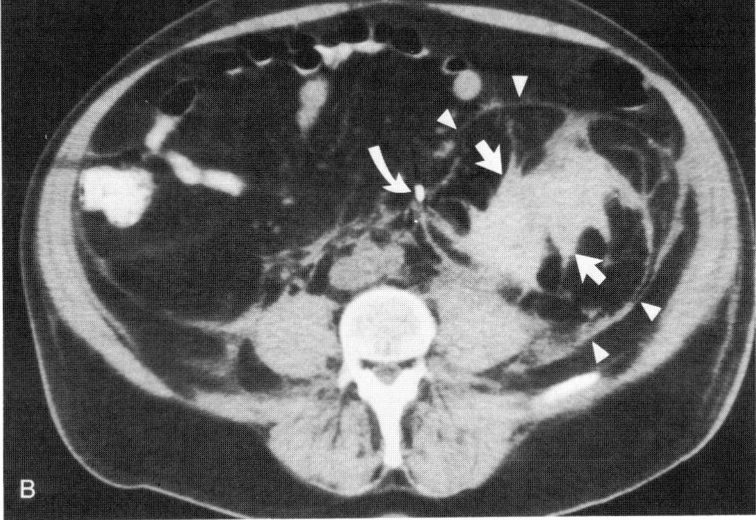

Figure 82–7. Perinephric hematoma complicating extracorporeal shock wave lithotripsy. *A*, An unenhanced CT scan shows anterior displacement of the left kidney *(black arrowheads)* by a high-density hematoma *(white solid arrow)*. Note a calculus *(black open arrow)* in the collecting system. The hematoma is limited posteriorly by the posterior renorenal bridging septum, which separates it from the thickened posterior renal fascia *(white arrowheads)*. The anterior renal fascia *(white open arrows)* is also thickened. *B*, CT shows extension of the hematoma *(straight arrows)* into the renal fascial cone below the kidney. Note thickening of the anterior and posterior renal fasciae *(arrowheads)*. The extension below the kidney confirms the perinephric location of the hematoma and distinguishes it from a subcapsular hematoma. The left ureter *(curved arrow)* contains a stent and is displaced anteriorly.

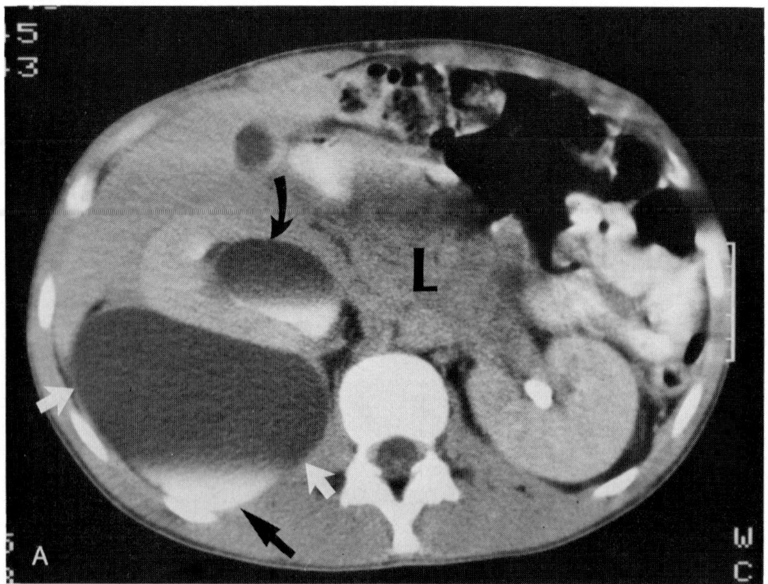

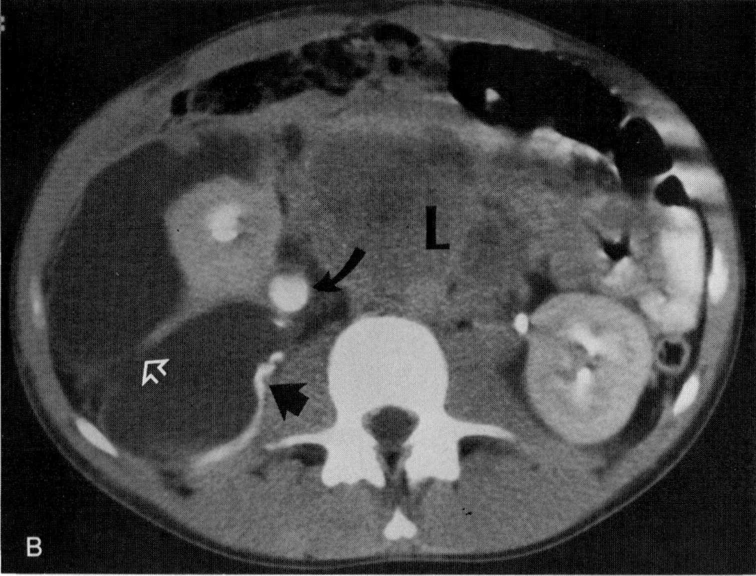

Figure 82–8. Right perinephric urinoma caused by ureteric obstruction secondary to retroperitoneal lymph node metastases from testicular carcinoma. *A,* A perinephric fluid collection *(white arrows)* causes anterior displacement of the right kidney. Note contrast material *(black arrow)* layering posteriorly in the perinephric space. The right renal pelvis *(curved arrow)* is dilated. (L = enlarged retroperitoneal lymph nodes.) *B,* A caudal scan exhibits contrast material *(straight arrow)* tracking posteriorly from a dilated and obstructed right ureter *(curved arrow)*. Note a bridging septum *(open arrow)* between the renal capsule and the posterior renal fascia. (L = lymph node metastases.)

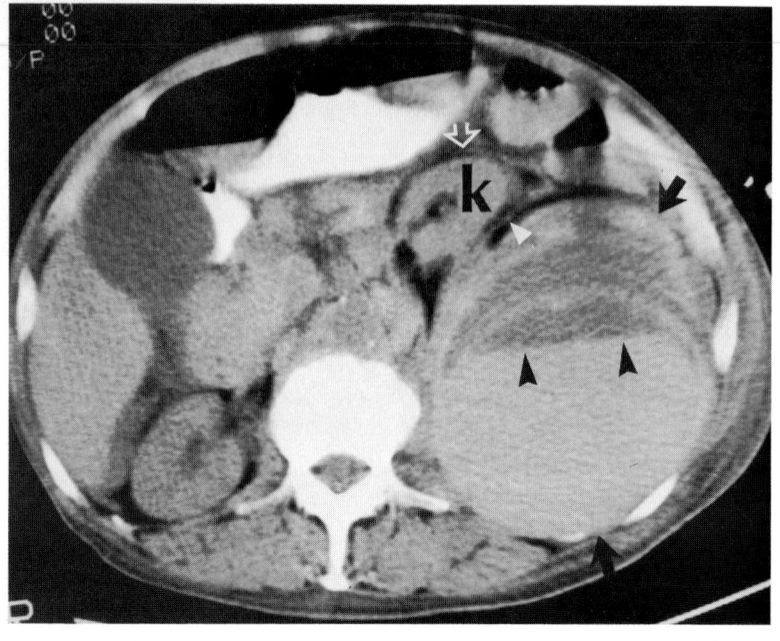

Figure 82–9. Hematoma in the left posterior pararenal space in a patient receiving heparin for deep venous thrombosis. Note a fluid-fluid level *(black arrowheads)* in the hematoma *(closed arrows)*. The left kidney (k) and the anterior *(open arrow)* and posterior *(white arrowhead)* renal fasciae are displaced anteriorly.

Posterior pararenal hematomas or effusions obliterate part of the psoas muscle border and cause anterior renal displacement. The perinephric fat and renal outline are usually preserved. Lateral extension of the fluid causes obliteration of the flank stripe.

PSOAS COMPARTMENT

Normal Anatomy

The psoas compartment consists of the psoas muscle and its covering fascia and various blood vessels and nerves. The compartment is bordered posteriorly by the quadratus lumborum muscle, medially by the spine, and laterally by the posterior renal fascia above the level of the renal vessels and by the perinephric space and its contents below the renal vessels (see Fig. 82–2). Anteriorly, the psoas muscle has close relationships with the pancreas, aorta, ureters, inferior vena cava, and retroperitoneal lymph nodes.

PATHOLOGIC CONDITIONS

The psoas compartment is generally involved secondarily by disease processes originating elsewhere. Psoas abscesses usually result from infections spreading from the kidney; from the perinephric or pararenal spaces; or from inflammatory bowel disorders, including diverticulitis, complicated appendicitis, and Crohn's disease. Tuberculous and pyogenic spondylitis and lumbar discitis may also cause a psoas abscess (Fig. 82–10). Neoplastic involvement of the psoas muscle may occur with metastatic lymph node disease originating in testicular, bladder, cervical, and ovarian tumors; in lymphoma; in renal cell carcinoma; and in retroperitoneal sarcoma. Primary neoplasms of the psoas muscle are rare. The psoas muscle is sometimes involved by benign and malignant neural neoplasms arising in the lumbar nerve plexus (Fig. 82–11). MRI is helpful in showing or excluding intraspinal extension of such neoplasms. Hemorrhage into the psoas compartment may result from bleeding disorders, trauma, a leaking aortic aneurysm or graft, or anticoagulation. CT and MRI facilitate early diagnosis of psoas compartment disease, although the findings are often nonspecific.

AORTA

Aortic Aneurysms

Abdominal aortic aneurysms occur in 1 to 3 per cent of the older population. Most aneurysms are associated with atherosclerosis, but occasionally syphilitic and mycotic aortic aneurysms are also encountered. The infrarenal aorta is the site of 95 per cent of abdominal aortic aneurysms. Untreated, these aneurysms enlarge and eventually rupture with a mortality of 50 to 90 per cent. Aortic aneurysms are identified on imaging studies as focal areas of aortic dilatation usually exceeding 3 cm in size. Recommendations vary, but surgery is considered necessary in most abdominal aortic aneurysms larger than 6 cm in diameter and unnecessary in those less than 4 cm in diameter. Individualized management is required for those abdominal aortic aneurysms with diameters of 4 to 6 cm.

About 55 to 85 per cent of abdominal aortic aneurysms contain enough calcium to be seen as curvilinear calcifications on plain abdominal radiography. Sonography provides an excellent technique for evaluating aortic aneurysms and for serial follow-up of patients who do not undergo aneurysm repair. However, CT and MRI are helpful in assessing the size and extent of aneurysms in cases in which sonography is unsuccessful owing to patient obesity or abundant bowel gas. Aneurysmal involvement of the renal and iliac arteries is well-shown by both CT and MRI. Angiography frequently underestimates the dimensions of an aneurysm because it shows only the blood flowing in the lumen and does not show mural thrombus, which is detected by CT in almost 90 per cent of aneurysms.

Aneurysmal rupture or leak is associated with a high morbidity and mortality if not promptly treated. When the classic clinical triad of abdominal pain, a pulsating abdominal mass, and hypotension is present, the diagnosis of ruptured aortic aneurysm is usually made clinically. In such cases, immediate surgery without intervening

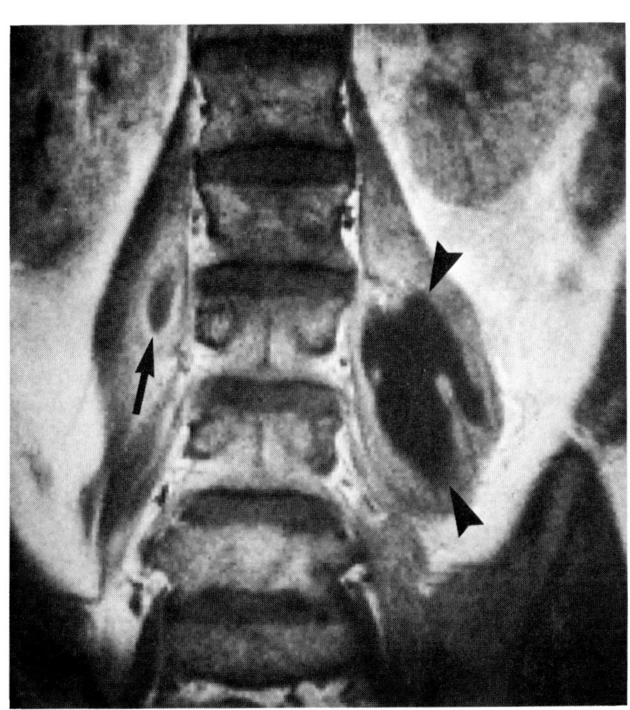

Figure 82–10. Bilateral psoas abscesses. A coronal T_1-weighted spin-echo MRI (500/17), obtained after intravenous injection of gadolinium-DTPA, shows a large left psoas abscess *(arrowheads)* with low signal intensity and a smaller right psoas abscess *(arrow)* complicating pyogenic discitis (not shown).

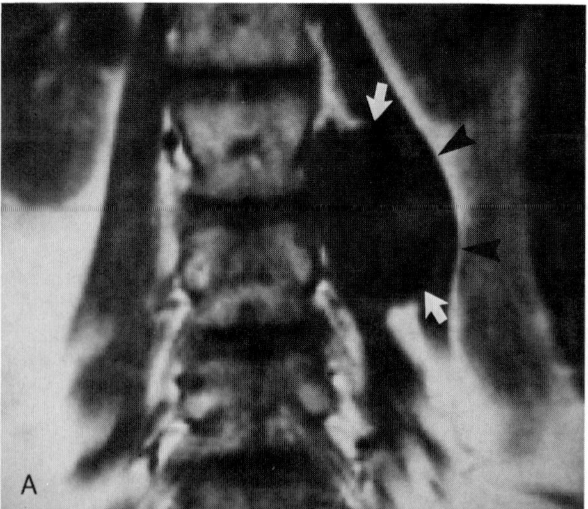

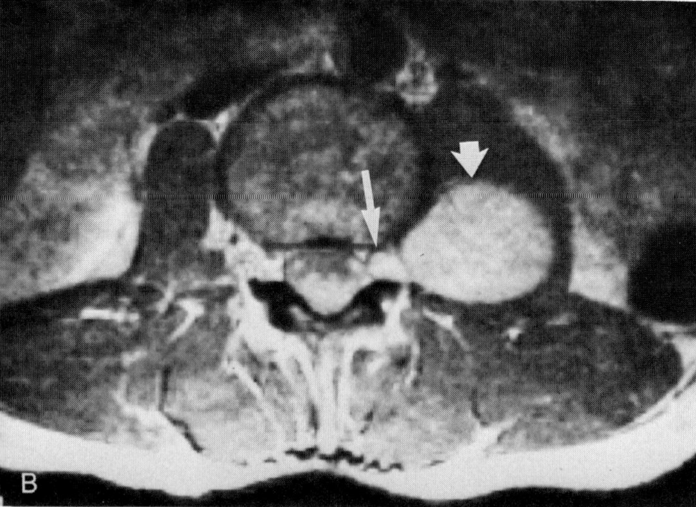

Figure 82–11. Paraspinous schwannoma. *A,* A coronal T_1-weighted spin-echo MRI (500/17) shows a well-defined mass *(arrows)* with a low signal intensity arising to the left of L2 and L3 and displacing the psoas muscle *(arrowheads)* laterally. *B,* On the axial proton density-weighted MRI (2500/35), the lesion *(short arrow)* has a high signal intensity. A small tumor component *(long arrow)* extends into the left L2-L3 neural foramen.

imaging procedures is indicated. In other cases, the clinical findings are less diagnostic and may mimic other disease processes. Such patients are often older men with acute or subacute back pain. CT is the imaging procedure of choice in stable patients with suspected aneurysm rupture for showing the size and extent of the hematoma.

Aortic Dissection

Aortic dissection usually originates in the thorax but sometimes extends into the abdomen. Contrast-enhanced CT with dynamic scanning is the examination of choice in many institutions for any patient suspected of having an aortic dissection. CT diagnosis requires the identification of opacified true and false lumina separated by an intimal flap (Fig. 82–12). The dissection usually ends in either the right or left common iliac artery. The false lumen is located in the left side of the aorta ending in the left iliac artery in 80 per cent of patients, the right side of the aorta ending in the right iliac artery in 10 per cent of patients, and either anteriorly or posteriorly with variable termination in 10 per cent of patients. The aortic branches may arise from the true or false lumen.

MRI provides much the same information as that obtained from CT without the need for intravenous administration of contrast medium. As is true with CT, a specific MRI diagnosis of aortic dissection requires the identification of a double lumen and an intimal flap. On spin-echo images the false lumen will often show a higher signal intensity than the true lumen because of slower movement of blood in the false lumen. Axial sections are best for determining whether the major abdominal vessels arise from the true or false lumen. The use of MRI in the acutely ill patient is limited because of the time required and because patients with life-support systems cannot be subjected to the magnetic field.

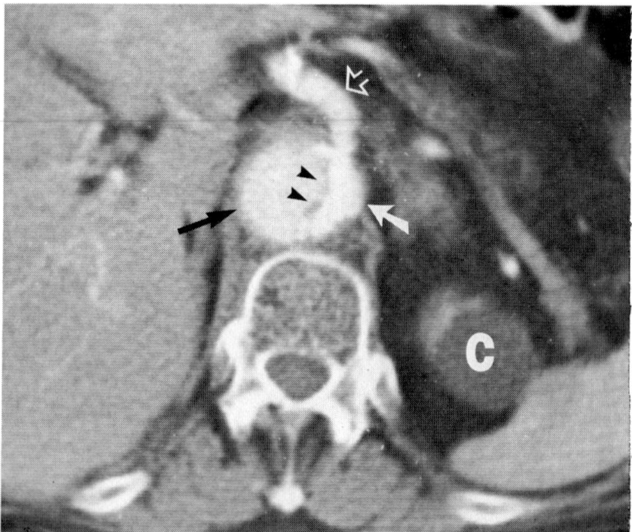

Figure 82–12. Aortic dissection shown by dynamic CT after an intravenous bolus contrast injection. There is enhancement of both the false *(black arrow)* and true *(white arrow)* lumina, which are separated by an intimal flap *(arrowheads).* The lower density of the false lumen indicates delayed filling. The patent celiac artery *(open arrow)* arises from the true lumen. (C = renal cyst.)

Postoperative Aorta

Prosthetic grafting of the abdominal aorta is often performed for patients with aortic aneurysms or occlusions. Complications of abdominal aortic graft surgery include graft infections, aortoenteric fistulas, pseudoaneurysms, and hemorrhage (Fig. 82–13). Graft infections and aortoenteric fistulas are life-threatening complications of aortic surgery, and prompt diagnosis is essential. Surgical repair, usually with graft resection, is indicated in any patient in whom graft infection, an aortoenteric fistula, or a pseudoaneurysm is identified. CT is the preferred technique for detecting these complications. In the immediate postoperative period, perigraft hematoma and retained gas at the anastomotic site are normal findings. Complete resolution of hematoma should occur in 2 to 3 months, and gas should not be present at 3 to 4 weeks after surgery. After this time, any amount of perigraft soft tissue, fluid, or gas should be considered a sign of graft infection.

In patients who have undergone aortic aneurysm repairs, graft infection is often indicated on CT by increased soft tissue, fluid, or gas between the graft and the original aneurysm. Also, focal discontinuity of the calcified aneurysmal wrap may be found when there is graft infection (Fig. 82–13). Aortoenteric fistulas usually develop as a result of both graft infection and mechanical factors and can be considered as part of the spectrum of manifestations of graft infec-

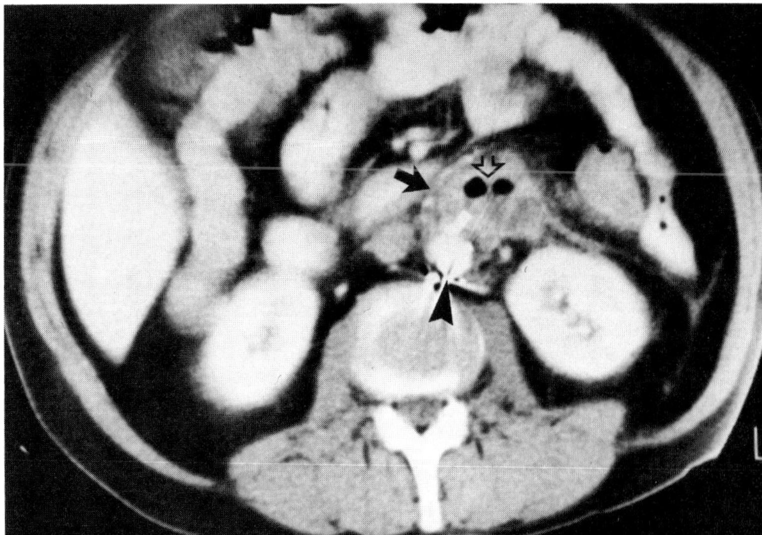

Figure 82–13. Graft infection 8 months after surgery for aortic aneurysm. The enhanced aortic graft *(arrowhead)* is contained in the original aneurysm, the calcified right wall *(closed arrow)* of which is still visible. A fluid collection with two gas pockets *(open arrow)* is present in the aneurysmal wrap. The left wall of the aneurysmal wrap is not seen.

tion. Their presence is suggested by acute or chronic gastrointestinal bleeding. CT often shows gas at the anastomotic site and contiguous focal bowel wall thickening.

INFERIOR VENA CAVA

Developmental Anomalies

Developmental anomalies of the inferior vena cava, although relatively uncommon, are well-shown by CT and MRI. Their recognition is important, because they may be confused on imaging studies with enlarged lymph nodes. Moreover, knowledge of the existence of these abnormalities is often helpful before surgery, particularly in patients undergoing shunt surgery for portal hypertension, kidney donation, placement of inferior vena caval filters for recurrent pulmonary emboli, abdominal aortic aneurysm repair, or nephrectomy. Some vena caval anomalies are associated with anomalies of the left renal vein.

INTERRUPTED INFERIOR VENA CAVA WITH AZYGOS/HEMIAZYGOS VEIN CONTINUATION

In this anomaly, which has a prevalence of 0.6 per cent, the suprarenal segment of the vena cava fails to develop, and blood returns to the heart through the azygos and hemiazygos systems. On CT, a normal inferior vena cava is seen from the confluence of the common iliac veins to the level of the kidneys. The intrahepatic segment of the inferior vena cava, which normally lies anterior to the right diaphragmatic crus and posterior to the caudate lobe of the liver, is absent. An enlarged azygos vein and sometimes also an enlarged hemiazygos vein are seen in the retrocrural space (Fig. 82–14). The enlarged azygos vein can be traced through the posterior mediastinum to its junction with the superior vena cava. The hepatic veins drain directly into the right atrium via the posthepatic segment of the inferior vena cava. Interruption of the inferior vena cava may occur as an isolated anomaly or may be associated with such abnormalities as asplenia, polysplenia, and abnormal abdominal and/or cardiac situs.

LEFT-SIDED INFERIOR VENA CAVA

In this anomaly, which has a prevalence of 0.2 to 0.5 per cent, imaging shows a single, right-sided inferior vena cava at levels cephalad to the renal veins and a single inferior vena cava to the left of the aorta in the infrarenal location. The left-sided vena cava ends by anastomosing with the left renal vein.

DUPLICATION OF THE INFERIOR VENA CAVA

In this anomaly, which has a prevalence of 0.2 to 3 per cent, imaging shows an inferior vena cava parallel to and on both sides of the infrarenal aorta (Fig. 82–15). Both cavas may be equal in size, although it is not uncommon for one vessel to be dominant. The left-sided cava usually ends by anastomosing with the left renal vein. Thus, only a single cava is usually seen above the level of the renal veins.

ANOMALIES OF THE LEFT RENAL VEIN

In the retroaortic left renal vein, imaging shows the left renal vein crossing posterior to the aorta (Fig. 82–16). This anomaly

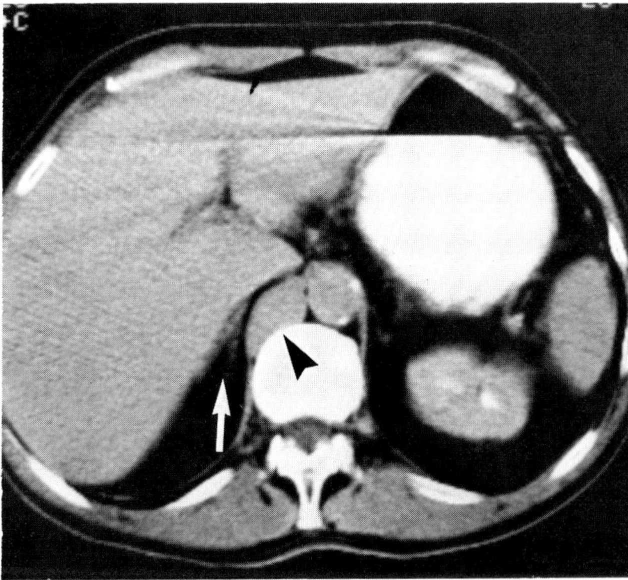

Figure 82–14. Interrupted inferior vena cava with azygos vein continuation. An enlarged azygos vein *(arrowhead)* is present in the retrocrural space to the right of the calcified aorta. The inferior vena cava is not seen in its usual location posterior to the caudate lobe and anterior to the right crus and right adrenal gland *(arrow)*.

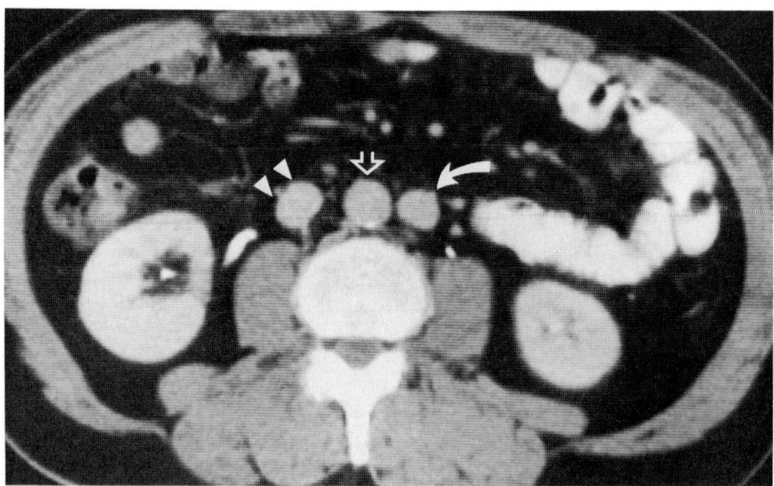

Figure 82–15. Duplication of the inferior vena cava. Three structures in the prevertebral space represent, respectively, the normal right inferior vena cava *(arrowheads)*, aorta *(open arrow)*, and left inferior vena cava *(curved arrow)*.

occurs in about 1.8 per cent of patients. A circumaortic renal vein is somewhat more common, occurring in about 4.4 per cent of patients. The ventral vein usually crosses the aorta anteriorly in the usual location, while the dorsal vein joins the inferior vena cava several centimeters more caudally.

RETROCAVAL AND TRANSCAVAL URETER

In retrocaval ureter, the proximal right ureter courses medially behind the inferior vena cava, usually at the L3 vertebral level, and then courses anteriorly around the cava to partially encircle it. The anomaly is characterized by hydronephrosis and extreme medial deviation (''fish hook deformity'') of the middle ureteral segment. In the transcaval ureter, the inferior vena cava is duplicated for a short distance and the deviated right ureter passes between the two components. The ureter is therefore surrounded by a venous ring at the level of L3 or L4. Ureteric obstruction often occurs. Surgical correction of hydronephrosis may be required in both anomalies. Both anomalies can be diagnosed by CT, although venacavography is sometimes also needed for diagnosis.

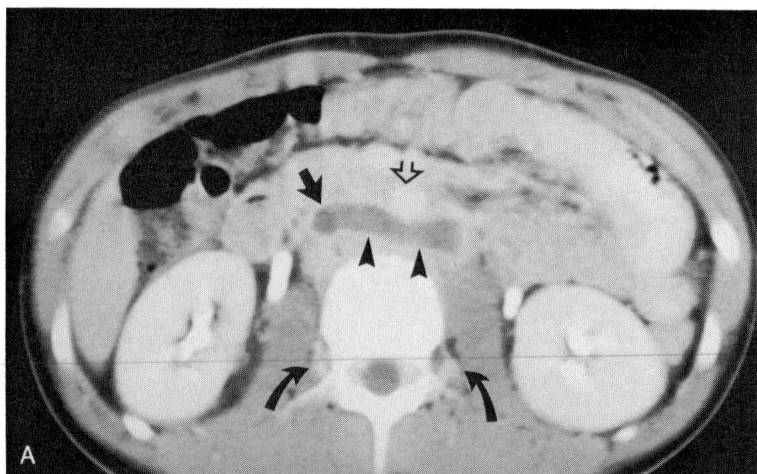

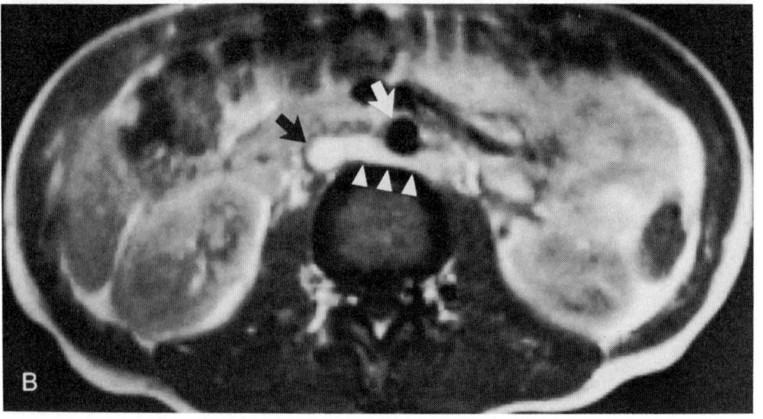

Figure 82–16. Thrombosed retroaortic left renal vein. Chronic vena caval and renal vein thrombosis of unknown cause occurring in a young male. *A,* CT scan shows thrombus in enlarged left renal vein *(arrowheads)* posterior to the aorta *(open arrow)* and caval thrombus *(closed arrow)*. Note enlarged ascending lumbar veins *(curved arrows)*. *B,* MR spin-echo image (600/30) reveals high-intensity thrombus in the retroaortic left renal vein *(arrowheads)* and in the inferior vena cava *(black arrow)*. The aorta *(white arrow)* shows a signal void indicating normal blood flow.

Thrombosis and Tumor Involvement of the Inferior Vena Cava

CT can detect thrombosis of the vena cava and its major tributaries (see Fig. 82–16). Caval thrombi may result from proximal extension of lower extremity, pelvic vein, or renal vein thrombi. Intracaval tumor extension may occur via veins draining such neoplasms as renal cell carcinoma, hepatoma, or adrenal carcinoma. Leiomyosarcoma may arise as a primary neoplasm of the caval wall. CT diagnosis of caval tumor extension depends on demonstration of intraluminal filling defects that may be associated with venous enlargement and enhancement of the caval wall. Collateral vessels, such as the azygos and hemiazygos veins, may be enlarged. MRI is somewhat more accurate than CT in showing venous tumor extension and in demonstrating the proximal extent of caval tumor thrombus relative to the hepatic veins and right atrium (Fig. 82–17).

RETROPERITONEAL LYMPH NODES

Normal Anatomy

The retroperitoneal lymph nodes may be evaluated by either CT or lymphography. The diagnosis of lymph node abnormality at CT is based on size criteria. Node size is best determined by measuring the short-axis diameter because this method has been proved to have the least variability in estimating node size on axial CT scans. The size of normal retroperitoneal lymph nodes varies by location. The upper limits of normal by location include retrocrural space, 6 mm; upper para-aortic region, 9 mm; and lower para-aortic region, 11 mm. Short-axis nodal diameters exceeding these values should be regarded as suspicious for lymph node abnormality, particularly if several nodes are present. However, the use of size alone as a criterion of disease causes diagnostic errors (Fig. 82–18). Lymphography is often more accurate than CT in diagnosing malignant disease of lymph nodes, because it can detect tumor deposits in normal-sized nodes. MRI does not currently enjoy any advantages over CT in detecting retroperitoneal lymph node involvement in patients with malignancy.

Pathologic Conditions

LYMPHOMA

Hodgkin's disease and non-Hodgkin's lymphoma are related diseases that, despite certain obvious similarities, manifest marked differences in clinical presentation, disease progression, response to treatment, and prognosis. Accurate anatomic staging is important in determining the appropriate therapy and prognosis in both diseases. In patients presenting initially with apparently isolated cervical, axillary, or mediastinal adenopathy, it is important to determine whether abdominal lymph nodes or organs are affected. Discussion in this section is limited to the retroperitoneum.

HODGKIN'S DISEASE. Retroperitoneal lymph nodes are involved in Hodgkin's disease in about 34 per cent of newly diagnosed, previously untreated cases. The affected nodes are either normal in size or only slightly enlarged (Fig. 82–18). However, with the use of good technique, some investigators have shown that CT achieves a sensitivity of 65 per cent, a specificity of 92 per cent, and an overall accuracy of 87 per cent in evaluating retroperitoneal lymph nodes in patients with newly diagnosed Hodgkin's disease undergoing staging laparotomy. In comparison, the overall accuracy of bipedal lymphography is 95 per cent, which represents a diagnostic superiority of only 8 per cent as compared with CT. However, in other centers, CT has been found to have a significantly lower sensitivity than lymphography, particularly in detecting abnormal lower abdominal lymph nodes.

Accordingly, in some centers, lymphography is the preferred method in the initial abdominal staging of patients with supradiaphragmatic Hodgkin's disease. Other centers perform CT first. If the CT scan is obviously positive, no further evaluation is undertaken. If CT is negative or equivocal, lymphography is performed to assess the nodal architecture (Fig. 82–18). A positive lymphogram in these circumstances may spare the patient an unnecessary staging laparotomy.

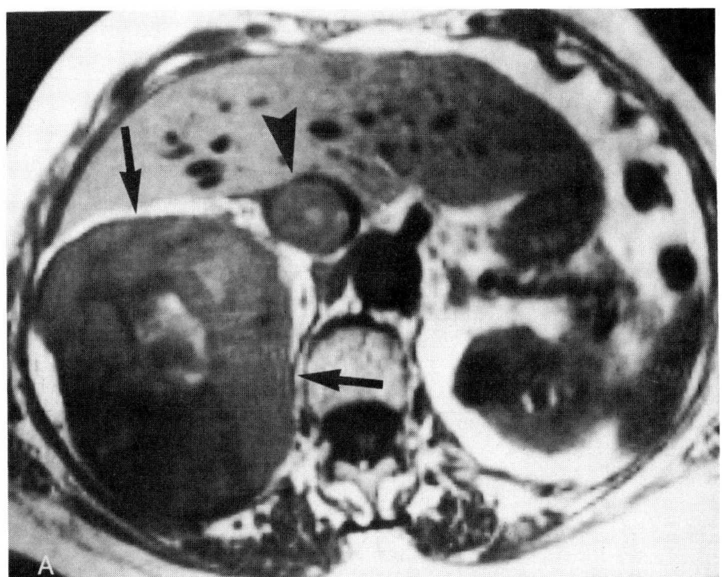

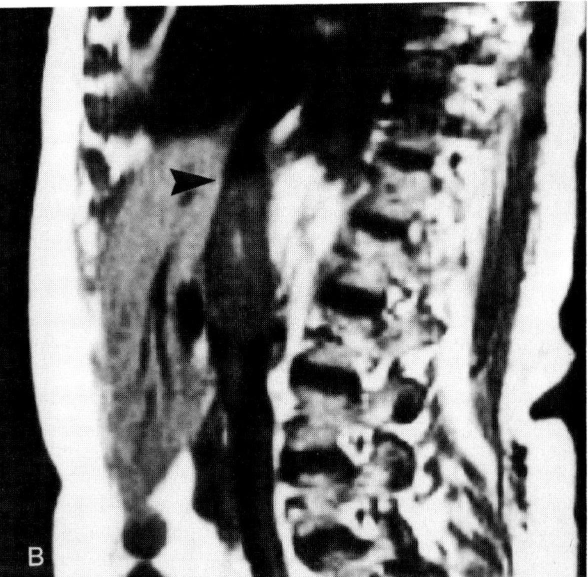

Figure 82–17. Renal cell carcinoma with caval extension. *A*, T_1-weighted spin-echo MR scan (500/15) shows a right renal cell carcinoma *(arrows)*. The inferior vena cava *(arrowhead)* contains tumor of signal intensity similar to that of the primary neoplasm. *B*, A sagittal MRI (500/15) reveals that the tumor extends proximally in the cava *(arrowhead)* to the confluence of the hepatic veins *(not shown)*, but does not extend above the level of the diaphragm.

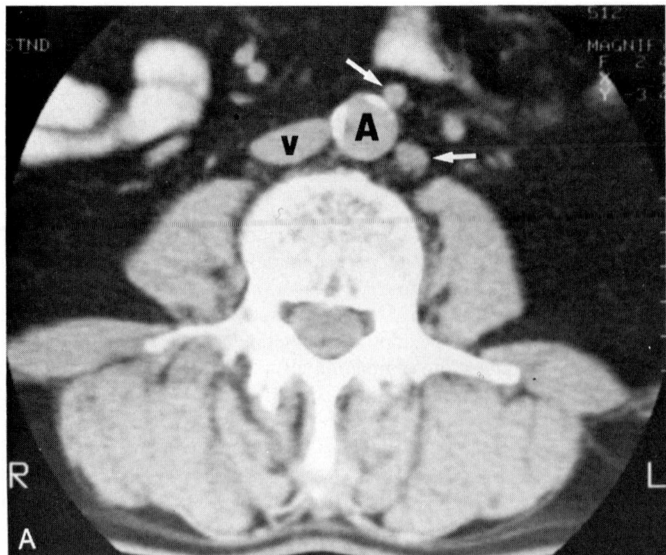

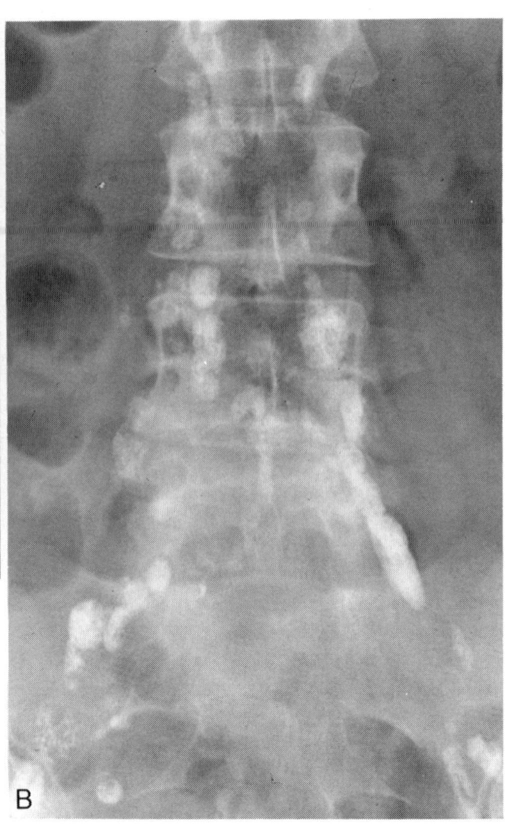

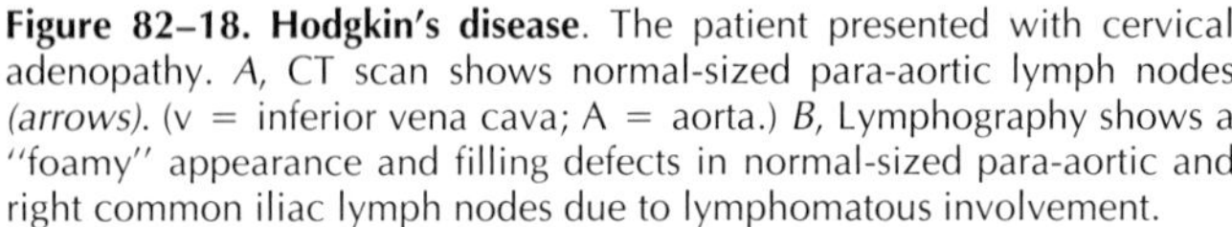
Figure 82–18. Hodgkin's disease. The patient presented with cervical adenopathy. *A*, CT scan shows normal-sized para-aortic lymph nodes *(arrows)*. (v = inferior vena cava; A = aorta.) *B*, Lymphography shows a "foamy" appearance and filling defects in normal-sized para-aortic and right common iliac lymph nodes due to lymphomatous involvement.

NON-HODGKIN'S LYMPHOMA. In previously untreated patients with non-Hodgkin's lymphoma undergoing laparotomy, there is a 49 per cent frequency of histologic involvement of the retroperitoneal lymph nodes and a 51 per cent frequency of involvement of mesenteric nodes. In general, when abdominal lymph nodes are affected with non-Hodgkin's lymphoma, they are usually bulky, and many node-bearing areas are affected. This is in contradistinction to Hodgkin's disease, in which only one or two subdiaphragmatic lymph nodes may be involved, and in which fewer than 5 per cent of patients have mesenteric lymph node involvement. Accordingly, CT is an excellent initial technique for evaluating abdominal involvement in patients with non-Hodgkin's lymphoma.

METASTATIC DISEASE

Neoplasms of the stomach, colon, pancreas, kidney, testis, ovary, uterus, bladder, and prostate may metastasize to retroperitoneal lymph nodes. The CT diagnosis of retroperitoneal adenopathy in such patients is based on the same criteria as have been outlined for malignant lymphoma. As in lymphoma, CT scans may be falsely negative for malignant disease when nodes occupied by metastases are not enlarged. Also, enlarged nodes are sometimes caused by benign reactive changes that may cause errors in neoplasm staging.

At most centers, abdominal CT has now replaced lymphography for staging and surveillance of patients with testicular neoplasms. Testicular lymphatics accompany the internal spermatic artery and vein and usually drain into the lumbar para-aortic and paracaval nodes from L1 to L3, so that nodal metastases from testicular neoplasms are usually first detected in the abdomen. Lymphography, followed by needle biopsy of abnormal or suspicious nodes, is still used for staging of carcinoma of the cervix at some centers, when patients are being considered for radical hysterectomy. Demonstration of retroperitoneal or pelvic nodal metastases by this technique after normal CT in patients with clinical Stage I B neoplasms may spare these patients unnecessary surgery, in favor of radiotherapy.

PRIMARY RETROPERITONEAL NEOPLASMS

Primary retroperitoneal neoplasms are rare. They may be benign or malignant. However, malignant lesions are more common, accounting for 77 to 90 per cent of all primary retroperitoneal neoplasms. Benign retroperitoneal neoplasms include schwannoma, paraganglioma, hemangioma, lymphangioma, lipoma, ganglioneuroma, teratoma, and desmoid tumor (Fig. 82–19). Malignant neoplasms include malignant fibrous histiocytoma, liposarcoma, leiomyosarcoma, malignant neural tumors, neuroblastoma, malignant neoplasms arising in ganglion cells, malignant germ cell tumors, hemangiopericytoma, fibrosarcoma, rhabdomyosarcoma, and undifferentiated sarcoma. Of these, malignant fibrous histiocytoma, liposarcoma, and leiomyosarcoma are the most common. CT is the preferred imaging method for any patient suspected of having a primary or recurrent retroperitoneal neoplasm. It provides clinically useful information about the presence, size, and extent of the tumors and also their effects on adjacent structures (Fig. 82–20). This information is particularly useful in surgical planning and in determining the feasibility of complete resection. MRI may also help in surgical planning by showing tumor extent and relationships in the sagittal and coronal planes and by revealing intraspinal neoplasm extension (see Fig. 82–11).

Most primary retroperitoneal neoplasms arise in front of the plane of the spine and psoas muscles, and, despite their retroperitoneal origins, some project forward to just beneath the anterior abdominal wall (Fig. 82–21). Less commonly, neoplasms arise in the paraspinal or posterior pararenal parts of the retroperitoneal space (Figs. 82–19 and 82–20). Both benign and malignant neoplasms of nerve sheath origin tend to occur in a posterior retroperitoneal location (see Fig. 82–11).

Apart from some liposarcomas, CT and MRI cannot usually predict the histologic type of retroperitoneal tumors. Tumor necrosis and hemorrhage are common among the larger tumors of most types

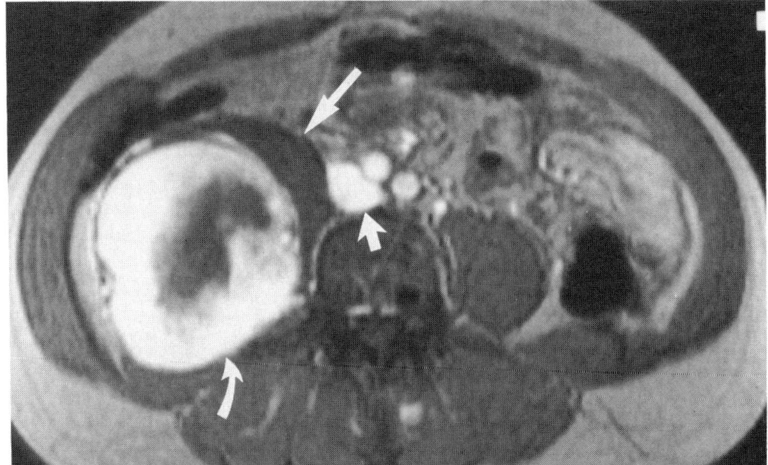

Figure 82–19. Desmoid tumor arising in right psoas compartment. Gradient-echo (FLASH) MRI (148/6/75 degrees) obtained during a bolus intravenous injection of gadolinium-DTPA and during breathholding shows a heterogeneously enhancing mass *(curved arrow)* displacing the right psoas muscle *(long arrow)* anteromedially. The enhanced inferior vena cava *(short arrow)* is seen medial to the psoas muscle.

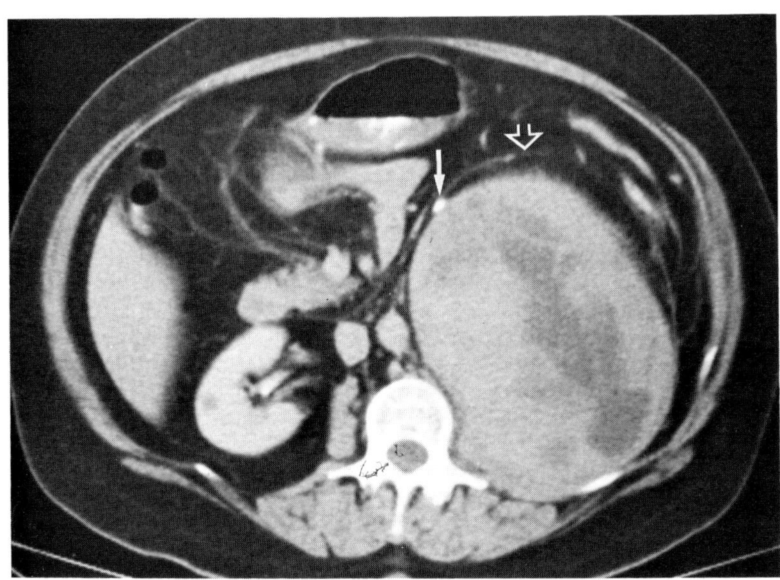

Figure 82–20. Retroperitoneal liposarcoma. The large left tumor mass contains low-density areas due to necrosis. Histologically, the tumor was predominantly a myxoid liposarcoma with some undifferentiated areas. The tumor probably arose in the left psoas muscle. The left ureter *(arrow)* and renal fascia *(open arrow)* are displaced anteriorly.

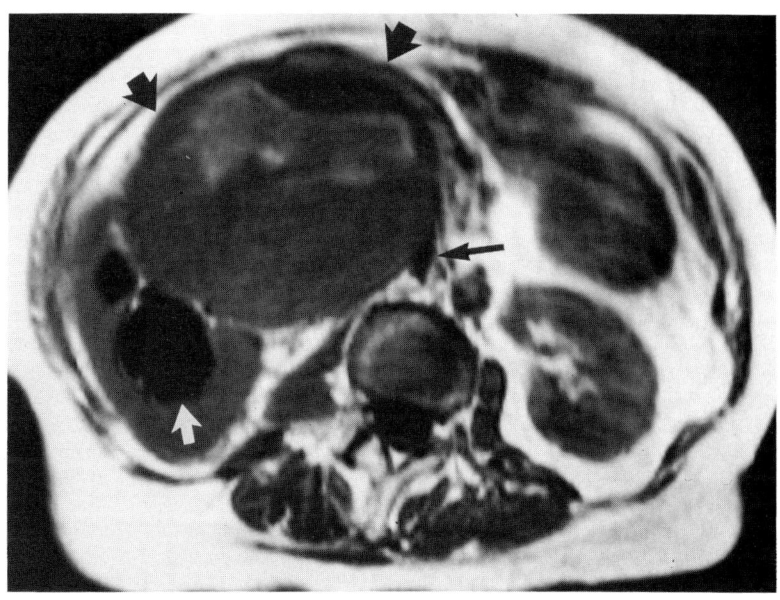

Figure 82–21. Retroperitoneal leiomyosarcoma. T_1-weighted spin-echo MRI (500/15) reveals large neoplasm *(short black arrows)* extending anteriorly to just beneath anterior abdominal wall. The lesion shows a large area of high signal intensity anteriorly due to hemorrhage. Note dilated calyces *(white arrow)* in the laterally displaced right kidney due to renal pelvic compression caused by the tumor. The inferior vena cava *(long black arrow)* is displaced medially by the neoplasm.

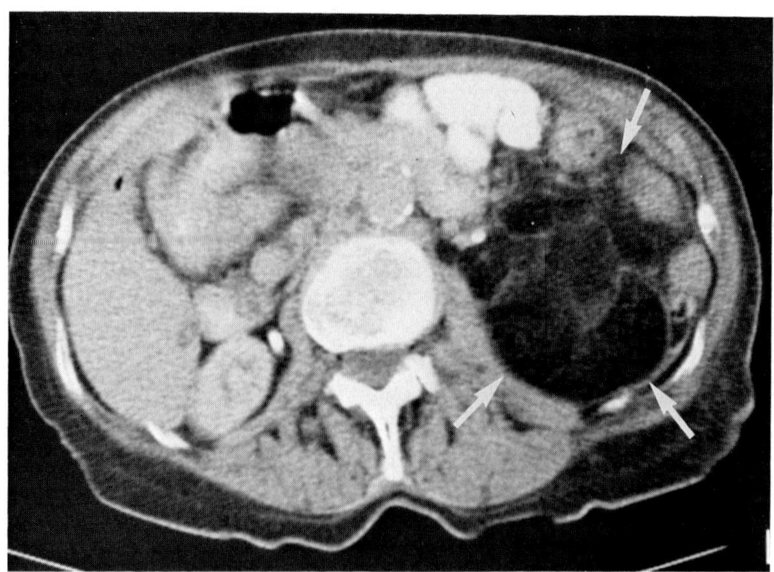

Figure 82–22. Lipogenic liposarcoma. The tumor *(arrows)* is composed predominantly of low-density (−85 HU) fat and contains linear, streaky densities.

and result in a range of appearances varying from slight heterogeneity to large cavities or cysts within the neoplasm (see Figs. 82–19 to 82–21). Cystic degeneration is particularly prevalent among leiomyosarcomas but may occur in any type of retroperitoneal sarcoma. Prominent calcification occurs in about 25 per cent of malignant fibrous histiocytomas.

Three types of retroperitoneal liposarcomas are encountered. Well-differentiated or lipogenic liposarcomas are predominantly of fat density on CT and contain irregular strands of higher density (Fig. 82–22). The tumors often merge imperceptibly with adjacent normal fat and usually displace rather than invade adjacent organs. Myxoid liposarcomas contain large amounts of connective tissue mucin and some fat cells. Their density is usually less than that of muscle, but greater than that of fat. Some myxoid liposarcomas have attenuation values near that of water. At the higher end of the density spectrum are those myxoid liposarcomas with densities similar to that of muscle (see Fig. 82–20). Undifferentiated liposarcomas show marked cellular pleomorphism and contain little lipid or mucin. They are indistinguishable on CT from non-fatty soft-tissue sarcomas.

RETROPERITONEAL FIBROSIS

Retroperitoneal fibrosis is an uncommon and ill-understood condition with a variety of causes and presenting features. About 70 per cent of cases are idiopathic. Other causes include various drugs (especially methysergide); previous abdominal surgery or radiation therapy; aortic aneurysm; and inflammatory bowel diseases such as Crohn's disease, ulcerative colitis, and diverticulitis. Retroperitoneal fibrosis may also be caused by a desmoplastic reaction that occurs in response to retroperitoneal spread of some neoplasms, notably lymphomas and carcinomas of the breast, stomach, lung, colon, and bladder.

Clinically, retroperitoneal fibrosis is insidious in onset, with poorly localized flank or abdominal pain occurring in about 90 per cent of cases. Most patients have impaired renal function, and some present with severe renal failure. Pathologically, retroperitoneal fibrosis is characterized by a mass of pinkish or grayish-white tissue with discrete margins covering the aorta and vena cava. It is usually centered on the lower lumbar spine and extends from the renal pedicles to the pelvic brim, where it bifurcates to follow the iliac vessels. Although the disease is midline or bilateral in 50 to 75 per cent of cases, it may involve one side more than the other or, less frequently, be entirely unilateral. The fibrosis may extend to involve the ureters, common bile duct, duodenum, mesentery, iliac vessels, bladder, and rectum and may extend through the diaphragmatic crura to cause fibrous mediastinitis. Idiopathic retroperitoneal fibrosis may be one component of multifocal fibrosclerosis, in which orbital pseudotumor, Riedel's sclerosing thyroiditis, sclerosing cholangitis, and cardiac valvular fibrosis may also occur.

On excretory urography, obstruction of one or both ureters is typically seen. Retrograde pyelography often depicts smoothly tapered narrowing of one or both ureters in the region of involvement. CT is the method of choice for evaluating suspected cases. Sometimes the fibrous tissue is minimal and barely discernible on CT, even in the presence of high-grade ureteric obstruction. However, CT often shows a soft-tissue plaque enveloping, but not displacing, the aorta and inferior vena cava (Fig. 82–23). Vena caval compression may occur. The fibrosis often extends laterally into the perinephric spaces to involve the ureters, causing hydronephrosis. Progressive ureteral obstruction may require ureterolysis—that is, surgical freeing of the ureters from the plaque. The ureter is then transplanted into the peritoneum or wrapped with omentum to provide a barrier against re-entrapment by fibrosis.

Similar CT findings occur in both idiopathic and malignant retroperitoneal fibrosis (Fig. 82–24). Accordingly, periureteral needle biopsy at the level of the ureteric obstruction or surgical exploration is sometimes necessary to establish a definitive diagnosis if there is no known primary neoplasm. MRI may sometimes help distinguish the two conditions. On T_1-weighted images, the fibrous plaque is of low or intermediate signal intensity in both benign and malignant retroperitoneal fibrosis. On T_2-weighted images, the benign variety usually maintains a somewhat low signal intensity and is homogeneous in appearance, whereas malignant retroperitoneal fibrosis often exhibits a high signal intensity and a heterogeneous appearance. However, overlap occurs and recently formed benign plaque may show a high signal on T_2-weighted images.

Retroperitoneal fibrosis may also be associated with aortic or iliac artery aneurysms. Fibrosis associated with such "inflammatory aneurysms" may be due to an immune response to leakage of an insoluble lipid from an atheromatous plaque into the periaortic tissue. On CT, the aneurysm may be surrounded by an enhancing soft-tissue mass. One or both ureters may be entrapped, causing hydronephrosis. Ureteric obstruction is not uncommon in Crohn's

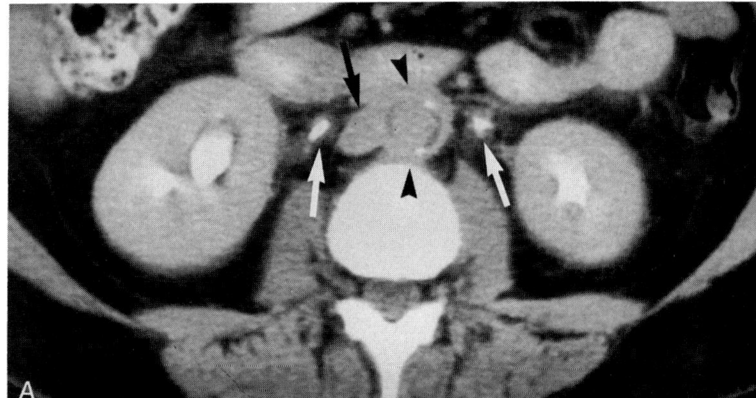

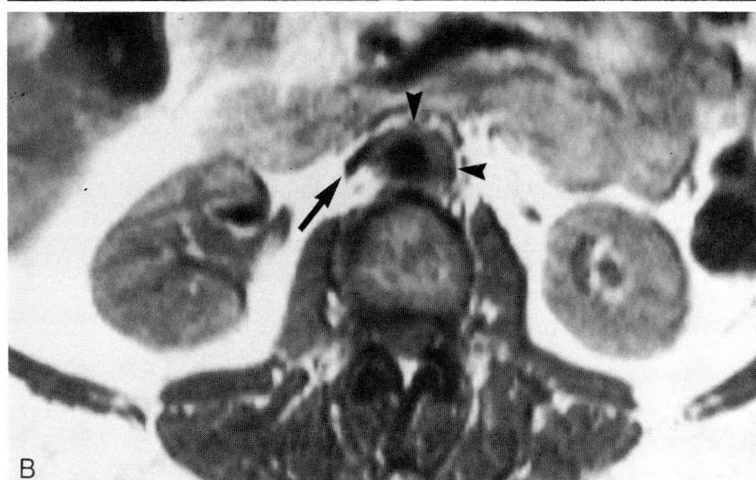

Figure 82–23. Idiopathic retroperitoneal fibrosis. *A,* A CT scan shows a rim of fibrous tissue *(arrowheads)* around the aorta, which contains calcified atherosclerotic plaques. The fibrous tissue obscures the plane between the aorta and vena cava *(black arrow).* Strands of fibrous tissue *(white arrows)* extend laterally to surround the ureters, which contain stents. Note bilateral calyceal dilatation. *B,* Proton density-weighted spin-echo MRI (1800/15) obtained six months after bilateral ureterolysis reveals a periaortic rim of fibrous tissue *(arrowheads)* with a signal intensity higher than that of muscle. The inferior vena cava *(arrow)* is patent but is attached to the fibrous tissue.

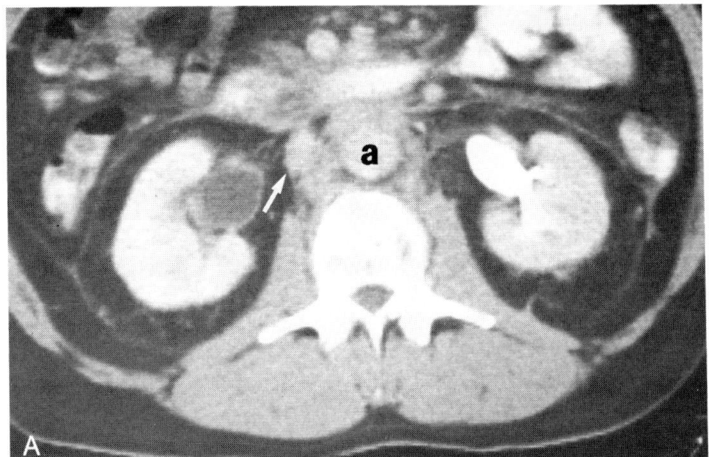

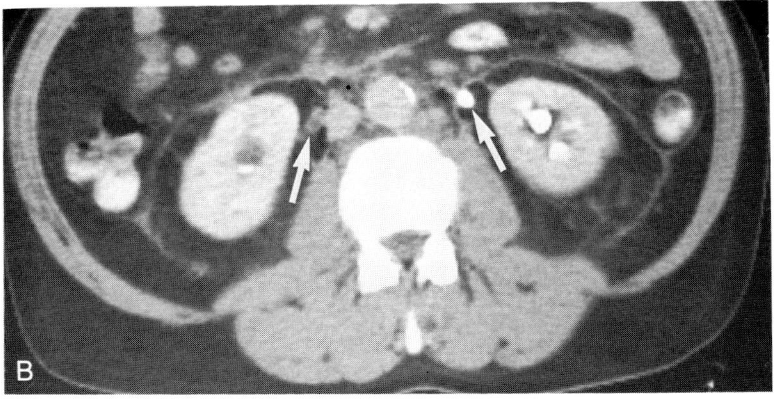

Figure 82–24. Malignant retroperitoneal fibrosis due to gastric carcinoma. *A,* There is bilateral hydronephrosis with no contrast excretion on the right. The contrast-enhanced aorta (a) is surrounded by an ill-defined mantle of tissue that displaces the inferior vena cava *(arrow)* to the right. There is bilateral thickening of the renal fascia. *B,* Caudal CT scan shows both ureters *(arrows)* entrapped by prevertebral fibrosis.

disease and may be caused by inflammatory fibrosis extending into the retroperitoneum. CT may provide the diagnosis by showing thickened bowel loops in the lower abdomen and pelvis.

Bibliography

Amis ES: Retroperitoneal fibrosis. AJR 157:321, 1991.

Belville JS, Morgentaler A, Loughlin KR, Tumeh SS: Spontaneous perinephric and subcapsular renal hemorrhage: Evaluation with CT, US, and angiography. Radiology 172:733, 1989.

Castellino RA: Hodgkin disease: Practical concepts for the diagnostic radiologist. Radiology 159:305, 1986.

Castellino RA: The non-Hodgkin lymphomas: Practical concepts for the diagnostic radiologist. Radiology 178:315, 1991.

Crawford ES: The diagnosis and management of aortic dissection. JAMA 264:2537, 1990.

Dorfman RE, Alpern MB, Gross BH, Sandler MA: Upper abdominal lymph nodes: Criteria for normal size determined with CT. Radiology 180:319, 1991.

Feldberg MAM, Koehler PR, van Waes PFGM: Psoas compartment disease studied by computed tomography. Analysis of 50 cases and subject review. Radiology 148:505, 1983.

Kellman GM, Alpern MB, Sandler MA, Craig BM: Computed tomography of vena caval anomalies with embryologic correlation. RadioGraphics 8:533, 1988.

Kneeland JB, Auh YH, Rubenstein WA et al: Perirenal spaces: CT evidence for communication across the midline. Radiology 164:657, 1987.

Kunin M: Bridging septa of the perinephric space: Anatomic, pathologic, and diagnostic considerations. Radiology 158:361, 1986.

Lane RH, Stephens DH, Reiman HM: Primary retroperitoneal neoplasms: CT findings in 90 cases with clinical and pathologic correlation. AJR 152:83, 1989.

Low RN, Wall SD, Jeffrey RB, et al: Aortoenteric fistula and perigraft infection: Evaluation with CT. Radiology 175:157, 1990.

Meyers MA: Dynamic Radiology of the Abdomen: Normal and Pathologic Anatomy, 3rd ed. New York, Springer-Verlag, 1988, p. 184.

North LB, Lindell MM, Jing BS, Wallace S: Current use of lymphography for staging lymphomas and genital tumors. AJR 158:725, 1992.

Raptopoulos V, Kleinman PK, Marks S, et al: Renal fascial pathway: Posterior extension of pancreatic effusions within the anterior pararenal space. Radiology 158:367, 1986.

Reed MD, Friedman AC, Nealey P: Anomalies of the left renal vein: Analysis of 433 CT scans. J Comput Assist Tomogr 6:1124, 1982.

Reuler JB, Kumar KL: Abdominal aortic aneurysm. J Gen Intern Med 6:360, 1991.

83 The Ureter

Robert F. Spataro, Fred T. Lee, Jr., and John R. Thornbury

The ureter may be involved by intrinsic primary disease or by extrinsic involvement by disease of the retroperitoneum and pelvis. Intrinsic diseases of the ureter include primary and metastatic tumors; infectious and inflammatory diseases; congenital and acquired obstructive lesions such as ureteropelvic junction obstruction, primary megaureter, and ureteral stricture; developmental abnormalities such as ureteral duplication; and trauma. Lesions extrinsic to the ureter may present primarily with ureteral obstruction and include diseases such as retroperitoneal fibrosis; primary and metastatic retroperitoneal tumors; primary and secondary pelvic malignancy; and inflammatory diseases such as Crohn's disease, diverticulitis, and abscesses.

Diseases of the ureter usually present primarily with hematuria, either microscopic or gross, or symptoms of obstruction. In calculus disease with ureteral obstruction, severe pain is usually present. However, with many primary and secondary diseases of the ureter, obstruction may be slowly progressive or intermittent, and vague or atypical flank or abdominal pain may be present. With slowly progressive ureteral obstruction, pain may be absent and the patient may present with an abdominal mass, hypertension, generalized constitutional symptoms, or uremia.

The diagnosis of ureteral abnormalities is quite accurate. Selection of the appropriate diagnostic imaging technique in a particular clinical situation is necessary. Intravenous excretory urography remains the best screening examination of the urinary system. Ultrasonography is particularly useful in the determination of ureteral obstruction. Computed tomography (CT) and magnetic resonance imaging (MRI) may be highly specific in differentiating intrinsic and extrinsic ureteral lesions as a cause of ureteral obstruction, particularly when poor function is present. CT is useful in the differentiation of benign and malignant lesions of the retroperitoneum that present with ureteral obstruction and in the differentiation of uric acid calculi and transitional cell carcinoma of the ureter. Percutaneous nephrostomy with antegrade pyelography is both therapeutic and diagnostic in patients presenting with ureteral obstruction and has significantly changed the approach to both acute and chronic obstruction. Retrograde pyelography is infrequently utilized in current practice but is sometimes necessary in the evaluation of obstructive lesions of the ureter. Radionuclide renography is usually not helpful in evaluating the etiology of ureteral disease but is helpful in determining renal function when chronic ureteral obstruction has been present. Ureteral brush biopsy and percutaneous thin-needle aspiration biopsy can be utilized to obtain cytology from primary ureteral and extrinsic masses affecting the ureter and allow specific preoperative diagnosis with minimal invasion. The use of magnetic resonance imaging (MRI) for the routine evaluation of ureteral disease is not widespread, although it may be used to image extrinsic lesions causing ureteral compression.

PATHOLOGY OF THE URETER

Ureteropelvic Junction Obstruction

Ureteropelvic junction (UPJ) obstruction is a common cause of ureteral obstruction in children and young adults but may be seen at any age. Typical presentation is one of multiple bouts of flank pain that spontaneously subside. Between acute episodes the urinary tract may be normal or nearly normal in appearance, and the diagnosis is often missed initially because of the episodic and effervescent nature of the symptoms and the absence of abnormal radiographic signs between acute obstructive episodes. UPJ obstruction is caused by a stricture that may be fibrotic or due to neuromuscular dysfunction or abnormal insertion of the ureter into the renal pelvis. Ultrasonography and intravenous urography show similar signs. There is dilatation of the calyces and renal pelvis with a collapsed ureter. In difficult diagnostic cases the use of diuretics in combination with intravenous urography, ultrasonography, or radionuclide renography may precipitate an obstructive episode and confirm the diagnosis. Although surgical repair by pyeloplasty is the current procedure of choice, percutaneous endopyelotomy or nonoperative percutaneous dilatation has led to some success.

Primary Megaureter (Megaloureter)

Congenital distal ureteral obstruction may be caused by an abnormality of the distal ureter in which a narrowed, poorly functioning distal ureteral segment is present. This distal narrowed ureter is aperistaltic, and there may be hypoplasia of the terminal muscle fibers resulting in functional obstruction of the ureter at this point. Congenital megaureter may present with a varying degree of obstructive uropathy. It may present early with severe obstruction requiring surgery to prevent renal destruction or present later with progressive obstruction (Fig. 83–1). In mild cases dilatation of the distal ureter is present without increased pressure within the renal pelvis, and the appearance may remain unchanged for many years.

Retrocaval Ureter

A retrocaval ureter is caused by abnormal embryogenesis of the inferior vena cava. A retrocaval ureter passes posteriorly behind the

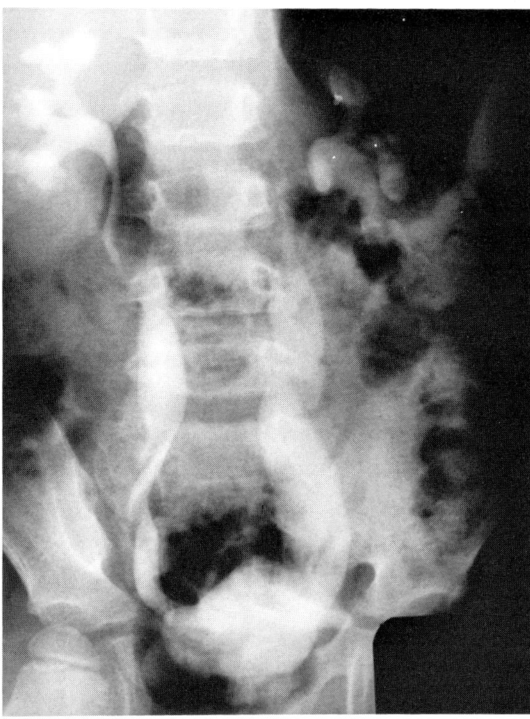

Figure 83–1. Primary megaureter. Excretory urogram in a four-year-old with recurrent urinary tract infection. Bilaterally, there is mild blunting and fullness of the calyces and renal pelvis, and the ureter becomes increasingly dilated to the region of the ureterovesical junction, where there is a narrowed aperistaltic segment just proximal to the ureterovesical junction typical of primary megaureter. There is no ureteral reflux present and no bladder outlet obstruction. Although in this case mild obstruction is present, in more severe cases high-grade obstruction may be present, and in less severe cases only minimal dilatation of the distal ureter may be present without upper urinary tract obstruction that may remain stable without symptomatology or progression. (Courtesy of Beverly P. Wood, M.D., Rochester, NY; currently at Children's Hospital UCLA Medical Center, Los Angeles, CA.)

vena cava, between the vena cava and the aorta, and then laterally to assume its normal position distally (Fig. 83–2). Occasionally, the retrocaval position of the ureter leads to ureteral obstruction. However, in many instances retrocaval ureter is a developmental anomaly without significant ureteral obstruction.

Hydronephrosis of Pregnancy

Dilatation of the ureters occurs with pregnancy. Although both ureters may be affected, the right ureter is more commonly affected and is usually more severely affected than the left. In hydronephrosis of pregnancy there is dilatation of the calyces, renal pelvis, and ureter to the pelvic brim. Compression of the ureters by the enlarged uterus is considered the most likely cause of the ureteral dilatation that is seen during pregnancy. Post partum, the dilatation may remain for several months, but eventually the collecting system returns to normal caliber.

Ureterocele

A ureterocele is a dilatation of the terminal ureter that prolapses into the bladder lumen. Ureteroceles may be seen with normal ureters inserting in a normal position within the bladder, and these are termed simple ureteroceles (Fig. 83–3). Ectopic ureteroceles may be seen with ectopic insertions of the ureter and with ureteral duplications with ectopic insertion of the ureter. When a ureterocele is present in a ureter with an abnormal insertion to the bladder or outside the bladder, it is termed an *ectopic ureterocele*. Ureteroceles may be of no significance and may be an incidental finding. However, ureteroceles may cause significant ureteral obstruction and may predispose to calculus formation. The ''typical'' cobra head appearance of a simple ureterocele with halo may be associated in adults with obstruction of the ureteral orifice by invasive tumor or calculus. These pseudoureteroceles caused by obstructing lesions must be differentiated from true simple ureteroceles.

Ureteral Duplication and Associated Anomalies

Partial duplications of the renal pelvis and ureters are common and are of no significance. Complete duplication of the ureters with two separate ureteral orifices is not an uncommon variant and may be of no significance. However, a number of significant functional anomalies are associated with ureteral duplication due to abnormality of the anatomy and position of the ureters. With complete duplication of the ureter, the ureter draining the lower aspect of the kidney enters the bladder in a normal or nearly normal location. The ureter draining the upper aspect of the kidney may enter the bladder in the region of the trigone, and the ureteral orifice opens inferior and medial to the ureter draining the lower portion of the kidney. When both ureters have ureteral orifices in the trigone with nearly normal tunnels, urinary drainage may be normal. However, one or both ureters of a ureteral duplication may have anomalies, including abnormal tunnels producing vesicoureteral reflux and ectopic ureteroceles causing obstruction. The ureter draining the upper aspect of the kidney is particularly prone to form an ectopic ureterocele with obstruction, and this may present in infancy or childhood with an upper-pole renal mass. This ectopic ureter is also more prone to vesicoureteral reflux and reflux nephropathy in the upper half of the kidney because of an abnormal ureteral tunnel. In addition, the ectopic ureter can insert anywhere along the mesonephric duct remnants. In males, insertion can be into the seminal vesicles, ejaculatory ducts, or low in the bladder. Because these insertion sites are always above the external sphincter, males with these

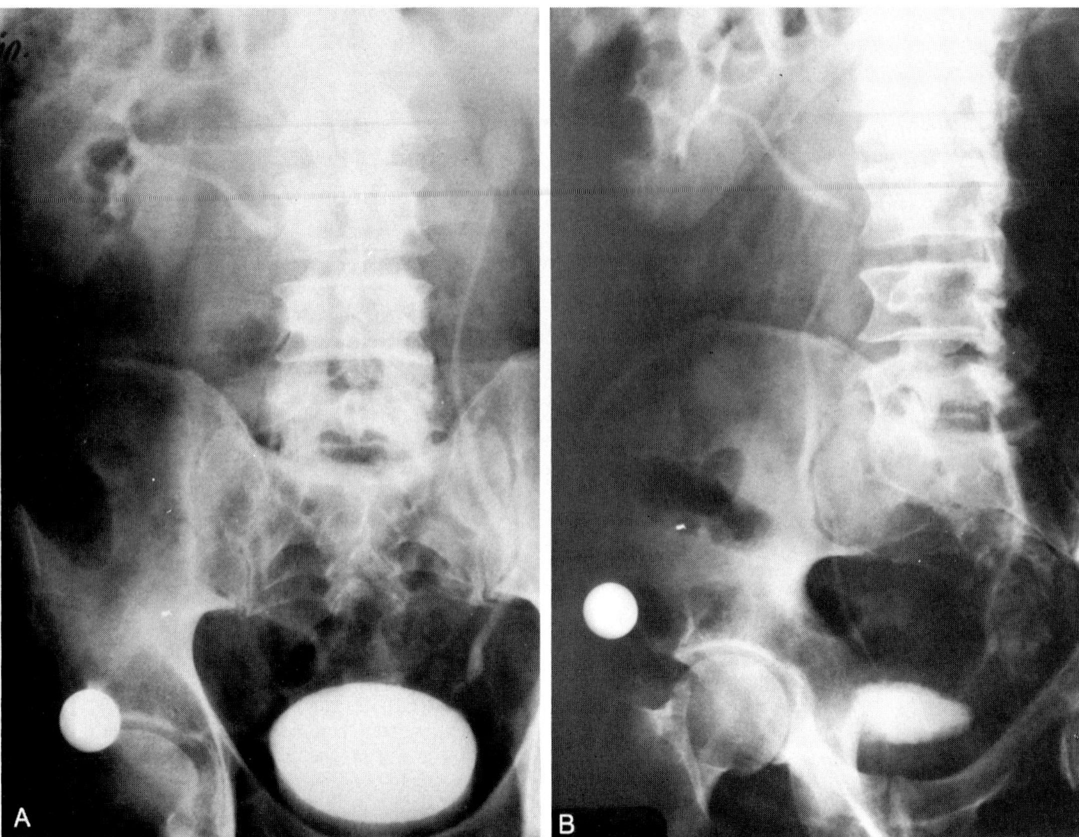

Figure 83–2. Retrocaval ureter. *A*, Frontal view from an excretory urogram shows abrupt medial deviation of the proximal right ureter, which lies well over the lumbar vertebral body. The ureter is passing behind the inferior vena cava at this point. The ureter then swings anteriorly and laterally and returns to its normal position in the region of the L5 vertebral body. *B*, A right posterior oblique view shows the medial, anterior, and then lateral course of the proximal right ureter behind the inferior vena cava to return to its normal position more distally. Its appearance is characteristic of retrocaval ureter.

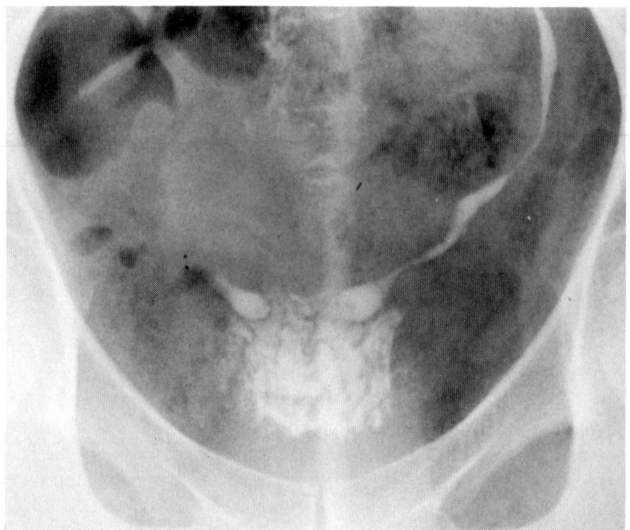

Figure 83–3. Bilateral simple ureteroceles. Post-void radiograph of the bladder during excretory urography shows the typical "cobra head" appearance of the dilated distal ureters, which are prolapsed into the bladder lumen. The outside of the ureterocele wall can be seen surrounded by contrast within the bladder. In this case there is no ureteral duplication, and these lesions represent true simple ureteroceles.

anomalies are continent. In females, the ureter can insert into the urethra below the external sphincter or vagina, and thus these females may present with urinary incontinence. The most common abnormality of the ureter draining the lower half of the kidney is vesicoureteral reflux with reflux nephropathy. Ectopic ureteroceles may prolapse into the urethra, causing bladder outlet obstruction.

Partial Ureteral Duplication

Blind-ending duplications from incomplete ureteral budding may occur and are usually of no significance. These are sometimes referred to as congenital ureteral diverticula (Fig. 83–4).

URETERAL LESIONS ASSOCIATED WITH INFECTIOUS AND INFLAMMATORY DISEASES

Mucosal Striations

Mucosal striations or ridges are redundant mucosal folds seen in the renal pelvis and proximal ureter that are often associated with vesicoureteral reflux and urinary tract infection but have been reported in patients without a history of either.

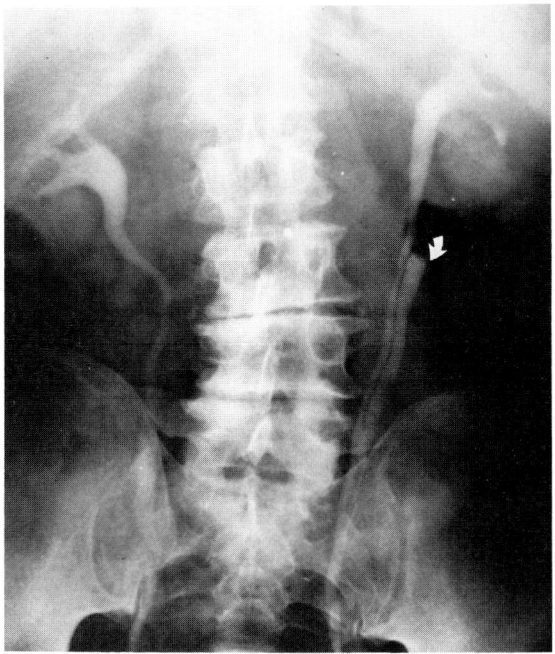

Figure 83–4. Blind-ending ureteral duplication (congenital ureteral diverticulum). A long blind-ending ureteral duplication can be seen arising from the mid-ureter and ending adjacent to the proximal ureter *(arrow)*. These may occur in any portion of the ureter and are most commonly seen in the distal ureter. They may vary from several millimeters to several centimeters in size. They are generally of no consequence but may predispose to infection or calculus formation if urinary stasis is present.

Pyeloureteritis Cystica

In pyeloureteritis cystica, small fluid-filled inflammatory cysts are produced as a result of invagination of mucosal cell buds of von Braun into the lamina propria of the ureter. These inflammatory cysts are usually associated with chronic uroepithelial inflammation due to urinary tract infection or stone disease. A typical radiographic pattern of multiple small, smooth-filling defects that involve the pelvis and ureter is characteristic (Fig. 83–5). These are benign lesions that should be differentiated from multicentric transitional cell carcinoma.

Ureteral Diverticula (Pseudodiverticula)

Multiple small ureteral diverticula (pseudodiverticula) are acquired lesions in which invaginations of hyperplastic epithelium project into the lamina propria of the ureter. This condition is also associated with chronic inflammatory disease of the urinary tract. There may be a higher incidence of transitional cell carcinoma of the ureter in patients with ureteral diverticula.

Cholesteatoma, Leukoplakia, and Squamous Metaplasia of the Renal Pelvis and Ureter

Cholesteatoma is a rare benign accumulation of keratinous tissue of the transitional epithelium due to a squamous metaplasia of the renal pelvis, ureter, or bladder that is frequently associated with chronic urinary tract infection or calculus disease. Cholesteatoma may appear as striations or irregular filling defects of the renal pelvis or ureter.

Leukoplakia is an uncommon severe form of keratinizing squamous metaplasia of the uroepithelium in which cellular atypia is present and is considered to be a premalignant condition eventually leading to squamous cell carcinoma of the ureter. The radiographic appearance is similar to that of cholesteatoma, with mucosal striations or ridges or irregular filling defects of the mucosa. Since radiographically it is impossible to differentiate cholesteatoma from leukoplakia, all keratinizing squamous metaplasia of the renal pelvis, ureter, and bladder should be considered premalignant and treated appropriately.

TUMORS OF THE RENAL PELVIS AND URETER

Transitional Cell Carcinoma of the Ureter

Transitional cell carcinoma accounts for 85 per cent of primary tumors of the renal pelvis and ureter. Transitional cell carcinoma of the renal pelvis and ureter may be primarily papillary, in which growth occurs into the lumen without significant invasion; papillary, with invasion; or primarily infiltrating in nature. Papillary tumors without invasion have a high cure rate with surgical resection, whereas the prognosis with infiltrating tumors is poor. Transitional cell carcinoma may present as a smooth or irregular intralu-

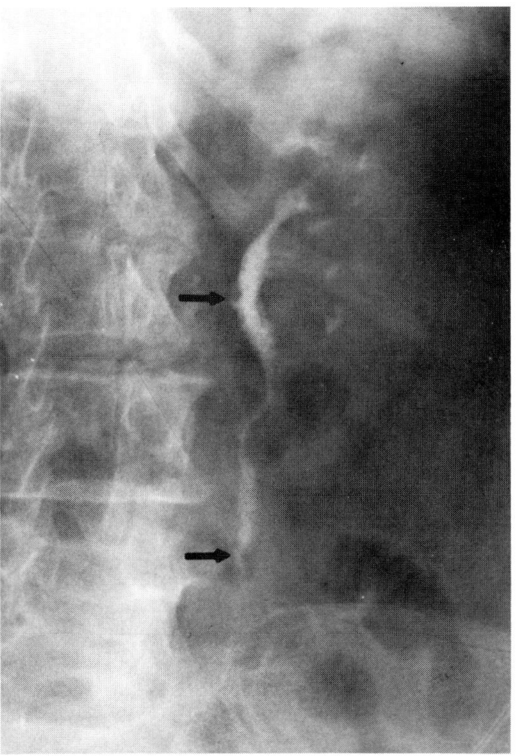

Figure 83–5. Pyeloureteritis cystica. Left posterior oblique view of the renal pelvis and ureter shows multiple small, smooth, round filling defects *(arrows)* projecting into the lumen of the left renal pelvis and ureter. This appearance is typical of pyeloureteritis cystica. Pyeloureteritis cystica is often seen in conjunction with recurrent urinary tract infection or urolithiasis.

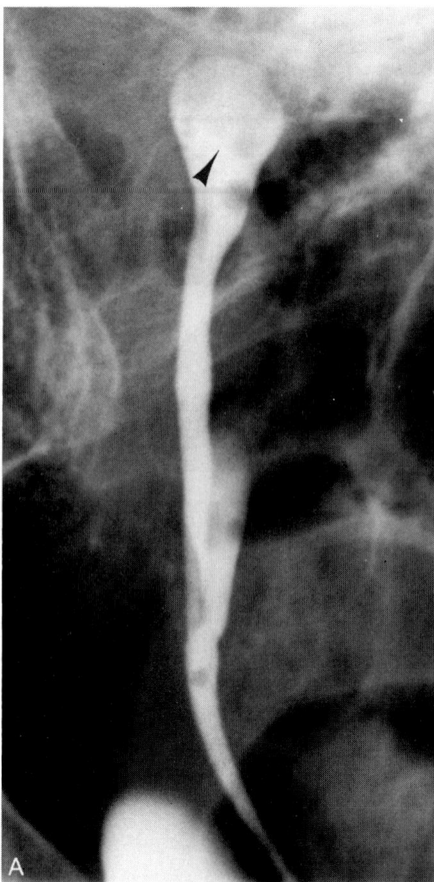

Figure 83–6. Invasive transitional cell carcinoma of the ureter. A patient presented with flank pain and a nonfunctioning right kidney on excretory urogram. *A,* A retrograde pyelogram shows an irregular intraluminal filling defect of the ureter typical of transitional cell carcinoma *(arrowhead).* A congenital blind-ending ureteral duplication is seen more distally. *B,* A CT scan shows a highly invasive transitional cell carcinoma with extensive invasion outside of the ureteral lumen into the retroperitoneum *(arrowheads).* This is not apparent on the retrograde pyelogram or excretory urogram. The CT scan clearly shows that this ureteral transitional cell carcinoma is not a resectable lesion. CT is currently the most accurate diagnostic imaging modality in the staging of transitional cell carcinoma of the ureter.

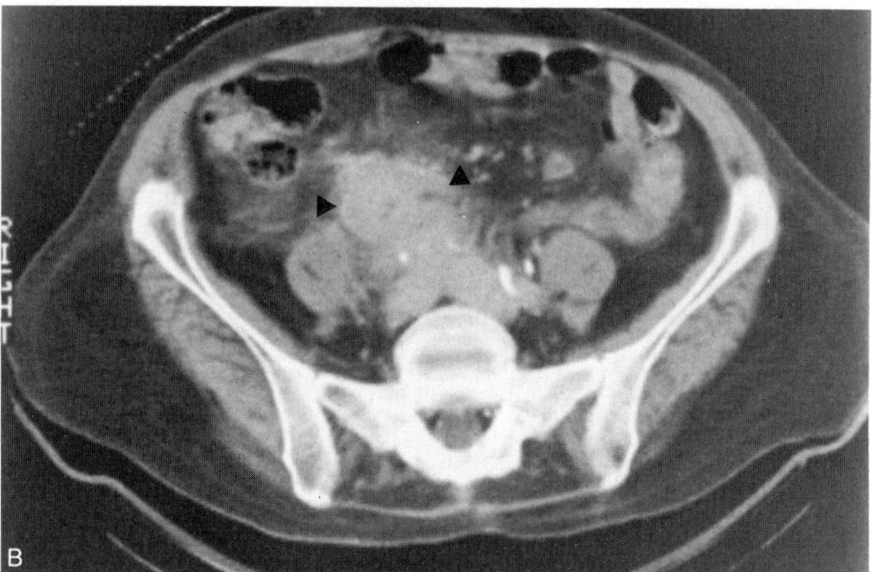

minal mass of the renal pelvis or ureter or as an area of thickening and stricture. Excretory urography will define many of these tumors. When high-grade or chronic obstruction is present, retrograde or antegrade pyelography may be necessary to define the etiology of the ureteral obstruction. CT is accurate in the diagnosis of transitional cell carcinoma of the ureter and is the most accurate imaging modality in the staging of transitional cell carcinoma. Extraureteral invasion and lymph node metastases are well-defined by CT (Fig. 83–6). CT can also clearly differentiate nonopaque uric acid calculi from transitional cell carcinoma of the ureter when the diagnosis is unclear or when high-grade ureteral obstruction is present. The spread pattern of transitional cell carcinoma of the ureter is initially by local invasion or lymphatic spread to regional lymph nodes. Metastases may occur to liver, lung, brain, or bone. When transitional cell carcinoma of the renal pelvis or ureters is present, there is a significantly increased risk of a synchronous transitional cell carcinoma occurring in the bladder or in the opposite renal pelvis or ureter, and the chance of a second transitional cell carcinoma arising at some time after the initial tumor in the bladder or opposite renal pelvis and ureter is significantly higher in patients with a previous transitional cell carcinoma. Thus, multiplicity of tumors and *de novo* development of second transitional cell carcinomas, as well as recurrence of tumor, must be searched for diligently in patients with transitional cell carcinoma and follow-up examinations obtained.

Squamous Cell Carcinoma

Squamous cell carcinoma of the renal pelvis and ureter is uncommon. These tumors are infiltrating tumors with early invasion and lymphatic spread and have a poor prognosis. Squamous cell carcinoma is frequently found in association with chronic inflammatory or infectious changes of the uroepithelium such as leukoplakia. Squamous cell carcinoma radiographically appears as an infiltrating tumor and cannot be differentiated from infiltrating transitional cell carcinoma.

Papilloma and Inverted Papilloma of the Ureter

Papillomas are slow-growing uroepithelial tumors that are either benign or low-grade malignant uroepithelial tumors. They are seen in a younger age group than is usually found with transitional cell carcinoma. Radiographically, they present as a smooth, round sessile filling defect of the ureter, but this cannot be differentiated from early transitional cell carcinoma, so surgical excisional biopsy is necessary.

Inverted papilloma of the ureter is a sessile or pedunculated polypoid lesion in which the epithelial fronds are surrounded by the fibromuscular stroma, the reverse of the usual pattern. Radiographically these lesions are indistinguishable from low-grade transitional cell carcinoma, and surgical excisional biopsy is necessary.

Fibroepithelial Ureteral Polyp

Fibroepithelial ureteral polyps are true benign lesions of the renal pelvis and ureter that are generally found in younger patients. The clinical presentation is usually that of intermittent pain caused by obstruction or microscopic or gross hematuria. A long, pedunculated, smooth-surfaced intraluminal tumor is characteristic of fibroepithelial ureteral polyps (Fig. 83–7). In these cases conservative

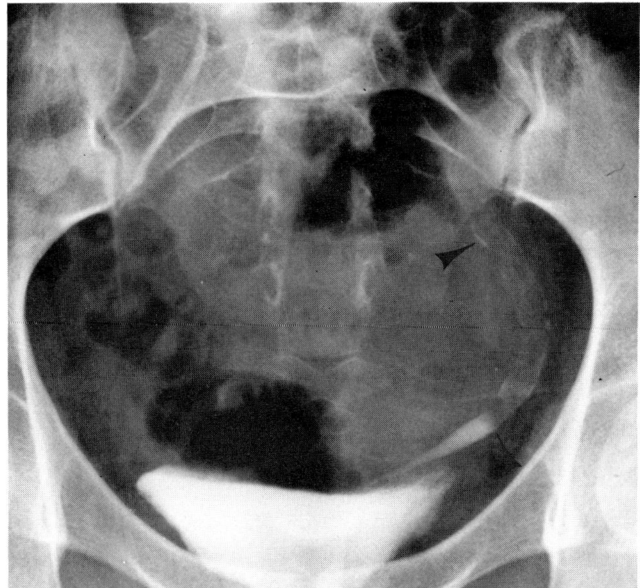

Figure 83–7. Benign fibroepithelial polyp. An excretory urogram shows a long smooth filling defect *(arrowheads)* of the distal left ureter in a young male. This has the typical appearance of a benign fibroepithelial polyp, which was confirmed at surgical resection. (Courtesy of Arthur W. Segal, M.D., Rochester General Hospital, Rochester, NY.)

surgical removal may be performed, since this is a benign lesion with no malignant potential.

Metastases to the Ureter

Primary malignancy of the breast, lung, colon, prostate, and stomach, and melanoma can metastasize directly to the ureter, although such metastases are rare. Radiologically the appearance is one of ureteral stricture with concentric ureteral tapering (Fig. 83–8). Occasionally an appearance identical to a primary ureteral transitional cell carcinoma may be seen with ureteral metastases.

Vascular Ureteral Notching

Ureteral notching—smooth extrinsic impressions on the proximal ureter—may be seen with dilatation of the periureteral arteries or veins that causes extrinsic impression upon the ureter. This may be acquired or congenital. Ureteral notching due to arterial dilatation is seen with main renal artery stenosis in which collateral flow through periureteral arteries occurs to supply the ischemic kidney and with hypervascular renal tumors or arteriovenous malformation. Ureteral notching may be seen with venous varicosities, either congenital secondary to collateral venous flow due to renal vein or inferior vena caval obstruction, or as an isolated finding without venous obstruction.

EXTRINSIC INVOLVEMENT OF THE URETER

Extrinsic involvement of the ureter by retroperitoneal or pelvic pathology may cause displacement, invasion, or obstruction of the ureter. Primary retroperitoneal tumors (most commonly lymphoma, liposarcoma, leiomyosarcoma, fibrous histiocytoma, teratoma, embryonal germ cell tumor, or neural tumor) may cause displacement, invasion, or obstruction of the ureter and are best diagnosed and imaged by ultrasonography, CT, or MRI. Metastatic retroperitoneal lymph node involvement from lymphoma or primary pelvic or other malignancies may also cause secondary changes in the ureter of displacement or obstruction. These retroperitoneal tumors affecting the ureter are discussed in Chapter 82.

A number of diseases that involve the ureter extrinsically but that may present primarily with ureteral obstruction, flank pain, hematuria, or other urinary symptoms will be discussed.

Ureteral Obstruction by Genitourinary and Pelvic Malignancies Other Than Primary Ureteral Tumors

Ureteral obstruction by direct invasion or pelvic metastatic involvement by malignancies is much more common than ureteral obstruction caused by primary ureteral uroepithelial tumors. Carcinoma of the bladder, carcinoma of the prostate, and carcinoma of the cervix may frequently cause ureteral obstruction by direct extension of an invasive tumor into the intramural or distal ureter. Staging of these tumors includes a determination of whether ureteral obstruction has occurred. Carcinoma of the rectosigmoid and ovarian carcinoma can also cause ureteral obstruction by direct invasion by locally invasive tumor.

After surgical resection, radiation therapy, or combinations of surgical, radiation, and chemotherapies, local recurrences of carcinomas of the bladder, prostate, cervix, ovary, and colon can cause ureteral obstruction that can be diagnosed by intravenous excretory urography, CT, ultrasonography, and antegrade or retrograde pyelography. Percutaneous transperitoneal thin-needle biopsy can provide cytologic confirmation of the etiology of ureteral obstruction. Percutaneous nephrostomy may provide life-extending urinary diversion in patients with noncurable malignancy.

Lymph node metastases from primary pelvic malignancies can

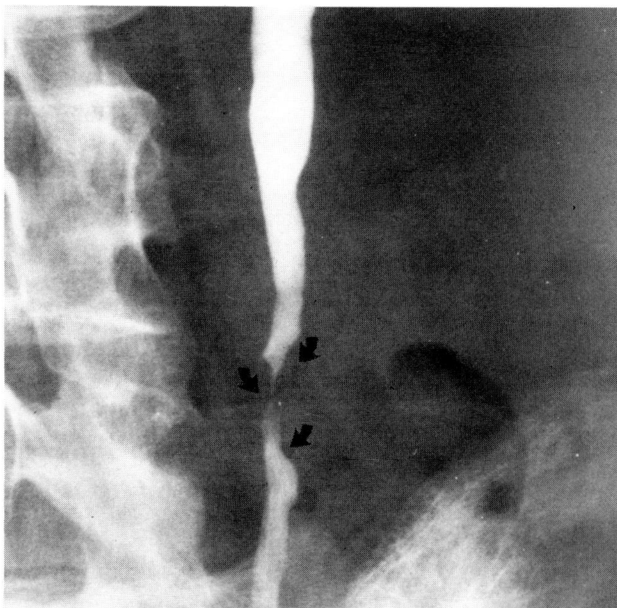

Figure 83–8. Metastasis to the left ureter. A woman presented with left flank pain and obstruction. She had a previous history of colon carcinoma. A percutaneous nephrostomy was performed. An antegrade pyelogram after percutaneous nephrostomy shows a sharply defined narrowing of the left mid-ureter due to direct metastatic involvement of the wall of the ureter from metastatic colon carcinoma *(arrows).*

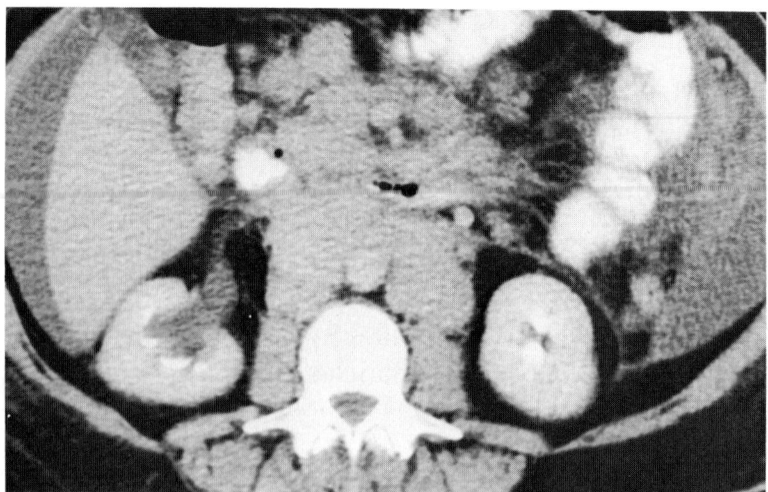

Figure 83–9. Ureteral obstruction due to lymphoma. Massive retroperitoneal adenopathy obstructs the right ureter, causing hydronephrosis.

cause secondary ureteral obstruction, most commonly in the region of the ureter just below the point where it crosses the common iliac artery (Fig. 83–9). The appearance of ureteral obstruction owing to metastatic lymph node involvement may show circumferential stenosis or a corkscrew or multiple fixed ureteral narrowings (Fig. 83–10).

Radiation Fibrosis of the Ureter

Treatment of pelvic malignancies frequently involves the use of radiation therapy. Fibrosis and stricture of the ureter secondary to irradiation can cause ureteral obstruction with an appearance that may be difficult to differentiate from metastatic involvement of the ureter by intravenous excretory urography or antegrade or retrograde pyelography. CT can be helpful when no large surrounding soft-tissue tumor mass is seen and when only ureteral thickening or localized periureteral mass may be seen. Percutaneous thin-needle periureteral biopsy is helpful in the determination of localized periureteral tumor involvement vs periureteral fibrosis.

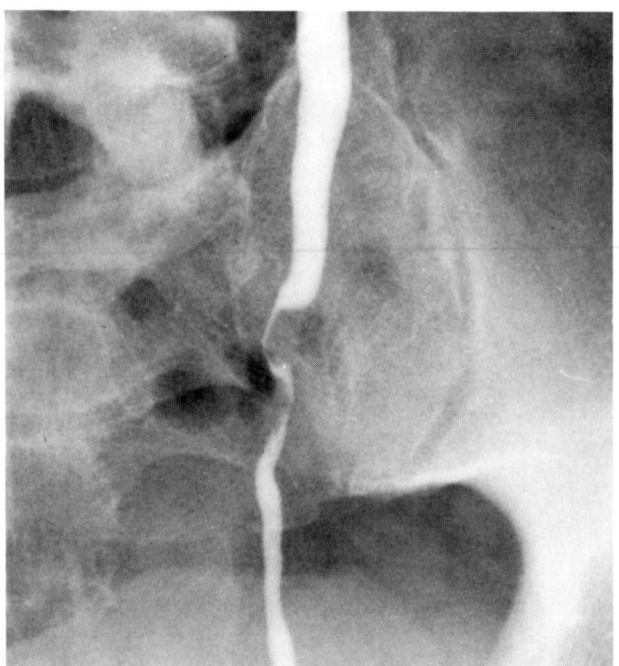

Figure 83–10. Ureteral obstruction due to pelvic lymph node metastases from adenocarcinoma of the sigmoid colon. Patient presented with left-sided ureteral obstruction. A percutaneous nephrostomy was performed, and antegrade pyelogram shows two areas of narrowing of the distal left ureter in the region of the common iliac lymph node chain. This corkscrew appearance of the distal left ureter is commonly seen with obstruction due to lymph node metastases.

Extrinsic Compression of the Ureter by Benign Pelvic Masses

Large benign pelvic masses such as large leiomyomas (fibroids) of the uterus, large benign ovarian cysts or teratomas (dermoid cysts) of the ovary, and pelvic fibrolipomatosis may cause partial ureteral obstruction by compression of the ureter between the large pelvic mass and the bony pelvis. Significant unilateral or bilateral ureteral obstruction may be produced, which is relieved with removal of the benign uterine, ovarian, or other pelvic mass.

EXTRINSIC INFLAMMATORY DISEASES AFFECTING THE URETER

Retroperitoneal Fibrosis

Idiopathic retroperitoneal fibrosis is a benign fibrotic reaction of the retroperitoneum of unknown etiology that may involve the ureters, causing unilateral or bilateral ureteral obstruction. One etiology proven to cause retroperitoneal fibrosis is the drug methysergide (Sansert). The diagnosis of retroperitoneal fibrosis may be difficult, since there may be little dilatation even when complete obstruction with anuria is present. Because of this, ultrasonography can be misleading, and the diagnosis of retroperitoneal fibrosis with minimal dilatation may be missed. Invasive retroperitoneal neoplasms and leaking aortic aneurysms may cause desmoplastic reactions and lead to retroperitoneal fibrosis. Idiopathic retroperitoneal fibrosis has no known etiology. Clinically, patients with retroperitoneal fibrosis may present with back or flank pain, hypertension, anuria, or uremia with constitutional symptoms of fatigue, malaise, anemia, or hypertension.

Since obstruction may occur with a minimal degree of dilatation, misdiagnosis can occur when this etiology is not considered in patients with undiagnosed nephropathy. Intravenous urography in retroperitoneal fibrosis will show a stricture of the ureter, with narrowing occurring generally in the middle third. Although the fibrotic process surrounds both ureters, only one ureter may be demonstrably involved at the time of presentation. Unilateral involvement should not dissuade the radiologist from considering retroperitoneal fibrosis as the most likely diagnosis when findings suspicious of retroperitoneal fibrosis are present. Although the ureters in retroperitoneal fibrosis may be deviated medially by the fibrotic process, this is usually not commonly seen at initial presentation. CT has proven to be accurate and sensitive in the diagnosis of idiopathic retroperitoneal fibrosis (Fig. 83–11). A plaque-like soft-tissue density surrounding the inferior vena cava, aorta, and ureters is characteristic of retroperitoneal fibrosis. MRI has also been used to diagnose and characterize the extent of retroperitoneal fibrosis. Whereas lesions of low signal intensity on both T_1- and T_2-weighted images are characteristic of benign retroperitoneal fibrosis, when high signal intensity is present on T_2-weighted images in the soft-tissue plaque, the malignant form of retroperitoneal fibrosis should be considered. However, overlap exists with the idiopathic form, particularly if associated with inflammatory edema. Occasionally, the differentiation of idiopathic retroperitoneal fibrosis from lymphoma or retroperitoneal metastatic neoplasm with desmoplastic reaction may require percutaneous thin-needle biopsy. In some cases the process of retroperitoneal fibrosis not only encases the ureter in the fibrotic process but also directly involves the ureteral wall. In these cases, the usual treatment of ureterolysis and intraperitonealization or omental wrapping of the ureter is inadequate, and segmental resection of the ureter is necessary as well. When obstruction is present, percutaneous nephrostomy allows temporization, and antegrade pyelography will define the ureteral stenosis and allow the correct diagnosis to be made and the correct surgical procedure to be performed in a patient who is stabilized and no longer obstructed.

Ureteral and Localized Periureteral Fibrosis

Localized ureteral stenosis can be caused by chronic infection or inflammation of the ureter or in the surrounding pelvis. Localized ureteral stenosis in the pelvis in these cases can cause significant obstruction. Intravenous urography will show an obstruction with a tapering ureter, usually in the pelvis. CT will show localized ureteral thickening, or a localized periureteral fibrotic mass, which may have to be differentiated from localized metastatic tumor or radiation fibrosis.

Aneurysmal Disease and Perianeurysmal Fibrosis

Retroperitoneal reaction and fibrosis may occur in association with abdominal aortic aneurysms, which may cause ureteral obstruction. In some cases the patient may present with ureteral obstruction as the initial clinical sign. Perianeurysmal fibrosis causes smooth tapering of the mid- to lower ureter typical of extrinsic ureteral encasement. CT is diagnostic in these cases, showing an aortic aneurysm that may contain clot surrounded by soft-tissue mass of reactive soft-tissue fibrosis (Fig. 83–12). Ultrasonography can also lead to the correct diagnosis when an abdominal aortic aneurysm is seen in a patient with acute ureteral obstruction. However, CT is more sensitive in the imaging of the perianeurysmal soft-tissue reaction and is highly specific in the diagnosis of perianeurysmal fibrosis with ureteral obstruction.

Crohn's Disease

Crohn's disease may cause obstruction of the ureter when an inflammatory mass due to Crohn's disease extends into the retroperitoneum. The right ureter below the pelvic brim is frequently involved by Crohn's disease of the terminal ileum when an extensive inflammatory mass occurs. Ureteral obstruction may be asymptomatic. Extrinsic tapering of the ureter is seen, and the diagnosis of Crohn's disease relies on clinical history, the determination of a pelvic inflammatory mass by CT or ultrasonography, and diagnostic gastrointestinal barium studies.

Endometriosis

The ureter may be involved by endometriosis within the pelvis, which may present as ureteral obstruction and/or microscopic or gross hematuria. An endometrial implant may involve the wall of the ureter without a large periureteral mass, and the diagnosis may be difficult if a positive clinical history is not present and may only be made during exploratory laparotomy.

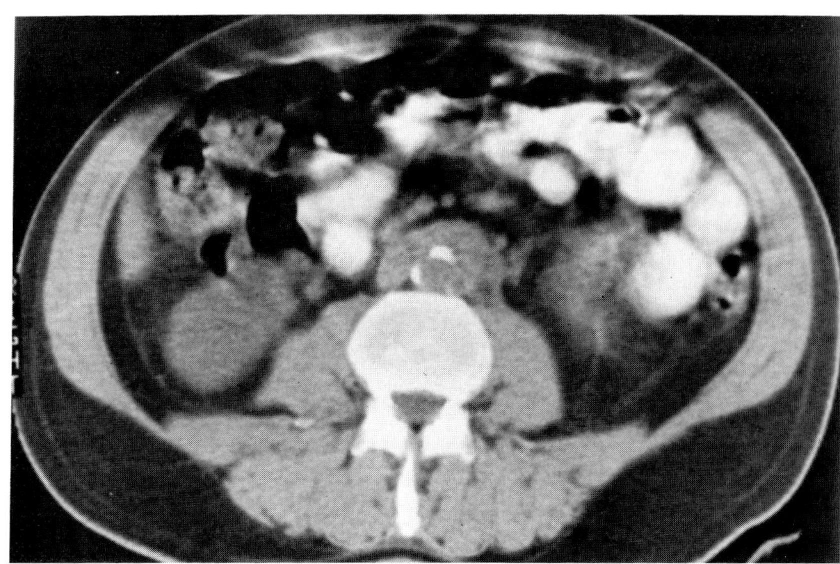

Figure 83–11. Retroperitoneal fibrosis. Bilateral ureteral obstruction for which percutaneous nephrostomy was performed. A CT scan shows a plaque-like soft-tissue density surrounding the aorta and inferior vena cava and involving the ureters. This appearance is seen with retroperitoneal fibrosis. Although this appearance is very characteristic of retroperitoneal fibrosis, occasionally metastatic malignancy with desmoplastic retroperitoneal reaction and treated lymphoma with recurrence may give a similar appearance.

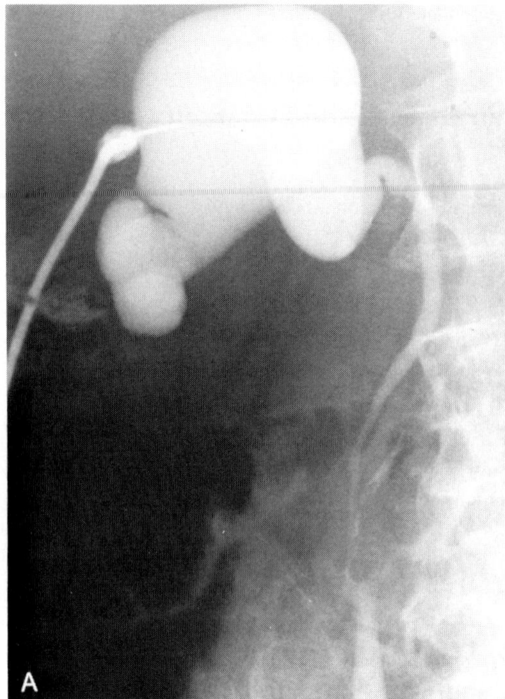

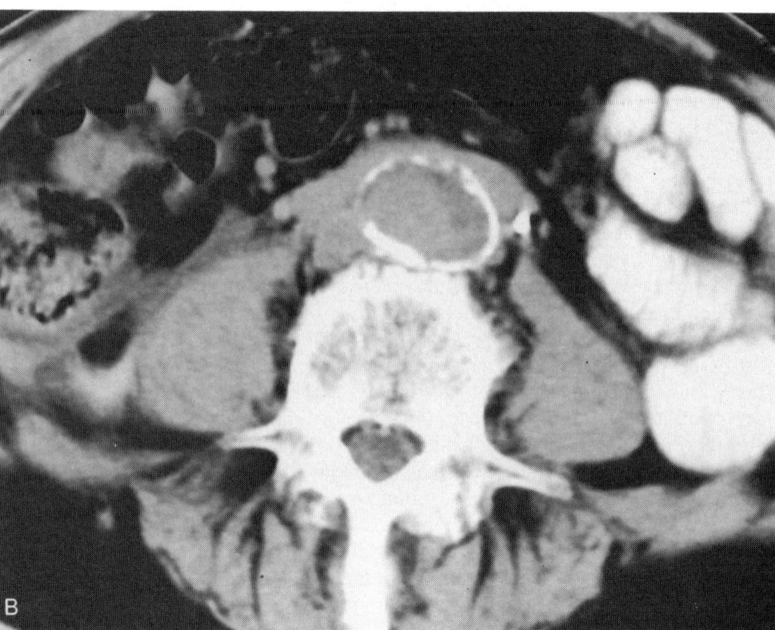

Figure 83–12. Ureteral obstruction due to aneurysmal disease and perianeurysmal fibrosis. *A*, An antegrade pyelogram during percutaneous nephrostomy shows dilated renal calyces and a dilated renal pelvis with extrinsic tapering of the right mid-ureter. Numerous retroperitoneal tumors, both primary and metastatic, as well as invasive transitional cell carcinoma and a variety of benign retroperitoneal abnormalities, including retroperitoneal fibrosis, might give a similar appearance on antegrade or retrograde pyelography. *B*, CT scan in a different patient shows an abnormal aortic aneurysm with perianeurysmal fibrosis surrounding the aorta and vena cava and involving both ureters. The left ureter was obstructed on lower slices. This CT appearance is characteristic of ureteral obstruction due to perianeurysmal fibrosis.

Diverticulitis and Pelvic Abscess

In diverticulitis, chronic or subacute diverticular abscess may involve the ureter, causing ureteral obstruction. If the ureteral involvement is not recognized preoperatively, ureteral injury at surgery may occur and go undetected. The distal left ureter is most commonly affected by diverticular abscess. Pelvic abscesses from other etiologies can also cause ureteral obstruction.

Bibliography

Amis ES Jr: Retroperitoneal fibrosis. AJR 157:321–329, 1991.

Arger PH, Stolz JL: Ureteral tumors. AJR 116:812, 1972.

Arger PH, Stolz JL, Miller WT: Retroperitoneal fibrosis: An analysis of the clinical spectrum and roentgenographic signs. AJR 119:812, 1973.

Banner MP, Pollack HM: Fibrous ureteral polyps. Radiology 130:73, 1979.

Bloom NA, Vidune RA, Lytton B: Primary carcinoma of ureter. J Urol 103:590, 1970.

Bosniak MA, Megibow AJ, Ambros MA, et al: Computed tomography of ureteral obstruction. AJR 138:1107, 1982.

Brito RR, Zulian R, Albuquerque J, Borges HJ: Retrocaval ureter. Br J Urol 45:144, 1973.

Bush WH, Brannen GE, Lewis GP: Ureteropelvic junction obstruction treatment with percutaneous endopyelotomy. Radiology 171:535–538, 1989.

Chair A, Matagas KW, Fabian CB, et al: Vascular impression on the ureters. AJR 111:729, 1971.

Cochran ST, Waisman J, Barbaric ZL: Radiographic and microscopic findings in multiple ureteral diverticula. Radiology 137:631, 1980.

Dalla-Palma L, Rosetti R, Possi S, et al: Computed tomography in the diagnosis of retroperitoneal fibrosis. Urol Radiol 3:77, 1981.

Fainstat T: Ureteral dilatation in pregnancy: A review. Obstet Gynecol Surv 186:845, 1963.

Freidland GW, Forsberg L: Striations of the renal pelvis in children. Clin Radiol 23:58, 1972.

Hartman GW, Hodson CJ: Duplex kidney and related anomalies. Clin Radiol 20:387, 1969.

Kadir S, White RI, Engel R: Balloon dilatation of a ureteropelvic junction obstruction. Radiology 143:263–264, 1982.

Peterson LJ, Grimes JH, Weinerth JL, et al: Blind ending branches of bifid ureters. Urology 5:191, 1975.

Pfister RC, Hendron VH: Primary megaureter in children and adults. Clinical and pathophysiologic features of 150 ureters. Urology 12:160, 1978.

Pfister RC, Newhouse JH: Radiology of the ureter. Urology 12:15, 1978.

Pistolesi GF, Procacci C, Candana R, et al: CT criteria of the differential diagnosis in primary retroperitoneal masses. Eur J Radiol 4:127, 1984.

Reece RW, Koontz WW: Leukoplakia of the urinary tract. A review. J Urol 114:165, 1975.

Sarajlic M, Durst-Zivkovic B, Svoren E, et al: Congenital ureteric diverticula in children and adults: Classification, radiological and clinical features. Br J Radiol 62:551–553, 1989.

Segal AJ, Spataro RF, Linke CA, et al: Diagnosis of non-opaque calculi by computed tomography. Radiology 129:447, 1978.

Slater JM, Fletcher GH: Ureteral strictures after radiation therapy for carcinoma of the uterine cervix. AJR 111:269, 1971.

Stiehm WD, Becker JA, Weiss RM: Ureteral endometriosis. Radiology 102:563, 1972.

Thornbury JR, Silver TM, Vinson RK: Ureteroceles vs pseudoureteroceles in adults. Radiology 122:81, 1977.

Wagle DG, Moore RH, Murphy GP: Squamous cell carcinoma of the renal pelvis. J Urol 111:453, 1974.

Wills JS, Pollack HM, Curtis JA: Cholesteatoma of the upper urinary tract. AJR 136:941, 1981.

Winalski CS, Lipman JC, Tumeh SS: Ureteral neoplasms. Radiographics 10:271–283, 1990.

84 Ureteral Obstruction and Dilatation

Ronald J. Zagoria

A variety of mechanisms can produce ureteral dilatation (Table 84–1). Determining the location and extent of dilatation may help to limit diagnostic considerations in the search for an underlying process (Table 84–2).

Increased intraluminal pressure, as with obstruction, and increased intraluminal volume, as with vesicoureteral reflux, are common explanations. Other causes include decreased or flaccid ureteral musculature, either acquired or congenital, and focal mechanical distention resulting from an intraluminal mass. Ureteral dilatation may be acute and may resolve after treatment of the underlying condition, or it may be a chronic problem that reflects a remote insult to the ureter. Ureteral dilatation may be subtle, as in acute or partial obstruction, or it may be obvious. In either case, detection of a dilated ureter requires explanation. The search for the underlying cause is usually best initiated with radiologic techniques described in this chapter.

CAUSES OF URETERAL DILATATION

Ureteral obstruction increases intraluminal pressure and results in ureteral dilatation. The development of ureteral dilatation may lag behind the onset of obstruction by a number of hours, and ureteral dilatation becomes pronounced with chronic high-grade ureteral obstruction.

To avoid misinterpretation of ureteral dilatation or ureteral narrowing, awareness of the normal anatomy is necessary. Relative ureteral narrowing at the ureteropelvic junction and the ureterovesical junction is normal. A mild, focal ureteral dilatation is often detected just above the point at which the ureter crosses the iliac vessels. This normal variant, referred to as the "ureteral spindle," is a transient accumulation of urine caused by a momentary delay in peristaltic wave transmission crossing the iliac blood vessels.

Ureteral obstruction can be caused by functional abnormalities that interfere with ureteral peristalsis or by mechanical processes that compromise the ureteral lumen. Mechanical processes may produce filling defects in a contrast-filled ureter. Other processes compromise the ureteral lumen circumferentially and lead to ureteral narrowing. Detecting obstructing lesions requires that attention be focused on the junction of the dilated ureteral segment and normal-caliber ureter.

Ureteral Filling Defects

Urolithiasis is the most common cause of ureteral obstruction. Once an obstructing radiopaque stone has been excluded by evaluation of the abdominal radiograph, other causes of obstruction should be considered. Ureteral filling defects may be caused by intraluminal processes such as radiolucent calculi (Fig. 84–1), blood clots, sloughed papillae, fungus balls, or tumors. Up to 10 per cent of urinary tract stones are radiolucent on abdominal radiographs. These stones are composed of uric acid or xanthine, or they may be unmineralized matrix stones. Their margins are usually well-demarcated, and they lodge most commonly at the ureterovesical junction (UVJ), at the ureteropelvic junction (UPJ), or at the point where the ureter crosses the iliac vessels.

Filling defects caused by ureteral blood clots generally have an elongated shape that forms a cast of the ureteral lumen. Blood clots can result from any cause of renal or ureteral hemorrhage and can cause acute obstruction, particularly when the urinary tract is already compromised by ureteral narrowing, as in some patients with congenital UPJ strictures. The presence of urokinase in the urine

TABLE 84–1. CAUSES OF URETERAL DILATATION

Increased Intraluminal Pressure
- Obstructing stone
- Ureteral neoplasm
- Pelvic/retroperitoneal abnormality (neoplasm, lymphadenopathy, abscess, lipomatosis)
- Retroperitoneal fibrosis
- Bladder outlet obstruction
- Uterine enlargement (pregnancy and postpartum)
- Strictures (acquired and congenital)
- Anomalies (retrocaval ureter, retroiliac ureter, ectopic or simple ureterocele, crossing vessels)

Mechanical Distention from Intraluminal Mass
- Mucosal neoplasm (goblet sign)

Decreased or Flaccid Ureteral Musculature
- Prune belly (Eagle-Barrett) syndrome
- Bacterial infection with endotoxin release
- Residual dilatation from remote obstruction

Increased Intraluminal Volume
- Vesicoureteral reflux (primary and acquired)
- Primary megaureter
- Diabetes insipidus
- Polydipsia

TABLE 84–2. LOCATION AND EXTENT OF URETERAL DILATATION

Entire Ureter
- Bilateral
  - Bladder outlet obstruction (mechanical and functional)
  - Extensive bladder neoplasm
  - Bladder inflammation
  - Pelvic malignancy (cervix, prostate, colon, lymphoma)
  - Pelvic lipomatosis
  - Prune belly (Eagle-Barrett) syndrome
  - Diabetes insipidus
  - Polydipsia
  - Primary megaureter
- Unilateral
  - Ureterovesical obstruction (stone, clot, neoplasm, stricture)
  - Vesicoureteral reflux (Grades II–IV)
  - Primary megaureter
  - Ectopic ureterocele
  - Ectopic ureter inserting below bladder
  - Simple ureterocele
  - Bacterial infection

Lower Ureter Only
- Primary megaureter
- Vesicoureteral reflux (Grade I)

Upper Ureter Only
- Intrinsic obstruction (stone, clot, neoplasm, stricture)
- Retroperitoneal abnormality (lymphadenopathy, neoplasm, fibrosis, abscess)
- Retrocaval or retroiliac ureter
- Enlarged uterus

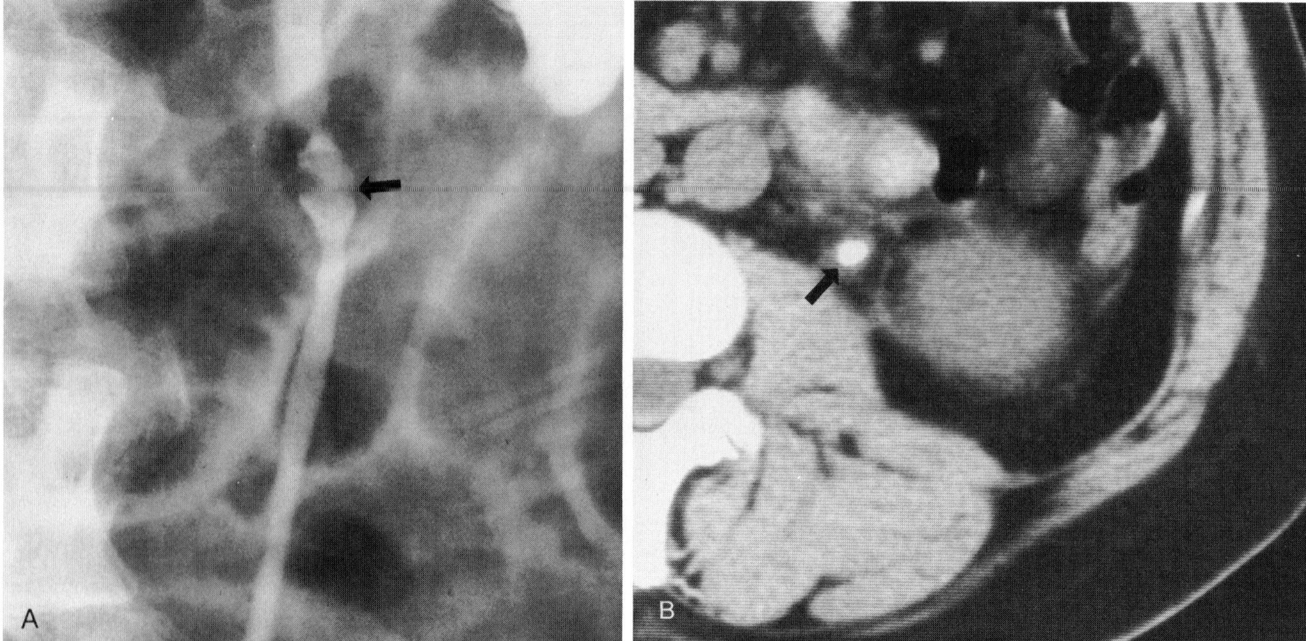

Figure 84–1. *A*, Urography demonstrates a **partially obstructing intraluminal mass** *(arrow)*. The lesion is well-circumscribed, forming acute angles as it interfaces with the contrast material in the ureter. *B*, An uninfused CT scan at the level of the obstruction demonstrates a **homogeneous, high-attenuation intraluminal lesion** *(arrow)*. This finding is diagnostic of a ureteral stone.

causes the appearance of blood clots to change with time. Therefore, contrast-enhanced examinations repeated hours or days after the initial demonstration of a blood clot usually demonstrate marked change or complete resolution in the appearance of the filling defect.

In patients who are susceptible to papillary necrosis, a segment or an entire papilla may be sloughed into the urinary tract, from which it may pass into the ureter and cause obstruction. Typically, a sloughed papilla has a triangular shape, and its perimeter may calcify with time. Demonstration of calyceal changes of papillary necrosis in combination with ureteral obstruction should suggest this diagnosis.

Fungus balls are usually caused by *Candida* or *Aspergillus* fungi and typically occur in patients who are immunocompromised or have diabetes mellitus. Although fungal infection of the urine may lead to a spherical fungus ball that obstructs the ureter, fungal debris more commonly mimics the appearance of a blood clot by forming an elongated cast of the ureteral lumen. Urine cultures positive for fungus can confirm the diagnosis.

Less commonly, infectious debris or frank pus can obstruct the ureter, particularly in patients who have a pre-existing narrowed segment. The appearance of these obstructing lesions mimics that of blood clots and fungal debris. Urine cultures are essential for establishing the correct diagnosis.

Obstructing mucosal lesions can also appear as ureteral filling defects with margins that form acute angles with the ureteral wall when seen in profile (Fig. 84–2). These mucosal lesions are often indistinguishable from intraluminal processes (Fig. 84–2). This category includes such processes as papillary urothelial neoplasms, mucosal edema, and leukoplakia.

Transitional cell carcinoma, the most common form of urothelial neoplasm, may be papillary or infiltrating. Two thirds of transitional cell carcinomas are papillary neoplasms that extend into the lumen of the urinary tract. When the ureter is involved, up to 40 per cent of patients have multifocal disease (Fig. 84–2); therefore, the entire length of urothelium should be examined for other foci of transitional cell carcinoma.

Transitional cell carcinomas typically arise in middle-aged or older adults and can be induced by numerous carcinogens. Prominent associations include exposure to aniline dyes and other benzene compounds, tobacco use, analgesic abuse, bone marrow transplantation, some chemotherapeutic agents used to treat malignant neoplasms outside the urinary tract, and, in rare cases, Balkan nephropathy. Other, less common urothelial neoplasms such as squamous cell carcinoma and adenocarcinoma have a similar appearance.

Ureteral edema usually results from direct mucosal irritation, either by passage of a ureteral stone or by iatrogenic insult to the ureter. Edema may appear bullous or somewhat striated. Although mucosal edema can lead to obstruction, removal of the inciting factor usually results in resolution within one to two days.

Leukoplakia, a premalignant squamous metaplasia of the urothelium, is an uncommon lesion that results from chronic irritation of the urothelium. Typically, leukoplakia is associated with urolithiasis or chronic urinary infection, such as schistosomiasis. Leukoplakia most commonly involves the bladder but may occur in other areas of the urinary tract, including the ureter.

Obstructing lesions with obtuse angles in the ureter are usually mural-based. The diagnostic considerations for this pattern include ureteritis cystica, intramural hemorrhage, malacoplakia, and implants from endometriosis. Ureteritis cystica is a relatively common cause of intramural filling defects that may obstruct the ureter and are virtually always associated with chronic urinary tract infections (Fig. 84–3). These benign, sterile fluid collections are caused by intramural inflammation leading to encystment and submucosal extension of transitional epithelium. Typically multicentric, these lesions resolve over a period of weeks or months after treatment of the underlying infectious process. Intramural hemorrhage is also generally multicentric. This diagnosis should be considered if the patient has ureteral filling defects or obstruction, has had extensive anticoagulation therapy, or has a coagulopathy.

Malacoplakia is a rare intramural ureteral lesion that occurs secondary to chronic urinary tract infection. These lesions are caused by excessive buildup of defective macrophages. Examination of the macrophages will demonstrate inclusion bodies containing incompletely phagocytized *Escherichia coli* bacteria. These inclusion bod-

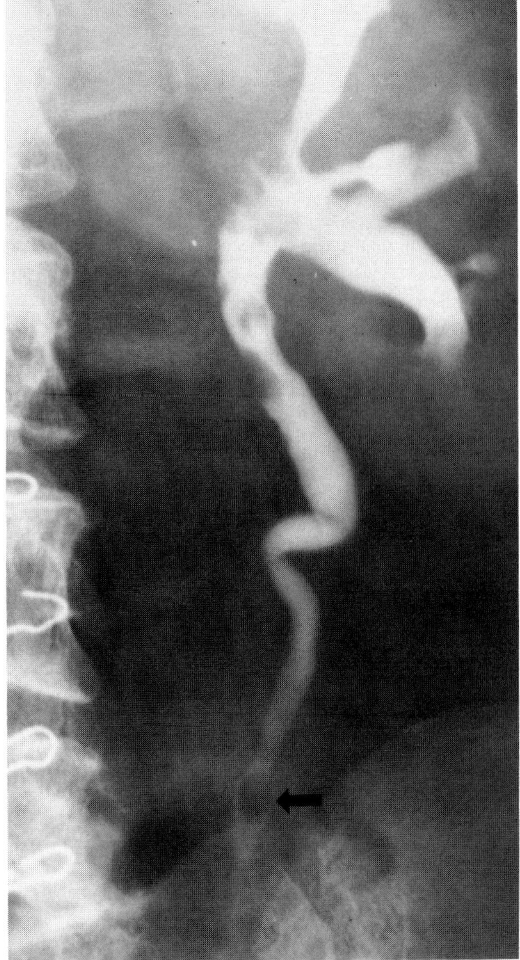

Figure 84–2. Urography demonstrates multiple pyeloureteral filling defects found to be **multicentric papillary transitional cell carcinomas.** In profile, the lesion–contrast material interface forms acute angles typical of mucosal lesions. The most caudal lesion that causes partial obstruction is viewed en face *(arrow).*

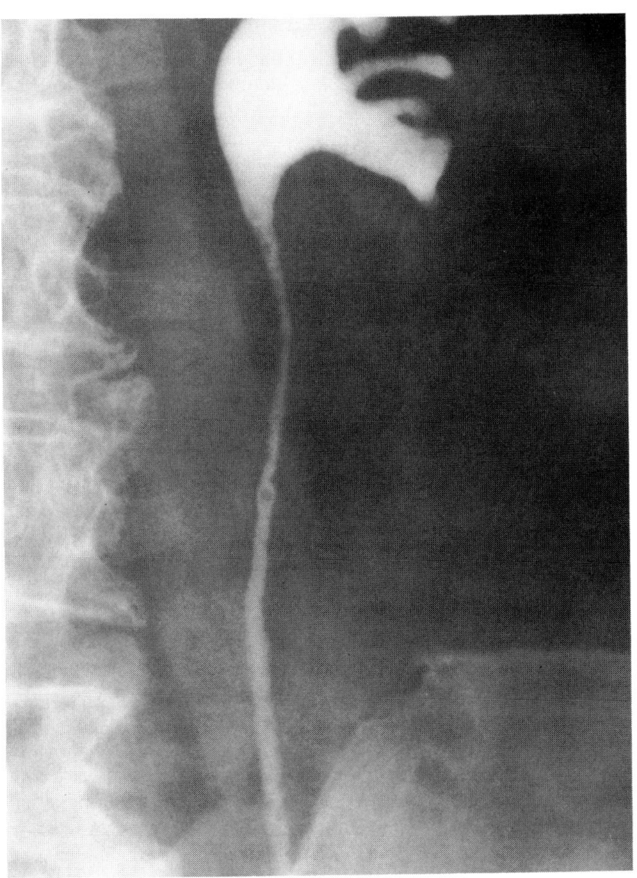

Figure 84–3. Urography demonstrates numerous small filling defects in this patient with **ureteritis cystica.** Lesions viewed in profile form obtuse angles with the contrast material.

ies, known as Michaelis-Gutmann bodies, are the sine qua non for the diagnosis of malacoplakia.

Rarely, endometriosis may spread to the intramural portion of the ureter and lead to filling detects and subsequent obstruction. The common form of endometriosis causes concentric narrowing of the lower portion of the ureter in proximity to the ureterotubal ligaments.

Finally, an obstructing process extrinsic to the ureter occasionally may appear as a ureteral filling defect. Generally, such processes form obtuse angles with the ureteral lumen and usually cause some deviation of the ureteral course as well. Focal extrinsic metastases and crossing vessels are the most common causes of this appearance.

Ureteral Narrowing

Ureteral obstruction may also be caused by an area of circumferential ureteral narrowing below the length of dilated ureter. The pattern and location of ureteral narrowing often aid in determining the underlying cause. If ureteral dilatation is limited to the upper third of the right ureter and the ureter courses abruptly toward the midline at the L3-L4 level in a ''fishhook'' configuration, the most likely diagnosis is retrocaval ureter, an abnormality resulting from anomalous development of the inferior vena cava. When focal ureteral narrowing is caused by an intrinsic ureteral process such as an infiltrating transitional cell carcinoma or stricture, the ureter has a characteristic appearance. An abrupt change occurs in the caliber of the ureter and usually produces a ''squared-off'' appearance as contrast material passes through the upper extent of the ureteral narrowing (Fig. 84–4). This appearance, sometimes called a ''shoulder,'' is caused by the impingement of an abnormally thick segment of ureteral wall upon the contrast material column.

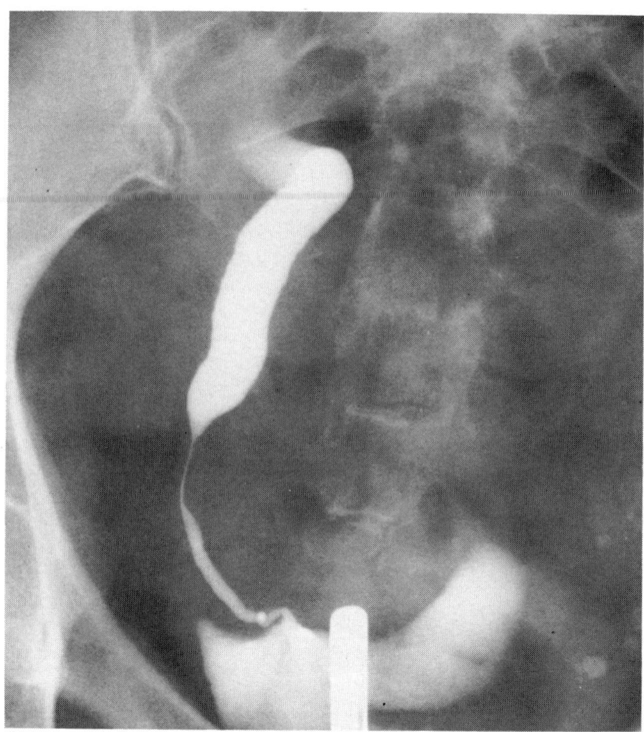

Figure 84–5. Retrograde ureterography demonstrates gradual tapering of the dilated ureter as it extends caudally into a segment narrowed by an **advanced carcinoma of the cervix.**

Ureteral narrowing caused by extrinsic processes generally results in a smooth, gradual tapering of the ureteral lumen and gives a conical or waist-like appearance to the ureteral lumen through the area of narrowing (Fig. 84–5). Common causes of this radiographic appearance include lymphadenopathy; primary malignancies; pelvic lipomatosis; retroperitoneal fibrosis; and inflammatory retroperitoneal or pelvic processes such as regional enteritis, diverticulitis, appendicitis, and endometriosis.

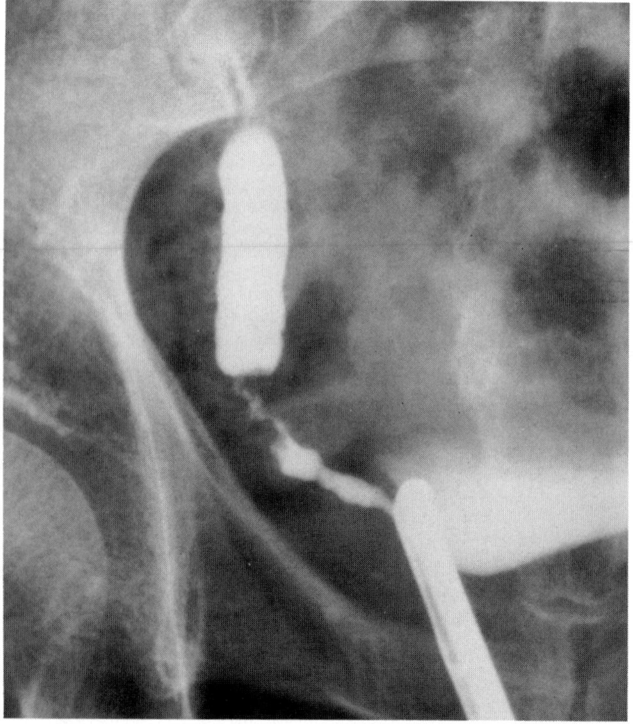

Figure 84–4. Retrograde ureterography demonstrates **abrupt caliber change of the obstructed ureter with a "squared-off" appearance** at the lower edge of the dilated ureter. The mucosa is irregular through the narrowed segment because of infiltrating transitional cell carcinoma.

Mechanical Distention

Infrequently, the ureteral lumen is dilated by a combination of obstruction and mechanical distention caused by an intraluminal mass. This appearance is typified by the ''goblet sign'' typically seen with a papillary transitional cell carcinoma but rarely seen with metastatic disease that seeds the ureteral mucosa (Fig. 84–6). Ureteral dilatation above the polypoid mass is caused by partial ureteral obstruction from the intraluminal extent of the neoplasm. However, in many cases ureteral dilatation extends over a short but discernible segment of ureter below the filling defect caused by the tumor. This condition is thought to result from repeated mechanical distention of the ureter from peristalsis of the polypoid mass into the lower ureteral segment. The curvilinear concave impression in the contrast material column is caused by the lower edge of the papillary transitional cell carcinoma. It resembles a partially filled wine goblet; hence the descriptive name for this finding.

Ureteral Flaccidity

Ureteral dilatation may be caused by functional abnormalities in the absence of mechanical obstruction. Nearly all patients with prune belly syndrome have decreased ureteral wall musculature that results in diffuse, bilateral ureteral dilatation. Also, certain bacteria may infect the urinary tract and release a neurologically active

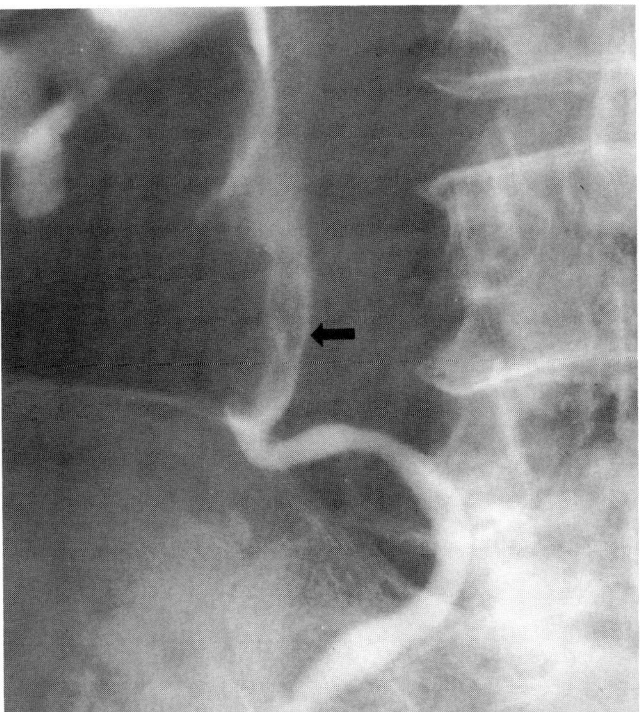

Figure 84–6. Urography demonstrates a **papillary transitional cell carcinoma** distending the upper right ureter *(arrow)*. The shape of the contrast material outlining the caudal edge of the mass is analogous to the appearance of liquid in a goblet.

endotoxin that causes flaccid paralysis of the ureteral musculature. As with other ureteral infections, this process is usually unilateral and is much more common in female patients than in male patients. Flaccid ureteral musculature is also seen in areas of the ureter that are exposed to long-standing high-grade obstruction. Although ureteral appearance generally returns to normal after treatment of acute ureteral obstruction, long-standing obstruction usually causes irreversible ureteral ectasia. Residual ureteral ectasia in a symptomatic patient can cause diagnostic difficulty and may require modifications in diagnostic examinations to exclude ongoing obstruction. This topic is discussed in greater detail later in this chapter.

Ureteral Hypervolemia

Finally, ureteral dilatation can be caused by increased ureteral pressure resulting from excessive intraluminal ureteral volumes. Among the underlying causes are vesicoureteral reflux, primary megaureter, and increased renal excretion, characteristic of diabetes insipidus and polydipsia syndromes. In most cases, vesicoureteral reflux is due to a congenitally short intramural portion of the ureter as it courses through the bladder wall. Vesicoureteral reflux is most common in young children and has a higher incidence in some families. Most mild cases resolve spontaneously with age. Acquired vesicoureteral reflux may be caused by bladder outlet obstruction, severe bladder inflammation, bladder diverticuli or neoplasms adjacent to the ureteral orifice, and iatrogenic manipulation of the ureteral orifice.

Regardless of its cause, vesicoureteral reflux can lead to ureteral dilatation. The ureteral lumen dilates in response to the increased pressure required to transmit the normal antegrade flow of urine in combination with the additional volume of urine flowing from the bladder in a retrograde direction. The degree of ureteral dilatation depends on the extent and volume of ureteral reflux. Grade I ureteral reflux is limited to the lower third of the ureter; therefore, the upper two thirds will have a normal appearance. More advanced grades of ureteral reflux result in increasing dilatation of the entire length of the ureteral lumen.

In primary megaureter, ureteral dilatation results from the collection of an increased volume of urine above a focal segment of aperistaltic ureter. This aperistaltic segment has a lumen of normal caliber, is generally several millimeters in length, and occurs just above the ureterovesical junction (Fig. 84–7). Lack of peristalsis in this ureteral segment is attributed to a focal muscular deficiency.

In rare cases, chronic high-volume renal output can lead to ureteral dilatation. This occurrence is most common in patients who have diabetes insipidus or other causes of polydipsia.

RADIOLOGIC DIAGNOSIS AND EVALUATION

In most cases, ureteral obstruction is the result of an acute process, and clinical symptoms will readily suggest a urinary tract abnormality. A wide array of radiologic examinations can assist in the diagnosis of ureteral obstruction and determination of the underlying cause. Currently there is some controversy as to which studies should be selected for evaluation of a patient with suspected ureteral obstruction. These imaging techniques are described in the following discussion.

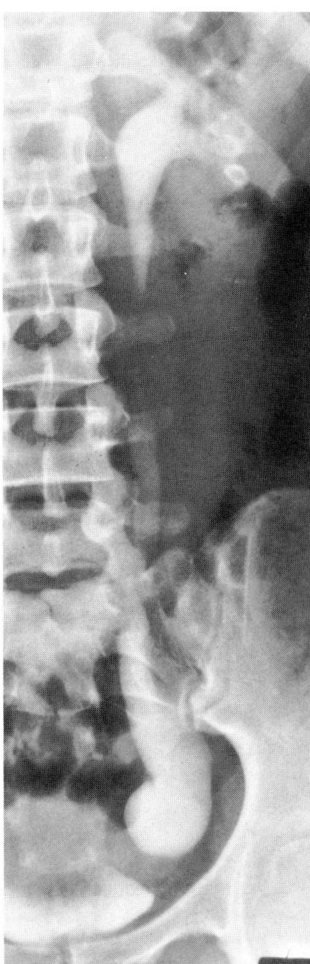

Figure 84–7. Urography demonstrates severe dilatation limited to the caudal third of the left ureter, typical of **primary megaureter;** the diagnosis was established after vesicoureteral reflux was excluded.

Excretory Urography

Excretory urography has for many years been the mainstay of the initial evaluation of suspected urinary tract obstruction because it is safe, relatively inexpensive, and readily available. It gives detailed anatomic and functional information about the urinary tract. It is not operator-dependent, and it is highly accurate in the detection of urinary tract obstruction, even in its earliest phases.

However, excretory urography does use ionizing radiation and intravenous contrast material administration. Furthermore, some abnormalities detected by urography, such as radiolucent filling defects, are nonspecific in appearance, necessitating the use of other examinations for further characterization.

In cases of acute obstruction, ureteral dilatation may be very mild or even absent for several days. Ureteral dilatation may also be minimized in the setting of acute obstruction by decompression of the collecting system via forniceal rupture and perinephric extravasation of urine. Even in these situations, urographic findings will indicate the presence of obstruction. Delayed entry of contrast material into the collecting system, a persistent nephrogram, and columnization of contrast material down to the level of obstruction are indicative of ongoing obstruction. Perinephric extravasation of contrast material is often visualized and indicates a high-grade ureteral obstruction.

Once the level of obstruction has been determined by urography, attention can be directed to determining the underlying cause. Radiopaque stones as small as 1 or 2 mm can be detected with the preliminary abdominal radiograph when present at the level of obstruction. Radiolucent stones are indistinguishable from other causes of radiolucent filling defects, and additional examinations are often required to establish the cause. Occasionally, the excellent depiction of the ureter that urography affords will allow the diagnosis of obstructing congenital anomalies such as retrocaval ureter or ureteral duplication anomalies.

With few exceptions, chronic obstruction will cause ureteral dilatation. Although in many cases urographic findings are obvious in the setting of chronic obstruction (i.e., marked nephographic and pyelographic delay, severe hydroureteronephrosis, demonstration of a causal ureteral lesion), in other cases, findings may be enigmatic. Patients with a previous diagnosis of ureteral obstruction who have had appropriate treatment may continue to have dilatation of the urinary tract. In these patients, ureteral dilatation persists, but usually in the absence of any temporal delay in opacification of the renal parenchyma or collecting system. Standard excretory urography may be augmented by the administration of a diuretic agent such as furosemide. Persistent accumulations of radiopaque contrast material in the dilated ureter, particularly when accompanied by increased dilatation after diuretic administration, suggest obstruction. The accuracy of urography augmented with diuretics remains controversial, and some authors have failed to demonstrate a correlation between this test and direct ureteral perfusion studies. Although the utility of urography is somewhat limited in the evaluation of chronic ureteral obstruction, it remains the best noninvasive radiologic technique to demonstrate detailed ureteral anatomy.

Ultrasonography

Ultrasonography is a relatively inexpensive, noninvasive technique for evaluating the urinary tract. It affords excellent demonstration of the renal parenchyma, the collecting system above the level of the ureteropelvic junction, and the urine-filled bladder. Ultrasound is considered completely safe for all patients. Limitations of ultrasonography in evaluation of the urinary tract include inability to demonstrate anatomy of the ureter and examination variability, which depends largely on the skill of the operator and the body habitus of the patient.

Traditionally, ultrasound has been limited to demonstration of anatomic detail, as it provides no information regarding urinary tract function. This limitation has been overcome to some extent by the increased use of Doppler and color-flow Doppler ultrasound technology. The diagnosis of chronic obstruction with ultrasonography is relatively easy; sensitivity approaches 98 per cent. However, before Doppler techniques came into general use, the rate of false-positive ultrasound examinations in the diagnosis of ureteral obstruction was unacceptably high. Doppler ultrasound techniques permit determination of the resistive index, an indirect measure of renal blood flow. In patients with ureteral obstruction, increased collecting system pressure leads to decreased renal diastolic pressures and usually results in an elevated resistive index. A resistive index in excess of 0.70 in conjunction with a dilated intrarenal collecting system indicates obstruction. This technique has greatly reduced the rate of false-positive examinations in some studies.

Color-flow Doppler ultrasonography of the bladder may be used to supplement renal ultrasound in cases of suspected ureteral obstruction. With color Doppler ultrasound, normal ureteral jets can be readily visualized as they enter the bladder. Ureteral obstruction generally decreases the rate and amplitude of ureteral jets on the affected side. This technique may be helpful in further improving the diagnostic accuracy of ultrasonography in the evaluation of the obstructed ureter.

Since ultrasonography does not require the injection of contrast material or the use of ionizing radiation, it is an excellent technique for follow-up examination of the urinary tract in patients with known urinary tract obstruction. Resolution of hydronephrosis can be readily demonstrated with ultrasonography, as can progression of hydronephrosis in cases of progressive obstruction.

When acute ureteral obstruction is suspected, the collecting system may not be dilatated. In these cases, ultrasonographic findings are normal in up to 50 per cent of patients. The usefulness of renal resistive indices in patients suspected of having acute obstruction despite a normal sonographic appearance has yet to be determined. Some authors advocate plain abdominal radiography in conjunction with standard renal ultrasonography in patients with acute renal colic. The correct approach to the evaluation of patients with acute renal colic and suspected ureteral obstruction remains unsettled pending further research. However, both excretory urography and ultrasonography augmented with plain abdominal radiography appear to be highly accurate.

Computed Tomography

Computed tomography (CT) can often characterize intraluminal ureteral filling defects and can greatly aid in the evaluation of extrinsic processes adjacent to the ureter. All urinary tract calculi, regardless of their calcium content, demonstrate homogeneous mineralization on CT scans. Since urate calculi are the most common cause of radiolucent ureteral filling defects on urography, an unenhanced CT scan of the ureter is often sufficient to complete the diagnostic evaluation of a ureteral filling defect. When a radiolucent calculus is not demonstrated on a CT scan of the abnormal ureter, other entities, such as ureteral neoplasm, blood clot, sloughed papilla, and fungus ball, must be considered. These lesions can be best diagnosed by either ureteroscopy with biopsy or by urine sampling with cytologic and microbial analysis.

Evaluation of the obstructed ureter with a demonstrated area of ureteral narrowing can also be enhanced by a CT study of the abnormal area. CT readily demonstrates extrinsic processes such as retroperitoneal fibrosis, pelvic lipomatosis, retroperitoneal and pelvic neoplasms, and lymphadenopathy, and provides evidence of adjacent inflammatory disease such as diverticulitis, appendicitis, and complicated regional enteritis. CT is also useful in guiding fine-needle biopsy of areas extrinsic to the ureter.

Percutaneous Pyelography and Ureteral Perfusion

Percutaneous antegrade pyelography is performed for opacification of the pelvocalyceal system and the ureter. The direct injection of radiographic contrast material into the renal collecting system yields excellent radiographic depiction of the ureter in cases of suspected obstruction. The radiographs are similar in quality to those obtained by means of retrograde pyelography. Percutaneous pyelography is most often used for clarification of a ureteral abnormality detected with either ultrasonography or excretory urography. It is also valuable for its detailed anatomic demonstration of the ureter in patients with poor renal function, for whom excretory urography would be inadequate, and for patients who have risk factors that contraindicate intravascular contrast agents. Antegrade pyelography is often used in the evaluation of hydronephrosis in a transplanted kidney. Commonly, percutaneous antegrade pyelography is performed as a prelude to nephrostomy drainage or percutaneous ureteral perfusion testing.

Both percutaneous pyelography and ureteral perfusion require fine-needle puncture of the renal collecting system and carry a very small risk of vascular injury or sepsis. Contraindications include coagulopathy and active urinary infection, which should be assessed and corrected prior to percutaneous puncture and distention of the urinary tract. The technique requires puncturing the pelvocalyceal system with a 22-gauge needle. Fluoroscopy, abdominal radiography, or ultrasonography can be used to demonstrate the kidney. If the kidney is not radiographically visible, a puncture site is initially selected empirically 2 to 3 cm lateral to the top of the L2 vertebral body. A vertical puncture is made with the 22-gauge thin-walled needle while the patient suspends respiration. The needle stylet is removed, and continuous aspiration is applied as the needle is gradually withdrawn. The aspiration of urine indicates that the location of the needle tip is within the pelvocalyceal system. Iodinated contrast material is injected through the needle and the needle's position confirmed by fluoroscopy. The collecting system and ureter are then opacified with additional contrast material injected under intermittent fluoroscopic monitoring. Overdistention of the collecting system should be avoided to minimize the risk of sepsis. Spot films are obtained as needed to demonstrate the entire pelvocalyceal system, ureter, and sites of suspected abnormality. At the end of the procedure, the needle is withdrawn and the patient monitored for several hours for signs of excessive bleeding or sepsis.

Percutaneous ureteral perfusion, also known as the Whitaker test, is performed for objective evaluation and quantification of the urodynamic significance of suspected ureteral obstruction. This test augments anatomic information with a functional evaluation of ureteral capacity by assessing the ability of the ureter to transmit varying volumes of urine from the renal pelvis to the bladder. Because percutaneous ureteral perfusion is reliable and reproducible, it is often recommended for further evaluation of the significance of ureteral abnormalities detected by other techniques such as excretory urography, ultrasonography, and retrograde pyelography.

The first step in percutaneous ureteral perfusion is puncture of the pelvocalyceal system with a 22-gauge needle in the manner described previously for antegrade pyelography. With the patient in a prone position and the needle in place, the bladder is emptied and the manometers, infusion lines, infusion pump, and bladder drainage conduit are connected as shown in Figure 84–8. Bladder and renal pelvic pressures are measured immediately prior to and immediately after each timed infusion. Dilute contrast material is infused into the pelvocalyceal system at varying rates. Initially, the infusion rate is 5 ml/minute for 10 minutes. Resulting pressures are then immediately recorded, and the infusion is repeated at a rate of 10 ml/minute for 10 minutes and, finally, at a rate of 15 ml/minute for 10 minutes. The test is discontinued immediately if renal pelvic pressures exceed 40 cm of water, or if extensive contrast material extravasation develops. If the results are equivocal or normal during this set of infusions, the test is repeated with the bladder distended.

Analysis of renal pelvic and bladder pressures indicates the urodynamic significance of ureteral lesions. Bladder pressure is subtracted from renal pelvic pressure to yield ureteral pressure corrected for intra-abdominal pressure. Corrected ureteral pressures less than 13 cm of water are normal. Pressures from 13 to 22 cm of water indicate mild or equivocal ureteral obstruction. Pressures from 23 to 40 cm of water indicate moderate ureteral obstruction. Pressures over 40 cm of water indicate severe ureteral obstruction. The patient should be instructed to notify personnel if symptoms are reproduced during the infusion procedure, as the reproduction of symptoms further supports the presence of urodynamically significant obstruction.

Percutaneous antegrade pyelography and ureteral perfusion are minimally invasive techniques for evaluating anatomy and function

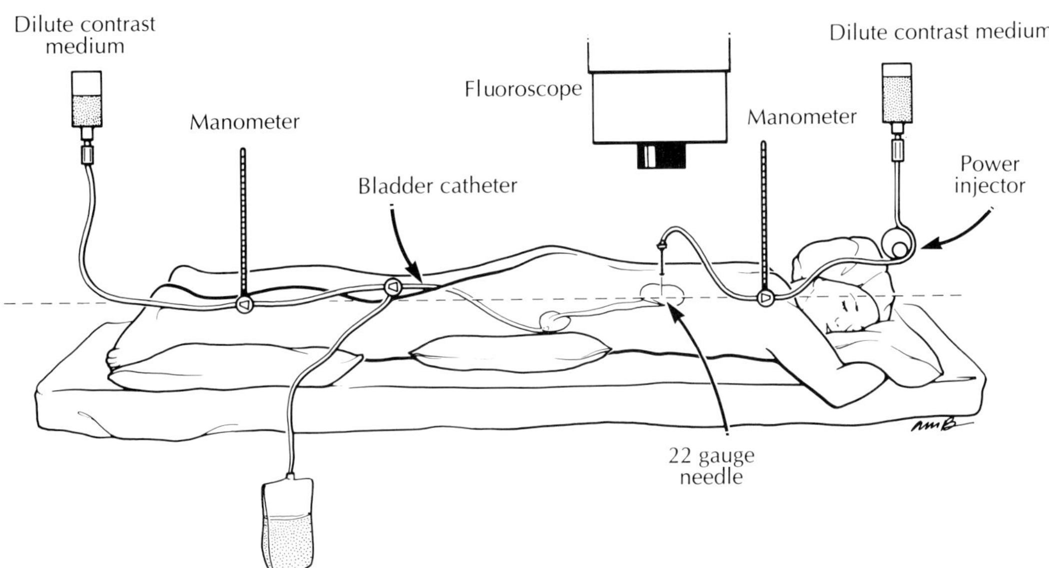

Figure 84–8. Diagrammatic depiction of equipment set-up used for ureteral perfusion testing.

of the ureter. These tests are generally performed after a ureteral abnormality is detected with another imaging technique. Ureteral perfusion testing is the most reliable method for assessing the urodynamic significance of a ureteral lesion. The results of this test are objective and reproducible and therefore reliable in determining the significance of ureteral lesions, as well as in follow-up of treatment. In addition, the performance of these tests is not dependent on normal renal function; in fact, these techniques are frequently used in the evaluation of the ureter of a poorly functioning kidney.

Diuresis Renography

Diuresis renography is a noninvasive test for the evaluation and follow-up of ureteral obstruction. It employs radionuclides augmented with the administration of a diuretic. Although less anatomic detail is derived from this nuclear medicine examination than from radiographic examinations, it does provide a simultaneous evaluation of individual renal function and an objective assessment of the significance of hydronephrosis.

Either technetium-DTPA or iodine-123–Hippuran can be used for initial renography. Diuresis renography requires a gamma camera–computer interface to monitor radionuclide progression through the urinary tract. Images of this progression are augmented by computer-generated renal blood flow data, relative functioning renal mass calculations, and a time-activity curve for radionuclide accumulation in each renal unit. A diuretic, generally furosemide, is injected intravenously after accumulation of the radionuclide in the collecting system of interest. Presumably, a dilated but unobstructed urinary system will demonstrate steady elimination of radionuclide in response to increased urine output stimulated by the injected diuretic. The obstructed system continues to accumulate the radionuclide even during diuresis. A radionuclide clearance half-time greater than 20 minutes indicates obstruction; half-times in the range of 15 to 20 minutes are equivocal.

Pitfalls in the interpretation of diuresis renography include improper definition of the region of interest used to calculate time activity curves and radionuclide clearance half-times. In addition, a poorly functioning renal unit may respond inadequately to the diuretic-stimulated washout of the accumulated radionuclide, leading to a false-positive study.

Retrograde Pyelography and Ureteroscopy

Retrograde pyelography and ureteroscopy require the introduction of a cystoscope into the bladder. Retrograde pyelography is then performed by cannulating the ureteral orifice and injecting radiographic contrast material while obtaining radiographic or fluoroscopic images. This technique yields detailed radiographic images of ureteral anatomy. Cannulation of the ureteral orifice also allows selective urine sampling for cytologic and bacteriologic analyses. With advanced endoscopic techniques, an experienced surgeon can evaluate areas of ureteral narrowing or radiolucent filling defects by means of a small-bore endoscope introduced into the ureteral lumen. This direct visualization of the abnormal area can be augmented by tissue sampling performed through the working port of the endoscope.

Voiding Cystourethrography

The complete evaluation of the dilated ureter often requires evaluation of the bladder. A dilated ureter in the absence of an area of ureteral obstruction, dilatation limited to the lower portion of the ureter, and bilateral ureteral dilatation suggest bladder abnormalities that may be demonstrated with voiding cystourethrography. Vesicoureteral reflux and causes of increased bladder pressure or volume may be demonstrated with this radiographic examination. Voiding cystourethrography is always recommended for patients thought to have a primary megaureter, as this diagnosis can be made only after the more common cause—vesicoureteral reflux—is excluded.

The degree of vesicoureteral reflux determines the degree and extent of ureteral dilatation. Grade I reflux is limited to the lower ureter. Grades II through IV involve the entire ureter, with progressive degrees of ureteral and pelvicalyceal dilatation. In most cases, vesicoureteral reflux is primary, and the cause is attributable to a congenital abnormality of the UVJ. The segment of ureter that tunnels through the bladder wall is abnormally short and therefore leads to an inadequate antireflux mechanism. Reflux is mild in most cases and generally subsides with age. Reflux may also be acquired. Diverticula or neoplasms adjacent to the ureteral orifice, severe bladder inflammation, and direct manipulation of the ureteral orifice can lead to vesicoureteral reflux.

In addition, ureteral dilatation may result from increased bladder pressure or increased bladder volumes, as is true of patients with mechanical or functional bladder outlet obstruction; or from a flaccid neurogenic bladder, which is typical in patients with a peripheral neuropathy. All of these conditions can be detected or suggested by means of radiographic voiding cystourethrography.

In voiding cystourethrography, the bladder is catheterized and filled with dilute radiographic contrast material. Radiographic films of both the partially filled bladder and the completely distended bladder are obtained. Films of the bladder and urethra are then obtained during voiding. With this technique, anatomy of the bladder can be evaluated in conjunction with assessment of bladder capacity, bladder function, and anatomy of the urethra. Contrast material entering the ureters is diagnostic of vesicoureteral reflux. The extent of ureter involved with the reflux, as well as the degree of reflux, can be documented with radiographic films.

Bibliography

Bergman H, Friedenberg RM, Sayegh V: New roentgenologic signs of carcinoma of the ureter. AJR 86:707, 1961.

Brooks AP: Computed tomography of idiopathic retroperitoneal fibrosis (''periaortitis''): Variants, variations, patterns and pitfalls. Clin Radiol 42:75, 1990.

Burge HJ, Middleton WD, McClennan BL, et al: Ureteral jets in healthy subjects and in patients with unilateral ureteral calculi: Comparison with color Doppler US. Radiology 180:437, 1991.

Choyke PL: The urogram: Are rumors of its death premature? Radiology 184:33, 1992.

Cronan JJ: Contemporary concepts for imaging urinary tract obstruction. Urol Radiol 14:8, 1992.

Djurhuus JC, Nielsen JB, Poulsen EU, et al: The relationship between pressure flow studies and furosemide urography in hydronephrosis. Scand J Urol Nephrol 21:89, 1987.

Ellenbogen PH, Scheible FW, Talner LB, et al: Sensitivity of gray scale ultrasound in detecting urinary tract obstruction. AJR 130:731, 1978.

Haddad MC, Sharif HS, Shahed MS, et al: Renal colic: Diagnosis and outcome. Radiology 184:83, 1992.

Herman TE, McAlister WH: Radiographic manifestations of congenital anomalies of the lower urinary tract. Radiol Clin North Am 29:365, 1991.

Heyns CF: Pelvic lipomatosis: A review of its diagnosis and management. J Urol 146:267, 1991.

Irby PB, Stoller ML, McAninch JW: Fungal bezoars of the upper urinary tract. J Urol 143:447, 1990.

Kamholtz RG, Cronan JJ, Dorfman GS: Obstruction and the minimally dilated renal collecting system: US evaluation. Radiology 170:51, 1989.

Kass EJ, Fink-Bennett D: Contemporary techniques for the radioisotopic evaluation of the dilated urinary tract. Urol Clin North Am 17:273, 1990.

Laing FC, Jeffrey RB, Wing VW: Ultrasound versus excretory urography in evaluating acute flank pain. Radiology 154:613, 1985.

Lyons K, Matthews P, Evans C: Obstructive uropathy without dilatation: A potential diagnostic pitfall. BMJ 296:1517, 1988.

Mulligan SA, Holley HC, Koehler RE, et al: CT and MR imaging in the evaluation of retroperitoneal fibrosis. J Comput Assist Tomogr 13:277, 1989.

Newhouse JH, Amis ES Jr, Pfister RC: Urinary obstruction: Pitfalls in the use of delayed contrast material washout for diagnosis. Radiology 151:319, 1984.

Pfister RC, Newhouse JH, Hendren WH: Percutaneous pyeloureteral urodynamics. Urol Clin North Am 9:41, 1982.

Pfister RC, Papanicolaou N, Yoder IC: The dilated ureter. Semin Roentgenol 21:224, 1986.

Platt JF, Rubin JM, Ellis JH: Distinction between obstructive and nonobstructive pyelocaliectasis with duplex Doppler sonography. AJR 153:997, 1989.

Platt JF, Rubin JM, Ellis JH: Duplex Doppler US of the kidney: Differentiation of obstructive from nonobstructive dilatation. Radiology 171:515, 1989.

Rodgers PM, Bates JA, Irving HC: Intrarenal Doppler ultrasound studies in normal and acutely obstructed kidneys. Br J Radiol 65:207, 1992.

Sarkar SD: Diuretic renography: Concepts and controversies. Urol Radiol 14:79, 1992.

Spital A, Valvo JR, Segal AJ: Nondilated obstructive uropathy. Urology 31:478, 1988.

Taha SA, Al-Mohaya S, Abdulkader A, et al: Prognosis of radiologically non-functioning obstructed kidneys. Br J Urol 62:209, 1988.

Winalski CS, Lipman JC, Tumeh SS: Ureteral neoplasms. Radiographics 10:271, 1990.

Young DW, Lebowitz RL: Congenital abnormalities of the ureter. Semin Roentgenol 21:172, 1986.

85 Lower Urinary Tract
The Bladder

Carl M. Sandler

ANATOMY

The bladder is a thick muscular organ located in the dependent portion of the pelvis behind the symphysis pubis whose function is to receive, store, and voluntarily empty urine produced by the kidneys. The superior portion (dome) of the bladder and the upper posterior portion are covered by peritoneum; the remainder of the bladder is encompassed by a loose areolar connective tissue that anteriorly is known as the space of Retzius. Inferiorly, the bladder and prostate gland are firmly attached to the pubis by the puboprostatic ligaments in the male. In children, the bladder is almost entirely an intra-abdominal organ; it does not descend into the pelvis until the age of puberty.

The size and contour of the bladder vary with the degree of filling; in its usual state of distention it has a roughly spherical, oblong shape, with its superior portion usually slightly indented by the overlying viscera. Complete filling, however, will usually erase this impression. The normal bladder is smooth in contour with rounded borders; straightening or asymmetry of the bladder margin is usually a sign of pathology.

RADIOLOGIC EXAMINATION

Excretory Urography

The bladder is most commonly evaluated on the cystographic phase of an excretory urogram. Although such an evaluation is fairly gross in nature, a reasonable amount of information about the shape and contour of the bladder can be obtained. This is especially true if the examination is started immediately after the patient has emptied the bladder; in this fashion the excreted contrast material will not be diluted by unopacified urine remaining in the bladder. The diuresis caused by the contrast agent usually will be sufficient to cause a moderate degree of bladder filling in the patient with normal renal function, especially when conventional ionic contrast media are used. When non-ionic contrast is used, a reduced diuresis will be present and the corresponding degree of bladder filling will be decreased. For this reason, some authorities recommend the routine use of a delayed radiograph specifically for the purpose of evaluating the bladder when non-ionic or low-osmolar contrast is used for urography. Because the contrast medium has a higher specific gravity than urine, it is not unusual to demonstrate a gradation in density in the bladder on supine radiographs, with the central portion of the bladder being more densely opacified. For this reason, erect and prone films of the bladder may occasionally be helpful in demonstrating its entire circumference. AP radiographs made with the bladder distended and following voiding will give adequate information in most cases; oblique films may be added as deemed necessary.

Mucosal lesions of the bladder are variably detected on urography, dependent on their size and location. Such lesions are best evaluated cystoscopically, but this fact does not relieve the radiologist of the responsibility to conduct a careful examination of the bladder even when cystoscopy is contemplated.

Cystography

Cystography is a radiologic examination of the bladder performed after direct instillation of a contrast agent into the bladder via a Foley catheter. In such an examination the degree of opacification and the degree of distention of the bladder can be controlled. Cystography with 20 to 25 per cent (wt/vol) contrast material is the examination of choice for the detection of bladder injuries and is the radiologic method of choice for the diagnosis of other bladder leaks and fistulas. It may also be of value in the evaluation of bladder contour abnormalities, diverticulae, filling defects, and calculi. A modification of the static cystogram, called the *voiding cystourethrogram,* in which fluoroscopic spot films of the bladder and urethra are made while the patient voids, is the method of choice for detecting the presence of posterior urethral valves in male infants and vesicoureteral reflux in both children and adults.

Ultrasonography

A distended bladder is an ideal sonographic "window" for the evaluation of the pelvis; however, the value of ultrasonographic evaluation of the bladder itself is limited to an evaluation of pelvic masses that either deform or invade its contour. Newer scanning techniques, such as transrectal real-time examinations, may extend the value of ultrasonography to the wall of the bladder.

Computed Tomography

Computed tomography (CT) is an important tool for the radiologic staging of bladder neoplasms. It is especially valuable in determining extravesical extension of the neoplasm.

Magnetic Resonance Imaging

Magnetic resonance imaging (MRI) has been shown to be of value for the evaluation of a variety of pelvic neoplasms and for the staging of bladder tumors. It may also be used to demonstrate the etiology of bladder contour abnormalities, but in general it has limited usefulness for the evaluation of benign bladder disease.

DIVERTICULA/HERNIAS/FISTULAS

Bladder Diverticula

Bladder diverticula are outpocketings of the bladder wall. They may be single or multiple and range in size from minor sacculations in the bladder wall to those that become larger than the bladder itself (Fig. 85–1). Congenital bladder diverticula are rare and have a complete muscular coat in contrast to the far more common acquired bladder diverticula, which represent protrusion of the mucosa of the bladder through its muscular wall. Diverticula occurring

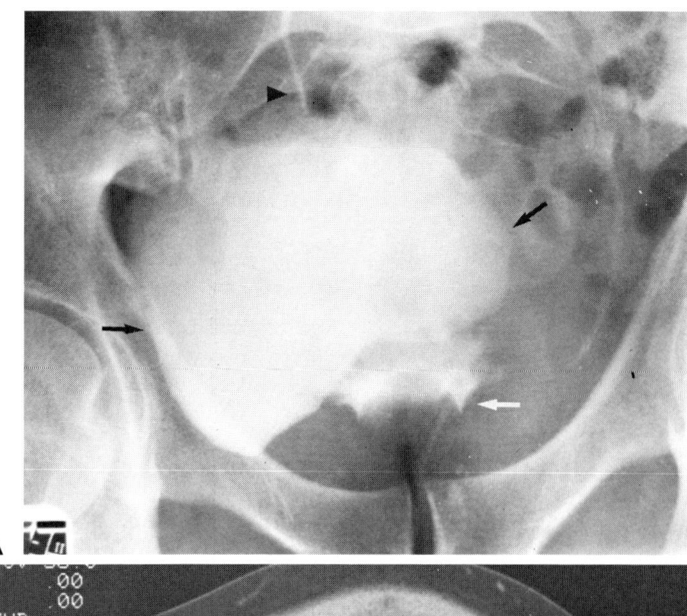

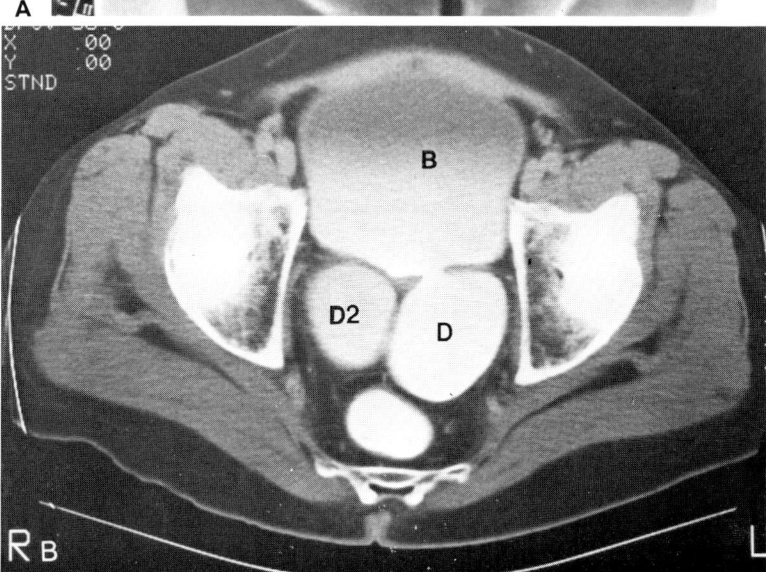

Figure 85–1. Bladder diverticulum. *A,* Large, poorly emptying bladder diverticulum *(arrows).* The bladder itself has been drained of contrast material through a Foley catheter *(white arrow).* Also note the medial deviation of the right ureter *(arrowhead). B,* CT scan of a different patient demonstrating the beak-like connection of a bladder diverticulum (D) to the bladder (B). Note the gradation of density within the bladder as the contrast material layers in the dependent portion of the bladder. A smaller diverticulum (D2) is also present whose connection to the bladder is not demonstrated on this slice.

near the ureteral orifices are commonly referred to as paraureteral or *Hutch* diverticula.

Acquired bladder diverticula are the result of either mechanical or functional bladder outlet obstruction as present in such conditions as benign prostatic hypertrophy and neurogenic bladder disease. They may be associated with infection, reflux, calculi, and neoplasms, presumably related to stasis of urine within the diverticulum. Posteriorly located bladder diverticula commonly cause medial deviation of the distal third of the ureter; this sign is a clue to the presence of the diverticulum even when it is not well-opacified with contrast material.

Hernias

Herniation of the bladder occurs most commonly into either the inguinal or femoral canals. These hernias usually do not cause specific symptoms; however, when the herniation is large, the patient may experience double voiding. Hernias may be discovered incidently on prone or erect films made as part of an excretory urogram or at the time of inguinal hernia surgery. Large bladder hernias that descend into the scrotum are termed scrotal cystoceles (Fig. 85–2). A forme fruste of bladder hernias, termed *bladder ears,* is found in approximately 10 per cent of normal infants and represents transitory extraperitoneal protrusion of the bladder in the region of the inguinal canal.

A cystocele is a prolapse of the anterior vaginal wall, with descent of a portion of the bladder into the vagina, as a result of childbirth. If the entire pelvic floor is weakened, the uterus itself may descend into the vagina along with the bladder, the urethra, and the ureters, a condition known as procidentia.

Fistulas

Fistulous communication between the bladder and a variety of pelvic and abdominal organs usually occurs as a result of a disease process or injury originating in that organ which has extended into the bladder. Most common is the vesicovaginal fistula (Fig. 85–3), which may occur as a result of gynecologic or obstetric surgery, particularly in association with abdominal or vaginal hysterectomy; tumors; trauma; or radiation therapy. Vesicocolic fistulas are usually secondary to diverticulitis, colon carcinoma, or Crohn's disease. Small bowel fistulas are almost always secondary to intestinal inflammatory disease. Vesicouterine fistulas may occur as a result of previous cesarean section involving the lower uterine segment. Such injuries present with recurrent urinary tract infection, infertility, and cyclic menouria (Youssef's syndrome).

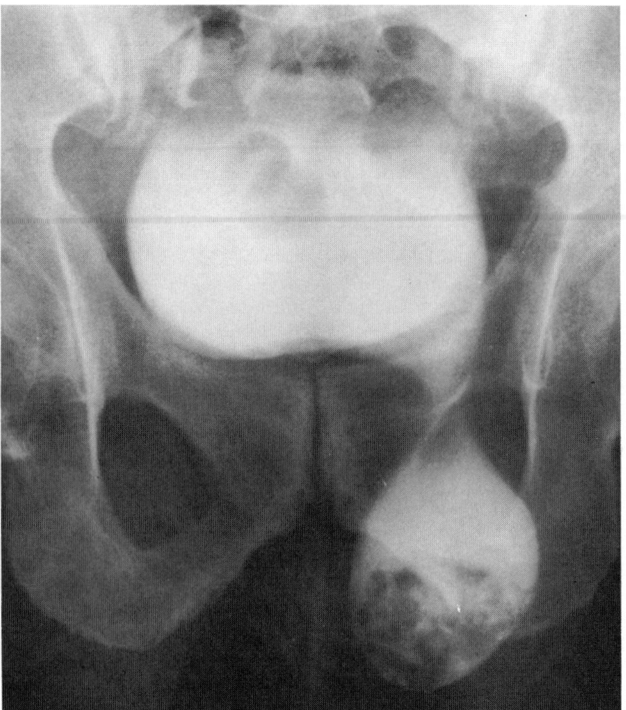

Figure 85–2. Scrotal hernia. A portion of the bladder has herniated into the scrotum. Multiple filling defects are present within the herniated portion of the bladder which represent multiple blood clots.

BLADDER OUTLET OBSTRUCTION/NEUROGENIC BLADDER

Bladder Outlet Obstruction

Long-standing mechanical obstruction of the flow of urine from the bladder results in muscular hypertrophy of the bladder wall, a condition that, when more advanced, is known as trabeculation. This results in an irregular, coarsened bladder outline. Bladder outlet obstruction may also lead to diverticulum formation, urinary stasis and infection, and acute urinary retention. Outlet obstruction is most commonly the result of benign prostatic hypertrophy in males but may also be produced by prostatic cancer and urethral strictures, tumors, and trauma. In infant males, bladder outlet obstruction may be the result of congenital posterior urethral valves.

Neurogenic Bladder

Neurogenic bladder is a term given to a variety of neurologic, muscular, and medical diseases that result in voiding dysfunction. These conditions include spinal cord injury, spinal anomalies, neurologic tumors, diabetes mellitus, Parkinson's disease, multiple sclerosis, and cerebral vascular accidents. In addition, a variety of drugs, particularly neurotrophic agents, may cause voiding dysfunction but rarely lead to radiologic changes.

Neurogenic bladders are classified by urodynamic studies into categories that define the site of the lesion and its therapy. These are (1) motor, (2) sensory, (3) autonomic, (4) reflex, and (5) uninhibited neurogenic bladders. In addition, patients with spinal cord injuries and occasionally neurologically normal children can exhibit detrusor-sphincter dyssynergia. In this syndrome the pelvic striated muscle contracts instead of relaxing when the bladder detrusor muscle contracts, producing a functional obstruction to the flow of urine in the region of the membranous urethra.

More recently, some urologists have adopted a functional classification of voiding dysfunction that groups patients into two basic categories: (1) failure to adequately store urine, and (2) failure to empty the bladder (Table 85–1).

The most common radiologic picture associated with neurogenic bladder disease is the triangularly shaped trabeculated bladder (Fig. 85–4). Other patients may exhibit small-volume trabeculated bladders; vesical diverticula; or, with sensory neurogenic bladders, smoothly marginated, poorly emptying bladders. While attempts to classify neurogenic bladder disease on the basis of its radiologic appearance have proven fruitless, radiologic studies nonetheless play a major role in the evaluation of such complications of neurogenic bladder as vesicoureteral reflux, stones, and hydronephrosis.

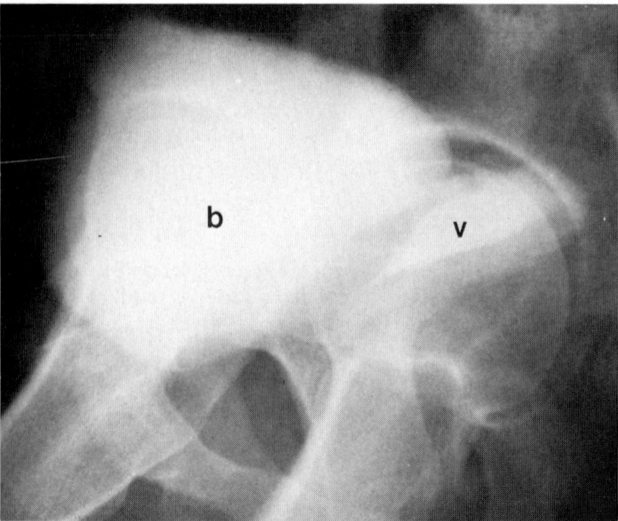

Figure 85–3. Vesicovaginal fistula. Lateral view of the bladder shows contrast material instilled into the bladder (b) outlining the vagina (v) through a fistulous communication.

TABLE 85–1. FUNCTIONAL CLASSIFICATION OF VOIDING DYSFUNCTION

FAILURE TO STORE
Because of the bladder
Detrusor hyperactivity
Decreased compliance
Sensory urgency
Because of the outlet
Stress incontinence
FAILURE TO EMPTY
Because of the bladder
Neurologic
Psychogenic
Idiopathic
Because of the outlet
Prostatic obstruction
Urethral stricture
Functional
Sphincter dyssynergia

Modified from Wein AJ: Overview of voiding function and dysfunction: Relevant anatomy, physiology, pharmacology, classification, definitions. In Pollack HM (ed): Clinical Urography. Philadelphia, WB Saunders Company, 1990, pp 1926–1934.

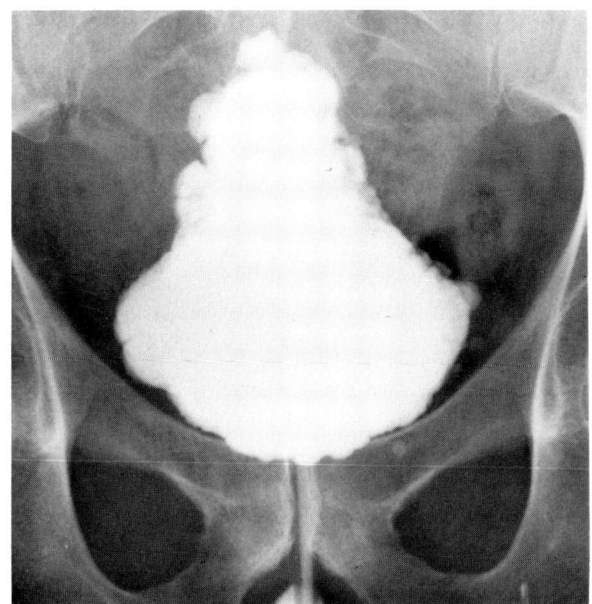

Figure 85–4. Neurogenic bladder. The bladder is irregularly shaped and there are multiple small bladder diverticula present in this patient with spinal cord injury.

BLADDER INFLAMMATION/ CALCULI/CALCIFICATIONS

Infection

Lower urinary tract infection is among the most common infectious disorders in mankind. The majority of cases of "simple" cystitis occur in women. Because of its short length, the female urethra provides little barrier to the retrograde inoculation of the bladder by perineal organisms; many cases are related to sexual activity—hence the name "honeymoon cystitis." The diagnosis is established on the basis of characteristic voiding symptoms and confirmed by laboratory studies. Radiologic investigation contributes little to the diagnosis of the infection but is utilized in patients with recurrent infection to exclude an anatomic abnormality that may have predisposed the patient to the infection or to exclude such complicating factors as vesicoureteral reflux or calculi. These studies assume an even greater significance when one realizes that the majority of bacterial renal infections are the result of the ascent of infected urine from the bladder to the kidney.

In the vast majority of patients with acute cystitis, the results of radiologic studies of the bladder will be normal. Occasionally, postvoiding films may demonstrate the presence of mucosal edema. In patients in whom the infection is a complication of underlying bladder pathology, radiologic abnormalities are most often attributable to that condition. Two complicated forms of bacterial cystitis deserve specific mention. Cystitis cystica is a form of bacterial infection of the bladder characterized by the appearance of numerous polypoid, fluid-filled cysts in the bladder mucosa. They are frequently found elsewhere within the urinary tract as well and are demonstrated radiographically as multiple smooth, rounded, 2 to 4 mm filling defects within the contrast-filled bladder. In the rare patient, these defects may persist months and even years following the eradication of the infection. Emphysematous cystitis results from infection of the bladder by a gas-forming organism that results in the presence of air within the wall of the bladder (Fig. 85–5). It is most commonly seen in diabetic patients, and gas may also be present in the bladder lumen.

Nonbacterial infections of the bladder include fungus and tubercular infections and schistosomiasis. Fungus infections are almost always secondary to *Candida albicans* and may result in the formation of mycetoma (fungus balls) within the bladder. Tuberculous cystitis is always the result of upper urinary tract infection. In advanced cases the bladder becomes small and scarred, and vesicoureteral reflux may be present. Schistosomiasis of the bladder is usually caused by the organism *Schistosoma haematobium*. Bilharzial infection of the bladder is characterized by calcification of the bladder wall and distal ureters and the presence of bladder calculi. In early stages of the disease the bladder appears thickened and edematous, while in advanced stages it becomes contracted with a rounded appearance. Unlike tuberculosis, bladder involvement in schistosomiasis precedes upper urinary tract involvement. There is an increased incidence of squamous carcinoma of the bladder associated with long-standing disease.

Non-infectious Inflammatory Conditions

Several non-infectious inflammatory conditions affect the bladder. In general, they are diagnosed by bladder biopsy or by a characteristic history. Their radiologic appearances are characterized by either increased bladder trabeculation or mucosal thickening, or both (Fig. 85–6). The bladder volume may be normal or decreased. These conditions include eosinophilic cystitis, cyclophosphamide (Cytoxan) cystitis, cystitis glandularis, and radiation-induced cystitis.

Interstitial cystitis (Hunner's cystitis) is a chronic bladder disease characterized by infiltration of the bladder wall by inflammatory cells in the absence of infection. Radiologic findings may be minimal or absent or may merely demonstrate a small capacity bladder.

Malacoplakia is a rare form of inflammatory disease of the urinary tract in which there is infiltration of the submucosa by inflammatory cells characterized histologically by the presence of basophilic staining Michaelis-Gutmann bodies. These inclusions are caused by a lysosomal enzymatic defect. There usually is a history of prior bacterial infection; however, acute infection need not be present. When the bladder is affected, yellowish lesions varying in diameter up to 3 cm will be visualized cystoscopically. On radiographic studies, malacoplakia will be demonstrated as multiple filling defects within the contrast-filled bladder.

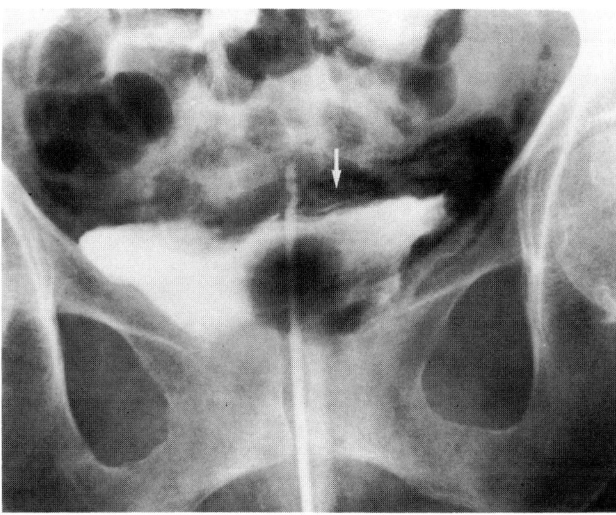

Figure 85–5. Emphysematous cystitis. A post-drainage film from a cystogram demonstrates air within the wall of the bladder *(arrow)*. A Foley catheter is in place.

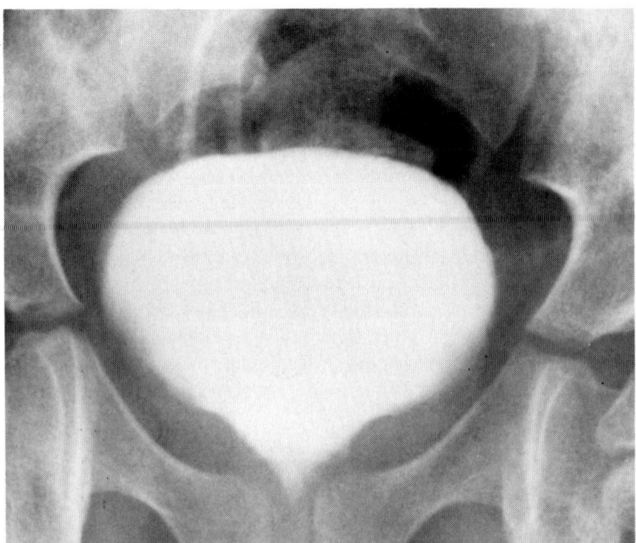

Figure 85–6. Cyclophosphamide cystitis. A ten-year-old patient being treated for acute leukemia demonstrating irregularity of the base of the bladder from cyclophosphamide cystitis. (Courtesy of Cynthia David, M.D.)

Bladder Calculi

Seventy per cent of bladder calculi occur as the result of poor bladder emptying, and therefore they are most common in patients with neurogenic bladder disease or bladder outlet obstruction. Foreign bodies may also serve as a nidus for bladder stone formation. Other conditions that predispose to bladder calculi include urethral strictures, bladder diverticula, cystoceles, and long-standing bladder catheterization. Bladder calculi vary in size from a few millimeters to several centimeters in diameter. While most bladder stones are radiopaque (calcium oxalate, calcium phosphate, and magnesium ammonium phosphate are most common), they can be easily overlooked because they may be obscured by the sacrum or by gas and feces in the rectum. Most bladder calculi have a rounded or oval appearance; however, one occasionally encounters a spiculated bladder stone known as a "jackstone" calculus (Fig. 85–7). Approximately one third of bladder stones occur in association with gram-negative urinary tract infections.

Bladder Calcification

Bladder wall calcification is considered characteristic of bilharzial infection; however, other lesions of the bladder may uncommonly also cause this finding. These conditions include transitional cell carcinoma, amyloidosis, tuberculosis, and alkaline encrusted cystitis.

BLADDER INJURIES

Injury of the bladder may occur as a result of blunt, penetrating, or iatrogenic trauma.

Clinical Features

Hematuria inevitably accompanies bladder rupture; gross hematuria is present in 95 per cent of the cases, while microscopic hematuria is present in the remainder. The urge to void may be absent or may be normal; in some forms of bladder rupture the organ may still act as a reservoir, and thus a normal urge to void may be present.

Radiologic Examination

Cystography is the examination of choice by which the presence of a bladder rupture is diagnosed. Although it is generally preferable to perform such an examination with fluoroscopic equipment, the procedure may be performed with fixed radiographic or even portable equipment when the clinical situation demands this be done. A minimum of 300 ml of diluted (30 per cent) contrast material must be utilized in order that adequate bladder distention is achieved. The use of 14 × 17 inch films, which will cover the upper abdomen, facilitates the diagnosis of intraperitoneal bladder rupture, and therefore should be utilized for at least one of the radiographs. The post-drainage radiograph is an essential component of the cystogram made for trauma and should not be omitted; the diagnosis of bladder rupture may be established by this film only in approximately 10 per cent of the cases.

Because CT has gained increased acceptance for the evaluation of patients suffering blunt abdominal and pelvic trauma, there has been interest in this modality for the initial evaluation of bladder injuries. Mee and coworkers demonstrated that CT cystography performed utilizing excreted contrast material after intravenous injection was unreliable for the detection of acute bladder injuries, when compared with conventional cystography. Subsequently, studies in which CT cystography was performed with retrograde filling of the bladder utilizing diluted contrast material report an accuracy comparable with that obtained with conventional cystography. It must be emphasized that this method of evaluation of the bladder is appropriate only for those patients in whom CT is to be performed for another purpose; in those patients with no other indication for CT, conventional cystography remains the most cost-effective and reliable method of diagnosis.

The accuracy of cystography for the diagnosis of bladder injury varies from 85 to 100 per cent in the reported series. A falsely negative cystogram may occur in patients who have suffered penetrating bladder injury, especially when caused by small-caliber bullets. In such cases it is assumed that the bladder rent seals with hematoma or by the surrounding mesentery and thus results in a falsely negative study.

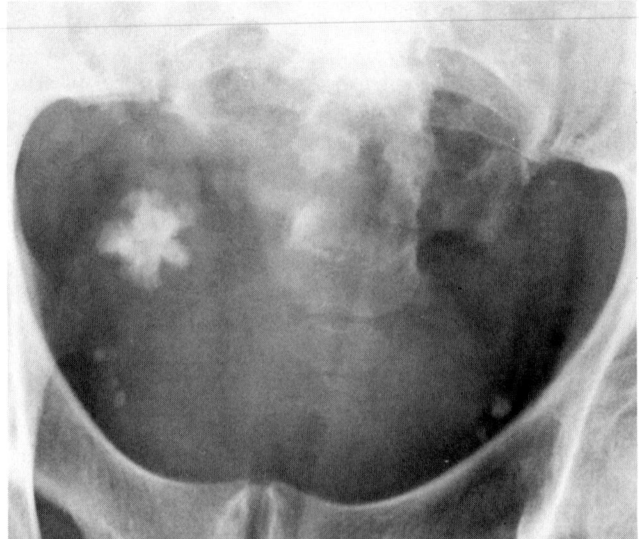

Figure 85–7. Jackstone calculus. A spiculated calculus is present, probably within a bladder diverticulum.

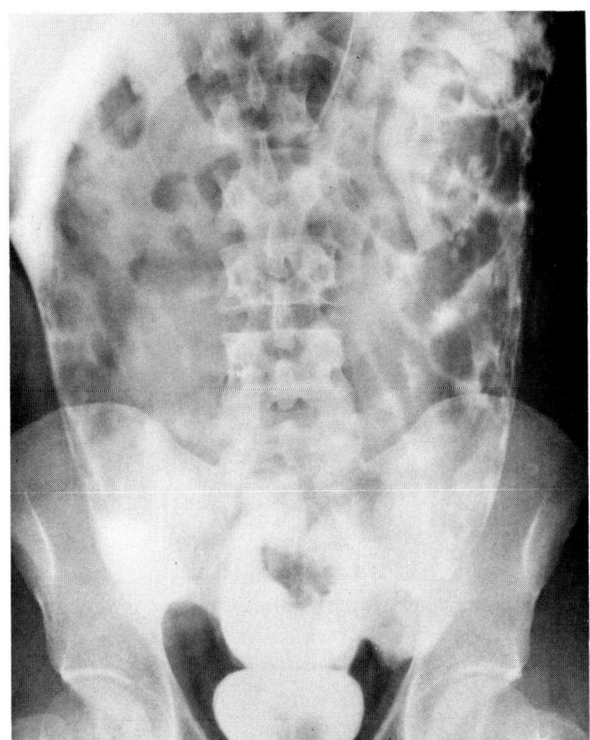

Figure 85–8. Intraperitoneal bladder rupture. Contrast is seen outlining the paracolic gutters and surrounding bowel loops within the peritoneal cavity.

Bladder Injury in Blunt Pelvic Trauma

Major bladder injury occurs in approximately 10 per cent of patients suffering a pelvic fracture. Injury of the bladder following blunt trauma may be classified as follows:

Type I	Bladder contusion
Type II	Intraperitoneal rupture
Type III	Interstitial bladder injury
Type IV	Extraperitoneal rupture
	a. Simple
	b. Complex
Type V	Combined bladder injury

Bladder contusion (type I) is an incomplete tear of the bladder mucosa following blunt injury. The injury results in an ecchymosis in a localized segment of the bladder wall. The results of cystography are normal. *Intraperitoneal bladder rupture (type II)* accounts for approximately one third of major bladder injuries (Fig. 85–8). It occurs when there is a sudden rise in intravesical pressure as a result of a blow to the lower abdomen in patients who have a distended bladder. The injury results in an approximately horizontal tear along the bladder dome. Intraperitoneal rupture commonly occurs as a seat belt or steering wheel injury. Approximately 25 per cent of the cases occur in patients without a pelvic fracture. On cystography, contrast material is seen in the paracolic gutters and outlining the abdominal viscera and loops of small bowel. *Interstitial bladder injury (type III)* occurs as a result of an incomplete perforation of the serosal surface of the bladder. On cystography, a mural defect in the bladder wall representing the site of injury is present; however, there is no extravasation of contrast material. *Extraperitoneal bladder rupture (type IV)* is associated with one or more fractures of the pubic rami or diastasis of the symphysis pubis in virtually every case. With *simple extraperitoneal rupture*, contrast material extravasation on cystography is limited to the pelvic extraperitoneal space. With *complex extraperitoneal rupture*, the contrast extravasation extends beyond the perivesical space to the thigh, the scrotum, the penis, or the perineum (Fig. 85–9). Complex extravasation implies that a disruption in the fascial boundaries of the pelvis has occurred as a result of the injury. *Combined bladder injury (type V)* results in both intraperitoneal and extraperitoneal bladder rupture.

External Penetrating Bladder Injury

Penetrating injury of the bladder may occur as a result of a bullet wound or as a result of impalement of the bladder by various objects. Penetrating bladder injury may result in intraperitoneal rupture, extraperitoneal rupture, or combined bladder injury.

Iatrogenic and Obstetric Bladder Injury

Injury of the bladder may occur in virtually any type of obstetric, gynecologic, urologic, or pelvic surgery, or as the result of migration of surgically placed devices.

Obstetric bladder injury may result from laceration of the bladder during cesarean birth, injury secondary to trauma from obstetric forceps, or pressure necrosis of the bladder wall during labor. Injury to the bladder has been reported during dilatation and curettage of the uterus, laparoscopy, or hysterectomy. Transurethral urologic procedures, especially transurethral biopsy of bladder tumors, result in bladder injury not infrequently. Migration of various surgically placed materials, including intrauterine devices, Penrose drains, and Foley catheters, has been associated with bladder injury.

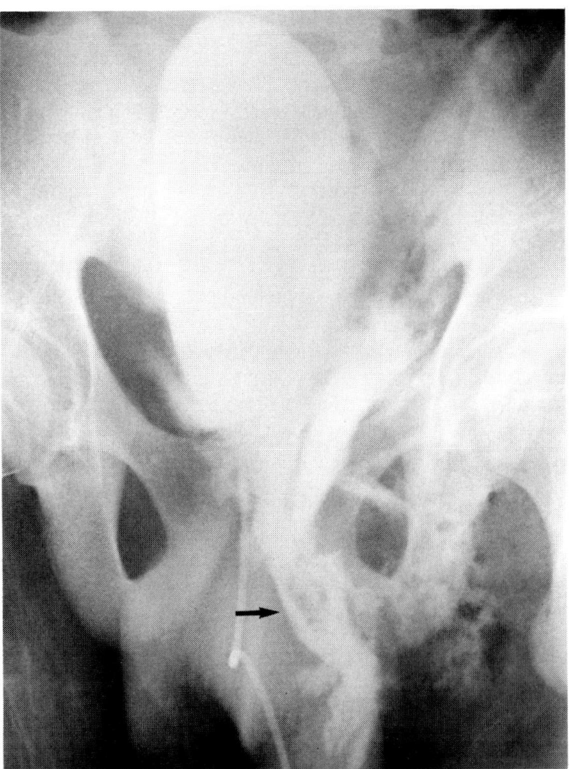

Figure 85–9. Extraperitoneal bladder rupture. A patient with an acute pelvic fracture suffered in a motor vehicle accident. Contrast extravasation is present from the base of the bladder into the scrotum *(arrow)*.

URINARY DIVERSION

A urinary diversion is performed to redirect urine flow in order to preserve renal function. It may be done at any level from the renal pelvis to the bladder. The ureter may be diverted to the skin (cutaneous ureterostomy), to the contralateral ureter (transuretero-ureterostomy), or to the bowel.

Ureterosigmoidostomy

Anastomosis of the ureters to the sigmoid colon is commonly performed on patients with bladder extrophy. Antireflux modifications of this procedure have helped to significantly reduce the complication of acute pyelonephritis. The most serious long-term complication is the development of adenocarcinoma of the colon at the site of the ureteral anastomosis. However, the long latency period of 15 to 25 years allows the ureterosigmoidostomy to be used as an interim procedure. Regular sigmoidoscopy examinations of the colon are recommended to look for the development of tumors.

Ileal Conduit

In 1950, Bricker described the construction of an ileal conduit for urinary diversion. Both ureters are anastomosed to an isolated segment of ileum. The proximal end is closed and the distal end is anastomosed to the skin. This procedure has been used successfully for many years, but an external prosthesis is required to collect the urine.

Since there is usually ureteral reflux, the entire collecting system can be examined by instilling dilute contrast material into the ileal loop. Mild ureteropelvicaliectasis is expected.

Kock Pouch

Modifications of Kock's continent ileostomy have resulted in a low-pressure, high-capacity urine reservoir. The ureteroileal anastomosis is formed with intussuscepted ureteral nipples to prevent reflux. The pouch is evacuated by intermittent self-catheterization, so that an external prosthesis is unnecessary. Numerous similar continent prostheses have been devised, including the Mainz, Indiana, King, and Le Bag pouches as well as the Camey ileocystoplasty and Malchior ileal bladder.

The radiographic evaluation consists of an initial study that is usually performed with bilateral ureteral stents extending from the renal pelves through the pouch into a drainage bag. A separate large-bore catheter is used to drain the pouch and stent the efferent limb.

The initial postsurgical study may be performed to look for extravasation or reflux. Follow-up studies require larger volumes of contrast, as the mature pouch has a large capacity.

BLADDER DISPLACEMENT/FILLING DEFECTS

Displacement of the bladder or distortion of its shape may occur as a result of a variety of intrapelvic processes that are extrinsic to the bladder itself. An impression on the base of the bladder is most commonly associated with the prostate gland in the male. When benign prostatic hypertrophy is present, such impressions can be quite extensive (Fig. 85–10); an irregular impression suggests the possibility of prostatic malignancy. An impression on the base of the bladder may be present in a variety of conditions in the female patient as well. These conditions include hypertrophy of the periurethral glands, urethral diverticuli, postoperative defects, degenerative change in the symphysis pubis, and pressure by the levator ani muscle.

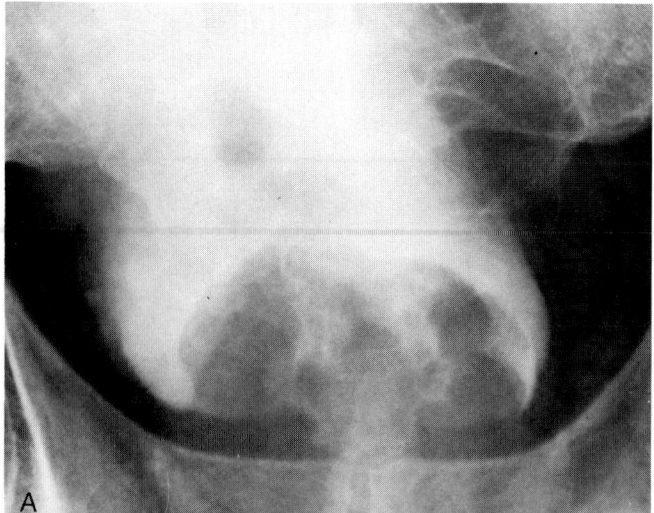

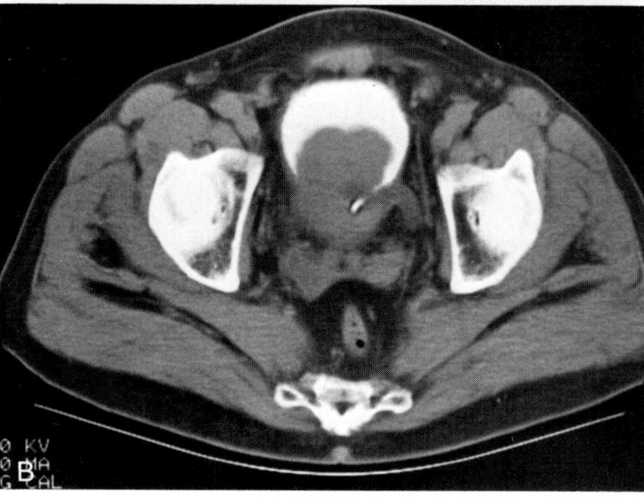

Figure 85–10. Benign prostatic hypertrophy. *A,* Cystographic phase from an excretory urogram shows a marked impression on the base of the bladder from benign prostatic hypertrophy. *B,* CT scan on the same patient showing a cross-sectional view of the enlarged prostate at the base of the bladder.

Displacement of the bladder from its usual midline position by a process lateral to it can occur from a variety of pathologic processes in the pelvis. Some of the more common causes of this finding are listed in Table 85–2. Symmetrical compression of the bladder from both sides is known as a "teardrop" bladder (Fig. 85–11). This is commonly the result of a pelvic hematoma and is frequently seen

TABLE 85–2. DIFFERENTIAL DIAGNOSIS OF AN EXTRINSIC COMPRESSION ON THE BLADDER

Aneurysm	Pelvic abscess or tumor
Hematoma	Fecal impaction
Lymphadenopathy	Prostatic tumor
Bladder diverticulum	Adnexal mass
Soft tissue or bone tumor	Extension of retroperitoneal process

Modified from Korobkin M, Minagi H, Palubinskas AJ: Lateral displacement of the bladder. AJR 125:337–347, 1975. © 1975 American Roentgen Ray Society.

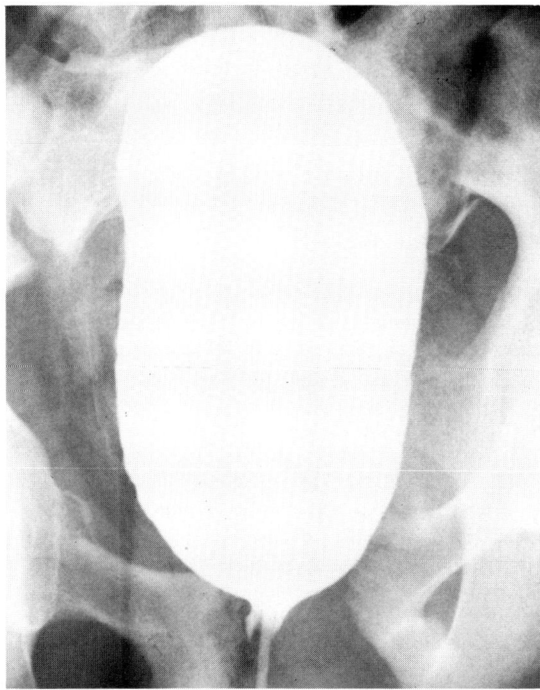

Figure 85–11. Teardrop bladder. The bladder has an elongated appearance secondary to symmetrical compression of the lateral walls by a pelvic hematoma. Note the grossly diastatic symphysis pubis in this patient with an acute pelvic fracture.

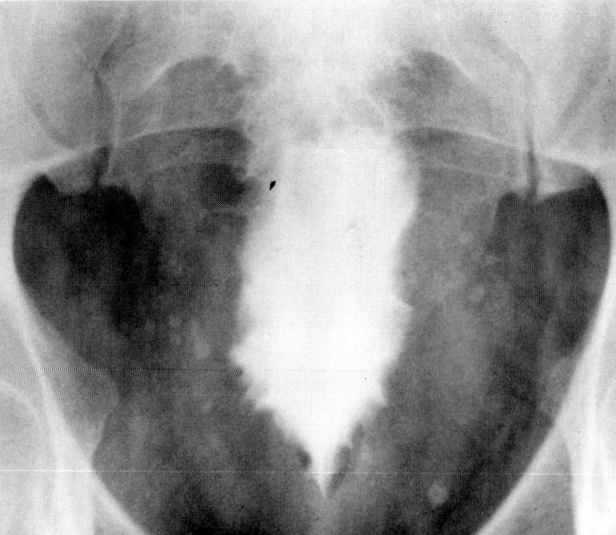

Figure 85–12. Intramural bladder filling defects. Numerous intramural filling defects present throughout the bladder were proven at cystoscopy to represent intramural hemorrhage secondary to anticoagulant therapy.

in patients with pelvic fractures. In addition, this deformity may be present with extensive bilateral pelvic lymphadenopathy, pelvic lipomatosis, retroperitoneal fibrosis, and iliopsoas muscle hypertrophy. Anterior displacement of the bladder is usually related to a variety of sacral or presacral conditions, including congenital anomalies and tumors. Pelvic masses, most commonly of gynecologic origin, produce impressions on the dome of the bladder. Leiomyomas of the uterus are the most common of these.

Filling defects are defined as mass impressions that distort the homogeneous distribution of contrast material within the bladder. Such defects may be produced by lesions within the bladder, by lesions in the mucosa or bladder wall, or by lesions extrinsic to the bladder. Filling defects extrinsic to the bladder have been dealt with in the preceding section. Filling defects within the wall or in the mucosa of the bladder are usually caused by tumors, hemorrhage (Fig. 85–12), or inflammatory conditions. Filling defects within the interior of the bladder may be either fixed or movable, single or multiple (Fig. 85–13). A list of some of the more common conditions that may cause intraluminal filling defects are listed in Table 85–3.

VESICOURETERAL REFLUX

Vesicoureteral reflux is the backward flow of urine from the bladder into one or both ureters. This condition is always considered abnormal in humans and is the primary mechanism for the ascent of lower urinary tract infection to the kidneys. The normal ureterovesical junction acts as a one-way valve to permit the free flow of urine into the bladder, but not in the reverse direction. Vesicoureteral reflux is diagnosed radiologically by voiding cystourethrography, as described earlier. Reflux is usually divided into primary reflux caused by a congenital abnormality of the ureterovesical junction and secondary or acquired causes of reflux.

Reflux is said to be primary when it is associated with the presence of an abnormal ureteral orifice on cystoscopy. With a normal ureterovesical junction, reflux is prevented by the length of the intramural ureter; the normal orifice is slightly medially placed and has a cone-like configuration. The refluxing orifice is more laterally placed owing to the shorter length of the intramural segment and has a concave or golf-hole appearance. Thus the normal valve-like mechanism of the intramural ureter is lost. Ectopic ureteral orifices associated with ureteral duplication are also prone to reflux. The ectopic ureter that inserts into the bladder caudally and more medi-

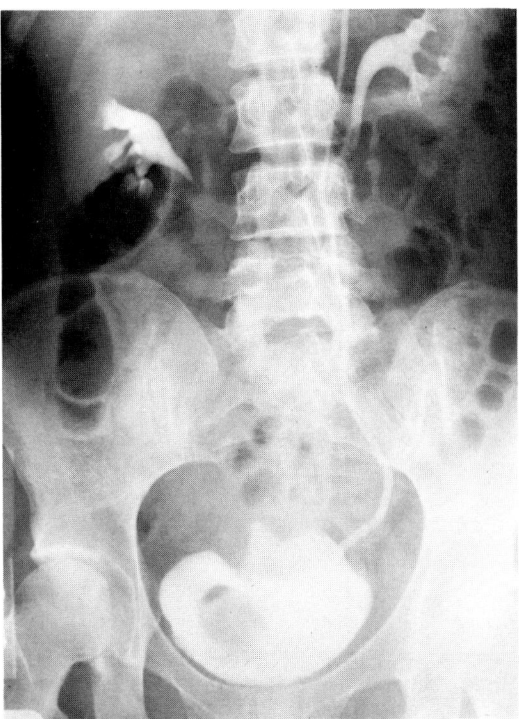

Figure 85–13. Ectopic ureterocele with an obstructed upper pole duplication on the right.

TABLE 85–3. DIFFERENTIAL DIAGNOSIS OF INTRALUMINAL FILLING DEFECTS

Blood clot	Ureterocele
Calculus	Fungus balls
Tumor	Foreign body
Cystitis cystica	Malacoplakia

ally (the Meyer-Weigert rule) is the ureter into which the reflux usually occurs.

Secondary reflux is that which occurs secondary to primary bladder pathology. First and foremost among its causes is inflammation of the bladder. Edema and cellular inflammation at the trigone reduce the efficiency of the valve-like mechanism of the ureteral orifice, especially in patients in whom the orifice is of marginal competency. Also included on the list of conditions that sometimes cause secondary reflux are neurogenic bladder disease, bladder diverticulum, postsurgical changes in the bladder, and lower urinary tract obstruction.

Classification

Vesicoureteral reflux is generally staged radiologically according to the degree of morphologic change in the upper urinary tract associated with it. While many schemes of classification have been devised, the most widely used grading system is divided into four categories as follows (Fig. 85–14):

Grade I—the reflux is confined to the lower ureter, which is nondilated.

Grade II—reflux extends into the renal pelvis and calyces without dilatation.

Grade III—mild ureteral, pelvic, and calyceal dilatation.

Grade IV—gross hydronephrosis.

Reflux is also described as being low pressure (that which occurs during passive bladder filling) or high pressure (that which occurs only during voiding). Some authors think that this distinction may have an effect on the degree of renal damage that may result from the deleterious effects of the reflux.

While the radiologic demonstration of the presence of reflux is an important factor in the management of the patient, it must be realized that reflux may be quite transitory in nature. In some patients, reflux may be demonstrated on one examination and not on another. Reflux is much more common in children than in adults, supporting the conclusion that reflux tends to disappear spontaneously with maturation. Many authorities recommend that reflux be followed in children with radionuclide rather than radiographic studies because the former is associated with a lower radiation dose. These factors notwithstanding, it must be remembered that vesicoureteral reflux is a diagnostic finding, not a disease, and that therapy should be directed toward controlling infection and the prevention of permanent upper urinary tract damage.

MISCELLANEOUS CONDITIONS

Pelvic Lipomatosis

Pelvic lipomatosis is a condition in which there is an accumulation of fat and fibrous tissue in the pelvis that deforms otherwise normal pelvic organs. The bladder and the rectum are the most commonly affected organs. The condition appears to be most common in middle-aged males with hypertension and is usually discovered incidentally during radiologic examination made for another purpose. It is associated with cystitis glandularis in approximately 75 to 80 per cent of the cases. Ureteral obstruction, which may result in renal failure in severe cases, is reported in 20 to 40 per cent of the cases. In other advanced cases, rectal obstruction and occlusion of the inferior vena cava have been reported.

The diagnosis of pelvic lipomatosis is usually established on radiologic studies (Fig. 85–15). Plain films of the pelvis typically reveal a pronounced radiolucency surrounding the bladder secondary to the fatty deposits. On contrast studies, the bladder is elongated with elevation of the bladder base. The abnormal configuration of the bladder has been variously described as teardrop, pear-shaped, gourd-shaped, or banana-shaped. There may be medial deviation of the distal ureters, and a variable degree of hydronephrosis may be demonstrated on urography. The rectosigmoid colon characteristically is straightened and elevated from the pelvis on barium enema. On ultrasonography, the abnormal configuration of the bladder surrounded by variably echogenic pelvic fat is demonstrated. Pelvic venography may show venous compression, which in severe cases may progress to frank venous occlusion. On MRI, an accumulation of fat within the pelvis with signal characteristics either identical to or of slightly lower intensity to those produced by subcutaneous fat on both T_1- and T_2-weighted images is present.

Endometriosis

Endometriosis is a common condition affecting perhaps 15 per cent of women during their menstrual years. Involvement of the urinary tract, while reported with increased frequency, is nonetheless considered rare. The bladder is the most commonly affected urinary organ. Classically, patients present with hematuria that occurs cyclically in relationship with menstruation, suprapubic pain, and dysuria. Vesical endometriomas are rarely demonstrated radio-

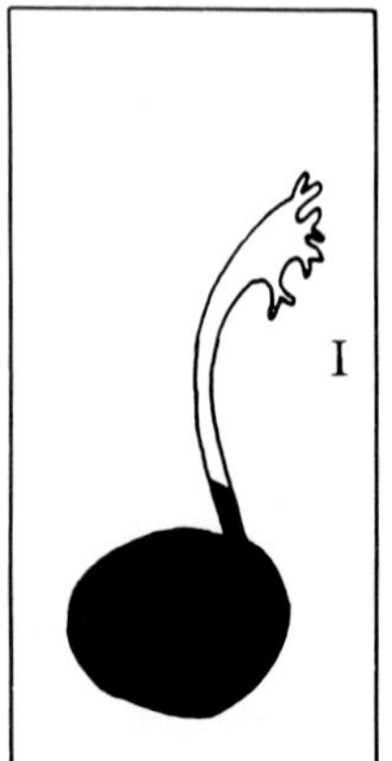

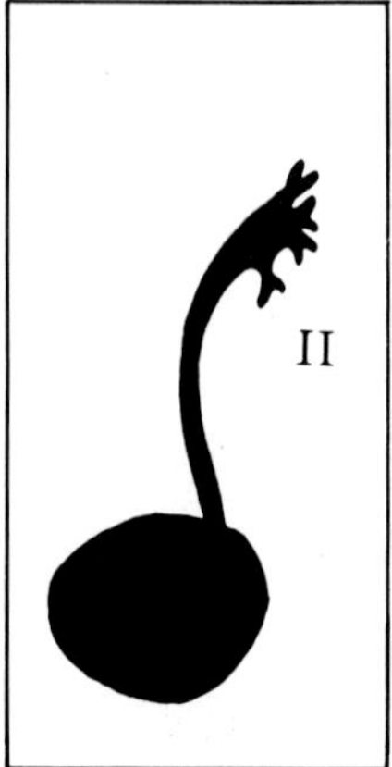

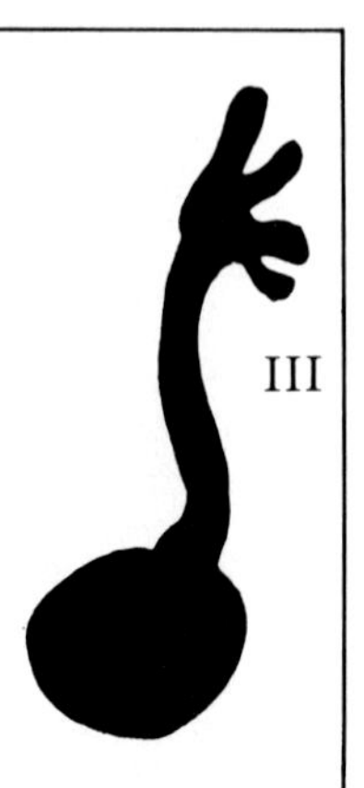

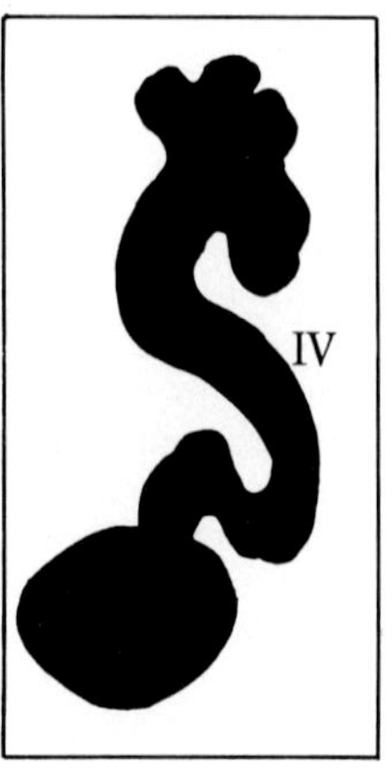

Figure 85–14. Grading of vesicoureteral reflux.

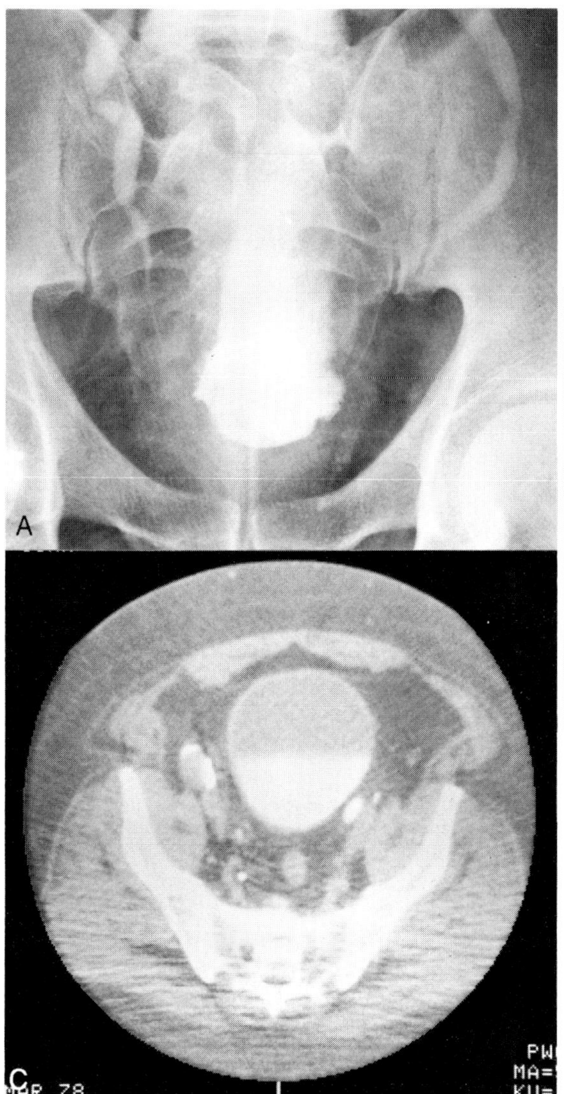

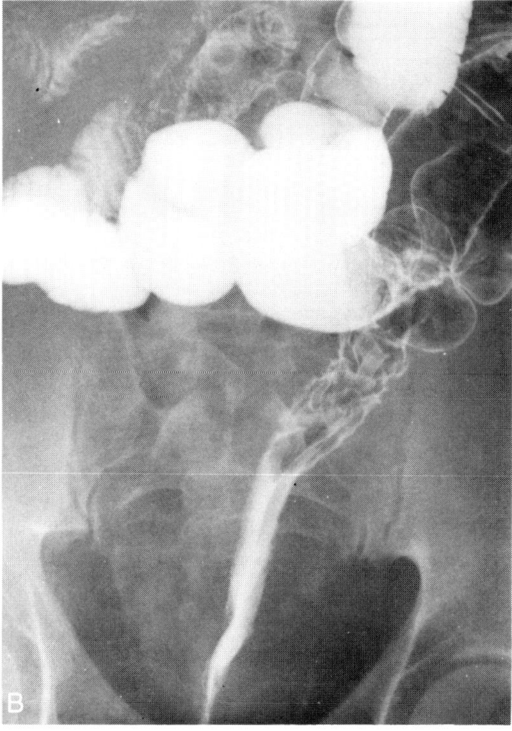

Figure 85–15. Pelvic lipomatosis. *A,* Excretory urogram demonstrating an irregular elongated bladder. *B,* Film from a barium enema demonstrating stretching of the rectum and sigmoid. *C,* CT scan shows that the perivesical mass is composed of fat.

logically. When present, the lesion appears as a poorly defined lesion that, while extrinsic to the bladder, appears to "pucker" the mucosa. Sonographic demonstration of vesical endometriosis has also been reported.

Bibliography

Abdou NI, NaPombejara C, Sagawa A, et al: Malakoplakia: Evidence for monocyte lysosomal abnormality correctable by cholinergic agonist in vitro and in vivo. N Engl J Med 297:1413–1419, 1977.

Al-Ghorab MM: Radiological manifestations of genitourinary bilharziasis. Clin Radiol 19:100–111, 1968.

Amis ES, Newhouse JH. Olsson CA. Continent urinary diversions: Review of current surgical procedures and radiologic imaging. Radiology 168:395–401, 1988.

Cohen JM, Weinreb JC: Teardrop bladder: Demonstration by magnetic resonance imaging. Urology 30:168–170, 1987.

Filmer RB, Spencer JR: Malignancies in bladder augmentations and intestinal conduits. J Urol 143:671–678, 1990.

Goodman JD, Macchia RJ, Macasaet MA, Schneider M: Endometriosis of the urinary bladder: Sonographic findings. AJR 135:625–626, 1980.

Hayes EE, Sandler CM, Corriere JN Jr: Management of the ruptured bladder secondary to blunt abdominal trauma. J Urol 129:946–948, 1983.

Husmann DA, Spence HM: Current status of tumor of the bowel following ureterosigmoidostomy: A review. J Urol 144:607–610, 1990.

Kane NM, Francis IR, Ellis JH: The value of CT in the detection of bladder and posterior urethral injuries. AJR 153:1243–1246, 1989.

Kenney PJ, Hamrick KM, Samuels LJ, et al: Radiologic evaluation of continent urinary reservoirs. RadioGraphics 10:455–466, 1990.

Korobkin M, Minagi H, Palubinskas AJ: Lateral displacement of the bladder. AJR 125:337–347, 1975.

Lamki N, Ruppert D, Madewell JE: Bladder diseases and imaging methods. Crit Rev Diagn Imaging 29(1): 13–101, 1989.

Lattimer JK, Apperson JW, Gleason DM, et al: The pressure at which reflux occurs, an important indication of prognosis and treatment. J Urol 89:395–404, 1963.

Liebeskind AL, Elkin M, Goldman SH: Herniation of the bladder. Radiology 106:257–262, 1973.

Lis LE, Cohen AJ: CT cystography in the evaluation of bladder trauma. J Comput Assist Tomogr 14(3):386–389, 1990.

Moss AA, Clark RE, Goldberg HI, Pepper HW: Pelvic lipomatosis: A roentgenographic diagnosis. AJR 115:411–419, 1972.

Pollack HM, Banner MP, Martinez LO, Hodson CJ: Diagnostic considerations in urinary bladder wall calcifications. AJR 136:791–797, 1981.

Pope TL Jr, Harrison RB, Clark RL, Cuttino JT Jr: Bladder base impressions in women: "Female prostate." AJR 136:1105–1108, 1981.

Ralls PW, Barakos JA, Skinner DG, et al: Imaging of the Kock continent ileal urinary reservoir. Radiology 161:477–483, 1986.

Sandler CM, Hall JT, Rodriguez MB, Corriere JN Jr: Bladder injury in blunt pelvic trauma. Radiology 158:633–638, 1986.

Sandler CM, Phillips JM, Harris JD, Toombs BD: Radiology of the bladder and urethra in blunt pelvic trauma. Radiol Clin North Am 19:195–211, 1981.

Spring DB, Deshon GE Jr: Radiology of vesical and supravesical urinary diversions. In Pollack HM (ed): Clinical Urography. Philadelphia, WB Saunders Company, 1990, pp 296–310.

Wechsler RJ, Brennan RE: Teardrop bladder: Additional considerations. Radiology 144:281–284, 1982.

Wein AJ: Classifications of neurogenic voiding dysfunction. J Urol 125:605–609, 1981.

Wein AJ: Overview of voiding function and dysfunction: Relevant anatomy, physiology, pharmacology, classification, definitions. In Pollack HM (ed): Clinical Urography. Philadelphia, WB Saunders Company, 1990, pp 1926–1934.

Yang A, Mostwin JL, Rosenshein NB, Zerhouni EA: Pelvic floor descent in women: Dynamic evaluation with fast MR imaging and cinematic display. Radiology 179:25–33, 1991.

86 Bladder Cancer

Richard L. Clark

Because the bladder is the most common location of urinary tract neoplasia, radiologists are frequently called on to participate in the diagnostic work-up and staging of patients with bladder cancer. The appropriate use of the many different imaging techniques available to assess the lower urinary tract is crucial for an accurate assessment of prognosis and for the development of rational treatment planning.

EPIDEMIOLOGY AND PATHOLOGY

There are approximately 40,000 new cases of bladder cancer each year, accounting for about 3 per cent of all human neoplasms. Three quarters of these tumors occur in men in their sixth or seventh decade. More than 90 per cent of these lesions are epithelial in origin, with transitional cell carcinoma by far the most common. A strong association between the development of transitional cell bladder tumors and industrial exposure to aromatic amines and cyclophosphamides has been documented. More recently, smoking, artificial sweeteners, and coffee have also been implicated as possible etiologies. In parts of the world where schistosomiasis is prevalent, the uncommon but aggressive squamous cell carcinoma of the bladder is frequently seen. Normally squamous tumors represent only about 2 per cent of all bladder cancer, but there is also an increased incidence of these more invasive lesions in patients with chronic cystitis or bladder stones. The even rarer adenocarcinoma (1 per cent of all bladder tumors) is the most common tumor seen with bladder extrophy. Adenocarcinomas, which occur most commonly on the trigone, are usually mucin-producing and are occasionally urachal in origin.

Transitional cell carcinoma (TCC) may present as superficial, invasive, or metastatic disease. Superficial TCC usually presents as papillary (Fig. 86–1) growths on or adjacent to the trigone or lateral walls. Occasional development in narrow-necked diverticula suggests that urine stasis may be another important etiologic factor (Fig. 86–2). Superficial bladder tumors may also be sessile or in situ. Histologic grade according to degree of differentiation is important for determination of prognosis and hence treatment. Rarely, TCC presents as disease invasive of submucosa or mucosa. As might be expected from experience with other neoplasms, the more anaplastic lesions tend to be more invasive. The crude five-year survival rate for all epithelial bladder cancer is 30 per cent but, depending on the stage and grade, may vary from 90 per cent in superficial, well-differentiated papillary tumors to 10 per cent in poorly differentiated locally advanced disease.

Although cystitis cystica or glandularis may be seen in patients with bladder cancer, these entities, which are frequently associated with chronic bladder inflammation, are not considered precancerous lesions. Malacoplakia is another benign mucosal process that is characterized by plaque-like infiltrates of histiocytes that are, for some unknown reason, unable to adequately digest and dispose of phagocytized bacteria. However, leukoplakia has been thought to represent premalignant changes. Unfortunately, none of these lesions produces distinct radiologic findings, and they are usually noted first at cystoscopy.

Besides the transitional, squamous, and adenocarcinomas mentioned above, there is a long list of very rare nonepithelial benign and malignant neoplasms, such as leiomyomas, pheochromocytomas, and rhabdomyosarcomas, that rarely are encountered even in large uroradiologic practices. In children without extrophy, embryonal rhabdomyosarcomas are the most common bladder neoplasm and are known as sarcoma botryoides because they present as grapelike masses protruding into the bladder.

DIAGNOSIS

Bladder tumors rarely calcify and may occasionally (1 per cent of lesions) be detected on plain abdominal films or at computed

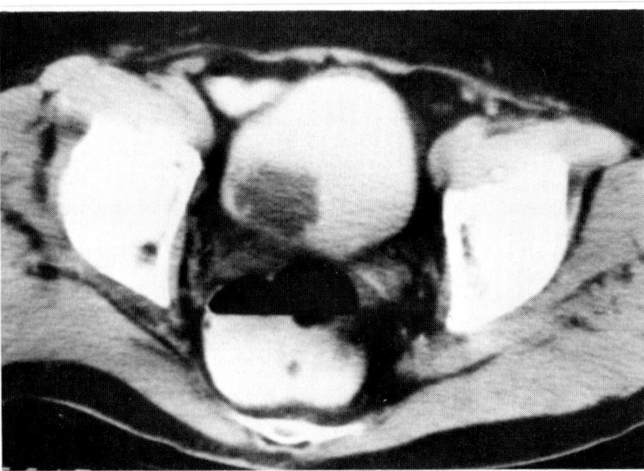

Figure 86–1. Papillary transitional cell carcinoma of the bladder, which at cystoscopy was attached to the right posterolateral wall by a stalk. Resection revealed no muscle invasion, making this a Stage A lesion.

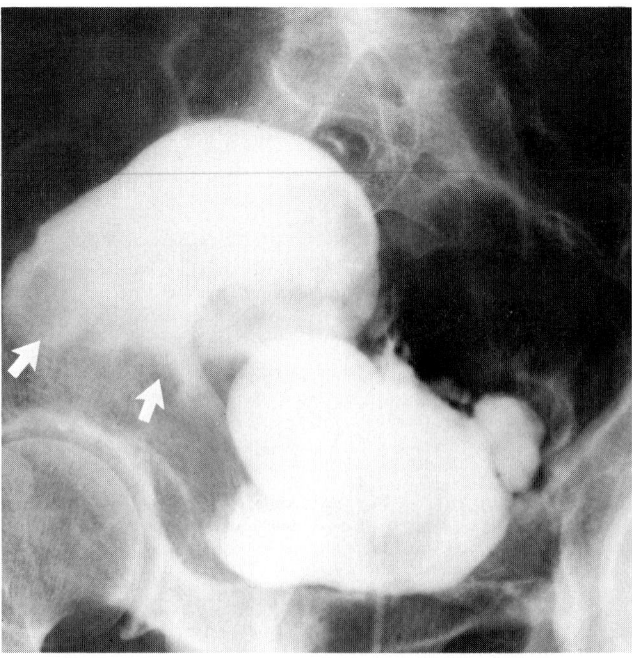

Figure 86–2. Large bladder diverticulum with an associated neoplasm *(arrows).* Cystography also revealed other diverticula and a small capacity bladder.

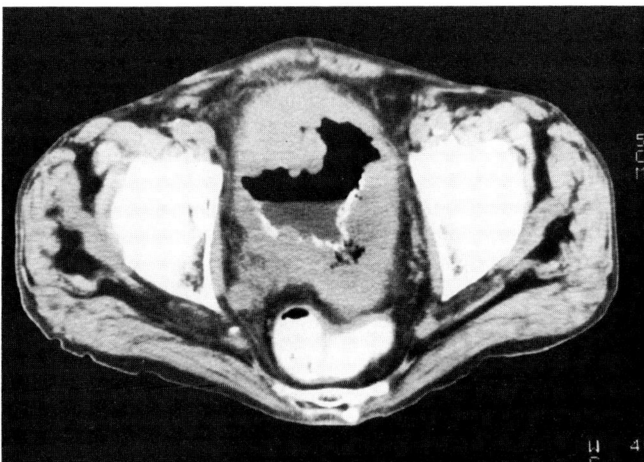

Figure 86–3. Calcification on the surface of a fungating bladder carcinoma. Infection and tumor necrosis were present. (Case courtesy of Dr. Adrian Dixon.)

tomography (CT) obtained for other medical reasons (Fig. 86–3). However, most patients who are subsequently shown to have bladder cancer present with total or terminal painless hematuria, although cystitis-like symptoms with or without hematuria may also be present. Large lesions may cause ureteral obstruction (Fig. 86–4). In the elderly patient with hematuria, an intravenous urogram is obtained prior to cystoscopy to evaluate the upper tracts despite the fact that a bladder cause is more likely. A cystogram may also be obtained, and if a sizable bladder cancer is present, these studies may demonstrate wall thickening and/or polypoidal filling defects. However, the search for the cause of lower genitourinary tract hematuria should never be the sole responsibility of the radiologist. Despite numerous attempts to increase the accuracy of urography and cystography with the use of multiple oblique projections, post-

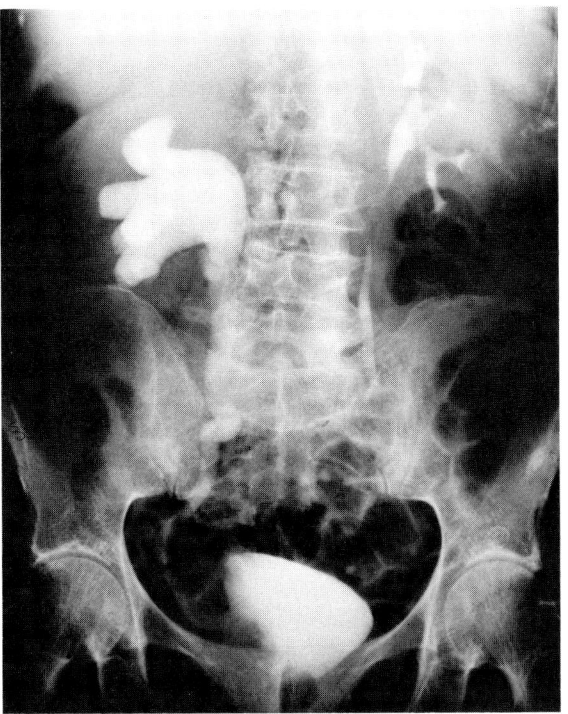

Figure 86–4. Invasion of the right ureter by a large bladder tumor has resulted in partial upper tract obstruction.

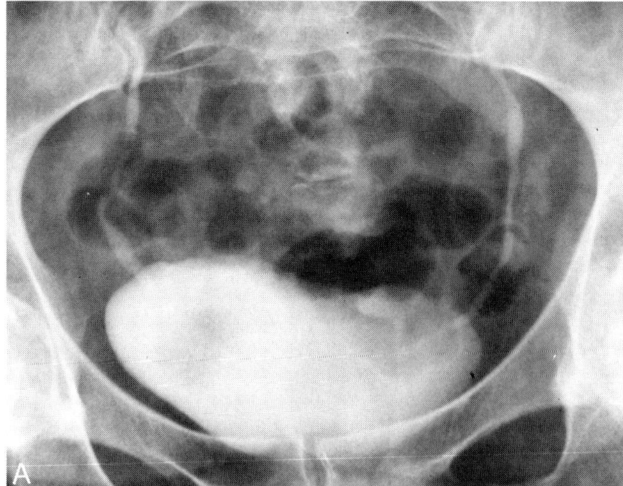

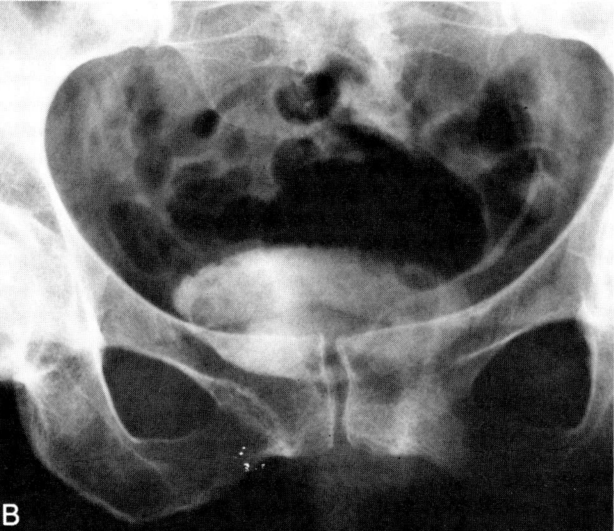

Figure 86–5. *A,* **Typical slightly irregular radiolucent filling defect in the right side of the bladder** is better seen and confirmed on a post-void film. *B,* Note how overlying bowel gas can make urographic or cystographic recognition of bladder tumors difficult.

void films (Fig. 86–5), double-contrast studies, and incremental or fractionated cystograms, only about 60 per cent of bladder tumors are detected. This is due in part to the fact that many bladder tumors are small when first coming to clinical attention (hematuria and irritative symptoms), and they are frequently located on or near the trigone, which is difficult to visualize radiographically. Cystography, therefore, besides being time-consuming and not cost-effective, may also give an inappropriate sense of security because of its high false-negative rate.

PATHOLOGIC STAGING

Two methods are commonly used for the staging of bladder neoplasms. The Jewett-Strong-Marshall system, developed over 35 years ago, is still the more popular classification, but the American Joint Commission's newer TNM system is gaining acceptance. Both of these schemes are presented in Figure 86–6 and Table 86–1. Note that, with either staging system, varying degrees of wall invasion result in different stages and consequently affect survival predictions. For example, Jewett found that five-year survival rates are

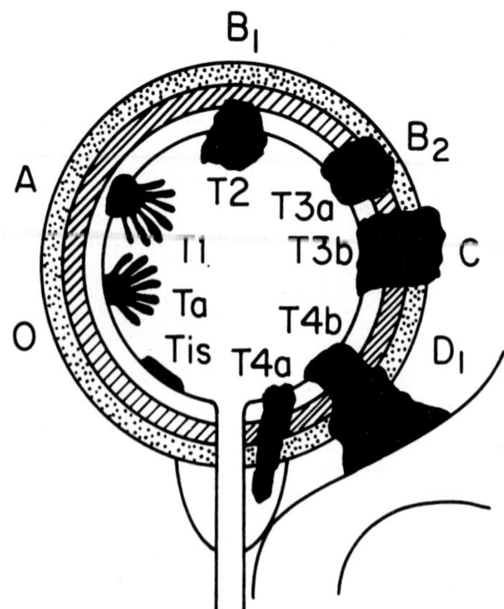

Figure 86–6. The TNM and Jewett-Strong-Marshall classifications of bladder tumors. See Table 86–1 for a description of each stage. (Modified from Wallace DM, Chisholm GD, Hendry WF: T.N.M. classification for urological tumours (U.I.C.C.)—1974. Br J Urol 47:1, 1975.)

greater than 50 per cent for stages less than B_2 and are less than 15 per cent for stages greater than B_2. Therefore, perivesical extension is an important staging milestone, as are invasion of adjacent organs and regional lymph node extension.

TREATMENT

Treatment varies greatly depending on clinical stage, local urologic practice, and patient preference. At the University of North Carolina Hospitals, for example, Stage 0 patients may receive transurethral resection and careful surveillance for recurrence. Recurrent high-grade Stage 0 tumors or Stage A lesions are frequently treated with bacille Calmette-Guérin intravesical immunotherapy. Muscle invasion, but clinically localized disease (Stage B_1 or B_2), is treated by radical cystectomy. The desirability of this procedure has been increased by the availability of potency preservation by nerve-sparing techniques and continent urinary reservoirs connected to the urethra in men or to cutaneous ostomies that avoid urinary appliances in men or women. More advanced local disease (Stage C) may be palliated with radiation therapy or treated on experimental protocol with combination chemotherapy prior to cystectomy. Metastatic disease (Stage D_1 or D_2) has a dismal prognosis, but occasional patients may respond to combination chemotherapy.

TABLE 86–1. STAGING OF BLADDER NEOPLASMS

TNM Classification (American Joint Committee on Cancer)	Description	Jewett-Strong-Marshall Classification (American Urologic System)
Tis	In situ: "flat tumor"	0
Ta	Papillary noninvasive	
T_1	Infiltration of submucosa but not beyond lamina propria	A
T_2	Infiltration of superficial muscle	B_1
T_{3a}	Infiltration of deep muscle	B_2
T_{3b}	Extension to perivesical fat	C
T_{4a}	Extension to adjacent organs (e.g., prostate, uterus)	
T_{4b}	Spread to pelvic side wall or anterior abdominal wall	D_1
N_1–N_3	Involvement of regional lymph nodes	
M_1	Distant metastases or nodes above aortic bifurcation	D_2

COMPARISON OF STAGING MODALITIES

Regardless of treatment, correct clinical staging is paramount. Therefore, radiologists and urologists alike have frequently studied and compared the accuracies of the many clinical and radiologic tools available for the assessment of bladder cancer. It is well-known that staging of bladder cancer by clinical methods alone (bimanual examination under anesthesia and transurethral resection biopsy) may under- or overstage up to 50 per cent of patients. Thus, through the years various imaging studies have been used in an attempt to improve this statistic by providing information regarding wall invasion, extravesical spread, ureteral obstruction, and extension to regional lymph nodes.

Angiography

Because 90 per cent of all bladder tumors have striking neovascularity, it is not surprising that angiography at one time was used in evaluation of patients with bladder cancer (Fig. 86–7). Historically, Lang took the lead in attempting to improve bladder cancer staging by applying newly developing angiographic techniques to assess bladder wall thickness and extravesical tumor spread. There can be no question that pelvic angiography, with or without the

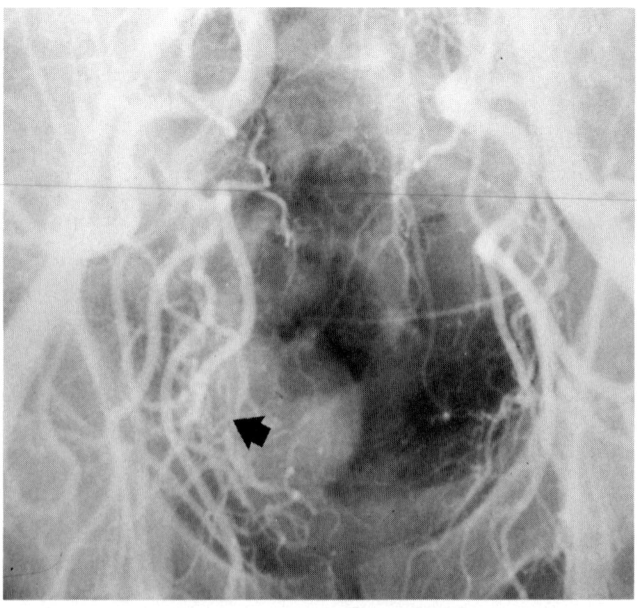

Figure 86–7. Angiographic manifestations of bladder cancer. Note the presence of air in the bladder to outline the tumor. There is evidence of hypervascularity and arterial encasement *(arrow)*. Although angiography is no longer used in the diagnosis of bladder cancer, therapeutic embolization is occasionally performed to control hemorrhage from these very vascular tumors.

additional help of peri- and/or intravesical gas, improved staging accuracy of B_2, C, and D lesions. Occasionally, pelvic phlebography was also used with similar improvements in staging accuracy documented. However, since the advent of CT, magnetic resonance imaging (MRI), and ultrasound, there seems to be little reason to persist in using invasive angiographic procedures in the evaluation of bladder cancer. Nevertheless, the treatment of potentially life-threatening bladder hemorrhage by therapeutic embolization is occasionally useful.

Lymphangiography

The normal lymphatic drainage from the bladder is via collecting trunks from the trigone and anterior and posterior walls. Flow is first to the medial (obturator) and middle groups of external iliac nodes and subsequently to the internal iliac and common iliac nodes. Studies correlating lymphangiography with pathologically determined stages have shown that approximately 25 per cent of patients with B lesions, 30 per cent of patients with C lesions, and 65 per cent of patients with D lesions will have positive lymphangiograms. Therefore, bilateral pedal lymphography continues to be popular in some institutions because CT and MRI cannot exclude tumor involvement in normal-sized nodes. Causes of false-positive lymphangiograms may be (1) collateral channels bypassing normal nodes simulating total replacement of these nodes; (2) fatty infiltration, especially in elderly patients; and (3) hyperplastic changes due to pelvic inflammation. The causes of false-negative lymphangiograms include (1) metastases that totally replace nodes and (2) the presence of microfocal deposits.

Lymphangiography can direct percutaneous lymph node biopsy (accuracy up to 95 per cent) and determination of response (or lack of response) to therapy and detection of disease relapse are also possible because contrast remains in the lymph nodes for several months, facilitating their follow-up evaluation with plain radiographs.

Computed Tomography

During the past 10 years there has been intense interest in the evaluation of bladder cancer with CT scanning. This is only appropriate considering the well-known inaccuracy of clinical staging of advanced disease and the invasive and technically more difficult alternatives, i.e., angiography, lymphangiography, and staging laparotomy. CT has also been recommended in the evaluation of post-cystectomy patients as being more sensitive than conventional radiography or sonography in detecting recurrent disease or postoperative complications.

With current, high-resolution "fast" scanners (less than 3-second scan time), diagnostic accuracy has improved dramatically. Slice thickness may vary from 5 to 10 mm, and table increments are usually 5 to 10 mm through the bladder and larger elsewhere. Adequate small bowel and rectal contrast and the use of vaginal tampons in females are recommended. Intravenous contrast may or may not be used, but bladder distention with or without low-dose contrast is essential. Some authors advocate gas insufflation and high-dose intravenous contrast to provide wall enhancement. Scanning in prone or decubitus positions may also help demonstrate certain intravesical lesions to better advantage. However, attempts to improve the CT recognition and assessment of intravesical lesions are reminiscent of earlier attempts to rival the cystoscope and have little to offer the staging procedure.

The real value of CT appears to be in the detection of (1) perivesical extension (Fig. 86–8), (2) adjacent organ invasion (Fig. 86–9), and (3) regional or remote lymph node spread. The overall accuracy of pelvic lymph node evaluation is approximately 80 per cent, which rivals lymphangiography but is accomplished without an invasive procedure. Information regarding tumor bulk necessary for accurate radiotherapy planning and the detection of hydronephrosis are additional advantages of CT.

False-positive scans are unusual but may be encountered if transurethral resectional biopsy precedes CT because of possible perforation and perivesical fluid accumulation, which may mimic peri-

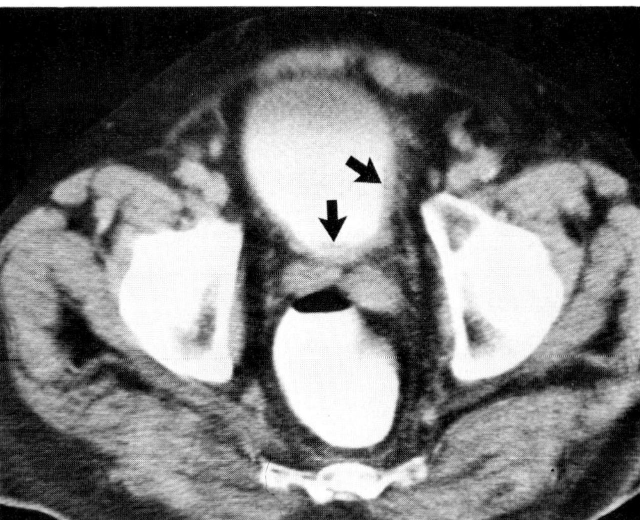

Figure 86–8. Posterior bladder wall thickening *(arrows)* without perivesical extension or involvement of rather prominent seminal vesicles in a patient with a Stage B neoplasm.

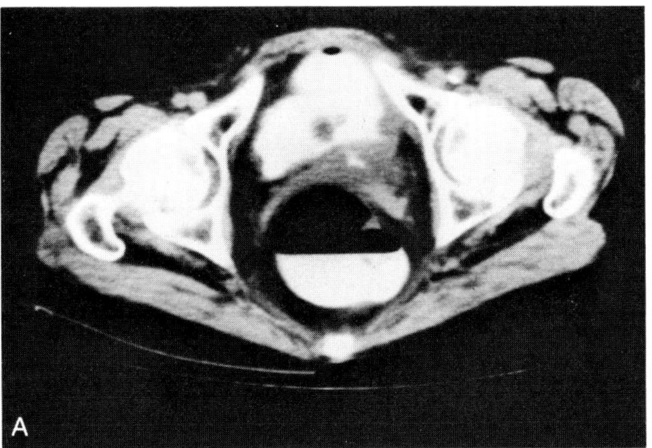

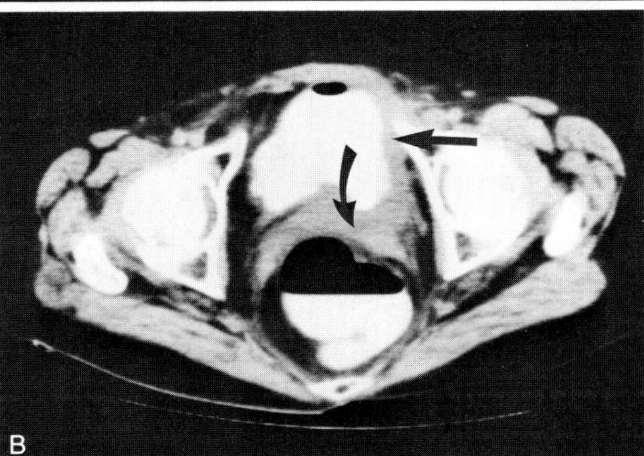

Figure 86–9. *A* and *B,* Two contiguous slices demonstrate **extravesical extension posteriorly into the uterus** *(curved arrow)* and anterolaterally to the pelvic side wall and anterior abdominal wall *(straight arrow).*

vesical tumor extension. Excessive dependence on the "normal" seminal vesicle angle, which may be obliterated or distorted by an enlarged rectum or the prone position, may also result in CT overstaging. False-negative CT studies usually result from the presence of histologically involved but normal-sized lymph nodes and from the difficulty of evaluating lymph nodes adjacent to variable vascular structures in the pelvis. This latter differentiation is now being facilitated by MRI. The inability of CT to detect microscopic invasion of the perivesical fat is also acknowledged.

Ultrasound

Despite recent advances in the evaluation of pelvic masses, with the use of transabdominal real-time ultrasound and transurethral and transrectal scanners, sonography still appears to have only a limited role in the staging of bladder tumors. Resolution in most situations does not approach that of CT or MRI, relegating ultrasound to the infrequent initial evaluation and follow-up of large lesions and, of course, the assessment of hydronephrosis. However, the recent development of higher megahertz transurethral transducers with their improved near-field resolution may rekindle interest in assessing bladder wall invasion with ultrasound.

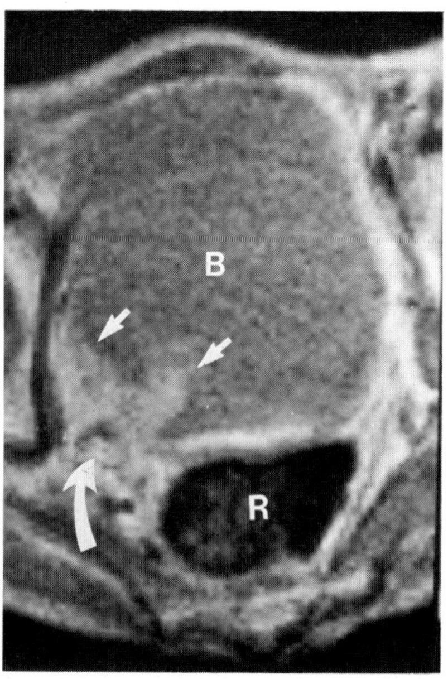

Figure 86–10. Magnetic resonance image of a transitional cell carcinoma arising from the posterior and lateral bladder wall *(small arrows)*. Extension of tumor into the dilated ureter *(curved arrow)* is also seen. Transverse image, 28 msec TE, 2 sec TR. (B = bladder; R = rectum.) (Courtesy of Hedvig Hricak, M.D.)

Scintigraphy

Although nuclear medicine studies such as iliopelvic lymphoscintigraphy generally lack the resolution needed for localized staging of bladder cancer, bone scans have been used routinely in some institutions to evaluate bladder tumor patients for disseminated disease prior to cystectomy. Recent data would suggest, however, that in the presence of a normal history (no bone pain) and physical examination as well as normal serum alkaline phosphatase, routine preoperative bone scanning is unnecessary.

Some workers have advocated the use of renal nuclear medicine studies in the follow-up of patients with bladder cancer as an ad-

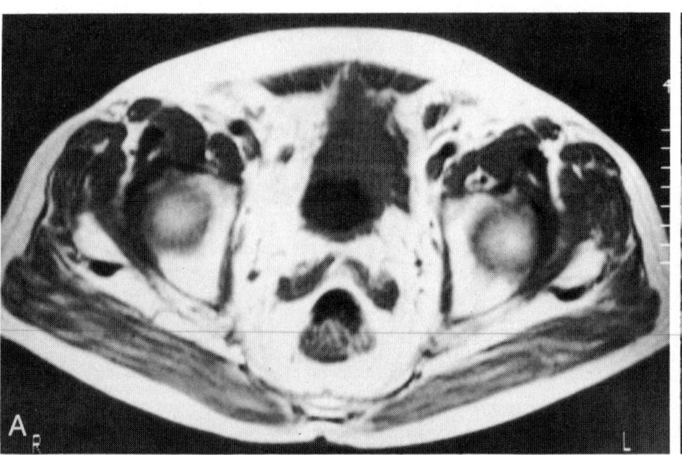

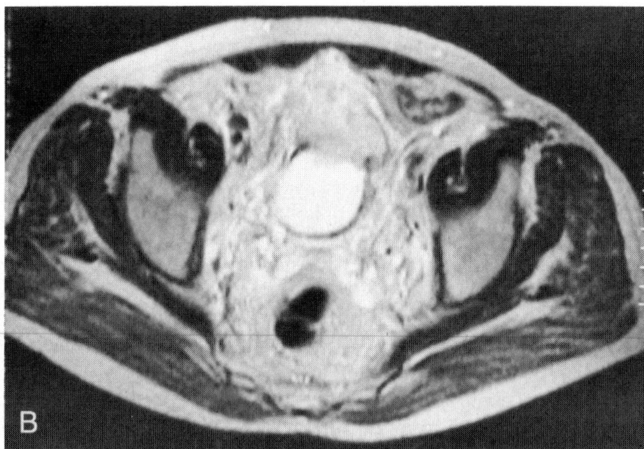

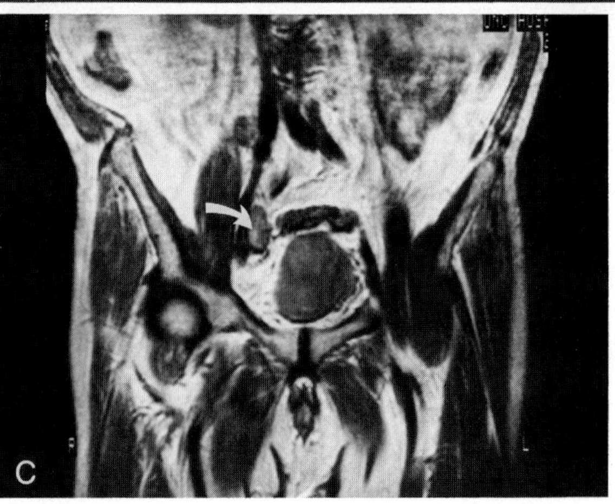

Figure 86–11. Magnetic resonance image of invasive bladder adenocarcinoma. T_1-weighted *(A)* and T_2-weighted *(B)* images nicely demonstrate tumor extending anteriorly into perivesicle space but stopping short of rectus muscle invasion (confirmed at surgery). Proton density coronal image *(C)* documents right iliac node enlargement *(arrow)* making this a Stage D_1 lesion.

junct to routine cystoscopy to rule out upper tract obstruction in high-risk cases. However, it would seem more prudent to follow these patients with intravenous urography and/or retrograde pyelography to exclude additional urothelial tumors, which develop in 5 per cent of upper collecting systems of patients with bladder carcinoma. Provided that the ureteroileostomies are refluxing anastomoses, periodic loopograms should also be performed in patients with cystectomy for the same reason.

Magnetic Resonance Imaging

During the past five years, MRI has assumed an increasingly important role in the evaluation of bladder cancer. Although initial promises of its ability to accurately distinguish normal from malignant tissue have not been completely fulfilled, MRI is contributing to the staging of locally invasive disease (Stage B vs Stage C) and in the assessment of pelvic lymph nodes (Stage C vs Stage D) (Fig. 86–10 and 86–11). It now rivals CT in accuracy in most series, and with newer pulse sequences and the increased use of contrast media, its pre-eminent role may soon be assured.

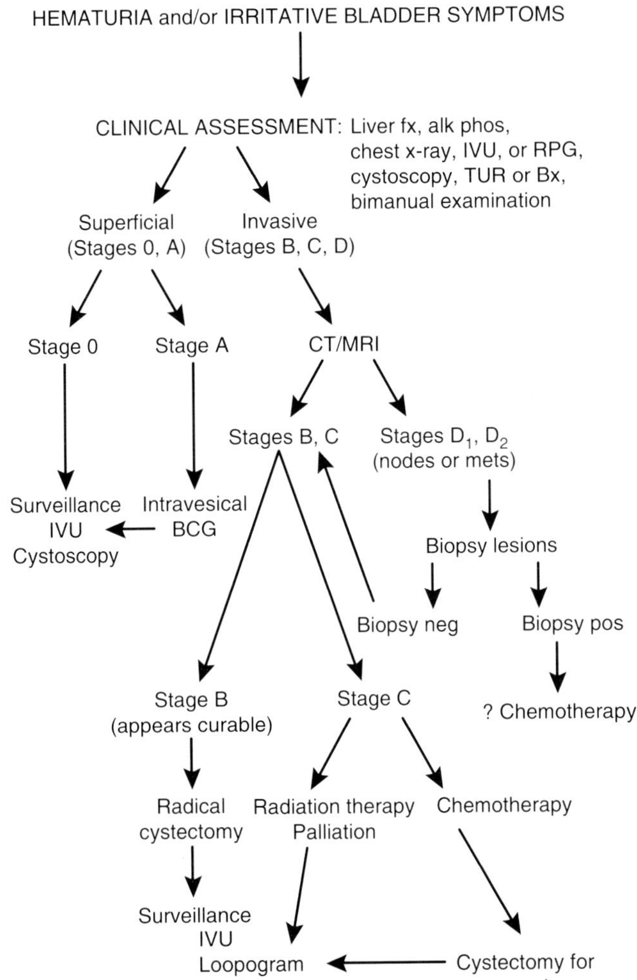

Figure 86–12. Management of bladder cancer.

SUMMARY

Epithelial bladder cancer is common and may be associated with chronic cystitis or environmental and occupational hazards. As Jewett has said, "The single most important characteristic of the tumor which influences its potential curability is depth, or stage, of infiltration." Nevertheless, despite the importance of cystoscopy for the initial diagnosis and assessment of local bladder wall extension, radiologists should also participate in the staging of bladder cancer, particularly in the evaluation of extravesical spread. Figure 86–12 offers a rational approach to the work-up of a typical patient with bladder cancer. It is acknowledged that there will always be many variations from institution to institution in the optimal diagnostic approach to patients with this difficult neoplastic condition.

Acknowledgment

The author wishes to thank Dr. James Mohler of the Division of Urology at University of North Carolina Hospitals for his advice and suggestions during the revision of this chapter.

Bibliography

Ahlberg N-E, et al: Computed tomography in staging of bladder carcinoma. Acta Radiol Diag 23:47, 1982.
Amendola MA, Glazer GM, Grossman HB, et al: Staging of bladder carcinoma: MRI-CT-surgical correlation. AJR 146:1179-1183, 1986.
Brick SH, Friedman AC, Pollack HM, et al: Urachal carcinoma: CT findings. Radiology 169:377-381, 1988.
Buy JN, Moss AA, Guinet C, et al: MR staging of bladder carcinoma: Correlation with pathologic findings. Radiology 169:695–700, 1988.
Castellino RA, Marglin SI: Imaging of abdominal and pelvic lymph nodes: Lymphography or computed tomography. Invest Radiol 17:433, 1982.
Chagnon S, Cochand-Priollet B, Gzaeil M, et al: Pelvic cancers: Staging of 139 cases with lymphography and fine-needle aspiration biopsy. Radiology 173:103-106, 1989.
Ege GN: Augmented iliopelvic lymphoscintigraphy: Application in the management of genitourinary malignancy. J Urol 127:265, 1981.
Hahn D: Neoplasms of the urinary bladder. In Pollack HM (ed): Clinical Urography. Philadelphia, WB Saunders Company, 1990, pp 1353–1380.
Hamlin DJ, et al: Updating computed tomography of bladder carcinoma in assessing response to immunotherapy and attenuated irradiation. Urology 17:622, 1981.
Hricak H, et al: Anatomy and pathology of the male pelvis by magnetic resonance imaging. AJR 141:1101, 1983.
Husband JES, Olliff JFC, Williams MP, et al: Bladder cancer: Staging with CT and MR imaging. Radiology 173:435-440, 1989.
Jewett HJ, Strong GH: Infiltrating carcinoma of the bladder. Relation of depth of penetration of the bladder wall to incidence of local extension and metastases. J Urol 55:366, 1946.
Jing B, et al: Metastases to retroperitoneal and pelvic lymph nodes: Computed tomography and lymphangiography. Radiol Clin North Am 20:511, 1982.
Koss JC, et al: CT staging of bladder carcinoma. AJR 137:359, 1981.
Lang EK: Assessment and staging of bladder tumors by roentgenographic techniques. In Ney C, Friedenberg R (eds): Radiographic Atlas of the Genitourinary System, 2nd ed. Philadelphia, JB Lippincott Company, 1981, pp 1481-1484.
Lee JKT, Marx MV: Pelvis. In Lee JKT, Sagel SS, Stanley RJ (eds): Computed Body Tomography with MRI Correlation. New York, Raven Press, 1989, pp 851–897.
Marshall VF: The relation of the preoperative estimate to the pathologic demonstration of the extent of vesical neoplasms. J Urol 68:714, 1952.
Neuerburg JM, Bohndoft K, Sohn M, et al: Urinary bladder neoplasms: Evaluation with contrast-enhanced MR imaging. Radiology 172:739-743, 1989.
Rholl KS, Lee JKTL, Heiken JP, et al: Primary bladder carcinoma: Evaluation with MR imaging. Radiology 163:177-121, 1987.
Sager EM, et al: The role of CT in demonstrating perivesical tumor growth in the preoperative staging of carcinoma of the urinary bladder. Radiology 146:443, 1983.
Sherwood T: Hematuria. In Eisenberg RL, Amberg JR (eds): Critical Diagnostic Pathways in Radiology: An Algorithmic Approach. Philadelphia, JB Lippincott Company, 1981, pp 212–221.
Wallace DM, Chisholm GD, Hendry WF: T.N.M. classification for urological tumours (U.I.C.C.)—1974. Br J Urol 47:1, 1975.
Weinerman PM: Pelvic adenopathy from bladder and prostate carcinoma: Detection by rapid sequence computed tomography. AJR 140:94, 1983.

87 The Prostate

E. Stephen Amis, Jr., and N. Reed Dunnick

The prostate is a pyramid-shaped glandular organ that is found fully developed in the adult male at the base of the bladder, surrounding the posterior urethra. It develops embryologically in the region of the entrance of the mesonephric duct by the outgrowth of five groups of urethral epithelial buds. The five prostatic lobes that are formed from the epithelial buds eventually become indistinct anatomically. The prostatic capsule merges with the bladder base cephalad and with the urethra caudad at the level of the urogenital diaphragm. The capsule further sends fibromuscular bundles into the glandular tissue of the prostate, resulting in separation of the external portion of the gland into lobules.

Two well-defined types of glands are found within the normal prostate. These include the external glands, which constitute the five lobes (and thus the bulk of the prostate), and glands in the periurethral region. The posterior, median, anterior, and two lateral lobes constitute the five basic lobes of the prostate. Further, submucosal glands may occur vestigially beneath the neck of the bladder and when hypertrophied become the subcervical lobe of Albarrán (the sixth lobe) and, if in the subtrigonal region, the subtrigonal lobe of Home (the seventh lobe).

Benign prostatic hypertrophy (BPH) results from small nodule proliferation in the periurethral glands. These nodules subsequently enlarge and compress the external glandular tissue into a progressively narrower fibroglandular structure. This compressed prostatic tissue becomes the surgical capsule of the prostate. A reasonably well-defined cleavage plane remains between the enlarging nodules and the surgical capsule. Adenocarcinoma of the prostate usually develops in the region of the posterior lobe.

Because of the intimate relation of the prostate to the bladder base and posterior urethra, it is optimally sited for causing urinary outlet obstruction when involved by a pathologic process. The most common cause of such pathologic obstruction is benign hypertrophy. Mechanically, the obstructive process may occur in one of two ways. Direct encroachment by the enlarging prostate on the urethra is the more common mechanism. However, intravesical growth of the prostate by hypertrophy of the median lobe or lobes of Albarrán or Home may produce a ball-valve effect on the bladder outlet. Either situation results in increased resistance to urine outflow.

DISEASES OF THE PROSTATE

Disease processes involving the prostate are generally inflammatory or neoplastic in origin. Both are more common in the aging male, although prostatitis, both acute and chronic, is not uncommon in younger men. Although there are many etiologies for prostatitis (Table 87–1), the most common is nonbacterial or nonspecific prostatitis, also known as prostatosis. Bacterial prostatitis may progress to frank abscess formation. Granulomatous prostatitis may be secondary to specific organisms or nonspecific secondary to a hypersensitivity type of reaction. The enlarged, firm gland seen in granulomatous prostatitis, coupled with its chronic course, may be confused with carcinoma of the prostate in the older male.

One of the most common pathologic entities causing restriction of urine flow in the male is BPH. Growth of the prostate, both normal and abnormal, appears to be mediated by testicular hormones. However, this hormonal action may be permissive rather than active. The development of BPH is a manifestation of aging, with greater than 80 per cent of males more than 50 to 60 years old having some degree of benign enlargement. It appears to be species specific, affecting only men and dogs. In cases of obstruction secondary to BPH it is generally the case that the larger the gland, the more severe the symptoms. However, acute urinary retention may result from minimal enlargement, whereas patients with larger glands may remain essentially symptom-free for many years. The normal weight of the prostate averages 20 g. Most glands requiring resection weigh 100 g or less, with glands weighing more than 200 g comprising less than 1 per cent of resected specimens.

Malignant disease of the prostate can be composed of various cell types, although by far the most common is adenocarcinoma (Table 87–1), which occurs more frequently in the region of the posterior lobe. It is the second most common malignancy in American men and the third most common cause of cancer death occurring in males over the age of 55. The diagnosis of carcinoma of the prostate is usually established by rectal examination and confirmed by transrectal or transperineal needle biopsy. A simple staging classification is as follows: Stage A—no palpable abnormality, carcinoma found in resected specimen performed for presumed BPH; Stage B—palpable nodule confined to prostate on rectal examination; Stage C—direct extension of carcinoma into the periprostatic tissues; and Stage D—distant metastases. Common channels of metastasis are lymphatics to the pelvic nodes and the periprostatic venous plexus of Batson to the bony pelvis and spinal column. Bony metastases are commonly blastic in nature. In far-advanced disease, rectal involvement may occur by direct extension, with resultant rectal mass or stricturing.

Failure to recognize metastases to the pelvic lymph nodes has been a major cause for understaging of carcinoma of the prostate and is discussed further in subsequent sections.

SYMPTOMATOLOGY RELATED TO PROSTATIC DISEASE

Patients suffering from inflammatory disease of the prostate, although occasionally complaining of restriction of urine flow, more

TABLE 87–1. DISEASE PROCESSES INVOLVING THE PROSTATE

Inflammatory
- Prostatitis
  - Bacterial (acute and chronic)
  - Viral
  - Parasitic (*Trichomonas vaginalis*)
  - Granulomatous
    - Specific (e.g., tuberculosis)
    - Nonspecific
- Prostatosis (nonspecific inflammation)
- Prostatic abscess

Neoplastic
- Benign
  - Benign prostatic hypertrophy
- Malignant
  - Adenocarcinoma (most common malignancy)
  - Squamous cell carcinoma
  - Transitional cell carcinoma
  - Sarcoma
  - Lymphoma
  - Metastases

frequently present with frequency, dysuria, perineal discomfort, and pain on ejaculation. In cases of acute bacterial prostatitis or abscess, high fever is the norm, and acute urinary retention may result from edematous swelling of the gland. Restriction of urine flow is often found with granulomatous prostatitis, BPH, and carcinoma of the prostate. Such patients usually present with a similar spectrum of symptoms, referred to as prostatism. Common complaints include hesitancy, weak or intermittent stream, post-void dribbling, frequency, and significant nocturia. There is often a feeling of incomplete emptying of the bladder. Prostatism, although usually due to prostatic disease, may be caused by other pathologic entities, such as neurogenic bladder, postoperative bladder neck contracture, urethral valves, and tumor or stricture of the urethra.

Specific upper tract symptoms are unusual in patients with prostatic disease. Hydronephrosis, even when present, is usually insidious in onset and therefore asymptomatic. If infection supervenes, fever and flank pain may occur. Progressive uremia is suggested by nausea and vomiting, weight loss, and malaise.

BLADDER AND UPPER TRACT CHANGES ASSOCIATED WITH PROSTATE DISEASE

Regardless of the outlet obstructive process, the bladder detrusor muscle responds by hypertrophy. Initially, in such cases, functional balance of the bladder is maintained by increased contractility. Muscular hypertrophy results in thickening of the bladder wall as well as enlargement of the trigonal muscle. Trabeculation occurs as cellules and saccules, and eventually diverticula, form as a result of herniation of the bladder mucosa between the hypertrophied muscle bundles. Long-term obstruction may result in detrusor decompensation with increasing residual urine as well as thinning and atony of the bladder wall. In early outlet obstruction, the increasing intravesical pressure is not transmitted to the upper tracts, as the ureterovesical valve mechanism maintains its competence. As intravesical pressure and residual urine increase, urine is not effectively delivered from kidney to bladder because of decreased ureteral peristalsis. The result is a functional obstruction of the upper tracts. In some cases, the ureterovesical valve mechanism may fail. Resultant reflux results in direct transmission of voiding pressure to the upper tracts. Either mechanism results in dilatation of the ureters and intrarenal collecting systems.

The late complications of urinary outflow obstruction, whatever the cause, are infection and/or calculus formation in the face of stagnant urine, hydroureteronephrosis due to vesicoureteral reflux or functional obstruction, and, as a final result, renal failure.

IMAGING THE DISEASED PROSTATE

In patients complaining of prostatism, imaging of the urinary system is performed in an effort to confirm the clinically suspected diagnosis and to determine associated pathologic urinary tract changes. If BPH is diagnosed, accurate determination of prostate size allows the surgeon to determine the optimal surgical approach, usually transurethral resection for mild to moderate prostate enlargement and open prostatectomy for larger glands. In cases of carcinoma of the prostate, various imaging modalities will be necessary for staging to allow the most satisfactory form of therapy. Regardless of the etiology of prostate disease, the integrity of the upper tracts should be evaluated.

Abdominal Radiography

The plain film of the abdomen may yield evidence of a distended bladder, urinary calculi, prostatic calcifications, or bony metastases. The prostate itself is not visualized. Prostatic calculi, when present, are not a reliable indicator of the actual size of the prostate. Although these calculi are often associated with chronic prostatitis, they may be idiopathic in origin. Their incidence in BPH is 7.9 per cent and in prostatic carcinoma 6.4 per cent, negating their use as a diagnostic sign to differentiate these two entities. In BPH, distribution of prostatic calculi is usually peripheral, as they are situated between the hyperplastic nodules and the surgical capsule. In carcinoma of the prostate without associated BPH, calcifications are likely to be small and visible in only one or two ductal systems. In chronic prostatitis, calculi may be numerous, large, and often fused to form large calculous masses owing to destruction of intervening prostatic tissue by the inflammatory process. Calcification may occur on the mucosal surface of an enlarged prostate and, if there is significant intravesical protrusion of the enlarged gland, the calculi may appear to originate within the bladder lumen or even the bladder wall (Fig. 87–1).

Bony structures should be carefully scrutinized for evidence of blastic metastatic disease associated with carcinoma of the prostate. These are usually homogeneously dense and have a rather smudgy appearance, although on occasion they may be well-defined. Particular attention should be paid to the pedicles of the lumbar vertebrae, as they are not uncommon sites of involvement. Occasionally, degenerative disease and Paget's disease are difficult to differentiate from metastatic carcinoma of the prostate.

Excretory Urography

The radiographic study most commonly used to evaluate the urinary tract is the excretory urogram. Anatomic detail and gross function of the entire urinary tract are depicted, along with complications of bladder outlet obstruction such as urinary calculi, bladder diverticula, and significant amounts of residual urine.

When filled with contrast, the base of the normal bladder on the standard anteroposterior view parallels the superior margin of the

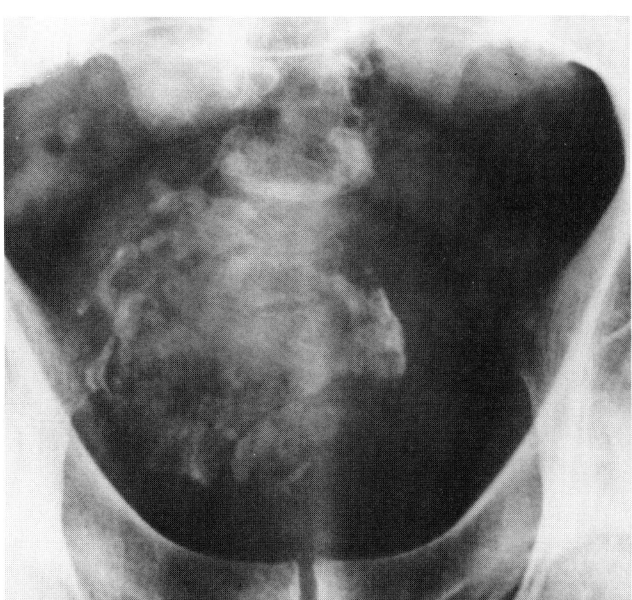

Figure 87–1. Plain film of pelvis showing significant **calcific encrustations on grossly enlarged prostate**.

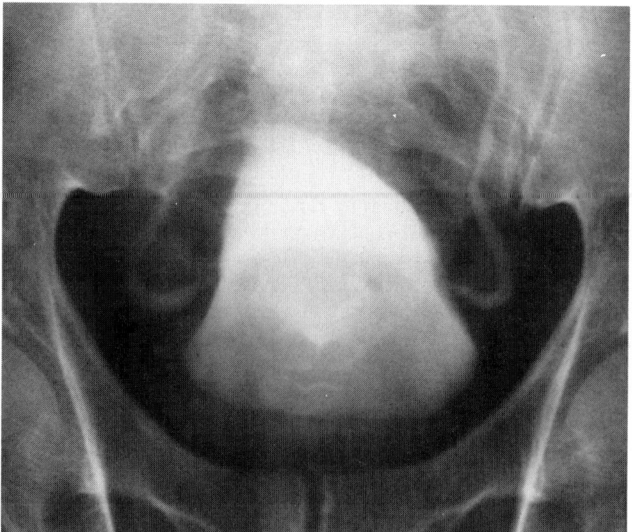

Figure 87–2. Ten-minute urogram film demonstrating "hooking" of both distal ureters due to significant **benign prostatic hypertrophy** causing elevation of the trigone.

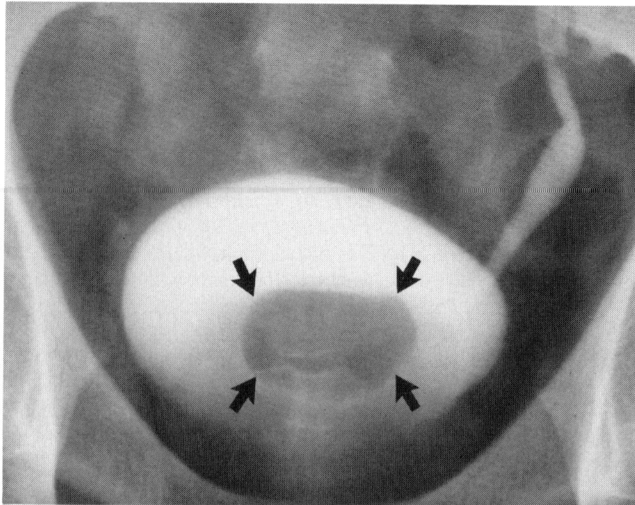

Figure 87–3. Ten-minute urogram film revealing smooth, round, apparently intravesical mass *(arrows).* Cystoscopy and sonography confirmed diagnosis of **intravesical prostate** (lobe of Albarrán).

pubis. Extravesical enlargement of the prostate, when significant, elevates the trigone and floor of the bladder. This extrinsic defect is somewhat posteriorly related to the bladder base, as can be easily demonstrated by oblique views. With progressive enlargement of the prostate, there may be significant elevation of the trigone and therefore the ureteral orifices. This results in "J-ing" or "fish hooking" of the distal ureters (Fig. 87–2). This abnormal ureteral course is the only reliable sign of significant prostatic enlargement. The degree of elevation of the bladder base has not otherwise been found to correlate with the weights of resected prostatic tissue.

Intravesical enlargement of the prostate, a less common presentation, occurs as a result of hypertrophy of the median, subcervical, or subtrigonal lobes. This appears as a smooth, rounded filling defect within the lumen of the bladder projecting from the floor or lower posterior wall on oblique views. Subtrigonal lobe enlargement may occur quite high on the posterior bladder wall and appear completely surrounded by contrast in the opacified bladder (Fig. 87–3). In such cases, the differential includes an inflated Foley balloon, a müllerian duct cyst invaginating the bladder posteriorly, and a large bladder calculus, although the last should be easily seen on the plain film. Less likely differential diagnoses include blood clot, bladder tumor, and urachal carcinoma, all of which usually exhibit an irregular margin. As opposed to the smooth impression on the bladder base associated with BPH, gross irregularity, lobulation, or asymmetry of the prostate should suggest the possibility of carcinoma. However, transitional cell carcinoma of the bladder base may have a similar appearance (Fig. 87–4).

In the opacified normal bladder, the wall is smooth and the detrusor thickness averages only 2 to 3 mm. Thickening of the bladder wall may become apparent as progressive outlet obstruction results in compensatory muscle hypertrophy. In the filled bladder, a feathery appearance of the luminal margin may suggest early trabeculation. However, in such cases cystoscopic confirmation is necessary. As intravesical pressure increases, trabeculation may become more apparent as the bladder mucosa herniates between the muscle bands, forming cellules and saccules. Once herniation progresses through the bladder wall, true diverticula result. These diverticula are commonly multiple, may be of varying sizes, and are located randomly around the bladder.

The failing bladder may exhibit dilatation due to decompensation of the detrusor with resultant fibrosis and thinning. In such cases, large volumes of residual urine are the rule. Once this point is reached, acute urinary retention may be imminent.

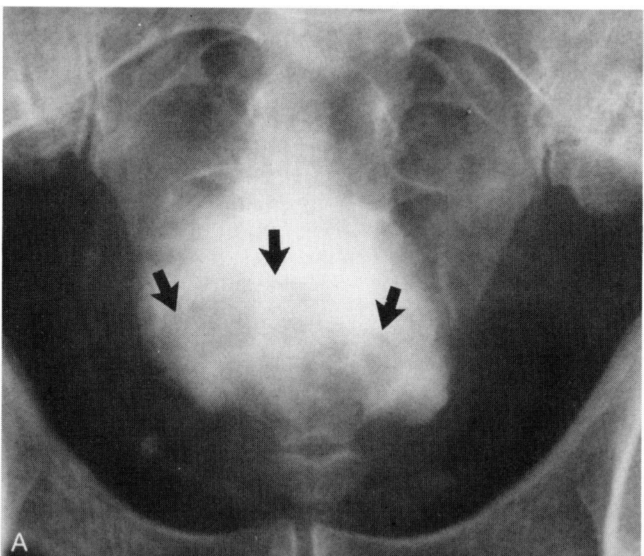

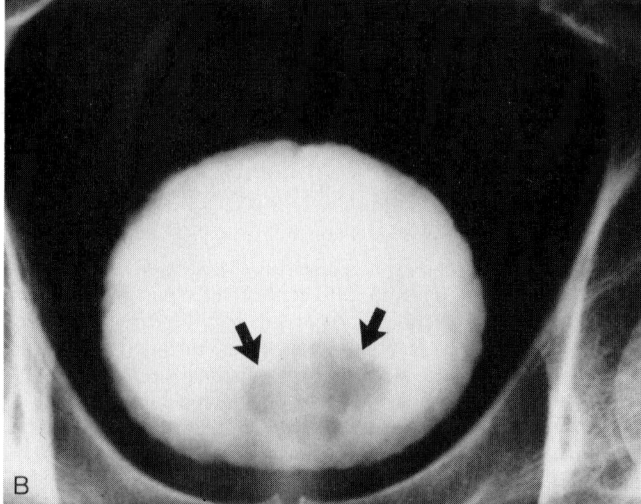

Figure 87–4. *A,* Nodular mass impressing bladder base *(arrows).* **Adenocarcinoma of prostate.** *B,* Nodular mass extending from bladder base *(arrows).* **Transitional cell carcinoma of bladder.**

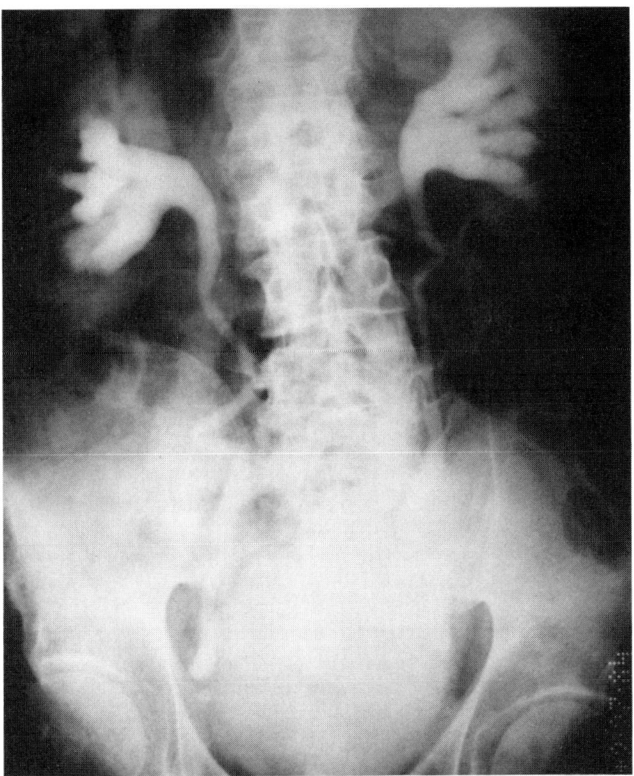

Figure 87–5. Thirty-minute urogram film demonstrating mild symmetrical bilateral hydroureteronephrosis and distended bladder in a case of **bladder outlet obstruction secondary to benign prostatic hypertrophy**.

Urographic estimates of residual urine commonly result in erroneous conclusions concerning the bladder's emptying ability. It should be remembered that the environment of the radiology department is often not conducive to normal voiding. Further, an unmeasurable error is introduced because of the time lapse that may occur between voiding and exposure of the post-void film. Urographically, therefore, in the patient with an otherwise normal-appearing bladder, the only valid clinical inference that can be drawn from the volume of contrast remaining in the bladder on a post-void film is limited to the patient whose film shows no residual.

When increased intravesical pressure and significant residual urine result in functional obstruction of the upper tracts, the degree of hydroureteronephrosis seen is almost invariably equal bilaterally (Fig. 87–5). This is most commonly secondary to BPH and usually resolves after removal of the obstructive process or following catheter drainage of the bladder. Carcinoma of the prostate, on the other hand, when invasive in the retrotrigonal area, may result in asymmetrical or unilateral hydronephrosis.

Medial deviation of either distal ureter may be caused by a nonopacified bladder diverticulum. In such cases, subsequent films usually demonstrate the diverticulum because of mixing of urine and contrast. Another consideration would be metastatic involvement of the pelvic nodes by carcinoma of the prostate or other tumors.

Voiding Cystourethrography

This study is useful for determining the patency of the ureterovesical valve mechanisms. Further, an exposure obtained while voiding provides visualization of the entire urethra. Although enlargement of the prostate in BPH generally increases the entire length of the prostatic urethra, granulomatous prostatitis has been noted to result in selective lengthening of the prostatic urethra in the region below the verumontanum. Also noted with granulomatous prostatitis has been a widening of the prostatic urethra, which helps in differentiating that process from the narrowing seen with carcinoma of the prostate. Median lobe benign hypertrophy often produces an anterior angulation of the prostatic urethra with respect to the bladder base.

Prostate Sonography

The development of the transrectal probe has improved prostate imaging such that it is now a practical modality. Examinations are most frequently done with 5.0 to 7.5 mHz transducers, and the prostate gland is routinely examined in both axial and sagittal planes. A single rectal probe with two transducers eliminates the need to insert a second probe to obtain images in the second plane.

The most common use for transrectal ultrasound (TRUS) examination of the prostate is the early detection of carcinoma. TRUS's proper place in the evaluation of men suspected of having prostate carcinoma is an area of intense investigation. Most investigators feel that it is most appropriately used as part of a protocol that includes not only TRUS but also a digital rectal examination (DRE) and measurement of serum levels of prostate-specific antigen (PSA). The sensitivity of TRUS for the detection of prostate cancer ranges from 60 per cent to more than 90 per cent. However, specificity rates are significantly lower and indicate the need for tissue confirmation. Furthermore, because the positive predictive value of TRUS is not significantly greater than that of DRE, TRUS is not routinely used as a screening modality. TRUS's ability to detect capsular invasion and involvement of the seminal vesicles has also been examined intensively. Although some reports show a high sensitivity, the specificities remain low. Furthermore, TRUS is not effective in detecting microscopic invasion.

The prostate gland can be clearly identified with TRUS and distinguished from surrounding fat, and the volume of the gland can be accurately measured. Differences in echogenicity allow distinction of the peripheral from central zones as well as identification of the seminal vesicles, urethra, and periprostatic venus plexus.

Prostatic carcinoma is most often detected as a hypoechoic area within the peripheral zone (Fig. 87–6). Although the majority of

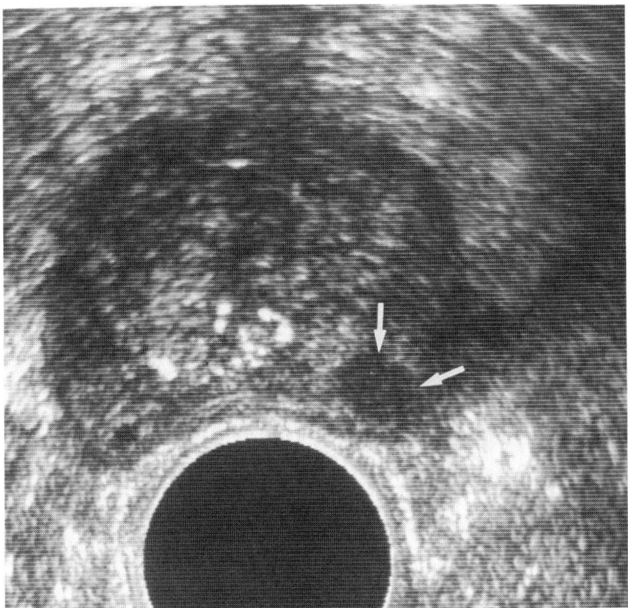

Figure 87–6. Transrectal ultrasound examination of the prostate. This transverse image demonstrates a hypoechoic lesion in the peripheral zone *(arrows)* which is suspicious for **adenocarcinoma**.

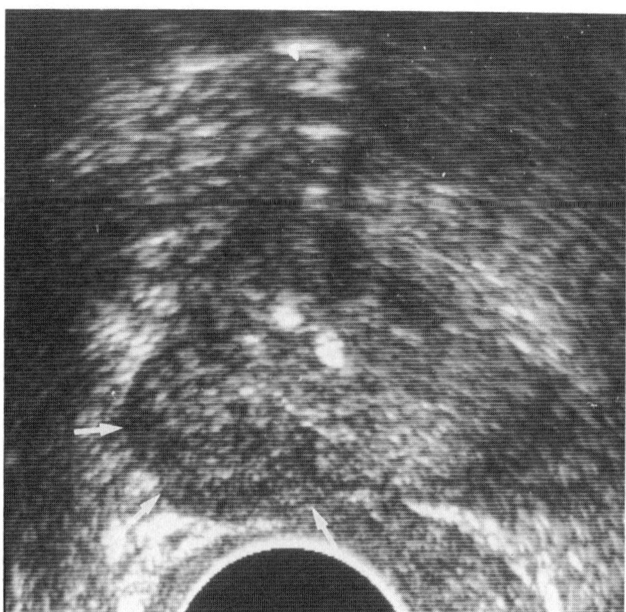

Figure 87–7. Transrectal ultrasound examination of the prostate. This longitudinal view reveals a larger **hypoechoic lesion with capsular bulging** *(arrows).*

carcinomas, especially small lesions, are hypoechoic, isoechoic and even hyperechoic lesions may be found. Larger lesions tend to be more echogenic, and secondary signs such as capsular bulging (Fig. 87–7) or direct extension may aid in their identification.

A hypoechoic lesion in the peripheral zone of the prostate gland is not specific for carcinoma as adenoma/hyperplasia may also give this appearance. Thus, biopsy is needed for confirmation of the diagnosis. Inflammatory lesions may also result in a hypoechoic focus, but most patients with inflammatory prostatitis can be identified by their clinical presentation. The gland is tender, and some patients are unable to tolerate even insertion of the rectal probe.

A completely anechoic lesion is unlikely to represent prostate carcinoma, but rather is usually a prostatic cyst. Cysts have no internal echos and increased through transmission. Prostatic cysts are easily recognized and seldom confused with a solid lesion.

TRUS may be used to monitor the response to treatment. However, it should be recognized that it may be difficult to define the tumor precisely within the prostate gland, particularly after therapy. Thus, total prostate volume is a much more reliable monitor. TRUS may also be used as a guide for the placement of radioactive seed implants into the prostate gland. This treatment technique offers some advantages to external beam irradiation because the radiation dose can be more precisely delivered to the tumor with less damage to normal tissue. Ultrasound guidance permits more satisfactory distribution of the seeds than can be obtained with the "blind" technique.

TRUS's most consistently valuable contribution is to guide the biopsy of suspicious prostate lesions. When an abnormality is detected by TRUS, a needle can be placed precisely within the suspicious area for tissue sampling. If no lesion is detected, TRUS can be used to direct systematic prostate biopsies to provide tissue sampling from all portions of the prostate gland.

Prostate biopsies can be easily performed at the same time as the diagnostic ultrasound examination. A tap-water enema is given prior to the ultrasound examination, but the rectum cannot be adequately sterilized. Thus, many advocate the prophylactic use of antibiotics prior to performing transrectal biopsy. An antibiotic may be given orally one day before the procedure or parenterally immediately prior to the prostate biopsy. Current transrectal probes contain needle guides for 14- to 18-gauge needles, which may be passed into the prostate gland under direct sonographic visualization.

The complications of ultrasound-directed transrectal biopsy are similar to those found when the needle is directed digitally and include local discomfort, fever, sepsis, and bleeding, both per urethra and per rectum. In most patients, these complications are minor and the procedure is appropriately done on an outpatient basis.

Computed Tomography

In imaging the prostate, computed tomography (CT) serves its most useful purpose in staging of malignant disease. The major disadvantage of CT is its inability to characterize various tissue changes occurring within the gland itself. The capsule cannot be differentiated from the adenomatous tissue in BPH, and there are no specific features of confined malignancy on CT sections. A nodular contour of the prostate has been reported to be specific for carcinoma. As prostatic carcinoma advances, CT is able to determine infiltration of the posterior bladder base. Changes in attenuation of prostatic tissue, change or obliteration of the angle between the prostate and seminal vesicles, and alteration of the pelvic fat

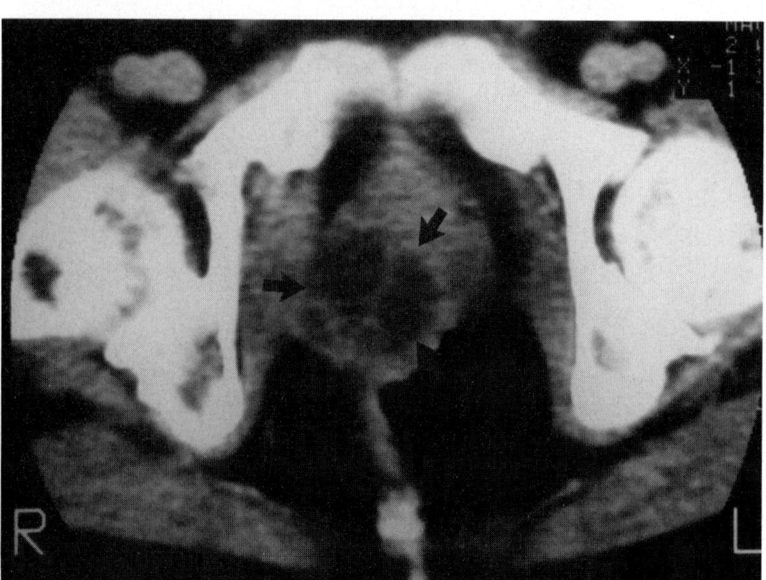

Figure 87–8. Computed tomographic section through prostate demonstrating large, loculated lucent area *(arrows).* **Prostatic abscess** *(Staphylococcus aureus).*

planes have been found in both carcinoma of the prostate and benign enlargement. Therefore, these changes are not helpful in differentiating benign from malignant processes. Calcifications of the prostate are easily detected by CT, as are prostatic abscesses (Fig. 87–8).

Changes in the bladder wall secondary to outlet obstruction may be seen if there is gross thickening. Bladder calculi may be seen in a non-contrasted bladder lumen but may be obscured by contrast material. Any obstructive changes present in the upper tracts are usually well-demonstrated.

Although CT is limited in recognizing minimal nodal disease or microscopic invasion of adjacent pelvic organs by prostatic carcinoma, it has demonstrated an accuracy ranging from 70 to 86 per cent in detecting significant malignant pelvic adenopathy and an accuracy of 47 per cent in detecting local extension.

Magnetic Resonance

Magnetic resonance (MR) has replaced CT as a cross-sectional imaging technique for examining the prostate gland. The spatial resolution of the two examinations is nearly equal, but MR is superior to CT in that it can distinguish among tissues within the prostate gland. The ability to provide direct multiplanar images and the absence of ionizing radiation are further advantages of MR.

MR may be used to detect prostate cancer. On T_1-weighted images, the signal intensity of cancer is equal to or slightly less than that of adjacent normal prostate tissue. However, on T_2-weighted images, the carcinoma usually has a low signal intensity compared with the high signal intensity of the peripheral zone (Fig. 87–9). It is difficult to detect tumors outside the peripheral zone because heterogeneous signal is normally present in the transitional zone.

MR's sensitivity is too low for it to be used as a screening modality for prostate cancer. In a study of 53 patients with clinically palpable prostate cancer reported by Carter et al., MR was able to detect 51 of the palpable tumors (96 per cent sensitivity) but only 19 of 33 unsuspected tumors (58 per cent sensitivity). MR is more accurate in detecting nonpalpable tumors when they are located posteriorly than when they are in the anterior portion of the gland. The posterior portion of the prostate is well-evaluated with TRUS. Approximately 70 per cent of prostate cancers arise in the peripheral zone; 20 per cent begin in the transitional zone and 10 per cent in the central zone. Furthermore, an area of fibrosis in the peripheral zone may result in a hypointense signal indistinguishable from that of carcinoma. A biopsy prior to the MR examination creates confusion by introducing blood into the area of interest.

The more practical application of MR is in the staging of prostate cancer. Accuracies over 80 per cent have been reported, and this rate should improve with the use of endorectal surface coils. Tumor confined to the prostate gland (Stages A and B) is amenable to treatment with radical prostatectomy and the possibility of cure. The abnormal signal is confined to the prostate gland, and the periprostatic fat remains normal. Disease that has spread beyond the capsule is more likely to be treated with radiation therapy and/or hormonal therapy. Extension beyond the gland is seen on MR as a contour bulge and a decrease in signal intensity on T_2-weighted images of the periprostatic fat or seminal vesicles.

Detection of tumor extension into the bladder or rectum is facilitated by imaging in the sagittal plane. An interruption of the bladder wall's low signal intensity indicates tumor invasion. Involvement of the rectum is uncommon in prostate cancer but can be detected by MR as obliteration of the perirectal fat plane, disruption of Denonvillier's fascia and a higher signal intensity of the anterior rectal wall.

Involvement of the pelvic lymph nodes by metastatic tumor can also be detected by MR using size criteria, similar to CT. MR may be particularly useful, however, in distinguishing potentially enlarged lymph nodes from the periprostatic venous plexus.

Interventional Radiology of the Prostate

The most frequently used interventional technique is transrectal biopsy. Automated biopsy devices have been adapted to transrectal ultrasound probes so the needle can be directed into suspicious lesions detected by TRUS. In addition, ultrasound-directed biopsies are a more reliable technique for obtaining biopsy samples from all portions of the gland when systematic or random biopsies are desired.

Percutaneous biopsy of enlarged lymph nodes to confirm metastatic tumor is usually guided by CT. This is not limited to enlarged regional lymph nodes, but may be applied to any area suspected of being involved by tumor.

Prostate abscess is amenable to transrectal catheter drainage. A

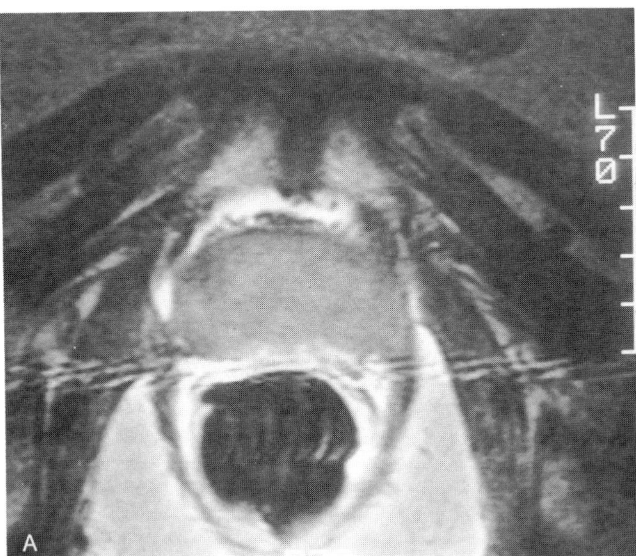

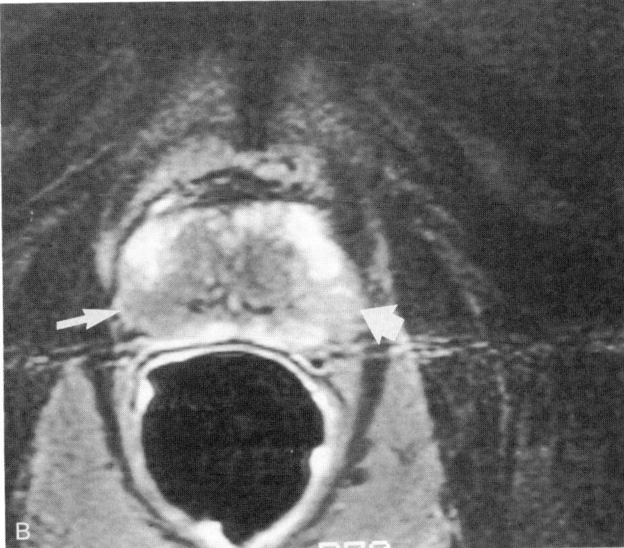

Figure 87–9. *A*, T_1-weighted magnetic resonance image of the prostate gland obtained using an endorectal coil. No tumor is seen. *B*, T_2-weighted image reveals low-signal intensity lesion on both sides of the gland. The lesion on the right *(arrow)* is **adenocarcinoma** while the left-sided lesion *(arrowhead)* is benign.

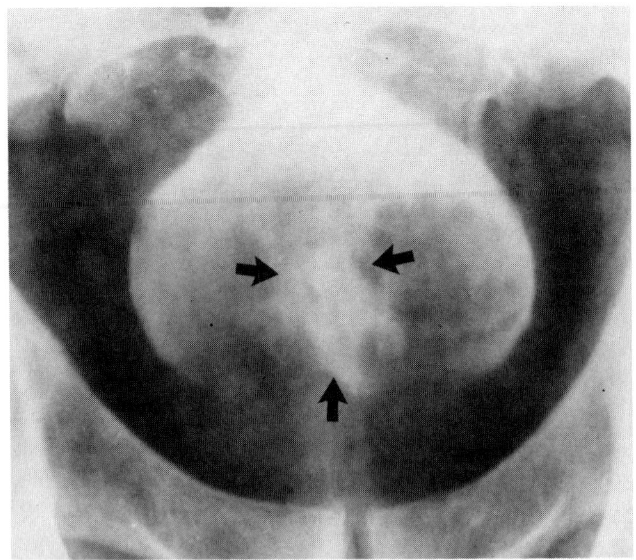

Figure 87–10. Bladder phase of urogram showing **large prostate (benign prostatic hypertrophy)** elevating bladder base and extending into lumen. The central collection of contrast *(arrows)* is typical of previous transurethral resection. In this case, 180 g of prostatic adenoma had been resected several years earlier and there is now significant regrowth.

tender, fluctuant prostate on DRE is the most characteristic finding. Transrectal ultrasound demonstrates an echopenic mass and may be used to direct needle placement.

Several reports have confirmed that bladder outlet obstruction secondary to BPH may be treated with balloon dilation of the posterior urethra. The position of the balloon must be monitored closely by fluoroscopy or ultrasound to prevent damage to the external sphincter. Although clinical success has been achieved, the durability of the technique has not yet been confirmed.

RADIOGRAPHIC CHANGES AFTER PROSTATECTOMY

Surgical intervention for benign obstructive disease of the prostate is common. For the moderate-sized gland, transurethral resection of the prostate is preferred by most urologists. For the grossly enlarged gland, an open simple prostatectomy with enucleation of the adenoma from the surgical capsule is performed. Either approach results in a fairly characteristic radiographic pattern. In such cases, contrast is usually seen in the region of the prostatic urethra on the bladder phase of the urogram (Fig. 87–10). This occurs as a result of the disruption of the internal sphincter mechanism at the bladder neck as a normal part of the prostatectomy. Contrast should not be seen below the region of the urogenital diaphragm, as the intact intrinsic sphincter continues to provide passive continence. Regrowth of adenomatous tissue in the posterior urethra may create a nodular appearance.

Carcinoma of the prostate in its early stages may be treated by a radical prostatectomy. This involves excision of the entire prostate, including the surgical capsule as well as the seminal vesicles. After resection, the free edges of the bladder neck are pulled down and anastomosed to the remaining stump of the membranous urethra as

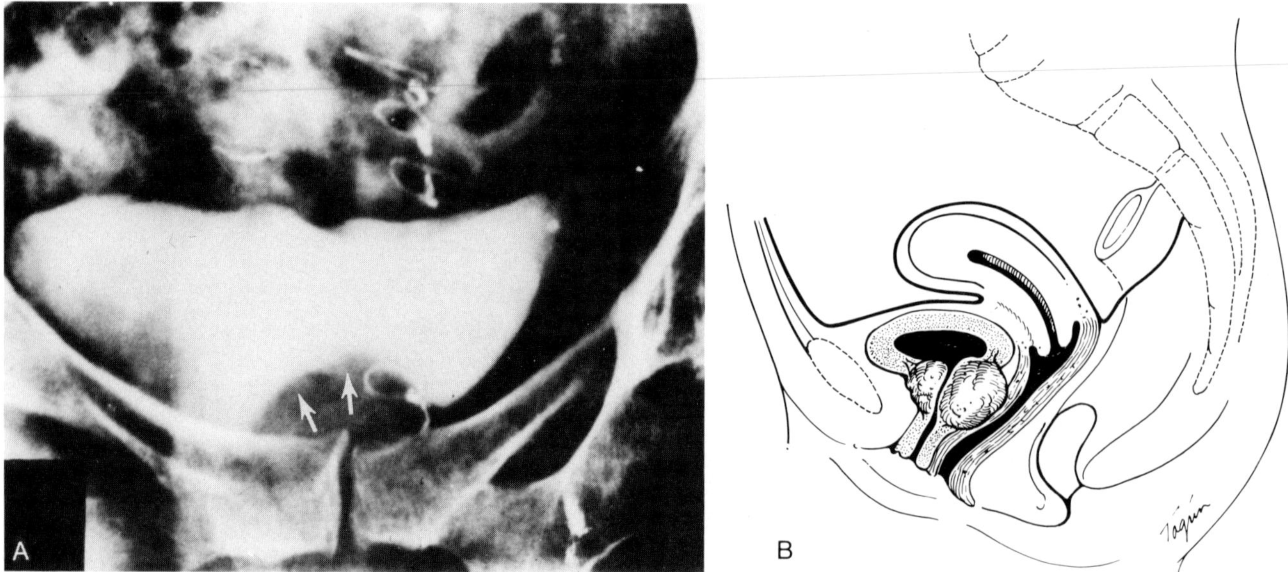

Figure 87–11. *A*, Bladder phase of urogram demonstrating a **female prostate** *(arrows)*. In this case the patient, an 85-year-old woman, suffered severe lower urinary tract irritative symptoms. Biopsy revealed only inflammatory tissue. *B*, Sagittal diagram of the female pelvis depicting the periurethral mass of inflammatory tissue adjacent to bladder neck. (Reprinted with permission from Amis ES Jr, Cronan JJ, Yoder IC, Pfister RC: Impressions on floor of female bladder: "The female prostate." Urology 19:441–446, 1982.)

TABLE 87–2. ETIOLOGIES OF THE "FEMALE PROSTATE"

Adjacent structures impressing bladder base
Cervix (retroverted uterus)
Levator ani muscle (postulated)
Inflammatory lesions
Periurethritis (female urethral syndrome)
Urethral diverticulum (proximal third of urethra)
Neoplastic lesions
Bladder floor tumors
Urethral tumors (proximal portion)
Anterior vaginal wall tumors
Bony lesions of pubic symphysis
Neoplastic
Degenerative joint disease
Miscellaneous lesions
Prostatic tissue (female pseudohermaphrodite)
Hematoma (post-traumatic or postoperative)
Urethral suspension surgery (for stress incontinence)
Ectopic ureterocele

it protrudes through the urogenital diaphragm superiorly. Again, as in simple prostatectomy, the intrinsic sphincter around the membranous urethra provides passive continence of urine. The postoperative appearance is classic in such patients, with funneling of the bladder base noted in the retropubic area to the level of the urogenital diaphragm. Also, in these cases, one will usually find multiple metallic clips in the pelvis resulting from the staging pelvic lymphadenectomy that precedes the actual resection of the carcinomatous prostate.

THE FEMALE PROSTATE

"Female prostate" is the term used to denote an impression on the female bladder base resulting in an appearance similar to that produced by benign prostate enlargement in the male (Fig. 87–11). As can be seen in Table 87–2, multiple etiologies for this finding have been reported. The more common causes include diverticula of the proximal urethra and significant degenerative changes of the pubic symphysis. Although these causes are benign, malignancy may rarely produce a similar picture. In reporting the finding, therefore, the possibility of a malignant etiology should be mentioned.

Bibliography

Amis ES Jr, Cronan JJ, Yoder IC, Pfister RC: Impressions on floor of female bladder: "The female prostate." Urology 19:441, 1982.

Amis ES Jr, Pfister RC, Yoder IC: Interventional radiology of the adult bladder and urethra. Semin Roentgenol 18:322, 1983.

Benson MC, Whang IS, Pantuck A, et al: Prostate specific antigen density: A means of distinguishing benign prostatic hypertrophy and prostate cancer. J Urol 147:815–816, 1992.

Carter HB, Brem RF, Tempany CM, et al: Nonpalpable prostate cancer: Detection with MR Imaging. Radiology 178:523–525, 1991.

Fox M: The natural history and significance of stone formation in the prostate gland. J Urol 89:716, 1963.

Hammerer P, Loy V, Dieringer J, Huland H: Prostate cancer in nonurological patients with normal prostates on digital rectal examination. J Urol 147:833–836, 1992.

Hricak H: Imaging prostate carcinoma. Radiology 169:569–571, 1988.

Labrie F, Dupont A, Suburu R, et al: Serum prostate specific antigen as prescreening test for prostate cancer. J Urol 147:846–852, 1992.

Lang EK: Neoplasms of the bladder, prostate and urethra. Semin Roentgenol 18:288, 1983.

McNeal JE: Normal and pathologic anatomy of prostate. Urology 17(Suppl):11, 1981.

Ney C, Miller HL, Levy JL: Granulomatous prostatitis. Urology 21:320, 1983.

Poon PY, Bronskill MJ, Poon CS, et al: Identification of the periprostatic venous plexus by MR imaging. J Comp Assist Tomogr 15:265–268, 1991.

Popovich MJ, Hricak H. The prostate and seminal vesicles. In Higgins CB, Hricak H, Helms CS (eds): Magnetic Resonance Imaging of the Body. New York, Raven Press, 1992, pp 911–938.

Rifkin MD, Dahnert W, Kurtz AB. State of the art: Endorectal sonography of the prostate gland. AJR 154:691–700, 1990.

Schiebler ML, McSherry S, Keefe B, et al: Comparison of the digital rectal examination, endorectal ultrasound, and body coil magnetic resonance imaging in the staging of adenocarcinoma of the prostate. Urol Radiol 13:110–118, 1991.

Schnall MD, Imai Y, Tomaszewski J, et al: Prostate cancer: Local staging with endorectal surface coil MR imaging. Radiology 178:797–802, 1991.

Shinohara K, Wheeler TM, Scardino PT: The appearance of prostate cancer on transrectal ultrasonography: Correlation of imaging and pathological examinations. J Urol 142:76–82, 1989.

Stamey TA: Editorial: Diagnosis of prostate cancer: A personal view. J Urol 147:830–832, 1992.

Terris MK, Freiha FS, McNeal JE, Stamey TS: Efficacy of transrectal ultrasound for identification of clinically undetected prostate cancer. J Urol 146:78–84, 1991.

Vallancien G, Prapotnich D, Veillon B, et al: Systematic prostatic biopsies in 100 men with no suspicion of cancer on digital rectal examination. J Urol 146:1308–1312, 1991.

Waterhouse RL, Resnick MI: The use of transrectal prostatic ultrasonography in the evaluation of patients with prostatic carcinoma. J Urol 141:233–239, 1989.

Weaver RP, Noble MJ, Weigel JW: Correlation of ultrasound guided and digitally directed transrectal biopsies of palpable prostatic abnormalities. J Urol 145:516–518, 1991.

88 The Urethra and Seminal Vesicles

Carl M. Sandler and Ronald W. McCallum

METHOD OF URETHROGRAPHY IN MALES

Dynamic retrograde and voiding urethrography are the methods by which the evaluation of the urethra is performed. Dynamic retrograde urethrography (DRU) implies motion of contrast medium through the urethra during exposure of the film. Exposure of the film during injection is the only way to visualize consistently the posterior urethra and verumontanum, which is an essential landmark for localization of the membranous urethra. The posterior urethra is rarely visualized in static retrograde urethrography (exposure of the film after the contrast medium has been injected into the urethra) because of the milk-back action of the intrinsic sphincter, which pushes into the bladder the few milliliters of contrast medium lying in the posterior urethra. DRU may be performed using a Brodney or Knudson clamp, but most authors prefer the Foley catheter technique. In this method, a Foley catheter is attached to a 50-ml syringe containing 30 per cent contrast medium and flushed to remove the air from the catheter lumen before the catheter is inserted into the penis. The catheter (size 14 to 16) is inserted 2 to 3 cm into the penis, and 1 or 2 ml of saline is injected into the balloon of the catheter, fixing it in the fossa navicularis. No lubricant should be used. Mild traction is applied to the catheter and syringe during the retrograde injection in order to straighten the penis at the penoscrotal junction. The patient should be positioned in the 25- to 30-degree oblique position; in the anteroposterior position, the bulbous urethra is superimposed on itself so that it cannot be satisfactorily imaged. Two or three films are obtained during the dynamic retrograde study, preferably done with fluoroscopy.

Voiding cystography is performed by advancing the Foley catheter into the urinary bladder and filling the bladder with 30 per cent contrast material. The catheter is then removed and the patient is asked to void. Once again, filming, particularly in the male, should be performed in the 25- to 30-degree oblique position. A spot film camera, set at two films per second, is helpful but not mandatory.

Both studies, voiding and retrograde, are useful in patients with extensive stricture disease, but the voiding procedure may be difficult to obtain if the stricture disease precludes the successful placement of the Foley catheter into the bladder.

Both voiding and retrograde studies should also be obtained in patients who have suffered urethral injuries prior to urethroplasty. In such cases, the studies should be performed simultaneously so that both the proximal and distal extents of the traumatic urethral stricture may be evaluated.

Occasionally, extra catheters are required when the patient presents with a perineal fistula. These extra catheters are inserted into the perineal fistulous tracts, and two or three catheters are injected at the same time in order to visualize the whole urethra. The Foley catheter method is also of value in evaluating the site of outlet obstruction in patients with neurogenic bladder. Obstruction may occur at the bladder neck or may be due to prostatic hypertrophy or sphincter dyssynergia. Sphincter dyssynergia is the most common cause of outlet obstruction in patients with upper motor neuron lesions.

The complications of the procedure are few. Extravasation of contrast medium into penile and perineal veins may occur either by overenthusiastic dilatation of the catheter balloon, causing a mucosal tear, or at the site of a severe stricture if too much pressure is applied during the retrograde injection. Although extravasation is rare if the examination is carefully performed under fluoroscopy, the possibility of extravasation into penile and perineal veins raises the same risk of reactions to contrast medium associated with any intravenous injection of contrast medium.

NORMAL ANATOMY ON URETHROGRAPHY IN MALES

Anatomically and on DRU, the male urethra is divided into the anterior and the posterior urethra by the inferior fascia or the urogenital diaphragm (Fig. 88–1). The anterior urethra is a simple tube of mucous membrane and connective tissue stroma surrounded by the cavernous tissue of the corpus spongiosum, on the dorsal aspect of which lie both corpora cavernosa. The anterior urethra is in turn subdivided into the penile urethra, which extends from the external meatus to the penoscrotal junction, and the bulbous urethra, from the penoscrotal junction to the inferior edge of the urogenital diaphragm. The most proximal bulbous urethra forms a symmetrical convex cone shape, the tip of which represents the inferior border of the membranous urethra. The posterior urethra is more complex because it is the site of the urinary sphincters, the verumontanum, and the prostate. It is divided into the membranous and prostatic urethras, respectively. The membranous urethra is located between the tip of the cone of the bulbous urethra and the inferior edge of the verumontanum in the urogenital diaphragm and is approximately 1.5 cm in length. It is seen as a thin 2-mm wisp of contrast medium continuous with the symmetrical cone of the proximal bulbous urethra extending to the verumontanum, a 1-cm filling defect in the posterior wall of the prostatic urethra. The prostatic urethra extends from the inferior border of the verumontanum to the bladder neck, which is recognized as a jet of contrast medium passing through the internal sphincter.

There are three urinary sphincters: two are smooth muscle, one is striated muscle (Fig. 88–2). The proximal smooth muscle sphincter is the internal sphincter adjacent to the bladder neck. The distal smooth muscle sphincter is the intrinsic sphincter that surrounds the membranous urethra in close proximity to the submucosa and mu-

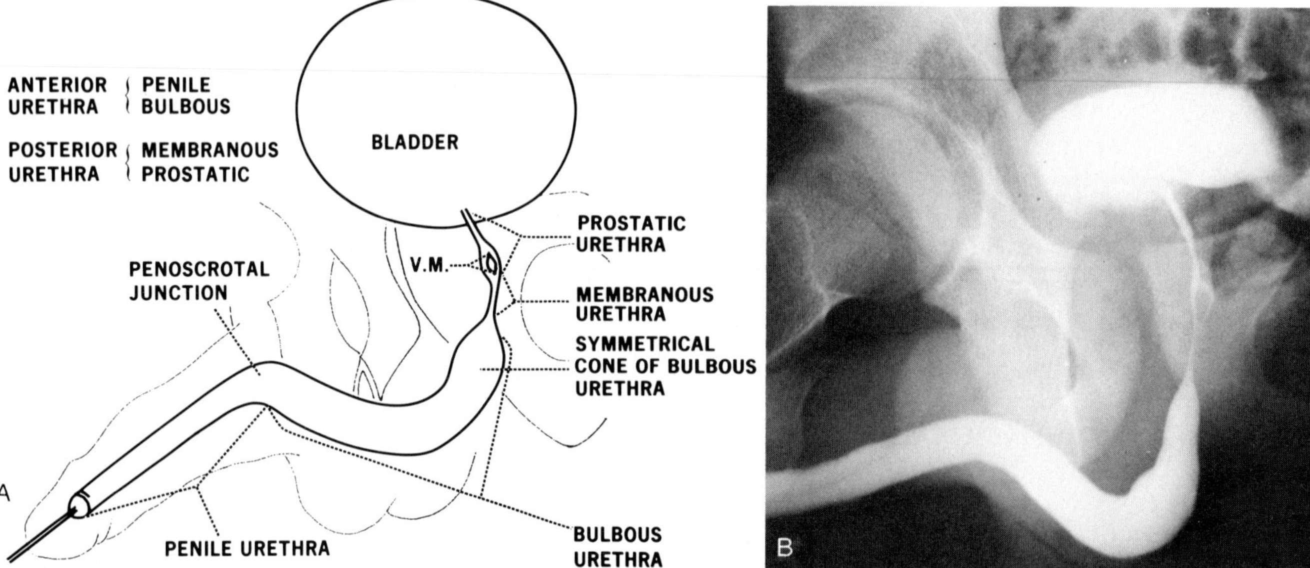

Figure 88–1. *A*, Tracing of a **normal dynamic retrograde urethrogram** showing important radiologic landmarks. (V.M. = verumontanum.) *B*, Normal dynamic retrograde urethrogram. (From McCallum RW, Colapinto V: Urological Radiology of the Adult Male Lower Urinary Tract. Springfield, IL, Charles C Thomas, Publisher, 1976, by permission.)

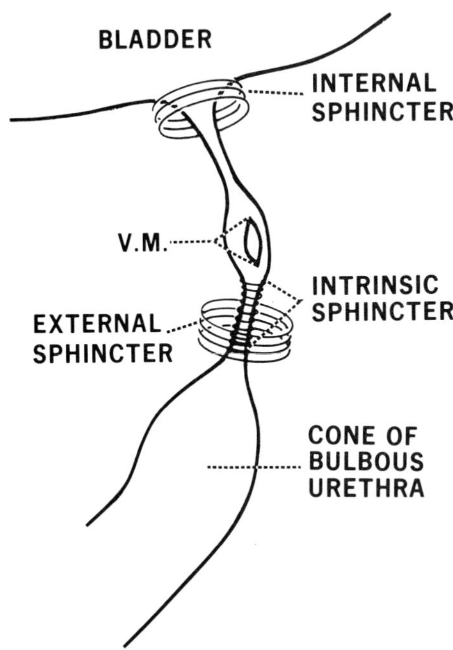

Figure 88–2. Diagrammatic representation of the **three urinary sphincters**. The internal and intrinsic sphincters are smooth muscle. The external sphincter is striated muscle. (V.M. = verumontanum.) (From McCallum RW: The adult male urethra: Normal anatomy, pathology and method of urethrography. Radiol Clin North Am 17:227, 1979.)

cosa. Both smooth muscle sphincters maintain passive continence and are governed by the sympathetic hypogastric nerves. The external striated muscle sphincter supplied by the pudendal nerve surrounds the intrinsic sphincter and membranous urethra and also passes arcuate fibers proximally within the prostatic capsule to the bladder neck. The external sphincter plays little if any part in passive continence but functions in active continence by interrupting micturition and inhibiting stress incontinence on increased intra-abdominal pressure. On DRU examination, all sphincters sustain normal tone to maintain passive continence.

The verumontanum contains three orifices. Midline is the orifice of the prostatic utricle, a vestigial remnant of the müllerian duct that is a short 1-cm blind-end tube extending into the medial lobe of the prostate. Inferior to the prostatic utricle orifice, the two orifices of the ejaculatory ducts lie close to the midline. The ejaculatory ducts are 1.5 cm in length and are formed by the ampullae of the vas deferens and the ducts of the seminal vesicles, which are paired convoluted structures inferior to the inferoposterior aspect of the bladder. In normal DRU, no reflux into the prostatic utricle or ejaculatory ducts is seen.

On the voiding study, some differences in the visualized anatomy can be appreciated (Fig. 88–3). The bladder neck is open and measures 1 to 1.5 cm in diameter. The prostatic urethra is filled with contrast medium, and the membranous urethra expands to 5 or 6 mm in diameter. The verumontanum lengthens, and the posterior urethra descends approximately 1 cm owing to relaxation of the urogenital diaphragm. Detrusor contraction is stimulated by the parasympathetic pelvic nerves, and sphincter relaxation is reciprocal. The cone of the proximal bulbous urethra disappears on the voiding study, and the bulbous urethra is well-visualized to the penoscrotal junction where the penile urethra bends downward. The radiologist should make sure that the urinal is not pressing against the urethra at the penoscrotal junction, since the penoscrotal junction is a common site of stricture. The edge of the urinal pressing against the urethra may cause reduction in flow and narrowing in this region, which may be mistaken for stricture.

ABNORMAL URETHROGRAPHY

Congenital Urethral Anomalies and Urethral Diverticula

Congenital urethral duplication, urethral valves, saccular or diffuse diverticulum, and congenital urethroperineal fistula have been

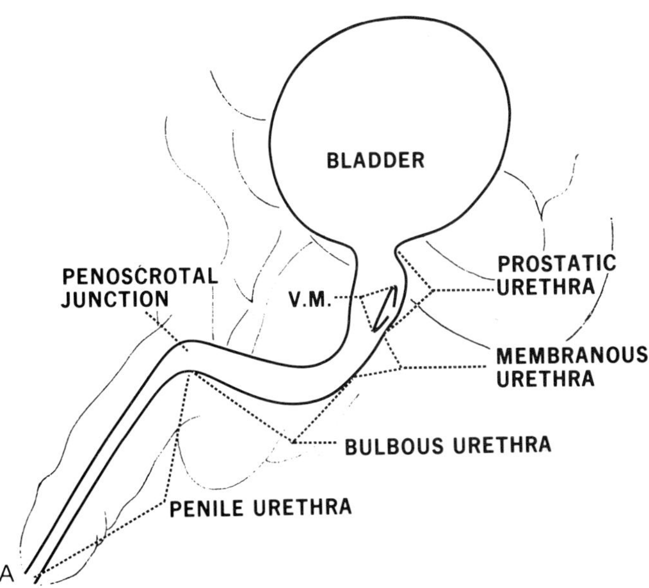

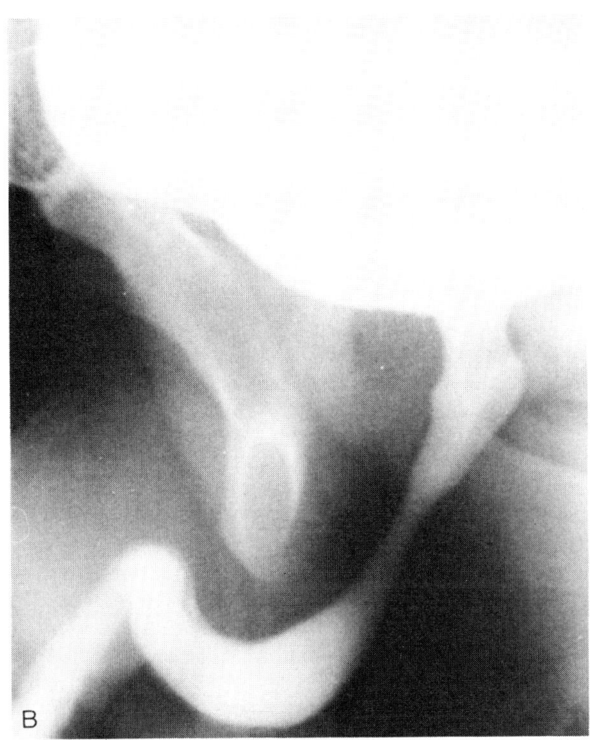

Figure 88–3. *A*, Tracing of a **normal voiding urethrogram** showing normal radiologic landmarks. (V.M. = verumontanum.) *B*, **Normal voiding urethrogram**. (From McCallum RW, Colapinto V: Urological Radiology of the Adult Male Lower Urinary Tract. Springfield, IL, Charles C Thomas, Publisher, 1976, by permission.)

reported in male infants and young male patients. Congenital urethral valves and fibrous bands have been reported in female infants. Anterior urethral diverticula, when congenital, are generally classified as diffuse or saccular. The diffuse variety is the same as megalourethra. Most anterior urethral diverticula in males and female diverticula are acquired. In males they are generally a consequence of long-term Foley catheterization, periurethral abscess, or trauma (discussed later).

Acquired Urethral Abnormalities

URETHRAL INFECTIONS

Infections affecting the urethra are the gonorrhea, tuberculosis, schistosomiasis (bilharziasis), viruses, and mixed bacterial infections associated with catheterization.

GONORRHEA. Gonorrhea is the major cause of urethral stricture in underdeveloped countries, since the majority of patients are untreated or inadequately treated. If adequate early antibiotic therapy is applied, urethral scarring is avoided. Only 40 per cent of urethral strictures are due to the gonococcus in North America. Gonococcal infection ascends the urethra, causing mucosal and submucosal inflammatory reaction in the anterior urethra, and involves the glands of Littre. Spread of the infection into the glands of Littre and corpus spongiosum causes venous thrombosis and eventual scarring. Urethrography usually shows a long irregular area of scarring in the mid-bulbous urethra, frequently with visualization of the glands of Littre. Of prime importance in the assessment of mid- or proximal bulbous urethral stricture is an evaluation of the cone of the proximal bulbous urethra, which in normal patients is symmetrical, smooth, and convex. If the cone of the proximal bulbous urethra is not symmetrical, smooth, and convex, but rather is narrowed, elongated, irregular, and asymmetrical, there is a strong indication that the proximal bulbous urethral disease extends into the membranous urethra and that transphincter urethroplasty will be required for complete eradication. This finding is not uncommon in gonococcal urethral scarring (Fig. 88–4). With extensive disease, multiple urethral perineal fistulas may develop, a phenomenon known as a "watering can perineum" (Fig. 88–5).

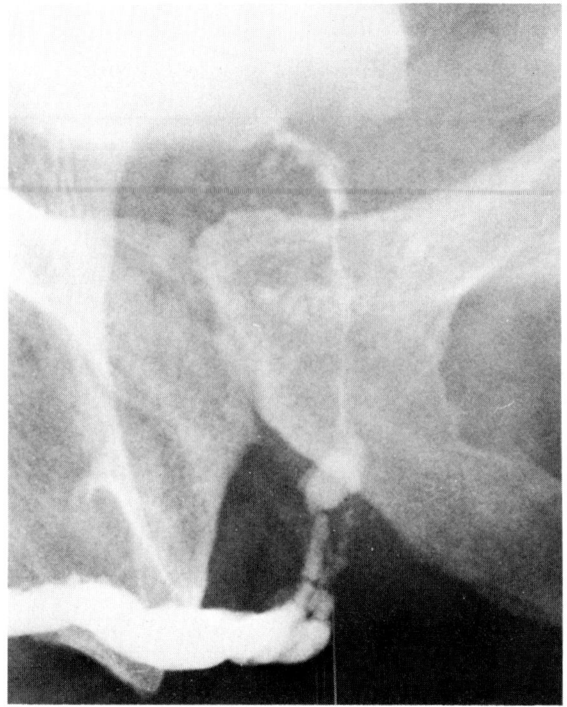

Figure 88–4. A patient with **gonococcal stricture in the mid-proximal bulbous urethra.** The cone of the proximal bulbous urethra is abnormal, being narrowed, elongated, and asymmetrical, indicating scarring that extends into the membranous urethra, confirmed at operation. Note the glands of Littre.

TUBERCULOSIS. Tuberculosis rarely affects the lower urinary tract. When present, it is a descending infection, most patients having concurrent manifestations of renal tuberculosis. Tuberculosis prostatitis and granulomatous prostatic abscess are the most common manifestations. Rarely, periurethral abscess, perineal fistula, and urethral scarring are seen. Antituberculous therapy promotes healing with calcification and fibrous tissue development, and treatment of the disease may lead to urethral stricture.

SCHISTOSOMIASIS (BILHARZIASIS). *Schistosoma haematobium* is a parasite prevalent in Africa and the Nile Valley. It is rare in Europe, and is unknown in North America. Abscess formation, calcification, and scarring affect the ureters, bladder, seminal vesicles, prostate, and urethra. Urethral fistulas are common and invariably result in urethral stricture. Fistulas between the bowel and urinary tract are common, and carcinoma of the bladder is a frequent complication in untreated cases.

CONDYLOMA ACUMINATUM. *Condyloma acuminata* (venereal warts) are caused by a papilloma virus infection on the skin of the genital region. Uncommonly such infections may spread into the urethra and result in an acute urethral discharge. Urethral involvement may be demonstrated by retrograde urethrography as multiple urethral filling defects ranging in size from 1 to 10 mm. Urethral strictures are generally not present.

PERIURETHRAL ABSCESS. Periurethral abscess is an acute life-threatening infection that originates in the periurethral glands of Littre. If the ostium of such a gland becomes occluded by inspissated pus or fibrosis, a periurethral abscess may form. A history of either venereal disease or previous urethral stricture disease is present in 80 per cent of the cases. The abscess tends to spread within the confines of Buck's fascia but may extend to the buttocks, thigh, or anterior abdominal wall. If the abscess drains spontaneously into the urethra, it may be demonstrated radiologically by retrograde urethrography (Fig. 88–6). The cavity of such an abscess may epithelialize after drainage, forming an acquired urethral diverticulum.

URETHRAL INFECTION ASSOCIATED WITH CATHETERIZATION. Bladder catheterization via the urethra may result in

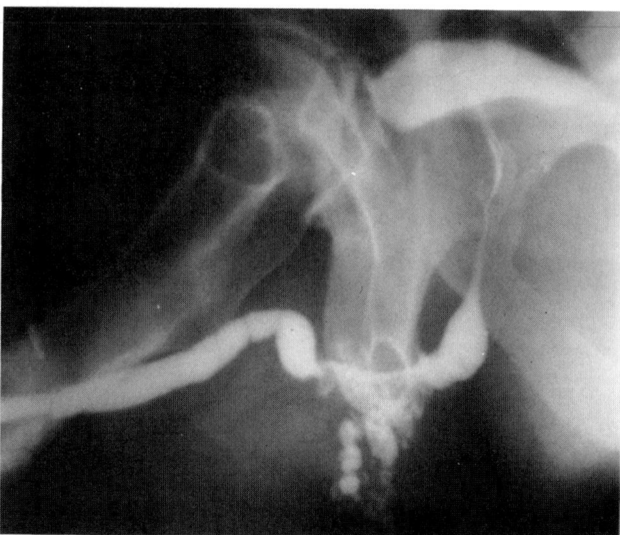

Figure 88–5. Watering-can perineum. Multiple urethral perineal fistulas are present in a patient with extensive stricture disease involving the bulbous urethra.

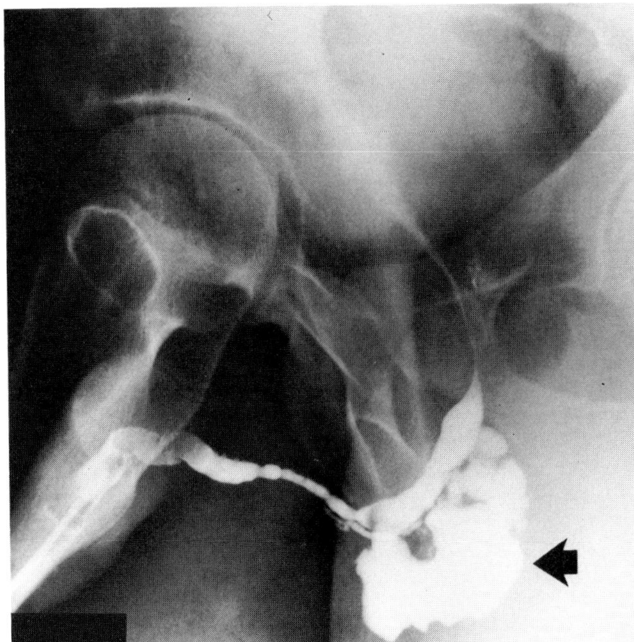

Figure 88–6. Periurethral abscess. A multiloculated periurethral abscess is present *(arrow)* in the perineum. Extensive urethral stricture disease is also present.

urethral infection, usually of mixed gram-negative organisms. The initial injury to the urethra is pressure necrosis that occurs at the fixed points of the urethra, i.e., the penoscrotal junction and the membranous urethra. In addition, if the penis is not strapped onto the anterior abdominal wall but is left to hang loose or is strapped to the thigh, pressure necrosis may occur at the penoscrotal junction. This latter situation is the most common cause of catheter strictures. It is almost inevitable that the area of pressure necrosis becomes infected, resulting in further urethral damage. Strictures due to pressure necrosis alone are generally short. Strictures due to pressure necrosis and superimposed infection are generally long and irregular, and glands of Littre are commonly visualized. Consequently, most catheter strictures occur at the penoscrotal junction and are long and irregular (Fig. 88–7). Occasionally a catheter stricture is due to pressure necrosis alone without superimposed infection and is short and well-defined.

REITER'S SYNDROME

The triad of urethritis, polyarthritis, and conjunctivitis is known as Reiter's syndrome. A number of patients also demonstrate a variety of mucocutaneous lesions. The disease generally affects males ages 15 to 30. In rare instances, urethritis may progress and result in extensive urethral necrosis and stricture disease.

URETHRAL DIVERTICULUM

In women, urethral diverticula are a common cause of frequency, dysuria, and post-void dribbling. They generally occur as a result of abscess formation in the periurethral glands. Urethroscopy may not reveal the orifice of a diverticulum consistently, and urethrography may be required for demonstration. A positive-pressure urethrogram can be obtained by the double-balloon catheter method. A Foley catheter balloon blocks the bladder neck, and a second balloon slides along the catheter to block the external meatus. Contrast medium fills the urethra and diverticulum from the catheter orifice between the balloons. More commonly, voiding cystourethrography in the erect, steep-oblique or lateral position is used and is generally successful in showing a urethral diverticulum (Fig. 88–8). Rarely, an ectopic ureteral orifice emptying into the female urethra may masquerade as a urethral diverticulum, and partial filling of the ectopic ureter may look like a urethral diverticulum. The radiologist should exclude this possibility by carefully scrutinizing the patient's excretory urogram to exclude a double collecting system with obstruction of the upper pole moiety.

Urethral Trauma

The urethra may be injured in pelvic fracture, straddle injury, and iatrogenic trauma.

URETHRAL INJURY IN PELVIC FRACTURE

Some degree of urethral injury occurs in 4 to 17 per cent of male patients sustaining a pelvic fracture. Urethral injury may be classified clinically as incomplete (urethral contusion), partial (a tear in the urethra), or complete (rupture of the urethra, usually with separation of the avulsed ends). Clinical criteria for the assessment of urethral injury in pelvic fracture include blood at the urethral meatus, inability to void, a high or hypermobile prostate on rectal examination, and inability to pass a catheter into the bladder.

In the past 10 years, urethrography has become accepted as the

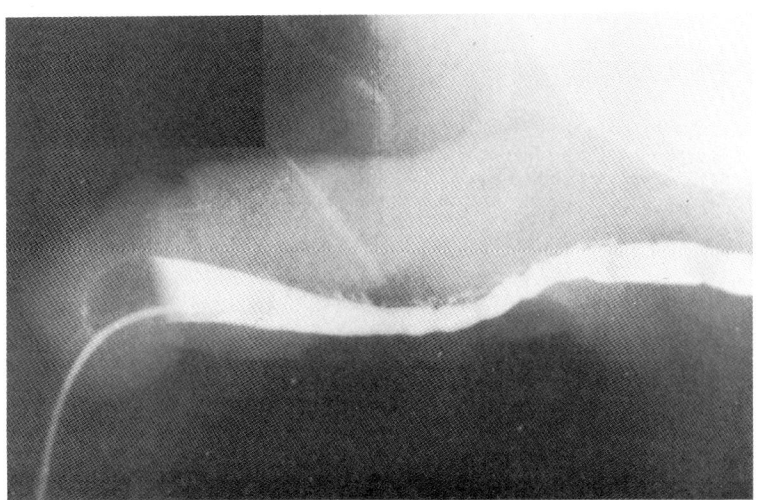

Figure 88–7. Irregular urethral scarring extending distally and proximally from the penoscrotal junction due to 10 days with an indwelling catheter. Note that the glands of Littre are well visualized.

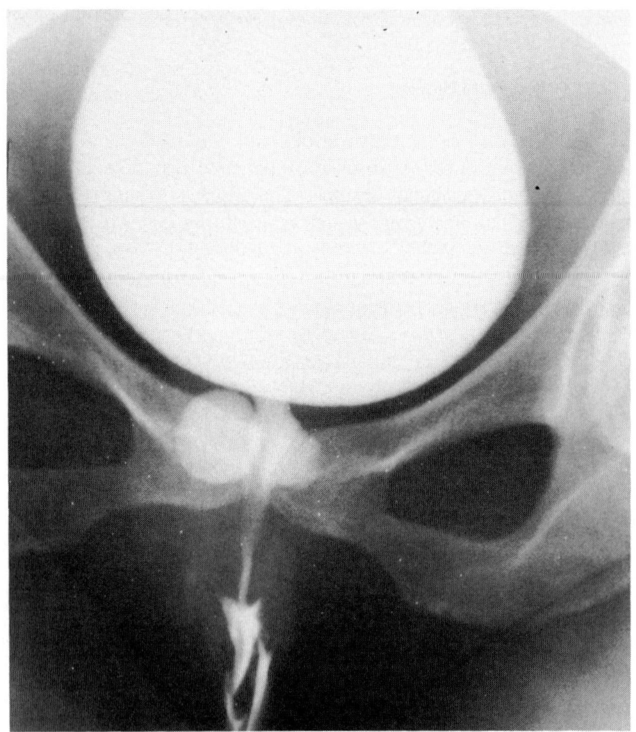

Figure 88–8. Urethral diverticula. A bilobed urethral diverticulum is demonstrated on voiding cystourethrography.

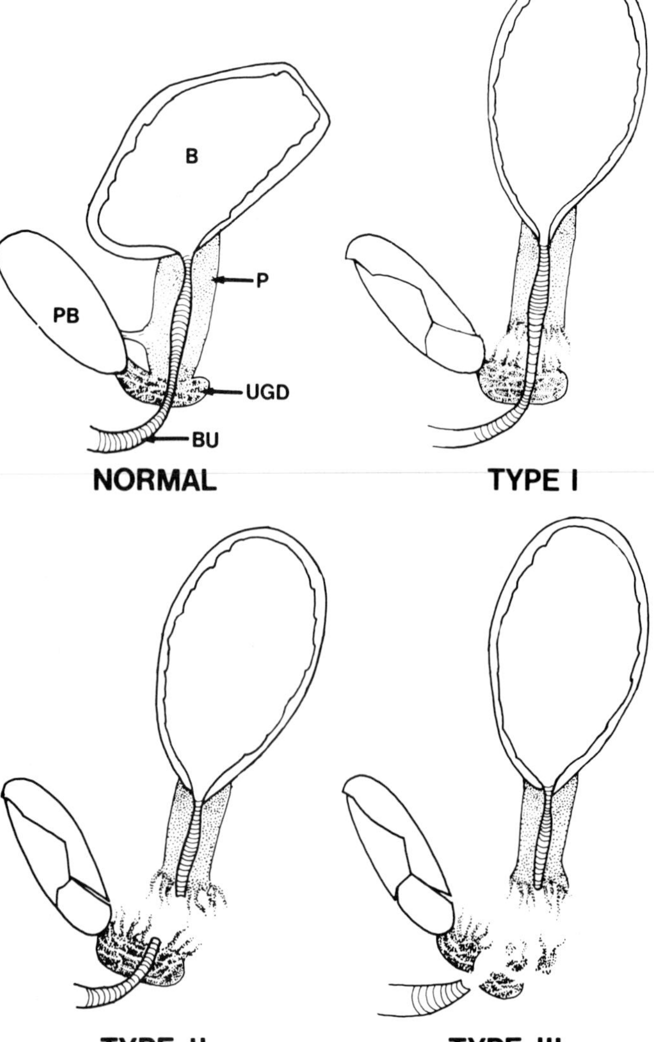

Figure 88–9. Diagrammatic presentation of the radiologic classification of acute urethral injury in pelvic fracture. (Modified from McCallum RW, Colapinto V: Urological Radiology of the Adult Male Lower Urinary Tract. Springfield, IL, Charles C Thomas, Publisher, 1976, by permission.)

most objective method by which accurate assessment of the extent of injury can be made. Urethral injuries associated with fractured pelvis are classified radiographically as follows (Fig. 88–9):

TYPE I. The posterior urethra is stretched because the puboprostatic ligaments are ruptured resulting in displacement of the bladder out of the pelvis. Although stretched, the urethra remains intact and there is no extravasation on urethrography. A Foley catheter may be carefully inserted, and no further therapy is typically required. Mere compression of the prostatic urethra by a pelvic hematoma should not be considered a type I injury.

TYPE II. The membranoprostatic urethra is ruptured above an intact urogenital diaphragm, which results in contrast material extravasation on urethrography into the pelvic extraperitoneal space *above* the position of the urogenital diaphragm.

TYPE III. The membranous urethra is disrupted; however, the injury extends into the proximal bulbous urethra and/or the urogenital diaphragm itself is ruptured. On urethrography, there is contrast material extravasation into the perineum *below* the level of the urogenital diaphragm (Fig. 88–10).

In studies reported by McCallum and by Sandler, more than 80 per cent of injuries were of the type III variety; type I injuries were the second most common, while true type II were seen only occasionally. Both types II and III may be either complete or incomplete. With complete disruption, no contrast material will enter the bladder, whereas with incomplete injuries, a portion of the continuity of the urethra remains intact, allowing some contrast material to enter the bladder. The incidence of partial ruptures varied in the reported studies from 19 to 90 per cent. The importance of partial ruptures should not be overlooked—although both complete and partial ruptures lead to subsequent urethral strictures, strictures that occur as a result of partial ruptures tend to be shorter and amenable to nonoperative or endoscopic management. Complete rupture generally requires a formal urethroplasty for repair. For this reason the importance of urethrography prior to Foley catheter placement in patients with pelvic fracture cannot be overstated. Placement of a Foley catheter blindly in a patient with a partial urethral tear may convert a partial tear into a complete disruption, increasing the morbidity of the injury.

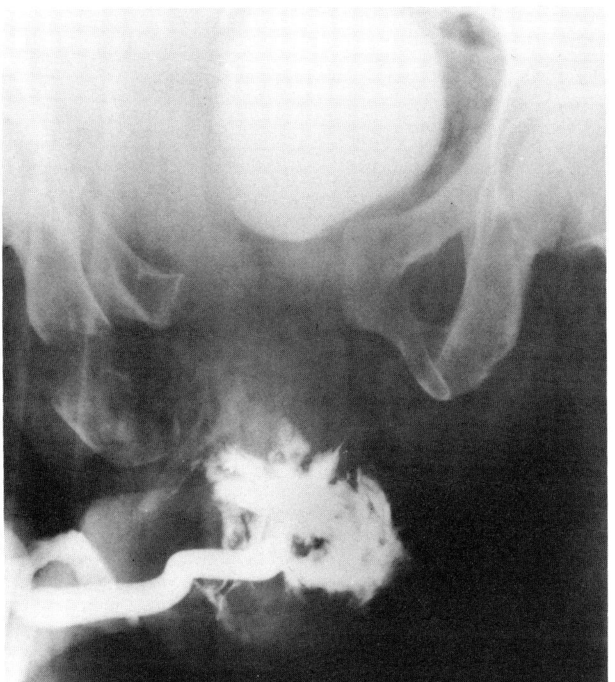

Figure 88–10. Type III urethral injury. Retrograde urethrogram demonstrates a complete type III urethral injury with contrast material extravasation into the perineum. There is contrast material in the bladder from a preceding excretory urogram.

In the past, immediate exploratory surgery to re-establish urethral continuity was considered to be the therapy of choice. In such a procedure, the pelvic hematoma is evacuated and the urethra is realigned over a Foley catheter. Unfortunately, the incidence of postoperative stricture may approach 100 per cent, up to one third of patients may suffer incontinence, and the rate of impotence approaches 60 per cent. Because of this high complication rate, many urologists prefer to manage such patients conservatively, delaying urethral reconstruction until after the patient has recovered from the acute injury. In such a procedure, only a suprapubic cystostomy is placed immediately and formal urethroplasty is delayed four to six months. By this time, the pelvic hematoma has resorbed, the prostate has redescended into the pelvis, and the pelvic fracture has stabilized.

STRADDLE INJURY

Straddle injury occurs when a patient falls astride a fixed object, crushing the urethra between the object and the inferior aspect of the symphysis pubis. The injury usually occurs in the proximal one third of the bulbous urethra and results in contusion and partial or complete urethral disruption. Clinically, there is blood at the urethral meatus and there may be a "butterfly" hematoma in the perineum on physical examination. On urethrography, both patients with partial injury and patients with complete injury demonstrate extravasation of contrast material into the corpus spongiosum (Fig. 88–11). Venous intravasation is also a common finding. Depending on the degree of urethral disruption present, many urologists treat patients with straddle injury with suprapubic urinary diversion. In many instances, such injuries result in a focal urethral stricture that may be managed easily with a visual internal urethrotomy.

IATROGENIC URETHRAL INJURY

Iatrogenic urethral injury is due to instrumentation, catheterization, or abdominoperineal resection. Urethral stricture is the end result of pressure necrosis produced by the passage of a straight metallic instrument along the S-shaped urethra. Pressure necrosis occurs at the fixed points of the urethra, namely, the penoscrotal junction and/or the membranous urethra (Fig. 88–12). This injury is therefore a complication of cystoscopy, transurethral resection of the prostate, transurethral resection of a bladder tumor, or transurethral removal of a ureteric stone. If the cystoscope or resectoscope is too large for the urethra, undue pressure is applied to straighten the urethra during the procedure, or the procedure takes a long time, pressure necrosis may occur at the fixed points, resulting in stricture. Strictures produced by pressure necrosis alone (without superimposed infection) are generally short and well-defined. Superimposed infection is uncommon after instrumentation. After transurethral resection, a catheter is usually left in the bladder and urethra for a maximum of three to four days, which is usually not long enough for infection to supervene, provided that the catheter has been placed with normal aseptic technique. A catheter left in place for more than three to four days increases the possibility of superimposed infection in the area of pressure necrosis, resulting in long, irregular strictures as discussed under Urethral Infection Associated with Catheterization. In a series of 88 traumatic strictures, 37 (42 per cent) were due to iatrogenic causes. In a retrospective study of 300 patients requiring transphincter urethroplasty, 135 injuries (45 per cent) were iatrogenic in origin and 109 (81 per cent) of these injuries were due to instrumentation.

In abdominoperineal resection for carcinoma of the rectum, occasionally, at the time of the pull-through part of the abdominoperineal resection, the posterior urethra is torn and may produce a

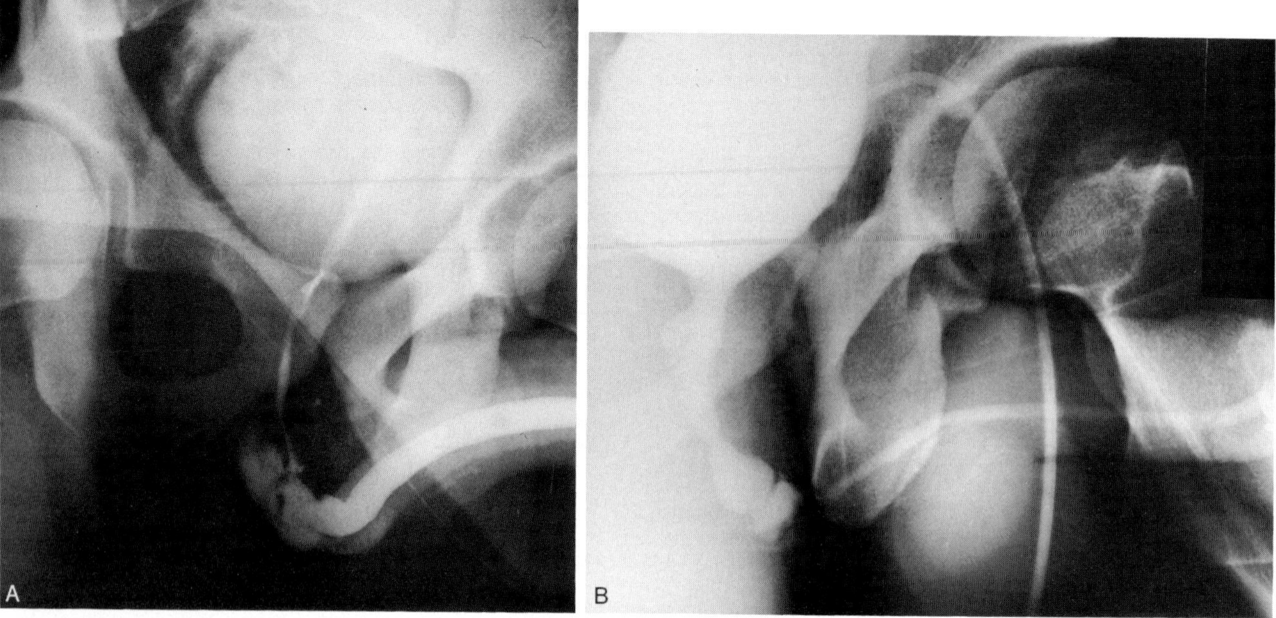

Figure 88–11. Straddle injury. *A*, Retrograde urethrogram demonstrates an incomplete straddle injury involving the proximal one third of the bulbous urethra. *B*, Follow-up voiding cystourethrogram one month after the acute injury demonstrates that a focal urethral stricture has developed at the site of injury.

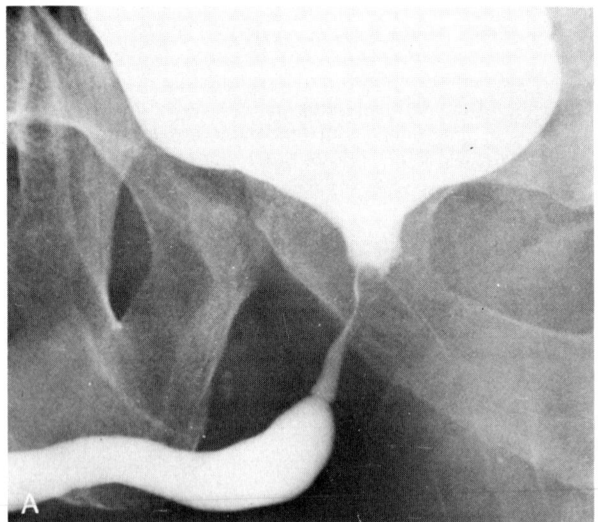

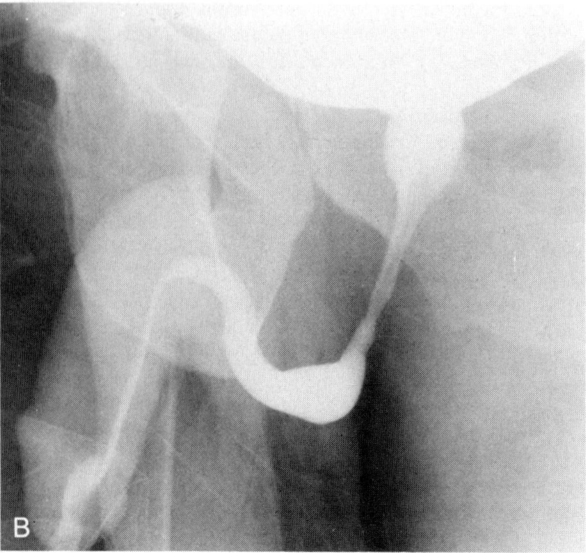

Figure 88–12. Iatrogenic injury of the urethra. *A*, Dynamic retrograde urethrogram one year after transurethral resection of the prostate. Note the resected prostate bed. Stricture in the proximal bulbous urethra with abnormal cone indicating scarring extends into the membranous urethra. *B*, Same patient voiding. The membranous urethra and proximal bulbous urethra are narrowed.

membranous urethral fistula or sufficient trauma to produce stricture at a later date.

Urethral Tumors

Urethral tumors are rare. Benign adenomatous and fibrous polyps are occasionally demonstrated in the anterior urethra and are usually associated with previous urethral infection. Primary amyloidosis of the urethra presents as a hard, palpable mass with urethral bleeding and is seen as an irregular filling defect in the anterior urethra on urethrography.

Malignant tumors of the urethra comprise only 1 per cent of all malignant urinary tract tumors. Squamous cell carcinoma typically occurs in the anterior urethra in men and women and accounts for 80 per cent of the cases overall (Fig. 88–13). Transitional cell carcinoma accounts for 15 per cent of the cases and is most commonly found in the prostatic urethra. The remainder of the cases are adenocarcinoma, metastatic lesions, and undifferentiated tumors. In patients with metastatic lesions, primary sites include carcinoma of the prostate, bladder, and testes, as well as malignant melanoma.

More than 60 per cent of cases of squamous cell carcinoma occur in the bulbous urethra and are related to squamous metaplasia, which occurs as a result of chronic irritation usually in association with long-standing urethral stricture disease. The disease progresses insidiously, with symptoms often attributed to the underlying benign stricture disease that is so often present. On urography, a long irregular stricture with or without a urethral perineal fistula is often found. Patients with transitional cell carcinoma often have a history of an antecedent bladder tumor.

Stress Incontinence

True stress incontinence is the result of incompetent sphincter function at the time of increased intra-abdominal pressure such as coughing or laughing. However, coughing or laughing may produce urinary incontinence if an unstable or irritable bladder is present when the patient experiences an urge to void. In true stress incontinence there is no urge to void. The distinction between true stress incontinence and urge incontinence is crucial. Cystography cannot distinguish stress from urge incontinence. Urodynamic studies recording detrusor pressure readily distinguish urge from stress incontinence. Only 40 per cent of women presenting with incontinence have true stress incontinence. Urge incontinence requires no operative intervention, whereas true stress incontinence requires some type of sling operative procedure, most often performed with a view to lengthening the urethra. The urethra usually is shorter in patients with stress incontinence, commonly less than 3 cm in length. The radiologic study for stress incontinence is bead chain cystourethrography, which is a static examination. The patient does not void. The bead chain is inserted into the bladder either through a polyethylene catheter or through a metal introducer. Both the polyethylene catheter and the metal introducer have an adaptor for the introduction of intravesical contrast medium. The bead and chain remain in the bladder and urethra; with the bladder almost filled with contrast medium, films are obtained with the patient in the erect lateral position. Resting and straining films are obtained. From these two films the anterior angle of inclination and the posterior urethrovesical angles are measured. The normal posterior urethrovesical angle is less than 100 degrees. The normal anterior angle of inclination is less than 40 degrees and is the angle made by the urethra and the vertical. Mild stress incontinence is shown by a posterior urethrovesical angle above 100 degrees and a normal anterior angle of inclination called Green type I deformity. More severe stress incontinence usually shows a posterior urethrovesical angle greater than 100 degrees and an anterior angle of inclination greater than 40 degrees. This is called the Green type II deformity. At the present time, this procedure is performed in many hospitals, but there are strong doubts about its usefulness. There is a trend toward using urodynamic studies in the assessment of all types of stress incontinence.

SEMINAL VESICLE RADIOLOGY

Normal Radiologic Anatomy

Seminal vesiculography in normal men (Fig. 88–14) shows considerable variation in appearance, but in general the average seminal

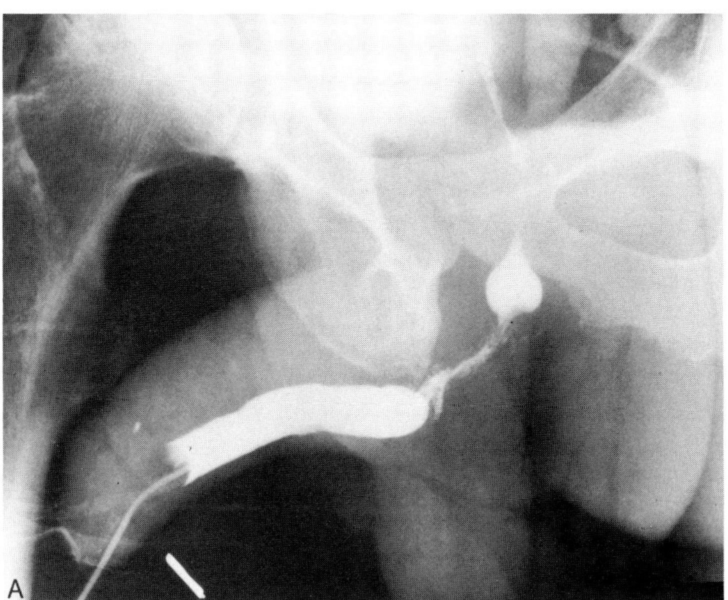

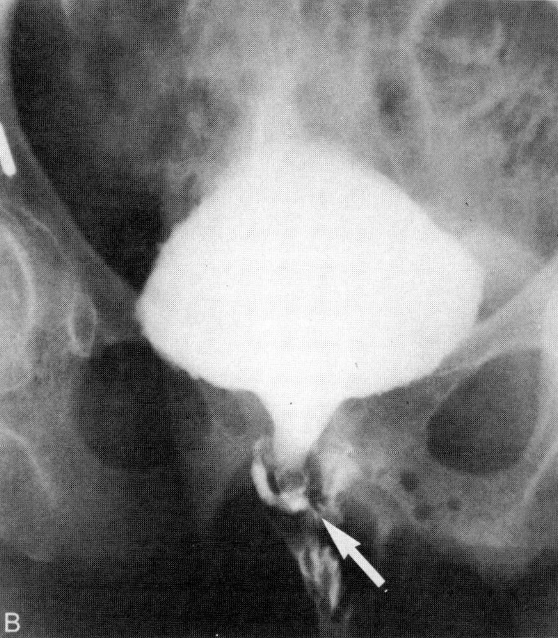

Figure 88–13. Squamous cell carcinoma of the urethra. *A,* Retrograde urethrogram shows a long irregular stricture in a male patient. *B,* Voiding cystourethrogram shows a stricture *(arrow)* at the distal one third of the urethra in a female that proved at biopsy to represent a squamous tumor.

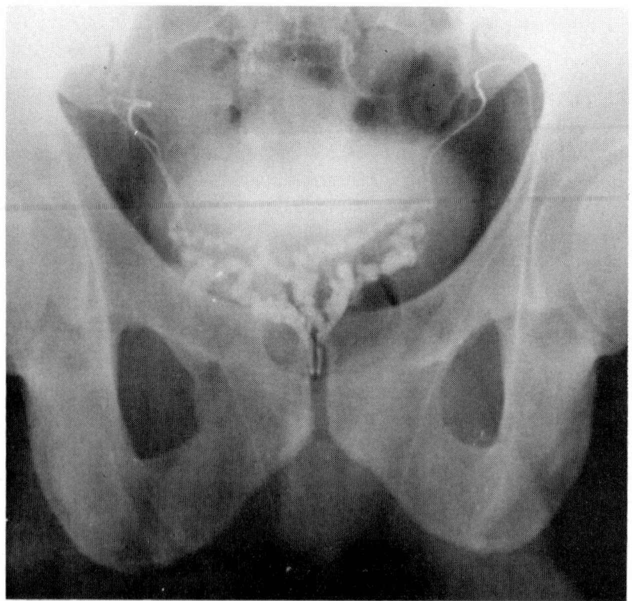

Figure 88–14. Normal bilateral vasoseminal vesiculography. Note the normal relationship of the seminal vesicle duct lying lateral to the neck of the ampulla of the vas deferens. The ampulla of the vas deferens is the convoluted portion, normally beginning adjacent to and above the superolateral aspect of the seminal vesicle.

vesicle is 2 cm wide, has a lumen of 6 mm, and is 5 cm long on the right and 4.6 cm long on the left. The seminal vesicle lies between the bladder and rectum anterior to Denonvilliers' fascia adjacent to the posteroinferior aspect of the bladder. The short excretory duct of the seminal vesicle joins the ampulla of the vas deferens to form the ejaculatory duct. The excretory duct lies lateral to the ampulla of the vas deferens at the junction. The vas deferens arises from the tail of the epididymis, ascends in the spermatic cord, and enters the abdomen through the external inguinal ring. It then sweeps up along the lateral pelvic wall before curving posteriorly, medially, and interiorly to form the ampulla of the vas deferens. The vas deferens becomes slightly dilated and convoluted in its medial inferior portion.

The seminal vesicles are readily imaged by transrectal sonography, computed tomography (CT), and magnetic resonance imaging (MRI). Transrectal sonography has become the technique of choice for the evaluation of cystic seminal vesicle abnormalities. The older technique of seminal vesiculography, which involves a scrotal incision and direct injection of contrast material into the vas deferens, should probably be reserved for the uncommon patient in whom a communication between the seminal vesicle and the urinary tract is suspected or for males in whom obstructive azoospermia cannot be confirmed with noninvasive techniques. Such patients will present with a low sperm count, a normal serum follicle-stimulating hormone assay, and normal seminiferous tubules on testicular biopsy.

Abnormalities of the seminal vesicles include congenital anomalies; acquired obstructions; tumors; and miscellaneous conditions, including inflammation, hemorrhage, and calcification.

Congenital seminal vesicle cysts are the most common congenital anomaly of the seminal vesicle and are associated with ipsilateral renal abnormalities, most commonly renal agenesis. Anomalies of other mesonephric duct derivatives, including ectopic insertion of the ureter into the bladder neck, the posterior urethra, ejaculatory duct, or the seminal vesicle itself, have also been reported. Typically, patients with seminal vesicle cysts do not present until 20 to 40 years of age. The most common presenting symptoms are perineal or flank pain, dysuria, and lower urinary tract infection.

The cysts are readily demonstrated on transrectal sonography,

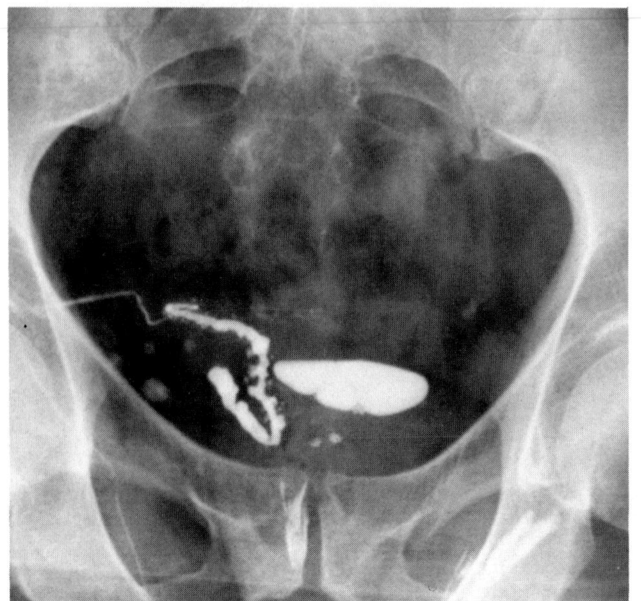

Figure 88–15. Tuberculosis involving the ampulla of the vas deferens and seminal vesicle. The vas deferens has a characteristic beaded appearance, and the seminal vesicle is shrunken and has lost most of the normal convoluted appearance

CT, and MRI. The finding of dilation of the ipsilateral ejaculatory duct on the imaging studies should raise suspicion of an ectopic ureteral insertion. The fluid in these cysts is reported to demonstrate increased signal intensity on both T_1- and T_2-weighted images. On CT a low attenuation mass posterior to the bladder is readily demonstrated.

Other congenital anomalies of the seminal vesicles include agenesis and dysgenesis; such abnormalities may be associated with cryptorchidism.

Acquired obstruction of the seminal vesicle occurs as a result of obstruction of the seminal vesicle itself or the ejaculatory duct. Most such cases are associated with benign prostatic hypertrophy or chronic infection that has resulted in scarring of the ejaculatory duct or seminal vesicle.

Most malignant tumors of the seminal vesicle occur as a result of invasion of the gland by direct extension of prostatic tumors. Tumor invasion may be global (involving the entire gland) or segmental. Invaded seminal vesicles generally show low signal intensity on T_2-weighted images. The reported accuracy for the detection of seminal vesicle invasion by prostate cancer on MRI is 78 per cent. Primary carcinomas of the seminal vesicles are rare, with fewer than 70 cases having been reported.

Most inflammatory conditions of the seminal vesicle are associated with prostatitis. In extreme cases, a seminal vesicle abscess may form. On MRI, high signal intensity on T_2-weighted images has been reported. In chronic inflammatory processes associated with hemorrhage, high signal intensity on both T_1- and T_2-weighted images may be found.

Tuberculosis produces a characteristic beaded appearance of the vas deferens on seminal vesiculography; the seminal vesicles themselves are commonly scarred and shrunken (Fig. 88–15). The granulomatous changes in the seminal vesicles commonly result in calcification that is visible on plain films. The most common cause of calcification in the vas, however, is underlying diabetes mellitus.

Bibliography

Abbit PL, Watson L, Howards S: Abnormalities of the seminal tract causing infertility: Diagnosis with endorectal sonography. AJR 157:337–339, 1991.

Amis ES Jr, Newhouse JH, Cronan JJ: Radiology of male periurethral structures. AJR 151:321–324, 1988.

Banner MP, Hassler R: The normal seminal vesiculogram. Radiology 128:339, 1978.

Baskin LS, Turzan C: Carcinoma of the male urethra: Management of locally advanced disease with combined chemotherapy, radiotherapy and penile-preserving surgery. Urology 39:21–25, 1992.

Brick AC, Shaw RC: Primary tumours of the retrovesicle region with special reference to the mesenchymal tumours of the seminal vesicles. Br J Urol 44:47, 1972.

Campbell JE, Sniderman KW: Urethral diverticula in the adult female. J Can Assoc Radiol 27:232, 1976.

Colapinto V, McCallum RW: Injury to the male posterior urethra in fractured pelvis: A new classification. J Urol 118:575, 1977.

Friedenberg RM: Abnormalities affecting structure and function of the bladder and urethra. Semin Roentgenol 18:307, 1983.

Friedland GW: The urethra—imaging and intervention in the 1990's. Clin Radiol 42:157–160, 1992.

Gibson GR: Urological management and complications of fractured pelvis and ruptured urethra. J Urol 111:353, 1974.

Gosling JA, Dixon JS, Crutchley HOD, Thompson SA: A comparative study of the human external sphincter and periurethral levator ani muscle. Br J Urol 53:35, 1981.

Green TH Jr: The problem of urinary stress incontinence in the female. Obstet Gynaecol Sum 26:603, 1968.

Hahn R, Krepart G, Malaker K: Carcinoma of female urethra. Manitoba experience: 1958–1987. Urology 37:106–109, 1991.

Holm L, Forsberg L: Computed tomography and ultrasound studies of prostatic utricle cyst associated with unilateral renal agenesis. Scand J Urol Nephrol 18:87, 1984.

Kenney PJ, Leeson MD: Congenital anomalies of the seminal vesicles: Spectrum of computed tomographic findings. Radiology 149:247, 1983.

King B, Hattery RR, Lieber MM, et al: Congenital cystic disease of the seminal vesicle. Radiology 178:207–211, 1991.

King B, Hattery RR, Lieber MM, et al: Seminal vesicle imaging. RadioGraphics 9:653–676, 1989.

Kirshy DM, Pollack AH, Becker JA, Horowitz M: Autourethrography. Radiology 180:443–445, 1991.

Lucon AM, et al: Congenital cyst of the seminal vesicle. Eur Urol 9:362, 1983.

Macpherson RI, Leithiser RE, Gordon L, Turner WR: Posterior urethral valves: An update and review. RadioGraphics 6:753–791, 1986.

McCallum RW: The adult male urethra: Normal anatomy, pathology, and method of urethrography. Radiol Clin North Am 17:227, 1979.

McCallum RW, Alexander MWT, Rogers JM: Etiology and method of radiologic assessment of male urinary incontinence. J Can Assoc Radiol 36:4–11, 1985.

McCallum RW, Colapinto V: Urological Radiology of the Adult Male Lower Urinary Tract. Springfield, IL, Charles C Thomas, 1976, p 13.

McCallum RW, Rogers J, Alexander M: Iatrogenic urethral injury. J Can Assoc Radiol 36:122–126, 1985.

Myers RP, DeWeerd JH: Incidence of stricture following primary realignment of the disrupted proximal urethra. J Urol 107:765, 1972.

Pollack HM, DeBenedictis TJ, Marmar JL, et al: Urethrographic manifestations of venereal warts (condyloma acuminata). Radiology 126:643, 1978.

Rimon U, Hertz M, Jonas P: Diverticula of the male urethra: A review of 61 cases. Urol Radiol 14:49–55, 1992.

Rubesin SE, Pollack HM, Banner MP: Simplified chain cystourethrography. Radiology 145:199, 1982.

Sandler CM, Corriere JN Jr: Urethrography in the diagnosis of acute urethral injuries. Urol Clin North Am 16:283–289, 1989.

Sandler CM, Harris JH Jr, Corriere JN Jr, Toombs BD: Posterior urethral injuries following pelvic fracture. AJR 137:1233–1237, 1981.

Sandler CM, Philips TM, Harris JD, Toombs BD: Radiology of the bladder and urethra in blunt pelvic trauma. Radiol Clin North Am 19:195, 1981.

Secaf E, Nuruddin RN, Hricak H, et al: MR imaging of the seminal vesicles. AJR 156:989–994, 1991.

Sue DE, Chicola C, Brant-Zawadzki MN, et al: MR imaging in seminal vesiculitis. J Comput Assist Tomogr 13:662–664, 1989.

Walter S, Olesen KP: Urinary incontinence and genital prolapse in the female: Clinical, urodynamic, and radiological examinations. Br J Obstet Gynaecol 89:393, 1982.

Walzer Y, Bear RA, Colapinto V, et al: Localized amyloidosis of urethra. Urology 21:406, 1983.

89 Impotence

Bernard F. King

Penile erection is a complex neurovascular event. Proper neurochemical stimuli initiate vascular changes that result in penile tumescence and ultimately rigidity. Adequate arterial inflow and sufficient restriction of venous outflow are the vascular changes that must be obtained to produce an erection. Because the most common cause of impotence is vascular, clinical evaluation of erectile dysfunction should always address the arterial supply of the penis as well as the veno-occlusive mechanism.

Arteriography of the penile and pelvic vasculature is considered the gold standard in the evaluation of impotence due to poor arterial inflow (arteriogenic impotence). Cavernosometry and cavernosography provide definitive evaluation of impotence due to excessive venous leakage (venogenic impotence). However, both arteriography and cavernosometry/cavernosography are invasive and expensive techniques. Because of this, much effort has been made to find an appropriate screening examination in patients with suspected vasculogenic impotence.

Duplex sonography of the penis was introduced in 1985 as a screening technique that could evaluate patients with suspected vasculogenic impotence. This technique allows for an estimation of velocity of blood flow and change in the diameter of the cavernosal artery in patients with possible arteriogenic impotence. In addition, evaluation of the arterial waveform and evaluation of the draining veins of the penis can provide a means of evaluating venogenic impotence.

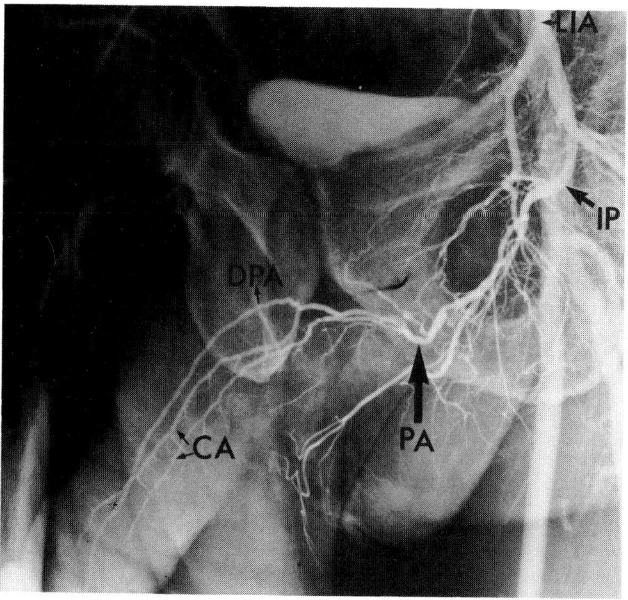

Figure 89–2. Angiogram (left anterior oblique position) depicting the left internal iliac artery (LIA), internal pudendal artery (IP), common penile artery (PA), right and left cavernosal arteries (CA), and left dorsal penile artery (DPA). Note the small helicine arteries arising from the cavernosal arteries and supplying the corpora cavernosa. Note the small areas of stenoses in the internal pudendal artery secondary to atherosclerotic disease.

ANATOMY

The penis is composed of three cylindrical structures. The two corpora cavernosa lie in the dorsal two thirds of the penis, and the single corpus spongiosum lies in the ventral one third of the penis and contains the urethra. The two corpora cavernosa are the main erectile structures of the penis. Although the corpus spongiosum becomes engorged during an erection, it adds little to the erectile status of the penis. Both of the corpora cavernosa and the corpus spongiosum are enveloped in a thick, facial sheath, the tunica albuginea (Fig. 89–1).

The corpora cavernosa and corpus spongiosum are composed of sinusoidal spaces lined by smooth muscle and endothelium. These small sinusoidal spaces in the corpora cavernosa distend with blood during an erection.

The blood supply to the penis is primarily via the right and left internal pudendal arteries, which originate from the right and left internal iliac arteries. The distal portion of the internal pudendal artery gives off a perineal branch, a bulbar branch, and a small urethral artery before continuing as the artery of the penis. The right and left common penile arteries enter the base of the penis and branch into a cavernosal artery and a dorsal artery. The cavernosal arteries are the primary source of blood flow to the erectile tissue of the penis (Fig. 89–2). Each cavernosal artery travels near the center of each corpus cavernosum and gives rise to small helicine arterial branches that communicate directly with the sinusoidal spaces. The paired dorsal penile arteries primarily supply blood to the skin and glans of the penis. Anastomotic branches frequently

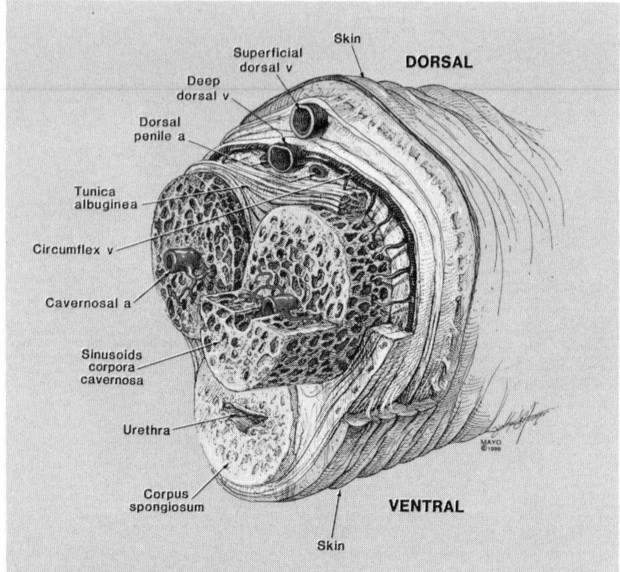

Figure 89–1. Cross-section of the penis. (From Quam JP, King BF, James EM, et al: Duplex and color Doppler sonographic evaluation of vasculogenic impotence. AJR 153:1141–1147, 1989. Used by permission.)

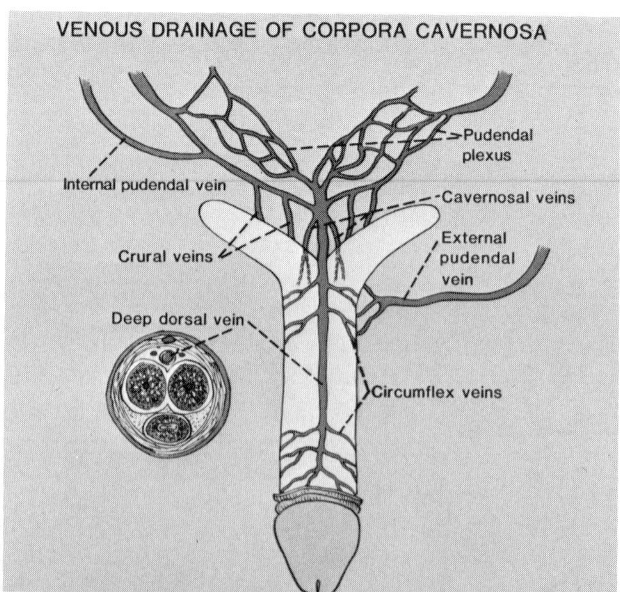

Figure 89–3. Drawing of the penis demonstrating various routes of venous drainage. The two major routes of venous efflux from the corpora cavernosa are the circumflex veins, which drain into the deep dorsal vein, and the crural veins near the base of the penis. Used with permission from Lippincott's Reviews: Radiology. Impotence and Infertility. Dec 1992.)

occur between the dorsal penile arteries and the deep cavernosal arteries and between right and left cavernosal arteries.

Venous drainage of the erectile tissue of the penis occurs primarily via small emissary veins that emanate from the corpus cavernosum and perforate the thick tunica albuginea. These emissary veins empty into circumflex veins surrounding the shaft of the penis. The circumflex veins ultimately travel to the dorsal aspect of the penis and empty into the deep dorsal penile vein (see Fig. 89–1). The deep dorsal vein then empties into the retropubic venous plexus. Venous drainage of the corpus cavernosum also can occur via crural veins near the base of the penis (Fig. 89–3). These crural veins are not accessible sonographically.

PHYSIOLOGY

Penile erection begins with a complex psychoerotic neurologic stimulus that results in smooth muscle relaxation in the walls of the sinusoids and helicine and cavernosal arteries of each corpora cavernosa. As the sinusoidal smooth muscle relaxes, the sinusoids distend with blood as a result of dramatically increased blood flow via the dilated cavernosal and helicine arteries. With sinusoidal distention, the small emissary veins draining the corpora cavernosa are compressed between the distended sinusoids and the unyielding peripheral tunica albuginea. This results in a veno-occlusive mechanism that maintains sinusoidal distention by limiting venous outflow from the sinusoidal spaces (Fig. 89–4). With continued arterial inflow and limited venous outflow, the sinusoidal spaces distend to such a degree that the cavernosal tissue becomes rigid.

The neurochemical mediators of sinusoidal relaxation are poorly understood. Acetylcholine, released by parasympathetic nerve terminals, appears to result in an inhibition of resting adrenergic tone and may also stimulate the production of an unknown neurotransmitter that produces direct smooth muscle relaxation in the sinusoidal spaces. Much attention has been given to substances that may act as neurotransmitters, such as endothelium-derived relaxing factor (EDRF). EDRF is released by endothelial cells of certain peripheral blood vessels and may also be released by endothelial cells lining the sinusoids in response to stimulation by neurotransmitters.

Prostaglandins are also produced by corporal tissues and are known to modulate autonomic nerve function. The release of prostaglandins in the corpora is under parasympathetic control and may be the important factor in the final step resulting in corporal smooth muscle relaxation. Recent evidence indicates that nitric oxide is the EDRF in the penile vascular tissues, and it is dependent on prostaglandin synthesis in the smooth muscle that lines the sinusoidal spaces. Adequate production of nitric oxide by endothelial cells may be the critical step in the normal physiologic response of an erection.

DUPLEX SONOGRAPHY

Duplex sonography should be performed in a quiet room without distractions. The patient is in the supine position with the penis on the anterior abdominal wall. High-frequency (7.5 to 10 mHz), linear-array, ultrasound transducers are used to image the penis in the longitudinal and transverse planes.

Duplex sonography of the cavernosal arteries is best accomplished in a longitudinal, parasagittal plane from a ventral approach (Fig. 89–5). In the flaccid state, the cavernosal arteries may follow a tortuous course and can be seen only intermittently on a single longitudinal plane. In the erect state, the cavernosal artery assumes a straighter course.

The first step is to measure the diameter of the cavernosal arteries prior to the injection of a vasodilating agent. This baseline measurement of each cavernosal artery diameter is necessary to determine the degree of change following the intracavernosal injection of the vasodilating agent. Magnified views of the cavernosal arteries are used for measurement purposes, and internal lumen diameter measurements are obtained. Because of the wide variability within each artery, multiple measurements on each side can be obtained and averaged.

After cavernosal artery diameter measurements are made, a vasodilating agent is injected into the penis. The types and doses of vasodilating agents that are used vary widely (Table 89–1). Initially, many investigators inject 60 mg of papaverine (2 ml) into either the left or right corpus cavernosum. Other investigators have used papaverine (40 mg) and phentolamine (2.5 mg) or a triple agent consisting of papaverine (4.4 mg), phentolamine (0.15 mg), and prostaglandin E_1 (1.5 μg) in 0.25 ml. The incidence of priapism varies from 3 to 10 per cent of patients and may be related to dose and combination of agents. We currently use prostaglandin E_1 (10 μg) alone in an attempt to minimize the risk of priapism.

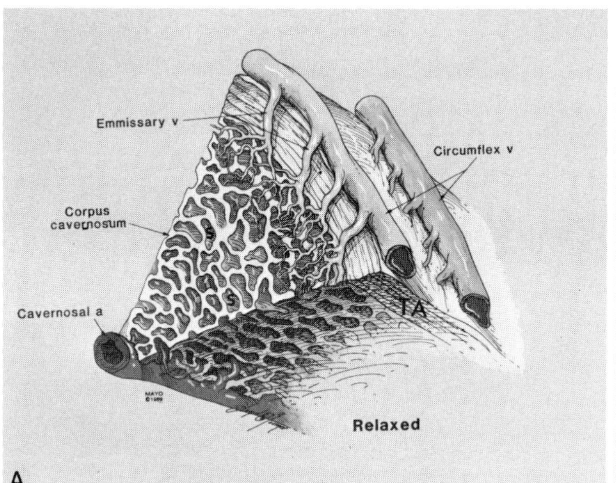

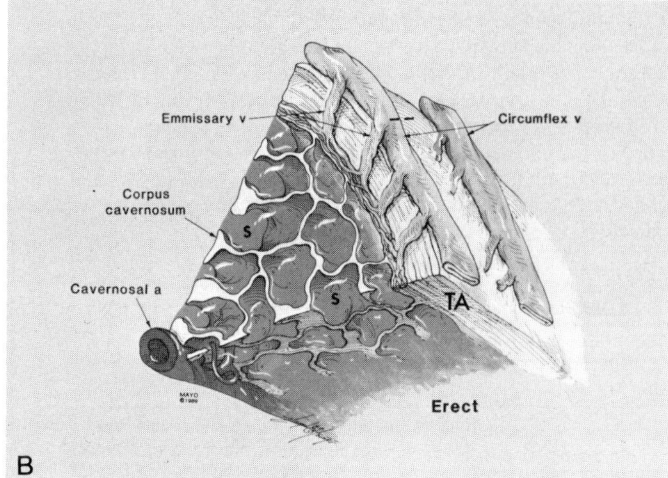

Figure 89–4. Corpora cavernosa in the flaccid and erect state. Cross-sectional wedge drawings of the corpus cavernosum in the flaccid *(A)* and erect *(B)* state. During the erectile process, the cavernosal arteries and sinusoids (S) distend with blood and compress the draining venules against the thick and rigid tunica albuginea (TA). The compression and near occlusion of these draining venules prevent venous efflux from the cavernosal tissues and allow for prolonged maximal distention of the cavernosal sinusoids, resulting in an erection. (By permission of Mayo Foundation.)

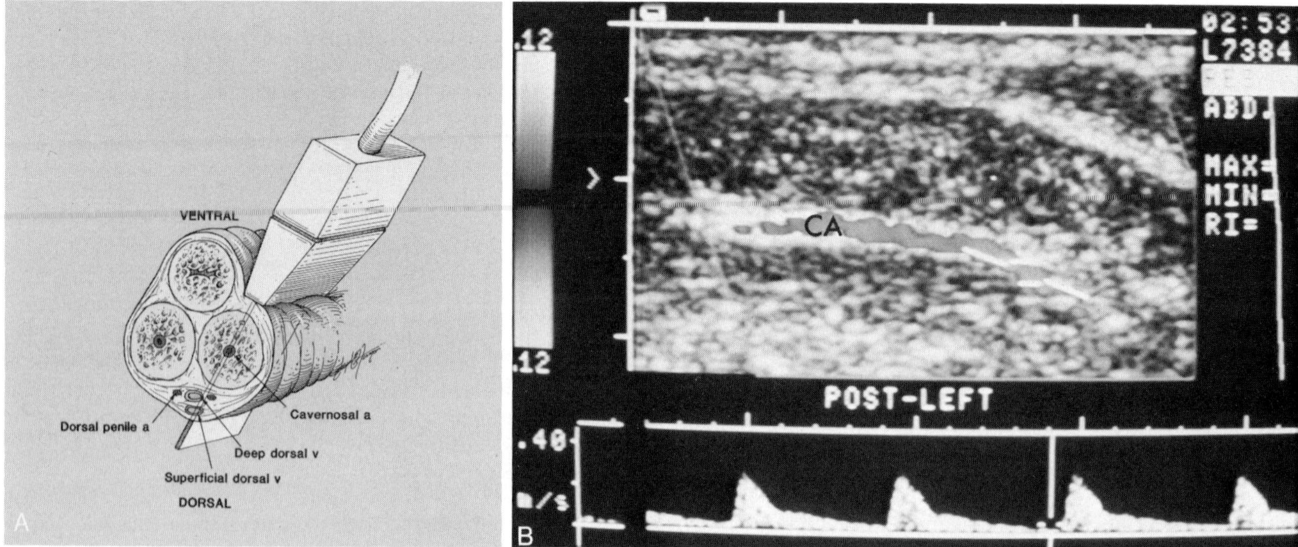

Figure 89–5. Transducer position for Doppler examination of the cavernosal artery. *A,* The transducer is placed in a parasagittal position along the ventral aspect of the penis for easy visualization of the cavernosal artery. Drawing depicts the medially directed position of the transducer. *B,* Longitudinal Doppler sonogram depicting the course of the left cavernosal artery (CA) within the corpora cavernosa. (*A* by permission of Mayo Foundation.)

After injection, the vasodilating agent diffuses readily from one corpus cavernosum to the other because of the fenestrations within the septum of the penis. It is, however, important to inject the vasodilating agent accurately into the dorsal two thirds of the proximal portion of the penile shaft so that the agent does not enter the corpus spongiosum, the urethra, or the glans. Care must be taken to avoid injecting the vasodilating agent into the subcutaneous tissue, which could result in massive swelling of the skin and possible necrosis. All patients should be instructed to contact their referring physician or go directly to an emergency room for evaluation and treatment of possible priapism if a painful erection occurs or if an erection does not subside after one to two hours. Pharmacologic-induced priapism is defined as persistent painful erection of the penis one to three hours after the intracavernosal injection of a vasodilating agent. Persistent priapism (longer than three to four hours) can result in ischemic necrosis and fibrosis of cavernosal tissue. Patients who are prone to priapism include those with a history of neurogenic impotence, those with sickle cell disease or trait, and patients on heparin therapy. The use of smaller doses of vasodilating agents or performance of the examination without pharmacologic agents may be warranted in these patients.

Treatment of priapism should be carried out by a trained urologist and usually consists of aspirating approximately 20 ml of blood from a corpus cavernosum. If this fails to relieve the priapism, a small dose of a vasoconstricting agent (i.e., phenylephrine hydrochloric acid) diluted in 1 ml of normal saline can be injected intracavernosally to facilitate mild vasoconstriction and cessation of the erection.

TABLE 89–1. VASODILATING AGENTS USED FOR EVALUATING IMPOTENCE

Agent	Mode of Action
Papaverine	Relaxes smooth muscle directly via interference with calcium flow during muscle contraction.
Phentolamine	Indirectly facilitates smooth muscle relaxation by blocking alpha-adrenergic receptors. Potentiates the action of papaverine.
Prostaglandin E_1	Relaxes smooth-muscle directly by possibly controlling the release of nitric oxide.

Following the intracavernosal injection of a vasodilating agent, the post-injection diameters of the cavernosal arteries are measured (Fig. 89–6) and dynamic velocity measurements are obtained at 5-minute intervals up to 20 minutes after injection. This Doppler analysis of the cavernosal artery is optimally obtained near the base of the penis, where the Doppler angle is the smallest. A Doppler angle of less than 60 degrees should always be achieved. Spectral analysis of the Doppler waveform in the cavernosal arteries should include measurement of peak systolic velocities (PSV) and end diastolic velocities (EDV) (Fig. 89–7).

There continues to be debate about the optimal time after pharmacologic enhancement to record cavernosal artery PSV and EDV measurements. In our experience, PSV can occur at any time between 5 and 20 minutes post-injection. Because of this time variation, we obtain velocity measurements at 5-minute intervals in both

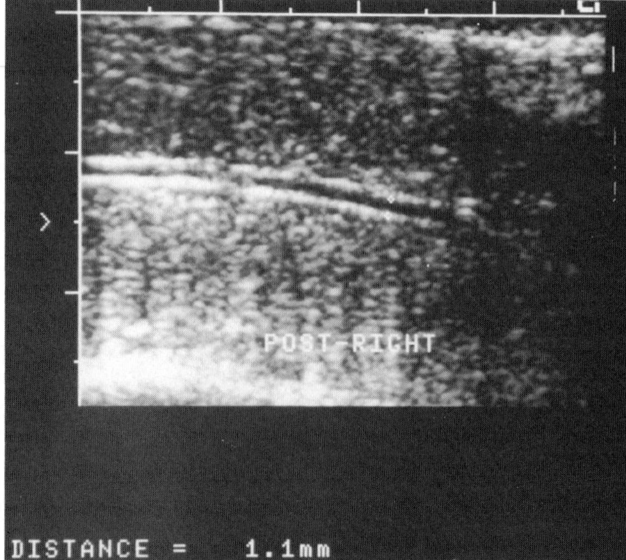

Figure 89–6. Longitudinal sonogram of the right cavernosal artery after the intracavernosal injection of a vasodilating agent. The internal lumen of the cavernosal artery measures approximately 1.1 mm.

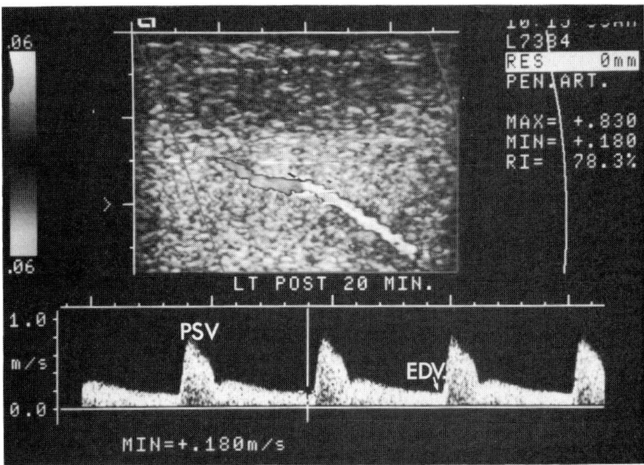

Figure 89–7. Doppler waveform in the left cavernosal artery 20 minutes after injection of a vasodilating agent. Peak systolic velocity (PSV) and end diastolic velocity (EDV) measurements are electronically calculated off the spectral waveform by a small electronic cursor.

cavernosal arteries for at least 20 minutes after the injection of a vasodilating agent.

The dynamic duplex sonographic evaluation of the cavernosal arteries after the intracavernosal injection of a vasodilating agent reveals a normal progression of the spectral waveform (Fig. 89–8). These dynamic changes in the Doppler waveform tend to occur within 20 minutes after the intracavernosal injection of a vasodilating agent and reflect the changes in intrapenile pressure during a normal erection. Dynamic evaluation of this waveform along with measurements of PSV, EDV, and diameter changes allows for the most accurate assessment of each patient for possible arteriogenic or venogenic impotence.

ARTERIOGENIC IMPOTENCE

According to most investigators, PSV following the intracavernosal injection of a vasodilating agent appears to be the most prom-

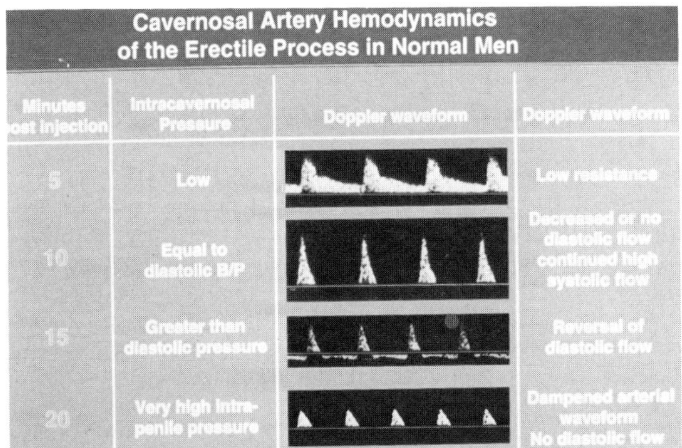

Cavernosal Artery Hemodynamics of the Erectile Process in Normal Men

Minutes Post Injection	Intracavernosal Pressure	Doppler waveform	Doppler waveform
5	Low		Low resistance
10	Equal to diastolic B/P		Decreased or no diastolic flow continued high systolic flow
15	Greater than diastolic pressure		Reversal of diastolic flow
20	Very high intrapenile pressure		Dampened arterial waveform No diastolic flow

Figure 89–8. Normal spectral waveforms in the cavernosal artery after the injection of a vasodilating agent. The Doppler spectral waveform changes from a low-resistance waveform to a high-resistance waveform during the process of an erection. This dynamic change in the waveform usually occurs within 20 minutes and corresponds to changes in intracavernosal pressure. (Used with permission. Adapted from Schwartz AN, Wang KY, Mack LA, et al: Evaluation of normal erectile function with color flow Doppler sonography. AJR 153:1155–1160, 1989.)

ising parameter for evaluating patients for possible arteriogenic impotence. In a study of normal male volunteers, it was found that the normal average PSV following the intracavernosal injection of a vasodilating agent is approximately 30 to 40 cm/sec. Subsequent studies have indicated that a PSV of 25 cm/sec or less suggests inadequate arterial inflow to permit clinically good erections.

Current data tend to group impotent patients into three subgroups based on cavernosal artery PSV. The first subgroup, which is considered to be normal, have a PSV above 35 cm/sec. The second subgroup of patients may have minimal to mild arterial insufficiency, with a PSV of 25 to 35 cm/sec. The third subgroup have severe arterial insufficiency and have a PSV of less than 25 cm/sec.

Again, it is paramount that PSV in the cavernosal arteries be studied for at least 20 minutes post-injection. This allows for the detection of high PSV that occur later in some individuals. Serial velocity measurements over time also allow for an evaluation of the dynamic changes in the waveform that should occur normally. Therefore, single measurements of PSV 5 or 10 minutes post-injection are inadequate. These sequential measurements should be made in *both* cavernosal arteries at 5, 10, 15, and 20 minutes post-injection (see Fig. 89–8).

It is our experience that even when performing a dynamic study up to 20 minutes post-injection, duplex Doppler sonography yields an 83 per cent sensitivity for the detection of bilateral hemodynamically significant arterial stenoses when compared to conventional angiography. Therefore, velocity measurements and waveform analysis alone may not detect all patients with arteriogenic impotence. This may be explained by the fact that arterial blood flow is not only a function of velocity in a particular vessel but also a function of the cross-sectional area of the lumen of the vessel. Therefore, the diameter of the cavernosal artery should also be evaluated. Measuring the initial size of the artery is probably not the best indicator of arterial disease and arterial compliance. It appears that a 75 per cent increase in vessel diameter is the best indicator of normal arterial compliance and vessel dilatation. Thus, assessment of cavernosal blood flow should include PSV as well as the degree of arterial dilatation. The additional evaluation of cavernosal artery diameter change may improve the sensitivity of the Doppler examination.

From these studies, it seems logical to assume that PSV in the cavernosal arteries of less than 25 cm/sec after administration of a vasodilating agent should suggest arterial inflow disease and should lead to a more definitive evaluation with selective internal pudendal arteriography if clinically warranted (Fig. 89–9). PSV values between 25 and 35 cm/sec along with a 75 per cent increase in vessel diameter should be considered borderline. PSV measurements greater than 35 cm/sec accompanied by a 75 per cent increase in vessel diameter should be considered normal.

Several other unique findings may also indicate arterial disease. If patients demonstrate a marked discrepancy (greater than 10 cm/sec) between the velocities of the two cavernosal arteries, unilateral arterial disease of the penis may be present. Adequate blood flow through one cavernosal artery may be all that is needed for adequate erection; however, unilateral disease of the penis may be significant in certain individuals, and appropriate arteriography may need to be pursued. Another unique indication of arterial disease occurs when the PSV is greatly elevated (i.e., over 100 cm/sec). This high velocity has been seen in patients with diffuse vascular spasm and/or small vessel disease (i.e., diabetes mellitus). Such patients demonstrate little or no change in cavernosal arterial diameter measurements before and after the injection of a vasodilating agent. Therefore, if normal or high velocities in the cavernosal arteries are detected, the caliber of the cavernosal arteries should be evaluated. If the caliber does not significantly increase following the vasodilating agent, the patient may have diffuse small vessel disease (i.e., diabetes) or diffuse vasospasm (nicotine abuse, medications) with artificially high velocities because of a small vessel lumen.

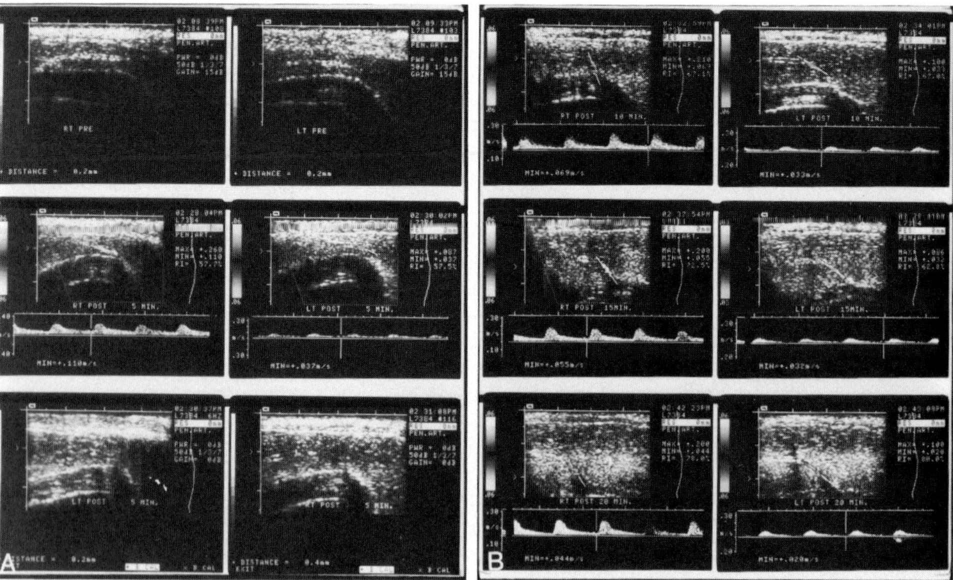

Figure 89–9. *A* and *B*, Abnormal duplex Doppler sonograms in a patient with arteriogenic impotence. Note that the change in cavernosal artery diameter is less than 75 per cent. This, in addition to suboptimal peak systolic velocities of less than 25 cm/sec in both cavernosal arteries, indicates probable arteriogenic disease. (MAX = peak systolic velocity; MIN = end-diastolic velocity.)

Recent evidence suggests that the sensitivity and accuracy of cavernosal artery duplex sonography may be increased by the evaluation of additional parameters such as systolic acceleration, pulsatility index, and resistive index. More work is needed to determine how these cavernosal artery Doppler waveform parameters relate to arterial inflow disease to the penis.

VENOGENIC IMPOTENCE

Venogenic impotence may be due to excessive venous leakage from the corporal bodies. Although the exact cause of excessive venous leakage is unknown, it may be due to stretching or thinning of the thick tunica albuginea, which prevents the adequate compression of emissary veins that drain the sinusoids during tumescence and rigidity. When these emissary veins are not adequately compressed, venous outflow from the cavernosa continues to occur during tumescence. Tumescence may be achieved but rigidity is never accomplished.

Traditionally, venogenic impotence has been evaluated with cavernosometry and cavernosography. However, these examinations are invasive and not suitable for screening purposes. Therefore, duplex sonography has been advocated as a screening examination for venogenic impotence.

During the duplex Doppler examination of the cavernosal arteries in the normal patient, there is an increase in EDV and PSV immediately following the intracavernosal injection of vasodilating agents. This corresponds to the physiologic dilatation of the cavernosal artery, helicine arteries, and sinusoidal spaces. As the sinusoidal spaces are dilating and filling, vascular resistance in the cavernosal artery is low and forward diastolic flow is prominent (see Fig. 89–8). However, when the veno-occlusive mechanism engages, the sinusoids become maximally distended and intracavernosal pressure dramatically increases. At this point, vascular resistance increases and diastolic flow ceases or even reverses. If a patient's veno-occlusive mechanism is not intact, excessive venous leakage persists and intracavernosal pressure remains low. The Doppler spectral waveform in this instance continues to exhibit the prominent forward diastolic flow of a low-resistance vascular bed throughout the examination. Therefore, patients who continue to have high EDV (over 3 cm/sec) throughout the examination (up to 15 to 20 minutes) despite normal arterial inflow (PSV of 35 cm/sec or greater) may have venogenic impotence. Cavernosometry and cavernosography should be considered in these patients to make a more definitive diagnosis. Incidentally, patients who demonstrate reversal of diastolic flow in both cavernosal arteries should have an intact veno-occlusive mechanism and should not have venogenic impotence.

The majority of venous efflux from the corpora cavernosa occurs via the deep dorsal vein. Some investigators have recommended measurements of velocity in the deep dorsal penile vein as a means of detecting excessive venous leakage. It appears that transient early dorsal vein flow is normal in many patients. However, persistent dorsal vein flow at 20 minutes post-injection may indicate excessive venous leakage. However, our experience suggests that both normal patients and patients with excessive venous leakage may have high deep dorsal vein velocities up to 20 minutes post-injection. In addition, some patients who have excessive venous leakage on cavernosometry and cavernosography may leak primarily via the crural veins near the base of the penis and not via the deep dorsal penile vein. These crural veins are not accessible to duplex sonographic evaluation. For these reasons, deep dorsal vein flow analysis does not appear to be a totally reliable method for the evaluation of a patient with possible venogenic impotence.

PITFALLS AND DUPLEX DOPPLER SONOGRAPHY FOR IMPOTENCE

Reversal of diastolic flow is a normal phenomenon in the later stages of erection (see Fig. 89–8). However, systolic flow reversal is not normal and usually indicates proximal penile artery occlusion with collateral flow in a retrograde fashion into the affected cavernosal artery. Proximal penile artery occlusion can result from trauma, corporal fibrosis, or atherosclerotic vessel disease. Reversal of systolic flow in the cavernosal artery warrants further evaluation with conventional angiography.

Collateral vessels from the contralateral cavernosal artery, dorsal penile artery, or spongiosal artery can often be seen with color Doppler sonography. These collateral vessels may be normal or may indicate proximal disease in the affected artery and should be noted.

Particular attention should also be given to the presence of arterial sinusoidal fistulas or arterial venous fistulas within the corporal tissue of the penis in patients who have developed erectile dysfunction following trauma. These lesions are often very amenable to surgical repair. Partial priapism can often be an accompanying sign in arterial sinusoidal fistulas, and color Doppler evaluation can often locate the fistula in question.

Although intracavernosal injection of vasodilating agents is supposed to bypass the psychologic stimulus needed for an erection, excessive psychologic overlay may result in an increase in adrenergic tone and ultimately lead to impaired response to these vasodilating agents. Suboptimal PSV (less than 25 cm/sec) can occur as a result of this excessive alpha-adrenergic tone in normal patients with excessive anxiety. Therefore, patients should be studied in an appropriate setting with the least amount of distraction.

The maximum response to an intracavernosal vasodilating agent varies among individuals, and PSV in normal males can occur at any time from 5 to 30 minutes post-injection. Therefore, in order to detect the absolute maximum velocities, PSV measurements should be taken at 5, 10, 15, and 20 minutes post-injection.

Because normal individuals may have high EDV early in the examination (5 to 10 minutes post-injection), EDV measurements should be assessed at the later time periods (15 to 20 minutes). Persistent low-resistance spectral waveforms at these later times in association with normal cavernosal artery PSV should indicate persistent and excessive venous leakage as a possible cause of the patient's impotence. If measurements are only made at 5 or 10 minutes post-injection, a false interpretation of excessive venous leakage could be made. Therefore, high EDV can only indicate excessive venous leakage when obtained 15 to 20 minutes post-injection and if there is adequate arterial inflow (PSV > 30 cm/sec).

Proper injection of the vasodilating agents is paramount to obtaining accurate results. If the vasodilating agent is injected into the corpus spongiosum, erection may not occur. In addition, the vasodilating agent may inadvertently enter the urethra and not have an effect on the cavernosa.

CAVERNOSOMETRY AND CAVERNOSOGRAPHY

Traditionally, cavernosometry and cavernosography have been used to evaluate patients further who have evidence of venogenic impotence and who are interested in possible surgery to correct their vasculogenic impotence. Cavernosometry is a method by which heparinized saline is infused into the corpora cavernosa and pressure measurements and flow measurements are made at the initiation and maintenance of an erection. These pressure measurements and flow measurements are then used to diagnose excessive venous leakage definitively. Cavernosography is a method by which contrast media is injected into the corpora cavernosa at a specified rate in order to detect excessive venous leakage and to identify the routes of venous efflux for future surgical ligation.

The techniques of cavernosometry and cavernosography vary widely and are most often performed by urologists in the operating room setting.

In our practice, maintenance flow rates greater than 100 ml/min usually indicate a significant venous leak on cavernosometry performed without a pharmacologic agent. When an intracavernosal vasodilating agent is given, maintenance flow rates greater than 50 ml/min are abnormal. Maintenance flow rates of 30 to 50 ml/min after the intracavernosal injection of a vasodilating agent are indeterminate. Maintenance flow rates less than 30 ml/min are considered normal.

If cavernosometry indicates excessive venous leakage, cavernosography is performed. Cavernosography should always be performed after a cavernosal pharmacologic agent has been injected to limit the volume of iodinated contrast that is to be used. In addition, arterial inflow and smooth muscle relaxation must be maximized pharmacologically for accurate demonstration of abnormal effluxing veins. Our technique for performing cavernosography uses 60 ml of a low-osmolar, iodinated contrast media agent. While the contrast is infusing at the previous maximum maintenance rate necessary to produce a pressure of at least 90 mmHg, anteroposterior and oblique films are taken of the penis.

Veins that commonly show efflux of contrast in patients with veno-occlusive dysfunction are the deep dorsal penile veins and the cavernosal or crural veins (Fig. 89–10). The deep dorsal penile veins and cavernosal veins drain into the retropubic venous plexus. The retropubic venous plexus drains into the pudendal veins. An alternative route of venous efflux from the penis is via the external pudendal system, which ultimately drains into the saphenous veins. Rarely, excessive venous efflux from the corpora cavernosa can occur via the corpus spongiosum and superficial venous system.

In summary, the definitive diagnosis of excessive venous leakage can only be made with cavernosometry data. The performance of cavernosometry after the injection of a vasodilating agent is more physiologic and more diagnostic in the evaluation of venogenic impotence. Cavernosography is used as a venous map for possible surgical ligation in patients who have demonstrated excessive venous leakage on cavernosometry.

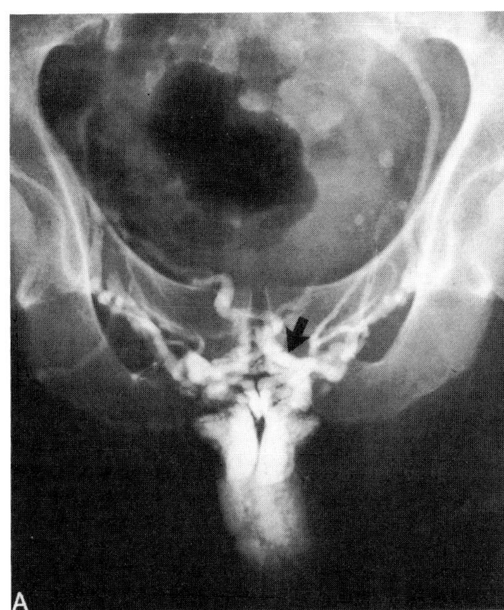

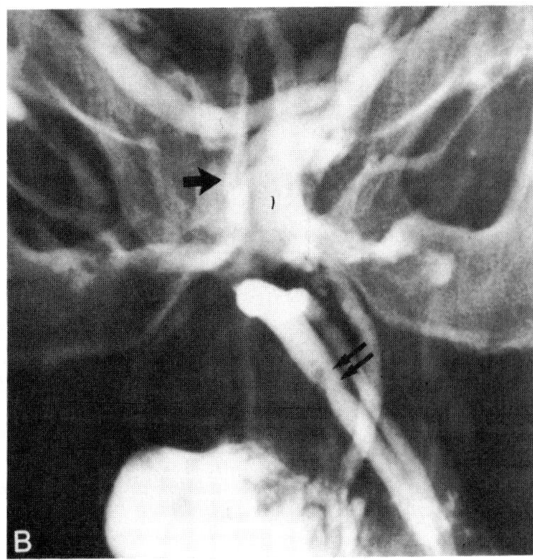

Figure 89–10. *A*, An anteroposterior image of the pelvis obtained during cavernosography depicting excessive venous leakage from the deep dorsal vein and crural veins into the retropubic venous plexus *(arrow)*. *B*, A magnified view of the base of the penis of another patient during a cavernosogram. Excessive venous leakage is occurring through the deep dorsal vein *(double arrows)* with ultimate drainage into the retropubic venous plexus *(arrow)*.

ANGIOGRAPHY

Only patients who are candidates for percutaneous balloon angioplasty or surgery should undergo more invasive arteriography in the evaluation of arteriogenic impotence. Certain patients are more likely to benefit from vascular surgery and, therefore, may be more appropriate candidates for arteriography. These patients include young men who are impotent and who have a history of severe pelvic trauma or older men who report symptoms and signs of small vessel disease, such as angina or claudication. In general, only patients under 60 years of age should be considered for angiography in the evaluation of impotence. All patients undergoing angiography should be screened first with duplex Doppler sonography of the cavernosal arteries.

Angiography in the evaluation of impotent men is challenging, and a proper understanding of arterial anatomy is important (see Fig. 89–2). The internal pudendal artery (IPA) is the major source of blood supply during an erection. This artery also supplies blood flow to the perineum and external genitalia. The IPA originates as a branch of the anterior division of the internal iliac artery. Several variations can occur at the origin of the IPA. In most patients, the IPA shares a common trunk with the inferior gluteal artery. The second most common presentation is the IPA as the terminal branch of the anterior division of the internal iliac artery. Rarely, the IPA arises as an isolated branch of the internal iliac artery or possibly as a branch of the obturator or hemorrhoidal arteries.

The IPA terminates in the common penile artery as it passes through the urogenital diaphragm. This terminal segment of the IPA is seen on an anterior oblique view of the pelvis at the inferior anterior margin of the obturator foramen just before the artery projects under the ischiopubic ramus. This segment of the artery gives rise to the artery of the penis, which then gives off the urethral branch, and finally terminates as the dorsal penile artery and cavernosal artery.

The best projection for the evaluation of the common penile artery branches is the ipsilateral anterior oblique projection usually from a 25 to 45 degree off axis with the penis stretched out over the media surface of the opposite thigh. The cavernosal artery is certainly the most important artery to visualize in angiography for impotence. Rarely, this artery may be bifid in one cavernous space. The cavernosal artery is usually 0.5 mm in diameter. The dorsal penile artery, which supplies the skin and glans of the penis, is usually more superior and larger, measuring 0.5 to 0.8 mm in diameter. As a normal variation, cavernosal arteries can be visualized as branches off the dorsal artery along the shaft of the penis.

It is not uncommon for both cavernosal arteries to arise from one penile artery. In addition, normal anastomotic bridges between both dorsal arteries, cavernosal arteries, or bulbar arteries can be appreciated at the base of the penis near the crura of the erectile bodies in the infrapubic region. For discussions of the variations in arterial anatomy and numerous collateral branches, the reader is referred to the reports by Bookstein (1987) and Ginestie (1978).

The angiographic technique in the evaluation of the impotent patient should begin with a nonselective pelvic angiogram with the catheter in the aorta above the bifurcation. This aortic flush study may demonstrate large vessel abnormalities that may be amenable to balloon dilatation or definitive pelvic vascular surgery. After this nonselective angiogram, selective internal pudendal arteriography is performed. Prior to selective internal pudendal arteriography, 40 to 60 mg of papaverine are injected into the left corpora cavernosa to aid in the visualization of the cavernosal artery. Taking a transfemoral approach, we use a 5.2 Fr, reverse curve, Bookstein-shaped catheter (Cordis Company, Miami, FL) for selective study of the internal pudendal artery. We generally inject 25 ml of a low–osmolar contrast agent at 4 ml/sec. Cut film techniques are used in the ipsilateral anterior oblique projection, and proper care is taken to position the penis so it is as stretched out as possible on the contralateral thigh. Patients are centered so that the field of view includes the penile tip in the lower corner of the film. We use a film series of two films every second for three seconds, one film every second for six seconds, and one film every three seconds for nine seconds for a total of 15 films.

Bookstein and associates have suggested that if normal penile arterial architecture is seen on the first selective study, the opposite side need not be investigated. However, we continue to evaluate both the right and left internal pudendal arteries in all patients.

Generally, abnormal lesions in arteriography can be grouped into three categories: obstructive, traumatic, or dysplastic. Obstructive lesions are often atheromatous lesions and generally occur in patients 50 to 60 years of age, usually affecting the ischiorectal segment of the internal pudendal artery. Traumatic and dysplastic lesions tend to involve the internal pudendal artery as it crosses the urogenital diaphragm.

Significant stenosis of these vessels has not been standardized. However, we feel that a 50 per cent reduction in diameter indicates significant arterial disease (Fig. 89–11). Failure to visualize the cavernosal arteries with pharmacoarteriography is indicative of arteriogenic disease. However, one must also be aware of anatomic variations, and if selective internal pudendal arteriography fails to visualize any penile arteries, more proximal studies of the hypogastric arteries are indicated to look for accessory pudendal arteries.

Attention should also be paid to the inferior epigastric arteries lying in the anterior abdominal wall, because they are often used for surgical revascularization of the penile arteries. Also, in patients who have experienced pelvic trauma, one must pay particular attention to the base of the corpora cavernosa for any evidence of arterial sinusoidal fistulas. All arteriograms should be correlated with the duplex Doppler sonography in order to correlate the physiologic velocity findings in the duplex Doppler examination with the anatomic findings of the arteriogram.

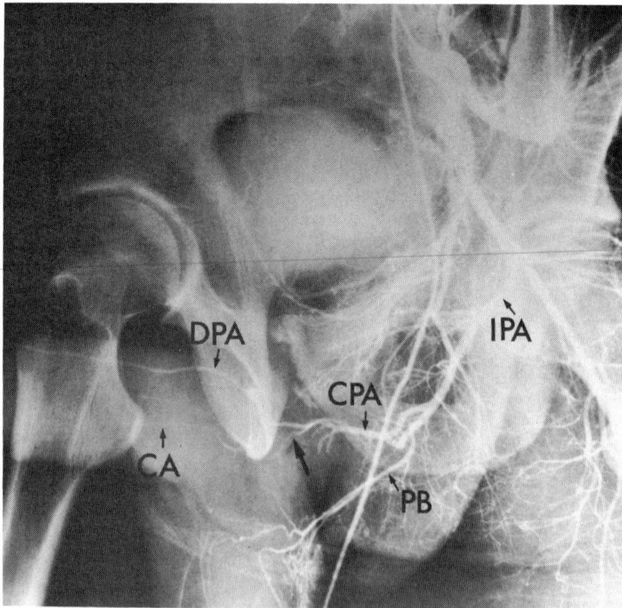

Figure 89–11. A selective injection of the left internal pudendal artery with subsequent reflux into the proximal internal iliac artery. This angiogram image demonstrates a normal internal pudendal artery (IPA) as it gives off the perineal branch (PB). However, as the internal pudendal artery terminates in the common penile artery (CPA), one notices adequate filling of the dorsal penile artery (DPA) but inadequate opacification and visualization of the cavernosal artery (CA). The inadequate opacification of the cavernosal artery is due to a significant stenosis at the origin of the cavernosal artery *(large arrow).*

TABLE 89–2. CLASSIFICATION OF PENILE PROSTHESES

Noninflatable: semirigid and malleable
Inflatable: multicomponent
Self-contained inflatable and mechanical prostheses

PENILE PROSTHESES

The treatment of impotence varies; however, the most common treatment is the placement of a penile prosthesis. Because impotence is a common problem, and because these devices are becoming more and more popular, it is important to have an understanding of the pelvic radiography of patients presenting with mechanical malfunctions of their prostheses. Because of potential malfunction, it is important to be familiar with the appearance of normal noninflatable and inflatable prostheses and to be able to recognize the radiographic appearance of the more common causes of malfunction in inflatable penile prostheses.

Classification

There are three major types of penile prostheses (Table 89–2; Fig. 89–12). The first penile prosthesis introduced consisted of a single semirigid acrylic or silicone rod placed into the penis. Subsequently, paired semirigid or malleable rods were developed for placement into each corpus cavernosum (Table 89–3). The AMS600, JONAS, and Mentor Malleable prostheses contain a central core of bendable, braided stainless steel or silver wires. The rest of the prostheses are only faintly radio-opaque.

Inflatable penile prostheses can either be self-contained in one single unit or can be made up of many components. Numerous types are available (Table 89–4). These inflatable penile prostheses represented an improvement over semirigid or malleable prostheses in that both erect and flaccid states could be achieved. Concealment by the patient was no longer an embarrassing problem, and the quality of erection was superior to that possible by noninflatable prostheses.

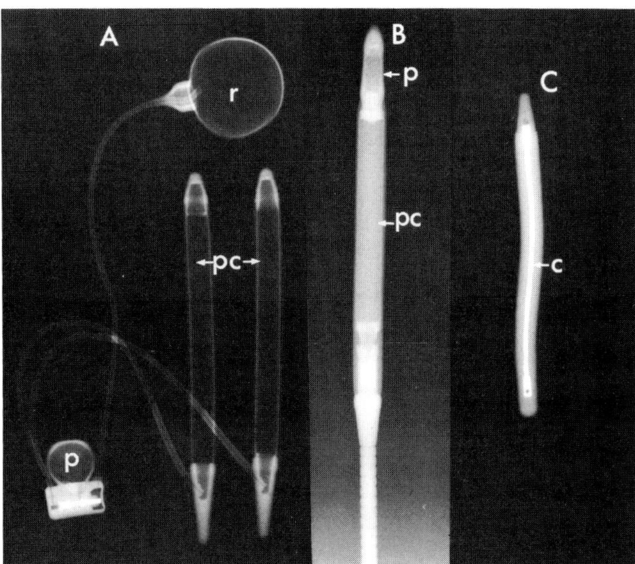

Figure 89–12. Radiographs of three different types of penile prostheses. *A*, Multicomponent inflatable prosthesis with reservoir (r), pump (p), and penile cylinders (pc). *B*, Self-contained inflatable prosthesis with pump (p) and penile cylinder (pc). *C*, Noninflatable, semirigid prosthesis with central core (c) of stainless steel.

TABLE 89–3. NONINFLATABLE: SEMIRIGID AND MALLEABLE PENILE PROSTHESES

Small carry-on prostheses (Heyer-Schultz Company, Minneapolis, MN)
Semirigid Finney prostheses (Surgitek Inc., Racine, WI)
AMS600 (American Medical Systems, Minnetonka, MN)
JONAS (Dacomed Company, Minneapolis, MN)
Mentor Malleable (Mentor Company, Goletta, CA)

Most current multicomponent inflatable prostheses contain four separate components interconnected by tubing. The major components are two penile cylinders made of extensile silicone rubber polymer so that they can widen and stiffen when inflated. These two cylinders are connected to a hydraulic pump implanted subcutaneously in the scrotum. This hydraulic pump is connected to a spherical reservoir usually placed just deep to the erectus abdominis muscle in the pelvis. The reservoir pump and cylinders are filled with diluted radiographic contrast media (12.5 per cent by weight) so that the integrity of the prosthesis can be checked easily with plain radiography should a malfunction occur.

Self-contained inflatable and mechanical prostheses have an advantage over the multicomponent inflatable prostheses in that surgical insertion and repair are technically easier. Preliminary reports indicate low surgical and medical complication rates and a reasonable degree of patient satisfaction. Some of these self-contained devices are changed from a flaccid to erect state by activation of a distal inflation pump (Hydroflex, American Medical Systems; Flexiflate 1 and 2, Surgitek Inc.), and others consist of a number of plastic segments connected by a spring-action cable (Omniphase and Duraphase from Dacomed) (Table 89–5).

Radiographic Manifestations of Malfunctioning Penile Prostheses

Mechanical malfunctions of penile prostheses occur most commonly with the inflatable penile prostheses. However, noninflatable semirigid and malleable prostheses can develop mechanical complications. Rarely, patients may present with complete breaks through the semirigid silicone prosthesis. Reports of erosion of a semirigid or malleable prosthesis through the skin or end of the urethra have been noted. This latter complication is usually obvious on physical examination. In addition, small breaks or fraying of the braided silver wire core in some malleable prostheses have been found. Despite the excellent radio-opacity of the silver core, many of the breaks or small areas of fraying have been underestimated on plain film radiography.

Malfunction of inflatable multicomponent prostheses is often difficult to evaluate with physical examination. Interestingly, most malfunctions of multicomponent inflatable prostheses can adequately be assessed with a single oblique pelvic radiograph with the prosthesis inflated.

One of the more common malfunctions that patients with mechanical inflatable penile prostheses present is inadequate inflation of the prosthesis to achieve a satisfactory erection. Pelvic radiogra-

TABLE 89–4. INFLATABLE MULTICOMPONENT PENILE PROSTHESES

AMS700 (American Medical Systems, Minnetonka, MN)
Mentor IPP (Mentor Company, Goletta, CA)
Uniflate* (Surgitek Inc., Racine, WI)
Mentor GFR* (Mentor Company, Goletta, CA)

*These models combine the pump and reservoir into one unit and, therefore, have fewer components.

TABLE 89–5. SELF-CONTAINED PROSTHESES

Inflatable
Hydroflex (American Medical Systems, Minnetonka, MN)
Flexi-flate 1 and 2 (Surgitek Inc., Racine, WI)
Mechanical
Omniphase (Dacomed Company, Minneapolis, MN)
Duraphase (Dacomed Company, Minneapolis, MN)

phy often reveals a marked decrease in the amount of fluid in the reservoir. The penile cylinders are often underinflated. The water-soluble iodinated contrast material that leaks out of the reservoir of cylinders is rapidly absorbed and excreted by the kidneys and is therefore not visible on plain film radiographs. Another complication of inflatable multicomponent prostheses is aneurysmal dilatation or buckling of the cylinder. This is often due to a structural deficiency within the cylinder or possibly due to pre-existing weakness in the tunica albuginea. These cylinder aneurysms are easily seen on plain film radiography. Patients often present with gradual loss of penile rigidity or may have erections that become angulated or asymmetrical.

Kinks or separation of the tubing of these multicomponent inflatable prostheses can occur and usually develop within the first few months after surgery. Kinking or separation of the tubing can easily be seen on plain film radiography.

Pump migration or malfunction should be considered in any patient with a nonfunctioning prosthesis whose pelvic radiograph is normal.

Erosion of the pump or reservoir has been known to occur. Reservoirs usually erode into the bladder. Pump erosions are usually easily detected on physical examination. Detection of reservoir erosion into bowel or the bladder is often difficult on a plain radiograph and often requires endoscopy or surgery for the diagnosis.

Inflatable self-contained prostheses also may malfunction. Fracture of the reservoir or mechanical malfunction of the spring-action cable (Omniphase) may occur. In some cases, there is no mechanical dysfunction but the patient has had difficulty in using the pump.

The wide variety of prostheses available and the constant change and improvement of many of these prostheses make it difficult to identify the exact type of prosthesis a patient has on plain film radiography; however, plain film radiography can aid in the problem solving for patients with a malfunctioning penile prosthesis.

Bibliography

Aboseif SR, Lue TF: Hemodynamics of penile erection. Urol Clin North Am 15:1–7, 1988.

Abozeid M, Juenemann K, Luo J, et al: Chronic papaverine treatment: The effect of repeated injections on the simian erectile response and penile tissue. J Urol 138:1263, 1987.

Benson CB, Vickers MA: Sexual impotence caused by vascular disease: Diagnosis with duplex sonography. AJR 153:1149–1153, 1989.

Bookstein JJ: Cavernosal veno-occlusive insufficiency in male impotence: Evaluation of degree and location. Radiology 164:175–178, 1987.

Bookstein JJ, Lang E: Penile magnification pharmacoarteriography: Details of intrapenile arterial anatomy. AJR 148:883–888, 1987.

Bookstein JJ, Valji K: The arteriolar component of impotence: A possible paradigm shift. AJR 157:932–934, 1991.

Brühlmann W, Pouliadis G, Zollikofer C: Cavernous hemangioma, et al: Arteriography of the penis in secondary impotence. Urol Radiol 4:243–249, 1982.

Buvat J, Bervat-Hertaut M, Dehaene JL, et al: Is intravenous injection of papaverine a reliable screening test for vasculogenic impotence? J Urol 135:476–478, 1986.

Collins JP, Lewandowski BJ: Experience with intracorporeal injection of papaverine and duplex ultrasound scanning for assessment of arteriogenic impotence. Br J Urol 59:84–88, 1987.

Curet P, Grellet J, Perrin D, et al: Technical and anatomic factors in filling of distal portion of internal pudendal artery during arteriography. Urology 20:333–338, 1987.

Desai KM, Gingell JC, Skidmore R, Follett OK: Application of computerized penile arterial waveform analysis in the diagnosis of arteriogenic impotence: An initial study in potent and impotent men. Br J Urol 60:5:450–456, 1987.

de Tejada IS, Goldstein I, Azadzoi K, et al: Impaired neurogenic and endothelium mediated relaxation of penile smooth muscle from diabetic men with impotence. N Engl J Med 320:1025, 1989.

Fallon B, Rosenberg S, Culp DA: Long-term follow-up in patients with an inflatable penile prosthesis. J Urol 132:270–271, 1984.

Fishman IJ, Scott FB, Light JK: Experience with inflatable penile prosthesis. Urology 23:86–92, 1984.

Fitzgerald SW, Erickson SJ, Foley WD, et al: Color Doppler sonography in the evaluation of erectile dysfunction: Patterns of temporal response to papaverine. AJR 157:331–336, 1991.

Fujita T, Shirai M. Mechanism of erection. J Clin Exp Med 148:249, 1989.

Gall H, Barhren W, Scherb W, et al: Diagnostic accuracy of Doppler ultrasound technique of the penile arteries in correlation to selective arteriography. Cardio Vasc Intervent Radiol 11:225–231, 1988.

Ginestie JF, Romieu A: Radiologic Exploration of Impotence. Boston, Martinus Nijhoff, 1978.

Jeremy JW, Thompson CS, Mikbalide DD, et al: Experimental diabetes mellitus prostocycline synthesis by the rat penis: Pathologic implications. Diabetologica 28:365, 1985.

Hattery RR, King BF, James EM, et al: Vasculogenic impotence: Duplex and color Doppler imaging. AJR 156:189–195, 1991.

Hattery RR, King BF, Lewis RW, et al: Vasculogenic impotence: Duplex and color Doppler imaging. Radiol Clinics North Am 29:629–645, 1991.

Hovsepian DM, Amis ES Jr: Penile prosthetic implants: A radiographic atlas. RadioGraphics 9:707–716, 1989.

Huguet JF, Clerissi J, Juhan C: Radiologic anatomy of pudendal artery. Eur J Radiol 1:278–284, 1981.

Juhan CM, Padula G, Huguet JF: Angiography in male impotence. In Bennett AH (ed): Management of Malignant Impotence. Baltimore, Williams and Wilkins, 1982, pp 73–107.

Kiely E, Williams G, Goldie L: Assessment of the immediate and long-term effects of pharmacologically induced penile erection in the treatment of psychogenic and organic impotence. Br J Urol 59:164, 1987.

King BF Jr: Color Doppler flow imaging evaluation of the deep dorsal penile vein in vascular impotence (abstract, scientific program). Radiologic Society of North America 1989 Scientific Program, Radiology, 173(P), p 371.

King BF Jr, Hattery RR, James EM, Lewis RW: Duplex sonography in the evaluation of impotence: Current techniques. Semin Intervent Radiol 7:215–221, 1990.

Krysiewicz S, Mellinger BC: The role of imaging in the diagnostic evaluation of impotence. AJR 153:1133–1139, 1989.

Lewis RW: This month in investigative urology: Venous impotence. J Urol 140:1560, 1988.

Lewis RW: Diagnosis and management of corporal veno-occlusive dysfunction. Semin Urol 8:113–123, 1990.

Lewis RW, Puyau FA: Procedures for decreasing venous drainage. Semin Urol 4:263–272, 1986.

Lue TF, Hricak H, Marich KW, Tanagho EA: Vasculogenic impotence evaluated by high-resolution ultrasonography and pulsed Doppler spectrum analysis. Radiology 155:777–781, 1985.

Lue TF, Hricak H, Marich KW, Tanagho EA: Evaluation of arteriogenic impotence with intracorporeal injection of papaverine and the duplex ultrasound scanner. Semin Urol 3:43–48, 1985.

Lue TF, Hricak H, Schmidt RA, et al: Functional evaluation of penile veins by cavernosography in papaverine induced erection. J Urol 135:479–482, 1986.

Lue T, Tanagho E: Physiology of erection and pharmacologic management of impotence. J Urol 137:829, 1987.

Mellinger BC, Fried JJ, Vaughan ED: Papaverine-induced penile blood flow acceleration in impotent men measured by duplex scanning. J Urol 144:897–899, 1990.

Paushter DM: Role of duplex sonography in the evaluation of sexual impotence. AJR 153:1161–1163, 1989.

Quam JP, King BF, James EM, et al: Duplex and color Doppler sonographic evaluation of vasculogenic impotence. AJR 153:1141–1147, 1989.

Rajfer J, Aronson WJ, Bush PA, et al: Nitric oxide as a mediator of relaxation of the corpus cavernosum in response to non-adrenergic, non-cholinergic neurotransmission. N Engl J Med 326:90–94, 1992.

Robinson LQ, Woodcock JP, Stephenson TP: Duplex scanning in suspected vasculogenic impotence: A worthwhile exercise? Br J Urol 63:432–436, 1989.

Roth JC, King BF, Hattery RR, et al: Vasculogenic impotence: Dynamic duplex and color Doppler penile sonography. (Submitted for publication.)

Saenz de Tejada IS, Goldstein I, Krane RJ: Local control of penile erection: Nerve, smooth muscle and endothelium. Urol Clin North Am 15:9–15, 1988.

Schwartz AN, Wang KY, Mack LA, et al: Evaluation of normal erectile function with color flow Doppler sonography. AJR 153:1155–1160, 1989.

Stackl W, Hasun R, Marberger M: Intracavernous injection of prostaglandin E1 in impotent men. J Urol 140:66, 1988.

Tanaka T: Papaverine hydrochloride in peripheral blood and the degree of penile erection. J Urol 143:1135–1137, 1990.

Virag R: About pharmacologically induced prolonged erection (letter to the editor). Lancet 1:519, 1985.

Witt MA, Goldstein I, de Tejada IS, et al: Traumatic laceration of intracavernosal arteries: The pathophysiology of non-ischemic, high flow, arterial priapism. J Urol 143:129–132, 1989.

90 Scrotal Imaging

Lynwood Hammers, Kenneth Bird, and Arthur T. Rosenfield

Many radiologic modalities are useful in the diagnostic work-up of disease involving the male external genitalia. Because modern ultrasound equipment can obtain high-resolution images within a few moments without pain, radiation, patient preparation, or the need for contrast material, scrotal evaluation is predominantly done utilizing Doppler color flow imaging (DCFI) technology (Fig. 90–1). DCFI combines high-resolution gray-scale imaging; qualitative hemodynamic blood flow information represented as color flow; and quantitative evaluation of blood flow presence, direction, and velocity with Doppler. Anatomic and physiologic information is now available with state-of-the-art ultrasound equipment.

DCFI equipment should be considered the primary modality for evaluation of the scrotum. Radionuclide scanning utilizing technetium-99m pertechnetate provides an accurate means for determining scrotal perfusion, thus complementing the anatomic data obtained by ultrasound. Computed tomographic (CT) scanning has proven to be of greatest value in detecting metastatic spread from primary testicular neoplasms. Scrotal plain-film radiography is seldom utilized except for confirming gas-filled loops in hernias or in detecting unusual calcifications such as calcified meconium peritonitis in infants. Testicular venography has use in locating undescended testes and in diagnosing varicoceles. Transvenous balloon occlusion techniques have been developed to successfully treat varicoceles nonoperatively. Magnetic resonance imaging (MRI) is a technique that can both define masses and demonstrate abnormalities in blood flow. Flow within vessels leads to an absence of signal, so those vessels without flow can be identified since they will generate a signal. Experience with MRI of the testis has shown that it is comparable with ultrasound.

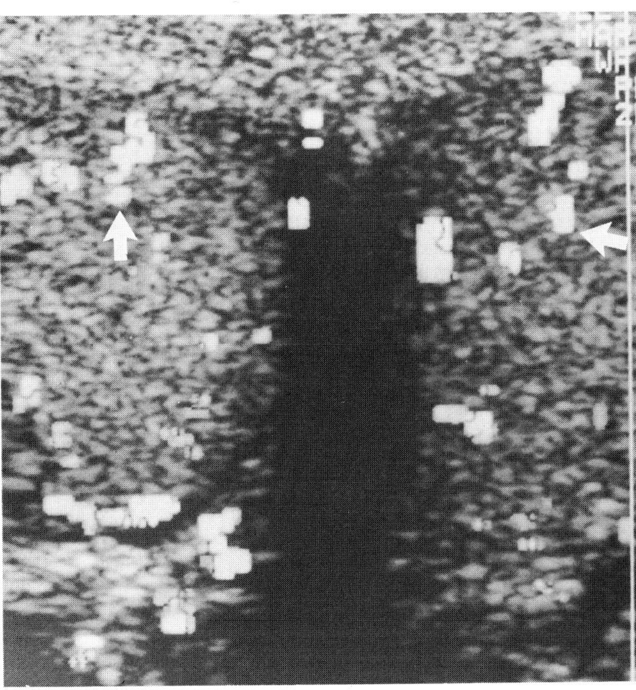

Figure 90–1. Transverse color flow image of testis demonstrates bilateral normal intratesticular flow (*arrows*).

SCROTAL ANATOMY

Radiologic and ultrasound imaging (Fig. 90–2) offers only limited resolution of intrascrotal anatomy when compared with the microscopist's view. However, high-frequency transducers provide sufficient detail to be diagnostically helpful with most clinicopathologic entities. The multiple individual layers of the scrotal skin are imaged as a single, relatively echogenic band surrounding the scrotal contents and extending into the median raphe separating the two hemiscrotal compartments. Increased scrotal skin thickening is most commonly observed with ischemic and inflammatory disorders and trauma. Lymphatic and venous obstructions are less frequent causes of skin thickening.

Small amounts of serous fluid are normally seen between the skin and testis, particularly in the crevices between the epididymis and testis in the polar regions. These are not diagnosed as hydroceles unless large and palpable.

The fibrous tunica albuginea that is closely adherent to the testis is not normally imaged except where it reflects into the testis proper

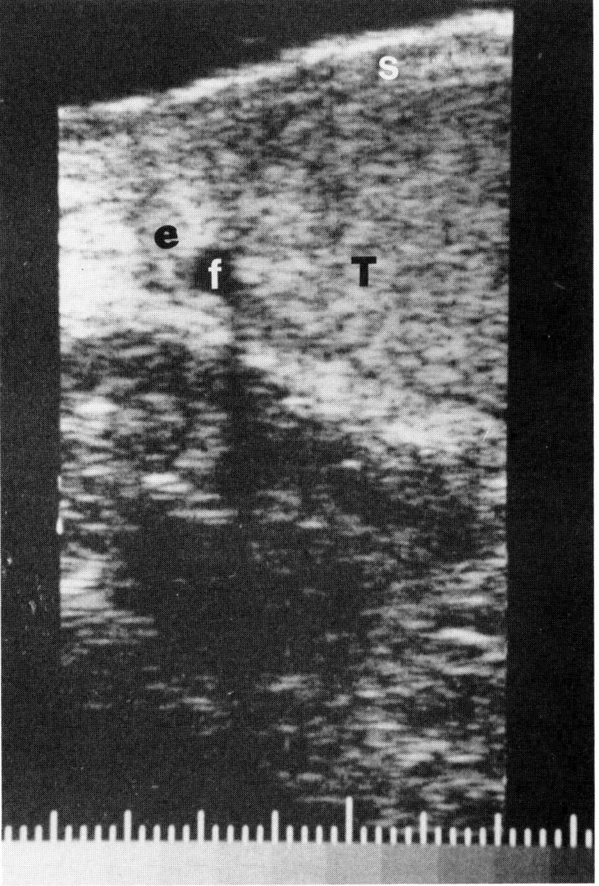

Figure 90–2. High-resolution 10-mHz longitudinal real-time sonogram of cephalic pole of normal testis. The mediastinum testis is not visualized on this single projection. (s = skin; T = testis; e = head of epididymis; f = intrascrotal fluid.)

as the mediastinum testis. This is identifiable as an echogenic band or plate extending into the otherwise uniform granular acoustic texture of the testis. The normal individual lobules of the testis are not imaged. Occasional small, bright reflecting foci are seen in otherwise normal testes as incidental findings.

The epididymis is somewhat crescentric in shape and is applied to the testis posterolaterally in most instances. The globus major is thicker than the body and tail of the epididymis and is usually, but not always, located at the cephalic pole. The epididymis is typically more echogenic than the testis, probably due to its connective tissue fascial linings. The tail of the epididymis is often difficult to discern from the lower pole of the testis unless enlarged and inflamed.

Veins of the pampiniform plexus can be imaged as branching, echo-free tubules posteriorly. Intratesticular veins are not always seen due to slow flow. The dilated veins of varicoceles are easily visualized with DCFI. The spermatic cord is seen as a moderately echogenic structure extending from the testis to the inguinal region.

The paired testicular arteries supply blood to the testes. Anastomoses occur between the testicular arteries and the differential and cremasteric arteries that supply the epididymis and peritesticular tissues, respectively. The testicular arteries branch into capsular arteries that lie beneath the tunica albuginea. The intratesticular arteries are the centripetal and recurrent rami. The arteries other than recurrent rami should consistently be seen with 7.5- or 10-mHz linear array color transducers. The arterial blood supply to the testes is of low impedance (Fig. 90–3). Normal color flow parameters of the testes have been established by Middleton et al (1989).

The indications for scrotal ultrasound are summarized in Table 90–1.

TABLE 90–1. USES OF SCROTAL ULTRASOUND

1. Evaluation of scrotal masses to determine if these are testicular or extratesticular and cystic vs solid
2. Assessment of acute scrotum
3. Evaluation of patients with epididymitis that do not respond to conservative treatment
4. Evaluation of patients with known metastatic disease and no known primary to localize occult tumors
5. Detection of testicular recurrence in patients with leukemia or lymphoma
6. Detection of varicoceles in fertility work-ups
7. Location of undescended testes
8. Evaluation of the traumatized scrotum

ULTRASOUND TECHNIQUE

Before scanning, patients are given a brief explanation of the examination, stressing its noninvasiveness. A brief history is obtained, and the scrotum is gently but thoroughly palpated unless there is severe pain. Patients are encouraged to volunteer pertinent history and to participate in localizing specific nodules, painful areas, or other abnormalities in the scrotum. This is helpful in allaying fears and in obtaining a better examination with full patient cooperation. The patient is most commonly scanned supine with the scrotum elevated and a towel tucked under the thighs. The coupling gel and the room should be warm to prevent cremasteric reflex contractions. The upright position may be helpful for confirming venous distention in varicoceles.

The scrotum is imaged utilizing a high-resolution (5, 7.5, or 10 mHz) dedicated ''small parts'' real-time scanner with Doppler color flow capabilities. A 3.5-mHz transducer may be used if the scrotum is massively enlarged. Satisfactory views can most easily be obtained by direct contact scanning. A stand-off gel pad can be utilized for a more global view of the scrotum. The asymptomatic side is scanned first to optimize the DCFI capabilities. The lowest pulse repetition frequency and wall filter are used. Color gain should be maximized for slow flow detection. Both longitudinal and transverse images are obtained. Comparison of right and left images, color flow, and Doppler signals should be noted.

The Acutely Painful Scrotum. An approach to imaging the acutely painful scrotum is summarized in Table 90–2.

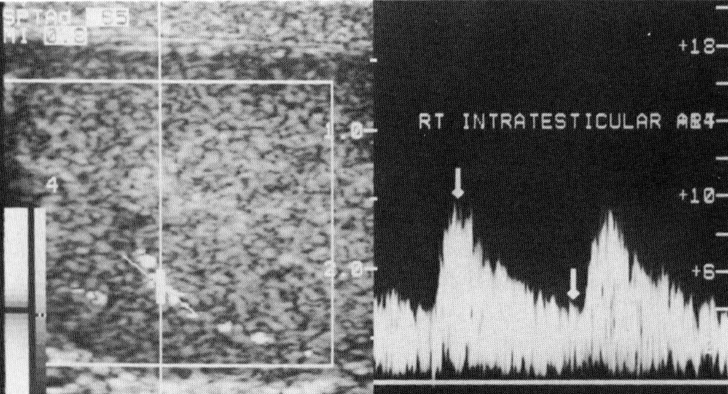

Figure 90–3. Normal intratesticular Doppler color flow imaging (DCFI) reveals low peak systolic velocity (PSV) (*arrow* at 10 cm/second) with prominent diastolic flow (*arrow* at 5 cm/second).

TORSION

Torsion of the testis is a relatively uncommon event, less common than neoplastic disease and much less common than epididymitis or epididymo-orchitis. Its importance lies in the urgency of rapid diagnosis so as to salvage a viable testis with prompt surgery.

Torsion can occur at any age from the fetus to the elderly. It most commonly occurs in young, prepubertal boys. The onset may occur during sleep, following minor trauma, or spontaneously. The pain associated with torsion is usually both immediate and intense. The scrotum is often swollen, erythematous, and exquisitely painful. The affected testis often sits higher in the scrotum than the contralateral side due to the twisting. Patients may give a history of one or more similar episodes of pain in the past with subsequent relief of symptoms due to transient torsion and detorsion. Occasionally, patients with torsion present with a less abrupt onset of symptoms and with less intense pain. These individuals may thus be incorrectly diag-

TABLE 90–2. RADIOLOGIC ALGORITHM FOR INITIAL EVALUATION OF THE PAINFUL SCROTUM

Acute Painful Scrotum (1–24 hours)
- A. Typical clinically
  1. Classic torsion: surgical exploration
  2. Classic epididymitis, epididymo-orchitis: conservative treatment, imaging not necessary
  3. Classic torsion appendix testis or appendix epididymis: surgical excision, imaging not necessary.
     a. Penetrating injury: surgical exploration and repair
     b. Blunt trauma: DCFI
- B. Indeterminate clinically or confirmation needed
  1. DCFI to determine testicular flow

Subacute Painful Scrotum (hours–few days)
- A. Typical clinical epididymo-orchitis: conservative treatment, imaging not necessary.
- B. Possible missed torsion: DCFI or ^{99m}Tc scan
- C. Possible tumor: ultrasound

Chronic Painful Scrotum (few days–weeks)
- A. Start with DCFI

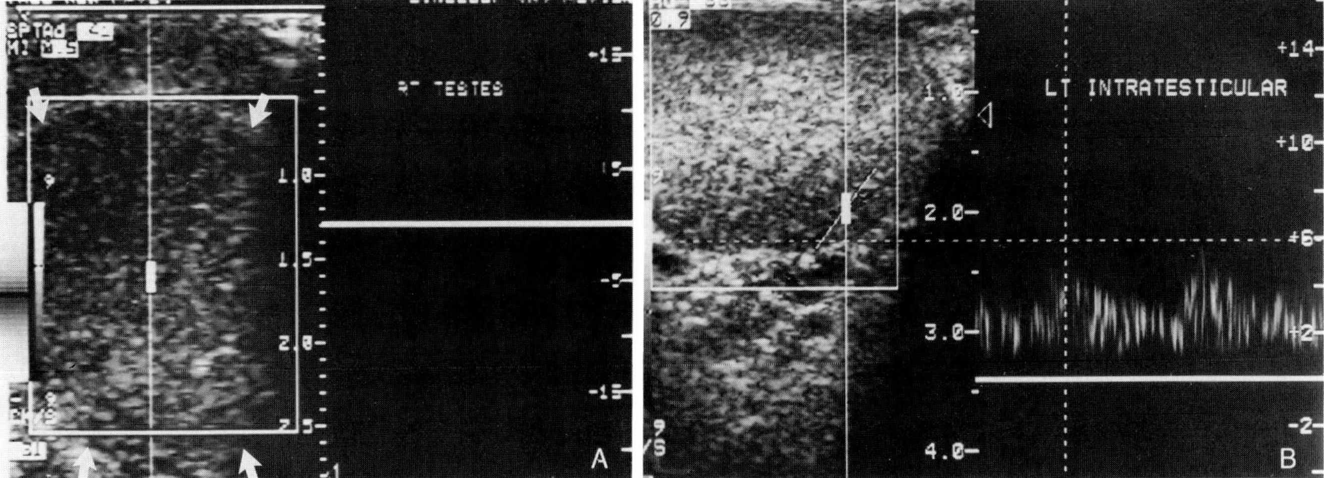

Figure 90–4. *A,* DCFI shows no flow with testis with right-sided torsion. Arrows outline testis. *B,* Normal intratesticular DCFI of asymptomatic side.

nosed as having epididymitis, given a trial of antibiotics, and unfortunately go on to infarct their testes as missed torsions.

When young men do present with classic clinical findings of acute torsion, one should proceed directly to surgery. If the clinical examination is equivocal or documentation is needed presurgically, DCFI or nuclear medicine is performed. DCFI reveals decreased or no flow when compared with the asymptomatic side (Fig. 90–4). The degree and duration of torsion are the most important factors in testicular salvage. DCFI can visualize decreased flow that nuclear medicine may miss. DCFI for torsion is a rapid examination requiring 5 to 10 minutes. At our institution, DCFI is the preferred examination. However, the examination performed—DCFI or nuclear medicine—should be the one most readily available. Radioisotope flow studies are diagnostically helpful not only with acute torsions but also with chronic missed torsions. These most often demonstrate a halo appearance with a central photon void surrounded by a reactive hyperemic rim of increased photon activity (Fig. 90–5).

The typical early ultrasound imaging findings of acute torsion are a subtle enlargement and sonolucency of the testis, which we have seen consistently within 3 to 4 hours after onset of symptoms. The epididymis is also slightly enlarged and usually more echogenic, presumably on the basis of hemorrhagic congestion. Early scrotal skin thickening may be present but becomes most intense during the subacute phase. If an acute torsion is not surgically corrected the testicle infarcts within 24 hours, and on ultrasound imaging this is seen as a further loss of echogenicity, a coarsening of the acoustic pattern with echo-free voids, and progressive swelling of the testicle. As infarcation progresses, further enlargement of the epididymis is noted with mixed areas of increased and decreased echoes due to hemorrhage and edema (Fig. 90–6). By 10 to 14 days, the

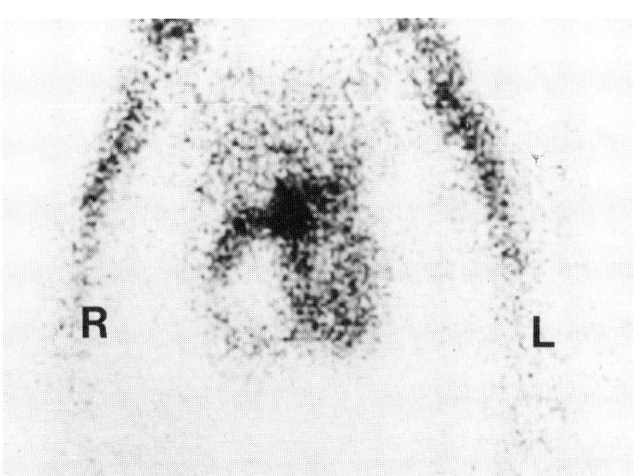

Figure 90–5. Static technetium-99m scintiphoto demonstrates a "cold" right testis in this patient with acute right testicular torsion. (R = right; L = left.)

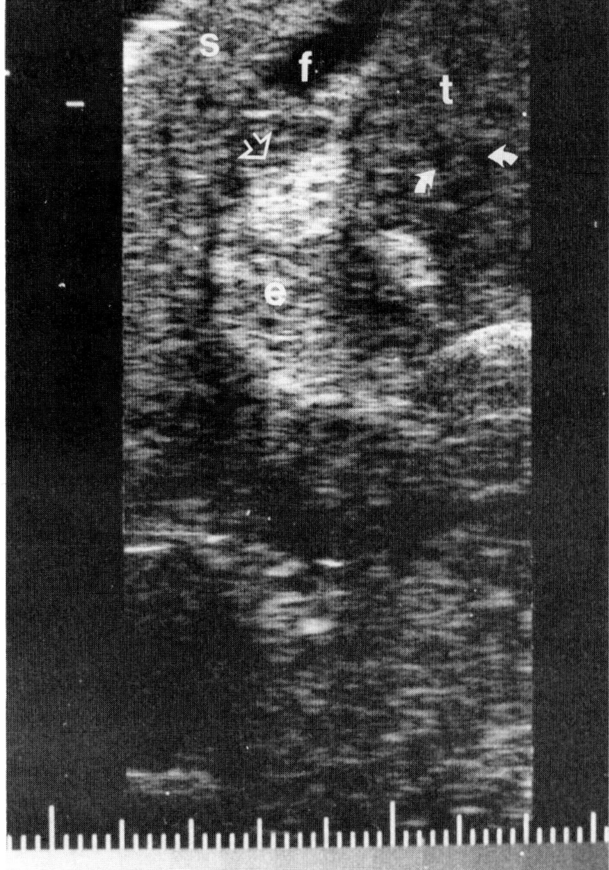

Figure 90–6. Missed torsion at 24 hours' duration of symptoms in 13-year-old boy. Note coarse acoustic texture in testis (t) with small echo-free voids (*curved arrows*), skin thickening (S), and foci of increased reflectivity (*open arrow*) in epididymis (e). Compare with Figure 90–2 same patient: unaffected testis.

testis starts to atrophy with complete loss of the normal acoustic pattern; skin thickening also begins to subside after 1 to 2 weeks. The epididymis remains relatively enlarged and echogenic in the late subacute phase. The DCFI findings of chronic missed torsion are that of profound testicular atrophy without flow loss of normal testicular echogenicity and globular echogenic scarring in the epididymis. The gray-scale findings of torsion overlap with epididymo-orchitis.

The "bell clapper deformity," which is the most common cause of torsion, represents a failure of a fixation of the testicle to the scrotal wall. Since the testicle is not fixed, the tunica vaginalis surrounds the testicle except for the region of the cord, creating the bell clapper deformity. The testicle resembles a clapper with the surrounding tunica representing the bell. This anomaly is typically bilateral even when it presents in a unilateral fashion. Clinically, it is important, therefore, not only to try to salvage the torsed testicle, but also to prevent subsequent torsion on the side that has not yet torsed with an orchiopexy. It is obviously important to accurately diagnose even missed and chronic torsions. Although these testes cannot be salvaged, the contralateral testis can be fixated by orchiopexy to prevent its undergoing torsion in the future.

Torsion of the appendix testes or epididymis occurs with the same order of frequency as testicular torsion in young males. These patients present clinically with a history similar to that of testicular torsion. DCFI or radionuclide studies are normal with torsion of the appendices. The swollen appendage may be recognized on gray-scale imaging as an extratesticular mass near the globus major. Reactive effusions are common with torsion of appendices. The diagnosis is most often made preoperatively on physical examination and trans-scrotal illumination by observing the twisted appendage as a pea-sized bluish scrotal nodule separate from the testis. Surgical excision of the infarcted appendage provides prompt symptomatic relief.

INFLAMMATORY DISEASE

In adults, inflammatory disease of the scrotum is far more common than neoplastic involvement or testicular torsion. Inflammatory changes may involve the epididymis, testis, or tunica cavity alone or in combination.

Most mild cases of epididymo-orchitits are treated conservatively by urologists or primary care physicians without any imaging procedure. DCFI or nuclear medicine is usually reserved for atypical or unusually severe cases in which there is suspicion for neoplasm, torsion, or complications of epididymo-orchitits. Other patients are imaged in the subacute or chronic phase when there is delayed or inadequate response to conservative antibiotic treatment, re-exacerbation of symptoms, or development of a focal palpable post-inflammatory mass. DCFI is often the imaging procedure of choice.

Even a severely inflamed scrotum can be comprehensively examined with ultrasound for detection of pathology when this is done in a gentle but thorough manner. Most commonly, acute inflammatory changes are confined to the epididymis with no apparent alteration in testicular architecture; somewhat less commonly focal or diffuse abnormalities are also seen in the testis.

Epididymitis and orchitis both reveal hyperemic increased color flow and velocity compared with the asymptomatic side when examined with DCFI (Fig. 90–7) and increased photon activity on dynamic and static technetium imaging. Failure to demonstrate these changes on DCFI or perfusion testing should cast suspicion on the diagnosis of epididymo-orchitis in the clinical setting of an acute painful scrotum. Tumors, appendiceal torsion, corrected testicular torsion, focal hematomas, and other lesions may all cause an acute painful scrotum.

Epididymitis is manifested on gray-scale imaging as focal or generalized enlargement of the epididymis. The texture usually becomes more lucent and coarse, probably reflecting edema. With severe hemorrhagic congestion, there may be foci of increased reflectivity. Focal epididymal abscesses and infarctions can occur, and these are seen as focal echo-poor epididymal masses. Concomitant skin thickening from one to several millimeters and reactive effusions are commonly observed.

Orchitis is manifested on ultrasound imaging as testicular enlargement and reduced echogenicity when compared with the contralateral testis. Usually orchitis involves the entire testis; somewhat less commonly, focal involvement is observed. Global orchitis and, to an even greater extent, focal orchitis can mimic tumor. Orchitis without epididymitis should raise suspicion for an underlying testicular tumor. When focal or diffuse echo-poor masses are seen with supporting ultrasound evidence for epididymo-orchitis (i.e., increased flow, epididymal enlargement, effusions, skin thickening) and with clinical evidence for epididymitis (i.e., prostatitis, pyuria, etc), such testicular lesions can be confidently ascribed to orchitis (Table 90–3). Follow-up ultrasound scans to observe for resolution or progression can be helpful. When echo-poor testicular masses are seen *without* good evidence for an inflammatory origin, they should be presumed to be neoplastic. The decision here to either promptly operate with radical orchiectomy or give an antibiotic trial with follow-up ultrasound scans rests with the urologist.

A limited scrotal biopsy of such unknown echo-poor masses is

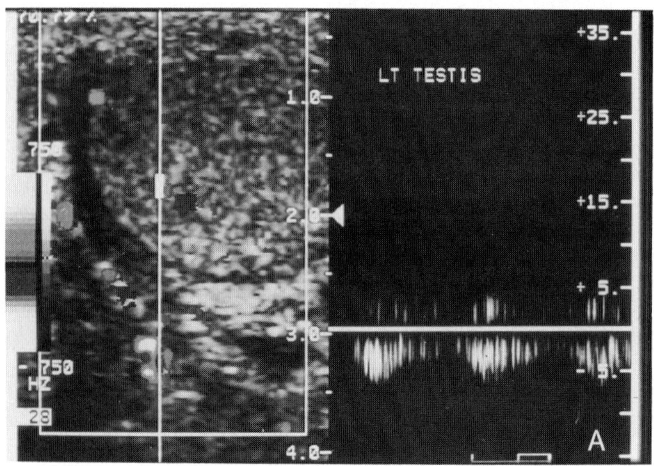

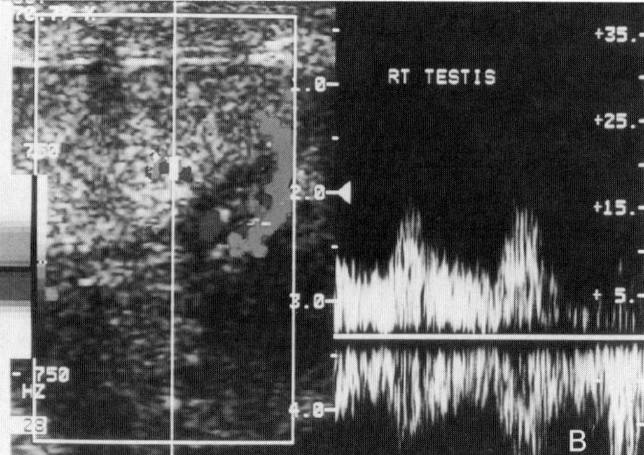

Figure 90–7. *A*, Normal DCFI to asymptomatic testis. PSV = 15 cm/second. *B*, Increased flow and increased PSV (15 cm/second) to symptomatic testis characteristic of orchitis.

TABLE 90–3. LIMITATIONS IN THE DIFFERENTIATION OF FOCAL ORCHITIS FROM NEOPLASM BY SERIAL ULTRASOUND STUDIES

1. Orchitis may increase in extent mimicking tumor growth.
2. Focal necrosis can occur that mimics tumor.
3. It may take weeks or months for focal orchitis to resolve (too long to observe a possible neoplasm—risk of metastases).
4. Focal orchitis may not resolve, but rather evolve into a chronic post-inflammatory mass.

also not generally done because (1) it is sometimes difficult grossly to tell a neoplastic from an inflammatory mass at surgery, and (2) tumor can be spread via such biopsies unless a radical inguinal orchiectomy is performed if indeed the mass in question is malignant. For these reasons, surgical intervention for solid testicular masses is both expeditious and appropriate when there is no firm evidence for an inflammatory basis despite the occasional sacrifice of a testicle for a noncancerous condition (see Table 90–3).

Since the ultrasound imaging findings of epididymo-orchitis overlap with those of testicular torsion, it is crucial that DCFI be performed. Indeed, since the testicular blood supply is in close apposition to the head of the epididymis and often compromised by epididymal swelling, infarctions of the testicle—either focal or diffuse—can occur without torsion.

Although the imaging appearance of infarction, whether due to torsion or severe epididymo-orchitis, will be similar, it is important to make this distinction surgically. The bell clapper deformity underlining torsion is always bilaterally present and can be corrected with orchiopexy to prevent contralateral torsion. No such deformity exists with inflammatory-induced infarction.

Clinical and laboratory differences between torsion and epididymitis exist but in a given circumstance cannot always make a firm distinction. The diagnosis of epididymo-orchitis in a child or adolescent should be made only after torsion has been unequivocally excluded with perfusion testing.

Ultrasound imaging can detect focal testicular or epididymal abscesses or generalized intratunical pyohydroceles, which may be seen with severe infections. Hyperemic peripheral flow is established with DCFI. These abscesses are generally treated promptly by surgery in an attempt to prevent more extensive intrascrotal necrosis. Testicular abscesses are seen ultrasonographically either as complex cysts or echo-poor masses indistinguishable from focal infarcts. Unlike simple hydroceles, pyohydroceles demonstrate low-level echoes in the surrounding testicular effusion due to cellular debris and often show areas of loculation or septation. Gas-forming abscesses have been reported and demonstrate specular echoes at the gas-tissue interface with typical artifactual echoes within the acoustic shadow distally.

MALIGNANT SCROTAL LESIONS

Testicular tumors represent the most common solid neoplasm in young adult males. The usual clinical presentation is either one of gradual painless enlargement of the entire testis or the development of a firm focal testicular nodule that is often associated with some vague discomfort. Minor trauma often focuses attention to an otherwise unnoticed scrotal mass. There may be sudden onset of pain due to hemorrhage or necrosis, thus mimicking torsion or epididymo-orchitis. It is not uncommon to see young men with rather massive scrotal enlargement when they first seek medical attention. In other instances, patients present with metastatic disease to the lungs, lymph nodes, or retroperitonum with no evident primary lesion until an occult testicular lesion is discovered by physical examination or on gray-scale ultrasound screening.

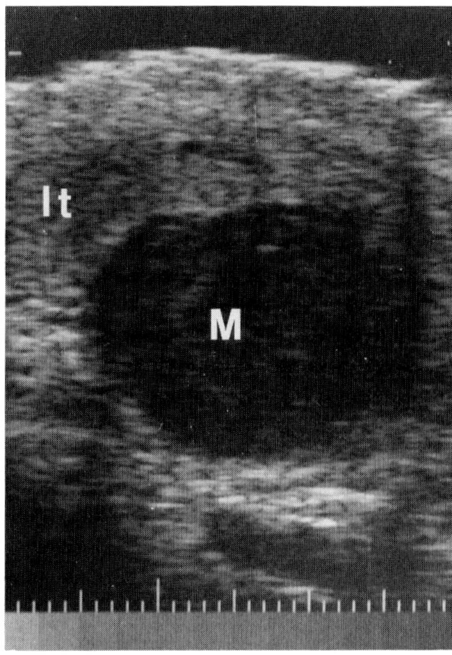

Figure 90–8. Surgically proven 2.2-cm seminoma is seen as an echo-poor solid mass (M) without epididymal enlargement. The remaining left testis (lt) appears normal and distinct from this well-demarcated focal mass. At other times, seminomas or other germ cell tumors will completely replace the testis.

Any solid testicular mass should be presumed to be neoplastic unless there is firm clinical evidence to the contrary. The typical ultrasound appearance is either a focal or a diffuse mass with reduced echogenicity and loss of the normal fine granular texture of a normal testicle (Fig. 90–8). Within the basically echo-poor mass, there may be foci of bright reflectors often due to hemorrhage or cystic areas of necrosis that yield a "tomato soup" type of fluid on gross sectioning. The ultrasound appearance of neoplasm is nonspecific and can be mimicked by benign tumors, focal orchitis, infarcts, hematomas, and, on occasion, even epididymal lesions such as spermatic granulomas. The diagnosis in any given case is made utilizing the clinical presentation and physical findings, pertinent laboratory tests, the ultrasound appearance, and, when appropriate, radionuclide studies.

The role of DCFI in evaluation of tumors is yet to be determined. Neoplastic lesions rarely show any significant epididymal enlargement or skin thickening such as is seen with inflammatory and ischemic pathology. The most common non-neoplastic lesion to mimic a primary malignancy on ultrasound is subacute focal orchitis. Follow-up ultrasound scans have only limited usefulness in distinguishing these two entities, as noted above.

The incidence of germ cell tumors (seminoma, embryonal cell carcinoma, teratocarcinoma, choriocarcinoma) greatly exceeds that of interstitial lesions (Sertoli cell, Leydig cell) in adults. Children have a higher incidence of interstitial tumors than adults. The testis is occasionally the site of metastatic lesions in adults (prostate, lung, kidney) and a common site for leukemia or lymphomatous infiltrates in children. Neuroblastoma also occasionally metastasizes to the testis in children.

Seminomas generally demonstrate a uniform level of reduced echogenicity, while the less common nonseminomatous lesions tend to be more complex in nature. With any given lesion, however, these generalizations have no firm diagnostic usefulness and the precise cellular diagnosis is always in the realm of the surgical pathologist. When malignant-appearing mass lesions are seen on ultrasound, it is advisable to perform a CT examination of the abdomen to search for metastastic lesions. Enlarged lymph nodes

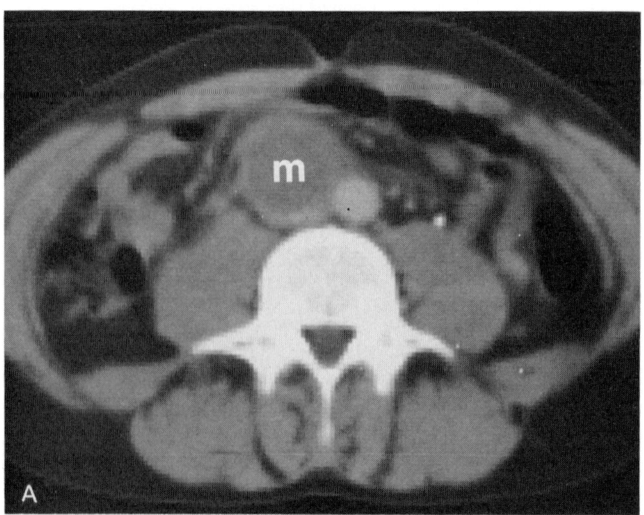

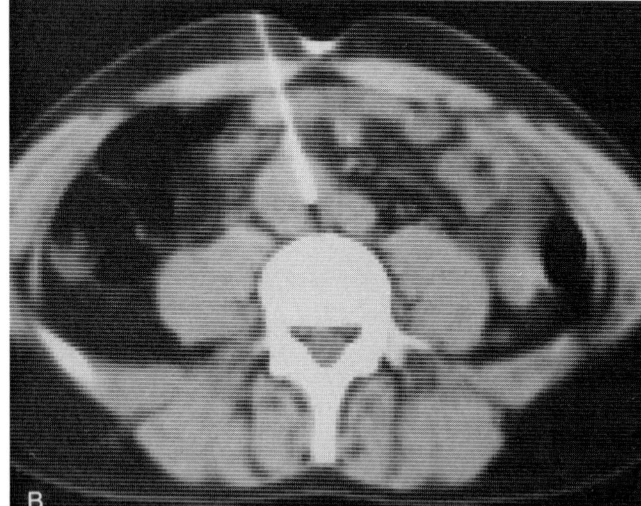

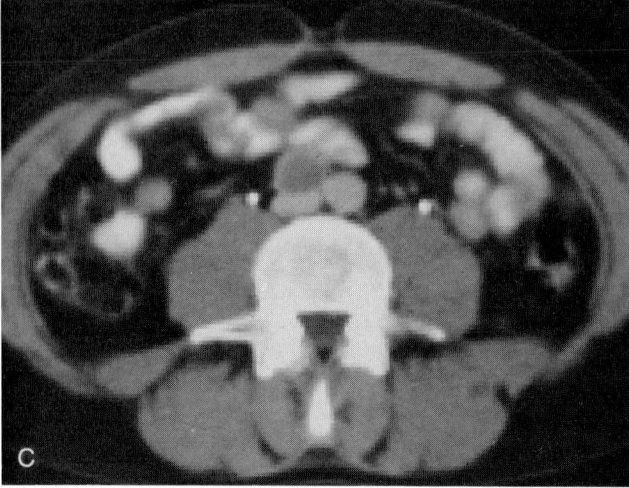

Figure 90–9. *A,* Contrast-enhanced CT scan reveals a 3.5-cm low-density, precaval, para-aortic mass (m) that suggests cystic degeneration in this 30-year-old male with known seminoma. *B,* Percutaneous CT-guided skinny-needle aspiration biopsy reveals a solid mass that yielded metastatic seminoma. *C,* Repeat CT following radiation therapy shows significant regression of tumor.

will most commonly be seen in the upper abdomen at, and just below, the level of the kidneys, reflecting the venous and lymphatic drainage of the testis. These involved lymph nodes may appear cystic on CT and ultrasound (Fig. 90–9).

"Burned out" primary testicular germ cell tumors have been shown to demonstrate a small, echogenic focus without associated mass. Similar small bright reflecting foci can also be seen in otherwise normal testes in patients without evidence for neoplasm. We presume most of these reflectors are scars from old trauma or inflammatory disease. The relationship of a mass to the mediastinum testis is easily determined by ultrasound and is important since tumors that invade the mediastinum carry a less favorable prognosis.

BENIGN SCROTAL LESIONS

High-resolution gray-scale ultrasound imaging of the scrotum has greater than 90 per cent accuracy in determining whether a given intrascrotal abnormality arises from the testis or extratesticular structures. Since the incidence of malignant extratesticular lesions is extremely rare, this distinction alone has great importance in distinguishing benign from malignant mass lesions. When there are difficulties in determining the origin of a lesion on ultrasound, it has been our experience that it is epididymal lesions, particularly if located in the globus minor, that may appear intratesticular. We have not had instances in which a intratesticular lesion appeared extratesticular.

The incidence of reported testicular cysts varies with the scanning equipment utilized. Leung et al noted small cysts in 8 per cent of 40 normal volunteers with a high-resolution real-time scanner. The origin of simple testicular cysts may be post-traumatic, postinflammatory, or congenital. Extratesticular cysts occur with greater frequency than testicular cysts and can be found in the spermatic cord, epididymis, tunica vaginalis, and tunica albuginea. The ultrasound distinction of solid lesions from simple cystic lesions in the scrotum is extremely accurate. Spermatoceles most typically occur in the head of the epididymis as 1 to 2 cm, rounded simple cystic lesions. Less commonly, they are multilocular. Differentiation from loculated hydroceles can be made by needle aspiration that yields milky semen with spermatoceles. Such aspirations are not usually needed clinically, and all such cysts are usually treated conservatively unless they cause pain, in which case they are surgically excised. These benign lesions are usually a sequela of previous epididymitis. There is an increased incidence of epididymal cysts in boys who were exposed to diethylstilbestrol in utero.

Hydroceles can occur as loculated lesions along the path of the processes vaginalis or as a generalized intratunical collection of fluid. Reactive effusions occur commonly with torsion and acute inflammatory processes. The presence of low-level echoes due to cellular debris often indicates secondary infection with intratunical pyohydrocele formation. Septations and loculations in effusions are common with inflammatory infusions. Although transillumination can detect most hydroceles, ultrasound is utilized to exclude underlying testicular pathology, especially if the hydrocele is of recent onset.

Although scrotal hernias can be positively confirmed on real-time scanning only if peristalsis is observed, they can be strongly suggested when extratesticular scrotal masses are seen in association with abnormalities along the plane of the inguinal canal that are due to contained bowel or omentum.

Fibrous plaques of the tunica albuginea are not uncommonly observed as flat focal echogenic lesions along the periphery of an otherwise normal testis. These are usually palpable on careful physical examination.

TRAUMA

DCFI has value in the acute and convalescent evaluation of the traumatized scrotum. The effects of trauma to the scrotum depend on both the severity and the mechanism of injury. Mild trauma may result in focal testicular contusion, may precipitate torsion in those with bell clapper deformity due to a strong cremasteric reflex, or may result in a post-traumatic epididymo-orchitis. More severe injuries result in intratesticular hematomas, testicular lacerations, or frank disruption of the globe. Hematomas can occur within the testis, within the tunica cavity (hematocele), or in the subcutaneous tissues of the scrotum.

At our institutions, penetrating scrotal injuries are treated by surgical exploration. With blunt trauma, lacerated or fragmented testes are surgically repaired to preserve function while small simple hematoceles are generally treated conservatively. The ability of imaging to discriminate between an intact or disrupted tunica albuginea is of great importance. Meticulous contact scanning is an accurate, noninvasive indicator of testicular rupture showing loss of the normal sharp testicular contour and intratesticular foci of altered parenchyma. Discrete avascular fracture planes are noted with severe injuries. Concomitant hematoceles are frequently but not invariably seen with laceration of the testis. Acute hematoceles are usually seen as echo-poor masses within the scrotum. Septations and low-level echoes are often seen with an organizing hematoma similar in appearance to a pyohydrocele. Thick septations can be seen with both acute or chronic hematoceles, and this finding should suggest hematoma when scrotal masses are evaluated even in the absence of recent documented trauma. The rare Sertoli cell tumor may also give a similar thick, multiseptated appearance.

Intratesticular hematomas are seen as slightly irregular, echo-poor, avascular masses within the otherwise uniform parenchyma. Differentiation from tumors is made by the history of recent trauma.

Chronic hematoceles may eventually calcify with bright reflecting curvilinear echoes from the calcified rim with acoustic shadowing beyond. Hemorrhage can also occur within the scrotal skin and muscle with marked resultant thickening of these tissues either on a postoperative or post-traumatic basis. Precise location of scrotal foreign bodies can be accomplished utilizing ultrasound.

VARICOCELES

Primary varicoceles of the testis represent dilatation of the veins of the pampiniform plexus secondary to incompetence of the internal spermatic vein. Much less commonly, secondary varicoceles arise because of thrombosis or neoplastic obstruction of the spermatic veins. Varicoceles are far more common on the left side. These lesions are associated with male infertility, and it is this symptom that often leads to requests for appropriate ultrasound studies. Large varicoceles are detected on physical examination by the "bag of worms" consistency. Varicoceles can cause scrotal pain, but this is uncommon.

The veins can be readily recognized as vessels on DCFI. DCFI is capable of demonstrating reversal of flow with the Valsalva maneuver or on upright imaging. The veins of the normal pampiniform plexus are less than 2 mm in diameter. While normal veins of the pampiniform plexus do not enlarge significantly in the upright position or with Valsalva maneuver, there is measurably increased venous distention with a varicocele.

While associated tumors are unlikely when varicoceles are noted, the abdomen and pelvis should be scanned when right-sided varicoceles alone are seen. Although somewhat invasive, testicular venography can also readily detect varicoceles with great accuracy. Venous angiography is often reserved either for treatment of vari-

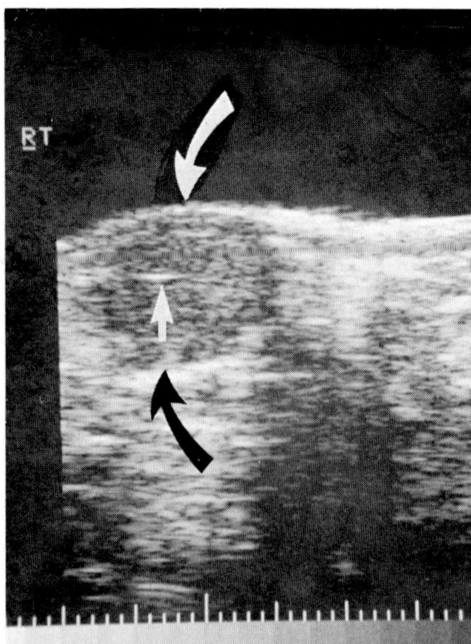

Figure 90–10. Ultrasonography of the undescended testis. Transverse sonogram through the right inguinal region in an adult with the testis in the right hemiscrotum and a normal testis in the left hemiscrotum. The undescended testis (*curved arrows*) is identified in the right inguinal region. Note the linear right line on this transverse scan (*straight arrow*), representing the mediastinum testis. In young children, the mediastinum testis is frequently not able to be appreciated in the undescended testis. When seen, however, it is important confirmatory evidence that the mass is a testis.

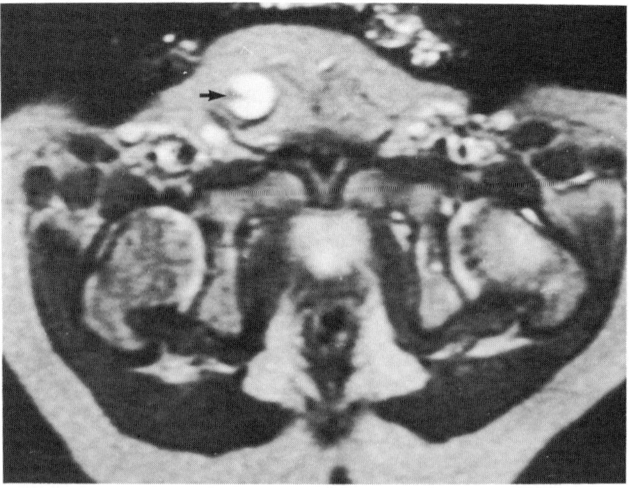

Figure 90–12. MRI axial image (2000/80). The mediastinum testis (*arrow*) is well-seen within the retractile right testis. (From Kier R, et al: Nonpalpable testes in young boys: Evaluation with MR imaging. Radiology 169:429–433, 1988.)

coceles via balloon occlusion techniques or performed preoperatively prior to surgical ligation of the internal spermatic vein.

UNDESCENDED TESTIS

The cryptorchid testis is a common anomaly, occurring in 0.7 per cent of full-term male newborns; 25 per cent of these cases are bilateral. In approximately 80 per cent of instances the testis is palpable, but in the remaining 20 per cent, identification is difficult. It is important to identify the undescended testis and surgically correct the abnormality because of the possibility of infertility and the much higher than expected incidence of carcinoma in the undescended testis. Also, it is crucial that the clinician be confident that failure to identify a testis on a specific imaging study is diagnostic of anorchia.

Ultrasound, CT, and MRI have been able to localize the undescended testis. On ultrasonography, a testis that is external to the inguinal ring can be readily identified as a mass with typical homogeneous echogenicity slightly greater than that seen in the normal liver and similar to that seen in the normally descended testis (Fig. 90–10). Lymph nodes tend to be smaller and are much less echogenic, so they generally do not cause confusion. In our own experience, sonography in the identification of the undescended testis above the inguinal ring has not been of great aid. All testes identified by sonography were able to be palpated by an experienced pediatric urologist, although referring pediatricians and urologists frequently failed to palpate these testes. Failure to identify the testis has not consistently correlated with anorchia.

CT can be used to locate the undescended testis. The spermatic cord can be followed into the inguinal canal and down to the scrotum. The undescended testis can be identified as a soft-tissue mass within the abdomen, pelvis (Fig. 90–11), or inguinal region.

In difficult cases, transfemoral gonadal venography can be used

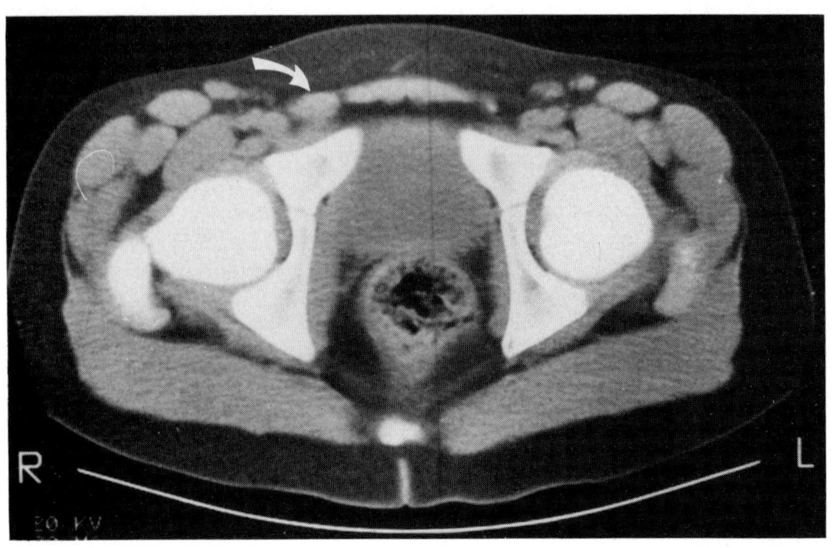

Figure 90–11. Computed axial tomographic scan through the superior inguinal region performed without the injection of intravenous contrast medium demonstrates the undescended right testicle (*arrow*).

to localize the nonpalpable descended testis. The left internal spermatic vein terminates in the inferior surface of the left renal vein, and the right internal spermatic vein typically terminates in the inferior vena cava. These veins can be catheterized and injected with contrast medium. The identification of the pampiniform plexus is a reliable predictor of the presence and site of a testicle. A blind-ending vein on a satisfactory venogram indicates absence of a testis. Failure to identify a gonadal vein on the side of the undescended testis is also consistent with anorchia. This technique is highly accurate but is invasive and should be reserved for those situations in which less invasive studies do not suffice. MRI offers the potential to accurately identify the testicle by imaging in both longitudinal and axial planes, thereby leading to accurate identification of the normal cord and its termination (Fig. 90–12). Vascular structures readily can be discriminated from a testicle on MRI because flowing blood does not generate a signal on MRI studies. A significant experience has not been obtained in this application of MRI.

Bibliography

Arger PH, Mulhern CB, Coleman BG, et al: Prospective analysis of the value of scrotal ultrasound. Radiology 141:763, 1981.

Bird K, Rosenfield AT: Testicular infarction secondary to acute inflammatory disease: Demonstration by B-scan ultrasound. Radiology 152:785, 1984.

Bird K, Rosenfield AT, Taylor KJW: Ultrasonography in testicular torsion. Radiology 147:527, 1983.

Bird KI: The testis. In Joseph AEA, Cosgrove DO (eds): Clinics in Diagnostic Ultrasound. Vol 11: Ultrasound in Inflammatory Disease. New York, Churchill Livingstone, 1983, pp 217–226.

Bird KI: Emergency testicular scanning. In Taylor KJW, Viscomi GN (eds): Clinics in Diagnostic Ultrasound. Vol 7: Ultrasound in Emergency Medicine. New York, Churchill Livingstone, 1981, pp 55–70.

Burks DD, Markey BJ, Burkhard TK, et al: Suspected testicular torsion and ischemia: Evaluation with color Doppler. Radiology 175:815–821, 1990.

Cunningham JJ: Sonographic findings in clinically unsuspected acute and chronic scrotal hematoceles. AJR 140:749, 1983.

Danielson KS, James EM, Kurtz SB: High-resolution sonographic detection of a gas-forming testicular abscess in a renal transplant patient. J Ultrasound Med 3:45–47, 1984.

Holder LE, Martire JR, Holmes ER, et al: Testicular radionuclide angiography and static imaging: Anatomy, scintigraphic interpretation, and clinical indications. Radiology 125:739, 1977.

Horstman WG, Middleton WD, Melson GL: Scrotal inflammatory disease: Color Doppler ultrasound findings. Radiology 179:55–59, 1991.

Kier R, McCarthy S, Rosenfield AT, et al: Nonpalpable testes in young boys: Evaluation with MR imaging. Radiology 169:429–433, 1988.

Lee JKT, McClennan BL, Stanley RJ, et al: Utility of computed tomography in the localization of the undescended testis. Radiology 135:121–125, 1980.

Leopold GR, Woo VL, Scheible FW, et al: High-resolution ultrasonography of scrotal pathology. Radiology 131:719, 1979.

Lerner RM, Mevorach RA, Hulbert WC, Rabinowitz R: Color Doppler US in the evaluation of acute scrotal disease. Radiology 176:355–358, 1990.

Leung ML, Gooding GAW, Williams RD: High-resolution sonography of scrotal contents in asymptomatic subjects. AJR 143:161–164, 1984.

Middleton WD, Melson GL: Testicular ischemia: Color Doppler sonographic findings in five patients. AJR 152:1237–1239, 1989.

Middleton WD, Siegel BA, Melson GL, et al: Acute scrotal disorders: Prospective comparison of color Doppler ultrasound and testicular scintigraphy. Radiology 177:177–181, 1990.

Middleton WD, Thorne DA, Melson GL: Color Doppler ultrasound of the normal testis. AJR 152:293–297, 1989.

Mostofi FK, Price EF: Tumors of the male genital system. In Atlas of Tumor Pathology. Washington, DC, Washington Armed Forces Institute of Pathology, 1973, 76.

Rifkin MD, Foy PM, Goldberg BB: Scrotal ultrasound: Acoustic characteristics of the normal testis and epididymis defined with high resolution superficial scanners. Med Ultrasound 8:91, 1984.

Sample WF, Gottesman JE, Skinner DG, et al: Gray scale ultrasound of the scrotum. Radiology 127:225, 1978.

Shawker TH, Javadpour N, O'Leary T, et al: Ultrasonographic detection of "burned-out" primary testicular germ cell tumors in clinically normal testes. J Ultrasound Med 2:477, 1983.

Subramanyam BR, Balthazar EJ, Raghavendra BN, et al: Sonographic diagnosis of scrotal hernia. AJR 139:535–538, 1982.

Weiss RM, Glickman MG: Venography of the undescended testis. Urol Clin North Am 9:387–395, 1982.

Williams CB, Litvak AS, McRoberts JW: Epididymitis in infancy. J Urol 121:125, 1979.

Willscher MK, Conway JF, Daly KJ, et al: Scrotal ultrasonography. J Urol 130:931, 1983.

Witherington R, Harper WM IV: The surgical management of acute bacterial epididymitis with emphasis on epididymotomy. J Urol 128:722, 1982.

Wolverson MK, Houttuin E, Heiberg E, et al: High-resolution real-time sonography of scrotal varicocele. AJR 141:775, 1983.

Wolverson MK, Houttuin E, Heiber E, et al: Comparison of computed tomography with high-resolution real-time ultrasound in the localization of the impalpable undescended testis. Radiology 146:133–136, 1983.

MUSCULOSKELETAL SYSTEM

The musculoskeletal system is often a frightening one to the beginning radiologist. Not only is the anatomy often unfamiliar, but the disease processes and orthopedic jargon often seem semi-obscure and even mystifying. The aspiring radiologist should take the time to learn the pertinent anatomy as well as to develop a sense of the wide range of normal appearances. Once this is accomplished, the disease processes are much easier to tackle.

Trauma can often be quite subtle. It can be of significant help to know the epidemiology of trauma relating to different parts of the musculoskeletal system as well as to different age groups. Thus, a fall-on-the-outstretched-hand (or FOOSH) injury most commonly results in a both-bone distal forearm fracture (often incomplete) in the 4 to 10 age range, in a Salter fracture in the distal radius in the 11 to 16 age range, in a nondisplaced scaphoid fracture in the 17 to 40 age range, and in a Colles' fracture in older patients. This knowledge leads the radiologist to look carefully for these sometimes subtle fractures in the appropriate age group. Similarly, injuries can often be associated with other specific injuries. For example, a bone bruise on the posterior aspect of the lateral tibial plateau is often associated with an anterior cruciate ligament disruption, which in turn is often associated with meniscal and/or medial collateral ligament injuries. Thus, finding one of these abnormalities on MRI should lead one to specifically search for the others. This kind of information is provided in the trauma chapter and should allow easier diagnosis of occult injuries.

Arthritides can at first appear confusing. However, the hallmark of each arthritic process is the distribution of abnormalities (which joints are involved, or even which parts of some joints), as well as the observation of whether the disease is erosive, productive, or mixed erosive-productive. This information alone usually leads to a correct diagnosis; the arthritis section will provide you with a guideline to these parameters for each disease process.

Tumors of the musculoskeletal system seem especially confusing to the uninitiated. However, there are a few determinants that, if properly assessed, will lead either to the correct diagnosis or at least to a reasonable differential, while pointing to an appropriate work-up. The tumor section will define these parameters and demonstrate them in the more common individual tumor varieties.

Finally, it should be remembered that advanced imaging of the musculoskeletal system usually requires careful attention. "Fishing" for an abnormality with CT or MRI is rarely productive, and can actually be detrimental because a real but subtle abnormality can be overlooked as a result of inadequate or incomplete imaging. Although planning imaging strategies is beyond the scope of an introductory textbook, one should simply remember that a carefully planned and monitored examination looking for a specific abnormality is always preferable to a wide-ranging fishing expedition.

B. J. Manaster

91 Basic Principles

SKELETAL GROWTH AND DEVELOPMENT

JOHN A. OGDEN

The radiographic evaluation of the skeleton, whether one is dealing with the multitude of skeletal dysplasias, the highly variable deficiency and duplication situations of congenital deformities, or the manifestations of acquired, traumatic, metabolic, or infectious problems, requires an adequate understanding of developmental and maintenance chondro-osseous biology and accepted common terminology. The terms used to refer to different regions and aspects of the skeleton are derived from the immature skeleton but also apply readily to the adult skeleton. The emphasis in the first part of this section will be on basic development and biologic parameters of the skeleton up to the stage of skeletal maturation. Once this occurs during adolescence (appendicular skeleton) and young adult years (axial skeleton), the skeletal components enter a phase of continued remodeling of the cortical and trabecular microanatomy. Disease states obviously affect these processes throughout the adult years. Diseases in which the articular cartilage is damaged, such as osteoarthritis, develop responsive chondro-osseous changes that are an attempt of the skeleton to redistribute joint reaction forces when normal patterns are not present. Even in the elderly individual the skeleton remains a relatively active organ system that is responsive to biologic demands (or lack of) and reflects the overall health of the individual.

SKELETAL FORMATION AND GROWTH

All skeletal elements initially form as genetically programmed mesenchymal condensations. Some cellular groupings modulate to fibrocellular tissue and ossify directly (membranous ossification), a mechanism that characterizes cranial bones, most facial bones, and the initial formation of the clavicle. In contrast, the appendicular and axial skeletal components are derived from the initial transformation of the mesenchymal model into a cartilaginous model with subsequent progressive transformation to an ossified structure. This integrated replacement of the pre-existent biologically plastic cartilaginous tissue by osseous tissue is termed endochondral ossification. These two basic types of osseous tissue formation—membranous and endochondral—refer *only* to the primary prenatal development of each individual structural unit, whether parietal

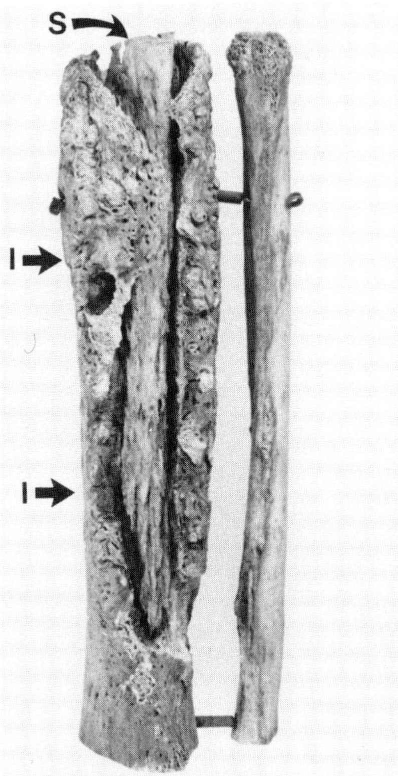

Figure 91–1. Diaphyses of the tibia and fibula from an adolescent with **severe osteomyelitis.** The periosteum has formed an involucrum (I) of new membranous bone surrounding the devascularized sequestrum (S).

bone, femur, or phalanx. Subsequent growth of any particular unit after its initial differentiation may involve discrete, juxtaposed, or interspersed areas of each basic pattern within the same bone. Endochondral-derived bones have concomitant membranous ossification by appositional bone growth from the periosteum (Fig. 91–1). Similarly, membrane-derived bone may undergo subsequent growth and elongation by an endochondral process, as in the clavicle.

Membranous Bone Formation

Primary membranous bone formation occurs in the cranial and facial bones, and, in part, in the clavicle and mandible, both of which subsequently develop epiphyses and physes (growth plates). The membranous bones are formed from mesenchymal condensations that are morphologic analogs of the eventual bone. At the site of presumptive primary ossification, small groups of cells elaborate a fibrous, extracellular matrix that is quickly calcified and ossified to form primary trabeculae. Ossification then spreads rapidly outward from this primary ossification center to cover relatively large areas. The trabecular orientation within the expanding centers is relatively random when first formed. Early remodeling ensues in response to mechanical stresses, both internal and external to the developing fetus. The internal and external surfaces of the cranial and facial bones form plates through selective trabecular orientation and thickening. Other mesenchymal tissue becomes established as periosteum, the tissue responsible for expansion of the membranous bones on their surfaces as well as at the sutures. The periosteum-mediated, membranous surface appositional deposition of bone may become quite active postnatally in diseases such as thalassemia. The sutures between the various cranial and facial bones represent a mechanism for integrated growth and expansion of adjacent bones, with growth occurring along each sutural area. The sutures per se remain biologically resilient to allow each bone to grow "away" from the adjacent one as intracranial and facial soft-tissue structures concomitantly expand. The sutures thus function for the membranous skeleton similar to the synchondroses of the endochondral skeleton (e.g., the triradiate cartilage of the acetabulum). Premature closure of these sutures, as in Apert's syndrome, leads to microcephaly. Multiple small bones (wormian bones) may form within the sutures. These intercalated bones may be normal or may be part of a pathologic process such as osteogenesis imperfecta.

The clavicle is the first fetal bone to undergo membranous ossification, followed rapidly by the mandible. The clavicle and mandible subsequently form hyaline epiphyseal cartilage, but only after primary ossification is well underway. This cartilage, sometimes referred to as secondary cartilage, forms a modified growth apparatus (physis) to modulate further growth. Histologically, such cartilaginous areas either resemble the nonepiphyseal ends of the small longitudinal bones (distal end of the clavicle and mandible) or form an epiphysis capable of secondary ossification (proximal clavicle).

All axial and appendicular skeletal elements are involved in secondary membranous ossification (Fig. 91–2). The diaphyseal cortex of each developing tubular bone is progressively formed (modeled) by the periosteum and modified (remodeled) by changing the woven trabecular bone to more dense cortical bone, which, in turn, is further refined by formation of osteon systems. This peripheral periosteal process of membrane-derived ossification can be extensive and rapid in some types of fracture healing, although the rate declines with increasing skeletal age. The replacement process may also be seen when portions of the developing metaphysis or diaphysis are removed for use as bone grafts.

Endochondral Ossification

Endochondral ossification is the primary formation process of the axial and appendicular skeletal components and may recur in selected areas of established bone as part of fracture repair through the formation and maturation of callus. Succinctly, this type of bone formation is the staged, synchronous replacement of mesenchymal tissue by cartilaginous tissue and the subsequent replacement of the cartilaginous model by osseous tissue. Although the overall process is a continuum, it may be divided arbitrarily into a number of steps: (1) the formation of a mesenchymal condensation representing the basic anlage of each bone; (2) increased extracellular matrix formation to create the precartilaginous model; (3) extensive ground substance elaboration to form the distinct chondral anlage; (4) further intracellular and extracellular enlargement of the entire chondral anlage, increasing hypertrophy of the central chondrocytes, formation of a trabeculated primary bone collar, associated periosteum, and rudimentary vascular supply at the presumptive diaphysis, and increased intracellular and extracellular biochemical activity, especially in the hypertrophied central chondrocytes, leading to calcification within this section of the cartilaginous anlage; (5) penetration of the primary osseous collar by the fibrovascular tissue, part of which will become the nutrient artery; (6) progressive central replacement of cartilage by bone, initially around the area of vascular invasion, followed by extension of the process (including the bone collar) longitudinally toward each end of the anlage, thereby forming the primary ossification center (which eventually will become the diaphysis and metaphysis), the establishment of an orderly arrangement to the growth mechanism (physis), and an actively remodeling metaphysis; (7) progressive vascularization of most of the chondroepiphyses by cartilage canal systems (some epiphyses, such as the distal ends of phalanges, are not vascularized and do not normally form secondary ossification centers); and (8) appearance of secondary ossification centers within the chondroepiphyses, which is primarily a postnatal process (Fig. 91–3).

Once the initial ossification center has formed and the nutrient

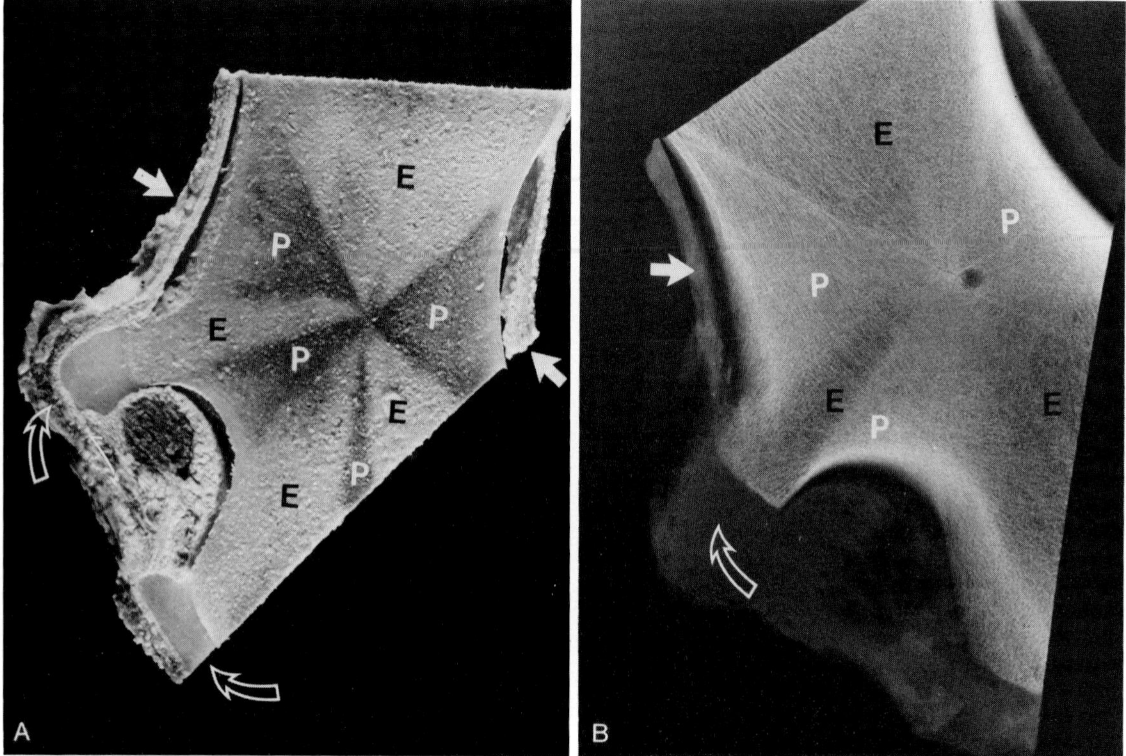

Figure 91–2. Slab section *(A)* and slab radiograph *(B)* of **the humerus from a leatherback turtle,** a unique reptile exhibiting some warm-blooded characteristics and forming large epiphyses that never form secondary ossification centers. Furthermore, this animal never forms a medullary cavity and retains the juxtaposed endochondral and membranous bone. In the slab section the light bone is endochondral bone formed by the epiphyses (E), whereas the dark bone is membranous bone formed by the periosteum (P). The radiograph also shows the demarcation between the endochondral (E) and membranous (P) bone. In both illustrations the *solid arrows* indicate periosteal tissue and the *open arrows* indicate epiphyseal/physeal tissue.

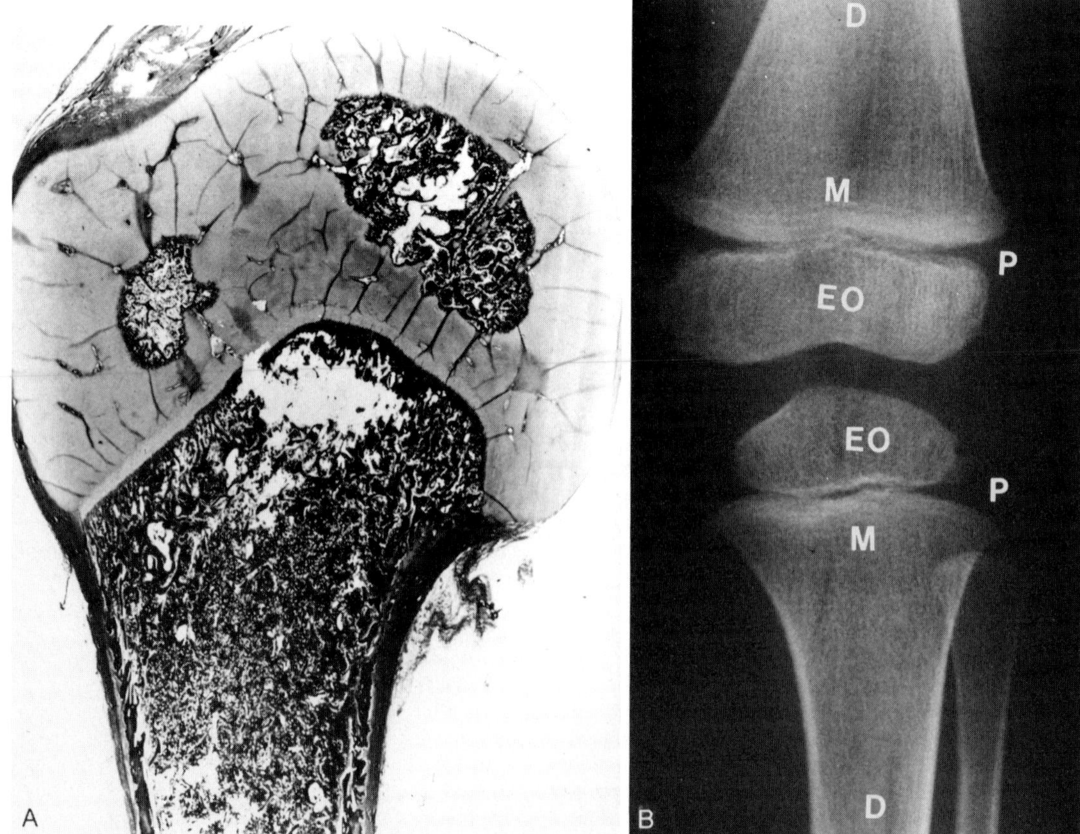

Figure 91–3. *A,* **Proximal humerus from a two-year-old child.** Two secondary ossification centers are present within the epiphysis. The physis is developing contour changes from the initially linearly transverse appearance in the neonatal period. A highly vascular medullary region is evident throughout the trabecular bone. The metaphyseal cortical bone blends progressively into the diaphysis. *B,* **Knee joint of a five-year-old child,** showing the characteristic regions of developing bone. (EO = epiphyseal ossification center; P = physis; M = metaphysis; D = diaphysis.) Note, in the tibia, how the thin metaphyseal cortex progressively thickens to become the diaphyseal cortex.

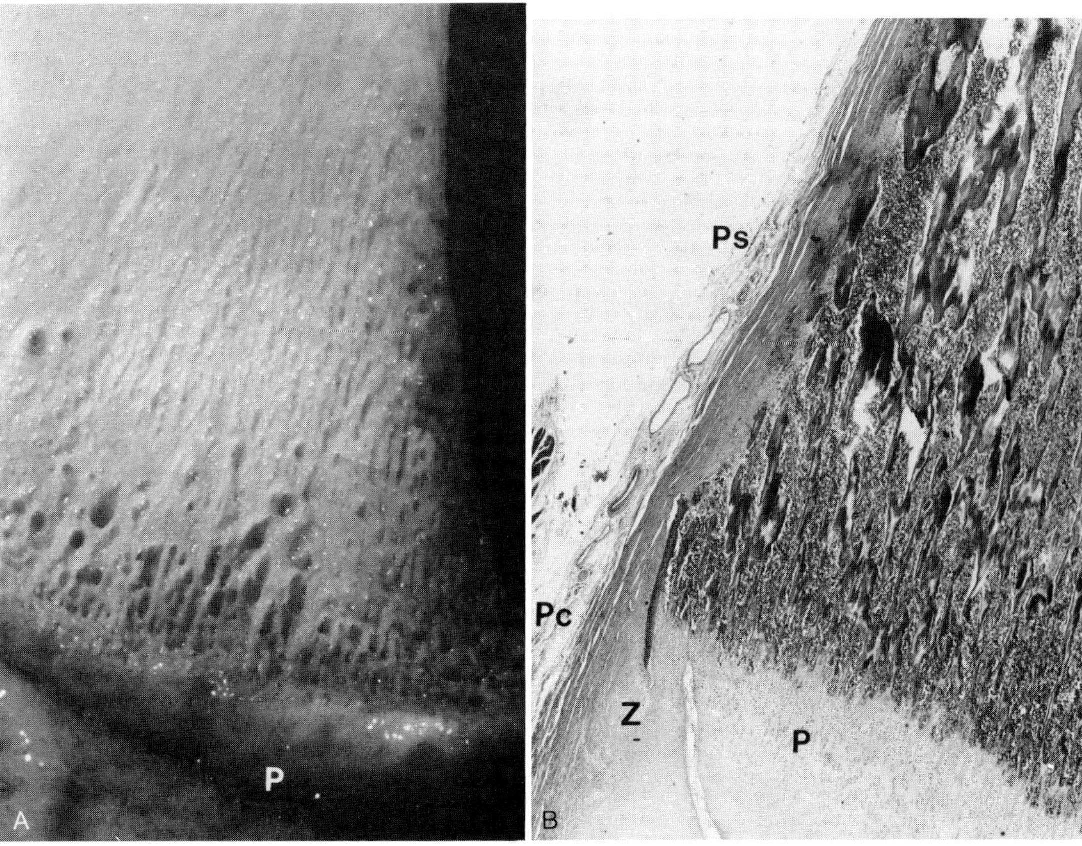

Figure 91–4. *A,* Osseous preparation of **the distal femur from a seven-year-old human** showing the physis (P) and the extensive porosity of the metaphyseal cortex. In contrast, the diaphyseal cortex is relatively smooth. *B,* Histologic section of **metaphyseal cortex from the distal femur of a two-year-old human** showing the physis (P), the zone of Ranvier with the fibro-osseous ring of Lacroix (Z), and the porous (fenestrated) cortex allowing fibrous communication between the periosteum (Ps) and the intertrabecular tissue. Also note how the periosteum (Ps) is continuous with the perichondrium (Pc).

artery has been established, expansile ossification progresses rapidly toward each end of the bone. The first bone formed is a loose trabecular network that fuses with the multilayered (laminated) periosteal shell. Initially, the endochondral ossification process extends at approximately equal rates toward each end of the bone. Postnatally, however, there are significant differences in the rates of physeal growth at each end of a given bone (e.g., 80 per cent of longitudinal growth in the humerus occurs from the proximal physis).

As the primary ossification center approaches each cartilaginous end, selected areas of the cartilaginous cells increasingly resemble a physis. This process usually occurs during the third and fourth gestational months. Concomitant with progression of the ossification center toward the cartilaginous ends, the primary periosteal collar also extends toward these regions, but slightly ahead of the more central endochondral ossification process. Once the physis is morphologically established (usually after 70 to 80 per cent of the initial cartilaginous anlage has been replaced by primary ossification), the periosteal ring stops further extension toward the epiphysis and remains level with the zone of hypertrophic cartilage (with which it continues growth in an integrated fashion), although it may extend further as osteoid tissue to reach the germinal zone. This periphyseal bone collar may be referred to as the fibro-osseous ring of Lacroix. The cellular association of periosteal ring, peripheral physis, and fibrovascular tissue is referred to as the zone of Ranvier, which is an important area of diametric (latitudinal) expansion of the physis.

As the individual bone elongates and widens in the metaphysis by the normal process of endochondral ossification, extensive remodeling begins. When the endochondral trabecular bone and the membranous bone collar initially unite, they form a shaft of relatively uniform diameter. However, the metaphysis must progressively widen to accommodate the diametrically expanding physis and epiphysis. Active remodeling occurs in two areas of the metaphysis—central and peripheral. Bone modeling and remodeling are so active that the metaphyseal cortex is relatively porous (Fig. 91–4). This porous bone is a factor in susceptibility of the immature skeleton to torus (buckle) fractures and also allows spontaneous "decompression" of a metaphyseal focus of osteomyelitis into the subperiosteal space. As the skeleton matures, especially during and after the stage of physeal closure, the metaphyseal cortex progressively "solidifies" with osteon bone. The central part of the metaphysis also remodels, with the primary spongiosa being replaced by secondary spongiosa.

SKELETAL COMPONENTS

The major long bones may be divided into distinct anatomic areas—the epiphysis, physis, metaphysis, and diaphysis (see Fig. 91–3*B*). Each region is prone to certain patterns of injury and disease responses, with the intrinsic susceptibility changing as physiologic and biomechanical capacities change in accord with postnatal developmental modifications at micro- and macroscopic levels. The four regions originate and become modified as a result of the basic endochondral ossification process. Subsequently, they are supplemented by membranous bone formation along the metaphyseal and diaphyseal shafts. Finally, the regions are remodeled to create mature cortical (osteon) bone.

Diaphysis

The diaphysis comprises the major portion of each long bone. It is a product of periosteal membranous osseous tissue apposition on the original endochondral model. This leads to the gradual replacement of the endochondrally derived primary ossification center and primary spongiosa, the latter being replaced by secondary spongiosa in the metaphyseal region. At birth, the diaphysis comprises laminar (fetal, woven) bone characteristically lacking in haversian systems. The neonatal femoral diaphysis appears to be the only area exhibiting any significant change from the fetal osseous state to more mature bone with osteon systems (lamellar bone). Periosteum-mediated, membranous appositional bone formation with concomitant endosteal remodeling leads to enlargement of the overall diameter of the shaft, variable increases in the width of the diaphyseal cortices, and formation of the marrow cavity. Mature lamellar bone with intrinsic but constantly remodeling osteonal patterns progressively becomes the dominant feature. The active remodeling osteon is referred to as a bone metabolic unit or bone modeling unit (BMU), and it is these units within the cortex that respond to physiologic and biomechanical conditions throughout life.

The developing bone in a neonate or young child is extremely vascular. When analyzed in cross-section it appears much less dense than the maturing bone of older children, adolescents, and adults. Subsequent growth leads to increased complexity of the haversian (osteonal) systems and the elaboration of increasing amounts of extracellular matrix, causing a relative decrease in cross-sectional porosity and an increase in hardness. These factors constantly change the susceptibility to fracture and the responses to metabolic diseases.

The inner surface of the cortex is called the endosteum, and it is also the site of continual remodeling throughout life. This inner surface is relatively irregular owing to the variable amount of adjacent trabecular bone and remodeling patterns. The outer cortical surface is usually smooth and covered with periosteum. This latter tissue, prior to skeletal maturation in adolescence, is highly osteogenic and progressively enlarges the bone diametrically while concomitant endosteal removal of the cortex maintains appropriate cortical thickness. The periosteum is relatively loosely attached to the bone and may be stripped away during trauma or elevated by pathologic processes such as osteomyelitis and tumors. When this occurs, the normal biologic response is new bone formation external to the cortical surface (Fig. 91–5).

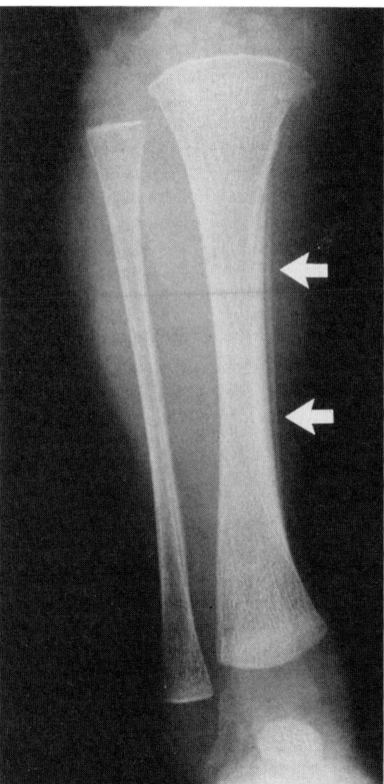

Figure 91–5. Disarticulated tibia and fibula from a seven-week-old baby victimized by child abuse. The antecedent violence had caused subperiosteal hemorrhage followed by new subperiosteal bone formation *(arrows)*. Similar processes occur in fracture callus, tumor-responsive bone, and osteomyelitis.

Metaphysis

The metaphysis is a variably contoured flare at each end of the diaphysis. The major characteristics are decreased thickness of the cortical bone and increased trabecular bone in the secondary spongiosa. Extensive endochondral remodeling, centrally and peripherally, initially forms the primary spongiosa, which is then transformed (remodeled) into more mature secondary spongiosa, a process that involves osteolytic, osteoclastic, and osteoblastic activity. The metaphyses exhibit considerable bone turnover compared with other regions of the bone, a factor responsible for the increased uptake of radionuclides during bone scans. The metaphysis, because of the high rate of bone modeling and remodeling, appears most susceptible to the development of lesions such as fibrous cortical defects (Fig. 91–6) and unicameral bone cysts.

Like the cortex of the diaphysis, the metaphyseal cortex changes with time. Relative to the confluent diaphysis, the metaphyseal cortex is thinner and has greater porosity. These cortical fenestrations contain fibrovascular soft-tissue elements interconnecting the metaphyseal marrow spaces with the subperiosteal region (see Fig. 91–4). The metaphyseal cortex exhibits greater fenestration near the physis than the diaphysis, with which it gradually blends as an increasingly thicker dense bone. As longitudinal growth continues, cortical fenestration becomes a less dominant feature and the overall width of the cortex increases, creating a greater morphologic transition between the juxtaphyseal cortices. The metaphyseal region does not develop secondary haversian systems until the late stages of skeletal maturation. The microscopic anatomic changes appear to be directly correlated with changing patterns of fracture occurrence, and undoubtedly influence the probability of torus fractures, as opposed to complete metaphyseal or epiphyseal/physeal fractures.

Although the periosteum is attached relatively loosely to the diaphysis, it becomes more firmly fixed to the metaphysis owing to the increasingly complex continuity of fibrous tissue through the metaphyseal fenestrations. Such intermingling of endosteal and interosseous fibrous tissues with periosteal tissue imparts additional biomechanical strength to the region. The periosteum subsequently attaches densely into the peripheral physis, blending into the zone of Ranvier as well as the epiphyseal perichondrium. The fenestrated metaphyseal cortex extends to the physis as the osseous ring of Lacroix.

The metaphysis is the site of extensive osseous modeling and remodeling, both peripherally and centrally. The metaphyseal cortex is fenestrated modified trabecular bone upon which the periosteum elaborates membranous bone to progressively thicken the cortex. Similar endosteal bone formation occurs. As this metaphyseal region thickens, the trabecular bone is progressively invaded by diaphyseal osteon systems, not unlike osteons traversing the fracture site in primary bone healing. This converts peripheral trabecular (woven) bone to lamellar (osteon) bone, which has different biomechanical capacities, and thus progressively transforms metaphyseal cortex into diaphyseal cortex as longitudinal growth continues.

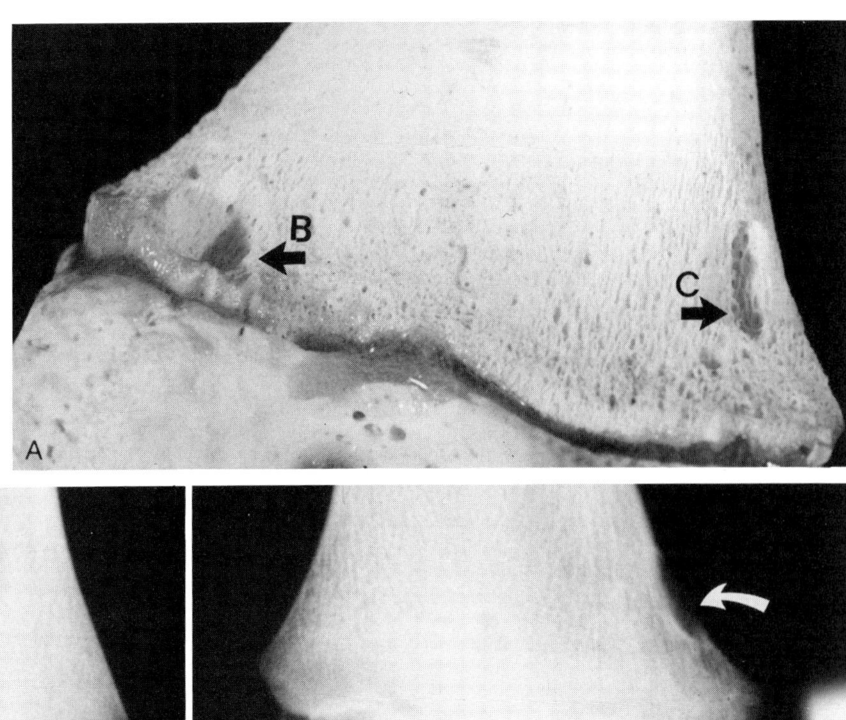

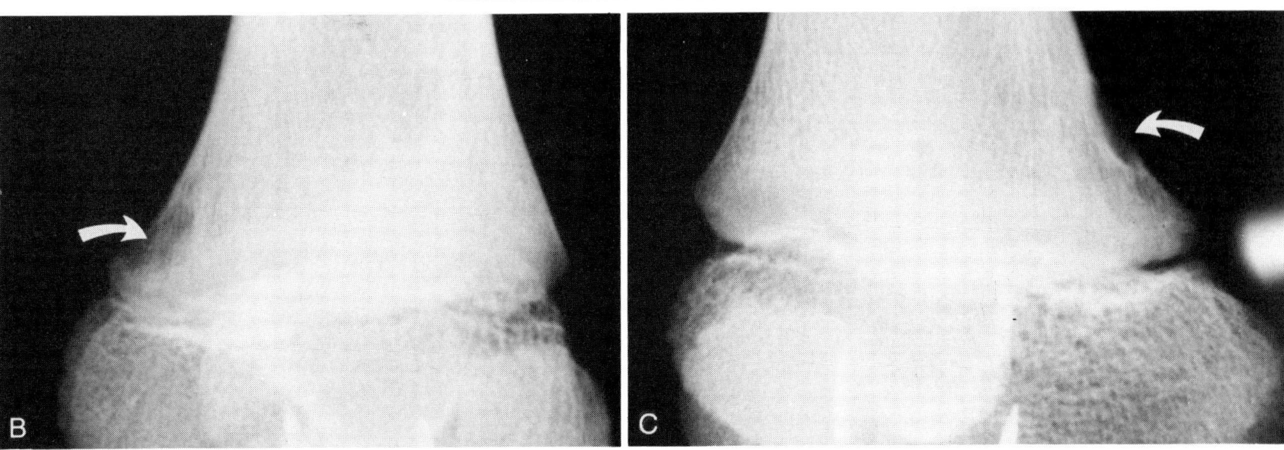

Figure 91–6. *A,* **Fibrous cortical defects** *(arrows)* **within the porous bone of the distal femur.** *B* and *C,* Oblique views of specimen showing the radiographic appearance of these lesions *(arrows).*

Another microscopic anatomic variation in the metaphysis occurs at the juxtaposition of primary spongiosa and the hypertrophic region of the physis. In most rapidly growing bones the trabeculae tend to be longitudinally oriented (Fig. 91–7). However, in shorter growing bones, such as the metacarpals and phalanges, trabecular formation is predominantly horizontal. As growth decelerates in adolescence, a similar horizontal orientation may be seen in the major long bones. Undoubtedly these variations in trabecular orientation affect the responsiveness of metaphyseal and physeal regions to abnormal stress and predispose to certain fracture modes.

Many bones exhibit transversely oriented, dense trabecular patterns in the metaphysis (Fig. 91–8). These usually duplicate the appropriate contiguous physeal contour. They may appear after trauma, particularly when the child has been immobilized (e.g.,

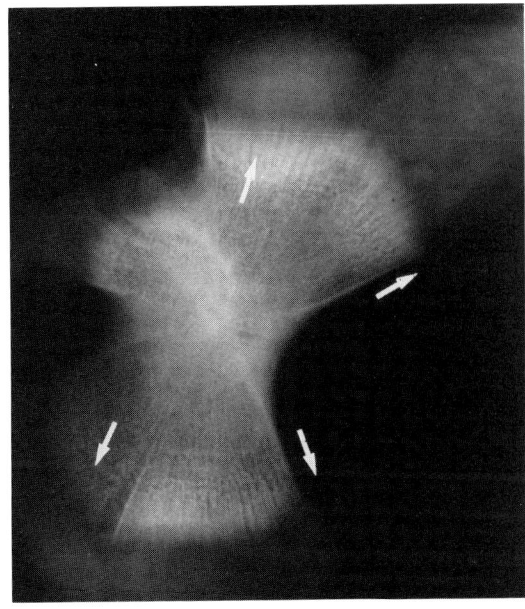

Figure 91–7. Specimen radiograph of **the humerus of a young leatherback turtle** showing the longitudinal orientation *(arrows)* of the trabecular bone formed by the physes. In this animal the orientation is retained permanently because of lack of remodeling. However, in terrestrial mammals this orientation pattern is rapidly lost by extensive remodeling and formation of the medullary cavity.

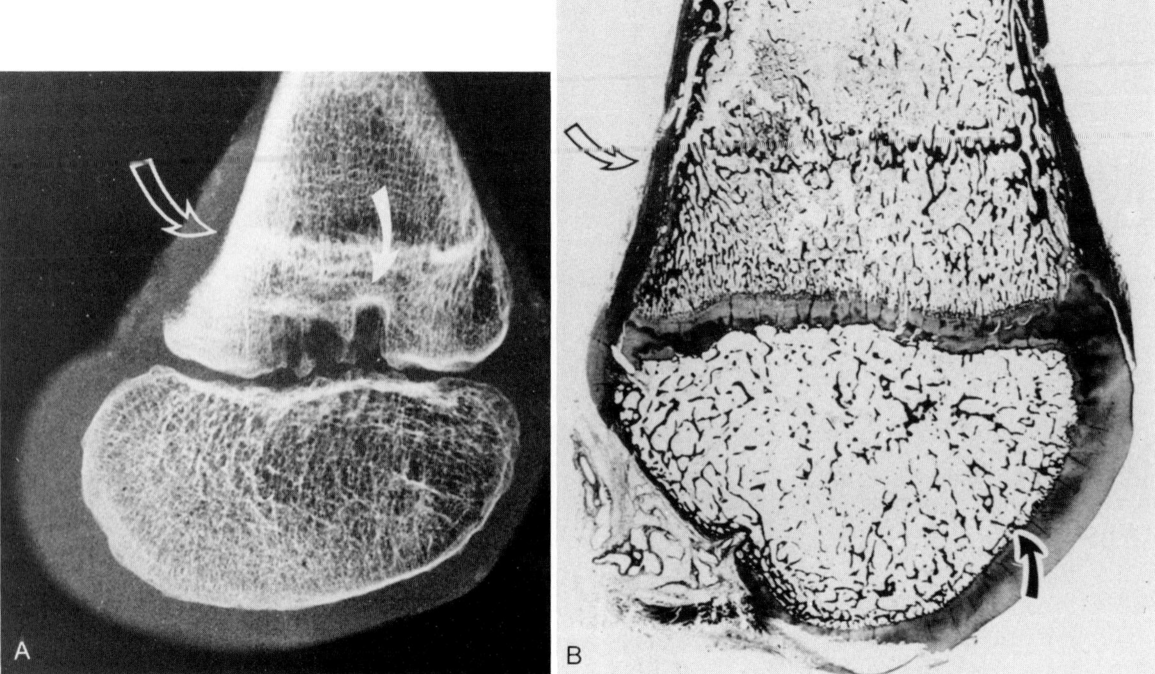

Figure 91–8. *A,* Radiograph of a distal femur exhibiting a **growth slowdown line** *(open arrow).* There are also some irregularities of the physis *(solid arrow).* This child had been on cyclic chemotherapy for leukemia. Note the appearance of the unossified epiphysis, the subchondral plate along the physis, and the subchondral plate along the articular region. *B,* Histologic specimen showing growth arrest line in the metaphysis *(open arrow)* and epiphyseal ossification center *(solid arrow).*

traction for a femoral fracture), and also may appear following generalized illness or even localized processes within the bone (e.g., osteomyelitis). They represent a temporary slowdown of normal longitudinal growth rates during the postinjury period or illness and often are referred to as Harris growth arrest lines. Because of the slowdown, the trabeculae of the primary spongiosa become more transversely than longitudinally oriented when they are initially formed, creating a *temporary* thickening in the primary spongiosa adjacent to the physis. Once normal longitudinal growth rates resume, the longitudinal trabecular orientation is restored. The thickened transverse osseous plate is "left behind" as the bone continues to elongate and is gradually remodeled as primary spongiosa becomes secondary spongiosa.

In the normal, constantly changing morphology of the different bones, the more rapidly growing ones are associated with longitudinally oriented trabeculae in the juxtaphyseal region (see Fig. 91–7), whereas the slower growing bones, particularly the proximal radius and the metacarpals, metatarsals, and phalanges, normally have a greater amount of transversely oriented primary spongiosa. Because this is the standard pattern of orientation in many smaller bones, transverse septa and their slower rates of growth are normal.

Epiphysis

At birth, with the exception of the distal femur, each epiphysis is a completely cartilaginous structure at the end of each long bone. This includes the small longitudinal bones of the hands and feet. Such a cartilaginous structure is referred to as the chondroepiphysis, whereas the corresponding ossifying structure is termed the chondro-osseous epiphysis. At a time characteristic for each chondroepiphysis, a secondary center of ossification forms (Fig. 91–9) and enlarges (see Fig. 91–3) until the cartilaginous model has been virtually completely replaced by bone at skeletal maturity (only articular cartilage will remain). With the exception of the distal femur, all secondary (epiphyseal) ossification is a postnatal phenomenon.

The epiphyseal cartilage enlarges by both cellular multiplication, particularly at the periphery through the perichondrium, and the elaboration of increasing amounts of extracellular matrix. Eventually a portion or portions of this cartilage hypertrophy and undergo chemical changes leading to the formation of a secondary ossification center. Such a center may be unifocal, as in the case of the distal femur, radius, or ulna, or it may be multifocal, as in the case of the distal humerus where separate secondary centers develop in the capitellum, medial epicondyle, trochlea, and lateral epicondyle.

As the ossification center expands, it undergoes structural modifications. In particular, the region adjacent to the physis forms a distinct subchondral plate parallel to the metaphysis demonstrated radiographically, as a characteristic lucent physeal line. Certain chondroepiphyses exhibit variations in the appearance and enlargement of the ossification centers, factors that must be considered in the appropriate diagnosis of biologic variation rather than disease within these regions. The appearance and progressive development of the secondary center of ossification within the chondroepiphysis undoubtedly play a role in the susceptibility to certain fracture patterns and deformation in dysplasias. The ossification center imparts increasing rigidity to the more resilient epiphyseal cartilage as the secondary osseous tissue expands. The secondary ossification center progressively enlarges in a pattern reasonably characteristic for each epiphysis.

The maturity of the growing skeleton can be assessed by examining the configuration of the epiphyses in the hand and identifying which secondary ossification centers have appeared. The bone age can then be compared with the chronologic age of the patient to identify delayed to accelerated skeletal maturation, which can occur with various diseases. The appearances of the secondary ossification centers, however, may often be variable when comparing one side

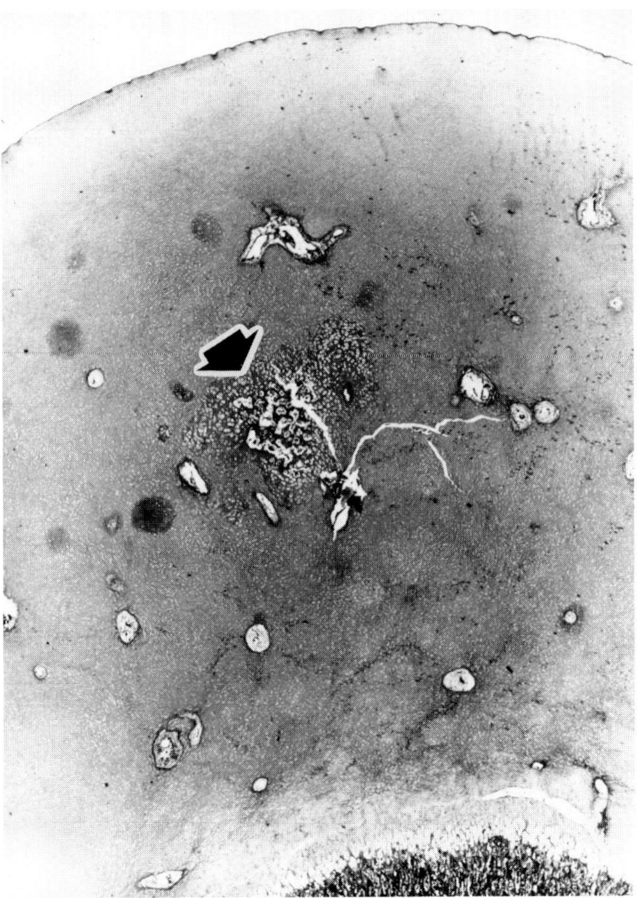

Figure 91–9. Proximal humerus from a neonate showing **early formation of the secondary ossification center** within the epiphyseal cartilage *(arrow).* Note the multiple cartilage canals throughout the epiphysis.

of the skeleton with the other, and one must be very careful in the evaluation of symmetry versus asymmetry. This process is related to biomechanics, and there often is increased maturation (i.e., ossification) in the epiphyses of the dominant side compared with the nondominant side.

The external surface of an epiphysis is composed of either articular cartilage or perichondrium. Muscle fibers, tendons, and ligaments attach directly into the perichondrium, which is densely contiguous with the underlying hyaline cartilage. Again, this anatomic arrangement imparts susceptibility to certain types of injury, particularly epiphyseal and physeal fractures. The perichondrium contributes to continued centrifugal enlargement of the epiphysis. It also blends imperceptibly into the periosteum. This perichondrial-periosteal tissue continuity contributes to the biomechanical strength of the region.

Physis

The growth plate, or physis, is the essential mechanism of endochondral ossification. The primary function of the physis is rapid, integrated longitudinal *and* latitudinal growth. Because the physeal cartilage remains radiolucent, except for the final stages of physiologic epiphysiodesis, the radiographic appearance often must be inferred from the metaphyseal contour, which follows the physeal contour. The changing size of the secondary ossification center more effectively demarcates the physeal contour on the epiphyseal (germinal layer) side. As this center of ossification enlarges centrifugally to approach the physis, the original spherical shape of the ossification center flattens and gradually develops a contour paralleling the metaphyseal contour. Similar contouring also occurs as the ossification center approaches the lateral and subarticular regions of the epiphysis. The region of the ossification center juxtaposed to the physis forms a discrete subchondral bone plate through which the epiphyseal blood vessels penetrate to reach the physeal germinal zone.

From a macroscopic viewpoint there are two basic types of growth plates—discoid and spherical (Fig. 91–10). Primary growth plates of the major long bones are discoid. They are characterized by a relatively planar area of rapidly differentiating and maturing cartilage that grades imperceptibly from the epiphyseal hyaline cartilage. Initially, most discoid physes are transversely planar, but with subsequent response to growth and biomechanical stresses, each physis assumes variable degrees of three-dimensional contouring while retaining the basic planar nature. Additionally, small interdigitations of cartilage extend into the metaphyseal bone. These are termed mamillary processes. Contouring and mamillary processes appear to contribute to the intrinsic stability of the physis, particularly when it is subjected to shearing forces.

Discoid (planar) growth plates also may be found between the metaphysis and an apophysis, which has been defined as an epiphysis subjected primarily to tensile, rather than compressive forces. The tibial tuberosity is such a structure. However, instead of the normal columnar cytoarchitecture, such a tension-responsive structure is characterized by variable amounts of fibrocartilage that represent a microscopic structural adaptation of the physis to the high tensile forces imparted by the quadriceps mechanism. Additionally, the growth of an apophysis leads to widening of bone but does not contribute to longitudinal growth as does the epiphysis.

In the short tubular bones (metacarpals, metatarsals, and phalanges) two discoid physes and contiguous chondroepiphyses initially

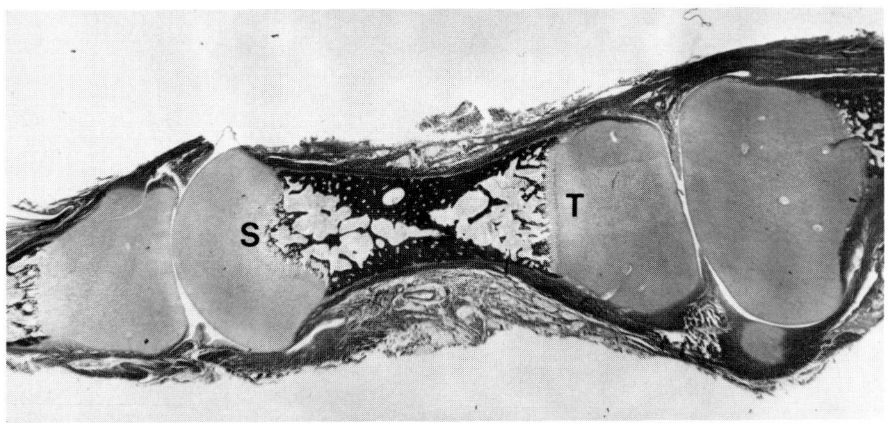

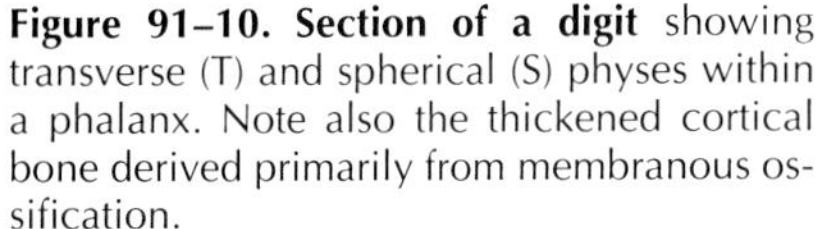

Figure 91–10. Section of a digit showing transverse (T) and spherical (S) physes within a phalanx. Note also the thickened cortical bone derived primarily from membranous ossification.

form, but with subsequent skeletal growth only one end maintains a true chondroepiphysis and physis, which become the primary mechanism for longitudinal growth of each bone. The epiphyseal hyaline cartilage of the opposite end is replaced relatively rapidly, until only a small amount remains between the articular surface and metaphysis. The associated physis assumes a spherical contour with decreased cell column length underneath the articular cartilage. This spherical physis contributes minimally to longitudinal growth but does allow contoured expansion. An epiphyseal ossification center rarely appears in the epiphysis associated with such a spherical growth plate, although a structural variation sometimes is encountered, the pseudoepiphysis. This commonly occurs in the distal end of the thumb metacarpal, where it should be considered a normal variant. However, when found in multiple small bones, it may be indicative of a pathologic situation such as hypothyroidism. The pseudoepiphysis is not a true ossification center, but rather an upward, and subsequently expansile, enlargement of metaphyseal ossification. The spherical growth plate, which is the major growth mechanism of the epiphyseal ossification center, is also found in the small bones of the carpus and tarsus. By progressive centrifugal expansion each spherical growth plate gradually assumes the contours of the cartilaginous anlage. Such enlargement of the secondary ossification center leads to juxtaposition of part of the spherical growth plate against the primary discoid physis, creating a bipolar growth zone. Similar bipolar growth zones are present in the acetabular triradiate cartilage, and between the proximal tibial and tuberosity ossification centers.

The physis has a characteristic and essentially unchanging basic cytoarchitecture from early fetal life until skeletal maturation. Histologic differences among the various physes are a reflection of growth rates and biomechanical stresses. These variations include the relative numbers of cells in each zone, the overall height of the physis, peripheral differences in the zone of Ranvier, and specific cellular modifications, such as replacement of the zone of hypertrophic cartilage by a zone of fibrocartilage. The basic patterns may be analyzed as either functional or morphologic zones.

The zone of growth is involved in both longitudinal and latitudinal (diametric) expansion of the bone. It is the area of most concern in any fracture involving the growth plate, because direct damage from trauma, or indirect damage by temporary or permanent vascular injury, in contrast to other zones of the physis, may have long-term ramifications for normal growth patterns. This is the cellular zone in which mitoses and new cell formation occur. The resting and dividing cells are intimately associated with blood vessels of the epiphysis.

Adjacent to the resting cell layer is the layer of active cell division. Mitoses appear in both longitudinal and transverse directions, although principally in the former, leading to the earliest evidence of cell column formation. In an active growth plate, such as the distal femur, cell columns may compose half the overall height of the physis. The randomly dispersed collagen of the resting and dividing regions becomes more longitudinally oriented between the cell columns.

Additional cells also may be added peripherally through a specialized region surrounding the physis—the zone of Ranvier. This zone contains fibrovascular tissue, undifferentiated mesenchymal tissue, differentiating epiphyseal and physeal cartilage, and the osseous ring of Lacroix.

The next functional area is the zone of cartilage maturation. Increased intercellular matrix is formed, principally between cell columns, rather than between successive cells in a given column. The cells remain separated by a thin transverse septum. This is composed of a distinct type of collagen that appears specifically related to endochondral ossification. The matrix exhibits cell-mediated biochemical changes, becoming metachromatic and subsequently calcifying, a necessary prelude for ossification. The chondrocytes hypertrophy.

The final functional zone is cartilage transformation. The cartilage matrix must be sufficiently calcified to allow vascular invasion by the metaphyseal vessels, which break down the transverse cartilaginous septa to invade the cell columns, laying down primary spongiosa along the preformed intercolumnar matrix. This initial cartilage/bone composite will be remodeled and removed, to be replaced by a more mature secondary spongiosa that no longer contains remnants of the cartilaginous precursor.

The regions of cellular hypertrophy and transformation appear to be the structurally weak zones most likely to be involved in a physeal fracture. In certain diseases, such as rickets, the hypertrophic zone may be widened significantly because the matrix fails to calcify. This prevents capillary invasion from the metaphysis, leading to a hypertrophic zone that cannot be replaced by osseous tissue. This hypertrophic cartilage zone continues to grow, resulting in a progressively wider region that becomes mechanically unstable and eventually may result in epiphyseal displacement.

Appositional growth of the diaphysis by the combined mechanisms of periosteal osteogenesis and endosteal remodeling has been described. The physis similarly expands in a diametric, or latitudinal fashion, a process that occurs by cell division and intercellular matrix expansion within the physis (interstitial growth) and by cellular addition (appositional growth) peripherally at the zone of Ranvier (Fig. 91–11). Interstitial growth within the physis appears directly related to enlargement of the secondary center of ossification. When the epiphysis is completely cartilaginous, or contains only a small, spherical ossification center, the biologically plastic cartilage does not present a total mechanical barrier to interstitial expansion of the juxtaposed physis. With increasing development of the epiphyseal ossification center, a discrete subchondral (cribriform) bone plate forms. Subsequent interstitial expansion of the physis is effectively precluded in the areas directly apposed to the subchondral plate. Latitudinal expansion thus becomes progressively limited to appositional growth from the peripheral zone of Ranvier, which remains peripheral to the enlarging cribriform plate.

Physiologic epiphysiodesis refers to the normal gradual replacement of the physis during adolescence. The process commences with the formation of small osseous bridges between the epiphyseal

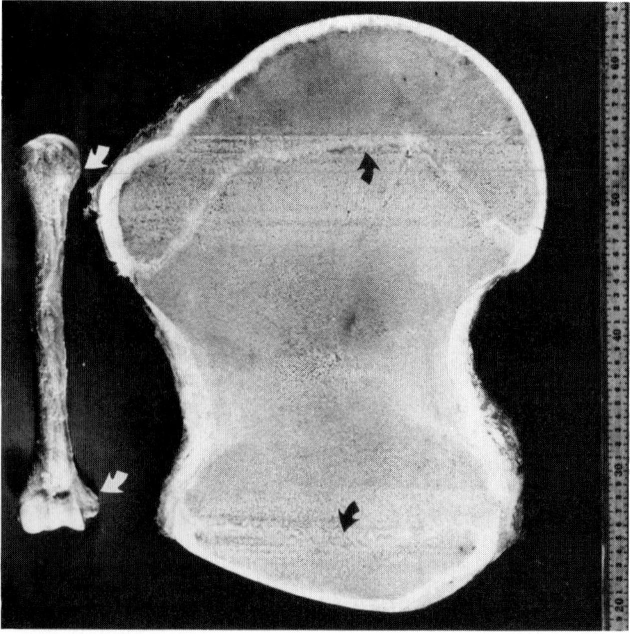

Figure 91–11. Proximal humeri from a 16-year-old human *(left)* and an "adolescent" fin whale *(right)*. The physes *(arrows)* of the human humerus are approximately the same distance apart as those in the whale. However, there is a massive difference in the amount of latitudinal growth in the whale.

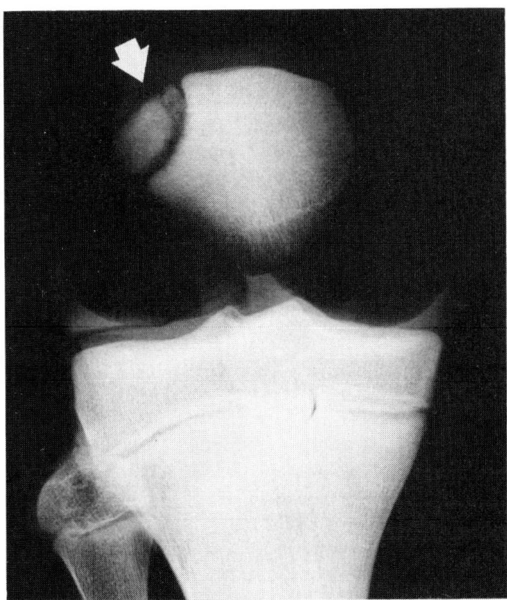

Figure 91–12. Specimen of **patella and tibia from a 15-year-old male.** Note the thickened subchondral plate adjacent to the physis preceding closure. Also note the bipartite patella *(arrow)*.

ossification center and metaphysis, and ends with the complete replacement of the cartilaginous physis by osseous tissue. This transversely oriented replacement may still be radiographically evident during adulthood, although it usually is progressively remodeled until it is no longer evident. Each physis appears to have its own pattern of closure, a factor that predisposes to certain types of fractures.

Several significant changes occur during normal epiphysiodesis. The epiphyseal cribriform bone plate thickens (Fig. 91–12). A similar thickening of the metaphyseal bone also occurs, with formation of the transverse osseous septa instead of the more characteristic longitudinal trabeculae. The basic cellular arrangement of the physis does not change significantly while these osseous plates initially are forming. However, there is a distinct cessation of cellular proliferation and altered biochemistry, with progressive calcification and mineralization extending into the germinal and resting zones to form multiple tide lines. The cell columns are rapidly replaced as they are progressively calcified. The extension of ossification from both sides leads to eventual perforation of the physis in several areas by small osseous bridges. Ossification then progresses outward from these perforations, replacing the cartilage and leaving a thick physeal ghost composed of coalesced thickened osseous plates of the metaphysis and epiphysis, which is evident on radiographs. The process usually starts centrally and proceeds centrifugally, so that small remnants of the physis may be found peripherally. However, certain physes show altered patterns. In particular, the distal tibial physis initially closes in the central and medial regions, and subsequently in the lateral region (Fig. 91–13), a factor predisposing to certain types of fracture (e.g., fracture of Tillaux).

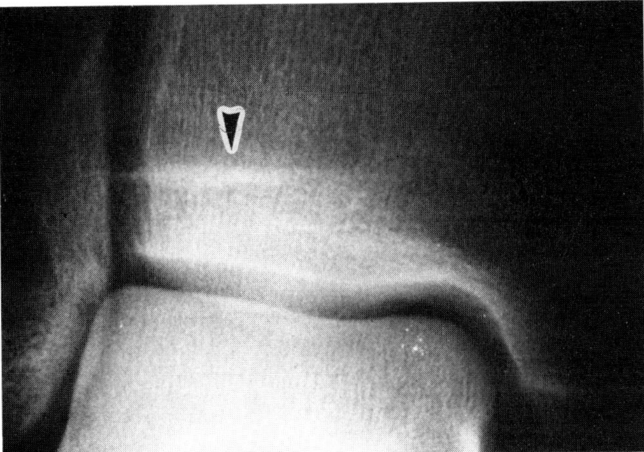

Figure 91–13. Distal tibia and fibula from a 16-year-old boy. Note that remodeling in the medial malleolar region has removed traces of physeal closure, whereas they are still readily evident in the lateral region *(arrow)*.

NORMAL VARIATIONS

The skeleton is subject to considerable variation in the ossification patterns (Fig. 91–14; see Fig. 91–12). This is particularly prevalent in the secondary ossification centers and the carpal and tarsal bones. Such variation in either the pattern or degree of ossification may even vary from side to side and should make one cautious about the interpretation of symmetry when observing comparison views. Ossification centers do not become smooth until the late stages of chondro-osseous maturation. Regions such as the distal femur can be very irregular, an appearance that probably reflects rapidity of chondro-osseous transformation rather than any discrete response to altered biomechanics or a specific disease state.

Care also must be taken in the arbitrary assignment of the term *variation*. There is increasing acceptance, particularly in the orthopedic community, that many of the lesions defined as osteochondroses actually may be chronic, stress-related responses (e.g., the residua of microfractures). Osgood-Schlatter's disease certainly fits such a category. Furthermore, disorders such as bipartite patella (Fig. 91–15; see Fig. 91–12) and accessory navicula, although usually being interpreted as radiographic variations, may be subject to injury, and when patients with such diagnostic findings happen to be acutely symptomatic in that region, the diagnosis of superimposed acute injury must be considered. The differentiation of an injury or disease process is difficult and necessitates that the physician be aware of the array of physiologic variants that can be extremely misleading in the assessment of the skeleton, no matter what the age of the patient. Radionuclide bone scans showing increased uptake can help distinguish the anatomic variation from an injury. These radiologic variations may represent nuances of chondro-osseous growth, alterations of individual development, or positional artifacts. All are potentially confusing and misleading. Of considerable help to the radiologist are a number of texts that provide detailed descriptions and illustrations of most anatomic variants.

BIOMECHANICS

During normal childhood activity and growth, the developing chondro-osseous skeleton is subjected to a complex pattern of forces that may cause microdeformations of the bone followed by appropriate biologic response patterns, such as replacement of epiphyseal and physeal cartilage by osseous tissues, increased amounts of osseous tissue, changing trabecular orientation, and varying amounts of different histologic types of bone. These local microdeformations are referred to as *strains*, and the local force concentrations at these points are termed *stresses*. The biologic relationships between stresses and strains at a particular point in the skeletal unit are governed by the material properties of the local chondro-osseous fibrous, or fibro-osseous, tissues; the direction and magnitude of imposed loads; and the geometric configuration of the region being loaded. The adult skeleton, no matter what the stage of maturation,

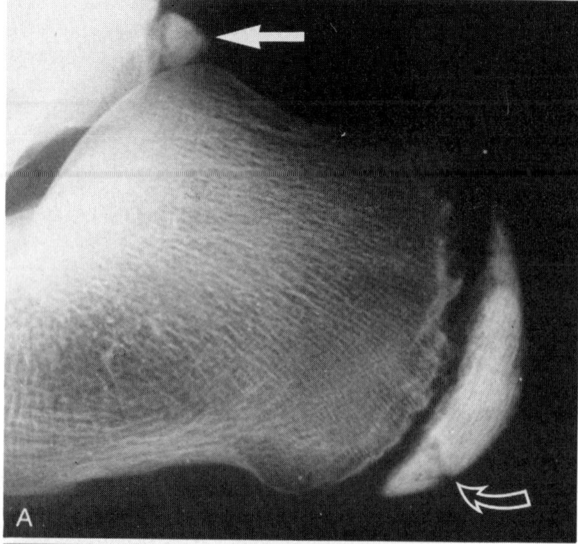

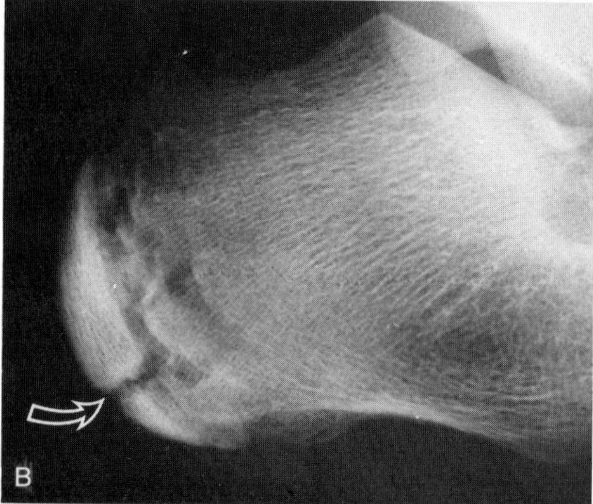

Figure 91–14. Variations in ossification within the secondary ossification center of the calcaneus in patients aged 11 *(A)* and 12 *(B)* years. Note the variably sclerotic appearance and the radiating lucencies *(open arrows).* Interpretation of these may be difficult when one is trying to diagnose Sever's disease. Also note the os trigonum *(solid arrow),* which is an accessory ossification center *within* the cartilaginous talus.

is always subject to varying stresses, and the microstructure is continuously altered in response. This occurs as part of the constant turnover of bone within the adult skeleton, and is accentuated in diseases such as osteoporosis (loss of bone) or osteoarthritis (irregular new bone).

The effects of normal biologic forces on the epiphysis are minimally understood. The development of the epiphyseal ossification center appears to be controlled both genetically and biomechanically. At a certain moment in time, summated joint reaction forces reach a maximum within a given region of the chondroepiphysis, stimulating osteogenesis in an area with appropriate vascular supply. If forces are abnormal, as in congenital hip dysplasia, this ossification process may be delayed, irregular, or eccentrically located. Physiologic stress appears necessary for the continued orderly development of both the physis and the secondary ossification center.

Stress is basically the internal resistance of bone and cartilage to deformation. It is not a directly measurable physical phenomenon but may be considered as force applied per unit area. Rate of application of the force is also important. Three types of stress involve bones under normal conditions: tension, compression, and shear. If these are increased beyond the physiologic response capacities for a given portion of the bone or cartilage, failure (fracture) may result. Compression and tension forces normally tend to act on bone at various angles. The growth plate develops undulations and mamillary processes, apparently as a means of aligning the physis either reasonably parallel or perpendicular to major force patterns of compression or tension. Similarly, trabecular patterns within the metaphysis and epiphysis, at any age, are a direct alignment and remodeling response to normal weight bearing and functional stresses (Fig. 91–16). Shear stress acts at any angle other than 90 degrees. The appearance of fibrocartilage rather than columnar cartilage is a biologic adaptation to minimize shear stresses in the apophysis. Extrinsic forces acting on cartilage and bone, therefore, may evoke a normal response (e.g., stimulation of growth and remodeling) or an abnormal response (e.g., fracture/failure or development of osteoarthritis), contingent upon the magnitude, duration, and direction of the evocative forces, as well as upon the rate at which the responsive tissue is loaded.

It is important to realize that there is a normal biologic range of compression/tension response within cartilage and bone and that a given region may be responsive to more than one type of stress. Within this physiologic limit, increased tension or compression accelerates modeling and remodeling. Compression appears to elicit a more rapid rate of modeling than tension. Beyond the physiologic limits of either stress, remodeling may be significantly altered. These principles may be referred to as the Heuter-Volkmann law of cartilage response and Wolff's law of osseous response.

Besides the effect of factors intrinsic to bone, four major intrinsic factors also affect the response of bone and cartilage to potentially injurious forces: (1) energy-absorbing capacity, (2) the modulus of elasticity, (3) fatigue strength, and (4) density. Each of these factors is influenced by the changes that occur in cartilage and bone over the period of progressive maturation. The increasing size of the secondary center of ossification affects the energy-absorbing capacity of the physis and contributes to the greater incidence of physeal injuries in older children. Increasing diaphyseal (and less so, metaphyseal) cortical width and the development of primary and secondary osteons affect the modulus of elasticity and relative density

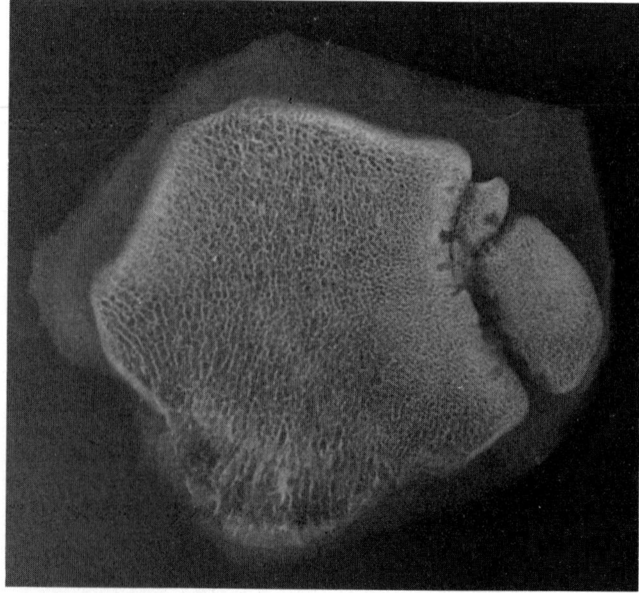

Figure 91–15. Radiograph of a specimen of a bipartite patella. Note the multiple centers and the irregular ossification margins. There was *complete* continuity of hyaline (epiphyseal) and articular cartilage. Thus, the "bipartite" nature may be osseous only, rather than involving contiguous cartilaginous separation.

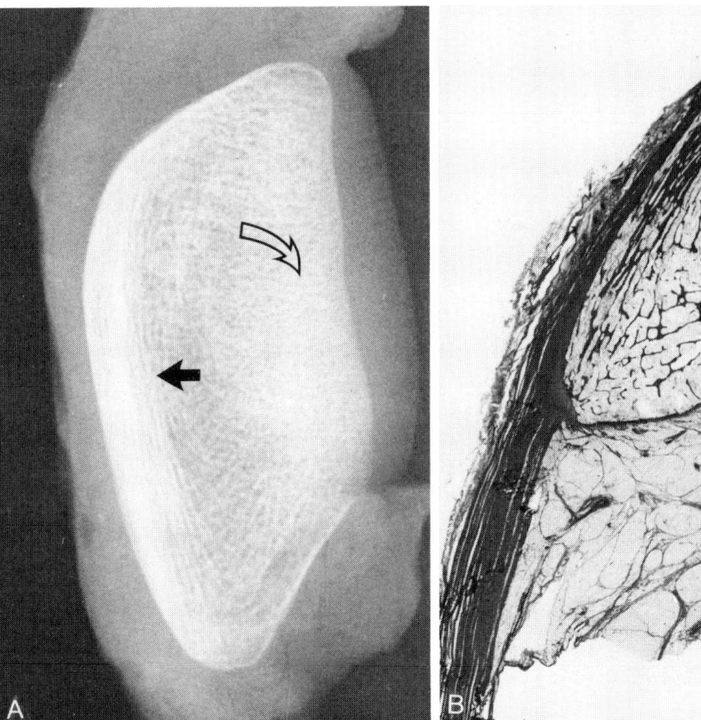

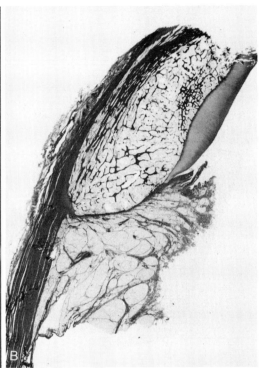

Figure 91–16. Radiograph *(A)* and histologic section *(B)* showing the **tensile** *(solid arrow)* **and compression** *(open arrow)* **responsive trabecular orientation and thickening within the patella.** Also, in *B,* note how the infrapatellar fat pad covers the lower third of the patella, which does not have a covering of articular cartilage.

and thereby cause different fracture patterns (e.g., greenstick, complete, or comminuted).

The progressive maturation of porous cortical bone causes a gradual shift in the distribution of bone strength and stiffness in the various regions of the bone, especially the metaphysis and diaphysis. In younger persons, bone in the cortical center is the strongest and stiffest, although with continued remodeling after physiologic epiphysiodesis, there is a gradual shift of strength and stiffness toward the periosteal surface. In addition to the varying distribution of porosity, a definite progressive change also takes place in the osseous microstructure from the endosteal to the periosteal surface. Bone near the endosteal surface undergoes more remodeling and thus contains more osteons. However, inherent to such osteonal structure are numerous cement lines that have been shown to be sites of weakness in cortical bone. In contrast, bone near the periosteal surface has undergone less remodeling and is often surrounded by a layer of circumferential laminar bone containing few cement lines.

Mechanical properties ultimately are determined by microstructure rather than macrostructure. The dynamic variations in microstructure throughout cortical bone undoubtedly reinforce the mechanical property distributions created by the porosity gradients. The strongest type of bone is circumferential lamellar bone, followed in order of decreasing strength by primary laminar, secondary haversian, and woven-fibered bone.

The effects of varying histology on bone mechanics have also been studied. The breaking strength and modulus of elasticity of bone are proportional to the quality and number of collagen fibers oriented in the plane of the applied force. The modulus of elasticity in tension and in bending is extremely dependent upon the vascular pattern within the bone, and an adequate functioning vascular supply is necessary to achieve a normal stress-pattern response. An obvious tissue discontinuity exists due to the multiple small vascular canals in mature cortical lamellar bone and in the fenestrated cortical bone of the metaphysis. The vascular pattern of bone varies considerably, not only among species, but among age groups and throughout regions of a single bone. It is evident that when a vascular gradient exists, Young's modulus of elasticity must vary progressively from the periosteal to the endosteal bone, and from the diaphysis to the metaphysis. In some bone, the vascular pattern is such that it causes a partial lamination of the tissues, with solid bone alternating with relatively porous layers. As the remodeling process becomes more extensive, the subdivision of the bone into vascular and nonvascular laminae becomes progressively less distinct until, in skeletally mature bones, it is no longer discernible.

Classically, bone has been considered a brittle material when loaded in tension. But over the past few years it has become evident that bone initially exhibits a type of ductile behavior, that is, elongation of bone tissue under tensile or elongating loads. Ductility depends upon the age of the individual and the area of the bone. Plastic deformation is essentially an irreversible ductile deformation. If a plastically deformed bone is subsequently cyclically loaded, total deformation will increase to result in failure. The clinical importance of this behavior of bone tissue is that bone as a structure can sustain permanent damage, even though *no* radiographically obvious fracture or decrease in load-carrying capacity is noted. The only detectable damage during plastic deformation appears to be the production of microvoids within the osseous tissue. Different bones exhibit different capacities for plastic deformation and strength, even in the same individual. For instance, between the third and eighth decades of life, femoral bone exhibits less plastic deformation and is somewhat weaker than tibial bone.

Bending stress in developing tubular bone often causes an incomplete fracture through only a portion of the cortical circumference (greenstick fracture). The remaining cortex is grossly intact but in actuality has microfractures. This "intact" cortex is invariably plastically deformed, whereas the fractured area has gone through the phase of plastic deformation to complete failure. Since plastic failure, by definition, means permanent deformation, this will have an effect on reducibility and ability to maintain longitudinal alignment. Some bones may undergo only plastic deformation, causing an increased bowing. This occurs most often in the ulna and the fibula.

Bending is not the only load situation that may cause permanent damage to bones without causing concomitant fracture. Axial or compressive loads, especially in the aging spine, may cause permanent injury even though no fracture is demonstrated radiographically. Because the predominant mode of loading of a long bone is axial compression, it is not surprising that overload conditions exist in which the compressive yield strength of bone tissue is exceeded, and upon further increasing the load, the tissue plastically deforms. Plastic deformation of cortical bone under a compressive load is a microfracture mechanism. These microfractures, due to the large shear stresses in oblique planes, may or may not coalesce into larger shear cracks or buckling as is characteristic of the torus fracture of the distal radius.

SKELETAL MAINTENANCE AND REPAIR

As discussed throughout the preceding sections, cartilage and bone are dynamic, mechanically responsive tissues that constantly model and remodel, no matter what the degree of skeletal maturation. Initial responses to stresses occur at a microstructural level and represent either a direct cellular response, as in trabecular bone, or a combined cellular and vascular response, as in cortical bone. The ability to model and remodel requires active physiologic mechanisms. For joint cartilage the physiologic status is maintained through joint motion and fluid dynamics. For the osseous tissues, as well as hyaline epiphyseal cartilage, maintenance is extremely dependent upon vascularity.

The developing osseous and cartilaginous components are both extremely vascular. The periosteum contains multiple small vessels that play a role in cortical osteogenesis and contribute to the increasingly complex haversian systems of the immature and mature diaphyseal cortices. The endosteal surfaces of the diaphysis and metaphyses receive blood through the nutrient artery, a major vessel that sends branches to each metaphysis and throughout the diaphysis. The epiphysis receives its blood supply from vessels that penetrate into and ramify through the cartilage and bone. The two major circulatory patterns—epiphyseal and metaphyseal vessels—appear to be functionally and anatomically separate, even after skeletal maturity is attained (Fig. 91–17).

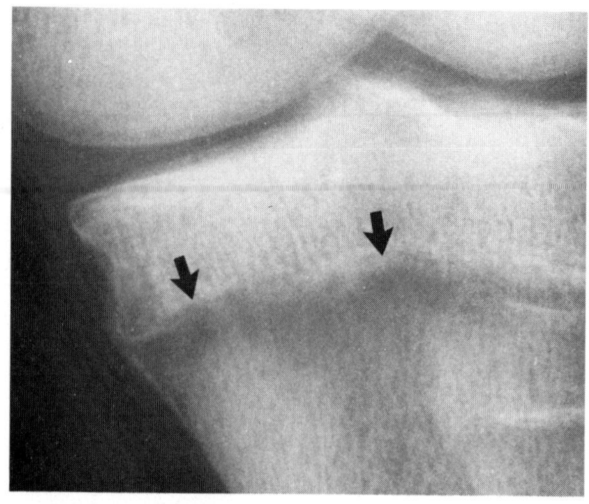

Figure 91–17. Proximal tibia from a 42-year-old woman four weeks after immobilization for a distal tibial fracture. Notice that the **relative osteoporosis** of the metaphysis has been demarcated by the old boundary between physis and metaphysis *(arrows).*

The epiphyseal circulation varies relative to the development and enlargement of the secondary center of ossification. Vessels initially enter the chondroepiphysis within specialized structures termed *cartilage canals.* These canals ramify throughout the chondroepiphysis and send branches to the resting/germinal zones of the physis (see Fig. 91–9). These canals have several important functional and morphologic characteristics: (1) they supply discrete regions of the

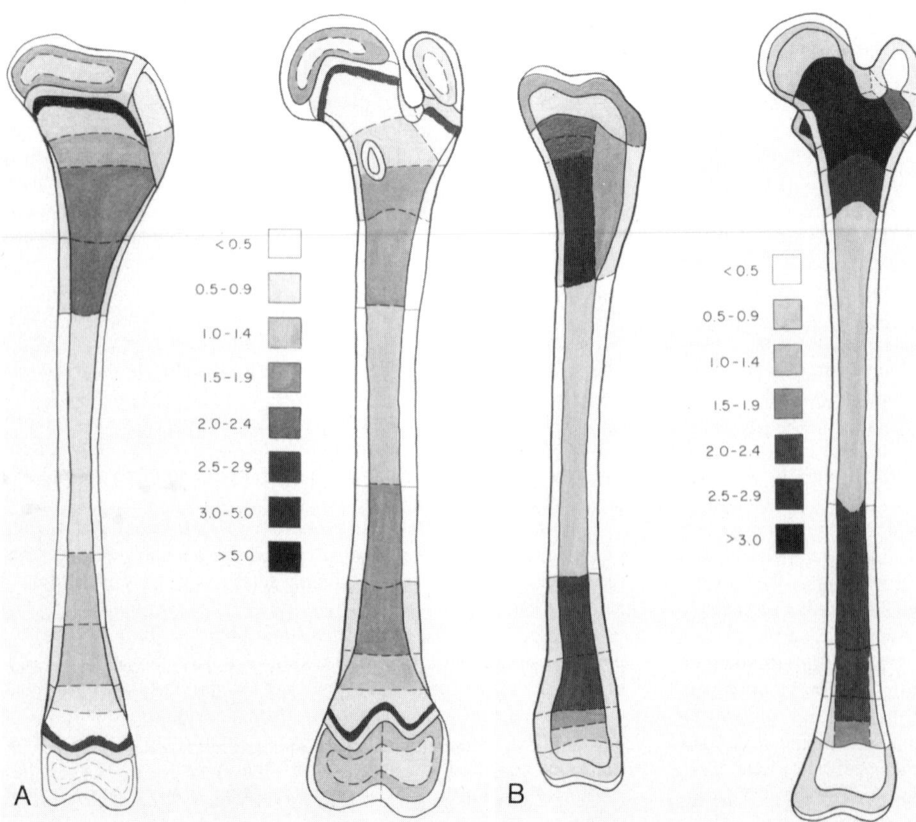

Figure 91–18. Schematics of **circulation to the canine femur and tibia** from animals aged four months *(A)* and two years *(B).* The white-gray-black colorations represent concentrations of radioactively labeled microspheres within discrete regions of bone and cartilage (black represents the highest concentration per volume).

epiphysis and physis, with no significant intraepiphyseal anastomoses; (2) the mesenchymal tissue within and around the canals may serve as a source of chondroblastic cells for continued interstitial enlargement of the chondroepiphysis; and (3) the canals play an integral role in the formation of the secondary center of ossification.

The vascular supply to the metaphysis comprises terminal ramifications of the nutrient artery, which constitutes about four fifths of the vessels reaching the growth plate. The other one fifth of the vasculature comes into the periphery through the metaphyseal fenestrations. This supply is also integral to the functioning of the physeal periphery (especially the zone of Ranvier) in the skeletally immature individual. The periosteal vessels create an essentially bipartite circulation to the metaphysis, the central portion being derived from the nutrient artery and the periphery from the periosteal vessels.

There are three functionally separate systems of circulation to the physis. One system supplies the epiphyseal surface of the physis, one supplies the peripheral portion (zone of Ranvier), and the other supplies the metaphyseal surface, with each system being essentially end-arterial. The vascular supply includes numerous branches of the epiphyseal arteries that reach the germinal and resting layers of the contiguous physis. These initially approach the physis directly through the chondroepiphysis. But with skeletal maturation and the appearance of a large ossification center, these branches eventually come through the maturing subchondral plate. The epiphyseal supply is quite abundant and necessary to normal development of the physis.

The degree of vascularity to the skeleton changes significantly over time. Major changes in flow distribution patterns are found in the developing canine tibia and femur (Fig. 91–18). In particular, there is a dramatic quantitative decrease of tibial circulation commensurate with increasing skeletal maturation. If this also occurs in humans, which is quite likely, it would explain the increasing delay in fracture healing and the high incidence of non-union characteristic of the tibia of an adult. Adequate vascularity is a major factor in fracture healing; thus, a poor vascular response would impair the early crucial stages of callus formation. These chronobiologic circulatory changes in distribution patterns also affect diagnostic tests such as radionuclide scans. Furthermore, there is a significant correlation between changing flow patterns and the likelihood of hematogenous osteomyelitis.

BONE METABOLISM

WILLIAM J. BURTIS and ROBERT LANG

Living bone is functionally a very dynamic tissue. It is constantly being turned over by means of a complex process of remodeling. There are approximately 30,000 cells per cubic millimeter of bone. These cells are interconnected to nearby cells and to the bone surface by long dendritic processes that run through bone canaliculi and are bathed in a special extracellular fluid. Bone is remarkably responsive to changes in plasma mineral concentration. In addition, throughout adult life bone retains an extraordinary capacity for complete and morphologically accurate regeneration following injury.

SKELETAL FUNCTION

The skeletal system provides two essential functions, one mechanical and the other biochemical. Bone is a specialized type of connective tissue in which the organic matrix, under the control of bone cells, undergoes calcification. This mineralization provides bone with rigidity and strength, important attributes of the mechanical aspect of skeletal function. Bones support the body, provide sites of muscular attachment for movement, and protect fragile soft tissues. Thus one important aspect of bone metabolism is to respond to changing demands for mechanical strength and to optimize bone structure while maintaining total skeletal mass, a process called skeletal homeostasis.

In addition to this mechanical role, bone also serves an important biochemical function as a mineral reservoir. The skeletal system contains over 99 per cent of the calcium in the body, and this skeletal calcium is continuously exchanged with calcium in the blood. The exchange is mediated by bone cells, which in turn are regulated by extracellular and plasma ion levels, local factors, and systemic hormones to maintain a plasma calcium level throughout the body essential for normal cell function. This second important aspect of bone metabolism is called mineral homeostasis.

BONE TISSUE

At the tissue level, bone is organized into two basic types: cortical and trabecular. The cortex, a thick vascularized layer of calcified matrix, forms the external aspect of all bones. For reasons of mechanical strength it is especially thick at the midshaft of the long bones. Remodeling of the cortex occurs not only on its surfaces but also in the interior along haversian canals. The periosteum covering the outer cortical surface continuously makes bone throughout adult life. The inner surface of the cortex is the endosteum. Resorption along this surface occurs during catabolic conditions that lead to thinning of the cortex (Fig. 91–19).

Trabecular bone, in contrast, is thinner and less compact than the cortex and is avascular. It is nourished by diffusion from the marrow space. Also known as spongy or cancellous bone, it is especially prominent in the flat bones, vertebral bodies, and the ends of the long bones. Remodeling occurs only on the trabecular surfaces because there are no haversian systems in trabecular bone.

Both cortical and trabecular bone consist of an organic matrix (33 per cent by weight) that has become mineralized. The matrix consists primarily (90 per cent) of type I collagen fibers, as well as a number of other proteins and glycosaminoglycans (e.g., osteonectin, osteoclacin, α2-HS-glycoprotein) thought to be structurally and/or functionally important in the calcification process. The mineral phase itself consists of spindle-shaped crystals of hydroxyapatite ($Ca_{10}(PO_4)_6 \cdot (OH)_2$) or some similar calcium-phosphate lattice. Both collagen and crystals are oriented in preferential directions (lamellae) in mature bone but are randomly oriented in immature (woven) bone.

This calcified matrix is metabolically responsive, containing bone cells called osteocytes that are situated in tiny osteocytic lacunae embedded throughout the mineralized bone. The osteocytes are in communication with one another and with surface cells via long cellular processes running through a network of osteocytic canaliculi. They are bathed in a special bone extracellular fluid that is relatively low in calcium and sodium compared to normal extracel-

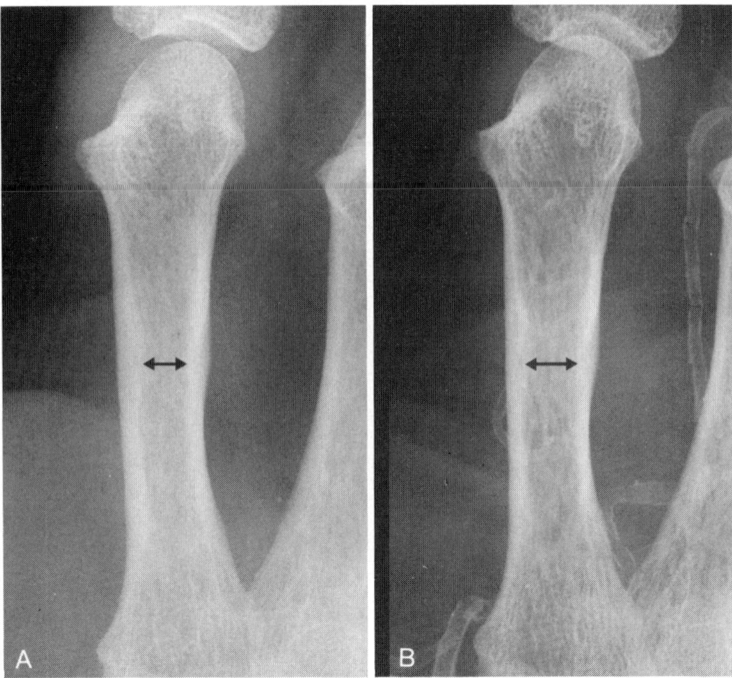

Figure 91–19. *A* and *B*, **Second metacarpal of a 60-year-old diabetic receiving chronic hemodialysis for renal failure.** Resorption of bone along the endosteal surfaces has led to thinning of the cortical bone *(arrows)*. Note the development of vascular calcification; this is a common occurrence in diabetics.

lular fluid. This fluid is separated from other tissue compartments by the bone envelope, a continuous layer of cells covering the bone surface. The osteocytic system is believed to play a significant role in bone mineral homeostasis and the regulation of plasma calcium concentration.

The bone surface is both morphologically and functionally diverse. Usually the greatest portion is covered by flat, metabolically less active lining cells of mesenchymal origin, constituting the bone envelope. In areas of new bone formation, plump cuboidal cells called osteoblasts, which are derived from mesenchymal marrow cells, overlie uncalcified osteoid matrix. These cells are rich in mitochondria and alkaline phosphatase and have long processes extending into the matrix. Osteoblasts actively synthesize and secrete collagen to form new organic matrix. The osteoblasts eventually become embedded within this matrix; they are then called *osteoid osteocytes* and they play a role in the process of mineralization. Finally, the same cells are surrounded by calcified bone and become the mature osteocytes described above.

In areas of active bone resorption a distinct type of bone surface cell called the *osteoclast* is found. One to several of these large, multinucleated cells may be seen in a scalloped area of resorption (Howship's lacuna). An osteoclastic ruffled border, surrounded by a sealing zone, contacts the calcified bone, and lysosomal enzymes and acids are released that degrade both apatite crystals and collagen. These resorption products are then phagocytized and the mineral ions and hydroxyproline-rich peptides are subsequently released into the marrow space from the other side of the cell. The origin of the osteoclast has only recently been determined. Unlike other bone cells that are of mesenchymal origin, the osteoclasts are of hematogenous origin and specifically appear to be derivative of circulating monocytes.

SKELETAL REMODELING

Skeletal remodeling is the process by which adult bone tissue is periodically resorbed and rebuilt. All remodeling of trabecular bone begins on the surface. In cortical bone, remodeling also occurs along the haversian canals, which are topologically an inward extension of the surface. A most important principle of skeletal homeostasis is that bone resorption and formation do not occur randomly along the bone surface, but are closely coupled sequential processes. That is, in the normal adult, new bone formation occurs in the location of and to the same magnitude as the previous bone resorption. Thus, functionally, the basic remodeling sequence consists of activation of osteoclast precursors, resorption by osteoclasts, and bone formation by osteoblasts. Spatially a bone remodeling unit (about 0.01 cu mm) extends inward from the surface and is bounded by a cement line. Eventually, bone remodeling units replace the entire bone tissue, with a turnover half-life of approximately 20 months.

The activation signal that initiates a bone remodeling sequence is not known. It may include some combination of effects from hormones (PTH, vitamin D), local ion levels, or mechanical stress (piezoelectric charge). Somehow bone lining cells part to allow osteoclast precursors access to the calcified matrix, and resorption begins. Active osteoclastic resorption is rapid, lasting only about 3 days, and is followed by an inactive reversal phase of 14 days. This, in turn, is followed by osteoblastic bone formation that over the next 70 days slowly fills the area of resorption with osteoid. This osteoid is then systematically mineralized 8 to 10 days following its elaboration by the osteoblasts. Thus the entire basic remodeling sequence of activation-resorption-formation requires approximately three months for completion. Once formed, this bone remodeling unit is then called a *bone metabolic unit* and it now assists in mineral homeostasis.

Cortical remodeling is somewhat more complex, taking place not only on the surface but internally along the haversian canals. Osteoclasts bore a longitudinal channel through the cortical bone and are followed by a blood vessel, which provides nutrition, and finally by osteoblasts that under normal circumstances fill in the hole. In conditions characterized by high bone turnover, such as renal osteodystrophy and hyperparathyroidism, the haversian canals are increased in size and number. These enlarged and more numerous canals can be demonstrated radiographically (Fig. 91–20). The increase in intracortical resorption will regress after the bone turnover returns to normal.

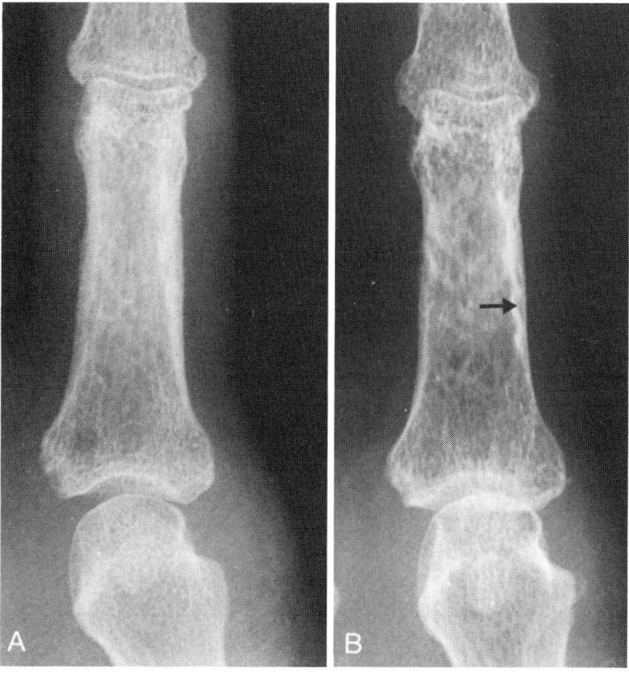

Figure 91–20. *A* and *B,* **Proximal phalanx of a 53-year-old woman with primary hyperparathyroidism.** Note the development of intracortical resorption, which appears as tunneling in the normally solid cortical bone *(arrow),* and the loss of cortical thickness due to endosteal resorption.

HORMONAL CONTROL OF BONE METABOLISM

Parathyroid hormone (PTH) is the most important hormone maintaining calcium homeostasis on a minute-to-minute basis in man. Secreted by the parathyroid glands in response to a decrease in ionized serum calcium, PTH acts directly on bone and kidney to raise the calcium level. In addition, PTH increases the synthesis of 1,25-dihydroxyvitamin D, which, in turn, stimulates calcium absorption from the intestine. In bone, PTH stimulation has several consequences. First, osteoblasts (which are rich in PTH receptors) respond with inhibition of collagen synthesis and (at least in vitro) separation of adjacent cells. Second, osteoclastic bone resorption is increased (an indirect effect, since osteoclasts lack PTH receptors) and activation of the basic remodeling sequence results in increased bone turnover. Third, there may be a rapid increase in osteocytic osteolysis, although this is controversial.

The net result of chronic PTH overstimulation, as seen in primary and secondary hyperparathyroidism, is greatly increased bone remodeling activity. This can be manifest radiographically as subperiosteal, endosteal, and intracortical resorption (Fig. 91–21; see Figs. 91–19 and 91–20). Bone cysts may occur in advanced disease. In hypoparathyroidism, by contrast, bone is relatively inactive with very little remodeling.

Vitamin D is metabolized to a number of more active compounds affecting bone metabolism. Vitamin D, obtained either from the diet or by the action of ultraviolet light on the skin, is hydroxylated to 25(OH)-vitamin D by the liver. This metabolite then undergoes hydroxylation in the 1 or 24 position, predominantly by the kidney. Calcitriol, or 1,25-dihydroxyvitamin D, is the most active D metabolite known, and its synthesis is stimulated by PTH or hypophosphatemia. The major actions of 1,25$(OH)_2$D on bone may be inhibition of osteoblast function and stimulation of osteoclastic resorption in a manner similar to PTH. Other vitamin D metabolites are important for calcification of the osteoid matrix, and may also have an effect on new bone formation. Clinically, lack of vitamin D results in rickets or osteomalacia and is characterized by inadequate mineralization of bone matrix and widened osteoid seams.

Calcitonin in lower animals acts as a calcium-lowering hormone, but it does not appear to play a major physiologic role in calcium metabolism in man. Osteoclasts do, however, have calcitonin receptors, and superphysiologic levels of calcitonin cause a rapid decrease in osteoclastic bone resorption.

Estrogen in women and androgen in men are necessary for maintenance of bone mass. Withdrawal of gonadal hormone can lead to relatively rapid bone loss and ultimately to osteoporosis. How the gonadal hormones exert this influence is not clear, because sex steroid receptors have not yet been found in bone cells. In general, estrogen appears to have a moderating influence with respect to the effects of PTH on bone.

Adrenocortical steroids have a marked osteolytic effect, with both increased bone resorption and decreased formation. The increased resorption is caused, at least in part, by a mild secondary hyperparathyroidism, consequent to direct steroid inhibition of intestinal calcium absorption as well as renal calcium wasting. The decreased bone formation has been attributed to decreased recruitment of active osteoblasts from their precursors.

Thyroid hormone stimulates bone metabolism, with increased activity of both osteoclasts and osteoblasts and an increased number of bone remodeling units. Hyperthyroidism, however, increases bone resorption to a greater degree than bone formation and can contribute to osteoporosis.

Growth hormone, acting via the somatomedins, is essential for normal linear bone growth in children. Both somatomedin-A and somatomedin-C have been shown to stimulate osteoblast function in vitro. Similarly, insulin stimulates osteoblast function in vitro,

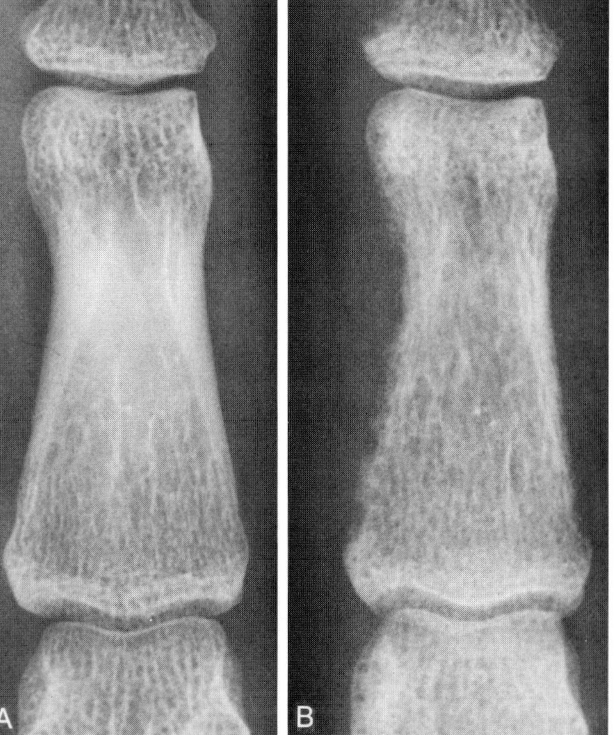

Figure 91–21. *A* and *B,* Middle phalanx of a 23-year-old man demonstrates the development of **advanced subperiosteal bone resorption in association with secondary hyperparathyroidism.** Note the loss of the sharp cortical margins and the lace-like pattern of resorption. Intracortical and endosteal resorption are also present.

and untreated diabetics have impaired growth in childhood and possibly an increased incidence of osteoporosis as adults.

IONIC INFLUENCES ON BONE METABOLISM

A constant ionized calcium concentration in the extracellular environment is critical for general cell function. With any perturbation of the calcium concentration, multiple hormonal responses occur to attempt to restore homeostasis. Thus, it is difficult to isolate direct effects of serum calcium from indirect ones in vivo. In vitro, osteoblast function (e.g., protein synthesis) and replication are slowed at low calcium concentrations.

Serum phosphate varies physiologically over a wider range and may have a greater direct influence on bone metabolism. In situations of phosphate depletion there is evidence of increased bone resorption, decreased bone formation, and impaired mineralization. A clinical correlate of this is the osteomalacic bone disease that occurs in association with renal phosphate wasting (e.g., familial hypophosphatemic rickets and tumor-associated osteomalacia). There is also evidence that hyperphosphatemia directly stimulates bone formation, although this is offset in vivo by the attendant hypocalcemia and secondary hyperparathyroidism.

Systemic acidosis has long been known to be associated with a negative calcium balance and bone demineralization. Although the mechanism has not been determined, it may involve an impairment of the renal 1α-hydroxylase activation of vitamin D. Magnesium deficiency leads to hypocalcemia with low serum PTH levels, probably due to a direct effect on parathyroid hormone synthesis and secretion.

LOCAL REGULATORS OF BONE METABOLISM

Besides systemic hormonal and ionic influences, bone metabolism is responsive to a variety of local factors that may be important in normal bone remodeling and response to injury. Prostaglandins, bone-derived growth factors, bone morphogenetic protein, osteoclast-activating factor, and noncollagenous bone proteins such as osteonectin and osteoclacin are examples of such locally active factors.

Bone mineral exhibits piezoelectric properties. When the hydroxyapatite crystal is deformed (such as with mechanical stress) it produces an electric charge. This electric activity orients osteoblastic bone formation and may be important in stimulating local bone cells to increase their remodeling activity. Clinical application of osteoblast stimulation by electricity has been successfully exploited for the treatment of delayed and non-united fractures.

Bibliography

Skeletal Development

Black J, Mattson R, Korotsoff E: Haversian osteons: Size, distribution, internal structure, and orientation. J Biomed Mater Res 8:299, 1974.

Carter DR, Spengler DM: Mechanical properties and composition of cortical bone. Clin Orthop 135:192, 1978.

Light TR, McKinstry MP, Schnitzer J, Ogden JA: Bone blood flow: Regional variation with skeletal maturation. In Arlet J, Ficat RP, Hungerford DS (eds): Bone Circulation. Baltimore, Williams and Wilkins, 1984.

Ogden J: Chondro-osseous development growth. In Urist M (ed): Fundamental and Clinical Bone Physiology. Philadelphia, JB Lippincott, 1981.

Ogden J: Radiology of postnatal skeletal development. X. Patella and tibial tuberosity. Skel Radiol 12:12, 1984.

Ogden J: Skeletal Injury in the Child, 2nd ed. Philadelphia, WB Saunders Company, 1990.

Ogden J: The uniqueness of growing bones. In Rockwood CA, Wilkins KE, King RE (eds): Fractures, 3rd ed. Vol. 3—Children. Philadelphia, JB Lippincott, 1991.

Ogden JA, Grogan DP, Light TR: Postnatal skeletal development and growth of the musculoskeletal system. In Albright JA, Brand RA (eds): The Scientific Basis of Orthopaedics, 2nd ed. New York, Appleton-Lange, 1987.

Simkin A, Robin G: Fracture formation in differing collagen fiber pattern of compact bone. J Biomech 7:183, 1974.

Smith JW, Walmsley R: Factors affecting the elasticity of bone. J Anat 93:503, 1959.

Normal Variants and Bone Age

Greulich WW, Pyle SI: Radiographic Atlas of Skeletal Development of the Hand and Wrist, 2nd ed. Stanford, CA, Stanford University Press, 1959.

Keats T: Atlas of Normal Roentgen Variants, 3rd ed. Chicago, Year Book Medical Publishers, 1984.

Kohler A, Zimmer EA: Borderlands of the normal and early pathology. In Wilk SP (ed): Skeletal Roentgenology. New York, Grune and Stratton, 1968.

Ozonoff MB: Pediatric Orthopedic Radiology. Philadelphia, WB Saunders Company, 1979.

Vogler JB, Helms CA, Callen PW: Normal Variants and Pitfalls in Imaging. Philadelphia, WB Saunders Company, 1986.

Bone Metabolism

Baron R, Vignery A, Lang R: Reversal phase and osteopenia: Defective coupling of resorption to formation in the pathogenesis of osteoporosis. In DeLuca HF, Frost HM, Jee WSS, Johnson CC Jr, Parfitt AM (eds): Osteoporosis: Recent Advances in Pathogenesis and Treatment. Baltimore, University Park Press, 1981, pp 311–320.

Canalis E: The hormonal and local regulation of bone formation. Endocrinol Rev 4:62–77, 1983.

Raisz LG, Kream BE: Regulation of bone formation. N Engl J Med 309:29–35, 83–89, 1983.

Rasmussen H, Bordier P: The Physiological and Cellular Basis of Metabolic Bone Disease. Baltimore, Williams and Wilkins, 1974.

Rodan GA, Martin TJ: Role of osteoblasts in hormonal control of bone resorption—a hypothesis. Calcif Tiss Int 33:349–351, 1981.

Urist MR, DeLange RJ, Finerman GAM: Bone cell differentiation and growth factors. Science 220:680–686, 1983.

92 Imaging Modalities

Carol L. Andrews and Gary S. Novick

Skeletal radiology can trace its history back to the very first x-ray film: a radiograph of the hand of Frau Roentgen taken in 1895. Much of the early radiographic literature was devoted to a description of the skeletal system because the high contrast that exists between bone and soft tissue was necessary to form images using the rudimentary equipment. With subsequent development of each new imaging modality some diagnostic use in the skeletal system has been discovered, and in many cases, this has also included imaging of the soft tissues. Although imaging with x-rays is based on the relative absorptive properties of the various tissues, these other modalities form images utilizing other tissue characteristics, such as metabolic, vascular, and acoustic properties. There is now a diverse assortment of powerful methods for examining the musculoskeletal system that must be judiciously employed in a timely fashion to arrive at both an accurate and an economical diagnosis.

PLAIN FILM RADIOGRAPHY

Plain film radiography remains the mainstay of musculoskeletal imaging despite the technical advances in new imaging modalities. It is the least expensive, most readily available, and quickest way of visualizing osseous and adjacent soft-tissue structures. Very small to very large areas can be imaged in a single exposure with good spatial resolution. The skeletal structures are relatively insensitive to hazardous effects of ionizing radiation, especially in the appendages, and image degradation from patient motion is only a minor technical problem.

The most important limitation of plain film imaging is poor contrast resolution for soft tissues—essentially restricted to air, fat, soft-tissue, and mineral densities. Soft-tissue radiographs serve as a screening tool and are useful for identifying fatty lesions such as lipomas, gas in some soft-tissue infections, and calcifications, and for localizing radio-dense foreign bodies. This poor contrast resolution contributes to plain film inaccuracy in judging bone destruction. As much as 50 percent of the trabecular bone can be lost before it can be identified radiographically.

Although the projected images of plain films are useful in covering large areas, more than one view is essential to adequately characterize pathology, and positioning the patient and equipment to obtain this three-dimensional image may be difficult. In fact, some lesions cannot be adequately visualized even with multiple projections, and other modalities, such as tomography, must be employed. There are also serious limitations in the measurement of sizes and angles on plain films as a result of complex magnification errors and divergent beam artifacts. Despite these weaknesses, the resolution of osseous detail is much better on plain film than computed tomography (CT) or magnetic resonance imaging (MRI). The use of more advanced plain film techniques, such as magnification radiography and low kilovoltage techniques, and the selected use of intra-articular and intravascular contrast agents can overcome some of these limitations.

Conventional Techniques

Frontal and lateral projections are the most common views obtained for evaluation of skeletal structures. These orthogonal views allow three-dimensional conceptualization of the anatomy and pathology. However, the complex spatial anatomy of most joints and certain bones, such as the small bones of the ankle and wrist, often make special views necessary. Careful attention to patient positioning, tube angulation, and technique is vital. Navicular, patellar and radial head fractures, tarsal coalitions, juxta-articular erosions, and congenital hip dislocations, among others, may go undetected without the proper view (Fig. 92–1).

Although plain film images are static, they can represent dynamic processes with proper positioning and technique. Stress views of certain joints—especially the acromioclavicular joint, ankle, wrist,

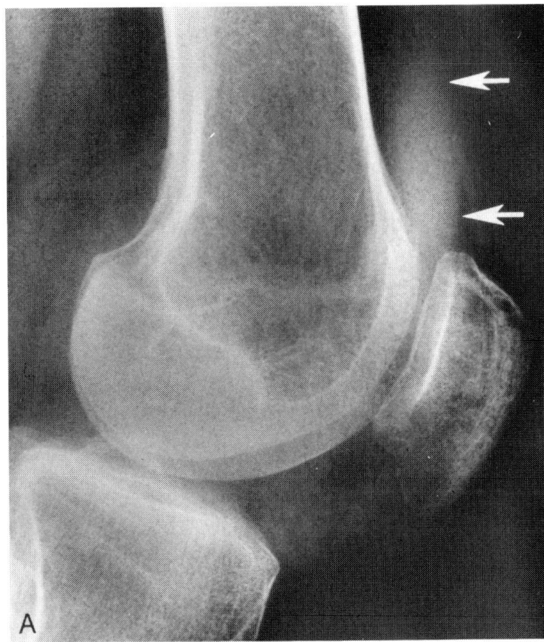

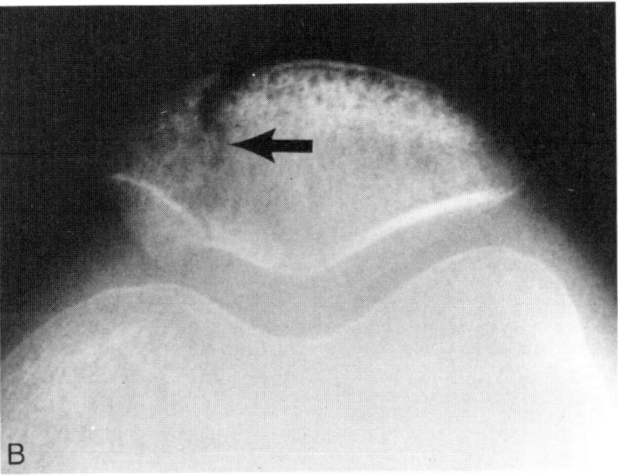

Figure 92–1. History of acute knee trauma. *A*, Lateral view of the knee demonstrates a suprapatellar effusion *(arrows)*. *B*, Sunrise view of the patella demonstrates a fracture *(arrow)* that can be seen only on this projection.

and the metacarpophalangeal joint of the thumb—can be diagnostic of ligamentous injuries that would be unsuspected on the routine views. Measurements of patellar stability are only accurate with the knee at the proper degree of flexion, and some pathology, such as congenital foot abnormalities, is demonstrated only with weight-bearing views.

Soft-tissue changes are often helpful in radiograph analysis. Displacement or obliteration of normal tissue planes can suggest the presence of underlying abnormalities. The presence of a joint effusion is a nonspecific sign of joint abnormality. The synovial space and joint capsule can be distended by a clear effusion, hemorrhage, or purulent material. In the elbow, the displacement of the fat adjacent to the joint capsule, called the *fat pad sign*, may be the only radiographic evidence of a radial head or supracondylar fracture. In the knee, fluid is demonstrated as an area of soft-tissue density where fat would normally be present (Fig. 92–1). If a joint effusion is noted after knee trauma in the absence of a discernible fracture, tangential beam views should be obtained to look for a fat-fluid level. This may be the only clue to an intra-articular fracture, where marrow fat is released and mixes with blood in the joint space. The fat is less dense than the blood and floats above it, creating a demonstrable interface radiographically.

Equally important as obtaining the appropriate views for each anatomic area is acquisition of the correct survey films for systemic processes. A knowledge of the disease process aids in determining which films are most appropriate. Surveys may be used for such diverse diseases as metastatic disease, hyperparathyroidism, multiple myeloma, vitamin deficiencies or excesses, skeletal dysplasias, and suspected child abuse. Ideally, the least number of radiographs should be obtained to make the diagnosis and aid in following the response to any therapy that is undertaken.

Low-Kilovoltage (kV) Technique

Both contrast and spatial resolution can be controlled and increased in skeletal radiography. Low-kilovoltage techniques increase contrast while special film/screen combinations may improve spatial resolution. The extremities are particularly favorable areas for these techniques. Their lack of bulk permits easy beam penetration with minimal scatter. Additionally, single emulsion "fine-detail" filming requires a higher radiation dose and is appropriately used where there is little risk of radiation damage but a high yield of diagnostic information is required (e.g., hand and wrist filming for evaluation of changes related to occult trauma, metabolic bone disease, or inflammatory arthropathies). Low-kilovoltage (25 to 35 kV) techniques for soft tissues of the extremities are similar to those used in mammography and are especially useful in the evaluation of soft-tissue masses, joint effusions, foreign bodies, soft-tissue calcifications, integrity of some ligaments and tendons (patellar and Achilles), and the periarticular edema, erosions, and calcifications of inflammatory joint disease. Abnormalities of calcium metabolism, calcium pyrophosphate deposition disease, and gout can also cause soft-tissue abnormalities.

Magnification Techniques

The relative absence of scatter and absorption permits the use of magnification radiography in the extremities, which is valuable for evaluating trabecular pattern, fine cortical detail, soft-tissue calcifications, and periosteal reaction. Magnification can be obtained by two methods. Optical magnification is achieved by using very fine-grained film and hand-held magnifiers. Although no special equipment is necessary, it is limited by body part thickness and radiation dosage. Direct radiographic magnification is achieved with the use of a very small focal spot (approximately 100 microns), which permits geometric enlargement. This requires special tubes that are quite expensive and are limited in penetration and field size. They offer the advantages of increased sharpness and less noise than the optical magnification method. Magnification radiography has been particularly helpful for detecting the earliest erosions in rheumatoid arthritis and its variants and in evaluating intracortical and subperiosteal resorption in metabolic bone disease.

CONVENTIONAL TOMOGRAPHY

Plain film radiography is a simple projection method that sometimes produces confusing overlapping shadows, even with excellent spatial and contrast resolution techniques and multiple views. Tomography is a technique of bringing a specific plane of interest into sharp focus by purposefully blurring the shadows of structures lying superficial or deep to that plane. This controlled image blurring is helpful in analyzing pathology involving joints where the anatomy is complex, such as ankle or knee. Subtle or complex fractures may be better characterized in this fashion. It can also facilitate the evaluation of osseous fusion of fractures, osteotomies, and arthrodeses and may prove particularly useful when overlying hardware makes the osseous structures difficult to see. Another occasional use is the characterization of solitary bone lesions, which may aid in suggesting the pathologic diagnosis. For example, in the proper clinical and anatomic setting, the detection of a central lytic nidus in a sclerotic bone lesion supports the diagnosis of an osteoid osteoma.

As with all imaging modalities, conventional tomography, whether linear or of a more complex motion, contributes its own set of artifacts. The major drawback is inherent in the technique: An area of interest is brought out by blurring the superimposed structures. Those ghost images are still present, however, and can mimic pathology. Simple linear tomography will emphasize linear patterns that parallel its direction of motion while blurring those perpendicular to that direction. This creates artifact in the bone image accentuating, for example, an otherwise normal trabecular pattern. Complex motion tomography, though requiring a higher radiation dose, can alleviate this problem and is the preferred method for bone evaluation. Radiation dose increases not only with more complex tube/film motion but with the number of sections required. It is not uncommon to need multiple sections in two orthogonal planes for adequate evaluation.

FLUOROSCOPY

Fluoroscopy is used as a method for localization during joint aspirations, contrast studies (such as arthrography and angiography), and closed percutaneous biopsy of some osseous and soft-tissue lesions. Joint motion and stability can also be evaluated fluoroscopically with the added benefit of later review if concomitant videotaping is performed. Digital subtraction arthrography is an additional fluoroscopic method that offers great contrast resolution while allowing very small amounts of dilute contrast material to be hand-injected through a small needle or catheter with far less morbidity and patient discomfort for evaluation of small joints, such as the wrist, and joints containing orthopedic hardware.

COMPUTED TOMOGRAPHY

Computed tomography (CT) allows cross-sectional imaging without the inherent artifact from surrounding structures found in conventional tomography. In CT, as in conventional tomography, a specific plane of the body is imaged. However, in CT, information about the region of interest is obtained through thin-section x-rays performed in multiple projections that are mathematically reconstructed to create an image of that plane of section. The relative differences in the tissues of the body are shown to advantage in this method. Fat, water-density fluid, muscle, air, bone, and blood can be differentiated based on density measurement. Density is reflected in terms of attenuation values (Hounsfield units—HU) ranging from 1000 HU for cortical bone to −1000 HU for air. This is particularly useful when characterizing the content of a lesion.

This technology is widely used in neuroradiology as well as chest and abdominal imaging and has multiple valuable uses in the musculoskeletal system as well. CT facilitates the evaluation of trauma; infectious processes; osseous and soft-tissue neoplasms; articular, metabolic, and congenital diseases; it also facilitates radiation therapy planning and can serve as guidance for fine needle aspiration and biopsy.

When planning use of CT in the musculoskeletal system, one must have a clear idea of the clinical question to be answered in order to properly direct the performance of the test. Ideally, access to plain films is essentially for protocol planning but the CT scanogram may also be used to localize the abnormality. Various software algorithms may be employed to emphasize the tissue in question and image it to best advantage. Bone algorithm may be preferred, for example, in evaluation of cortical integrity of a possible aneurysmal bone cyst, whereas a soft-tissue algorithm may be more appropriate for characterizing a soft-tissue mass.

CT is limited, particularly in the axial skeleton, with regard to the obtainable plane of section (limited to a transverse/axial section), although this can be offset by image reconstruction in a different plane (i.e., coronal or sagittal plane). The resulting reformatted image quality is less than that of the original scan but can add useful information regarding alignment, location of a lesion, or presence and position of bony fragments or hardware. Appendicular imaging is more flexible because the patient can position hands, wrists, elbows, knees, ankles, and feet in orientations other than the axial plane. The thickness of image slices can vary from 1.5 mm to 10 mm slices or thicker, and the area of image acquisition can be overlapped if reformation in another plane is planned. Thin-section imaging is preferred for such reformation and when subtle pathology is being evaluated. Imaging of both extremities simultaneously often provides a "built-in" normal for comparison when assessing a lesion in one extremity.

The use of contrast in CT examination of the musculoskeletal system must also be tailored to the exam and may not be necessary when imaging complex fractures but is essential for identifying and characterizing soft-tissue lesions. It is useful for distinguishing scar from recurrent herniated disc in the patient with low back pain who has previously undergone surgery. Intra-articular contrast and intrathecal contrast are two additional routes of administration that can contribute to the diagnostic value of the examination.

Fractures, subluxations, and dislocations of cervical, thoracic, and lumbar vertebrae are well-evaluated with CT. Likewise, the presence and spatial localization of fracture fragments in other anatomic regions can be demonstrated. This is of particular importance in fractures of the pelvis and acetabulum in which position of the bone fragments is important to surgical management and may not be readily apparent on plain film imaging (Fig. 92–2). Hematoma and rupture of pelvic viscera can be visualized at the same time. Three-dimensional reformation of the images may be valuable for determining the surgical approach to complex fractures such as facial fractures. CT also aids in determining bone fusion in complex fractures, following osteotomy, and in congenital coalitions (Fig. 92–3).

The scan image is unaffected by plaster casts, an advantage over conventional tomography, but is seriously degraded by any metal appliances in the plane of section. Artificial joint replacements can also cause image degradation. This streak artifact may be minimized, however, by using a bone algorithm, imaging in the plane of the hardware (when possible—especially in the hand or wrist) or thin-section imaging (3 mm or less) with reconstruction of the images in a different plane. An additional disadvantage is patient motion. The movement of an agitated patient will not only degrade the axial images obtained but also make reformation in other planes or into a three-dimensional image impossible.

In evaluation of osseous and/or soft-tissue lesions, CT or MRI can be used following plain film imaging and radionuclide examination. CT provides excellent spatial resolution and detailed information about the bony cortex, trabecular pattern, and mineralization within or adjacent to a lesion. It can demonstrate the extent of the lesion and its involvement with the surrounding structures, although its multiplanar capabilities are limited in comparison with MRI.

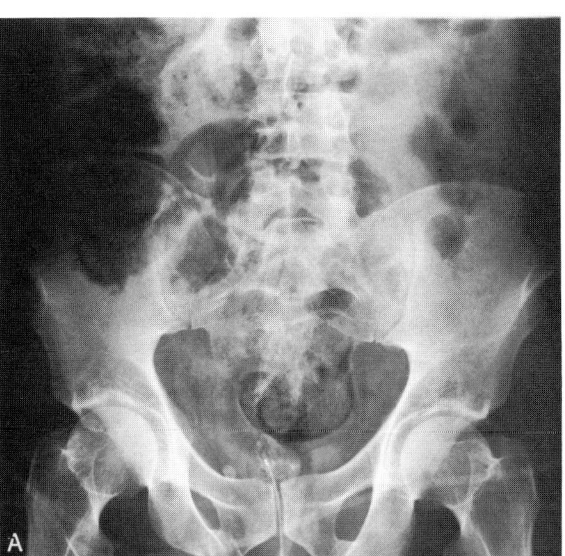

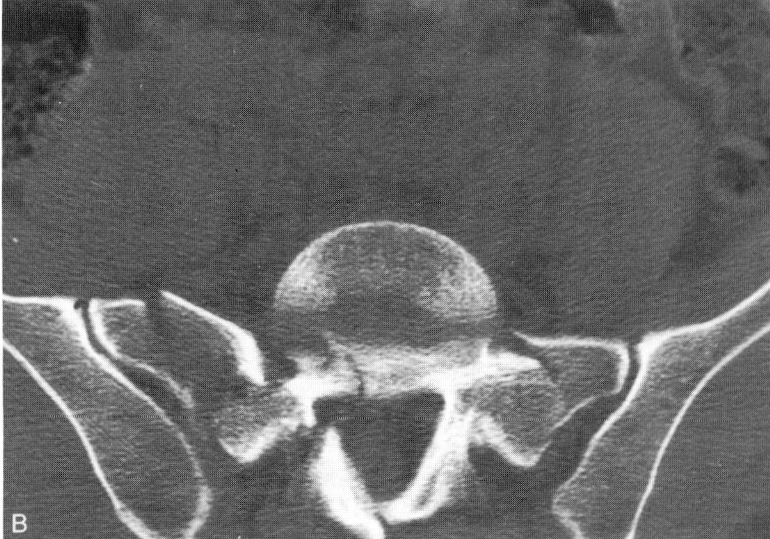

Figure 92–2. History of fall from a height. *A,* AP view of the pelvis demonstrates a minimally displaced fracture of the right inferior pubic ramus. The sacrum and sacroiliac joints are obscured by overlying soft tissue and bowel gas. *B,* Axial CT, performed in bone algorithm, delineates comminuted fractures of the sacral ala bilaterally.

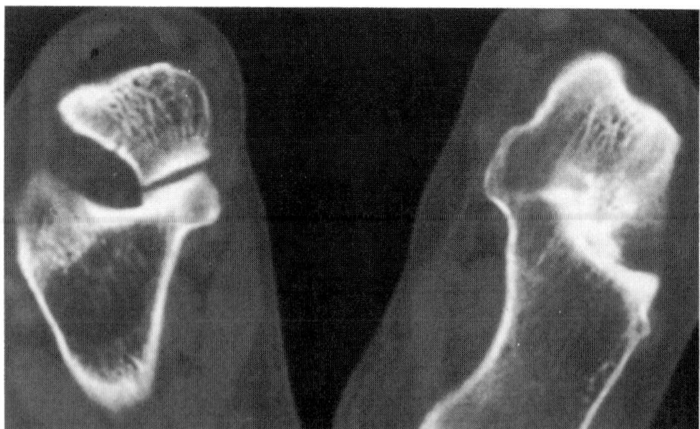

Figure 92–3. History of foot pain. Axial CT demonstrates congenital coalition of the the anterior and medial facets of the left subtalar (talocalcaneal) joint.

Measurement of attenuation values, such as fat density in a lipoma, or fluid density in a cystic, soft-tissue mass may be useful in developing an appropriate differential diagnosis. Blood attenuation values suggest the presence of a recent or remote hemorrhage within a lesion. The use of intravenous contrast in the CT evaluation of soft-tissue masses is indispensable, both for direct tumor enhancement and for localization of major vessels adjacent to or surrounded by the mass. Without contrast enhancement, solid masses may mimic fluid collections or be indistinguishable from normal muscle. The presence of circular densities within it may suggest the presence of phleboliths within an hemangioma. If a biopsy is indicated, CT offers excellent localization and confirmation of needle position during the procedure. Additionally, CT may be used in treatment planning including surgical approach or radiation port planning and for following the outcome of various treatments such as radiation and chemotherapy.

CT is useful in other settings as well. Changes of inflammation and/or infection of soft tissues as well as osteomyelitis may be demonstrable with CT. Although scintigraphy is highly sensitive to acute changes related to infection and inflammation, it is nonspecific, and the extra-osseous extent of the process and associated problems such as abscesses are better delineated on CT. Bony sequestra may be identified in chronic infection. Information about congenital abnormalities such as tarsal coalition and congenital hip dislocation can be provided by CT. Digital pelvimetry aids in clinical decisions regarding vaginal versus cesarean delivery in breech presentation labor. By obtaining frontal and sagittal scanograms as well as a transverse scan at the ischial spines, one can measure the bony pelvis dimensions and assess the fetal position with minimal radiation dose to both mother and fetus (Fig. 92–4).

ULTRASONOGRAPHY

Diagnostic ultrasonography uses high-frequency (1 to 10 mHz) sound to produce cross-sectional images in multiple planes. By sampling the returning echoes from tissue interfaces, ultrasonography can produce useful anatomic images in real time. Mechanical and electronic scanners with sector or linear array scanning patterns allow rapid examination and observation of the anatomy in real time as well as observation of vascular pulsations and other movements. Doppler ultrasonography allows analysis of high-frequency sound waves as they reflect off moving fluid, especially blood. When real-time ultrasonography is combined with Doppler ultrasonography, the result is a duplex scanner that allows the scan operator to know where the pulsed Doppler beam is sampling anatomically. This markedly increases the sensitivity of vascular sonography and allows evaluation of masses for vascularity and quality of pulsatility as well as assisting in general assessment of venous and arterial flow in an extremity.

Because of the intrinsic inability of sound to penetrate bone, ultrasound is used mainly for soft-tissue imaging. Cartilage is relatively sonolucent but in most areas is hidden by bone. A notable exception is in the neonate and infant, in whom the ends of the bones are still cartilaginous and have a distinct echotexture sonographically. Sonography has been successfully used in evaluating the infant hip for dislocation, and synovial fluid collections have been localized in the septic hip (Fig. 92–5). Arthrosonography can detect effusions in the adult joints and can evaluate the rotator cuff of the shoulder.

Although sonography can image neoplasms of the extremities, CT and MRI are more effective in evaluation of the extent of disease and in treatment planning. However, ultrasonography is useful in determining whether a soft-tissue mass is cystic or solid and whether vascular pulsations are adjacent to or within the mass. A popliteal mass may be effectively evaluated by ultrasonography, for example, to determine whether it is a synovial cyst or a popliteal aneurysm. The synovial cyst tends to have a simple wall and a classic location. Hemorrhage or rupture of the cyst may mimic symptoms of a deep vein thrombosis. Doppler examination of the adjacent venous system may help to distinguish this. A popliteal artery aneurysm will be also be cystic, but pulsatile (if not filled with clotted blood) and have characteristics of arterial flow on Doppler examination.

If a mass proves to be solid and nonvascular by ultrasonography, the image also serves as an accurate guide for biopsy. Although nonspecific, the sonographic appearance may suggest a pathologic diagnosis. For example, lipomatous tumors are often quite echogenic. Simple cysts and hemorrhagic masses can usually be differentiated from solid masses. This is of particular importance in bleeding diatheses, in which hematomas of the iliopsoas muscle or

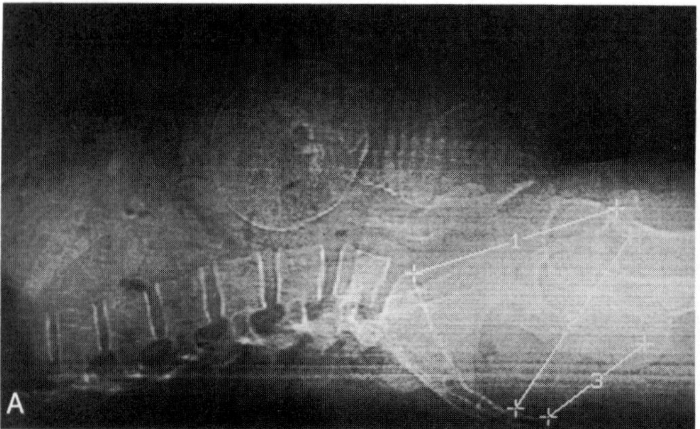

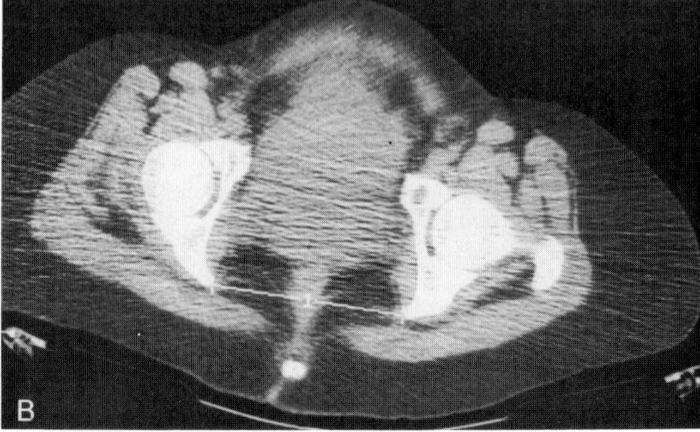

Figure 92–4. Breech presentation. *A,* CT sagittal scanogram allows measurement of the pelvic inlet and outlet. *B,* A transverse scan at the level of the fovea allows measurement of the narrowest portion of the pelvis, the ischial spines.

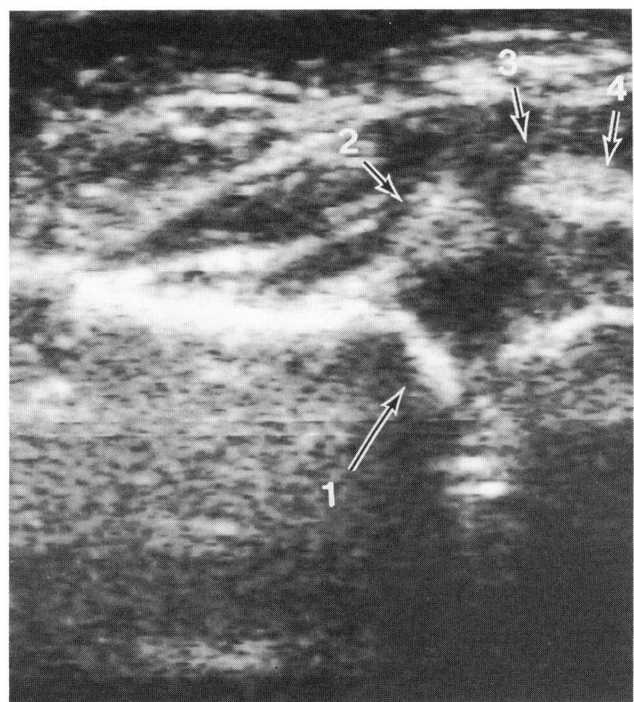

Figure 92–5. Congenital hip dysplasia. Coronal ultrasonography demonstrates a shallow, hypoplastic acetabulum (1) with the femoral head (2) subluxated posterolaterally and only partially covered by the dysplastic acetabulum. (3 = greater trochanter; 4 = femoral shaft).

rectus sheath are easily imaged. Abscesses can be differentiated from cellulitis, and localization for aspiration and drainage is relatively straightforward with ultrasonography.

Ultrasonography has other advantages: It uses non-ionizing energy, is noninvasive, has multiplanar ability, and allows real-time imaging. The equipment is readily available, relatively portable, and less expensive than many other cross-sectional imaging modalities such as CT and MRI.

There are disadvantages in addition to the inability to penetrate bone. Ultrasonography of the musculoskeletal system can be quite confusing because of the uneven topography of the skin and the resulting complex imaging planes. Although higher-frequency transducers afford better spatial resolution, these higher frequencies have a decreased depth of sound wave penetration resulting in poor visualization of deeper structures, particularly in the obese. Even at lower frequency, poor visualization of deeper structures may result from the higher natural reflectance of sound wave from the interposed adipose tissue.

ARTHROGRAPHY AND TENOGRAPHY

The soft tissues of the joints, including articular cartilage, are not well imaged with conventional plain film techniques. Although cartilage destruction can be inferred from joint space narrowing and effusions can be suggested directly or indirectly, these are only a rough estimate of pathology. Diarthrodial joints are surrounded by synovium and fibrous capsules. The joint "space" is actually only a potential space unless it is filled with fluid. Imaging of this space and its contents has been achieved by injecting iodinated contrast material, either alone or with air, to produce single- or double-contrast arthrograms, respectively. Arthrographic techniques have been described for every joint in the body. After obtaining informed consent, positioning is done fluoroscopically. A needle is inserted into the joint and any fluid present is drained; this can be sent for appropriate chemical, microscopic, or bacteriologic examination. Contrast is then introduced into the joint. Intra-articular epinephrine, used to delay absorption of the contrast, is to be avoided in the hypertensive individual. Rigid adherence to sterile technique should preclude infection, but inflammatory synovitis, particularly after wrist arthrography, is not uncommon but fortunately is self-limiting.

The views obtained following the injection of contrast depend on the joint injected and the clinical question. For instance, after a single-contrast injection into the radiocarpal joint, pre- and post-exercise films may be desired to evaluate the integrity of the triangular fibrocartilage complex as well as the radioulnar and proximal carpal ligamentous attachments (Fig. 92–6). If instability of the shoulder is in question, a double-contrast shoulder arthrogram is often combined with CT to evaluate the glenoid labrum (Fig. 92–7).

While MRI is used in evaluating the complex anatomy of many joints, arthrography still remains useful in the claustrophobic patient, in the patient who requires a joint aspiration as part of the diagnostic work-up, in the patient with possible complications related to a prosthesis, and in the patient who needs dynamic study of the joint as it is placed through a full range of motion. Commonly studied joints include the wrist, shoulder, hip, and ankle with the elbow and knee also studied occasionally. In addition to the applications listed above, arthrography can be used for evaluation of suspected ligamentous disruption following trauma, intra-articular cartilaginous and osseous loose bodies, presence and extent of synovial inflammation or soft-tissue masses and possible adhesive capsulitis. Prostheses can also be evaluated by injecting contrast material deep to the pseudocapsule that forms after such surgery. If the contrast passes between the methylmethacrylate and the bone or the prosthesis, this may be indicative of loosening.

Significant complications are rare but an occasional patient will have an idiosyncratic allergic reaction to the contrast. More commonly, the patient may experience a vasovagal reaction during the procedure and one should try to anticipate this when positioning the patient prior to the beginning of the examination.

Other periarticular structures can be studied after contrast injection. Tenography, achieved by injecting the synovial tendon sheaths, is used primarily about the wrist and ankle to locate areas of restriction to tendon motion. Damage to the peroneal tendon sheath can occur following calcaneal fracture and may be a cause of subsequent foot pain. Ganglions, most common in the wrist and ankle, are cystic structures usually in communication with the joint space; they may be imaged prior to removal by injecting the adjacent joint.

ANGIOGRAPHY

In the extremities, arteriography is used primarily in imaging the effects of atherosclerosis. It may serve as a road map for surgical intervention or percutaneous angioplasty. Arteriography is invaluable in the evaluation of vascular integrity after trauma, especially in the detection of arteriovenous malformation and aneurysms. Arteritis, small-vessel disease, and aseptic necrosis can be imaged angiographically, but these diagnoses are usually arrived at by other means. Although it may be helpful in the localization and characterization of soft-tissue and osseous tumors, CT and/or MRI can better achieve these functions. It may be used to demonstrate the vascular supply of a tumor unless it is "avascular" and can be detected only by its mass effect. Arteriovenous connections are best detected angiographically. With selective and superselective techniques, angiography can be used for embolization of some vascular malformations or large malignant lesions prior to surgery. Suspected aneurysms of the popliteal artery are as well or better studied with sonography.

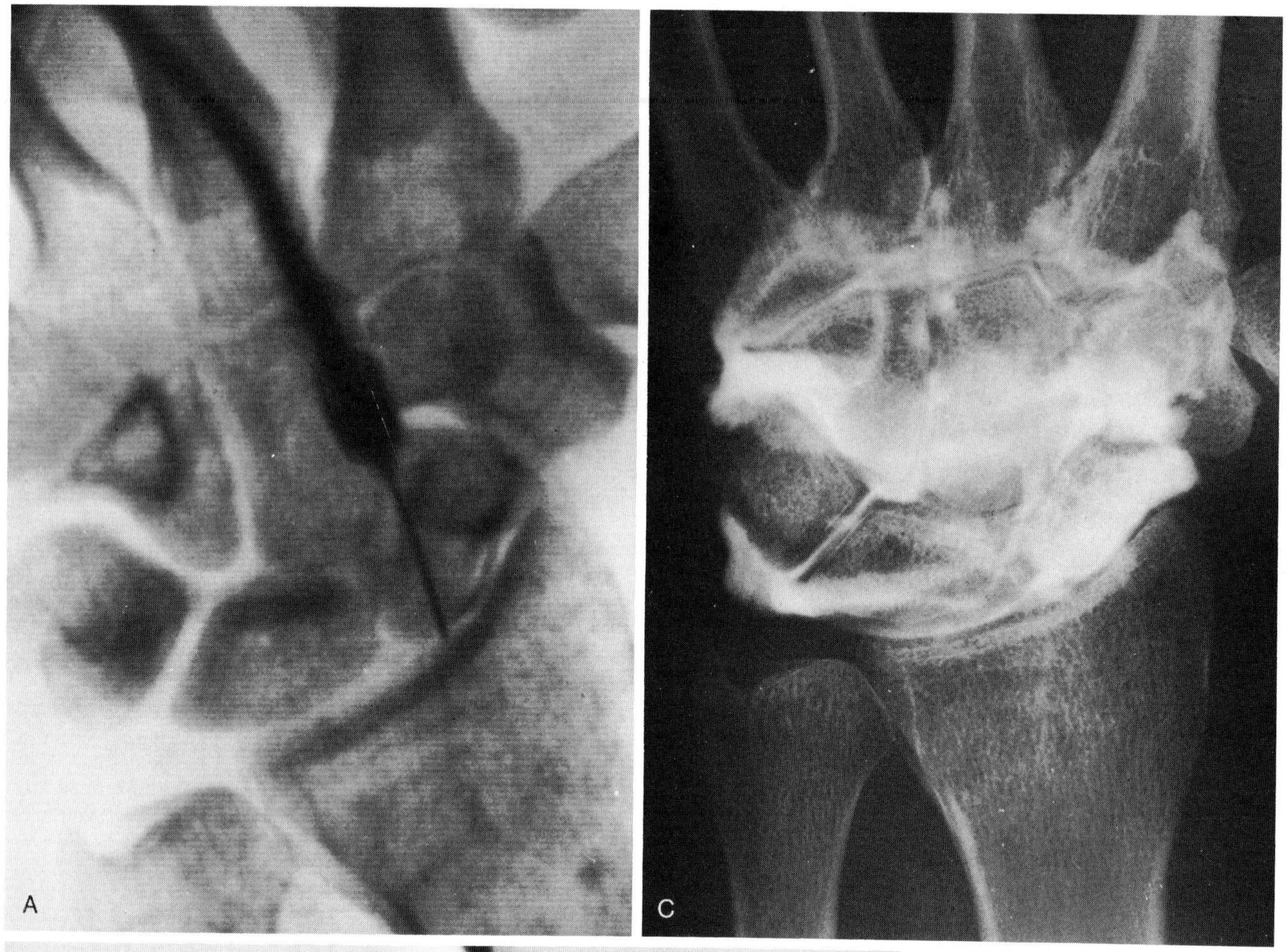

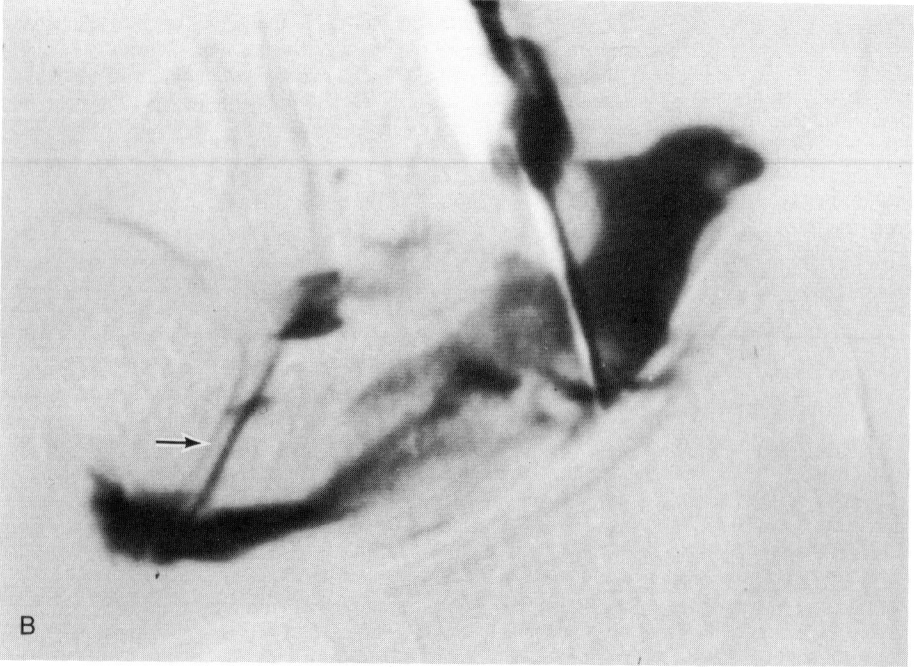

Figure 92–6. Wrist pain. *A,* Digital radiograph of the left wrist with needle positioned for contrast injection into the radiocarpal joint. *B,* Digital subtraction arthrography "subtracts" the osseous structures and overlying tubing allowing visualization of contrast flow into the midcarpal row via a lunate triquetral joint space *(arrow)*. *C,* Post-exercise plain film demonstrates contrast in the midcarpal row as well as the radiocarpal joint, confirming disruption of the lunate triquetral ligament.

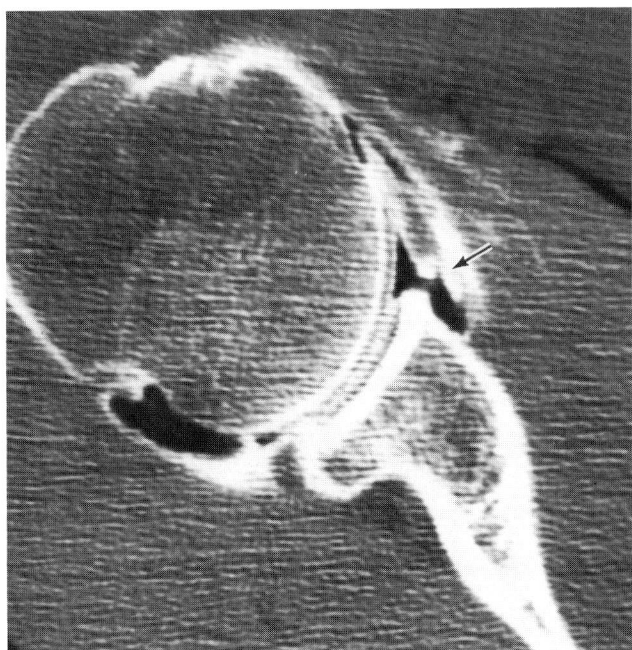

Figure 92–7. Shoulder injury. Axial CT, performed with right shoulder in external rotation after performing a double-contrast arthrogram, demonstrates separation of the anterior glenoid labrum from the glenoid itself *(arrow)*.

The amount of intra-arterial contrast and its concentration can be substantially decreased using digital fluoroscopy, which has greater contrast resolution. This permits the use of smaller catheters and hand injections, leading to better patient tolerance and fewer complications of hematoma or vascular spasm. The breathing, swallowing, and peristaltic motion that can limit high-quality intravenous angiograms in other parts of the body are not significant factors in the extremities.

RADIONUCLIDE IMAGING

The use of bone-seeking isotopes for imaging began with the use of strontium-85 in 1961. Since then, other agents with better biologic and physical properties for imaging at the lowest possible radiation exposure have come into use. Technetium-99m (^{99m}Tc) is an ideal isotope for imaging because of its half-life of six hours, inexpensive production from molybdenum generators, and ease of binding to organ-specific compounds. Its keV of 140 is excellent for gamma camera imaging. In the case of bone agents, a series of inorganic and organic phosphate compounds have come into use, each new compound offering a better bone-to-blood pool distribution.

Bone scintigraphy is an extremely sensitive but nonspecific means of imaging the entire skeleton rapidly and inexpensively. Within two hours after the intravenous injection of 15 mCi of a ^{99m}Tc phosphate bone imaging agent, an osseous survey can be obtained in approximately 30 to 40 minutes. Both the rate of bone turnover and the integrity of the blood supply to the bone determine the scintigraphic activity; the effect of the latter is probably of greater importance because if the labeled blood can't reach the area of interest, no uptake will occur. The addition of multiplanar imaging has improved the localization of increased or decreased scintigraphic activity. Single-photon emission computed tomography (SPECT) surpasses planar bone imaging in detecting lesions, especially in the low back and pelvis.

The most common use of the bone scan is to detect metastatic disease, frequently due to breast, prostate, lung, or renal carcinoma. Lymphoma, neuroblastoma, and multiple myeloma are also commonly evaluated with radionuclide scanning. Although bone scans are far more sensitive than radiographs for detecting bone lesions, some aggressive tumors, such as multiple myeloma and certain anaplastic carcinomas, may produce either no increased uptake or "cold" lesions. Even though a smaller percentage of multiple myeloma lesions are picked up by bone scan, it is still a larger number than may be identified on a radiographic skeletal survey and the two modalities should be used in a complementary fashion to identify bony abnormalities and anatomic areas of potential fracture (Fig. 92–8).

When bone disease, metastatic or metabolic, is extensive, a bone scan may present as a "superscan" with much more than the expected 50 per cent uptake in the bones and minimal soft-tissue activity as well as absent renal uptake. This is most commonly seen with breast or prostate metastases and in secondary hyperparathyroidism.

Scintigraphy may be used to follow bone metastases during therapy. However, dramatic improvement evidenced by less activity in bony metastatic disease may not mean the tumor cells have been ameliorated. Conversely, when treatment is withdrawn, there may be a transient "flare" of increased uptake on bone scan that may simply represent bone in a reparative state rather than worsening metastatic disease. Sensitivity is also problematic in surveys for metastatic disease in which mild arthritis, degenerative spine changes, old fractures, and recent trauma can all produce areas of increased radionuclide uptake. This is particularly common in the spine and ribs, which are also frequent sites of metastases.

Bone scanning is useful in the evaluation of primary bone neoplasms. Demonstration of the polyostotic or monostotic nature of a lesion will assist in developing an appropriate differential diagnosis and treatment plan. The appearance may, occasionally, support a particular diagnosis but scintigraphic appearance is not reliable for distinguishing a malignant lesion from a benign one, nor is it a good estimate of the full extent of the process.

Non-neoplastic conditions with multiple areas of increased uptake include Paget's disease of bone, fibrous dysplasia, multiple enchondromatosis, osteochondromatosis, and eosinophilic granuloma. Metabolic disorders affecting bone, such as hyperparathyroidism, vitamin D and C deficiencies, and hypervitaminosis A, may produce abnormal scans. Hypertrophic osteodystrophy can cause a distinct pattern of increased cortical uptake along the diaphyses of long bones, particularly in the lower extremities, and may be the first sign of a lung neoplasm. However, although this has been associated with lung neoplastic or inflammatory processes, it can also be seen (occasionally) with non-lung processes such as ulcerative colitis.

Another important diagnosis aided by bone scintigraphy is the early detection of acute osteomyelitis or the reactivation of its chronic form. The bone scan will usually demonstrate increased uptake within 24 hours, and plain film lags far behind in detecting abnormalities. (On rare occasion there can be decreased activity resulting from impairment of the blood supply to the affected area.) Imaging in three or four phases with ^{99m}Tc methylene diphosphonate (MDP) will increase the overall sensitivity and help to distinguish osteomyelitis from cellulitis, thus increasing the specificity as well. Septic joints and loosened or infected joint prostheses can be evaluated as well.

In multiphase bone scanning, the first phase is a series of images obtained over the area of interest immediately after injection of the imaging agent with filming every two seconds for 60 seconds and a static blood pool image taken at 60 seconds. The second phase is a static image at two to three hours after injection. A third static image at six to seven hours after injection constitutes the third phase, with an additional static image taken at the same time using a specific number of counts (e.g., 100 K). This low-count image

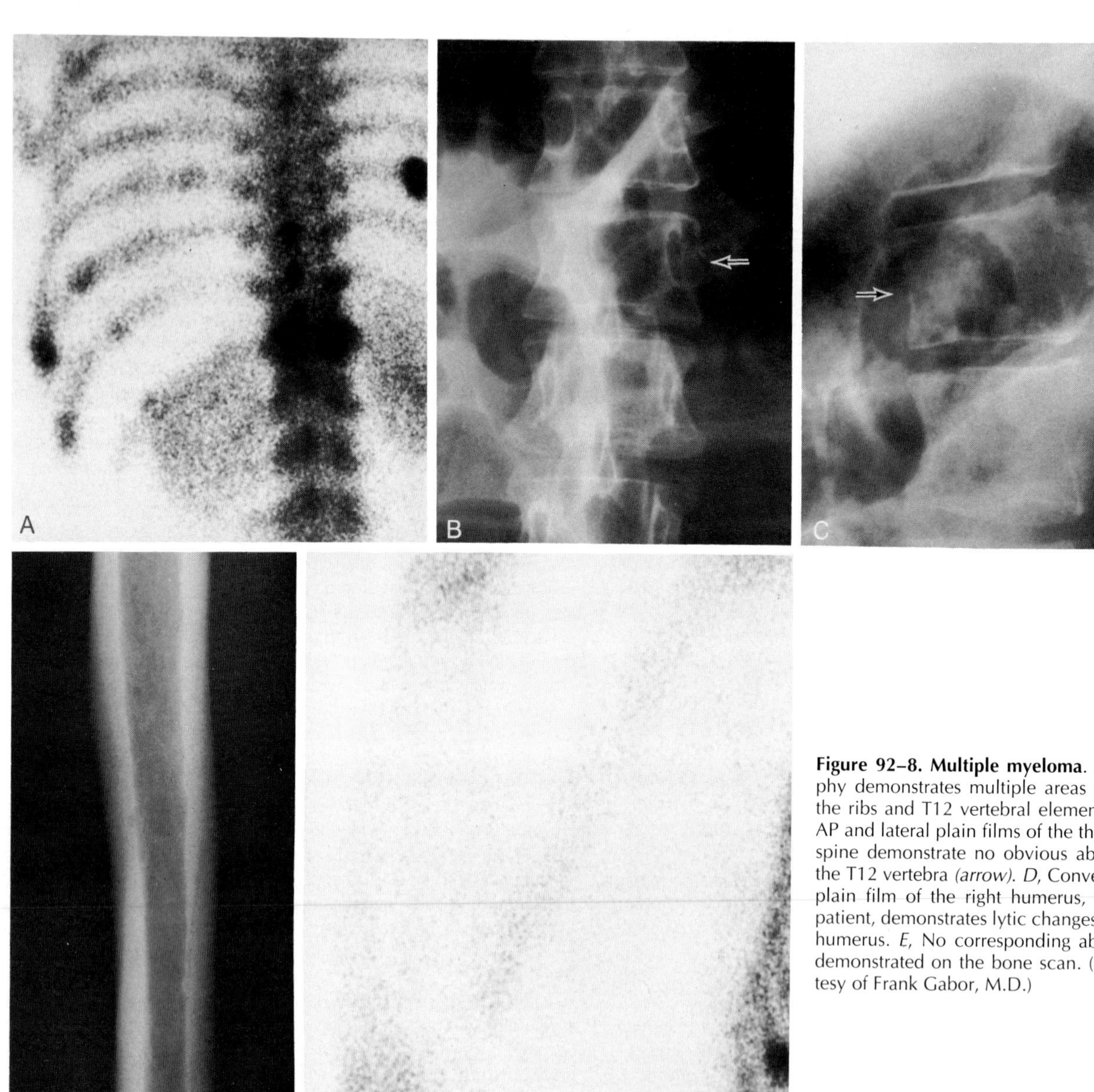

Figure 92–8. Multiple myeloma. *A,* Scintigraphy demonstrates multiple areas of uptake in the ribs and T12 vertebral elements. *B* and *C,* AP and lateral plain films of the thoracolumbar spine demonstrate no obvious abnormality of the T12 vertebra *(arrow). D,* Conversely, an AP plain film of the right humerus, in the same patient, demonstrates lytic changes in the distal humerus. *E,* No corresponding abnormality is demonstrated on the bone scan. (*A* to *E* courtesy of Frank Gabor, M.D.)

will be compared with a 24-hour static image of the same number of counts, which is the fourth phase. An inflammatory process, whether due to bone or soft-tissue infection, will result in increased blood flow to the affected area and increased activity on the angiographic phase of imaging. However, over time the soft-tissue activity will decrease (even in cellulitis), whereas uptake in the bone will increase in osteomyelitis, resulting in increased bone activity with minimal soft-tissue activity at 24 hours. Thus, multiphase bone scans can differentiate cellulitis from osteomyelitis.

Multiphase bone imaging may not always be diagnostic, and imaging with other agents such as gallium-67 can assist, particularly when used in combination with ^{99m}Tc. Gallium is a valuable means of identifying periepiphyseal infections in the pediatric population because these areas normally display tremendous uptake of technetium at the growth plates on routine bone scans. However, the use of indium-111–labeled leukocytes in combination with ^{99m}Tc has a greater overall sensitivity and specificity for osteomyelitis than any of these agents individually or in other combinations (Fig. 92–9). It should be noted that the sensitivity and specificity of any of these agents will vary with the location of the infection and its chronicity as well as patient factors such as age, renal function, and hydration status. These same agents can be used for monitoring response to therapy and are more sensitive in following changes than plain radiographs.

Trauma is usually well-evaluated with plain film. However, an incomplete fracture such as a toddler's fracture or a fracture in a certain location, such as in the tarsals, carpals, or proximal hip, may be difficult to identify. Stress fractures, either of insufficiency (a fracture resulting from a normal stress through an abnormal bone — e.g., the occult subcapital hip fracture in the elderly) or fatigue (a fracture from abnormal repetitive stresses on normal bone— e.g., the tibial stress fracture of the long-distance runner) may also be hidden. Scintigraphy is useful for identifying these occult fractures as well in screening for fractures of varying ages in the victim of suspected nonaccidental trauma if its limitations are recognized (e.g., completely healed fractures may not have increased uptake and metaphyseal/epiphyseal injury can be masked by the normal increased uptake of the epiphyseal growth plate).

Assessment of complications related to trauma such as avascular necrosis and fracture non-union is possible. Avascular necrosis, whether the result of trauma or other causes, such as steroid use, sickle cell anemia, or alcoholism, will vary in appearance depending on its acuity and may appear "cold" initially because of lack of blood flow and "hot" as microfractures and collapse occur with subsequent healing. In non-union of a fracture (failure of healing within six to eight months with radiographic evidence of sclerotic, rounded fracture ends), the degree of scintigraphic activity may guide clinical decisions about the use of electrical stimulation (e.g., the more activity present on bone scan, the more likely that fracture healing will be stimulated with electrical therapy).

Radionuclide bone scans are a sensitive and inexpensive means for screening skeletal abnormalities but suffer from poor specificity, low spatial resolution, and whole-body radiation with increased exposure to the pelvis as a result of the renal excretion of the radioisotope.

Advances in tracer chemistry have helped to produce a greater signal from the target organ, technologic improvements have produced sharper images, and tomographic techniques have allowed better spatial localization of abnormal area. Use of computers for acquisition and display has led to quantitation in some disorders. Bone turnover in metabolic diseases including osteoporosis has been studied using multicompartmental models of calcium metabolism and other methods for measuring bone mineralization using radionuclides include photon absorptiometry (^{125}I and ^{153}Gd) and in vivo neutron activation analysis to measure whole-body calcium.

MAGNETIC RESONANCE IMAGING

Magnetic resonance provides an excellent means of producing diagnostic images. Nuclear magnetic resonance spectroscopy has been an important tool in chemical analysis for more than 40 years, but it was not until the early 1970s that images were produced using this property. Although this is not the place for a detailed physics discussion, a basic description follows: Nuclei with odd numbers of

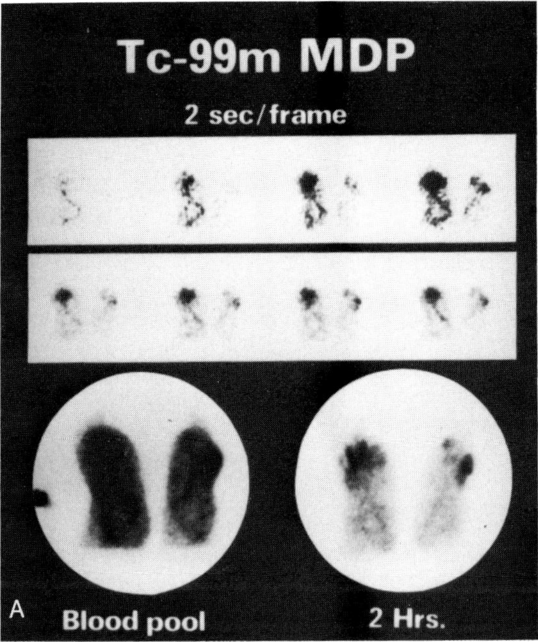

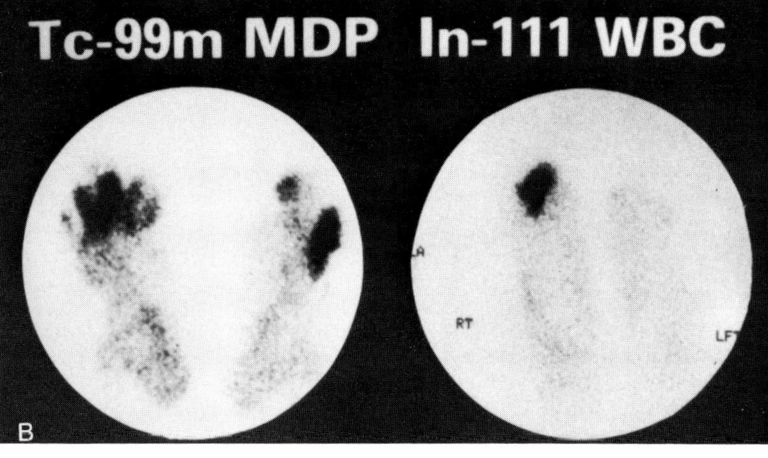

Figure 92–9. Cellulitis osteomyelitis. *A,* A patient with extensive peripheral vascular disease and prior bilateral transmetatarsal amputations presents with swelling and pain of the feet. Bone scan demonstrates uptake in bones and soft tissues of both feet (right greater than left) and angiogram phase, blood pool, and two-hour imaging. *B,* Twenty-four hour ^{99m}TC image shows increased uptake in the metatarsals bilaterally. Leukocyte scan (^{111}In), however, pinpoints a focus of osteomyelitis in the right mid-metatarsals only. (*A* and *B* courtesy of Frank Gabor, M.D., and Kathryn Morton, M.D.)

protons, such as hydrogen, sodium, phosphorus, and carbon, can be made to align as tiny magnetic dipoles in large magnetic fields. This alignment can be perturbed with radio pulses of particular frequencies determined by the strength of the static aligning field and an intrinsic property of the nucleus, its gyromagnetic ratio. Once perturbed, the nucleus will attempt to realign its axis with that of the static field by giving off the energy that it absorbed when knocked out of alignment. The released energy can be detected by an antenna and the rate of energy release is a function of the chemical environment of the nucleus. Images are formed by encoding the spatial position of the released signal using frequency and phase information. Most imaging to date has been of the hydrogen nucleus because of its relatively high concentration in tissues. This high concentration is important because MRI has an intrinsically low signal-to-noise ratio.

The exceptional contrast resolution obtained in MRI is due in part to the inherent differences in the tissue. Each contains a varying amount of hydrogen. Once the hydrogen is stimulated (perturbed), it returns to its resting state by releasing its excess energy. The time in which it does this is referred to as a "relaxation time." T_1 relaxation time is defined by the amount of time it takes nuclei to release energy to the adjacent environment (thus creating a signal), and T_2 relaxation time is defined by the amount of time it takes the nuclei to release their energy among themselves to return to their random resting state (again, creating a signal). These interactions are the basis for spin-echo imaging and its many variations. The "weighting" toward the T_1 or T_2 relaxation is determined by the TR (time to repetition — the interval between excitation pulses) and the TE (time to echo — measured from the excitation pulse to the peak of the detected echo from the released energy).

Signal strength depends upon concentration, rate of signal decay, and blood flow. Cortical bone has a very low concentration of hydrogen and has essentially no signal in proton imaging. This is of value in imaging the posterior fossa, in contrast to CT, in which artifacts caused by surrounding bone may be a problem. When the cortex is destroyed by tumor or other disorders, the soft tissue replacing the cortex is easily imaged by MRI. Trabecular bone, on the other hand, is a source of increased signal on proton images because bone marrow contains fat.

The magnetic field strength and style of acquisition are fixed for a given magnet. However, variables including radiofrequency (RF) coils, imaging planes, matrix size, section thickness and gap, pulse sequences, total number of sections, and field of view are set by the operator. One must be very careful about setting protocols, or even the largest lesions can actually be masked by the wrong pulse sequence, field of view, etc. On the other hand, the ability to change these variables allows excellent contrast resolution with or without contrast administration. Additionally, with software advancements, evaluation of blood flow with magnetic resonance angiography (MRA) may be possible. Although a number of inherent problems including direction and type of flow as well as tortuosity of vessels must be considered in determining a protocol and interpreting the resulting images, MRA may make other methods of angiographic evaluation and their attendant morbidity less necessary (Fig. 92–10).

As with CT, the MRI examination should be tailored to the patient's and clinician's needs and whenever possible should be performed with plain film findings for comparison and guidance. The key goal of imaging should be to demonstrate the full extent of the lesion and its relationship to the surrounding tissues. In general, an initial short duration pulse sequence should be performed in the plane perpendicular to the expected axis of the lesion. Attempts should be made to position the patient so that imaging is in one of the standard planes (sagittal, coronal, or axial), parallel to or perpendicular to the lesion. Use of surface coils allows for increased spatial resolution.

Tissue contrasts are controlled by pulse-sequence selection, and imaging should, generally, be performed with at least two different pulse sequences. Tissues containing fat (such as subcutaneous fat and fatty marrow) have increased signal on T_1-weighted imaging. Muscle and hyaline cartilage will have slightly less intense signal and ligaments, tendons, and mineralized bone will have little or no signal. Water-density fluid such as a joint effusion will have little signal. T_2-weighted images will make ligaments, tendons, and bone appear to have little signal. But water-density fluid will now have increased signal, with subcutaneous fat, fatty marrow, and muscle being less intense. Bone detail will be best demonstrated with proton density imaging.

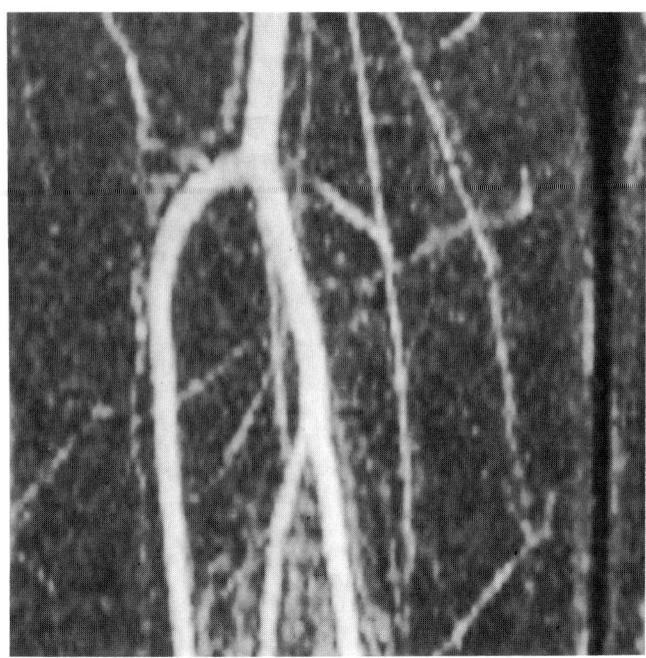

Figure 92–10. Normal trifurcation. Two-dimensional time-of-flight imaging of the right lower extremity exquisitely maps normal trifurcation vasculature.

Imaging of the various joints provides remarkable information about the integrity of the joint with its related ligaments, tendons, muscular attachments, and cartilage. It has essentially replaced arthrography in the examination of many joints, especially the knee (Fig. 92–11). With slight angulation of the knee, the cruciate ligaments can be well-illustrated (Fig. 92–12). The hip can easily be evaluated for avascular necrosis. Although there is a slight false-negative rate, this may still be the modality of choice after plain film to show the extent of a vascular abnormality and subsequent change in the femoral head.

Imaging of osseous and soft-tissue neoplasms is excellent with MRI. The multiplanar capabilities allow one to fully characterize the extent of the abnormality and define its relationship to adjacent structures such as the neurovascular bundle and adjacent joints, muscles, and bones. The image is exquisite but the appearance, unfortunately, is nonspecific and can be used only rarely to suggest histopathologic diagnosis. The most critical use for MRI in bone tumors is in staging the lesion, as further delineated in the chapter covering musculoskeletal tumors.

Bone marrow imaging can also be performed with MRI but abnormalities can only be identified if the normal evolution of marrow from infancy to adulthood is understood. Intramedullary extent of tumor or tumor replacement (such as in leukemia) may be demonstrated with carefully selected sequences that emphasize the difference between the tumor and adjacent normal marrow. Bone marrow edema from trauma can be demonstrated as can bone marrow ischemia (avascular necrosis as described above). However, bone marrow imaging is also nonspecific and may require needle aspiration/biopsy for full evaluation.

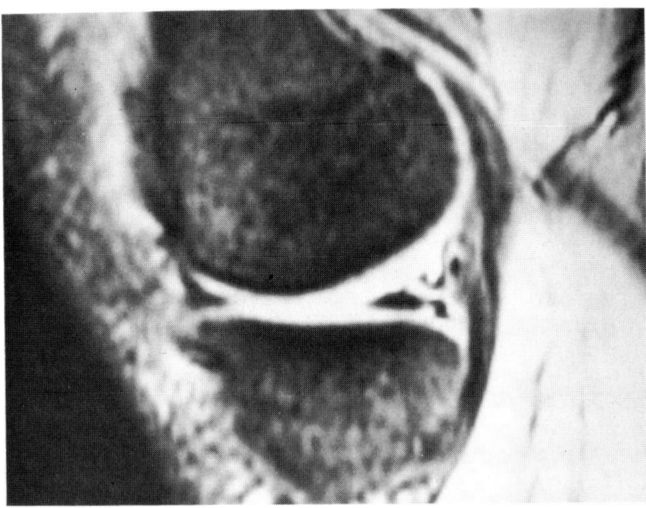

Figure 92–11. Skiing injury. Sagittal GRE MRI of the right knee demonstrates a complex tear of the posterior horn of the medial meniscus with irregularity along both superior and inferior surfaces as well as the obvious tear.

The presence of a metal object in the field will result in degradation of the image especially in the area immediately surrounding the metal. Potential difficulties related to metal include possible movement of the metal object, such as a wire or clip, or malfunction of the object, such as an electronic pacemaker. Although there is generally no contraindication for use of MRI with the patient with orthopedic hardware, patients with known cerebral aneurysm clips, pacemakers, or metal within the orbit are usually not imaged with MRI. Screening orbital CT or a Waters' view plain radiograph may serve as a screening mechanism for patients who report possible ocular exposure to metal without known complication.

At present, MRI offers several advantages over other modalities.

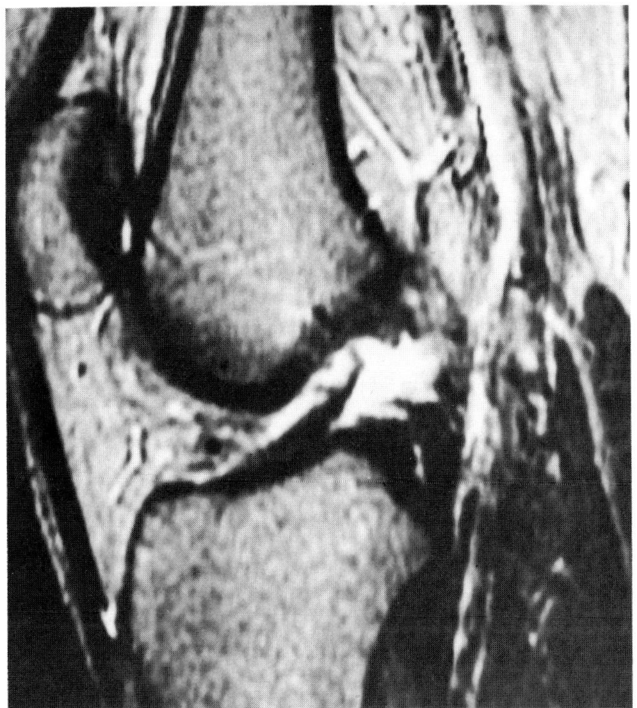

Figure 92–12. Knee pain. Sagittal GRE MRI of the left knee demonstrates discontinuity in the anterior cruciate ligament with fluid surrounding the retracted fibers.

The first is the lack of any known biologic hazard. Another advantage is the ability to maximize contrast differences by changing machine factors rather than by intravenous contrast injection with its attendant risks and discomfort. Injectable paramagnetic contrast agents, such as gadolinium compounds, which achieve their effect by altering the relaxation times of abnormal structures relative to normal ones, may be used for specific indications in musculoskeletal imaging.

Disadvantages in MRI include the expense of the equipment and the somewhat time-consuming nature of the examinations, although newer software is markedly shortening the time required to obtain a diagnostic examination. Motion can decrease spatial resolution considerably, and the long examination time makes repeat imaging burdensome. The lack of signal from cortical bone, periosteum, and soft-tissue calcifications can be a handicap in differential diagnosis as well.

QUANTITATIVE METHODS

Quantitative measurements of various image parameters are sometimes of value. These measurements must be approached with caution because there is invariably a technical reason for inaccuracy associated with each one. An understanding of these pitfalls is essential to accurate interpretation of the results of these measurements.

Quantitation in routine radiographic studies usually consists of the measurements of size or angle. Although the absolute dimension of a lesion is not of much diagnostic utility, the change from one study to the next is commonly questioned, especially during therapy. The growth of an osteochondroma after epiphyseal closure may indicate malignant degeneration. The determination of size may also be necessary for presurgical planning of joint replacement or other reconstructive methods. The major cause of inaccuracy in these measurements is magnification, which is an unavoidable artifact caused by beam spread. Magnification can be reduced by lengthening the tube-subject distance, and rulers with radiographically detectable markings can be placed in the field so that magnification will affect the marks in the same way as it affects the anatomic region in question. CT scanograms also provide accurate linear and angular measurement.

Angle measurements are frequently determined radiographically but are also prone to errors due to projection as well as magnification. One important point is that an angle can never be made artifactually acute by projection or positioning. For example, in the determination of the neck-shaft angle of the femur prior to corrective osteotomy, rotation of the hip can make this angle appear artifactually valgus, but never varus. Other common angle measurements are for scoliosis and genu valgum or varus deformities. Erect views are obtained to accurately reflect the physiologic state. Angle measurements are also necessary in other congenital and acquired deformities such as congenital hip and foot anomalies and hallux valgus. Again, in measuring foot deformities, weight-bearing views are a necessity to describe the abnormalities accurately. Fracture alignment is critical in some locations. Dorsal tilt of the articular surface of the distal radius may lead to hand dysfunction. Some calcaneal fractures are only detected by measuring the angle between the anterior and posterior superior surfaces (Boehler's angle).

Quantification of bone mineral density (BMD) has been approached in various methods over the years and has had mixed success. Single-photon absorptiometry uses a monoenergetic photon source (iodine-125) for evaluation of BMD but can be used only in the appendicular skeleton, such as the radius, and is not felt to accurately reflect bone loss in potential fracture sites. Dual-photon absorptiometry uses gadolinium-153, which emits photons at two different energy levels and can be used in the lumbar spine and proximal femur. However, this method includes both trabecular and cortical bone in its measurement and it may not accurately reflect true BMD, especially if there are adjacent osteophytes or vascular calcifications present resulting in overestimation of bone density. Quantitative computed tomography of the axial skeleton allows separation of trabecular from cortical bone. Although the single-energy CT has variable accuracy depending on the content of fat within the marrow spaces, dual-energy CT offers a more accurate determination. Measurements are performed with a mineral reference calibration and compared with age-matched normals. It requires a much higher radiation dose than absorptiometry, and sophisticated data processing is necessary to evaluate such structurally complex areas as the proximal femur. Anatomic factors that affect the accuracy of the other approaches contribute to problems with computed tomography methods as well. The normal amount of trabecular bone in the midportion of a vertebral body is extremely variable, owing to the unpredictable extent of basivertebral venous plexus. Compression fractures and microfractures are frequent complications of osteoporosis of the spine. Although they occur as a result of bone loss, these fractures stimulate callus formation; the compression of the remaining trabeculae into a smaller volume also increases the density of the bone, yielding false results with any quantitative volume measurement. Finally, dual-energy x-ray equipment now allows highly accurate measurement of BMD with a significantly lower radiation dose to the patient.

The digital format of CT allows various parameters such as organ or lesion size or attenuation to be determined. These numbers are readily available and are often displayed to multiple-decimal accuracy. Nevertheless, profound inaccuracies may be associated with these. In the seemingly straightforward measurements of linear distance, substantial errors can result from the choice of inappropriate window and level settings. Although a range of greater than 4000 Hounsfield units is generally used for storage of pixel values, only 16 levels of gray are actually displayed. The borders of an object generally encompass a wide range of numbers. The perceived border and, therefore, the measurable size of an object are a function of the window and level chosen for display. This will affect the measurement of length, perimeter, area, and volume. Additionally, the use of Hounsfield units in characterizing different tissues must be tempered with the knowledge that there can be significant variation in absolute numbers from scanner to scanner and even in various locations within the same patients.

The digital capability of CT is advantageous in identifying the depth and angular location of a lesion relative to the skin surface during percutaneous needle biopsy. CT can also be used in radiation treatment planning because location of ports and dosimetry can be calculated directly from the CT slices using special software.

Ultrasonography can be used to obtain dimensions or depths of structures either by comparison with a graticule on the screen or by direct measurement with digital cursors. These measurements are accurate so long as the machine has been correctly calibrated. The depth of an object is determined by the length of time to signal detection, which assumes uniform speed in all tissue. This assumption is incorrect in fat, which has a decreased speed of sound; tissue beyond an area of fat may be depicted as farther from the transducer than it actually is. Attempts have been made to quantitatively characterize tissue sonographically using various properties of reflected sound energy. These methods range from simple mapping of amplitudes to digital texture analysis and other pattern recognition techniques. There is hope that tissue specificity can be achieved, perhaps obviating the need for biopsy; however, as with other methods of quantitative imaging, results have been disappointing to date.

Radionuclide bone imaging can also be used to derive data rather than just images. The chief use in skeletal imaging lies in metabolic measurements of rates of mineralization as noted above. Unfortunately, the kinetics of bone radionuclides is not a trivial problem and requires a complex multicompartmental system for modeling.

Magnetic resonance, whether by imaging systems or those designed for spectroscopy, also offers some promise for quantitation leading to tissue characterization as well as measurement of metabolic activity. T_1 and T_2 relaxation times can be calculated using special imaging sequences, and some indication of tissue type can be made. However, there is significant overlap of these values among various normal and diseased tissues, thus limiting their usefulness to date. Work in the measurement of chemical shifts in muscle is encouraging, especially in evaluating diffuse disease such as muscular dystrophy, and in differentiating between neurologic and muscular disorders. This does not replace biopsy of tissue and confirmatory histopathology. Vascular flow evaluation with MRA is promising but is also limited at present as newer software is being developed that can deal with the complexities of various flow patterns encountered in vascular analysis.

Bibliography

Berquist TH: MRI of the Musculoskeletal System, 2nd ed. New York, Raven Press, 1990.

Curry TS, Dowdey JE, Murry RC: Christensen's Physics of Diagnostic Radiology, 4th ed. Philadelphia, Lea and Febiger, 1990.

Lee JKT, Sagel SS, Stanley RJ: Computed Body Tomography with MRI Correlation, 2nd ed. New York, Raven Press, 1989.

Manaster BJ (ed): Magnetic Resonance Imaging of Joints. Semin Ultrasound CT MRI 11(4), 1990.

Montana MA, Richardson ML (eds): Ultrasonography of the musculoskeletal system. Radiol Clin North Am 26(1), 1988.

Resnick D, Niwayama G: Diagnosis of Bone and Joint Disorders, 2nd ed. Philadelphia, WB Saunders Company, 1988.

Taylor A, Datz FL: Clinical Practice of Nuclear Medicine. New York, Churchill Livingstone, 1991.

93 Congenital and Developmental Anomalies

Andrew K. Poznanski

Congenital abnormalities of bone are relatively common and may occur through various means, including (1) *malformations*, in which there is an intrinsically abnormal developmental process (e.g., cleft lip or extra digits); (2) *deformation*, in which abnormalities are due to intrauterine changes such as mechanical compression or deviation (e.g., clubfoot, plagiocephaly, and abnormal sutural closure); and (3) *disruption*, which is due to the breakdown of an otherwise normal developmental process (e.g., aberrant tissue bands in the fingers, amputations of digits, or some brain anomalies such as porencephalic cysts). Any of these processes may be combined. Poor formation of tissues may produce a single malformation or a combination of malformations known as a malformation sequence. A single localized abnormality in early morphogenesis can cause secondary anomalies, which can then result in a pattern of multiple anomalies in later morphogenesis. Approximately 3 per cent of newborns have significant malformations; 1 per cent have multiple malformations.

TERMINOLOGY

The term *syndrome* refers to a combination of abnormalities that often occur together. There are various types of syndromes: (a) *dysmetabolic syndromes*, in which metabolic abnormality results in an anomaly of bone or a congenital malformation syndrome (e.g., the mucopolysaccharidoses such as Hurler's syndrome); (b) *dyshistogenic syndromes*, in which abnormal tissue is formed (e.g., Marfan's syndrome or achondroplasia); (c) *general malformation syndromes*, in which a constellation of anomalies seem to occur together (e.g., Rubinstein-Taybi syndrome); and (d) *deformation syndromes* due to a variety of intrauterine factors (e.g., amniotic band syndrome).

THE IMPORTANCE OF A CORRECT DIAGNOSIS

The study of the congenital malformation syndromes is somewhat complicated because of the large number of entities that have been described. As a result, many radiologists and other physicians are discouraged. In addition, some feel that these conditions are too rare, too hard to remember, or not worth diagnosing because nothing can be done about them. They may also believe that it is better to identify these disorders with other methods, such as chromosome or enzyme studies. However, these thoughts are incorrect. The congenital disorders are not as rare as many other disorders that are studied with great diligence. For example, the incidence of bone tumors is approximately 20 per million and that of malignant bone tumors is only 5.6 per million. On the other hand, the incidence of congenital malformations with multiple malformations is approximately 7,000 per million.

It is true that many of these malformation syndromes are too difficult to remember. However, there are now many reference books available, and even expert radiologists who deal with these conditions daily find it necessary to use a variety of books to identify some syndromes. It is important to diagnose these conditions for various reasons. First, making the correct diagnosis is essential in determining prognosis. If a newborn has a form of short-limbed dwarfism, it is very important to be able to correctly differentiate achondroplasia from other forms of dwarfism such as thanatophoric dwarfism, which is usually fatal at birth, or homozygous achondroplasia, which is usually fatal in several years. The differentiation of these entities can be securely made only on radiologic grounds. A correct diagnosis can be very important in deciding how to treat the patient. Achondroplastic dwarfs usually have a normal life span and, although they are short, they usually have relatively few medical problems. On the other hand, thanatophoric dwarfism, which at one time was confused with achondroplasia, is usually fatal at birth or shortly thereafter. Thus, if a neonate with achondroplasia suffers a potentially life-threatening experience, vigorous attempts should be made to keep the child alive because this infant has a good prognosis. In contrast, these efforts would be futile in attempting to treat a thanatophoric dwarf.

The correct diagnosis is also essential in directing the clinician to look for the presence of associated malformations. In chondroectodermal dysplasia, congenital heart disease is relatively common, whereas it is not common in achondroplasia. In spondyloepiphyseal dysplasia congenita there is a high incidence of myopia with retinal detachment; therefore, these infants and children should be carefully followed with ophthalmologic examinations to identify early retinal detachment. One of the forms of metaphyseal chondrodysplasia is associated with immunity problems; thus, the parents must be advised about the risk of vaccination and exposure to other children with viral infections. The correct diagnosis is also essential in genetic counseling. If two normal parents have an achondroplastic baby, they will have an almost negligible chance of having another such baby because achondroplasia, when inherited, is an autosomal dominant. On the other hand, if the baby has diastrophic dwarfism, which is inherited as an autosomal recessive, they have a 25 per cent chance of producing another such infant.

Although some of the forms of congenital malformation, such as the mucopolysaccharidoses, can be diagnosed by enzyme studies, most cannot. Even in those conditions in which the diagnosis can be based on chromosomal or enzyme studies, the radiologic examination is extremely useful because positive radiographic findings often stimulate the clinician to obtain the proper biochemical test.

TRIANGULATION IN THE EVALUATION OF CONGENITAL MALFORMATION SYNDROMES

Because of the complexity and presence of many different anomalies, the approach to the congenital malformation syndromes should include an attempt to simplify, to identify the major findings, to determine the extent and pattern of abnormality, and then to triangulate these findings using standard texts and various gamuts of anomalies. In order to be able to discover anomalies, of course, it is essential to have a good understanding of the normal anatomy and normal variations of bones in children.

Triangulation involves comparing lists of disorders having the same radiologic findings to determine which disorder is present in several gamuts. The following examples illustrate the method: Figure 93–1 is a radiograph of a girl who has congenital heart disease and an abnormal hand with a finger-like thumb, as well as abnormal carpals with extra carpal bones. Using the gamuts that list conditions having a triphalangeal thumb (Table 93–1) and conditions associated with accessory carpal ossicles (Table 93–2), it is evident that both of these findings are present only in the Holt-Oram syndrome. One can then more closely look at the other clinical findings to see if the diagnosis fits; this child did have a left-to-right cardiac shunt, which is also part of the Holt-Oram syndrome. Another example of the use of triangulation is illustrated in Figure 93–2, which shows the hand of a child with multiple carpal bones that appear to be arranged in an unusual pattern. This youngster also had a history of multiple dislocations, including dislocated hips. Looking at the list of malformations associated with accessory ossicles (see Table 93–2) and the list of conditions with multiple dislocations (Table 93–3), one can find by triangulation that both lists intersect at Larsen syndrome, which is indeed what this youngster had. These conditions are further discussed under the specific congenital malformation syndromes. The solution is not always so simple; sometimes several lists of gamuts have to be consulted to narrow the differential diagnosis. The gamuts can consist of radiographic or clinical signs. A good source of clinical gamuts is in *Smith's Recognizable Patterns of Human Malformation.* Radiologic gamuts can be found in Taybi and Lachman's *Radiology of Syndromes* and those in the hand in Poznanski's *The Hand in Radiologic Diagnosis.* Recently, a computer program has become available that facilitates diagnosis (OSSUM).

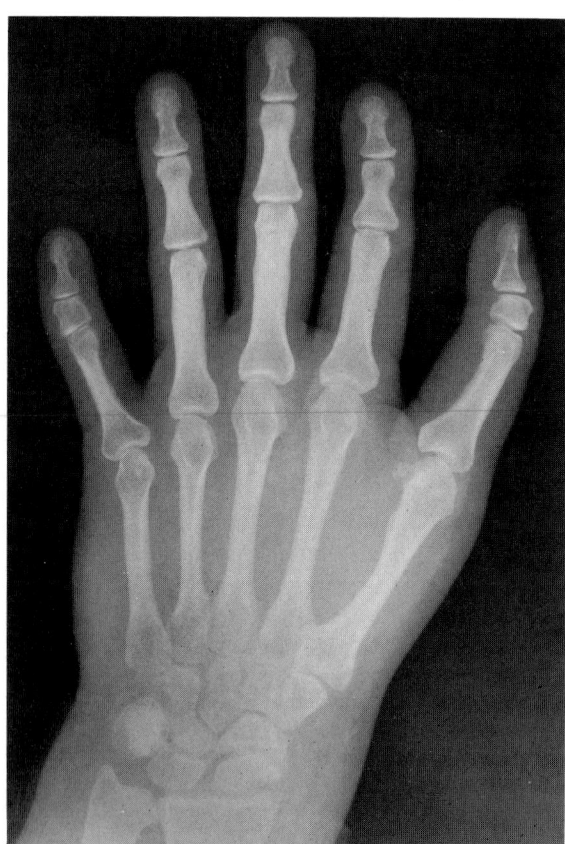

Figure 93–1. Triphalangeal thumbs and extra carpal bones (Holt-Oram syndrome). Left hand of a teenage girl with congenital heart disease and finger-like thumbs. The thumb has a finger-like appearance and has an extra phalanx; normally the thumb has only two phalanges. There are two additional carpals present, one between the scaphoid and the trapezium and one in the central part of the wrist (os centrale).

TABLE 93–1. SYNDROMES AND OTHER ANOMALIES ASSOCIATED WITH TRIPHALANGEAL THUMB

Syndromes
Blackfan-Diamond anemia
Cardiomelic (Holt-Oram)
Duane
Fetal thalidomide
Goodman's
IVIC
Juberg-Haywood
LADD (lacrimo-auriculo-deuto-digital)
Townes'
Trisomy 13 (occasionally)
Other Associated Anomalies
Absent pectoral muscle
Absent tibia
Deafness
Duplication of great toe
Imperforate anus, deafness
Lobster claw hand
Onychodystrophy
Preaxial polydactyly
Polydactyly, fifth toe

From Poznanski AK: The Hand in Radiologic Diagnosis, 2nd ed. Philadelphia, WB Saunders Company, 1984, p 264.

In many congenital disorders and particularly in the bone dysplasias, radiologic examination is usually essential; however, the diagnosis should not be made on radiologic grounds alone. One has to correlate radiologic findings with the history and other clinical information, including the size of the individual. Another important point is that not all of the findings are necessarily present in each case. It is possible to have a syndrome without having one or two of its major findings: a three-legged dog is still a dog! In general, evaluation of congenital malformation syndromes requires a thorough review of the clinical history and findings, as well as a total skeletal survey. Although in many of these disorders, one or two bones may have a classic appearance, often that is not enough to be certain of the diagnosis. From the standpoint of remembering the conditions, however, it is useful to know the most important and characteristic radiographic features associated with the various disorders.

TABLE 93–2. MALFORMATION SYNDROMES ASSOCIATED WITH ACCESSORY CARPAL OSSICLES

Distal Row
Arthro-ophthalmopathy
Brachydactyly A-1
Diastrophic dysplasia
Ellis–van Creveld
Larsen
Otopalatodigital
Os Centrale—Remnants of Central Row
Gorlin-Schlorf-Paparella
Hand-foot-genital
Hollister-Hollister
Holt-Oram
Larsen
Otopalatodigital
Other
Grebe's
Larsen
Oto-spondylo-megaepiphyseal
Ulnar dimelia

From Poznanski AK: The Hand in Radiologic Diagnosis, 2nd ed. Philadelphia, WB Saunders Company, 1984, p 198.

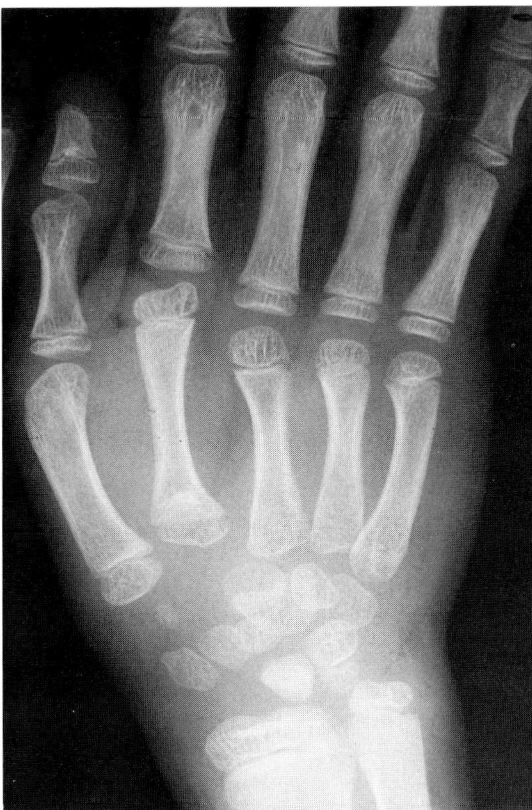

Figure 93–2. Extra carpal bones and dislocations (Larsen syndrome). Right hand and wrist of a child with a history of many dislocations. The carpal bones are very atypical in shape, and more than the normal number are present. They appear scattered rather than being in their normal position. There is shortening of the distal phalanx of the thumb, and there is widening of the distal portion of the proximal phalanges. The metacarpals are short, particularly the third and fourth. The distal phalanx of the thumb is short, and the distal ends of the proximal phalanges are broad.

DIAGNOSTIC FEATURES

In evaluating a bone dysplasia, one must look at a variety of factors (Table 93–4). The relative length and shape of each bone must be assessed. Alterations at the growth plate and in the epiphysis and metaphysis are extremely important in the characterization of the various abnormalities. Many of these radiographic findings disappear in the adult, making the diagnosis more difficult. Similarly, in the neonate, diagnosis of disorders affecting the epiphyses may be difficult because very few are ossified.

TABLE 93–3. SYNDROMES WITH JOINT DISLOCATION

Frequent in
- Beals auriculo-osteodysplasia syndrome (hip)
- Coffin-Siris syndrome (elbow)
- Distal arthrogryposis syndrome (hip)
- Fetal hydantoin effects (hip)
- Hajdu-Cheney syndrome
- Langer-Giedion syndrome
- Larsen's syndrome (elbow, knee, hip)
- Léri-Weill dyschondrosteosis (wrist, elbow)
- Otopalatodigital syndrome type I (elbow, hip)
- Otopalatodigital syndrome type II (elbow, knee)
- Stickler syndrome (hip)
- Trisomy 9 mosaic syndrome (hip, knee, elbow)
- XO syndrome (hip)

From Jones KL: Smith's Recognizable Patterns of Human Malformation, 4th ed. Philadelphia, WB Saunders Company, 1988, p 747.

TABLE 93–4. DIAGNOSTIC FEATURES OF CONGENITAL ANOMALIES

- Bone length
- Appearance of the bone
  - Epiphysis: size, shape, regularity
  - Metaphysis: good modeling, splaying, regularity
  - Diaphysis: diameter, cortical thickness, straight/bowed
  - Growth plate: width, regularity, premature closure
- Bone density
- Lucent lesions within the bones
- Spinal involvement
- Number of digits
- Fusion of bones
- Symmetry of abnormality
- Skeletal maturation
- Age of onset
- Pattern of anomalies

In assessing the density of the bones, one must be aware of the exposure factors that were used to obtain the radiograph. A high-kV technique can make the bones look more lucent than they are; a low-kV technique will make them look more dense. In addition, bone density may appear decreased if single-emulsion high-detail films are used as is common in the hands and feet. Lucent defects within the bones can be circumscribed or patchy. Identification of spinal abnormalities can be helpful. There is a major subgroup of bone anomalies that is associated with flat vertebrae. Not only does this finding help differentiate this subgroup from the others; it is also important because individuals with flattening of the vertebrae have a higher incidence of subluxation at the atlantoaxial area and they should be watched more carefully for possible dislocations, particularly if undergoing anesthesia or participating in active sports.

Symmetrical anomalies such as polydactyly or absence of digits are usually associated with a familial type of inheritance, whereas unilateral changes are more likely to be sporadic and not part of a major syndrome. This generalization has exceptions but is correct most of the time. Fusions of various bones may also be diagnostic in certain conditions. Carpal or tarsal fusion may occur as a sporadic anomaly or may be syndrome-associated. In otherwise normal individuals, carpal fusions usually involve bones in the same carpal row (Fig. 93–3). Fusions between carpals of the proximal row and ones in the distal row are almost invariably associated with a congenital malformation syndrome (Fig. 93–4). Fusions in congenital malformation syndromes, however, may involve carpals in the same row. In the foot, the syndrome-associated fusions involve the distal portion of the forefoot, including the cuneiforms, navicular, and cuboid, which may be fused to one another or to the metatarsals (Fig. 93–5). This type of fusion almost never occurs as an isolated abnormality. Fusion of the more proximal tarsals, such as the calcaneus and navicular, is more often isolated and not syndrome-associated, but it may be seen in the syndromes as well.

In a majority of syndromes skeletal maturation is delayed, so it is of little diagnostic value. However, in those conditions in which skeletal maturation is advanced, it can be an important clue to the diagnosis. Also, certain patterns of maturation are important. In cerebral gigantism, the relative advancement of maturation of the phalanges when compared with the carpals is helpful in the diagnosis of this condition; this syndrome is associated with mental retardation. Other rare syndromes associated with advanced skeletal maturation include the Marshall syndrome, in which there is advancement of skeletal maturation in infancy. In dealing with bone dysplasias, one can also separate them into those that are seen in

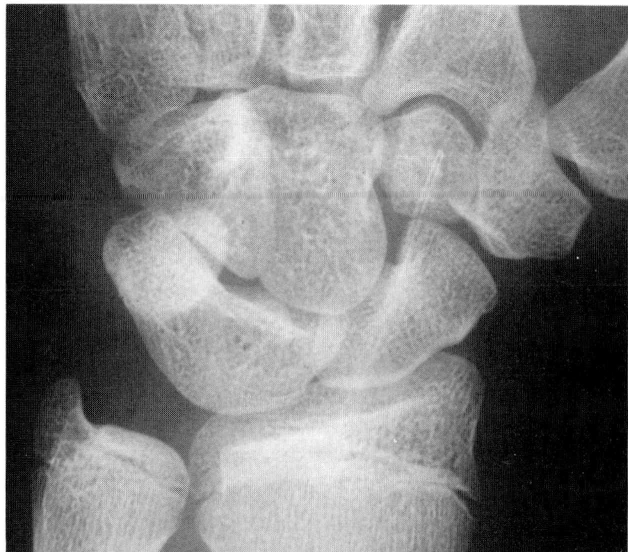

Figure 93–3. Carpal fusion involving carpals in the same row. The left wrist of a normal individual has a triquetral-lunate fusion. This fusion is common, particularly in blacks, in whom it occurs in 1.6 per cent of individuals.

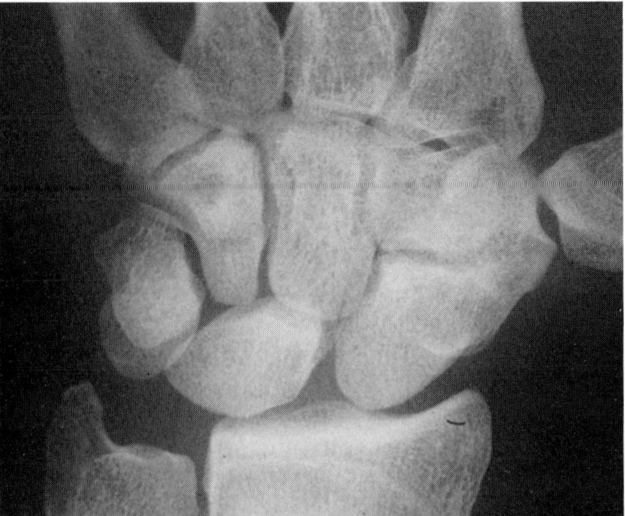

Figure 93–4. Syndrome-associated carpal fusion. The left wrist of a patient with the otopalatodigital syndrome has a fusion of the scaphoid and trapezium. This fusion involves carpals in the proximal and distal rows. Presence of a fusion going across rows is indicative of a congenital malformation syndrome.

early infancy and those that are noted in later life. In this fashion one can separate pseudoachondroplasia from true achondroplasia.

Many of the malformations are themselves nonspecific. However, when associated with other anomalies, they suggest a diagnosis. Clubfoot can be seen as an isolated abnormality, or it may be seen in a variety of syndromes including chromosomal abnormalities such as trisomy 18 or the sequence-associated meningomyeloceles or familial syndromes such as the whistling face syndrome. By considering the pattern, one can make the correct diagnosis.

NOMENCLATURE OF THE BONE ABNORMALITIES

In the subsequent parts of this chapter on congenital and developmental anomalies, the various disorders will be considered using the general categories adopted by the Committee for the International Nomenclature of Constitutional Diseases of Bone (Table 93–5). The problem with many of these bone conditions and syndromes is that various names have been used to describe them. The International Conference Nomenclature has been adopted to try to minimize this problem. Only a few of the entities in the list can be described in this chapter. The majority of entities discussed have been chosen because they have important radiologic manifestations; the description of findings in each of the disorders has been limited to the most important features. For greater detail, the reader is referred to the reference texts listed in the bibliography.

OSTEOCHONDRODYSPLASIA

Defects of Growth of Tubular Bones and/or Spine

The following entities are identifiable at birth and are usually lethal shortly before or following birth.

ACHONDROGENESIS. This is a fatal form of neonatal dwarfism. At least two types are now recognized. The head is very large, the extremities are small, and the trunk is markedly diminished in size. The condition probably has an autosomal recessive inheritance. The most characteristic finding in achondrogenesis is in the spine, where there is almost complete absence of ossification of the vertebral bodies (Fig. 93–6). There is also lack of sacral ossification, and the iliac bones are very small. All of the long bones are markedly shortened, particularly in type I achondrogenesis and less so in type II. There is often cupping at the ends of the bone, which is most marked in type II. The skull is poorly ossified, particularly in type I.

THANATOPHORIC DYSPLASIA. The name thanatophoric means "death dealing." This is a condition that was initially confused with achondroplasia; however, it is a completely different

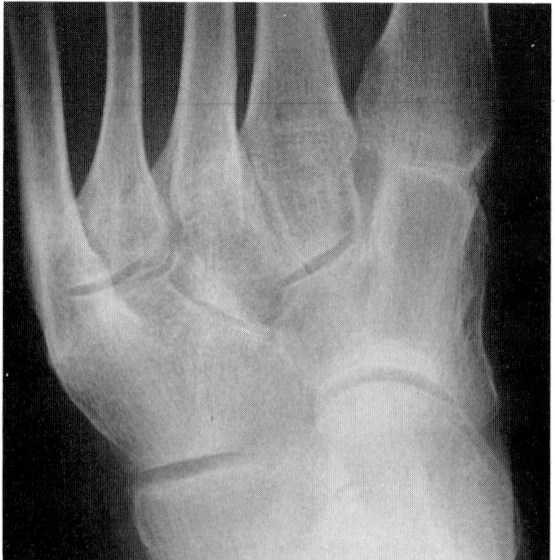

Figure 93–5. Syndrome-associated tarsal fusion. The left foot of a patient with the otopalatodigital syndrome. Some of the distal tarsals are fused to one another as well as to the metatarsals. Cuneiforms and cuboid are all involved. This type of fusion involving the distal portion of the forefoot is not seen in normal individuals and is indicative of a syndrome.

TABLE 93–5. INTERNATIONAL NOMENCLATURE OF CONSTITUTIONAL DISEASES OF BONE (1992)

Osteochondrodysplasias	Inheritance
Defects of the Tubular (and Flat) Bones and/or Axial Skeleton	
1. Achondroplasia group	
Thanatophoric dysplasia	AD
Thanatophoric dysplasia-straight femur/cloverleaf skull type	AD
Achondroplasia	AD
Hypochondroplasia	AD
2. Achondrogenesis	
Type IA	AR
Type B	AR
3. Spondylodysplastic group (Perinatally lethal)	
San Diego type	Sp
Torrance type	Sp
Luton type	Sp
4. Metatropic dysplasia group	
Fibrochondrogenesis	AR
Schneckenbecken dysplasia	AR
Metatropic dysplasia	AD
5. Short rib dysplasia group (with/without polydactyly)	
SR(P) Type I Saldino Noonan	AR
SR(P) Type II Majewski	AR
SR(P) Type III Verma-Naumoff	AR
SR(P) Type IV Beemer-Langer	AR
Asphyxiating thoracic dysplasia	AR
Ellis-van Creveld dysplasia	AR
6. Atelosteogenesis/Diastrophic dysplasia group	
Boomerang dysplasia	Sp
Atelosteogenesis type 1	Sp
Atelosteogenesis type 2 (de la Chapelle)	AR
Omodysplasia I (Maroteaux)	AD
Omodysplasia II (Borochowitz)	AR
Oto-palato-digital syndrome type 2	XLR
Diastrophic dysplasia	AR
Pseudodiastrophic dysplasia	AR
7. Kniest-Stickler dysplasia group	
Dyssegmental dysplasia—Silverman Handmaker type	AR
Dyssegmental dysplasia—Rolland-Desbuquois type	AR
Kniest dysplasia	AD
Oto-spondylo-megaepiphyseal dysplasia	AR
Stickler dysplasia (heterogeneous, some not linked to Cole CoL2A)	AD
8. Spondyloepiphyseal dysplasia congenita group	
Langer-Saldino Dysplasia (Achondrogenesis type II)	AD
Hypochondrogenesis	AD
Spondyloepiphyseal dysplasia congenita	AD
9. Other spondylo epi-(meta)-physeal dysplasias	
X-linked spondyloepiphyseal dysplasia tarda	XLD
Other late onset spondyloepi-(meta)-physeal dysplasias (i.e., Namaqualand d., Irapa d.)	
Progressive pseudorheumatoid dysplasia	AR
Dyggye-Melchior-Clausen dysplasia	AR
Wolcott-Rallison dysplasia	AR
Immunoosseous dysplasia	AR
Pseudachondroplasia	AD
Opsismodysplasia	AR
10. Dysostosis multiplex group	
Mucopolysaccharidosis I-H	AR
Mucopolysaccharidosis I-S	AR
Mucopolysaccharidosis II	XLR
Mucopolysaccharidosis III-A	AR
III-B	AR
III-C	AR
III-D	AR
Mucopolysaccharidosis IV-A	AR
Mucopolysaccharidosis IV-B	AR
Mucopolysaccharidosis VI	AR
Mucopolysaccharidosis VII	AR
Fucosidosis	AR
α-Mannosidosis	AR
β-Mannosidosis	AR
Aspartylglucosaminuria	AR
g_{M1} Gangliosidosis, several forms	AR
Sialidosis, several forms	AR

Table continued on following page

TABLE 93–5. INTERNATIONAL NOMENCLATURE OF CONSTITUTIONAL DISEASES OF BONE (1992) *Continued*

Osteochondrodysplasias	Inheritance
Sialic storage disease	AR
Galactosialidosis, several forms	AR
Mucosulfatidosis	AR
Mucolipidosis II	AR
Mucolipidosis III	AR
Mucolipidosis IV	AR
11. Spondylometaphyseal dysplasias	
Spondylometaphyseal dysplasia—Kozlowski type	AD
Spondylometaphyseal dysplasia—corner fracture type (Sutcliffe)	AD
Spondyloenchondrodysplasia	AR
12. Epiphyseal dysplasias	
Multiple epiphyseal dysplasia—Fairbanks/Ribbing	AD
13. Chondrodysplasia punctata (Stippled epiphyses) group	
Rhizomelic type	AR
Conradi-Hünermann type	XLD
X-linked recessive type	XLR
MT-type	Sp
Others including CHILD syndrome; Zellweger syndrome; Warfarin embryopathy, Chromosomal abnormalities; Fetal alcohol syndrome	
14. Metaphyseal dysplasias	
Jansen type	AD
Schmid type	AD
Spahr type	AR
McKusick type (CHH)	AR
Metaphyseal anadysplasia	XLR?
Shwachmann type	AR
Adenosine deaminase deficiency	AR
15. Brachyrachia (Short spine dysplasia)	
Brachyolmia, several types	
16. Mesomelic dysplasias	
Dyschondrosteosis	AD
Langer type	AR
Nievergelt type	AD
Robinow type	AD
17. Acro/acro-mesomelic dysplasias	
Acromicric dysplasia	Sp
Geleophysic dysplasia	AR
Acrodysostosis	AD
Tricho-rhino-phalangeal dysplasia type 1	AD
Tricho-rhino-phalangeal dysplasia type 2	AD
Saldino-Mainzer dysplasia	AR
Pseudohypoparathyroidism several types	AD AR? XLD?
Cranioectodermal dysplasia	AR
Acromesomelic dysplasia	AR
Grebe dysplasia	AR
18. Dysplasias with significant (but not exclusive) membraneous bone involvement	
Cleidocranial dysplasia	AD
Osteodysplasty, Melnick-Needles	XLD
19. Bent bone dysplasia group	
Campomelic dysplasia	AR
Kyphomelic dysplasia	AR
Stüve-Wiedemann dysplasia	AR
20. Multiple dislocations with dysplasias	
Larsen syndrome	AD
Desbuquois syndrome	AR
Spondylo-epi-metaphyseal dysplasia with joint laxity	AR
21. Osteodysplastic primordial dwarfism group	
Type 1	AR
Type 2	AR
22. Dysplasias with decreased bone density	
Osteogenesis-Imperfecta (several types)	AD AD AR
Osteoporosis with pseudoglioma	AR
Idiopathic juvenile osteoporosis	Sp
Bruck syndrome	AR
Homocystinuria	AR
Singleton-Merten syndrome	Sp
Geroderma osteodysplastica	AR
Menkes syndrome	XLR

TABLE 93–5. INTERNATIONAL NOMENCLATURE OF CONSTITUTIONAL DISEASES OF BONE (1992) *Continued*

Osteochondrodysplasias	Inheritance
23. Dysplasias with defective mineralization	
Hypophosphatasia	AD
Hypophosphatemic rickets	XR
Pseudodeficiency rickets, several types	AR
Neonatal hyperparathyroidism	AR
24. Dysplasias with increased bone density	
Osteopetrosis	
a) precocious type	AR
b) delayed type	AD
c) intermediate type	AR
d) with renal tubular acidosis	AR
Dysosteosclerosis	AR
Pyknodysostosis	AR
Osteosclerosis—Stanescu type	AD
Axial osteosclerosis including	
a) Osteomesopyenosis	AD
b) with bamboo hair (Netherton Syndrome)	AR
c) Tricho-thiodystrophy	AR
Osteopoikilosis	AD
Melorheostosis	Sp
Osteopathia striata	Sp
Osteopathia striata with cranial sclerosis	AD
Diaphyseal dysplasia—Camurati-Engelmann	AD
Craniodiaphyseal dysplasia	AD
	AR
Lenz-Majewski dysplasia	Sp
Craniometadiaphyseal dysplasia	Sp
Endosteal hyperostoses	
a) van Buchem disease	AR
b) Sclerosteosis	AR
c) Worth disease	AD
d) with cerebellar hypoplasia	AR
Pachydermoperiostosis	AD
Fronto-metaphyseal dysplasia	XLR
Craniometaphyseal dysplasia	
a) severe type	AR
b) mild type	AD
Pyle (disease) dysplasia	AR
Osteoectasia with hyperphosphatasia	AR
Oculo-dento-osseous dysplasia	
a) severe type	AR
b) mild type	AD
Familial infantile cortical hyperostosis—Caffey	AD
Disorganized Development of Cartilaginous and Fibrous Components of the Skeleton	
Dysplasia epiphysealis hemimelica	Sp
Multiple cartilaginous exostoses	AD
Enchondromatosis (Ollier)	Sp
Enchondromatosis with hemangiomata (Maffucci)	Sp
Metachondromatosis	AD
Osteoglophonic dysplasia	Sp
Fibrous dysplasia (Jaffe-Lichtenstein)	Sp
Fibrous dysplasia with pigmentary skin changes and precocious puberty (McCune-Albright)	Sp
Cherubism	AD
Myofibromatosis (Generalized fibromatosis)	AR
Idiopathic Osteolyses	
1. Predominantly phalangeal	
Hereditary acrosteolysis, several forms	
Hajdu-Cheney type	AD
2. Predominantly carpal/tarsal	
Carpal-tarsal osteolysis with nephropathy	AD
François syndrome (Dermochondro-corneal dystrophy)	AR
3. Multicentric	
Winchester syndrome	AR
Torg type	AR
Mandibulo-acral dysplasia	AR
4. Other	
Familial expansile osteolysis	AD

AD = Autosomal dominant; AR = autosomal recessive; XLD = X-linked dominant; XLR = X-linked recessive; Sp = sporadic.

From the International Working Group on Constitutional Diseases of Bone: International classification of osteochondrodysplasias. Eur J Pediatr 151:407–415, 1992. © 1992, Springer-Verlag.

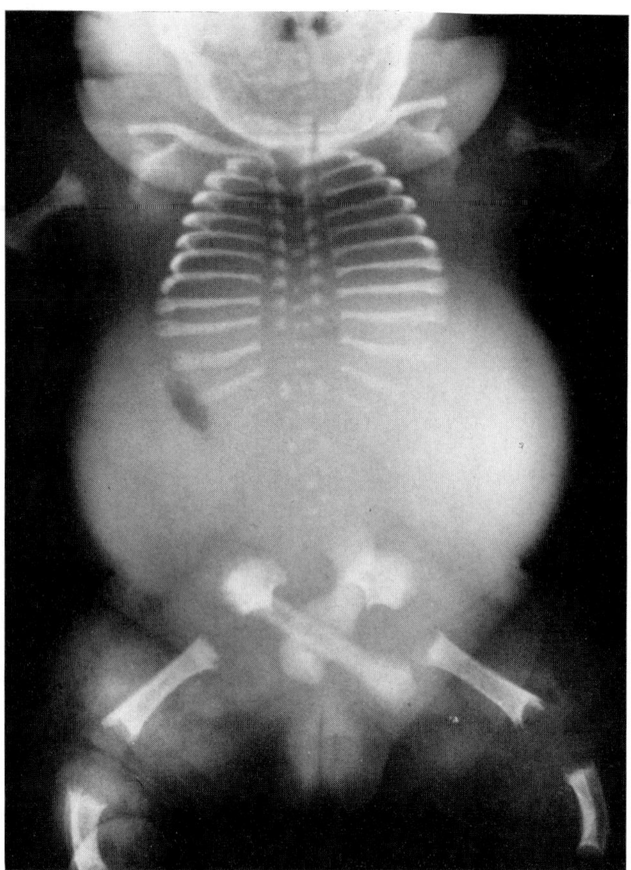

Figure 93–6. Achondrogenesis type II. Frontal view of a stillborn infant. There is lack of ossification of many of the vertebral bodies. The only ossification on the spine is in the posterior elements. The pelvis is poorly developed and the long bones are short and cupped. (The umbilical cord and clamp are superimposed on the pelvis.)

entity both histologically and prognostically inasmuch as most achondroplasts live and all infants with thanatophoric dwarfism die. They are either stillborn or usually die a few days after birth. Although clinically there may be some difficulty in differentiating this condition from other forms of neonatal dwarfism, the radiographic distinction is very clear. The most characteristic finding is the flat vertebral bodies with wide spaces between them (Fig. 93 7*A*). This is not present in achondrogenesis or other neonatal dysplasias. All of the long bones are short and cupped, and there is marked bowing of the femora and humeri (Fig. 93–7*B*).

The following entities are also identifiable at birth but are usually nonlethal.

Chondrodysplasia Punctata (Stippled Epiphyses). This condition is heterogeneous and is characterized by calcifications in the region of the epiphyses that appear as dense white dots on the radiograph (Fig. 93–8). There are probably three main forms of this condition: one inherited as an x-linked autosomal dominant, one as an autosomal recessive, and a milder form with relatively few findings. There are also several other disorders and syndromes that have punctate epiphyses associated with them. These include the children of mothers who received warfarin or similar anticoagulants during pregnancy; a rare condition called the cerebrohepatorenal syndrome, which can be differentiated radiographically by the presence of calcifications in the patella; and some of the chromosomal disorders, as well as some mucopolysaccharide disturbances. The flecks of calcification may occur in a variety of locations. In some forms, the disease has associated shortening of the femur and the humerus; in others, the findings are quite mild. Any of the bones affected by the calcifications may be foreshortened.

Campomelic Dysplasia. In this syndrome, which is usually fatal in early life, bowed extremities are noted in infancy. Characteristically, anterior bowing of the tibias with pretibial dimples is often evident. The children have the classic clinical appearance of a flat nasal bridge, small mouth, and micrognathia; they may also have a cleft palate. Airway problems may be present. Clubfoot deformities are seen in many patients. The infants are usually very hypotonic. The condition is inherited as an autosomal recessive

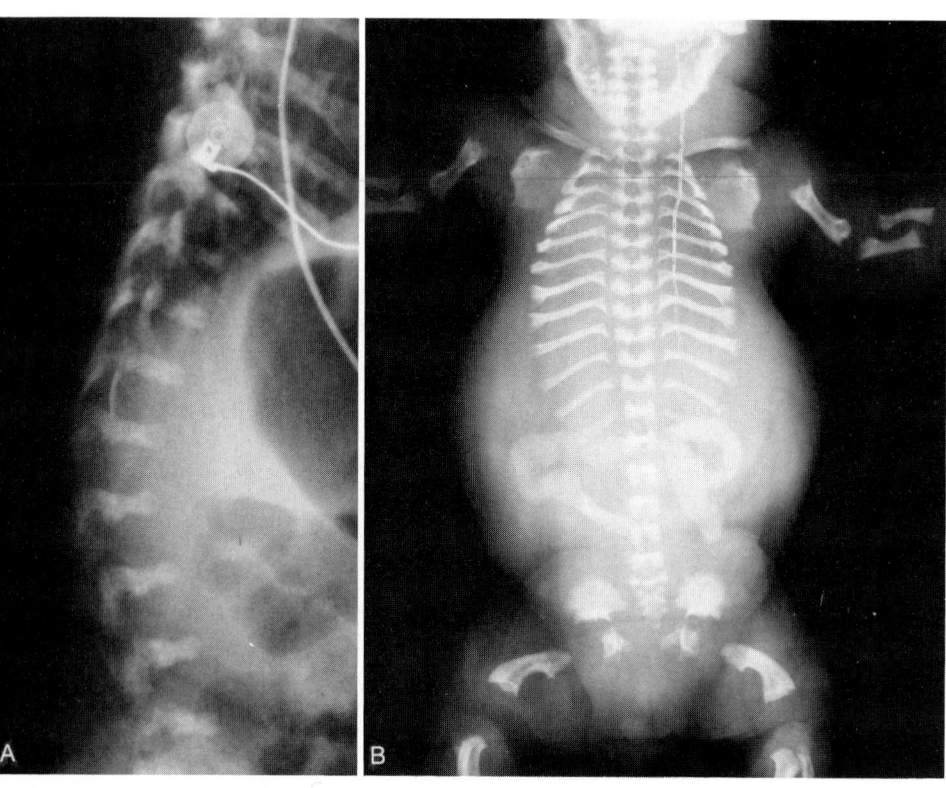

Figure 93–7. Thanatophoric dysplasia. *A,* Lateral view of the thoracolumbar spine. There are flattened vertebrae with wide spaces between them characteristic of this syndrome. *B,* The pelvis of a stillborn infant (the lungs are not inflated) is hypoplastic, with small iliac wings and absence of the lower iliac segment. It has an appearance similar to that of achondroplasia (illustrated in Figure 93–10*A*) but with much more pronounced findings. The femora are shortened and curved, and the ribs are very short.

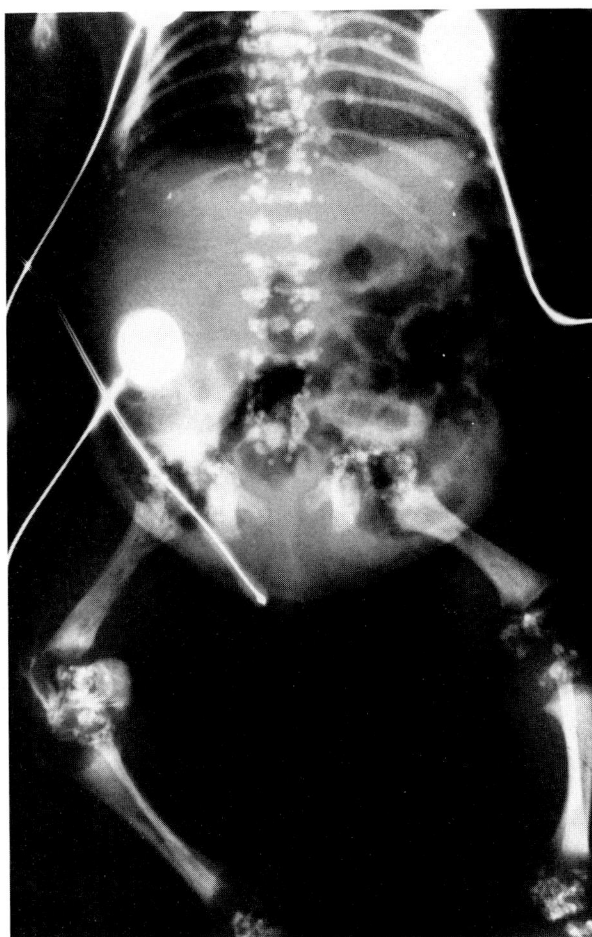

Figure 93–8. Chondrodysplasia punctata. Multiple flecks of calcification are present adjacent to the spine and in the epiphyseal regions of the long bones.

disorder. In addition to the anterior bowing of the tibia, which is often severe (Fig. 93–9*A*), there may be mild femoral bowing. Another characteristic radiographic finding is the marked separation of the ischia, which are wider inferiorly than superiorly because the inferior ischia point downward instead of medially as happens in a normal child (Fig. 93–9*B*). There is a substantial delay in skeletal maturation with the absence of the epiphyses about the knees. There may be mild bowing of humeri and radii. The ribs are very slender, and the scapulae are severely hypoplastic.

ACHONDROPLASIA. This is the best known and probably most

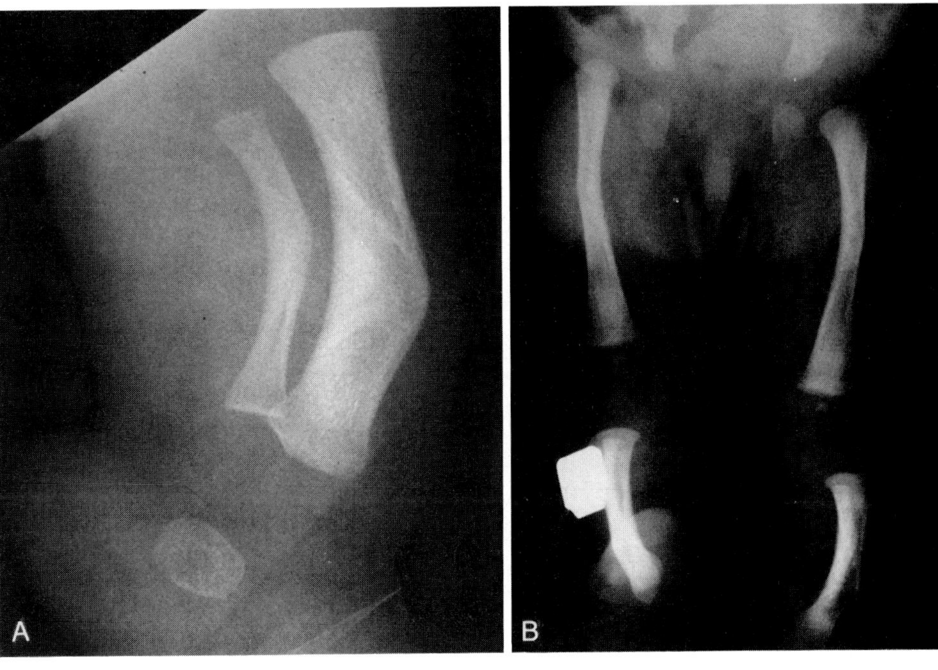

Figure 93–9. Campomelic dysplasia. *A,* Characteristic bowing of the tibia with the apex protruding anteriorly. This is clinically palpable. *B,* There is some bowing of the femora as well as the tibias. The separation of the ischia is another defining characteristic in this syndrome. The inferior tips of the ischia point medially in normal infants (see Fig. 93–10*B*).

common form of short-limbed dwarfism that is evident at birth. The term in the past included many other entities that have now been classified separately. The affected individuals are usually of normal intelligence and have normal activity. The facial configuration is abnormal, with a depressed nasal bridge and a prominent forehead. The condition is inherited as an autosomal dominant disorder. However, most cases are due to mutations. Occasionally one sees the homozygous form of the disease in a child of two achondroplastic parents. In contradistinction to the usual heterozygous form, those infants are very severely affected and usually die in infancy. The most typical radiographic abnormality of achondroplasia is the pelvic wings (Fig. 93–10*A*), which have the appearance of a paddle without a handle; this is due to a flat acetabular angle and a square ilium with shortening of the lower portion. Another important finding is the narrowing of the interpediculate distances from L1 to L5; normally, the distances between the pedicles on the frontal view progressively increase as one descends in the lumbar spine. There is some narrowing of the anteroposterior (AP) diameter of the chest and of the spinal canal. There is shortening of the extremities, which is usually more significant proximally than distally (rhizomelic). The metaphyses may be cupped, but they have smooth margins (Fig. 93–10*C*). Skeletal maturation is delayed. Because the condition is due to failure of enchondral bone formation, the base of the skull, which is formed in cartilage, is usually small. This results in a relatively large calvarium, since calvarial size is dependent on brain size, which is usually normal. Some affected children may have hydrocephalus and a small foramen magnum. The hands may have a trident shape, particularly in infancy, with inability to approximate the fingers when the fingers are extended. In the homozygous form, the findings are more severe, but not as severe as in thanatophoric dwarfism. The vertebrae are also not as severely flattened in homozygous achondroplasia as in thanatophoric dwarfism.

DIASTROPHIC DYSPLASIA. The term *diastrophic* means "bent" or "twisted." This is a form of short-limbed dwarfism that is noted at birth but clinically differs from achondroplasia by a normal facial appearance and by the presence of clubfoot deformity. Scoliosis may be present in older children but is not usually present at birth. There is deformity of the pinna of the ears in 82 per cent of cases, and the affected children may also have cleft palate. Intelligence is usually normal. The condition is inherited as an autosomal recessive. The hand findings are probably the most important radiographically. The thumb is very short with a short first metacarpal, and in some patients the thumb projects laterally in a "hitchhiker" configuration (Fig. 93–11). The first metacarpal may appear simply as a round ossicle. Multiple epiphyseal abnormalities may be present, with growth plates that run along the axis of the

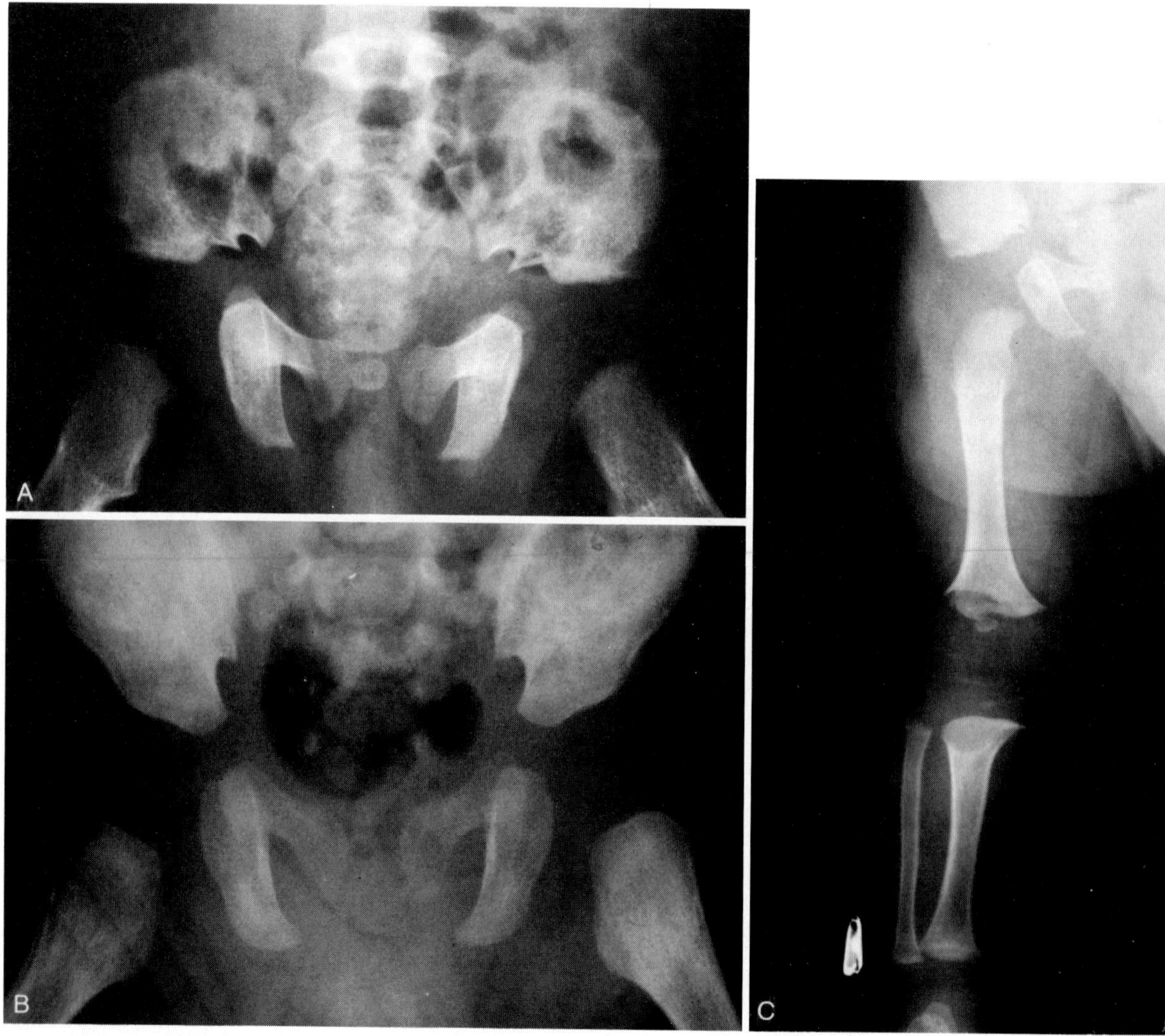

Figure 93–10. Achondroplasia. *A,* Typical pelvis demonstrating the square iliac wings and absence of the lower iliac segment. Small projections are seen at the bottom of the ilia. *B,* Pelvis of a normal infant. Note the lower iliac segment, which looks like a handle. The achondroplastic pelvis has been described as a paddle without a handle or as having the appearance of Mickey Mouse ears. *C,* Lower extremity. The long bones are short, and the distal femur and proximal tibia show some beaking and small indentations. Otherwise, the structure of the bone is unremarkable.

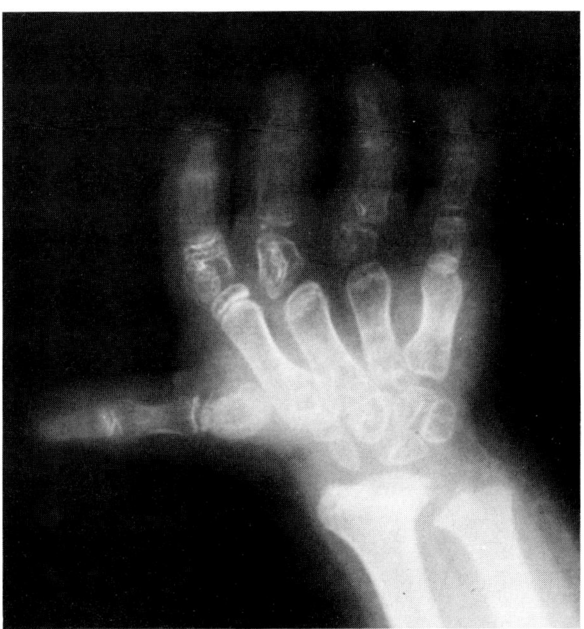

Figure 93–11. Diastrophic dysplasia. The thumb is short, with a short first metacarpal that points outward like that of a hitchhiker. Note the abnormal epiphyses in the proximal phalanges. Some of the growth plates are along the axis of the phalanges rather than perpendicular to them. There is marked shortening of the metacarpals.

bone rather than at right angles to it (Fig. 93–11). There may also be abnormality of the carpals, which may be precocious in appearance. The long bones are short and thick, and there is flattening of the epiphyses about the knees. This epiphyseal involvement leads to early arthritis, and older children and adults have considerable joint problems. The presence of clubfoot and scoliosis is helpful in diagnosis.

METATROPIC DYSPLASIA. This is another form of neonatal dwarfism that again somewhat resembles achondroplasia. There is, however, marked flattening of the vertebrae. A scoliosis usually develops later, although it may not be present initially. The joints appear prominent and stiff. Some patients have a small caudal appendage that looks like a tail. The condition is inherited as an autosomal recessive disorder. The most characteristic radiographic finding in the neonate is the prominent bulbous ends of the long bones, which have the appearance of drumsticks. There is marked flattening of the vertebral bodies, which could be confused with thanatophoric dysplasia, but the extremities are different. The pelvis also is fairly characteristic with a flattened acetabular angle.

CHONDROECTODERMAL DYSPLASIA (ELLIS–VAN CREVELD SYNDROME). The major clinical feature of this condition that differentiates it from the other forms of short-limbed dwarfism is the presence of polydactyly and dysplastic nails. The shortening of the limbs is most marked in the distal portion of the extremities rather than the proximal. Congenital heart disease is seen in 60 per cent of the cases; the most common lesion is a single atrium or large atrial defect. Other clinical findings include genu valgum, abnormalities of the hair and teeth, and a short upper lip bound by a small frenulum. The condition is inherited as an autosomal recessive disorder. The most characteristic radiographic findings are in the hand. The bones of the hand are short, and the distal phalanges appear very slender (Fig. 93–12). Cone-shaped epiphyses are present in the middle and proximal phalanges, and there may be fusion of the carpal bones. There is polydactyly on the ulnar side of the hand. Polydactyly of the feet is less common than in the hands. Other radiographic findings include a pelvis that is similar to an achondroplastic pelvis but has an extra notch along its base. There may be early ossification of the proximal femoral epiphyses.

ASPHYXIATING THORACIC DYSPLASIA (JEUNE DISEASE). This syndrome is characterized by a very small thorax, which in some patients may cause difficulty with respiration. There is considerable variation in severity among affected individuals. The child who survives infancy with this disorder may develop juvenile nephronophthisis. The most characteristic finding is the very small thoracic cage, which is often bell-shaped. This appearance may be similar to that seen in chondroectodermal dysplasia. The pelvis is small but relatively normal and does not have the appearance seen in chondroectodermal dysplasia. There may also be premature ossification of the proximal femoral epiphyses. In the hand, the initial findings are unremarkable; later, cone-shaped epiphyses that indent deeply into the metaphyses are seen (Fig. 93–13).

SPONDYLOEPIPHYSEAL DYSPLASIA CONGENITA. The main clinical characteristics of this disorder are short trunk and neck with a normal head. Important clinical associations include myopia and retinal detachment, which occurs later in childhood. Inheritance is autosomal dominant. The most characteristic radiographic findings include flattening of the vertebral bodies, which may appear pinched-in posteriorly; the vertebrae have an ovoid or almost pear-shaped configuration during infancy. The odontoid is often hypoplastic. There is marked delay in ossification of the pubis, and the iliac wings appear broad and flared (Fig. 93–14). Marked retardation of ossification of the femoral head and neck is also present. In the hand, the findings are relatively mild in the neonate; later, there is flattening of epiphyses.

CLEIDOCRANIAL DYSPLASIA. Clinically, these individuals are able to move their shoulders anteriorly, which is related to the absence of the clavicle. The whole skeleton is involved, with a brachycephalic head, prominent forehead, and a small face. There is often persistence of an open anterior fontanelle. Multiple tooth abnormalities may be seen. The condition is inherited as an autosomal dominant disorder. The most important radiographic finding is an absence of the whole or part of the clavicle (Fig. 93–15*A*); usually it is only a portion of the clavicle that is absent. The skull is poorly ossified and has multiple wormian bones (ossicles within

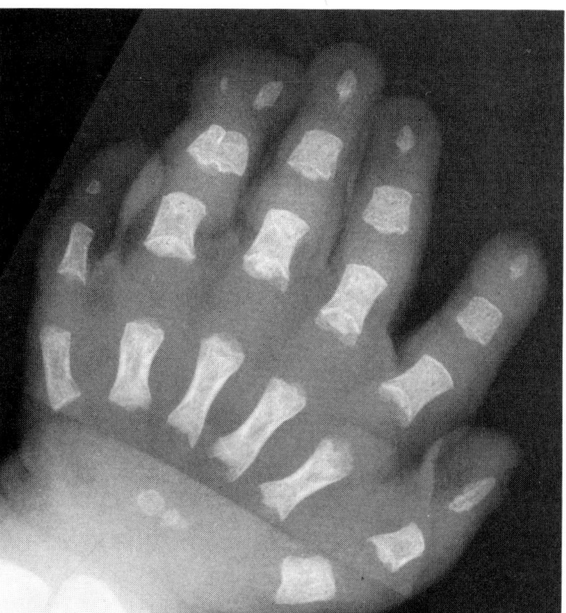

Figure 93–12. Chondroectodermal dysplasia (Ellis–van Creveld syndrome). Typical configuration of the hand with polydactyly, short bones, and slender, spindle-shaped distal phalanges. The capitate and hamate are very close together, which indicates that their cartilage model is fused. There are cone-like indentations in the bases of the proximal phalanges. All of these findings are typical of chondroectodermal dysplasia.

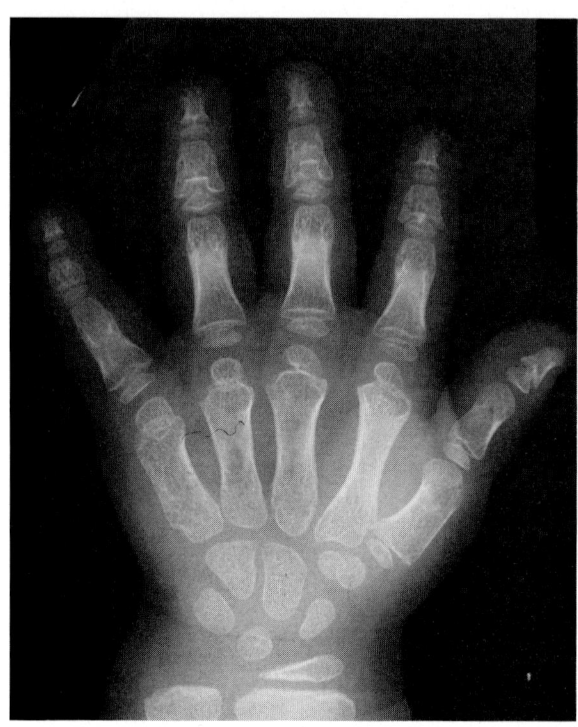

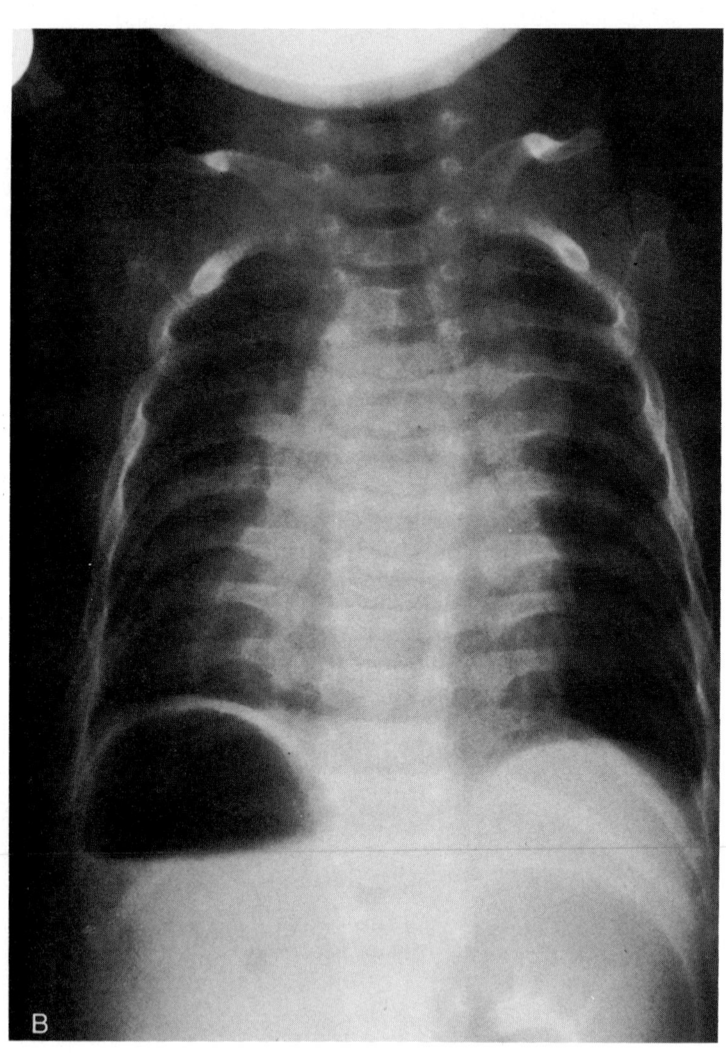

Figure 93–13. *A,* **Asphyxiating thoracic dysplasia (Jeune disease).** Prominent cone epiphyses in the middle phalanges that deeply indent the metaphyses are present in this older child. *B,* Narrow thorax.

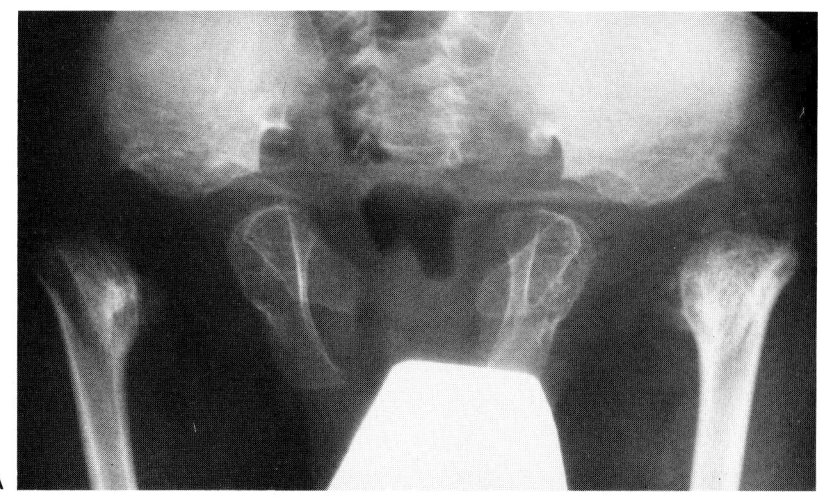

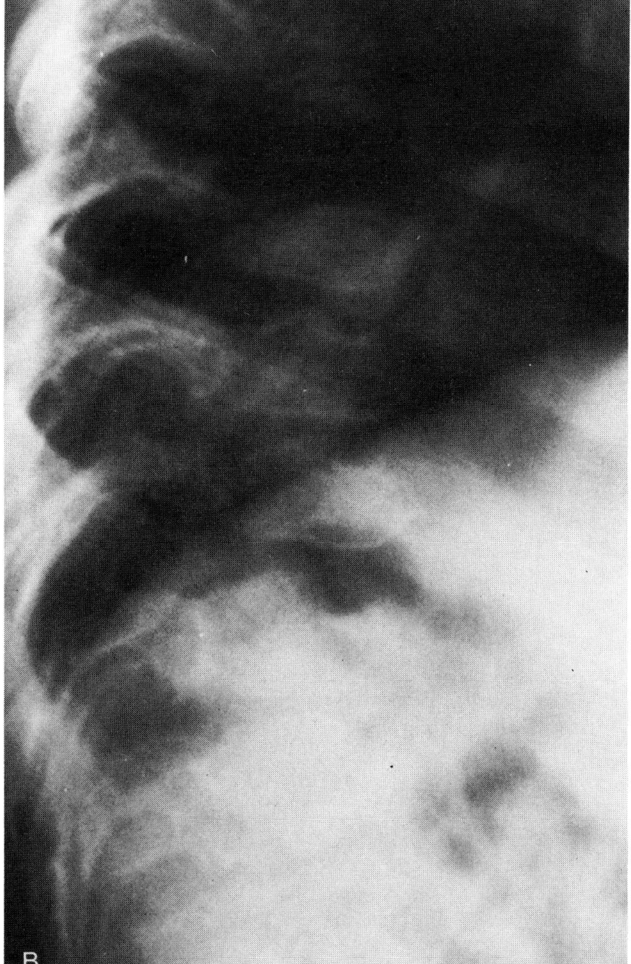

Figure 93–14. *A,* **Spondyloepiphyseal dysplasia congenita.** The acetabulae are almost horizontal. There is delayed ossification of the pubis, femoral heads, and necks. *B,* Flattening of multiple vertebral bodies.

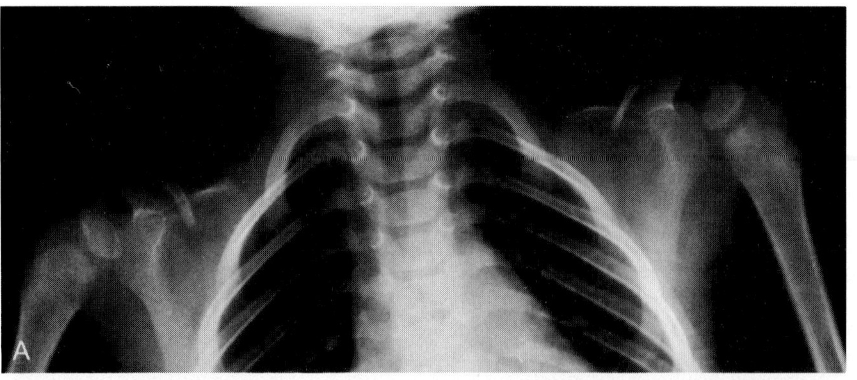

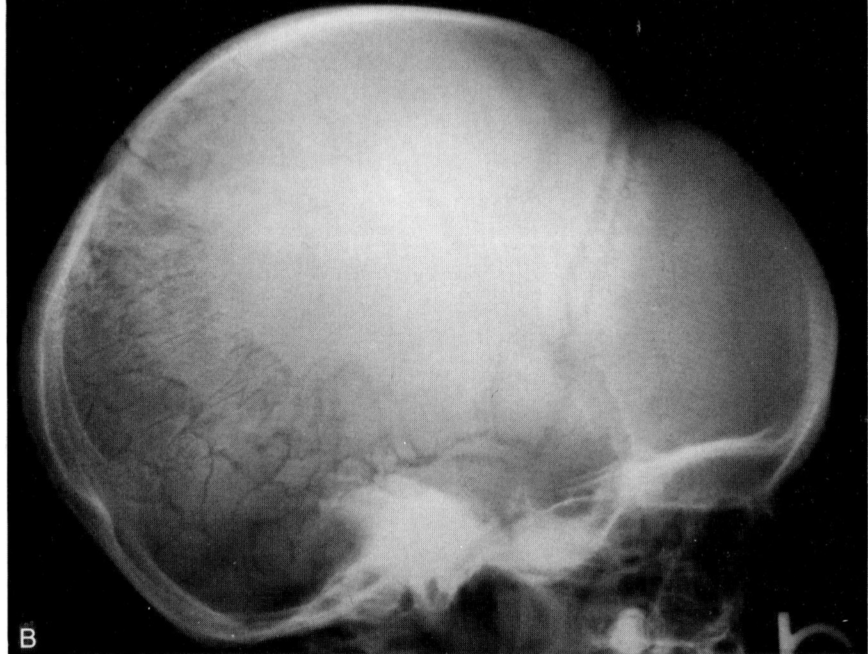

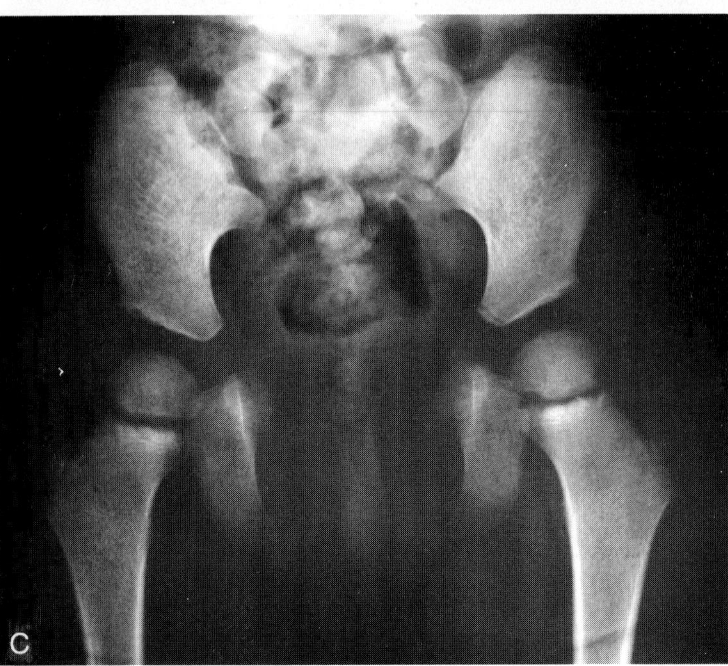

Figure 93–15. Cleidocranial dysplasia. *A,* There is almost complete absence of the clavicles, with only small remnants seen laterally. *B,* There are multiple wormian bones (sutural bones) present, particularly in the lambdoid sutures. The anterior fontanelle is still open in this older child. *C,* There is lack of ossification of the pubis and ischium.

the sutures) (Fig. 93–15*B*). The fontanelles persist long after they should have closed. There is a marked delay in tooth maturation. The pelvis is poorly ossified, with a wide gap at the symphysis pubis (Fig. 93–15*C*). In the hand, there is shortening of the distal phalanges, and the epiphyses of the phalanges are often thick.

Otopalatodigital Syndrome. This is a disorder associated with a cleft palate in males, whereas females usually have a normal palate. The children have a broad nasal bridge and an appearance suggestive of hypertelorism. Deafness is present in some cases, but this is usually secondary to ear infections, which are often associated with cleft palate. The great toe is very short in some; when this is extreme, it gives the foot a tree frog–like appearance. The most characteristic findings are in the hand and foot. The base of the second metacarpal is pointed and protrudes adjacent to the trapezoid, which has a comma shape (Fig. 93–16*A*). The capitate is often transverse, and the distal phalanges of the thumb are often broad. In older individuals, carpal fusion may be seen going from proximal to distal rows (see Fig. 93–4). The foot has a very short great toe involving both phalanges (Fig. 93–16*B*), and multiple tarsal fusions are seen in older individuals, particularly affecting the distal tarsals and the metatarsals (see Fig. 93–5). Prominent frontal and occipital areas of the skull are present.

Larsen Syndrome. This is a syndrome of multiple dislocations, with bilateral dislocations of the knees being commonly present. This helps to differentiate it from some of the other dislocation syndromes. The hips, feet, elbows, and other joints may also be dislocated. The facial appearance is fairly characteristic, with a flat face, prominent forehead, and widely spaced eyes. Both dominant and recessive forms of inheritance have been seen. This disease has two very characteristic radiographic findings, which when present are very helpful in diagnosis because these changes are not seen in very many other conditions. The first is a double ossification center in the calcaneus, which is demonstrated on the lateral view (Fig. 93–17). The two centers eventually fuse, so this finding is seen only in early childhood. The other finding is a very bizarre appearance of the carpals, with multiple extra bones that appear to be placed in the wrist in random fashion (see Fig. 93–2). Other findings in the hand include shortening of the metacarpals and distal phalanges. The various dislocations can also be seen but are nonspecific; however, the presence of a knee dislocation should suggest this diagnosis.

The following entities are identifiable in later life.

Hypochondroplasia. This is a form of dwarfism that is clinically similar to achondroplasia but has much milder manifestations. Findings include disproportionately short limbs when compared with the trunk, but the face does not show the depressed nasal bridge and frontal bossing that is present in achondroplasia. Inheritance is autosomal dominant. Radiographically this is a very difficult condition to diagnose because the skeleton is often unremarkable. It is almost a diagnosis of exclusion. The most positive finding is the lack of progressive widening of the interpediculate distances from L1 to L5. There may be some decrease in the AP diameter of the spine, but the changes are considerably milder than those seen in achondroplasia. The skull has a normal configuration. It is difficult to separate the relatively short limbs seen in these patients from those of just normally short persons.

Dyschondrosteosis (Leri-Weill Syndrome). This form of dwarfism is associated with abnormalities of the wrist, which has a dinner-fork configuration. There is some shortening of the radius and ulna, and the tibias and fibulas may also be short. Radiographically the deformity of the wrist (Fig. 93–18) is due to a V-shaped appearance of the distal radius and ulna, a decrease in

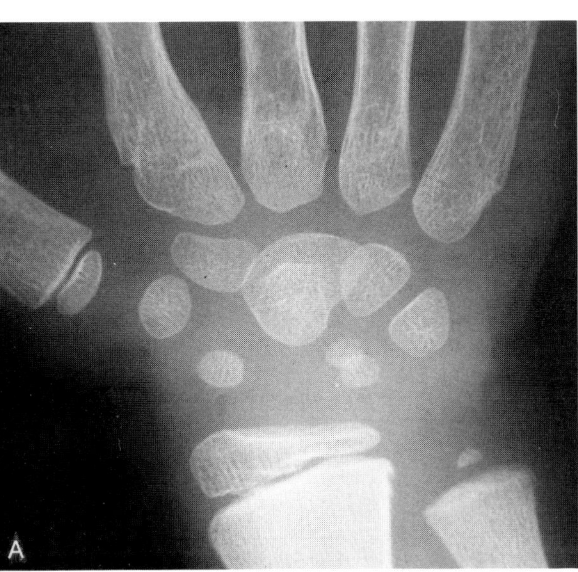

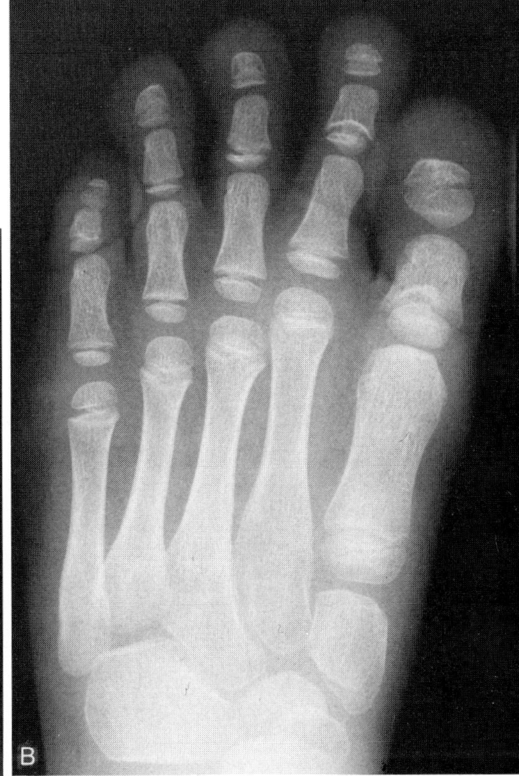

Figure 93–16. Otopalatodigital syndrome. *A,* The transverse capitate, a somewhat prominent pointed base of the second metacarpal, and a comma-shaped trapezoid adjacent to it are characteristic. The double ossification of the lunate is common but not invariably present in this syndrome. Other manifestations in the wrist are illustrated in Figure 93–4. *B,* Short great toe with particularly short distal phalanx. In many affected children, the toes are much shorter than illustrated here. Note also the fusion of the middle and lateral cuneiform to their adjacent metatarsals. This type of fusion is always associated with syndromes and does not occur as an isolated finding. Other manifestations in the foot are illustrated in Figure 93–5.

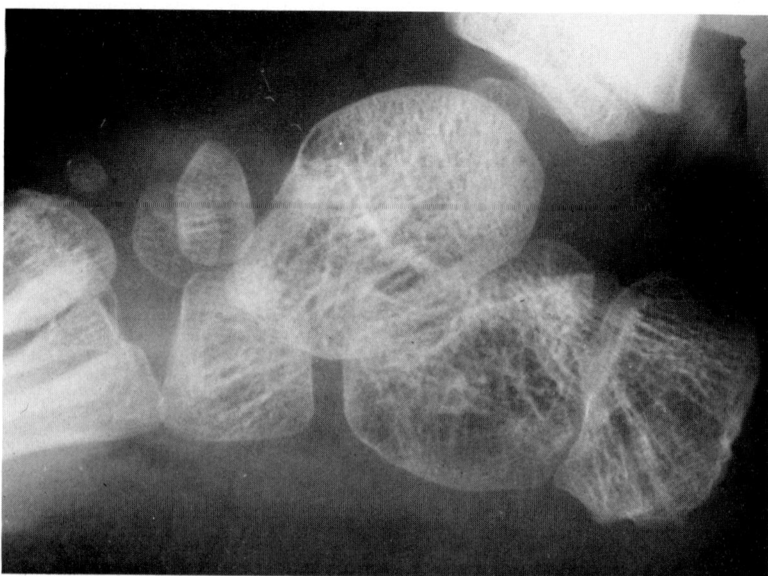

Figure 93–17. Larsen syndrome. Double ossification of the calcaneus is a finding that rarely occurs in otherwise normal individuals but is common in the Larsen syndrome (although it is not seen in all affected individuals). Other manifestations of the Larsen syndrome are illustrated in Figure 93–2.

carpal angle, an anterior position of the wrist, and bowing of the radius. The wrist deformity is called a Madelung deformity, and when associated with dwarfism, it is called dyschondrosteosis.

Metaphyseal Chondrodysplasias (Dominant Types, Jansen and Schmid; Recessive Type, McKusick). These are forms of dwarfism associated with irregularity of the metaphyses of bone, which appear cupped and may mimic rickets. The metaphyseal chondrodysplasia with the most typical radiographic findings, although one of the rarer ones, is the Jansen type. At birth, the bones have a rachitic appearance (Fig. 93–19*A*), but later in life there is irregular calcification in the metaphyseal ends of the bones (Fig. 93–19*B*). This appearance is seen in no other disorder and is pathognomonic of the entity. Later on in life, these calcified areas are incorporated into the bone, leaving the individual with widened deformed ends of the bone, which appear short and irregular, but the flecks of calcification are no longer apparent. In other forms of metaphyseal chondrodysplasia, the metaphyseal changes are milder. One form of this disease—the hair-cartilage hypoplasia, or McKusick form—is important because it is associated with abnormalities in cellular immunity in some patients. Children with this disorder may have a very violent reaction to chickenpox and other viral diseases. The metaphyseal changes in this form may be confused with rickets at all ages in children.

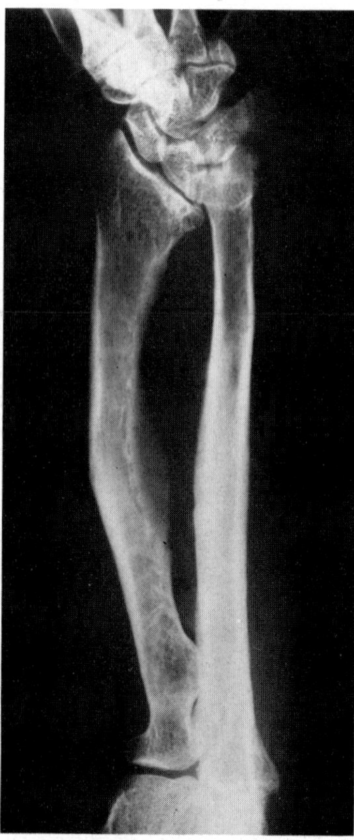

Figure 93–18. Dyschondrosteosis. Note the sharp angulation of the distal radius and ulna, giving the wrist a cup-like configuration. There is bowing of the radius, and the forearm is short.

Multiple Epiphyseal Dysplasia. This probably represents several different conditions. However, they are all characterized by an abnormality of the epiphyses which leads to a short stature that is usually not very severe. The important clinical manifestations include joint pain in older individuals, particularly in the hips. Radiographically, most epiphyses are flattened, and in older individuals, articular irregularity is seen. The condition may be confused with bilateral Legg-Perthes disease. Evaluation of the hands and knees is helpful in making the correct diagnosis. A coronal cleft in the patella is a helpful diagnostic sign (Fig. 93–20*A*). In the hand, there is flattening of the epiphyses, and the carpals are irregular in configuration (Fig. 93–20*B*). The carpal area is smaller than normal.

Pseudoachondroplasia. This form of short-limbed dwarfism resembles achondroplasia; however, the findings are not present at birth. It is characterized by the presence of flat vertebrae (Fig. 93–21*A*), which are not seen in achondroplasia. The trunk is relatively large compared with the limbs. Atlantoaxial dislocation may occur, causing cord compression. Epiphyses may be irregular. The hand is often diagnostic, having short broad phalanges with cone epiphyses and cupping of the metaphyses, which have a characteristic configuration (Fig. 93–21*B*). The pelvis is also very different from that in achondroplasia (Fig. 93–21*C*, compare with Fig. 93–10*A*).

Trichorhinophalangeal Dysplasia. This syndrome is characterized by a bulbous nose, hypoplasia, slow growth of the hair, and in some cases, short stature. The patients are occasionally mentally retarded. The condition is inherited as an autosomal dominant disorder. The findings in the hand are pathognomonic of this condition. Typical cone-shaped epiphyses are seen in the middle

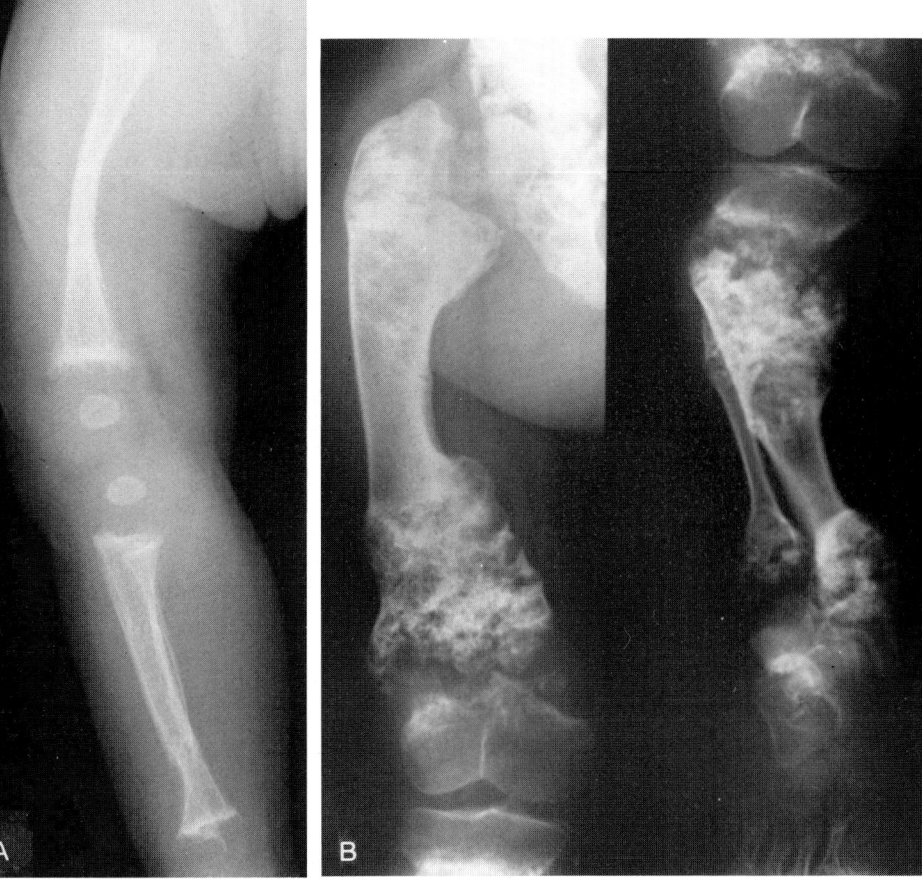

Figure 93–19. Metaphyseal chondrodysplasia—type Jansen. *A,* Newborn infant. The appearance is somewhat similar to rickets, although rickets is almost never seen in the neonatal period. There is marked widening of the growth plate, which is wider than expected in rickets. The metaphysis appears ragged. Fractures of the tibia and fibula are seen. The marked separation of the epiphyses and the demineralized condition of the bone are characteristic of the neonatal form of this disease. *B,* More typical findings in this disorder later in childhood. Large areas of calcification are seen in the metaphyses. At this stage, the findings are pathognomonic of the Jansen form of metaphyseal chondrodysplasia.

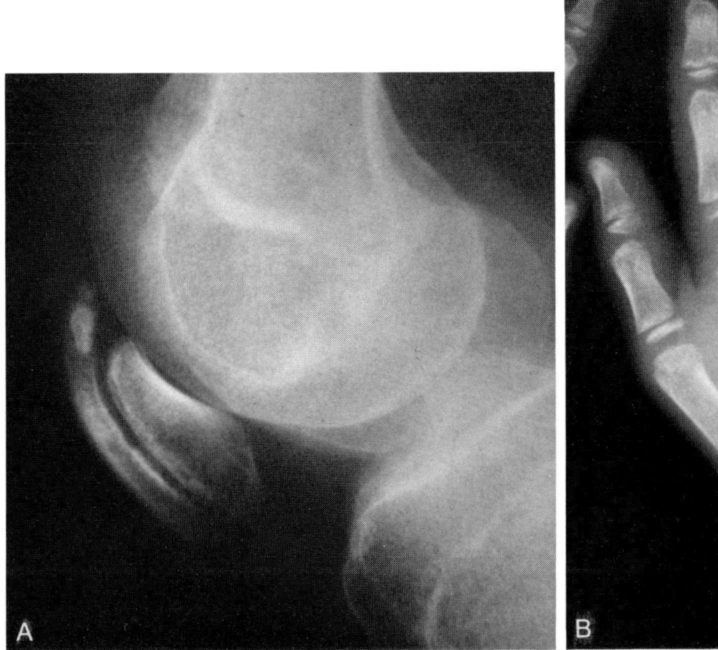

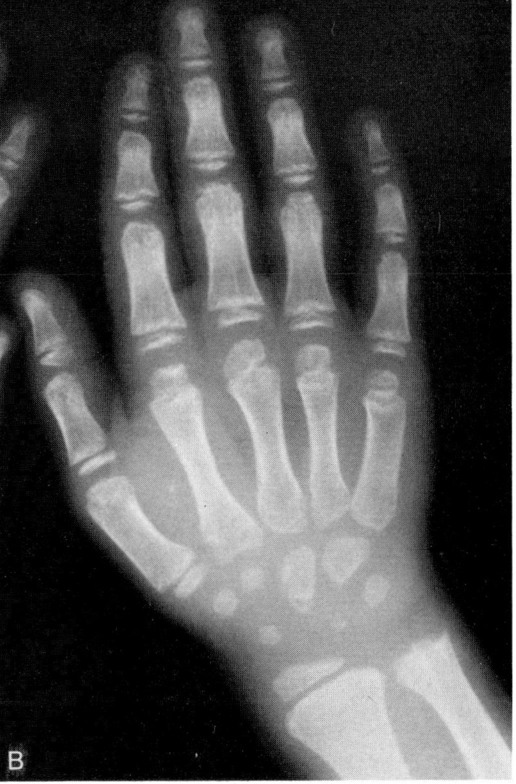

Figure 93–20. Multiple epiphyseal dysplasia. *A,* Double ossification of the patella. This is seen in some patients with multiple epiphyseal dysplasia and, when present, is helpful in diagnosis. *B,* There is flattening and irregularity of the epiphyses. The carpals are irregular in contour, and the whole area of the carpus occupies less space than normal.

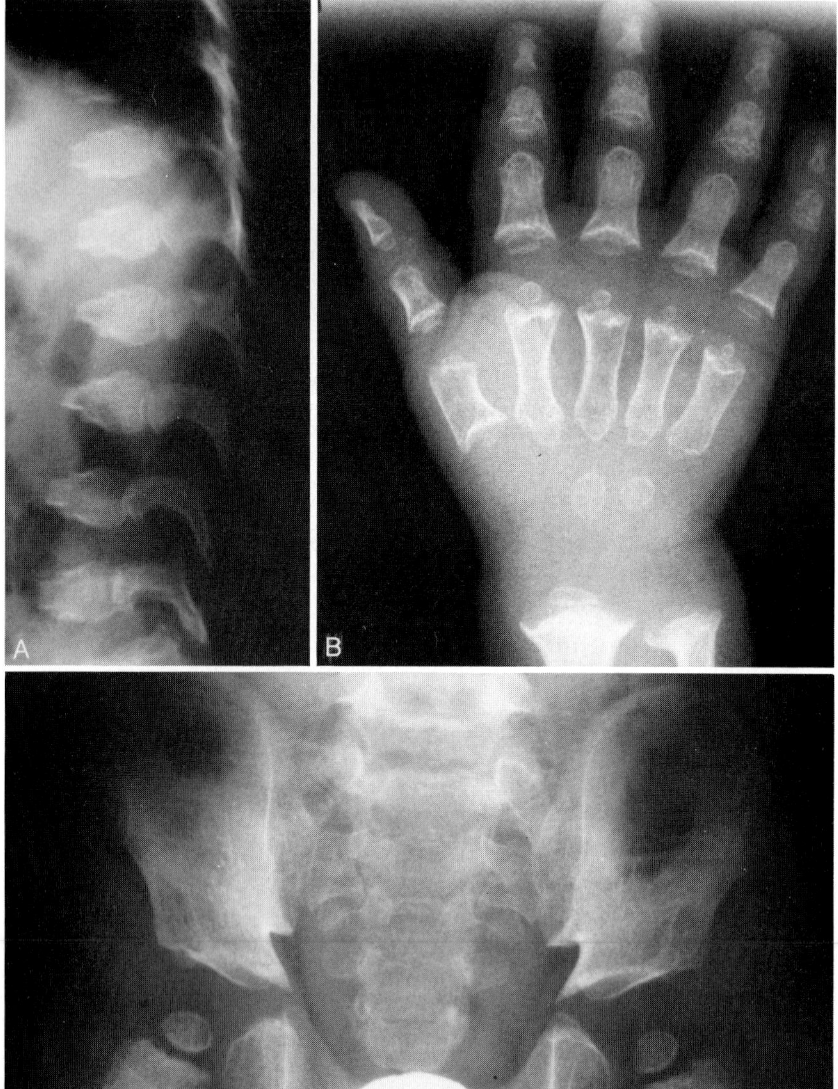

Figure 93–21. Pseudoachondroplasia. *A,* Flattening of the vertebrae with some beaking anteriorly. *B,* The bones of the hand are short. The phalanges are broadened, and the metaphyses are cupped. *C,* The acetabulum is unusual in shape, with a sharp beak-like projection medial to the lower iliac segment. The appearance is very different from that of achondroplasia (see Fig. 93–10*A*).

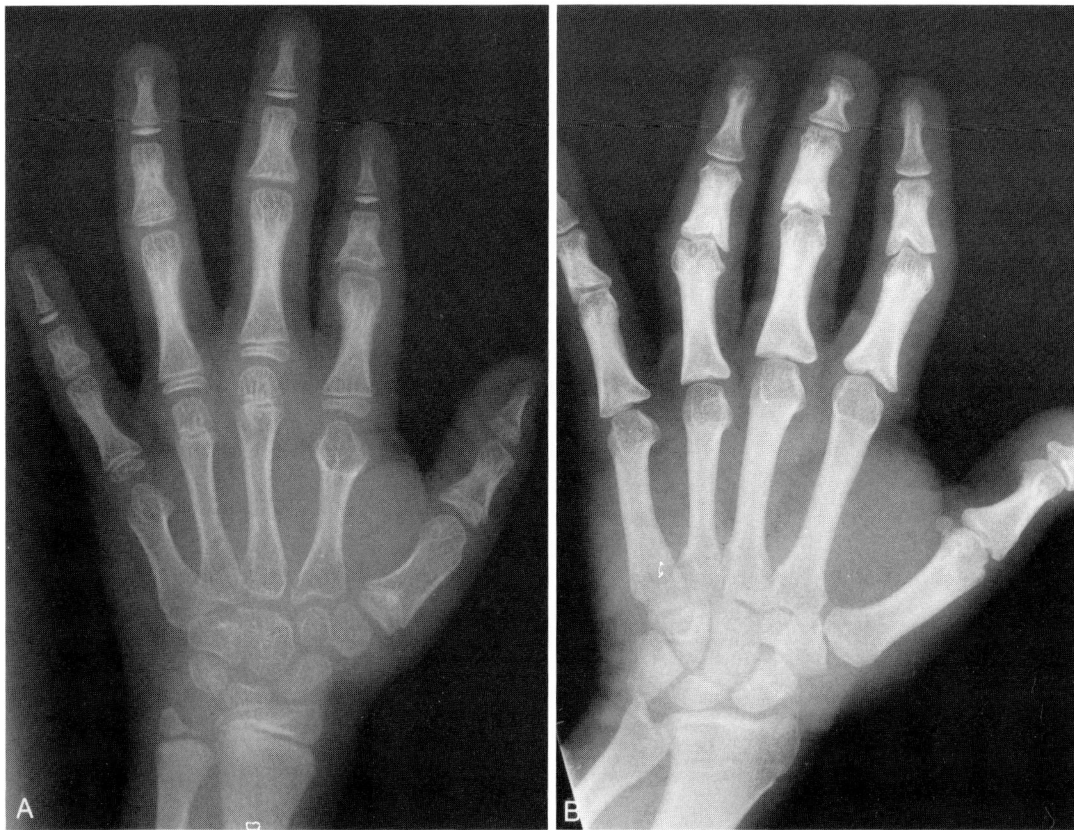

Figure 93–22. Trichorhinophalangeal syndrome. *A,* The cone epiphysis and splaying of the metaphyses involving the middle phalanges are characteristic. In this patient the middle phalanx of the index finger is most affected. A similar appearance is seen in the middle finger, but here the growth plate is closed. There are also sclerotic flat epiphyses in the distal phalanges; these have been called ivory epiphyses. The second and fifth metacarpals are short owing to early closure of their growth plates. Various patterns of shortening may be seen in this condition. *B,* Hand of an adult with similar metaphyseal findings in the middle and proximal phalanges, which are the result of the cone epiphyses.

phalanges (Fig. 93–22*A*), and there is splaying of the metaphyses, with the central portion of the cone fused to the metaphysis. In adults, the cone epiphyses leave a deformity on the articular surface of the phalanges; these are most pronounced in the middle phalanges (Fig. 93–22*B*). During growth, very dense epiphyses in the distal phalanges (ivory epiphyses) are common. The proximal femoral epiphyses sometimes appear flatter than usual. Legg-Perthes–like changes in the hips may occasionally be seen and cause considerable clinical problems. If exostoses are associated with this condition, it is a another entity called trichorhinophalangeal syndrome type II, or the Langer-Giedion syndrome; this syndrome has different clinical manifestations and is associated with a chromosomal abnormality.

Disorganized Development of Cartilage and Fibrous Components of Skeleton

The following diseases are characterized by abnormalities of bone growth. They involve the skeleton focally and usually asymmetrically; however, sometimes symmetrical findings may be present.

Dysplasia Epiphysealis Hemimelica (Trevor's Disease). This disorder of asymmetrical cartilaginous overgrowth is quite rare but has typical radiographic findings. It involves only the lower extremities in most cases and is unilateral. The tarsus is most commonly affected, and the radiographic appearance is of calcific masses that disrupt the usual architecture and have an appearance similar to osteochondromas. They project into the joint and interfere with function. Other bones, including the knee and sometimes the wrist, may be involved.

Multiple Cartilaginous Exostoses. This disorder is characterized by projections from bone that clinically appear as bumps that may protrude through the skin. It is a relatively common bone disorder and is inherited as an autosomal dominant disorder. Radiographically these exostoses or projections may be seen near the ends of any bone (Fig. 93–23). They can result in shortening of the bones, particularly when they involve the wrist, although almost any bone may be affected. They can cause deformity of growth and bowing of the bones as well. Widening of the femoral neck is a common manifestation of this disorder. Displacement and pressure upon nerves and the spinal cord may result. Involvement with arteries can lead to pseudoaneurysms.

Enchondromatosis. Enchondromatosis refers to cartilaginous growths that are present inside the bone. The severity of this disorder is quite variable, ranging from an occasional enchondroma to marked changes causing considerable bone deformity and disfiguration. When associated with hemangiomas, the condition is called Maffucci's syndrome. Multiple enchondromas without hemangiomas have been termed Ollier's disease. Most of the cases are sporadic, but familial cases have been described. In Maffucci's syndrome, brain tumors, ovarian teratomas, and sarcomas may occur. In Ollier's disease there is also an increased incidence of bone neoplasm but less than in Maffucci's syndrome. The enchondromas cause localized expansions of bone, which are often central but may be eccentric. They often start in the region of the growth plates and, in very young children, may appear as punched-out metaphyseal defects (Fig. 93–24*A*). They may also produce linear streaks in

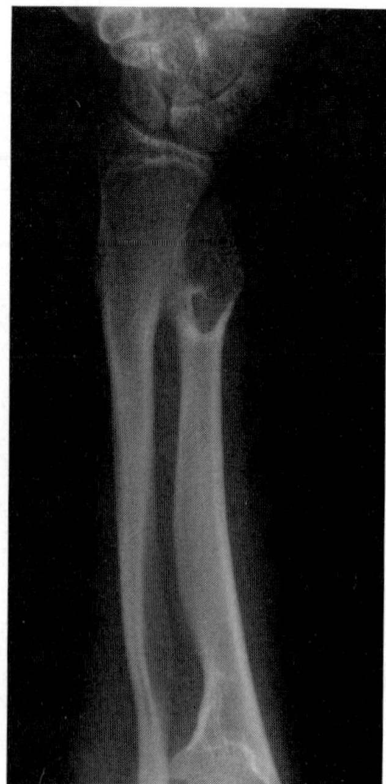

Figure 93–23. Multiple exostoses. Bony projections along the distal radius with mild bowing and shortening of the ulna due to exostoses.

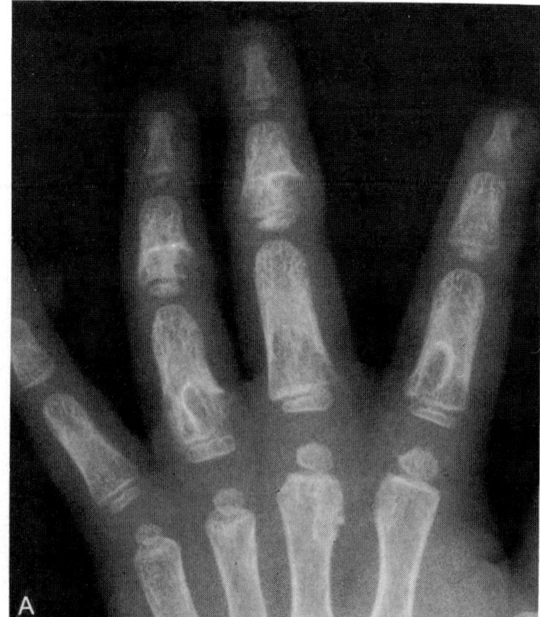

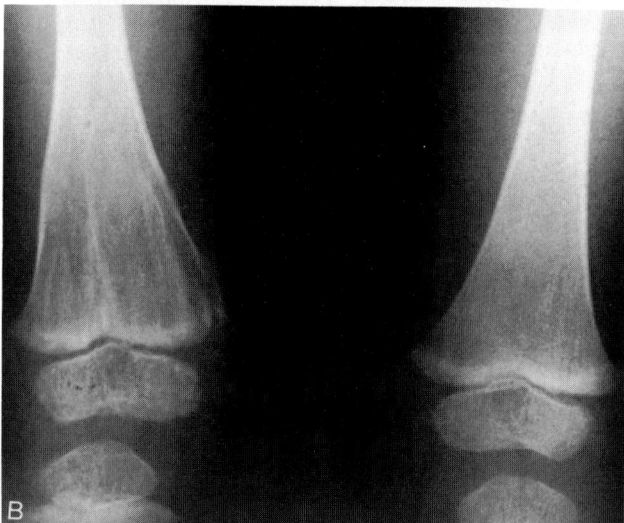

Figure 93–24. Enchondromatosis. *A,* Multiple punched-out defects with well-defined sclerotic margins are present, particularly in the region of the metaphyses. These are due to multiple enchondromas of bone. *B,* Lucency and linear streaks are seen in the distal femur on the right. This is another manifestation of multiple enchondromas.

metaphysis of bone (Fig. 93–24*B*). Involvement is often, but not always, asymmetrical. When associated with hemangiomas, calcifications may also be apparent.

Fibrous Dysplasia. This is a condition in which fibrous tissue occupies portions of the medullary cavities of bone. It may involve one or multiple bones. The clinical symptoms may be due to the expansion of bone or may be related to fracture, which occasionally occurs. In the polyostotic form, there is often an association with café-au-lait spots on the skin. Sexual precocity is seen in 20 per cent of cases, in which case the disorder is called the McCune-Albright syndrome. Without sexual precocity, the entity has been termed Jaffe-Lichtenstein disease. Radiographically many bones may be affected. There may be local lucent lesions, thinning or expansion of the cortex, and bowing. In some, the osseous lesion has the appearance of ground glass (Fig. 93–25). There may be considerable thickening of the skull or facial bones. The affected areas exhibit increased uptake of isotope with radionuclide bone scanning.

Abnormalities of Density of Cortical Diaphyses and/or Metaphyseal Modeling

The cortex of long bones may be excessively lucent, dense, thin, or thick. The main entity with an excessively lucent cortex is osteogenesis imperfecta, whereas the main conditions with greater density are osteopetrosis and pyknodysostosis. Osteopoikilosis, osteopathia striata, and melorheostosis have spotty areas of increased density in the skeleton.

Osteogenesis Imperfecta. This is a heterogeneous group of disorders that are due to faulty collagen I formation. A very severe form is seen in the neonate and is manifest by multiple fractures in utero; this may present as short-limbed dwarfism. The skull is often soft in these babies. At the other end of the spectrum, there is a tarda form in which the findings are very mild, with only occasional fractures; the only other clinical sign that may be apparent is blue sclera. The skin in some affected individuals is translucent. Deafness may occur, and there may be tooth abnormalities. There are at least four distinct forms of this disease. Most are

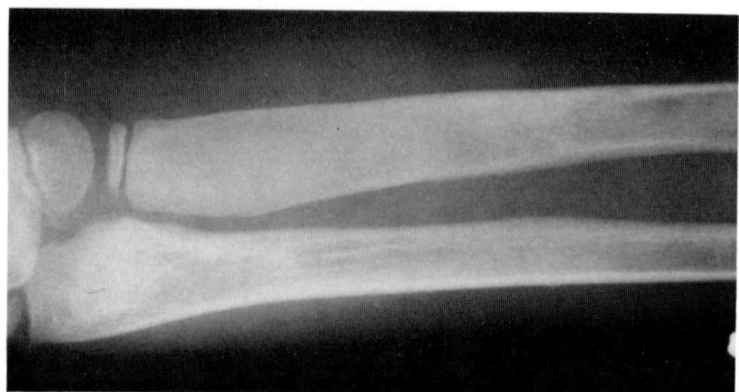

Figure 93–25. Fibrous dysplasia. There is sclerosis and thickening of the trabeculae in the proximal ulna. The proximal radius is widened and there is loss of the normal trabecular structure, leading to a ground-glass appearance.

inherited as autosomal dominant and a few as recessive disorders. In the severe juvenile form, the most characteristic radiographic finding is the marked shortening of the long bones, which may have an accordion-like configuration due to telescoping (Fig. 93–26*A*). In older children, there may be bowing of the long bones (Fig. 93–26*B*). The most important clue, particularly in the older children with milder involvement, is the cranial ossification that is often markedly delayed (Fig. 93–26*C*). There may be multiple bones within the sutures (wormian bones) (Fig. 93–26*D*). The skull findings help differentiate the tarda form of osteogenesis imperfecta from other causes of osteoporosis. Osteogenesis imperfecta is, in reality, a form of congenital osteoporosis. Fractures can be seen in any bone and usually heal well. The vertebrae may appear flat from compression fractures; this may be the presenting symptom. Occa-

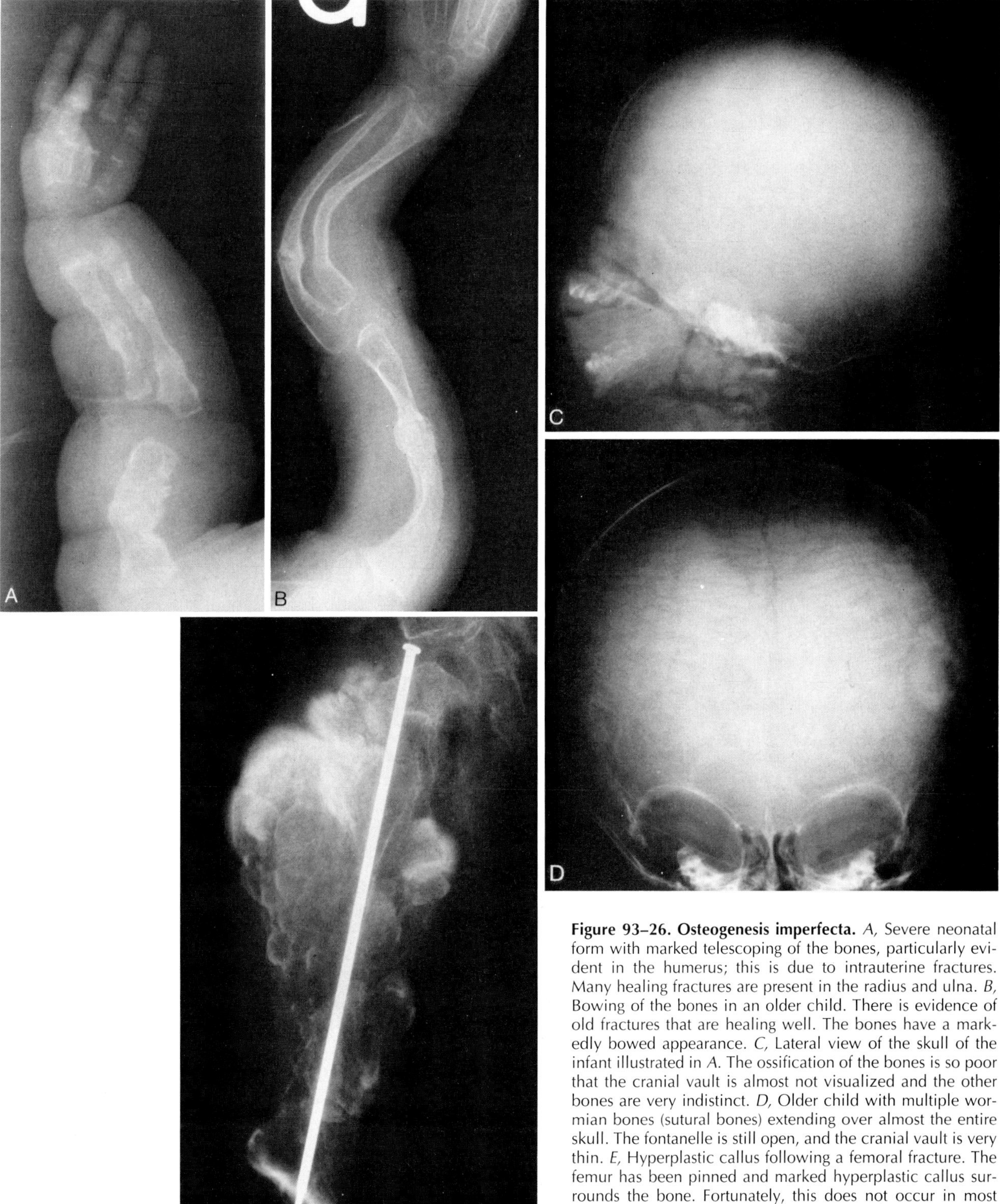

Figure 93–26. Osteogenesis imperfecta. *A,* Severe neonatal form with marked telescoping of the bones, particularly evident in the humerus; this is due to intrauterine fractures. Many healing fractures are present in the radius and ulna. *B,* Bowing of the bones in an older child. There is evidence of old fractures that are healing well. The bones have a markedly bowed appearance. *C,* Lateral view of the skull of the infant illustrated in *A*. The ossification of the bones is so poor that the cranial vault is almost not visualized and the other bones are very indistinct. *D,* Older child with multiple wormian bones (sutural bones) extending over almost the entire skull. The fontanelle is still open, and the cranial vault is very thin. *E,* Hyperplastic callus following a femoral fracture. The femur has been pinned and marked hyperplastic callus surrounds the bone. Fortunately, this does not occur in most cases. (*E* courtesy of Dr. E. Miller, Shriners Hospital for Crippled Children, Chicago, IL.)

sionally osteogenesis imperfecta with fractures may be misdiagnosed as child abuse. This is an important distinction! The skull radiograph is often useful in differential diagnosis. Occasionally, after fracture or surgery, an overabundant callus formation may occur (Fig. 93–26*E*), which can mimic a tumor.

OSTEOPETROSIS. This condition has also been called marble bone disease or Albers-Schönberg disease. It is due to persistence of calcified cartilage and slowing of bone resorption. There may be significant encroachment upon the marrow spaces, which may result in anemia. The enlargement of bones in the skull can impinge upon the cranial nerves with resulting nerve dysfunction. The bones, although they appear very dense, are brittle and susceptible to fracture. There is a spectrum of severity varying from the very severe form in infancy, which may be fatal, to a benign form that is usually identified as an incidental finding radiographically. The severe infantile form is usually inherited as an autosomal recessive disorder, whereas the more benign forms have an autosomal dominant inheritance. Radiographically the bones are dense and there is failure of modeling seen throughout the skeleton (Fig. 93–27*A*). Sometimes a bone-within-bone appearance may be seen (Fig. 93–27*B*). Fractures may occasionally be present. In infancy, the sclerosis has to be differentiated from the physiologic sclerosis that is present in some normal infants.

PYKNODYSOSTOSIS. This condition has some similarity to osteopetrosis but differs from it in that the individuals usually have a very short stature and a relatively large head with open fontanelles and sutures. The condition is believed to have affected the painter Toulouse-Lautrec. The main radiographic findings include a greater-than-normal density of the bones and an increased number of wormian bones in the skull. There is an obtuse angle to the mandible (Fig. 93–28*A*). One of the important differentiating signs from osteopetrosis is erosion of the tufts of the distal phalanges (Fig. 93–28*B*), which may have a pointed configuration, or there may be a loss of a major portion of the distal phalanx. The combination of sclerosis, tuft erosion, and an abnormal mandibular angle is characteristic of pyknodysostosis.

OSTEOPOIKILOSIS. This is an abnormality characterized by multiple foci of sclerosis within the skeleton. Although these have an interesting radiographic appearance, they are of little clinical significance and are usually asymptomatic. They may be associated with osteopathia striata and melorheostosis (Fig. 93–29).

OSTEOPATHIA STRIATA. This is a disorder characterized by longitudinal sclerotic streaks in the long bones that are usually asymptomatic (Fig. 93–30). Occasionally it has been associated with focal dermal hypoplasia and absence of the digits.

MELORHEOSTOSIS. In this disorder, there are dense linear streaks, mostly on the inner cortex of affected bones in children (see Fig. 93–29). In adults, irregular ossification may also be seen along the outside of the cortex mimicking candle drippings. The findings are minimal in infancy and the disease progresses later in childhood. The cortical thickening may encroach on the medullary canal of bones. The disease is usually limited to a single limb, with the sclerotic streaks affecting several bones in a distribution that usually follows the sclerotomes.

DIAPHYSEAL DYSPLASIA (CAMURATI-ENGELMANN DISEASE). This is a sclerotic disorder affecting the diaphyses of the bones. Clinically, the patients appear straight legged, with spindle-shaped limbs that appear widened in their middle portions owing to the increased thickness of the bone. The musculature is usually poor. The condition is inherited as an autosomal dominant disorder. The classic radiographic appearance is a fusiform enlargement of the diaphysis of the long bones (Fig. 93–31). The skull is also

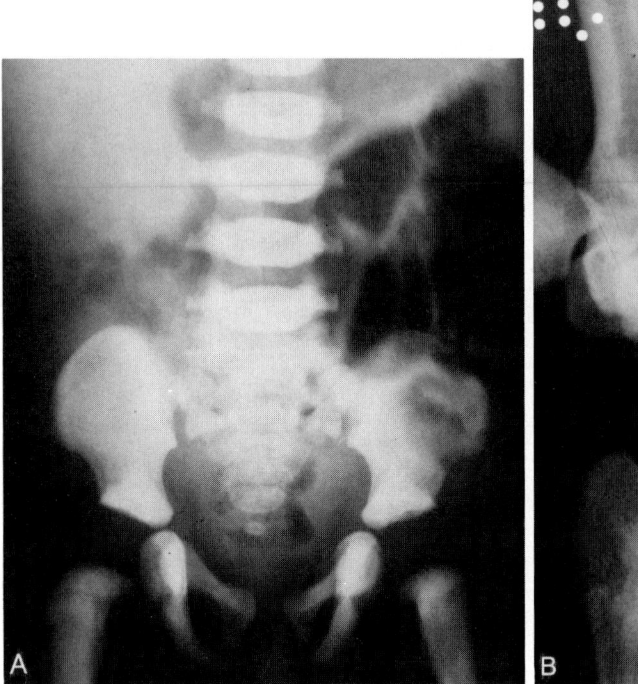

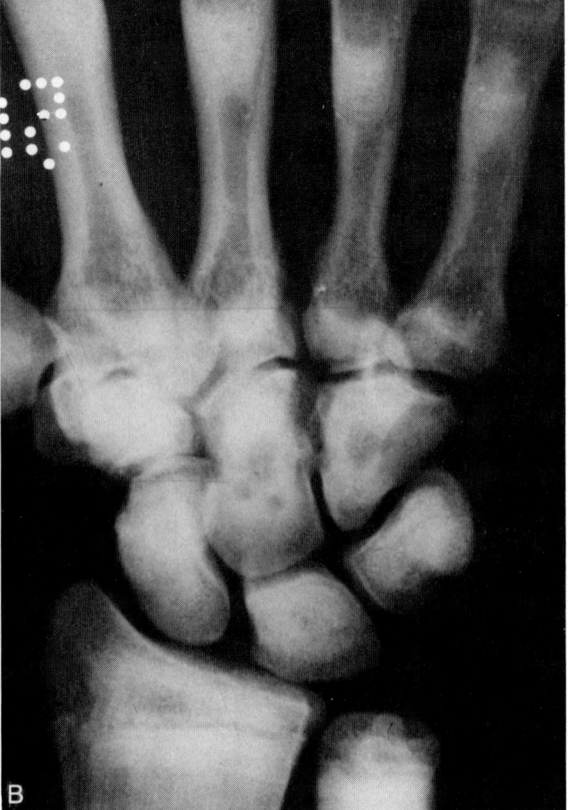

Figure 93–27. Osteopetrosis. *A,* Infant with increased density of all bones. *B,* The bone-in-bone appearance of some of the carpals suggests an extra carpal within each carpal. Dense bone fills the medullary cavities of a portion of the metacarpals and ulna.

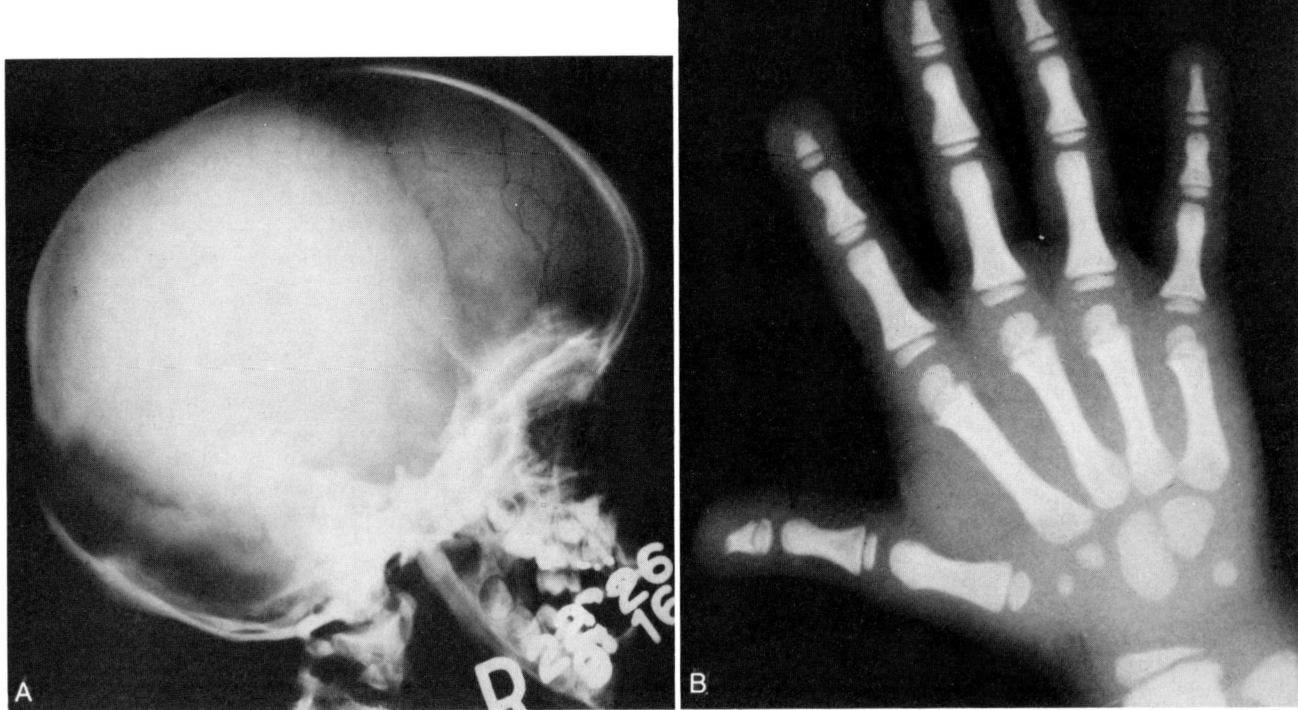

Figure 93–28. Pyknodysostosis. *A,* The angle between the body and ramus of the mandible is almost 180 degrees. This increase in mandibular angle is common in this condition. The fontanelles are still open. *B,* There is sclerosis of all of the bones and erosion of the tufts, which is most marked in the index finger. The combination of sclerosis and tuft erosion plus an abnormal mandibular angle is characteristic of pyknodysostosis.

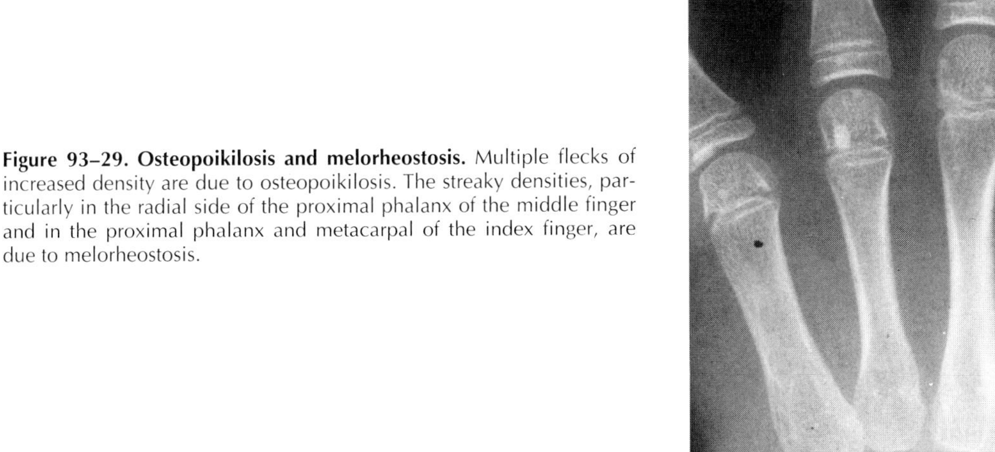

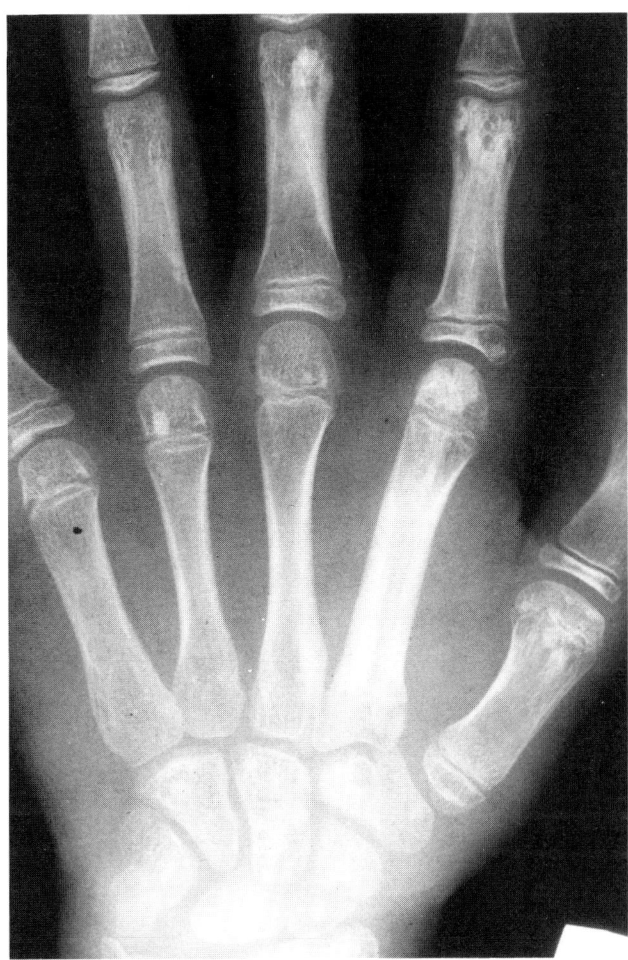

Figure 93–29. Osteopoikilosis and melorheostosis. Multiple flecks of increased density are due to osteopoikilosis. The streaky densities, particularly in the radial side of the proximal phalanx of the middle finger and in the proximal phalanx and metacarpal of the index finger, are due to melorheostosis.

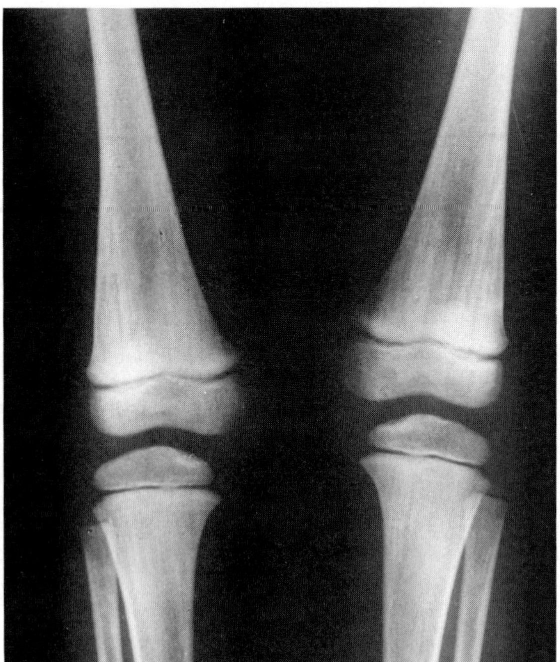

Figure 93–30. Osteopathia striata. There are longitudinal streaks in the distal femora and proximal tibia. Compare this with the normal left femur illustrated in Figure 93–24*B*. This was an otherwise normal child.

usually affected. Other bones including the spine are only occasionally affected. The involved areas have increased activity on radionuclide bone scans.

INFANTILE CORTICAL HYPEROSTOSIS (CAFFEY'S DISEASE). This is a condition of unknown etiology that causes periosteal thickening of the bones. It may occasionally be familial, although in most cases no familial history is evident. Symptoms, which occur at birth or in early infancy, include irritability, pallor, fever, and soft-tissue swelling along the affected bones. Occasionally, pseudoparalysis may be present. The condition may mimic infection or tumor. Radiographically there is marked thickening of the cortex of the affected bones. The mandible is frequently involved, as are various long bones and ribs. Typically only a few bones are affected in most infants, and the involvement is often asymmetrical. New lesions rarely occur after nine months, and the disorder is self-limiting. It is questionable whether this is really a bone dysplasia or some other type of problem such as infection, although an infective agent has not been identified.

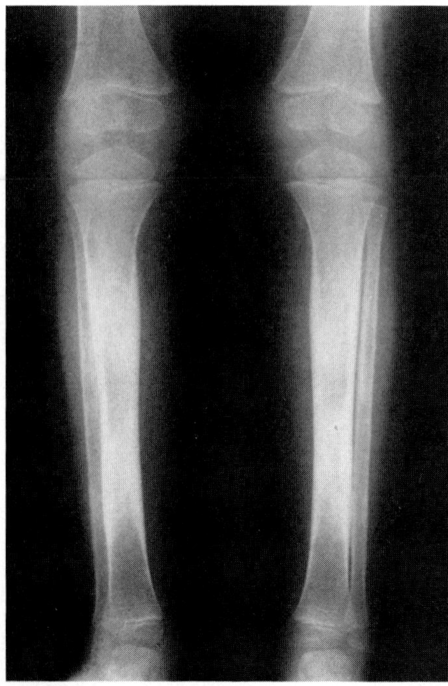

Figure 93–31. Diaphyseal dysplasia (Camurati-Engelmann disease). There is sclerosis and increased thickness of the bones in the diaphyses of the femora.

DYSOSTOSES

Dysostoses with Cranial and Facial Involvement

There are a large number of disorders that affect primarily the face, sometimes in conjunction with involvement of the extremities. The following are two relatively common forms of these conditions that involve much of the skeleton.

ACROCEPHALOSYNDACTYLY (APERT'S SYNDROME). Affected children have a flat face, shallow orbits, hypertelorism, and osseous and cutaneous syndactyly, with hands and feet that appear as if they are in mittens and socks. The thumbs are usually broad. The patients are often mentally retarded. The condition when inherited is an autosomal dominant disorder; however, most cases represent new mutations. The most important radiographic findings are in the skull, hands, and feet. In the skull, there is premature fusion of the coronal suture, which results in a decreased AP diameter of the skull or brachycephaly (Fig. 93–32*A*). In the hand, there are osseous and cutaneous syndactyly and a very broad thumb (Fig. 93–32*B*). In infants, the fusions are actually more extensive than is apparent radiographically because the cartilaginous portions are also fused. Similar findings are seen in the feet. There are other forms of acrocephalosyndactyly, including the Pfeiffer form, in which there are much milder changes in the hands, and little or no syndactyly and only a broad thumb; in the skull, there may be brachycephaly or other craniosynostoses.

ACROCEPHALOPOLYSYNDACTYLY (CARPENTER'S SYNDROME). This is a syndrome of acrocephaly, peculiar facies with mild syndactyly of the fingers, preaxial (on the medial side) polydactyly of the feet, hypogenitalism, obesity, and mental retardation. Congenital heart disease is seen in a significant proportion of these cases, as are abdominal hernias. It is important to differentiate this syndrome from Apert's syndrome because the inheritance is autosomal recessive. This condition is differentiated from Apert's syndrome by the presence of preaxial polydactyly of the feet and by the much milder changes in the hands with very little syndactyly. The fingers are short and the middle phalanges of the hand are most affected. The thumbs are broad, as they are in the other acrocephalosyndactyly syndromes. Coronal suture synostosis may be present, but often other sutures are also affected. The skull findings are much more variable in Carpenter's syndrome than they are in Apert's syndrome.

Dysostoses with Predominant Axial Involvement

VERTEBRAL SEGMENTATION DEFECTS. These include anomalies of vertebral formation, including hemivertebrae and block vertebrae. Some of these are isolated abnormalities, but they are seen more frequently in association with various other anoma-

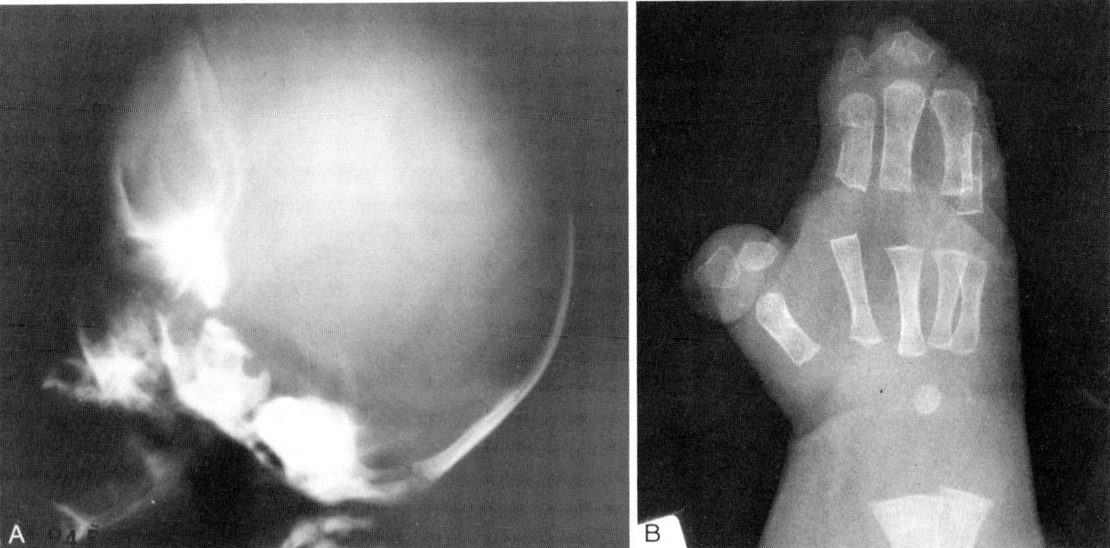

Figure 93–32. Acrocephalosyndactyly (Apert's disease). *A,* There is a shortening of the skull in the AP diameter (brachycephaly) that is due to early closure of the coronal sutures. Sclerosis of the coronal sutures is evident. *B,* There is fusion of the soft tissues of the hand, which has a mitten-like configuration. There are also some osseous fusions of the distal phalanges. The thumb is short and broad and angulates radially. The proximal phalanx of the thumb is round in configuration.

lies, such as congenital heart disease, anal atresia, renal anomalies, esophageal anomalies, and radial defects (Fig. 93–33).

KLIPPEL-FEIL ANOMALY. The term *Klippel-Feil syndrome* usually refers to any congenital lack of segmentation of vertebrae in the cervical spine. Although the appearance is that of a progressive fusion, the entity is present at birth with fusion of the cartilaginous model; as the ossified portions enlarge, they coalesce and the fusion appears to be progressive. The classic description by Klippel and Feil was of a patient with a very short neck, low posterior hairline, and limitation of movement of the head and neck. The condition is usually painless. It may rarely be associated with cord compression or with symptoms of the Arnold-Chiari malformation. Three types of Klippel-Feil syndrome are evident radiographically. In type I, the vertebrae are fused massively into blocks (Fig. 93–34). Type II fusions involve only one or two interspaces, and the patients are usually normal in appearance and usually asymptomatic. The most common site of localized fusion is at the C2-C3 interspace; the fusions are discovered only incidentally. Type III deformity includes cervical fusion together with coexisting fusion of the lumbar or thoracic spine. The affected vertebrae have a decreased AP diameter (Fig. 93–34). In very severe forms, the whole cervical spine may appear as a single block vertebra, which can resemble a long bone. Acquired fusions of the spine can mimic

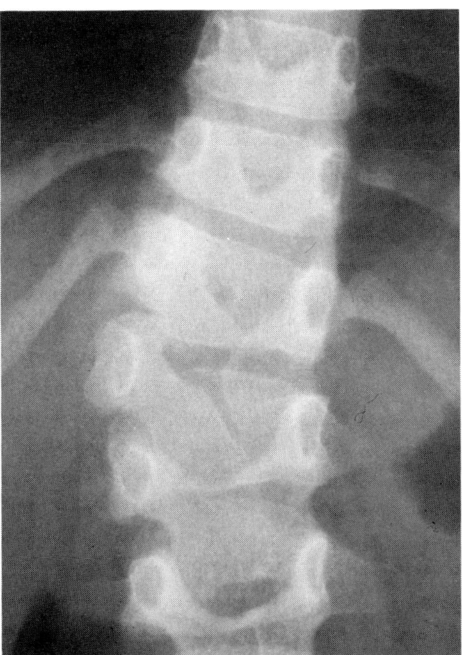

Figure 93–33. Hemivertebra. The left side of L1, including the pedicle, is absent. An acute scoliosis is evident. The child also had tetralogy of Fallot.

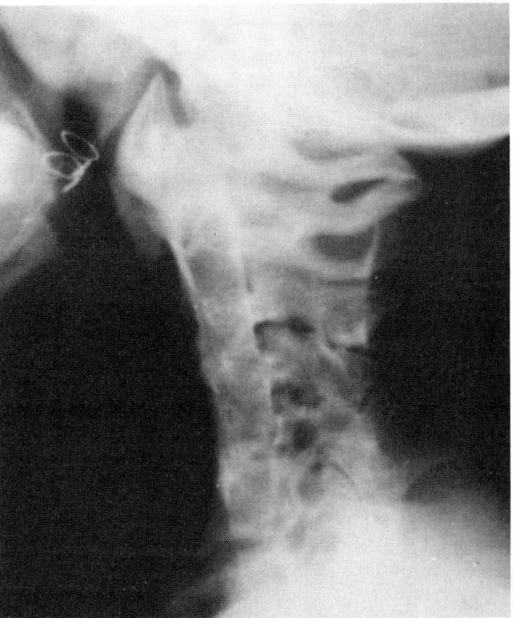

Figure 93–34. Klippel-Feil anomaly. This is a classic form of the disorder with all of the vertebral bodies appearing fused and decreased in AP diameter. The posterior elements are not fused.

Klippel-Feil syndrome and may be seen in rheumatoid arthritis and fibrodysplasia ossificans progressiva and with some other acquired lesions. Differentiation is sometimes difficult; however, many acquired fusions such as rheumatoid arthritis usually begin along the posterior aspects of the spine, involving the arches and laminae primarily, and only later do the vertebral bodies fuse. With the congenital fusions, it is usually the opposite. Fusion of the spine also occurs as part of other syndromes, including the acrocephalosyndactyly syndromes (particularly Apert's) and fibrodysplasia ossificans progressiva. The Klippel-Feil anomaly is associated with a large number of other anomalies of the skeleton, including other anomalies of the spine. Sprengel's deformity, congenital heart disease, and many visceral abnormalities may be seen with any segmentation defect.

SPRENGEL'S DEFORMITY. This deformity consists of an elevated scapula and is associated with the Klippel-Feil anomaly. In some cases of Sprengel's deformity, an omovertebral bone may be seen (Fig. 93–35). Hemivertebrae with scoliosis are also common.

SCOLIOSIS. The term scoliosis is derived from a Greek term meaning "crooked." It is a common deformity of the spine. Scoliosis is defined as a lateral deviation of the vertebrae from the midline anatomic position. Usually the deformity is not only in the lateral plane, but there is often a rotatory component as well. Scoliosis may be simply postural and may be associated with pain in the spine or abdomen. Structural scoliosis may be caused by congenital anomalies of bone, in which case it is considered congenital, or it may be acquired. The latter is the more common variety, and it is usually idiopathic. This type of scoliosis can occur at any age and has been classified into infantile, juvenile, and adolescent forms. It is most common in adolescence and is much more common in girls than in boys. A variety of congenital and acquired disorders may also be associated with scoliosis. Neurofibromatosis, for example, is commonly associated with scoliosis, often with a sharp angular bend. Scoliosis is seen in certain forms of dwarfism, such as diastrophic dysplasia, and in certain conditions, such as arthrogryposis. It may be secondary to problems in innervation, such as may be seen with spinal defects or poliomyelitis, or it may be secondary to an intraspinal tumor. It may be iatrogenic (e.g., radiation therapy involving only one side of the vertebrae), or it may be related to trauma, tumors, or inflammatory processes. Scoliosis may be associated with other abnormalities, particularly with congenital heart disease and with anomalies involving asymmetry of the face. Idiopathic scoliosis usually occurs before the age of 14 years. The incidence in the population is approximately 1.9 per cent. Two thirds of these are postural or functional in type, one fourth are idiopathic, and the remaining 10 per cent are divided among congenital, paralytic, and post-thoracoplasty. Idiopathic scoliosis is a familial disorder. Although the incidence in the family is relatively small, scoliosis is 20 times more common in families of scoliotic patients than in the general population.

The radiologic evaluation of the patient with scoliosis includes PA and lateral views of the entire spine from the pubis to the cervical region. The PA view rather than AP is used because it significantly reduces the radiation to the breast, which is a potentially sensitive tissue, especially given that most patients affected are girls. Also, the fastest available film/screen combination is used to further decrease the radiation dose because those children often have repeat films and fine detail is not necessary. The film is usually obtained upright. Sometimes recumbent films as well as films with lateral flexion are also obtained. The angle of the curve is usually measured by the method of Cobb (Fig. 93–36): one identifies the top vertebra of the curve—it is the one whose superior surface has the greatest tilt to the side of the concavity of the curve being measured—and a line is drawn parallel to the superior cortical plate; next, the bottom or distal vertebra is identified—it is the one whose inferior surface tilts maximally to the side of the concavity of the curve to be measured—and a line is drawn parallel to the inferior cortical plate of this distal end vertebra. Occasionally the end-plates cannot be clearly identified and the line is drawn at the inferior border of the pedicles. A line is erected perpendicular to each of these lines, and the angle of intersection of the perpendiculars is the angle of the curve. On the first evaluation of the scoliotic spine, great care has to be taken to look for various anomalies of the spine, particularly a spinal cord or bone tumor, which may present as scoliosis. Also, congenital anomalies such as diastematomyelia must be considered because if these are undetected prior to treatment considerable problems may result from surgery. MRI may be useful in children with congenital scoliosis to rule out diastematomyelia or tethered cord.

Dysostoses with Predominant Involvement of the Extremities

ECTRODACTYLY. The term ectrodactyly refers to various anomalies of the hand, including a split hand and transverse defects. A variety of forms may be seen. Many of them are inherited as autosomal dominant disorders; others are associated with a variety of syndromes.

BRACHYDACTYLY. A variety of brachydactyly syndromes are known and are generally characterized by the phalanges that are shortened. For example type A brachydactyly affects the middle

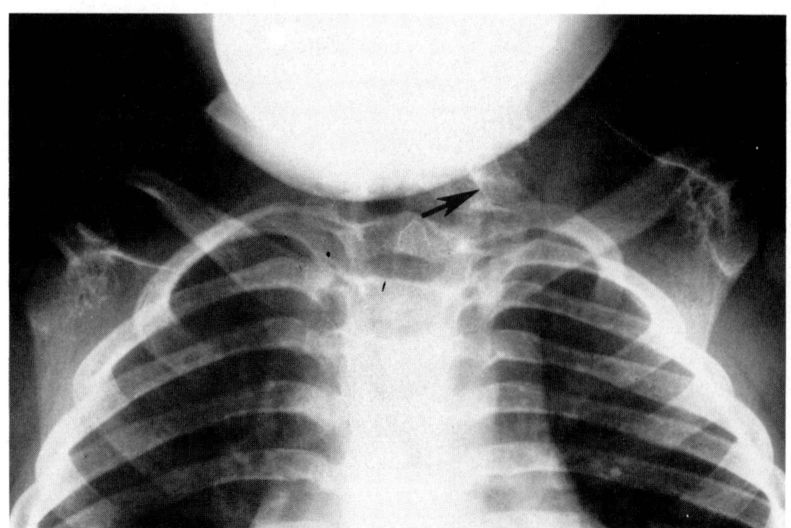

Figure 93–35. Sprengel's deformity. The left scapula is higher than the right. There is an unusual tubular bone between the spine and left scapula *(arrow)*. This bone is called the omovertebral bone and has been seen in association with this deformity. Klippel-Feil anomaly is often associated with the Sprengel deformity.

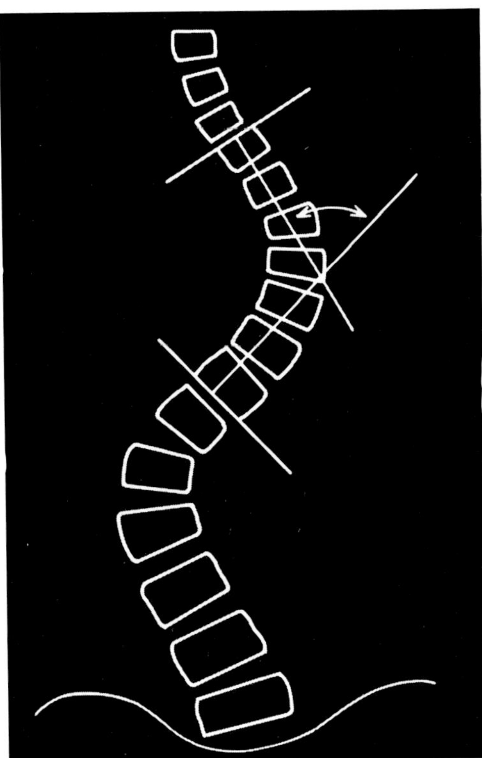

Figure 93–36. Measurement of scoliosis using the Cobb method. See text for details. (From Kittelson AC, Lim LW: Measurement of scoliosis. AJR 108:775, 1970. © 1970 American Roentgen Ray Society.)

phalanges and type B the distal phalanges. Most of the brachydactyly conditions are inherited as autosomal dominant disorders.

SYMPHALANGISM. This is a fusion of the phalanges of the same ray. The condition can be inherited as an autosomal dominant disorder. It is associated with carpal and tarsal fusions as well.

POLYDACTYLY. Extra toes and fingers can be seen as a sporadic abnormality or may be associated with familial disorders. The familial forms are inherited as autosomal dominant disorders. Polydactyly can be on the thumb side (preaxial) or on the side of the fifth finger (postaxial). Polydactyly adjacent to the fifth digit is a common finding in otherwise normal individuals, particularly in American blacks, in whom it is present in over 1 per cent of individuals. It may also be associated with a number of syndromes.

CAMPTODACTYLY AND CLINODACTYLY. These are curvatures of the fingers. Camptodactyly means curvature with a flexion configuration, whereas clinodactyly refers to curvature in the plane of the hand. The fifth finger is most commonly affected. Both camptodactyly and clinodactyly can be inherited as autosomal dominant disorders in otherwise normal individuals but can also be associated with a large number of syndromes.

POLAND'S SYNDROME (PECTORAL APLASIA–DYSDACTYLY SYNDROME). This is a disorder involving unilateral absence of part of the pectoralis major muscle, which is associated with hypoplasia and syndactyly of the ipsilateral hand. The condition is usually sporadic, and affected individuals are usually otherwise normal. Three fourths of the cases occur in males and are most common on the right side. There may be absence of the nipple or breast on the affected side. Radiographically there is hypoplasia of the affected hand with particular hypoplasia of the middle phalanges. There may also be hypoplasia of the forearm or of the arm, and the chest may appear unilaterally lucent because of lack of pectoral muscle. Rib anomalies have also been noted.

RUBINSTEIN-TAYBI SYNDROME. This is a syndrome of mental retardation associated with broad thumbs and great toes. The proximal phalanx of the thumb is sometimes comma-shaped and the distal phalanx is wide (Fig. 93–37). Other findings are less typical and include angulation deformity of the foot and an abnormal proximal phalanx of the first metatarsal, which may also be duplicated. Occasionally, pelvic anomalies are seen, with a flat acetabular angle and flaring of the ilia.

PANCYTOPENIA-DYSMELIA SYNDROME (FANCONI'S ANEMIA). Congenital anemia with pancytopenia may be identified at about five to ten years of age. It is associated with a hypoplastic marrow, and the patients may develop leukemia. Most of the affected children are of small stature and have hypoplastic genitalia. The condition is transmitted as an autosomal recessive disorder. The most characteristic radiographic findings are in the hand, where there is hypoplasia or aplasia of the radial side of the hand. The carpal bones on the radial side of the wrist may be absent, and the radius may be absent or hypoplastic (Fig. 93–38). The spectrum of findings varies from a small thumb to a vestigial or absent thumb. Occasionally, bifid thumbs may be present. Other radiologic findings include hip dislocation, Klippel-Feil deformity, and renal anomalies.

THROMBOCYTOPENIA–ABSENT RADIUS SYNDROME (TAR SYNDROME, THROMBOCYTOPENIA-PHOCOMELIA SYNDROME). This is an association of hypomegakaryocytic thrombocytopenia with bilateral absence of the radius. The hematologic findings occur at birth or during infancy and usually become less severe if the patient survives. The condition can be differentiated both clinically and radiologically from Fanconi's anemia, in which pancytopenia and other symptoms appear later in life. Although in most situations with radial absence there is significant hypoplasia or absence of the thumb, in the TAR syndrome, the thumb is usually present and may be normal in appearance (Fig. 93–39). This presence of the thumb when the radius is absent also helps to differentiate the TAR syndrome from Holt-Oram syndrome, Fanconi's anemia, or other situations in which the radius may be absent. Clinodactyly of the fifth finger is a common finding. Other skeletal findings include delay in ossification of the distal

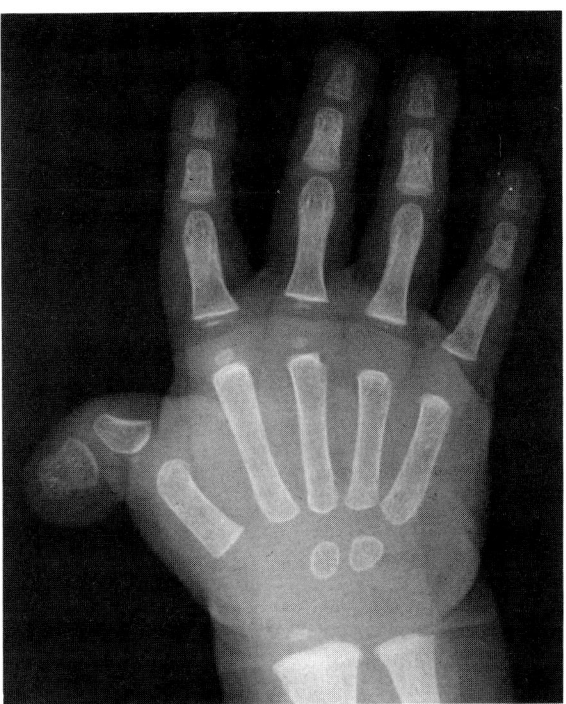

Figure 93–37. Rubinstein-Taybi syndrome. The thumb is short and radially deviated. The proximal phalanx has a comma shape.

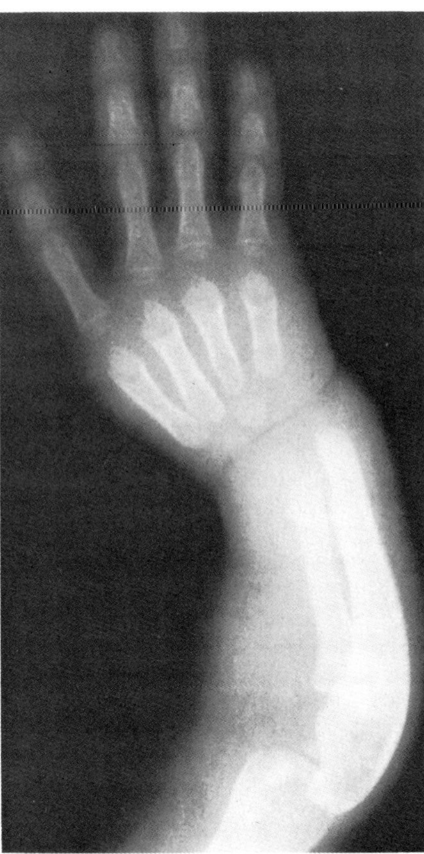

Figure 93–38. Fanconi anemia (pancytopenia-dysmelia syndrome). There is hypoplasia of the radius and absence of the thumb. These findings are not specific for Fanconi anemia and may be seen in association with a wide range of other anomalies, including anomalies of the heart, kidneys, and spine, as well as imperforate anus and esophageal atresia.

femoral epiphysis and abnormalities of the feet, including an overriding fifth toe, calcaneus valgus, clubfoot, or other deformity.

Holt-Oram Syndrome. This disorder consists of characteristic upper-limb abnormalities associated with congenital heart disease. The heart disease is usually an atrial or ventricular defect. However, pulmonary hypertension and arrhythmic disturbances are also common. It is inherited as an autosomal dominant disorder. The most characteristic radiographic findings are in the hand, where there is a wide spectrum of abnormalities. A triphalangeal thumb may be seen (see Fig. 93–1). This is uncommon in other disorders and should suggest the entity when associated with congenital heart disease. There may, however, be hypoplasia or absence of the thumb, in which case the condition may be difficult to differentiate from other disorders. It must also be differentiated from a simple association of radial absence and heart disease, which can occur in a sporadic way (the VATER association: *V*, vertebral; *A*, anal atresia; *T*, tracheoesophageal fistula; *E*, esophageal atresia; *R*, radial or renal anomaly). There is often a crooked fifth finger with a short middle phalanx. Carpal fusions may occur. Another interesting radiographic finding in the hand in this disorder is the presence of accessory carpals, particularly as os centrale in the middle row (see Fig. 93–1). Because this is a very rare normal variant, its presence is helpful in the diagnosis of this condition. The shoulders are often abnormal, with outwardly rotated scapulae and prominent coracoid processes of the clavicles that may articulate with the coracoid process of the scapula. The clavicles are thick in older individuals and sharply curved in infants. Accessory ossicles are also seen about the shoulder. Frequently the medial epicondyles of the humeri project medially and posteriorly, and occasionally there may be abnormalities of the humeral head. The lower extremities are usually not involved.

Proximal Focal Femoral Deficiency (PFFD). This is a disorder of shortness of the femur that is usually unilateral. It may be associated with focal abnormality when bilateral. It varies in severity from mild hypoplasia to complete absence of the proximal femur, including the femoral head. In the milder cases, these may be associated with coxa vara (a decrease in the angle between the femoral neck and shaft). MRI or ultrasonography is useful in determining the presence and position of the cartilaginous femoral head and neck in affected infants.

De Lange's Syndrome (Cornelia de Lange's). This is a syndrome of mental retardation, growth failure, microbrachycephaly, small mandible, small nose, characteristic down-turned upper lip, low-pitched growl and cries, eyebrows meeting in the middle, curly eyelashes, and hirsutism. Clinically, the thumb is often hypoplastic and may have a proximal insertion. A simian crease may be present. There is a wide spectrum of skeletal abnormalities in this condition, ranging from minor defects to phocomelia. The most characteristic finding, which is not seen in all cases, is hypoplasia of both the radial and ulnar sides of the hand (Fig. 93–40). This type of involvement is not seen in very many other disorders and is, therefore, diagnostically useful. The thumb is usually very short or completely absent. The first metacarpal may simply be a small nodule. There may be some shortening of the distal phalanx of the thumb. Clinodactyly of the fifth finger occurs in a large percentage of cases. When phocomelia is present, the findings are nonspecific. Other findings include foot deformities and rib anomalies.

Arthrogryposis. This is a disorder of multiple contractures

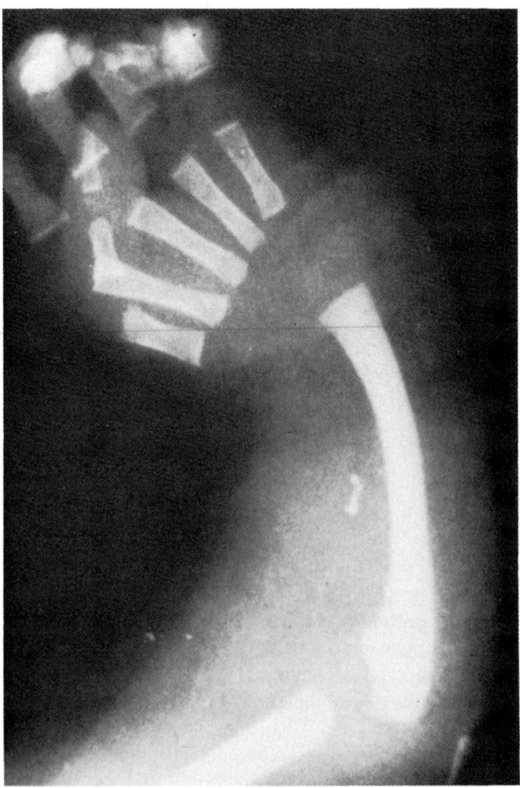

Figure 93–39. Thrombocytopenia–absent radius syndrome. Most disorders having an absent radius have absent thumbs as well. When the thumb is present with an absent radius, it is very suggestive of the thrombocytopenia–absent radius syndrome. (Compare with Figure 93–38.)

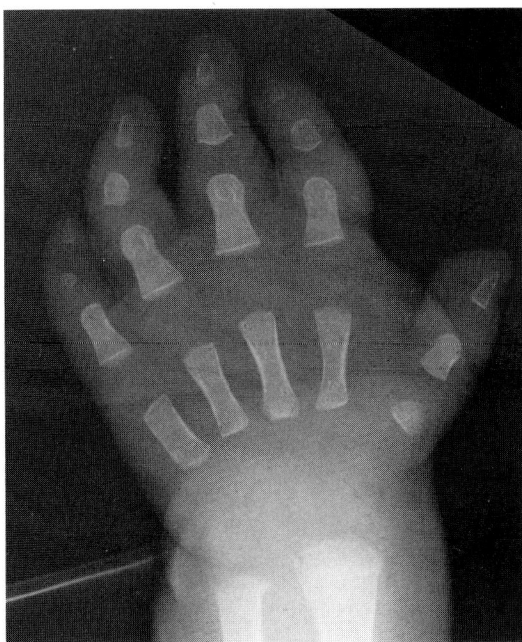

Figure 93–40. de Lange syndrome. Although various patterns can be seen in this condition, the pattern illustrated here is almost diagnostic of the disease. Hypoplasia of both the radial and ulnar sides of the hand with a very short first metacarpal and a very short fifth finger is characteristic.

that are present at birth and appear nonprogressive; these may be associated with bone anomalies. Although many conditions produce contractures, the term *arthrogryposis* is used primarily for those situations in which a specific condition cannot be identified. The pathogenesis of arthrogryposis is related to lack of movement of the fetus in utero. The cause of lack of motion is not clear, and it may be due to a primary agent, such as a virus, that damages the spine or causes neurogenic or myogenic damage. The radiographic findings include abnormalities of the extremities, including dislocations of various joints, diminished muscle mass, ulnar flexion and ulnar deviation of the hand, and clubfeet. There may be progressive fusion of the carpal and/or tarsal bones.

IDIOPATHIC OSTEOLYSES

Phalangeal Osteolysis (Hajdu-Cheney Syndrome). Individuals with this disorder have short fingers that may be broad distally, slightly clubbed, and often tender. Nails are often short and broad. Other features include some increased mobility of the joints, bones that are prone to fractures, and coarse, stiff hair. The condition is inherited as an autosomal dominant disorder. The most characteristic radiographic findings are erosions of the tips of the tufts of the distal phalanges of the hands and feet. The erosion may vary from slight loss of the tuft to destruction of most of the distal phalanx, with only the base of the phalanx remaining. The distal phalanx of the ring finger is often spared. The osteolytic lesions are usually progressive. The erosions are indistinguishable from other causes of acro-osteolysis, including those seen in pyknodysostosis, in acquired forms such as that occurring in chemical workers, and in scleroderma. The familial history is useful in differentiation. An additional radiologic finding in some affected individuals is an elongation of the skull, which often has a dolichocephalic configuration (increased AP diameter), and there may be a significant basilar impression and delayed closure of the cranial sutures with multiple wormian bones (Fig. 93–41).

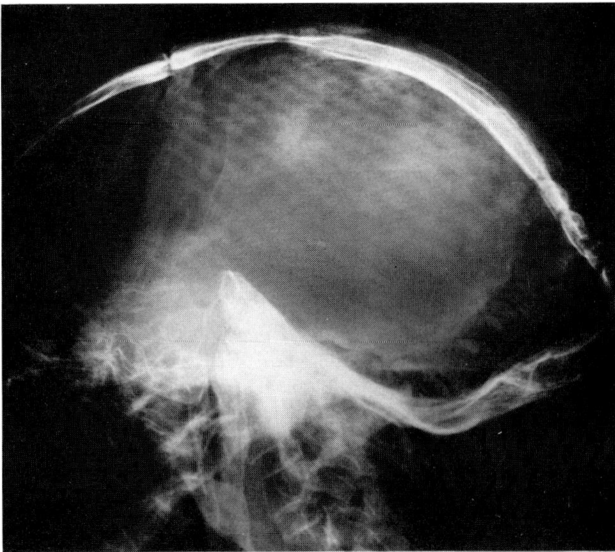

Figure 93–41. Phalangeal osteolysis (the Hajdu-Cheney syndrome). There is increased AP diameter and marked basilar impression of the skull with multiple sutural bones. (Courtesy of Dr. Scott Dunbar, Cincinnati, OH.)

Carpal-Tarsal Osteolysis. This is a heterogeneous group of disorders in which there is lysis of the carpal and tarsal bones. The symptoms are difficult to differentiate from those of an acute arthritis, and some forms are associated with renal disease and hypertension. Both dominant and recessive forms of this disorder have been described. Destruction of the carpal and tarsal bones occurs during childhood. The carpals diminish in size and become markedly distorted (Fig. 93–42). In the early stages, the findings can mimic juvenile rheumatoid arthritis, but later they are much

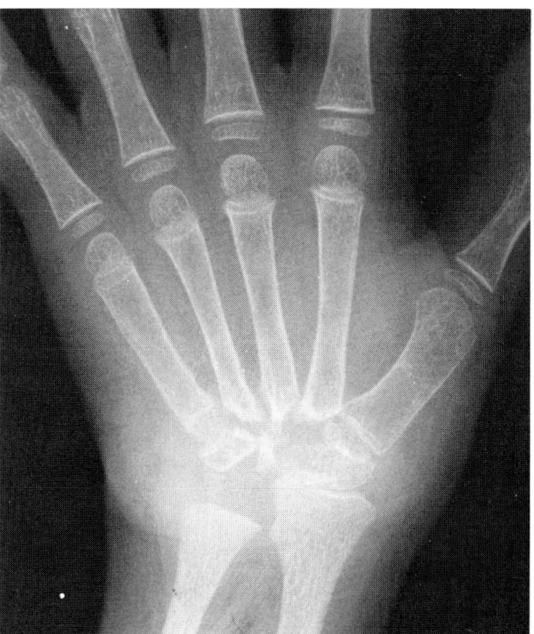

Figure 93–42. Carpal-tarsal osteolysis. There is a marked loss of all of the carpal bones, with the radius virtually articulating to the proximal portions of the metacarpals. The proximal metacarpals are also eroded. This condition can be confused with rheumatoid arthritis; however, the findings illustrated here are much more severe than are usually seen with juvenile rheumatoid arthritis.

more severe. In the severe cases, there may even be erosion and loss of portions of the metatarsals and metacarpals as well as other bone ends, particularly the elbow. The disease may become quiescent in adult life but usually results in permanent deformity and scarring.

MISCELLANEOUS DISORDERS WITH OSSEOUS INVOLVEMENT

Marfan's Syndrome. This is a connective tissue disorder. The clinical findings include long fingers and hyperextensibility associated with lens subluxation, aortic dilatation, and other forms of congenital heart disease. Affected individuals have a tendency to be tall. The condition is inherited as an autosomal dominant disorder with variable degrees of expression. The radiographic manifestations in the skeleton include long bones, particularly those of the hands. Bones of the feet are thin and long with prominent elongation of the first metatarsal and great toe. Sometimes there is a severe flatfoot deformity. Dislocations, kyphoscoliosis, and sternal deformities ranging from pectus excavatum to pectus carinatum occur.

Fibrodysplasia Ossificans Congenita (Myositis Ossificans Progressiva). This is an unusual disorder characterized by progressive ossification adjacent to striated muscle. The condition begins in early childhood and is of unknown origin. Initially, there is swelling and pain, mostly around the shoulders and paravertebral areas. Clinically, one sees the hypoplasia of the great toe and sometimes of the thumb, which is present at birth. The most characteristic radiographic finding is the peculiar appearance of the short great toe, with lateral deviation associated with hypoplasia of the proximal phalanx (Fig. 93–43*A*). This has been seen in all cases of the disease and occurs prior to the calcification and ossification. The thumb may be hypoplastic as well. The areas of ossification are first seen around the shoulder girdle (Fig. 93–43*B*) but eventually involve all of the body. Exostoses are common around many of the bones. Fusion of the cervical vertebrae, particularly the posterior aspects, can mimic the Klippel-Feil syndrome.

Neurofibromatosis. This is a disorder with many radiographic findings. It includes multiple neurofibromas involving various organs, as well as many mesenchymal defects involving both bone and soft tissue. There may be café-au-lait spots on the skin. Inheritance is autosomal dominant, with high penetrance and a wide variability in expression. The clinical findings vary with the organs that are involved. Many different abnormalities may be present in the skeleton. There may be absence of various portions of the cranial vault, particularly the lesser or greater wings of the sphenoid. There may be defects along the lambdoid sutures and enlargement of foramina, particularly the optic or auditory canal, which may be associated with tumors of the cranial nerves. The skull is usually large. A sharply angulated kyphoscoliosis is one of the hallmarks of this disease, although it is not present in all cases. Tumors of nerves may enlarge intervertebral foramina. There may also be involvement of the cord itself, or the cord may be compressed by external tumors. Scalloping of the posterior aspect of the vertebrae is a common finding (Fig. 93–44*A*) and is sometimes associated with dural ectasia. In the long bones in children, particularly in the leg, there may be pseudarthroses (Fig. 93–44*B*). Hypoplasia or hyperplasia of bones may occur, or the bones may have a dysplastic appearance. Erosion of bones may also be seen. In the chest, masses may project from the spine. Rib notching can be present, or the ribs may be thin or ribbon-like in configuration. Occasionally, bilateral apical densities may be seen as a result of neurofibromas. In the kidneys, renal arterial narrowing may be present, which can be associated with hypertension. The renal arterial lesions are mesenchymal defects not necessarily associated with neurofibromas. Other vascular abnormalities have also been seen, and almost any part of the body can be affected by this disease.

Cerebrohepatorenal Syndrome (Zellweger's Syndrome). This is a severe, usually fatal, congenital syndrome that involves multiple body systems. It is a disorder of peroxisomes. The infants are severely hypotonic, and the condition may be clinically confused with Down's syndrome. They have a characteristic facial appearance. The pathologic findings include multiple small cortical renal cysts (which are usually not seen radiologically), liver fibrosis, lissencephaly, and evidence of excessive iron storage. The

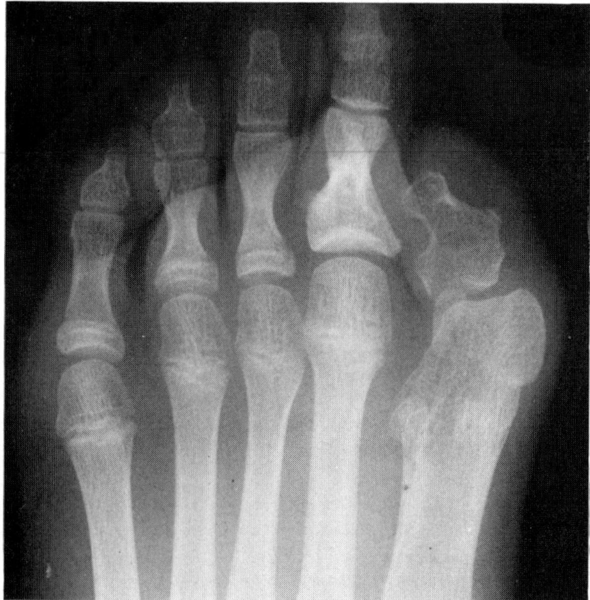

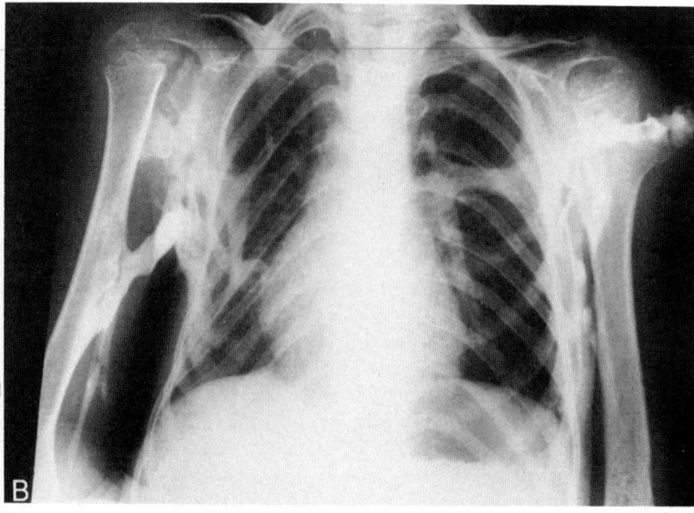

Figure 93–43. Fibrodysplasia ossificans progressiva. *A,* The great toe is short and deviated laterally. The proximal phalanx of the great toe is not a separate bone but appears to be fused to the metatarsals and produces a prominent bulge along the medial part of the foot. This configuration of the great toe is seen in all cases of this disorder. It is present at birth before the onset of calcification. There are also some exostoses of the proximal phalanx of the second toe; this is a less common manifestation. *B,* Extensive ossification around the shoulder girdle, which limits the motion of the humeri.

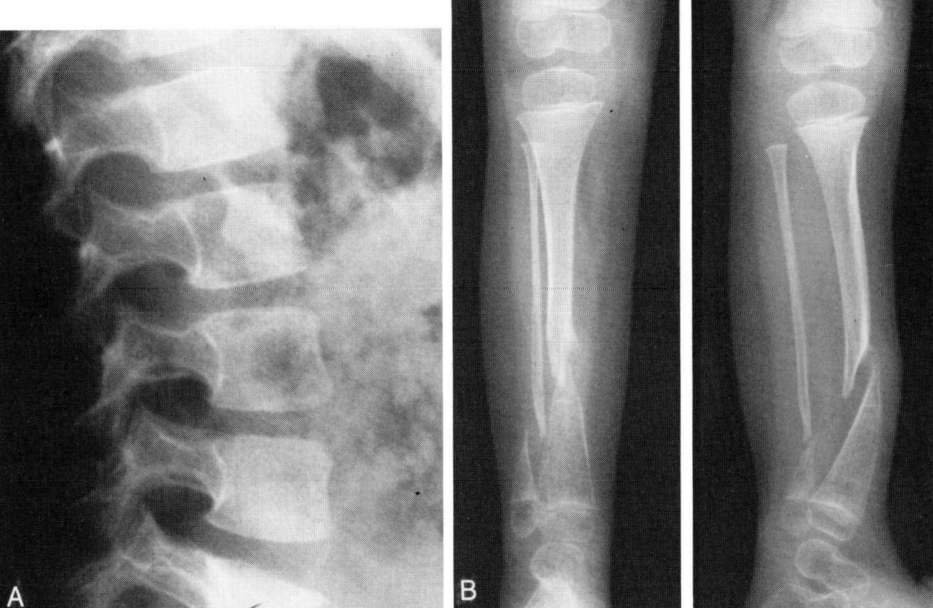

Figure 93–44. Neurofibromatosis. *A,* There is prominent scalloping of the posterior aspects of the vertebral bodies. *B,* Pseudarthrosis of the tibia and fibula. This pseudarthrosis can sometimes occur as an isolated finding but is commonly associated with neurofibromatosis. There is usually no neurofibromatous tissue in the affected area.

cerebral ventricles may be dilated. The condition is inherited as an autosomal recessive disorder. The main diagnostic radiographic finding in bone is the presence of calcification of the patella. The stippled calcification is similar to that seen in chondrodysplasia punctata, but in the cerebrohepatorenal syndrome it seems to occur most frequently in the patella, where it is best visualized in the lateral view. Calcification in other areas may also be seen. There is often an associated clubfoot or other deformity of the foot, and crooked fingers may be present.

CHROMOSOMAL ABERRATIONS

Although many chromosomal disorders have radiographic findings, they are nonspecific. Diagnosis is made on the basis of the clinical findings and the karyotype. Several of the disorders, however, have fairly characteristic patterns of manifestations. These include trisomy 21, trisomy 18, and Turner's syndrome.

TRISOMY 21 (DOWN'S SYNDROME). This is the most common of the chromosomal abnormalities and is due to an extra chromosome 21. The condition was described by Down long before the advent of karyotypes. The clinical findings include hypotonia, mental retardation, slanted palpebral fissures (thus the term *mongolism*), and relatively small stature. Other clinical findings include Brushfield spots in the eye and fine lens opacities. Congenital heart disease is common, with an incidence somewhere between 40 and 60 per cent; the most common defect is an atrioventricular canal defect. The children affected with this disorder have a greater incidence of other congenital anomalies. Although the crooked fifth finger (clinodactyly) was the first radiographic finding to be described in this condition, having been identified only one year after the discovery of x-rays, this sign is not very specific. Other radiologic clues that help to establish the diagnosis are a relative increase in the height of the vertebral bodies in the lumbar region in infants affected with this condition, and a double ossification center of the sternum. Although the latter occurs in approximately 90 per cent of young children affected with this condition, it also occurs occasionally in the normal population. Probably the most characteristic radiographic findings are in the pelvis, where there is flattening of the acetabular angle, large flared ilia, and reduction of the iliac index (Fig. 93–45*A*). Anomalies of the upper cervical spine with subluxation at the atlantoaxial joint and odontoid abnormalities may be seen in a small percentage of children with Down's syndrome. Because of the potential for cord compression, flexion and extension views of the spine should be obtained on these patients if they are to undergo anesthesia or be involved in active sports.

TRISOMY 18. This condition is due to an extra chromosome in the 18 position. Congenital heart disease is common. Foot deformities are also common, with the great toe usually short and dorsiflexed. A multitude of other organ abnormalities is also present. Most of the infants die within the first year of life. The radiographic manifestations most suggestive of this disease are very small pelvic wings that appear anteriorly rotated (Fig. 93–46) and are the opposite of the large flared ilia seen in trisomy 21 (see Fig. 93–45*A*). The ribs are very thin. The association of very thin ribs and an antimongoloid pelvis should suggest the diagnosis of trisomy 18. Other findings include an unusual clenched appearance of the hand, which, when straightened, leaves a V between the fingers.

TURNER'S SYNDROME (XO). This condition is due to an absence of one of the X chromosomes in patients of female phenotype. The children have a broad chest with wide spacing of the nipples, and they may have a webbed neck. At birth, lymphedema of the extremities may be present. There is absence of ovaries in most cases. The important cardiac finding associated with this disease is coarctation of the aorta. The most characteristic and well-known finding is the relative shortening of the fourth metacarpal (Fig. 93–47). If a line is drawn through the heads of the fifth and fourth metacarpals in normal individuals, it does not intersect the third. In adults and older children affected with Turner's syndrome, the third metacarpal is sometimes intersected (a positive metacarpal sign); the finding is not usually present in very young infants. It also may not be abnormal if other metacarpals are affected; for example, if the third metacarpal is short, it will not be intersected. In addition, the sign is not specific for Turner's syndrome; it can occur in other conditions such as pseudopseudohypoparathyroidism. Osteoporosis is common in Turner's syndrome. Skeletal maturation is usually delayed, but only in older patients because closure of epiphyses is sex hormone–dependent and these children lack estrogens. Other findings include renal anomalies such as horseshoe

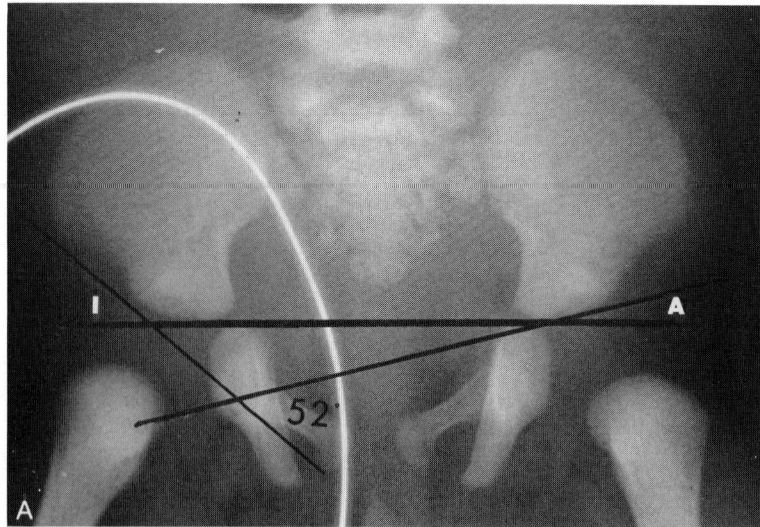

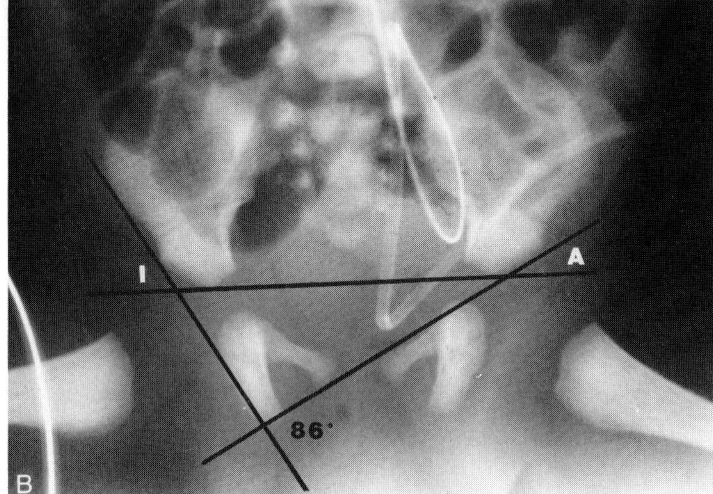

Figure 93–45. Trisomy 21 (Down's syndrome, mongolism). *A,* The appearance of the pelvis is characteristic, with flat acetabular angles and broad iliac wings. Compare this with the normal pelvis illustrated in Figure 93–10*B*. This appearance can be quantitated by measuring the sum of the acetabular angle (A) and the iliac angle (I), which has been called the iliac index. The angle made by intersection of the iliac angle on one side and the acetabular angle on the other is equal to the sum of these two angles and therefore equal to the iliac index. The child with Down's syndrome has an angle of 52 degrees. *B,* Normal value for the iliac index in the neonate is 84 degrees, with the ± two standard deviation range being 72 to 95 degrees. This normal child has an angle of 86 degrees.

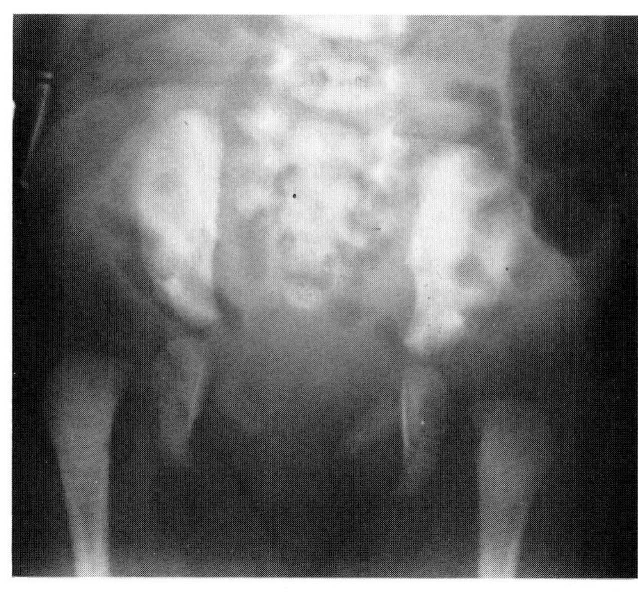

Figure 93–46. Trisomy 18. The pelvic wings are very small and anteriorly rotated. The opposite configuration is seen in trisomy 21. This appearance has been termed antimongoloid.

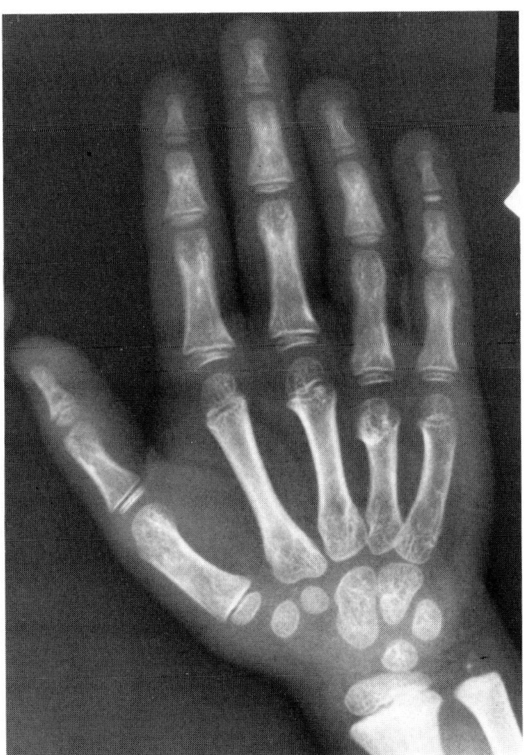

Figure 93–47. Turner's syndrome. There is shortening of the fourth metacarpal with early closure of the growth plate of that bone. There is no shortening of the distal phalanges, in contradistinction to pseudohypoparathyroidism, in which they are frequently short (see Fig. 93–48).

kidney and duplication. Absence of ovaries can usually be demonstrated with ultrasonography.

PRIMARY METABOLIC ABNORMALITIES

Calcium and Phosphorus Abnormalities

HYPOPHOSPHATASIA. This is an inherited metabolic abnormality that is characterized by low serum and tissue alkaline phosphatase and the presence of excess phosphoethanolamine in the urine. The condition is inherited as an autosomal recessive disorder. The characteristic radiographic finding is the irregularity of the metaphyses of various bones. There may be cupping and fraying of the metaphyseal margin. The appearance of the metaphyses differs somewhat from that in rickets in that the metaphyseal abnormalities are often more punched out and discrete than is seen in rickets. Fractures of the long bones and premature synostosis of cranial sutures occur. The severity of this disorder may vary from almost totally absent bones to very mild rachitic indentations in the skeleton.

PSEUDOHYPOPARATHYROIDISM. This is a disorder characterized by hypocalcemia and hyperphosphatemia similar to that seen in hypoparathyroidism, but the affected individuals do not respond to parathyroid hormone. The patients are usually short, obese, and mentally retarded, and have small hands. The metacarpals are short, particularly the fourth (Fig. 93–48), but any of the metacarpals may be affected; thus, the metacarpal sign may not be useful. There is also shortening of the distal phalanges, particularly the thumb, and this occurs more frequently than the shortened metacarpals. There may be soft-tissue calcification in the extremities, and occasionally small exostoses are seen in the hand. Intracranial calcification in the basal ganglia also occurs.

Complex Carbohydrate Abnormalities

MUCOPOLYSACCHARIDOSES. This is a large group of disorders that now contains at least eight well-defined forms. They are separated on the basis of the enzyme defect. The Hurler form (type I), which is the most severe and best known, is associated with severe mental retardation. The Hunter form (type II) is a sex-linked form that occurs only in males and generally appears milder, although some severe forms are also recognized. In the Sanfilippo form (type III), the patients have severe mental defects but relatively mild somatic and bony features. The Scheie form (also type I) is very mild and yet has the same enzyme defect as the Hurler form. The Maroteaux-Lamy form (type VI) has marked osseous and corneal changes that are similar to those in the Hurler form, but there is no intellectual abnormality. The Morquio form (type IV) also has no intellectual impairment; in contrast to the other mucopolysaccharidoses, however, there is no abnormality of bone modeling, but there are severe spinal changes with flattening of all the vertebrae. All of these conditions are inherited as autosomal recessive disorders, except for the Hunter form, which is inherited as a sex-linked recessive disorder. In most of these disorders (except Morquio), the radiographic findings include wide short bones with lack of normal modeling, and pointing of the proximal ends of the metacarpals (Fig. 93–49*A*). The skull is usually enlarged and elongated and has

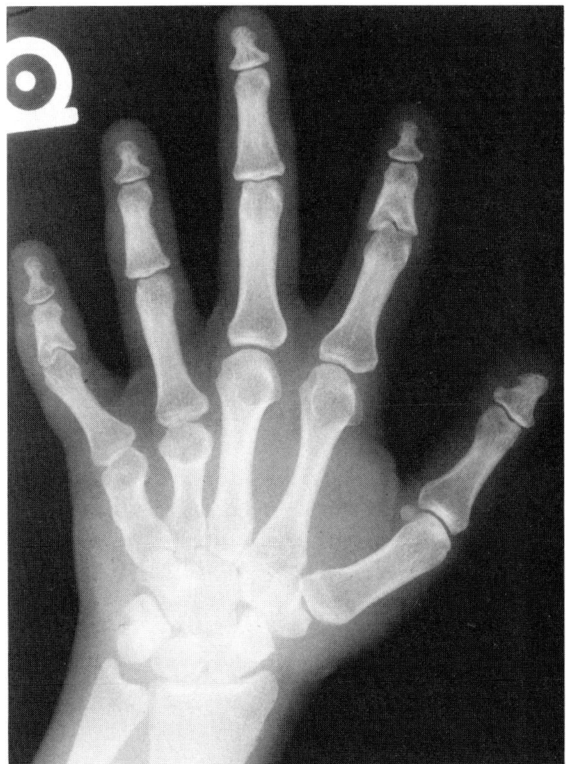

Figure 93–48. Pseudohypoparathyroidism. There is shortening of the fourth and fifth metacarpals. There is also shortening of many of the distal phalanges. There is cupping of the middle phalanges of the index and fifth fingers, which is the result of previous cone epiphyses at this level. The association of shortened metacarpals, short distal phalanges, and cone epiphyses is very characteristic of pseudohypoparathyroidism or pseudopseudohypoparathyroidism and helps to differentiate this from Turner's syndrome, in which metacarpal shortening may be seen but distal phalangeal shortening is rarely present (see Fig. 93–47).

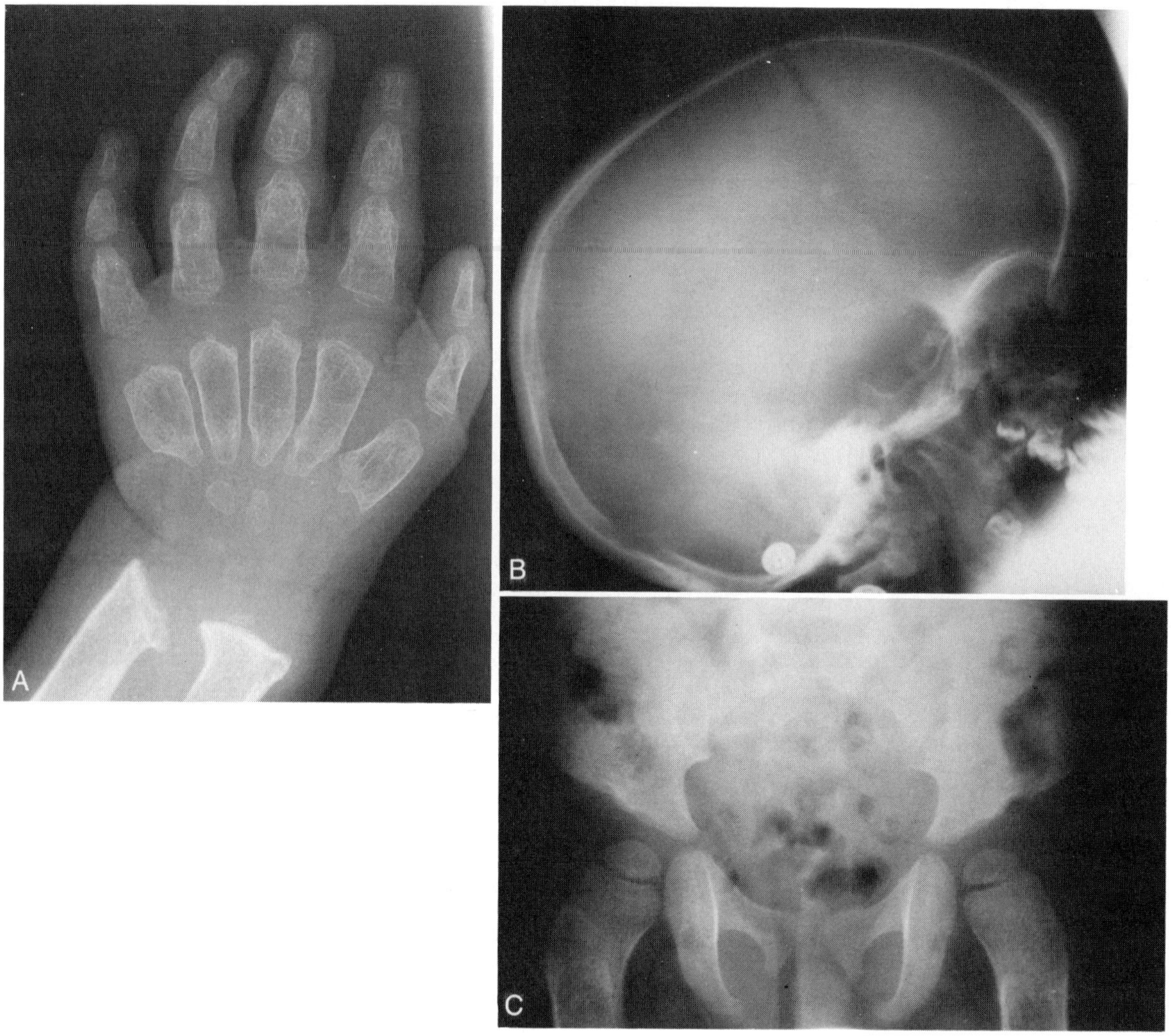

Figure 93–49. Hurler's syndrome (mucopolysaccharidosis type I). *A,* The metacarpals are wide and short, lacking the normal tubular shape, and are pointed at the proximal ends. There is also some pointing of the ulna and radius. The other phalanges appear broad. This appearance is characteristic of the mucopolysaccharidoses. *B,* There is a J-shaped sella, and the head appears elongated with some separation of the coronal sutures. *C,* There is thinning of the lower iliac segment at the part between the acetabulum and the lateral margin of the pelvic inlet. (Compare this to the normal ilium illustrated in Figure 93–10*B*.) This appearance has been a useful radiographic sign in the mucopolysaccharidoses and may occur when other signs are not present.

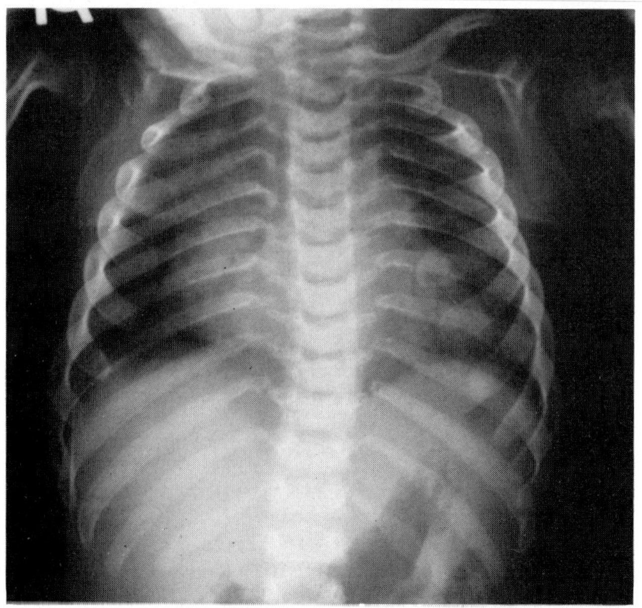

Figure 93–50. Mucolipidosis II (I-cell disease). The ribs are broad in their midportion but become narrow and pointed in the region where they join the vertebral bodies. This appearance has been described as "oar-shaped." This is also seen in the Hurler syndrome.

a large sella turcica (Fig. 93–49*B*). The pelvis often has a characteristic indentation with a narrow lower iliac segment (Fig. 93–49*C*). In the spine, there is anterior beaking of a few vertebral bodies around L1 except in Morquio's disease, where all of the vertebral bodies are flat (platyspondyly). The ribs are often thick, with a relatively narrow segment near the spine. The characteristic changes of mucopolysaccharidoses are seen most commonly in the Hurler and Maroteaux-Lamy forms, with very mild changes seen in the other types. The condition may be difficult to differentiate from the mucolipidoses, particularly mucolipidosis II.

Mucolipidosis II (I-Cell Disease). This is a Hurler-like condition that differs clinically from Hurler's syndrome in that its onset is much earlier and may even be apparent at birth, whereas Hurler's syndrome is usually not apparent until two years of age. There is no increased excretion of the mucopolysaccharides in the urine. However, there are striking findings in cell culture in which multiple inclusions are seen. It is for this reason that the condition is known as I-cell disease. It is inherited as an autosomal recessive disorder. The radiographic findings are similar to those of Hurler's syndrome but are more severe and occur at an earlier age (Fig. 93–50).

Lipid Abnormalities

Gaucher's Disease. This is a disorder of lipid metabolism involving the cerebrosides. It is due to absence or deficiency of glucosyl ceramide beta-glucosidase. Clinically, there is considerable variability depending on whether the findings are in a young or old patient. In young children, there may be hepatosplenomegaly, abdominal fullness, bone pain, and tenderness. The radiographic findings are also different depending upon the age of the patient affected. In infants, lucent erosive changes are present with some sclerosis. This occurs particularly around the hips, where an aseptic necrosis–like configuration may be present in either the head or the neck of the femur; fractures can occur. Subperiosteal resorption may also be present. In children, in addition to fractures, collapse of the vertebrae may also be seen. In older individuals, there is expansion of the bones with a lack of normal modeling and some sclerotic changes (Fig. 93–51). Early marrow changes can be seen with MRI.

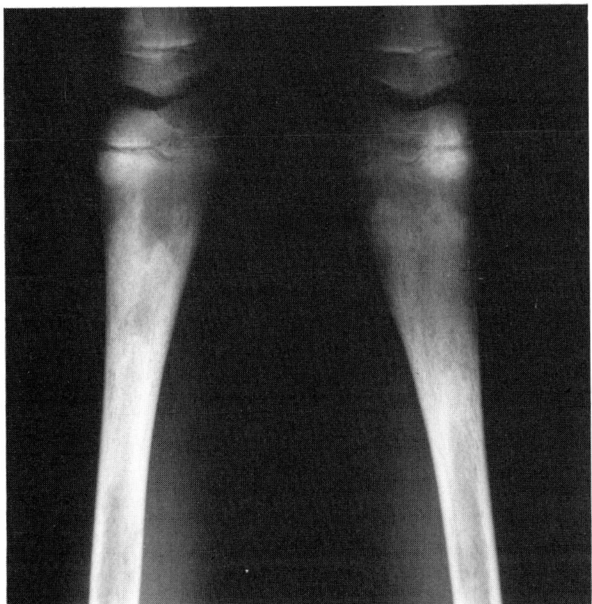

Figure 93–51. Gaucher's disease. There is lack of normal modeling of the distal femora with areas of sclerosis within the bone. The shape of the distal femur resembles an Erlenmeyer flask. These findings are typical of Gaucher's disease.

DEVELOPMENTAL DYSPLASIA OF THE HIP (CONGENITAL DYSPLASIA OF THE HIP)

The term *developmental dysplasia of the hip* (DDH) has been substituted for the old term *congenital dysplasia* (or *dislocation*) *of the hip* (CDH) because it is felt that the disorder is developmental and not congenital. DDH is most effectively treated when identified in the neonatal period. The hip may be subluxed or completely dislocated. Unfortunately, routine radiographs of the hips and pelvis at birth reveal only a partially mineralized skeleton with the femoral heads consisting of cartilage. This makes identification of subluxation of the hip more difficult. Lines projected from various portions of the ossified skeleton can be used to locate indirectly the position of the unossified femoral head. These include measurement of the acetabular angle, which is increased in DDH; assessment of lateral and superior migration of the femoral metaphysis in relation to the acetabulum; and determination of the relationship between the medial side of the femoral neck and the obturator foramen (Shenton's line) (Fig. 93–52). Subluxation in the neonatal period is much more common than dislocation. If not identified at this time, progressive subluxation can lead to frank dislocation. Because the femoral head is no longer within the acetabulum in the dislocated hip, formation of the normal acetabulum ceases and a false acetabulum begins to form. The femur continues to grow, and reduction becomes progressively more difficult.

If a subluxed or dislocated hip is suspected and the plain radiographs do not reveal this, ultrasonography (Fig. 93–53*A*) can be used to further delineate the anatomy. It is imperative, once DDH

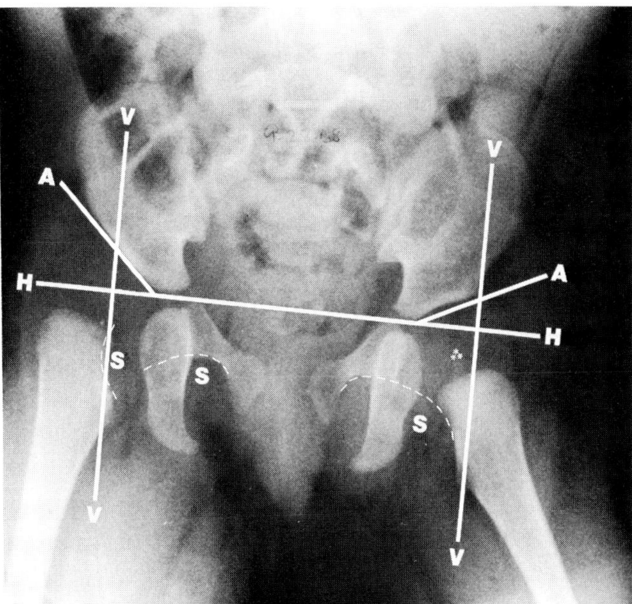

Figure 93–52. Developmental dysplasia of the hip. The left hip is normal, the right dysplastic. The horizontal line (H), or Hilgenreiner's line, is drawn through the triradiate cartilage of the acetabulum. The vertical line (V), or Perkin's line, is drawn perpendicular to the horizontal line through the lateral margin of the ossified acetabular roof. The acetabular line (A) is drawn along the slope of the ossified acetabulum. In the normal neonatal hip, the acetabular angle (angle between lines A and H) is 27 to 30 degrees; in the dysplastic hip the angle is increased. The capital femoral epiphysis normally lies below the horizontal line and medial to the vertical line in the medial lower quadrant demonstrated on the left *(asterisks)*. Shenton's line (S) is a curved line drawn along the medial border of the femoral metaphysis and the superior border of the obturator foramen. In the normal hip this is a smooth curve; in the dysplastic hip the curve is broken.

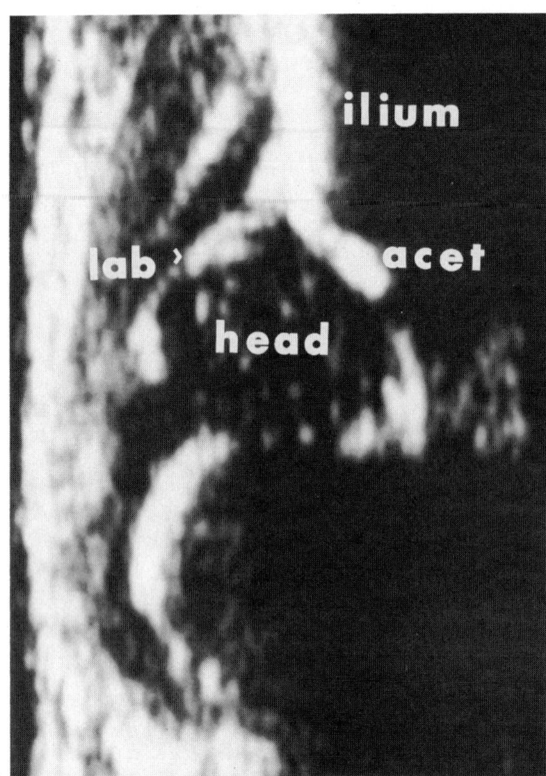

Figure 93–53. *A,* **Ultrasound of normal hip.** The labrum (lab) is echogenic and covers the femoral head. In dislocation the acetabular angle (acet) is usually abnormal and dislocation of the femoral head can be clearly seen. *B,* and *C,* Hip arthrograms in infant with developmental dysplasia of the hip. *B,* The normal beak-like configuration of the cartilaginous acetabular labrum is demonstrated *(arrow). C,* The cartilaginous acetabular labrum has been inverted into the acetabulum, forming a large limbus *(arrow)* in this dysplastic hip.

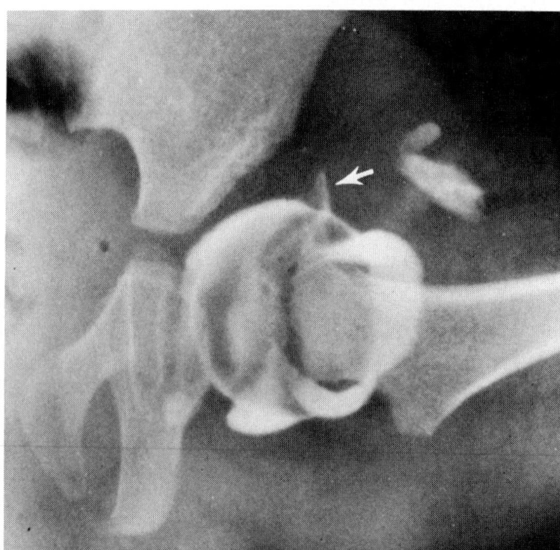

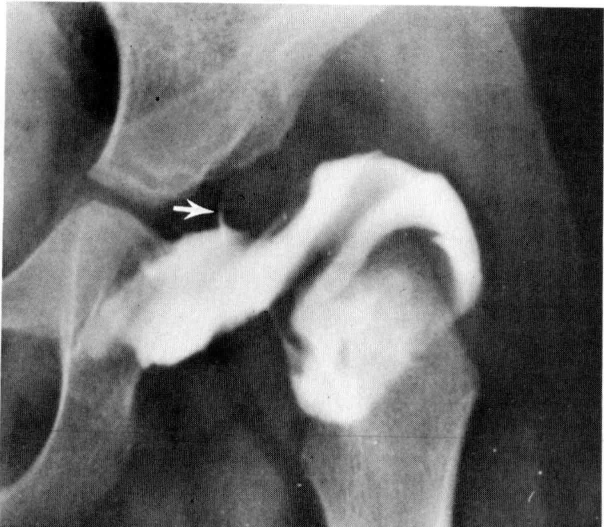

is identified, that the cartilaginous rim (labrum) of the acetabulum be identified (Fig. 93–53*B*). As the hip subluxes upward and outward, it may also merely push the labrum ahead of it. In this situation, the hip can be reduced and good apposition of the articular surfaces of the femur and acetabulum will be achieved. If, on the other hand, the labrum is inverted into the acetabulum, forming a limbus, the hip cannot be fully reduced owing to the interposition of this dysplastic tissue (Fig. 93–53*C*). With hip arthrography, ultrasonography, or CT, assessment of the acetabular labrum can be accomplished. In addition, the laxity of the hip joint can be assessed by stabilizing the pelvis and manipulating the femoral head to determine the extent to which it can be located, subluxed, or dislocated. Treatment of a mild DDH in the neonate can often be accomplished by keeping the hips in flexion and abduction (triple diapering). In the older infant a Pavlik harness, which also keeps the hips flexed, may be used. When adequate reduction cannot be achieved, surgery is required. CT and MRI are useful techniques for determining whether the hip has been reduced after surgery. The plain film in a cast is very inaccurate in determining whether reduction has occurred. (In our experience it is accurate only 50 per cent of the time.) Ultrasonography may also be used if a window is cut in the cast but is not as definitive in some cases.

FOOT ANOMALIES

Weight-bearing views of the foot in the frontal and lateral projections are needed to assess the alignment of the hindfoot and forefoot in congenital and developmental anomalies of the foot. Only the more common are discussed here.

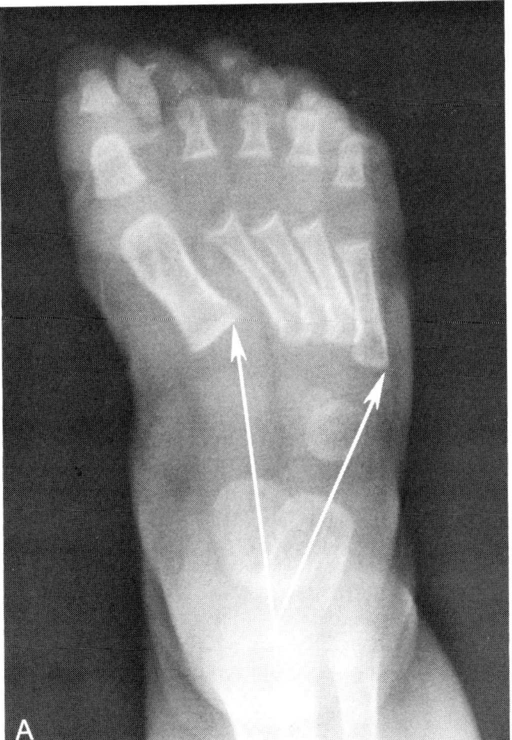

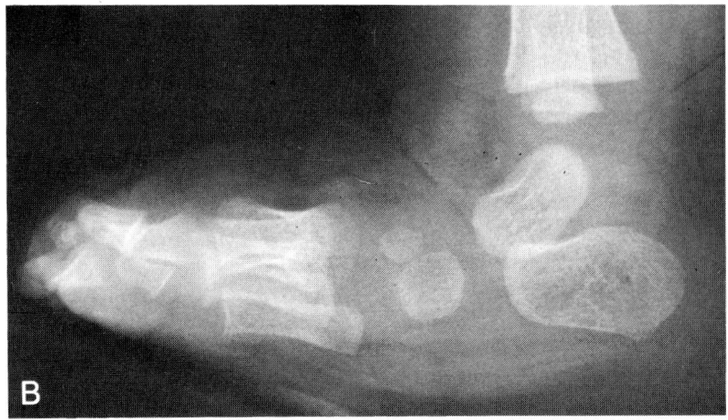

Figure 93–54. Metatarsus varus. *A,* A line drawn through the long axis of the calcaneus falls lateral to the midportion of the base of the fourth metatarsal, and the talar line is lateral to the midportion of the base of the first metatarsal. With a weight-bearing view, the talar line would fall even more laterally. *B,* The step-ladder configuration of the metatarsals is evident on the lateral projection.

Metatarsus Varus

In the normal foot, a line projected through the long axis of the talus on the frontal projection will intersect the base of the first metatarsal in its midportion. Similarly, a line drawn through the long axis of the calcaneus will intersect the midportion of the base of the fourth metatarsal (Fig. 93–54).

Talipes Equinovarus (Clubfoot)

This is a more severe deformity. The talar line lies lateral to the first metatarsal, and the calcaneal line lies very much lateral to the fifth. In the lateral projection, the calcaneus and tolus are parallel and there is plantar flexion of the foot.

Heel Valgus

On the frontal projection, when the lines drawn through the long axes of the talus and calcaneus pass medial to the bases of the first and fourth metatarsals, respectively, heel valgus (flatfoot) is present. On the lateral projection the arch of the foot is flattened and the talus is more vertical than usual.

Vertical Talus

A congenital vertical talus can be demonstrated on the lateral projection of the foot along with the associated dislocation of the talonavicular joint. Because the tarsal navicular is not ossified at birth, subluxation between it and the talus cannot be determined on radiographs. The cartilaginous bones however are clearly seen with MRI. Metatarsus valgus is also usually present, resulting in a rigid flatfoot deformity.

Bibliography

Cohen MM Jr: The Child with Multiple Birth Defects. New York, Raven, 1982.

Cremin BJ, Beighton P: Bone Dysplasias of Infancy: A Radiological Atlas. Berlin, Springer-Verlag, 1978.

Gorlin RJ, Cohen MM, Levin LS: Syndromes of the Head and Neck, 3rd ed. New York, Oxford University Press, 1990.

Jones KL: Smith's Recognizable Patterns of Human Malformation, 4th ed. Philadelphia, WB Saunders Company, 1988.

Novick G, Ghelman B, Schneider M: Sonography of the neonatal and infant hip. AJR 141:639–645, 1983.

OSSUM, Parkville Victoria Murdoch Institute, 1991.

Poznanski AK: The Hand in Radiologic Diagnosis: With Gamuts and Pattern Profiles, 2nd ed. Philadelphia, WB Saunders Company, 1984.

Spranger JW, Langer LO Jr, Wiedemann H-R: Bone Dysplasias: An Atlas of Constitutional Disorders of Skeletal Development. Philadelphia, WB Saunders Company, 1974.

Tachdjian MO: Pediatric Orthopedics, 2nd ed. Philadelphia, WB Saunders Company, 1990.

Taybi H, Lachman RS: Radiology of Syndromes, Metabolic Disorders, and Skeletal Dysplasias. Chicago, Year Book Medical Publishers, 1990.

Warkany J: Congenital Malformations: Notes and Comments. Chicago, Year Book Medical Publishers, 1971.

Wynne-Davies R, Fairbank TJ: Fairbank's Atlas of General Affections of the Skeleton, 2nd ed. Edinburgh, Churchill-Livingstone, 1976.

94 Infectious Diseases

Murray K. Dalinka,
Bradford A. Yeager,
Michael G. Velchik,
and Kevin E. McCarthy

The presentation, diagnosis, and treatment of infectious disease of the osteoarticular system have undergone considerable changes in the past few decades. Newer and more refined diagnostic techniques, including radionuclide bone scanning, computed tomography (CT), magnetic resonance imaging (MRI), arthrography with joint aspiration, and percutaneous aspiration and biopsy, have led to earlier diagnosis. The more aggressive use of antibiotics and judicious surgical therapy have improved treatment.

PYOGENIC OSTEOMYELITIS AND SEPTIC ARTHRITIS

The incidence of classic acute osteomyelitis has decreased, but subacute presentations have become more common. The use of immunosuppressive agents and antibiotics has affected the organisms involved and led to antibiotic-resistant strains. The increasing use of prosthetic joints has created additional problems in the diagnosis and management of low-grade infections. Musculoskeletal infections have not been eradicated; in fact, the complexity and scope of the problems encountered in diagnosis and therapy have increased.

Classification and Pathophysiology

Osteomyelitis, or septic arthritis, may be subclassified pathophysiologically into infection secondary to hematogenous spread, direct extension from soft-tissue infection, and infection following open fracture or penetrating wounds. Postsurgical infections are a subclassification of the latter.

A knowledge of the vascular anatomy in different age groups provides an adequate explanation for the pathophysiology and helps in understanding the radiologic appearance. The blood supply to bone is mainly through nutrient vessels that make sharp, hairpin turns adjacent to the epiphyseal plate where they enter large sinusoidal venous plexi in the medullary canal (Fig. 94–1). In children below the age of one, some of the capillaries perforate the epiphyseal plate and allow spread of infection into the epiphyses and joints. Between the age of one and epiphyseal closure, there is no direct connection between the epiphyses and the metaphyses. The capillary loops are, therefore, end vessels. In adults, the growth cartilage is resorbed and epiphyseal anastomoses occur. The afferent capillaries lack phagocytic lining cells, and the efferent loops contain functionally inactive phagocytic cells. The metaphyseal capillaries are end vessels with stagnation of blood flow. The slow blood flow and lack of phagocytosis make the metaphysis the major focus of hematogenous dissemination of osteomyelitis. In children below the age of one and in adults, because of the epiphyseal anastomoses, osteomyelitis may extend into the epiphyses and the adjacent joint. In the hip and knee, the joint capsule is attached to the metaphyseal end of the bone, enabling direct communication with the adjacent joint in all age groups.

Hematogenous osteomyelitis may be subdivided into acute, subacute, and chronic types, depending upon the clinical presentation. It is often associated with a known focus of infection or underlying predisposing factor. Predispositions include skin and upper respiratory infections, intravenous drug abuse, umbilical catheterization, disordered immune function, and underlying systemic disease. Classically, acute osteomyelitis is found mostly in the pediatric age group. Patients present with rapid onset of pain; tenderness; and associated signs of systemic toxicity, including high fever and leukocytosis. In the preantibiotic era, the mortality rate was 15 to 25 per cent, and those who survived were often plagued by chronic complications, including deformity, growth disturbance, draining sinuses, secondary amyloidosis, and neoplasm.

In the past few decades, the clinical spectrum of osteomyelitis has broadened considerably. The prevalence has not decreased and indeed may be rising. In neonates, infection often follows an invasive procedure such as umbilical catheterization. Involvement of multiple bones and effusions in the adjacent joints are common. In children and adults, osteomyelitis often presents in a subacute fashion. Clinical signs and symptoms are relatively mild with local pain,

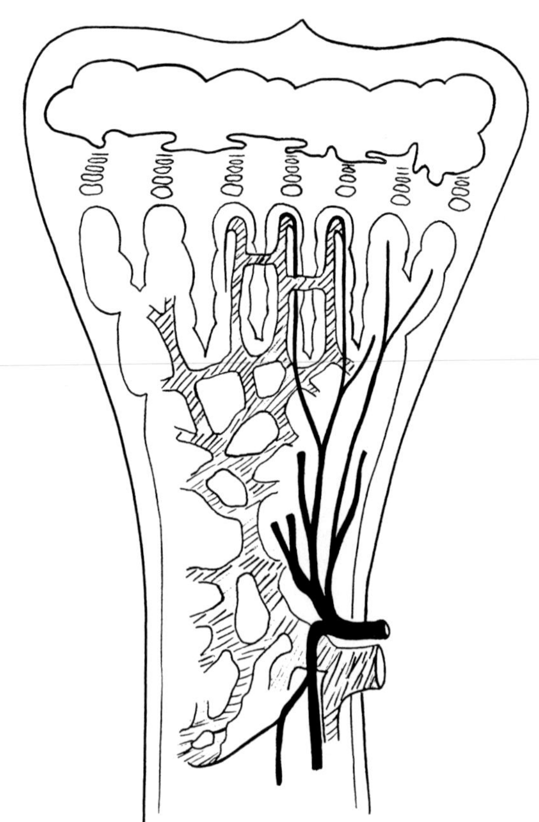

Figure 94–1. Diagrammatic representation of the **vascular supply at the end of a long bone** in a growing rabbit. (Reprinted with permission from Dalinka MK, Lally JF, Koniver G, Coren GS: The radiology of osseous and articular infections. CRC Crit Rev Clin Radiol Nucl Med 7:1, 1975, with permission. Copyright, CRC Press, Inc., Boca Raton, FL.)

normal temperature, and the absence of systemic toxicity. The erythrocyte sedimentation rate is frequently slightly elevated, and blood cultures are often normal. Approximately 20 per cent of the lesions show no growth on direct culture. The incidence of chronic osteomyelitis following acute hematogenous osteomyelitis has decreased considerably. Chronic osteomyelitis now most often follows infected fractures or prosthetic joint replacement.

Osteomyelitis and septic arthritis may be secondary to direct extension from a soft-tissue infection. This may be seen in patients with skin ulcerations or nailbed infections. Patients with decubitus ulceration are prone to contiguous infection. Occasionally, patients with decubitus ulcers and spastic paraplegia may develop septic dislocation of the hip. Open fractures, penetrating wounds, or animal bites, with or without foreign body penetration, may lead to osteomyelitis or septic arthritis. Surgical procedures, particularly those associated with the use of inert avascular devices such as joint replacements, may be followed by insidious infections that are often difficult to diagnose and treat.

Radiologic Appearance and Diagnosis

The radiologic findings in acute hematogenous infection mirror the evolving pathophysiologic changes. In the first three days following the onset of symptoms the radiologic findings are limited to local, deep soft-tissue swelling in the metaphyseal region continuous with the underlying bone. The findings are frequently very subtle, with displacement of the deep muscle planes best appreciated when a comparison view is available. Pathologically, the periosteum is thickened with increased vascularity. Pus is frequently absent at this stage, although bone aspirate cultures are often positive. Early diagnosis with treatment at this time often results in a significant decrease in morbidity with resolution of the inflammatory process without significant bone destruction. Swelling of the deep muscles with obliteration of the fascial planes between them is the next radiologic change, and it is followed by involvement of the superficial muscles with subcutaneous edema (Figs. 94–2 and 94–3). Early focal metaphyseal rarefaction and trabecular destruction may be present at this time, secondary to hyperemia.

When the osseous changes are absent or minimal, radioisotope bone scanning is extremely helpful. Scintigraphic abnormalities precede the osseous changes by approximately 10 to 14 days, and the diagnostic accuracy approaches 100 per cent (Fig. 94–4). Bone scanning is performed by intravenous injection of 10 to 20 mCi of ^{99m}Tc MDP (technetium methylene diphosphonate) in adults or 200 μCi/kg in children. A three-phase scan includes a radionuclide angiogram or blood flow study consisting of 20 serial three-second images obtained while injecting the isotope. At the conclusion of the injection the second phase, or blood pool scan, is obtained and consists of images of 300,000 counts. After the injection, intake of fluids is encouraged and the patient is instructed to void. Static scans consisting of 300,000 count images are obtained two to three hours later, completing the study. The use of three-phase scanning does not increase the radiation dose to the patient, although it causes a slight increase in the imaging time required for completion of the study. Its main advantage derives from the ability to differentiate cellulitis from osteomyelitis. In patients with cellulitis, the first two phases are typically positive and the third stage is negative or minimally positive. The radiation dose in rad/mCi is as follows: total body dose 0.013, testes 0.034, ovaries 0.10, bone marrow 0.35, and bladder wall (which is the critical organ) 0.13.

The use of ^{67}Ga citrate or ^{111}In-labeled white blood cell scanning may increase the level of confidence in the diagnosis of infection in patients with positive ^{99m}Tc bone scans. It may also be helpful in the presence of a high clinical suspicion of infection when the bone scans are normal or nondiagnostic. Gallium or indium scintigraphy is particularly useful in patients with underlying bone disease, postoperative changes, and trauma. Gallium is complexed to citrate and injected intravenously in a dose of 3 to 6 mCi. Approximately 25 per cent of the injected dose is excreted in the first 24 hours by the kidneys, and 10 per cent is excreted via the intestines. Gallium is not specific for infection, since it localizes in certain tumors, particularly lymphoma and hepatoma. Its bowel excretion interferes with the detection of abdominal infections, leading to the necessity for delayed images and delayed diagnosis. The target organs of localization are primarily the liver, spleen, bone marrow, and skeleton. The radiation dose in rad/mCi to various organs is as follows: stomach 0.22, small intestines 0.36, distal colon 0.90, gonads 0.25, kidneys 0.41, liver 0.45, bone marrow 0.58, spleen 0.53, and total body 0.26. Indium does not localize in tumors or surgical wounds, and bowel and urinary tract activity is absent. Indium has greater localization than gallium at sites of infection. This suggests an inherent advantage with regard to sensitivity and diagnosis because of the greater target-to-background ratio. However, indium is not readily available and requires an extensive preparation time. It is more expensive than gallium and gives a higher radiation dose to the spleen.

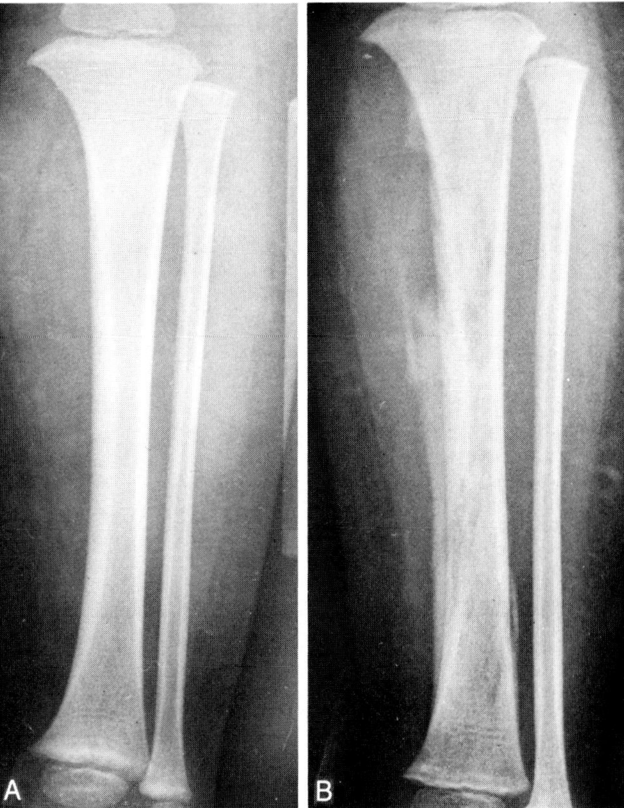

Figure 94–2. Acute osteomyelitis. *A,* Swelling and obliteration of the deep soft-tissue planes, particularly about the proximal tibia. *B,* Progression of infection with osseous destruction along the tibial shaft and associated florid periosteal new bone formation. (Courtesy of Dr. Orlando Cordero, New Jersey College of Medicine and Dentistry, Newark, NJ.) (Reprinted with permission from Dalinka MK, Lally JF, Koniver G, Coren GS: The radiology of osseous and articular infections. CRC Crit Rev Clin Radiol Nucl Med 7:1, 1975, with permission. Copyright, CRC Press, Inc., Boca Raton, FL.)

CT may occasionally be of value in the early diagnosis of osteomyelitis. Although CT is not specific, osteomyelitis can cause increased attenuation of the medullary canal, even in the presence of normal radiographs (Fig. 94–5). CT may be helpful in the demonstration of cortical destruction or sequestrum formation. The presence of medullary involvement may help differentiate between soft-tissue and bony abnormality. Therapy can be monitored by CT, as

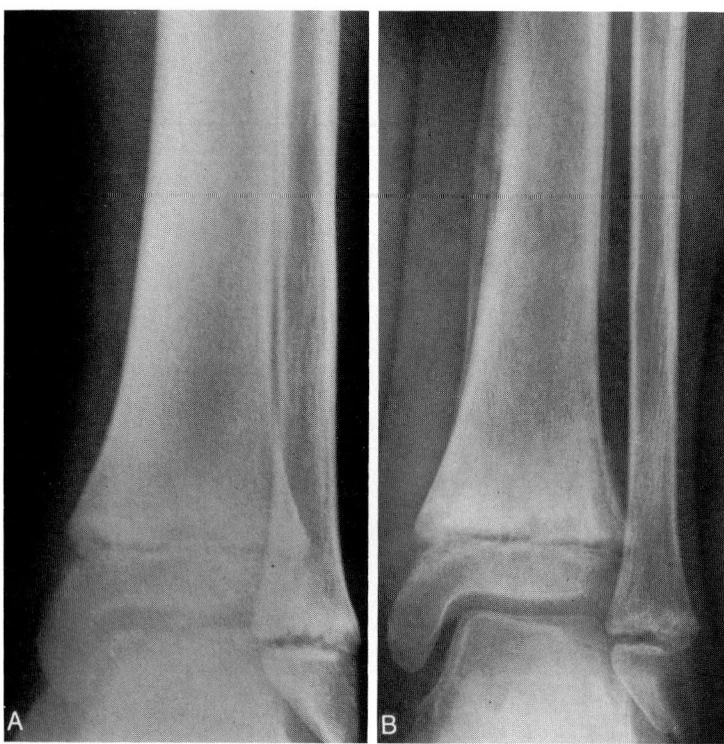

Figure 94–3. Acute osteomyelitis. *A,* Loss of the superficial and deep soft-tissue planes due to subcutaneous edema. *B,* Diffuse periosteal reaction along the distal tibial shaft. There is a metaphyseal destructive focus and a smaller area of periostitis adjacent to the metaphysis laterally. (Courtesy of Dr. Orlando Cordero, New Jersey College of Medicine and Dentistry, Newark, NJ.) (Reprinted with permission from Dalinka MK, Lally JF, Koniver G, Coren GS: The radiology of osseous and articular infections. CRC Crit Rev Clin Radiol Nucl Med 7:1 1975, with permission. Copyright, CRC Press, Inc., Boca Raton, FL.)

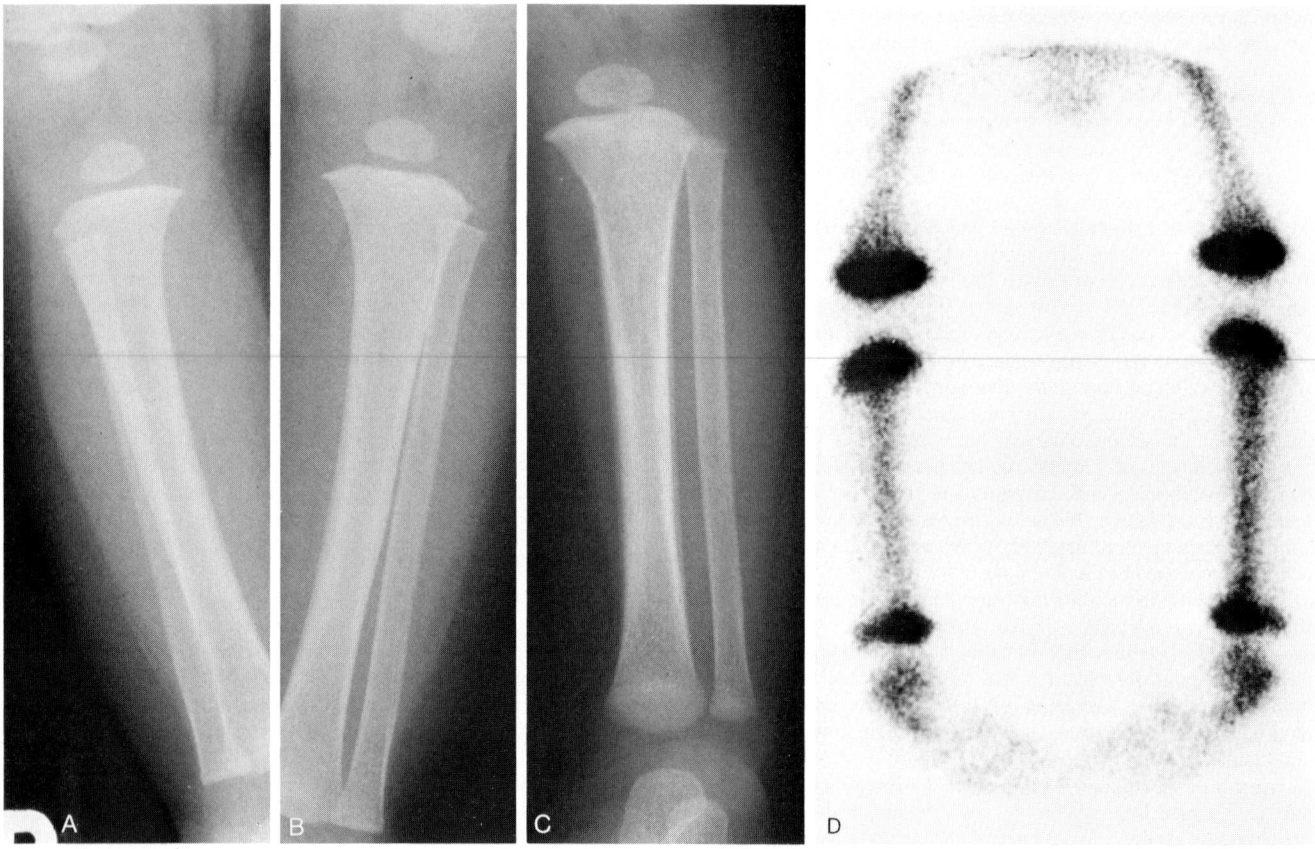

Figure 94–4. Acute osteomyelitis. *A,* Radiograph of the normal right leg (comparison view). *B,* Left leg demonstrating the loss of deep soft-tissue planes about the tibia. *C,* Anterior technetium MDP scan of the same patient showing diffuse increased activity along the left tibial shaft. *D,* Radiograph of the left leg taken 19 days following the original radiograph demonstrating periosteal new bone formation. (Courtesy of Dr. S. Mahboubi, Children's Hospital, Philadelphia, PA.)

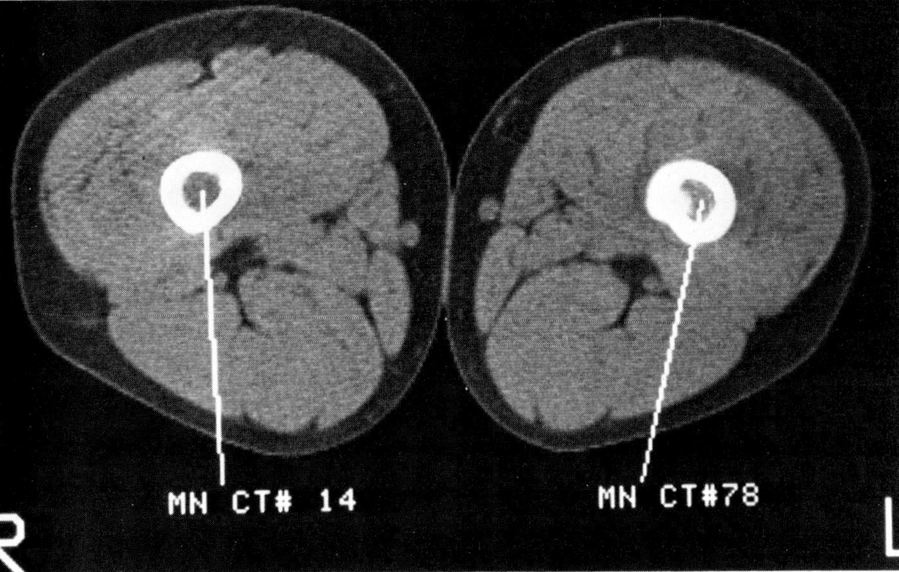

Figure 94–5. Acute osteomyelitis. CT scan showing increase in attenuation (increased CT number) of the medullary canal of the left femur. Periosteal new bone formation is present medially. (Courtesy of G. Mandel, A. I. Dupont Hospital, Wilmington, DE.)

the size of the soft-tissue mass and CT numbers both decrease with treatment. However, CT is expensive and may not be readily available on an emergency basis. CT is nonspecific and cannot distinguish between intramedullary infection and tumor. Density measurement errors occur and the axial extent of infection cannot be accurately assessed because of the cross-sectional format.

At the present time, MRI is considered to be more specific and as sensitive as nuclear medicine techniques in the diagnosis of osteomyelitis. The multiplanar imaging capabilities and high contrast resolution of MRI can be used to distinguish osteomyelitis from soft-tissue infection and may demonstrate the presence of sinus tracts. It is extremely valuable in the diabetic foot, where it can distinguish edema, effusions, localized soft-tissue collections, and ulcers from osteomyelitis. In most patients, chronic neuroarthropathy can also be differentiated from active infection; however, patients with acute neuropathic fractures may have signal characteristics similar to that of osteomyelitis. The absence of high signal on T_2 weighing suggests a chronic, inactive process. The same criteria may be helpful in differentiating inactive from chronic complicated osteomyelitis.

Marrow infection usually causes a decrease in signal intensity on T_1-weighted images, which increases on T_2 weighing. Fat suppression techniques, including short-tau inversion recovery (STIR) and fat saturation pulse sequences, increase the sensitivity of MRI in the detection of marrow abnormalities.

In the spine, the use of paramagnetic contrast agents such as gadolinium–diethylenetriaminepenta-acetic acid (DTPA) has been proported to increase the delineation of epidural abscess, help increase diagnostic confidence in equivocal cases of osteomyelitis, and localize areas for biopsy. It has also been stated, but not proven, that gadolinium-enhanced MRI can differentiate active infection from infection that has responded to antibiotic therapy.

Bone destruction usually occurs 10 to 14 days following infection. The earliest findings are a poorly defined area of metaphyseal destruction that may enlarge secondary to the presence of an inflammatory exudate. The pus penetrates the cortex and elevates the periosteum. In infants and young children, the loosely adherent periosteum leads to widespread periosteal new bone formation. In adults, the periosteum is more tightly adherent to bone and its response is limited. When the periosteal new bone formation is exuberant and envelops a focus of necrotic bone, it is termed an *involucrum*. A *sequestrum* is an area of dead bone isolated from living bone by a surrounding bed of granulation tissue. Sequestra may be very small or as large as the entire diaphysis; they usually appear denser than the surrounding osteoporotic living bone. Sequestra may harbor viable organisms for many years and may be responsible for clinical flare-ups following long periods of dormancy. Occasionally, they may be extruded through perforations in the involucrum, termed *cloaca*.

Subacute osteomyelitis has an entirely different radiologic appearance based on a complex interplay of reduced bacterial virulence, host response, and incomplete therapy. The lesion may be localized to the metaphysis or metaphyseal equivalent sites. There is usually a well-defined area of bone destruction with a fading margin (Fig. 94–6). The destruction frequently extends to the epiphyseal plate and occasionally crosses into the epiphysis (Fig. 94–7). Periosteal response is minimal to absent, and the border of the lesion may be sclerotic. The organism is frequently difficult to culture. These well-defined areas may contain a tract extending from the abscess cavity to the cortex (Fig. 94–8). This serpiginous tract represents the radiologic appearance of the host response to the infection as it spreads along the path of least resistance in an attempt to decompress by penetrating through the cortex. The eponym *Brodie's abscess* has also been used to describe a circumscribed focus of bone destruction surrounded by a variable amount of bone reaction. Subacute osteomyelitis may occur in the shaft of a long bone beginning at the site of penetration of the nutrient vessels. Cortical and medullary destruction and periosteal reaction may on occasion simulate a round cell tumor (Fig. 94–9). These diaphyseal lesions are often associated with little or no systemic symptoms.

In patients with chronic osteomyelitis, the radiologic diagnosis is frequently difficult. Multiple factors may be responsible, including inadequate therapy for acute osteomyelitis, altered immunity or repair processes, draining sinuses, and large sequestra. It may be extremely difficult to differentiate active chronic osteomyelitis from inactive osteomyelitis and to assess response to therapy from continued infection. The presence of sequestra enables one to unequivocally make the diagnosis of osteomyelitis. Since these sequestra are avascular, they serve as a continuing focus of active infection (Fig. 94–10). Gallium- or indium-labeled white blood cell scans may be particularly helpful in this circumstance, since they are positive in areas of active infection but not at sites of treated osteomyelitis. Subacute or chronic symmetrical osteomyelitis may also present as multiple sclerotic lesions with soft-tissue swelling and slight periosteal reaction. In these patients, a plasma cell infiltrate is frequently present. Sclerosing osteomyelitis of Garré was first described in 1893. Lack of purulent exudate and bone necrosis

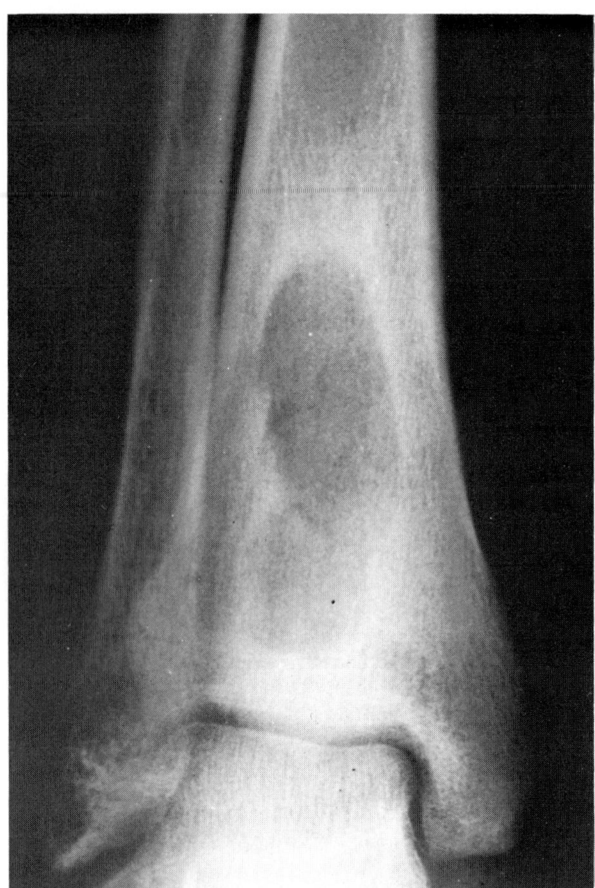

Figure 94–6. Subacute osteomyelitis. AP radiograph of the ankle reveals a large destructive lesion surrounded by a sclerotic margin that fades into the periphery.

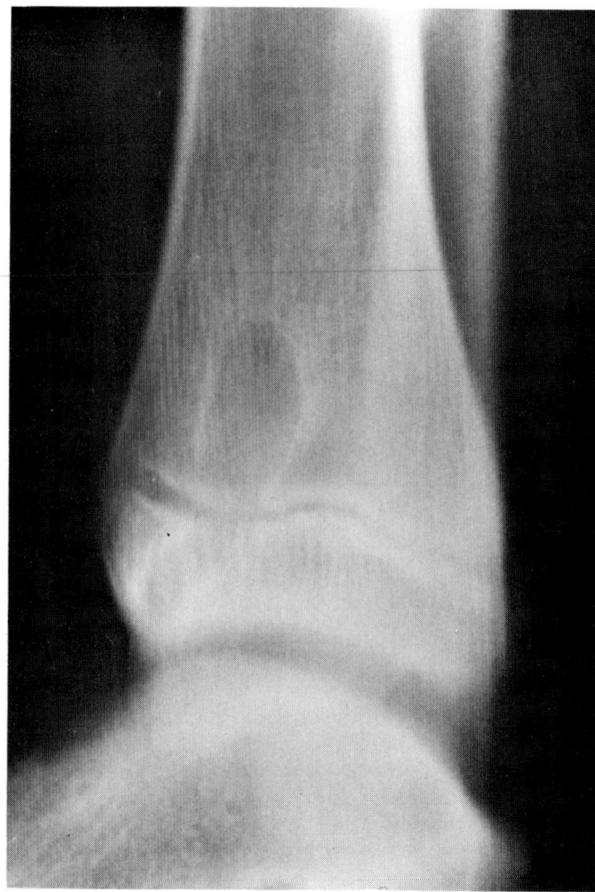

Figure 94–7. Subacute osteomyelitis. Lateral tomogram of the ankle demonstrates a destructive metaphyseal lesion with extension through the epiphyseal plate.

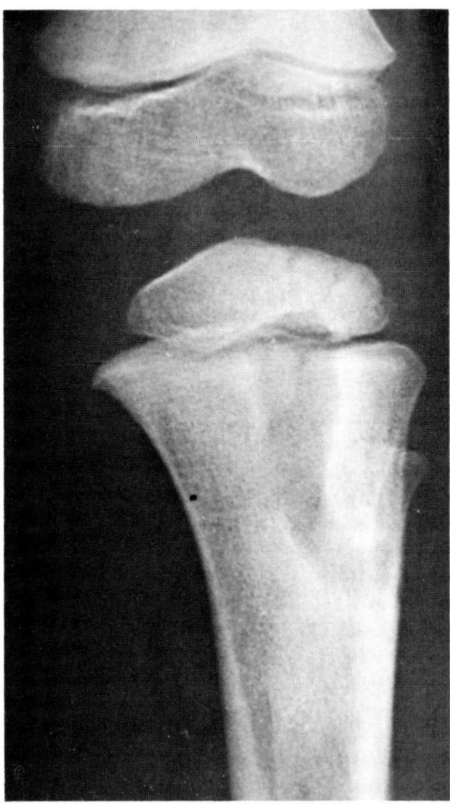

Figure 94–8. Subacute osteomyelitis. AP radiograph of the knee demonstrating a metaphyseal lesion with a serpiginous tract extending to the cortex. The epiphysis is also involved. (Reprinted with permission from Dalinka MK, Lally JF, Koniver G, Coren GS: The radiology of osseous and articular infections. CRC Crit Rev Clin Radiol Nucl Med 7:1, 1975, with permission. Copyright, CRC Press, Inc., Boca Raton, FL.)

were explained on the basis of infection by an organism of low virulence. Radiographically, there is thickening and increased density in cortical and cancellous bone without significant areas of rarefaction. It is now believed that many of the cases reported in the older literature as sclerosing osteomyelitis of Garré were erroneously diagnosed and actually represented other lesions, most notably osteoid osteoma. This rare form of osteomyelitis is most commonly seen in the mandible.

Vertebral osteomyelitis deserves special mention because of its increasing incidence and potential for serious complications, including paraplegia, meningitis, and atlantoaxial dislocation. The earliest changes on plain radiographs may not appear for several months and are characterized by narrowing of the disc space with irregular destruction of the neighboring vertebral end-plates (Fig. 94–11). Paravertebral soft-tissue swelling is often seen.

The radiologic diagnosis of postoperative infection, particularly following prosthetic replacement, is often extremely difficult. A zone of lucency at the metal-cement or bone-cement interface should raise the possibility of loosening and/or infection. This is particularly true if it is larger than 2 mm in size or enlarges over time. Scalloped irregularity of the lucent zone or cortex and periosteal reaction are other suggestive findings. Radioisotope bone scanning or joint aspiration followed by arthrography is extremely helpful in patients with painful prosthetic joints. The bone scan normally shows increased radionuclide uptake about the prosthesis for four to six months following surgery secondary to reactive bone formation related to the surgery and stress of the prosthesis. After the initial postoperative period, increased uptake about the entire prosthesis suggests infection. Loosening is indicated by abnormal focal areas of increased uptake in the region of the distal tip of the

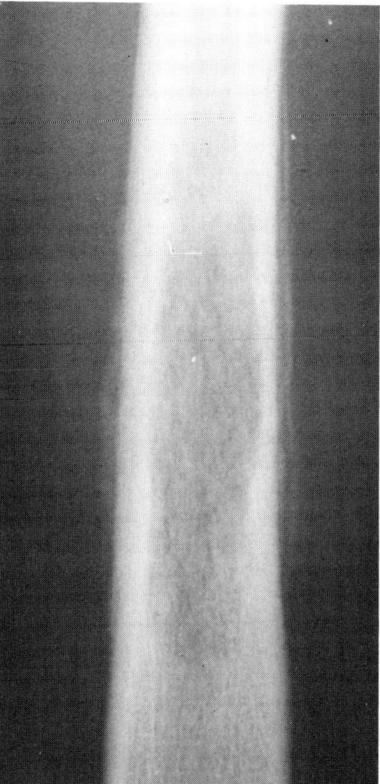

Figure 94–9. Subacute osteomyelitis. Destructive lesion in the diaphysis of the femur, with periosteal reaction simulating a round cell tumor.

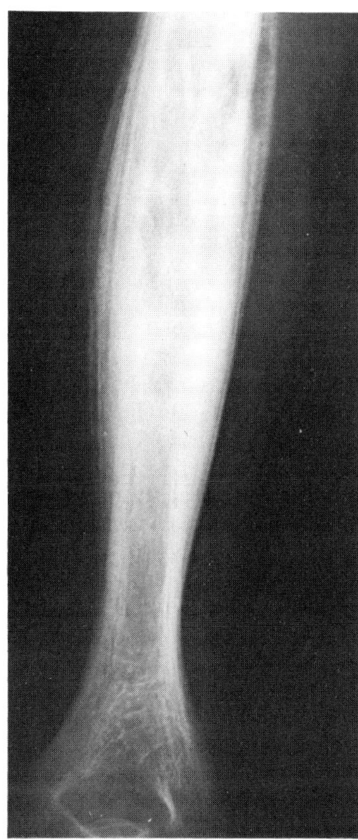

Figure 94–10. Chronic osteomyelitis. Large destructive focus within the humeral shaft with periosteal new bone formation and dense areas of bone within the area of medullary destruction due to sequestra formation.

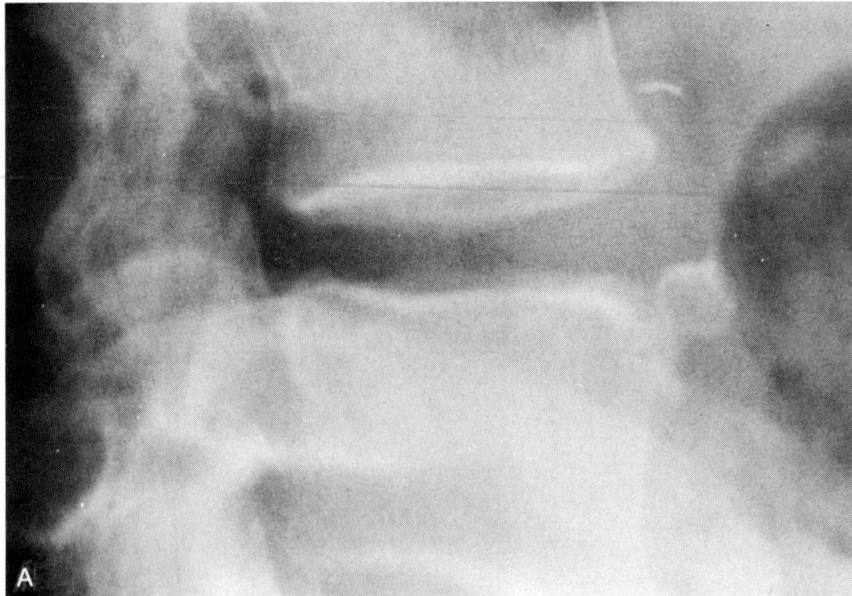

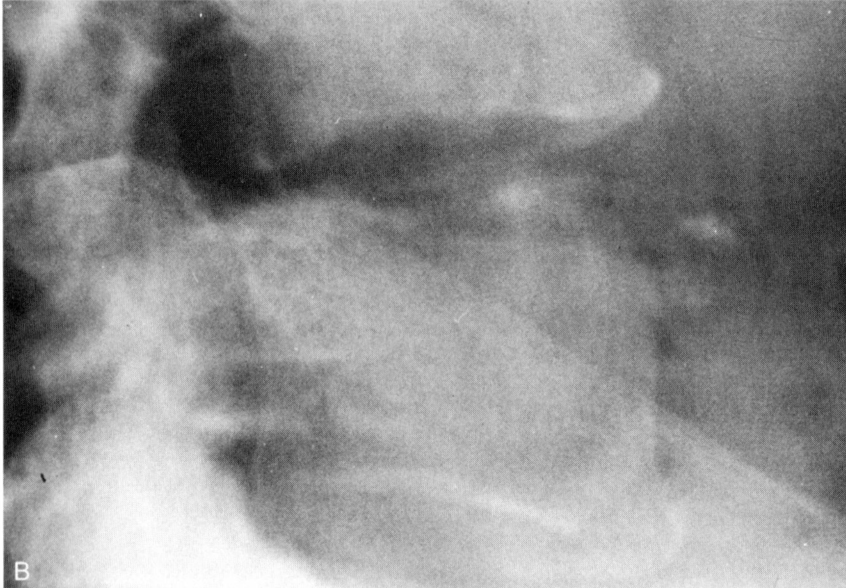

Figure 94–11. Pyogenic spondylitis. *A,* Normal lateral view of the lumbar spine in a patient with acute spondylitis. *B,* Same patient approximately three weeks later showing destruction of the end-plates of L3-L4 and narrowing of the intervertebral disc.

prosthesis or about the greater trochanter owing to increasing motion. The use of gallium-67 citrate or indium has been advocated as a subsequent imaging procedure to increase the specificity of the examination. Gallium or indium uptake that is greater than the technetium uptake is strongly suggestive of infection (Fig. 94–12). Hip aspiration followed by arthrography enables one to culture the aspirate and confirm the intra-articular needle placement and may demonstrate loosening of the prosthesis or abscess cavities communicating with the pseudojoint.

The diagnosis of septic arthritis does not and should not depend upon radiologic findings. Any patient with suspected septic arthritis should have the joint aspirated and cultured, as delay in diagnosis may lead to severe, early joint destruction, particularly in infancy and childhood. Involvement is most often monoarticular. In infants and children, the hip or knee is involved in greater than 75 per cent of patients. In adults, the knees, hips, and shoulders account for over 70 per cent of the cases. A predisposing factor is often present in adults; these factors include trauma, diabetes mellitus, infection elsewhere, and intra-articular steroid injection. Blood cultures are positive in approximately 50 per cent of cases, but recovery of the organism by aspiration of the joint is crucial to the diagnosis.

In childhood, the onset of septic arthritis is usually acute with fever, erythema, localized pain, tenderness, swelling, and limitation of joint motion. In infants, signs and symptoms may occasionally be minimal or absent, making diagnosis difficult. While a fixed flexed position or lack of movement of an extremity may raise the possibility of a septic joint, sometimes the only clues are nonspecific ones such as increased irritability or loss of appetite. *Staphylococcus aureus* is the most common organism isolated. In infants, *Streptococcus* and gram-negative organisms are also important. Gonococcal arthritis should be considered in any sexually active individual. Three-phase bone scanning is helpful. A diffuse increase in soft-tissue activity is present in the first two stages, with osseous uptake on both sides of the joint in the third stage.

The earliest radiographic sign of septic arthritis is adjacent soft-tissue swelling, most easily appreciated in the hip and knee. Accumulation of intra-articular fluid may lead to subluxation or dislocation. This is an important finding in neonatal septic arthritis of the hip, although this observation is sometimes difficult to make because of the lack of ossification in most of the proximal capital femoral epiphysis. Joint space narrowing may become radiographically apparent several days after the onset of symptoms and reflects

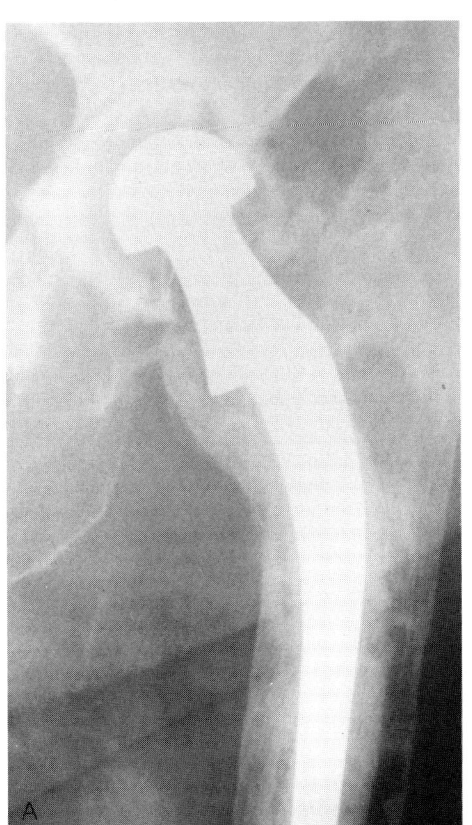

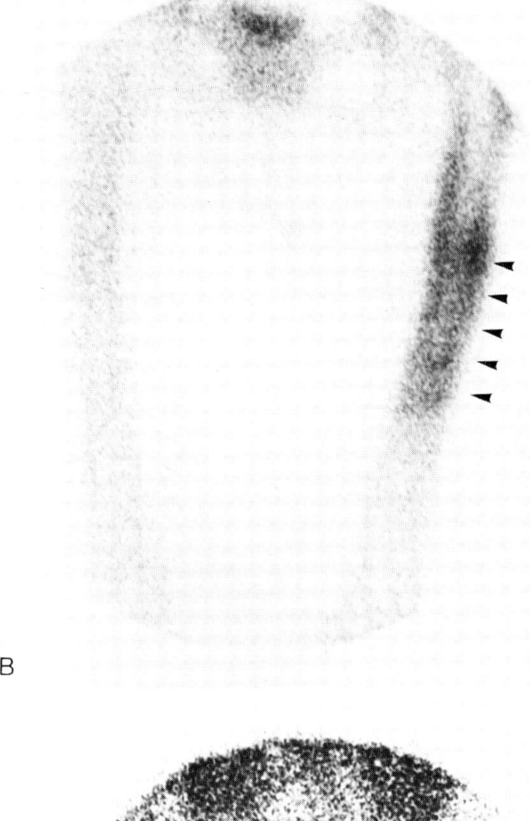

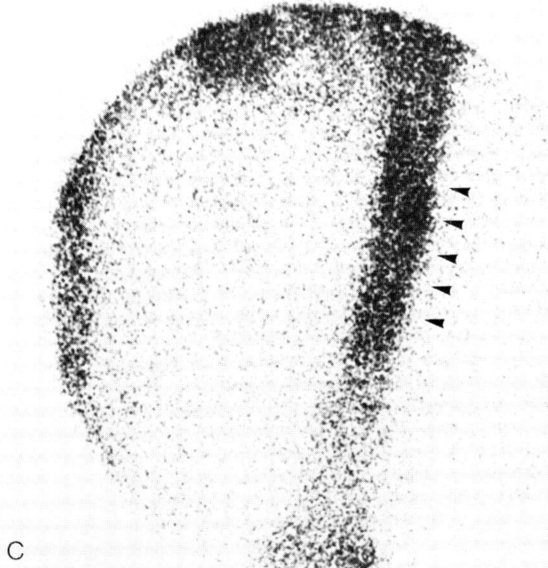

Figure 94–12. Infection following total hip replacement. *A*, AP radiograph four years following a left total hip replacement, demonstrating irregular cortical destruction about the femoral component of the prosthesis. A lucency is present about the acetabular component, which is vertical rather than obliquely oriented. *B*, Anterior image of the same femur two hours following intravenous injection of 20 mCi of technetium MDP. There is a diffuse abnormal focal uptake about the left hip prosthesis. *C*, Anterior image of the same left femur obtained 24 hours after intravenous injection of 500 μCi of ^{111}In-labeled white blood cells, showing an abnormal accumulation of activity diffusely surrounding the distal portion of the hip prosthesis, corresponding to the abnormality seen on the bone scan. Intraoperative bone biopsy confirmed the presence of infection.

the destruction of cartilage. The first osseous changes are ill-defined erosions of the articular cortex that appear within eight to ten days.

It should be apparent from the above discussion that the radiologic diagnosis of septic arthritis is a late diagnosis. Clinical suspicion of a septic joint mandates prompt arthrocentesis. With early diagnosis and treatment, radiographic abnormalities may never develop. Unfortunately, the radiologist is all too often given the unenviable task of documenting secondary degenerative changes or even ankylosis resulting from joint destruction when diagnosis and treatment are delayed.

Complications

Destruction of bone by osteomyelitis may lead to pathologic fracture and/or gross deformities. Involvement of the epiphyses may lead to growth arrests. Septic arthritis may lead to degenerative arthritis and fibrous or bony ankylosis. Secondary amyloidosis may complicate chronic osteomyelitis, but its incidence is considerably less common than in the past. Squamous cell carcinoma may occur in patients with long-standing osteomyelitis and draining fistulas. Fibrosarcomas and other neoplasms may also occur in the drainage tract or the involved bone. This usually follows long-standing infection, with an average duration of approximately 30 years. Clinically, pain, mass, lymphadenopathy, and increased drainage may help suggest the diagnosis.

Modifying Factors

The radiologic appearance of osteomyelitis is obviously altered by the age-dependent blood supply of bone and variations in host response. Underlying systemic disease is another factor that leads to great variation in the radiologic appearance.

Vascular Insufficiency. A combination of factors, including poor vascular supply, neurologic impairment, soft-tissue infection, and osteomyelitis is common in patients with diabetes mellitus. The obvious response to infection is significantly altered by poor vascular supply and microangiographic changes, and it may be paradoxic. Patients with bone resorption in association with infection may respond to conservative therapy, while those with little or no osseous alteration often have severe vascular disease and require amputation. The presence of pedal pulses or vascular calcification does not correlate with the adequacy of blood supply to the distal extremity. Three-phase bone scanning may be helpful in differentiating osteomyelitis from soft-tissue infection, and the addition of gallium or indium may aid in the specificity (Fig. 94–13). Bone scanning, however, is of no value in differentiating osteomyelitis from diabetic neuropathic osteopathy. Multifocal involvement, bilaterality, and absence of soft-tissue involvement favor the osteopathy.

Altered Immune Response. Patients with altered immunity have a decreased resistance to infection. This may occur in patients with hereditary immunologic deficiencies such as chronic granulomatous disease of childhood or patients with an acquired immunologic deficiency due to immunosuppressive drugs, radiation therapy, steroids, or narcotic addiction. The infection in these patients is often due to unusual or gram-negative organisms and may occur in unusual sites (Fig. 94–14). The appearance is typically more like that of subacute or chronic infection.

Sickle Cell Disease. Patients with sickle cell disease have an unusual propensity for *Salmonella* osteomyelitis. This osteomyelitis is often diaphyseal (Fig. 94–15), and differentiation of osteomyelitis from infarction in these patients is often difficult. The final diagnosis is dependent upon culturing the organism. Bone scanning, followed by bone marrow scanning with technetium sulfur colloid, may be of value in this regard.

TUBERCULOSIS AND OTHER MYCOBACTERIA

Tuberculosis

The incidence of tuberculosis has decreased dramatically over the last few decades. Multiple osseous and extraosseous sites of involvement have been reported in narcotic addicts, and osteoarticular tuberculosis remains a major cause of joint destruction in many parts of the world. In one large series, tuberculous arthritis was the most common osseous manifestation, with spondylitis second and osteomyelitis third.

Articular involvement most commonly affects the large joints, particularly the hip and knee. The infection is often primarily synovial with synovial hypertrophy and effusion. Monoarticular involvement predominates. Marginal erosions in the non–weight-bearing areas of weight-bearing bone are typical. Predisposing factors include narcotic addiction, intra-articular steroid injection, systemic illness, and direct trauma. Tuberculosis should be considered in any patient with a monoarticular arthritis, even in the absence of tuberculous involvement elsewhere. The tuberculin skin test is usually positive. Early diagnosis is essential to prevent severe deformity. Radiographic changes usually require months to develop but are frequently present when the initial radiograph is obtained.

The radiographic combination of peripherally located osseous erosions, juxta-articular osteoporosis, and relative preservation of the articular cartilage, known as Phemister's triad, is strongly suggestive of tuberculous arthritis (Fig. 94–16). Wedge-shaped areas of necrotic bone may appose one another on opposite sides of the joint; these have been termed "kissing sequestra." Cartilage destruction is slow in comparison with that in pyogenic arthritis. Large joint effusions and synovial calcification may be present.

Tuberculous Spondylitis. In most series, tuberculous spondylitis is more common than tuberculous arthritis. It commonly involves the thoracic and lumbar spine and often begins in the anterior portion of the vertebral body. The disc is usually involved at the time of presentation. When the dorsal spine is involved, a paraspinous mass is frequent. Involvement of the appendages is uncommon. Usually the disease is confined to one interspace, although multiple contiguous or noncontiguous lesions may occur. Destruction of the vertebral body may lead to a characteristic gibbus deformity (Fig. 94–17). Prominent paraspinal extension may occur and involve a multitude of organs and tissues. Psoas abscesses are common and may be calcified or extend to involve the sacroiliac joint. Bony proliferation and ligamentous calcification may cause bony bridging. Fusion indicates healing and may occur spontaneously. The differentiation of tuberculous from pyogenic osteomyelitis is best made clinically. Involvement of long segments of the spine, a long clinical history, or calcified paraspinal mass should suggest a tuberculous etiology.

Cystic Tuberculosis. This is a rare form of tuberculosis usually seen in young malnourished infants with massive infection. In these patients, multiple, frequently symmetrical areas of circumscribed bone destruction occur with little or no reactive sclerosis. These lesions are often peripheral in location.

Tuberculous Dactylitis. Occasionally, tuberculosis may involve the phalanges, metacarpals, or metatarsals, causing diffuse expansion of the diaphysis; this has been termed *spina ventosa* (Fig. 94–18). It is particularly common in infants and young children and may be associated with multiple areas of involvement and fusiform soft-tissue swelling. Extension into the epiphysis may lead to deformity and brachydactyly.

Caries Sicca. This form of tuberculosis consists of multiple large cystic lesions about a joint, usually the shoulder (Fig. 94–19). The lesions are predominantly fibrous and hence the term *caries sicca,* or dry tuberculosis.

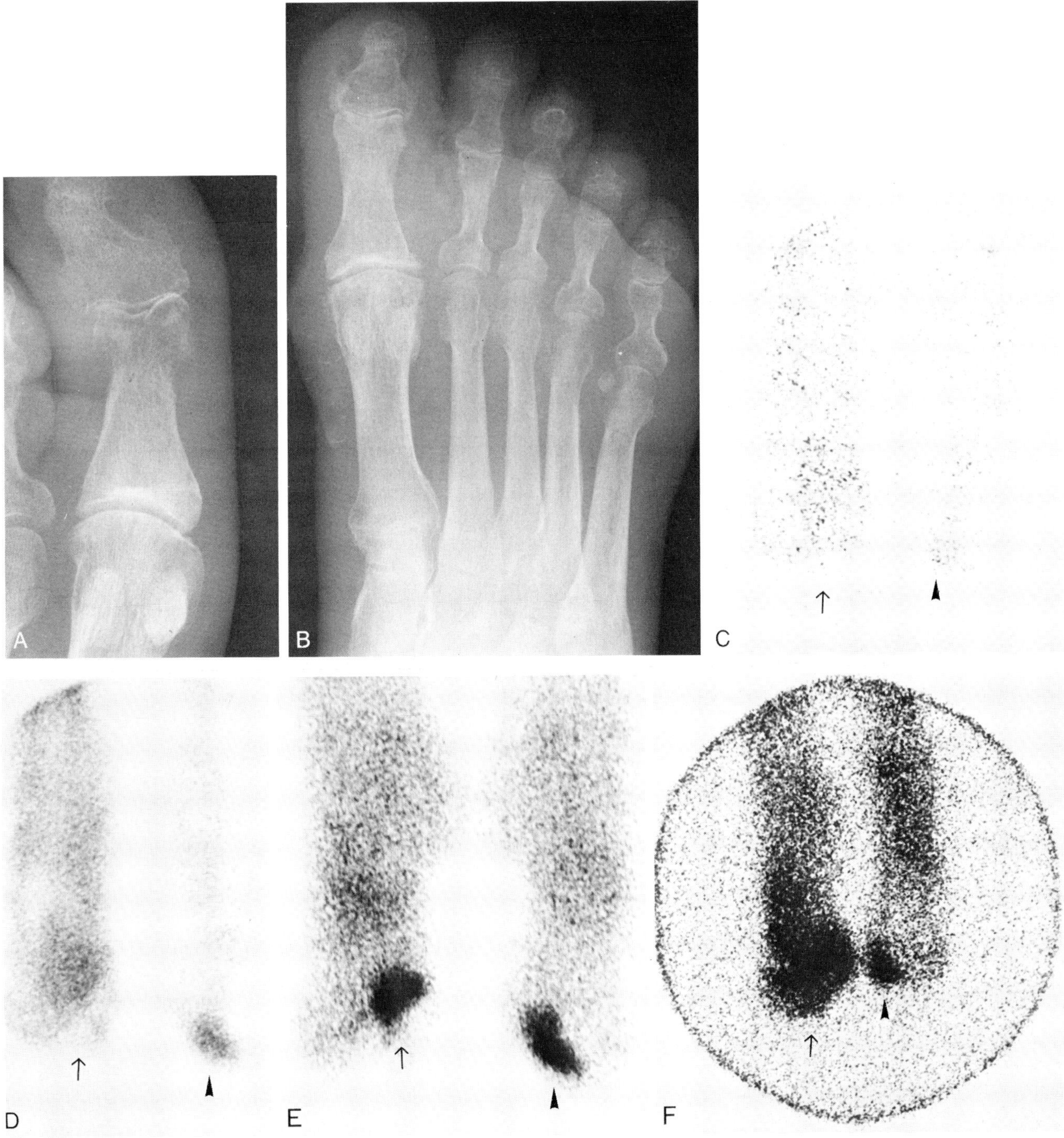

Figure 94–13. Osteomyelitis and cellulitis. *A,* AP radiograph of the left great toe. There is cortical destruction plus an area of irregular lucency throughout the distal portion of the proximal phalanx suggestive of osteomyelitis. There is a break in the articular cortical surface due to a pathologic fracture. *B,* AP radiograph of the right foot demonstrating diffuse osteopenia with irregular soft-tissue swelling about first metatarsophalangeal joint. *C* to *E,* Three-phase bone scan following injection of 20 mCi of technetium MDP. An image selected from the radionuclide angiogram *(C)* demonstrates increased blood flow in the region of the left great toe *(arrowhead)* and diffusely in the region of the first and second metatarsals and toes of the right foot *(arrow).* The blood pool image *(D)* demonstrates the same abnormalities to better advantage owing to the greater number of counts per image. The static image *(E)* obtained two hours following injection demonstrates an intense abnormal focal accumulation of technetium MDP in the region of both great toes *(arrowhead* and *arrow).* All three phases of the bone scan were positive in both great toes, suggestive of osteomyelitis in these areas. The diffuse activity in the right foot should suggest the presence of superimposed cellulitis. *F,* Indium-111 white blood scan obtained 24 hours following an intravenous injection of 500 μCi of ^{111}In-labeled white cells demonstrates an abnormal focal area in the region of the left great toe and diffusely throughout the distal right foot, suggestive of infection. The right foot was amputated because of gangrene, and a biopsy of the left great toe demonstrated osteomyelitis.

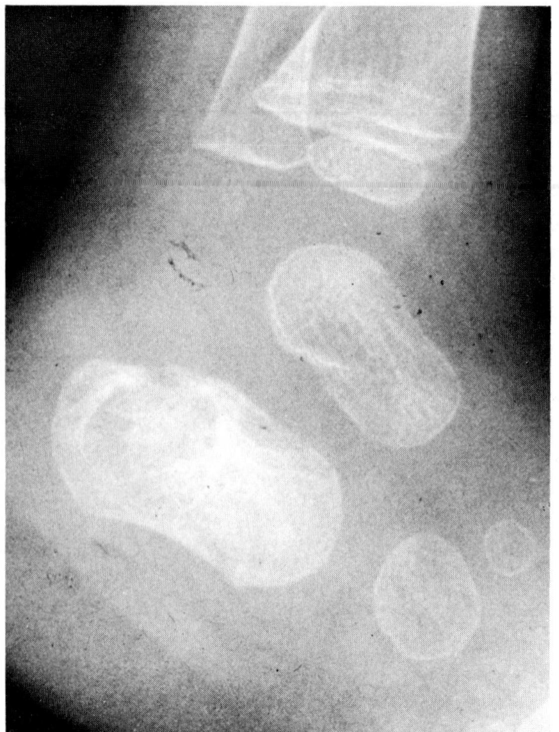

Figure 94–14. Osteomyelitis. Lateral view of the ankle of a child with chronic granulomatous disease of childhood. There is a destructive lesion in the os calcis associated with considerable surrounding sclerosis.

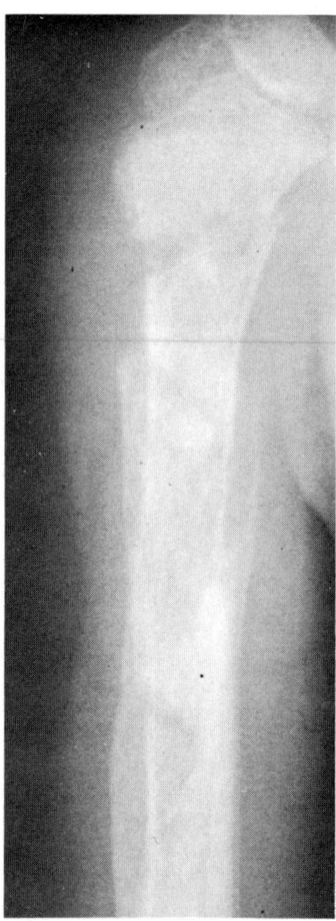

Figure 94–15. *Salmonella* osteomyelitis in sickle cell disease. Destructive diaphyseal lesion in the humerus with a pathologic fracture and periosteal new bone formation.

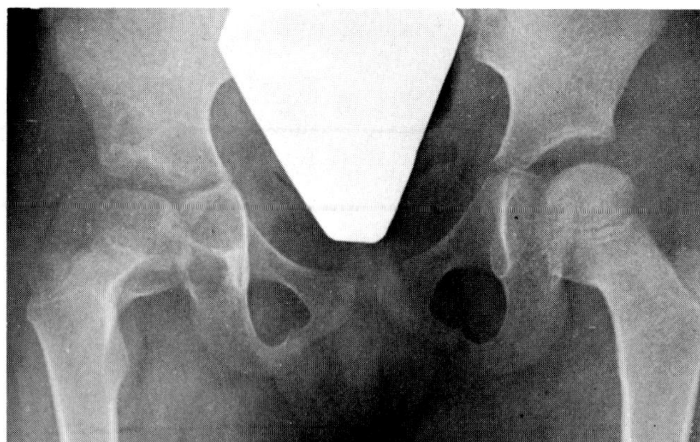

Figure 94–16. Phemister's triad. Radiograph of the pelvis in a child with tuberculosis of the right hip. Despite the extensive acetabular lesions and femoral head deformity, the joint space is preserved. (Courtesy of Dr. G. D. MacEwen, Wilmington, DE.)

BCG Vaccine–Related Osteomyelitis

Bacille Calmette-Guérin is a vaccine produced from the attenuated bovine tubercular bacillus. Approximately one in 80,000 vaccinated patients will develop bone or joint involvement as a complication of the vaccine. This usually occurs at least two months following inoculation, and the findings are nonspecific.

Other Mycobacterial Infections

Atypical Mycobacterial Osteomyelitis. Occasionally, the atypical mycobacteria have been implicated in bone and

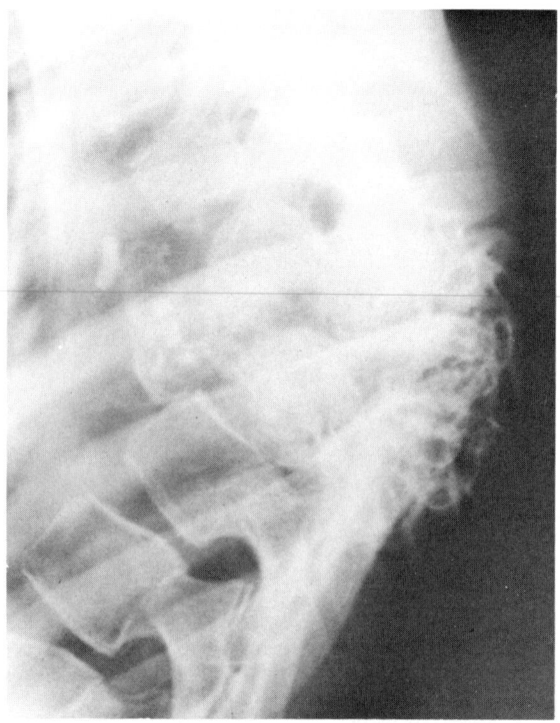

Figure 94–17. Tuberculous spondylitis. Gibbus deformity in a patient with tuberculous spondylitis. Note the destruction of multiple vertebral bodies, soft-tissue calcification, and the acute kyphosis. (Reprinted with permission from Dalinka MK, Lally JF, Koniver G, Coren GS: The radiology of osseous and articular infections. CRC Crit Rev Clin Radiol Nucl Med 7:1, 1975, with permission. Copyright, CRC Press, Inc., Boca Raton, FL.)

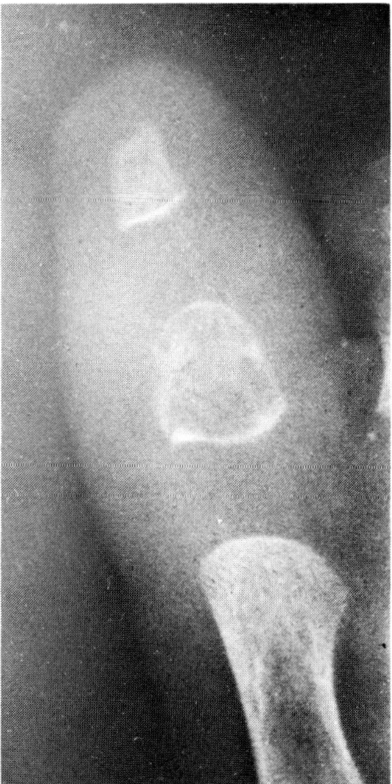

Figure 94–18. Tuberculous dactylitis. A young child with an expansile lesion of the proximal phalanx of the first digit and fusiform swelling. This is called spina ventosa. (Courtesy of Dr. George Wohl, Philadelphia, PA.) (Reprinted with permission from Dalinka MK, Lally JF, Koniver G, Coren GS: The radiology of osseous and articular infections. CRC Crit Rev Clin Radiol Nucl Med 7:1, 1975, with permission. Copyright, CRC Press, Inc., Boca Raton, FL.)

joint disease. The disease frequently pursues an indolent course. The abnormalities are often multiple and the organism may be difficult to culture. The lesions most commonly occur in the pediatric age group and, on occasion, may resemble spina ventosa.

LEPROSY. Leprosy is a chronic granulomatous infection caused by *Mycobacterium leprae.* Osseous involvement occurs in 3.5 per cent of patients and is usually due to extension of the infection from the overlying skin or mucous membrane. The fingers and toes are commonly involved. Intraosseous granulomatous tissue reaction leads to trabecular destruction and resorption of the endosteal cortex. A cystic or lace-like pattern may evolve. Periostitis, reactive sclerosis, and soft-tissue swelling may also occur. Resorption of the nasal spine is typical with destruction of the maxilla, nasal bone, and alveolar ridge. Most bony changes in leprosy are secondary to the associated neurologic abnormalities rather than direct infection of bone. These include osteoporosis, atrophy of the digits, neuropathic joints, and secondary osteomyelitis. Nerve calcification is considered characteristic of this disorder (Fig. 94–20).

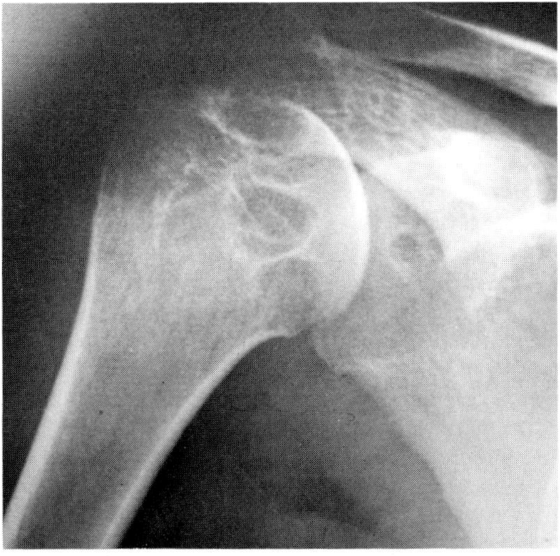

Figure 94–19. Caries sicca. Multiple cystic lesions in the humeral head with small juxtaglenoid lesions in the scapula. (Reprinted with permission from Dalinka MK, Lally JF, Koniver G, Coren GS: The radiology of osseous and articular infections. CRC Crit Rev Clin Radiol Nucl Med 7:1, 1975, with permission. Copyright, CRC Press, Inc., Boca Raton, FL.)

BRUCELLA. Brucellosis is endemic in the midwestern United States. A subacute or chronic disease may be caused by many varieties of the *Brucella* species, including *B. abortus, B. melitensis,* and *B. suis.* It is not uncommonly seen in farmers, meat packers, and those who drink unpasteurized milk. *Brucella* osteomyelitis most often involves the spine, followed in frequency by the long tubular bones of the extremities and the flat bones of the trunk. Joints and bursae may be involved alone or in combination with osteomyelitis. The radiologic findings develop after the clinical symptoms abate and closely resemble those of tuberculosis. The organism may be cultured from synovial tissue. Diagnosis is often difficult, since titers are frequently negative. Pathologically, granulomas are present, which may caseate.

OTHER BACTERIAL INFECTIONS

Spirochetes

SYPHILIS. Syphilis is a systemic infection caused by the spirochete *Treponema pallidum,* a spiral-shaped bacterium. Infection may be acquired transplacentally (congenital syphilis) or by direct contact with lesions of the skin or mucous membranes (acquired syphilis). The osseous manifestations of congenital syphilis are common and may be present in infancy or be delayed until later in life. Early lesions of congenital syphilis may be dystrophic rather than inflammatory and are thought to represent a pathophysiologic disturbance in bone formation. Its symmetrical nature and appearance are striking; metaphysitis, diaphysitis, and periostitis are characteristic. Bony mineralization is affected with widening of the zone of provisional calcification and the growth plate. Erosions at the medial portion of the proximal tibial metaphysis (Wimberger's sign) are characteristic of syphilis, but similar lesions may occur elsewhere.

Less commonly, congenital syphilis may present in childhood, adolescence, or early adult life. In these patients, the osseous lesions are often due to a gumma or an endarteritis and are manifestations of tertiary syphilis. While the radiologic changes occasionally may resemble those of infantile syphilis, they more frequently appear similar to those of acquired syphilis. The most frequent site of these changes is the anterior aspect of the tibia, leading to periosteal new bone formation and a "saber shin" appearance. Osseous lesions associated with acquired syphilis are rare. The most common manifestation is an irregular proliferative periostitis. There may be scattered areas of bone destruction associated with gumma formation, with reactive sclerotic changes predominating. The most frequent changes of tertiary syphilis are in the skull.

YAWS. Yaws is a spirochetal infection caused by *Treponema pertenue.* Bone lesions may be seen in the secondary and tertiary stages resembling those of syphilis. Changes resembling neuropathic joints may also occur.

LYME DISEASE. Lyme disease, initially identified in 1975, is caused by the spirochete *Borrelia burgdorferi,* which is transmitted by the deer tick *Ixodes dammini* and related ixodid ticks. It is called Lyme disease after the small town in Connecticut where the disease was first noted. Although the disease is common along Long Island

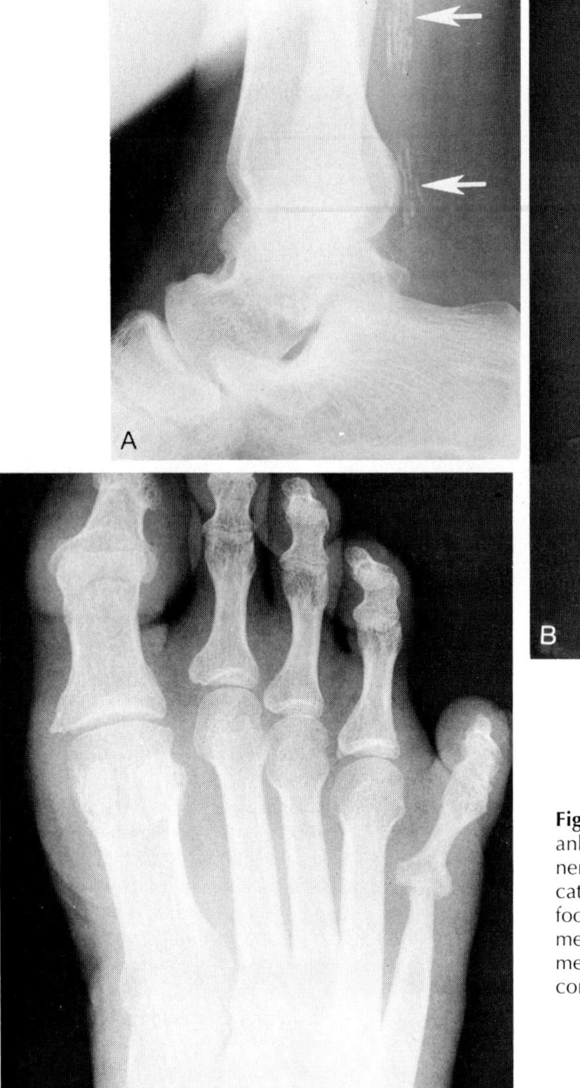

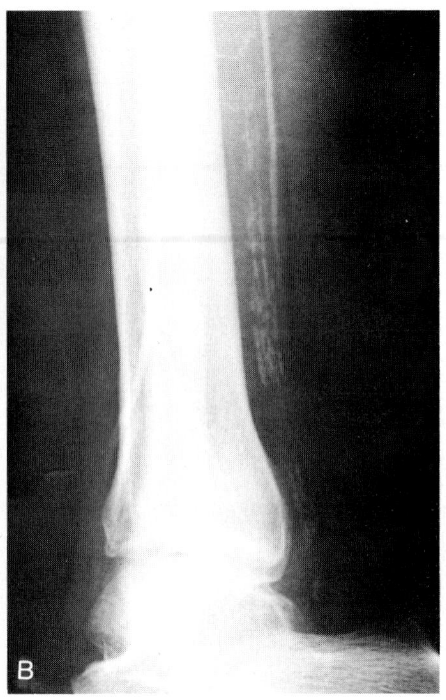

Figure 94–20. Leprosy. *A,* Lateral view of the ankle showing calcification in the sural nerve. *B,* Angiogram showing that the calcification is not vascular. *C,* AP view of same foot showing neuropathic changes in the fifth metatarsophalangeal joint. Atrophy of the metatarsal head and distal shaft has led to considerable shortening of the digit.

Sound, it has now been found in 24 states and 18 countries. Lyme disease typically begins with the unique skin lesion erythema chronicum migrans (ECM), which may be accompanied by headache; stiff neck; fever; myalgias; malaise; fatigue; and a brief but often recurrent asymmetrical oligoarticular swelling and pain in the large joints, particularly the knee. ECM may not be noted or may not occur in some patients. Weeks or months later, some patients develop meningoencephalitis, cranial or peripheral neuropathies, myocarditis or AV node block, or migratory musculoskeletal pain. Frank arthritis may occur following recurrent attacks over several years accompanied by synovial proliferation and joint effusions. Cartilage and bone erosion occur rarely. The entity has been confused with juvenile rheumatoid arthritis. Diagnosis is relatively easy when the early clinical symptoms are accompanied by ECM. In the absence of ECM or later in the course of the disease, the diagnosis can be confirmed by antibody titers. Presence of the antibody is specific for the infection, but false-negative titers may be encountered early in the disease. Penicillin or tetracycline, given early in the illness, shortens the duration of ECM and may prevent or attenuate the subsequent arthritis. High-dose intravenous antibiotic therapy in chronic disease can also be effective, indicating that spirochetes are still alive in the chronically affected joints where they elicit an immune response.

Gram-Positive Cocci

Staphylococcus aureus. This is the most common pathogen in childhood and adult hematogenous osteomyelitis. It is also the most common organism responsible for septic arthritis. In older series, this organism accounted for as many as 90 per cent of cases of osteomyelitis. More recent data suggest 50 to 60 per cent as a more accurate figure. The explanation for this apparently decreased prevalence is not entirely clear, but the earlier institution of antibiotic therapy may be a contributing factor. Most typically, staphylococcal osteomyelitis affects preteenagers, boys more than girls, and localizes in the metaphyses of the most rapidly growing bones. An infectious source, such as the skin or respiratory tract, can be found in more than one third of cases.

Streptococcus pyogenes. This is the most common cause of neonatal osteomyelitis. Group B streptococcal osteomyelitis tends to affect otherwise healthy neonates in the first few weeks of life and often involves only a single bone of the upper extremity. In contrast, *Staphylococcus aureus* and *Escherichia coli* tend to afflict high-risk infants and are more likely to involve multiple bones. Osteoarticular infection with pneumococcal organisms is rare. In almost all cases, a predisposing factor can be identified.

Gram-Negative Cocci

Neisseria gonorrhoeae. Gonococcal arthritis is the most common form of infectious arthritis. Women are more frequently affected; pregnancy and menstruation are predisposing factors. Patients present with fever, chills, multiple painful joints, and distinctive cutaneous lesions thought to be caused by vascular embolization with the *Neisseria gonorrhoeae* organism. Polyarthalgias due to circulating immune complexes give way to one or several septic joints, most commonly involving the knee, ankle, and wrist.

Gram-Negative Bacilli

Osteomyelitis and septic arthritis due to gram-negative bacilli are unusual in the uncompromised host. Usually a predisposing factor can be identified such as pre-existing joint disease, drug abuse, or chronic illness. Such infection may also occur in atypical sites. Osteoarticular infections due to enteric organisms such as *Escherichia coli* and *Aerobacter aerogenes* are usually secondary to gastrointestinal or genitourinary tract disease. Such organisms account for about one third of cases of vertebral osteomyelitis.

For unknown reasons, infection with *Pseudomonas* species accounts for the majority of cases of osteomyelitis in intravenous drug abusers. In addition to the spine, there is a propensity toward involvement of the sacroiliac, sternoclavicular, and acromioclavicular joints, which are unusual locations for other organisms. *Pseudomonas aeruginosa* osteomyelitis of the calcaneus has also been described following puncture wounds of the foot. Osteomyelitis due to *Klebsiella pneumoniae* has also been seen in drug abusers; preliminary evidence suggests this organism causes more widespread bone destruction than other gram-negative species.

Salmonella typhi is the organism responsible for typhoid fever. Before antibiotics, osteomyelitis occurred in approximately 1 per cent of cases. Typhoid osteomyelitis is currently quite rare but should be suspected in a patient with prolonged fever and multiple bones involved with chronic diaphyseal osteomyelitis. The association between *Salmonella* osteomyelitis and sickle cell disease or other hemoglobinopathies is well known. Indeed, *Salmonella* species, such as *S. choleraesuis, S. paratyphi,* and *S. typhimurium,* are the most common causes of bone infection in patients with hemoglobinopathies. The risk of *Salmonella* osteomyelitis in patients with sickle cell disease is several hundred times that of the normal population. The reason for this association is unknown. Suggested theories include deficiencies in the immune mechanism; minute infarctions of the bowel wall promoting diffusion of organisms; and the presence of red blood cell byproducts in areas of bone infarction, leading to an environment conducive to the growth of organisms. With a combination of bone destruction and reaction, *Salmonella* osteomyelitis is radiographically difficult to distinguish from the frequently present infarctions, and, indeed, they may coexist.

FUNGAL INFECTIONS

It is unusual to make the diagnosis of fungal disease purely on the basis of the radiographs. The clinical information is particularly important. The presence of draining sinus tracts, indolent ulcerations, and chronic osteomyelitis in association with mixed lytic and sclerotic changes may be present in patients with long-standing infection. With systemic fungal infection, other organs are frequently involved, in particular the lungs, skin, and central nervous system.

Actinomycosis

Actinomycosis does not represent a true fungal infection, but it has many clinical and radiographic similarities. The offending organisms, usually *Actinomyces israelii,* are gram-positive anaerobic bacteria that are part of the normal flora of the mouth and pharynx. Cervicofacial involvement is characteristic of actinomycosis and may complicate a dental abscess or tooth extraction. Spinal involvement is common, with relative disc sparing. When the thoracic spine is affected, the neighboring ribs are almost always involved. Cutaneous fistulas are present. The contiguous involvement of lung, pleura, spine, and ribs should suggest the diagnosis of actinomycosis.

Aspergillosis

Aspergillus fumigatus is a mold with septate hyphae about 4 mm in diameter. It is usually a noninvasive fungus but can cause disease, particularly in immunosuppressed patients or following massive inoculation due to inhalation of spores. When it involves bone, it is usually secondary to contiguous infection. A pulmonary focus may lead to rib or spine involvement; the skull may be affected following extension from sinus or orbital infection.

Blastomycosis

The organism *Blastomyces dermatitidis* has a predilection for bone. Bone involvement is more frequent than with the other fungi. Blastomycosis is endemic to the Mississippi and Ohio River Valley and the southeastern United States. The primary lesions are usually in the skin, with the respiratory tract serving as the alternate site of infection. Osteomyelitis may result from hematogenous spread or by direct extension from an overlying skin lesion. Bony prominences are particularly susceptible, and symmetrical lesions are common. Findings are almost indistinguishable from those of tuberculosis. The skin test is unreliable; however, the organism is relatively easy to culture.

Candidiasis

Osteomyelitis and septic arthritis are rare manifestations of disseminated disease due to *Candida albicans* and related species. A predisposing factor such as diabetes mellitus, drug abuse, or immunosuppressive therapy is very common. The large weight-bearing joints are most frequently involved; multiple bone involvement may occur.

Coccidioidomycosis

The fungus *Coccidioides immitis* is endemic to the southwestern United States, particularly the San Joaquin Valley, as well as portions of Central and South America. Infection occurs primarily via inhalation of the airborne arthrospores. Approximately 60 per cent of infected humans remain asymptomatic, even in the presence of an abnormal radiograph. Approximately 0.5 per cent of patients with coccidioidomycosis have disseminated disease, and about 20 per cent of patients with disseminated disease will have involvement of the osseous system. Infection is most commonly hematogenous, although it may occur via direct extension from the skin or the synovium. Multiple bone involvement and symmetrical lesions are not infrequent (Fig. 94–21). There is a predilection for bony prominences. With spinal involvement, discs are preserved until relatively late in the course of disease. The lesions are usually lytic and well-defined, with occasional periostitis and sclerosis. Joint involvement is typically the result of extension from the involved bone and occurs most commonly in the knee or ankle.

Cryptococcosis

Cryptococcosis is caused by the organism *Cryptococcus neoformans* or *Torula histolytica.* There is no endemic area for cryptococcosis. It occurs three times as often in males and particularly in young adults. Seventy per cent of patients with disseminated disease will have a predisposing factor, including Hodgkin's disease, sarcoidosis, pregnancy, or steroid treatment. Osseous involvement occurs in 4 per cent of patients. Characteristically there are osteolytic lesions with sharply scalloped margins and little or no periosteal reaction. As with other fungal infections, there is a tendency for involvement of bony prominences.

Histoplasmosis

The dimorphic fungus *Histoplasma capsulatum* is endemic to the great river valleys of the central and southeastern United States. Bony involvement due to this organism is extremely rare. Osseous involvement is common in patients with *Histoplasma duboisii,* which is seen in tropical Africa. The ribs are most frequently infected, and periosteal reaction leads to an expanded appearance. Multiple well-defined skull lesions are also characteristic.

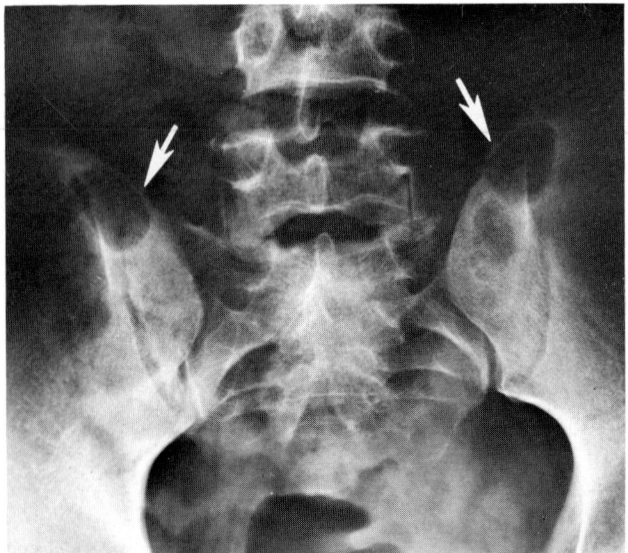

Figure 94–21. Coccidioidomycosis. There are symmetrical lesions in the ilium *(arrows),* with an additional lesion on the left side of the sacrum. (Reprinted with permission from Dalinka MK, Lally JF, Koniver G, Coren GS: The radiology of osseous and articular infections. CRC Crit Rev Clin Radiol Nucl Med 7:1, 1975, with permission. Copyright, CRC Press, Inc., Boca Raton, FL.)

Mucormycosis

Mucormycosis is an infection caused by fungi of the order Mucorales, with *Rhizopus* and *Mucor* species being the principal pathogens. Mucormycosis infection may originate in the paranasal sinuses and nose or lungs. Vascular invasion may lead to hemorrhagic necrosis. Extension from the sinuses to the craniofacial bones leads to osteomyelitis and vascular thrombotic destruction.

Maduromycosis

The characteristic mycetoma due to *Monosporium apiospermum* is seen in tropical and subtropical countries. Local injury to bare feet is followed by infection (Madura foot). In the United States, infection is largely confined to patients with seriously debilitating conditions such as poorly controlled diabetes mellitus, hematologic malignancy, and uremia.

Sporotrichosis

Infection of the subcutaneous soft tissue by the fungus *Sporothrix schenckii* leads to sporotrichosis. This is an occupational disease of veterinarians and horticulturists. Most commonly, the disease begins as a painless ulcer extending along proximal lymphatic channels. Osteoarticular involvement is rare and is most common in the knee, hand, wrist, and foot.

PARASITIC INFECTIONS

Cysticercosis

Cysticercosis is caused by the ingestion of food, water, or feces containing eggs of the pork tapeworm *Taenia solium.* The larvae migrate throughout the body, most notably to skeletal muscle and the brain. The parasites live three to six years. After death, they act as irritant foreign bodies; cellular response leads to calcification, which takes approximately three years in body tissues, longer in the brain. The radiographic findings are distinctive. There are numerous oval calcifications in the soft tissues and muscles, with the long axes in alignment with the plane of the muscle bundles (Fig. 94–22).

Echinococcosis

Echinococcosis or hydatid disease results from infection with the larval stage of the cestode *Echinococcus granulosus.* Infection occurs by contact with infected dogs or by ingestion of food, water, or soil contaminated by egg-containing feces of the dog, wolf, or other canine. The larvae migrate through the intestinal mucosa, enter the mesenteric venules and lymphatics, and are dispersed throughout the body, leading to cyst formation in multiple organs. Osseous involvement occurs in approximately 1.5 per cent of patients; the spine and pelvis account for the majority of cases. The lesions begin in the medullary canal and produce an expansile multilocular appearance resembling a "bunch of grapes." With eventual cortical breakthrough, there is abundant growth in the adjacent soft tissues. Complications include pathologic fracture, secondary pyogenic infection, and neurologic damage from spinal cord compression.

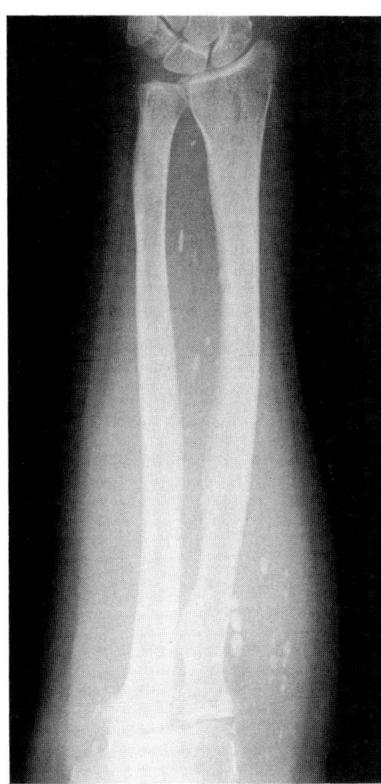

Figure 94–22. Cysticercosis. Note the orientation of the calcified lesions along the muscle planes of the forearm.

Filariasis

Filarial disease is endemic to the equatorial regions of the world. Infection by the adult worm of *Wuchereria bancrofti* or *Brugia malayi* is termed filariasis. Chronic fibrosis and obliteration of the lymphatics lead to massive lymphedema or elephantiasis. The microfilariae are under 4 mm in size and are rarely seen as faint calcifications. Loiasis is due to infection with the filaria *Loa loa* and is generally confined to the equatorial rain forest regions in West Africa. The dead worms may calcify and are best seen in the hands and feet. They may appear linear, coiled, or beaded. Bloodsucking black flies transmit *Onchocerca volvulus* to human beings. Onchocerciasis affects more than 50 million people and is responsible for the blindness of at least a half million Africans. Subcutaneous nodules on the head, hip, and extremities harbor adult nematodes and microfilariae. Soft-tissue calcifications indistinguishable from *Loa loa* may be seen.

Dracunculiasis

Dracunculiasis is an infection in the soft tissues due to the presence of the guinea worm *Dracunculus medinensis.* The disease is endemic to tropical Africa, the Middle East, and India. Calcified guinea worms may be identified radiographically. The adult male guinea worm is only 3 to 4 cm long and is rarely seen. The female worm may reach lengths of 30 to 120 cm. These long linear, coiled, or serpiginous soft-tissue calcifications present no problem in diagnosis (Fig. 94–23).

Porocephalosis

Porocephalosis, or tongue worm infestation, is caused by *Armillifer armilatus.* The disease is common in West Africa and parts of Asia. The parasites inhabit the respiratory tracts of snakes and other reptiles.

Radiologically, the dead calcified parasites are found in the thorax and abdomen. They are crescent- or comma-shaped and vary from 3 to 7 mm in size. Calcifications are frequently multiple and can be differentiated from cysticercosis, since they are not seen in the extremities.

VIRAL DISEASES OF BONE

Variola (Smallpox)

This disease is now mainly one of historic interest. Most cases of smallpox osteomyelitis involve the elbow, either unilaterally or bilaterally. Primary osseous or articular involvement has been reported with frequent secondary infection and draining sinuses. Epiphyseal involvement with deformity, symmetry, and joint fusion is characteristic.

Vaccinia

There have been rare reports of vaccinial osteomyelitis, most of which demonstrate periostitis. In one case, the findings were characteristic of infantile cortical hyperostosis.

Other Viral Infections

Radiographically demonstrable lesions of bone have been described in rubella and cytomegalic inclusion disease. The findings consist of irregular metaphyseal lesions with lucent defects that resemble "celery stalks." They usually heal spontaneously in one to three months but can persist in infants that fail to thrive. These changes may be related to intrauterine stress, as they have not been reported after infancy. The rubella virus has been isolated from the lymphoreticular cells of some children with chronic rheumatic disease, including those diagnosed as having juvenile rheumatoid arthritis.

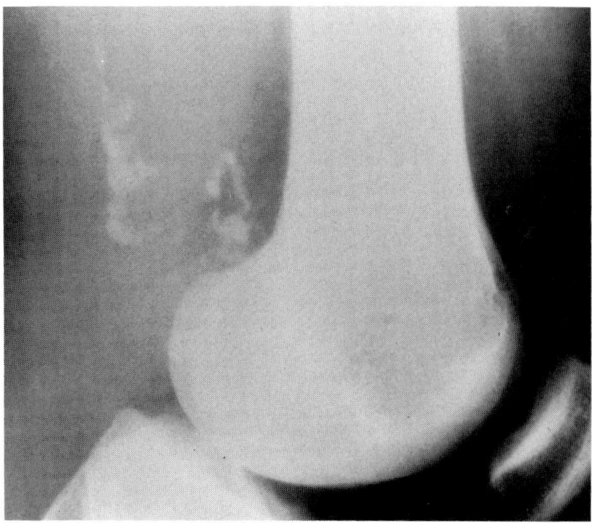

Figure 94–23. Dracunculiasis. Lateral radiograph of the knee revealing the long tubular calcifications characteristic of dracunculiasis. (Courtesy of Dr. Melvin Turner, Philadelphia, PA.)

CONDITIONS OF UNDETERMINED ETIOLOGY

Pamela S. Jensen

Sarcoidosis

Sarcoidosis is a systemic granulomatous process of undetermined etiology. Any organ or tissue can be affected, but there is a predilection for the thoracic lymph nodes and the lungs. The major discussion of this entity will be found in the pulmonary section. Polyarthritis without joint changes occurs. Muscle involvement is uncommon, but when it occurs the muscles of the extremities are the ones usually involved. Less than 10 per cent of patients with sarcoidosis experience bone abnormalities, and these are usually asymptomatic. Osseous involvement is typically limited to the hand or foot. A lace-like or honeycombed appearance of the trabecular bone is characteristic. Cystic punched-out lesions at the ends of the phalanges also occur and may coalesce to form large areas of destruction.

Paget's Disease

In 1876, Sir James Paget described a disease he characterized as a chronic inflammation of bone causing considerable structural alteration of the affected parts of the skeleton. A portion of his description follows:

> It begins in middle age or later, is very slow in progress, may continue for many years without influence on the general health, and may give no other trouble than those which are due to the changes of shape, size, and direction of the diseased bones. Even when the skull is hugely thickened, and all its bones exceedingly altered in structure, the mind remains unaffected.

Distribution and Etiology. Paget's disease, or osteitis deformans, as it is also known, is found with greatest frequency in Great Britain, Australia, New Zealand, Germany, France, and the United States, where as many as 3 per cent of the population are identified as affected. The prevalence is undoubtedly greater, since the disease can be asymptomatic. The disease is rare in India, China, Japan, the Middle East, Africa, and Scandinavia. The disease is identified primarily in people over the age of 40 years, with men and women nearly equally affected.

The etiology of Paget's disease has not been fully established. It does not appear to be hereditary, although horizontal family clustering has been reported. Metabolic etiologies, including calcitonin deficiency and abnormal function of the pituitary, adrenal, and parathyroid glands, have been excluded. The affected bone during the active stage of the disease can be highly vascular, but a neoplastic process has not been established. Nuclear inclusions have been identified in the osteoclasts of a number of patients with Paget's disease, suggesting that a slow virus may be the cause. This would account for the long latent period that occurs before the diagnosis of Paget's disease is made.

Pathophysiology. In the normal adult, remodeling of the bone begins with formation of osteoclasts from osteoprogenitor cells. Osteoclasts resorb previously formed bone. This is followed by a reversal phase during which the osteoclasts disappear and the osteoblasts subsequently appear. The osteoblasts make the collagen matrix or osteoid, which is organized in a lamellar fashion. This arrangement gives the bone its strength. In Paget's disease, there is a high rate of bone turnover and the phases of bone resorption and formation are grossly exaggerated. Initially there is excessive osteoclastic resorption of bone. This osteolytic phase is followed by a period of greatly increased bone formation. The bone formed is abnormal because the collagen is not organized in the usual lamellar fashion. Instead, woven or fibrous bone is made, which is composed of very disorganized collagen, and this weakened bone is susceptible to fractures and bowing deformities (Fig. 94–24). The marrow becomes highly vascular.

Clinical and Laboratory Features. There is a wide range of clinical findings in Paget's disease. The disease may be asymptomatic, being recognized by routine radiographic examinations, blood studies, or autopsies. Serum alkaline phosphatase, an indicator of osteoblastic activity, is elevated; very high levels can be seen when the bone formation phase of the disease is most active. Increased urinary secretion of hydroxyproline, an amino acid found in bone collagen, occurs during the resorptive phase.

Pain is a frequent complaint and may be quite severe. Progressive changes in the hip and pelvis leading to protrusio acetabuli are often accompanied by medial or concentric joint narrowing (Fig. 94–25). Affected vertebral bodies may collapse (Fig. 94–26). The bone itself may be painful, possibly owing to stimulation of somatic nerve endings secondary to the stretching of the periosteum at sites of bony expansion and new bone formation. The temperature of the skin over the affected bone may be increased.

Deformity is another common problem; it is manifested by bowing of the bone, which in turn leads to potential degenerative changes of the adjacent joints as well as shortening of the limb. Marked enlargement of the skull may occur, sometimes to such an

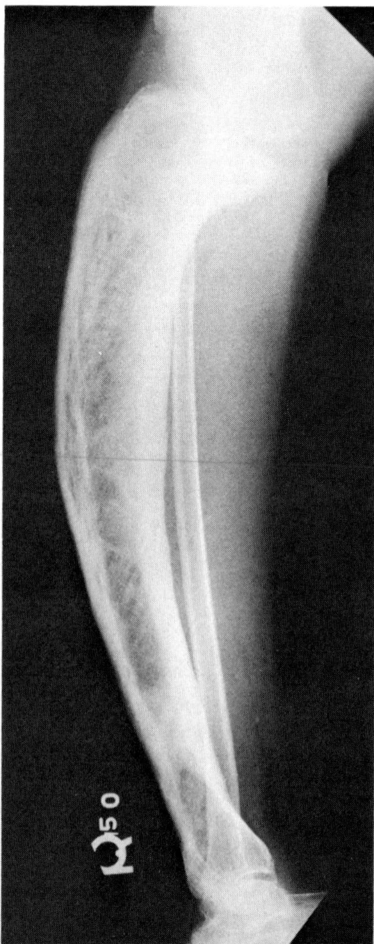

Figure 94–24. Paget's disease. Lateral view demonstrates the characteristic findings, including expansion of the shaft of the proximal tibia, considerable bowing, and thickening of the cortex on the concave side of the curve. The fibula is unaffected.

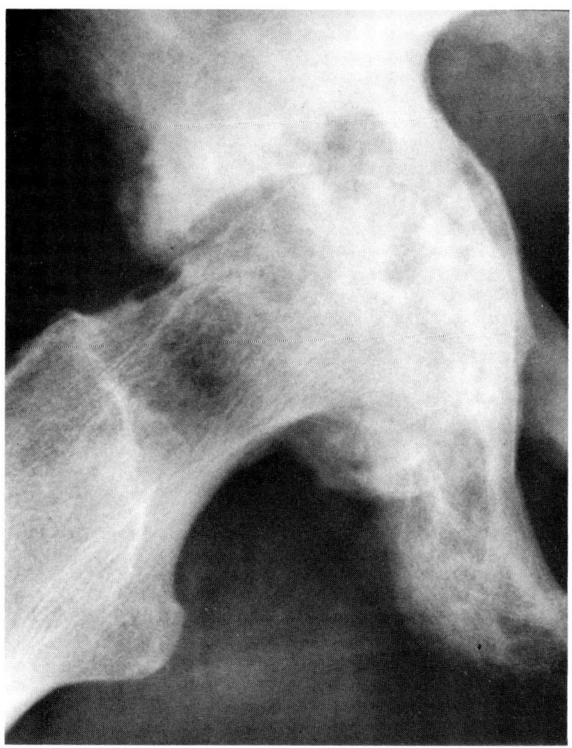

Figure 94–25. Paget's disease. Narrowing of the hip joint with bowing of the medial acetabular wall (protrusio acetabuli) occurs frequently with advanced Paget's disease. Sclerosis and widening of the ischium are also typical findings.

extent that patients have noted an increase in hat size. Pathologic fractures are the most common serious complication of Paget's disease. The demineralization of bone during the resorptive phase, as well as the haphazard deposition of new bone in the sclerotic phase, produces a structurally weakened bone that has increased susceptibility to fracture. Fractures of the femur and tibia are most common. The fracture may be complete or incomplete. Incomplete fractures, resembling the pseudofractures associated with osteomalacia, occur along the convex side of the cortex (Fig. 94–27). Complete fractures may be transverse instead of having the typical spiral configuration, since the underlying bone is abnormal (Fig. 94–28).

Neurologic complications include hearing loss due to pagetic overgrowth of the temporal bone; less commonly, impingement upon the auditory nerve due to deformity of the internal auditory canal can occur. Basilar invagination of the skull can affect cranial

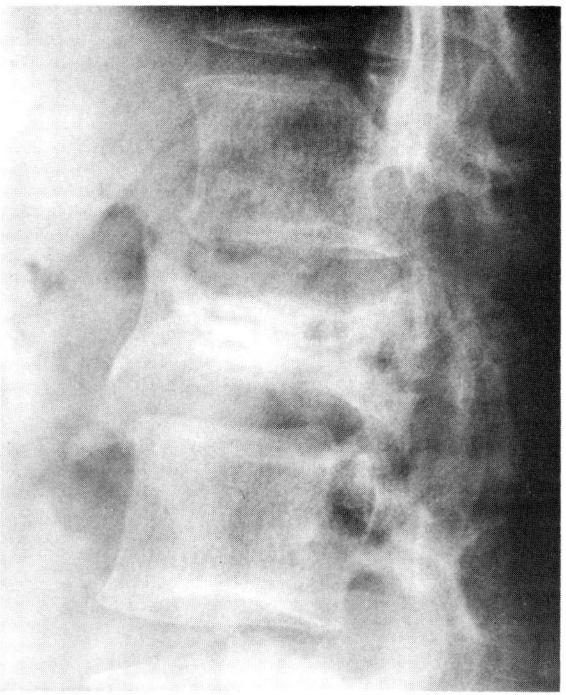

Figure 94–26. Paget's disease. Extensive collapse of a pagetic vertebra can result in the appearance of vertebra plana.

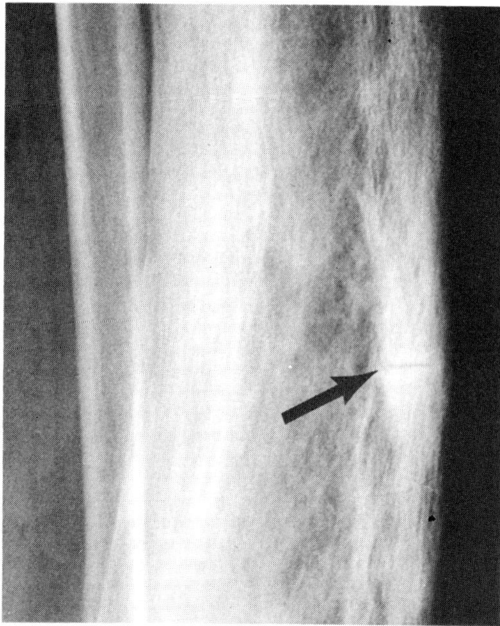

Figure 94–27. Paget's disease. The midshaft of a tibia demonstrates expansion of the diameter of the shaft, coarsening of the trabecular pattern, bowing, and thickening of the cortex. An incomplete or pseudofracture in the convex cortex is evident *(arrow)*. Compare the appearance of the pagetic tibia with that of the normal fibula.

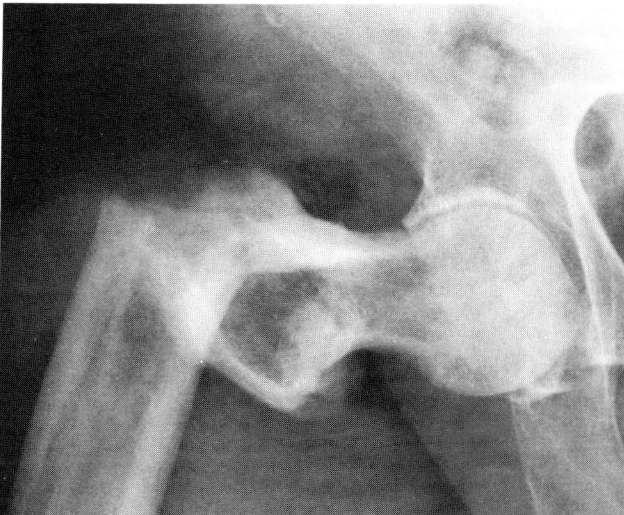

Figure 94–28. Paget's disease. A transverse or "chalk stick" fracture of a femur affected with Paget's disease can occur owing to the weakened and abnormally modeled bone. The pattern of fracture in a normal femur is spiral.

nerves, brain stem, and cerebellum. Vertebral body changes can result in spinal cord compression. Other clinical manifestations include congestive heart failure due to the marked increase in the vascularity of pagetic bone in severe polyostotic disease, which can occur in patients with underlying heart disease. An increased incidence of hyperuricemia and gout have been observed. Calcium homeostasis is usually normal despite the high rate of bone turnover. Occasionally hypercalcemia and hypercalciuria occur in patients with extensive bone disease who are put to bedrest, usually for a fracture; kidney stones may also result.

Malignant degeneration, usually in the form of osteosarcoma or fibrosarcoma, occurs in less than 1 per cent of patients. When this happens the prognosis is very poor; most patients die within a year despite intensive therapy. In general, however, Paget's disease is a slowly progressive disease—patients die *with* the disease, but only rarely *because* of it.

RADIOGRAPHIC MANIFESTATIONS. The bones most commonly affected by Paget's disease are the pelvis and spine, followed by the femur, skull, tibia, humerus, clavicles, and ribs. Usually the involvement is polyostotic, but occasionally only one bone is affected. The smaller bones of the hands and feet are less commonly involved. In the pelvis, the earliest radiographic finding is thickening of the pelvic rim along the iliopectineal line. Another early change, best seen in the proximal femur, is demineralization demonstrated by increase in prominence of the primary trabeculae along lines of stress (Fig. 94–29). Later findings include the development of protrusio acetabuli due to the loss of strength of the medial acetabular wall when the normal bone is replaced by pagetic bone. Increased density of the bone is often accompanied by widening of the pubic and ischial bones. This expansion of the bones along with preservation of the trabecular pattern is helpful in identifying the process as that of Paget's disease and not metastases or other diffuse processes.

A classic demonstration of the osteolytic phase of the disease is the development of osteoporosis circumscripta in the skull (Fig. 94–30*A*). This usually begins as a sharply defined area of demineralization in the frontal or occipital regions, which may with time extend to involve the whole calvarium. In the bone formation phase, the skull expands and there is marked thickening of the inner and outer tables; chaotic bone deposition has a "cotton wool" appearance, and in advanced stages basilar invagination occurs (Figs. 94–30 and 94–31). The facial bones are less often involved; when deformity occurs, there is anterior expansion of the maxilla and mandible, leading to a snout-like appearance called leontiasis ossea.

In the long bones, the osteolytic phase begins at one end of the bone and often has a wedge- or V-shaped leading edge (Fig. 94–32). Bowing of the long bones, particularly the tibia, is characteristic (see Fig. 94–24). Thickening of the cortex and expansion of the bone may occur. The trabeculae may be thickened and coarse in appearance but remain sharp, thus distinguishing the disease from other processes. Involvement of the vertebral bodies may be mani-

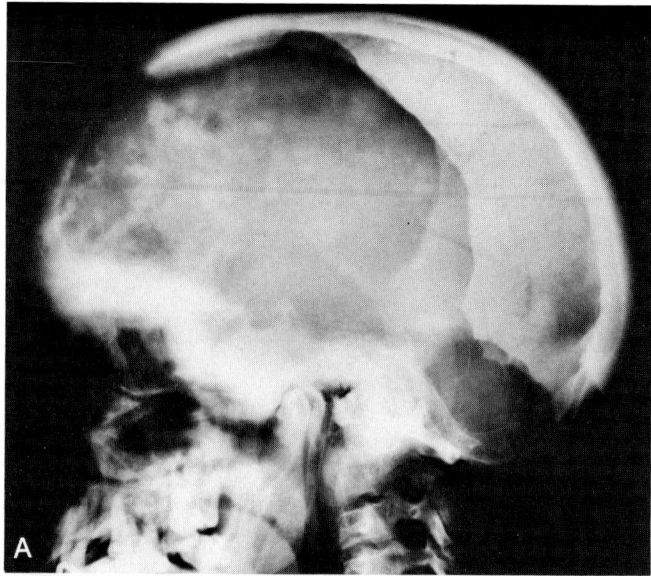

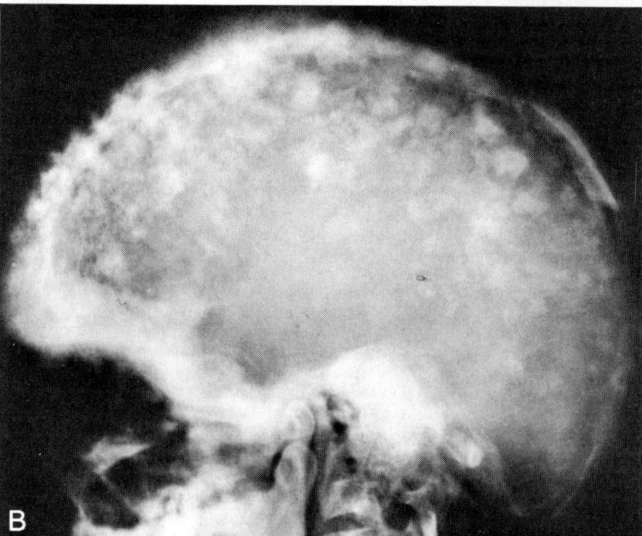

Figure 94–30. Paget's disease. *A*, A large, sharply defined area of resorption involving the calvarium (osteoporosis circumscripta) plus thickening and sclerosis of the base of the skull is characteristic of early pagetoid changes. *B*, Seven years later bone has formed in the area of previous resorption and has a "cotton wool" appearance. A line drawn from the posterior portion of the hard palate to the inferior base of the occiput transects the lower part of the body of C2, indicating the presence of basilar invagination.

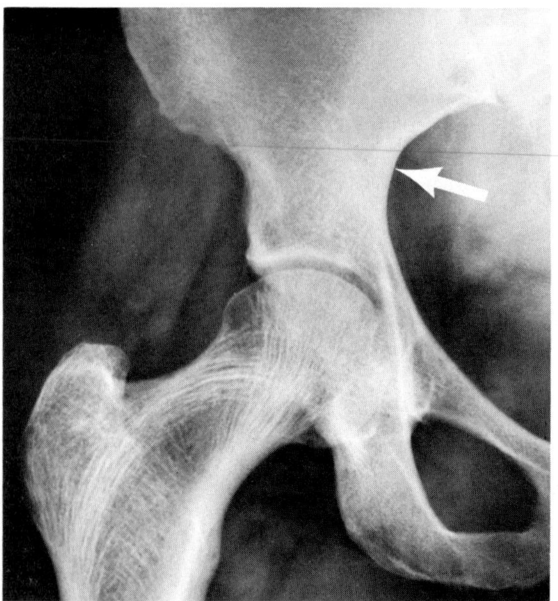

Figure 94–29. Paget's disease. The early resorptive phase can be identified in the proximal femur when there is increased prominence of the primary trabeculae; this occurs because these trabeculae are being reinforced along the lines of stress as the secondary trabeculae are resorbed. Thickening of the bone along the iliopectineal line *(arrow)* is also present.

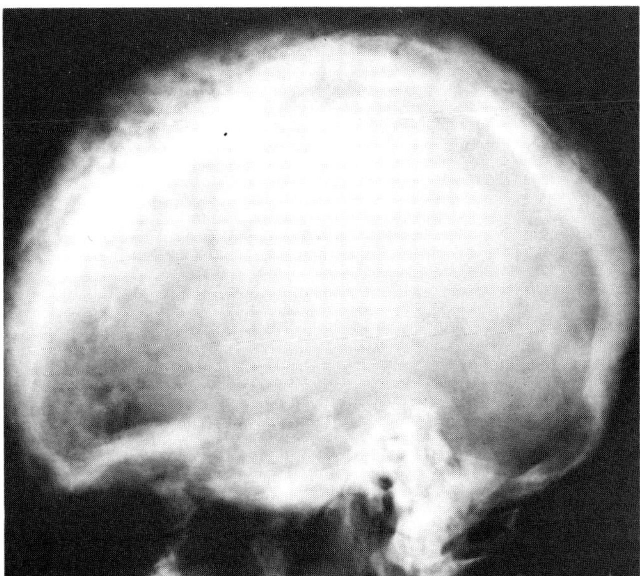

Figure 94–31. Paget's disease. There is extensive thickening and expansion of the calvarium. This highly vascular pagetic bone will exhibit marked increased uptake of radionuclide on a bone scan.

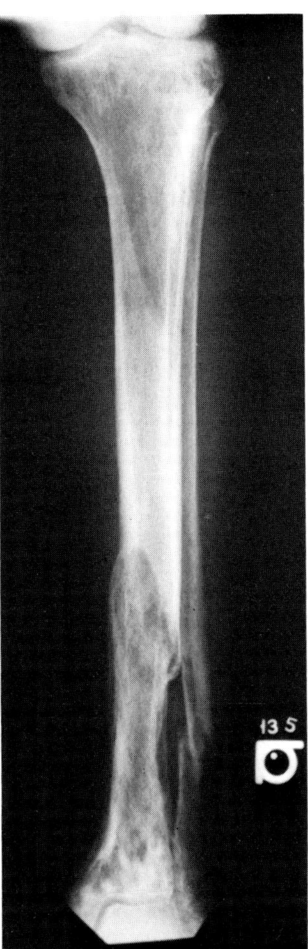

Figure 94–32. Paget's disease. The V-shaped advancing edge of pagetic bone is present at both ends of the tibia; only the midshaft is unaffected. Expansion of the shaft at the edge of the lower area of involvement is evident.

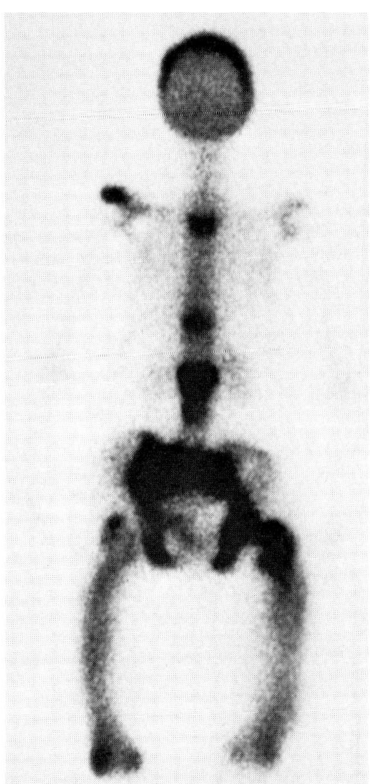

Figure 94–33. Paget's disease. This whole-body technetium bone scan has the distribution of increased radionuclide uptake characteristic of Paget's disease—pelvis and sacrum, vertebrae, femora, skull, and clavicle. Expansion and bowing of the femora are also evident.

fested as demineralization or osteosclerosis, with or without expansion. Severe compression of expanded demineralized vertebrae can lead to the appearance of vertebra plana (see Fig. 94–26).

The ^{99m}Tc radionuclide bone scan is a major diagnostic tool in Paget's disease. Areas of increased bone turnover are readily identified by increased uptake of the isotope. The bone scan can identify areas of early involvement that are not evident on the routine radiographs. A bone scan demonstrating multiple areas of increased uptake is most compatible with widespread bony metastases or Paget's disease. The typical distribution of Paget's disease—pelvis, vertebrae, skull, long bones of the lower extremities, and long lesions of the ribs when they are involved—suggests the diagnosis (Fig. 94–33). Routine radiographs of the affected bones usually confirm the diagnosis. When the distribution of the lesions is atypical or limited to only one bone, the radiographic examination will usually be sufficient to make the diagnosis.

DIAGNOSIS AND TREATMENT. Characteristic radiographic manifestations plus elevated serum alkaline phosphatase and urinary hydroxyproline are diagnostic in most cases. Monostotic disease may resemble osteomyelitis or a primary bone tumor; polyostotic disease in a distribution not typical for Paget's disease may resemble metastatic disease. Bone biopsy in these cases may be needed to confirm the diagnosis. Treatment of the disease process has focused on inhibiting bone resorption with drugs such as mithramycin, diphosphonates, and, more recently, calcitonin. Mithramycin is toxic to the osteoclasts. The diphosphonates appear to inhibit bone resorption and formation by forming a film over the exposed bone surface (chemabsorption), which results in a marked decrease in mineral uptake and release. Calcitonin, a hormone produced by the thyroid gland, has a hypocalcemic effect in patients with a high metabolic turnover of bone. In patients with Paget's disease, the administration of calcitonin inhibits bone resorption. Numbers of osteoclasts and hydroxyproline levels decrease with chronic use of the drug. Salmon and porcine calcitonin can lose effectiveness with time, probably owing to the development of neutralizing antibodies. This does not appear to happen with synthetic human calcitonin.

Bibliography

Aegerter EA, Kirkpatrick JA Jr: Orthopedic Diseases: Physiology, Pathology, Radiology, 4th ed. Philadelphia, WB Saunders Company, 1975.

Barry HC: Paget's Disease of Bone. Baltimore, Williams and Wilkins, 1969.

Beltran J, Noto AM, McGhee RB, et al: Infections of the musculoskeletal system: High-field-strength MR imaging. Radiology 164:449–454, 1987.

Bonakdarpour A, Gaines VD: The radiology of osteomyelitis. Orthop Clin North Am 14:1, 1983.

Butt WP: The radiology of infection. Clin Orthop 96:20, 1973.

Capitanio MA, Kirkpatrick JA: Early roentgen observations in acute osteomyelitis. AJR 108:488, 1970.

Dalinka MK, Lally JF, Koniver G, Coren GS: The radiology of osseous and articular infections. CRC Crit Rev Clin Radiol Nucl Med 7:1, 1975.

Edeiken J: Roentgen Diagnosis of Diseases of Bone, 3rd ed. Baltimore, Williams and Wilkins, 1981.

Enarson DA, Fujii M, Nakielna EM, Grzybowski S: Bone and joint tuberculosis: A continuing problem. Can Med Assoc J 120:139, 1979.

Goldenberg DL, Reed JI: Bacterial arthritis. N Engl J Med 312:764–771, 1985.

Jaffe HL: The classic Paget's disease of bone. Clin Orthop 127:4, 1977.

Krane SM: Skeletal metabolism in Paget's disease of bone. Arthritis Rheum 23:1087, 1980.

Mason MD, Zlatkin MB, Esterhai JL, et al: Chronic complicated osteomyelitis of the lower extremity: Evaluation with MR imaging. Radiology 173:355–359, 1989.

Miller WB Jr, Murphy WA, Gilula LA: Brodie abscess: Reappraisal. Radiology 132:15, 1979.

Moore TE, Yuh WTC, Kathol MH, et al: Abnormalities of the foot in patients with diabetes mellitus: Findings on MR imaging. AJR 157:813–816, 1991.

Post MJD, Gordon S, Quencer RM, et al: Gadolinium-enhanced MR in spinal infection. J Comput Assist Tomogr 14(5):721–729, 1990.

Reeder MM, Palmer PES: The Radiology of Tropical Diseases with Epidemiological, Pathological and Clinical Correlation. Baltimore, Williams and Wilkins, 1981.

Resnick D, Niwayama G: Diagnosis of Bone and Joint Disorders with Emphasis on Articular Abnormalities. Philadelphia, WB Saunders Company, 1981.

Silverman FN: Virus diseases of bone. Do they exist? AJR 126:677, 1976.

Steere AC, Green J, Schoen RT, et al: Successful parenteral penicillin therapy of established Lyme arthritis. N Engl J Med 312:869–874, 1985.

Waldvogel FA, Medoff G, Swartz MN: Osteomyelitis: A review of clinical features, therapeutic considerations and unusual aspects. N Engl J Med 181:198, 260; 182:316, 1970.

Waldvogel FA, Vasey H: Osteomyelitis: The past decade. N Engl J Med 303:360, 1980.

95 Arthropathies

GENERAL APPROACH TO JOINT DISEASE

D. M. FORRESTER

Appropriate evaluation of a patient with joint pain includes assessment of the clinical history, the laboratory data, and the radiographic studies. In some of the arthropathies the clinical diagnosis is well established at the time the radiographic evaluation is performed. Examples include psoriasis, gout, and hemophilia. The purpose of the studies is to assess the extent of disease, monitor response to therapy, identify underlying complications, and, on occasion, determine if the joint symptoms are due to the known diagnosis. In some arthritides the symptoms are minimal or nonspecific, and the radiographic examination provides the appropriate differential diagnosis; ankylosing spondylitis, calcium pyrophosphate dihydrate (CPPD) deposition disease, and osteoarthrosis are examples. Of the many imaging modalities that reveal the secrets of a joint, the plain radiograph remains the simplest, least expensive, and most useful tool. In specific clinical situations, additional information may be obtained by the use of arthrography, scintigraphy, computed tomography (CT), and magnetic resonance imaging (MRI).

PLAIN FILM RADIOGRAPHY

If a systematic approach in evaluating the plain radiograph is not used, important subtle clues are frequently overlooked. Information pertaining to joint disease may be compartmentalized to three anatomic regions: the soft tissues, the bones, and the joint itself. Observing changes in the soft tissue is most critical if the early stages of arthritis are to be detected. Subsequent alteration in alignment and bone mineralization may suggest an underlying arthritis, and eventually the joint space itself will be altered if there is continued progression of the disease.

A straightforward systematic approach—the "ABCs"—leads to an orderly scheme for reviewing the radiograph. The ABCs of plain film analysis are: *A*—Alignment, *B*—Bone mineralization, *C*—Cartilage space, and *S*—Soft tissue. The features to be evaluated are the following:

Soft Tissue. There may be diffuse swelling of all the soft tissue surrounding the joint or there may be a local swelling indicating the presence of a joint effusion or synovial proliferation (Fig. 95–1). Palpable subcutaneous lumps and nodules can be assessed. Soft-tissue atrophy, calcification, or ossification can be identified.

Alignment. Features to be evaluated include deviation, subluxation or dislocation, and flexion or extension deformities (Fig. 95–2).

Bone Mineralization. Demineralization may be diffuse, localized, or juxta-articular (Fig. 95–3). Cortical bone loss may be subperiosteal, intracortical, or endosteal. Serial studies may demonstrate rapid bone loss over time. Bone loss may be minimal or absent, or there may be new bone formation and periostitis (Fig. 95–4).

Cartilage Space. The joint may be widened, narrowed, or ankylosed. There may be articular or periarticular erosions. The location and nature of erosions are often important in suggesting a diagnosis. Erosions may be difficult to identify if they are not tangential to the x-ray beam. Oblique views often reveal the lesions

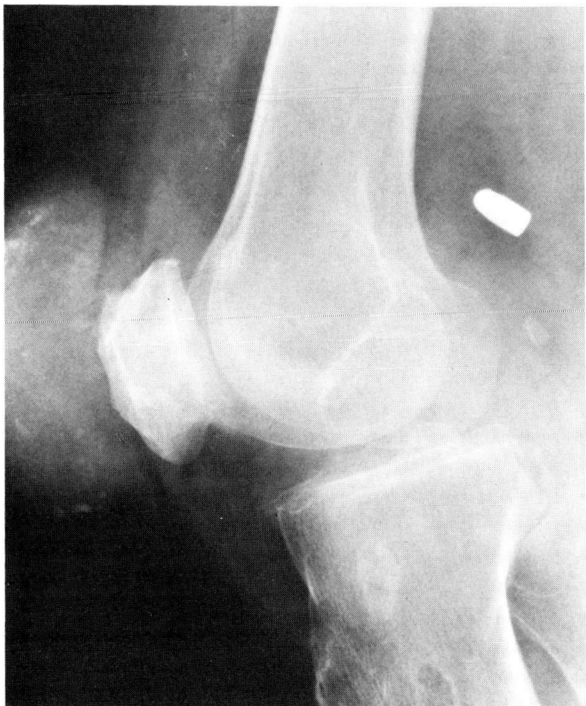

Figure 95–1. Soft-tissue abnormalities. Distention of the suprapatellar space with anterior displacement of the quadriceps tendon indicates a joint effusion. Prepatellar bursitis is reflected by massive soft-tissue swelling. The calcific densities reflect urate deposits in this patient with tophaceous gout.

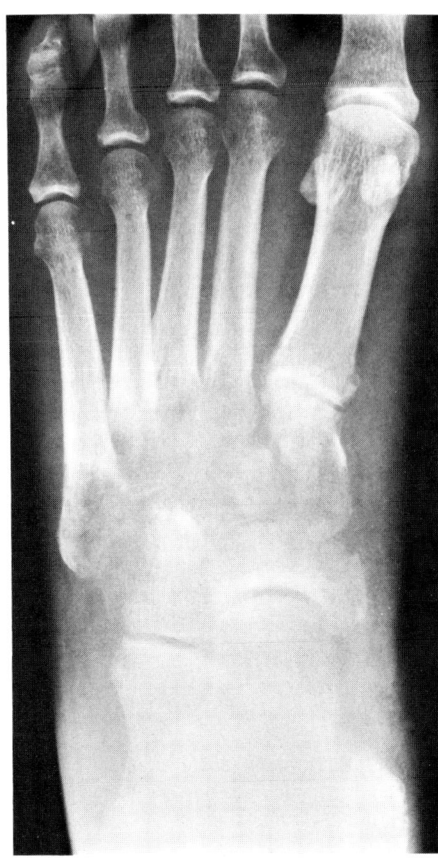

Figure 95–3. Demineralization. Severe juxta-articular demineralization of the mid-foot reflects focal hyperemia in a patient with gonococcal arthritis.

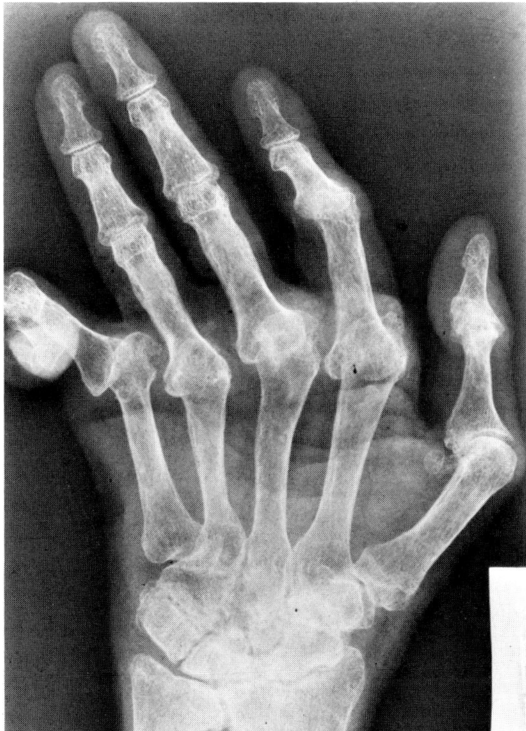

Figure 95–2. Alignment abnormalities. Subluxation of the metacarpophalangeal joints and bouttoniere deformities of the second and fifth digits reflect chronic inflammatory arthritis in a patient with advanced destructive changes of rheumatoid arthritis. Note the severe, generalized osteoporosis and joint destruction of the wrist.

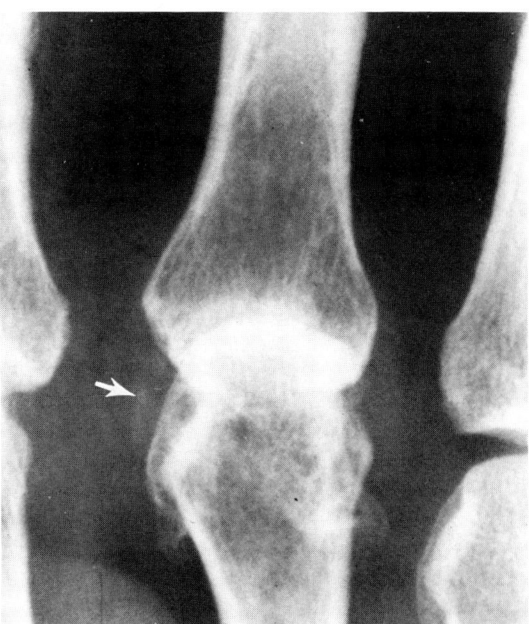

Figure 95–4. Chondrocalcinosis. Calcification of the cartilage of the metacarpophalangeal joint *(arrow)* has resulted in secondary osteoarthrosis. Note the narrowed joint space, eburnation, and osteophyte formation of the metacarpal head.

when the frontal projection does not. Calcification of the cartilage or synovium may be present (Fig. 95–5). Osteophytes may or may not be present.

RADIOGRAPHIC CRITERIA OF ARTHRITIS

Five radiographic features establish the presence of joint disease. These reflect the underlying pathophysiologic disease conditions. The five major criteria are (1) joint effusion, (2) joint space narrowing, (3) erosion, (4) chondrocalcinosis, and (5) osteophyte formation. Four additional radiographic changes develop as a consequence of arthritis. Unfortunately, they may also occur in diseases other than joint disease (neuromuscular disease, trauma, disuse, etc.). When present, these changes may suggest the presence of arthritis or confirm the clinical diagnosis, but by themselves they do not allow the diagnosis of arthritis to be made. The four minor criteria of arthritis are (1) alignment changes, (2) juxta-articular demineralization, (3) periosteal reaction, and (4) diffusely swollen digit.

THE THREE TYPES OF ARTHRITIS

The lengthy list of arthritides falls conveniently into three easily distinguished categories: inflammatory, degenerative, and metabolic arthritis. Each has characteristic clinical and radiographic features.

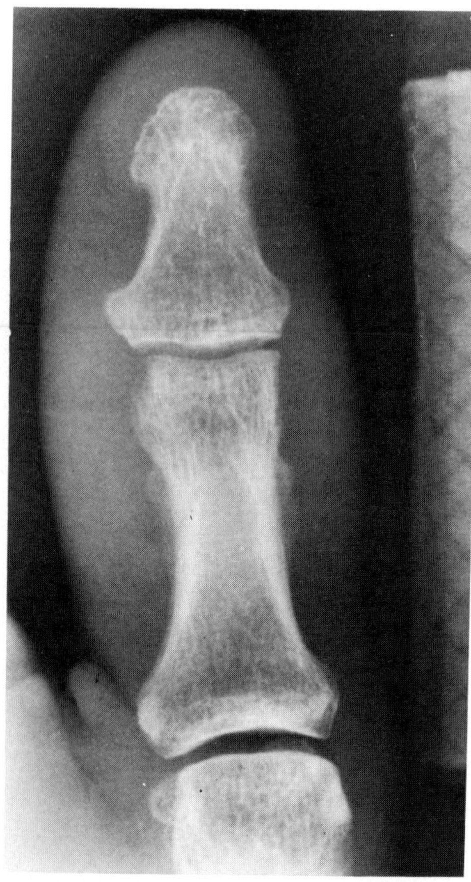

Figure 95–5. Periostitis. Diffuse soft-tissue swelling of the thumb and solid periosteal new bone along the proximal phalanx are seen in a patient with Reiter's syndrome.

Inflammatory Arthritis

The target of inflammatory arthritis is the synovium. Its distinguishing features include excessive synovial fluid or synovial hypertrophy, uniform joint space destruction, and erosions of the articular bone. Rheumatoid arthritis affects the small joints of the hands and feet in a symmetrical fashion (see Fig. 95–2). Identical radiographic changes occur in the seronegative spondyloarthropathies; however, the distribution is not symmetrical and the process frequently involves the axial skeleton (Fig. 95–6).

Degenerative Joint Disease

Wear of the cartilage results in focal areas of joint space narrowing. This leads to stimulation of the adjacent articular bone, which, in turn, reacts by forming osteophytes and reactive sclerosis (eburnation). When it occurs in the interphalangeal joints of the hands or the articulation of the base of the thumb, it is called primary osteoarthrosis or Kellgren's disease because no predisposing factor has been discovered. Secondary osteoarthrosis results from a specific insult to the cartilage such as trauma or crystal deposition diseases (see Fig. 95–5).

Metabolic Arthritis

Deposition of a substance, most commonly uric acid, in and around joints causes destruction in a pattern completely different from inflammatory arthritis. Masses with adjacent sharply marginated pressure erosions and intraosseous deposits resulting in lytic lesions are a hallmark of deposition disease (Fig. 95–7). Unlike inflammatory arthritis, the joint space is preserved until late in the disease.

ADVANCED IMAGING MODALITIES

There are specific situations in which additional imaging modalities add information to the data from the plain film.

Arthrography

Direct visualization of the joint by injecting water-soluble contrast material is useful in the diagnosis of adhesive capsulitis, cartilage or ligamentous damage, or disruption of the joint capsule (Fig. 95–8). Filling defects within the contrast material indicate synovial proliferation or loose bodies. Arthrography is also used to confirm the intra-articular position of a needle during aspiration of a joint.

Scintigraphy

The two most useful isotopes that are used to evaluate joint disease are technetium phosphate compounds and gallium-67 citrate. Technetium phosphate is taken up by bone in areas of increased turnover. It is a very sensitive but nonspecific marker and is useful in confirming the presence of an abnormal joint when plain films are normal. Unlike technetium compounds, gallium is very specific. It is taken up in areas of inflammation and in certain tumors. Its usefulness in the diagnosis of joint disease is to confirm the presence of infection when cultures are unobtainable or have negative results (Fig. 95–9).

Computed Tomography

Computed tomography (CT) is used to evaluate joint problems that are difficult to image by plain radiography, such as the sacroiliac joints, spine, and hips. Soft-tissue masses, osteochondromata, and bone fragments within joints are readily identified (Fig. 95–10).

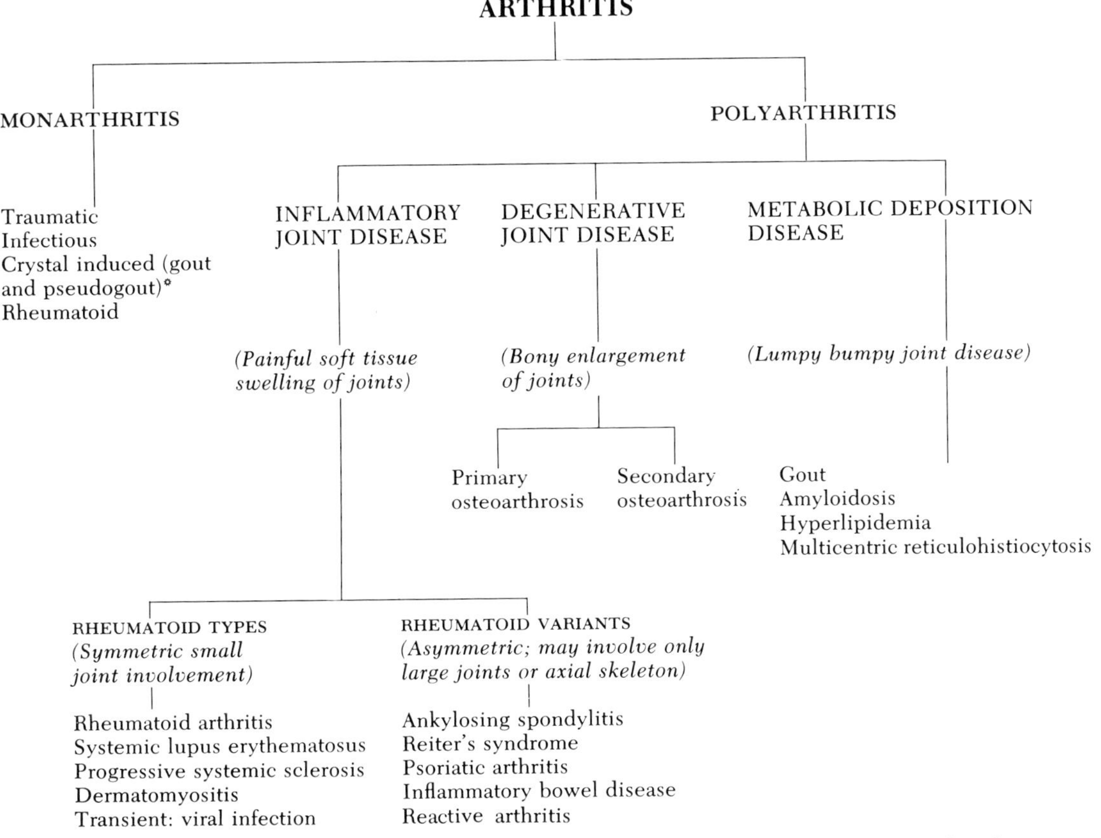

°Occasionally, more than one joint may be involved by an infectious process, or acute crystal induced synovitis. These are differentiated by joint aspiration, followed by Gram's stain, culture, and examination of the aspirate by compensated polarizing microscopy for crystals.

Figure 95–6. The differential diagnosis of arthritis.

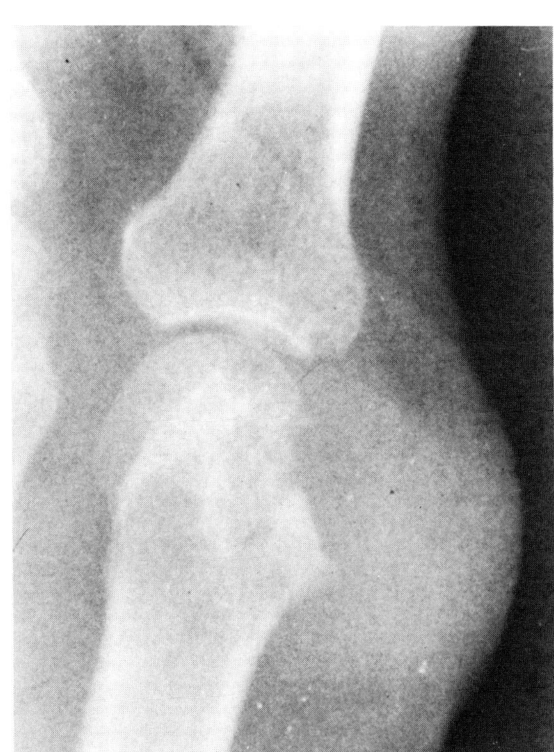

Figure 95–7. Gout. Soft-tissue mass adjacent to the metacarpophalangeal joint with a sharply marginated erosion. Note the normal joint space.

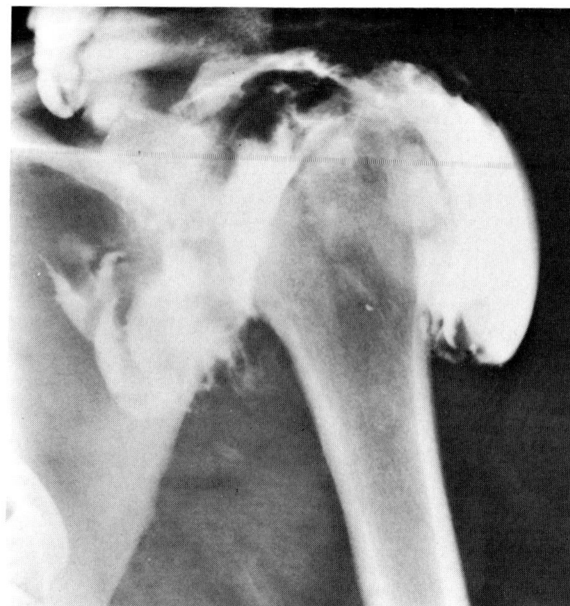

Figure 95–8. Arthrography. Injection of contrast material outlines the glenohumeral joint and its communication with the subacromial-subdeltoid bursa in a patient with syringomyelia and a neuropathic shoulder. Dissection of the joint into the supraclavicular space is also apparent.

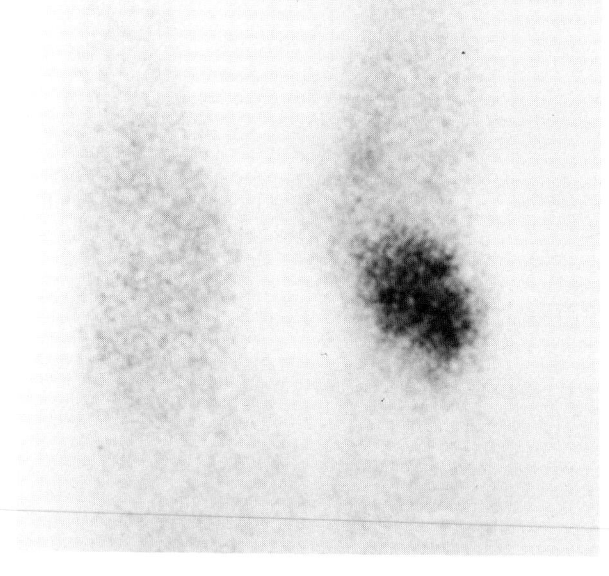

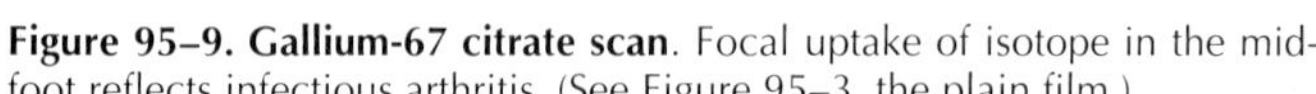

Figure 95–9. Gallium-67 citrate scan. Focal uptake of isotope in the midfoot reflects infectious arthritis. (See Figure 95–3, the plain film.)

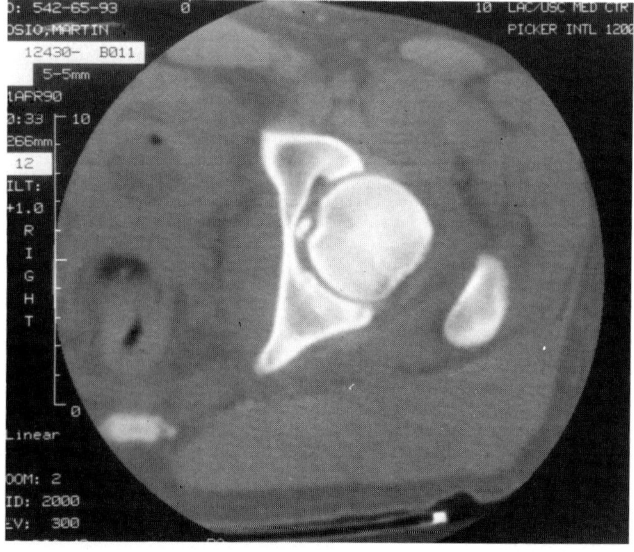

Figure 95–10. Intra-articular fracture fragment. Computed tomography demonstrates a small bony fragment in the hip joint. This unrecognized fragment resulted from a posterior hip dislocation.

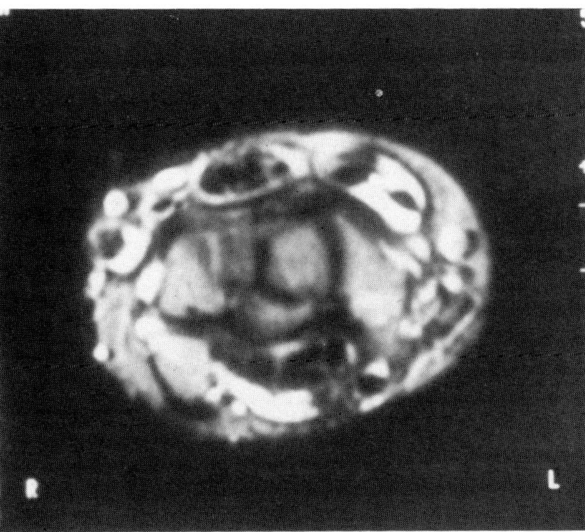

Figure 95–11. Acute tenosynovitis. A T_2-weighted axial image demonstrates markedly distended flexor and extensor tendon sheaths. Bright signal of the synovial fluid surrounds the black tendons.

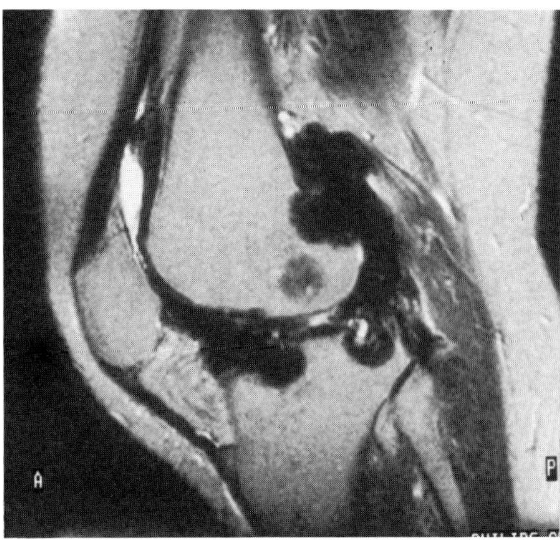

Figure 95–12. Pigmented villonodular synovitis. A T_2-weighted sagittal image illustrates the decreased signal of the synovium, characteristic of hemosiderin. Note the large erosions of the articular margins.

Magnetic Resonance Imaging

Magnetic resonance imaging (MRI) has the ability to image bone marrow, ligaments, and articular cartilage. This complements the plain radiograph's exquisite delineation of cortical bone and mineralization. Because of the sensitivity of marrow evaluation, initial use of MRI focused on the early detection of osteonecrosis. In specific situations it is now playing an increasing role in the evaluation of joint pathology. Because of its ability to image tendons, ligaments, and cartilage, it is replacing arthrography in the evaluation of the knee, shoulder, and ankle joints. The diagnosis of ligamentous injury, meniscal tears and rotator cuff injury and impingement syndrome can be made easily, avoiding invasive procedures and radiation exposure.

Joint or tendon effusions are obvious on MRI as a bright signal on T_2-weighted images (Fig. 95–11). Synovial hypertrophy may have a more nonhomogeneous signal. The signal characteristics of pigmented villonodular synovitis may be identical to fluid or synovial hypertrophy (low signal on T_1, high signal on T_2). In many cases, however, there is a decreased signal of the joint contents on the T_2-weighted image. This is due to the high hemosiderin content. Thus the MRI may suggest a specific diagnosis of PVNS. Articular erosions can be detected as irregularity of the cortical margins. These may be difficult to see on plain films but are easily detected on MRI (Fig. 95–12).

Anatomic detail of joints becomes more exquisite as coils improve. Information pertaining to cartilage width, once surmised by the proximity of articular bony margins, can now be directly observed. Cartilage has an intermediate signal on T_1, higher than the signal of adjacent cortical bone. In the presence of a joint effusion, T_2-weighting delineates the cartilage-effusion interface.

Small intra-articular fragments of bone or cartilage are invisible owing to their signal void; large osseous fragments are apparent on plain radiographs. MRI may have a role in localizing an obvious osseous density by demonstrating its position within the joint capsule or in the surrounding soft tissues.

Because of the sensitivity of MRI to directly image the bone marrow, incorrect assumptions may be made. A common error is the assumption that changes in marrow signal of the articular bones in patients with infectious arthritis indicate osteomyelitis. In fact, in most cases, they reflect edema (Fig. 95–13). Serial radiographs will document the absence of destructive bony changes.

A careful physical examination and correct interpretation of plain films, in most cases, provide the clinical information needed to care for a patient. In special circumstances, the exquisite anatomic detail provided by MRI alters the diagnosis or treatment.

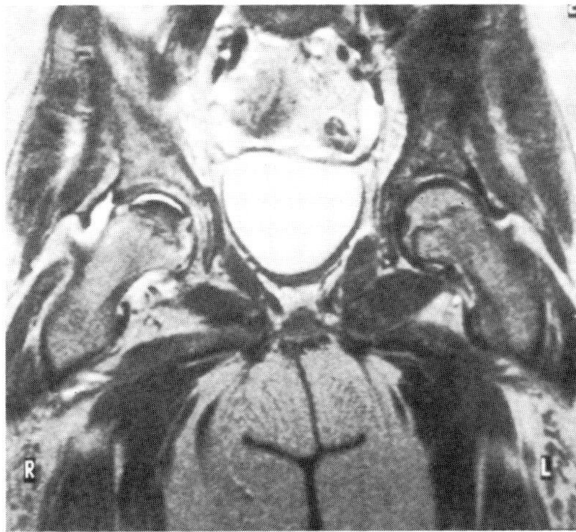

Figure 95–13. Infectious arthritis. A T_2-weighted coronal image demonstrates high signal of the marrow of the proximal right femur and adjacent ilium, as well as a joint effusion. Biopsy of the femur to document osteomyelitis demonstrated only edema, reflecting the inflammatory arthritis.

INFLAMMATORY ARTHRITIS

RHEUMATOID ARTHRITIS

Pamela S. Jensen

Rheumatoid arthritis (RA) is a subacute or chronic inflammatory disorder affecting many joints and periarticular structures. The joints of the extremities are most frequently involved, usually in a symmetrical distribution. Exacerbations and remissions associated with systemic abnormalities characterize the disorder.

Incidence and Diagnosis

Although rheumatoid factor is present in the serum of most affected individuals, RA does not have a specific biologic marker. The diagnosis is dependent upon signs and symptoms and fulfillment of a number of criteria. Incidence varies depending upon the criteria used, but the disorder probably affects less than 1 per cent of the adult population in the United States. In Great Britain, the incidence appears to be higher. RA is three times more common in women. Men with the disease generally tend to be more severely affected. The etiology has not been established; however, the possibility that an infective agent such as a virus is responsible is being seriously considered. The diagnosis is based on the exclusion of other arthritides and the presence of a minimum number of criteria including the following: morning stiffness, joint pain, swelling, symmetrical joint involvement, subcutaneous nodules, typical radiographic manifestations, presence of rheumatoid factor, poor synovial fluid mucin precipitate, and characteristic histologic changes in the synovial membrane or nodules. The American Rheumatoid Association indicates that a definitive diagnosis of RA can be made if five of the above criteria are present in a patient experiencing joint symptoms of greater than six weeks' duration.

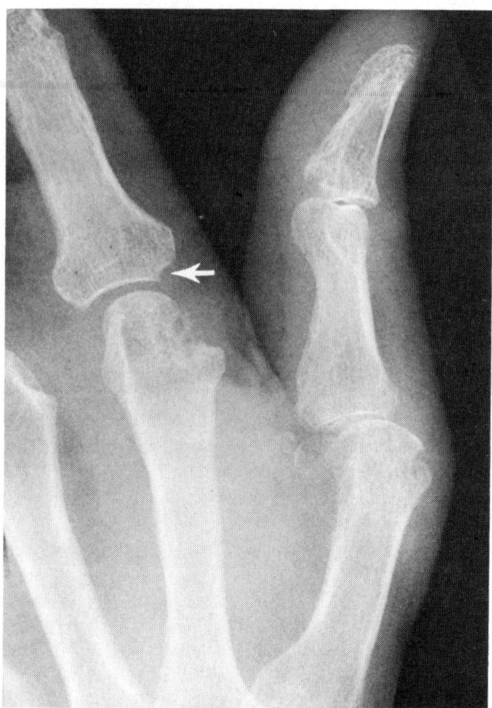

Figure 95–14. Early rheumatoid arthritis (RA). Bony erosions are present in the joint recesses of the second metacarpophalangeal joint adjacent to the articular surface in the area not covered by cartilage. The proximal portion of the capsule attaches to the bone at a distance from the articular surface in contrast to its distal attachment. This accounts for the much larger size of the proximal erosion and the smaller size of the distal erosion *(arrow)*. The joint space is preserved, but demineralization (cortical thinning) is present. The increased density around the first metacarpophalangeal joint is due to a joint effusion. Erosion in the first metacarpal head and narrowing and ulnar subluxation of the metacarpophalangeal joint of the thumb are common features of RA.

Pathophysiology

The initial process in RA involves proliferation of the synovial membrane, particularly in the recesses of the joints. If the disease is mild and remits, the inflammatory process may subside. Chronic synovitis is accompanied by further inflammation of the synovium, with the proliferative tissue mass extending over the articular cartilage to form a pannus. Similar proliferative changes in the tendon sheaths occur. Synovial fluid increases in volume and changes in character. The protein content increases, the white blood count is elevated, and the fluid becomes turbid. Lysosomal enzymes and proteases appear, which can cause cartilage destruction. The proliferative tissue mass erodes bone initially in the joint recesses where the bone is not covered by cartilage (Fig. 95–14). With cartilage loss, erosion extends across the articular surface and joint narrowing ensues. Juxta-articular demineralization occurs at both affected and nonaffected joints. Generalized skeletal demineralization is also a common feature of progressive disease. Subcutaneous rheumatoid nodules remote from joints and tendon sheaths can develop in areas subjected to external pressure such as on the extensor surfaces of the arms; they are also found in the viscera.

Clinical Manifestations

The onset of RA is variable. It may be acute or insidious, affecting one or multiple joints. Articular involvement may be preceded by constitutional symptoms of anorexia, malaise, fatigue, weight loss, low-grade fever, or by myalgias, Raynaud's phenomenon, or paresthesias. Most commonly, the small joints of the hands or feet are intially involved. If the presentation is monoarticular, the knee is most commonly affected. Progressive disease may eventually involve nearly every joint, although the joints of the thoracic and lumbar spine are usually spared. Joint stiffness, with or without pain or swelling, is indicative of disease activity.

Extra-articular manifestations in addition to the constitutional symptoms mentioned above include the sicca, or Sjögren's, syndrome, consisting of decreased tear formation; dryness of the nose, mouth, vagina, and rectum; and enlargement of the lacrimal and salivary glands. Pleural effusion, pleural or pulmonary nodules, empyema, and pulmonary fibrosis may occur. Pericarditis is the most significant cardiac lesion. Myopathies and neuropathies, including peripheral nerve entrapment such as carpal tunnel involvement, also occur. Widespread vasculitis tends to occur in advanced disease in association with high titers of rheumatoid factor and multiple rheumatoid nodules. Felty's syndrome consisting of RA plus splenomegaly and leukopenia is also associated with severe disease.

Laboratory Findings

Although there is no specific biologic marker for RA, up to 90 per cent of affected individuals have a positive rheumatoid factor (seropositive RA). However, rheumatoid factor is not specific for RA. It can be present in significant titers in systemic lupus erythematosus, progressive systemic sclerosis (scleroderma), dermatomyositis, and in a variety of nonarthritic conditions such as hepatic cirrhosis, pulmonary fibrosis, and sarcoidosis. High titers of rheumatoid factor in patients with RA are frequently associated with progressive unremitting disease and greater systemic manifestations. Although classic RA can occur in the absence of rheumatoid factor, many rheumatologists now consider seronegative RA to be a separate entity. Elevated sedimentation rate and presence of C-reactive protein are also nonspecific findings. The mucin clot produced by the addition of dilute acetic acid to the synovial fluid of an affected joint does not produce the tight ropy mass seen in normal individuals but instead results in a precipitate that is easily disrupted by agitating the solution. This finding is also not specific for RA and can be seen in infectious and crystal-induced arthritis.

Treatment

Management of RA is directed at relieving pain and discomfort, preserving mobility and joint function, preventing deformities, and relieving systemic manifestations. Drug therapy includes the use of analgesics, anti-inflammatory agents, and cytotoxic and immunosuppressive drugs. Aspirin is the most common drug for initial therapy. Nondrug therapies include procedures that deplete T-lymphocytes (lymphoplasmapheresis) and total lymphoid irradiation. Physical therapy is of major importance in the management of RA. Surgical procedures include synovectomy, carpal tunnel release, capsule and tendon repair, and joint replacement or fusion.

Radiographic Manifestations

The joints most commonly affected in RA include the metacarpophalangeal and metatarsophalangeal joints, proximal interphalangeal joints of the hand, wrists, toes, knees, elbows, ankles, shoulders, hips, temporomandibular joints, cervical spine, and sacroiliac joints.

Soft-Tissue Findings

Joint effusion and soft-tissue swelling are the earliest manifestations of RA and are often more readily detected by physical examination than by radiography. Outward displacement of the subcutaneous fat surrounding a joint capsule indicates the presence of an effusion or synovial proliferation. This is often best seen at the interphalangeal joints of the hands (Fig. 95–15). Effusions in the prepatellar or suprapatellar bursa of the knee, displacement of the fat pad in the elbow, and fluid in the olecranon bursa are evident on the lateral radiograph. When there is a communication between the gastrocnemius-semimembranosus bursae and the knee joint, the presence of a joint effusion will lead to distention and sometimes rupture of the connecting bursae. The clinical presentation may suggest thrombophlebitis. In the hip, distention of the iliopsoas bursa may displace the cecum, ureter, or other viscera. Subcutaneous rheumatoid nodules can also be identified radiographically.

Osteoporosis

Juxta-articular demineralization can occur at both affected and nonaffected joints. Although this may occur early in the disease, it is often difficult to identify with certainty until a substantial amount of trabecular bone is lost. In contrast, thinning of the cortical bone due to endosteal resorption is more easily identified. Generalized demineralization is common in RA and may be quite pronounced in progressive disease. Loss of bone in the acetabulum often leads to protrusio acetabuli.

Periosteal Changes

Periosteal new bone formation can occur in association with inflammatory changes in a joint or owing to an overlying tenosynovitis. It does not occur with the frequency of periosteal new bone

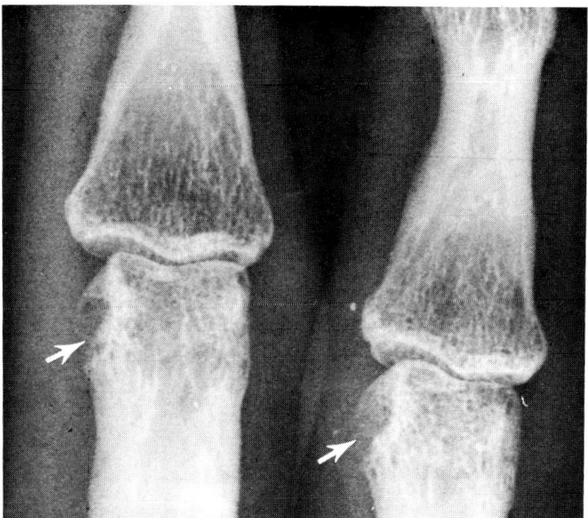

Figure 95–15. Early rheumatoid arthritis. There is fusiform swelling about the right second and third proximal interphalangeal joints due to effusion and marginal erosions at the radial side of the proximal phalanges *(arrows)*.

formation seen with psoriatic arthritis, Reiter's syndrome, and ankylosing spondylitis. In addition, the periosteum is usually elevated in a single layer along the shaft of the bone and is not the exuberant fluffy periosteal new bone formation seen with the seronegative arthropathies mentioned above. Periosteal changes can occur before erosive changes are evident. Ultimately, the periosteal new bone becomes incorporated into the cortex.

Bony Erosions

Erosive destruction of the bone characteristically begins at the margin of the joint in the recesses at the junction of the articular cartilage, in capsular and ligamentous attachments, and in the synovial reflection (Figs. 95–14 to 95–16). The earliest radiographic sign is a loss of definition of the sharp margin of the cortex. Ultimately the erosion becomes a cup-shaped defect, often having overhanging edges (Fig. 95–16). The margins of the erosions are often irregular during active disease and may become smooth when the disease remits. Large cystic defects with smooth borders can occur some distance from the joint surface (Fig. 95–17*A*). They are often synovium-lined and communicate with the joint. Extra-articular erosions occur at ligamentous and tendinous insertions. These are commonly noted at the dorsal and plantar surfaces of the calcaneus, dorsal processes of the lower cervical spine where the nuchal ligament attaches, crest of the ilium, lateral margin of the scapula, greater trochanter of the femur, inferior and distal surfaces of the clavicle, and along the posterior and dorsal surfaces of the second to ninth ribs.

Cartilage Space Loss

Narrowing of the articular cartilage is usually uniform and most commonly affects the interphalangeal joints of the hand and feet and the carpal, tarsal, knee, and hip joints (Figs. 95–17 to 95–20). Even in the presence of marked cartilage loss, there is virtually no hypertrophic osteophyte formation while the disease is active. Secondary changes due to superimposed osteoarthrosis can occur at joints damaged by RA when the latter becomes quiescent (Fig. 95–20). The cartilage loss is often symmetrical and this finding, in addition to the uniform nature of the loss and the absence of hypertrophic changes, helps distinguish RA from other arthritides. In the wrist, the cartilage loss involves nearly all the joints and is not limited to the joints about the trapezium as it is with osteoarthrosis.

Text continued on page 1384

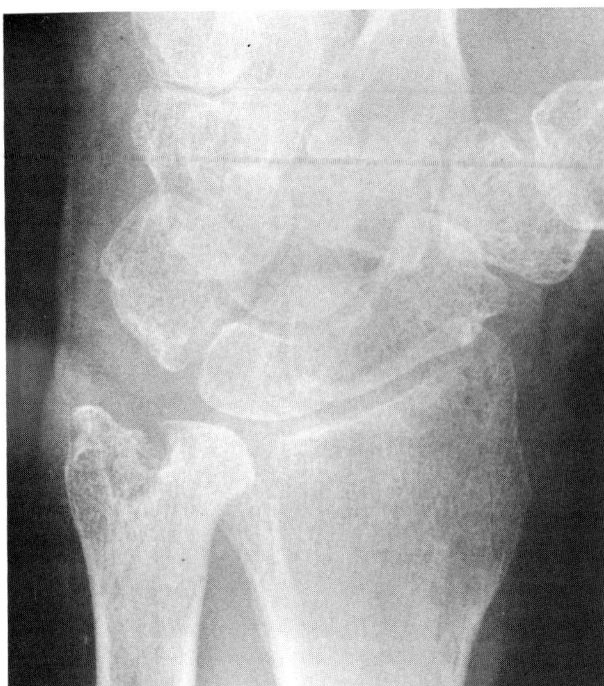

Figure 95–16. Early rheumatoid arthritis. There is a large erosion in the fovea of the ulna and swelling of the extensor carpi ulnaris tendon adjacent to the ulnar styloid. The scaphoid and proximal carpal row are rotated medially toward the radius.

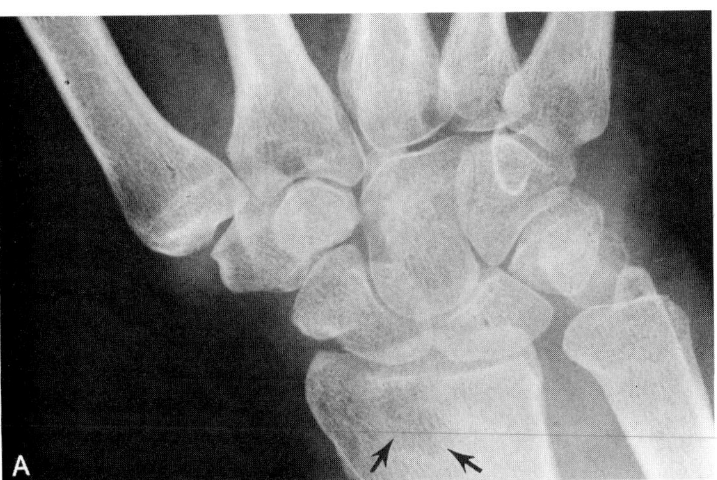

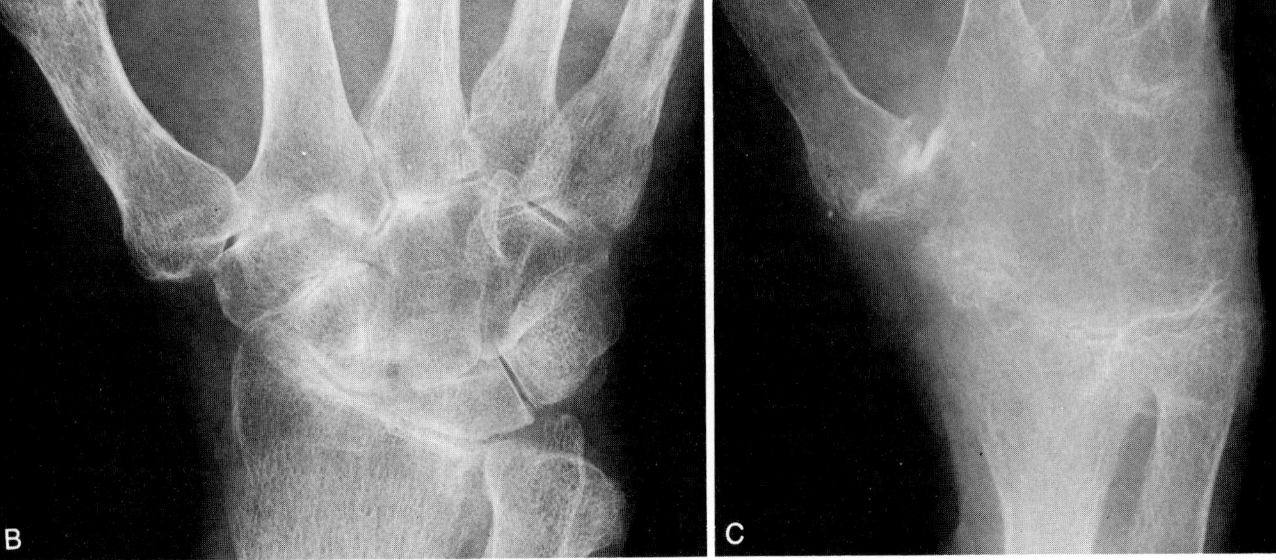

Figure 95–17. Progressive changes in rheumatoid arthritis. *A,* Diastasis of the radioulnar joint, medial rotation of the proximal carpal row, and early joint narrowing about the carpal bones are typical of early RA. A large cyst in the distal radius *(arrows)* communicates with the joint. The cortical thickness of the metacarpals is still preserved. *B,* Moderately advanced RA with generalized demineralization, carpal rotation, and extensive joint space loss. *C,* End-stage disease with severe osteoporosis, carpal fusion, and fusion of the second to fourth carpometacarpal joints. Erosion of the articular surface of the radiocarpal joints is also evident.

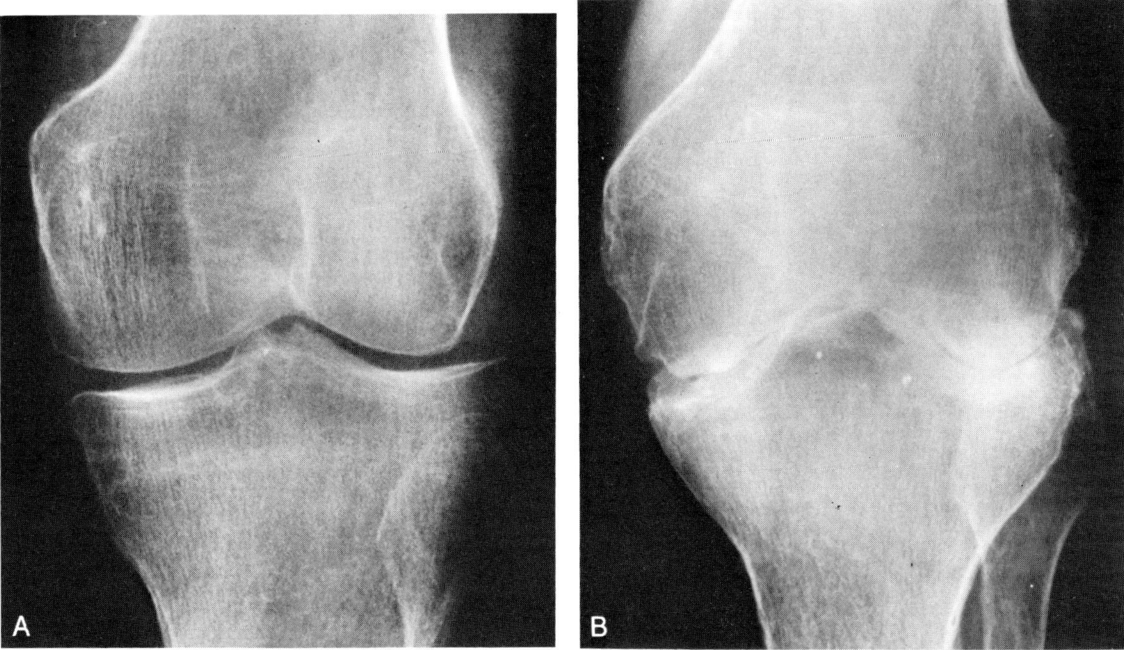

Figure 95–18. Progressive rheumatoid arthritis. *A,* Early uniform cartilage narrowing of the knee without hypertrophic osteophyte formation. *B,* Total loss of the joint space with indentation of the femoral condyles into the osteoporotic tibial plateaus.

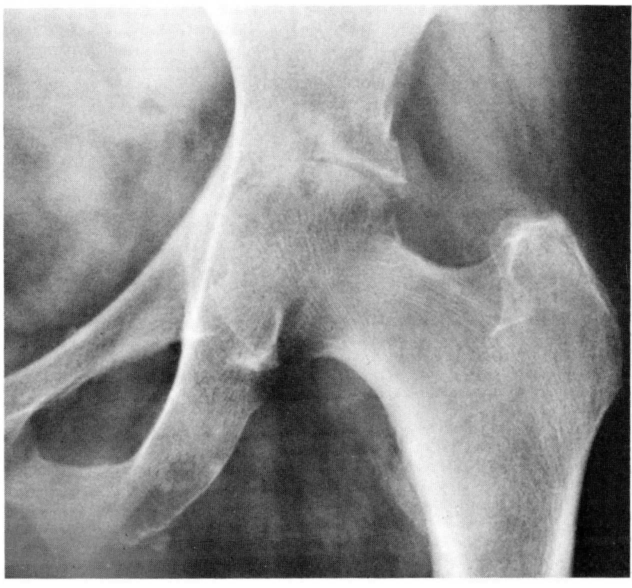

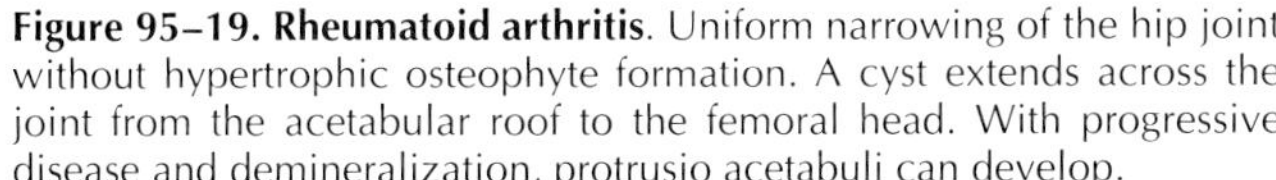

Figure 95–19. Rheumatoid arthritis. Uniform narrowing of the hip joint without hypertrophic osteophyte formation. A cyst extends across the joint from the acetabular roof to the femoral head. With progressive disease and demineralization, protrusio acetabuli can develop.

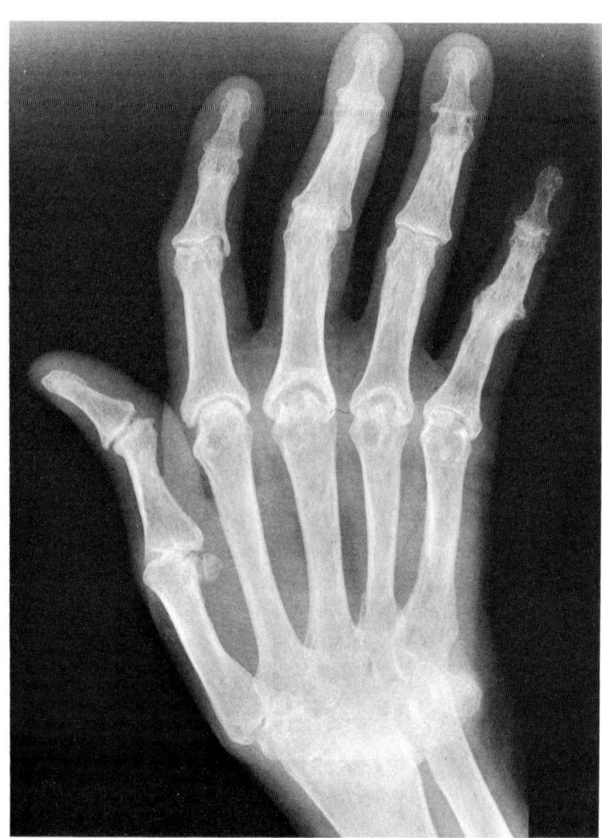

Figure 95–20. Quiescent rheumatoid arthritis. End-stage ("burned-out") disease with fusion of the wrist, sclerotic margins about the metacarpal head erosions, and bony overgrowth at the metacarpophalangeal joints. Fusion of the interphalangeal joints is not common in RA, and the possibility of psoriatic arthritis must be considered.

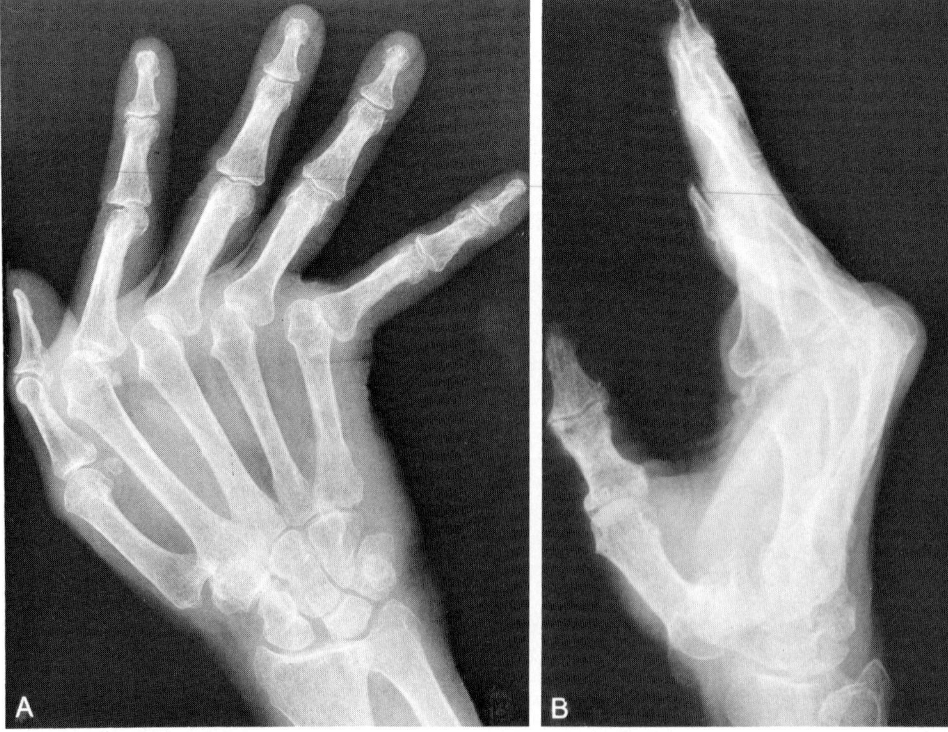

Figure 95–21. Rheumatoid arthritis. *A*, Ligamentous laxity with diastasis of the scapholunate joint and ulnar subluxation of the second to fifth metacarpophalangeal joints. Generalized osteoporosis with thinning of the cortical bone is evident. Minimal joint space narrowing or erosion is present. *B*, Lateral view of the hand demonstrates volar subluxation at the metacarpophalangeal joints.

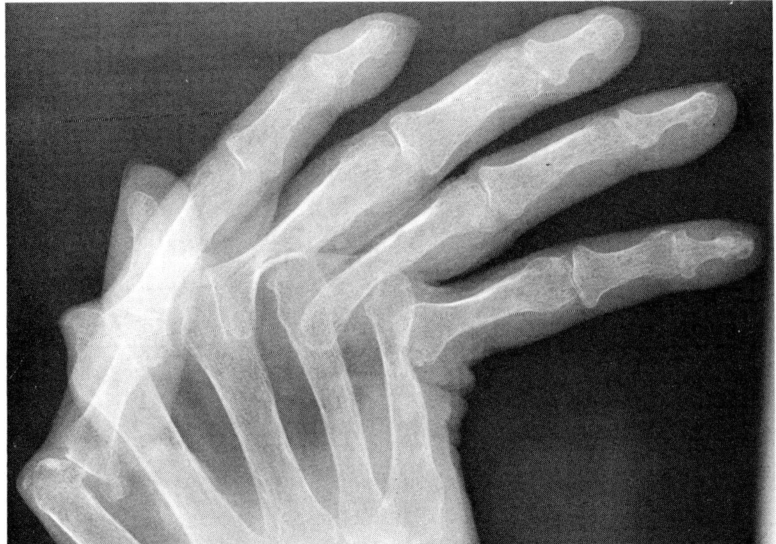

Figure 95–22. Rheumatoid arthritis. Marked ligamentous laxity with dislocation of the metacarpophalangeal joints. Pressure erosion along the shaft of the third proximal phalanx is due to contact with the head of the fourth metacarpal. Another pressure erosion is present along the shaft of the fifth metacarpal.

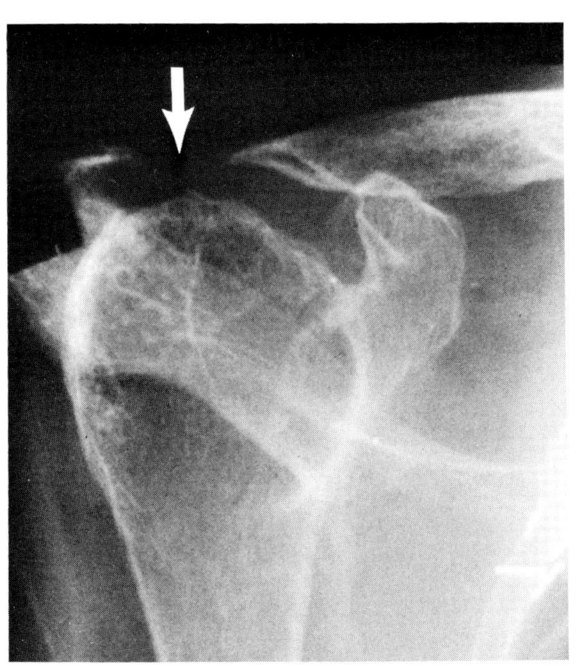

Figure 95–23. Advanced rheumatoid arthritis. Superior subluxation of the humerus, destruction of the rotator cuff, erosion of the humeral head and the acromioclavicular joint *(arrow)*, and generalized demineralization are all characteristic of RA.

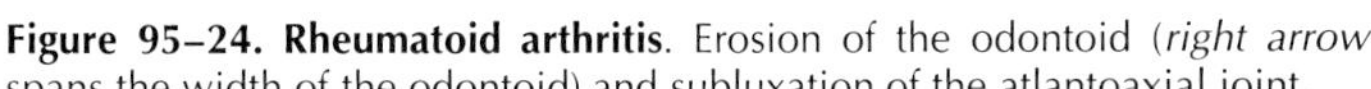

Figure 95–24. Rheumatoid arthritis. Erosion of the odontoid (*right arrow* spans the width of the odontoid) and subluxation of the atlantoaxial joint.

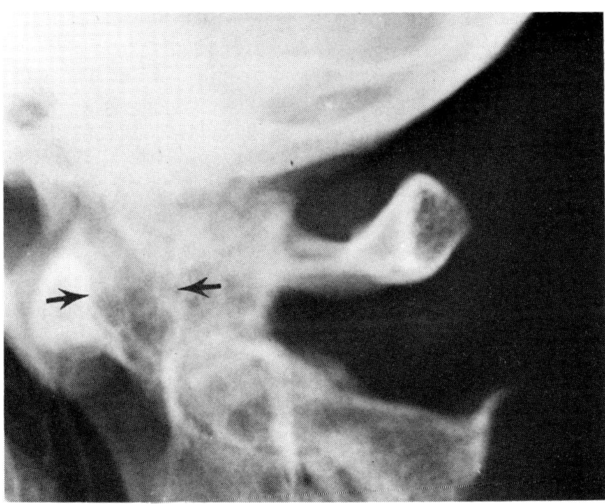

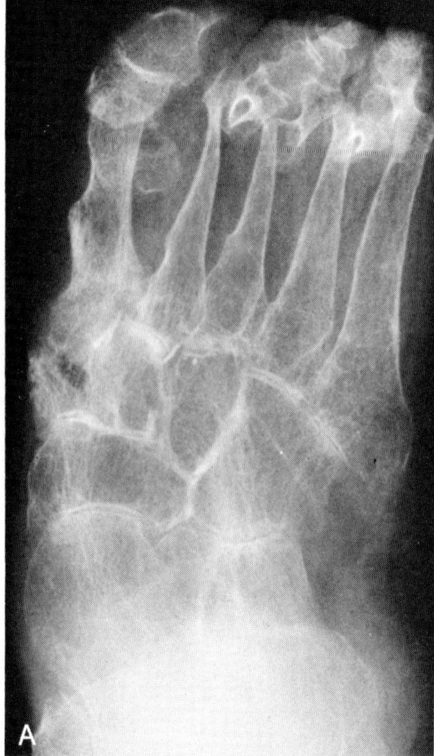

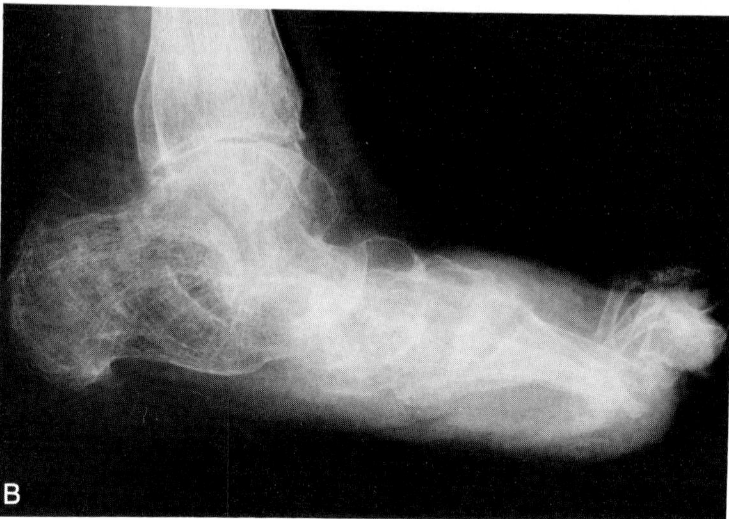

Figure 95–25. Advanced rheumatoid arthritis. *A,* Arthritis mutilans of the foot with extensive joint narrowing, loss of the metatarsal heads, tapering of the distal ends of the metatarsals, dislocation of the toes, and marked osteoporosis. *B,* Lateral view demonstrates the gross dislocation of the metatarsophalangeal joints and the dorsiflexion of the toes.

Fusion of the carpal and tarsal bones following cartilage loss is common. Fusion of the interphalangeal joints, metacarpophalangeal joints, knees, or hips despite extensive cartilage loss is uncommon.

Abnormalities of Alignment

Multiple subluxations due to ligamentous laxity are common. Diastasis of the distal radioulnar, carpal, acromioclavicular, and sternoclavicular joints occurs frequently (Figs. 95–21 to 95–25). Ulnar deviation and volar subluxation or dislocation of the fingers are common, as is superior subluxation of the shoulders with narrowing or destruction of the rotator cuff (see Fig. 95–23). Subluxation of the atlantoaxial joint is often accompanied by erosion of the odontoid (see Fig. 95–24). Multiple subluxations of the upper cervical intervertebral discs are also a common feature. Narrowing of the disc space is not accompanied by hypertrophic osteophyte formation, thus distinguishing RA from osteoarthrosis. Osteoarthrosis also typically affects only the lower cervical spine. Fusion of the articulating facets can occur with progressive disease. However, calcification in the anterior and posterior spinal ligaments and ankylosis of the vertebral bodies is uncommon, thus distinguishing RA from ankylosing spondylitis and the other seronegative arthropathies. In addition, the thoracic and lumbar spine are usually spared, and if the sacroiliac joints are involved the changes are generally mild.

Bibliography

Krane SM: Rheumatoid arthritis. In Rubenstein E, Federman DD (eds): Scientific American Medicine. New York, Scientific American, 1986.

Resnick D, Niwayama G: Diagnosis of Bone and Joint Disorders. Philadelphia, WB Saunders Company, 1981.

Steinbach HL, Jensen PS: Roentgenographic changes in the arthritides. Semin Arthritis Rheum 5:167–202, 1975.

JUVENILE RHEUMATOID ARTHRITIS

Barbara N. Weissman

Juvenile rheumatoid arthritis (JRA) is a disorder of unknown etiology characterized by chronic synovial inflammation that develops before the age of 16. Although George Frederic Still described and attempted to classify chronic polyarthritis in children, the term *Still's disease* is not usually used in the United States. The term *juvenile chronic polyarthritis* is used in the United Kingdom and includes JRA and other types of chronic childhood arthritis.

Incidence and Diagnosis

JRA is a relatively common chronic condition of childhood affecting between 60,000 and 200,000 children in the United States. It is about 5 per cent as common as adult rheumatoid arthritis. In 1977, a subcommittee of the American Rheumatism Association published revised criteria for the diagnosis of JRA consisting of the presence of persistent arthritis of one or more joints for at least six weeks' duration, provided a variety of other conditions that can also cause chronic arthritis in juveniles are excluded (Table 95–1). Arthritis was defined as swelling of a joint or limitation of motion with increased warmth, pain, or tenderness. Pain or tenderness alone was not sufficient for the diagnosis of arthritis.

In addition to establishing criteria for diagnosis, three subtypes—systemic, pauci/oligoarticular, and polyarticular—were defined based on the manifestations present within the first six months of disease. In systemic-onset JRA, persistent intermittent fever is present with or without the rheumatoid rash or other organ involvement. In some cases, joint manifestations are minimal and the typical fever pattern and rash make the diagnosis of systemic-onset JRA probable. If arthritis is also present, a definitive diagnosis can be

TABLE 95–1. EXCLUSIONS IN THE DIAGNOSIS OF JUVENILE RHEUMATOID ARTHRITIS

A. **Other Rheumatoid Diseases**
  1. Rheumatic fever
  2. Systemic lupus erythematosus
  3. Ankylosing spondylitis
  4. Polymyositis and dermatomyositis
  5. Vasculitis
    a. Anaphylactoid purpura (Henoch-Schönlein)
    b. Polyarteritis
    c. Serum sickness and other allergic reactions
    d. Mucocutaneous lymph node syndrome: infantile polyarteritis
    e. Other
  6. Scleroderma
  7. Psoriatic arthritis
  8. Reiter's syndrome
  9. Sjögren's syndrome
  10. Mixed connective tissue disease
  11. Behçet's syndrome

B. **Infectious Arthritis**
  1. Bacterial arthritis (including tuberculosis)
  2. Viral, fungal, and mycoplasmal arthritides
  3. Nonbacterial arthritis associated with bacterial infections
  4. Other

C. **Inflammatory Bowel Disease**

D. **Neoplastic Diseases Including Leukemia**

E. **Nonrheumatic Conditions of Bones and Joints**
  1. Osteochrondritis
  2. Toxic synovitis of the hip
  3. Slipped capital femoral epiphysis
  4. Trauma
    a. Battered child syndrome
    b. Fractures
    c. Joint, ligamentous, and muscular injuries
    d. Congenital indifference to pain
    e. Acute chondrolysis
  5. Chondromalacia of the patella
  6. Congenital anomalies and genetically determined abnormalities of the musculoskeletal system (including inborn errors of metabolism)
  7. Idiopathic tenosynovitis

F. **Hematologic Diseases**
  1. Sickle cell anemia
  2. Hemophilia

G. **Psychogenic Arthralgia**

H. **Miscellaneous**
  1. Immunologic abnormalities
  2. Sarcoidosis
  3. Hypertrophic osteoarthropathy
  4. Villonodular synovitis
  5. Chronic active hepatitis
  6. Familial Mediterranean fever

From Brewer EJ Jr, Bass J, Baum J, et al: Current proposed revision of JRA criteria. Proceedings of the Conference on the Rheumatic Diseases of Childhood. Reprinted from Arthritis and Rheumatism Journal, 20:195–199, copyright 1977. Used by permission of the American Rheumatism Association.

made. This subgroup accounts for about 20 per cent of patients. Pauciarticular or oligoarticular JRA refers to involvement of four or fewer joints initially, with the exclusion of systemic-onset disease. This occurs in approximately 40 per cent of patients. Polyarticular-onset JRA refers to involvement of five or more joints initially; patients with systemic onset are excluded. Joints are counted individually except for the cervical spine, carpals, and tarsals, which are each counted as one joint. Forty per cent of children have this type of disease onset.

Clinical Manifestations

Any type of fever may be seen in patients with JRA, but the characteristic picture is one of persistent intermittent fever with diurnal variation from normal to 103° F or more. The characteristic rash is an evanescent, pale erythematous macular eruption that appears predominantly on the chest, axillae, thighs, and upper arms. Iridocyclitis is found most often in young females with monoarticular and pauciarticular onset disease. The onset of iridocyclitis may be insidious and asymptomatic and, since blindness is a possible consequence, frequent ophthalmologic follow-up is necessary. Pericarditis has been found on echocardiography in 47 per cent of children with JRA and is most often associated with systemic-onset disease. Cardiac tamponade, constrictive pericarditis, and congestive heart failure are uncommon sequelae. Hepatosplenomegaly and lymphadenopathy are most severe and frequent in patients with active systemic-onset JRA. Amyloidosis is a rare complication in patients with JRA reported from the United States, although in Europe the incidence may be considerably higher (4 to 6 per cent). The importance of amyloidosis is documented by the fact that renal disease is responsible for the largest number of deaths in patients with JRA, and this is most often due to amyloidosis. Renal amyloidosis may be manifested by normal, enlarged, or small renal size. Ultrasound examinations may demonstrate nonspecific increased echogenicity of the cortex and prominence of the corticomedullary junction.

Laboratory Findings

There are no specific diagnostic laboratory tests for JRA. Presence of rheumatoid factor is less frequent in patients with JRA than in adults with rheumatoid arthritis; between 5 and 20 per cent of JRA patients have positive agglutination tests. Rheumatoid factor is found more frequently in older children with polyarticular onset disease and appears to be a poor prognostic factor with regard to joint destruction. Between 10 and 40 per cent of children with polyarticular- and pauciarticular-onset disease have positive tests for antinuclear antibody (ANA); patients with JRA and chronic iridocyclitis also tend to have positive tests for ANA. Anemia and leukocytosis occur most frequently in systemic-onset disease.

Treatment

Nonsteroidal anti-inflammatory drugs and a program of physical therapy are typically the initial treatment for newly diagnosed JRA. This is effective in 50 per cent or more of patients, particularly those with pauciarticular disease. Slower-acting antirheumatic drugs such as gold, antimalarial agents, or penicillamine are often added in patients who do not respond to the initial therapy. A recent study, however, did not demonstrate that the addition of hydrochloroquine or penicillamine to the nonsteroidal anti-inflammatory therapy resulted in superior treatment when compared with the nonsteroidal therapy alone.

Radiographic Features

Radiographic features of JRA are usually nonspecific. Characteristic growth abnormalities and cervical spine fusions may, however, suggest the diagnosis.

Soft-Tissue Findings

In most cases soft-tissue swelling is nonspecific and identical to that seen in adults with rheumatoid arthritis. Subcutaneous nodules are less frequent in patients with JRA than in adults with rheumatoid arthritis and are more often associated with polyarticular disease; they generally indicate a poor prognosis. Soft-tissue calcification is an uncommon finding in patients with JRA. It is usually periarticular and is occasionally extensive enough to suggest a diagnosis of dermatomyositis. In a recent study, soft-tissue calcifica-

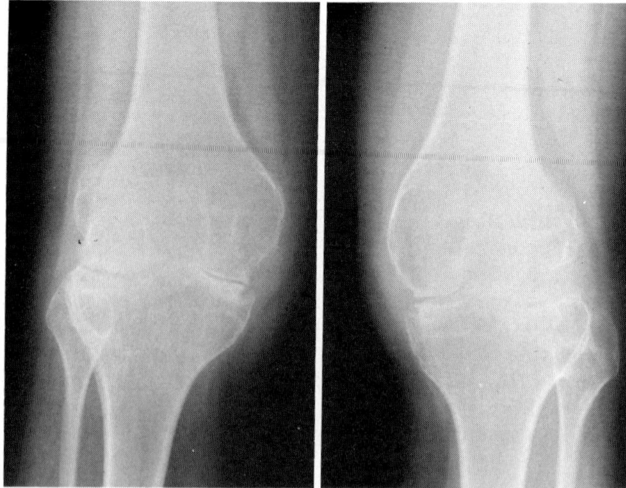

Figure 95–26. Juvenile rheumatoid arthritis (JRA) knees. AP views show enlargement of the epiphyseal centers near the metaphyseal ends and tapering of the epiphyses at the joint. The appearance is exaggerated by flexion deformities. There is bilateral cartilage space narrowing. The tibial erosions are well-defined, suggesting that they are old. There is secondary osteoarthritis with hypertrophic lipping from the joint margins.

tion was found to be associated with a history of one or more prior injections of intrasynovial corticosteroids. Calcification was periarticular in most cases, and synovial or intra-articular in fewer instances. As in adults, rupture of a popliteal cyst may present with symptoms mimicking thrombophlebitis; however, this is an uncommon finding in JRA.

Periosteal Reaction

Periosteal reaction is noted most frequently along the shafts of proximal phalanges, metacarpals, and metatarsals adjacent to affected joints. It may be seen as early as two weeks after the onset of symptoms.

Cartilage Space Abnormalities

Cartilage space narrowing is a late finding in patients with JRA, particularly in young children and in patients with monoarticular arthritis. In one series, children under seven years of age with severe disease required one or two years until cartilage space narrowing was evident. Improvement in cartilage space narrowing and reconstitution of adjacent subchondral bone have been demonstrated radiographically in both the small joints of the hands and wrists and in large joints such as the hips.

Erosions

Articular erosion is a late finding in JRA, particularly in the large joints of young children. Erosion may occur within the unossified portions of the epiphyses and remain invisible on radiographs until ossification occurs (Fig. 95–26). Therefore, the appearance of erosion in children may not correlate with the current disease activity. Patients with rheumatoid factor may show earlier erosive changes and more severe chronic arthritis than patients who are rheumatoid factor–negative. Bony ankylosis may follow complete cartilage loss. This most commonly occurs in the wrists, particularly the carpometacarpal articulations of the index and middle fingers and the intercarpal articulations. Ankylosis of the apophyseal joints of the cervical spine may result in a characteristic radiographic appearance. Usually segments of two, three, or four vertebrae are involved, although diffuse ankylosis may occur (Fig. 95–27). If the joints are fused early, growth abnormalities of the vertebral bodies may be prominent, producing a decrease in the anteroposterior dimensions as well as in the heights of the involved vertebrae. At the junction with more normal vertebrae where motion occurs, the underdeveloped vertebrae flare. Disc spaces at the involved levels are decreased in size and a secondary calcification may occur. Facet joint fusion has been noted in 35 per cent of patients with polyarticular disease, 20 per cent of patients with systemic-onset disease, and 10 per cent of patients with monoarticular disease.

Abnormalities of Alignment

C1-C2 subluxation due to inflammatory damage to the transverse ligament of the atlas is less frequent in patients with JRA than in

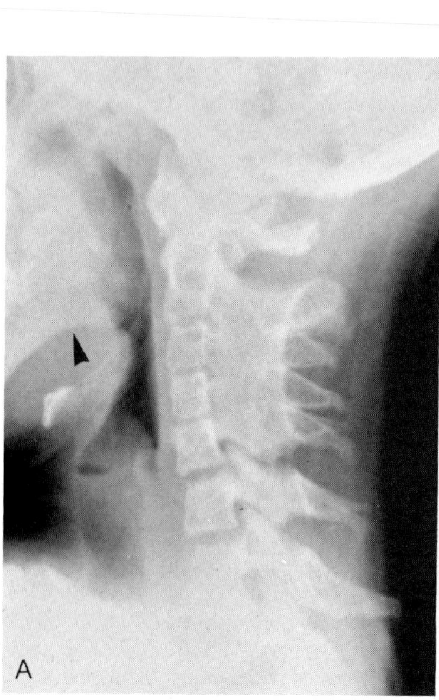

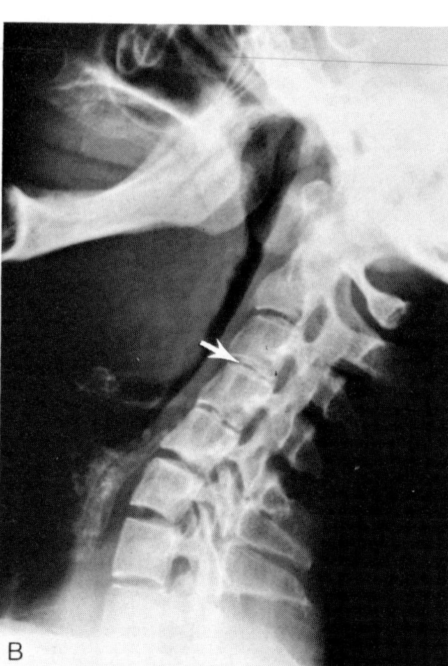

Figure 95–27. The cervical spine in juvenile rheumatoid arthritis. *A,* This patient developed fusion of the facet joints from C2 to C5 during growth. This resulted in undergrowth of the involved vertebrae. Decreased mandibular growth resulted in micrognathia and a prominent mandibular curve *(arrowhead). B,* An older patient developed C2 through C5 facet fusion after growth was achieved, and the vertebral shapes are normal. Disc narrowing and calcification *(arrow)* occurred subsequently. There is mild C1-C2 subluxation. The enlargement of the base of the tongue is due to amyloidosis.

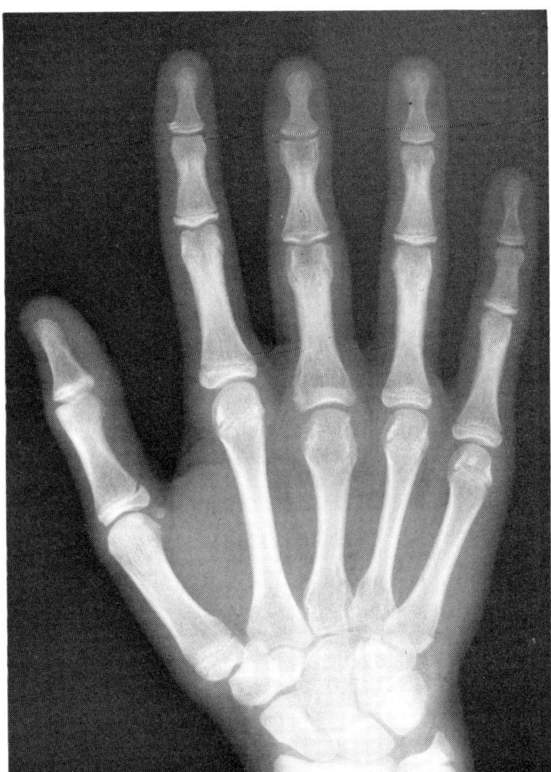

Figure 95–28. Early epiphyseal fusion. There has been early closure of the third metacarpal epiphysis, resulting in marked metacarpal shortening. The other epiphyses of that digit are fusing early. The phalanges of the middle finger are broader than normal, and periosteal reaction is present at the base of the third proximal phalanx.

adult RA and is more frequent in patients who are seropositive than those who are seronegative. C1-C2 subluxation is very uncommon in patients with monoarticular JRA.

Abnormalities of Growth

Accelerated maturation may result in an asymmetrical increase in maturation and is particularly prominent in the affected carpals. Ultimately, however, carpal size is decreased in comparison with the unaffected side. In the long bones, enlargement of the secondary centers of ossification is particularly prominent at their metaphyseal ends, with relative tapering of the ossification center at its articular surface (see Fig. 95–26). The metaphyses appear flared and the shafts relatively reduced in diameter. Overgrowth of an extremity may accompany enlargement of the secondary centers of ossification. Eventually, these epiphyses may undergo premature fusion, resulting in shortening of the affected limb. Early epiphyseal closure has been noted in 15 to 30 per cent of patients with JRA and most frequently affects the metacarpals and metatarsals (Fig. 95–28). When the mandibular condyles are affected, decreased growth may result in muscular imbalance and an up-curving of the inferior margin of the mandible just anterior to its angle; this appearance is termed *antegonial notching*. Generalized decrease in growth may also occur as a consequence of the disease itself or as a consequence of prolonged corticosteroid therapy. An irregular, angular appearance of the epiphyses may occur, particularly in the carpals but also in the epiphyses of the larger joints.

Bibliography

Ansell BM, Kent PA: Radiological changes in juvenile chronic polyarthritis. Skel Radiol 1:129–144, 1976.

Brewer EJ, Giannini EH, Kuzmina N, Alekseev L: Penicillamine and hydrochloroquine in the treatment of severe juvenile rheumatoid arthritis. N Engl J Med 314:1269–1276, 1986.

Cassidy JT, Martel W: Juvenile rheumatoid arthritis: Clinicoradiologic correlation. Arthritis Rheum 20:207–211, 1977.

Gilsanz V, Bernstein BH: Joint calcification following intraarticular corticosteroid therapy. Radiology 151:647–649, 1984.

Hensinger RN, DeVito PD, Ragsdale CG: Changes in the cervical spine in juvenile rheumatoid arthritis. J Bone Joint Surg 68A:189–198, 1986.

Martel W, Holt JF, Cassidy JT: Roentgenologic manifestations of juvenile rheumatoid arthritis. AJR 88:400–423, 1962.

Rodnan GP, Schumacher HR (eds): Rheumatic disease of childhood. In Primer on the Rheumatoid Diseases. Atlanta, The Arthritis Foundation, 1983.

Stillman JS, Barry PE: Juvenile rheumatoid arthritis: Series 2. Arthritis Rheum 20:171–175, 1977.

THE SPONDYLOARTHROPATHIES

Ethan M. Braunstein

The association of different histocompatibility antigens with various rheumatic diseases has had a profound effect upon our understanding of the pathogenesis and clinical manifestations of these diseases. The HLA-B27–positive spondyloarthropathies share many radiologic characteristics. As with other inflammatory arthropathies, there is involvement of the synovial tissue. Often there is early sacroiliac erosion, followed by progressive sacroiliac destruction and ankylosis. This may be followed by ankylosis of the apophyseal joints of the spine. In contrast to rheumatoid arthritis and other seropositive (rheumatoid factor–positive) disorders, there is often exuberant bony proliferation at the site of ligamentous and capsular attachments to the bone (entheses). New bone proliferation bridging adjacent vertebrae (syndesmophytes or parasyndesmophytes) is characteristic. In the appendicular skeleton, the entheses of large and small joints may be involved with erosive and sometimes exuberant proliferative change. This latter feature frequently enables the radiologist to distinguish the appendicular manifestations of a spondyloarthropathy from rheumatoid arthritis. Rheumatic conditions that are B27-related include ankylosing spondylitis, Reiter's syndrome, psoriasis, enteropathic arthropathy, and some forms of juvenile chronic arthritis.

Histocompatibility Antigen HLA-B27

The most striking correlation to date between the HLA antigens and disease has been the association of B27 and ankylosing spondylitis. Over 90 per cent of patients with ankylosing spondylitis are HLA-B27–positive. It is unclear just how this relationship accounts for the manifestation of the disease; however, it has been hypothesized that B27 is a marker for an immune response gene that determines the susceptibility to an environmental insult, or that B27 itself is a receptor site for an infectious agent. If one examines the relationship between diseases that may or may not have spondylitis, the link becomes apparent. The presence of the HLA-B27 antigen in patients with psoriasis is as follows: psoriasis without skeletal involvement (5 to 10 per cent), psoriatic arthropathy without sacroiliitis (18 to 22 per cent), and psoriatic arthropathy with sacroiliitis (50 to 60 per cent). The frequency of HLA-B27 in healthy whites is 6 to 14 per cent and in American blacks 0 to 4 per cent. The frequency of the B27 gene in Japanese is less than 1 per cent, and the incidence of ankylosing spondylitis in this population is very low. However, over 90 per cent of the Japanese who do develop ankylosing spondylitis are HLA-B27 positive.

Ankylosing Spondylitis

Ankylosing spondylitis has a prevalence similar to that of rheumatoid arthritis, with 1 to 1.5 per cent of whites having the disease.

About 10 to 20 per cent of B27-positive individuals have sacroiliitis. It was once thought to occur predominantly in males, but it now appears that there is a more uniform sex distribution. Women tend to present with appendicular involvement, and they are less likely to have progressive spinal involvement. Because it was thought that ankylosing spondylitis was rare in women, many of these individuals were given the diagnosis of seronegative rheumatoid arthritis. Diagnosis is based upon the presence of symptomatic sacroiliitis and positive radiographic findings. In contrast to mechanical spinal disorders, mobility is decreased in both the anteroposterior and lateral planes. Other clinical manifestations may include fatigue, weight loss, low-grade fever, uveitis, pulmonary fibrosis, cardiac disease, and amyloidosis. Therapy is directed at relieving the pain, decreasing inflammation, and increasing mobility and strengthening the muscles through exercise. Early diagnosis is critical for therapy to be most effective.

Radiographic Manifestations

In about 99 per cent of cases of ankylosing spondylitis, the sacroiliac joints are involved before any other portion of the skeleton. In most cases, this involvement is bilaterally symmetrical from disease onset. In some cases, the disease does not progress after causing sacroiliac change, but in many cases the spine becomes involved as well. The sacroiliac joints may be adequately examined in an anteroposterior projection with the x-ray tube at a 20-degree cephalad angle. This provides a tangential view through the anterior, synovium-lined portion of the joints (Fig. 95–29). Rarely are oblique projections necessary. High-resolution computed tomography has been suggested for more detailed information; this may show erosions, subchondral sclerosis, and narrowing earlier than conventional radiographs. The earliest sacroiliac findings may consist simply of indistinctness of the cortical margins of the joint, without any cartilage loss or subchondral sclerosis. As the disease progresses, such sclerosis may become profound, and finally bony ankylosis may occur (Fig. 95–30). In ankylosing spondylitis, this evolution typically is bilaterally symmetrical.

There may be characteristic findings at the entheses, the sites of insertion of ligaments, tendons, and articular capsules into bone. These findings often take the form of proliferative changes, particularly at the entheses of the bony pelvis. Cartilaginous articulations such as the symphysis pubis and discovertebral joints, syndesmoses, and sites of extra-articular tendon insertions, such as the greater and lesser trochanters, may become involved along with synovial joints (Fig. 95–31). Particularly common locations for these changes are the tendon insertions on the ischial tuberosities (Fig. 95–32).

In the spine, the earliest findings are at sites of greatest spinal motion, particularly the thoracolumbar and lumbosacral junctions. As the disease progresses, the remainder of the spine becomes involved. The spinal erosions may occur in the synovium-lined posterior apophyseal joints, and resultant fusion of the posterior elements may be seen before there are significant radiographic changes in the vertebral bodies (Fig. 95–33). Erosions of the bodies occur at the anterosuperior and anteroinferior entheses. If there is reactive sclerosis to these erosions, a typical "shining corner" may appear (Fig. 95–34). As the erosions become larger, enough bone may be destroyed at the vertebral corners to give a square appearance to the vertebral body (Fig. 95–35). This "squaring" may be further enhanced by proliferative bony changes along the anterior vertebral margins. Ultimately, reactive bone may bridge vertebral bodies, causing ankylosis of the entire spine (Fig. 95–36). These reactive ossifications spanning disc spaces and connecting vertebrae are called syndesmophytes. They are thin, delicate struts of bone extending from the margin of one vertebral body to the margin of an adjacent vertebral body (Fig. 95–37). In contrast, in psoriatic arthritis and Reiter's syndrome, the bony buttresses may be larger and appear bulkier, extending from the middle of one vertebral body to another (Fig. 95–38); these are called nonmarginal syndesmophytes or parasyndesmophytes. As ankylosis of the spine progresses, motion is curtailed, and there may be either straightening of the spine or progressive kyphosis.

Another phenomenon related to spinal ankylosis is the development of pseudarthrosis of a discovertebral joint secondary to a posterior element fracture (Fig. 95–39). This sort of fracture occurs through fused apophyseal joints, usually near the thoracolumbar junction, since this is a site of much motion of the spine. The pseudarthrosis is the result of movement at the fracture site and the adjacent disc, with destruction of the end-plates of the contiguous vertebrae and subchondral sclerosis. The disc space between the involved vertebrae may also be widened. Pseudarthrosis should not be mistaken for infectious discitis, in which a paravertebral soft-tissue mass may be evident, and which develops over a shorter time

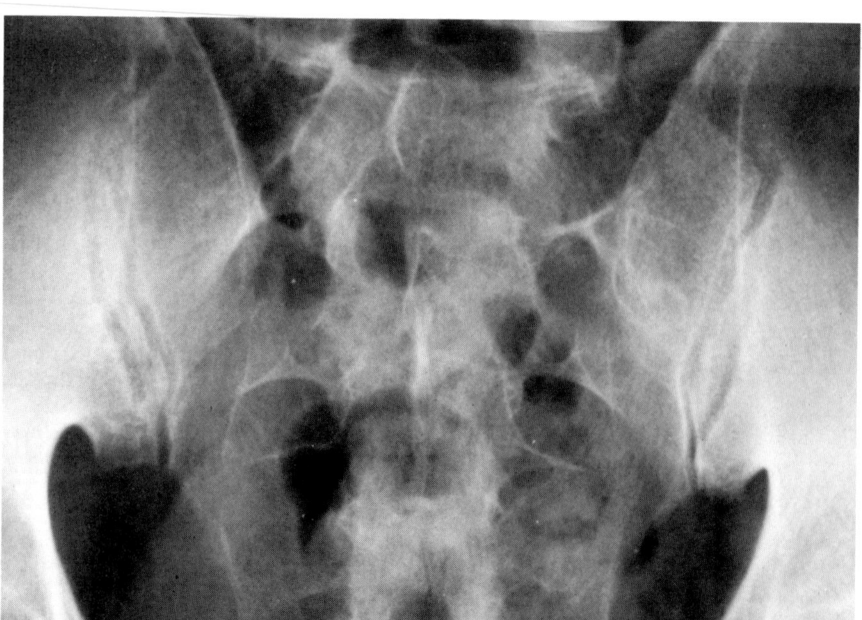

Figure 95–29. Frontal view of **normal sacroiliac joints** with a 20-degree cranial angle of the x-ray tube. The normal joints have well-defined cortex.

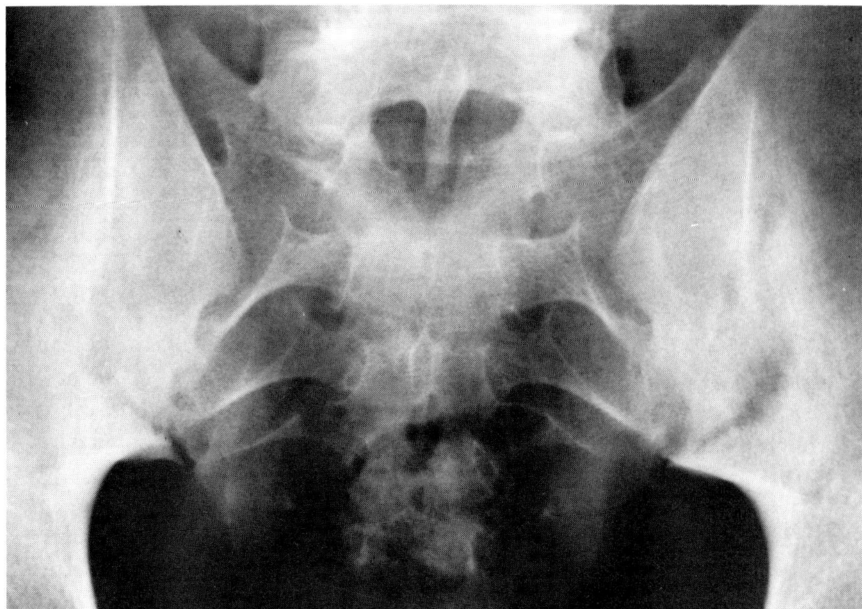

Figure 95–30. Bilateral sacroiliac erosions in a patient with ankylosing spondylitis. The joint margins are indistinct and sclerotic in a nearly symmetrical pattern.

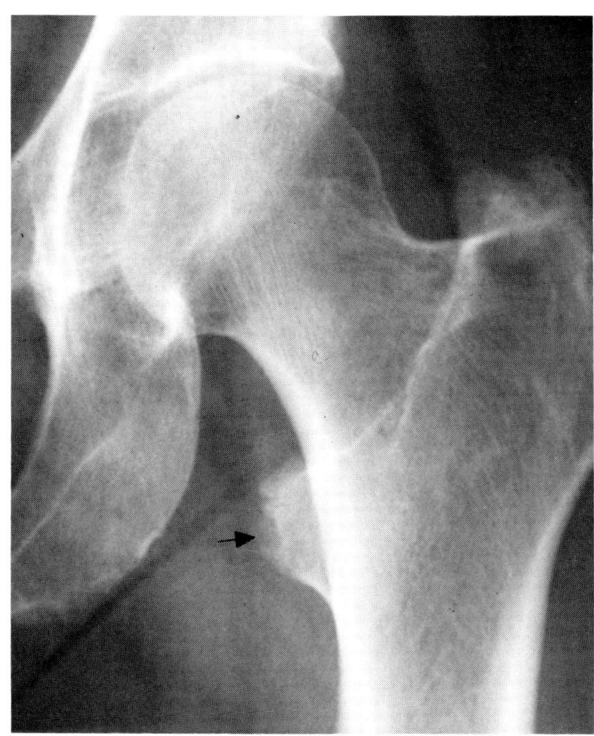

Figure 95–31. Erosion and bony proliferation at the iliopsoas insertion on the lesser trochanter of the femur in a patient with ankylosing spondylitis *(arrow)*.

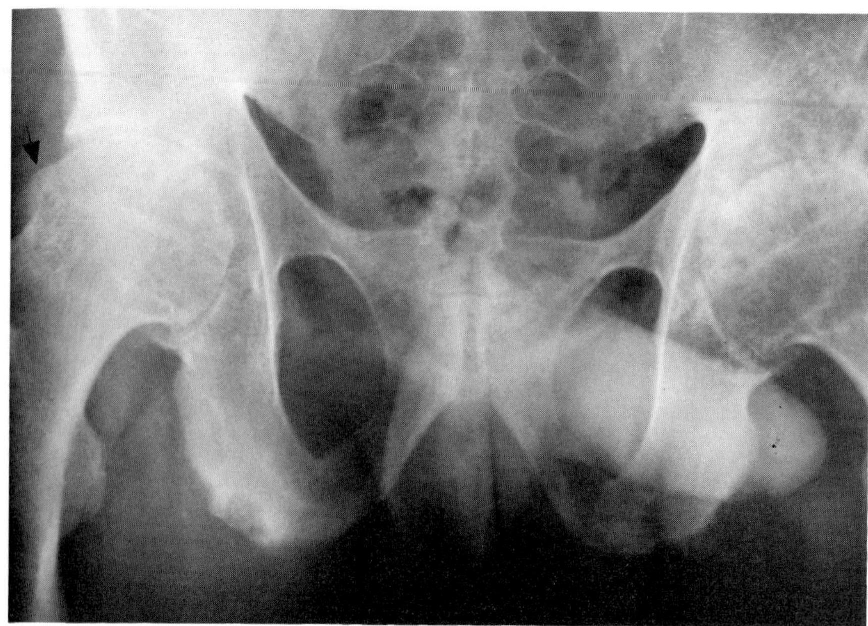

Figure 95–32. Ankylosing spondylitis with sclerosis, new bone apposition, and erosion at the entheses of the ischial tuberosities. Notice also the uniform cartilage loss of the hips and the small osteophyte at the capsular insertion of the right femoral head *(arrow).*

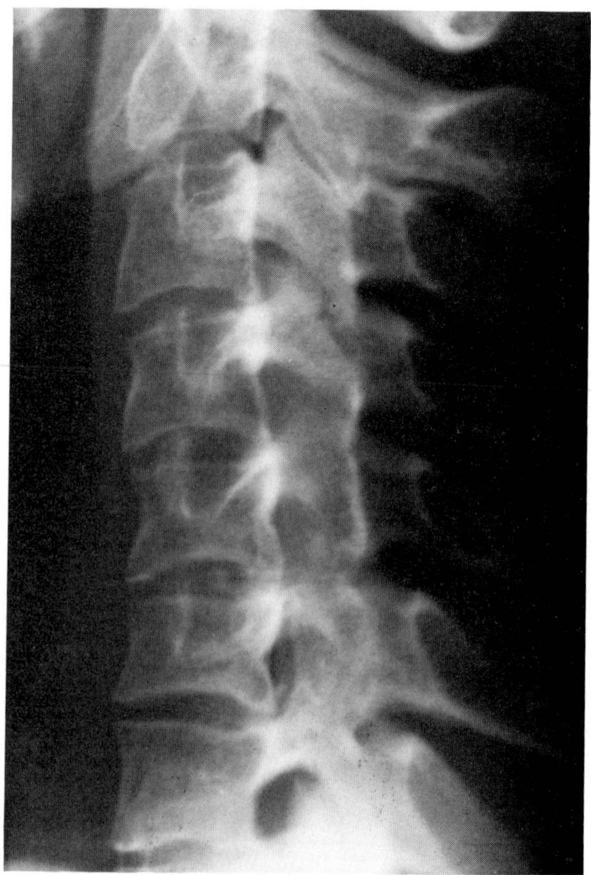

Figure 95–33. Fusion of the apophyseal joints with relative sparing of the cervical vertebral bodies in ankylosing spondylitis.

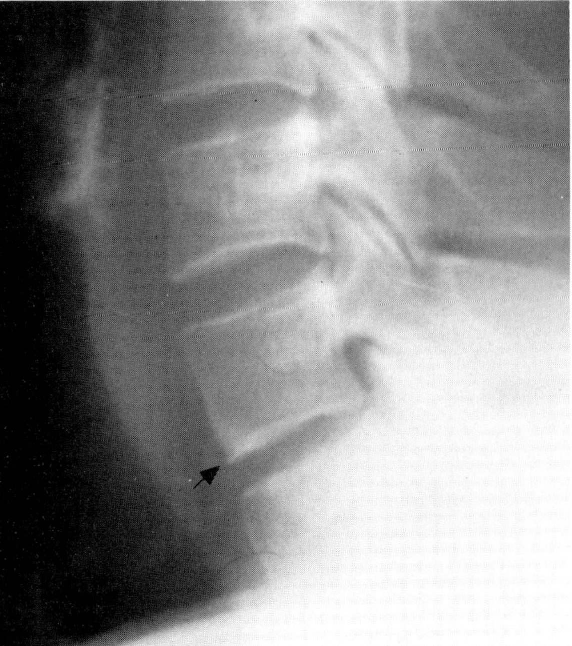

Figure 95–34. "Shining corner" *(arrow)* due to **reactive sclerosis** at the site of a small vertebral body erosion in ankylosing spondylitis.

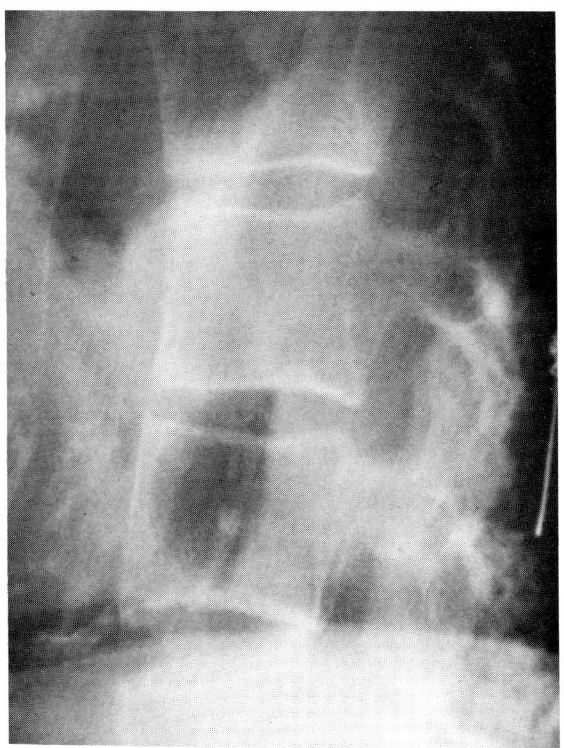

Figure 95–35. Vertebral body "squaring" due to erosions at the corners in advanced ankylosing spondylitis.

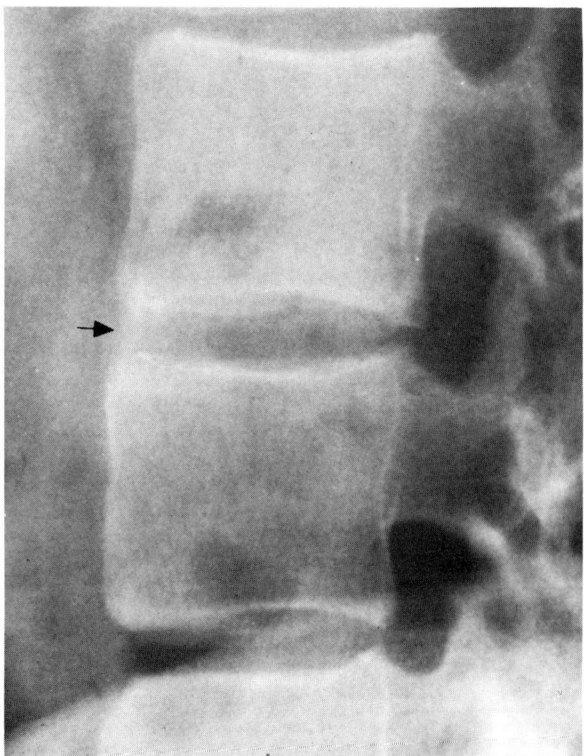

Figure 95–36. Reactive bone formation bridging two vertebral bodies anteriorly *(arrow)*.

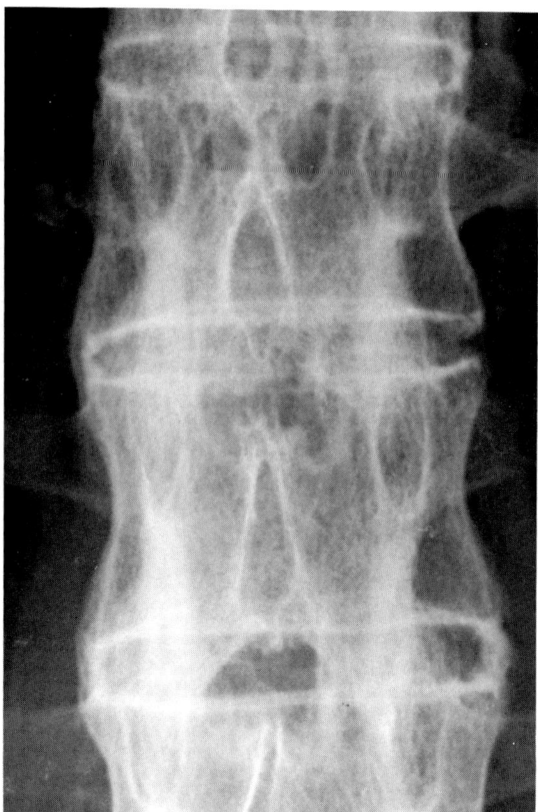

Figure 95–37. Syndesmophytes in ankylosing spondylitis. These gracile bony struts extend from the margin of one vertebral body to the margin of the next.

span. Occasionally, spinal canal block with cord impingement may develop in patients with ankylosing spondylitis and pseudarthrosis, presumably owing to reactive epidural inflammation.

In the appendicular joints, symptomatic involvement is out of proportion to the usually mild radiologic changes. Many radiographic findings in the extremities may be due to inflammation of tendon sheaths and bursae, and they are manifested simply by soft-tissue swelling. There may be some secondary bony reaction. In large joints such as the shoulders and hips; there is uniform cartilage loss with superficial erosions near the margins of the joint capsules. The reactive sclerosis to these erosions may resemble small osteophytes at the capsular insertions, particularly on the femoral head (see Fig. 95–32). In smaller joints, radiologic findings are minimal. Appendicular skeletal involvement appears to be more common in women than men, but erosions may not be radiographically demonstrable.

Women may also be more likely to have involvement of the cervical spine and sacroiliac joints, with sparing of the intervening spinal segments. Juvenile ankylosing spondylitis may begin with severe appendicular involvement, particularly of the hips and knees, and it may be difficult to differentiate clinically from juvenile rheumatoid arthritis. However, most patients have progressive disease that is ultimately indistinguishable from adult ankylosing spondylitis. They may be positive for HLA-B27 antigen in up to 90 per cent of cases.

Enteropathic Arthropathy

There is an association between inflammatory bowel disease and spondyloarthropathy well recognized in ulcerative colitis, but also occurring in Crohn's disease. Indeed, there may even be two distinct types of arthropathy, one an HLA-B27–negative form usually affecting large joints of the lower extremities, and the other an entity indistinguishable from ankylosing spondylitis. The former has a migratory pattern and mirrors the clinical course of the inflammatory bowel disease. It may appear even before the clinical onset of gastrointestinal disease, and it is apparently cured by surgical resection of the diseased sections of bowel. Radiologic changes in this "colitic arthropathy" are nonspecific and are secondary to inflammatory changes in the affected areas.

In about 5 per cent of patients with inflammatory bowel disease, a spondyloarthropathy radiologically identical to ankylosing spondylitis is present. In these patients, the ankylosing spondylitis may precede gastrointestinal findings by years, and the pattern of disease progress is identical to that of patients with ankylosing spondylitis who have no bowel disease. Approximately 60 per cent of these patients are HLA-B27 positive. As in ankylosing spondylitis, the sacroiliac joints are involved initially. If the disease progresses, the spine may become involved, followed by changes in the shoulders, hips, and occasionally small appendicular joints. Men and women are equally affected.

Other gastrointestinal diseases, such as Whipple's disease, may be associated with a similar picture of spondyloarthropathy. Infectious gastrointestinal organisms such as *Shigella, Salmonella,* and *Yersinia* may cause an inflammatory but sterile arthritis in large joints such as the knee. Some speculate that the histologic changes in these inflammatory bowel diseases may allow organisms to pass from the gastrointestinal tract into the circulatory or immune system, raising the possibility that the enteropathic arthritides may represent a series of similar immune responses to an initial insult by a variety of microorganisms, including those mentioned above.

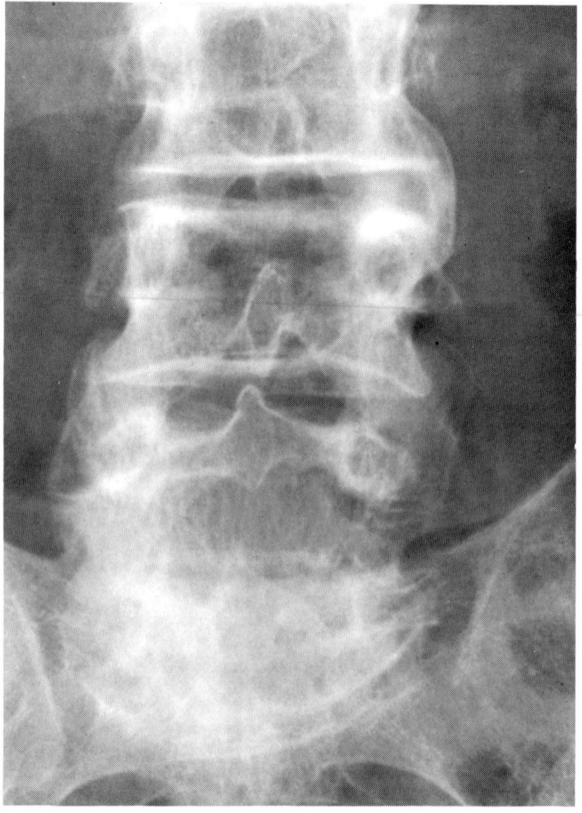

Figure 95–38. Nonmarginal syndesmophytes in psoriatic spondylitis. These larger bridges of bone usually extend from the middle of one vertebral body to the middle of the next vertebral body.

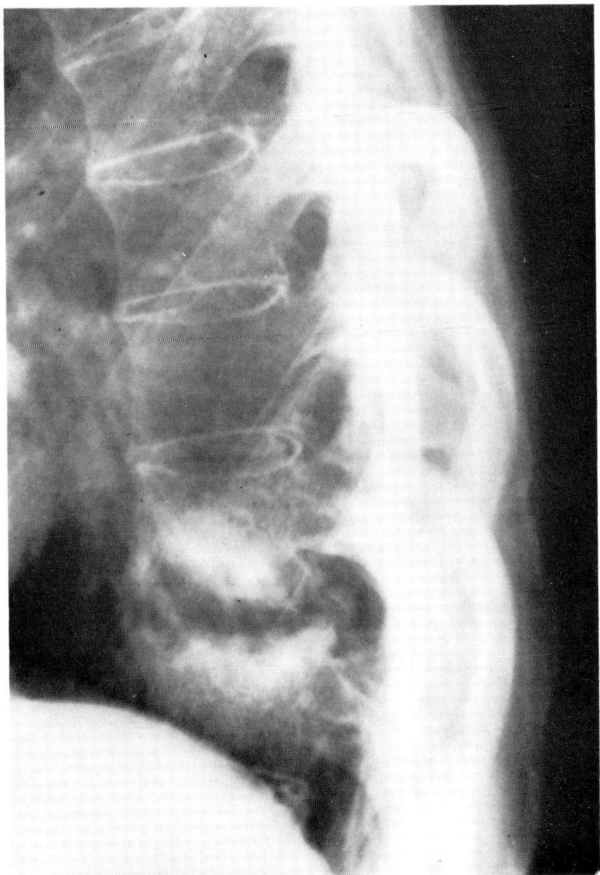

Figure 95–39. Pseudarthrosis in ankylosing spondylitis. There is endplate erosion, sclerosis, and disc widening at the affected level. The posterior element fracture is inapparent in this case.

Reiter's Syndrome and Psoriatic Arthritis

Reiter's syndrome is characteristically manifest as the triad of urethritis, conjunctivitis, and arthritis. In fact, this syndrome is the most common cause of an inflammatory oligoarthropathy in a young male. Seventy to 90 per cent of individuals are HLA-B27 positive. *Shigella* has been established as an infective agent in epidemic dysenteric and venereal infection. The sex distribution is difficult to assess because the syndrome is not easy to diagnose in women or children. In addition, Reiter's syndrome may present with only two components of the triad being manifest. Approximately 20 per cent of patients with Reiter's syndrome develop sacroiliitis and ascending spinal disease. The disorder is incurable, and therapy is directed to symptomatic management.

Psoriatic arthropathy is present in approximately 20 per cent of patients with psoriasis. As many as 10 per cent of patients with the arthropathy present before the skin lesions are manifest, and a small number may never develop skin disease. In contrast to rheumatoid arthritis, in which inflamed joints are painful, there may be a disparity between the symptoms and the extent of joint disease. Severely affected joints may be asymptomatic, and this should suggest the diagnosis of psoriatic arthritis. The distribution of joint involvement is variable. Oligoarthropathy, symmetrical polyarthropathy resembling rheumatoid arthritis, and arthritis mutilans occur. About 20 per cent of patients with psoriatic arthropathy have sacroiliitis. Therapeutic improvement of the skin disease may be associated with amelioration of joint inflammation.

Radiographic Manifestations

The spondyloarthropathies of Reiter's syndrome and psoriatic arthritis are indistinguishable. In the small number of cases in which the sacroiliitis and syndesmophytes are bilaterally symmetrical, both closely resemble ankylosing spondylitis. Usually, in psoriatic arthritis and Reiter's syndrome the sacroiliac arthritis is asymmetrical or unilateral, facilitating radiologic differentiation from ankylosing spondylitis. The sacroiliac changes in these entities are manifested by early cortical blurring of the joints, followed by reactive subchondral sclerosis (Fig. 95–40). As the disease progresses, cartilage loss becomes more apparent, and at the end stage there may be ankylosis of the sacroiliac joints. As with ankylosing spondylitis, the progress of the disease may halt before the spinal arthropathy is apparent. When present, spinal inflammatory changes may take the form of massive bony buttresses connecting vertebral bodies, sometimes sparing the anterior cortex. As with sacroiliac changes, buttresses are likely to be asymmetrical or unilateral. They have been termed parasyndesmophytes or nonmarginal syndesmophytes because they often extend from the middle of one vertebral body to the middle of the next, unlike the marginal syndesmophytes of ankylosing spondylitis (see Fig. 95–38). This new bone represents reaction to an inflammatory process and should not be confused

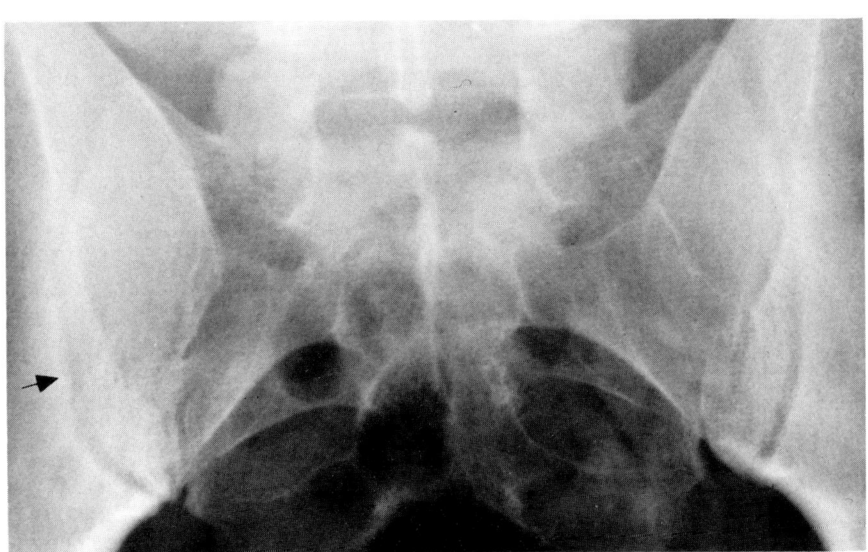

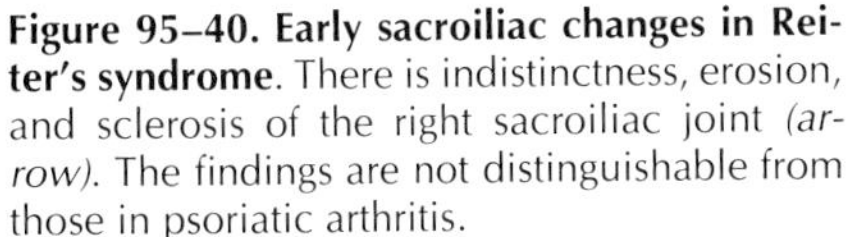

Figure 95–40. Early sacroiliac changes in Reiter's syndrome. There is indistinctness, erosion, and sclerosis of the right sacroiliac joint *(arrow)*. The findings are not distinguishable from those in psoriatic arthritis.

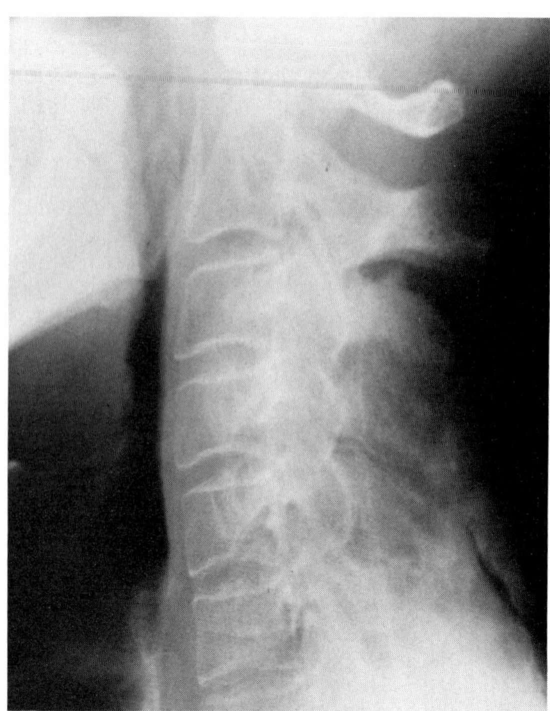

Figure 95–41. Posterior element involvement in psoriatic spondylitis. Notice the florid new bone apposition posteriorly as well as ankylosis of the facet joints.

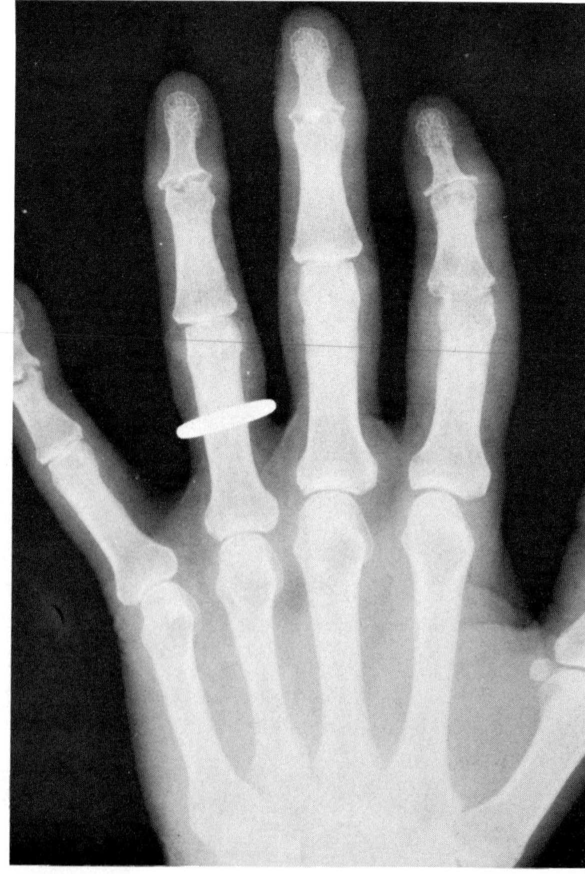

Figure 95–42. Psoriatic arthropathy with involvement of distal interphalangeal joints and fusiform soft-tissue swelling. Destruction of the second proximal interphalangeal joint as well gives rise to a "sausage" appearance of the second digit.

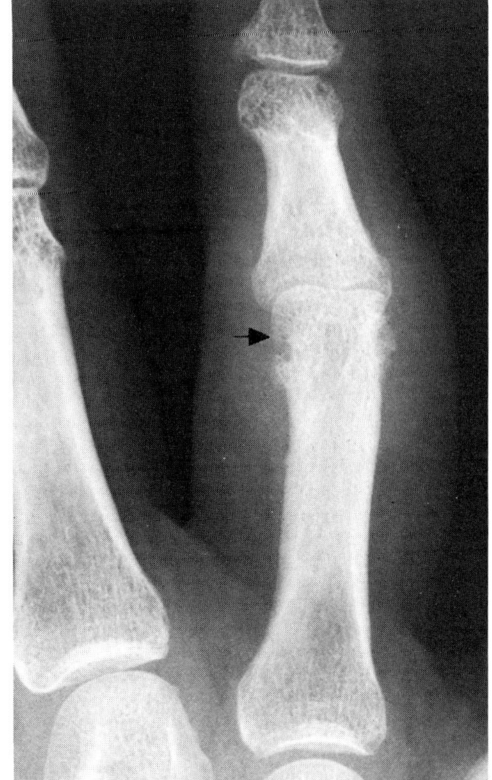

Figure 95–43. Indistinct erosion at the capsular insertion of the proximal interphalangeal joint in a patient with psoriatic arthritis *(arrow)*. There also is marked soft-tissue swelling.

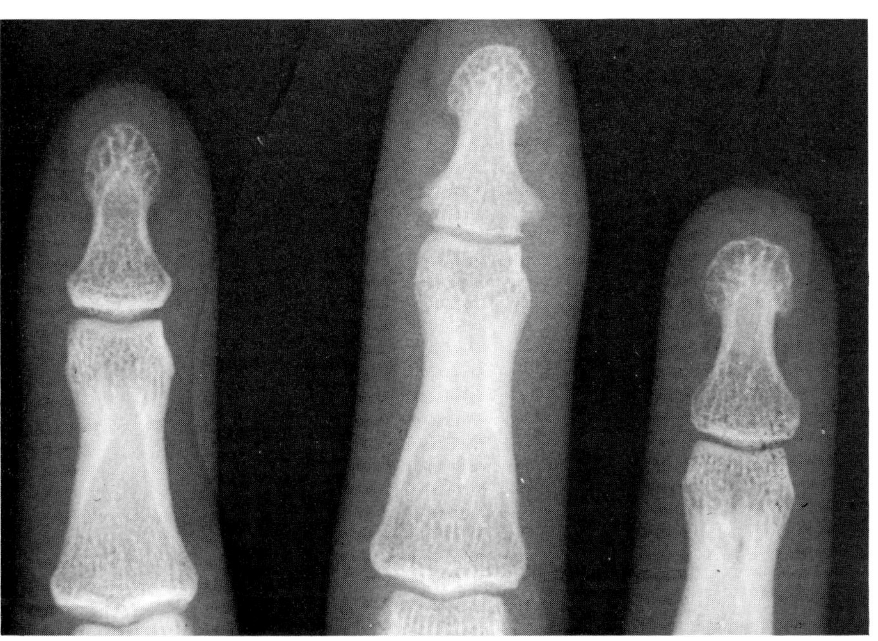

Figure 95–44. Cortical erosion with blurring giving a "mouse ear" appearance at the distal interphalangeal joint in psoriatic arthritis.

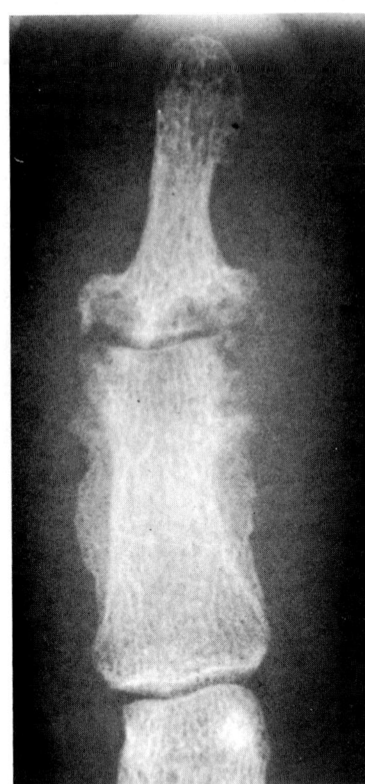

Figure 95–45. Psoriatic arthritis. The erosions have extended to the entheses beyond the capsular margin. There is much reactive new bone formation near the erosions.

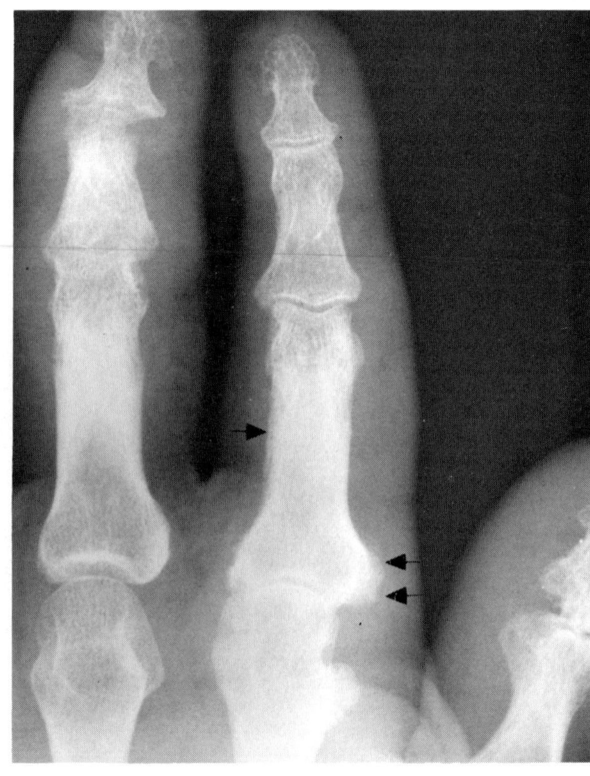

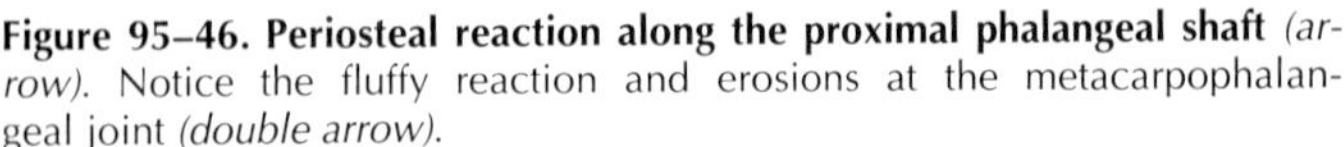

Figure 95–46. Periosteal reaction along the proximal phalangeal shaft *(arrow)*. Notice the fluffy reaction and erosions at the metacarpophalangeal joint *(double arrow)*.

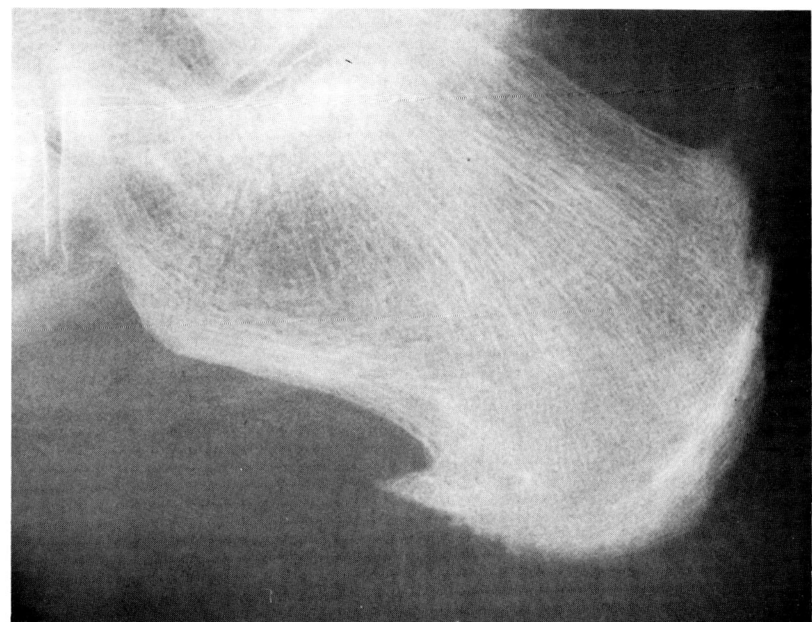

Figure 95–47. Fuzzy, indistinct new bone along the posterior border of the calcaneus in a patient with Reiter's syndrome. There also are a prominent inflammatory plantar spur and an erosion at the Achilles tendon insertion.

with the osteophytes of degenerative arthritis of the spine. Although true marginal syndesmophytes and squaring of vertebral bodies may be seen as in ankylosing spondylitis, these changes are not generalized, particularly in those patients who have large nonmarginal syndesmophytes. Patients may also have progressive involvement of posterior element synovial joints leading to ankylosis (Fig. 95–41).

The appendicular arthropathies of psoriasis and Reiter's syndrome closely resemble each other, and it may be impossible to tell them apart radiographically in a given case. Even additional clinical information may not aid in making the diagnosis. In patients with Reiter's syndrome keratoderma blennorrhagica may produce crusty, pustular skin lesions resembling those of psoriasis. Radiologic similarities in the appendicular skeleton include cartilage destruction, reactive sclerosis to the bony erosion, and relative lack of osteopenia. Soft-tissue swelling is also present, but this is nonspecific and may be due to tenosynovitis. Cartilage destruction and bony erosion may be distributed along a single digital ray with complete sparing of one or more of the other digits. Destruction of the distal interphalangeal, proximal interphalangeal, and metacarpophalangeal joints of an isolated digit may be seen. With soft-tissue swelling in the same distribution, the characteristic "sausage digit" results (Fig. 95–42). Destruction within a joint is analogous to that in rheumatoid arthritis, in which the earliest bony erosions are seen near the margins of the joint capsule in areas unprotected by articular cartilage (Fig. 95–43). These erosions, in association with periosteal new bone and cortical indistinctness, may give a so-called mouse-eared appearance to the joint (Fig. 95–44). As cartilage is destroyed, there is further deterioration of subchondral bone, particularly along the convexity of the proximal bone within the capsule. Ultimately, there may be arthritis mutilans, with extensive bone resorption and utter destruction of the joint. The erosions may extend beyond the limits of the capsule to the sites of the tendon attachment along the shafts of the small tubular bones (Fig. 95–45). Reactive sclerosis or true periosteal reaction along the shaft of these bones may be exuberant in both psoriatic arthritis and Reiter's syndrome, but it is rare in adult rheumatoid arthritis (Fig. 95–46). Entheses elsewhere may also display this prominent, fluffy, reactive new bone formation, particularly at the calcaneus and the ischial tuberosities (Fig. 95–47). As with ankylosing spondylitis, the proliferative changes at the entheses may be quite striking. Psoriatic arthritis and Reiter's syndrome also share a predilection for involvement of the interphalangeal joint of the first toe (Fig. 95–48). Although bone mineral loss on the basis of reactive hyperemia and inflammation should not exclude the diagnosis of psoriatic arthritis or Reiter's syndrome, osteoporosis is often conspicuously absent in spite of severe bone and joint destruction.

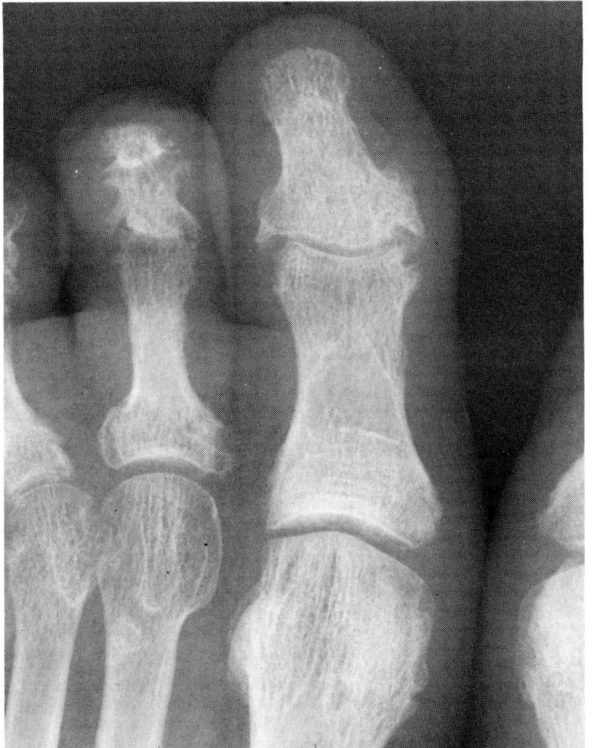

Figure 95–48. Erosion, cartilage loss, and fluffy new bone at the interphalangeal joints with relative sparing of the metatarsophalangeal joints in Reiter's syndrome.

Certain findings may help to differentiate psoriatic arthritis from Reiter's syndrome. Although any joint in the hand may be involved in either disease, commonly there is involvement of multiple distal interphalangeal joints of the fingers only in psoriatic arthritis. If the feet are involved much more extensively than the hands, the patient is more likely to have Reiter's syndrome. Resorption of distal tufts of the fingers may also be a differentiating feature in favor of psoriatic arthritis. Finally, a polyarticular unilateral pattern in which multiple joints of one hand only are involved has also been described in psoriatic arthritis, but not in Reiter's syndrome.

Bibliography

Braunstein EM, Martel W, Moidel R: Ankylosing spondylitis in men and women: A clinical and radiographic comparison. Radiology 144:91–94, 1982.

Good AE, Keller TS, Weatherbee L, Braunstein EM: Spinal cord block with a destructive lesion of the dorsal spine in ankylosing spondylitis. Arthritis Rheum 25:218–222, 1982.

Martel W: Spinal pseudoarthrosis: A complication of ankylosing spondylitis. Arthritis Rheum 21:485–490, 1978.

Martel W: Diagnostic radiology in the rheumatic diseases. In Kelly WN, Harris ED, Ruddy S, Sledge CB (eds): Textbook of Rheumatology. Philadelphia, WB Saunders Company, 1981, pp 580–621.

Martel W, Braunstein EM, Borlaza G, et al: Radiologic features of Reiter disease. Radiology 132:1–10, 1979.

Martel W, Stuck KJ, Dworin AM, Hylland RG: Erosive osteoarthritis and psoriatic arthritis: A radiologic comparison in the hand, wrist, and foot. AJR 134:125–135, 1980.

Resnick D, Niwayama G: Entheses and enthesopathy. Radiology 146:1–9, 1983.

SYSTEMIC LUPUS ERYTHEMATOSUS

Barbara N. Weissman

Systemic lupus erythematosus (SLE) is a connective tissue disease involving multiple organ systems. The etiology is unknown. Prevalence rates of about one case per 2000 individuals have been noted, with young women affected about eight times more often than men and black women almost three times as often as white women.

Pathogenesis

SLE is an autoimmune disease in which antibodies to a variety of nuclear and cytoplasmic elements are present. Among the antinuclear antibodies (ANA) found are those directed against deoxyribonucleoprotein, DNA, RNA, histone, nucleoli, and Sm (a component of extractable nuclear antigen). The indirect immunofluorescence test for ANA is abnormal in 99 per cent of patients with SLE but this is nonspecific; positive titers are also found in some normal individuals and in patients with other collagen diseases. However, the presence of antibody to native (double-stranded) DNA is essentially diagnostic of the disease. Antibodies to the Sm antigen are found in up to 30 per cent of patients with SLE. Antinuclear antibody cannot penetrate healthy cells but can affect the nuclei of injured cells, causing them to swell and be extruded, producing an LE body (called a hematoxylin body when seen in vivo). In the presence of complement, this LE body is phagocytized by a neutrophil or macrophage to form an LE cell. In addition to being a marker for disease, the autoimmune process is responsible for some of the clinical features of the disorder, including the immune complex–mediated vasculitis and glomerulonephritis. Tissue damage also occurs owing to other antibodies such as those directed against red blood cells or neurons.

Joint disease is a frequent finding in SLE. Unlike the changes in rheumatoid arthritis, synovial proliferation is not marked and inflammation is slight or absent. Occasionally, thin layers of granulation tissue are found at the margins of finger joints associated with erosion of adjacent articular cartilage, but deeper involvement is minimal. A layer of eosinophilic, fibrin-like material deposited on or just beneath the synovial lining and along tendon sheaths has been noted. Inflammatory changes with infiltration by lymphocytes and plasma cells occur more often along tendon sheaths than within joints.

Clinical Manifestations

Clinical findings are varied. The most frequent symptom is arthralgia or arthritis, which occurs in 90 per cent of patients. Other common findings include fever, weight loss, and skin lesions. Lymphadenopathy and renal, pulmonary, and cardiac disease occur in about 50 per cent of affected individuals, and central nervous system involvement is present in about one third. Hepatomegaly and splenomegaly may also be present.

The diagnosis of SLE is based on the clinical and laboratory findings. Patients are said to have SLE if they display four or more of the following criteria at any time during their illness:

1. Butterfly rash
2. Discoid lupus
3. Photosensitivity
4. Oral ulcers
5. Arthritis (nonerosive arthritis of one or more peripheral joints, characterized by tenderness, swelling, or effusion)
6. Serositis (pleuritis or pericarditis)
7. Renal disease (persistent proteinuria of >0.5 gm/day (or 3+) or cellular casts
8. Neurologic disorder (seizures or psychosis)
9. Hematologic abnormalities (hemolytic anemia, leukopenia [<4000 WBC/cu mm] or thrombocytopenia [<100,000 platelets/cu mm])
10. Immunologic abnormalities (positive LE cell preparation, anti-DNA antibodies, or anti-Sm nuclear antigen antibodies, or false-positive serologic test for syphilis)
11. Antinuclear antibody

These criteria result in a specificity of 99.5 per cent and a sensitivity of 91 per cent.

Radiographic Manifestations

The most prominent skeletal manifestations include abnormalities of alignment and soft-tissue changes.

Abnormalities of Alignment

Deformity of the joints in the absence of articular erosion is characteristic of SLE, although this occurs in only a small percentage of patients (Fig. 95–49). The hands and feet are the most frequently affected sites, although similar disabling knee involvement may occur. Proximal interphalangeal joint deformity is most common. Alignment abnormalities are usually due to periarticular inflammatory changes with ligamentous laxity and muscular weakness rather than due to articular destruction. The deformity may be correctable early in the course.

Soft-Tissue Abnormalities

In the hands, periarticular swelling frequently occurs. Soft-tissue calcification is uncommon but when present it may be periarticular, diffuse, or distal (Fig. 95–50); it most often occurs in the subcutaneous and deeper soft tissues of the legs. Premature vascular calcification is also seen. Calcified nodules have been noted at sites of skin inflammation or ulceration. The calcification is the result of tissue damage (dystrophic calcification) rather than abnormalities of serum calcium or phosphorus (metastatic calcification).

Tendon ruptures may occur in patients with SLE following little or no trauma (Fig. 95–51). The patellar tendon is most often in-

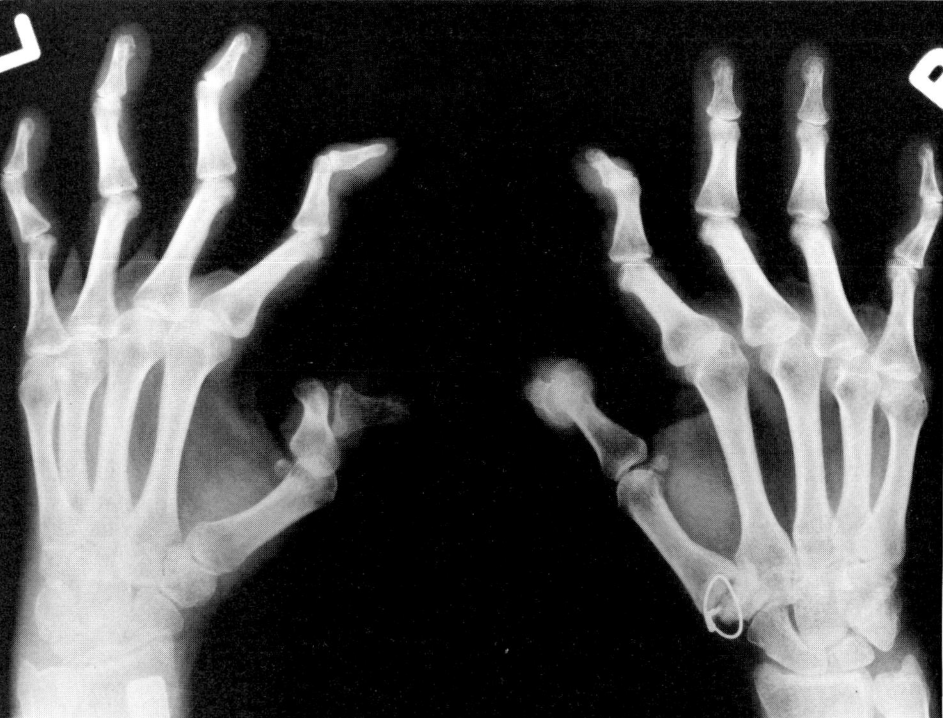

Figure 95–49. Deformity without erosion. There are multiple swan-neck deformities but no evidence of erosion or cartilage space narrowing. The thumb interphalangeal malalignment is a typical finding. Surgical changes are noted at the right thumb base.

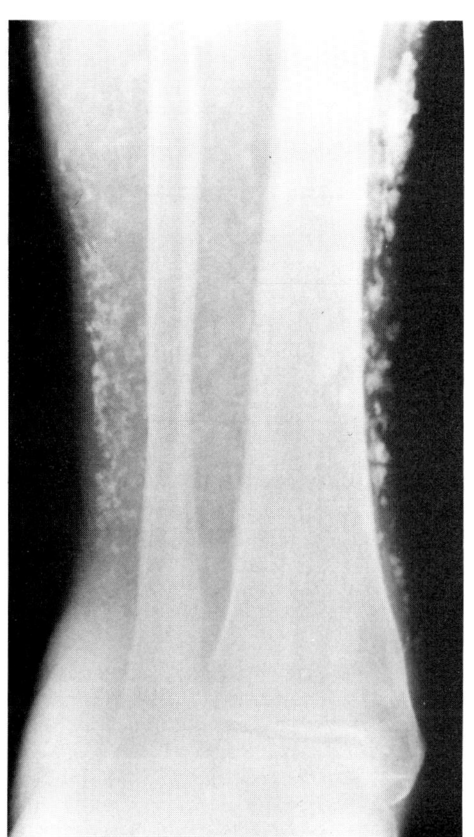

Figure 95–50. Soft-tissue calcification in systemic lupus erythematosus (SLE). The AP view of the lower leg shows extensive subcutaneous and vascular calcification. There is soft-tissue swelling over the lateral malleolus.

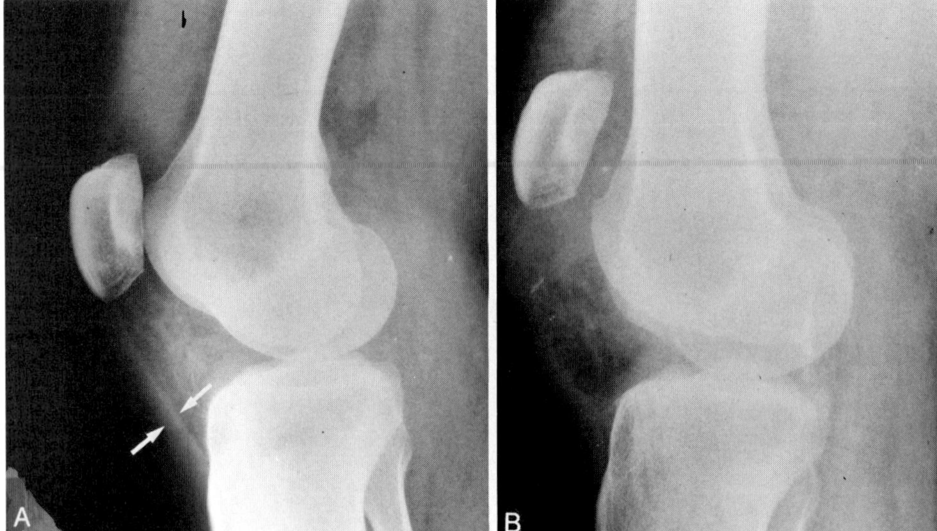

Figure 95–51. Patellar tendon rupture in SLE. *A,* A baseline lateral view in mild flexion shows normal patellar position and a normal patellar tendon shadow *(arrows).* A joint effusion is present. *B,* Years later, acute patellar tendon rupture occurred with swelling about the proximal portion of the patellar tendon and an abnormally high patellar position.

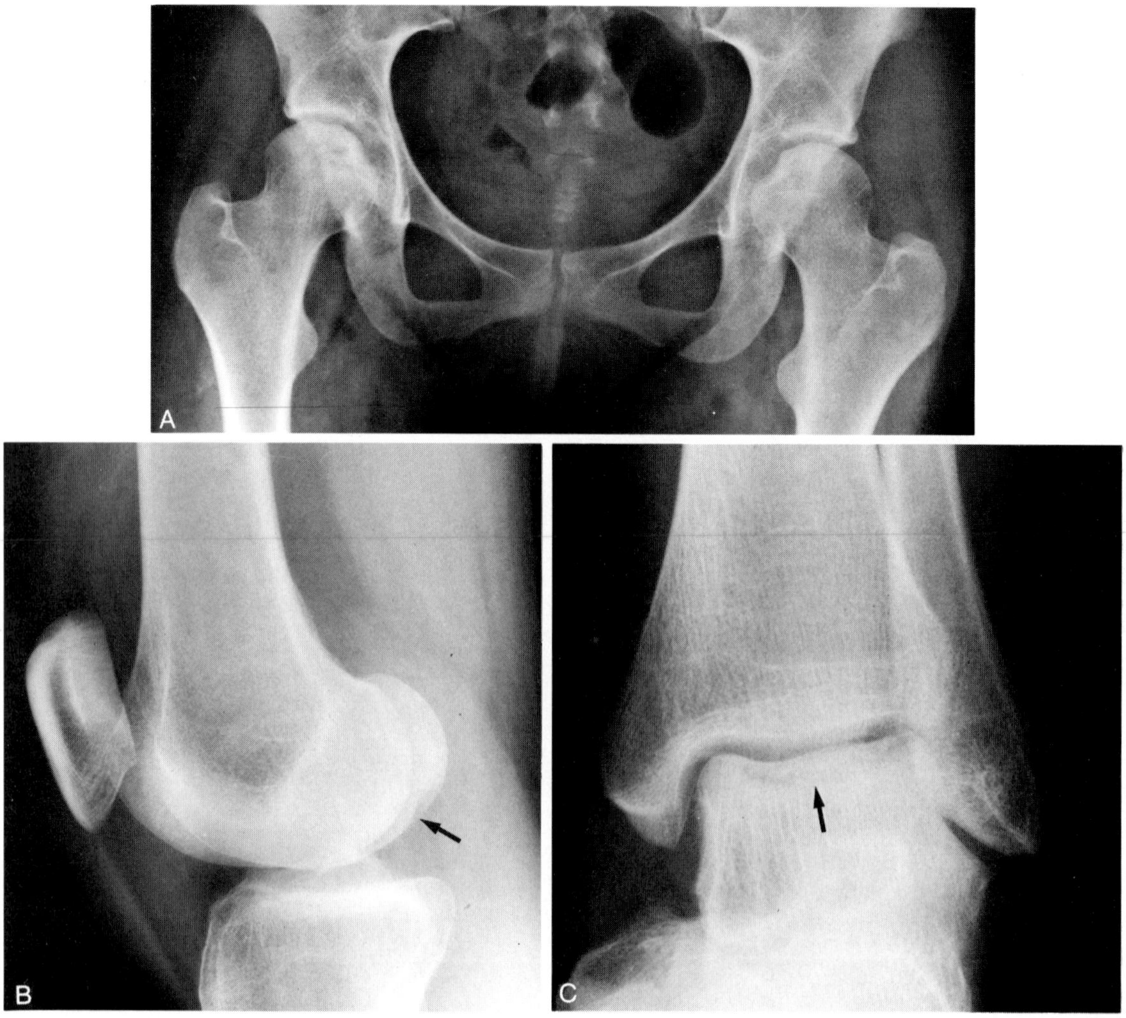

Figure 95–52. Ischemic necrosis of hips, ankle, and knee. *A,* There is irregularity of the right femoral head with underlying sclerosis and lucency, all typical features of ischemic necrosis. Histologic evidence of ischemic necrosis was also present on the radiographically normal left side. *B,* The lateral view of the knee shows irregularity *(arrow),* sclerosis, and lucency of the femoral condyle. *C,* The mortise view of the ankle shows flattening of the articular surface and the crescent sign *(arrow)* of ischemic necrosis.

volved. Tendon rupture occurs most often in patients taking oral corticosteroids; thus the role of the disease itself versus the treatment is unclear. The disease is likely to be a decisive factor in the etiology because tendon rupture is very uncommon in asthmatic patients receiving corticosteroids.

Bone Changes

Juxta-articular osteoporosis is a frequent although nonspecific finding in the hands of patients with SLE. Sclerosis of the terminal tufts of the distal phalanges may also occur. This abnormality does not correlate with the presence of Raynaud's phenomenon and is nonspecific because it has been described in normal individuals as well as in patients with scleroderma, dermatomyositis, rheumatoid arthritis, and sarcoidosis. Erosions of the bone and cartilage space narrowing are unusual features of SLE. Well-defined cyst-like lesions have been noted in periarticular regions of the phalanges, metacarpals, and wrists. Resorption of the tufts of the distal phalanges may occur in association with Raynaud's phenomenon.

Ischemic or avascular necrosis (AVN) may occur. Because this most commonly occurs in patients treated with corticosteroids, the relative roles of the treatment and the underlying disease in the production of AVN have been a controversial issue. Standard radiographic studies have shown the hips and knees to be the most frequent sites of AVN in patients with SLE (Fig. 95–52). Examination of radionuclide bone scans, however, has shown the shoulder to be involved in 47 per cent, the knee in 34 per cent, and the hip in 19 per cent; almost 80 per cent of cases had bilateral involvement. Using bone marrow pressure measurements as the final indicator of AVN, the sensitivity of the bone scan was 89 per cent and that of plain film radiography only 41 per cent. In addition to involvement of large joints, ischemic necrosis may affect the small bones of the hands and feet in patients with SLE.

Nonskeletal Manifestations

Renal impairment has been found in patients who have had small, normal, or large kidneys on imaging studies. Increased cortical echogenicity by ultrasound and abnormal renal size correlate well with the clinically documented severity of renal insufficiency owing to SLE. In patients with uncomplicated lupus nephritis, however, sonography added little information not already available from laboratory data. Angiographic examination has demonstrated renal microaneurysms.

The heart valves or myocardium are affected in about one half of cases of SLE. A verrucous, nonbacterial endocarditis (Libman-Sacks endocarditis) occurs with microscopic or macroscopic vegetations present on the valves and occasionally on the mural endocardium or the chordae tendineae. Identification of calcification in a Libman-Sacks lesion was made on standard chest radiographs and at fluoroscopy. Subsequent angiocardiography confirmed an irregular, multilobulated intraventricular mass between the posterior mitral leaflet and the adjacent left ventricular wall. Pericarditis occurs in about 25 per cent of patients. Pleuritis and pleural effusion are the most frequent pulmonary abnormalities. Acute lupus pneumonitis occurs in less than 5 per cent of cases and has a predilection for the lung bases. Infection is a more frequent cause of pulmonary infiltrates and is an important diagnosis to exclude. Diffuse interstitial fibrosis is uncommon.

Neurologic manifestations include psychosis, organic brain syndromes, seizures, cranial nerve palsies, motor weakness, and peripheral neuropathy. Major pathologic patterns of CNS involvement include vasculopathy, infarction, hemorrhage (usually intracerebral and subarachnoid), and infection. Computed tomography (CT) has demonstrated enlargement of sulci and ventricles, infarction, and intracranial hemorrhage. It has been suggested that magnetic resonance imaging (MRI) may be more accurate than CT in determining the extent of CNS involvement in patients with SLE. MRI changes in SLE include areas of decreased intensity involving white matter at sites where corresponding CT scans reveal areas of hypodensity consistent with infarction. MRI has also demonstrated small areas of increased signal intensity in the white matter, not visible on CT scans and possibly representing microinfarcts. Focal areas of increased signal intensity in cortical grey matter have also been noted, with no corresponding abnormality identified by CT.

The majority of patients with SLE suffer from recurrent abdominal pain. In some cases, vasculitis resulting in reversible or irreversible ischemia is responsible. Some patients have radiographic findings consistent with vasculitis, including pseudo-obstruction, effacement of mucosal folds, and thumbprinting. Gas in the bowel wall (pneumatosis intestinalis) has been described in its benign form as well as in conjunction with necrotizing enterocolitis due to vasculitis. Gastrointestinal ulceration, protein-losing enteropathy, ascites, and pancreatitis may also occur.

Bibliography

Abeles M, Urman JD, Rothfield NF: Aseptic necrosis of bone in systemic lupus erythematosus. Relationship to corticosteroid therapy. Arch Intern Med 138:750–754, 1978.

Budin JA, Feldman F: Soft tissue calcifications in systemic lupus erythematosus. AJR 124:358–364, 1975.

Conklin JJ, Alderson PO, Zizic TM, et al: Comparison of bone scan and radiograph sensitivity in the detection of steroid-induced ischemic necrosis of bone. Radiology 147:221–226, 1983.

Leskinen RH, Skrifvars BV, Laasonen LS, Edgren KJ: Bone lesions in systemic lupus erythematosus. Radiology 153:349–352, 1984.

Passas CM, Wong RL, Peterson M, et al: A comparison of the specificity of the 1971 and 1982 American Rheumatism Association criteria for the classification of systemic lupus erythematosus. Arthritis Rheum 28:620–623, 1985.

Robbins SL, Cotran RS, Kumar V (eds): Diseases of immunity. In Pathologic Basis of Disease, 3rd ed. Philadelphia, WB Saunders Company, 1984, pp 158–213.

Rodnan GP, Schumacher HR (eds): Systemic lupus erythematosus. In Primer on the Rheumatic Diseases, 8th ed. Atlanta, Arthritis Foundation, 1983, pp 49–59.

Weissman BN, Rappoport AS, Sosman JL, Schur PH: Radiographic findings in the hands in patients with systemic lupus erythematosus. Radiology 126:313–317, 1978.

PROGRESSIVE SYSTEMIC SCLEROSIS

Barbara N. Weissman

Progressive systemic sclerosis (PSS), also called systemic scleroderma, is a generalized disorder of connective tissue characterized by symmetrical fibrous thickening and hardening of the skin (scleroderma) and fibrosis and vascular changes of various viscera and the synovium. Limited manifestations, including more localized skin involvement, occur in the CREST syndrome (*C*alcinosis, *R*aynaud's phenomenon, *E*sophageal hypomotility, *S*clerodactyly, and *T*elangiectasia). Localized scleroderma may also occur (e.g., morphea and linear scleroderma) without visceral involvement. PSS is an uncommon disease with between three and five new cases per million population appearing each year. In most cases, the diagnosis is made in patients between the ages of 35 and 55. The disease is three times more common in females than in males.

Diagnosis

Criteria for the diagnosis of PSS have been developed from population studies. The diagnosis may be made if the major criterion and at least two of the three minor criteria are present. The major criterion is proximal scleroderma defined as symmetrical thickening, tightening, and induration of the skin of the fingers and tissue proximal to the metacarpophalangeal and metatarsophalangeal joints. Minor criteria include sclerodactyly, digital pitting scars or loss of substance, and bilateral basilar pulmonary fibrosis.

Pathophysiology

Skin changes consist of an early edematous phase accompanied by perivascular lymphocyte aggregation, capillary damage and partial occlusion, and swelling and degeneration of collagen fibers. This is followed by a fibrotic phase in which there is fibrosis of the dermis, thinning of the epidermis, and hyalinization and thickening of the walls of capillaries and arterioles. A similar sequence of events occurs in other tissues. In the GI tract there is atrophy followed by fibrosis of the muscularis. Interstitial and alveolar fibrosis may occur in the lungs. The interlobular arteries in the kidneys are narrowed by deposits of mucinous or fine collagenous material in their walls and by intimal proliferation.

Fibrosis of the skin and internal viscera results from the overproduction of collagen. The cause of this is unknown. Abnormalities in humoral and cellular immunity have been found, supporting the hypothesis that fibrosis in PSS results in part from abnormalities in the immune system. According to this theory, T-cells are sensitized to collagen, resulting in a delayed hypersensitivity reaction and the release of lymphokines. The lymphokines then attract fibroblasts and stimulate them to produce collagen with resultant additional lymphokine production. A number of autoantibodies have been identified, including rheumatoid factor (20 to 30 per cent) and antinuclear antibodies. An anticentromere antibody has been found particularly in patients with the CREST syndrome.

Clinical Features

Usually PSS is insidious in its onset and slow in its course. Raynaud's phenomenon is often an early or initial symptom of the disease and develops in about 95 per cent of patients. In fact, absence of Raynaud's phenomenon makes a diagnosis of PSS suspect. Cutaneous involvement begins with diffuse edema of the hands. In full-blown cases, the skin of the fingers and hands becomes tight and thickened and firmly bound to the subcutaneous tissue. The normal skin folds and knuckle creases are obliterated. The digits become shorter owing to terminal tuft resorption, and distal ulceration develops, which may be associated with subcutaneous calcification. Involvement of the skin about the mouth restricts the size of its aperture.

Muscular involvement is usually mild but occurs in up to 70 per cent of cases and may be difficult to distinguish on biopsy from dermatomyositis. Muscle wasting and weakness are greatest proximally. Articular abnormalities are common. These are due both to periarticular skin changes and muscle weakness, and to inflammatory and fibrotic synovial changes. The latter may lead to limitation of motion and to clinical and radiographic findings that mimic rheumatoid arthritis. The fingers, wrists, knees, and ankles are most often affected. Nearly one half of patients experience polyarthralgias or arthritis within the first year of disease.

Dyspnea is present in more than half of patients with PSS and in some, severe respiratory insufficiency develops. Pulmonary function tests may show abnormalities in diffusing capacity prior to symptoms or before changes are evident on the chest radiographs. There is evidence that an inflammatory alveolitis may precede restrictive and/or obstructive disease. Increased pulmonary vascular resistance may develop in some cases without associated fibrotic pulmonary parenchymal changes. Scleroderma heart disease may be seen in association with myocardial fibrosis.

Gastrointestinal abnormalities are common and involve all areas of the GI tract. Sjögren's syndrome is common. Esophageal motility abnormalities produce dysphagia, heartburn, nausea, and substernal fullness in many patients. Distal esophageal strictures may occur as a result of reflux esophagitis. Small bowel motility disturbances may produce malabsorption from stagnation of intraluminal contents and bacterial overgrowth. Renal disease is a major cause of death in individuals with PSS. Characteristically, renal disease is manifest by the acute development of malignant arterial hypertension requiring prompt treatment to avoid rapidly progressive and irreversible renal insufficiency. The course of PSS varies, with almost all patients eventually demonstrating visceral involvement. The prognosis is said to be worse when there is clinical evidence of renal, cardiac, or pulmonary involvement at the time of diagnosis. The prognosis for the CREST syndrome is considerably better than that for PSS.

Radiographic Manifestations

Loss of soft tissue from the fingertips is a characteristic feature of PSS (Fig. 95–53). Terminal digit soft-tissue loss may be documented by visual inspection or by comparing the thickness of the soft tissue measured from the distal phalanx to fingertip to the width of the base of the distal phalanx. A ratio of 20 per cent or less is considered abnormal. Atrophy is more frequent in patients with Raynaud's phenomenon than in those without this symptom. The characteristic location for soft-tissue calcification is in the fingertips, usually on the ventral or lateral aspects of the terminal phalanges. Such calcification may be apparent within six months of the onset of disease. More than one half of patients with PSS have one or more of the classic findings of fingertip calcification, erosion of the distal tufts, and soft-tissue atrophy. Calcification in the fingertips is also seen in calcinosis universalis, Raynaud's syndrome, dermatomyositis, systemic lupus erythematosus, and epidermolysis bullosa. Rarely, calcification occurs within joints, and in some cases a chalk-like effusion is present in which hydroxyapatite crystals can be identified. Presumably, this intra-articular calcification is due to the shedding into the joint of dystrophic calcification present in the synovial lining. Large collections of calcific material may be noted adjacent to joints and bony prominences and may involve tendons and bursae.

Bone resorption of the terminal tufts of the fingers is particularly characteristic of PSS (see Fig. 95–53). Resorption has also been reported, however, in other phalanges, the radius, ulna, distal clavicle and acromion, ribs, cervical spine, mandible, and base of the fifth metacarpal. Tuft resorption in PSS generally begins on the palmar surface of the terminal phalanges and therefore is best seen on oblique or lateral radiographs. The erosion may progress proximally, leading to extensive loss of substance of the distal, middle, or proximal phalanges. Sometimes a distal portion of the terminal tuft remains separated from the base of the phalanx by an area of bone resorption. Occasionally, reconstitution of distal tufts may occur. Bone resorption from terminal tufts may be seen in other collagen vascular diseases, but it is much less frequent than in PSS. Selective resorption at the first carpometacarpal joint has been noted in patients with PSS. Subluxation occurs at this joint, and intra-articular calcification may coexist. Resorption at the angle of the mandible is related to the tightness of the skin of the face and atrophy of the masseter and pterygoid muscles. Bone resorption and superior notching of posterior ribs have been seen in association with PSS. Bone loss from the posterior elements of the cervical spine in association with disc narrowing and severe subluxation may also occur.

Radiographic findings simulating those of rheumatoid arthritis (RA) occur in patients with PSS (Table 95–2). The most common manifestations are cartilage space narrowing, generally localized to the wrists and radiocarpal articulations, and bone erosion. The erosion has been attributed to the inflammatory changes that occur in the synovial lining. Initially there is infiltration of the synovial lining with lymphocytes and plasma cells. Subsequently, rather than progression to pannus formation as is seen in rheumatoid arthritis, fibrosis occurs. In rare instances, erosion or bony ankylosis occurs at the distal and proximal interphalangeal joints, with relative sparing of the metacarpophalangeal and wrist articulations. These findings suggest psoriatic or erosive osteoarthritis. In addition to bare

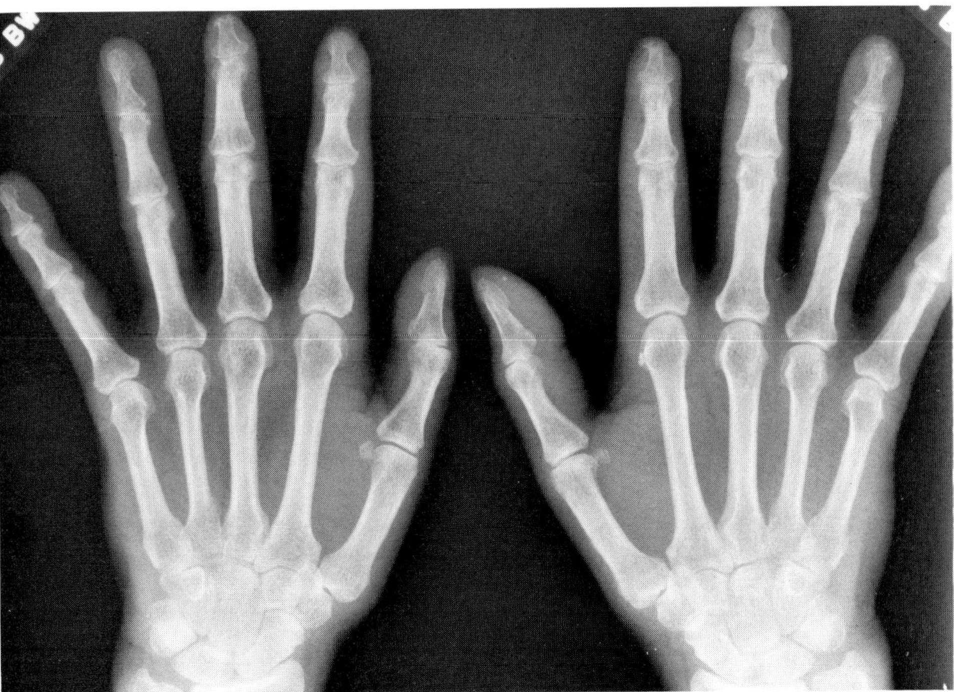

Figure 95–53. Early hand changes in progressive systemic sclerosis (PSS). There is severe atrophy of the distal soft tissues of the index and middle fingers bilaterally. On the right, this is accompanied by diffuse swelling with loss of the normal skin folds at the knuckles. Several areas of soft-tissue calcification are noted. There is resorption of the tips of the distal phalanges of the right index and left middle fingers. The combination of distal soft-tissue and tuft atrophy and calcification is characteristic of PSS.

area erosions, compressive erosions due to muscular forces across subluxed osteoporotic joints also occur. Pressure by extensor tendons on the dorsal aspects of joints may be responsible for producing an unusual dorsal erosion of the metacarpophalangeal joints.

Widening of the periodontal membrane is a characteristic feature of PSS. The periodontal membrane is normally apparent on radiographs as a 0.2 mm-wide lucency between the root of the tooth and the lamina dura. It is widened in up to 60 per cent of patients with PSS, and this is most prominent around the posterior teeth. Radiographic abnormalities of the esophagus are present in over 75 per cent of patients with PSS (Table 95–3). Increased amounts of collagen in the lamina propria and submucosa and atrophy of the muscularis are most severe in the lower two thirds of the esophagus and are responsible for the characteristic diminution or absence of peristalsis noted in this region. Other radiographic abnormalities include dilatation of the esophagus, hiatus hernia, esophageal stricture, reflux, and delayed emptying. Several instances of esophageal carcinoma (squamous cell, adenocarcinoma, and adenoacanthoma) have been reported, and candidiasis has been noted as a complication of obstruction. Gastric involvement is unusual, but dilatation, abnormal peristalsis, and delayed emptying may be seen. The most common small bowel abnormalities are pseudo-obstruction and malabsorption. Dilatation of the duodenum may suggest obstruction. There may be thickening of mucosal folds. A decrease in the distance between the valvulae conniventes owing to submucosal fibrosis may be present. Transient nonobstructing intussusception has been noted and is most likely a consequence of the abnormal motility. Characteristic sacculations of the small bowel (pseudodiverticula) may occur (Fig. 95–54). These are differentiated from true diverticula by their broad opening and square contour.

In the colon, wide-mouth sacculations (pseudodiverticula) that are located along the antimesenteric border, particularly in the transverse and descending colon, are characteristic findings in PSS. The wall of the pseudodiverticulum is composed of hypertrophied elastic tissue and collagen and the muscular contractions of this portion of the colon are deficient, leading to retention of barium and better visibility of the sacculations on the post-evacuation rather than on the filled films of the barium enema. Complete loss of colonic haustrations accompanied by an increased length of the colon can occur in patients with PSS; these patients also have abnormalities in the esophagus and small bowel, which helps in differentiating the changes from those of ulcerative colitis or cathartic colon. Pneumatosis cystoides intestinalis is a rare condition in which multiple gas-containing thin-walled cysts are present in the intestinal wall

TABLE 95–2. INCIDENCE OF VARIOUS RADIOGRAPHIC ABNORMALITIES IN THE HANDS OF PATIENTS WITH PSS

Finding	Incidence (%)
Typical of PSS	
Flexion contracture	89
Osteopenia	40–42
Acral sclerosis	9
Subcutaneous calcification	17–54*
Soft-tissue atrophy	38–93
Tuft resorption	33–51
Rheumatoid-like	
Erosion	9–54
Dorsal erosion	6–9
Cartilage narrowing	13–46
Bony ankylosis	2–4
Severe malalignment	8

*Seventy per cent in CREST syndrome.

TABLE 95–3. INCIDENCE OF RADIOGRAPHIC FINDINGS IN PATIENTS WITH PSS (EXCLUDING THE HANDS)

Finding	Incidence (%)
Wide lamina dura	54
Mandibular erosion	17
Rib erosion	13
Pulmonary abnormalities	22–44
Cardiomegaly	20–40
Esophageal abnormalities	47–84
Stomach and duodenal abnormalities	18
Small bowel abnormalities	20–22
Colon abnormalities	25–51

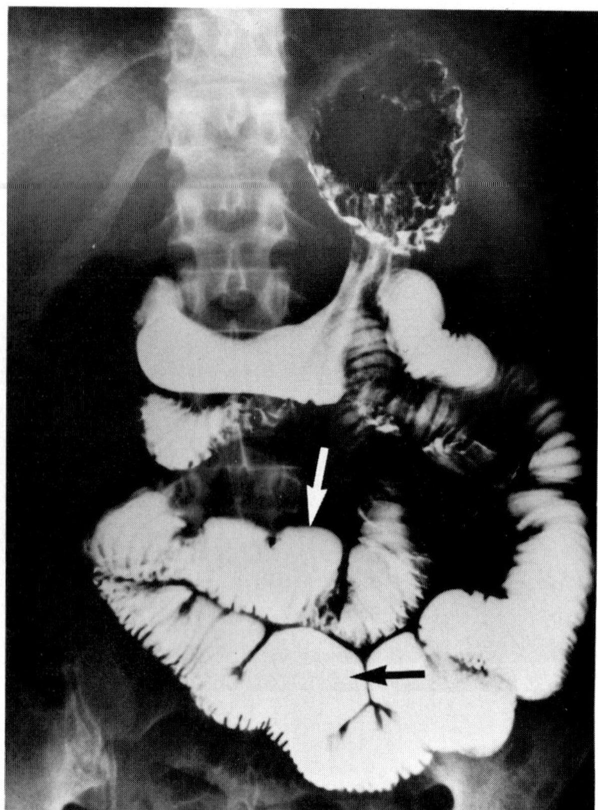

Figure 95–54. Small bowel abnormalities in PSS. This film was obtained 90 minutes after the ingestion of barium. The residual barium in the esophagus attests to its abnormal motility. The bowel is dilated, and the valvulae are slightly thickened. Pseudodiverticula *(arrows)* are present. Basilar pulmonary changes are visible. (Courtesy of Dr. Herbert Gramm, New England Deaconess Hospital, Boston, MA.)

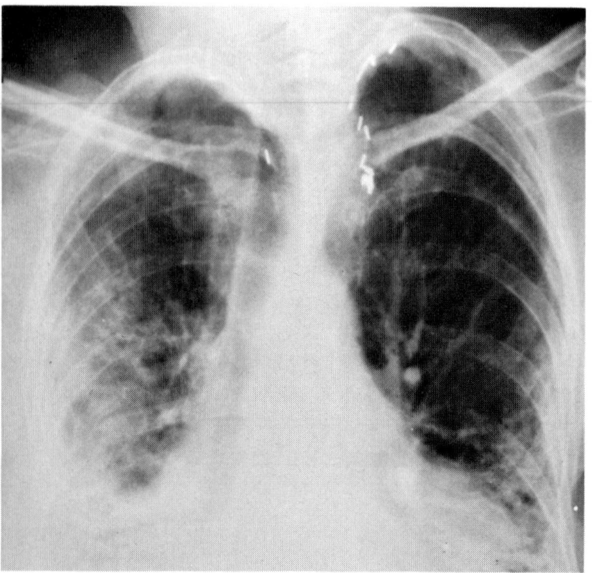

Figure 95–55. Pulmonary fibrosis. This patient had severe Raynaud's phenomenon and underwent bilateral sympathectomies (note the surgical clips and upper rib resections). There is a honeycomb pattern peripherally at both bases, a typical although nonspecific finding in patients with PSS.

and mesentery. Pneumoperitoneum may occur. Although radiographically striking, pneumatosis cystoides is usually asymptomatic in patients with PSS. Barium impaction after upper GI examination can occur. This complication can be avoided by the use of cathartics after examination. However, administration of mineral oil by mouth should not be used because patients with esophageal dysfunction may aspirate the oil.

Renal size is normal. Angiographic studies may demonstrate irregular arterial narrowing, tortuosity of interlobular arteries, delayed transit of contrast material through the kidneys, lack of definition of the corticomedullary junction, and an abnormal (spotted) nephrogram with areas of decreased density in the absence of major arterial abnormality. Cardiac abnormalities are due to the presence of myocardial fibrosis, pericardial effusion, or right ventricular hypertrophy due to pulmonary artery hypertension. Radiographically, cardiac enlargement is the major manifestation of disease. Pulmonary abnormalities include diffuse bilateral fibrosis most prominent at the lung bases (Fig. 95–55), pulmonary hypertension, bilateral pleural effusions due to congestive heart failure, pneumothorax, recurrent pneumonia, and alveolar or bronchiolar cell carcinoma. Pulmonary artery hypertension is secondary to pulmonary fibrosis in some cases, but, particularly in the CREST syndrome, progressive pulmonary vascular obliteration may lead to pulmonary artery hypertension in the absence of pulmonary fibrosis.

Bibliography

Bassett LW, Blocka KLN, Furst DE, et al: Skeletal findings in progressive systemic sclerosis (scleroderma). AJR 136:1121–1126, 1981.

Blocka KLN, Bassett LW, Furst DE, et al: The arthropathy of advanced progressive systemic sclerosis. A radiographic survey. Arthritis Rheum 24:874–884, 1981.

Brower AC, Resnick D, Karlin C, Piper S: Unusual articular changes of the hand in scleroderma. Skeletal Radiol 4:119–123, 1979.

Lawson JP: The joint manifestations of the connective tissue diseases. Semin Roentgenol 17:25–38, 1982.

Massi AT, Rodnan GP, et al: Preliminary criteria for the classification of systemic sclerosis (scleroderma). Bull Rheum Dis 31:1–6, 1981.

Robbins SL, Cotran RS, Kumar V: Pathologic Basis of Disease. Philadelphia, WB Saunders Company, 1984.

Rodnan GP, Schumacher HR: Progressive systemic sclerosis and related disorders. In Primer on the Rheumatic Diseases, 8th ed. Atlanta, Arthritis Foundation, 1982, pp 59–65.

Shanks MJ, Blane CE, Adler DD, Sullivan DB: Radiographic findings of scleroderma in childhood. AJR 141:657–660, 1983.

MIXED CONNECTIVE TISSUE DISEASE

Barbara N. Weissman

In some individuals characteristic clinical, radiologic, and laboratory features of a particular rheumatologic disorder may coexist with features typical of another rheumatic disorder. Many combinations or overlap syndromes can be seen (Fig. 95–56). Mixed connective tissue disease (MCTD) is a disorder characterized clinically by features of systemic lupus erythematosus (SLE), scleroderma (PSS), and polymyositis, and in many cases by the presence of a high titer of circulating antibody to the ribonucleoprotein (RNP) component of extractable nuclear antigen (ENA). It is somewhat controversial whether MCTD is a separate entity, an overlap syndrome, or a variant of SLE, PPS, or polymyositis.

Clinical Features

The prevalence of MCTD is not known, but it is probably more common than polymyositis and less common than SLE. More than 80 per cent of patients with this disorder are women. Symptoms and signs are those of SLE, PSS, and polymyositis and most often

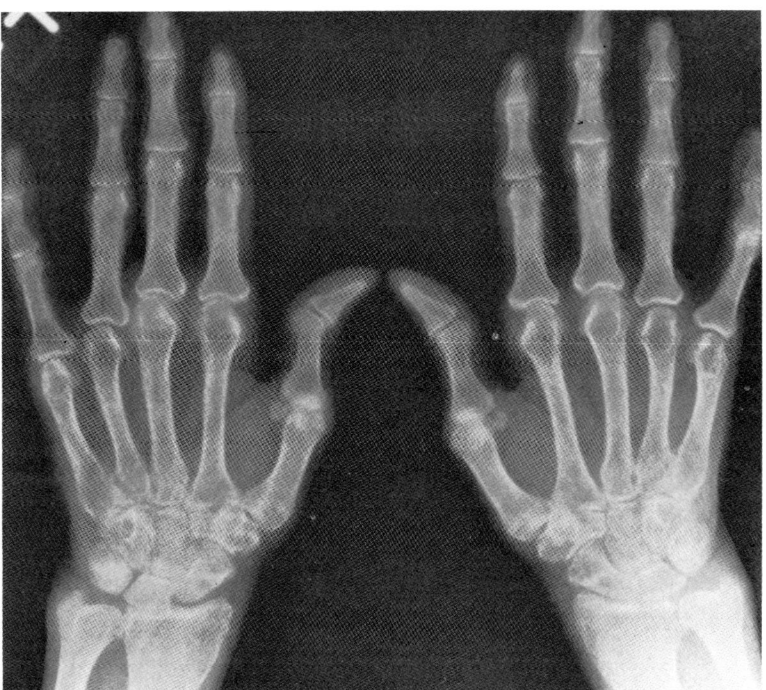

Figure 95–56. Overlap syndrome (mixed connective tissue disease [MCTD]). This patient had clinical features of rheumatoid arthritis. Radiograph of the hands shows mild changes of rheumatoid arthritis (intercarpal cartilage space narrowing in the left wrist, erosion of a few MCPs and carpals), but patient also has terminal tuft resorption in the index and middle fingers typical of scleroderma (PSS).

include polyarthralgias or arthritis, diffuse swelling of the hands, Raynaud's phenomenon, symptoms related to abnormal esophageal motility, proximal muscle weakness, and dyspnea on exertion (Table 95–4). The skin is typically taut and thick owing to edema plus an increase in dermal collagen. Diffuse sclerodermatous involvement of the skin is rare. Some individuals have a rash similar to that of SLE, whereas others have the violaceous eyelids and the skin changes over the knuckles typically associated with dermatomyositis. Proximal muscle weakness, tenderness, and elevated muscle enzymes are due to an inflammatory myositis. Lymphadenopathy may be prominent. Pleuritis and/or pericarditis may occur. Renal disease is less common in MCTD than in SLE and occurs more often in patients with anti-Sm antibodies but rarely in those with anti-RNP antibodies. Cardiac and renal involvement are more frequent in children than in adults.

TABLE 95–4. CLINICAL FEATURES OF MCTD

	100 Patients*: Frequency (%)	10 Children with MCTD: Frequency (%)
Polyarthralgia/polyarthritis	95	100
Raynaud's phenomenon	85	70
Diminished esophageal motility	67	50
Decreased pulmonary diffusing capacity	67	
Swollen hands	66	
Myositis	63	50
Lymphadenopathy	39	50
Skin rash	38	
Sclerodermatous changes	33	80
Fever	33	80
Serositis	27	
Splenomegaly	19	50
Hepatomegaly	15	50
Neurologic abnormality	10	30
Salivary gland enlargement, xerostomia, and/or keratoconjunctivitis sicca	7	20
Hashimoto's thyroiditis	6	
Renal disease, definite	5	40
Renal disease, possible	5	
Cardiac involvement		70

*Hemagglutinating antibodies to RNP. Most of the patients (74 per cent) in this multicenter study had the clinical features typical of mixed connective tissue disease, whereas 26 per cent had more limited disease consistent with SLE, scleroderma, or an undifferentiated connective tissue disorder. (Reprinted from the Bulletin on the Rheumatic Diseases copyright 1975. Used by permission of the Arthritis Foundation; and Singsen BH, Kornreich HK, Koster-King K, et al: Mixed connective tissue disease in children. Arthritis Rheum 20:355–360, 1977.)

Laboratory Findings

Anemia, leukopenia, an elevated erythrocyte sedimentation rate, and hypergammaglobulinemia are common but not specific findings. Muscle enzymes (SGOT, CPK) may be elevated. Rheumatoid factor is present in about one half of the patients. The characteristic laboratory abnormality in patients with MCTD, however, is the presence of high titer in the blood of a particular hemagglutinating antibody. It has been shown that a nuclear antigen that is extractable in isotonic buffers from isolated nuclei, called extractable nuclear antigen (ENA), has two components—one sensitive to trypsin and RNase (termed RNP) and one resistant to RNase (termed Sm) (Table 95–5). Seventy-four per cent of patients with precipitating antibodies to the RNP antigen and not the Sm antigen have typical features of MCTD, whereas 85 per cent of patients with antibodies to Sm have typical SLE. About 25 per cent of patients with SLE

TABLE 95–5. ANTIGENIC COMPONENTS OF ENA

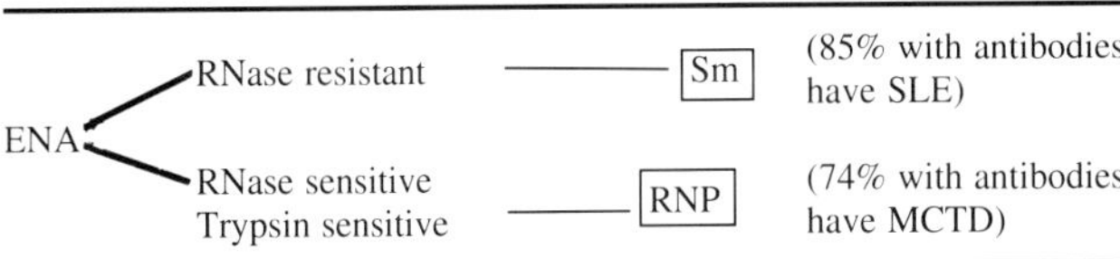

ENA	RNase resistant	Sm	(85% with antibodies have SLE)
	RNase sensitive Trypsin sensitive	RNP	(74% with antibodies have MCTD)

SLE = Systemic lupus erythematosus; MCTD = mixed connective tissue disease; RNP = ribonucleoprotein; ENA = extractable nuclear antigen.

also have anti-RNP, and the presence of this antibody may be a good prognostic sign. Pulmonary abnormalities are common and are usually accompanied by abnormal pulmonary function tests and abnormal chest radiographs in symptomatic patients. In addition, some asymptomatic patients also have abnormal pulmonary function tests. Decreased diffusion capacity with or without reduced lung volumes is a frequent finding. Progressive restrictive lung disease occurs in some cases, even in the absence of symptoms.

Treatment

In mild cases, nonsteroidal anti-inflammatory drugs or low doses of corticosteroids may be used. With more severe involvement, corticosteroids are generally employed, often leading to improvement in esophageal and pulmonary disturbances. The importance of distinguishing MCTD from PSS and other disorders seems to be the generally more favorable prognosis of MCTD, although the mortality rate from MCTD is comparable to that of SLE and only slightly better than that for PSS.

Radiographic Manifestations

The radiologic features are generally those of SLE, PSS, polymyositis, and/or rheumatoid arthritis (RA). No distinctive radiographic features differentiate patients with MCTD from those with a clinical overlap syndrome of PSS and SLE.

In the hands, soft-tissue swelling is common. Atrophy of the distal soft tissues occurs in about one third of patients and may be accompanied by tuft erosion. Periarticular calcification seems to be uncommon. Erosive changes reminiscent of RA are the most frequent findings in many series. In some cases metacarpal and interphalangeal joint erosions differ from those of classic RA by being small, well-defined, and asymmetrically distributed. Severe erosion may occur at the distal interphalangeal joints and may involve much of the middle phalanges. Multiple subluxations with mild erosion similar to the appearances in SLE may be seen.

Findings on barium examination generally mimic those of PSS, with abnormal esophageal motility, esophageal dilatation, and colonic pseudodiverticula occurring most often. Atrophy of the parotid glands has been noted on sialography and is compatible with Sjögren's syndrome. Chest radiographs in patients with MCTD characteristically demonstrate lower lobe interstitial infiltrates identical to those seen in patients with PSS. Less common findings are volume loss and pleural disease. Severe pulmonary arterial hypertension may occur. Pericardial effusion may also be present.

Bibliography

Halla JT, Hardin JG: Clinical features of the arthritis of mixed connective tissue disease. Arthritis Rheum 21:497–503, 1978.

Reichlin M: Problems in differentiating SLE and mixed connective tissue disease. N Engl J Med 295:1194–1196, 1976.

Sharp GC: Mixed connective tissue disease. Bull Rheum Dis 25:828–831, 1974–75.

Silver TM, Farber SJ, Bole GG, Martel W: Radiological features of mixed connective tissue disease and scleroderma—systemic lupus erythematosus overlap. Radiology 120:269–275, 1976.

Singsen BH, Kornreich HK, Koster-King K, et al: Mixed connective tissue disease in children. Arthritis Rheum 20:355–360, 1977.

DEGENERATIVE JOINT DISEASE

ROBERT O. CONE and DONALD L. RESNICK

Degenerative joint disease is the most common articular process. In the past it has been considered to be a normal result of the aging process and accorded little attention. Improved medical and surgical therapeutic regimens have sparked increased interest in understanding the etiology and natural history of this ubiquitous disorder. Radiographic studies provide the cornerstone for the diagnosis of degenerative joint disease as well as an important tool in treatment planning and monitoring disease progression.

The nomenclature applied to degenerative joint disease varies widely and includes the terms *arthritis deformans, osteoarthritis,* and *osteoarthrosis.* The term *degenerative joint disease* refers to degenerative alterations involving any type of articulation, including synovial joints, cartilaginous joints, syndesmoses, and entheses. The term *osteoarthritis* should be reserved to describe degenerative joint disease involving synovial articulations. In the European literature the synonymous term *osteoarthrosis* is used in place of *osteoarthritis* and is actually more accurate because since the suffix "-itis" implies inflammation that is not common nor prominent in this disorder. However, in deference to the accepted terminology in the United States we will use the term *osteoarthritis.* Entheses are anatomic sites where tendons or ligaments attach to bone. Enthesopathy refers to pathologic alterations at these sites. Degenerative enthesopathy refers to a specific pattern of abnormality associated with degenerative joint disease. Other more specific terms are in common usage to describe degenerative joint disease involving certain anatomic regions or those with specific clinical patterns. Many of these will be mentioned at appropriate points in the text.

The classic concept of degenerative joint disease involves primary and secondary varieties of disease. Primary degenerative joint disease is considered to be a disorder that occurs de novo in the absence of predisposing sources of abnormal stress or articular abnormalities. Secondary degenerative joint disease refers to degenerative changes in association with pre-existing abnormalities. A wide variety of traumatic, congenital, metabolic, and primary articular abnormalities may subsequently lead to degenerative joint disease. A more modern concept is that degenerative joint disease is a nonspecific response to primary abnormalities of force distribution or pathologic alterations of articular and/or juxta-articular anatomic components. Thus, all forms of degenerative joint disease may be considered to be secondary phenomena. It has been suggested that degenerative joint disease can be subgrouped into two main categories: (1) disorders in which there are abnormal forces exerted on an otherwise normal articulation and (2) disorders in which normal forces are exerted on an abnormal articulation.

In most instances there appears to be no genetic predisposition to degenerative joint disease. The one apparent exception is generalized osteoarthritis with Heberden's nodes, a condition that appears to be familial. In general, the incidence of degenerative joint disease is directly proportional to age. This may relate to repeated episodes of microtrauma as well as to endogenous changes in bone, cartilage, and soft tissues associated with aging. Men tend to demonstrate degenerative changes at a younger age than women but are less likely to develop severe deforming disease. Generalized osteoarthritis with Heberden's nodes is more common in females, whereas inflammatory (erosive) osteoarthritis is seen almost exclusively in women. Occupational and certain sporting activities are associated with localized degenerative joint disease related to repetitive trauma. Hypertension and atherosclerosis have also been reported as predisposing to degenerative joint disease; however, the significance of these associations is not entirely clear.

CARDINAL RADIOGRAPHIC FEATURES OF DEGENERATIVE JOINT DISEASE

Although there is a tremendous variation in the radiographic appearance of degenerative joint disease, certain features are characteristic of this disorder. These include (1) joint space narrowing, (2) subchondral sclerosis (eburnation), (3) subchondral cyst formation, (4) osteophytosis, and (5) enthesopathy. These key features will be discussed individually prior to an anatomically oriented discussion of degenerative joint disease.

Joint Space Narrowing

The joint space narrowing that accompanies degenerative joint disease is the radiographic counterpart of articular cartilage destruction. Characteristically joint space narrowing in degenerative joint disease occurs in the portion of the articulation exposed to the greatest amount of physical stress. Thus in some articulations, such as the interphalangeal joints, the entire articulation may be involved diffusely, whereas in others, such as the knee or hip, the changes may be segmental or focal (Fig. 95–57). Pathologically the earliest abnormality consists of thinning and discoloration of the involved cartilaginous segment. As the process advances the articular surface becomes roughened, and irregular cracks and crevices appear. Large cartilaginous ulcerations follow that may penetrate to the subchondral bone plate. In advanced degenerative joint disease entire segments of subchondral bone may be completely denuded of their cartilaginous coat. The presence of cartilage destruction as manifested by joint space narrowing as well as the predilection for involvement of stressed segments of an articulation are key to the radiographic identification of degenerative joint disease of synovial articulations (osteoarthritis). Appreciation of these features is important in differentiating osteoarthritis from other arthritides such as rheumatoid arthritis (in which joint space narrowing is diffuse) and osteonecrosis (in which the cartilaginous coat is spared until late in the disease process).

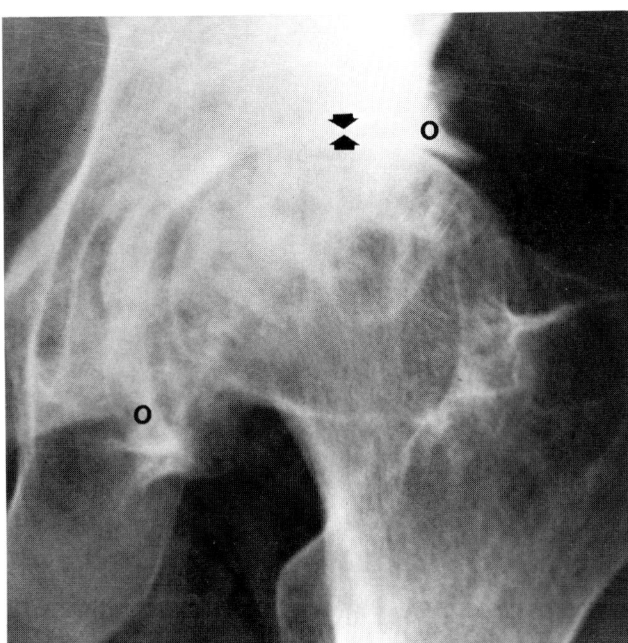

Figure 95–57. Osteoarthritis. In this patient with advanced osteoarthritis of the hip, there is asymmetrical narrowing of the superior portion of the joint space *(between arrows).* Marginal osteophytes (O) are present, as well as numerous subchondral cysts, within both the femoral head and the adjacent acetabulum.

Subchondral Sclerosis (Eburnation)

Subchondral sclerosis refers to an abnormal increase in density of the subchondral bone plate (Fig. 95–58). Although prominent in degenerative joint disease, subchondral eburnation is a nonspecific response to articular cartilage destruction of any etiology. In the presence of denudation of overlying articular cartilage, the subchondral bone plate increases in density because of a combination of fracture and collapse of trabeculae and reparative callus formation. Some investigators feel that intraosseous venous congestion is important in stimulating the reparative response. Eburnation of the subchondral bone plate, which is especially prominent in stressed segments of the articulation, is a characteristic radiographic finding in degenerative joint disease and indicates the presence of concomitant articular cartilage destruction. Frequently, in weight-bearing articulations such as the knee, standard radiographic projections may reveal prominent subchondral sclerosis with an apparently normal joint space. In these instances, radiographs obtained as the patient bears weight on the involved extremity more accurately define the true extent of cartilage loss.

Subchondral Cysts

Subchondral cysts are rounded or ovoid radiolucent lesions that are identified in the subarticular bone in degenerative joint disease. On pathologic examination, the subchondral cysts in degenerative joint disease possess a gelatinous fibromyxoid matrix or demonstrate central cavitations filled with proteinaceous debris and articular cartilage fragments. They are surrounded by a wall of fibrous tissue containing foci of metaplastic cartilage. The pathogenesis of these lesions remains uncertain, but two fundamental concepts have been developed to explain these lesions. In one (synovial fluid intrusion theory), it is suggested that the presence of joint effusions and chronically elevated intra-articular pressure results in synovial fluid and cartilage fragments being driven into cracks and ulcerations in degenerating cartilage. Secondary resorption of subchondral trabeculae results in subchondral cysts that communicate with the articular cavity. The other theory (bony contusion theory) proposes that, with the loss of the protective cartilaginous coat, the subchondral bone plate is exposed to excessive trauma resulting in contusion and cystic necrosis of trabeculae. This results in a primary cystic lesion that initially does not communicate with the articular space, but, if collapse of the overlying cartilage covering occurs, such communication develops.

Radiographically the cysts in osteoarthritis tend to be small (<2 mm), multiple, and surrounded by a thin rim of condensed sclerotic bone. Rarely do they attain sufficient size to allow significant collapse of the articular surface. The largest subchondral cysts in osteoarthritis are found at the lateral margin of the acetabulum. Cysts are also observed in a variety of other articular processes and possess characteristics that enable accurate differential diagnosis. In rheumatoid arthritis subchondral cysts are frequent and may become extremely large (>5 cm). These giant rheumatoid cysts are most common in the ulnar olecranon, the femoral neck, and about the knee and may predispose to pathologic fracture. A characteristic

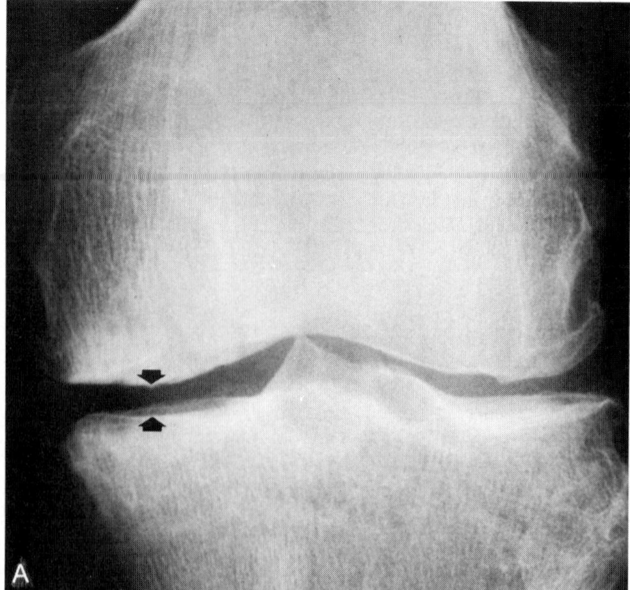

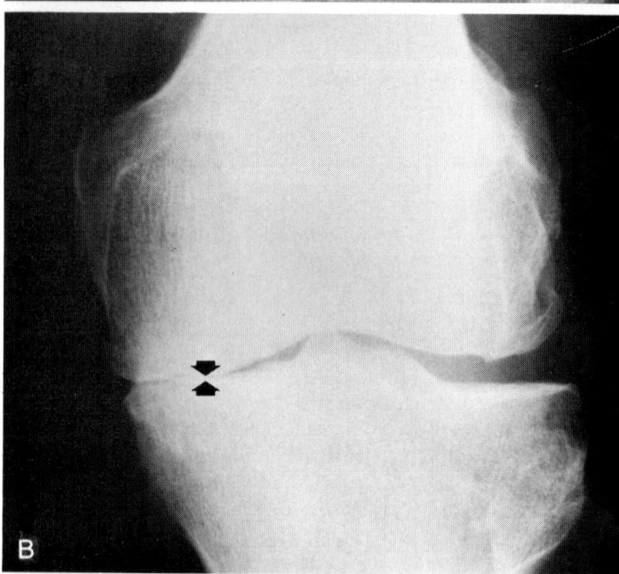

Figure 95–58. Osteoarthritis. In this patient with osteoarthritis of the knee, supine frontal radiograph of the knee *(A)* demonstrates marginal osteophyte formation and subchondral sclerosis, which is most prominent in the medial portion of the joint. However, there does not appear to be significant medial joint space narrowing *(between arrows)*, in this radiograph. A repeat frontal radiograph with the patient bearing weight *(B)* demonstrates a marked narrowing of the medial portion of the joint space *(between arrows)*, which was not visible on the supine radiograph.

feature of rheumatoid subchondral cysts is the lack of a sclerotic margin. In calcium pyrophosphate dihydrate (CPPD) crystal deposition disease, subchondral cysts are numerous, large, and frequently associated with collapse and deformity of the articular surface. In osteonecrosis the subchondral cysts are irregular with thick sclerotic margins and often associated with articular surface flattening or collapse with sparing of the articular cartilage coat. Intraosseous ganglia are solitary unilocular or multilocular lesions with a sclerotic margin. They are usually located in non–weight-bearing segments of the articulation. The presence of a contiguous soft-tissue mass is a helpful diagnostic feature in some patients with an intraosseous ganglion.

Osteophytosis

The presence of osteophytes constitutes the single most characteristic feature of degenerative joint disease. An osteophyte is a bony excrescence arising in relation to a synovial articulation. Bony outgrowths arising at tendon or ligament insertions are more properly termed enthesophytes.

Pathologically, osteophytes consist of spongy marrow-containing bone with a thin cortical shell and are usually covered with hyaline cartilage. In most instances, osteophytes develop from islands of metaplastic cartilage, although origin from periosteum or synovium may occur. It should be emphasized that osteophytes represent a response by articular cartilage to pathologic alteration. In highly stressed areas of the joint, cartilage fibrillation and denudation occur, whereas in low-stress areas of the articulation, islands of intact cartilage undergo bony metaplasia to form osteophytes. Two types of osteophytes form by this mechanism: marginal osteophytes (Fig. 95–59) and central osteophytes (Fig. 95–60). Marginal osteophytes, as their name implies, arise from the edge or periphery of an articulation where ''free'' articular cartilage is in contact with synovium. They grow along the path of least resistance and may eventually become large, filling the articular cavity. Central osteophytes arise from islands of metaplastic cartilage in the interior of the joint. These osteophytes tend to be flat and broad. Both types of osteophyte possess a thin radiodense line at their base that represents the original zone of calcified cartilage.

Periosteal or synovial osteophytes develop by osteogenic transformation of synovium or periosteum in response to mechanical factors. These osteophytes appear on radiographs as a smooth thickening of the cortical surface of the involved bone and are most common along the medial surface of the femoral neck (''buttressing'') (see Fig. 95–59). Osteophytes are also produced by traction phenomena at sites of capsular and intra-articular ligamentous attachments. In degenerative joint disease, such osteophytes are most characteristic at the margins of the interphalangeal joints of the hands and at the insertion points of the cruciate ligaments of the knee.

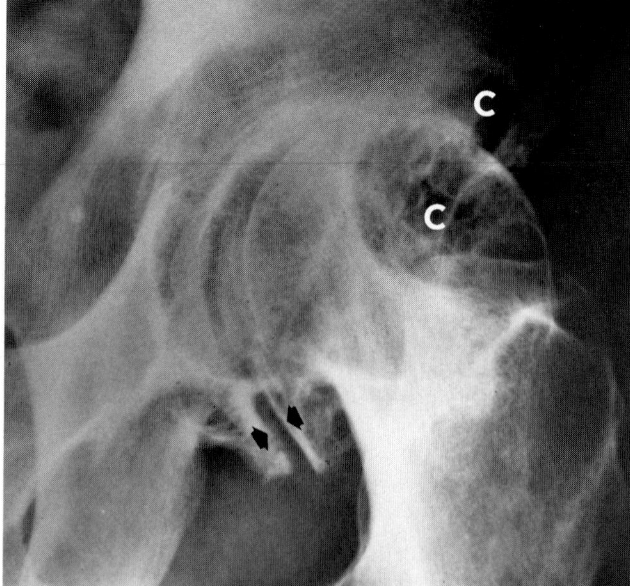

Figure 95–59. Osteoarthritis. In this patient with advanced degenerative joint disease of the hip, note the prominent osteophytes arising from the medial margins of the femoral head as well as the medial margin of the acetabulum *(arrows)*. This patient also demonstrates a pronounced thickening in the medial margin of the femoral neck (''buttressing'') as well as unusually large subchondral cystic lesions (C) in the lateral portion of the femoral head and acetabulum.

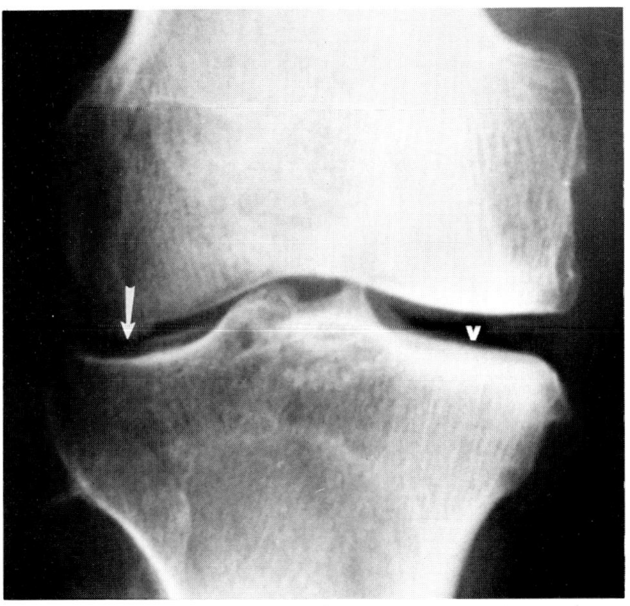

Figure 95–60. Osteophytosis. In this patient with degenerative disease of the knee, a central osteophyte *(arrow)* is present arising from the articular portion of the lateral femoral condyle. The medial portion of the joint demonstrates a vacuum phenomenon (V) with subchondral sclerosis and small-margin osteophytes.

Enthesopathy

Enthesopathy is a generic term referring to pathologic alterations at extra-articular sites of tendon or ligament insertion to bone. The enthesopathy of degenerative joint disease appears to represent a reparative response, with new bone produced by metaplastic transformation of chondrocytes as a response to repetitive trauma. The precise stimulus may be an overstress of a normal enthesis or a normal stress of an abnormal enthesis. The former is commonly seen in athletes or persons whose occupation results in significant physical stress. The latter may occur in an elderly patient in whom biochemical changes have occurred in the ground substance of the connective tissue.

Radiographically, degenerative enthesopathy is characterized by thick, rounded, well-corticated bony outgrowths occurring at a tendon or ligament insertion (Fig. 95–61). This pattern should be differentiated from the fine, spiculated, indistinct bony proliferation that is associated with acute inflammation in certain inflammatory arthritides such as ankylosing spondylitis, psoriatic arthritis, and Reiter's syndrome. The most common site of degenerative enthesopathy is the plantar surface of the calcaneus at the insertion point of the plantar aponeurosis of the foot. Other common sites include the posterior surface of the calcaneus, the patella, the femoral trochanters, pelvic ligamentous attachments, and the ulnar olecranon.

Other Radiographic Signs in Degenerative Joint Disease

The previously mentioned radiographic signs are common to virtually all varieties of degenerative joint disease. There are other radiographic findings that are occasionally encountered in certain specific situations or at specific anatomic sites. Intra-articular erosions are distinctly unusual in typical osteoarthritis and, in most instances, comprise an important finding in excluding this diagnosis. However, in patients with inflammatory (erosive) osteoarthritis, marginal or central erosions in the interphalangeal joints of the hand are common (Fig. 95–62). Malalignment or subluxation is frequently encountered in the knee, where genu varus and lateral subluxation of the tibia are common in advanced osteoarthritis. Superolateral migration of the femoral head is also frequently seen in degenerative joint disease of the hip. Intra-articular bony ankylosis is very rare in typical osteoarthritis but may be encountered in the interphalangeal joints of the hand in inflammatory (erosive) osteoarthritis (Fig. 95–63). Extra-articular bony ankylosis is relatively common at certain sites such as the sacroiliac joints. It is also observed in the vertebral column in spondylosis deformans and diffuse idiopathic skeletal hyperostosis (DISH). Intra-articular osteocartilaginous bodies are frequent in osteoarthritis, especially in the knee (Fig. 95–64). Radiolucent cartilage fragments may grow in size and ossify. Such bodies may remain free in the articular cavity or become embedded in the synovial membrane.

DEGENERATIVE JOINT DISEASE OF THE PERIPHERAL SKELETON

Osteoarthritis can affect virtually any articulation in the peripheral skeleton. The most commonly involved articulations are the interphalangeal joints of the hand, first carpometacarpal joint, acromioclavicular joints, hip, knee, and first metatarsophalangeal joints.

Hand and Wrist

The interphalangeal joints of the hand and, in particular, the distal interphalangeal articulations are very common sites of involvement in osteoarthritis. Radiographic abnormalities include joint space narrowing, subchondral sclerosis, and prominent marginal osteophytes (Fig. 95–65). Adjacent articular surfaces are closely applied, producing an undulating contour. Occasionally osteophytes may be identified arising from the central portion of one articular surface and interdigitating with a defect in the apposing surface (Fig. 95–66). In advanced cases, intra-articular osseous bodies may be present. Metacarpophalangeal joint involvement is usually seen only in the presence of prominent distal interphalangeal joint involvement. Nonerosive uniform joint space loss is the most typical finding. Osteophyte formation is much less prominent at this site than in the interphalangeal articulations. In the wrist the most commonly involved articulations are the first carpometacarpal and trapezioscaphoid articulations. At the former site, the characteristic changes include joint space narrowing, subchondral sclerosis and cyst formation, osteophytosis, and fragmentation. Radial subluxation of the first metacarpal base may occur in advanced cases. Trapezioscaphoid joint involvement is virtually always associated with first carpometacarpal joint involvement. In fact, abnormalities at the trapezioscaphoid joint without first carpometacarpal joint involvement should suggest another disorder, especially CPPD crystal deposition disease. Other sites in the wrist may be involved in osteoarthritis but generally in patients with a history of trauma or occupational stress.

Although other diseases affect the wrist, accurate differential diagnosis is not difficult. The seronegative spondyloarthropathies, including ankylosing spondylitis, psoriatic arthritis, and Reiter's syndrome, feature prominent interphalangeal joint disease. However, in contrast to osteoarthritis, irregularity of terminal tufts as well as articular erosions and diaphyseal periostitis is usually present. Rheumatoid arthritis is associated with osteoporosis, marginal erosions, and extensive metacarpophalangeal joint involvement with relative sparing of the distal interphalangeal joints. Osteophytosis is not a feature of rheumatoid arthritis. CPPD crystal deposition disease may closely resemble osteoarthritis, especially in the first carpometacarpal and trapezioscaphoid joints. However, this disease

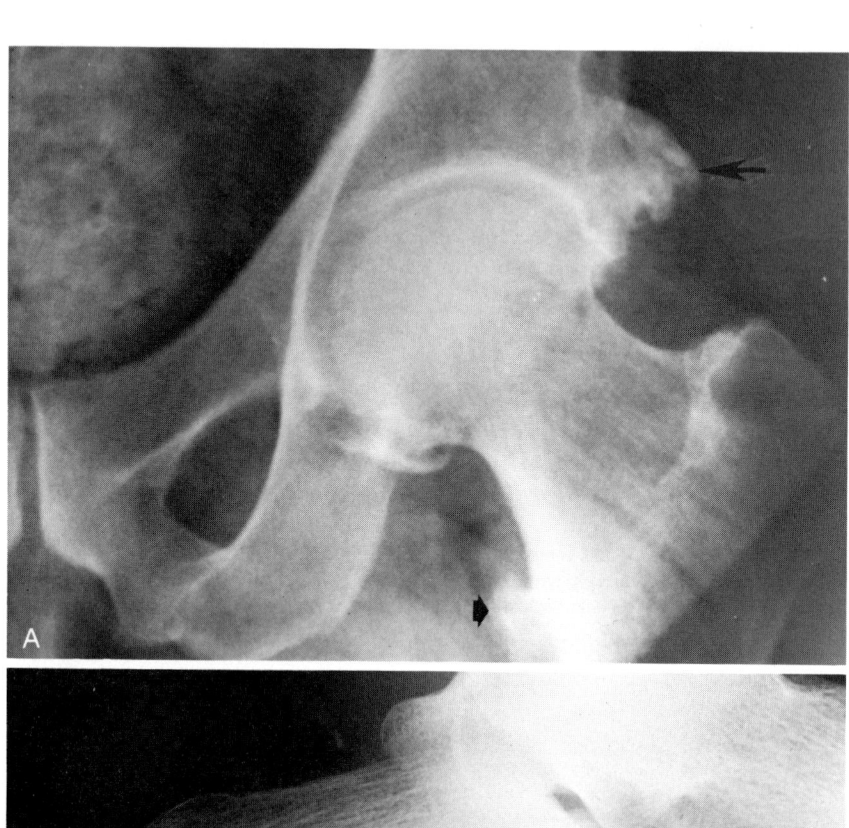

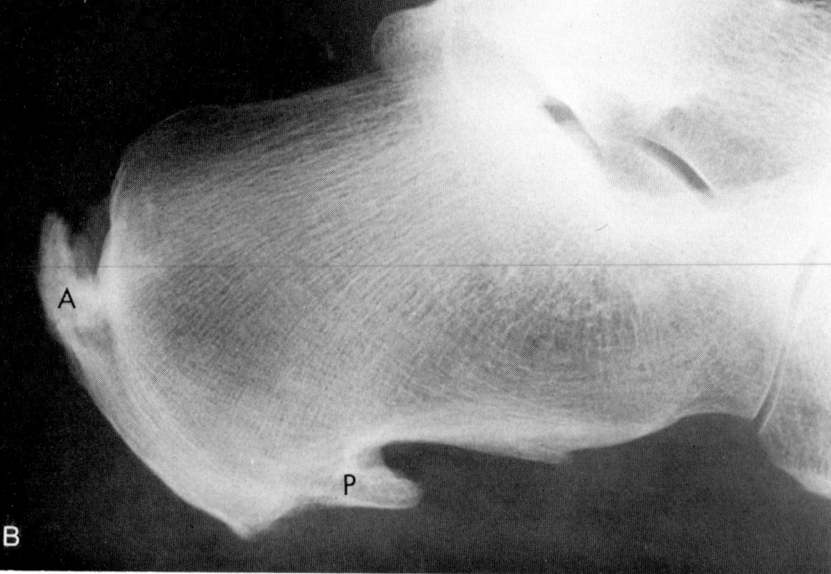

Figure 95–61. Enthesopathy. In this patient with diffuse idiopathic skeletal hyperostosis, there is pronounced bony proliferation at the sites of tendon and ligament insertion about the hip *(A)* and calcaneus *(B)*. Enthesophytes are present at the lateral portion of the acetabulum *(large arrow)* and at the lesser trochanter *(small arrow)*. Calcaneal enthesophytes are prominent at the insertions of the plantar aponeurosis (P) and the Achilles tendon (A).

Figure 95–62. Central erosion. In this patient with inflammatory (erosive) osteoarthritis, note the large central erosion *(arrows)* involving the distal subarticular region of the middle phalanx. In the proper clinical setting, this finding is virtually pathognomonic of inflammatory (erosive) osteoarthritis.

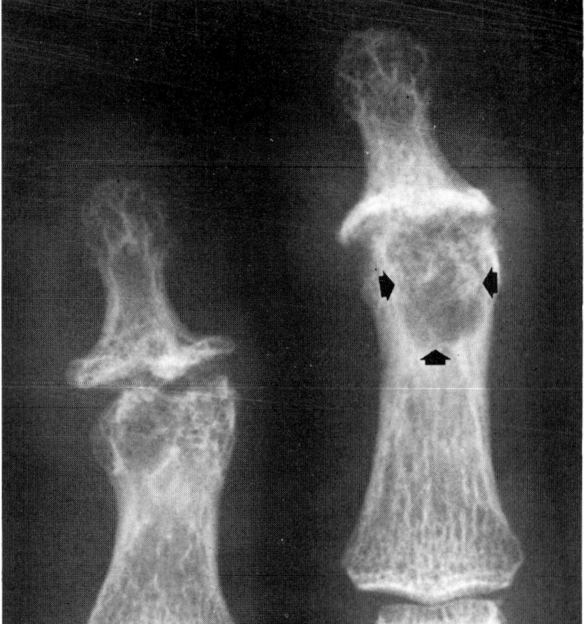

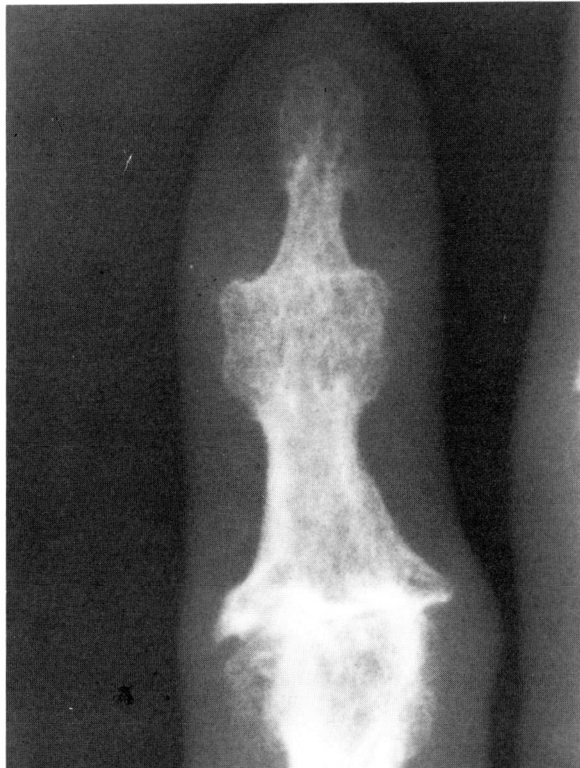

Figure 95–63. Intra-articular ankylosis. In this patient with inflammatory (erosive) osteoarthritis, there is bony intra-articular ankylosis at the distal interphalangeal joint. Typical osteoarthritic changes are also present at the proximal interphalangeal joint, with joint space narrowing, subchondral sclerosis, and osteophyte formation.

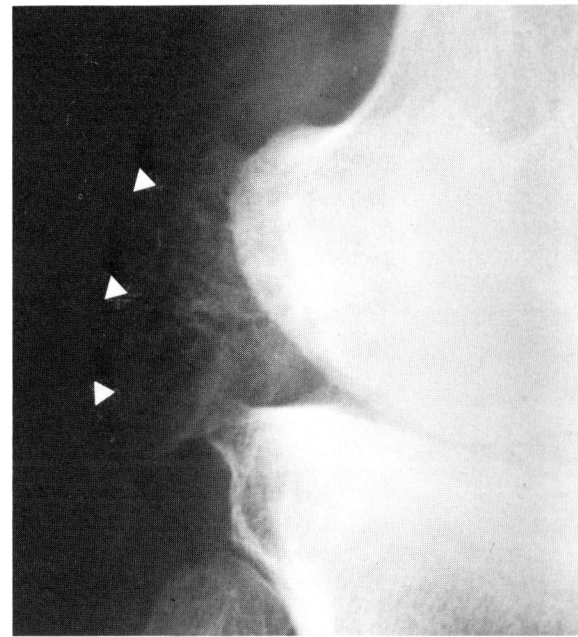

Figure 95–64. Intra-articular loose body (joint mouse). In this patient with advanced degenerative joint disease of the knee, a large loose body *(arrowheads)* is present posterior to the articulation.

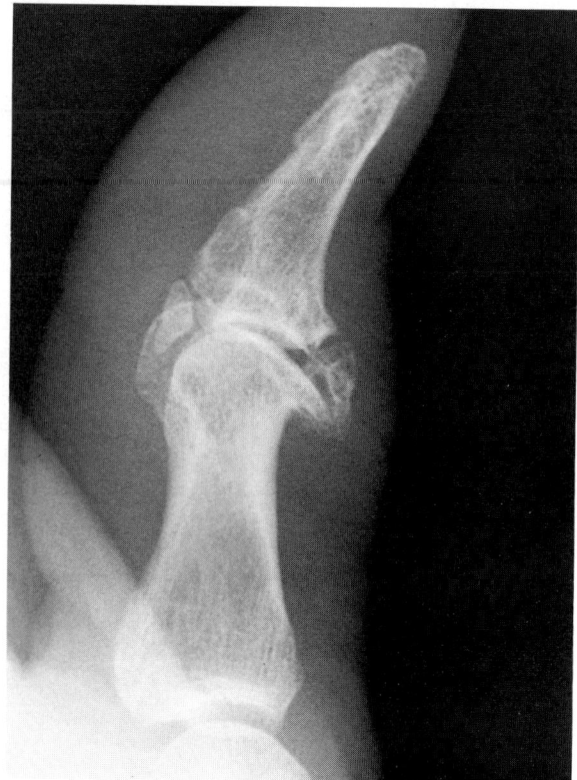

Figure 95–65. Osteoarthritis. In this patient, there is advanced osteoarthritic change of the distal interphalangeal joint of the thumb. Note the prominent marginal osteophyte formation. This finding is a hallmark of degenerative joint disease in this location.

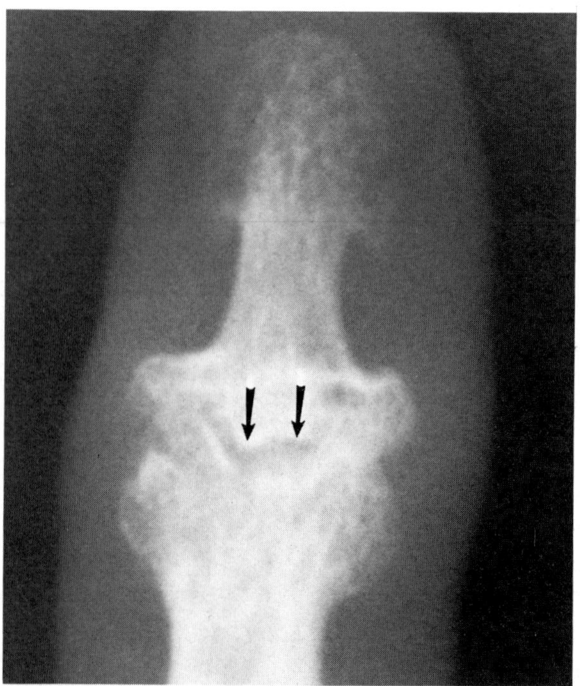

Figure 95–66. Osteoarthritis. In this patient with prominent interphalangeal joint involvement, note the central osteophyte *(arrows)* arising from the articular surface of the distal phalanx, which interdigitates with the articular surface of the middle phalanx.

produces extensive radiocarpal joint involvement and selective involvement of the second and third metacarpophalangeal joints. Furthermore, subchondral cysts tend to be quite numerous and prominent, and chondrocalcinosis is usually present, especially in the triangular fibrocartilage. Inflammatory (erosive) osteoarthritis may be indistinguishable from typical noninflammatory osteoarthritis on radiographic studies. However, there are two features that, if present, suggest the diagnosis: interphalangeal joint erosions, especially erosions of the central articular surface, and intra-articular bony ankylosis of an interphalangeal joint.

Elbow

Osteoarthritis is rare in the elbow except in association with a history of accidental or occupational trauma. The radiographic changes are similar to those at other sites, with joint space narrowing, subchondral sclerosis, subchondral cysts, and osteophyte formation. Degenerative enthesopathy consists of an extra-articular bony spur arising from the ulnar olecranon at the insertion of the triceps tendon.

Glenohumeral Joint

Degenerative joint disease of this articulation is infrequent in the absence of trauma or other predisposing condition such as a chronic tear of the rotator cuff, CPPD crystal deposition disease, hemophilia, alkaptonuria, acromegaly, and various epiphyseal dysplasias. Radiographic findings consist of joint space narrowing with subchondral sclerosis and cysts. Large hook-like osteophytes characteristically form on the medial margin of the humeral head (Fig. 95–67). Elevation of the humeral head with a smooth scalloped erosion of the undersurface of the acromion indicates the presence of a tear of the rotator cuff that may be either a primary or a secondary factor in glenohumeral degenerative joint disease (Fig. 95–68).

Acromioclavicular Joint

Degenerative joint disease involving the acromioclavicular joint is a very common radiographic finding, especially in the elderly. The radiographic findings consist of joint space narrowing with subchondral sclerosis and marginal osteophyte formation.

Hip

Osteoarthritis of the hip is one of the most frequent causes of debility in the elderly population. The cardinal radiographic features of osteoarthritis of the hip are asymmetrical joint space narrowing, subchondral cysts and sclerosis, and osteophytosis (see Fig. 95–57). Cartilage loss with joint space narrowing is focal in distribution, leading to movement or migration of the femoral head in one of several characteristic directions: superior (80 per cent), medial (20 per cent), or axial (1 per cent) (Fig. 95–69; see Fig. 95–57). Osteophytes are prominent in osteoarthritis of the hip, especially in the medial margin of the femoral head and in the lateral acetabular margin. Hypertrophy of the cortex of the femoral neck ("buttressing") tends to be most prominent in the medial aspect of the femoral neck. Cysts are usually prominent in the subchondral region, underlying areas of cartilage loss. A large subchondral cyst in the superolateral margin of the acetabulum is especially characteristic of degenerative joint disease. In long-standing osteoarthritis of the hip, collapse of the subarticular bone occurs, resulting in a pattern difficult to distinguish from that of advanced osteonecrosis.

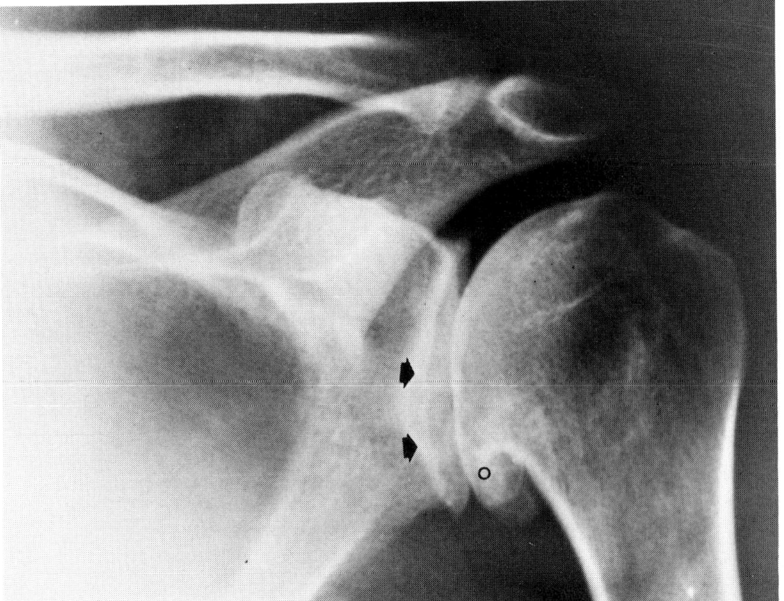

Figure 95–67. Glenohumeral osteoarthritis. In this patient with a history of prior anterior glenohumeral dislocation, the changes of secondary degenerative joint disease are present. The most prominent finding is the large hook-like osteophyte at the medial margin of the humeral head (O). Subchondral sclerosis is also prominent in the subarticular portion of the glenoid *(arrows)*.

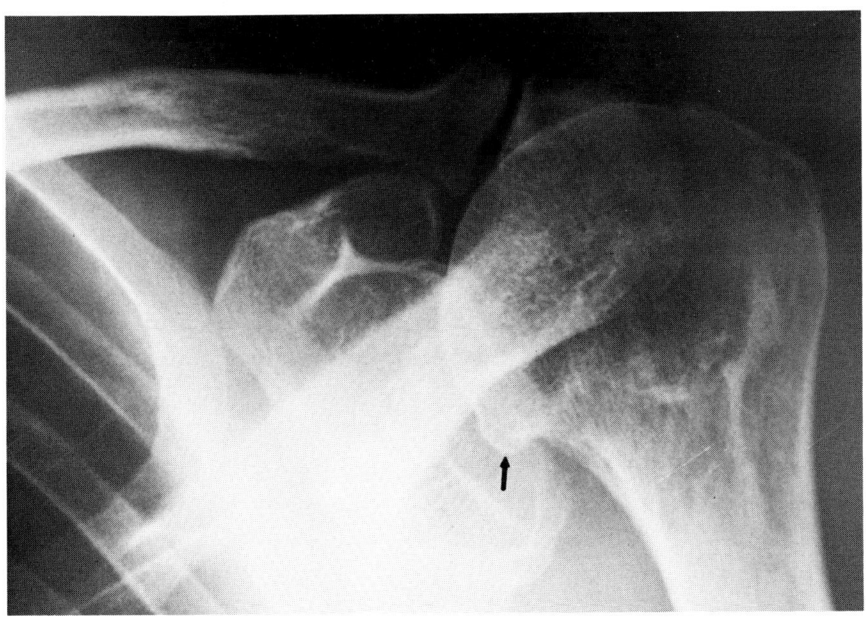

Figure 95–68. Rotator cuff arthropathy. In this patient with a long-standing tear of the musculotendinous rotator cuff of the shoulder, there is elevation of the humeral head as well as a small osteophyte at the medial margin of the humeral head *(arrow)*.

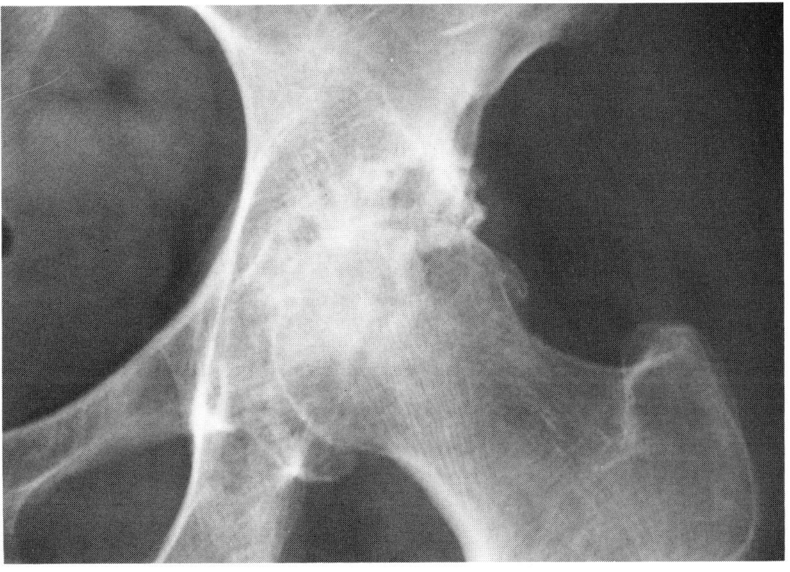

Figure 95–69. Osteoarthritis of the hip. In this patient with advanced osteoarthritis of the hip, there is virtually complete obliteration of the superomedial portions of the joint space with marginal osteophytes and subchondral cyst formation.

With regard to differential diagnosis, axial joint space narrowing and the lack of osteophytes are typical of the inflammatory arthropathies such as rheumatoid arthritis, ankylosing spondylitis, and psoriatic arthritis. CPPD crystal deposition disease may simulate osteoarthritis radiographically in some cases, although subchondral cysts tend to be more numerous and larger in CPPD crystal deposition disease, and chondrocalcinosis may be present in the acetabular labrum or symphysis pubis.

Knee

The knee is the most common site of degenerative joint disease. As in other weight-bearing joints, the presence of asymmetrical involvement of the articulation with joint space narrowing, subchondral sclerosis, subchondral cysts, and osteophytes is characteristic of osteoarthritis in the knee. In decreasing order of frequency, the medial femorotibial, the patellofemoral, and the lateral femorotibial compartments of the knee demonstrate radiographic abnormalities. In some instances joint space narrowing may not be apparent on standard anteroposterior supine radiographs but quite apparent in the tunnel view or on radiographs obtained during weight bearing (see Fig. 95–58). In advanced osteoarthritis, multiple, large intra-articular osseous bodies may be identified. In advanced disease, instability of the knee joint is prominent with varus angulation and lateral subluxation of the tibia (Fig. 95–70).

Ankle

Osteoarthritis of the ankle is unusual in the absence of prior trauma. Radiographic findings include joint space narrowing with subchondral sclerosis and cyst formation in the distal tibia or talar dome. Often the talar dome appears somewhat flattened in the lateral radiographic projection. Osteophytes are prominent along the margins of the distal tibia, and a large irregular osteophyte may be noted on the anterior surface of the talar neck at the site of insertion of the anterior margin of the joint capsule.

Foot

The most common sites of degenerative disease in the foot are the plantar and posterior surfaces of the calcaneus and the first metatarsophalangeal joint. Sharply marginated spurs (enthesophytes) are common at plantar (plantar aponeurosis) and posterior (Achilles tendon) tendinous and ligamentous insertion sites. These spurs may or may not be associated with clinical abnormality. Very large well-marginated osseous spurs at the same site may also be seen in patients with diffuse idiopathic skeletal hyperostosis (DISH) or acromegaly. Ill-defined calcaneal spurs are seen in the seronegative spondyloarthropathies such as ankylosing spondylitis, psoriatic arthritis, or Reiter's syndrome.

Degenerative abnormalities of the first metatarsophalangeal articulation are very common. Hallux rigidus is a disorder of unknown etiology that may affect adolescents and young adults. Clinically, it is manifest by a painful limitation of dorsiflexion of the great toe (Fig. 95–71). Radiographic changes include joint space narrowing, sclerosis, and marginal osteophytes. Hallux valgus is characterized by valgus angulation at the first metatarsophalangeal joint with lateral subluxation of the proximal phalanx (Fig. 95–72). Degenerative changes about the articulation and in the adjacent sesamoid bones are present as well as reactive sclerosis and cystic change in the medial aspect of the first metatarsal head, which may simulate the changes of gout.

DEGENERATIVE JOINT DISEASE OF THE AXIAL SKELETON

Degenerative joint disease of the spine is very common, especially in the older age group. The spinal column consists of a

Figure 95–70. Osteoarthritis of the knee. Frontal *(A)* and lateral *(B)* projections of the knee in this patient with advanced osteoarthritis reveal obliteration of the medial portion of the joint space with subchondral sclerosis and marginal osteophyte formation. This patient also demonstrates several of the complications of advanced degenerative joint disease, with lateral subluxation of the tibia, genu varus, and loose bodies (L). Observe the enchondroma in the femur.

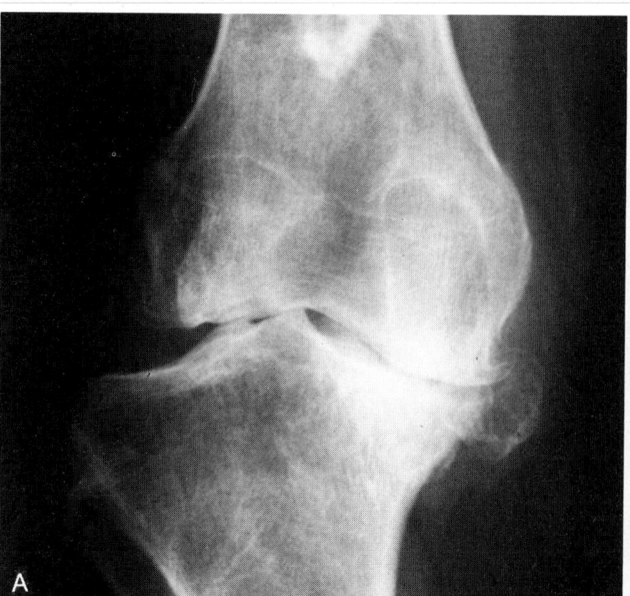

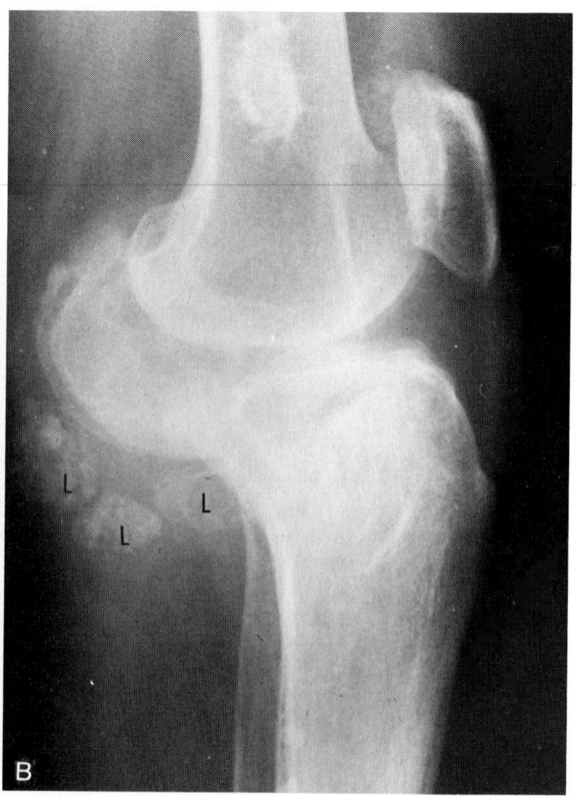

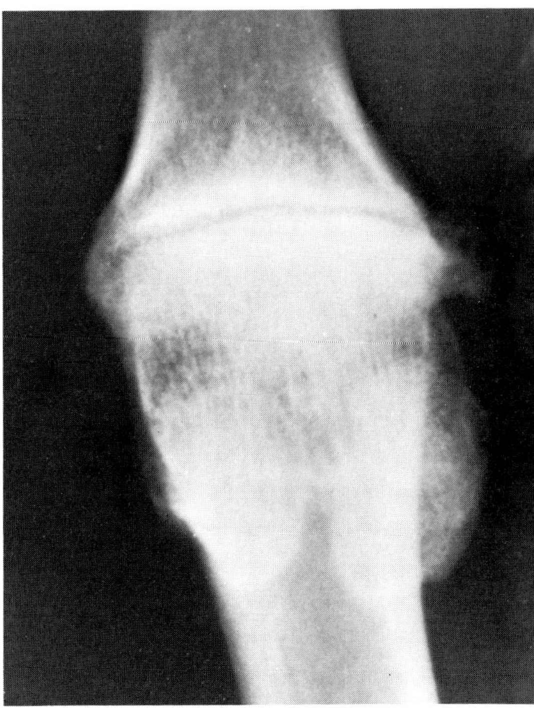

Figure 95–71. Hallux rigidus. In this patient with hallux rigidus, there is narrowing of the first metatarsophalangeal joint with subchondral sclerosis. No alignment abnormality is present.

complex arrangement of synovial, cartilaginous, and fibrous articulations, each of which may demonstrate distinctive radiographic alterations in degenerative joint disease.

Intervertebral Discs

Intervertebral osteochondrosis is a primary degenerative disorder of the intervertebral disc, particularly the nucleus pulposus. The earliest pathologic changes consist of desiccation, cleft formation,

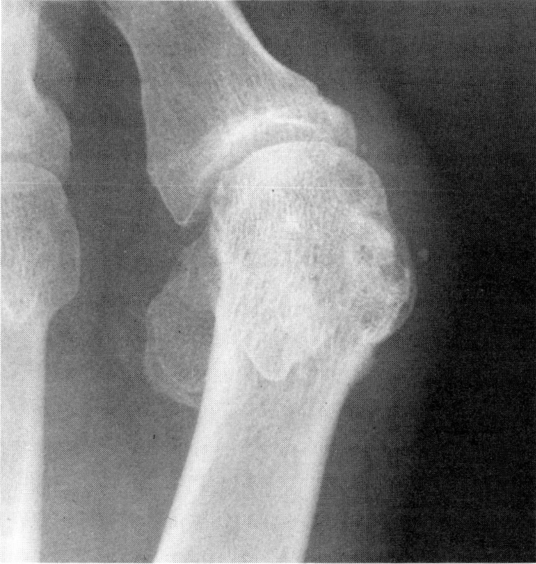

Figure 95–72. Hallux valgus. In this patient with hallux valgus, note the prominent lateral deviation of the proximal phalanx of the great toe. Cystic changes are present at the medial margin of the metaphysis of the metatarsal with adjacent soft-tissue swelling.

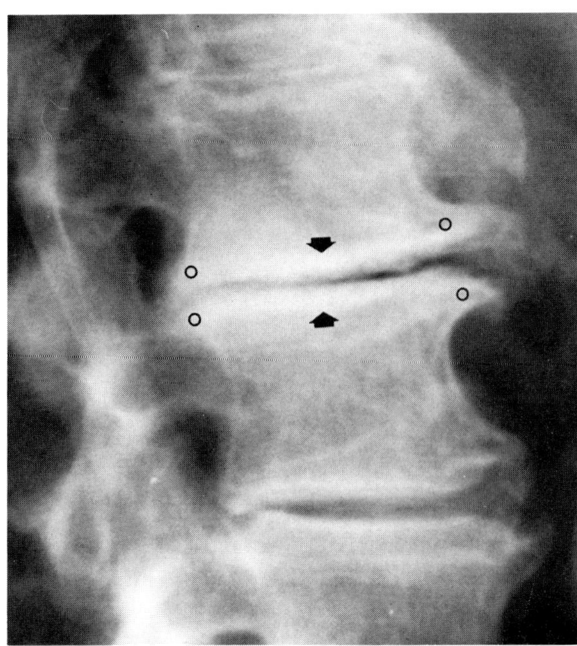

Figure 95–73. Intervertebral osteochondrosis. In this patient with primary disc degeneration (intervertebral osteochondrosis), there is narrowing of the intervertebral disc spaces with adjacent sclerosis *(arrows)* of the vertebral end-plates. Small triangular osteophytes are also present at the anterior and posterior vertebral margins (O).

and loss of elasticity in the nucleus pulposus. At this early stage, the only radiographic abnormality is the identification of linear or circular radiolucent gas collections (''vacuum'' phenomenon) in the substance of the intervertebral disc. This gas is principally nitrogen, and its demonstration may be accentuated in radiographs obtained with the spine in the extended position. As the disorder progresses, narrowing of the intervertebral disc space is noted and secondary abnormalities of the vertebral end-plates are identified (Fig. 95–73). Sclerosis of the subchondral vertebral bone may be seen in association with small triangular spurs arising from the margins of the vertebrae. In some patients herniation of a portion of the intervertebral disc (cartilaginous node) into the vertebral body is evident as a round or oblong radiolucent lesion bordered by a hemispherical rim of sclerotic bone.

Spondylosis deformans is also a manifestation of intervertebral disc degeneration but, in contrast to intervertebral osteochondrosis, predominantly involves the peripheral fibers of the annulus fibrosus. It is manifested radiographically by the presence of multiple large anterior and anterolateral spinal osteophytes (Fig. 95–74). In this disorder the earliest abnormality appears to consist of breakdown of the peripheral fibers of the annulus fibrosus (Sharpey's fibers), which anchor the disc to the vertebral rim. The nucleus pulposus remains relatively normal, at least initially, such that gelatinous nuclear material under pressure displaces the outer portion of the annulus fibrosus. The bony attachments of the paraspinal ligaments superficial to the annulus are exposed to abnormal pressure and stretching resulting in the formation of bony outgrowths. These bony outgrowths are commonly referred to as osteophytes (but are more accurately termed enthesophytes). Radiographic analysis reveals that the spinal osteophytes arise from the anterior and lateral margins of the vertebral body adjacent to, but separate from, the discovertebral junction. As the osteophytes grow, they demonstrate an initial horizontal segment with a subsequent vertical one that extends superiorly or inferiorly around the intervertebral disc space. Spinal osteophytes at adjacent levels will either interdigitate, remaining separate from each other by a thin radiolucent space, or completely fuse. In the thoracolumbar spine, osteophytes are relatively unusual on the left side of the vertebral body, presumably

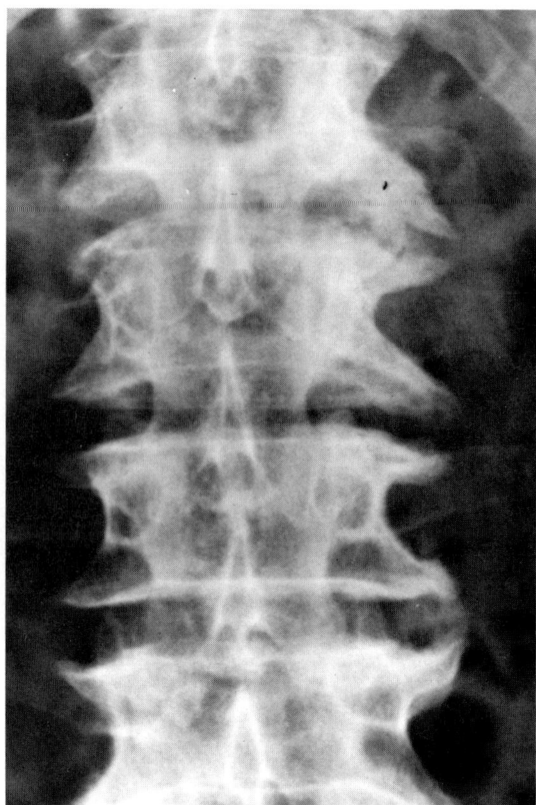

Figure 95–74. Spondylosis deformans. In this patient with spondylosis deformans, the heights of the intervertebral discs are preserved. There are multiple osteophytes arising from the margins of the vertebral bodies.

owing to inhibition of their growth by the pulsations of the adjacent aorta. In the cervical spine, large anterior cervical osteophytes may encroach on the upper esophagus, resulting in dysphagia. In spondylosis deformans associated with scoliosis, the osteophytes tend to be most prominent on the concave side of the curve and relatively small or absent on the convex side.

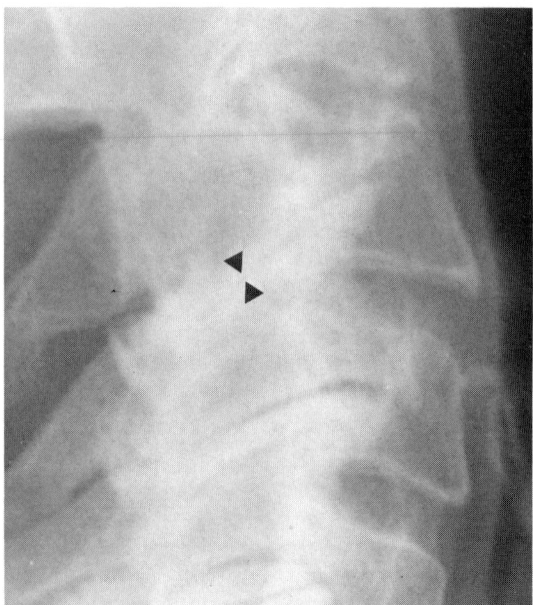

Figure 95–75. Apophyseal joint osteoarthritis. In this patient with advanced apophyseal joint osteoarthritis of the cervical spine, there is narrowing of the cervical apophyseal joints *(between arrows)* with adjacent subchondral sclerosis.

Synovial Articulations

The apophyseal joints of the vertebral column are true synovial joints, existing between adjacent vertebral arches from the level of the third cervical vertebra to the top of the sacrum. Osteoarthritis occurring in these articulations is commonly associated with prior trauma or abnormal spinal curvature and is accompanied by pathologic and radiographic changes that are identical to those evident in osteoarthritis in peripheral articulations. Joint space narrowing, eburnation, and osteophytosis are the major aberrations (Fig. 95–75). Osteophytes may encroach on the spinal canal or neural foramina, resulting in symptoms and signs of spinal cord or nerve root compression. Occasionally, instability of the facet joints is evident, leading to degenerative spondylolisthesis or degenerative scoliosis.

Spinal Ligaments

Calcification and ossification of the anterior longitudinal ligament of the spine in elderly individuals is the cardinal roentgenographic finding in the ossifying enthesopathy known as diffuse idiopathic skeletal hyperostosis (DISH, Forestier's disease, ankylosing hyperostosis of the spine). Flowing ossification in the anterior longitudinal ligament connecting four adjacent vertebral bodies is one diagnostic criterion of the disease. Other criteria are presentation of the height of intervertebral discs at the involved levels and the absence of apophyseal and sacroiliac joint intra-articular ankylosis, erosions, or sclerosis.

The earliest and most frequent site of involvement is the lower thoracic spine. In this area as well as in the lumbar spine, two types of osseous lesions are identified (Fig. 95–76). The most typical abnormality consists of a bumpy, flowing osseous band that parallels the anterior and anterolateral margins of the vertebral body and intervertebral disc. It is thicker than the syndesmophytes seen in ankylosing spondylitis, and a radiolucent shadow separates the ossified ligament and anterior vertebral margins. A second type of spinal lesion consists of large marginal osteophytes identical to those seen in spondylosis deformans. In the cervical spine, large, irregular deposits of bone contiguous with the anterior margin of the cervical vertebral bodies may be seen. These bony outgrowths may produce dysphagia. Although the key to the radiographic diagnosis of DISH resides in the identification of characteristic spinal changes, the sacroiliac joints and peripheral skeleton may also be involved. Calcification and ossification of the para-articular sacroiliac ligaments result in bridging extra-articular osteophytes that may simulate true intra-articular bony ankylosis. In the peripheral skeleton, bone proliferation involves sites of ligament and tendon insertions such as the plantar and posterior surfaces of the calcaneus, the ulnar olecranon, and the anterior surface of the patella.

The most important differential diagnosis of spine abnormalities in DISH is ankylosing spondylitis. In this latter disorder, ossification in the outer layers of the annulus fibrosus produces a syndesmophyte that is readily identified as a thin, slender, vertically oriented bone outgrowth on frontal radiographs of the involved spinal segment. In DISH, larger areas of ossification are best seen in the lateral radiographic projection of the spine. Sacroiliitis is not present in DISH, in contrast to ankylosing spondylitis. In the cervical spine the changes of a rare disorder known as sternocostoclavicular hyperostosis resemble those of DISH. Coarse bony proliferation along the anterior margins of the cervical vertebral bodies is evident.

Ossification of the posterior longitudinal ligament (OPLL) is a relatively rare occurrence that may be an isolated phenomenon or may be seen in association with DISH (Fig. 95–77). Radiographi-

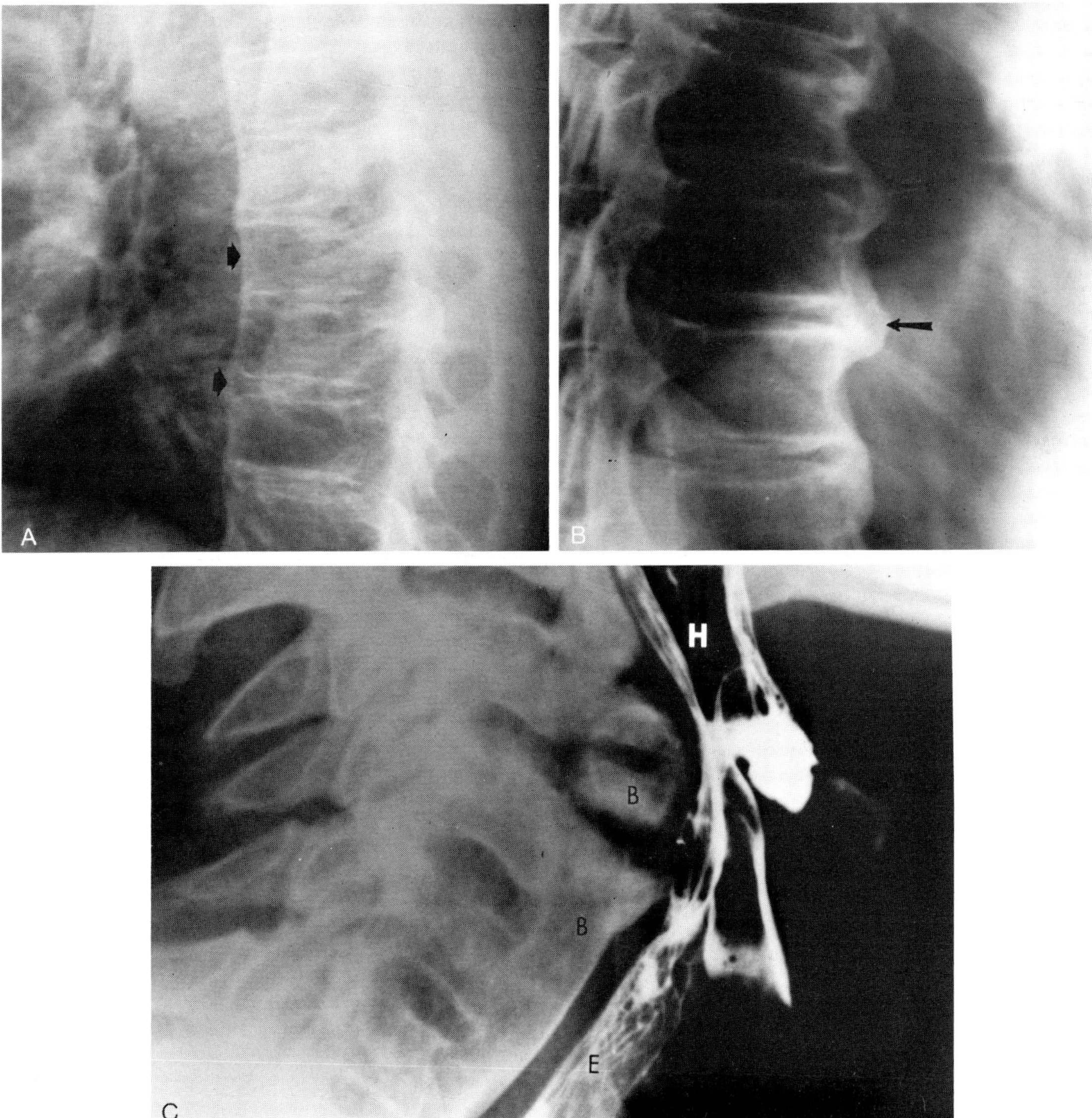

Figure 95–76. Diffuse idiopathic skeletal hyperostosis. The patient in *A* demonstrates the most typical findings in this disorder, with smooth-flowing calcification and ossification of the anterior longitudinal ligament *(arrows)* of the thoracic spine. The patient in *B* demonstrates a second type of radiographic finding. There are bridging ossifications *(arrows)* extending over more than four contiguous vertebral levels; however, the ossifications are larger and more irregular than in the patient in *A* and more reminiscent of the osteophytes in spondylosis deformans. In *C,* the cervical spine changes of this disorder are well-demonstrated on a film from a barium swallow. Large masses of bone (B) are present contiguous with the anterior margin of the lower cervical spine, with prominent encroachment upon the hypopharynx (H) and upper esophagus (E).

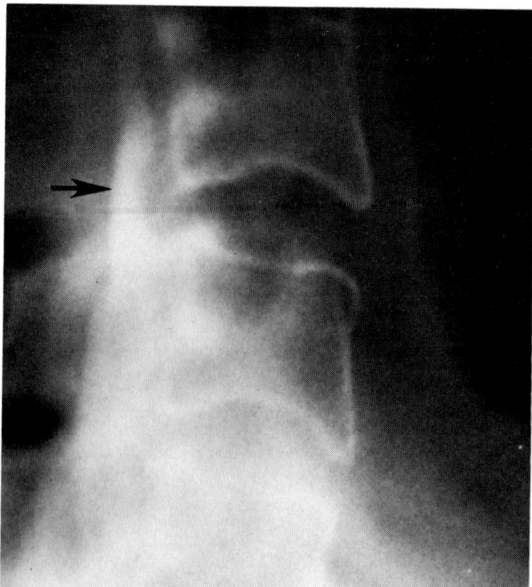

Figure 95–77. Ossification of the posterior longitudinal ligament. In this patient with diffuse idiopathic skeletal hyperostosis, there is also ossification of the posterior longitudinal ligament *(arrow)* of the cervical spine, which is manifested by a smooth osseous linear density parallel to the posterior margins of the vertebral bodies.

cally a well-defined linear band of osseous density paralleling the posterior margin of one or more vertebral bodies, especially in the cervical spine, is apparent. The changes may be quite subtle on plain radiographs and require polytomography or computed tomography for confirmation.

Other Sites

The uncovertebral (Luschka) joints are located between the uncinate processes of the third through seventh cervical vertebral bodies and the inferolateral margin of the adjacent cephalad vertebra. The precise anatomic nature of these articulations is a matter of some debate. Arthrosis of these articulations is roentgenographically manifested by joint space narrowing, sclerosis, and osteophytes that frequently project posteriorly into the adjacent cervical neural foramina, resulting in radiculopathies.

Osteoarthritis is occasionally identified at the synovium-lined costovertebral articulations. This finding is more frequent than is commonly appreciated because these articulations are quite difficult to visualize utilizing conventional roentgenographic techniques.

Bibliography

Ahlback S: Osteoarthritis of the knee. A radiographic investigation. Acta Radiol (Suppl) 227:7, 1968.

Bick EM: Vertebral osteophytosis. Pathologic basis of its roentgenology. AJR 73:979, 1955.

Cameron HU, Macnab I: Observations of osteoarthritis of the hip joint. Clin Orthop Rel Res 108:31, 1975.

Cooper RR, Misol L: Tendon and ligament insertion. A light and electron microscopic study. J Bone Joint Surg 52A:1, 1970.

Coventry MB, Ghormley RK, Kernohan JW: The intervertebral disc: Its microscopic anatomy and pathology. II. Changes in the intervertebral disc concomitant with age. J Bone Joint Surg 27:233, 1945.

Epstein JA, Epstein BS, Lavine LS, et al: Lumbar nerve root compression at the intervertebral foramina caused by arthritis of the posterior facets. J Neurosurg 39:362, 1973.

Ferguson AB: The pathological changes in degenerative arthritis of the hip and treatment by rotational osteotomy. J Bone Joint Surg 46A:1337, 1964.

Forestier J, Lagier R: Ankylosing hyperostosis of the spine. Clin Orthop Rel Res 74:65, 1971.

Forestier J, Rotes-Querol J: Senile ankylosing hyperostosis of the spine. Ann Rheum Dis 9:321, 1950.

Fort LT, Gilula LA, Murphy WA, Gado M: Analysis of gas in vacuum lumbar disc. AJR 128:1056, 1977.

Freund E: The pathological significance of intra-articular pressure. Edinburgh Medical J 47:192, 1940.

Gershon Cohen J, Schraer H, Sklaroff D, Blumberg N: Dissolution of the intervertebral disc in the aged normal. The phantom nucleus pulposus. Radiology 62:383, 1954.

Goldberg RP, Carter BL: Absence of thoracic osteophytosis in the area adjacent to the aorta: Computed tomography demonstration. J Comput Assist Tomogr 2:173, 1978.

Gorton T: Osteoarthrosis in United States adults. In Bennett PH, Wood PHN (eds): Population Studies of the Therapeutic Diseases. International Congress Series No. 148. Amsterdam, Excerpta Medica Foundation, 1968, p 391.

Greenway GD, Danzig L, Resnick D, Haghighi P: The painful shoulder. Med Rad Photog 58:56, 1982.

Haines RW, McDougall A: The anatomy of hallux valgus. J Bone Joint Surg 36B:272, 1972.

Havdrup J, Hulth A, Telhag H: The subchondral bone in osteoarthritis and rheumatoid arthritis of the knee. A histological and microradiographic study. Acta Orthop Scan 47:345, 1976.

Hernbort JS: The natural course of untreated osteoarthritis of the knee. Clin Orthop Rel Res 123:139, 1977.

Hiramatsu Y, Nobechi T: Calcification of the posterior longitudinal ligament of the spine among Japanese. Radiology 100:307, 1971.

Kambolis C, Bullough PG, Jaffe HL: Ganglionic cystic defects of bone. J Bone Joint Surg 55A:496, 1973.

Kellgren JH, Lawrence JL: Osteoarthrosis and disk degeneration in an urban population. Ann Rheum Dis 17:388, 1958.

Kellgren JH, Lawrence JS, Bier F: Genetic factors in generalized osteoarthrosis. Ann Rheum Dis 22:237, 1963.

Kidd KL, Peter JB: Erosive osteoarthritis. Radiology 86:640, 1966.

Knuttson F: The vacuum phenomenon in the intervertebral discs. Acta Radiol 23:173, 1942.

Landells JW: The bone cysts of osteoarthritis. J Bone Joint Surg 35B:643, 1953.

Lawrence JS: Hypertension in relation to musculoskeletal disorders. Ann Rheum Dis 34:451, 1975.

Leach RE, Gregg T, Siber FJ: Weight-bearing radiography in osteoarthritis of the knee. Radiology 97:265, 1970.

Macnab I: Cervical spondylosis. Clin Orthop Rel Res 109:69, 1975.

Magyar E, Talerman A, Feher M, Wouters HW: Giant bone cysts in rheumatoid arthritis. J Bone Joint Surg 56B:121, 1974.

Mann RA, Coughlin MJ, DuVries HL: Hallux rigidus. A review of the literature and a method of treatment. Clin Orthop Rel Res 142:57, 1979.

Marklund T, Myrnerts R: Radiographic determination of cartilage height in the knee joint. Acta Orthop Scand 45:752, 1974.

Martel W, Sitterley BH: The diagnostic value of buttressing of the femoral neck. Arthritis Rheum 12:161, 1978.

McEwen C: Osteoarthritis of the fingers with ankylosis. Arthritis Rheum 11:734, 1968.

Meachim G: Age changes in articular cartilage. Clin Orthop Rel Res 64:33, 1969.

Milgram JW: The development of loose bodies in human joints. Clin Orthop Rel Res 124:292, 1977.

Miller EJ, Vanderkorst JK, Sokoloff L: Collagen of human articular and costal cartilage. Arthritis Rheum 12:21, 1969.

Mitchell NS, Cruess RL: Classification of degenerative arthritis. Can Med Assoc J 117:763, 1977.

Ondrouch AS: Cyst formation in osteoarthritis. J Bone Joint Surg 47B:755, 1963.

Ono K, Ota H, Tada K, et al: Ossified posterior longitudinal ligament. Spine 2:126, 1977.

Peter JB, Pearson CM, Marmor L: Erosive osteoarthritis of the hands. Arthritis Rheum 9:365, 1966.

Rennell C, Mainzer F, Multz CV, Genant HK: Subchondral pseudocysts in rheumatoid arthritis. AJR 129:1069, 1977.

Resnick D: Patterns of migration of the femoral head in osteoarthritis of the hip. AJR 124:62, 1975.

Resnick D: Sternocostoclavicular hyperostosis. AJR 135:1211, 1980.

Resnick D, Guerra J Jr, Robinson CA, Vint VC: Association of diffuse idiopathic skeletal hyperostosis (DISH) and calcification and ossification of the posterior longitudinal ligament. AJR 131:1049, 1978.

Resnick D, Niwayama G: Ankylosing spondylitis. In Resnick D, Niwayama G (eds): Diagnosis of Bone and Joint Disorders. Philadelphia, WB Saunders Company, 1981, p 1040.

Resnick D, Niwayama G: Degenerative disease of extraspinal locations. In Resnick D, Niwayama G (eds): Diagnosis of Bone and Joint Disorders. Philadelphia, WB Saunders Company, 1981, p 1270.

Resnick D, Niwayama G: Degenerative disease of the spine. In Resnick D, Niwayama G (eds): Diagnosis of Bone and Joint Disorders. Philadelphia, WB Saunders Company, 1981, p 1368.

Resnick D, Niwayama G: Diffuse idiopathic skeletal hyperostosis (DISH): Ankylosing hyperostosis of Forestier and Rotes-Querol. In Resnick D, Niwayama G (eds): Diagnosis of Bone and Joint Disorders. Philadelphia, WB Saunders Company, 1981, p 1416.

Resnick D, Niwayama G: Entheses and enthesopathy: Anatomical, pathological, and radiological correlation. Radiology 146:1, 1983.

Resnick D, Niwayama G: Intervertebral disc herniations: Cartilaginous (Schmorl's) nodes. Radiology 126:57, 1978.

Resnick D, Niwayama G: Osteonecrosis: Diagnostic techniques, specific situations, and complications. In Resnick D, Niwayama G (eds): Diagnosis of Bone and Joint Disorders. Philadelphia, WB Saunders Company, 1981, p 2832.

Resnick D, Niwayama G: Radiographic and pathologic features of spinal involvement in diffuse idiopathic skeletal hyperostosis (DISH). Radiology 119:559, 1976.

Resnick D, Niwayama G, Coutts RD: Subchondral cysts (geodes) in arthritic disorders: Pathologic and radiographic appearance of the hip joint. AJR 128:799, 1977.

Resnick D, Niwayama G, Goergen TG, et al: Clinical, radiographic and pathologic abnormalities in calcium pyrophosphate dihydrate deposition disease (CPPD): Pseudogout. Radiology 122:1, 1977.

Resnick D, Shaul SR, Robins JM: Diffuse idiopathic skeletal hyperostosis (DISH): Forestier's disease with extraspinal manifestations. Radiology 115:513, 1976.

Rhaney K, Lamb DW: The cysts of osteoarthritis of the hip. A radiological and pathological study. J Bone Joint Surg 37B:663, 1955.

Schmorl G, Junghanns H: The Human Spine in Health and Disease, 2nd ed. Translated by EF Basemann. New York, Grune and Stratton, 1971, p 138.

Solomon L: Patterns of osteoarthritis of the hip joint. J Bone Joint Surg 58B:176, 1976.

Thomas RH, Resnick D, Alazraki NP, et al: Compartmental evaluation of osteoarthritis of the knee. A comparative study of available diagnostic modalities. Radiology 116:585, 1975.

Thompson RC, Bassett CA: Histological observations on experimentally induced degeneration of articular cartilage. J Bone Joint Surg 52A:435, 1970.

Utsinder PD, Resnick D, Shapiro RE: Diffuse skeletal abnormalities in Forestier's disease. Arch Intern Med 136:763, 1976.

Weiss C, Mirow S: An ultrastructural study of osteoarthritic changes in articular cartilage of human knees. J Bone Joint Surg 54A:954, 1972.

Zanca P: Shoulder pain: Involvement of the acromioclavicular joint (analysis of 1,000 cases). AJR 12:493, 1971.

CRYSTAL-INDUCED AND RELATED ARTHROPATHIES

CHARLES S. RESNIK and DONALD L. RESNICK

Articular and periarticular abnormalities can result from the deposition of a variety of crystals and other related substances. The most commonly recognized disorder of this type is gouty arthritis secondary to deposition of monosodium urate crystals. Other frequently identified crystals are calcium pyrophosphate dihydrate (CPPD), which may cause "pseudogout," and calcium hydroxyapatite (HA), which is the cause of calcific tendinitis. Cartilage destruction may also be related to abnormal accumulation of iron in hemochromatosis, copper in Wilson's disease, or homogentisic acid in alkaptonuria. This chapter describes the clinical, pathologic, and radiologic manifestations of the arthropathies associated with deposition of these various substances.

GOUTY ARTHRITIS

Clinical Features

Gout is a disease that has been recognized for many centuries. The clinical features of gouty arthritis are related to the periarticular and intra-articular deposition of monosodium urate crystals. A convenient classification of gout divides idiopathic disease from that associated with any of a number of known disorders or enzymatic defects. Hereditary diseases that may lead to hyperuricemia include type I glycogen storage disease (glucose-6-phosphatase deficiency), Lesch-Nyhan syndrome (hypoxanthine-guanine phosphoribosyltransferase deficiency), and, occasionally, Down's syndrome. Gout may also be associated with a variety of other clinical disorders, including myeloproliferative diseases (polycythemia vera, leukemia, lymphoblastoma, myeloid metaplasia, hemolytic anemia, sickle cell anemia, pernicious anemia, thalassemia, multiple myeloma, Waldenström's macroglobulinemia), endocrine disorders (hyperparathyroidism, hypoparathyroidism, myxedema, hypoadrenal states), obesity, idiopathic hypercalciuria, cirrhosis, myocardial infarction, vascular disease, renal disease, starvation, lead poisoning, and drug therapy (diuretics, pyrazinamide, salicylates).

The vast majority of cases of gout are idiopathic. Men are affected approximately 20 times more frequently than women. The first attack of arthritis generally occurs between the ages of 40 and 50 years, although primary juvenile gout has been reported to occur as early as five weeks of age. Patients with gout, particularly premenopausal women and others with early onset of findings, often have a familial history of the disease. Certain racial groups, such as inhabitants of the Mariana Islands and the Maori of New Zealand, have a high incidence of gout; black patients are infrequently affected.

Hyperuricemia is often present for prolonged periods of time before the onset of symptoms or signs. Acute gouty arthritis may be quite severe. Pain, tenderness, and swelling may occur within several hours and persist for days to weeks. The disease usually begins as a monoarticular or oligoarticular process, with the lower extremities most commonly affected. The first metatarsophalangeal joint is the most frequent site of initial involvement and is eventually altered in up to 90 per cent of patients. Upper extremity involvement occurs in gouty arthritis of longer duration, whereas the axial skeleton is usually spared. An asymptomatic interval phase of gout may last from months to years. With recurring attacks, the arthritis commonly becomes longer in duration, more frequent in occurrence, and polyarticular in distribution. Asymmetry of articular involvement is common. Recovery between acute attacks may be incomplete.

Chronic gouty arthritis occurs in fewer than half of patients who experience recurrent acute attacks. Tophaceous deposits of monosodium urate generally do not become evident until many years after the initial attack. Tophi may be observed in subcutaneous and tendinous tissues about the foot, knee, hand, forearm, and elbow as well as in synovium and subchondral bone and on the helix of the ear. These deposits appear as irregular hard masses that produce ulceration of the overlying skin, which may lead to extrusion of chalky tophaceous material.

Pathologic Features

The diagnosis of gouty arthritis is based on the demonstration of monosodium urate crystals in synovial fluid. These crystals show strong negative birefringence when examined under polarized light. They can be identified in synovial lining cells as well as within leukocytes in the synovial fluid. These crystals invoke an acute inflammatory response in skin, subcutaneous tissues, and joints, with polymorphonuclear leukocytic infiltration as well as accumulation of chronic inflammatory cells. During the interval phase of gout, urate crystals may still be identified in synovial fluid although they are usually extracellular.

In chronic tophaceous gout, urate deposits may be identified in articular cartilage, subchondral bone, synovial membrane, and periarticular tissues. The initial deposits in cartilage are located in superficial layers. Nonspecific degenerative changes occur with cartilage fibrillation, fragmentation, and erosion. Adjacent areas of cartilage may be relatively spared. As urate deposits penetrate the entire thickness of cartilage, subchondral and deeper osseous collections may become evident. Direct deposition in the bone marrow may also occur. This produces cystic defects within the bone or erosions along the osseous contour.

Urate deposits within synovial villi cause thickening with infiltration of giant cells, macrophages, and other inflammatory cells. This inflammatory synovial tissue, or pannus, may grow across the entire cartilaginous surface. Sequestered fragments of cartilage and bone may become embedded within the synovium. Complete ankylosis of a joint is only rarely encountered.

Tophi may also be observed in periarticular tissues such as the joint capsule, tendons, ligaments, and bursae, particularly in the olecranon and prepatellar regions. Various other tissues may contain urate deposits including the skin, the aorta, and the heart. Tophaceous nodules are composed of urate crystals, intercrystalline matrix, and foreign body granulomatous reaction. Calcification or ossification of these nodules may occur.

Radiologic Features

General Findings

The radiologic features of gouty arthritis usually do not become evident until the disease has been present for many years. During an acute attack of arthritis, soft-tissue swelling about an involved joint may reflect synovial inflammation, capsular distention, and soft-tissue edema. These findings disappear as the attack subsides, and permanent abnormalities develop only during the stage of chronic tophaceous gout.

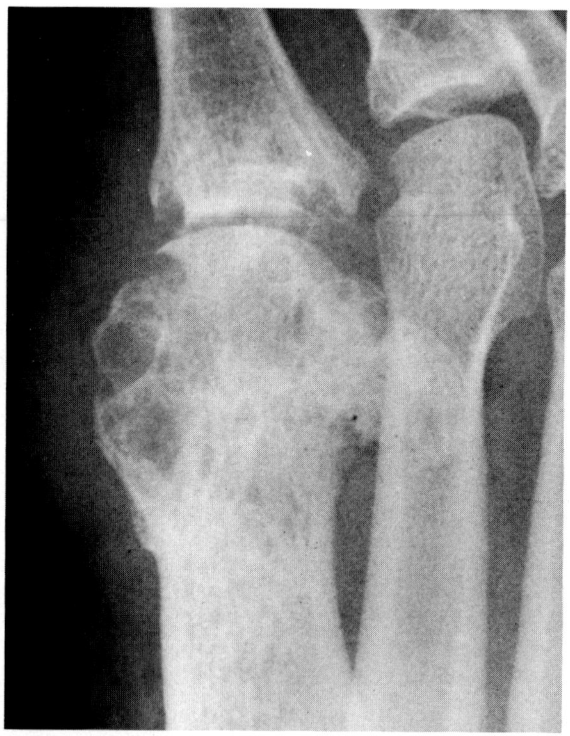

Figure 95–78. Gouty arthritis. There are several well-defined erosions of the metatarsal head and proximal phalanx with preservation of the intervening joint space.

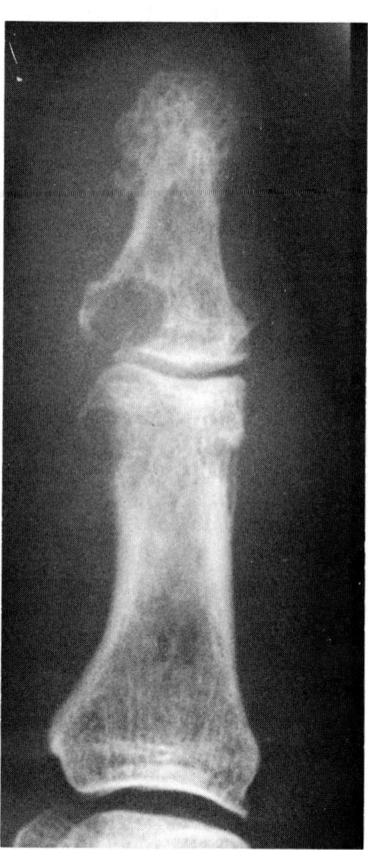

Figure 95–79. Gouty arthritis. The well-defined erosion in the distal phalanx has a characteristic "overhanging edge" of bone.

Radiologic soft-tissue abnormalities in gouty arthritis are characterized by eccentric or asymmetrical nodular prominences, particularly in the olecranon region and about the dorsum of the foot. Calcification of tophi is an unusual finding, often associated with an abnormality in calcium metabolism. Calcific deposits appear as irregular or cloud-like areas of radiodensity typically in the peripheral portion of the soft-tissue mass. Ossification of tophi may also rarely occur.

Preservation of joint space until late in the course of articular disease is one of the hallmarks of gouty arthritis. This relates to the sparing of some areas of cartilage adjacent to other areas of extensive destruction (Fig. 95–78). As the entire cartilaginous surface eventually becomes involved, uniform joint space narrowing may be observed. This is most frequently seen in the hands, wrists, feet, and knees.

The bony erosions seen in gout are produced by tophaceous deposits. These may be intra-articular, where they usually commence along the margins of the joint, periarticular, where they are usually eccentric in location, or at a considerable distance from the joint, usually beneath soft-tissue nodules. Gouty erosions are generally round or oval in shape and oriented in the long axis of the bone. They are variable in size and often have a "punched-out" appearance owing to a well-defined sclerotic margin. An elevated bony margin or lip characteristically extends outward in the soft tissues, creating an "overhanging edge" that covers a portion of the overlying tophaceous nodule (Fig. 95–79). This finding may relate to bone resorption beneath the gradually enlarging tophus with periosteal bony apposition at the outer aspect of the involved cortex. Subchondral lytic bone lesions may reveal communication with the joint cavity or may appear as discrete cystic radiolucent areas apparently unrelated to the joint. In advanced gout, extensive osseous destruction may be evident.

Osteoporosis is not a characteristic feature in gout. In long-stand-

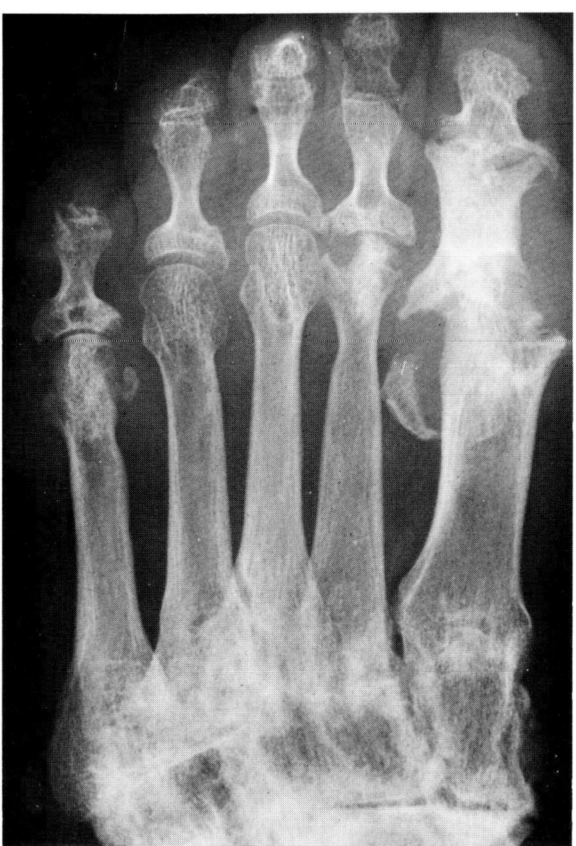

Figure 95–80. Gouty arthritis. There is extensive involvement of the metatarsophalangeal joints with multiple well-defined erosions. The tarsometatarsal and intertarsal joints are also affected.

ing disease, osteoporosis may occur secondary to disuse atrophy of bone. Secondary changes of osteoarthritis commonly develop in joints affected by gouty arthritis. Bony proliferation is occasionally observed with enlargement of the ends and shafts of involved bones. Malalignment and subluxation also occasionally occur.

Findings at Specific Sites

Gouty arthritis shows a predilection for the joints of the lower extremity, particularly those in the foot. The most characteristic site of abnormality is the first metatarsophalangeal joint. Erosions are frequently present on the medial and dorsal aspect of the first metatarsal head and, to a lesser extent, on the adjacent proximal phalanx. Enlargement of the metatarsal head may be identified, and soft-tissue swelling and hallux valgus deformity are common. Other metatarsophalangeal joints may be similarly affected, particularly the fifth, as well as any of the interphalangeal joints (Fig. 95–80). Swelling on the dorsum of the foot may be associated with extensive destruction of the tarsometatarsal joints. Other sites of abnormality include the intertarsal, talocalcaneal, and ankle joints.

Radiographs of the hand and wrist often reveal widespread asymmetrical abnormalities that may involve any of the articulations (Fig. 95–81). Large erosions of the carpometacarpal joints are a frequent finding. In the knee, marginal erosions occur on the medial or lateral aspect of the femur and the tibia. Articular space narrowing is usually absent. Prepatellar tophi produce soft-tissue masses with or without calcification. A popliteal cyst is rarely present. Articular changes in the elbow itself are not so common as inflammation of the olecranon bursa, leading to bilateral soft-tissue swelling over the extensor surface of the joint. Radiologic abnormalities in the glenohumeral articulation and hip are uncommon.

Gouty involvement in the axial skeleton is also uncommon. Erosion of vertebral end-plates with disc space narrowing has been reported, but reports of osteophytosis in patients with gout probably reflect the common occurrence of this radiologic finding in the general population. Similarly, sclerosis of the sacroiliac joints is most often due to coexistent degenerative disease. True gouty erosions in this location have an appearance similar to those elsewhere in the skeleton. Additional sites rarely involved with gout include the temporomandibular joints, the sternoclavicular joints, and the innominate bones.

Differential Diagnosis

The initial diagnosis of gout is rarely made by the radiologist; the clinical diagnosis is usually well established before radiologic abnormalities become evident. Although the roentgenographic features are often characteristic, diagnostic confusion may sometimes arise, particularly in the presence of coexisting disorders.

Calcium pyrophosphate dihydrate (CPPD) crystal deposition disease can produce the ''pseudogout syndrome,'' an acute arthritis clinically identical to that of gout. Radiologic abnormalities in this disorder consist of articular and periarticular calcification and pyrophosphate arthropathy, with findings similar to but distinct from degenerative arthritis. Chondrocalcinosis (cartilage calcification) in CPPD crystal deposition disease is often widespread, involving hyaline cartilage and fibrocartilage. Chondrocalcinosis can also be

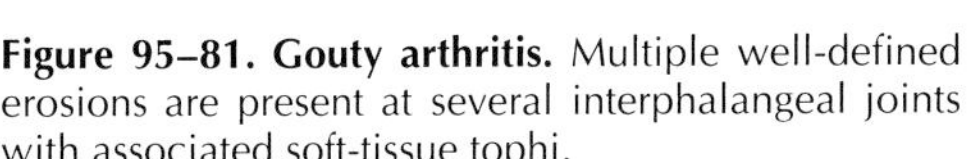

Figure 95–81. Gouty arthritis. Multiple well-defined erosions are present at several interphalangeal joints with associated soft-tissue tophi.

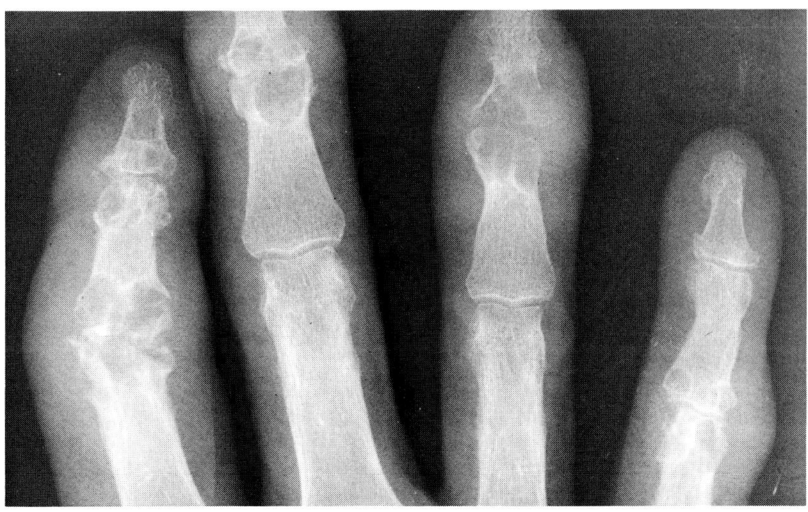

seen in gout, but this is generally localized to fibrocartilage in one or two joints. Both monosodium urate and CPPD crystals may occasionally be present within the same joint. The arthropathy of gout should easily be differentiated from that of CPPD crystal deposition disease by the presence of lobulated soft-tissue masses, intact joint spaces, and osseous erosions.

The radiologic manifestations of rheumatoid arthritis differ significantly from those of gout in most instances. Joint involvement is usually symmetrical, soft-tissue swelling is often fusiform, osteoporosis is prominent, and joint space loss occurs relatively early. Rheumatoid arthritis erosions occur at the margins of involved joints and may be poorly defined, whereas gouty erosions are often extra-articular and have well-defined sclerotic margins. Rheumatoid nodules may have an appearance similar to gouty tophi, but calcification is quite rare. Occasionally, particularly in men, the radiologic abnormalities of rheumatoid arthritis simulate those of gout with extensive erosions and a lack of osteoporosis and joint space loss. Also, the two diseases may rarely coexist.

The radiologic features of psoriatic arthritis include progressive articular destruction of the peripheral joints of the extremities with periosteal proliferation at the margins of the joints. Although the first metatarsophalangeal joint and the interphalangeal joint of the great toe are common sites of involvement, the pattern of destruction in psoriasis is usually easily differentiated from that in gout. Another disease that causes destructive changes of interphalangeal joints is multicentric reticulohistiocytosis, a rare systemic disorder primarily affecting skin and synovium. Radiologic features similar to those in gout include sharply marginated erosions and a lack of osteoporosis, but the distribution is usually symmetrical, and the articular spaces may be rapidly narrowed.

Many other disorders should be considered in the differential diagnosis of gout. Degenerative joint disease is often superimposed on gouty arthritis, and the resulting osteophytosis and sclerosis may obscure the destructive changes characteristic of gout. Inflammatory (erosive) osteoarthritis causes destruction of interphalangeal joints, but the erosions in this disorder usually begin in the central portion of the joint with subsequent involvement of marginal bone. Amyloid infiltration of articular structures may cause soft-tissue masses and cystic and erosive osseous lesions indistinguishable from those of gout. Finally, xanthomatosis secondary to disorders of lipid metabolism may produce masses about the extensor tendons in the hand and foot and the Achilles tendon. Xanthomas may also occur in the subcutaneous tissues of the elbows and knees, and the resultant eccentric nodular soft-tissue masses simulate gouty tophi.

CALCIUM PYROPHOSPHATE DIHYDRATE (CPPD) CRYSTAL DEPOSITION DISEASE

Terminology and Diagnostic Criteria

Many terms have been used to describe the entity originally reported as articular chondrocalcinosis. Perhaps the most familiar of these is the "pseudogout syndrome," but the most accurate term is *CPPD crystal deposition disease,* which describes the presence of CPPD crystals in or around joints. *Pseudogout* is only one of a variety of clinical patterns that may be associated with CPPD crystal deposition disease. *Chondrocalcinosis* is a term reserved for pathologically and radiologically evident cartilage calcification. Finally, *pyrophosphate arthropathy* is the term used to describe the pattern of structural joint damage occurring in CPPD crystal deposition disease.

A definite diagnosis of CPPD crystal deposition disease can be made by demonstration of CPPD crystals by x-ray diffraction or chemical analysis or if typical weakly positive birefringent crystals are identified by polarized light microscopy and characteristic calcifications are present radiologically. The diagnosis is suggested by acute or chronic arthritis occurring in common "target" areas which produces typical radiologic features including subchondral cyst formation, severe degeneration, variable osteophyte formation, or tendon calcification. These latter features may at times be so characteristic that a diagnosis of CPPD crystal deposition disease can be made confidently despite the absence of chondrocalcinosis or the inability to recover CPPD crystals on joint aspiration.

Clinical Features

CPPD crystal deposition disease can be classified into cases that are hereditary, those that are sporadic, and those associated with other diseases. Although patients with the hereditary form of the disease may have an earlier onset of clinical symptoms, the vast majority of cases are idiopathic, affecting middle-aged and elderly patients. The prevalence of chondrocalcinosis as a radiologic finding has been reported to be as high as 34 per cent, but a reasonable estimate of the incidence of CPPD crystal deposition disease is about 5 per cent.

A large number of diseases have been reported in association with CPPD crystal deposition disease. Many metabolic conditions, including hyperparathyroidism, hemochromatosis, hemosiderosis, gout and hyperuricemia, hypothyroidism, hypophosphatasia, hypomagnesemia, Wilson's disease, amyloidosis, alkaptonuria, and hemophilia, may directly or indirectly relate to the deposition of CPPD crystals. Other disorders, such as degenerative joint disease, diabetes mellitus, rheumatoid arthritis, and hypertension, probably coexist with CPPD crystal deposition disease on an incidental basis. As chondrocalcinosis is quite common in primary hyperparathyroidism and hemochromatosis, and many patients with these disorders also demonstrate evidence of CPPD crystal deposition disease, a significant association in these instances appears likely.

CPPD crystal deposition disease has been called a great mimic because of its clinical resemblance to many other arthritides. The various clinical presentations that may occur can be summarized as follows: Approximately 25 per cent of patients in large clinical series have acute or subacute attacks of arthritis separated by asymptomatic intervals. This pattern has been designated "pseudogout" (type A) because of its resemblance to attacks of gouty arthritis. Approximately 5 per cent of patients with CPPD crystal deposition disease have "pseudorheumatoid arthritis" (type B) with almost continuous acute or subacute attacks of arthritis in multiple joints. Approximately 50 per cent of symptomatic patients demonstrate progressive degeneration of multiple joints resembling osteoarthritis (pseudo-osteoarthritis), either with (type C) or without (type D) superimposed acute inflammatory episodes. Various additional clinical patterns include pseudoneuroarthropathy, monoarthropathy, and "traumatic" arthritis. It should be noted that clinical findings in an articulation do not correlate well with the presence or extent of pathologic and radiologic findings, and it is likely that most patients with CPPD crystal deposition disease remain relatively asymptomatic (type E).

Pathologic Features

CPPD crystal deposition is the basic microscopic process underlying the macroscopic features of articular and periarticular calcification and pyrophosphate arthropathy. There is no conclusive evidence that indicates whether crystal deposition is a primary or secondary phenomenon; in many patients calcification precedes arthropathy, but in some instances, arthropathy develops in patients without evidence of local or distant calcification. It has been well established that CPPD crystals can cause an acute inflammatory response. Their presence in synovial fluid may occur by a process (crystal "shedding") in which crystalline deposits are sloughed into the joint cavity secondary to either cartilage destruction or an alteration in the characteristics of surface crystals. This latter mechanism might explain the increased incidence of acute attacks of "pseudogout" following medical illnesses or surgical procedures.

CPPD crystal deposits may be identified in articular cartilage around chondrocyte lacunae in the midzonal area. As accumulation of crystals progresses, they are evident also at the cartilaginous surface. Focal hyaline and myxoid degeneration is accompanied by cartilage fibrillation, erosion, and denudation. The subchondral bone displays sclerosis and thickened trabeculae. Multiple subchondral cysts contain fibrous tissue or proteinaceous material and may or may not communicate with the adjacent joint cavity. Fracture of these cysts may lead to bony fragmentation, collapse, and intra-articular osteocartilaginous bodies. Marginal osteophytosis is usually evident. All of these structural joint changes closely resemble those of degenerative joint disease.

Deposits of CPPD crystals may also be present in other articular and periarticular locations, particularly the synovial membrane. It is unclear if crystals are deposited directly in these tissues or if they migrate from adjacent cartilage. Synovial membrane crystals are located primarily near the surface and are concentrated in poorly vascularized areas with little or no associated synovial hyperplasia. Acute and chronic inflammatory reaction is variable; infiltration of lymphocytes, plasma cells, and histiocytes may be evident. Small pieces of bone or cartilage may become embedded in synovium with associated villous or nodular synovial proliferation and cellular infiltration. During acute attacks of inflammation, crystals may be present within neutrophils and mononuclear cells in the synovial fluid and in surface exudate.

Radiologic Features

General Findings

Many of the radiologic features of CPPD crystal deposition disease are common to all articulations in the body. The general findings in this disorder consist of calcification of articular and periarticular structures (including cartilage, synovium, capsule, tendons, bursae, ligaments, and soft tissues) and pyrophosphate arthropathy, which describes the characteristic pattern of structural joint changes. These abnormalities are usually bilateral and symmetrical in distribution. It is important to note that any individual articulation may be the site of both calcification and arthropathy or of either feature alone (i.e., calcification without arthropathy or arthropathy without calcification). Similarly, characteristic radiologic features of pyrophosphate arthropathy may sometimes occur in the absence of calcification anywhere in the body.

Fibrocartilage calcification is most common in the menisci of the knee, the triangular cartilage of the wrist, and the symphysis pubis. It may also be observed in the acetabular and glenoid labra, the annulus fibrosus of the intervertebral disc, and the discs of the acromioclavicular and sternoclavicular articulations. This calcification appears as thick, shaggy, irregular radiodense collections (Figs. 95–82 to 95–84). Hyaline cartilage calcification is most common in the wrist and knee, although it may be seen in the glenohumeral joint and other articulations. This type of calcification appears thin and linear and parallels the subjacent subchondral bone (see Figs. 95–82 and 95–83). Either hyaline or fibrocartilage calcification may be designated as chondrocalcinosis.

Synovial calcification is usually associated with chondrocalcinosis but may be seen in the absence of cartilage involvement. Synovial deposits are most commonly demonstrated in the knee and in the metacarpophalangeal and metatarsophalangeal joints. They may also be recognized in the wrist, shoulder, elbow, and hip. Their appearance is cloud-like, especially at the margins of the joint (Figs. 95–85 and 95–86). Capsular calcification is most commonly observed in the elbow and metatarsophalangeal articulations; other sites of involvement are the metacarpophalangeal and glenohumeral joints. This appears as fine or irregular linear calcification that spans the articulation.

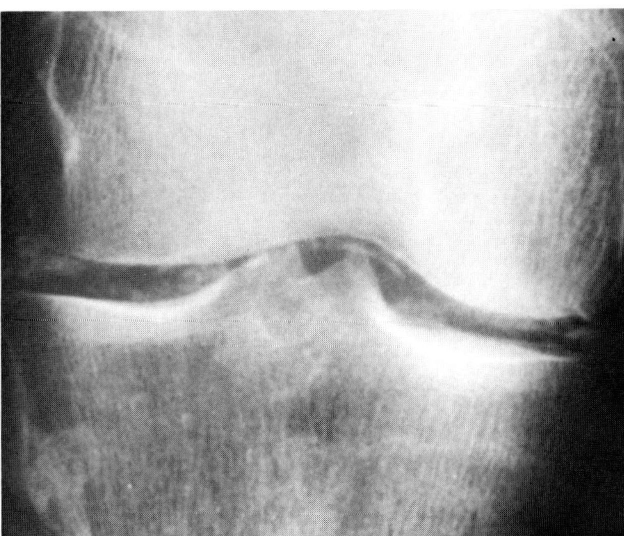

Figure 95–82. Calcium pyrophosphate dihydrate (CPPD) crystal deposition disease. There is fibrocartilage calcification in the medial and lateral menisci as well as calcification in hyaline articular cartilage along the midportion of the distal femur.

Calcification is commonly seen in the quadriceps, triceps, Achilles, and supraspinatus tendons. Such calcification is thin and linear in appearance and may extend for considerable distances from the osseous margins. Cloud-like bursal calcification and linear ligamentous calcification are additional patterns that are observed in various locations. Ill-defined calcification may occasionally occur within the soft tissues, and amorphous calcified masses, known as "tophaceous pseudogout," are rarely identified.

The structural joint changes of pyrophosphate arthropathy are most common in the knee, wrist, and metacarpophalangeal joints, but any articulation may be involved. The general radiologic fea-

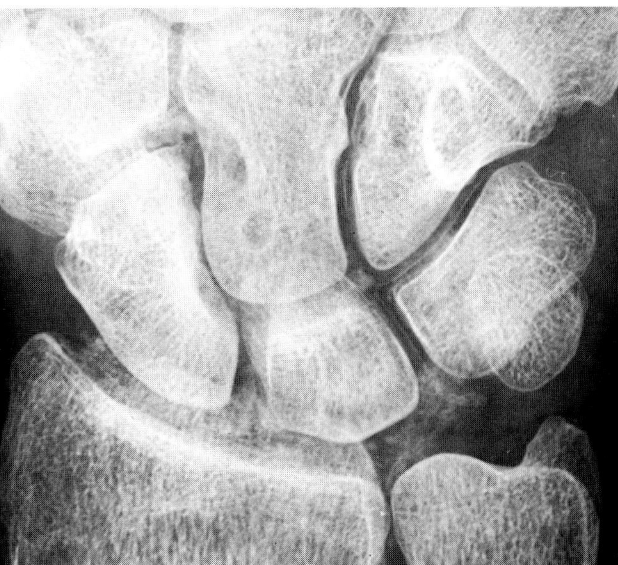

Figure 95–83. CPPD crystal deposition disease. Note calcification in the triangular fibrocartilage and extensive hyaline cartilage calcification involving multiple carpal bones.

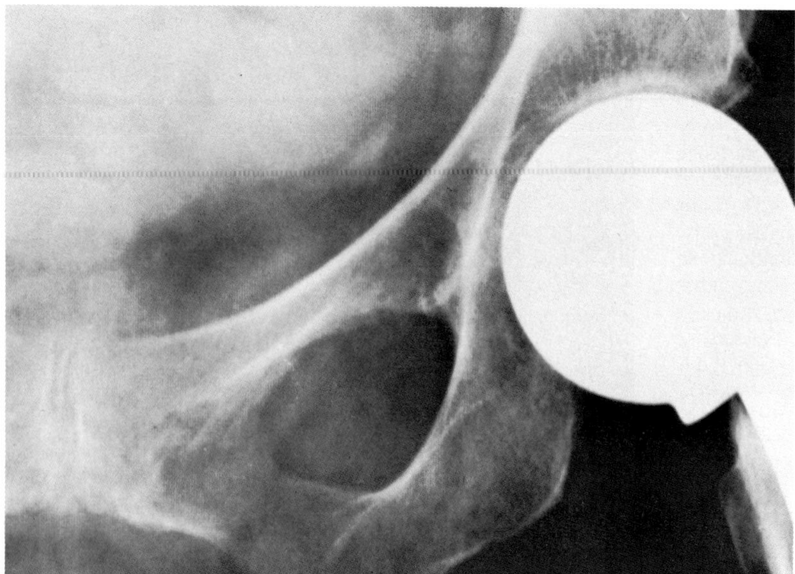

Figure 95–84. CPPD crystal deposition disease. Fibrocartilage calcification in the symphysis pubis.

tures of this arthropathy include joint space narrowing, bone sclerosis, and subchondral cyst formation. These findings are similar to those seen in degenerative joint disease, but there are five distinctive features of pyrophosphate arthropathy that differentiate it from osteoarthritis:

1. Unusual articular distribution: In addition to the large weight-bearing joints of the knees and hips that are commonly involved in degenerative joint disease, non–weight-bearing joints, such as the wrist, elbow, and shoulder, are often affected in pyrophosphate arthropathy.
2. Unusual intra-articular distribution: Involvement of characteristic compartments in certain articulations, such as the patellofemoral compartment of the knee and the radiocarpal compartment of the wrist, distinguish pyrophosphate arthropathy from degenerative joint disease.
3. Prominent subchondral cyst formation: Although subchondral cysts are often present in degenerative joint disease and other articular disorders, the cysts associated with pyrophosphate arthropathy tend to be more numerous and may reach considerable size. These cysts may be round, oval, bilobed, aligned like a ''string of beads,'' or clustered and coalescent. Well-defined sclerotic margins are often evident.
4. Severe and progressive destructive bone changes: Rapid, extensive subchondral bone collapse and fragmentation with joint disorganization may sometimes occur in pyrophosphate arthropathy. These features resemble those of neuroarthropathy but are not typically seen in degenerative joint disease.
5. Variable osteophyte formation: Large, irregular bony excrescences that are characteristic of degenerative joint disease may be seen in pyrophosphate arthropathy, but many joints involved in CPPD crystal deposition disease show only narrowing and sclerosis unaccompanied by osteophyte formation.

If findings suggestive of CPPD crystal deposition disease are discovered in one location, a search should be made to discover the presence of more widespread involvement in order to establish a firm radiologic diagnosis. This can easily be accomplished by obtaining radiographs of the knees, the pelvis, and the hands and wrists. This combination should identify essentially all patients with

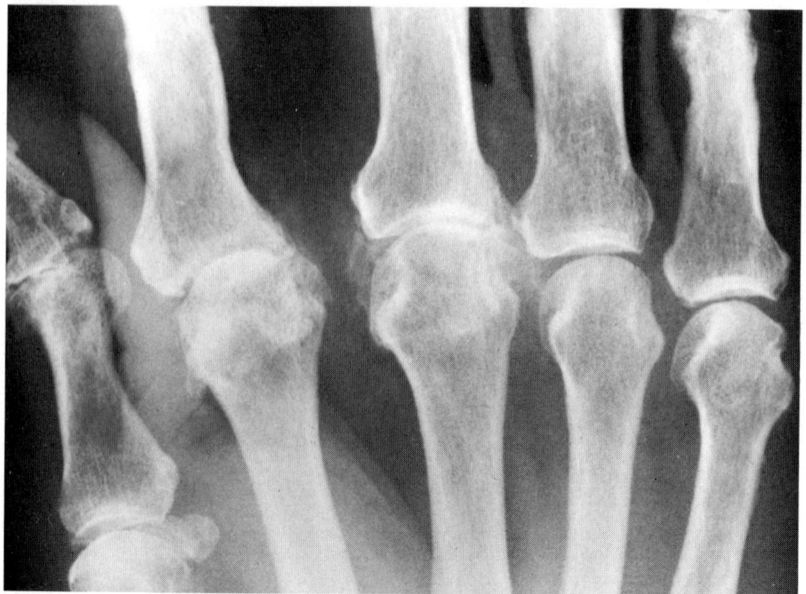

Figure 95–85. CPPD crystal deposition disease. There is sclerosis, narrowing, and osteophyte formation at the second and third metacarpophalangeal joints along with synovial calcification involving the radial aspect of the third metacarpophalangeal joint.

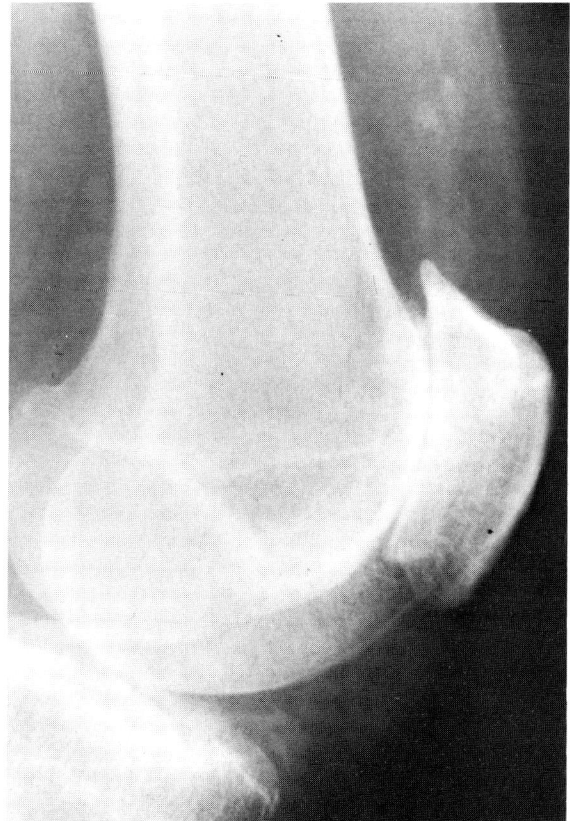

Figure 95–86. CPPD crystal deposition disease. There is complete loss of the patellofemoral joint space with preservation of the femorotibial space. Note also synovial calcification in the suprapatellar region.

radiologically evident calcification, and this also evaluates the areas most commonly involved with pyrophosphate arthropathy.

Findings at Specific Sites

The knee is the most commonly involved joint in CPPD crystal deposition disease. Fibrocartilage calcification in the medial and lateral menisci appears as wedge-shaped radiodensities (see Fig. 95–82). Hyaline cartilage calcification is less frequently observed, paralleling the femoral condyles or tibial plateau (see Fig. 95–82). Synovial and quadriceps tendon calcification may also be seen, and a joint effusion is often present.

Pyrophosphate arthropathy in the knee consists of joint space narrowing, sclerosis, and osteophyte formation. Severe and rapid destruction with fragmentation of bone and intra-articular osseous bodies simulating neuroarthropathy may occasionally occur. In this location, the compartmental distribution of arthropathy may strongly suggest the diagnosis of CPPD crystal deposition disease. Although the medial femorotibial compartment is most commonly affected, as in degenerative joint disease, isolated or severe patellofemoral compartment involvement is characteristic of pyrophosphate arthropathy (see Fig. 95–86). At times, erosion of the anterior cortex of the distal femur may occur secondary to mechanical pressure and remodeling.

Involvement of the hand and wrist is common in CPPD crystal deposition disease. Chondrocalcinosis of the triangular fibrocartilage appears as punctate or amorphous radiodensities extending in a horizontal fan-like fashion from the medial aspect of the distal radius to the ulnar styloid (see Fig. 95–83). Hyaline cartilage calcification in the carpus, synovial or capsular calcification in the metacarpophalangeal joints, and intercarpal ligament calcification are additional manifestations (see Figs. 95–83 and 95–85). Disruption of the scapholunate ligament leads to separation of these bones, known as scapholunate dissociation (Fig. 95–87).

Pyrophosphate arthropathy in the wrist characteristically involves the radiocarpal compartment with joint space narrowing, sclerosis, and subchondral cyst formation. There may be proximal migration of the scaphoid with compression of this bone and corresponding deformity of the distal radius. This, combined with narrowing of the lunate-capitate portion of the midcarpal compartment, creates a "step-ladder" configuration that is characteristic of CPPD crystal deposition disease (Fig. 95–87). Joint space narrowing may also be identified in the trapezioscaphoid articulation. In the hand, pyrophosphate arthropathy predominantly affects the metacarpophalangeal joints, particularly the second and third, with less prominent changes in the interphalangeal joints (see Fig. 95–85). Joint space loss may be complete, but osseous erosions do not occur.

Radiologic features of CPPD crystal deposition disease in the ankle and foot include capsular calcification in the metatarsophalangeal joints, Achilles tendon calcification, and pyrophosphate arthropathy, particularly in the talonavicular articulation. In the elbow, hyaline cartilage, capsule, synovium, and triceps tendon calcification may be accompanied by joint space narrowing, sclerosis, and cyst formation. In the shoulder, sites of calcification include the hyaline cartilage of the humeral head, the fibrocartilage of the glenoid labrum, the disc of the acromioclavicular joint, the supraspinatus tendon, and the subacromial bursa. A rotator cuff tear may be identified by an unusually high position of the humeral head.

In the pelvis, calcification of the fibrocartilage of the symphysis pubis is common (see Fig. 95–84). Joint space narrowing, sclerosis, cyst formation, osteophytosis, and subchondral erosions may be identified in the sacroiliac joints. Hyaline cartilage calcification about the femoral head and fibrocartilage calcification of the acetabular labrum are additional abnormalities. Joint space narrowing may produce either superolateral or axial migration of the femoral head with respect to the acetabulum. Subchondral cyst formation may be extensive, rapid destruction of bone may occur, and protrusio acetabuli may develop.

Spinal involvement in CPPD crystal deposition disease consists of intervertebral disc calcification, most prominently in the annulus fibrosus, disc space narrowing at multiple levels with associated sclerosis, osteophytosis, and "vacuum" phenomena, and narrowing

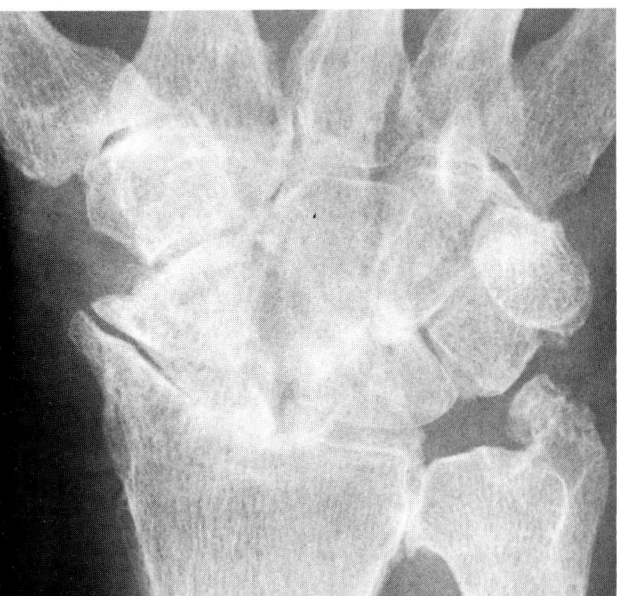

Figure 95–87. CPPD crystal deposition disease. There is narrowing and sclerosis between the radius and scaphoid and between the lunate and capitate, creating a "step-ladder" configuration. Scapholunate dissociation is also evident.

and sclerosis of apophyseal joints. In the cervical spine, atlantoaxial subluxation, with an increased distance between the anterior arch of the atlas and the odontoid process, is rarely encountered and is probably related to calcific deposits within the transverse ligament of the atlas.

Differential Diagnosis

CPPD crystal deposition disease is usually easily differentiated from all other arthritides by radiologic evaluation. Although chondrocalcinosis can be related to deposition of other types of crystals, widespread cartilage calcification is caused exclusively by deposition of CPPD crystals. Chondrocalcinosis secondary to calcium hydroxyapatite or dicalcium phosphate dihydrate deposition is usually limited to a single articulation and commonly a single meniscus. Other causes of intra-articular radiodense shadows, such as primary or secondary synovial osteochondromatosis, do not have the same appearance as the calcifications of CPPD crystal deposition disease. Only rarely will an intra-articular neoplasm display calcification. Periarticular calcification, which is usually related to hydroxyapatite crystal deposition, is seen in a variety of disorders, including renal osteodystrophy, collagen vascular diseases, idiopathic tumoral calcinosis, the milk-alkali syndrome, and hypervitaminosis D, but these diseases all lack the other associated findings that are present in CPPD crystal deposition disease. Finally, tendon calcification is most commonly caused by the deposition of calcium hydroxyapatite crystals, but such calcification is usually focal and round or oval rather than extensive and linear as seen in CPPD crystal deposition disease.

Degenerative joint disease simulates pyrophosphate arthropathy, although distinguishing characteristics of the latter condition include an unusual articular distribution, an unusual intra-articular distribution, prominent subchondral cyst formation, severe and progressive destructive bone changes, and variable osteophyte formation. Prominent involvement of the wrist, elbow, and shoulder and isolated involvement of the patellofemoral compartment of the knee or the radiocarpal compartment of the wrist are characteristic of pyrophosphate arthropathy. So, too, is the ''step-ladder'' appearance in the wrist, although the same combination of narrowing of the radioscaphoid and lunocapitate articulations can be seen in the scapholunate advanced collapse (SLAC) wrist, a post-traumatic degenerative condition. Articular and periarticular calcification would not be expected in degenerative joint disease. Differentiation of these two disorders may be more difficult in the spine, but the degree of destruction is usually less in degenerative joint disease, and widespread involvement with multiple intradiscal ''vacuum'' phenomena is more typical of pyrophosphate arthropathy.

CPPD crystal deposition disease can be differentiated from rheumatoid arthritis and the seronegative spondyloarthropathies (psoriatic arthritis, Reiter's syndrome, and ankylosing spondylitis) by the lack of bone erosions. Uniform joint space loss, which is seen in the knee and wrist in rheumatoid arthritis, is not evident in CPPD crystal deposition disease. The degree of bone sclerosis and osteophytosis that is present in CPPD crystal deposition disease does not generally occur in rheumatoid arthritis. Pyrophosphate arthropathy can sometimes be difficult to differentiate from neuroarthropathy. When a severe destructive arthropathy manifest as extensive bone collapse, fragmentation, and joint disorganization is present, it may be necessary to obtain radiographs of other articulations to identify calcification or characteristic features of pyrophosphate arthropathy. Gouty arthritis can be differentiated from CPPD crystal deposition disease by the presence of lobulated soft-tissue masses, intact joint spaces, and osseous erosions. Finally, the arthropathy of hemochromatosis is almost identical to that of CPPD crystal deposition disease. Subtle differences between these two disorders include more prominent osteoporosis, more prevalent hyaline cartilage calcification, more significant metacarpophalangeal joint involvement (particularly the fourth and fifth), and peculiar hook-like osteophytes of the metacarpal heads in hemochromatosis.

CALCIUM HYDROXYAPATITE (HA) CRYSTAL DEPOSITION DISEASE

Classification

HA crystal deposition may be a primary or secondary phenomenon. Periarticular calcification may occur in many disorders, including collagen vascular diseases, renal osteodystrophy, hyperparathyroidism, hypoparathyroidism, hypervitaminosis D, the milk-alkali syndrome, idiopathic tumoral calcinosis, idiopathic calcinosis universalis, and sarcoidosis. In many of these disorders, the calcified masses contain calcium phosphate and calcium carbonate; HA crystals are identified in the calcific deposits that are evident in scleroderma and renal osteodystrophy. Also, secondary deposition of HA within the intervertebral disc is seen in alkaptonuria. Primary deposition of HA crystals occurs commonly in various periarticular locations as calcific tendinitis and, less commonly, in an intra-articular location as a cause of inflammatory arthritis.

Clinical Features

Periarticular deposition of HA crystals, which has been called a variety of names including peritendinitis calcarea and calcific tendinitis, is a disorder that affects men and women most commonly between the ages of 40 and 70 years. Involvement is usually monoarticular, although multiple joints may be involved simultaneously or successively. A history of trauma is often but not invariably present. Acute symptoms include pain, tenderness to palpation, local swelling, and restriction of motion. Fever and malaise may sometimes be present, and the erythrocyte sedimentation rate may be elevated. Recurrence of symptoms is common, and mild pain and tenderness may be chronically present. However, most patients with radiologically evident calcific deposits remain entirely asymptomatic.

Intra-articular HA crystal deposition disease is a rarely encountered arthropathy that may produce symptoms of acute inflammation. Chronic abnormalities such as disruption of the rotator cuff associated with the demonstration of intra-articular HA crystals and various enzymes have also been described.

Pathologic Features

The pathogenesis of HA crystal deposition in periarticular tissues is unknown. A commonly suggested etiology is a primary degenerative process of tendon fibers leading to secondary dystrophic calcification. On gross examination, the calcific deposits have a milky or cheesy appearance and may be inspissated or chalk-like in quality. Microscopically, a combination of findings may be present, including focal fibrocartilaginous transformation of tendinous tissue, deposition of nonbirefringent crystals, phagocytic resorption of some calcific deposits, and reconstitution of tendinous tissue following this resorption. Other histologic features include inflammation, necrosis, cellular proliferation, giant cell reaction, neovascularity, and small vessel occlusion.

Radiologic Features

The initial radiologic appearance in periarticular HA crystal deposition disease is a thin, cloud-like, poorly defined area of increased

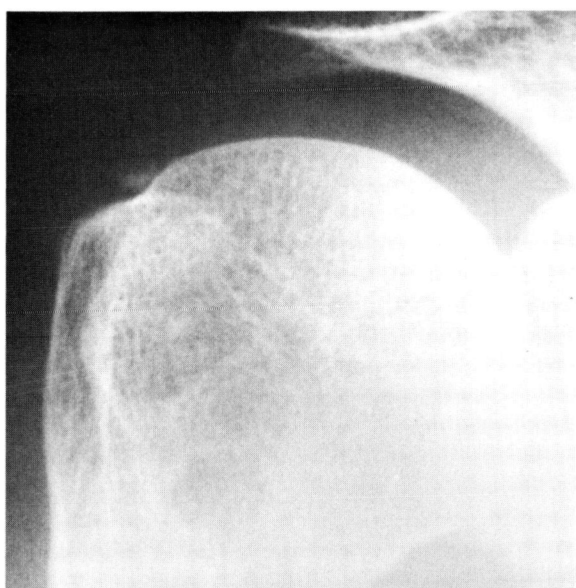

Figure 95–88. Hydroxyapatite (HA) crystal deposition disease. Faint calcification is present in the position of the supraspinatus tendon adjacent to the greater tuberosity.

radiodensity (Fig. 95–88). This eventually becomes denser, homogeneous, and more sharply defined, often with a circular or oval configuration (Fig. 95–89). A fluffy appearance may be related to pathologically evident resorption; this is often associated with acute pain (Fig. 95–90). Over a period of time, the crystal deposit may disappear completely.

The periarticular tissues about the shoulder are the most common sites of HA crystal deposition. The supraspinatus tendon is the single structure most frequently affected, with calcific deposits located at the tendinous insertion on the greater tuberosity. Other sites of involvement are the tendons of the infraspinatus, teres minor, subscapularis, biceps, triceps, and deltoid muscles and the subacromial bursa.

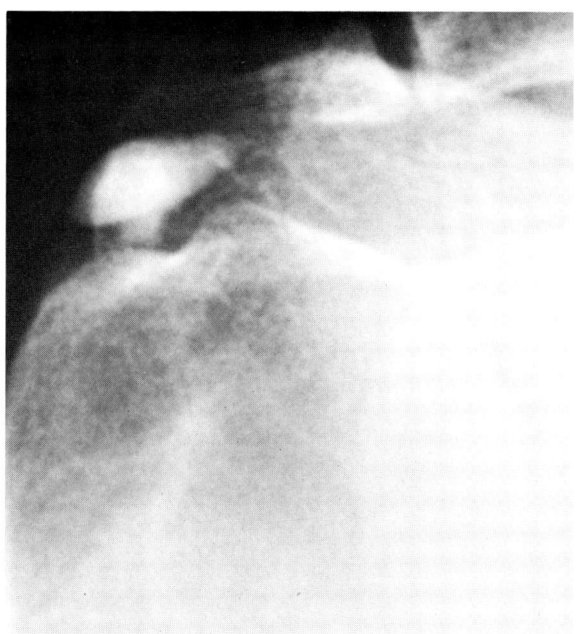

Figure 95–89. HA crystal deposition disease. There is dense, homogeneous, well-defined calcification in the position of the supraspinatus tendon.

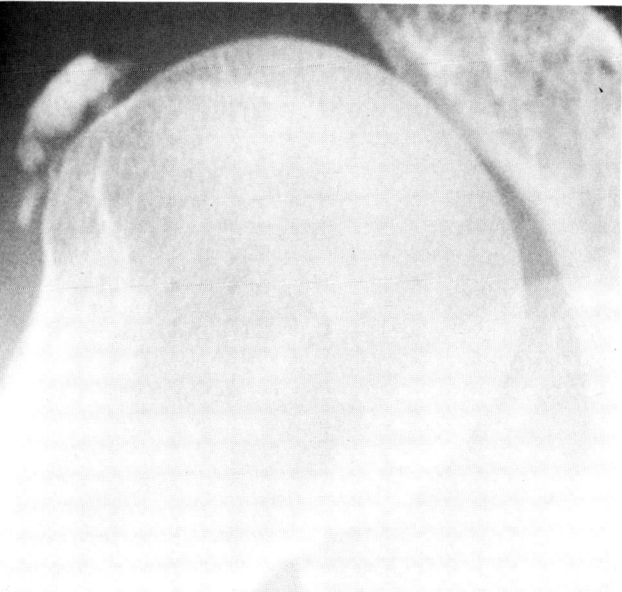

Figure 95–90. HA crystal deposition disease. There are several loculations of calcification with somewhat fluffy margins in the position of the infraspinatus or teres minor tendon.

Less commonly affected locations include the elbow, wrist, hand, knee, ankle, and foot. In the hip, the gluteal insertions at the greater trochanter and the surrounding bursae often contain calcific deposits. Calcification within the longus colli muscle in the neck, known as retropharyngeal tendinitis, may cause acute neck pain, rigidity, and dysphagia. Prevertebral soft-tissue swelling may be evident radiologically as well as calcification, usually seen anterior to the second cervical vertebra just inferior to the body of the atlas.

The radiologic features of HA crystal deposition within a joint include an amorphous pattern of intra-articular calcification in addition to occasional meniscal, synovial, or capsular calcification. A destructive arthropathy characterized by irregularity of bone contours, sclerosis, and multiple osteocartilaginous bodies may be observed.

HEMOCHROMATOSIS

Clinical Findings

Hemochromatosis is a rare disorder in which tissue damage is produced by iron deposition. A classic triad of clinical features consists of bronze pigmentation, cirrhosis, and diabetes mellitus that is related to the abnormal accumulation of iron in the skin, liver, and pancreas. Cardiac failure secondary to deposition of iron in the heart is also common, and a specific arthropathy often occurs. The disease is diagnosed by detection of elevated serum iron concentration, increased transferrin saturation, and a typical histologic appearance on liver biopsy.

Hemochromatosis can be classified into a primary form, probably the consequence of a genetically determined error of metabolism allowing increased absorption of iron from the gastrointestinal tract, and a secondary form, associated with an increased intake and accumulation of iron due to multiple blood transfusions, chronic excess oral iron ingestion, alcoholic cirrhosis, or refractory anemia. The onset of disease is generally recognized between the ages of 40 and 60 years because significant iron overload occurs only after an extended period of time. Men are much more frequently affected, perhaps because iron levels in women are influenced by menstrual blood loss.

The arthropathy associated with hemochromatosis generally occurs late in the disease. The hands are most commonly involved, particularly the second and third metacarpophalangeal joints, with the knees, hips, and shoulders being affected less frequently. Symmetrical distribution is usually present. Symptoms and signs reflecting a noninflammatory arthritis include mild joint pain, swelling, and stiffness without warmth, erythema, or significant deformity. The arthropathy is often chronic and progressive in nature, although attacks of acute arthritis, probably related to the presence of CPPD crystals, may be superimposed. Joint aspiration demonstrates noninflammatory synovial fluid and, occasionally, iron present within mononuclear cells.

Pathologic Features

Synovial membrane abnormalities in hemochromatosis are characterized by hemosiderin granules in synovioblasts or perivascular histiocytes. This is most likely due to deposition from circulating iron-containing macrophages and is related to the degree of total body iron overload. Increased synovial tissue iron deposition may be seen in other disorders that produce chronic hemarthrosis, such as hemophilia or pigmented villonodular synovitis, but the location of iron in these instances is generally within deep macrophages as opposed to the localization in synovial lining cells in hemochromatosis. Mild villous synovial hyperplasia may be seen in hemochromatosis, but significant synovial inflammation is generally absent. CPPD crystal deposition may also be noted in the synovium as well as in fibrocartilage and hyaline cartilage, and the pathologic features of the arthropathy in hemochromatosis are identical to those of CPPD crystal deposition disease described earlier in this chapter. The exact relationship between CPPD deposition and iron deposition in cartilage remains unknown.

Radiologic Features

The radiologic articular abnormalities in hemochromatosis are almost indistinguishable from those of idiopathic CPPD crystal deposition disease. Only minor differences exist that allow differentiation of the two arthropathies. The most commonly reported of these is osteoporosis, which may occur in half of patients with primary hemochromatosis as well as some with the secondary form of the disease. This may be diffuse with involvement of both the axial and the appendicular skeleton. The exact etiology of osteoporosis in hemochromatosis is unknown.

As in CPPD crystal deposition disease, articular calcification is commonly observed in hemochromatosis. In the latter disorder, there may be more prominent involvement of the fibrocartilage of the symphysis pubis and of hyaline cartilage in various locations; periarticular structures may be less commonly affected. Subtle differences between the arthropathy of hemochromatosis and pyrophosphate arthropathy may be detected in the hand and wrist. Metacarpophalangeal joint involvement, particularly the fourth and fifth, is more significant in the former disease, whereas scapholunate dissociation is more common in the latter. A characteristic feature of hemochromatosis is the development of peculiar hook-like osteophytes that occur along the radial aspect of the metacarpal heads (Fig. 95–91). Although these may occur in other disorders, their presence with or without associated calcification should suggest a diagnosis of hemochromatosis.

WILSON'S DISEASE

Clinical Features

Wilson's disease, or hepatolenticular degeneration, is a rare disorder with autosomal recessive inheritance characterized by degenerative changes in the brain, particularly the basal ganglia, and cirrhosis of the liver. A diagnostic feature is the presence of a greenish-brown Kayser-Fleischer ring at the limbus of the cornea. The clinical manifestations of this disease relate to progressive accumulation of copper in tissues throughout the body. Men are slightly more commonly affected than women, with the age of onset varying from 5 to 40 years. Neurologic symptoms in Wilson's disease include tremor, rigidity, dysarthria, incoordination, and personality change. Clinical evidence of hepatic disease is usually minimal. Renal tubular abnormalities may lead to aminoaciduria, proteinuria, phosphaturia, glucosuria, and uricosuria. Joint abnormalities, which occur in up to 50 per cent of adults, are often asymptomatic, with occasional episodes of pain and swelling. Fractures leading to pain and deformity may occur.

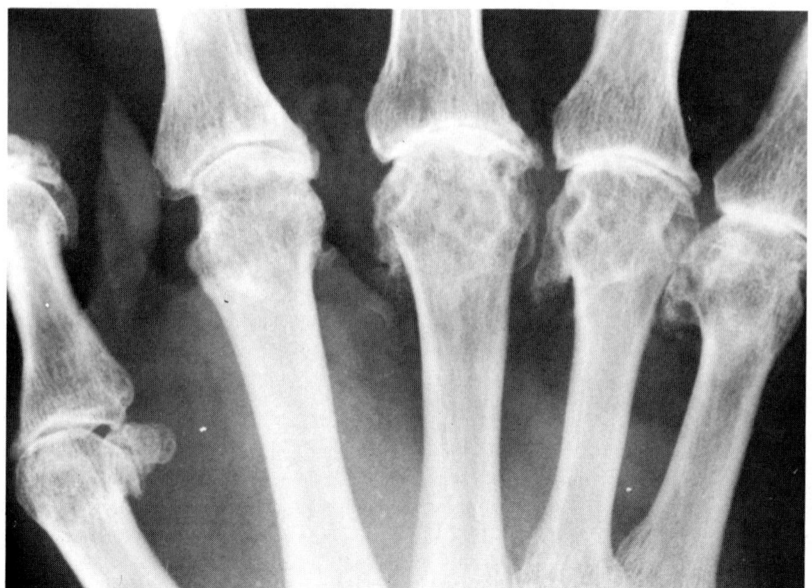

Figure 95–91. Hemochromatosis. There is extensive joint space loss and sclerosis of the metacarpophalangeal joints with associated hook-like osteophytes along the radial aspect of the metacarpal heads.

Pathologic Features

The pathologic features of articular involvement in Wilson's disease have not been thoroughly described. Changes in the synovium include microvillus formation, hyperplasia of the lining cells, inflammation, and vasculitis. Copper accumulation is not necessarily demonstrated by synovial biopsy. Fragmentation of bone is commonly present, but this feature has been better delineated by radiologic studies.

Radiologic Features

The two major radiologic manifestations of Wilson's disease in the skeleton are osteopenia and arthropathy. Loss of bone density, which may occur in as many as 50 per cent of patients, is most apparent in the hands, feet, and spine. The most likely cause of this decreased bone density is rickets or osteomalacia due to loss of calcium and phosphorus in the urine. In addition to osteopenia, radiologic features include widening and irregularity of growth plates, retarded skeletal maturation, "pseudofractures," and true pathologic fractures.

The arthropathy associated with Wilson's disease is characterized by subchondral bone fragmentation, cyst formation, cortical irregularities, and sclerosis. These changes may occur in any of the joints of the extremities as well as in the spine. Fragmentation of subchondral bone involving large areas of the osseous surface may resemble osteochondritis dissecans. Distinct ossicles with complete cortices may be present. There may also be a "paint brush" appearance to the articular bony surface with fine irregularity and indistinctness. Joint space narrowing is sometimes present, and tongue-like osteophytes and fluffy periostitis may be seen at bony prominences and sites of tendon and ligament attachment to bone. Finally, chondrocalcinosis has been noted in some patients with Wilson's disease, but a significant association with CPPD crystal deposition disease has not been established.

ALKAPTONURIA

Clinical Features

Alkaptonuria is a rare metabolic disorder that may demonstrate autosomal dominant or recessive inheritance. An absence of the enzyme homogentisic acid oxidase leads to accumulation of homogentisic acid in various tissues with eventual bluish-black pigmentation, termed *ochronosis,* of the skin, sclerae, and ears. This pigmentation generally does not become evident until 20 to 30 years of age, and men and women are affected about equally. When the urine of patients with alkaptonuria is allowed to stand, the homogentisic acid is oxidized to a melanin-like product, and the urine gradually turns dark. Symptoms and signs of alkaptonuria relate to ochronotic deposition in a variety of organs, including the cardiovascular, genitourinary, and upper respiratory systems as well as articular structures.

Ochronotic arthropathy generally becomes evident by the age of 40 years. Pain and limitation of motion in the hips, knees, and shoulders may be present, as well as low back pain and stiffness. Acute exacerbations of arthritis may occur, and joint effusions may be evident. Progressive deformity of the spine may develop with obliteration of the normal lumbar curve, thoracic kyphosis, restriction of spine motion and chest expansion, and loss of height. Intervertebral disc herniation may cause acute symptoms, particularly in men.

Pathologic Features

The pathologic features of alkaptonuria relate to abnormal pigmentation of connective tissue in organs throughout the body. Intercellular and intracellular deposition is seen in a granular or homogeneous distribution. Within joints, fibrocartilage and hyaline cartilage may be affected, with pigment first occurring in deeper layers between chondrocytes and later appearing at cartilaginous surfaces. The cartilage then becomes brittle, with fibrillation, fissuring, and fragmentation leading to a shaggy, irregular surface and exposure of severely pigmented deeper layers and sclerotic subchondral bone. Necrotic cartilage may become embedded within the marrow and surrounded by granulation tissue, resulting in cystic collections. Cartilage and bone may also become embedded in the synovial membrane and stimulate synovial metaplasia and foreign body reaction.

In the spine, pigmentation may be evident in the hyaline cartilage between the intervertebral disc and the vertebral body as well as in the annulus fibrosus. The discs become hard and brittle, and fragments may become separated and surrounded by histiocytes. Bony proliferation of the vertebral bodies may lead to ankylosis. Disc calcification secondary to hydroxyapatite deposition may be extreme, and pigment may be identified in various vertebral ligaments.

Radiologic Features

The most characteristic radiologic abnormality in alkaptonuria is intervertebral disc calcification. This may be distributed solely within the fibers of the annulus fibrosus, giving an appearance similar to the syndesmophytes of ankylosing spondylitis, or may

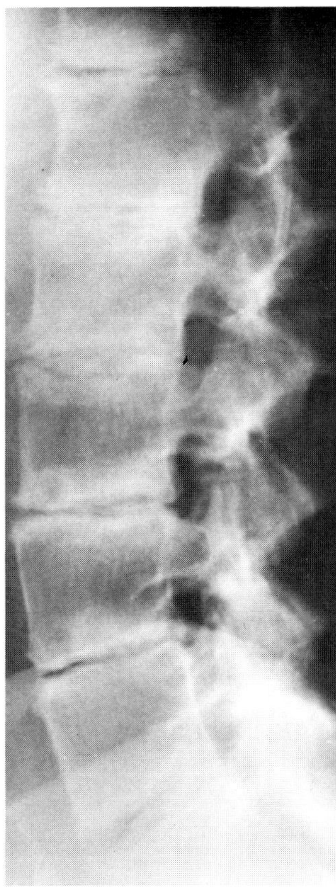

Figure 95–92. Alkaptonuria. There is extensive narrowing of disc spaces with associated sclerosis, "vacuum" phenomena, and faint calcification.

involve the entire disc diffusely. The lumbar spine is most frequently affected. Narrowing of the disc spaces and "vacuum" phenomena are common accompanying features, and bony eburnation of apposing vertebral bodies and small osteophytes may be present (Fig. 95–92). As the disease progresses, disc calcification may be obscured by total obliteration of the disc space and bony bridging that produces a "bamboo" spine, again reminiscent of ankylosing spondylitis. The apophyseal joints in the spine may also demonstrate articular space narrowing, bony sclerosis, and ankylosis.

Peripheral involvement in alkaptonuria occurs in the knees, hips, and shoulders, and less commonly in the symphysis pubis, sacroiliac joints, and other articulations. Radiologic findings are similar to those of degenerative joint disease with interosseous space narrowing and bone sclerosis; characteristic features in alkaptonuria include relatively symmetrical cartilage loss within an articulation, bony collapse and fragmentation with multiple radiopaque intra-articular bodies, limited osteophytosis, and tendinous calcification. These abnormalities are also evident in CPPD crystal deposition disease, and differentiation of this disorder from alkaptonuria may be difficult. Capsular and synovial calcification, widespread chondrocalcinosis, and an absence of diffuse disc calcification are features of CPPD crystal deposition disease that would not be expected in alkaptonuria. These two disorders may occasionally coexist.

Bibliography

Adamson TC III, Resnik CS, Guerra J Jr, et al: Hand and wrist arthropathies of hemochromatosis and calcium pyrophosphate deposition disease: Distinct radiographic features. Radiology 147:377, 1983.

Atkins CJ, McIvor J, Smith PM, et al: Chondrocalcinosis and arthropathy: Studies in haemochromatosis and in idiopathic chondrocalcinosis. Q J Med 39:71, 1970.

Barthelemy CR, Nakayama DA, Carrera GF, et al: Gouty arthritis: A prospective radiographic evaluation of sixty patients. Skel Radiol 11:1, 1984.

Bassett ML, Halliday JW, Powell LW: Hemochromatosis—newer concepts: Diagnosis and management. DM 26:1, 1980.

Bloch C, Hermann G, Yu T-F: A radiologic reevaluation of gout: A study of 2000 patients. AJR 134:781, 1980.

Bonavita JA, Dalinka MK, Schumacher HR Jr: Hydroxyapatite deposition disease. Radiology 134:621, 1980.

Bosworth BM: Calcium deposits in the shoulder and subacromial bursitis: A survey of 12,122 shoulders. JAMA 116:2477, 1941.

Dieppe PA, Huskisson EC, Crocker P, Willoughby DA: Apatite deposition disease. A new arthropathy. Lancet 1:266, 1976.

Doherty M: Pyrophosphate arthropathy—Recent clinical advances. Ann Rheum Dis 42(Suppl):38, 1983.

Dymock IW, Hamilton EBD, Laws JW, Williams R: Arthropathy of haemochromatosis. Clinical and radiological analysis of 63 patients with iron overload. Ann Rheum Dis 29:469, 1970.

Faure G, Daculsi G: Calcified tendinitis: A review. Ann Rheum Dis 42(Suppl):49, 1983.

Genant HK: Roentgenographic aspects of calcium pyrophosphate dihydrate crystal deposition disease (pseudogout). Arthritis Rheum 19(Suppl):307, 1976.

Golding DN, Walshe JM: Arthropathy of Wilson's disease. Study of clinical and radiological features in 32 patients. Ann Rheum Dis 36:99, 1977.

Hamilton E, Williams R, Barlow KA, Smith PM: The arthropathy of idiopathic haemochromatosis. Q J Med 37:171, 1968.

Holt PD, Keats TE: Calcific tendinitis: A review of the usual and unusual. Skeletal Radiol 22:1, 1993.

Justesen P, Andersen PE Jr: Radiologic manifestations in alcaptonuria. Skel Radiol 11:204, 1984.

Kaklamanis P, Spengos M: Osteoarticular changes with synovial biopsy findings in Wilson's disease. Ann Rheum Dis 32:422, 1973.

Kuntz D, Naveau B, Bardin T, et al: Destructive spondylarthropathy in hemodialyzed patients. A new syndrome. Arthritis Rheum 27:369, 1984.

Laskar FH, Sargison KD: Ochronotic arthropathy. A review with four case reports. J Bone Joint Surg 52B:653, 1970.

Lichtenstein L, Kaplan L: Hereditary ochronosis: Pathologic changes observed in two necropsied cases. Am J Pathol 30:99, 1954.

Markel SF, Hart WR: Arthropathy in calcium pyrophosphate dihydrate crystal deposition disease. Pathologic study of 12 cases. Arch Pathol Lab Med 106:529, 1982.

Martel W, Champion CK, Thompson GR, et al: A roentgenologically distinctive arthropathy in some patients with the pseudogout syndrome. AJR 109:587, 1970.

McCarty D: Crystals, joints, and consternation. Ann Rheum Dis 42:243, 1983.

McCarty DJ Jr: Arthritis and Allied Conditions, 9th ed. Philadelphia, Lea and Febiger, 1979.

McCarty DJ Jr: Calcium pyrophosphate dihydrate crystal deposition disease—1975. Arthritis Rheum 19(Suppl):275, 1976.

McCarty DJ Jr, Halverson PB, Carrera GF, et al: "Milwaukee shoulder"—Association of microspheroids containing hydroxyapatite crystals, active collagenase, and neutral protease with rotator cuff defects. I. Clinical aspects. Arthritis Rheum 24:464, 1981.

McCarty DJ Jr, Kohn NN, Faires JS: The significance of calcium phosphate crystals in the synovial fluid of arthritic patients: The "pseudogout syndrome." I. Clinical aspects. Ann Intern Med 56:711, 1962.

McKendry RJR, Uhthoff HK, Sarkar K, Hyslop PSG: Calcifying tendinitis of the shoulder: Prognostic value of clinical, histologic, and radiologic features in 57 surgically treated cases. J Rheumatol 9:75, 1982.

O'Brien WM, LaDu BN, Bunim JJ: Biochemical, pathologic and clinical aspects of alcaptonuria, ochronosis and ochronotic arthropathy. Am J Med 34:813, 1963.

Pomeranz MM, Friedman LJ, Tunick IS: Roentgen findings in alkaptonuric ochronosis. Radiology 37:295, 1941.

Resnick D: The radiographic manifestations of gouty arthritis. CRC Crit Rev Diag Imag 9:265, 1977.

Resnick D, Niwayama G, Goergen TG, et al: Clinical, radiographic and pathologic abnormalities in calcium pyrophosphate dihydrate (CPPD) deposition disease: Pseudogout. Radiology 122:1, 1977.

Resnick D, Niwayama G: Diagnosis of Bone and Joint Disorders with Emphasis on Articular Abnormalities. Philadelphia, WB Saunders Company, 1981.

Resnik CS, Resnick D: Calcium pyrophosphate dihydrate crystal deposition disease. Curr Probl Diagn Radiol 11:1, 1982.

Resnik CS, Resnick D: Crystal deposition disease. Semin Arthritis Rheum 12:390, 1983.

Sandstrom C: Peritendinitis calcarea. A common disease of middle life: Its diagnosis, pathology and treatment. AJR 40:1, 1938.

Schumacher HR Jr: Hemochromatosis and arthritis. Arthritis Rheum 7:41, 1964.

Schumacher HR, Smolyo AP, Tse RL, Maurer K: Arthritis associated with apatite crystals. Ann Intern Med 87:411, 1977.

Sokoloff L: The pathology of gout. Metabolism 6:230, 1957.

Warrington G, Palmer MK: Retropharyngeal tendinitis. Br J Radiol 56:52, 1983.

Watt I, Middlemiss H: The radiology of gout. Clin Radiol 26:27, 1975.

Yarze JC, Martin P, Munoz SJ, Friedman LS: Wilson's disease: Current status. Am J Med 92:643, 1992.

Yu-Zhang X, Xue-Zhe Z, Xian-Hao X: Roentgenologic study of 41 cases of Wilson's disease. Chinese Med J 95:674, 1982.

Zitnan D, Sit'aj S: Chondrocalcinosis articularis. Section I: Clinical and radiological study. Ann Rheum Dis 22:142, 1963.

SURGICAL TREATMENT OF JOINT DISEASE

RICHARD R. PELKER

The surgical treatment of joint disease is often equated with total joint replacement. Given the enormous relief these procedures have offered, this perception is easy to understand. A large share of this chapter will be devoted to these procedures. However, it is important to keep in perspective that joint replacement surgery represents only one end of the spectrum of procedures that the orthopedic surgeon must consider in optimizing the choices for the patient. Among these are arthrodesis, interposition or resection arthroplasties, osteotomy, and synovectomy.

It is beyond the scope of this text to detail all the special considerations involved in the selection of each procedure for each joint. However, some of the more pertinent features of each are outlined for the major joints. A short glossary of the more common terms is presented immediately below for those not already familiar with them.

Definitions of Terms

Arthrodesis (synonym: fusion, ankylosis): The ablation of a joint with bony union of the opposing bones.
Arthroplasty: The reconstruction of one side (hemiarthroplasty) or both sides (total joint arthroplasty; TJA) of a joint.
Arthroscopy: The visualization of the interior of a joint, usually by means of a fiberoptic scope.
Hemiarthroplasty: The replacement of only one side of a joint.
Interposition arthroplasty: The removal of a joint surface and replacement with a lining substance (e.g., fascia).
Osteotomy: The surgical production of a cut in the bone and realignment of the joint surfaces to improve either the weight distribution across the joint surfaces or the congruency of the opposing articular surfaces.
Replacement arthroplasty (synonym: total joint replacement, TJR): The reconstruction of a joint with a foreign substance, usually nonbiologic.
Resection arthroplasty: The removal of a joint surface without replacement with a biologic or nonbiologic substance.
Synovectomy: The removal of the synovial lining of a joint or tendon sheath.

SYNOVECTOMY

Removal of the synovial lining of joint and tendons has a considerable amount of applicability in the inflammatory arthritides. Tenosynovectomy of the hand in rheumatoid arthritis is aimed at preventing the tendon rupture that occurs in this disease. Synovectomy of the large weight-bearing joints is useful when the disease is confined to one major joint that has been unresponsive to adequate medical management, usually after four to six months. To be successful, there should be little roentgenographic evidence of disease, such as joint space narrowing. Although the procedure can arrest the course of cartilage and bone destruction and offer significant pain relief, the motion in the joint is usually diminished and the rheumatoid synovium does regenerate.

ARTHROSCOPY

The arthroscope has made the diagnosis and treatment of many abnormalities and injuries to the knee much less traumatic and disabling. The scope of procedures that can now be done through the arthroscope or guided by it has expanded from being merely a diagnostic aid or ablative tool to include the repair of meniscal tears, cruciate ligament reconstruction, and repair of osteocartilaginous defects. It also has commonly been utilized to perform "closed" synovectomies of the knee for inflammatory diseases and to perform "débridements" of degenerative disease in attempt to avoid joint arthroplasty. Although the therapeutic value of the arthroscope has continued to expand, its utility as a diagnostic aid has been supplanted to a degree by less invasive imaging techniques such as magnetic resonance imaging, which can rival the arthroscope's ability to detect meniscal tears or cruciate ligament injuries.

The most explosive growth of the arthroscope's use has occurred in its expansion to most of the other joints in the body. Currently the shoulder joint is probably the next most common joint where the arthroscope is used. At that site it is commonly used to perform repairs of shoulder instabilities and treat impingement syndromes. In the ankle it is used to address osteochondral lesions and even perform arthrodeses. Small-diameter arthroscopes are utilized to arthroscope the wrist and even perform carpal tunnel release.

CORE DECOMPRESSION AND BONE GRAFTING

Avascular necrosis can be a devastating problem, especially in the young patient in whom the reconstructive options are limited. Therefore, every attempt is made to preserve the original bone in as congruent a geometry as possible. In the femoral head this is done by initially unweighting the load placed on the joint by placing the patient on crutches. Unfortunately, this conservative type of management often is followed by progressive collapse of the joint and subsequent degenerative changes.

Some authors have reported remarkably good results with a simple procedure for avascular necrosis in the proximal femur. This consists of drilling a hole up through the intertrochanteric region and the femoral neck into the femoral head. This theoretically serves to decompress the elevated bone marrow pressures that have been reported to be associated with avascular necrosis. Although this technique has prevented the usual collapse in the early radiographic stages (spherical head contour with normal trabeculae [stage I] or diffuse porosis/sclerosis or wedge sclerosis [stage II]), it has not been able to reverse the collapse in stage III (early collapse with sequestrum) and IV (marked collapse of the head with trabecular destruction) lesions. It also has not had much success in joints other than the hip.

Some authors recommend supplementing the decompression by shoring up a collapsed head with a bone graft. This can take the form of a conventional graft or a vascularized piece of bone with its own blood supply.

OSTEOTOMY

When applied to arthritis surgery, an osteotomy is simply a cut in the bone and realignment of the joint surfaces to improve either the weight distribution across the joint surfaces or the congruency of the opposing articular surfaces. Although these principles can be applied to any joint, the most popular are the large weight-bearing joints of the hip and knee.

Numerous types of osteotomies about the knee have been devised, but the "Coventry," or high tibial, osteotomy has gained the most acceptance. The preoperative evaluation for this type of operation usually includes anteroposterior and lateral weight-bearing roentgenograms of the knee. These are assessed for the extent of medial compartment versus lateral or patellofemoral compartment narrowing as well as the degree of varus deformity. A bone scan is occasionally obtained as well to assess this (Fig. 95–93*A*). The surgical correction consists of the removal of a wedge of bone from the tibia to restore the normal (approximately 7 degrees) valgus alignment of the knee joint and thus redistribute the load across the joint to the lateral side (Fig. 95–93*B*).

Although less common, a varus osteotomy can be performed for lateral joint disease. However, because of the neurovascular constraints of this region, if the osteotomy is more than 10 to 15 degrees, the surgery is usually performed in the distal femur rather than the proximal tibia.

Similarly, the patellofemoral articulation can be realigned by soft-tissue releases and transfers to properly align the patella in the femoral groove. If there is significant patellofemoral disease a pa-

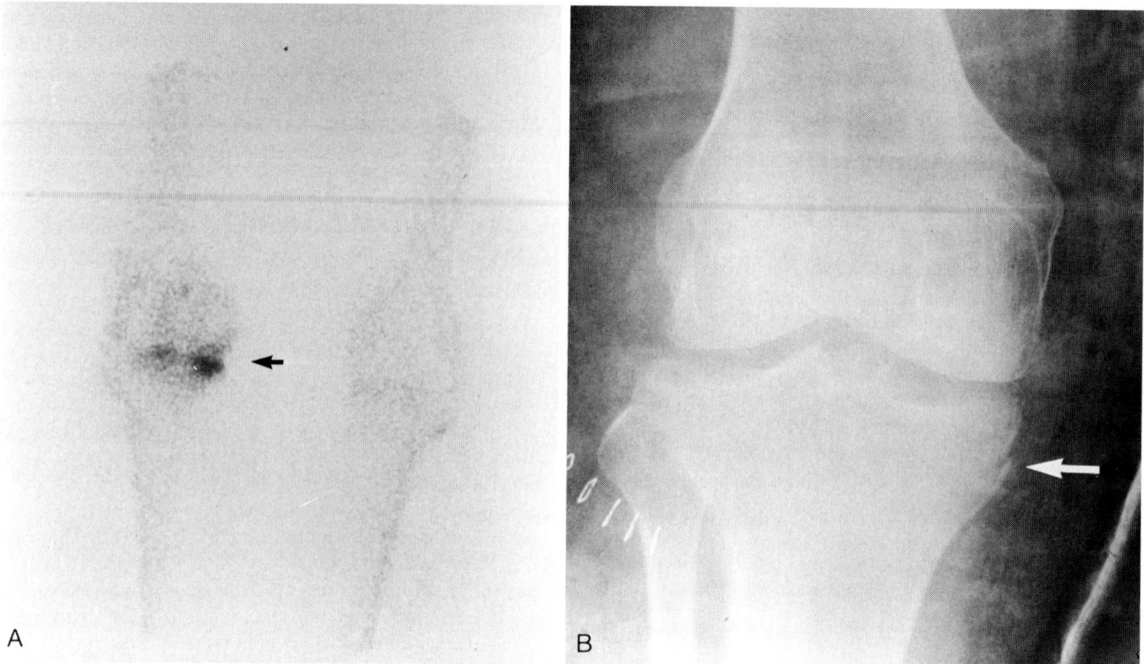

Figure 95–93. *A,* **Preoperative technetium bone scan** for osteotomy reveals primarily medial compartment uptake in the symptomatic knee *(arrow)*. *B,* **Postoperative anteroposterior roentgenogram** shows the high tibial osteotomy *(arrow)* with medial joint space improved and approximately 7 degrees of valgus alignment of the knee.

tellectomy can be considered. However, removal of this structure should not be done without due regard to the quadriceps' reserve strength. The expected loss of approximately 30 per cent of extensor strength after patellectomy has helped popularize tibial elevation osteotomies such as that advocated by Maquet. In this type of procedure the tibial tubercle and anterior spine are osteotomized. A bone graft is used to elevate the patellar tendon insertion approximately 1.5 cm. This results in a decrease in the patellofemoral contact stresses (Fig. 95–94).

Before the advent of an acceptable total joint replacement, osteotomy was the mainstay of reconstructive surgery of the hip joint. It is still a useful alternative, especially in the younger patient. As with the other osteotomies, the basic principle is to transfer the load bearing to that portion of the joint surface that has been least affected by the disease. Several different osteotomies have been devised for this purpose. Most authors recognize the need for a residual range of motion in the hip of at least 70 degrees of flexion and have experienced poor results in hips that did not have this mobility as well as in those with inflammatory disease, dysplastic acetabulum, coxa magna, and bone destruction. The main complication with this procedure is a delayed union or non-union of the osteotomy (3 to 4 per cent), bony ankylosis (up to 34 per cent), and a residual limp.

Frequently the osteotomy is held in place with a rigid internal fixation device. Reportedly, this decreases the incidence of non-union. In joints other than the knee and hip, osteotomies are used more to correct a deformity that may be the underlying cause for a degenerative process.

ARTHRODESIS

A useful alternative to joint replacement, the ablation and union between two joint surfaces results in a construct that produces a highly reliable relief of pain. In the hip this procedure is well suited for the younger patient, the overweight patient, and the patient who wishes to return to heavy labor. The adult hip is usually fused in a position of less than 20 degrees of flexion, slight adduction, and 5 to 15 degrees of external rotation. The main complication is non-union, which occurs in the hip in approximately 10 per cent of the cases. In fusion of the major weight-bearing joints of the lower

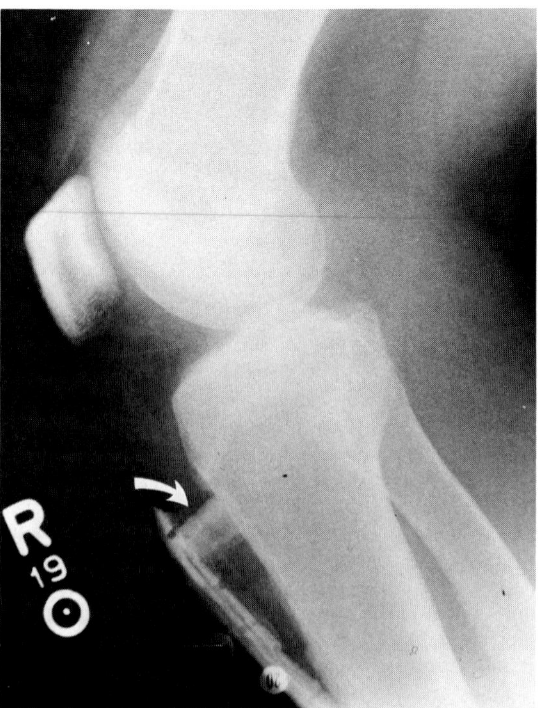

Figure 95–94. Postoperative lateral roentgenogram of a **Maquet type osteotomy** demonstrating the elevation of the tibial tubercle with a bone graft *(arrow)*. This graft is occasionally held in place with a metal screw.

extremity it is important to consider the status of the spine and ipsilateral and contralateral joints, because arthrodesis of one joint will produce an increased load on the other joints. These potential functional limitations, including sexual, must be balanced against the highly durable and reliable result.

Arthrodesis of the shoulder joint is harder to achieve than that of other joints, and therefore combined intra- and extra-articular techniques are often used in combination with internal fixation of the joint to increase the probability of union. The position in which the shoulder is fused is especially critical to the continued utility of the upper extremity. Generally, the shoulder is positioned in 50 degrees of abduction, 20 degrees of flexion, and 25 degrees of internal rotation.

Similarly, it is difficult to obtain a bony fusion in the elbow. However, since the mobility of the elbow is of great importance to the function of the upper extremity, the indications for elbow fusion are few. The general position of the fused elbow is 90 degrees of flexion.

Arthrodesis of the ankle is an important salvage procedure for badly fractured ankles with traumatic arthritis, etc., especially since it is a major weight-bearing joint in which replacement arthroplasties have not had the same success as in the hip and knee. If the remainder of the foot has normal mobility and musculature, the ankle should be fused in a neutral position. The remaining motion in the midfoot will compensate for the lost motion in the ankle and give an almost normal gait pattern.

In joints in which the intrinsic stability of the joint is not as good as in the hip (e.g., the wrist in inflammatory arthritis), arthrodesis has the added advantage of providing a more stable base for the surrounding joints. Thus, the functional strength can be increased.

ARTHROPLASTY

Reconstruction surgery is often equated with total joint replacement. However, it is possible to reconstruct a joint or portion of it without replacing it. Usually this involves the removal of one portion of the bone and using another substance interposed between the two bones of the joint to form a new lining surface for the joint. These ''interposition'' arthroplasties have limited use. However, in certain joints in which the replacement prostheses have not had widespread success, these types of relining arthroplasties can give good functional results. This is true in the elbow joint, where the bone is recontoured and relined with a piece of fascia. Unlike other types of arthroplasties, there is very little correlation between radiographic appearance of these arthroplasties and the clinical results.

Another type of arthroplasty is the resection arthroplasty. Here, the entire bony component of the joint is resected without the surgical interposition of a new lining surface. One of the better-known examples of this is the Girdelstone type of resection in the hip joint. These procedures depend on the formation of scar tissue to act as a new ''joint.'' The resection and interposition arthroplasties leave the joint relatively unstable, and in the hip requires the continued use of crutches.

Replacement Arthroplasties

The replacement of body organs with fabricated substitutes has been a goal of many medical disciplines. The orthopedist has been able to realize this, with replacements available for just about every possible joint. One must remain cognizant that any prosthetic implant is still an inferior substitute for the original. One of the most significant advances in this area was the use of ''bone cement'' (polymethylmethacrylate, PMM) to firmly anchor the prosthesis to the bone. However, loosening at this bone-cement interface also poses one of the serious problems to the long-term survival of the prosthesis (see below).

The problem of aseptic loosening of cemented arthroplasties has led to the advent of several types of prostheses that seek to secure long-term fixation through a direct anchoring of the prosthesis to bone by means of either a macrointerlock on the surface of the prosthesis to bone or a microinterlock of the bony trabeculae growing into a porous coating or to a ''bioactive'' material (e.g., hydroxyapatite) on the surface of the prosthesis (Fig. 95–95). At the same time improvements have been made in the design and technique of cemented arthroplasties. Many orthopedists believe that the cemented femoral component, using current design and cementing techniques, is still the recommended choice for the older and sedentary patient. The combination of this with a noncemented acetabulum or ''hybrid'' replacement is advocated by those who feel that long-term acetabular loosening is a continuing concern despite contemporary cemented techniques.

When evaluating a patient for a replacement arthroplasty, the choice must be made whether to replace one or both sides of the joint (i.e., total vs hemiarthroplasty). This decision is based on multiple factors, including the patient's age, disease, etc. However, the radiographic appearance of the joint is often the key.

In order for a hemiarthroplasty to be successful, the disease process should be confined mainly to one side of the joint. In general, one would be more inclined to do a hemiarthroplasty on a younger patient. This is especially true in the hip joint where every attempt is made to preserve the bone stock. One method of achieving this uses a conventional type of femoral component of the hip replacement system and places a concentric head on top of this to fit the acetabular diameter. This ''biarticular'' system allows conversion to a total hip system at a later date if the acetabulum needs to be replaced without having to revise the femoral component of the system. It is usually this wearing down of the articular surface of the acetabulum with protrusio that has caused the conventional ''Austin Moore'' type of hemiarthroplasties of the hip to fail. By providing a second bearing surface, this procedure theoretically diminishes the shear stresses that cause this acetabular wear.

Another attempt at preserving bone stock in the younger patient is the resurfacing type of hip arthroplasty. Basically, this entails placing a metal cup over the femoral head, similar to the old cup or mold arthroplasty with a matching acetabular replacement. This has the theoretical advantage of retaining much of the femoral bone stock (at some sacrifice of acetabular bone). However, after some initial reports of good success, these types of prostheses are failing at a rather high rate.

The gold standard of reconstructive hip joint surgery in the older patient remains the conventional, cemented total hip replacement. This procedure has excellent initial results with increased range of motion and pain relief and acceptable longevity for the older sedentary patient. A most useful tool in evaluating the hip joint replacement is the plain anteroposterior roentgenogram of the pelvis. This should be evaluated for the position of the prosthesis and cement technique. Although there are myriad different types of hip prostheses (besides the cemented and uncemented discussed above), some general guidelines apply to most of them. The femoral component should be placed with its stem in neutral to slight valgus position (within the femoral canal on anteroposterior and lateral). If the prosthesis has a collar at its femoral neck, it should be resting squarely on the calcar femoralis without any interposing methacrylate. An evaluation of the relative leg lengths may be made by comparing the level of the lesser trochanter in regard to the inferior pubic rami on both sides. The acetabular portion should be in approximately 45 degrees of inclination and 15 degrees of anteversion with good bone coverage over the prosthesis. The radiographic evaluation of the noncemented hip replacement should include the methods mentioned above as well as an evaluation of the amount of intramedullary space filled by the prosthesis, presence of bead or coating shedding/association, cortical hypertrophy or thinning, and evidence of distal bony bridging.

Total knee replacements initially did not have the same success

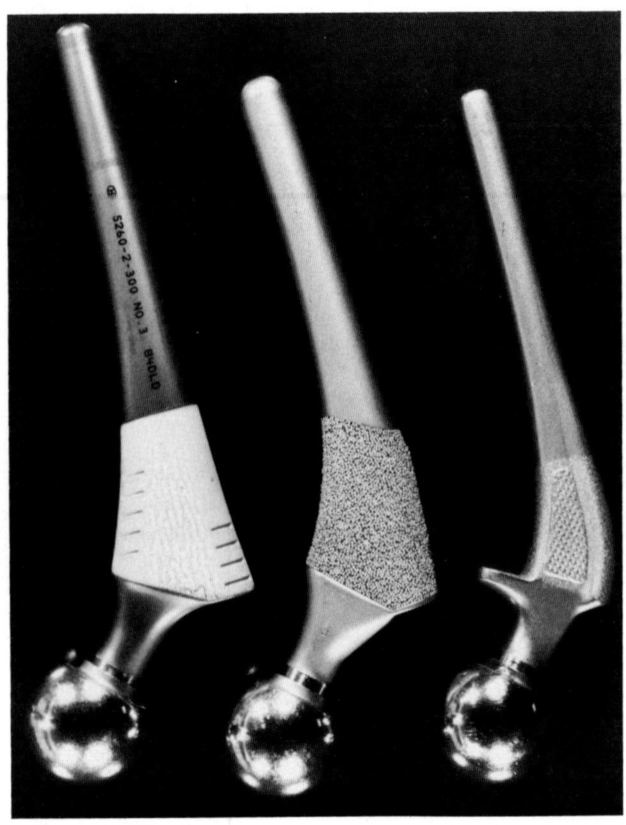

Figure 95–95. Examples of three types of femoral components. *Left,* A textured proximal surface design for cemented use. *Center,* A beaded porous ingrowth type prosthesis. *Right,* An HA-coated surface.

as the hip replacements. Unlike the ball-and-socket hip joint, the knee has an irregular, three-dimensional contour and is very dependent on this and soft-tissue constraints to provide stability to the joint. Initially, attempts were made to provide this stability within the knee replacement itself with such devices as hinged joints. These protheses suffered high failure rates because they confined the usually multiplanar motion to one plane, resulting in increased stresses on the prostheses and the bone cement interface. The majority of the knee replacements currently placed are unconstrained or semiconstrained, relying on preserved soft-tissue structures and joint contour to maintain the stability of the joint. Radiographically, these prostheses should have the joint surfaces aligned parallel to each other and with the ankle.

Joint replacement in the hand has had the most success at the metacarpophalangeal joint. Unlike the majority of the other joint implants, which are composed of metal and high-density polyethylene, these prostheses are usually composed of a radiolucent silicone rubber. Radiographic evidence of fracture of these prostheses does not imply a clinical failure.

Current designs, surgical techniques and postoperative rehabilitation have improved the success and utilization of replacement arthroplasties for the shoulder and to a lesser extent the elbow. Although implants are available for other joints, the anatomic constraints, biomechanical considerations, and physical demands have precluded high clinical success for joints such as the ankle and hence their clinical utilization has been limited.

Evaluation of a Painful Arthroplasty

In view of the large number of joint replacements being performed each year (100,000 total hip replacements per year in the United States), the problem of determining the etiology of continued pain after arthroplasty has become increasingly important. This is brought out by the reported long-term revision rates for total joint replacements ranging between 9 and 40 per cent. The standard procedures for evaluating a painful total hip replacement are provided below. The same general principles may be applied to the other joint arthroplasties.

The main consideration in evaluating pain after a total hip replacement is determining whether it is due to loosening of the prosthesis (either septic or aseptic). Several clues in the patient's history may suggest that the prosthesis is loose, especially if there was no pain-free interval after surgery. Then the question of a septic process or faulty technique must be raised. A deep, aching pain of the thigh radiating down to the knee and increasing with weight bearing is suggestive of femoral component loosening, whereas groin or buttock pain increasing with weight bearing and relieved by rest is suggestive of acetabular loosening.

After total joint arthroplasty, the relative pain relief allows most patients to markedly increase their physical activities. This places an augmental stress on the neighboring anatomy. If the surrounding structures are not able to remodel themselves adequately, this can result in stress fractures of the pelvis or other bones; these structures should be evaluated for radiographic signs of this.

Evaluation of the cement is key to interpreting the status of the components. There should be a 2-mm-thick glue mantle behind the entire acetabular component and surrounding the femoral component and extending 2 cm past the distal tip of the femoral prosthesis. No radiolucency should be apparent between the prosthesis and cement or bone and cement, although up to 2 mm may be seen without associated loosening if it is not progressive (Fig. 95–96*A*).

In the cementless arthroplasty, some of the above evaluations are not as useful. However, subsidence or change in the prosthesis is an indication of a loose component. The evaluation of the painful cementless arthroplasty should include observation for shedding of beads or other surface coatings, cortical hypertrophy or stress shielding, and distal bony bridging. A certain percentage (4 to 24 per cent) will have anterolateral thigh pain that can be transient. A higher incidence has been associated with larger (stiffer) and longer prostheses and is not necessarily associated with a loose prosthesis.

Polyethylene wear has been reported as relatively low (mean 0.1

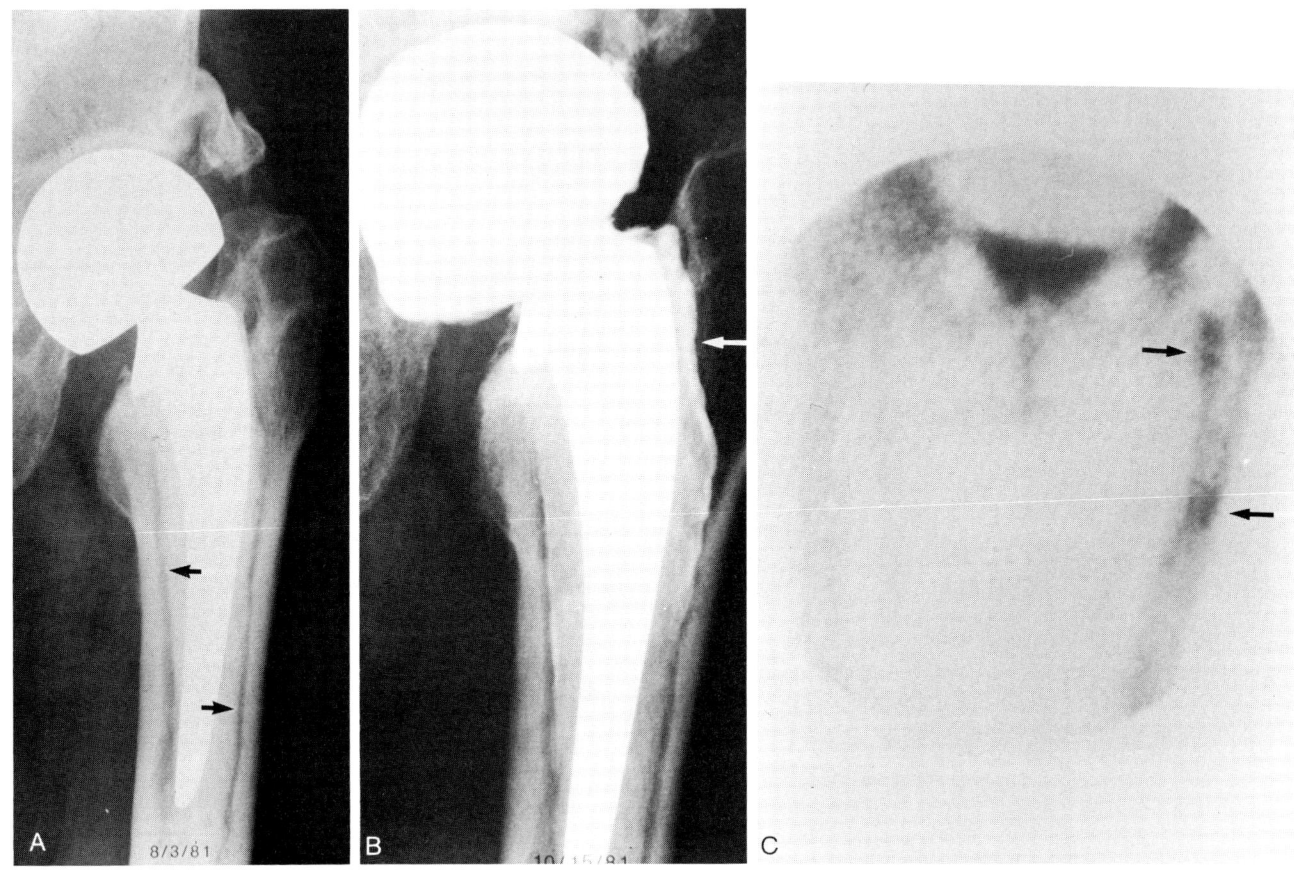

Figure 95–96. Loose hip replacement. *A,* Anteroposterior roentgenogram of a loose hip replacement demonstrating a radiolucent line between the bone and cement *(arrows). B,* Arthrogram of a loose cemented hip replacement. Dye can be seen tracking laterally between the cement and bone *(arrow). C,* Technetium bone scan of a loose total hip replacement demonstrating increased uptake at the tip and calcar regions *(arrows).*

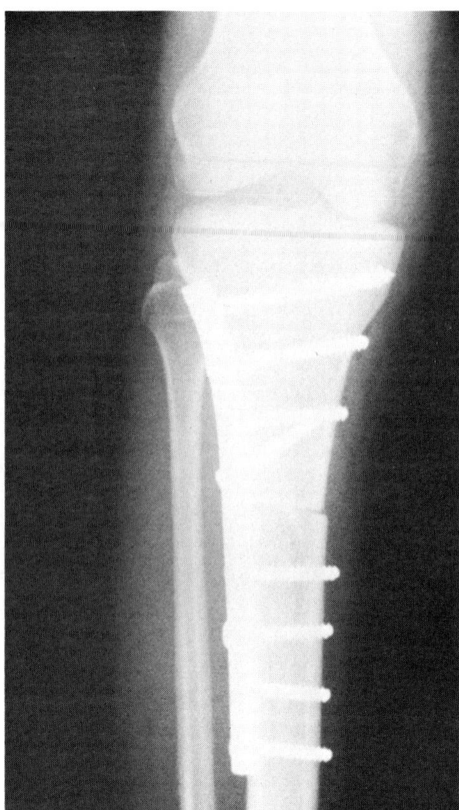

Figure 95–97. Replacement of the tibial portion of the knee joint with an allograft held in place with a plate and screws. (Courtesy of G. E. Friedlaender, M.D., and H. J. Mankin, M.D.)

mm per year in the acetabulum). The wear rate has been reported to depend upon the size of the femoral head (the smallest femoral head size, 22 mm, had the highest linear wear rate whereas the largest head size, 32 mm, had the highest volumetric wear rate and the highest revision rate). Metallic wear of components has not been a significant problem except for titanium bearing surfaces, which can produce significant wear debris. It is currently believed that wear particle debris from the cement, polyethylene, etc., may contribute to the cascade of events causing loosening by triggering macrophages and foreign body type giant cells. A synovium-like membrane containing high levels of prostaglandin-E_2 has been found at the bone-cement interface that may contribute to the osteolysis associated with loosening.

This emphasizes the necessity for comparison with initial films, looking specifically for changes in the position of the prosthesis or progressive widening of any bone-cement lucency. With current metallurgy and design standards, failure of the prosthesis itself has become uncommon. However, the structural integrity of the implant should also be assessed.

With attention to these details, the correct fixation status of 92 per cent of the femoral components but only 63 per cent of the acetabular components can be ascertained. Arthrography can increase the accuracy of detecting loose acetabular components to 84 per cent, but without any increased accuracy in determining femoral loosening. This is best done under fluoroscopic control with local anesthesia. The region should be thoroughly prepped and draped and a large-bore spinal needle introduced into the joint space. One of the major reasons for performing an arthrogram is to determine whether or not the joint is infected; therefore every attempt should be made to obtain a specimen of joint fluid for culture and sensitivity (aerobic and anaerobic) before the radiopaque dye is instilled. If no joint fluid can be aspirated, several milliliters of nonbacteriostatic saline may be injected and aspirated back. Initial and delayed films are obtained after compression and distraction and evaluated for extension of the contrast into the bone-cement or cement-prosthesis interface (Fig. 95–96*B*) as well as for filling of abscess cavities or fistulae.

Nuclear imaging is a useful adjunct in determining prothesis loosening and differentiating septic loosening. The ^{99m}Tc pyrophosphate bone scan may normally show increased uptake up to six months after total joint replacement but is considered abnormal after that time. The pattern of the scan is also valuable in assessing loosening, specifically increased uptake at the stem tip (Fig. 95–96*C*). Osteomyelitis has a more diffuse uptake than aseptic loosening. While the technetium scan is felt to be 100 per cent sensitive, its specificity is only 72 per cent. Therefore, the ^{67}Ga scan is often used in conjunction with the ^{99m}Tc scan; if the relative distribution patterns are incongruent, osteomyelitis is likely. Indium-labeled leukocyte scans can also be useful in detecting infected joint arthroplasties.

ALLOGRAFTS

An alternative to replacing joints with metal or plastic parts is to use cadaver material. Although the use of allografts has become increasingly more common, their use for joint replacements still faces many problems. In order for the new joint to avoid early degenerative changes, the two opposing surfaces must have matching contours. Thus, the surgeon must have access to a bone bank with a sufficient supply of various sizes to match the fit of the recipient. Because the graft is initially avascular, one has all the problems of avascular necrosis to deal with as well as problems of cartilage cell viability, stress fractures, fixation, etc. Despite these obstacles, several centers are reporting satisfactory initial results (Fig. 95–97). They are currently done mainly as limb salvage procedures for tumor patients but hold promise as a reconstructive alternative.

Bibliography

Edmonson AS, Crenshaw AH: Campbell's Operative Orthopaedics, 6th ed. St. Louis, CV Mosby, 1980.

Flatt AE: Care of the Arthritic Hand, 4th ed. St. Louis, CV Mosby, 1983.

Friedlaender GE, Mankin HJ, Sell KW: Osteochondral Allografts: Biology, Banking and Clinical Applications. Boston, Little, Brown, 1983.

Hungerford DS: Bone Marrow Pressure, Venography and Core Decompression in Ischemic Necrosis of the Femoral Head. Proceedings of the 7th Meeting of the Hip Society, 1979, pp 218–237.

O'Neil D, Harris W: Failed total hip replacement: Assessment by plain radiographs, arthrograms and aspiration of the hip joint. J Bone Joint Surg 60A:540–546, 1984.

Rosenthall L, Linbona R, Hernandez M, Hadjipavlou A: ^{99m}Tc-PP ^{67}Ga imaging following insertion of orthopaedic devices. Radiology 133:717–721, 1979.

Turner RH, Scheller AD: Revision Total Hip Arthroplasty. New York, Grune and Stratton, 1982.

Weiss PE, Mall JC, Hoffer, PB, et al: ^{99m}Tc-Methylene diphosphonate bone imaging in the evaluation of total hip prosthesis. Radiology 133:727–729, 1979.

Williamson BR, McLaughlin RE, Wang GJ, et al: Radionuclide bone imaging as a means of differentiating loosening and infection in patients with a painful total hip prosthesis. Radiology 133:723–725, 1979.

96 Hematologic Disorders

HEMOGLOBINOPATHIES

JACK P. LAWSON

The hemoglobinopathies constitute a heterogeneous group of genetically determined abnormalities of hemoglobin synthesis. Hemoglobin consists of an iron-containing pigment called heme, conjugated to a protein, globin. The globin component is formed from two pairs of unlike polypeptide chains. In normal individuals above one year of age, the major component of hemoglobin is HbA ($\alpha_2\beta_2$), in which the globin component consists of two alpha and two beta polypeptide chains. In addition to HbA, normal adult hemoglobin contains small amounts of HbA_2 ($\alpha_2\delta_2$) and fetal hemoglobin, HbF ($\alpha_2\gamma_2$).

Although over 300 structural variants of hemoglobin have been identified, only a very small number are associated with clinical abnormalities. These may be divided into two groups. The thalassemic syndromes are the result of retarded production of a globin chain. In the other group, which includes sickle cell anemia, there are structural abnormalities of the globin polypeptides.

THE THALASSEMIC SYNDROMES

In 1927, Cooley and his coworkers described an "anemia in children with splenomegaly and peculiar changes in the bones." Clinically, these children were noted to have a muddy, yellowish discoloration of the skin, prominence of the malar eminences, distortion of the alignment of the teeth, and a profound anemia. These children were mainly from Italian and Greek families, and it was soon realized that this disorder occurred frequently in families living near, or originating from, the eastern Mediterranean ("thalassa" = sea). The incidence of the thalassemic trait is approximately 2.5 per cent in Italian-Americans and 7 to 10 per cent in Greek-Americans. There are an estimated 800 to 1000 patients suffering from homozygous beta-thalassemia in the United States.

Etiology and Diagnosis

In the thalassemic syndromes, retarded production of a globin chain, most frequently the beta chain, leads to a decreased synthesis of total hemoglobin and a severe hypochromic anemia. The excess alpha chains are precipitated within the erythrocytes and their precursors, resulting in hemolysis and diminished hematopoiesis. The end result of these processes is a profound anemia and a marked increase in marrow activity, which has been estimated to be increased 5- to 30-fold.

In thalassemia major, severe hypochromic anemia with splenomegaly occurs in infancy. Thalassemia intermedia occurs in a subset of patients with homozygous beta-thalassemia, composing 5 to 10 per cent of the patients with thalassemia major (Figs. 96–1 to 96–3). These patients are able to maintain levels of hemoglobin compatible with an active life (6 to 9 gm/100 ml) without regular transfusion, but often at the expense of marrow hypertrophy and skeletal deformity.

Pathophysiology

The profound anemia leads to marrow hypertrophy and extramedullary hematopoiesis, resulting in hepatosplenomegaly, facial deformities, and pathologic fractures. Retardation of growth and secondary sexual characteristics is common. In addition, the longstanding hemolysis results in the accumulation of the breakdown products of heme, predisposing to the formation of pigmentary gallstones and to hemosiderosis from deposition of the excess iron in the reticuloendothelial system. Secondary hemochromatosis may ensue, leading to hepatic, pancreatic, or cardiac failure and an arthropathy similar to primary hemochromatosis. In the untransfused patient, death may occur in the first five years of life, although life can be prolonged by regular blood transfusions.

Radiographic Features

The skeletal changes result from the response of the medulla, cortex, or periosteum to the proliferating marrow; this response is dependent on the type of the transfusion therapy and the age of the patient at its commencement. The most pronounced changes occur in the axial skeleton and in the proximal portions of the femur and humerus, which house the hematopoietic marrow. Marrow proliferation causes expansion of the medulla, thinning of the cortex, and resorption of the trabeculae, resulting in a generalized loss of bone density and, frequently, small focal lucencies demarcated by coarsened residual trabeculae. A frequent finding is the presence of a lucency, which is adjacent to the endosteal aspect of the cortex. This is thought to represent resorption at the margin of the proliferating marrow. In weight-bearing bones, the primary trabeculae are preserved. In the spine this results in a vertical striated appearance.

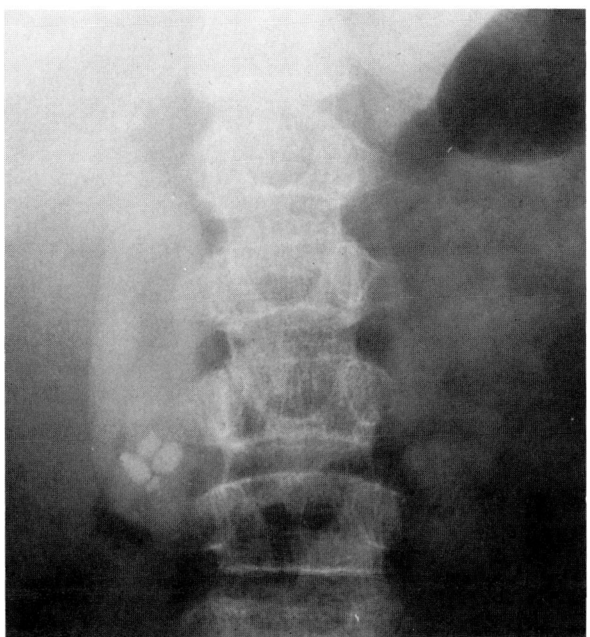

Figure 96–1. Seventeen-year-old female with **thalassemia intermedia.** The vertebral bodies are osteoporotic and demonstrate prominence of the vertical trabeculae. Gallstones are present.

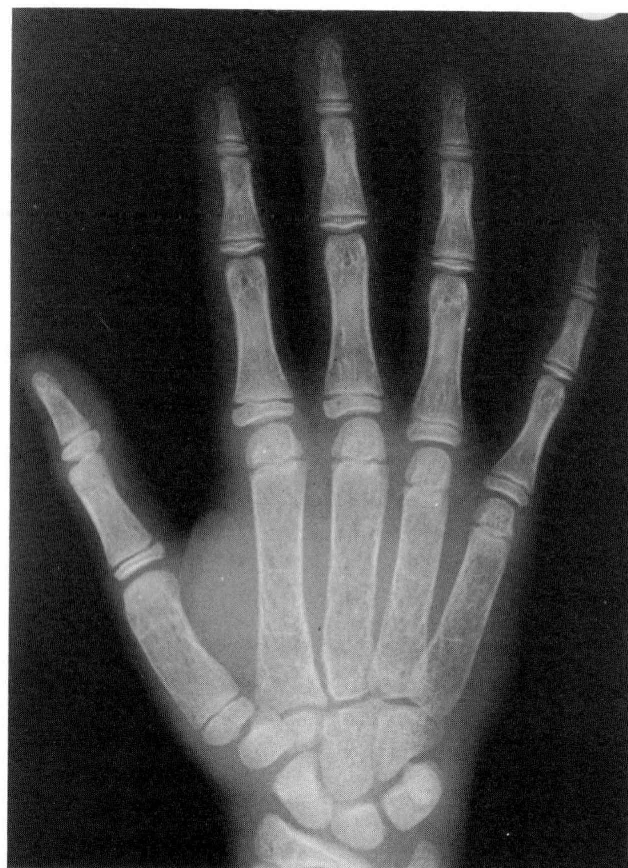

Figure 96–2. Sixteen-year-old male with **thalassemia intermedia.** Marrow proliferation in the medulla has resulted in cortical thinning, focal lucencies, and the loss of the normal tubulation. The nutrient foramina of the second to fourth proximal phalanges are enlarged.

With more profound anemia the changes may be noted more distally in the extremities, and in the most severe cases there is loss of the normal tubulation of the phalanges. Fractures are common in both the axial skeleton and the extremities.

The appearance of the skull is characteristic and results from the marrow proliferation in the diploë. In severe cases there is widening of the diploë with loss of the outer cortex. New bone formation, at right angles to the inner table, develops in response to the proliferating marrow, leading to the classic "hair-on-end" appearance. Characteristically the occipital bone is not involved, owing to the absence of hematopoietic marrow in this bone. Proliferation of marrow within the maxilla will result in hypertrophy of the lateral margins of the malar eminences and anterior and medial displacement of the developing teeth.

Focal subperiosteal proliferation of marrow may lead to cortical erosions, which in the ribs may simulate notching due to coarctation. Extensive proliferation, involving vertebral bodies, the pelvis, and particularly the anterior and posterior margins of the ribs, will result in extramedullary hematopoiesis. Ossification of the latter is the explanation of the costal osteomas, which are occasionally identified, whereas ossification of a linear zone of subperiosteal marrow produces a "rib within a rib" appearance.

Premature fusion of the epiphyses occurs most commonly in the proximal humerus and results in shortening and a humeral varus deformity. Less commonly, the distal femur or proximal tibia may be involved and occasionally there is premature fusion of multiple epiphyses.

The hyperplasia and hypertrophy of bone marrow are associated with an increase in vascularity, which may be identified as enlarged nutrient foramina in the phalanges or vascular impressions in the calvarium.

Therapy

Current therapy consists of transfusions of 15 ml/kg of packed red blood cells every three to five weeks to maintain the hemoglobin level above 9.5 to 10 gm/100 ml. This is given in conjunction with long-term chelation therapy.

Patients who have been maintained on this hypertransfusion regimen from an early age appear free from osseous abnormalities because the profound anemia associated with the disease is avoided. The skeletal changes are more pronounced in those patients not treated with a hypertransfusion regimen or not started on such a regimen until after the age of five years. The most dramatic changes occur in the patients with thalassemia intermedia, who are able to maintain a reasonable hemoglobin without transfusion but appear to do so at the price of severe skeletal changes.

It has been demonstrated that the administration of high subcutaneous doses of deferoxamine to young children with thalassemia before iron overload is established may be associated with a rickets-like syndrome.

Before the introduction of a hypertransfusion regimen, gallstones were noted in approximately 25 per cent of patients with homozygous beta-thalassemia. However, following the introduction of this therapy, which reduces marrow activity and the production of fragile erythrocytes, there has been a dramatic reduction in the percentage of cases demonstrating biliary calculi. Iron deposition may be demonstrated by computed tomography or by magnetic resonance imaging.

SICKLE CELL ANEMIA AND VARIANTS

In 1910, Herrick drew attention to a young black male with anemia in which there was a characteristic red cell deformity, which

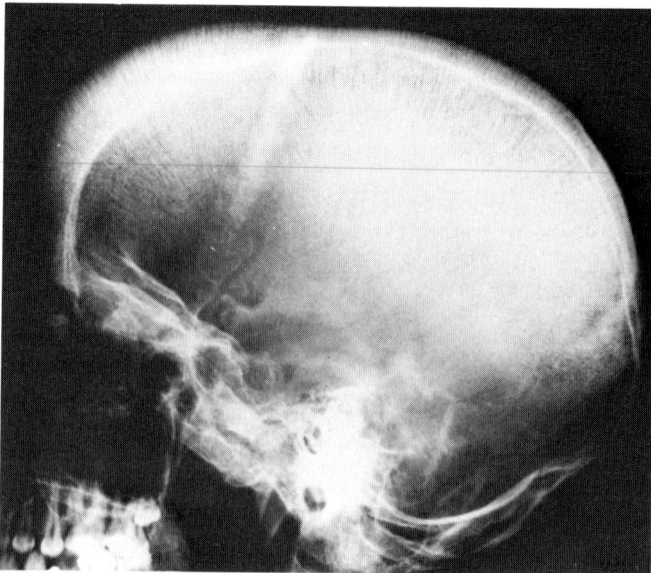

Figure 96–3. Twenty-one-year-old male with **thalassemia intermedia.** The diploë of the frontal and parietal bones is widened. Loss of the outer table and new bone formation in the diploë have resulted in a "hair-on-end" appearance. The occipital bone is uninvolved. The calvarial vascular impressions are enlarged.

he likened to a sickle. It was soon discovered that sickle cell anemia has a worldwide distribution in people of black ancestry. In the United States, the homozygous state affects one in 500 black children and the heterozygous state, called sickle cell trait, is present in approximately 8 per cent of Americans of African origin.

Pathophysiology

The molecular structure of the hemoglobin in sickle cell disease (HbS) differs from that of normal adult hemoglobin and allows distortion of the erythrocytes to occur when the hemoglobin is deoxygenated. With oxygenation, the red cells will return to a normal configuration, only to sickle again under further conditions of deoxygenation. This results in a reduced half-life of the sickle cell. In addition, vaso-occlusive changes may occur owing to the inability of the rigid and deformed erythrocytes to negotiate the small vessels.

The severity of these processes is dependent on the concentration of hemoglobin S in the cells. The changes are most severe in the homozygous state, less pronounced in the sickle cell variants (hemoglobin SC disease and sickle-thalassemia), and rare in the heterozygous or carrier state.

Radiographic Features

The hemolysis and anemia are associated with marrow proliferation and the accumulation of the breakdown products of heme, resulting in the same physiologic and radiographic manifestations as in the thalassemic syndromes (Fig. 96–4).

The radiographic features of the vaso-occlusive phenomena that occur in the osseous system are dependent on multiple factors: age of the patient, acute or chronic nature of the vaso-occlusive phenomena, site of the occlusion, extent of the collateral circulation, and the interval between the occlusion and the radiographic examination.

The most common site for infarction is the medullary cavity. The earliest clinical manifestation of sickle cell anemia is frequently the "hand-foot" syndrome due to avascular necrosis of the small bones of the hands and feet. The onset, which has a peak incidence at two years of age, may occur from six months to eight years of age. It is rare in the first months of life because 95 per cent of the hemoglobin at birth is HbF and it is not until four to five months of age that the hemoglobin becomes predominantly HbS. This syndrome is characterized by soft-tissue swelling and tenderness over the hands and feet. Seven to 10 days later, periosteal new bone formation can be demonstrated radiographically in one or more bones. In addition, medullary expansion, cortical thinning, trabecular resorption, and resultant focal lucencies may occur. These changes usually resolve within weeks. However, involvement of the physis may produce cone-shaped epiphyses or premature fusion of the epiphysis, resulting in shortening or angular deformity of the involved bone. A similar process involving the secondary ossification centers of the vertebral bodies will result in angular defects in the central portions of the end-plates, causing a characteristic H deformity of the vertebral body.

Three anatomic sites in bone appear to be particularly vulnerable to vaso-occlusive disease. The first is that zone between the areas supplied by the nutrient artery and metaphyseal vessels. Radiographically this appears as an area of focal or permeative osseous destruction with associated periosteal reaction. These changes may be identical to those produced by acute infection and, even clinically, it may not be possible to make the distinction between infarction and the infection. The area of infarction may heal completely or result in the characteristic medullary calcification.

A second area of vulnerability is the zone between the areas supplied by the nutrient artery and the periosteal vessels, the latter normally providing the blood supply to the outer one third of the cortex. When this blood supply is compromised, a periosteal reaction may be produced. This can be quite pronounced in the young infant, since the periosteum is loosely attached. Consolidation of the periosteal reaction, particularly in association with an adjacent area of linear lucency from necrosis, may result in a "bone within a bone" or "tramline" appearance characteristic of sickle cell disease.

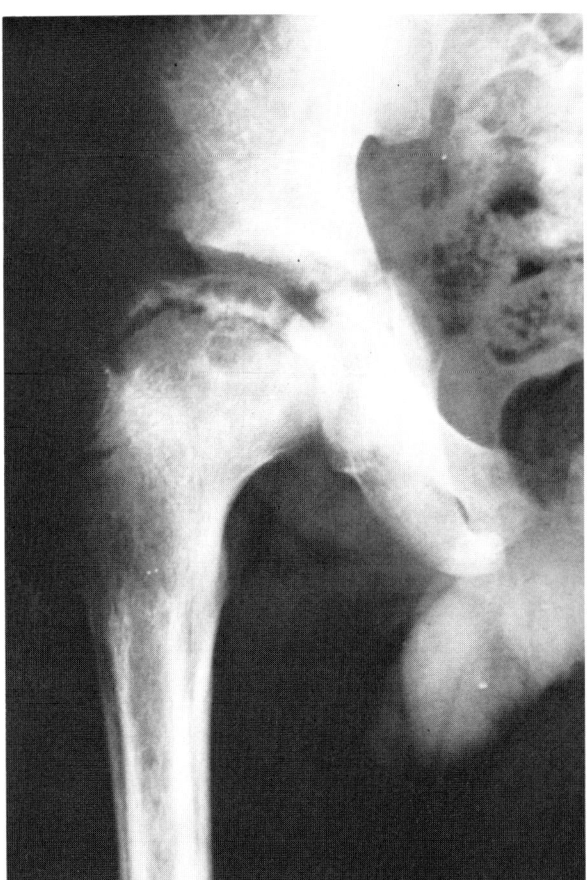

Figure 96–4. Ten-year-old black male with **sickle cell disease.** Avascular necrosis of the proximal femoral epiphysis has resulted in osseous resorption and new bone formation in the ossification center, which is flattened. Widening of the ossification center and femoral neck is present. Diaphyseal infarction has produced subperiosteal new bone, resulting in a "tramline" appearance. (Courtesy of S. P. Bohrer, M.D.)

The third area, which is affected in 15 to 30 per cent of patients, is the epiphysis. Avascular necrosis of the epiphyses, uncommon prior to 10 years of age, produces the characteristic changes of necrosis, repair, and deformity, manifesting radiographically as areas of sclerosis and/or lucency with loss of the normal bone contour. The associated skeletal abnormalities of sickle cell disease allow differentiation from Perthes' disease in the unilateral cases. The onset of bilateral avascular necrosis in sickle cell disease is usually synchronous on both sides, in contrast to Perthes' disease, in which the two sides usually show differing stages of development.

Osteomyelitis

Patients with sickle cell disease develop pneumococcal and *Salmonella* osteitis more frequently than patients with normal hemoglobin, particularly after acute infarction. Clinical and radiographic differentiation between acute infection and infarction may not be possible. During the first seven days following the onset of the process, it may be possible to make a distinction between aseptic necrosis and osteomyelitis by utilizing both bone and marrow scans.

An acute infarct will reveal diminished uptake of both radionuclides, the negative defect being much larger on the marrow scan. In contrast, an area of osteomyelitis will demonstrate a normal marrow scan and an area of increased uptake on the bone scan. After approximately seven days both lesions will show decreased activity on a marrow scan and increased activity on a bone scan.

Variants

In addition to occurring in the homozygous state, either the thalassemia or sickle cell gene may occur in combination with HbA (the trait or carrier), with one another, or with some other abnormal hemoglobin. Hemoglobin SC disease and hemoglobin S–thalassemia disease may be associated with the radiographic changes of both marrow proliferation and ischemia. The thalassemia gene in combination with hemoglobin E or Lepore may be associated with changes that are indistinguishable from thalassemia major. When this gene is in combination with hemoglobin A, C, or H, the radiographic changes are usually minimal or absent, as are the changes associated with the sickle cell trait.

Bibliography

Bohrer SP: Acute long bone diaphyseal infarcts in sickle cell disease. Br J Radiol 43:685–697, 1970.
Cooley TB, Witwer ER, Lee P: Anemia in children with splenomegaly and peculiar changes in bones. Am J Dis Child 34:347–363, 1927.
Currarino G, Erlandson ME: Premature fusion at the epiphyses in Cooley's anemia. Radiology 83:656–664, 1964.
Herrick JB: Peculiar elongated and sickle shaped red blood corpuscles in a case of severe anemia. Arch Intern Med 6:517–522, 1910.
Lawson JP, Ablow RC, Pearson HA: The ribs in thalassemia: I. The relationship to therapy. Radiology 140:663–672, 1981.
Lawson JP, Ablow RC, Pearson HA: The ribs in thalassemia: II. The pathogenesis of the changes. Radiology 140:673–679, 1981.

MYELOPROLIFERATIVE DISORDERS

NANCY S. ROSENFIELD

BONE LESIONS IN LEUKEMIA

Incidence. Acute lymphocytic and acute undifferentiated leukemias are the most common malignancies of childhood. The skeletal lesions of childhood leukemia were described in 1948 by Silverman in a classic paper. Bone lesions are seen more frequently in leukemic children than in adults and are more common in younger children than in older ones. Studies have found no correlation among the cell type of the leukemia, the age or sex of the patient, and the presence of bone lesions on radiography. Some reports found no correlation between the presence of bone pain and the existence of radiologic bone lesions and reported that cortical or periosteal radiologic lesions occur three times more frequently in patients with severe bone pain. In other studies, there was no correlation between the presence of bone pain and the existence or site of radiographic lesions. This is presumably because small pain-causing bone lesions may not be demonstrable radiologically. It has been found that the presence of bone lesions in a child with leukemia does not influence the prognosis of that child.

In series of children with leukemia, bone involvement has been reported in 21 to 100 per cent at the time of diagnosis. The bone lesions appeared as early as four weeks after the onset of symptoms and became more numerous as the disease progressed.

Radiographic Findings Before Treatment

Four pretreatment bone lesions are seen: (1) leukemic lines (transverse bands of decreased density); (2) generalized and focal osteoporosis; (3) subperiosteal new bone formation; (4) osteosclerosis.

The classic "leukemic line" is the most common bone lesion seen in children with leukemia. These bands of decreased density are seen most readily at the knee, where most rapid growth takes place, but they may be seen at all metaphyses. Under age two, these lines are not specific for leukemia and have been seen in children with neuroblastoma, scurvy, and chronic conditions such as juvenile rheumatoid arthritis and generalized sepsis. When seen in a child who is over age two, the line is virtually pathognomonic for leukemia and may help to distinguish leukemia from aplastic anemia (Fig. 96–5).

Another common radiologic finding in the bones of leukemic children is generalized osteoporosis. Wide-spread vertebral body collapse has been seen in the severe osteoporosis that may precede clinical diagnosis of leukemia. When these children go into hema-

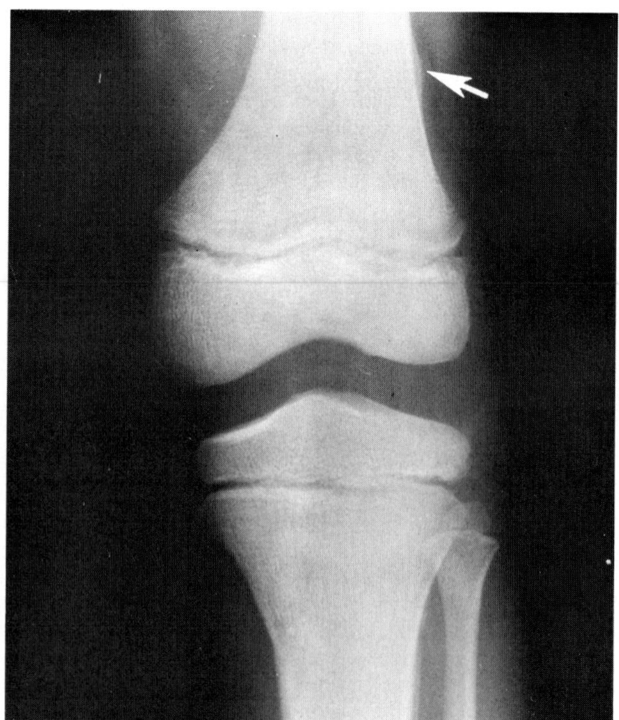

Figure 96–5. Classic "leukemic line." The femoral and tibial metaphyses of a child with newly diagnosed leukemia contain a transverse line of decreased density. Periosteal new bone formation *(arrow)* is also noted.

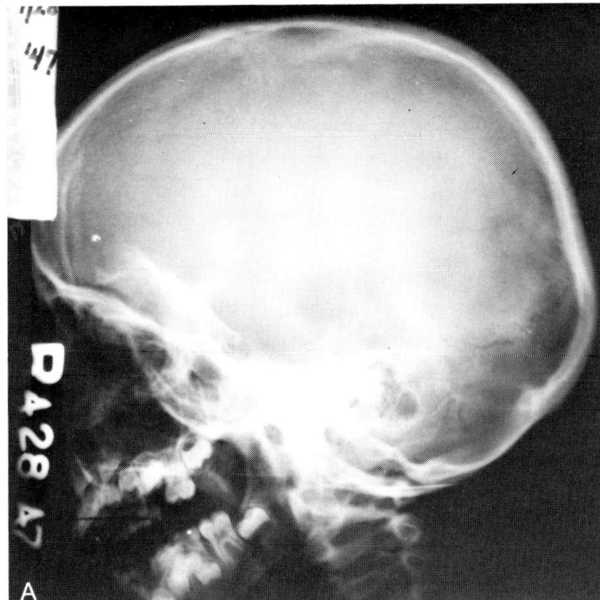

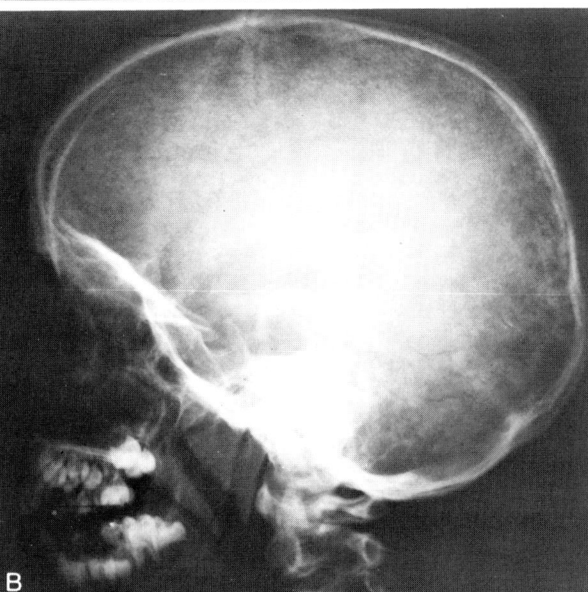

Figure 96–6. Osteoporosis. *A,* Normal skull radiograph in a seven-year-old boy. *B,* The same child's skull, 10 months later, at the time of diagnosis of leukemia. Demineralization is present. (Reproduced from Rosenfield N: The Radiology of Childhood Leukemia and Its Therapy. St. Louis, Warren H. Green Inc, 1982, with permission from the author and publisher.)

tologic remission, they often have relief of their back pain, but radiologic evidence of healing is rare (Fig. 96–6).

Focal osteolytic areas that mimic neuroblastoma metastases may be seen. This is the most common bone lesion seen radiographically in infants under one year of age and also in adults with leukemia (Fig. 96–7).

Periosteal new bone formation may be smooth or irregular when seen in association with leukemia and may be due to actual leukemic cells infiltrating under the periosteum or to subperiosteal bleeding (see Fig. 96–5). Osteosclerosis is a late bone manifestation of childhood leukemia, and although it was described in early reports, it is very rarely seen today.

MRI may be used to study the bone marrow in children with leukemia. Dr. Mervyn Cohen was the first to do this, with a recent excellent study from Babies Hospital in New York. The T_1 relaxation time is prolonged when leukemia cells have infiltrated the marrow, and there may be a bright marrow signal on T_2-weighted scans (Fig. 96–8).

Histology of Bone Lesions

In some leukemic children, in areas in which radiographic leukemia lines were seen, autopsy bone specimens of these metaphyseal areas revealed leukemic cells. Perhaps that accounts for the fact that metaphyseal lucent bands are seen more commonly in leukemic children than in adults because in children, there is more marrow-bearing bone, and replacement of normal marrow cells by leukemia cells would be visible at an earlier stage. However, in other patients, the areas corresponding to the metaphyseal lucent bands were found to show only demineralization with thin trabeculae. This explains the occasional appearance of the "leukemic line" in other disease entities because the line is probably due to a generalized disturbance of enchondral bone formation.

In areas of bone in which periosteal new bone formation was seen on a radiograph, histologic examination has shown leukemic cells under the periosteum. In areas of bone in which there was generalized osteoporosis on radiography, histologic examination has shown a reduction in the size and number of trabeculae with an enlargement of the haversian and Volkmann's canals. In the presence of patchy lytic foci in the bones, enlargement of these canals was found as well as leukemic infiltration of bone.

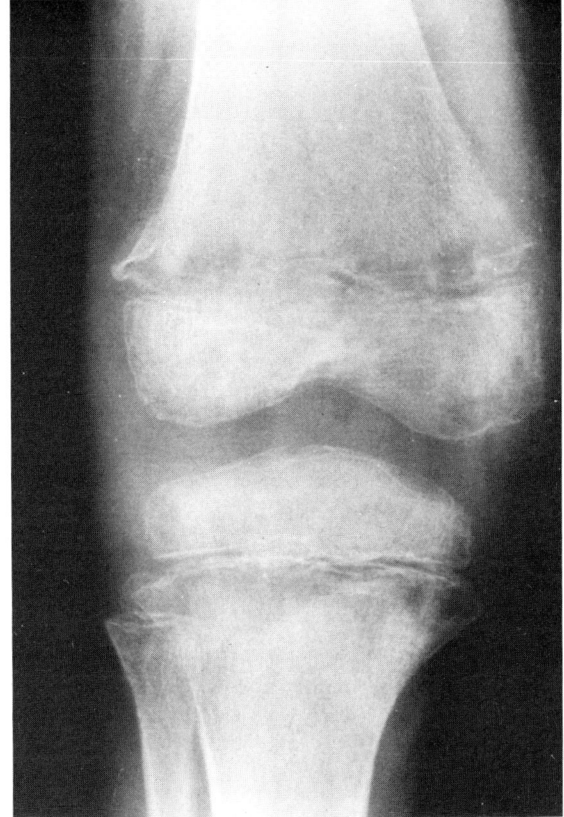

Figure 96–7. Patchy osteolysis. Focal areas of bone destruction in the knee of an eight-year-old child with newly diagnosed leukemia. (Reproduced from Rosenfield N: The Radiology of Childhood Leukemia and Its Therapy. St. Louis, Warren H. Green Inc, 1982, with permssion from the author and publisher.)

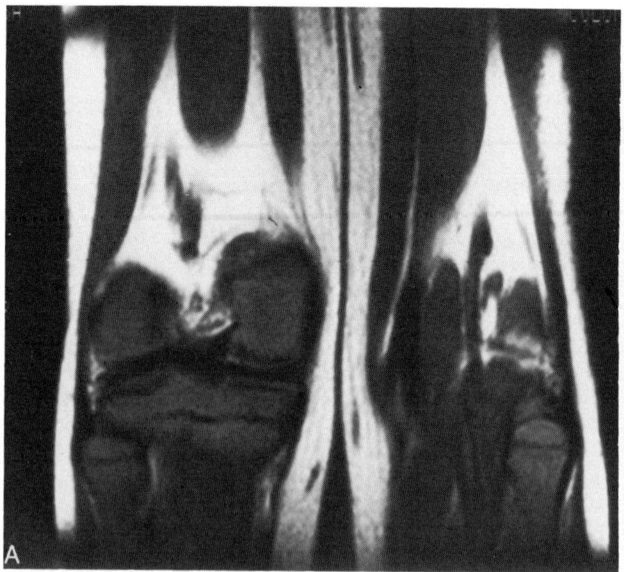

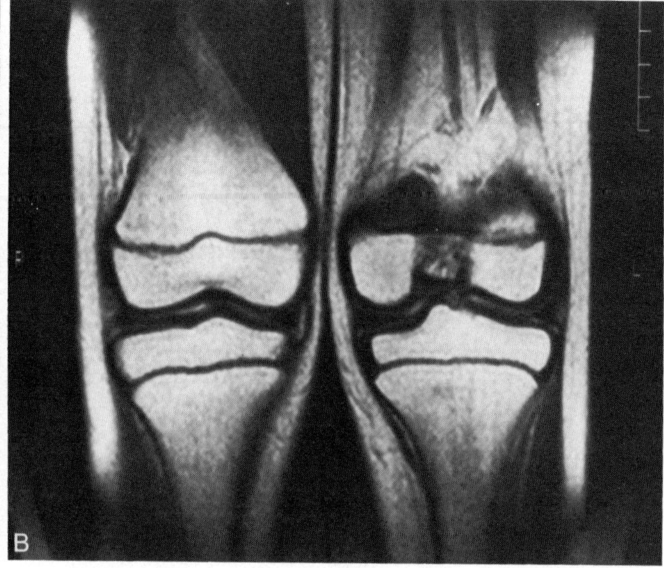

Figure 96–8. *A,* T_1-weighted MRI scan of the knees of a child with **leukemia.** The normal bright marrow signal is not seen. *B,* T_2-weighted scan of the same child. The marrow signal is unusually bright. (From Ruzal-Shapiro C, et al: MR imaging of diffuse bone marrow replacement in pediatric patients with cancer. Radiology 181:587–589, 1991.)

The rarely seen sclerotic changes may be due to necrosis of trabecular bone, with increase in marrow connective tissue, or to reactive bone formation in response to the leukemia along with some bone infarction.

Therapy and Prognosis

As recently as 1967, the prognosis for children with acute leukemia was grim. After years of modern treatment regimens, more than 50 per cent of such children remain disease-free and are potentially cured.

Induction of remission of leukemia is accomplished with a combination of chemotherapeutic drugs, usually prednisone and vincristine. Once remission is achieved, other drugs are used to maintain it, usually 6-mercaptopurine and methotrexate. There is periodic reinduction with vincristine and prednisone every six months.

Bone Changes After Treatment

Silverman reported the reversibility of leukemic bone changes during treatment with folic acid inhibitors over 30 years ago. He found that when "leukemic lines" were present at the time of diagnosis, the lesions regressed during periods of hematologic remission. In a study of serial knee radiographs of children with leukemia, radiographs were taken at the time of diagnosis and every six months during treatment. In 10 of 58 children, bone abnormalities were found at the time of diagnosis and persisted for as long as 10 months after therapy was initiated. All of these children went into hematologic remission, and in all of them the bone lesions were seen to fade gradually.

There have been two reports of the reappearance of leukemic bone lesions in children who had hematologic relapse of their leukemia. However, these bone changes reappeared quite late in the relapse. Rosenfield and McIntosh found that children on the modern treatment regimen for leukemia did not have reappearance of their "leukemic lines" before or at the time of hematologic relapse. Therefore, the bone changes of leukemia could not be used to predict the likelihood of occurrence of relapse.

Silverman reported transverse bands of increased density in the metaphyses of long bones of leukemic children treated with aminopterin. The 1977 series of Rosenfield and McIntosh found that 20 of the 58 children studied developed dense metaphyses during treatment. The fibular metaphysis, which is not usually dense in growing children, was also quite dense, simulating the appearance of lead poisoning (Fig. 96–9). The dense bands seen in the metaphyses of treated children have been thought to result from chemotherapy-related changes in enchondral bone formation. However, dense bands have also been reported in one patient who exhibited a spontaneous remission of leukemia and in another untreated patient. The dense bands have been found to become less prominent with prolonged survival. Rosenfield and McIntosh found that the bands gradually faded from 6 to 24 months after their initial appearance.

Fifty per cent of leukemic children were found to have growth arrest lines in one study. These thick strands of bone trabeculae are seen in patients who are ill from any cause and are therefore nonspecific. Rosenfield and McIntosh reported the appearance of one growth arrest line at the time of each elective reinduction of leukemia. These lines then moved up the shaft of the bone as subsequent new lines were formed. The lines were found to fade gradually.

Dr. Sheila Moore has used the calculated T_1 from spine MRI to predict the recurrence of leukemia in the bone marrow.

LYMPHOMA

Hodgkin's Disease

Incidence. In the United States, Hodgkin's disease and non-Hodgkin's lymphoma account for 10 per cent of malignancy in children. The prognosis of Hodgkin's disease is gradually improving, and the vast majority of children do well. One rarely sees Hodgkin's disease in a child under one year of age, and its peak incidence is in young adulthood. It is more common in boys. Most children with Hodgkin's disease present with cervical lymphadenopathy. Other lymph nodes may also be involved, as may the liver, spleen, lung, pleura, and bone marrow. Kidney, heart, and bone lesions are rare in newly diagnosed Hodgkin's disease in children.

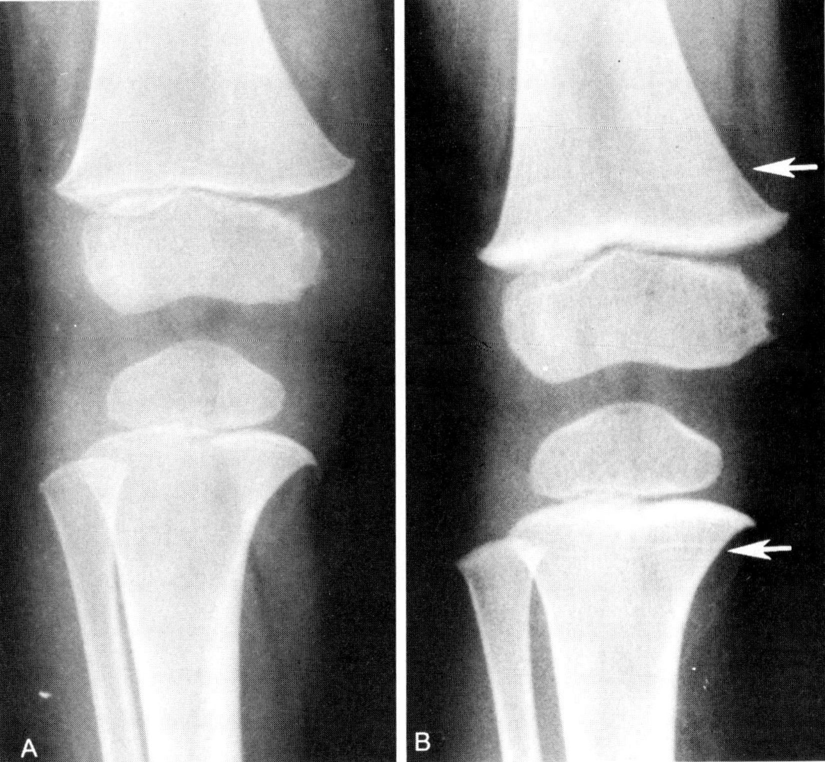

Figure 96–9. Bone changes after treatment. *A,* The knee of a two-year-old child at the time of initial remission of leukemia. *B,* The knee of the same child, six months later, during treatment. Growth arrest lines *(arrows)* are seen. The metaphyses are dense. (Reproduced from Rosenfield N: The Radiology of Childhood Leukemia and Its Therapy. St. Louis, Warren H. Green Inc, 1982, with permission from the author and publisher.)

Radiographic Findings of Bone in Hodgkin's Disease

Skeletal lesions have been found in only 1 to 5 per cent of children at the time of diagnosis of Hodgkin's disease. The lesions have been seen in the pelvis and thoracic and lumbar spine. Bone lesions are rarely seen at the time of relapse of Hodgkin's disease. These lesions appear the same on radiographs as those in newly diagnosed patients.

The radiographic findings are usually lytic bone lesions with accompanying periosteal new bone formation (Fig. 96–10). Occasionally osteoblastic lesions are seen; classically "ivory vertebrae" in the spine are seen (Fig. 96–11). Soft-tissue tumors have been reported to grow into the sternum.

Osseous Histology in Hodgkin's Disease

Osteolytic lesions usually are the result of continuous spread from involved marrow rather than hematogenous metastasis. Hodgkin's disease may be found in histology sections of osteoblastic

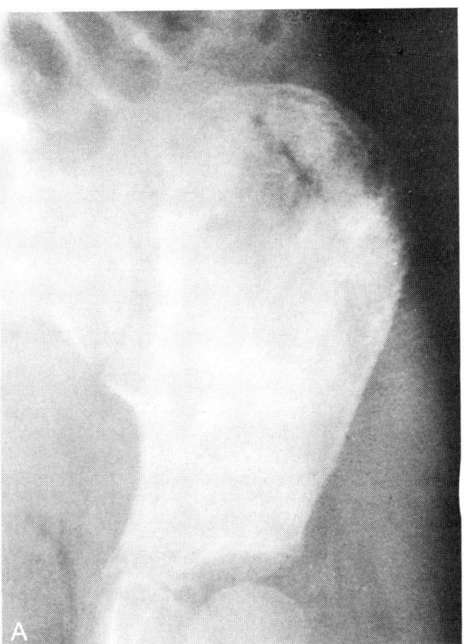

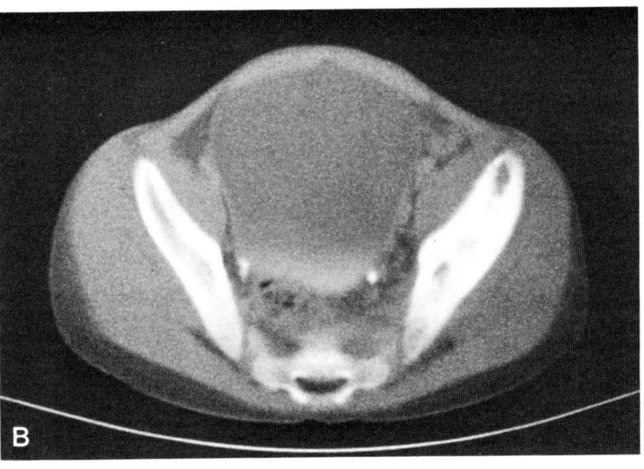

Figure 96–10. Hodgkin's disease of bone. Mixed lytic and sclerotic lesion of the iliac bone in a young boy. *A,* Radiograph. *B,* CT scan.

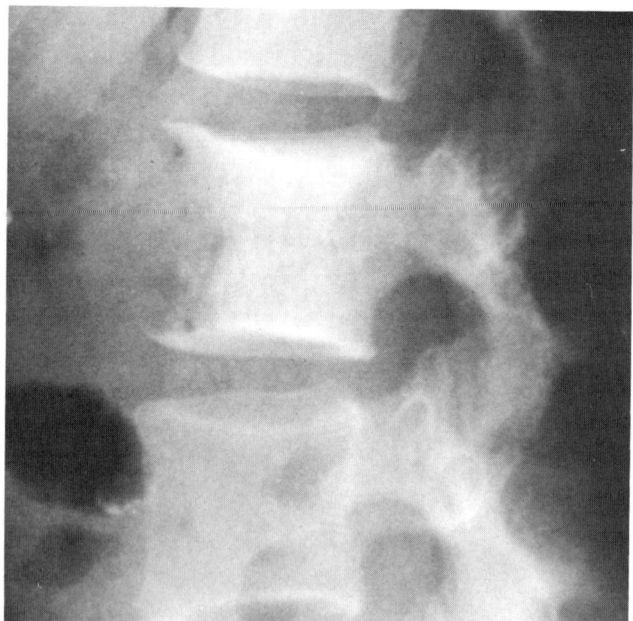

Figure 96–11. "Ivory vertebra" at L3 in a young woman with Hodgkin's disease. An anterior destructive lesion is also evident.

bone, but more commonly there is stimulation of bone formation by soft-tissue lesions near the involved bone. Myelofibrosis caused by bone infiltration may cause diffusely dense bones.

Non-Hodgkin's Lymphoma

INCIDENCE. The childhood "non-Hodgkin's lymphomas" are a mixed group of disorders that are rapidly progressive and have a high mortality rate. More males are affected than females.

CLINICAL MANIFESTATIONS. In children, most tumors originate in lymphomatous tissue. The GI tract, mediastinum, central nervous system, and bone may be involved.

RADIOGRAPHIC FINDINGS. Destructive lesions of the mandible and sinuses are not uncommonly seen in children, particularly in Burkitt's lymphoma. Other bones of the face may be affected as well. About 20 per cent of newly diagnosed non-Hodgkin's lymphoma patients have bone lesions on radiographs. Adults have a very low incidence of bone lesions. These lesions are usually symptomatic and are radiographically nonspecific. They are usually lytic, mottled, and moth-eaten. Blastic lesions are also seen.

Diffuse Histiocytic Lymphoma

Isolated lymphomatous bone lesions may also be seen. This tumor is the third most common primary malignant tumor of childhood. The children present with pain and swelling. It is more common in males than in females. Fifty per cent of patients with this diagnosis are under 40 years of age, 7 per cent under 20 years of age, and 2 per cent under 10 years of age. Lesions in the long bones are most common, although they can occur anywhere in the skeleton. Forty to 50 per cent occur in the lower femur and upper tibia. Pathologic fractures may be found in 18 to 21 per cent of these cases, and the tumor may also develop in an area of chronic osteomyelitis. The prognosis for this tumor is better than that for any other primary malignant bone tumor.

PATHOLOGY. The tumor usually involves a large portion of the long bone and extends into the soft tissues. Reactive sclerosis of the bone is common.

RADIOGRAPHIC FINDINGS. Isolated lymphomatous bone lesions classically show a combination of bone destruction and reactive change. There is a permeative destructive pattern with ill-defined margins. Occasionally sclerosis is the predominant feature, causing thick periosteal new bone formation. The medullary canal may be narrowed. The soft-tissue component may be seen on radiographs, but it rarely calcifies. Pathologic fractures may be seen. Case reports have described a relatively "benign" appearance of this tumor and a "bubbly" appearance.

MASTOCYTOSIS

INCIDENCE. Mastocytosis is a disease characterized by mast cell infiltration of a number of organs. It is also called urticaria pigmentosa. In young children, there is a benign form characterized by skin involvement alone. Rarely, mastocytosis may progress to the systemic form. In the adult-onset type of the disease, 50 per cent of the patients have the systemic form, and there is a fatal outcome in 30 per cent. Bone is frequently involved in systemic mastocytosis.

RADIOGRAPHIC FINDINGS. Bone lesions of mastocytosis are radiographically either mixed lytic and sclerotic or diffusely osteoporotic. The latter type, which may include pathologic features, is rare in the United States. The lytic and sclerotic lesions are most commonly found in the central skeleton and at the ends of the long bones. There may be coarse trabeculae interspersed with small osteoporotic areas, giving a "cystic" appearance. The lesions are usually asymptomatic (Fig. 96–12).

A characteristic appearance of mastocytosis on ^{99m}Tc-phosphate bone scan has been reported. The scintigraphs show markedly in-

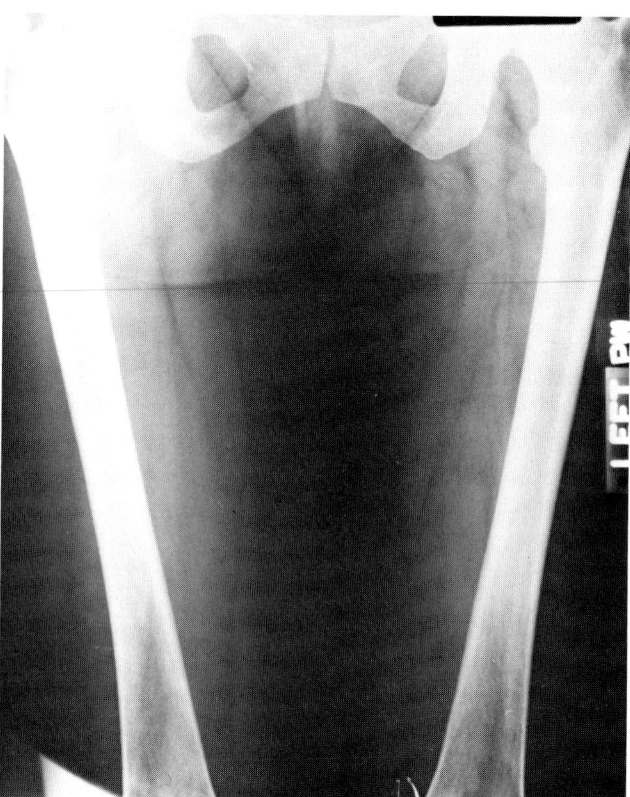

Figure 96–12. Mixed lytic and sclerotic lesions in a 29-year-old woman with mastocytosis.

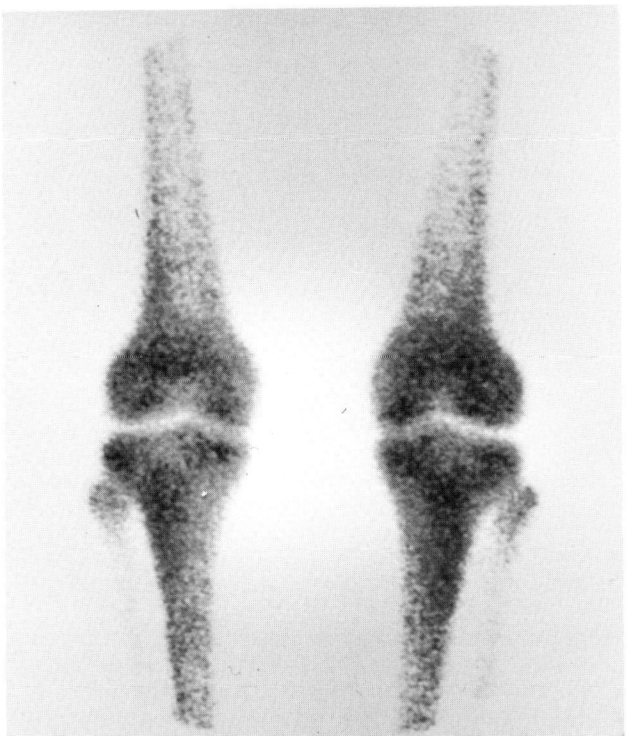

Figure 96–13. "Superscan." Increased bone uptake of ^{99m}Tc phosphate in a 45-year-old man with mastocytosis.

creased bone activity ("superscan") (Fig. 96–13). Gallium scans have also been reported to show increased bone activity.

HISTOLOGY. A large portion of the patients with systemic mastocytosis have bone marrow infiltration by mast cells. The lytic bone lesions have been found to be due to collections of mast cells (granulomata) in the bone marrow and hyperplasia of marrow elements. Sclerotic reaction may be due to mast cell enzymes or to the effect of circulating histamine.

MYELOFIBROSIS

Myelofibrosis is an uncommon disorder of unknown etiology that is characterized by fibrosis of the bone marrow and extension of hematopoiesis into areas usually not involved. It has also been known as myelosclerosis and agnogenic myeloid metaplasia.

In general, this is a disease of middle-aged and elderly men and women who present with generalized symptoms of malaise. They may have bone pain, but this is uncommon. The prognosis is variable, but ultimately the disorder is fatal. The patient develops a profound anemia, and death comes from anemia or infection. In some cases leukemia may develop owing to abnormal proliferation of the remaining marrow elements. The role of radiation therapy in treating this disorder is not certain.

RADIOGRAPHIC FINDINGS. This disorder usually affects the spine, pelvis, skull and ribs, humerus, and femur. Extramedullary hematopoiesis may also be seen as soft-tissue masses. About 40 per cent of patients who have myelofibrosis have radiographic abnormalities. As fibrosis overtakes the bone marrow, one sees areas of sclerosis with coarse trabeculae and thick cortices. Osteolytic lesions are rare.

HISTOLOGY. The dense areas seen on radiography correspond histologically to myeloid fibrosis and atrophy. The medullary architecture of the bone is obliterated. The marrow is incapable of maturation to normal blood cells.

Bibliography

Bone Lesions in Leukemia

Aur RJA, Westbrook HW, Riggs W Jr: Childhood acute lymphocytic leukemia. Am J Dis Child 124:653–654, 1972.

Baty JM, Vogt EC: Bone changes of leukemia in children. AJR 34:310–313, 1935.

Benz G, Brandeis WE, Willich E: Radiological aspects of leukemia in childhood. An analysis of 89 children. Pediatr Radiol 4:201–213, 1976.

Brunner S, Gudbjerg CE, Iversen T: Skeletal lesions in leukemia in children. Acta Radiol 49:419–424, 1958.

Cohen MD, Klatte EC, Bachner R, et al. Magnetic resonance imaging of bone marrow disease in children. Radiology 151:715–718, 1984.

Dresner E: The bone and joint lesions in acute leukemia and their response to folic acid antagonists. Q J Med 29:339–351, 1950.

Epstein BS: Vertebral changes in childhood leukemia. Radiology 68:65–69, 1957.

Erb IH: Bone changes in leukemia: Pathology. Arch Dis Child 9:319–326, 1934.

Frei E III, Sallan SE: Acute lymphoblastic leukemia: Treatment. Cancer 42:828–838, 1978.

Griffiths D: Bone changes and blood diseases. In Wilkinson JF (ed): Modern Trends in Blood Disease. London, Butterworth, 1955, pp 1–21.

Karpinski FE, Martin JF: The skeletal lesions of leukemic children treated with aminopterin. J Pediatr 37:208–223, 1950.

Lightwood R, Barrie H, Butler N: Observations on 100 cases of leukemia in childhood. Br Med J 5175:747–752, 1960.

Moore SG, Gooding CA, Brasch RC, et al: Bone marrow in children with acute lymphocytic leukemia: MR relaxation times. Radiology 160:237–240, 1986.

Newman AJ, Melhorn DK: Vertebral compression in childhood leukemia. Am J Dis Child 125:863–865, 1973.

Nixon GW, Gwinn JL: The roentgen manifestations of leukemia in infancy. Radiology 107:603–609, 1973.

Pinkel D: Treatment of acute leukemia. Pediatr Clin North Am 23:117–130, 1976.

Rosenfield NS, McIntosh S: Prospective analysis of bone changes in treated childhood leukemia. Radiology 123:413–415, 1977.

Ruzal-Shapiro C, Berdon WE, Cohen MD, Abramson SJ: MR imaging of diffuse bone marrow replacement in pediatric patients with cancer. Radiology 18:587–589, 1991.

Shackelford GD, Bloomberg G, McAlister WH: The value of roentgenography in differentiating aplastic anemia from leukemia masquerading as aplastic anemia. AJR 116:651–654, 1972.

Silverman FN: The skeletal lesions in leukemia. Clinical and roentgenographic observations in 103 infants and children, with a review of the literature. AJR 59:819–844, 1948.

Silverman FN: Treatment of leukemia and allied disorders with folic acid antagonists; effect of aminopterin on skeletal lesions. Radiology 54:665–678, 1950.

Simmons CR, Harle TS, Singleton EB: The osseous manifestations of leukemia in children. Radiol Clin North Am 6:115–130, 1968.

Snelling CE, Brown A: Bone changes in leukemia. Am J Dis Child 49:810–812, 1935.

Thomas LB, Fornker CE Jr, Frei E III, et al: The skeletal lesions of acute leukemia. Cancer 14:608–621, 1961.

Wilson JKV: The bone lesions of childhood leukemia. Radiology 72:672–681, 1959.

Lymphoma

Castellino RA, Parker BR: Non-Hodgkin's lymphoma. In Parker BR, Castellino RA (eds): Pediatric Oncologic Radiology. St. Louis, CV Mosby, 1977.

Parker BR, Castellino RA: Hodgkin's disease. In Parker BR, Castellino RA (eds): Pediatric Oncologic Radiology. St. Louis, CV Mosby, 1977.

Raymond HK, Unni KK: Case report: Primary non-Hodgkin's lymphoma of bone. Skel Radiol 8:153, 1982.

Rodman E, Raymond AK, Philips WC: Case report: Primary lymphoma of bone. Skel Radiol 8:235, 1982.

Sherman CS, Wolfson SL: Roentgen diagnosis of lymphosarcoma and reticulum cell sarcoma in infancy and childhood. AJR 86:693, 1961.

Stark P: Invasion of the sternum by lymphoma—role of CT. Radiology 24:130, 1984.

Steinbach HL, Parker BR: Primary bone tumors. In Parker BR, Castellino RA (eds): Pediatric Oncologic Radiology. St. Louis, CV Mosby, 1977.

Mastocytosis

Ensslen R, Jackson F, Reid A: Bone and gallium scans in mastocytosis: Correlation with count rates, radiography and microscopy. J Nucl Med 24:586–588, 1983.

Rafii M, Firooznia H, Golimbu C, Balthazar E: Pathologic fracture in systemic mastocytosis. Clin Orthop 180:260–267, 1983.

Myelofibrosis

Aegerter E, Kirkpatrick JA: Orthopedic Disorders. Philadelphia, WB Saunders Company, 1975.

Leimert JT, Armitage JO, Dick FR: Myeloid metaplasia and osteolytic lesions. Am J Clin Pathol 70:706–708, 1978.

Resnick D: Myeloproliferative disorders. In Resnick D, Niwayama G (eds): Diagnosis of Bone and Joint Disorders. Philadelphia, WB Saunders Company, 1981.

BLEEDING DISORDERS

PAMELA S. JENSEN

Skeletal abnormalities due to intra-articular and intraosseous hemorrhage are most commonly seen with two forms of hemophilia: classic hemophilia A, due to a deficiency of or defect in antihemophilic factor (Factor VIII), and hemophilia B, also known as Christmas disease, which is due to a deficiency of plasma thromboplastic component (Factor IX). These are both sex-linked, recessive diseases in which women are carriers and men are affected. Clinical manifestations are variable and correlate with the level of factor VIII or IX activity. Gastrointestinal and genitourinary bleeding, hemorrhage into the soft tissues and retroperitoneum, and hemarthrosis are typical manifestations. Children and adolescents experience the greatest frequency of hemarthrosis, probably associated with their increased level of physical activity. Characteristically, joints most susceptible to trauma are affected, the knee most commonly, followed by the elbow, ankle, hip, and shoulder.

Pathophysiology

Recurrent bleeding into a joint results in absorption of hemosiderin by the synovial membrane. This in turn leads to synovial proliferation and increased vascularity. Granulation tissue may then form in the synovium and adjacent soft-tissue structures. Pannus can form over the articular cartilage, following which cartilage loss ensues. Subchondral bone becomes osteoporotic, and osseous cystic lesions commonly appear. Communication between these bone cysts and the joint cavity is common. Late joint changes include the complete loss of articular cartilage and associated deformity. Hemophilic pseudotumors occur when there is massive hemorrhage under the periosteum, at muscle attachments, within the medullary cavity of the bone, or in the soft tissues.

Radiographic Manifestations

Initially, hemorrhage into the joint or soft tissues is manifest as a joint effusion or tissue swelling. The effusion may appear quite dense owing to the presence of hemosiderin (Fig. 96–14). Hyperemia can lead to periarticular osteoporosis, and in young children bony enlargement or overgrowth of the affected epiphysis occurs (Fig. 96–15). Recurrent episodes of bleeding initially may lead to irregular bone erosion and subchondral cyst formation (Fig. 96–16). Ultimately, cartilage destruction may occur, leading to joint space loss. Should the process continue to progress to the end stage, considerable deformity occurs owing to abnormal growth of the epiphysis, complete cartilage loss, extensive bony erosion, and cyst formation (Fig. 96–17). Contractures may develop, but despite the extensive cartilage loss bony ankylosis is uncommon.

Other complications include osteonecrosis, fracture of the osteoporotic bone, soft-tissue ossifications, and (rarely detected) chondrocalcinosis. Hemophilic pseudotumors occur infrequently and most often affect the femur or iliac wing. Before factor concentrates were available, these pseudotumors could reach prodigious proportions. The periosteum in a child is readily separated from the cortex by an intervening collection of blood. New bone forms in the outer edge of the expanded periosteum, leading to the radiographic appearance of a tumor mass. Pressure erosion of the underlying cortical bone can also occur. Intraosseous hemorrhage may produce well-demarcated radiolucent lesions within the medullary canal or may cause expansion of the bone. Extension into the subperiosteal space and the soft tissue may follow. Computed tomography is very helpful in demonstrating the extent of the lesion and its relationship to the various tissues involved.

Diagnosis of a hemophilic pseudotumor is usually not difficult in a patient whose underlying disease is known. Differential diagnosis includes malignancy and infection. The articular manifestations of hemophilia most closely resemble those of juvenile rheumatoid arthritis (JRA). When only the knee is involved, it is not possible to distinguish between these two entities on the basis of the radiographic manifestations alone. With multiple joint involvement, the typical distribution of hemophilia (knee, elbow, ankle) distinguishes it from JRA, in which the hands and wrists as well as the spine are also often involved.

Therapy

Good results with replacement of the deficient factor (VIII or IX) can be achieved, thereby preventing many of the late-stage compli-

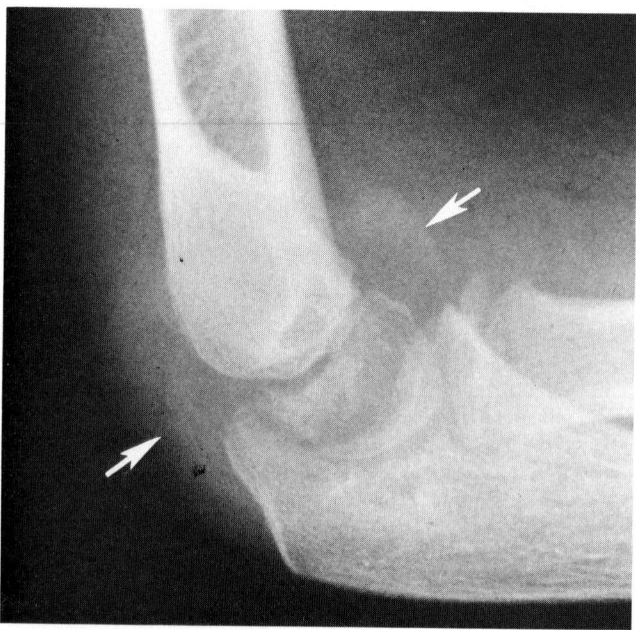

Figure 96–14. Hemophilia. Lateral view of the elbow demonstrates an effusion *(arrows),* which is increased in density owing to the presence of hemosiderin in the blood.

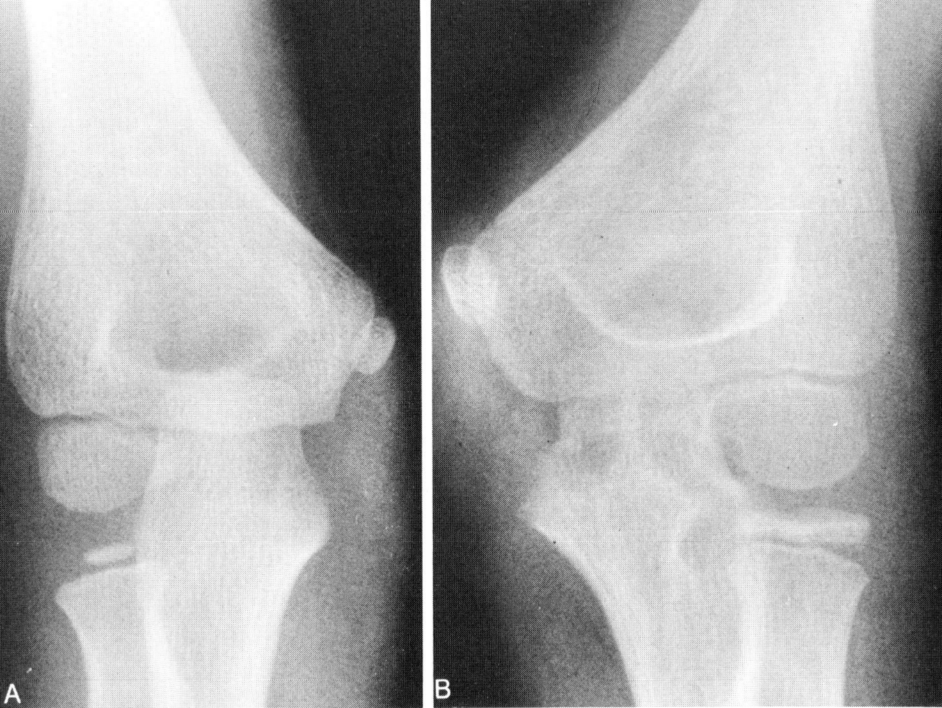

Figure 96–15. Hemophilia. *A,* Normal right elbow. *B,* Recurrent hemarthroses in the elbow of a nine-year-old boy have led to enlargement of the epiphyses and advancement of the bone age (compare with *A*). Erosive lesions are present in the olecranon fossa of the ulna.

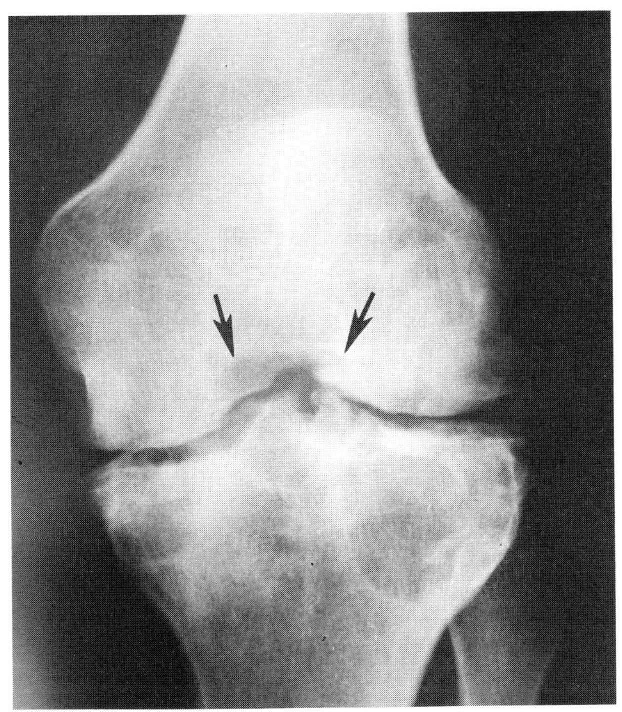

Figure 96–16. Characteristic features in the knee include cartilage space narrowing, irregular erosion of the articular surfaces, widening of the intercondylar notch of the femur *(arrows)*, presence of multiple cysts, and osteoporosis. The other knee and both elbows were also involved.

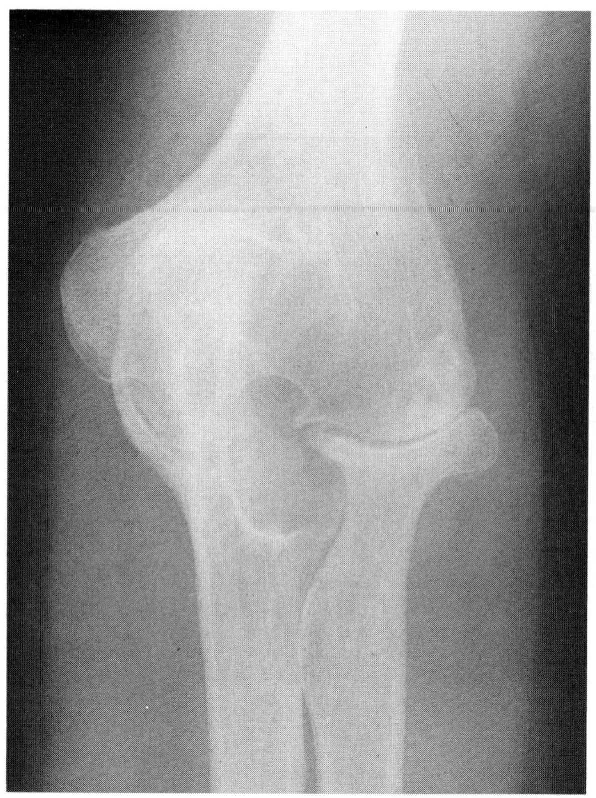

Figure 96–17. Hemophilia. Advanced changes in the elbow include marked cartilage space loss, deformity of the proximal ulna and radial head, erosion of the intercondylar area of the humerus and the olecranon fossa, and osteoporosis.

cations of hemophilia. Hemarthrosis can be successfully treated by limited transfusion early in the course of the episode. Patients requiring repeated transfusions and blood replacement due to hemorrhage are at risk for contracting hepatitis B. The recent possibility of developing acquired immune deficiency syndrome (AIDS) has led some hemophiliacs to refuse transfusion therapy, thereby leading to an increase in the incidence of the more severe complications. A new potentially effective therapy may be the administration of the androgenic steroid danazol, which has raised the levels of Factors VIII and IX in patients with classic hemophilia and Christmas disease, respectively.

Bibliography

Arnold WD, Hilgartner MW: Hemophilic arthropathy. Current concepts of pathogenesis and management. J Bone Joint Surg 59A:287, 1977.

Jensen PS, Putman CE: Hemophilic pseudotumor. Diagnosis, treatment and complications. Am J Dis Child 129:717, 1975.

Johnson JB, Davis TW, Bullock WH: Bone and joint changes in hemophilia. Radiology 63:64, 1954.

MULTICENTRIC RETICULOHISTIOCYTOSIS

PAMELA S. JENSEN

Proliferation of histiocytes in the skin, subcutaneous tissues, mucosa, and synovium characterizes multicentric reticulohistiocytosis. Of unknown etiology, this uncommon condition affecting adults has been called by a number of other terms, including lipoid dermatoarthritis and reticulohistiocytoma. Polyarthritis or the development of skin nodules is typically the initial manifestation of this disorder. Joint manifestations are characteristically symmetrical and most commonly involve the interphalangeal joints of the hands. Other joints involved are similar to those affected in rheumatoid arthritis, including the knees, shoulders, wrists, hips, ankles, feet, elbows, spine including the atlantoaxial joint, and the temporomandibular joints. The clinical findings of soft-tissue swelling, stiffness, and tenderness also resemble rheumatoid arthritis. In contrast to rheumatoid arthritis, multicentric reticulohistiocytosis has a much greater predilection for the distal interphalangeal joints of the hand, and joint space loss and periarticular osteoporosis are not typical early findings. Diagnosis can be established by biopsy of a skin or subcutaneous nodule.

Radiographic Manifestations

The erosive lesions of multicentric reticulohistiocytosis begin at the margins of the joint and spread centrally, producing separation of the articular surfaces. This is not accompanied by juxta-articular demineralization or periosteal new bone formation. Nodules can often be identified in the soft tissues. Progression of the disease to arthritis mutilans is much more common in multicentric reticulohistiocytosis than in rheumatoid arthritis. Atlantoaxial subluxation and severe destructive changes in the spine can occur early. Differential diagnosis includes rheumatoid arthritis, psoriasis, erosive osteoarthritis, and hyperuricemic gout.

Bibliography

Gold RH, Metzger AL, Mirra JM, et al: Multicentric reticulocytosis (lipoid dermatoarthritis). An erosive polyarthritis with distinctive clinical, roentgenographic, and pathologic features. AJR 124:610, 1975.

Mickelson MR, Bonfiglio M: Eosinophilic granuloma and its variations. Orthop Clin North Am 8:933, 1977.

97 Endocrine Disorders

PITUITARY

ROBERT A. LEVINE,
ROBERT A. GELFAND,
and PAMELA S. JENSEN

The pituitary gland is divided into two developmentally, anatomically, and functionally distinct parts: the anterior pituitary, or adenohypophysis, and the posterior pituitary, or neurohypophysis. The posterior pituitary is composed of the terminal portions of hypothalamic neurons. It stores and releases antidiuretic hormone (ADH) and oxytocin, which are synthesized in the hypothalamic neurons. ADH functions to conserve body water by allowing the formation of a concentrated urine. Oxytocin stimulates milk release in the lactating breast and contraction of the uterus at parturition. Although the anterior pituitary has no direct neural connection with the brain, blood from the hypothalamus flows down a portal venous system that surrounds the anterior pituitary. Hypothalamic neurons produce releasing and inhibiting hormones that flow through this portal system and regulate the secretion of anterior pituitary hormones. The anterior pituitary synthesizes, stores, and releases six well-characterized hormones: adrenocorticotropic hormone (ACTH), luteinizing hormone (LH), follicle-stimulating hormone (FSH), thyroid-stimulating hormone (TSH), growth hormone (GH), and prolactin.

ACTH is produced in response to hypothalamic corticotropin-releasing factor (CRF). There is a normal diurnal pattern of ACTH release, which is increased by stress and other stimuli and inhibited by feedback to the pituitary by serum cortisol. ACTH stimulates steroid hormone production by the adrenal cortex. TSH stimulates all phases of thyroid hormone synthesis and release. TSH production in turn is stimulated by hypothalamic thyrotropin-releasing hormone (TRH) and inhibited by circulating thyroid hormones.

The neuroendocrine control of LH and FSH has not been completely elucidated. Both LH and FSH are stimulated by hypothalamic gonadotropin-releasing hormone (GnRH). In the male, LH stimulates testosterone synthesis by the Leydig cells of the testes. FSH acts on Sertoli cells, promoting spermatogenesis. Circulating testosterone affects the pituitary, inhibiting further LH release, whereas "inhibin," a polypeptide produced by the testes, suppresses FSH release. In the female, LH stimulates ovulation and formation of the corpus luteum and FSH stimulates follicle development. Feedback inhibition of LH and FSH are far more complex in the female, influenced by duration of exposure, rate of change, and absolute levels of circulating estrogens and progestins.

Prolactin is a peptide hormone that acts along with other hormones to stimulate development of mammary glands and lactation. Unlike the other pituitary hormones, prolactin is primarily under inhibitory control by the hypothalamus. Prolactin-inhibitory factor appears to be dopamine.

PITUITARY TUMORS

Adenomas comprise over 90 per cent of all pituitary neoplasms. Pituitary tumors may be classified by their cells of origin, secretory capabilities, or size. Microadenomas are less than 10 mm in diameter, and all larger tumors are referred to as macroadenomas. The most common hormone produced is prolactin and may be due to a lactotroph cell tumor or a tumor of another cell type that blocks the transport of hypothalamic prolactin-inhibitory factor. Pituitary tumors also commonly produce ACTH and GH, but overproduction of TSH, LH, or FSH is exceedingly rare. Any pituitary tumor may cause hormone deficiencies by compression of surrounding normal tissue. Pituitary tumors are occasionally associated with parathyroid hyperplasia and pancreatic neoplasms in the multiple endocrine neoplasia syndrome, type 1.

Craniopharyngiomas are benign tumors that probably arise from remnants of Rathke's pouch. They most commonly appear above the sella turcica at the upper end of the pituitary stalk, but 10 per cent may arise directly from the anterior pituitary. Those arising above the sella may cause pressure on the anterior pituitary, but more commonly they compress the pituitary stalk and hypothalamus, resulting in deficiency of posterior pituitary hormones. About one half show characteristic calcification on radiography.

Skeletal abnormalities due to pituitary tumors may be manifest either by local effects on the sella turcica or by remote effects of

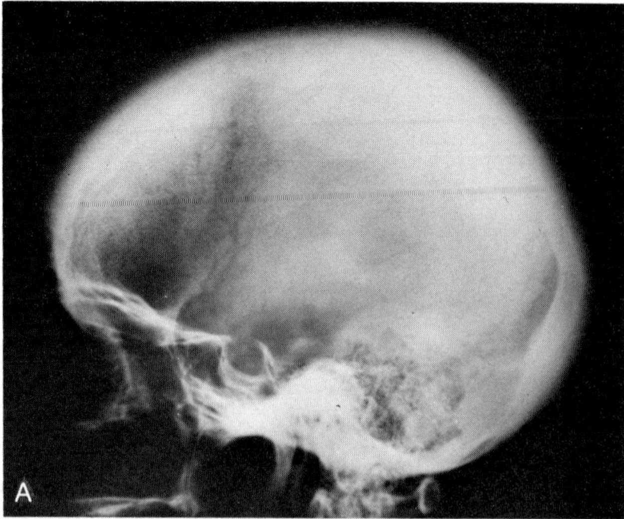

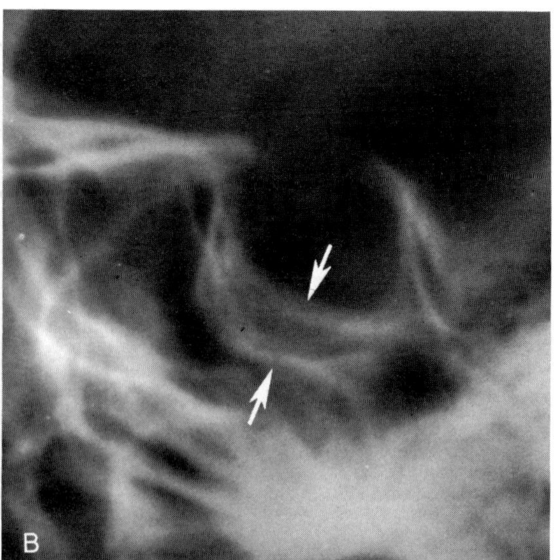

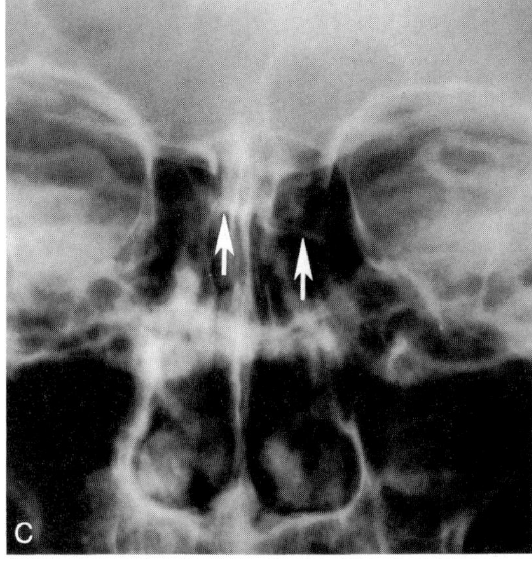

Figure 97–1. Acromegaly. *A,* Lateral view of the skull reveals an enlarged sella turcica and thickening of the calvarium. *B,* Lateral view of the sella turcica demonstrates a double floor *(arrows)* due to unequal expansion of the pituitary tumor. *C,* Frontal view of the sella also demonstrates the double floor *(arrows).*

pituitary hormone excess or deficiency. Pituitary tumors may cause enlargement of the sella turcica, distortion or disruption of its architecture, or, infrequently, intrasellar calcification. Many tumors erode the sella asymmetrically and produce the image of a double floor of the sella on skull radiographs (Fig. 97–1). Because conventional skull radiographs are often entirely normal in patients with pituitary adenomas, computed tomography or magnetic resonance imaging is necessary for complete structural evaluation of the pituitary.

ACROMEGALY AND GIGANTISM

Prior to puberty and the closure of the epiphyseal growth plates, hypersecretion of GH results in gigantism, characterized by excessive and accelerated linear growth. Hypersecretion of GH subsequent to epiphyseal closure produces the clinical syndrome of acromegaly. Gigantism can also occur with normal GH levels if insufficiency of gonadotrophic hormones delays epiphyseal closure, prolonging the period during which linear growth may occur.

Clinical Manifestations

Acromegaly occurs most commonly in the third and fourth decades and has an insidious onset and progression. Coarsening of the facial features and soft-tissue swelling of the hands and feet are among the earliest features. Other early signs include oiliness of the skin due to sebaceous gland hypersecretion, excessive sweating, and an increase in body hair. Headache is an extremely common symptom, occurring in approximately 80 per cent of patients. As the disease progresses the classic features appear. The skin thickens owing to connective tissue proliferation and development of interstitial edema. It becomes coarse and leathery, with prominent skin folds and occasionally increased pigmentation. Soft-tissue and bone changes give rise to the characteristic acromegalic facies. There is elongation of the mandible and prominence of the forehead, with growth of the frontal, nasal, and malar bones.

As the name acromegaly suggests (acral = extremity), enlargement of the hands and feet is characteristic. Acral bone thickening and soft-tissue swelling produce hands that are broad and spadelike, with thick fingers that have blunted ends. Overgrowth of bone and cartilage results in arthralgias and occasionally in severe deforming osteoarthritis. Lower back pain is a common complaint, and arthropathy of the larger joints frequently occurs. Carpal tunnel syndrome and other compressive neuropathies are common, but peripheral neuropathy may also result from GH-stimulated proliferation of perineural and endoneural connective tissue. Generalized visceromegaly occurs, and the kidneys, lungs, and liver may increase to over twice their normal size and weight. Organ enlargement is generally uniform and therefore not clinically apparent. Cardiomegaly is a common finding, and acromegalics have a higher incidence of hypertension. Although the existence of a distinct acromegalic cardiomyopathy is controversial, cardiovascular disease represents an important cause of increased mortality in untreated acromegaly. Abnormal glucose tolerance or even frank diabetes mellitus occurs in about one fourth of acromegalics owing to the insulin-antagonistic actions of GH. Decreased libido, amenorrhea, and impotence also occur commonly, most often due to prolactin hypersecretion.

Patients with gigantism frequently also manifest many of the characteristics of acromegaly. Prior to puberty, excess GH causes the bones to increase in length although normal proportions are maintained. In many cases appositional growth also occurs. Gigantism is more common in men but does occur in women. Growth continues until epiphyseal closure at puberty, with final height often being between seven and eight feet. The muscles and viscera increase in size in proportion to the height. If excess GH persists after puberty, further characteristics of acromegaly will appear in addition to the excess height already achieved. Although patients with gigantism may be unusually strong early in the course of the disease, as it progresses they are apt to develop pituitary insufficiency, weakness, and debility. Laboratory confirmation of the diagnosis of acromegaly is provided by demonstrating elevated plasma GH levels that do not suppress normally in response to oral glucose ingestion. Recently, measurements of somatomedin-C by radioimmunoassay have become available and may play a greater role in the diagnosis of acromegaly.

Pathophysiology of Skeletal Changes

GH increases the rate of protein synthesis in virtually all cells of the body. Its effects on bone and cartilage are mediated by somatomedins, which are peptides produced in the liver in response to GH stimulation. Prior to closure of the epiphyseal growth plate, GH stimulation results in endochondral ossification and longitudinal growth of the skeleton. Following epiphyseal closure, elongation no longer occurs. Excessive GH secretion then results in increased periosteal bone formation, most commonly along the diaphyses of long bones. This increase in periosteal and endosteal bone formation is coupled with increased bone resorption, and while increased cortical thickness is most common, local areas of decreased bone thickness may occur. Under the influence of excess GH, normal appositional growth of bone is greatly accentuated. Appositional growth of the zygomatic arches and supraorbital ridges is in part responsible for the typical facial appearance. Appositional growth occurs mainly at areas of tendon or ligament attachment or in areas of normal bony prominence.

Excess GH is a strong stimulus for cartilage proliferation. Joint spaces, especially in the hands and feet, initially appear widened. Early in the course, as the cartilage hypertrophies, range of joint motion is preserved or even excessive, especially in the spine. As the new, structurally inferior cartilage begins to break down and be replaced, osteoarthritic changes occur. Cartilage proliferation at the costochondral junctions gives rise to the so-called acromegalic rosary.

In addition to the overgrowth of bone and cartilage, diffuse soft-tissue hypertrophy develops as fibroblasts are stimulated to produce excess collagen and connective tissue. Unlike the bony changes, which are permanent, the soft-tissue changes are largely reversible when the excess GH stimulation ceases. While osteoporosis is mentioned as a characteristic of acromegaly, studies have suggested that it occurs infrequently. Bone biopsies of acromegalics generally show increased bone resorption and normal bone formation; cortical thickness and trabecular width are normal or increased. Radiographs usually do not show extensive osteoporosis unless debilitation or arthritis causes impaired mobility.

Radiographic Manifestations

Soft-tissue enlargement is one of the characteristic abnormalities seen in acromegaly. Acral soft-tissue widening is usually clearly evident on radiographs of the hands and feet (Fig. 97–2). Thickening of the heel pad of the foot occurs. Heel pad thickness is defined as the shortest distance between the posterior inferior border of the calcaneous and plantar surface of the skin measured on a true lateral radiograph. A value greater than 23 to 25 mm in men or 21.5 to 23 mm in women is highly suggestive of acromegaly, whereas a value less than 20 mm is rarely encountered in acromegaly. Other causes of soft-tissue thickening that must be excluded include infection, injury, massive obesity, edema, or myxedema.

The classic description of ''spade hands'' refers to the soft-tissue changes consisting of widened digits with blunted ends. The most characteristic radiographic changes include widening of the joint spaces due to cartilaginous hypertrophy and widening and squaring of the ends of the phalanges and metacarpals. The shafts of the phalanges typically also show widening, but in a few cases they may exhibit narrowing. The tufts of the distal phalanges typically enlarge, with pointing of the proximal edges. Exostoses may be seen at points of tendon or ligament attachment, particularly at the heads of the metacarpals (Fig. 97–3). The sesamoid index is another measurement that may have diagnostic value. The index is calculated by measuring the longest axis of the medial sesamoid of the thumb and multiplying it by the diameter perpendicular to this line. An index greater than 40 sq mm in men or 32 sq mm in women strongly suggests acromegaly, whereas an index less than 30 sq mm argues against, but does not exclude, the diagnosis.

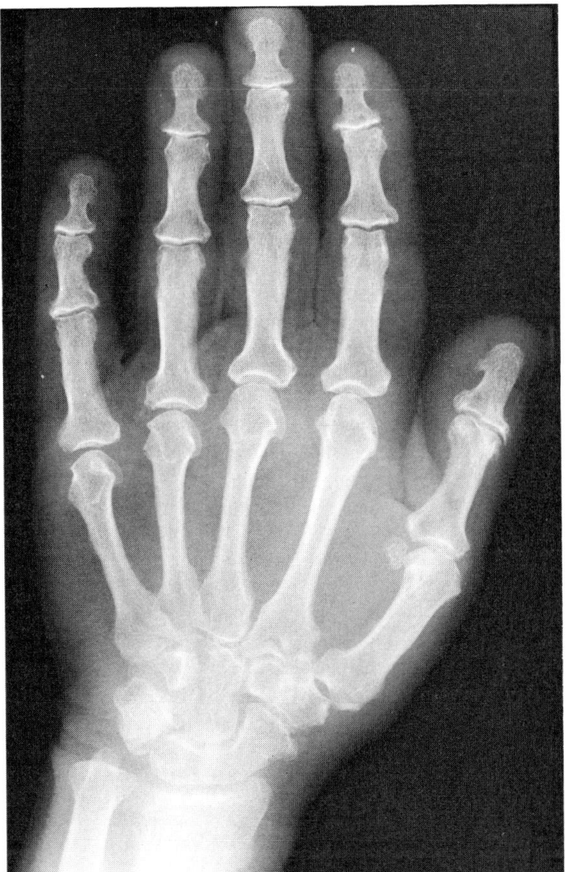

Figure 97–2. Acromegaly. Thickening of the soft tissues with characteristic widening of the palm, enlargement of the ungual tufts, and hook-like bony spurs at the metacarpal heads.

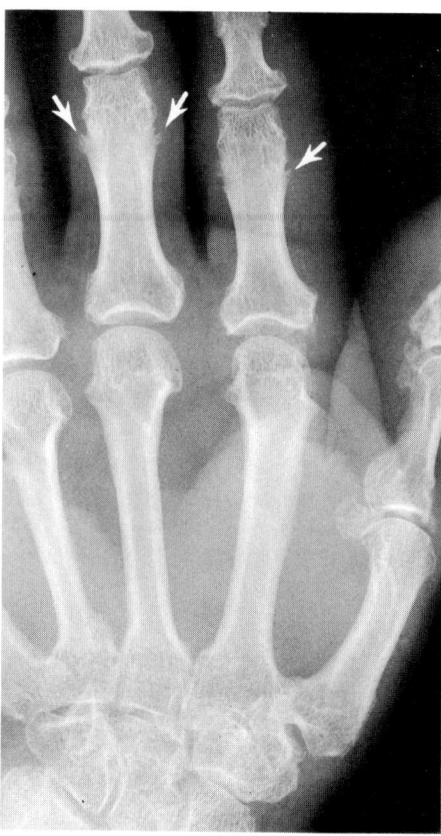

Figure 97–3. Acromegaly. There is widening of the metacarpophalangeal cartilage spaces, exostoses along the shafts of the proximal phalanges *(arrows),* thickening of the cortex along the shaft of the second metacarpal, and enlargement of the sesamoid bone adjacent to the first metacarpophalangeal joint.

Acromegalic changes in the feet are similar to those of the hands, with soft-tissue thickening, widening of the joint spaces (particularly the metatarsophalangeals), and widening and squaring of the ends of the metatarsals and phalanges. In contrast to the hands, however, resorptive changes are more prominent with narrowing of the shafts of the phalanges.

Radiographs of the skull may disclose striking abnormalities. In most cases the sella turcica is enlarged, often with signs of erosion or destruction. The frontal sinuses are enlarged and prominent, with bossing of the frontal bones. Increased pneumatization of the mastoid air cells and other sinuses is commonly seen, and the mastoid tip is often very prominent. The mandible enlarges in both length and thickness, resulting in a characteristic prognathism. The teeth may become widely separated, and pressure from the enlarged tongue may cause them to tilt outward. Thickening of the cranial vault is commonly seen. Involvement may be generalized or localized to the frontal and parietal regions. Localized thinning of the parietal bones may infrequently occur. When thickening ocurs, the frontal or parietal bones may measure up to 2 cm in width. The portion of the occipital bone just above the foramen magnum is usually not involved. As with other areas of ligamentous attachment, a large exostosis may be seen at the occipital protuberance, at the insertion of the nuchal ligament. Appositional growth of the zygoma and the supraorbital ridge may cause them to be especially prominent.

Vertebral changes in acromegaly vary in different regions of the spine. The thoracic vertebrae widen in the AP diameter owing to apposition of new bone along the anterior aspects of the vertebral bodies. Anterior and lateral osteophytes are common and may be extensive, especially in the thoracic and lumbar spine. In contrast to the bony apposition occurring in the thoracic spine, resorption predominates in the lumbar spine, producing posterior concavity of the vertebral bodies. It has been suggested that this posterior scalloping is due to pressure by the hypertrophic soft tissues of the spinal canal and adjacent areas. Hypertrophy of the intervertebral discs results in increased height of the disc spaces, especially in the lumbar region. An increase in the normal physiologic thoracic kyphosis occurs, often with a compensatory hyperlordosis of the lumbar spine. Many acromegalic patients show the typical changes of degenerative osteoarthritis of the spine, including spurring and disc space narrowing, but there is rarely the sclerosis of the end-plates of the vertebral bodies that is commonly seen in degenerative disc disease not associated with acromegaly.

Skeletal changes in the pelvis also occur most commonly at sites of tendon and ligament attachment. "Beaking" of the superior border of the pubic ramus at the pubic symphysis is characteristic. In women the pubic bones may be abnormally narrowed. The hip joints are among the earliest to show degenerative changes and are among the most severely involved. Bony spurs are often seen along the margin of the acetabulum. Cartilage hypertrophy also occurs (Fig. 97–4).

The AP diameter of the thorax is increased owing to a ventral displacement of the sternum. The costochondral junctions may appear prominent secondary to endochondral ossification. Widening of the anterior ends of the first ribs and medial halves of the clavicles may provide an important diagnostic clue on standard chest radiographs.

Differential Diagnosis

When advanced, the constellation of clinical and radiographic abnormalities of acromegaly is easily recognized. In isolation, each

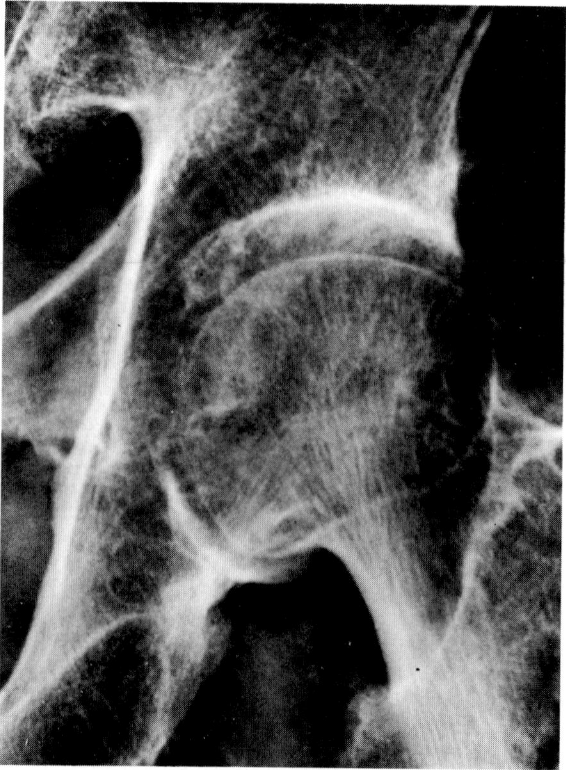

Figure 97–4. Acromegaly. There is widening of the hip joint due to cartilage hypertrophy.

of the radiographic features may suggest a variety of diagnostic possibilities. Several features of acromegaly are shared by pachydermoperiostosis. This rare disorder is inherited in an autosomal dominant pattern with incomplete penetrance or occurs as an acquired form, usually seen in men over 40 with bronchogenic carcinoma. The patients may resemble acromegalics with thickening of the skin of the face, hands, arms, and legs. The facial features coarsen, with deepened facial and scalp folds. As with acromegaly, there is increased sebaceous gland secretion and oiliness of the skin. Radiographically the disorders share increased periosteal bone formation, enlarged sinuses, prominent supraorbital ridges, and thick phalanges. Unlike patients with acromegaly, those with pachydermoperiostosis do not have pituitary or sellar abnormalities, joint space enlargement, or increased GH levels.

The differential diagnosis of soft-tissue thickening includes edema of any etiology, obesity, myxedema, injury, and infection. Enlargement of the tufts of the terminal phalanges may be seen in patients who engage in heavy labor. It is unusual to see a third digit distal phalanx tuft wider than 12 mm in men or 10 mm in women except in acromegaly.

Scalloping or concavity of the posterior aspects of the vertebrae can be seen in a variety of disorders that increase intraspinal pressure, such as neoplasms or syringomyelia. Posterior scalloping is also seen in neurofibromatosis, achondroplasia, and the Marfan, Morquio, Hurler, and Ehlers-Danlos syndromes. Abundant osteophytoses along the anterior aspect of the spine may appear similar to those seen in diffuse idiopathic skeletal hyperostosis (DISH, Forestier's disease). The arthropathy seen in acromegaly is initially very characteristic, with joint space widening. Later in the course it may look like other forms of degenerative joint disease. Features that may suggest acromegaly as the etiology include excessive spurring and early involvement of non–weight-bearing joints such as the shoulder and elbow.

An enlarged sella is also seen in the empty sella syndrome. Pituitary function is normal. Sellar enlargement is a result of extension of the subarachnoid cistern into the sella turcica. The pathogenesis is unclear. CT and MRI are helpful in demonstrating the actual size of the pituitary. Hyperprolactinemia plus an apparently empty sella may indicate the presence of a microprolactinoma.

HYPOPITUITARISM

Pituitary hypofunction may result from a primary pituitary abnormality or may be secondary to hypothalamic dysfunction. The etiologies of hypopituitarism include compression of the pituitary by a primary tumor (chromophobe adenoma most commonly), craniopharyngioma, metastasis (breast or lung most commonly), postpartum infarction (Sheehan's syndrome), hypothalamic glioma, suprasellar tumors, and destruction of the pituitary by granuloma or infection. Surgery and radiation to neighboring structures can also lead to pituitary hypofunction. Either single or multiple hormone deficiencies may occur. Partial hormone deficiencies are seen only after loss of 70 to 75 per cent of the pituitary gland, but complete hypopituitarism does not occur until more than 90 per cent of the gland has been destroyed.

Clinical Manifestations

Patients with hypopituitarism frequently experience fatigue, weakness, and headaches. The skin appears pale and waxy with fine wrinkling. There is a decrease in axillary and pubic hair. Deficiency of each of the specific pituitary hormones produces characteristic changes. Loss of gonadotropic hormones (LH and FSH) leads to gonadal atrophy, resulting in loss of libido, decreased potency in men, and menstrual abnormalities in women. Deficient TSH causes the usual manifestations of hypothyroidism, including weakness, lethargy, cold intolerance, and dry skin. If TSH deficiency occurs during childhood, growth retardation that is not responsive to exogenous GH ensues. Decreased prolactin results in failure to lactate following parturition and is often the first indication of Sheehan's syndrome.

Loss of ACTH causes fatigue, orthostatic hypotension, anorexia, and nausea. In contrast to primary adrenal insufficiency, the skin becomes pale rather than hyperpigmented, and abnormalities of sodium and potassium usually do not occur. Diabetes insipidus (DI) may arise if hypothalamic destruction impairs ADH secretion. If ACTH deficiency occurs with DI, the urine volume may not be as large because cortisol plays a permissive role in excretion of free

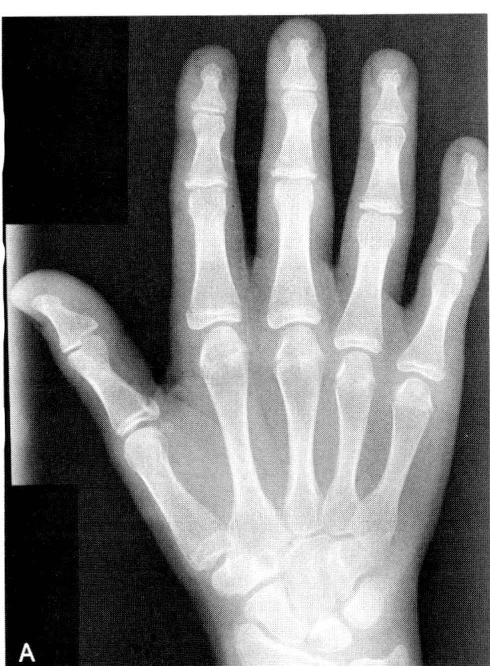

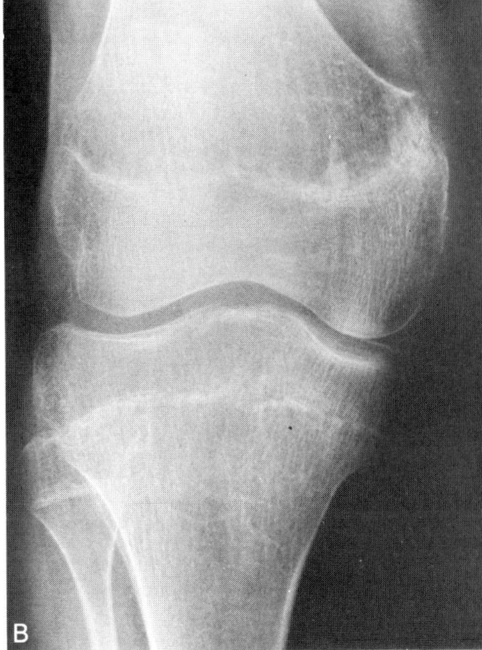

Figure 97–5. Hypopituitarism. *A,* A 44-year-old woman with short stature, incompletely fused epiphyses, and a bone age of 14 years. The cortical bone is thin, and the bones appear osteoporotic. *B,* Same patient as in *A*; the growth plates of the knee are still evident, and the bones are osteoporotic.

water. When GH is deficient prior to puberty, growth retardation and short stature occur. After puberty, growth hormone deficiency may be apparent only in a decrease in insulin requirement and a greater propensity to hypoglycemia in insulin-dependent diabetics.

Radiographic Manifestations

(Fig. 97–5)

When hypopituitarism occurs after puberty, there may be no radiographic findings other than a relatively small heart and kidneys. Occasionally calcification of the pinnae may be seen. When hypopituitarism occurs prior to puberty, the radiographic manifestations are primarily those of growth hormone deficiency. Ossification centers appear late, bone age is retarded, endochondral ossification is delayed, and closure of the epiphyses may not occur until the fourth or fifth decade. Short stature with normal body proportions ensues. However, if growth arrest occurs during childhood there may be a disproportion between the cranial vault and the facial bones. The juvenile pattern of the vault, being substantially larger than the face, may then persist. The permanent teeth erupt late and are of normal size, resulting in crowding and malocclusion. Pharmacologic GH administered prior to epiphyseal closure may be curative.

Differential Diagnosis

Short stature is most frequently familial, with normal GH levels being present. Laron dwarfism is a syndrome in which resistance to GH is seen. GH levels are high but somatomedin levels are low and are not responsive to GH administration. Resistance to somatomedins is seen in African pygmies. Other endocrine causes of delayed growth include hypothyroidism and Cushing's syndrome. Thyroid hormone appears to be permissive for GH action. Precocious puberty causes early epiphyseal fusion, and although these patients initially are relatively tall, they never attain normal height. Other causes of short stature include intrauterine disturbances, malnutrition, chronic illness, metabolic disorders including diabetes, skeletal dysplasia, and chromosomal abnormalities.

ADRENAL

ROBERT A. LEVINE,
ROBERT A. GELFAND,
and PAMELA S. JENSEN

The adrenal gland is composed of two physiologically different components, the medulla and the cortex. The adrenal medulla consists of chromaffin tissue of neuroectodermal origin that synthesizes the catecholamines epinephrine and norepinephrine. Its only significant pathologic condition is the tumor pheochromocytoma. The adrenal cortex converts cholesterol into three categories of steroid hormones. It is the sole endogenous source of glucocorticoids and mineralocorticoids and, in women, is a major source of androgens.

Cortisol, the principal glucocorticoid, is secreted at a rate of 15 to 30 mg per day, with a diurnal variation peaking in the early morning. In times of stress, cortisol production may reach 250 to 300 mg per day. Its secretion is regulated by adrenocorticotropic hormone (ACTH), a peptide hormone produced in the pituitary. ACTH production, in turn, is regulated by corticotropin-releasing factor (CRF) produced in the hypothalamus. Circulating cortisol exerts negative feedback on the pituitary, suppressing ACTH production.

Aldosterone, the primary mineralocorticoid, acts on the kidney to cause sodium retention and to enhance the excretion of potassium and hydrogen ions. It plays a major role in fluid and electrolyte homeostasis and blood pressure control. ACTH plays a minor role in stimulating aldosterone production, which is controlled primarily by circulating levels of potassium and angiotensin II.

Androstenedione and dehydroepiandrosterone (DHEA) are the primary androgens produced by the adrenal gland. They are relatively weak androgens and exert most of their effects after peripheral conversion to testosterone and dihydrotestosterone. In women the adrenals are the major source of androgens, whereas in men they account for less than 5 per cent of circulating testosterone. Androstenedione can be converted to the potent estrogen estrone by adipose tissue and the liver. This is the major source of estrogen in children and postmenopausal women.

Glucocorticoids have a variety of functions in homeostasis, metabolism, immune regulation, and response to stress. As the name implies, they play a role in glucose metabolism, increasing gluconeogenesis and decreasing glucose uptake and utilization by peripheral tissues. In large amounts they exert a pronounced net catabolic effect on protein metabolism, evidenced by negative nitrogen balance and wasting of muscle and other lean body tissues. Glucocorticoids increase lipolysis, play a permissive role in catecholamine-induced fatty acid mobilization, and, in excess, result in redistribution of fat in a characteristic truncal pattern. They block many of the signs of acute inflammation and, in excess, impair cell-mediated immunity.

CUSHING'S SYNDROME

Cushing's syndrome results from excess adrenal corticosteroid activity. To some degree, its characteristics reflect an exaggeration of many of the normal actions of steroids. Among the most common manifestations is obesity, which occurs in a typical central (truncal) pattern with round ("moon") facies, enlarged supraclavicular and dorsocervical fat pads, and abdominal protuberance. The combination of central obesity and muscle wasting makes the extremities appear disproportionately thin. Epidermal and connective tissue atrophy gives rise to thinning of the skin, plethora, easy bruisability, poor wound healing, and characteristic purple striae. Forty per cent of patients exhibit psychologic disturbances, which include depression, mania, irritability, and impaired concentration. Proximal muscle weakness with a myopathic EMG pattern may be seen. Glucose intolerance due to insulin resistance is common, and frank diabetes mellitus may occur in susceptible individuals. Calcium wasting may be manifest clinically as osteoporosis or nephrolithiasis. Glucocorticoid effects on the humoral and cell-mediated immune systems lead to an increase in the frequency and severity of infections. Mineralocorticoid excess causes hypertension in the majority of patients with Cushing's syndrome and may result in edema and congestive heart failure. Excess adrenal androgen production causes hirsutism in two thirds of female patients and frequently produces acne and seborrhea. True virilization is usually seen only with adrenal carcinomas that produce large amounts of androgens. Amenorrhea, impotence, and decreased libido are common.

The majority of cases of Cushing's syndrome are a consequence of exogenous glucocorticoid administration. The most common cause of endogenous Cushing's syndrome is pituitary ACTH hypersecretion (Cushing's disease). The next most common cause is ectopic ACTH secretion by nonpituitary tumors. Small cell carcinoma of the lung is the most frequent tumor type, followed by thymomas, pancreatic islet cell tumors, carcinoid tumors, medullary carcinoma of the thyroid, and pheochromocytomas. Cushing's disease occurs most commonly in women in the third and fourth decades, whereas the ectopic ACTH syndrome tends to occur in men in their fifth and sixth decades. In both situations the excess ACTH stimulates adrenal overproduction of cortisol, deoxycorticosterone (with mineralocorticoid activity), and androgens. Finally, endogenous Cushing's syndrome may be caused by autonomous production of steroids by adrenal adenomas and carcinomas. Both occur with approximately equal frequency. Adenomas generally secrete either cortisol or aldosterone but rarely produce significant amounts of androgens. Adrenal carcinomas frequently secrete multiple steroids, most often cortisol and androgens.

As in adults, iatrogenic administration of steroid hormones is the most common cause of Cushing's syndrome in children. In addition to the clinical features described above, Cushing's syndrome in childhood is characterized by growth failure and delayed onset of puberty.

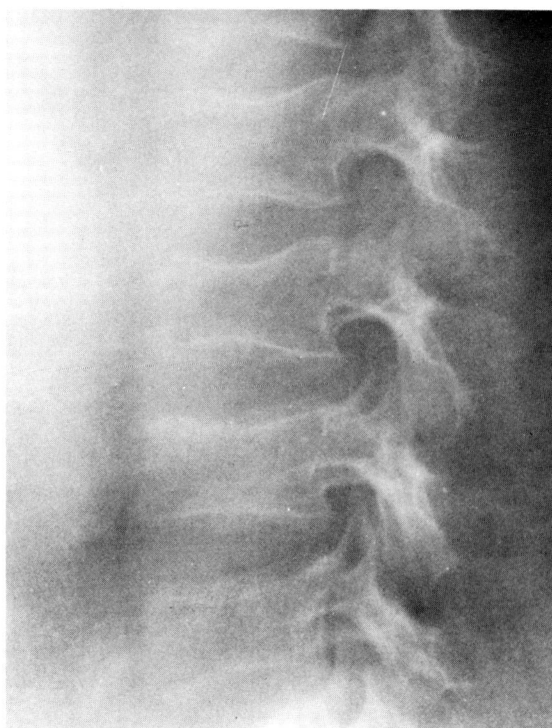

Figure 97–6. Cushing's syndrome. Advanced osteoporosis of the spine with loss of height of the vertebral bodies and increased concavity of the end-plates due to remodeling of the osteoporotic bone in response to the nucleus pulposus resuming its spherical shape within the intervertebral disc ("codfish vertebrae").

Calcium and Bone Metabolism

Corticosteroids have major effects on calcium and bone metabolism. Corticosteroid osteopenia is seen in almost all cases of clinically evident endogenous Cushing's syndrome and can be induced by modest doses of exogenous steroids. The effects on bone are due to several mechanisms, including decreased intestinal calcium absorption, increased urinary calcium loss, secondary effects of parathyroid hormone (PTH), and direct effects on bone formation. Bone biopsy specimens demonstrate both decreased bone formation and increased bone resorption. In vitro, corticosteroids decrease protein synthesis by osteoblasts, and it is believed that corticosteroids may impair the conversion of osteoprogenitor cells to functioning osteoblasts. The increased osteoclastic activity can be blocked by parathyroidectomy in most experimental animals treated with steroids, and likely reflects a PTH-mediated effect.

Corticosteroids markedly inhibit intestinal calcium absorption, although the mechanism remains controversial. In addition, corticosteroids have a calciuric effect, decreasing tubular resorption of calcium by the kidney. The combination of decreased intestinal absorption and increased renal loss of calcium leads to a secondary increase in PTH in an effort to maintain normal serum calcium. This rise in PTH causes increased resorption of bone and worsening of the osteopenia.

Radiographic Manifestations

The skeletal manifestations of Cushing's syndrome include osteoporosis, osteonecrosis (aseptic necrosis), pathologic fractures, abnormal callus formation, delayed skeletal maturation, and increased infections of bones and joints. Radiographic loss of bone mass frequently precedes clinical symptoms. Osteoporotic changes are most evident in the axial skeleton, femoral neck, and metacarpals. The vertebral bodies demonstrate decreased bone density, compression fractures, and "codfish deformities," and the spine frequently develops kyphoscoliosis (Fig. 97–6). It is difficult to distinguish between the osteoporotic changes secondary to Cushing's syndrome and other causes of osteopenia, but several characteristics are suggestive of a corticosteroid etiology. There may be increased radiographic density of the superior and inferior margins of compressed vertebral bodies (subchondral end-plate sclerosis). This is usually not seen with most other causes of osteoporosis. In addition, early involvement of the skull and ribs may help to differentiate Cushing's from postmenopausal osteoporosis. The degree of osteopenia seen in Cushing's syndrome is highly dependent on preexisting bone density and concurrent factors such as immobilization or the presence of an underlying condition such as rheumatoid arthritis.

Osteonecrosis (Fig. 97–7) is more often associated with exogenous than endogenous Cushing's syndrome. The etiology remains uncertain and is most likely multifactorial. Theories regarding pathogenesis include vascular infarcts secondary to microemboli or vasculitis, loss of vascular supply due to traumatic compression secondary to osteoporosis, and development of increased pressure in a relatively closed anatomic space such as the femoral head or head of the mandible due to hypertrophy and hyperplasia of fat cells. The infarctions can be either subarticular or, less often, diaphyseal. They most commonly affect the femoral and humeral heads, the distal femur, and the proximal tibia and may occur in any other location where the blood supply is vulnerable. Because infarcted bone has the same radiographic density as living bone, initially there may be no radiographic signs of osteonecrosis. If pain limits mobility, disuse osteopenia of the vascularized segment may develop so that the avascular segment appears relatively sclerotic. However, in many cases the necrosis is initially painless, and disuse osteopenia does not occur. The earliest radiographic sign may be a thin subarticular line of lucency ("crescent sign") that represents a fracture through the trabecular bone supporting the subchondral plate. As repair occurs, intermixed areas of lucency and sclerosis may be seen. Resorption around the margins or within the infarcted segment may produce areas of structural weakness, and the segment may break off or develop localized foci of collapse. Diaphyseal

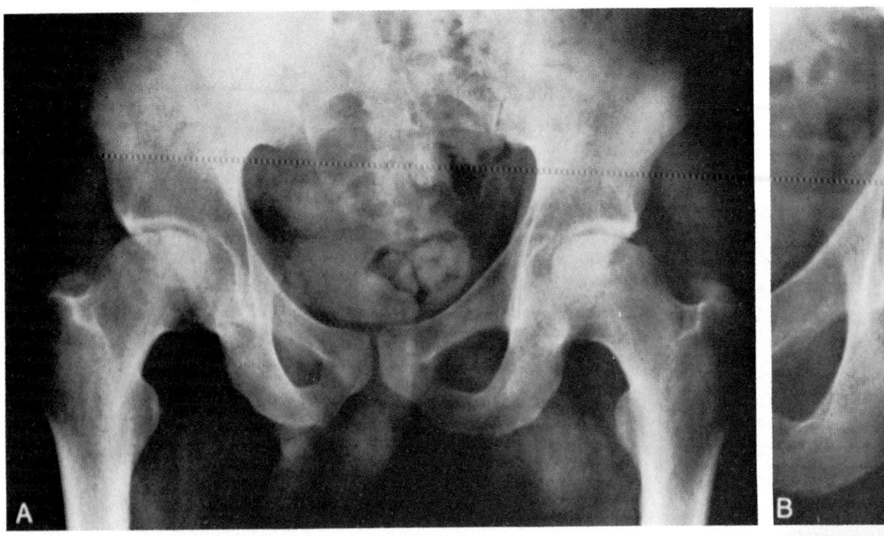

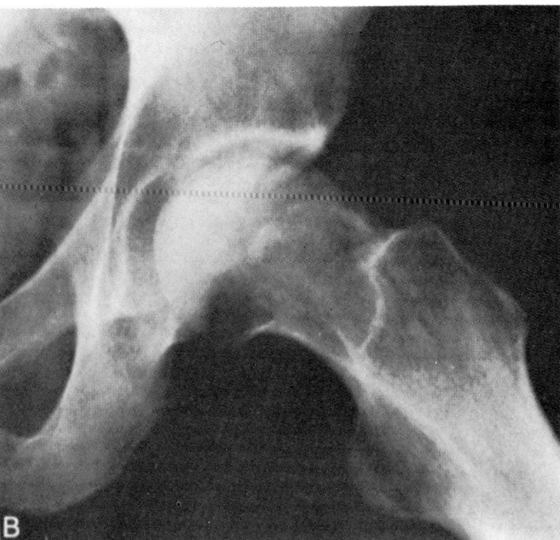

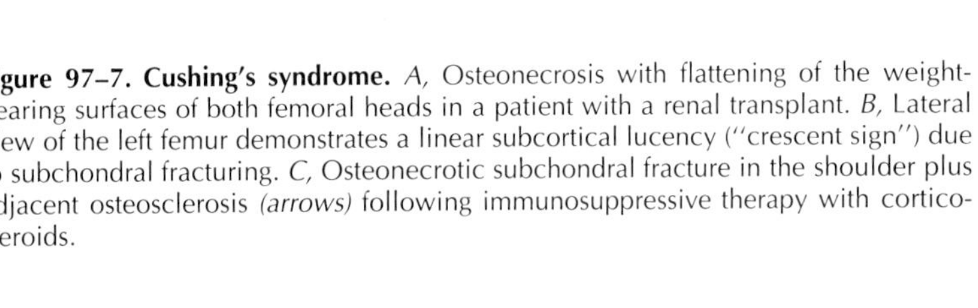

Figure 97–7. Cushing's syndrome. *A,* Osteonecrosis with flattening of the weight-bearing surfaces of both femoral heads in a patient with a renal transplant. *B,* Lateral view of the left femur demonstrates a linear subcortical lucency ("crescent sign") due to subchondral fracturing. *C,* Osteonecrotic subchondral fracture in the shoulder plus adjacent osteosclerosis *(arrows)* following immunosuppressive therapy with corticosteroids.

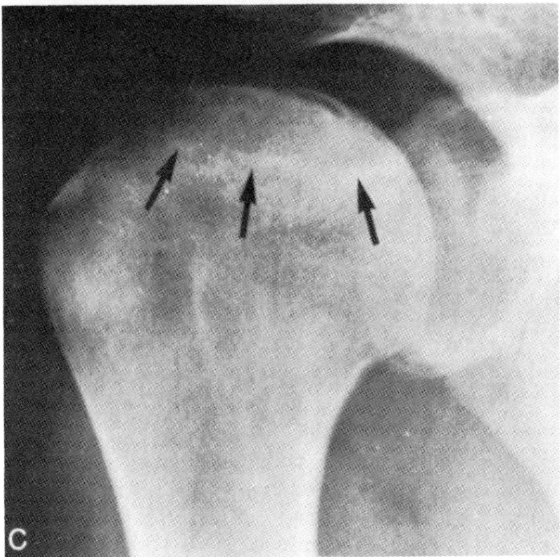

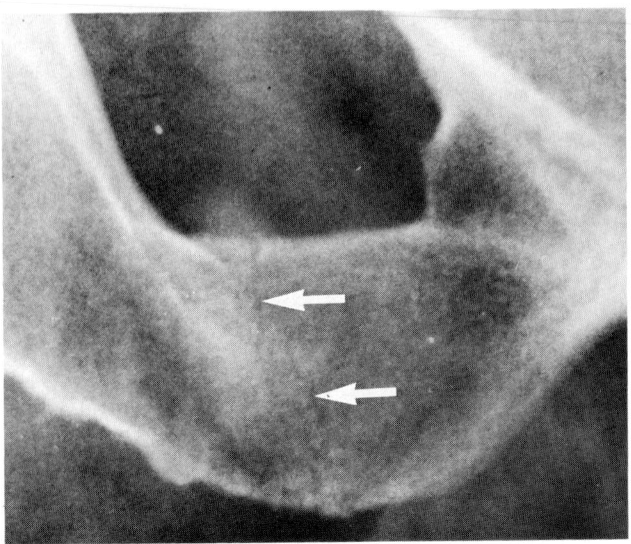

Figure 97–8. Cushing's syndrome. Pathologic fracture through the inferior pubic ramus *(arrows)* with early callus formation. There was no history of trauma.

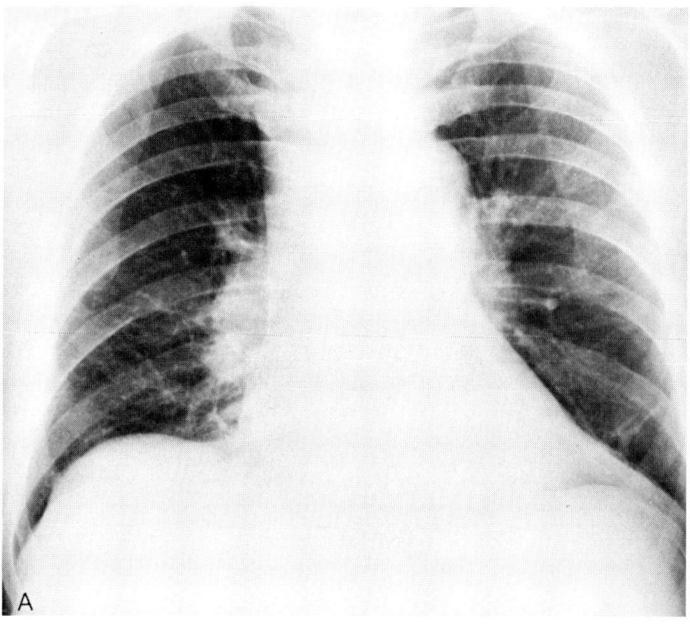

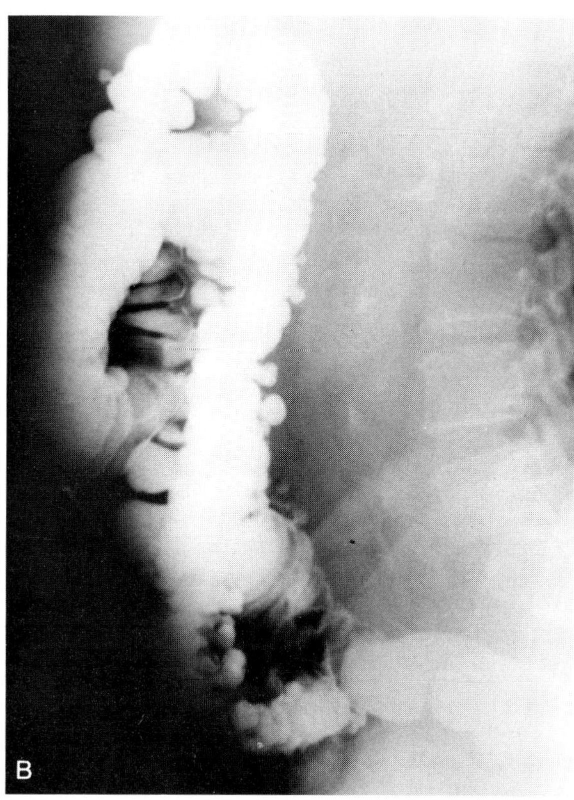

Figure 97–9. Cushing's syndrome. *A,* Mediastinal widening is present as a result of fat hypertrophy. *B,* Marked anterior displacement of the colon is due to the development of 2000 g of retroperitoneal fat following very high dose corticosteroid therapy.

infarcts present as radiolucent lesions, usually surrounded by a sharp, thin serpiginous margin. At later stages, formation of new bone may cause the diaphyseal infarct to become a sclerotic lesion.

Pathologic fractures (Fig. 97–8) may occur in any location. The ribs, spine, ischeal and pubic rami, and long bones are commonly affected. Vertebral compression fractures usually involve multiple vertebral bodies of the middle and lower thoracic spine and upper lumbar spine, and they may be relatively asymptomatic. Rib fractures often exhibit exuberant callus formation, but the callus may be poorly defined and healing is frequently delayed or incomplete. In severe cases some bones may soften to such a degree that deformation may occur.

The elevated pain threshold and compromised immune system in patients with Cushing's syndrome result in an increased incidence of osteomyelitis and septic arthritis. The radiographic appearance of osteomyelitis is usually not distinctive in Cushing's syndrome, although the lesions may be much more advanced than would be expected by their clinical presentation. Infections may be caused by the usual pyogenic organisms or may be due to a variety of opportunistic organisms.

Other common radiographic findings that occur with increased frequency in Cushing's syndrome include soft-tissue edema, cardiac enlargement and congestive heart failure secondary to fluid retention, nephrolithiasis, and vascular and soft-tissue calcifications. Excess fat tissue may accumulate in the mediastinum and epicardial fat pad spaces and can lead to widening of the mediastinum or the development of a discrete mediastinal mass demonstrated on the lateral chest radiograph (Fig. 97–9). Computed tomography can reveal the fat density of the lesion.

Differential Diagnosis

Osteopenia may be seen in many situations, including idiopathic and senile osteoporosis, juvenile osteoporosis, primary hyperparathyroidism, immobilization, heparin therapy, osteomalacia, multiple myeloma, Turner's syndrome, and Gaucher's disease. Osteonecrosis may be seen in a wide variety of disorders besides hypercorticism, including trauma, rheumatoid arthritis, hyperuricemic gout, systemic lupus erythematosus, alcohol abuse, caisson disease (decompression sickness), sickle cell disease, pancreatitis, polycythemia vera, Fabry's disease, Gaucher's disease, and Chandler's disease (idiopathic osteonecrosis).

THYROID

ROBERT A. GELFAND

The normal human thyroid gland is composed of two lateral lobes, one on either side of the trachea, connected by a thin isthmus of thyroid tissue that crosses the trachea anteriorly just below the cricoid cartilage. At birth the normal gland weighs about 2 g, by puberty about 14 g, and in the adult varies between 15 and 25 g. The right lobe is usually slightly larger than the left and tends to enlarge more in disorders causing a diffuse increase in the size of the thyroid (Fig. 97–10). Occasionally in normal adults, but particularly when the gland is goitrous, a finger-like pyramidal lobe may be discernible extending upward from the isthmus, representing a remnant of the embryologic path along which the thyroid developed (Fig. 97–11). Histologically, the thyroid is made up of multiple spherical follicles filled with colloid, a proteinaceous material consisting largely of thyroglobulin, the unique protein within which thyroid hormone is stored.

Embryologically, the thyroid originates as an evagination of the pharyngeal epithelium, which elongates inferiorly as the thyroglossal duct. As the thyroid anlage migrates caudally to its cervical position, it assumes a bilobar shape, and the thyroglossal duct, which connects the developing isthmus to the base of the tongue, normally disappears by about the eighth week of intrauterine life. By about 10 to 12 weeks of gestation the fetal thyroid begins to concentrate iodide, and significant accumulation of radioactive iodine given to the mother is evident in the fetal thyroid by end of the first trimester.

Developmental anomalies of the thyroid include agenesis of one or both lobes (the latter causing athyreotic cretinism) and conditions that arise from defective migration of the thyroid in utero. Ectopic thyroid tissue may be located anywhere between the base of the tongue and the normal site of the gland and is usually recognized as a lingual or midline neck mass that concentrates radioiodine. In such cases the ectopic thyroid may represent the sole functioning thyroid tissue, and its secretion may or may not be sufficient to maintain a euthyroid state. Infrequently, thyroid tissue progenitors may descend to occupy a location within the anterior mediastinum, usually remaining contiguous with thyroid tissue in the neck. Substernal goiter formation in later life may lead to compression of adjacent mediastinal structures. The most common clinically apparent developmental anomaly is the persistence of thyroglossal duct tissue in the neck, giving rise to thyroglossal cysts. Occasionally the site of recurrent infection and very rarely of thyroid carcinoma, a thyroglossal duct remnant should be excised when discovered.

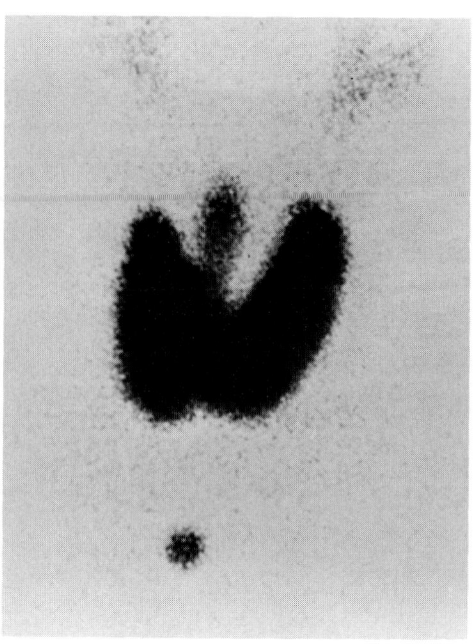

Figure 97–11. Thyrotoxicosis. Enlarged gland with marked homogeneous ^{99m}Tc uptake diffusely throughout both lobes and in the pyramidal lobe located between the lobes. Radioactive iodine uptake (RAIU) was 72 per cent in this patient with Graves' disease.

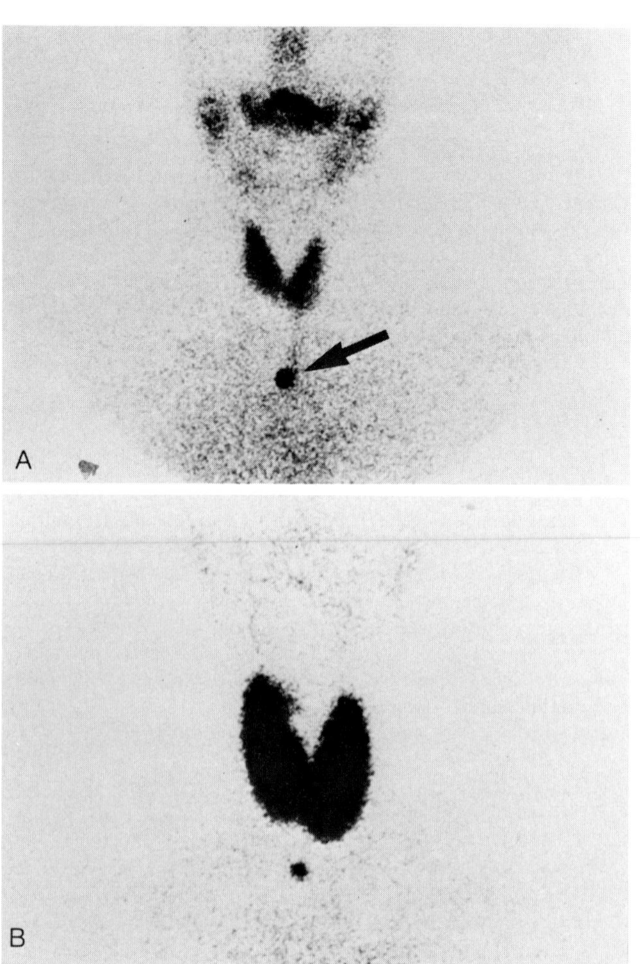

Figure 97–10. Diffuse toxic goiter. *A,* Technetium-99m scan of a normal thyroid gland for comparison. A radioisotope marker has been placed at the top of the sternum at the sternal notch *(arrow).* Salivary gland uptake is also evident. *B,* Enlarged gland with increased ^{99m}Tc uptake in a patient with Graves' disease. Very little radionuclide has been taken up by the salivary glands.

PHYSIOLOGY AND LABORATORY TESTS

The thyroid gland regulates overall body tissue metabolism by virtue of its secretion into the bloodstream of two iodinated amino acid hormones, thyroxine (T_4) and triiodothyronine (T_3). The biosynthesis of these hormones begins with the active transport of iodide from the plasma into the thyroid cell (trapping) followed by the iodination of tyrosyl residues in the follicular thyroglobulin (organification). Pairs of iodotyrosyl residues are subsequently joined to form the active iodothyronine hormones. Finally, the hydrolysis of thyroglobulin within the thyroid cell liberates the active hormones for release into the circulation. The central role of iodine in thyroid hormone biosynthesis provides the basis for the radionuclide evaluation of thyroid function using radioactive iodine.

In normal individuals, the thyroid secretes predominantly T_4 but relatively little T_3, which is produced primarily by extrathyroidal deiodination of T_4. In the blood, over 99 per cent of circulating T_4 and T_3 is bound to serum proteins, primarily thyroid-binding globulin (TBG), and less than 1 per cent is unbound or free. Nevertheless, it is only this small free fraction that appears to be readily available to tissues and therefore metabolically active. Consequently, the laboratory evaluation of thyroid status is aimed primarily at determining the circulating concentration of this small unbound fraction of T_4.

As might be anticipated from its central role in metabolism, thyroid function is closely regulated to maintain free thyroid hormone levels within a narrow range. If the hormone supply to tissues diminishes, the reduction is sensed by the pituitary, which increases its secretion of thyroid-stimulating hormone (TSH). TSH, in turn, stimulates all steps in the synthesis and secretion of hormone by the thyroid, until circulating thyroid hormone levels rise sufficiently to suppress TSH. Chronic stimulation by TSH also causes hypertrophy and hyperplasia of the gland. Clinically, the documentation of increased circulating TSH levels is essential to confirm a diagnosis of primary hypothyroidism. Finally, the hypothalamus participates in the thyroid regulatory feedback loop with its production of thyrotropin-releasing hormone (TRH), a tripepetide that stimulates the pituitary secretion of TSH. The stimulatory effect of TRH on the pituitary is enhanced by concomitant thyroid hormone deficiency and is completely blocked when thyroid hormone concentration is even slightly elevated. Clinically, measurement of the serum TSH response to administered exogenous TRH is now commonly performed to evaluate the pituitary-thyroid axis. The test is probably most useful in situations of suspected mild hyperthyroidism; in this circumstance an absent TSH response provides confirmatory evidence, whereas a normal response virtually excludes the diagnosis. A diminished or absent response is also characteristic of autonomous thyroid function without frank thyrotoxicosis.

DIAGNOSTIC IMAGING MODALITIES

Radionuclide Techniques

Radionuclide studies of the thyroid were the first clinically important procedures in nuclear medicine, and they continue to play a major role in modern thyroid evaluation. These techniques are unique in providing not only anatomic and localization information, but also in allowing a quantitative assessment of thyroid function.

The thyroid radioactive iodine uptake (RAIU) measures the fractional uptake by the thyroid of a tracer dose of radioiodine. Using a nonimaging probe detector, the RAIU is generally determined 24 hours after oral administration of isotope, by which time it has reached a plateau. Concern regarding the high radiation exposure from ^{131}I has made ^{123}I, with its shorter half-life, the radioisotope of choice for this application. In general, the RAIU is assumed to reflect the rate of thyroid hormone synthesis and, by inference, the rate of thyroid hormone release into the bloodstream. Although this is justified in most instances, there are important exceptions, such as the low RAIU observed in thyrotoxicosis due to thyroiditis and the high RAIU seen in hypothyroidism due to iodine deficiency. It should be emphasized that the RAIU will vary inversely with the size of the endogenous stable iodide pool in which the isotope is diluted. Thus, the widespread increase in dietary iodide intake among the general population in recent years has substantially lowered the normal RAIU to approximately 5 to 25 per cent at 24 hours. This, combined with the wide variation in individual iodide intake, has greatly reduced the ability of the RAIU to distinguish between the normal and hypothyroid states. Similarly, although clearly elevated values generally indicate thyroid hyperfunction, many mildly thyrotoxic patients now exhibit an RAIU in the high normal range. Thus, interpretation of the RAIU must be performed cautiously and only in conjunction with the clinical assessment of the patient and tests of circulating hormone concentrations.

The RAIU is of unique value in the diagnosis of several thyrotoxic states in which the uptake is characteristically low rather than elevated (Table 97–1). Another special circumstance in which the RAIU may be useful is in the calculation of treatment doses of radioiodine for hyperthyroidism. Finally, a number of interventional modifications of the RAIU have been designed: the T_3 suppression test in which nonsuppression by exogenous T_3 administration indicates autonomous thyroid function; the TSH stimulation test, which is a measure of thyroid reserve; and the perchlorate discharge test, which can be used to diagnose defects in iodide organification. Although this last test is still occasionally used in the investigation of thyroid failure or familial goiter, the first two tests have now been largely supplanted by, respectively, the TRH stimulation test (an absent TSH response indicting autonomous thyroid function) and the direct measurement of basal circulating TSH levels (elevated levels indicating diminished thyroid reserve). The TSH stimulation test may be used in conjunction with nuclear imaging techniques to demonstrate normal thyroid tissue that has been suppressed by a hyperfunctioning thyroid nodule or by exogenous thyroid hormone administration.

TABLE 97–1. THYROTOXIC STATES ASSOCIATED WITH A LOW RAIU

Thyroiditis with transient hyperthyroidism (subacute or silent thyroiditis)
Iodine-induced thyrotoxicosis (Jod-Basedow)
Thyrotoxicosis factitia
Hyperfunctioning ectopic thyroid tissue (rare) (struma ovarii, metastatic follicular carcinoma)

Imaging of the thyroid by radionuclide scanning gives an objective assessment of thyroid anatomy, including the presence and functional activity of thyroid nodules. Scanning may be performed using either radioiodine or technetium-99m pertechnetate (^{99m}Tc), a monovalent anion that is trapped by the thyroid but not significantly organified. Pertechnetate offers the particular advantages of low cost, wide availability, low radiation dose to the thyroid, and convenience because scanning is performed shortly after an intravenous bolus; the procedure can therefore be completed in a single visit.

The most frequent clinical indication for thyroid scanning is to define the functional activity of palpable thyroid nodules, which, when compared on the scan with surrounding thyroid tissue, may appear less active (cold), more active (hot), or of comparable activity (warm). Although the majority of nonfunctioning nodules are benign, lack of function increases the likelihood of malignancy, particularly if only a single nodule is present. Conversely, nodules that have greater activity than surrounding tissue are very unlikely to be malignant. An important caveat in this regard is the occasional malignant lesion that appears hot with ^{99m}Tc but cold with radioiodine owing to preserved anion trapping function but impaired organification. Finally, radionuclide scanning is also useful in detecting substernal goiter or ectopic thyroid tissue using ^{123}I, and whole body scanning with ^{131}I plays an important role in the detection of functioning metastases of thyroid carcinoma. Because both radioiodine and ^{99m}Tc readily cross the placenta and also appear in breast milk, use of these pharmaceuticals is contraindicated in women who are pregnant or nursing.

Ultrasonography

Thyroid ultrasonography allows assessment of pathologic alterations in thyroid anatomy independent of glandular function. The technique can demonstrate diffuse abnormalities or localized enlargements of the gland and is particularly useful as an objective means of assessing changes in size over time, such as in response to suppressive therapy with thyroid hormone. Perhaps its greatest value lies in distinguishing nodules that are cystic (Fig. 97–12) from those that are solid or mixed solid-cystic (Fig. 97–13). The demonstration that a nodule is purely cystic reduces, but does not entirely eliminate, the likelihood of malignancy. Mixed lesions have the same significance as solid lesions, but benign and malignant lesions cannot be reliably differentiated from one another.

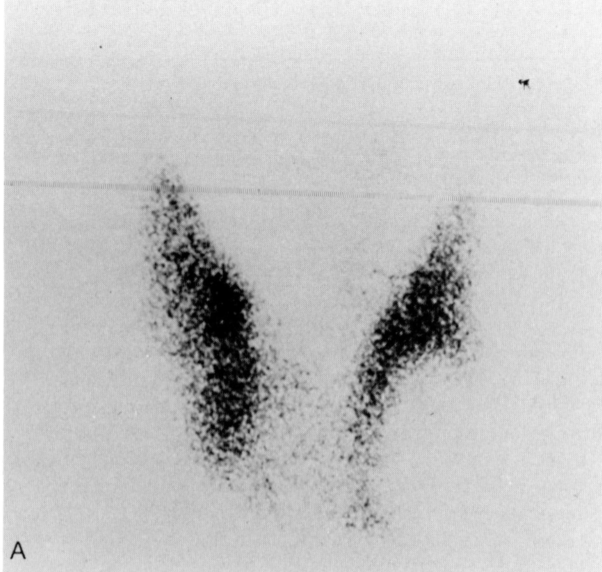

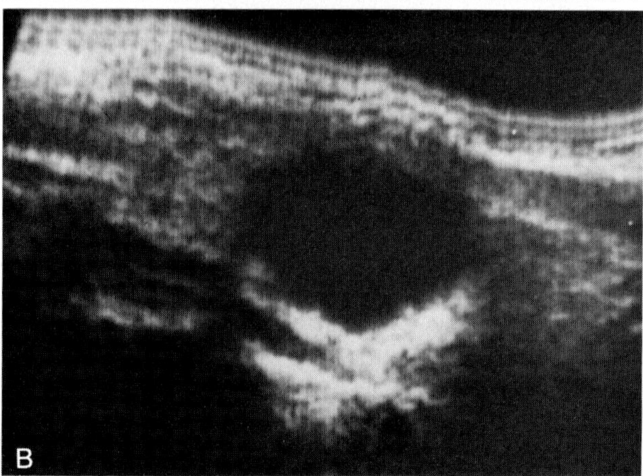

Figure 97–12. Thyroid cyst. *A,* There is a large palpable nodule in the left lower lobe of the thyroid that does not take up the ^{99m}Tc (cold nodule). *B,* Ultrasound reveals a cystic lesion characteristic of a thyroid cyst.

THYROTOXICOSIS (HYPERTHYROIDISM)

Thyrotoxicosis is the clinical syndrome resulting from sustained elevation of circulating thyroid hormone levels. The condition may result from a number of etiologically distinct disorders summarized in Table 97–2. Graves' disease, the most common cause, is a systemic autoimmune disorder characterized by diffuse thyrotoxic goiter, infiltrative ophthalmopathy, and occasionally infiltrative dermopathy (pretibial myxedema). Although it most often affects women in the third and fourth decades, Graves' disease may occur in either sex at any age. In toxic multinodular goiter, the second most common cause of persistent thyrotoxicosis, hyperthyroidism results from the gradual development of foci of autonomous hyperfunction in a pre-existing, usually long-standing, nontoxic multinodular goiter. Presumably reflecting the natural history of this condition evolving over a period of years, toxic multinodular goiter is usually a disease of the elderly. Toxic uninodular goiter, also more common in older age groups, represents the autonomously hyperfunctioning thyroid adenoma. In some forms of thyroiditis, hyperthyroidism may develop transiently as the inflammatory process leads to follicular disruption with leakage of preformed hormone into the blood. ''Painless'' or ''silent'' thyroiditis has recently gained increasing recognition as a relatively common cause of hyperthyroidism. Exogenous thyroid hormone excess, as with surreptitious self-administration (thyrotoxicosis factitia), produces a clinical syndrome indistinguishable from endogenous hyperthyroidism. Iodine-induced (Jod-Basedow) hyperthyroidism, originally described following dietary iodine supplementation in regions of endemic iodine deficiency, may also occur in areas of iodine sufficiency in patients with nontoxic multinodular goiter who have received large doses of iodine. Radiographic contrast media containing substantial quantities of iodine can cause thyrotoxicosis following routine diagnostic studies in patients with nodular goiter. The other causes of thyrotoxicosis listed in Table 97–2 are all exceedingly rare.

Clinical Manifestations and Laboratory Findings

In keeping with its ubiquitous actions, thyroid hormone excess may result in abnormalities involving virtually every organ system.

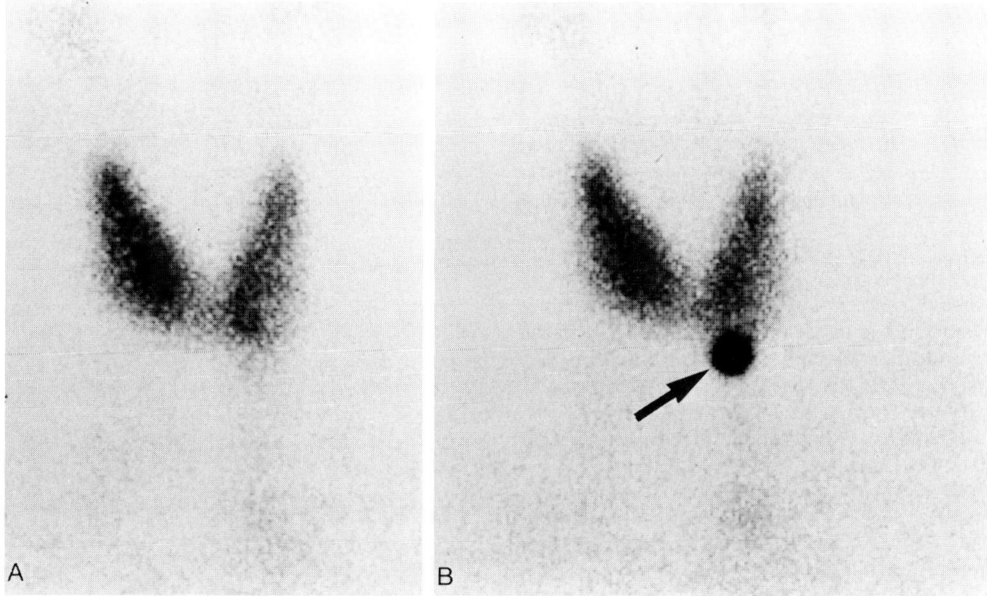

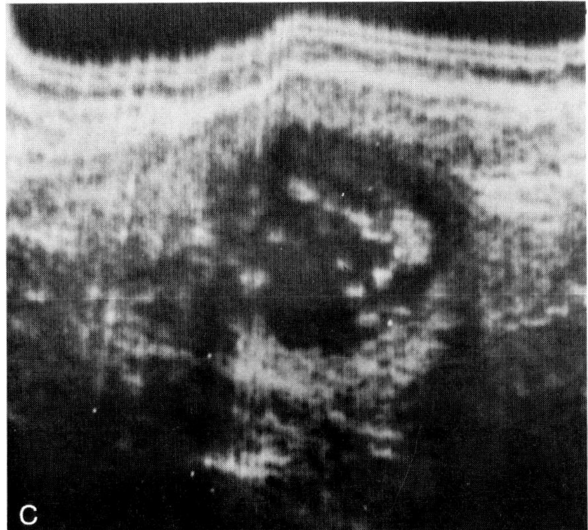

Figure 97–13. Thyroid carcinoma. *A,* A palpable nodule is present at the lower pole of the left thyroid gland, but it is not demonstrated on the ^{99m}Tc scan. *B,* A radioisotope marker is placed over the palpable nodule *(arrow)* and the gland rescanned. A cold nodule is present under the marker. *C,* Ultrasound demonstrates a complex mixed solid-cystic mass. Biopsy revealed a carcinoma of the thyroid.

Clinical manifestations generally reflect an increase in organ function and metabolism but are quite variable and are modified considerably by such factors as the age of the patient and the presence of underlying disease, particularly those affecting the heart. Common manifestations include nervousness, tremor, excessive sweating, heat intolerance, dyspnea, palpitations, hyperdefecation, weakness, fatigue, and weight loss, often occurring despite increased appetite.

TABLE 97–2. CAUSES OF THYROTOXICOSIS

Common
Graves' disease (diffuse toxic goiter)
Toxic multinodular goiter (Plummer's disease)
Toxic uninodular goiter (toxic adenoma)
Thyroiditis (esp. silent or painless thyroiditis)
Unusual
Exogenous thyroid hormone excess (factitious or iatrogenic)
Iodide-induced hyperthyroidism (Jod-Basedow)
Metastatic follicular thyroid carcinoma
Struma ovarii with hyperthyroidism
Pituitary TSH hypersecretion
Trophoblastic neoplasms (circulating thyroid stimulator)

Atrial tachyarrhythmias occur frequently, and patients with underlying cardiac disease may develop frank congestive heart failure. In general, cardiovascular and myopathic symptoms tend to dominate in the elderly, whereas nervous symptoms predominate in younger individuals.

Most patients with thyrotoxicosis have increased serum concentrations of both T_4 and T_3, although occasionally one or the other of these may be normal. Measures or estimates of free hormone concentration are elevated. TSH concentrations are, with very rare exception, undetectable; however, because most assays cannot distinguish between normal and low values, basal TSH determinations are not helpful in the diagnosis of hyperthyroidism. Although the diagnosis of hyperthyroidism is not difficult in advanced cases, mild hyperthyroidism may be associated with few or no symptoms and only marginal abnormalities in laboratory tests. In such instances, the TRH stimulation test assumes critical importance.

Radiographic Manifestations

The diagnosis of thyrotoxicosis rests primarily on the laboratory studies discussed above. Although the finding of an elevated RAIU may provide helpful confirmatory evidence, thyroid hyperfunction is not excluded by a normal uptake, and in some thyrotoxic states the RAIU is actually depressed (see Table 97–1). Because biochemical studies can more sensitively discriminate between the hyperthyroid and euthyroid states, nuclear scintigraphic techniques are of relatively limited usefulness as primary diagnostic modalities. However, these techniques are extremely valuable in distinguishing among the various causes of thyrotoxicosis (see Table 97–2). Because the therapeutic approach to each of these disorders differs, it is critical that a specific etiologic diagnosis be made in all cases of thyrotoxicosis.

In thyrotoxicosis due to Graves' disease and, to a lesser extent, in toxic uni- or multinodular goiter, the RAIU is characteristically increased. These conditions may be readily differentiated by their appearance on radionuclide scans. The Graves' gland exhibits a diffuse, homogeneous distribution of radionuclide, whereas the latter conditions display either a patchy, heterogeneous uptake (multinodular goiter) (Fig. 97–14) or an accumulation of isotope within one or more discrete nodules, the remainder of the gland appearing nonfunctional (uni- or multinodular goiter).

The finding of a low RAIU in a thyrotoxic patient is extremely useful in signaling the presence of one of the causes of thyrotoxicosis shown in Table 97–1. Of these, the recently recognized entity termed *painless* or *silent thyroiditis* deserves special emphasis as a relatively common cause of thyrotoxicosis, accounting for as many as 20 per cent of all newly diagnosed cases of hyperthyroidism. Thyrotoxicosis caused by thyroiditis runs a self-limited course, typically of several months, and conventional antithyroid therapy is contraindicated. Finally, it should always be remembered that the RAIU may also be low in other hyperthyroid conditions, such as Graves' disease, if the patient has recently received iodine-containing drugs or radiographic contrast agents.

Thyrotoxicosis may be associated with radiographically demonstrable osteopenia and increased incidence of fractures, particularly in elderly thyrotoxic patients. Bone turnover is accelerated, with resorption exceeding formation, and urinary and fecal calcium excretion are increased, leading to negative calcium balance. The relative rarity of clinical osteoporosis probably reflects the short duration of the disease in most patients. A rare extrathyroidal manifestation of Graves' disease is the syndrome of thyroid acropachy (Fig. 97–15), which occurs in 1 per cent of Graves' patients and is nearly always associated with infiltrative dermopathy (pretibial myxedema and exophthalmos). Its main freatures are clubbing of the fingers and toes, subcutaneous edema and fibrosis of the hands and feet, and a peculiar type of periosteal proliferative bone formation involving the phalanges and metacarpal and metatarsal bones. The new bone formation involves the diaphysis and has a characteristic fluffy, spiculated, or feathery appearance.

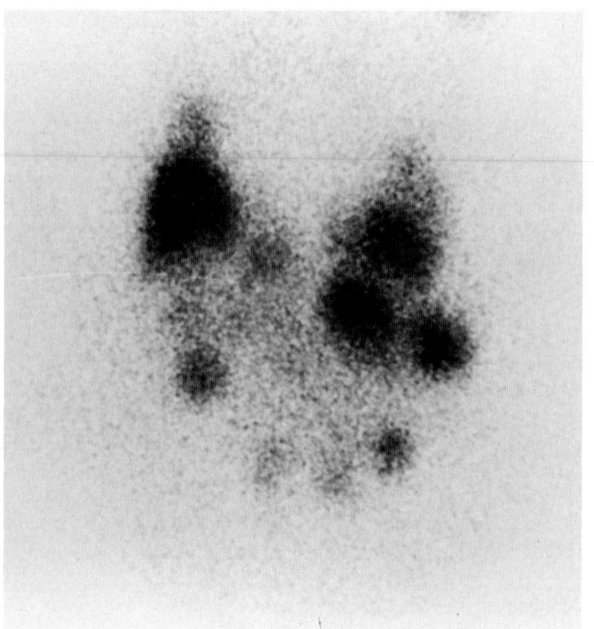

Figure 97–14. Thyrotoxicosis. A multinodular gland demonstrated patchy heterogeneous ^{99m}Tc uptake with some hot, warm, and cold nodules. The gland is enlarged in size.

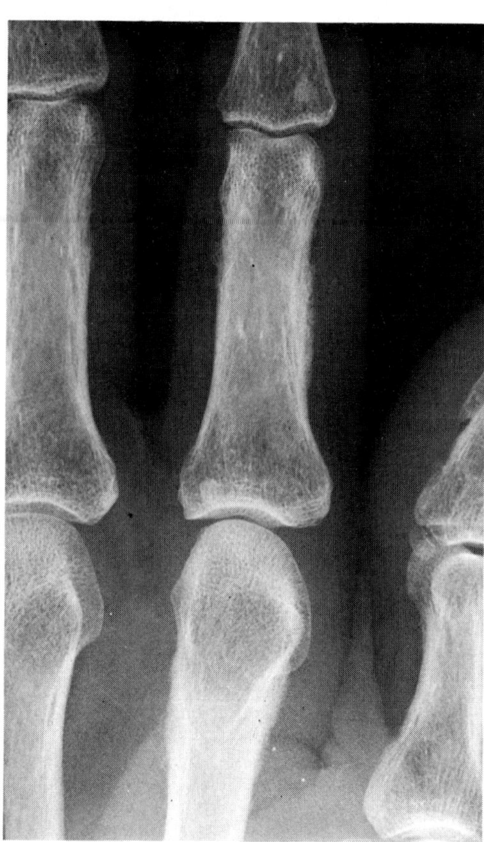

Figure 97–15. Thyroidacropachy. Characteristic thick periosteal new bone formation is present along the diaphysis of the proximal phalanx and the diametaphyseal area of the distal metacarpal.

HYPOTHYROIDISM

Hypothyroidism is the condition resulting from inadequate peripheral tissue levels of thyroid hormone; in severe cases, it is termed *myxedema*. Hypothyroidism is most commonly caused by disorders of the thyroid itself (primary hypothyroidism) but may also result from deficient pituitary TSH secretion due to either pituitary or hypothalamic disease (secondary and tertiary hypothyroidism, respectively). A rare syndrome of peripheral resistance to thyroid hormone has also been described. The causes of hypothyroidism are listed in Table 97–3. Iatrogenic causes (radioiodine therapy for hyperthyroidism and thyroidectomy) and chronic lymphocytic thyroiditis (Hashimoto's disease) are the most common conditions causing thyroid failure in the adult. Thyroid dysgenesis accounts for the great majority of cases of infantile hypothyroidism, followed by congenital biosynthetic defects. Severe thyroid failure beginning in infancy and resulting in developmental abnormalities is termed *cretinism*.

TABLE 97–3. CAUSES OF HYPOTHYROIDISM

I. Thyroidal (primary) (95 per cent of cases)
  A. Goitrous
    1. Chronic autoimmune thyroiditis (Hashimoto's disease)
    2. Iodine deficiency
    3. Heritable biosynthetic defects
    4. Goitrogens (iodine, antithyroid drugs, others)
    5. Infiltrative diseases (rare)
    6. Subacute or "silent"* thyroiditis
  B. Nongoitrous
    1. Primary idiopathic atrophy
    2. Postablative (radioiodine, surgery)
    3. Following external radiotherapy (for head/neck cancer)
    4. Thyroid dysgenesis
II. Pituitary failure (secondary)
  A. Tumor, infiltrative disease
  B. Postablative (surgery, radiotherapy)
  C. Postpartum necrosis (Sheehan's syndrome)
  D. Idiopathic TSH deficiency (rare)
III. Hypothalamic dysfunction (tertiary)
IV. Peripheral resistance to thyroid hormone (rare)

*Goiter may be minimal or absent.

Clinical Manifestations and Laboratory Findings

In adults, the clinical syndrome of hypothyroidism generally develops insidiously with initially nonspecific symptoms that include lethargy, constipation, cold intolerance, weakness or apathy, dry skin and hair, modest weight gain, and menorrhagia. Ultimately, the clinical picture of florid myxedema appears, with dull puffy facial features, slow hoarse voice, enlarged tongue, sparse brittle hair, and coarse doughy skin with nonpitting peripheral edema. Sluggish reflexes and bradycardia are present, and effusion may develop in pleural, pericardial, and abdominal cavities, as well as in various joints. Left untreated, long-standing hypothyroidism may progress into a life-threatening hypothermic and stuporous state termed *myxedema coma*.

In children, deficiency of thyroid hormone results in skeletal and neurologic retardation in addition to the changes associated with adult hypothyroidism. The clinical picture varies with the age of onset and the severity of thyroid failure. Severe hypothyroidism in infancy, if untreated, leads to permanent growth retardation and skeletal deformities with severe mental retardation (cretinism). Because early recognition and treatment provide a reasonable expectation for normal development, routine biochemical screening of the neonate is now widely practiced. Thyroid failure in the older child produces a syndrome intermediate between infantile and adult hypothyroidism, with growth failure, delayed sexual maturation, and variable degrees of intellectual impairment.

The laboratory hallmark of hypothyroidism, regardless of etiology, is a reduction in circulating free hormonal levels, established by measurements of total T_4 together with some index of serum protein binding. In primary or thyroidal hypothyroidism, which composes the vast majority of cases (95 per cent), serum TSH is invariably increased and represents the single most sensitive index of thyroid failure. Serum TSH is normal or low in the far less common suprathyroidal causes of hypothyroidism.

Radiographic Findings (Fig. 97–16)

Lack of thyroid hormone during development markedly retards the growth and maturation of the skeletal system and causes distinctive skeletal abnormalities that have a characteristic radiographic appearance. In cretinism, the skull has a poorly developed base, delayed ossification of the sphenoid bone, widened frontal suture, enlarged anterior fontanelle, widely set orbits, and a short flat nasal bone. Delayed skeletal ossification and absent distal femoral epiphyses may be noted at birth. Linear growth is severely impaired, leading to dwarfism with infantile skeletal proportions (disproportionately short limbs relative to the trunk). Dental maturation is delayed. A characteristic radiographic feature of hypothyroidism in infancy or childhood is epiphyseal dysgenesis. This abnormality may affect any endochondral ossification center but is usually most apparent in the larger centers such as the femoral and humeral heads and the tarsal navicular bone. Centers of ossification appear late, leading to a retarded bone age. When the center eventually appears, it develops from multiple foci of scattered calcifications that gradually coalesce within a misshapen epiphysis, forming a single center with an irregular outline and a stippled appearance (stippled epiphysis).

In juvenile hypothyroidism, linear growth plateaus, dental development is delayed, and sexual maturation is retarded. On radiographic examination, epiphyseal dysgenesis may be present in centers that undergo ossification after the age of onset of the thyroid deficiency. Epiphyseal fusion is always delayed, resulting in a bone age that is retarded in relation to chronologic age.

In adult hypothyroidism, bone turnover is diminished and bone density may be increased. Articular involvement causing joint aching and stiffness is common with synovial thickening and noninflammatory effusions affecting the small joints and knees. Radiographs may show periarticular osteoporosis, occasional erosions and joint space narrowing without osteophytes, and, rarely, avascular necrosis. Although the pathophysiologic basis for the joint involvement is unknown, the articular symptoms abate with thyroid hormone therapy.

THYROID GOITER

Nontoxic diffuse goiter, often referred to as a simple goiter, may be defined as an enlargement of the thyroid that does not result from an inflammatory or neoplastic process and that is not initially associated with either thyrotoxicosis or hypothyroidism. When long-standing, the diffuse goiter becomes multinodular. Pathogenetically, the nontoxic goiter represents a compensatory hyperplastic response, presumably driven by TSH, to any impairment in the efficiency of thyroid hormonogenesis. Thus, the disorder differs only in degree from goitrous hypothyroidism and may be presumed to result from the same specific etiologic factors. However, in the majority of cases of nonendemic (sporadic) goiter, a specific etiology is not apparent, and vigorous efforts at its elucidation are probably unjustified. Once a multinodular goiter has developed, patients often display evidence of functional thyroid autonomy, and thyrotoxicosis may ultimately develop spontaneously (toxic multinodular goiter) or in response to exogenous iodine administration. Nontoxic goiter may be cosmetically disturbing to the patient but generally causes no symptoms and is usually discovered during a routine examination. Pressure symptoms such as coughing, stridor, dysphagia, or hoarseness should suggest malignancy but may occur in a large goiter low in the neck that is compressed by the sternum or grows around behind the trachea. Narrowing of the thoracic inlet may produce venous engorgement of the head, neck, and upper limbs, which is accentuated when the patient's arms are raised (Pemberton's sign). Hemorrhage into a nodule or cyst may produce sudden painful enlargement locally and, if crucially situated, may exacerbate or induce obstructive symptoms.

Patients with nontoxic goiter should undergo radioisotopic thyroid scanning to identify nodularity and potential areas of autonomous function. Although goiter per se does not appear to predispose to malignancy, the demonstration of a large, dominant nonfunctioning nodule or the recent growth of a cold nodule should arouse

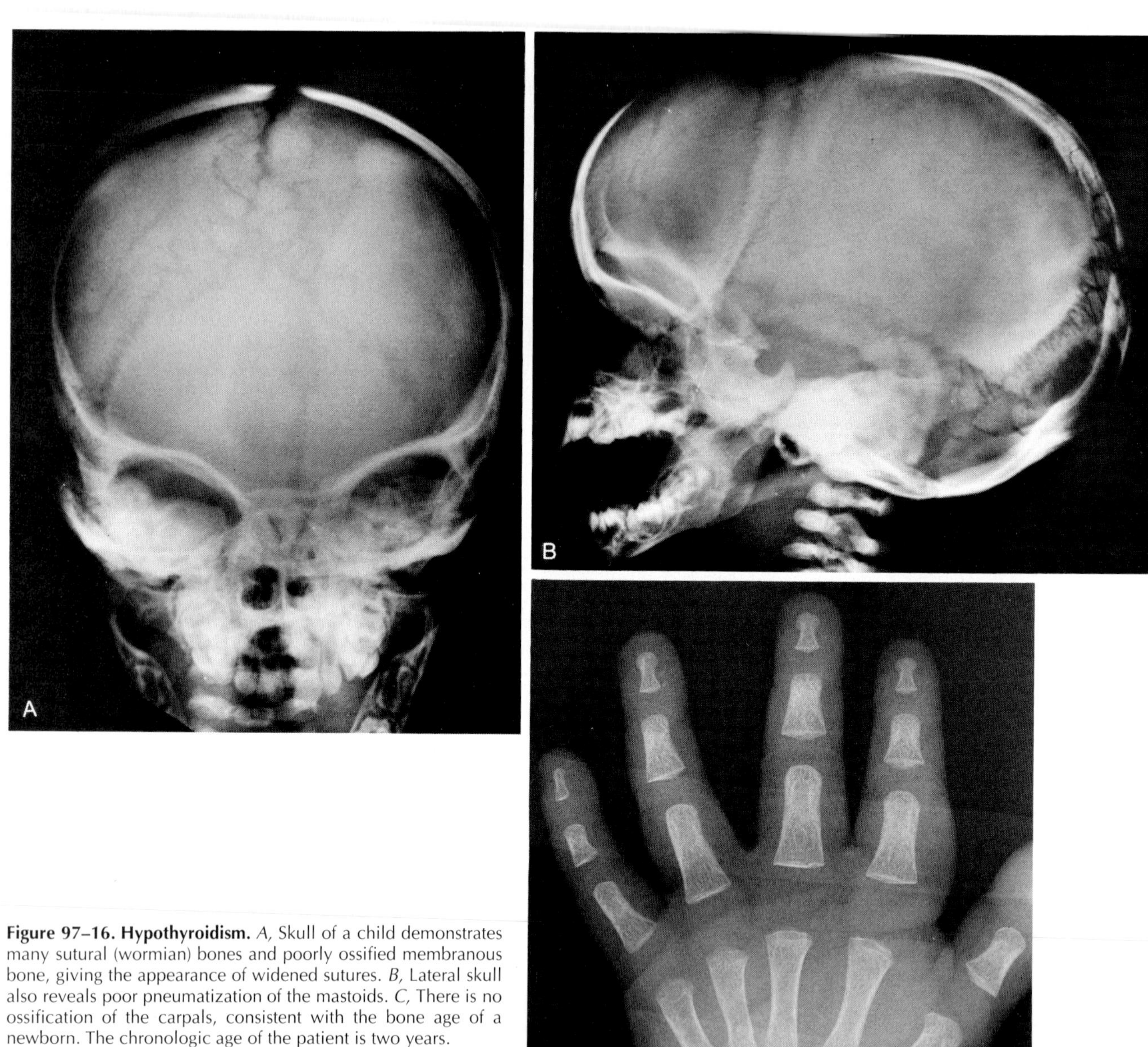

Figure 97–16. Hypothyroidism. *A,* Skull of a child demonstrates many sutural (wormian) bones and poorly ossified membranous bone, giving the appearance of widened sutures. *B,* Lateral skull also reveals poor pneumatization of the mastoids. *C,* There is no ossification of the carpals, consistent with the bone age of a newborn. The chronologic age of the patient is two years.

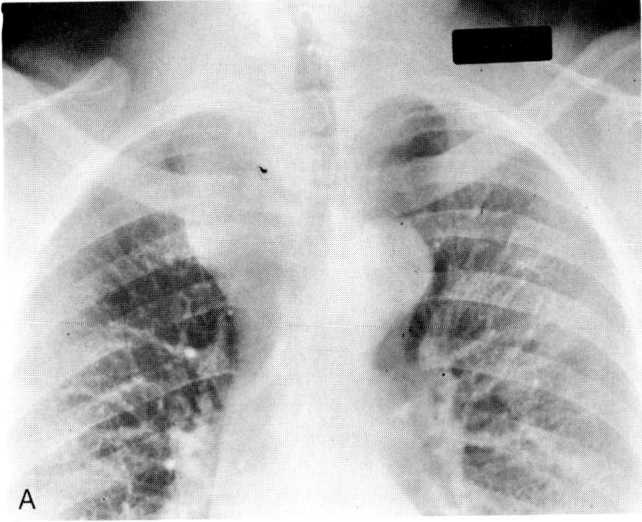

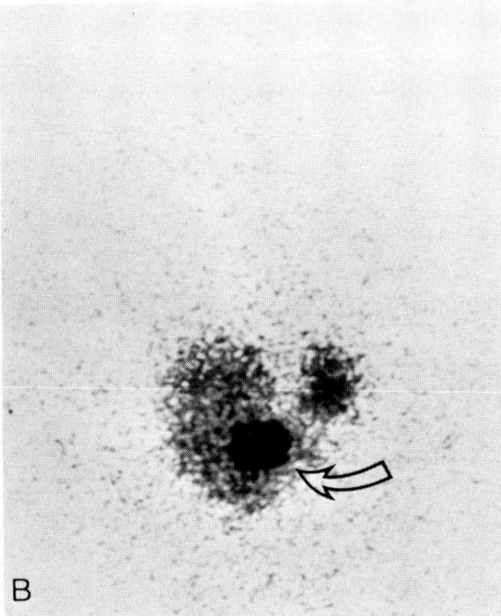

Figure 97–17. Substernal thyroid goiter. *A,* A right paratracheal mass is deviating the trachea to the left. *B,* Iodine-123 scan at 24 hours demonstrates the location of the thyroid to be directly under the radioisotope marker *(arrow),* which was placed at the sternal notch. No thyroid tissue is demonstrated in the normal location in the neck.

suspicion. Functional autonomy is suggested on scan by areas of disproportionately intense isotope accumulation and would be further supported by the finding of a blunted or absent serum TSH response to exogenous TRH. Nontoxic goiter is sometimes difficult to differentiate on the radionuclide scan from chronic autoimmune thyroiditis (Hashimoto's disease). The demonstration of circulating antithyroid antibodies in high titer would indicate the presence of Hashimoto's disease. The RAIU in nontoxic goiter is usually normal, but it may be increased in some patients, such as those with mild iodine deficiency or a biosynthetic defect.

A special circumstance that arises not infrequently is the use of thyroid scanning to identify substernal goiter in the patient with an undiagnosed mediastinal mass (Fig. 97–17). For this application radioiodine (usually ^{123}I), which allows delayed imaging at 24 hours, is considered preferable to ^{99m}Tc, because at the 20- to 30-minute imaging time for ^{99m}Tc, the high mediastinal blood pool activity makes visualization of a substernal thyroid difficult. An additional advantage of radioiodine is its higher-energy photons, which are attenuated less by the sternum than those of ^{99m}Tc. When the thyroid extends substernally it almost always does so in contiguity with the cervical portion of the gland. Thus, the demonstration of a normal thyroid gland in the neck markedly reduces the probability that a substernal mass represents a goiter.

THYROIDITIS

Several etiologically distinct inflammatory disorders of the thyroid are subsumed under the heading *thyroiditis.* Included in this category are two extremely rare entities—acute suppurative thyroiditis, caused by bacterial infection involving one or occasionally both lobes, and fibrous (Riedel's) thyroiditis, a chronic process of unknown etiology characterized by extensive fibrosis of the thyroid and adjacent structures. Reidel's thyroiditis may be difficult to differentiate from thyroid cancer because it presents clinically as a palpably hard, painless goiter, which on scan shows reduced radionuclide uptake over the involved area.

Subacute (nonsuppurative) thyroiditis (Fig. 97–18), also known as granulomatous, giant cell, or de Quervain's thyroiditis, is a disorder of probable viral origin and is the most common cause of thyroid pain and tenderness. Frequently following an upper respiratory infection, its onset is usually fairly abrupt, with neck pain radiating to the ears or lower jaw accompanied by systemic manifestations such as fever and malaise. On physical examination the thyroid is tender and mildly to moderately enlarged, usually asymmetrically, and it may contain distinct nodules.

On laboratory testing, the two hallmarks of the disease are an inordinately elevated erythrocyte sedimentation rate (ESR) and a markedly suppressed RAIU. Early in the course of the disease, disruption of follicular epithelium leads to release of preformed hormone, often in quantities sufficient to cause mild thyrotoxicosis, with a resultant suppression of TSH that contributes to the reduced RAIU. Rarely, in milder cases, some uptake of radioiodine may persist in unaffected portions of the gland, and radionuclide scanning may disclose a patchy irregular pattern or no uptake over the involved area, which may simulate a cold nodule. Later in the disease, depletion of preformed hormone may lead to transient hypothyroidism, with low serum T_4 and T_3 levels and high TSH levels. As the disease becomes inactive, the RAIU rises to normal or even transiently elevated values, as glandular hormone stores are replenished. Ultimately, with very rare exception, all tests return to normal as complete spontaneous healing occurs after a clinical course lasting an average of two to five months.

A late recognized form of thyroiditis termed *painless* or *silent thyroiditis* follows a pathophysiologic and clinical course that is

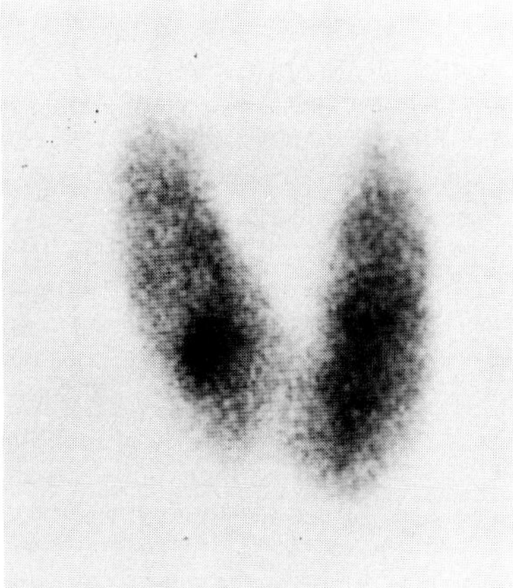

Figure 97–18. Subacute thyroiditis. Heterogeneous ^{99m}Tc uptake in a mildly enlarged tender thyroid gland in a patient who had a viral illness one month before.

virtually identical to that of subacute thyroiditis—namely, an early thyrotoxic phase with a low to absent RAIU, sometimes followed by a transient phase of hypothyroidism, but proceeding ultimately to complete recovery with a normal radioiodine uptake. Clinical features differentiating this entity from subacute thyroiditis include the absence of pain and tenderness (hence the term silent), the frequent absence of goiter, and the absence of any clinical evidence suggesting a viral infectious etiology such as fever, lassitude, elevated ESR, or prior respiratory illness. Moreover, thyroid biopsy in silent thyroiditis discloses not the acute inflammatory changes seen with subacute thyroiditis, but rather a lymphocytic infiltration resembling chronic lymphocytic (Hashimoto's) thyroiditis. Silent thyroiditis also has a unique predilection for the postpartum period. Although the balance of evidence favors an autoimmune etiology, as in Hashimoto's disease, it remains controversial as to whether silent thyroiditis should be considered a variant of Hashimoto's disease, from which it is clinically, if not histologically, quite distinct. With the increasing recent awareness of its distinctive clinical features, silent thyroiditis has been shown to represent a relatively common, previously unrecognized cause of thyrotoxicosis. It should be suspected in any thyrotoxic patient without a palpable goiter and is probably the most common cause of thyrotoxicosis with a low RAIU (see Table 97–1).

In chronic lymphocytic (Hashimoto's) thyroiditis, the thyroid is infiltrated by lymphocytes that form germinal centers with varying degrees of fibrosis, leading to goiter, parenchymal destruction, and thyroid hormone insufficiency. Circulating antithyroid antibodies, an association with other immune disorders, and evidence of cell-mediated immunity all support an autoimmune etiology for this disease, which is sometimes termed *chronic autoimmune thyroiditis.* A common disorder that may be increasing in frequency, Hashimoto's disease is the most common cause of goitrous hypothyroidism in areas of iodine sufficiency. Although occurring most frequently in women of middle age, it is also one of the most common causes of sporadic nontoxic goiter in children. The gradual onset of a painless goiter is the outstanding clinical feature of the disease. The diagnosis is made by demonstrating circulating antithyroid antibodies in high titer. Thyroid function tests are usually abnormal but unpredictable. Early in the disease the patient may be euthyroid but may have an elevated serum TSH (so-called compensated or subclinical hypothyroidism). Rarely, transient hyperthyroidism may develop, or the disorder may coexist with Graves' disease, causing sustained hyperthyroidism (''Hashitoxicosis''). Some patients may remain euthyroid for many years. Most commonly, however, with the passage of time frank hypothyroidism of increasing severity supervenes and is permanent.

Radionuclide studies yield markedly variable results, reflecting a spectrum of pathophysiologic defects that depend in part on the stage of the disease process. The RAIU may be low, normal, or elevated. Prior to the development of end-stage hypothyroidism, the Hashimoto's gland typically traps iodide normally, but subsequent organification and biosynthetic steps are impaired. Because of the faulty hormone synthesis, hypersecretion of TSH occurs, producing functional evidence of thyroid hyperactivity (high RAIU) without thyrotoxicosis (normal circulating T_4 and T_3). With the passage of time, progressive destruction of thyroid parenchyma impairs the response to TSH, and both the RAIU and circulating hormone concentrations gradually decline to subnormal values. Finally, in the rare patient with persistent thyrotoxicosis associated with histologic Hashimoto's thyroiditis, the RAIU is elevated. This contrasts with the low RAIU seen transiently in silent thyrotoxic thyroiditis.

Radionuclide scanning in Hashimoto's thyroiditis usually shows an enlarged gland with a patchy or mottled uptake. Although activity is usually present throughout the gland, occasionally the pattern may masquerade as a solitary cold nodule. Recent studies have challenged the previously held notion that the prevalence of thyroid carcinoma is increased in this disorder. However, because a definite association with lymphoma of the thyroid has been established, needle biopsy has been recommended for demonstrated cold nodules in Hashimoto's thyroiditis.

THYROID NEOPLASMS

Thyroid adenomas are benign epithelial neoplasms that usually present clinically as a painless thyroid nodule. The chief importance of these tumors lies in the need to differentiate them from carcinoma and in their ability occasionally to induce a thyrotoxic state (toxic adenoma). By far the most common variety is the follicular adenoma, a well-differentiated tumor that may mimic the function of normal thyroid tissue and concentrate radioiodine, a feature that helps distinguish it from most carcinomas. However, the greatest majority of adenomas are hypofunctional on the radionuclide scan compared with surrounding thyroid tissue. Follicular adenomas commonly undergo hemorrhagic infarction, often with calcification that may be visible on plain film radiographs. Together with thyroid cysts, degenerated adenomas compose the majority of nonfunctioning nodules of the thyroid.

Thyroid carcinomas may be broadly subdivided into two general types: those arising from the thyroid follicular epithelium and those arising from the parafollicular (C cell) elements. In the former category the tumors are classified into three general histologic types, which differ in their biologic behavior and clinical course. The rare anaplastic carcinoma is an undifferentiated, highly malignant tumor that usually afflicts the elderly and is rapidly fatal owing to extensive local invasion. Follicular carcinoma, comprising about 15 to 20 per cent of all thyroid malignancies, is a slow-growing tumor that tends to undergo early hematogenous spread with distant metastases to lung, bone, or other sites. The third and most common type, accounting for well over half of all thyroid cancers, is papillary carcinoma. This is the most slowly growing and indolent of all thyroid malignancies. It may remain localized for many years, and its spread is typically confined to regional lymph nodes. Carcinoma arising from the parafollicular or C cells (calcitonin-secreting) of the thyroid is termed *medullary carcinoma*, an aggressive tumor that spreads both to local lymph nodes and via the bloodstream to distant sites and that tends to be intermediate in biologic malignancy between follicular and anaplastic carcinoma. Finally, the thyroid may be secondarily involved by lymphoma or metastases from various extrathyroidal carcinomas such as kidney, lung, breast, and melanoma.

Thyroid-imaging studies figure prominently in the diagnostic evaluation of potentially malignant palpable thyroid nodules. Although the distinction between benign and malignant nodules can never be made with absolute certainty, with appropriate evaluation one can minimize the likelihood of performing surgery for a benign nodule or of leaving a carcinoma in place. The importance of a selective surgical approach is underscored by the very high prevalence of palpable thyroid nodules in the general United States population (about 4 per cent), in contrast to the exceedingly low incidence of clinical thyroid cancer (less than 4 cases per 100,000 yearly).

Clinical and radiographic features (Fig. 97–19) suggesting malignancy in a thyroid nodule are listed in Table 97–4. Because carcinomas almost invariably concentrate less radioiodine than surrounding thyroid tissue, the demonstration on radionuclide scanning of a solitary, hypofunctioning (cold) nodule in an otherwise normal gland should arouse suspicion. Unfortunately, this finding is nonspecific, since the great majority of benign thyroid nodules are also hypofunctional. The likelihood of malignancy in any solitary cold nodule is probably no greater than 20 per cent. Most such nodules represent cysts, adenomatous colloid nodules, areas of localized thyroiditis, or true thyroid adenomas. When radionuclide scanning reveals a diffusely abnormal thyroid with multiple imaging defects, as in multinodular goiter, the likelihood of malignancy is markedly

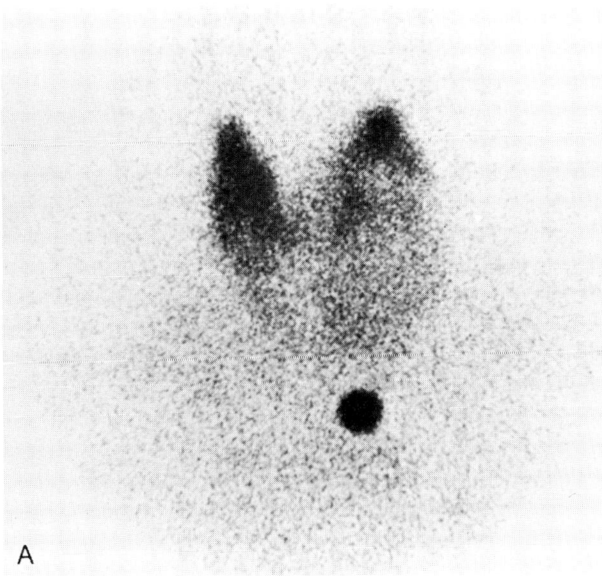

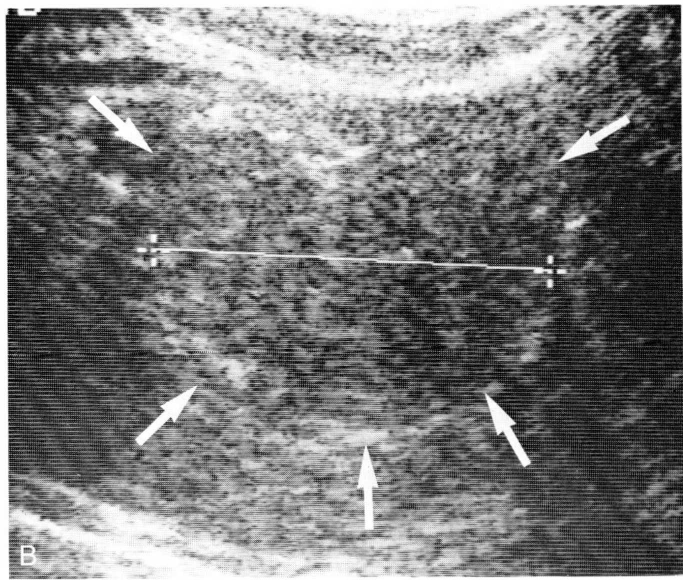

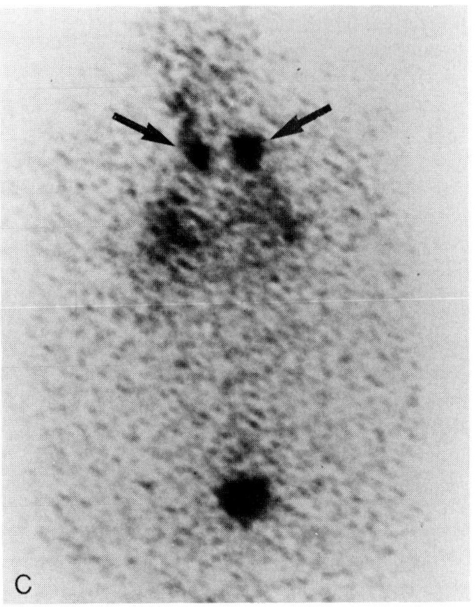

Figure 97–19. Thyroid carcinoma and multinodular goiter. *A,* Multinodular goiter with a dominant hypofunctioning mass present in the lower left lobe above the radioisotope marker placed at the sternal notch. *B,* Ultrasound reveals a large solid mass *(arrows)* in the lower left portion of the gland, which proved to be a carcinoma on biopsy. The patient had radiation to the neck as a child. *C,* Iodine-131 scan demonstrates two metastatic lesions in the superior mediastinum *(arrows)*. Isotope is also present in the liver and bladder.

TABLE 97–4. THE THYROID NODULE: FEATURES INCREASING THE LIKELIHOOD OF MALIGNANCY

A. Clinical / historical
1. Age < 40
2. Male
3. History of neck irradiation
4. Family history of medullary thyroid carcinoma or pheochromocytoma
5. Recent growth
6. Symptoms of local growth (hoarseness, dysphagia)

B. Anatomic / radiographic
1. Solitary
2. Hypofunctional (''cold'') on radionuclide scan
3. Solid or complex on ultrasound
4. Failure to regress with thyroid hormone suppression

C. Physical examination
1. Hard
2. Fixed to surrounding tissue
3. Lymphadenopathy

reduced. Similarly, a nodule that exhibits greater function than normal thyroid tissue by radioiodine scanning may be assumed to be a benign adenoma. However, because an occasional malignant lesion will actively accumulate ^{99m}Tc but not radioiodine, the appearance of hyperfunction on technetium scanning requires confirmation with radioiodine.

The presence of a cold nodule on nuclear imaging may indicate either a solid nodule that does not accumulate isotope or a cystic area of the gland. Ultrasonography permits the differentiation of the solid from the cystic nodule. Simple cysts, comprising about 20 per cent of cold nodules, are very rarely malignant, especially if smaller than 4 cm in diameter. Solid or mixed lesions can be either benign or malignant, but there are no firm criteria on which to base a diagnosis of malignancy. An advantage of sonography over both isotope imaging and physical examination is its superior spatial resolution. Consequently, ultrasound provides the most sensitive discrimination between solitary lesions and the multinodular goiter, and it also permits the most accurate assessment of change in nodule size over time, as, for example, in response to suppressive therapy with thyroid hormone. Ultrasound has also been used to help localize lesions for needle biopsy.

Needle biopsy of the thyroid has recently been adopted in an effort to enhance the diagnostic evaluation of thyroid nodules. The most commonly employed technique is fine-needle aspiration. Disadvantages include the requirement for a specifically experienced cytopathologist, the problem of nonrepresentative tissue sampling, and the inability of the technique to differentiate follicular carcinoma from benign follicular neoplasms. Despite these shortcomings this method has the potential of yielding improved diagnostic accuracy when the technique is used to complement conventional radiographic studies.

PARATHYROID

PAMELA S. JENSEN

The parathyroid gland is responsible for the regulation of calcium. It actually consists of four separate glands located in the region of the upper and lower poles of the thyroid. Embryologically the glands originate from the third and fourth pharyngeal pouches. The superior glands migrate caudally with the thyroid. The inferior glands move with the thymus, coming to rest in the lower poles of the thyroid about 95 per cent of the time. Ectopic locations of the parathyroid gland include the thymus, the mediastinum, between the thyroid and esophagus, and within the carotid sheath.

PARATHYROID HORMONE

Parathyroid hormone (PTH) is synthesized in the parathyroid gland as a large molecule, and it is in this form that it is stored in the gland. This pro-hormone must be enzymatically cleaved prior to release into the circulation, where it is again broken into two fragments, creating active PTH. The fragment with the amino terminal has a short half-life and is the biologically active portion. The carboxyl-terminal fragment has a longer half-life but no biologic activity.

PTH synthesis and release are controlled by the ionized serum calcium level. Low serum calcium stimulates and high serum calcium suppresses PTH synthesis and release. Elevated serum phosphate levels also promote PTH secretion by reducing the ionized serum calcium level. PTH maintains the serum calcium level in the following ways: it promotes the intestinal absorption of calcium by stimulating the renal synthesis of active vitamin D; PTH promotes calcium release from the bones by inhibiting osteoblasts, stimulating osteocytes, and favoring osteoclast formation; and it enhances the renal tubular resorption of calcium and the excretion of phosphate. Measurement of the circulating level of PTH is difficult, particularly in the presence of renal failure, because of the various forms that are present. Radioimmunoassays that measure the biologically active amino-terminal fragment are probably preferable to the standard measurement of the nonactive carboxyl-terminal fragment. PTH activity can also be assessed by measuring the production of nephrogenous cyclic AMP (cAMP). In addition to PTH, vitamin D and calcitonin are also regulators of calcium metabolism.

VITAMIN D

Vitamin D is an important hormone that is involved with the regulation of bone mineral metabolism. Vitamin D_3 (cholecalciferol) is formed when sterols in the skin are exposed to ultraviolet light. This vitamin D_3 and dietary D_3 are then hydroxylated in the liver to form 25-hydroxy vitamin D_3, which, in turn, is hydroxylated in the kidney to form the active metabolite 1,25-dihydroxy vitamin D_3 (calcitriol). The activity of the renal enzyme responsible for the final hydroxylation is enhanced by PTH, hypocalcemia (via increased PTH secretion), and hypophosphatemia. Liver and renal disease impair the activation of vitamin D_3. The major function of calcitriol is promoting the intestinal absorption of both calcium and phosphorus. This activity enhances bone formation by raising both serum calcium and phosphorus levels, thereby making these minerals available for mineralization of the osteoid matrix to form hydroxyapatite. In high pharmacologic concentrations, calcitriol can actually promote the breakdown of hydroxyapatite, leading to bone loss.

CALCITONIN

Calcitonin is secreted by the parafollicular cells of the thyroid gland. Its pharmacologic action is to reduce bone resorption, whereby it may have a role in reversing hypercalcemia. However, its actual physiologic role in humans has not yet been defined.

PRIMARY HYPERPARATHYROIDISM

Excess PTH production can occur as a result of adenoma, hyperplasia, or carcinoma of the parathyroid gland. Primary hyperparathyroidism is caused by a single adenoma in nearly 90 per cent of cases. Large adenomas are usually associated with high serum calcium levels, a short course, and discernible bone disease. Smaller adenomas have a longer history and lower levels of hypercalcemia and may cause renal stones. Parathyroid hyperplasia usually involves all four glands and typically has a longer history. Less than 1 per cent of primary hyperparathyroidism is due to carcinoma of the gland. Carcinoma is often associated with very high levels of serum calcium (greater than 15 mg/dl), a finding that is uncommon with the more common causes of primary hyperparathyroidism.

Clinical and Laboratory Manifestations

The clinical manifestations of primary hyperparathyroidism are diverse. Prior to multiphasic screening, the disease was usually identified only in the advanced stages. Severe bone disease (osteitis fibrosa cystica) (Fig. 97–20), increased kyphosis and loss of height due to multiple vertebral compression fractures, weakness, anemia, renal impairment with or without renal stones, and neurologic, mental, gastrointestinal, and musculoskeletal disorders were common presenting features. With multiphasic screening, patients with asymptomatic hypercalemia are being identified. Increased aware-

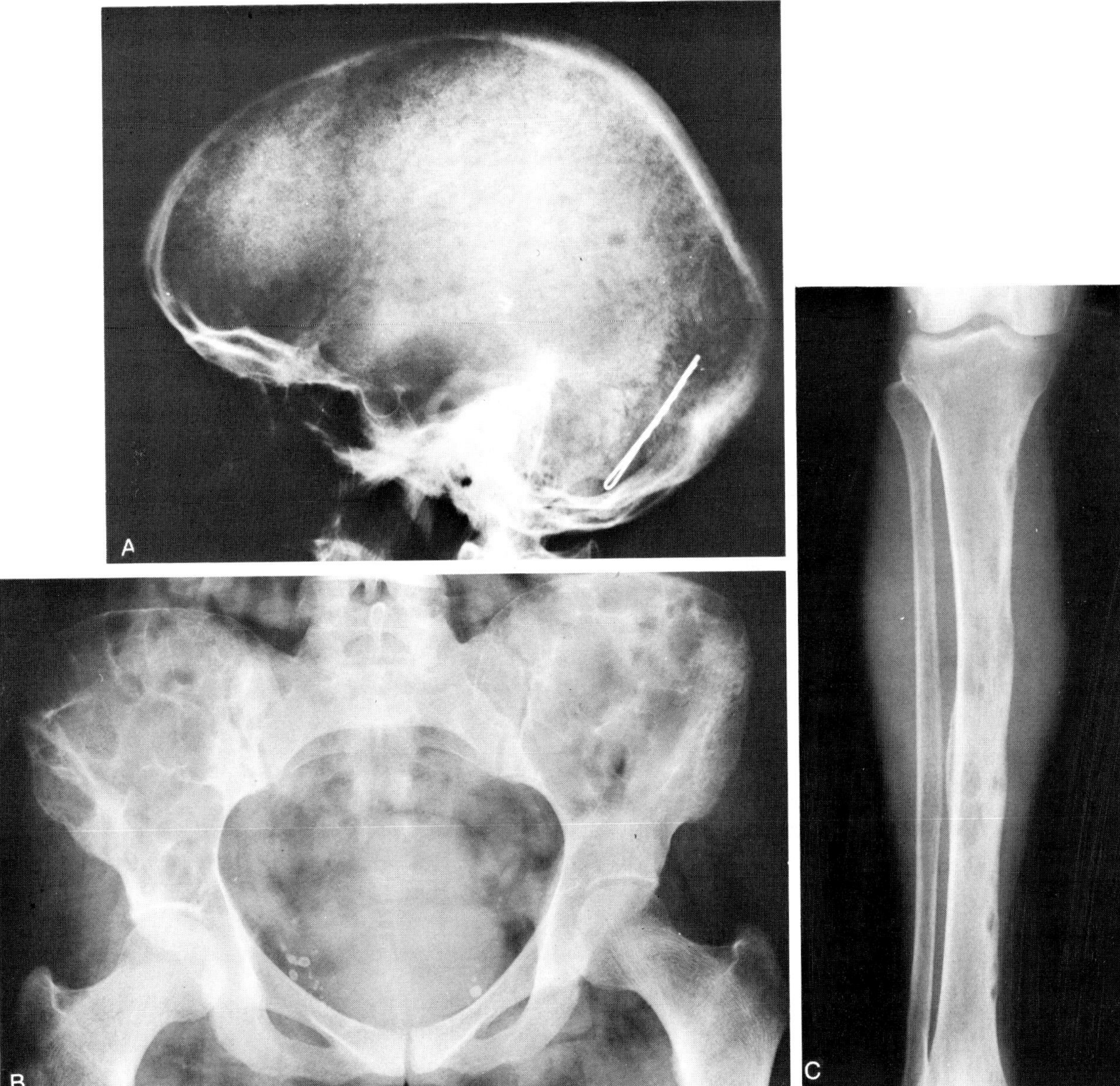

Figure 97–20. Advanced primary hyperparathyroidism. *A,* The calvarium has a mottled "salt and pepper" appearance because areas of resorption are adjacent to areas of preserved bone. *B,* Very large cystic bubbly osteoclastomas (secondary giant cell tumors or brown tumors) are present in both ilia. *C,* Multiple well-demarcated cystic lesions are present in the tibia (osteitis fibrosa cystica). Intracortical lesions have caused expansion of the cortex and bowing of the bone.

ness and concern regarding osteoporosis are also leading to the identification of asymptomatic hyperparathyroidism. The serum calcium is elevated in over 95 per cent of patients. Repeated samples are sometimes needed to establish the diagnosis in mild hyperparathyroidism because the hypercalcemia can be intermittent. In addition, hyperparathyroidism can be present without demonstration of an elevated serum calcium despite repeated sampling because other factors can reduce the calcium level, including vitamin D deficiency, intestinal malabsorption of calcium, magnesium deficiency, and hyperphosphatemia, usually in association with chronic renal insufficiency.

Multiple endocrine neoplasia types I and II (MEN I and II), formerly termed multiple endocrine adenomatosis (MEA), usually exhibits hyperparathyroidism with the initial presentation. MEN I has variable involvement of the following glands: pituitary with resultant acromegaly, hyperprolactinemia, hypopituitarism, or normal function; parathyroid with resultant hyperparathyroidism; pancreas with resultant hyperinsulinism, hypergastrinism (Zollinger-Ellison syndrome), or pancreatic cholera; and peptic ulcer disease. With MEN II, medullary carcinoma of the thyroid, which secretes increased levels of calcitonin leading to secondary hyperparathyroidism, and pheochromocytoma are present. These disorders are inherited as an autosomal dominant; thus, first-order family members have a 50 per cent chance of having the disease.

Because measurement of PTH is difficult owing to the various fragments and uncleaved hormone present in the serum, it is often of little utility in suspected mild hyperparathyroidism. Urinary cAMP is elevated in patients with hyperparathyroidism but not with other causes of hypercalcemia. The only curative therapy is surgical resection of the abnormal parathyroid tissue. However, patients with mild disease and no clinical symptoms often remain asymptomatic for many years.

Radiographic Manifestations

The radiographic manifestations are diverse, reflecting the variable extent of the clinical disease. In advanced stages marked skeletal changes can be present. Findings include extensive bone loss, compression fractures of the spine, pathologic fractures, brown tumors, arthropathy, renal stones, and nephrocalcinosis. With early detection of the disease there may be no radiographic findings. In longstanding mild disease endosteal cortical bone loss most readily detected at the midshaft of the second metacarpal (Fig. 97–21) and intracortical resorption (tunneling) demonstrated by fine-detail radiography may be the only indicators of bone loss on plain film radiography (Fig. 97–22). Subperiosteal resorption, the hallmark of hyperparathyroidism, is often not detectable in mild or slowly progressive disease. If it is present, it may be limited to the radial sides of the bases of the middle phalanges at the site of the ligamentous attachment; the index and middle digits of the hand are often first affected. Loss of the cortical margins of the phalangeal tufts also can be frequently identified in early stages of the disease. Only in more rapidly progressive hyperparathyroidism with higher PTH levels will subperiosteal resorption of bone be a prominent feature. In addition to the cortical surfaces of the digits, resorption can involve the sites of ligamentous attachments at the medial side of the proximal tibia, trochanter, and ischial and humeral tuberosities. Subchondral bone resorption can occur at many sites but is most often detected at the acromioclavicular and sternoclavicular joints, sacroiliac joints, and the symphysis pubis. Less often the joints of the appendicular skeleton are involved, leading to weakening of the bone and collapse of the articular surface. With the increasing utilization of laboratory screening of serum calcium, hyperparathyroidism is now usually identified early in the course of disease and the dramatic manifestations of advanced bone loss are rarely seen today. Although subperiosteal resorption is virtually pathognomonic of increased PTH secretion, the source may not be the parathyroid. Some tumors secrete a PTH-like substance that can also lead to

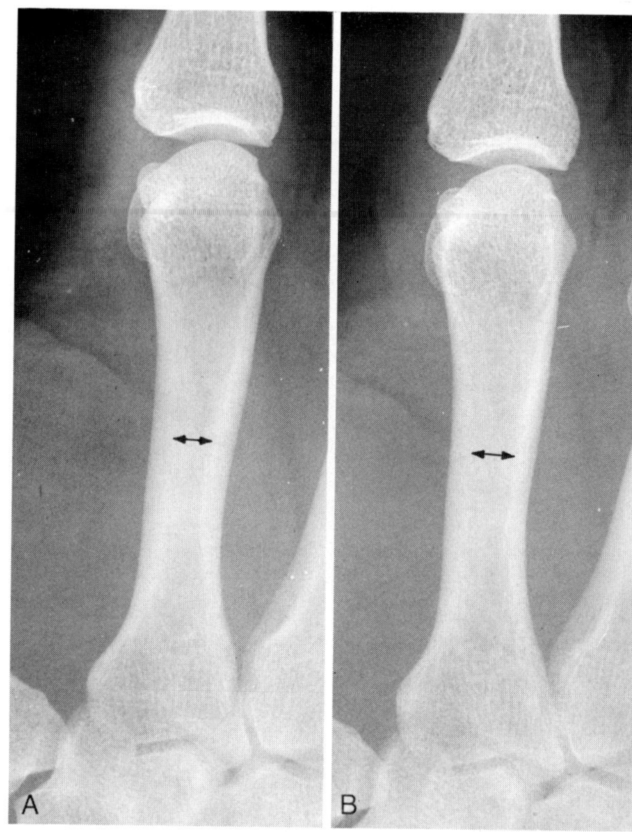

Figure 97–21. Hyperparathyroidism. *A,* Good preservation of the cortical thickness prior to the onset of disease is evident. *B,* Endosteal cortical resorption has led to widening of the medullary cavity *(arrows)* and thinning of the cortical bone.

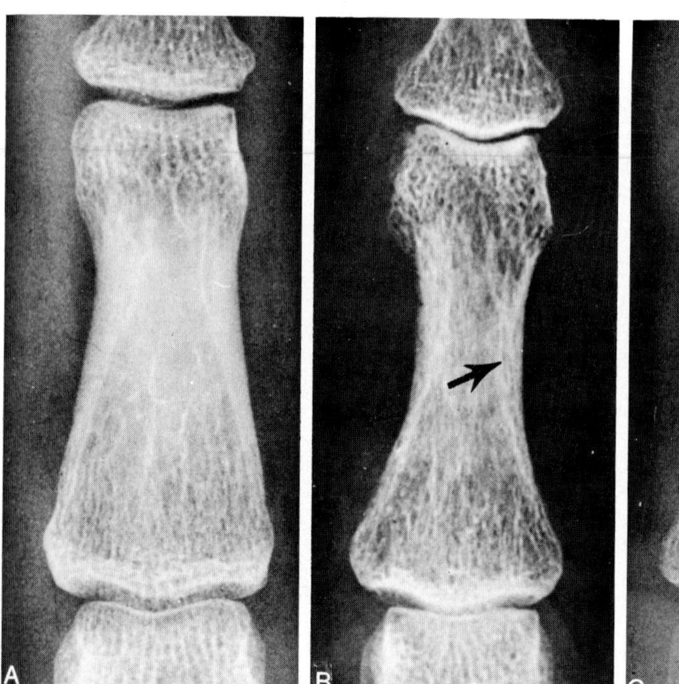

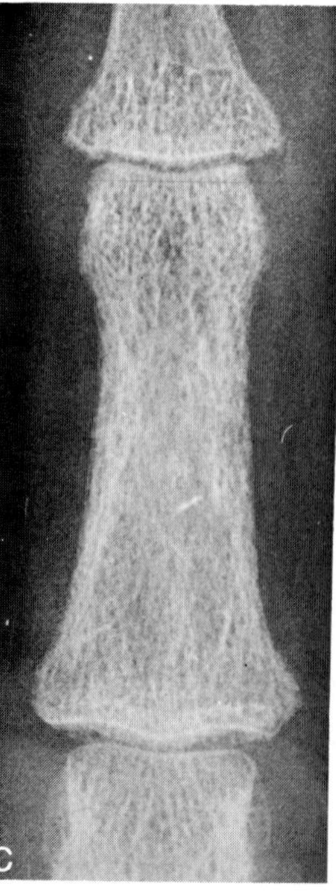

Figure 97–22. Primary hyperparathyroidism. *A,* Normal right middle phalanx for comparison. *B,* Intracortical resorption *(arrow)* or tunneling in the cortex is often present without subperiosteal resorption in primary hyperparathyroidism. *C,* Advanced intracortical resorption is demonstrated. It is hard to identify the endosteal surface of the cortex. Early subperiosteal resorption along the radial side of the phalanx is present in this patient with rapidly progressive primary hyperparathyroidism.

subperiosteal resorption identical to that associated with hyperparathyroidism. Arthropathy and calcium pyrophosphate deposition (CPPD) disease can also occur in association with hyperparathyroidism (Fig. 97–23).

Quantitative computed tomography of the distal radius reveals two main patterns. Younger patients, including premenopausal women, are often able to keep pace with the increased bone turnover induced by the elevated PTH and have normal or sometimes even increased bone mass. In contrast, older people typically demonstrate both cortical and trabecular bone loss. Postmenopausal women often have a loss that is greater than would be predicted for their age, indicating the added effect of PTH in causing bone loss in this group.

Radionuclide imaging with technetium-thallium ($^{99m}Tc/^{201}Tl$) sub-

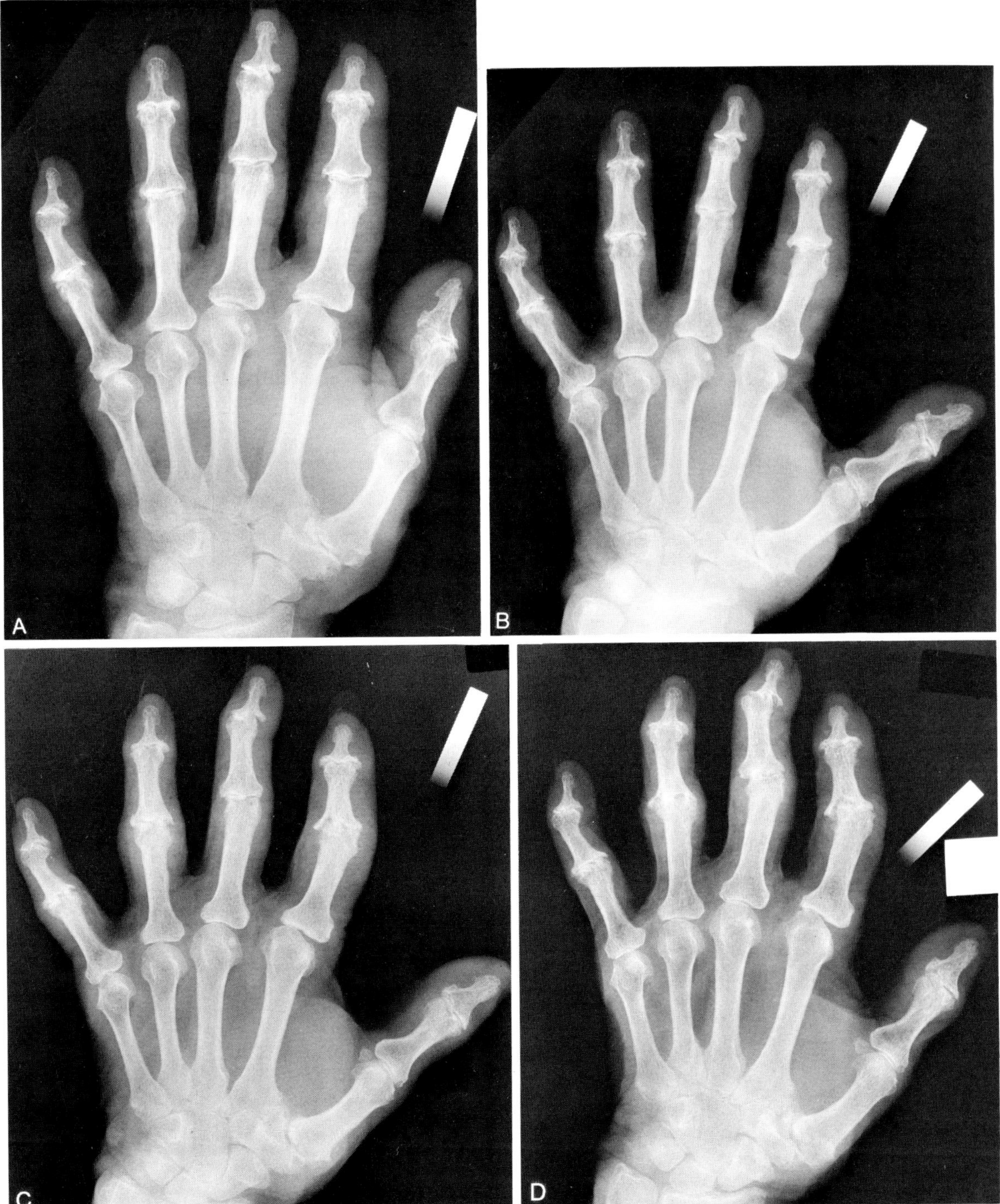

Figure 97–23. Arthropathy of hyperparathyroidism. *A,* The initial study of a patient with renal failure prior to the institution of hemodialysis reveals joint changes of primary osteoarthrosis. *B,* Two years later, there is further narrowing of the joints and increased subluxation of the second proximal interphalangeal joint. *C,* Subchondral erosion and collapse of the base of the second middle phalanx and the third distal interphalangeal joint have occurred in the following year. *D,* Six years following the initial study, there have been further erosion and subluxation of most of the interphalangeal joints. Cortical thinning and osteoporosis are evident.

traction can be used to localize parathyroid adenomas. The thyroid traps both ^{99m}Tc and ^{201}Tl, whereas the parathyroid adenoma takes up only ^{201}Tl. Subtracting the ^{99m}Tc image from the ^{201}Tl image reveals areas of ^{201}Tl concentration corresponding to the parathyroid adenomas.

High resolution, real-time ultrasonography can be used to detect abnormally enlarged parathyroid glands. Adenomas, hyperplasia, and carcinomas of the parathyroid demonstrate a sonographic texture that is less echogenic than the surrounding thyroid tissue. Normal parathyroid glands can only occasionally be detected owing to their small size. Enlargement of multiple glands is most consistent with hyperplasia. False-negative studies may occur when the gland is in an unusual location such as retrosternal or mediastinal.

Magnetic resonance imaging (MRI) is comparable to high-resolution ultrasonography in the detection of parathyroid adenomas in the initial evaluation of hyperparathyroidism. It has a more significant role in detecting aberrant parathyroid tissue in patients with persistent hyperparathyroidism following surgery.

SECONDARY HYPERPARATHYROIDISM

Secondary hyperparathyroidism is due to increased secretion of PTH occurring as an appropriate response to the reduction of ionized serum calcium. The most common cause of secondary hyperparathyroidism in the United States is chronic renal failure. Loss of renal function leads to hyperphosphatemia, which in turn leads to hypocalcemia and stimulation of the parathyroid gland. Ultimately loss of renal parenchyma causes diminished formation of active vitamin D_3, which leads to decreased intestinal absorption of calcium. Progressively increasing levels of PTH are secreted to try to maintain the serum calcium. Less commonly, malabsorption due to gastrointestinal disease can also result in a low serum calcium and increased PTH secretion. Chronic stimulation of the parathyroid leads to hyperplasia of the gland. With significant hyperplasia, sustained increase in PTH secretion can occur even after the stimulus for the increased PTH secretion has been removed. This has led some to postulate the development of autonomy of the gland (tertiary hyperparathyroidism). Considerable hyperplasia can develop in patients with chronic renal failure. Although dialysis improves the serum chemistries, the hyperparathyroidism can persist unabated. Total parathyroidectomy with reimplantation of a portion of the gland under the skin of the forearm (autotransplant) has been effective in reducing PTH levels to the normal range. If excess gland was reimplanted, only a minor surgical procedure is required to remove another portion of the tissue owing to its accessible location in the forearm.

An uncommon cause of secondary hyperparathyroidism is hypocalcemia caused by tumors that produce excessive amounts of calcitonin, such as medullary carcinoma of the thyroid. Calcitonin production has also been reported with other tumors including pancreas, lung, prostate, uterus, breast, and melanoma.

Radiographic Manifestations

Patients with secondary hyperparathyroidism often have readily demonstrable bone loss. Endosteal and intracortical resorption is seen as with primary hyperparathyroidism, but subperiosteal bone resorption is also usually present owing to the sustained higher levels of PTH. The use of fine-detail high-resolution film and optical magnification permits the detection of early changes in the hands. Early subperiosteal resorption, not detectable by conventional plain film radiography, is often present along the radial sides of the cortical bone (Fig. 97–24); cortical loss from the ungual tuft is also easily identified (Fig. 97–25). Other areas of resorption include the acromioclavicular and sternoclavicular joints, along the proximal tibial, humeral, and femoral shafts, the edges of the ribs, and the lamina dura. Areas subjected to increased stress and bone turnover, such as ligamentous attachments, also undergo resorptive changes.

Secondary hyperparathyroidism is a prominent feature of renal osteodystrophy. Osteomalacia may also predominate when vitamin D deficiency is present. In countries where the population is exposed to reduced sunlight and food products are not fortified with vitamin D, adults with chronic renal failure will manifest their bone loss as osteomalacia. Growing children, who have a greater need for vitamin D, will also exhibit the changes of rickets as the predominant feature of renal osteodystrophy (Fig. 97–26). If vitamin D or one of its metabolites is administered in the presence of increased serum phosphate levels, calcification of the vessels and soft tissues will ensue. This calcification is reversible if the calcium × phosphate product is lowered (Fig. 97–27). Calcification of vessels without vitamin D administration is frequently quite extensive in diabetics treated with chronic dialysis. If treatment leads to conditions favoring bone mineralization, increased bone density will be seen at sites of osteomalacia-induced bone loss when the excessive amounts of osteoid are mineralized (Figs. 97–28 and 97–29). Other radiographic findings that may also be associated with dialysis include the development of small cystic lesions (dialysis cysts) in the bones of the hands and wrists. Tenosynovitis and pseudogout (with or without detectable chondrocalcinosis) can also occur. A new form of dialysis-induced osteomalacia due to aluminum accumulation in the bones has also been identified.

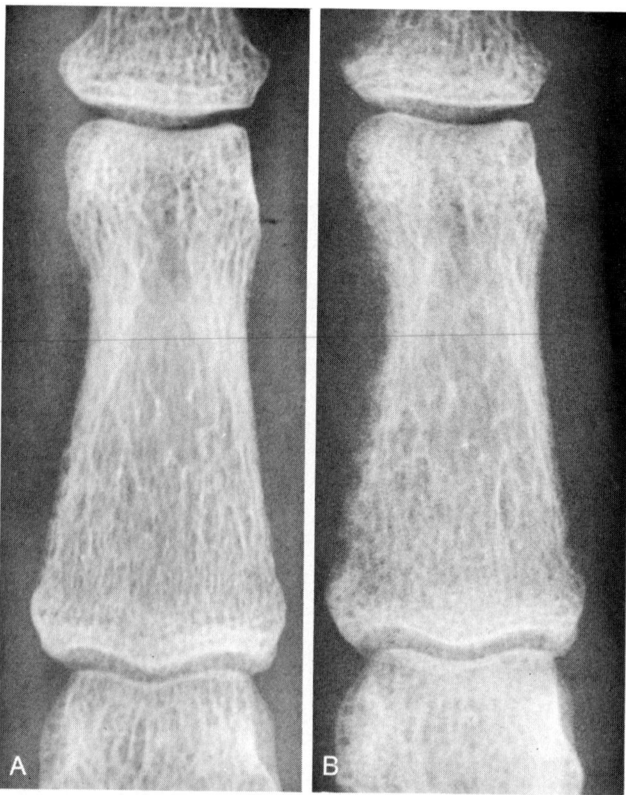

Figure 97–24. Secondary hyperparathyroidism. *A,* Early subperiosteal resorption is present along the radial side of the right middle phalanx. Intracortical resorption is also present. *B,* Advanced subperiosteal resorption is now present on the radial surface, and resorption has developed along the ulnar surface. The extent of the intracortical resorption has increased, and cortical thinning is also evident.

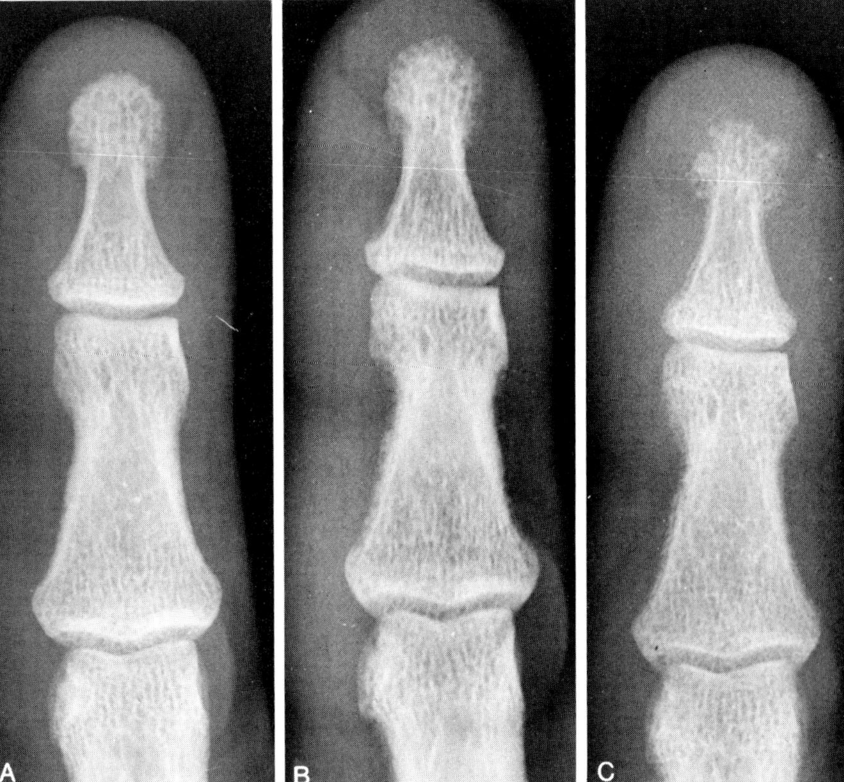

Figure 97–25. Secondary hyperparathyroidism. *A,* Early intracortical resorption without subperiosteal resorption is present. The cortical bone around the ungual tuft is intact. *B,* Subperiosteal resorption is now present along the shaft of the middle phalanx, and resorption of the cortex about the ungual tuft is evident. *C,* There has been further progression of the subperiosteal and intracortical resorption plus increased bone loss from the ungual tuft.

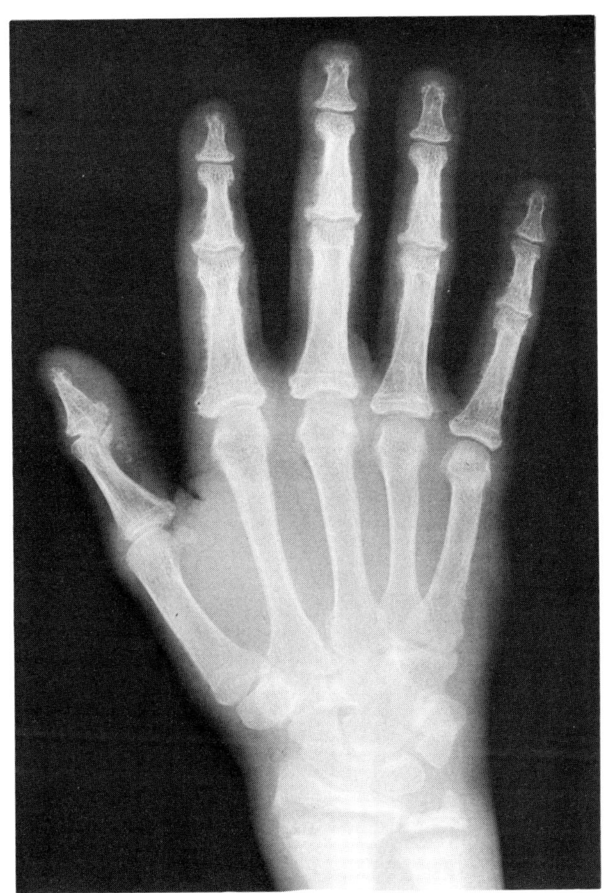

Figure 97–26. Secondary hyperparathyroidism and rickets. Renal failure in a child has led to extensive subperiosteal, intracortical, and endosteal bone resorption due to hyperparathyroidism. Widening and fraying of the growth plates of the wrist are due to rickets.

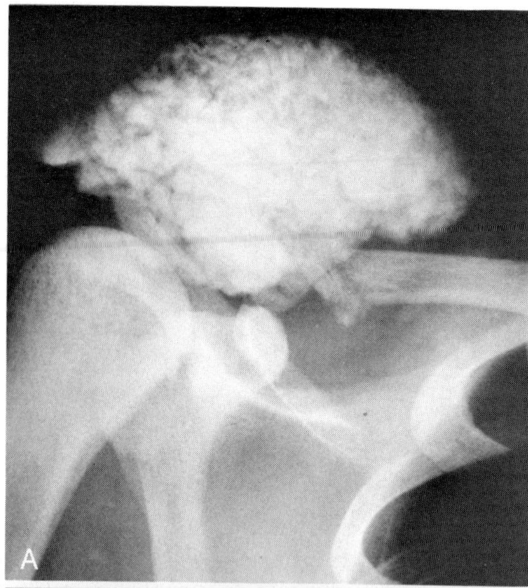

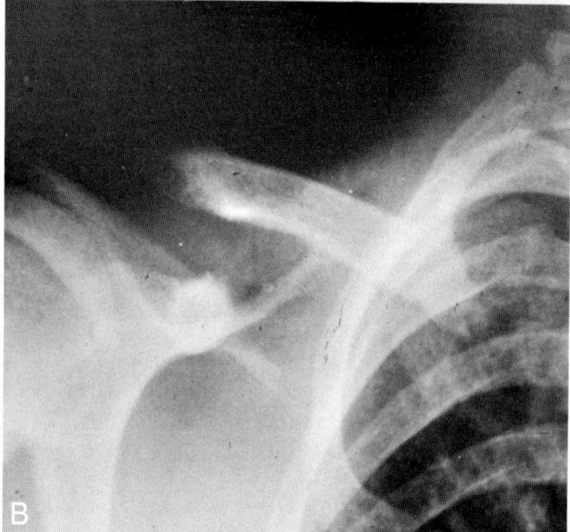

Figure 97–27. Renal osteodystrophy. *A*, Large soft-tissue calcification is present in a hemodialysis patient with an elevated serum phosphate who was treated with an active vitamin D metabolite. *B*, Resolution of the calcification followed the cessation of the vitamin D therapy. Extensive resorption of the distal clavicle due to hyperparathyroidism is now evident.

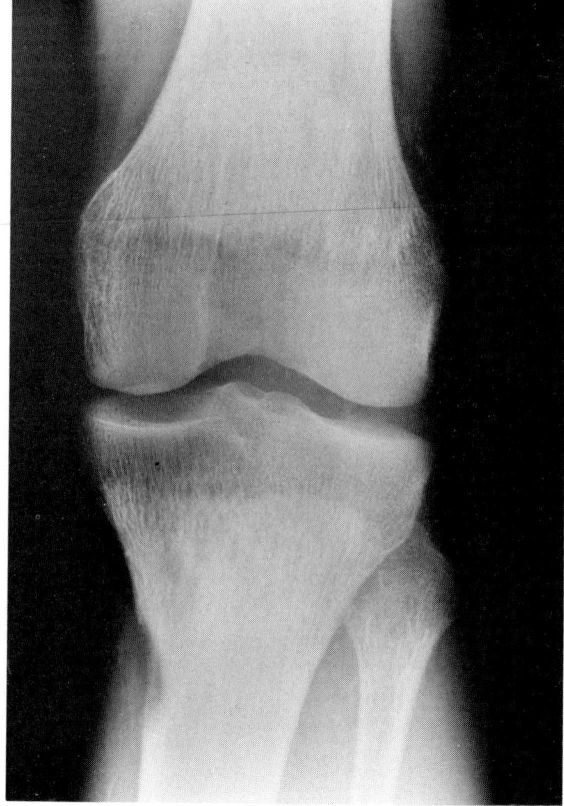

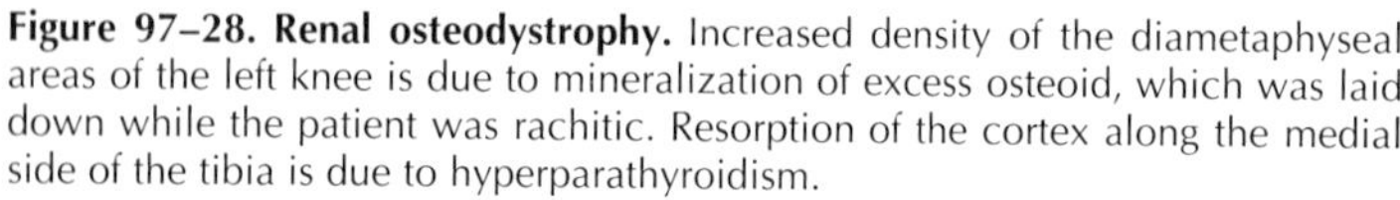

Figure 97–28. Renal osteodystrophy. Increased density of the diametaphyseal areas of the left knee is due to mineralization of excess osteoid, which was laid down while the patient was rachitic. Resorption of the cortex along the medial side of the tibia is due to hyperparathyroidism.

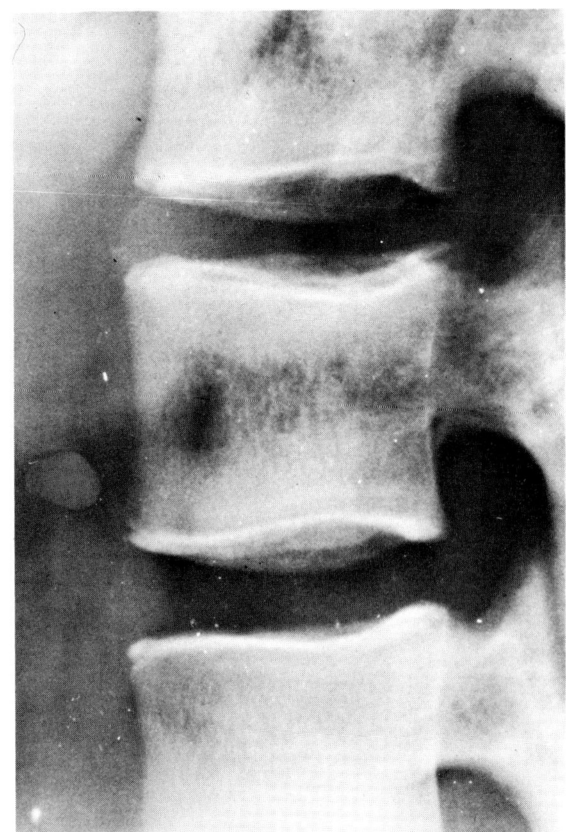

Figure 97–29. Renal osteodystrophy. "Rugger jersey" appearance of the vertebral body is due to mineralization of excess osteoid adjacent to the end-plates and resorption of bone from the midportion of the body.

HYPOPARATHYROIDISM

Hypoparathyroidism (Fig. 97–30) is the result of failure of the parathyroid glands to secrete PTH or failure of the target tissue to respond to the hormone (pseudohypoparathyroidism). Thyroid surgery is the most common cause of loss of PTH secretion resulting in hypocalcemia. Other acquired causes of hypocalcemia include hypomagnesemia, anticonvulsant therapy, and malabsorption and chronic renal failure with vitamin D deficiency. Idiopathic hypoparathyroidism is usually associated with circulating antibodies to the parathyroid as well as to other endocrine glands. Resistance to PTH is seen with pseudohypoparathyroidism (PHP). Hypocalcemia, hyperphosphatemia, parathyroid gland hyperplasia due to hypersecretion of PTH plus short stature, short metacarpals and metatarsals, and basal ganglia calcification characterize this disease. Pseudopseudohypoparathyroidism is the normocalcemic form of this disease.

Radiographic Manifestations

Widespread osteosclerosis with calvarial thickening, hypoplastic dentition, and calcification of the basal ganglia and soft tissues is characteristic. In PHP, the metacarpal sign may be positive due to shortening of the fourth and fifth metacarpals (a line drawn tangential to the heads will intersect with the third metacarpal if the sign is positive). If the third metacarpal is also shortened, this line will not intersect the third metacarpal and the sign will be falsely negative. None of these features is specific for hypoparathyroidism, but taken together they support the diagnosis.

Bibliography

Pituitary

Bluestone R, Bywaters EGL, Hartog M, Holt PJL: Acromegalic arthropathy. Arthritis Rheum 14:371, 1971.

George AE: Radiologic diagnosis of pituitary tumors. Sem Reproduc Endocrinol 2:47, 1984.

Steinbach HL, Feldman R, Goldberg MB: Acromegaly. Radiology 72:535, 1959.

Valenta LJ, Sostrin RD, Eisenberg H, et al: Diagnosis of pituitary tumors by hormone assay and computed tomography. Am J Med 72:861, 1982.

Adrenal

Bondy PK: Disorders of the adrenal gland. In Wilson JD, Foster DW (eds): Williams' Textbook of Endocrinology, 7th ed. Philadelphia, WB Saunders Company, 1985.

Cruess RL, Ross D, Crawshaw E: The etiology of steroid induced avascular necrosis of bone. Clin Orthop Rel Res 113:178, 1975.

Krieger DT: Pathophysiology of Cushing's disease. Endocr Rev 4:22, 1983.

Thyroid

Felig P, Baxter JD, Broadas AE, Frohman LA (eds): Endocrinology and Metabolism. New York, McGraw-Hill Book Company, 1981, pp 281–382.

Gross MD, Shapiro B, Thrall JH, et al: The scintigraphic imaging of endocrine organs. Endo Rev 5:221–281, 1984.

Mazaferri EL: The thyroid. In Mazaferri EL (ed): Endocrinology. New York, Medical Examination Publishing Company, 1980, pp 79–292.

Van Herle AJ: The thyroid nodule. Ann Intern Med 96:221–232, 1982.

Williams RH (ed): Textbook of Endocrinology. Philadelphia, WB Saunders Company, 1981, pp 117–247.

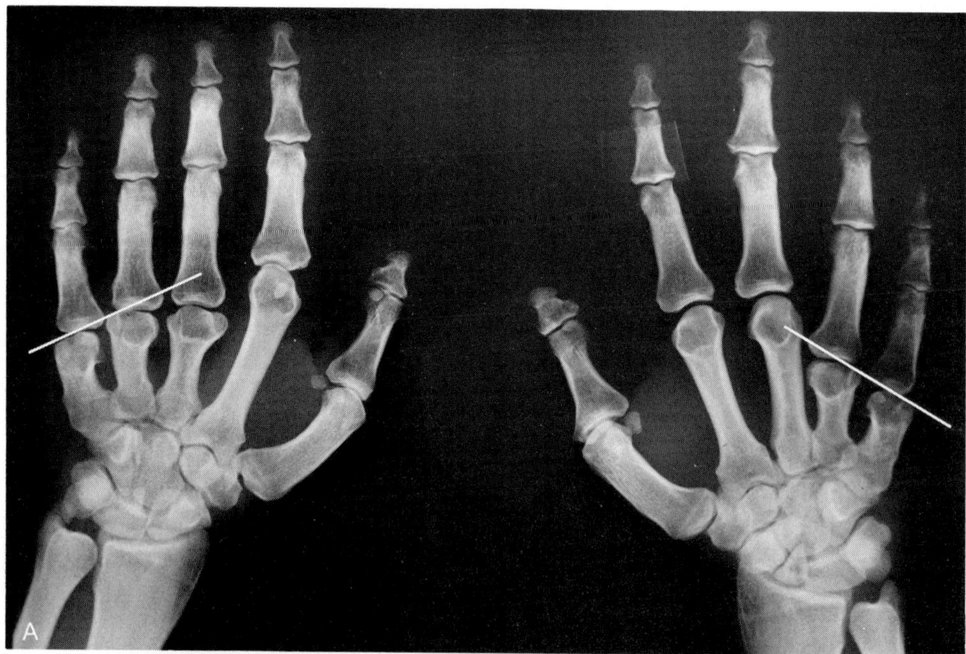

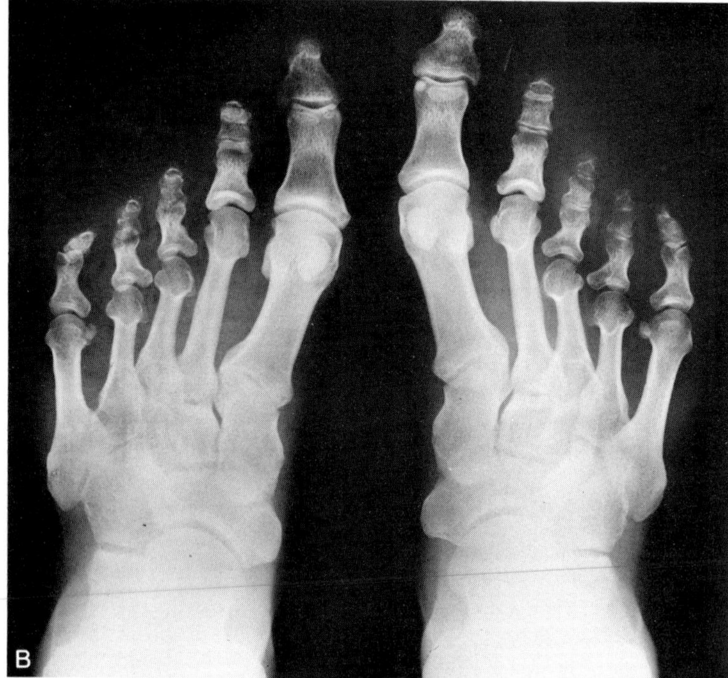

Figure 97–30. Pseudohypoparathyroidism. *A,* The right hand demonstrates a positive metacarpal sign due to shortening of the fourth and fifth metacarpals. The left hand demonstrates a false-negative metacarpal sign because the third metacarpal is also shortened. *B,* Similar shortening of the metatarsals is also evident in the feet.

Parathyroid

Jensen PS, Kliger AS: Early radiographic manifestations of secondary hyperparathyroidism associated with chronic renal disease. Radiology 125:645–652, 1977.

Resnick D: Erosive arthritis of the hand and wrist in hyperparathyroidism. Radiology 110:263, 1974.

Sandler MP, Patton JA, Partain CL: Thyroid and Parathyroid Imaging. East Norwalk, CT, Appleton-Century-Crofts, 1986.

Steinbach HL, Rudhe U, Jonsson M, Young DA: Evolution of skeletal lesions in pseudohypoparathyroidism. Radiology 85:670, 1965.

98 Metabolic Disorders

OSTEOPOROSIS

WILLIAM J. BURTIS and ROBERT LANG

Albright and his coworkers first clearly described the syndrome of osteoporosis in 1941. However, progress in determining its cause and developing effective therapy has been slow until the past decade. In spite of evidence to the contrary, osteoporosis has often been considered to be an inevitable accompaniment of aging. This, coupled with its obscure pathogenesis and unproven treatment, has led many physicians to ignore the underlying condition and treat only the complications. With research and improved understanding, this clinical resignation is changing. Although there clearly remain large gaps in our knowledge, efficacious programs of prevention and treatment are becoming available, resulting in much greater awareness of osteoporosis by both the medical community and the public.

DEFINITION

Osteoporosis is a condition in which there is decreased bone mass per unit volume, with the composition of the bone remaining essentially normal. This is to be contrasted with osteomalacia, in which there is deficient mineralization of organic matrix. Osteoporosis, when sufficiently advanced, will always give the radiologic appearance of decreased density (osteopenia) whereas with osteomalacia the radiographic density will depend on the amount of organic matrix present. For example, in hypophosphatemic rickets the presence of a normal amount of mineralized matrix plus a large amount of unmineralized matrix results in an increased bone mass, whereas osteomalacia associated with other etiologies results in radiographic osteopenia.

Osteoporosis is not a single disease, but rather a syndrome having many possible contributing causes. When bone density falls to some critical level, fractures begin to occur, resulting in the clinical picture of pain, deformity, and loss of mobility. Most of the bone loss occurs on the trabecular and endosteal surfaces of the cortex. Until fracture occurs, the bone retains its normal size and configuration but exhibits decreased density and mechanical strength.

INCIDENCE

Osteoporosis is a major health problem, affecting an estimated 15 to 20 million older Americans and causing over 700,000 fractures per year. The current economic cost of osteoporosis is estimated to be over $6 billion annually. Following the menopause, all women experience an acceleration of normal bone loss, and over 25 per cent of white women will experience a fracture due to osteoporosis. The incidence is even higher in Asians and much lower in blacks. Men are relatively protected until later in life, but after the age of 80 the incidence of osteoporosis is equal in both sexes. Osteoporosis secondary to other medical conditions is relatively less common and tends to affect younger individuals.

PATHOGENESIS

Although postmenopausal estrogen withdrawal is clearly the most important cause of bone loss in women in industrialized countries, it should be stated at the outset that osteoporosis is a heterogeneous disorder. Many risk factors (Table 98–1) can contribute to the clinical picture. Normal individuals lose skeletal mass at a rate of about 5 per cent per decade starting at 35 years of age; in the first few years after menopause this rate is closer to 10 per cent. In established osteoporosis, either there was insufficient bone mass to begin with, or the rate of loss is accelerated, or both. In some cases the loss results primarily from increased bone resorption and in others from decreased bone formation, but in all cases there must be some net uncoupling of the normally tightly interconnected processes of bone resorption by osteoclasts and bone formation by osteoblasts. Factors that may influence these processes include hormonal, nutritional, physical, and genetic effects (see Chapter 91 on Bone Metabolism).

Intestinal calcium absorption, known to decrease with age, is even lower in osteoporotics than in age-matched controls. Some investigators have found that levels of 1,25-dihydroxyvitamin D (calcitriol), a metabolite that stimulates calcium absorption from the intestine, are lower than age-matched normals but still in the normal range. Others have suggested that there may be impaired renal conversion of 25-hydroxyvitamin D to calcitriol in response to parathyroid hormone (PTH) in these patients. PTH levels in normals generally increase slightly with age, but in osteoporotics they are somewhat lower than in age-matched controls; however, a subgroup of osteoporotics has higher-than-normal PTH levels. It has been hypothesized that with postmenopausal estrogen deficiency there is a loss of the estrogen-induced inhibition of calcium release from bone. The resultant calcium loss from bone suppresses PTH, leading to decreased calcitriol and decreased intestinal calcium absorption. In other osteoporotics, relative renal insufficiency may cause mild secondary hyperparathyroidism with PTH-mediated bone loss, and/or impaired renal production of calcitriol.

Nutritional factors are important contributors to the maintenance of a healthy skeleton. Dietary deficiency of calcium or excess of phosphate may lead to secondary hyperparathyroidism and skeletal loss. A diet high in protein may accelerate renal insufficiency, and the acid residue may be a direct stimulant of bone resorption and renal calcium excretion.

Alcoholics have decreased bone density, possibly due to a toxic effect of ethanol on bone metabolism. Cigarette smoking has also been shown to increase the risk of osteoporosis, although the mechanism is unknown. Complete immobilization causes a dramatic increase in bone resorption, and a sedentary lifestyle may contribute to the gradual bone loss in many osteoporotics. Generally athletic individuals have a higher bone mass than the spectators!

Several endocrinologic conditions are known to be associated with osteoporosis, including hyperthyroidism, Cushing's syndrome, hyperparathyroidism, and hypogonadism. Although less common than postmenopausal osteoporosis, they are important in that they frequently affect individuals at a younger age, and they can be

TABLE 98–1. RISK FACTORS FOR OSTEOPOROSIS

I. Hormonal
- A. Hypogonadism
  - 1. Congenital, i.e., Turner's, Klinefelter's
  - 2. Hypopituitarism
  - 3. Ovarian failure
  - 4. Hyperprolactinemia
- B. Hyperparathyroidism
- C. Hyperthyroidism
- D. Cushing's syndrome
- E. Diabetes mellitus
- F. ? Calcitonin deficiency

II. Nutritional
- A. Calcium deficiency
- B. High acid-ash (protein) diet
- C. Excess phosphate intake
- *D. Malabsorption
- E. Scurvy
- F. Malnutrition

III. Drugs and toxins
- A. Corticosteroids
- B. Anticonvulsants
- C. Heparin
- D. Chemotherapeutic agents
- E. Alcohol
- F. Tobacco

IV. Physiologic and other stress
- A. Pregnancy
- B. Lactation
- C. Lack of exercise
- D. Immobilization
- E. ? Emotional stress

V. Race: Caucasian and Mongoloid

VI. Sex: Female

VII. Congenital
- A. Osteogenesis imperfecta
- B. Ehlers-Danlos syndrome
- C. Gaucher's disease

VIII. Miscellaneous
- A. Metabolic acidosis (e.g., renal tubular acidosis)
- *B. Post-gastrectomy
- C. Malignancy in bone marrow, especially multiple myeloma
- D. Mast cell disease
- E. Rheumatoid arthritis
- *F. Renal failure
- *G. Liver disease, especially primary biliary cirrhosis
- H. Juvenile osteoporosis
- I. ? Aging

*Also associated with osteomalacia.

Modified from Lang R: Osteoporosis. In Bollet AJ (ed): Harrison's Principles of Internal Medicine. Patient Management Problems; Pretest, Self-Assessment and Review, Vol II. New York, McGraw-Hill, 1984.

effectively treated. The most common of the endocrine causes of osteoporosis is iatrogenic, as a side-effect of glucocorticoid therapy. With chronic hypercortisolism there is decreased recruitment of osteoblast precursors, as well as an inhibition of osteoblast function. In addition, there is a steroid-induced inhibition of intestinal calcium absorption and augmentation of renal calcium excretion, causing a mild secondary hyperparathyroidism with increased bone resorption. The combination of these steroid-associated effects causes a relatively rapid decrease in skeletal mass. Parathyroid hormone stimulates both osteoblasts and (indirectly) osteoclasts, producing a state of increased bone turnover with some net resorption. Although severe primary hyperparathyroidism causes the radiologic findings of bone cysts and subperiosteal resorption, this is uncommon today, and most cases of primary hyperparathyroidism affecting the bone appear as accelerated osteoporosis in postmenopausal women.

A number of genetic diseases are associated with osteoporosis because of collagen defects in the organic matrix. These include osteogenesis imperfecta, Ehlers-Danlos syndrome, Marfan's syndrome, and the Menkes syndrome. Hematologic malignancies, particularly multiple myeloma and some lymphomas, can lead to rapid skeletal loss through local release of osteoclast-activating factor, a lymphokine, by the tumor cells. Rheumatoid arthritis, diabetes mellitus, and systemic mastocytosis can occasionally cause decreased bone density by unknown mechanisms.

PATHOLOGY

Trabecular bone is generally diminished to a greater extent than cortical bone in osteoporosis. Individual trabeculae become thinned, eventually perforate, and ultimately become fewer in number. The common result is fractures occurring after minimal stress in the vertebral bodies and other areas high in cancellous bone. There may be endosteal resorption leading to thinning of the cortex, but except in severe hyperparathyroidism, subperiosteal resorption is rare and there may even be periosteal apposition. Cortical width and density may be diminished secondary to endosteal resorption and intracortical resorption (haversian remodeling), and the strength of the cortical shafts of the long bones may be affected enough to lead to a fracture.

Quantitative bone histomorphometry is a technique in which undecalcified sections from a bone biopsy are studied under the light microscope, usually after the patient has taken tetracycline to label areas of newly mineralized bone at two discrete points of time. Osteoporosis (in contrast to osteomalacia) usually shows normal amounts of unmineralized osteoid, and at least some areas of double tetracycline banding indicating new bone formation. The degree of bone remodeling (turnover), however, varies from patients with few osteoclasts and flattened, inactive osteoblasts, to others with above-average osteoclastic and osteoblastic activity. Furthermore, in osteoporotic patients, there seems to be little correlation between the amount of bone turnover and clinical or biochemical parameters. In general, bone histomorphometry has underscored the heterogeneity of osteoporosis.

CLINICAL MANIFESTATIONS

Osteoporosis may remain asymptomatic, or it may be complicated by fractures, depending on the amount of bone loss and such other factors as muscle mass and general physical conditioning. It is assumed that there is a subclinical phase of variable duration, during which the patient has no symptoms, and conventional radiographs appear normal, but quantitative measurements would show progressive loss of bone density.

The first clinical manifestation of osteoporosis is usually back pain, caused by a compression fracture of the vertebral body. The pain is frequently of sudden onset after bending or lifting a heavy object. The discomfort is steady, is made worse by movement or weight bearing, and may be severe. It is usually well-localized to the area of the vertebral body involved, most frequently in the thoracic or upper lumbar region. In addition, associated spasm of the paravertebral muscles often produces a more diffuse back pain. Because it is not practical to splint or immobilize the spine, the fracture remains painful for four to six weeks until it heals. It is important to realize that osteoporosis itself (in contrast to osteomalacia and other bone diseases) is not painful. It is quite common to see radiographs of patients with severe osteoporosis who have not complained of back pain. In fact, radiographs with multiple vertebral fractures, in patients who have not had more than a mild backache, are also not rare. Back pain persisting more than two months following vertebral crush fracture either represents continuing paraspinal muscle spasm (common) or new compression fracture or is of some unrelated etiology. Nerve compression is rare in osteoporosis, and neuropathy should suggest back pain caused by degenerative joint disease, disc disease, or an infiltrative process.

Untreated, a common course of osteoporosis consists of recurring acute episodes of back pain from vertebral compression fractures and paravertebral muscle spasm. The latter pain may become self-perpetuating because in addition to trauma, spasm may be precipitated by inactivity (poor muscle tone) and emotional stress, both of which frequently occur following a fracture. Spinal deformity, with dorsal kyphosis and loss of height, occurs progressively as multiple vertebral bodies are crushed. Frequently this deformity will evolve without severe pain. Eventually in the most severe cases, the kyphosis may become crippling or interfere with pulmonary function.

The long bones most often clinically affected by osteoporosis are the distal radius and the proximal femur. The incidence of Colles' fracture of the distal radius begins to rise with the onset of menopause. Fractures of the proximal femur begin occurring at about the age of 60 years in women. The delay in onset of hip fractures, also seen with compression fractures of the spine, probably reflects the ability of weight-bearing bones to reinforce the cortical bone and trabeculae along lines of stress when bone loss first ensues. These fractures often occur in the elderly following minimal trauma owing to both the bone loss and a decrease in muscle mass and tone. Whereas Colles' fractures usually heal without sequelae, hip fractures in the elderly, because of constant immobilization, may lead to complications including pneumonia, pulmonary emboli, and depression. Estimates indicate that the fatality rate following osteoporotic hip fracture is between 12 and 20 per cent.

LABORATORY FINDINGS

All laboratory parameters usually remain within the normal range in uncomplicated postmenopausal osteoporosis. Serum and urine calcium and phosphorus are invariably normal. Alkaline phosphatase is normal except for transient elevations during bone repair following fractures. Parathyroid hormone and 1,25-dihydroxyvitamin D levels, although slightly different from those of age-matched controls in some studies, remain within the normal range.

The main use of laboratory tests is to screen for other conditions or secondary causes of osteoporosis. The extent of the diagnostic work-up should be tailored to the individual patient. Serum calcium, phosphate, alkaline phosphatase, creatinine, and protein electrophoresis should be obtained in most patients to rule out hyperparathyroidism, osteomalacia, Paget's disease, renal insufficiency, and multiple myeloma. Endocrine dysfunction suggested by the clinical findings should be investigated with the appropriate hormonal assays. A 24-hour urine collection for calcium may be elevated from any condition that is associated with rapid bone resorption, such as cancer, hypercortisolism, or hyperparathyroidism, but will be normal in uncomplicated osteoporotics.

RADIOGRAPHIC MANIFESTATIONS

Losses of as much as 30 to 50 per cent of bone mass must occur before osteoporosis appears as decreased density on routine radiographs. Lateral views of the thoracic and lumbar spine can demonstrate changes in the normal configuration of the vertebral bodies which indicate the presence of bone loss. These include increased prominence of the end-plates, increased concavity of the end-plates if the nucleus pulposus is not degenerated (codfish vertebrae), anterior wedging, and in later stages significant loss of height of the bodies and compression fractures (Figs. 98–1 and 98–2). In the hip, increased prominence of the primary weight-bearing trabeculae indicates the loss of the horizontal secondary trabeculae (Fig. 98–3).

Cortical bone loss can also be assessed. Standards are available for the midshaft thickness of the cortical bone of the second metacarpal. Identification of a decreased thickness on a single study does not indicate when the loss occurred or if the reduction might be due to decreased formation of the cortical bone during growth. Many factors affect the midshaft cortical thickness during development, including health and nutrition as a child and adolescent, physical activity and strength, and endocrine status.

The lack of sensitivity of conventional radiography, coupled with normal laboratory parameters and the asymptomatic nature of early osteoporosis, creates a major problem for early diagnosis and institution of therapy. In the past, it has been difficult to quantitate the extent of disease or measure response to therapy, except in the crudest fashion by counting the number of vertebral compression fractures. More sensitive methods to evaluate bone mineral content have been refined and are becoming widely available. Single-photon absorptiometry (SPA) is suitable for measuring the density of cortically enriched bone with little overlying tissue, such as the distal radius or calcaneus, but it is not clear that measurements at these sites correlate well with the risk of osteoporotic fractures. Dual-photon absorptiometry (DPA), by considering the differential absorption of soft tissue and bone at two different wavelengths and then subtracting the soft tissue component, is capable of measuring the lower density of bones that are primarily trabecular, such as spine and hip, but there are problems with the accuracy of comparison of repeated measurements over time because of variations in the photon source. A more recent adaptation, dual x-ray absorptiometry (DEXA), overcomes this problem by substituting an adjustable x-ray source. With proper calibration this technique is precise ($\pm$ 0.5 to 2%), has the lowest radiation dose (1 to 3 mrem), and has become the most popular method of bone density determination. Attention must be taken in interpreting DEXA measurements to avoid reading vertebral crush fractures, osteophytes, or soft-tissue calcifications (visible on plain films) as an increased bone density. Finally, quantitative CT is the only widely available method that can distinguish between cortical and trabecular components of density in a single bone (e.g., vertebral body), but the higher cost and radiation dose (100 to 1000 mrem) make this technique less suitable for routine measurements.

TREATMENT

The treatment of osteoporosis encompasses various modalities, including elimination of risk factors, diet, drugs, and physical therapy. In general, it is much easier to retard loss of skeletal mass than to stimulate new bone formation, so treatment is most effective when begun relatively early in the course of the disease.

The major dietary intervention is to increase calcium intake to a total of 1500 mg of elemental calcium daily (approximately triple that of the average American diet). The high intake overcomes the

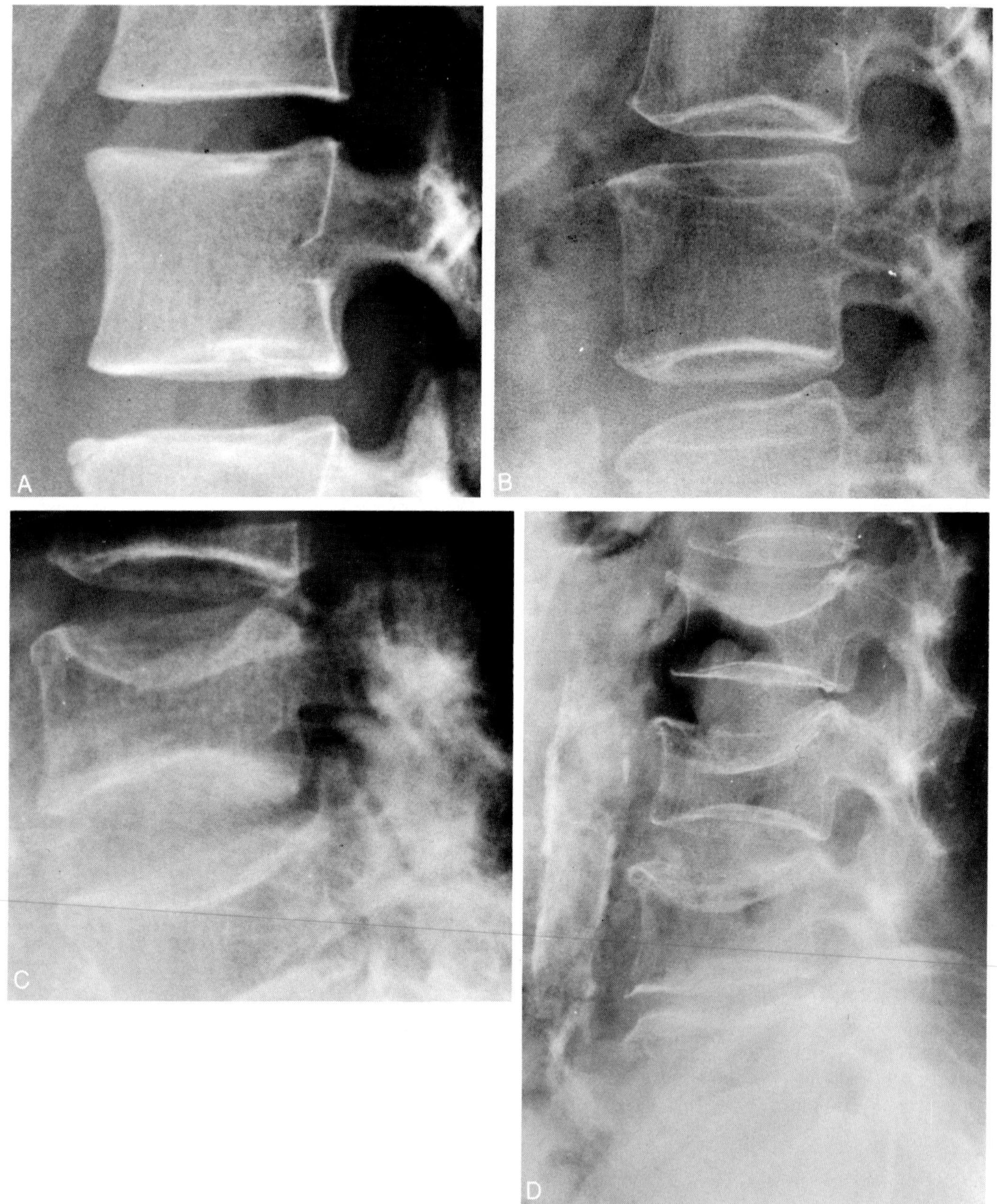

Figure 98–1. Osteoporosis. *A,* Normal lateral lumbar vertebral body for comparison. *B,* Bone loss is demonstrated by the increased prominence and increased concavity of the end-plates. Decreased overall bone density is also evident, but this must be evaluated with caution because differences in technical exposure factors can produce apparent changes in density. *C,* Markedly increased concavity of the end-plates leads to "codfish" vertebrae. This can happen only if the nucleus pulposus is intact; if it is not, a more uniform loss of height of the vertebrae occurs. *D,* Advanced osteoporosis with extensive loss of height of the lumbar vertebrae is present.

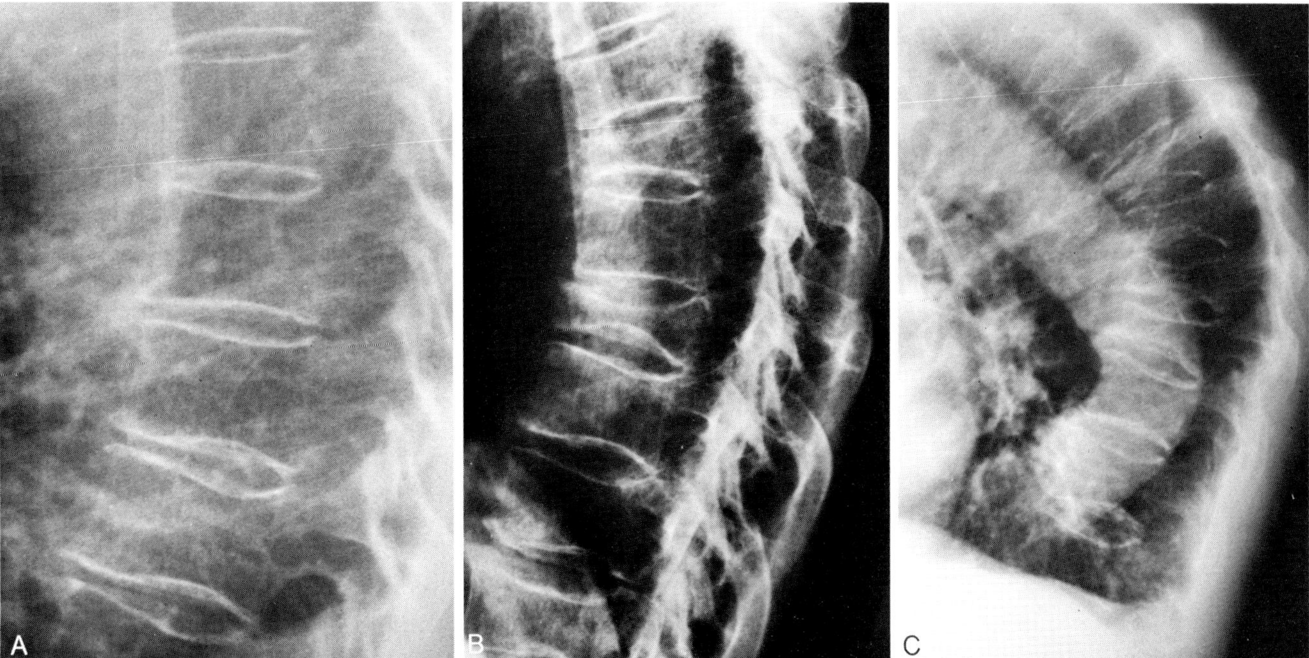

Figure 98–2. Osteoporosis. *A,* Generalized demineralization with increased concavity of the end-plates and mild anterior wedging of the thoracic vertebral bodies is present. *B,* Further bone loss with the development of compression fractures and an increasing kyphosis is demonstrated. *C,* Advanced osteoporosis with multiple compression fractures and a prominent kyphosis (dowager's hump) is present.

relative inefficiency of intestinal absorption and has been demonstrated to correct negative calcium balance and inhibit bone loss. Calcium carbonate tablets are the most convenient and economical means to supplement dietary calcium, although in achlorhydric patients calcium carbonate is insoluble. Calcium gluconate tablets are more soluble but contain only 9 per cent elemental calcium by weight; thus it takes 11 pills daily to supplement the diet with 1.0 g of calcium. Other dietary manipulations are more controversial, but excessive amounts of protein, sodium, phosphate, and alcohol should probably be avoided.

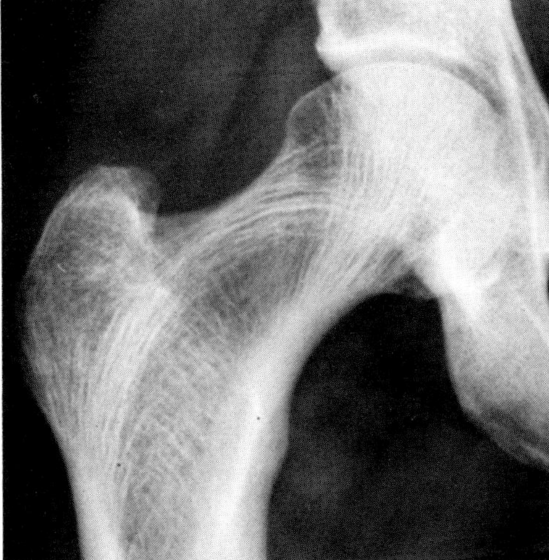

Figure 98–3. Early bone loss in a weight-bearing bone. Increased prominence of the primary vertical trabeculae along lines of stress is due to reinforcement of these weight-bearing trabeculae following loss of the horizontal or secondary trabeculae.

Vitamin D supplementation at the recommended allowance of 400 units daily is always advisable in patients with a poor diet and little exposure to sunlight. Use of higher doses or more active forms of vitamin D, such as calcitriol, is controversial. Studies have shown variable benefit from such therapy, and the long-term clinical consequences of the hypercalciuria that commonly results from such therapy are unknown.

Early estrogen replacement therapy in postmenopausal women is the most effective means of preventing bone loss. Obviously, the earlier it is started the greater the benefit. Estrogen will prevent the accelerated bone resorption that occurs with low estrogen levels and should probably be continued for life. Modest doses such as 0.625 mg of conjugated equine estrogens are sufficient to protect the bones and often do not cause endometrial hyperplasia or menstrual bleeding. These doses of estrogen also appear to substantially lower the incidence of atherosclerosis by favorably impacting on lipid ratios, but conversely they have been associated with a slightly increased risk of breast and uterine malignancies. They are usually given in monthly cycles with or without progestogens to avoid endometrial hyperplasia. Any unexpected vaginal bleeding must of course be evaluated by a gynecologist, and a history of breast cancer is a contraindication to their use.

Therapy using antiresorptive agents such as calcitonin and bisphosphonates is more controversial. Although these agents often increase the bone density slightly during the first year of use, the long-range benefits are less clear cut. Calcitonin therapy has been shown to protect against corticosteroid-induced bone loss if begun concurrently and continued as long as the steroids are given. Initial enthusiasm for cyclical therapy with the bisphosphonate etidronate in postmenopausal osteoporosis has been dampened by the report of an increased number of fractures in these patients, although the numbers are small and additional data should be forthcoming shortly from ongoing clinical trials with this and other bisphosphonates. Similarly, fluoride therapy has fallen from favor because, at least at the doses used in a recent large multicenter trial, there was a statistically significant increase in the fracture rate despite a documented increase in bone density, suggesting that fluoride-induced bone growth is mechanically deficient.

Physical therapy is as important as medication in preventing disability from osteoporosis. Too often patients become inactive following the onset of fractures, because of both pain and fear of additional fractures. The inactivity hastens bone resorption and weakens the paravertebral muscles, leading to increased risk of fracture and painful muscle spasm. When the pain of acute vertebral fracture has subsided, the patient should begin progressive back exercises (particularly extension), initially under the direction of a physical therapist or other health professional, and later include a daily regimen of exercise, such as swimming, walking, or biking.

In cases of osteoporosis secondary to another disorder, treatment should be directed at the underlying abnormality. Correction of hyperthyroidism or hypercortisolism ameliorates bone loss. Patients requiring long-term glucocorticosteroid therapy for other diseases pose a difficult problem; certainly the dose and duration should be limited to the absolute minimum required. It is not known whether alternate-day steroid therapy will slow the development of osteoporosis. Hypogonadal men and amenorrheic women should be given testosterone and estrogen, respectively, if appropriate for their medical condition.

PREVENTION

For osteoporosis an ounce of prevention is worth well over a pound of cure. Good nutrition with an appropriate calcium intake and regular meaningful exercise will help assure attainment of maximal skeletal mass as a young adult and will retard bone loss in middle age and beyond. Prevention is particularly important in women with a positive family history or with other risk factors. Many physicians today routinely prescribe estrogen therapy to white or Asian postmenopausal women to prevent osteoporosis, although this is still somewhat controversial. Exercise, adequate calcium intake with supplementation if necessary, and avoidance of smoking and excess alcohol can be recommended to all normal postmenopausal women at risk for bone disease.

OSTEOMALACIA AND RICKETS

PAMELA S. JENSEN

Osteomalacia occurs when the bone matrix made by the osteoblasts fails to be mineralized to form hydroxyapatite. This leads to excessive amounts of osteoid demonstrable on bone biopsy. In the immature skeleton, the disorder is termed *rickets*. Many factors can cause inadequate osteoid mineralization, including deficiency of vitamin D or its active metabolites, insufficient calcium and/or phosphorus for mineralization, acidosis that inhibits hydroxyapatite synthesis, the presence of abnormal ions in the matrix such as aluminum, and defective matrix production as with fibrogenesis imperfecta ossium.

CLINICAL MANIFESTATIONS

Many diseases and conditions are associated with osteomalacia. In contrast to osteoporosis, bone pain is a common feature of osteomalacia. In a patient with bone pain, evidence of bone loss, and a disorder that is known to cause abnormal mineral metabolism, the possibility of osteomalacia should be considered. Deficiency of vitamin D can result from inadequate dietary intake or lack of sufficient exposure of the skin to ultraviolet light. Dietary deficiency is most common in countries that do not fortify food products with vitamin D. Rickets in premature newborns resulting in part from insufficient dietary supplementation of vitamin D has also been noted. Intestinal malabsorption due to disorders of the bowel, hepatobiliary system, or pancreas can lead to vitamin D loss. Liver and kidney disease can lead to failure of hydroxylation of vitamin D whereby the active metabolites are not made. Administration of anticonvulsants can also lead to interference with vitamin D metabolism.

Renal tubular disease, including renal tubular acidosis and hypophosphatemia (Fanconi's syndrome) as well as chronic renal failure, is also associated with osteomalacia. In dialysis-related aluminum-induced osteomalacia (Fig. 98–4), the presence of aluminum in the osteoid inhibits calcification of the mineralization front, leading to increasing amounts of unmineralized matrix. Aluminum is present in the water, but most is removed before it is used for dialysis; the aluminum is believed to accumulate over time from intestinal absorption of small amounts of the orally administered aluminum hydroxide that is given to reduce intestinal absorption of phosphate. In addition to impaired renal reabsorption of phosphate, hypophosphatemia can be due to an inadequate dietary intake of phosphate. Some tumors, usually vascular in nature such as hemangiopericytomas, secrete a substance that also leads to hypophosphatemia. These patients often present with proximal muscle weakness simulating polymyositis. Laboratory findings are variable depending upon the etiology. Treatment is directed at correcting the underlying pathology.

RADIOGRAPHIC MANIFESTATIONS

In untreated osteomalacia, bone density is generally decreased. In some areas, such as the spine and pelvis, there is so much osteoid that partial mineralization leads to areas of increased density. The secondary horizontal trabeculae are resorbed and the primary trabeculae may appear thickened and have indistinct fuzzy edges (Fig. 98–5). Cortical bone is usually reduced in thickness, although occasionally osteoid can be deposited along the subperiosteal surface of the cortex. Mineralization of this osteoid results in thickening of the cortical bone. Intracortical resorption due to the uncoupling of the normal bone resorption-formation sequence is a common feature. Osteoid lines the widened haversian canals within the cortex. Should conditions change to favor hydroxyapatite formation, the excess osteoid in all areas of the skeleton will mineralize, leading to increased density of the trabecular bone and improvement or resolution of the intracortical resorption. Subperiosteal resorption may occasionally be present if secondary hyperparathyroidism is also a component of the disease. However, if the cortical surfaces are covered with osteoid, subperiosteal resorption will not be evident radiographically because osteoclasts cannot break down unmineralized matrix.

Characteristic pseudofractures, also called Looser's zones or Milkman's fractures, are incomplete fractures that heal poorly, lead-

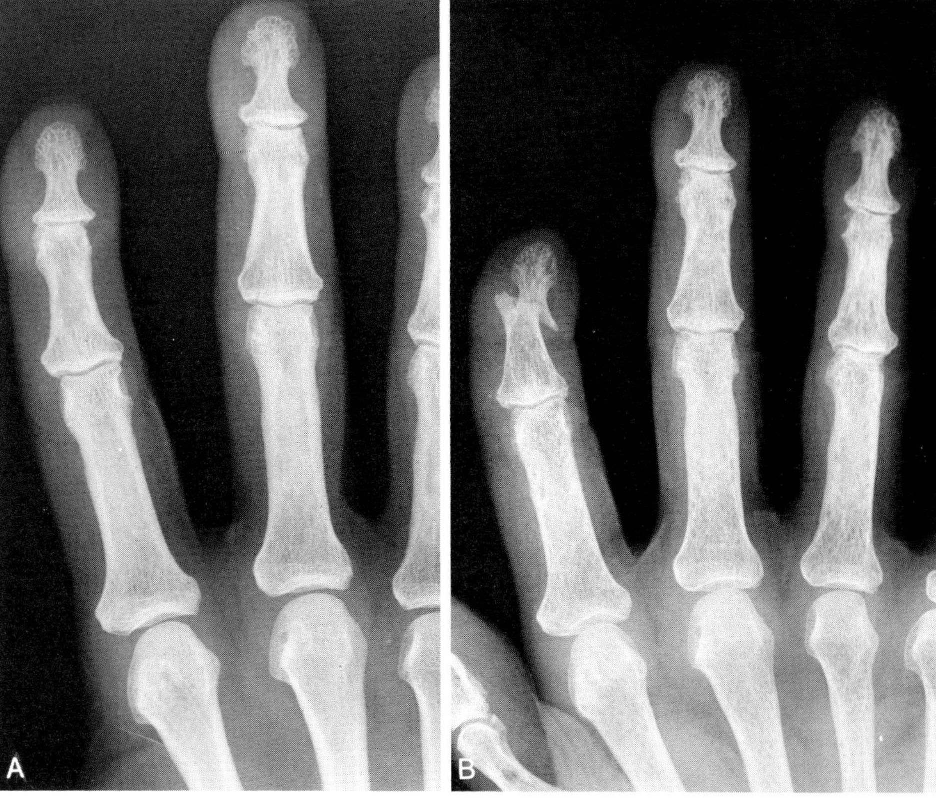

Figure 98–4. Aluminum-induced osteomalacia. *A,* Initial study of a patient with renal failure prior to the institution of hemodialysis. *B,* Eight years later, the changes at the distal interphalangeal joint of the second digit are secondary to hyperparathyroidism. The pattern of resorption with increased thickening of some of the trabeculae is due to osteomalacia.

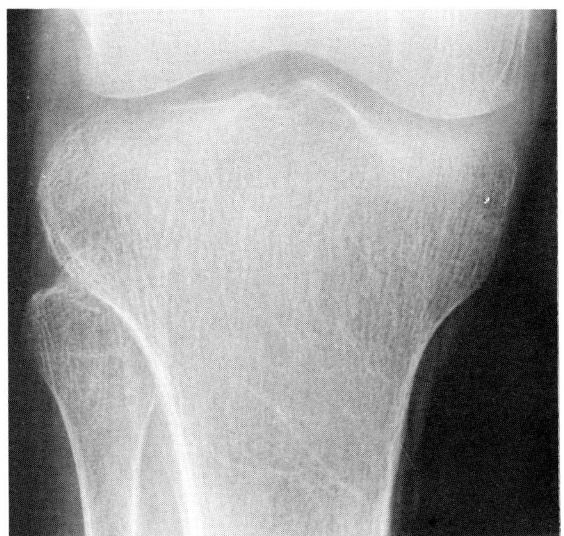

Figure 98–5. Osteomalacia. Generalized demineralization is present. The trabeculae along lines of stress have been preserved and have somewhat fuzzy edges.

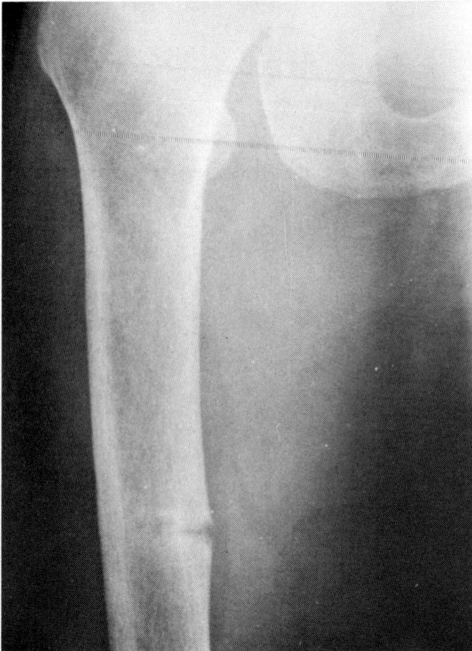

Figure 98–6. Osteomalacia. Pseudofracture (stress fracture) along the concave side of the femoral shaft with little evidence of healing is present. Intracortical resorption is also evident.

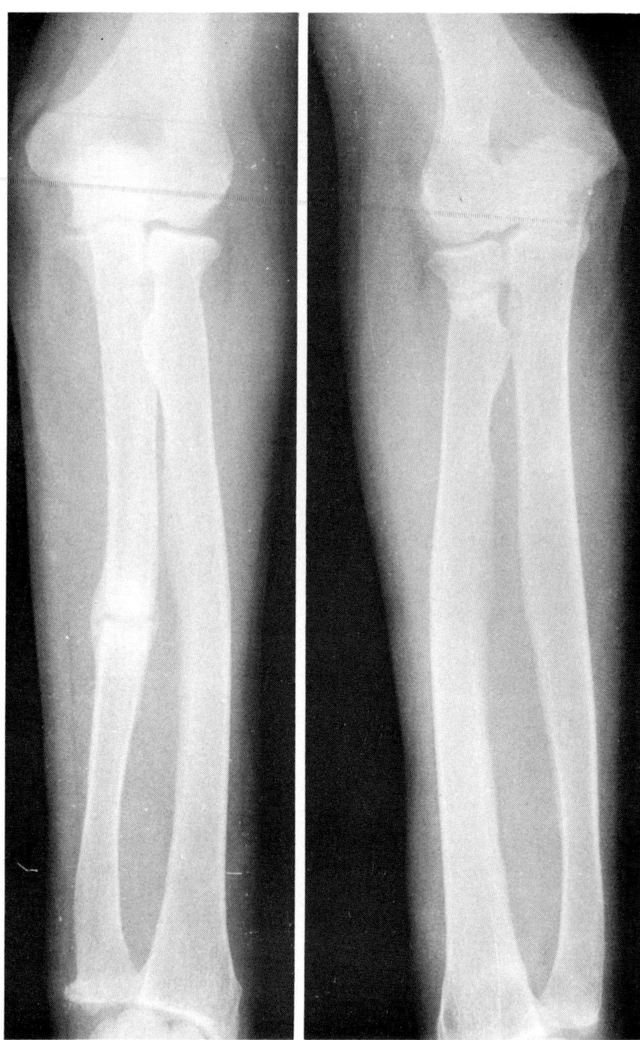

Figure 98–7. Osteomalacia. Stress fracture of the ulna at the midshaft with evidence of healing and a fracture below the radial head in the other arm are demonstrated.

ing to persistent radiolucent areas in the cortical bone. Bones most commonly affected include the medial cortex of the femur (Figs. 98–6 to 98–8), the pubic and ischial rami, the axillary border of the scapula, and the ribs. They are often symmetrical in distribution. Extension of the fracture across the entire bone can also occur. The incomplete fractures are frequently asymptomatic despite the fact that they take up increased radionuclide on bone scans. They probably represent slowly healing stress fractures or areas of erosion caused by adjacent blood vessels. Although they are characteristic of osteomalacia, they can be seen in any disease of disordered bone formation, including Paget's disease and osteogenesis imperfecta.

In children, the failure of normal mineralization is most pronounced at the growth plates. Disorganization of the normally well-ordered process of bone formation occurs. The zone of provisional calcification and the zone of primary spongiosia do not mineralize, and the cellular components continue to grow and expand, leading to a markedly elongated and widened area on the metaphyseal side of the growth plate (Figs. 98–9 and 98–10). The ends of the bones undergoing the greatest rate of growth exhibit the greatest abnormality. These include the costochondral junctions (rachitic rosary) (Fig. 98–11), distal femur, proximal tibia and humerus, and distal tibia, ulna, and radius. This distribution aids in distinguishing diseases of a metabolic origin from the battered child syndrome. The metaphyseal side of the growth plate becomes progressively more demineralized, longer and wider. In addition to the cupping and ballooning of the metaphyses, structural weakness leads to bowing of the long bones. Weight bearing leads to greater bowing of the lower extremities, scoliosis, upward protrusion of the femurs into the pelvis (Fig. 98–12), and basilar invagination of the skull. A skeletal dysplasia, metaphyseal chondrodysplasia type Schmid, has radiographic manifestations similar to rickets; however, laboratory values are normal. Nevertheless, some of these children have been treated with high-dose vitamin D to the level of intoxication; the skeletal abnormalities demonstrated in this syndrome do not change in response to this therapy. Dramatic improvement of the rachitic changes can occur when the underlying etiology is successfully treated (Fig. 98–13).

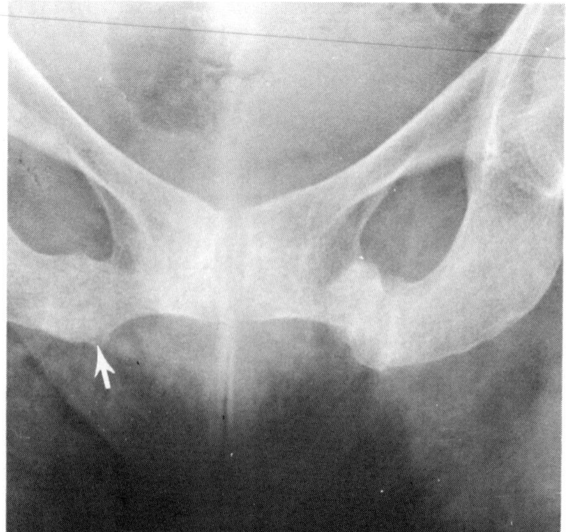

Figure 98–8. Osteomalacia. There is an incomplete fracture (*arrow*) of the right inferior pubic ramus and a complete fracture of the inferior pubic ramus on the left.

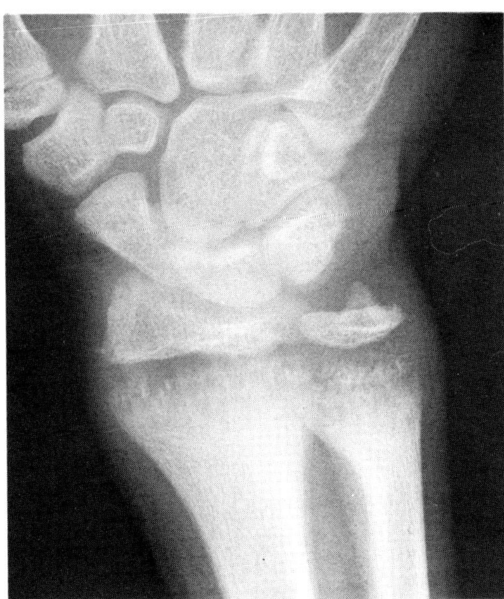

Figure 98–9. Rickets. Widening of the metaphysis, fraying of the metaphyseal side of the growth plate, and increased thickness of the growth plates due to nonmineralization of the zone of provisional calcification of the wrist are characteristic.

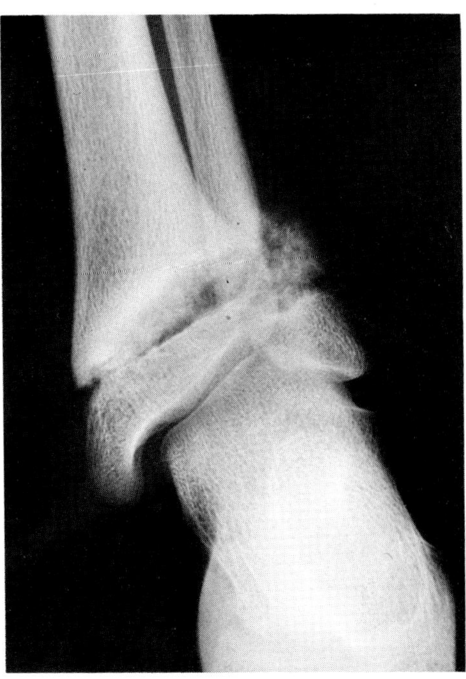

Figure 98–10. Rickets. Characteristic changes of rickets are present at the growth plates of the ankle. Nonuniform growth has led to an angular deformity.

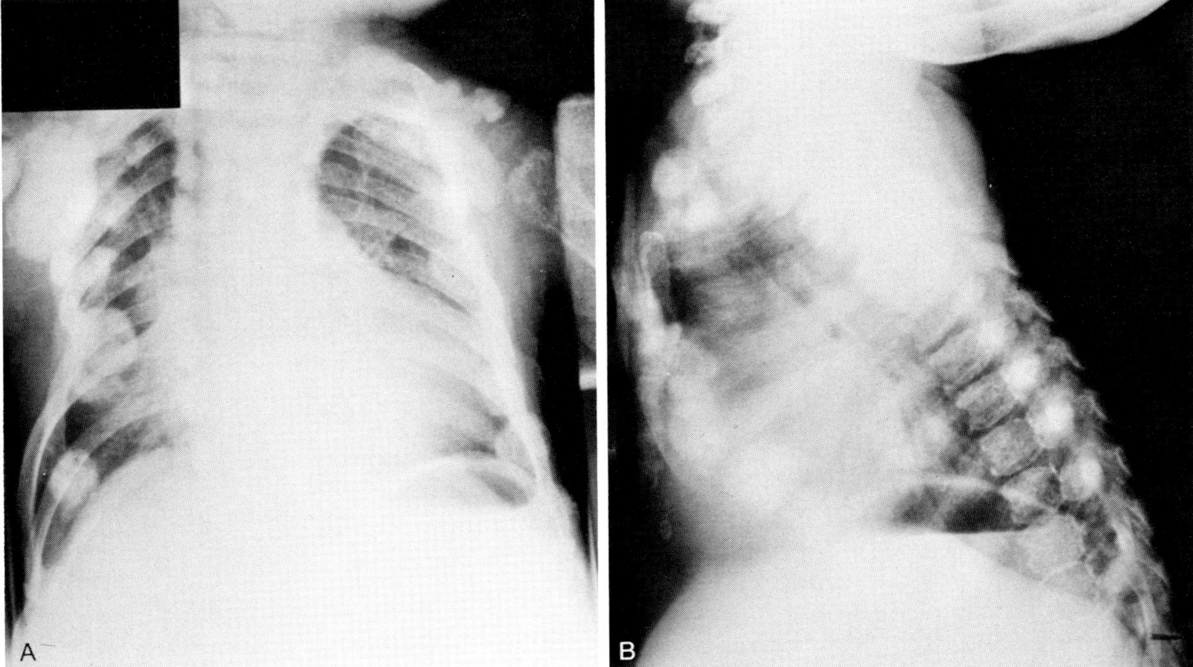

Figure 98–11. Rickets. *A,* Frontal projection of the chest in an infant with advanced renal failure demonstrates overgrowth of the costochondral junctions of the anterior ribs (rachitic rosary). *B,* Lateral projection shows overgrowth of the cartilaginous portions of the posterior elements of the spine as well as the costochondral junctions of the ribs.

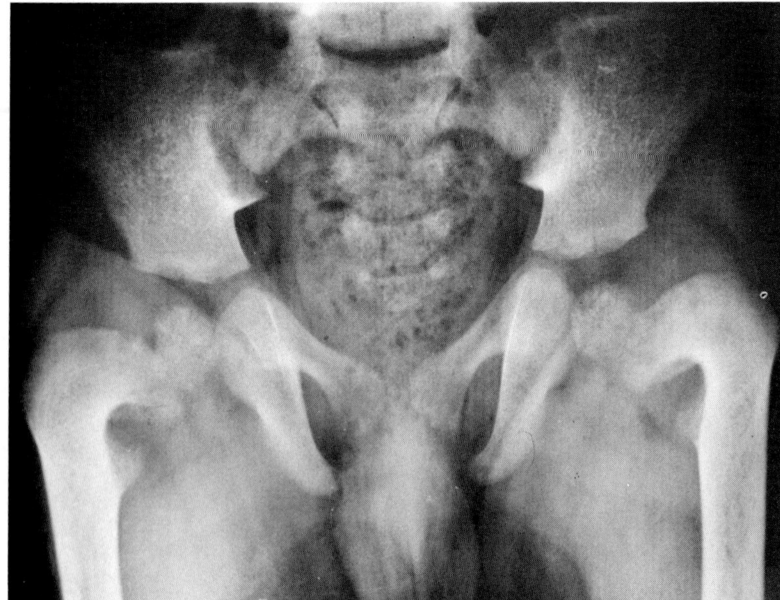

Figure 98–12. Rickets. Marked coxa vara of the proximal femora is present bilaterally.

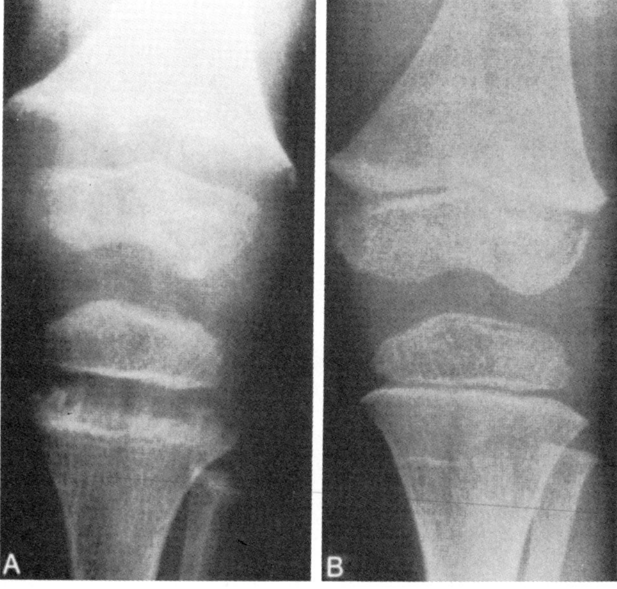

Figure 98–13. Rickets. *A,* Characteristic widening of the growth plate and widening and fraying of the metaphyses of the knee are present in a child on anticonvulsant therapy. *B,* Addition of vitamin D to the anticonvulsant therapy has reversed the bone changes due to rickets.

HYPERVITAMINOSES AND HYPOVITAMINOSES

LEE D. KATZ

It had been known for centuries that liver cures night blindness and the juice of oranges and lemons cures scurvy, but it wasn't until 1912 that the term *vitamin* appeared in the literature. In that year two significant observations were made. First, F. G. Hopkins proved experimentally that animals needed more than protein, fat, and carbohydrate for normal growth. He postulated that certain ''accessory factors'' were required in the diet for proper nutrition. Second, Casimir Funk demonstrated that a concentrate made from rice husks and polishings could alleviate the symptoms of beri-beri in Japanese sailors. He postulated that a ''vital-amine'' was needed, from which the term *vitamine* (*vitamin*) was coined. In the 1930s, the molecular structures of several vitamins were derived, including thiamine (B_1), riboflavin (B_2), and nicotinic acid.

Vitamins are now better defined as certain organic substances that function in trace amounts to promote cellular function. The role of certain vitamins, for example, may actually cross the strict definition given above and approach that of a hormone. Because the latter is defined as a trace substance that is produced by an endocrine gland and serves as a chemical messenger to target organs where it helps regulate physiologic and metabolic activities, it may not be too long before vitamin D is referred to as hormone D.

As we approach the twenty-first century, the world food supply demonstrates the dichotomy of malnutrition and gluttony. In addition, alternate lifestyles in diet still require the radiologist to be aware of skeletal changes of vitamin (hormone) lack and excess. This section will concentrate on the clinical and radiologic manifestations of vitamins A, C, and D. Hypovitaminosis D has been discussed earlier in this chapter.

VITAMIN A

Vitamin A is one of the fat-soluble vitamins, along with vitamins D, E, and K. It exists in nature as alicyclic diterpene alcohol and is found in vegetables as carotene or in the liver. Vitamin A is a necessary dietary requirement. Its absorption from the bowel depends on the presence of bile salts and normal gastrointestinal transport across small bowel mucosa.

Hypervitaminosis A

"... it made us all sicke, specially three that were exceeding sicke, and we verily thought we should have lost them all, for all their skins came off from the foote to the head; but yet they recovred again for which we gave God heartie thanks."

This quote from Gerrit De Veer in 1597 recorded his observations of the toxic effects of polar bear liver eaten during an arctic expedition. Both acute and chronic intoxication of vitamin A has been described in children and adults. The clinical and radiographic presentations differ depending on the age of the patient and time course after ingestion. Vitamin A intoxication is a diagnosis that will go unrecognized unless a detailed dietary history, including medications, is obtained. In addition, vitamin A intoxication from hyperalimentation solutions and from 13 *cis*-retinoic acid, a medication used to treat such dermatologic abnormalities as ichthyosis, can occur.

Acute vitamin A intoxication in children manifests itself between 12 and 24 hours. The children may present with agitation, vomiting, insomnia, and bulging of the anterior fontanelle, which has a typical mushroom cap appearance. These symptoms usually disappear within 36 to 48 hours. Radiographically, skull films may demonstrate widening of the sutures. These findings are consistent with increased intracranial pressure (Fig. 98–14). Whether this represents overproduction or decreased reabsorption of cerebrospinal fluid (CSF) is not known.

In adults, the clinical signs of acute vitamin A intoxication include abdominal pain, nausea and vomiting, severe headache, dizziness, irritability, and a strong desire to sleep. This is followed in 24 hours by desquamation of the skin beginning at the fingertips. There are no radiographic findings of acute vitamin A intoxication in adults.

Children with chronic vitamin A ingestion are usually ill-appearing with dry skin, coarse hair, anorexia, hepatosplenomegaly, and sometimes painful subcutaneous nodules over their long bones. In addition, ascites and pleural effusion have been described secondary to the hepatic disease.

Radiographically, chronic vitamin A intoxication induces periosteal new bone formation involving tubular bones. This is seen mainly in the metatarsals and the ulna. In addition, there may be widening of the sutures of the skull with decalcification of the dorsum sella consistent with increased intracranial pressure. Splaying or cupping of the metaphysis and enlargement of the ossification centers with premature fusion may lead to growth abnormalities, including short stature, disparity of growth of paired bones, and flexion deformities of the lower extremities. Chronic vitamin A intoxication must be differentiated from Caffey's disease (infantile cortical hyperostosis) and the battered child syndrome.

The use of 13 *cis*-retinoic acid to treat ichthyosis, has been shown to produce a disorder resembling diffuse idiopathic skeletal hyperostosis. In children, premature fusion of growth centers may occur (Fig. 98–15). Retinyl acetate in animals produces calcification at tendinous insertions which may be irreversible.

In adults, chronic vitamin A intoxication produces a clinical picture not remarkably different from what has been described in children. The patients suffer from fatigue, alopecia, dryness and fissuring of the skin, anorexia, and hepatosplenomegaly. The patient may also manifest a migratory pattern of bone and joint pain.

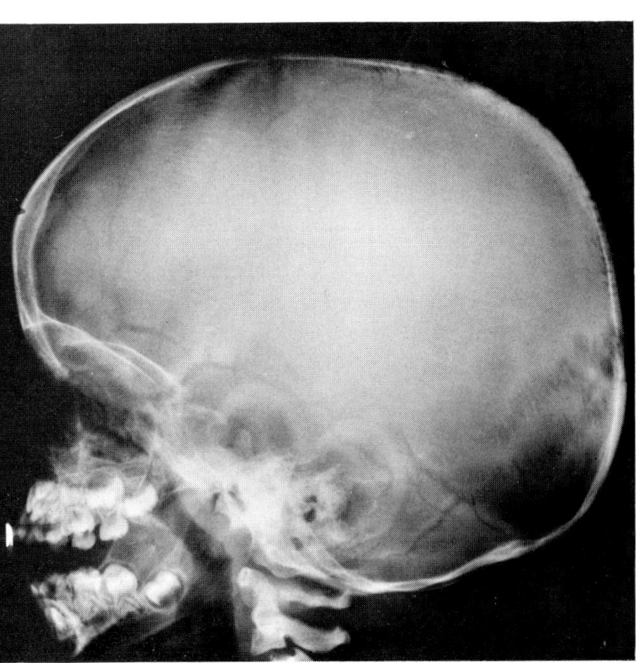

Figure 98–14. Hypervitaminosis A. Eighteen-month-old child with increased intracranial pressure due to excess vitamin A ingestion. There are widening of the sutures, increased size of the skull, and thinning of the calvarium. There is no erosion of the dorsum sella.

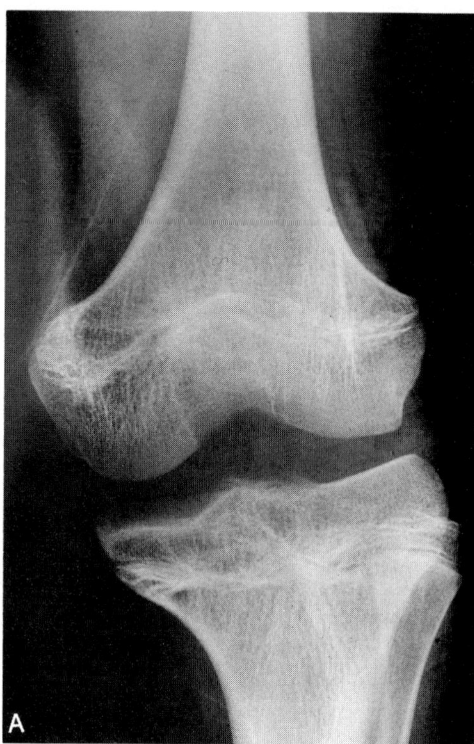

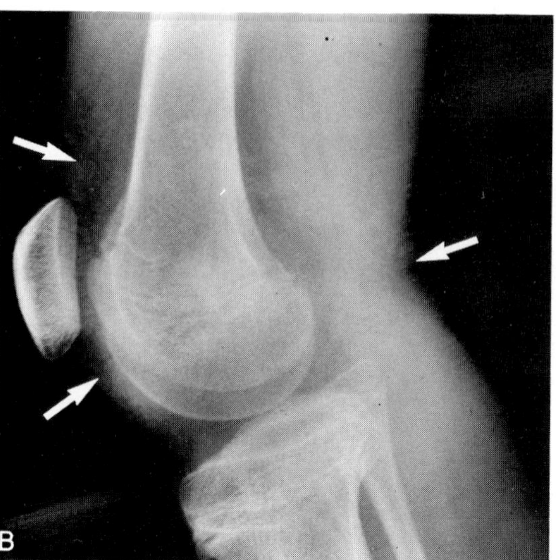

Figure 98–15. Hypervitaminosis A. *A,* A 13-year-old treated with 13 *cis*-retinoic acid for ichthyosis. Frontal view of the left knee reveals widening of the metaphyses, angular deformity, and premature fusion of the growth plates centrally. *B,* The skin changes of ichthyosis can be seen on the lateral view (*arrows*).

Although uncommon, vitamin A intoxication has been shown to be responsible for unexplained hypercalcemia. Jacques reported a case of an adult who had documented hepatic fibrosis and portal hypertension with ascites secondary to vitamin A intoxication but who continued abusing the drug and progressed to cirrhosis. Liver biopsy demonstrated that the hepatomegaly was from perisinusoidal fibrosis, with sclerosis of the central veins and obliteration of the space of Disse by fat-storing Ito cells. There are typically no radiographic findings of chronic vitamin A intoxication in adults.

Hypovitaminosis A

Hypovitaminosis A is not well documented in the literature and there appears to be a paucity of radiographic findings. Clinically, these patients mainly have alterations in epithelial layers as evidenced by dry skin, keratomalacia of the eye, hematuria, and cornified vaginal epithelium. There may be evidence of anemia and splenomegaly in children. Central nervous system manifestations of hypovitaminosis A in infants include bulging of the fontanelles with widening of the intracranial sutures secondary to increased intracranial pressure of unknown etiology. Cranial nerve injury has been reported. Hypovitaminosis A in pregnancy has been reported to result in abortion. If the deficiency is not severe, the fetus may be stillborn. If still less, there may be no skeletal defects, but ophthalmologic abnormalities have been described. No other radiographic abnormalities have been noted in the adult.

VITAMIN C

Vitamin C, ascorbic acid, is a necessary requirement in the diet of man and other primates, certain birds, and fish. Other mammalian species can synthesize the vitamin from D-glucose and D-galactose. The lack of vitamin C in the diet has been of great historic significance. The first classic description of scurvy dates back to the Crusades in the thirteenth century. By the end of the fifteenth century, with the tremendous increase in sea travel, scurvy was the most dreaded malady. It wasn't until 1753 that Lind, an English naval surgeon, studied various types of treatment and showed that those whose diet was supplemented with "2 oranges and one lemon given every day" responded dramatically. These sailors, who once had putrefied gums, the spots, and weakness in their knees, became known as limeys.

Hypovitaminosis C (Scurvy)

Vitamin C in normal bone metabolism is a necessary requirement for production of normal bone matrix. In its absence, a generalized decrease in bone density becomes manifest as generalized osteoporosis. It is important to differentiate this from rickets, in which the lack of vitamin D results in defective mineralization of a normal organic matrix. In scurvy, mineralization of the osteoid continues normally, but the overall amount is decreased.

The lack of vitamin C also increases capillary fragility and may lead to hemorrhage from minor trauma with the formation of subperiosteal or soft-tissue hematoma. Other signs of increased capillary fragility include bleeding in joints (hemarthrosis), epidermis (petechiae), or mucous membranes (bleeding gums).

Infantile scurvy usually does not manifest itself during the first six months because of the maternal contribution of vitamin C, assuming that the mother had normal vitamin stores. The child classically presents after nine months with irritability, pallor, anemia, tenderness and swelling at the distal ends of the limbs, and bleeding abnormalities. The radiographic changes (Figs. 98–16 to 98–18) seen in infantile scurvy are (a) a generalized osteoporosis of the bones that gives a characteristic ground glass appearance with thin cortices (pencil-point cortex); (b) thickening of the zone of provisional calcification secondary to normal deposition of calcium and phosphate in the osteoid that is present (Frankel's line); (c) a lucent zone on the diaphyseal side of Frankel's line secondary to poorly formed trabeculae known as Trummerfeldzone, which is prone to fracture; (d) fractures of the Trummerfeldzone may present as small, beak-like projections off the metaphysis (Pelkan spurs);

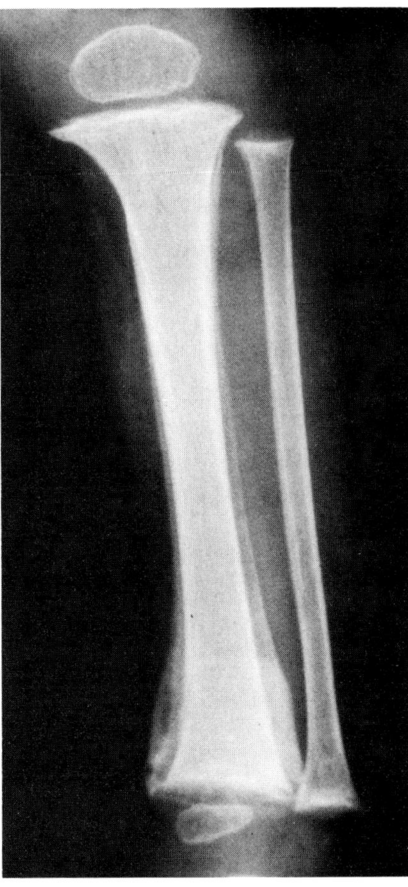

Figure 98–16. Hypovitaminosis C (scurvy). Periosteal elevation along the tibial shaft is due to subperiosteal hemorrhage. Increased density along the metaphyseal sides of the growth plates is due to calcification of the thickened zone of provisional calcification (Fränkel's line).

(e) a ring of increased density formed around the ossification center (Wimburger's sign); and (f) periosteal reaction secondary to subperiosteal hemorrhage.

Although the above radiographic signs are classic for scurvy, Kato found that the only reliable sign of infantile scurvy was evidence of periosteal reaction secondary to hemorrhage. The increase in the zone of provisional calcification can also be seen in congenital syphilis, healed rickets, and heavy metal poisoning. Zones of decreased bone density can be seen in congenital syphilis, neuroblastoma, and leukemia. The dense line around the ossification centers of the epiphysis may be seen in a limb with a residual palsy from polio. Finally, the spurring seen extending from the metaphysis may also be seen in rickets.

Vitamin C deficiency in the adult is seen in patients who are severely malnourished for a considerable length of time. These patients present with nonspecific constitutional symptoms including weight loss and fatigue or with hemorrhagic complications as described in children including tender subcutaneous nodules from focal hemorrhage. The radiographic findings are nonspecific. In a study by Jaffe, 50 per cent of adults with the clinical diagnosis of scurvy had no radiographic findings. The most common abnormality noted in the remaining group was confined to the spine and bones of the lower extremity. Osteoporosis of the spine, usually associated with a compression fracture of a vertebral body without history of trauma, is typical. Other changes of the bones included osteoporosis of the lower extremities, periosteal new bone formation along the shaft of the long bone associated with subperiosteal hemorrhage, and changes seen in the joints secondary to hemarthrosis.

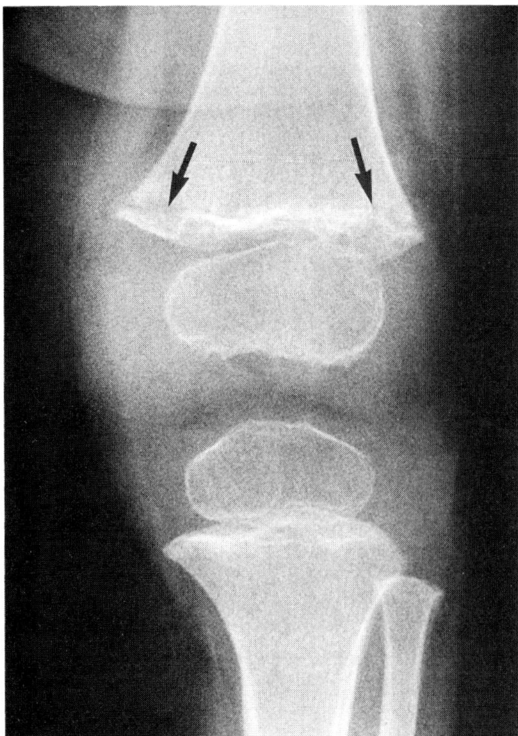

Figure 98–17. Hypovitaminosis C (scurvy). Generalized demineralization is present. A lucent zone (Trummerfeldzone) on the diaphyseal side of the zone of provisional calcification (*arrows*) is due to poorly formed trabecular bone and is prone to fracture.

Hypervitaminosis C

Over the last 10 years, it has been suggested that massive doses of vitamin C taken daily may prevent or at least speed up the recovery time from the common cold. This therapy has not resulted in any gross radiographic evidence of vitamin C intoxication. Smith

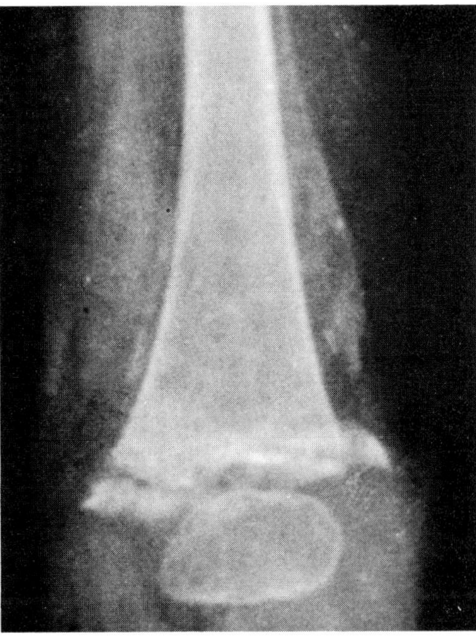

Figure 98–18. Hypovitaminosis C (scurvy). Fractures of the Trummerfeldzone appear as beak-like projections off the metaphysis (Pelkan spurs). Periosteal elevation is also evident.

has reported that with greater than 4 g of vitamin C taken daily, there is a statistically significant increase in oxalic acid excretion. In a small series of patients with inactive renal stone disease, those who increased their vitamin C intake became active renal stone formers. If the vitamin C was discontinued, the urinary excretion of oxalic acid returned to normal and the stone disease resolved.

VITAMIN D

Vitamin D is one of the fat-soluble vitamins and its effects have been studied for centuries, especially in the states of deficiency producing bowing deformities of growing bones known clinically as rickets (see Osteomalacia and Rickets earlier in this chapter).

Hypervitaminosis D

The initial reports of hypervitaminosis D were in infants and children who had been given large doses of vitamin D for the treatment of rickets. In adults, vitamin D has been given to treat rheumatoid arthritis and Paget's disease without success. The main use of vitamin D today is in trying to correct the abnormal calcium-phosphate metabolism in patients with renal insufficiency. Acute hypervitaminosis D is rare and is characterized by CNS symptoms including headache, convulsions, and even coma. The patient may be dehydrated, febrile, and complaining of pain at multiple skeletal sites. There are no radiographic signs of acute hypervitaminosis D.

Manifestations of chronic hypervitaminosis D, as with any other chronic ingestant, depend on several contributing factors. Primary considerations include the source and concentration of vitamin D, the length of time supplementation has occurred, the dose and activity of the ingestant, renal and hepatic function, calcium and phosphate intake, and the route of administration. Clinically these patients present with fever, abdominal pain, thirst, and dehydration. Frequently neurologic dysfunction prevails, ranging from headache to coma. Frequency and nocturia are common. Chemistry evaluation demonstrates elevated levels of calcium, phosphate, alkaline phosphatase, and BUN. There may be gross bony deformities secondary to metastatic calcifications. Radiographically in infants and children, metaphyseal bands of increased density, cortical thickening, and metastatic calcifications of the viscera, cartilage, and the falx cerebri may be present.

In adults, the radiographic finding is that of generalized osteopenia involving mainly the spine. There may be soft-tissue calcifications involving the tendon sheaths, bursae, and joint capsules. Discontinuation of vitamin D leads to slow resorption of these soft-tissue calcifications. Other considerations of metastatic calcifications, aside from hypervitaminosis D, include metastatic disease to the skeleton, hyperparathyroidism, milk-alkali syndrome, plasma cell myeloma, and tumoral calcinosis.

HEAVY METAL AND CHEMICAL EXPOSURES

LEE D. KATZ

Over the past 25 years, there have been tremendous advancements in terms of education of the lay public as well as improvements in the workplace so that the incidence of bone disease secondary to chemical exposure has been greatly reduced.

LEAD INTOXICATION

Lead may be transferred transplacentally from mother to fetus from the twelfth week of gestation until term, resulting in congenital lead poisoning. This may be manifested by delayed dental and skeletal development, dense metaphyseal bands (so-called lead lines), and osteosclerosis. Lead intoxication during pregnancy may occur by ingestion of red clay, which is high in lead content.

Although the incidence of lead poisoning in children has been dramatically reduced with the removal of lead-based paints from the market, there still exist walls covered with lead-based paint as well as old children's furniture and toys, which are all readily accessible to a child's mouth. In adults, lead intoxication can also occur by inhalation of fumes from burning storage batteries. Bullet buckshot fragments have been implicated in lead poisoning by direct contact.

Clinically, the patients present with crampy abdominal pain, central nervous system symptoms including peripheral neuritis, encephalopathy, delirium, and even coma. Profound anemia may be present. Serum lead levels may be obtained for verification.

Radiographically, lead poisoning manifests itself as radiodense lines at the metaphyses of growing bones (Fig. 98–19). In children, if lead poisoning is suspected, a radiograph of the abdomen is helpful in detecting radiodensities in the intestine, which may represent flakes of lead-based paint. Other etiologies of dense metaphyseal lines include stress, other heavy metal ingestion, healing stages of leukemia or scurvy, hypervitaminosis D, hypothyroidism, and hypoparathyroidism.

RADIUM

In the days before quartz watches with LED readouts were available, watch faces were painted with radium so they would be luminescent at night. The radium dial painters would moisten the tips of their brushes with their tongues to obtain a sharp point necessary to do the intricate work. Martland and Humphries in 1921 described squamous cell carcinoma of the mastoids and paranasal sinuses in radium dial workers. In addition, osteosarcoma and fibrosarcoma have been reported (Fig. 98–20). In 1924, Blum described "radium jaw," which was a form of osteomyelitis in radium dial workers. Many of the deaths of these workers resulted from aplastic anemia as a direct effect of the radium on the bone marrow.

BISMUTH

Parenteral bismuth was used at the turn of the twentieth century to treat syphilis. It could cross the placenta and become deposited

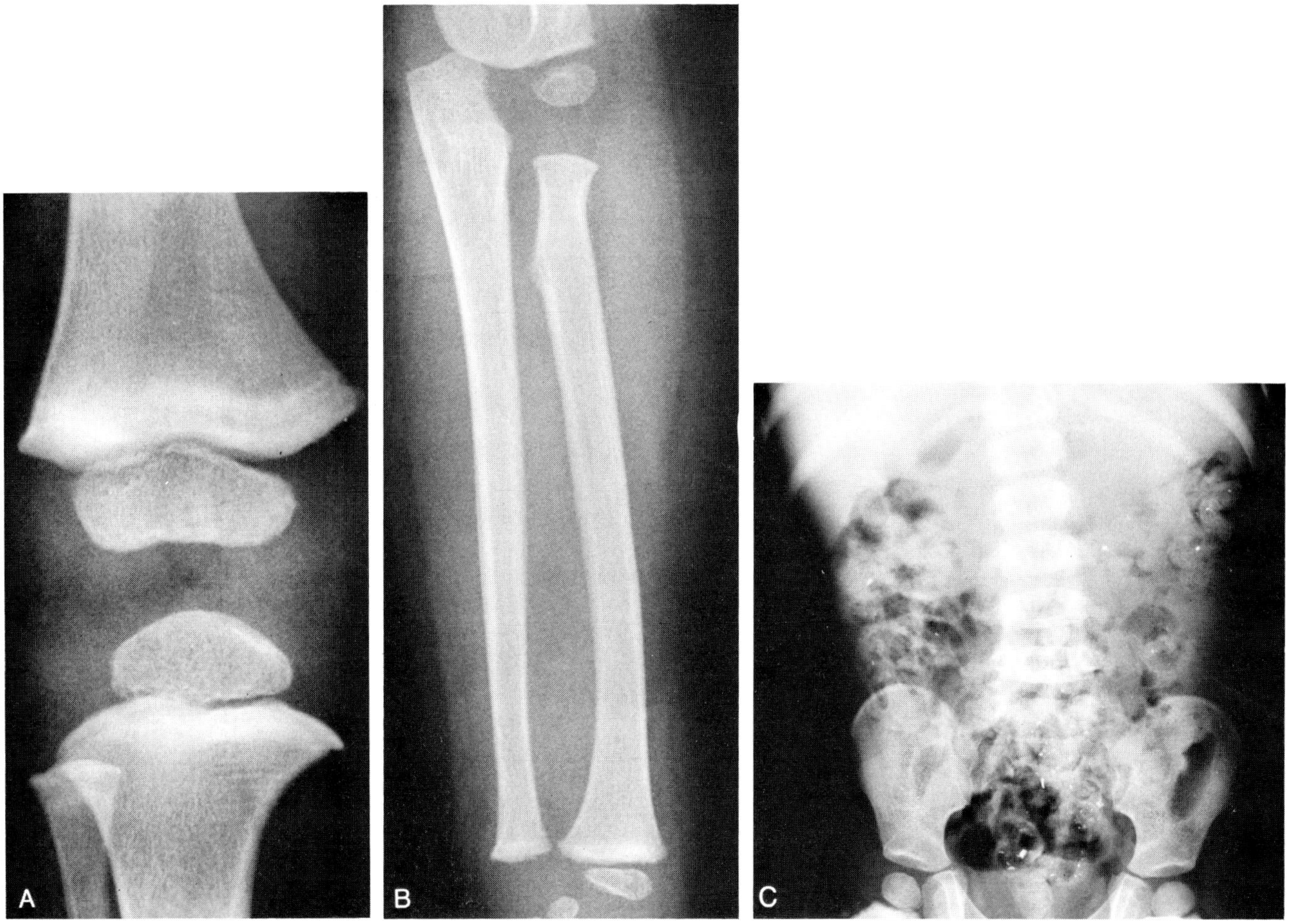

Figure 98–19. Lead intoxication. *A,* Transverse radiodense lines or bands are present in the metaphyses of the femur, tibia, and fibula. *B,* Radiodense bands are present in the metaphyses of the distal radius and ulna, where the rate of growth is the greatest. The proximal ends of these bones grow more slowly and do not exhibit lead lines. *C,* Metallic radiodensities are present throughout the intestine. The patient ate the lead paint off his crib.

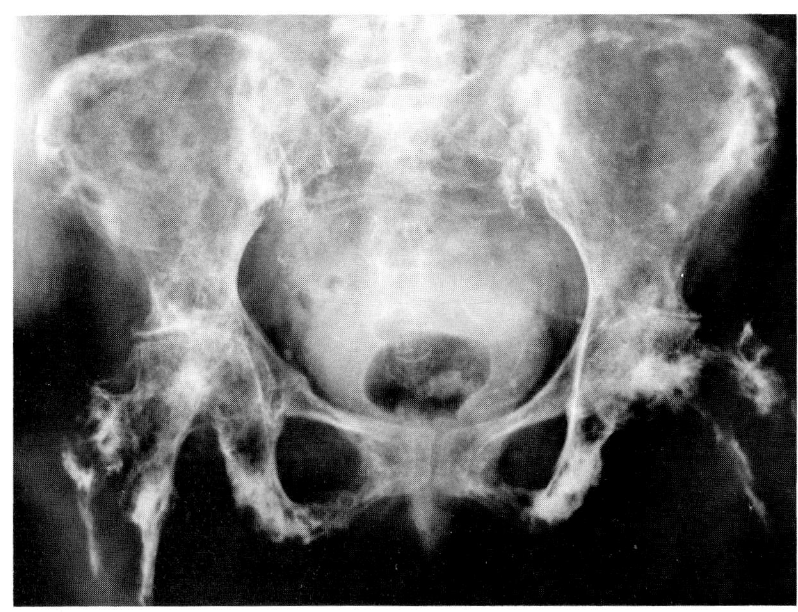

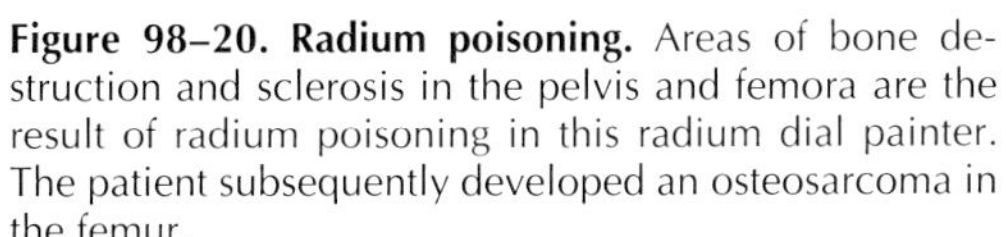

Figure 98–20. Radium poisoning. Areas of bone destruction and sclerosis in the pelvis and femora are the result of radium poisoning in this radium dial painter. The patient subsequently developed an osteosarcoma in the femur.

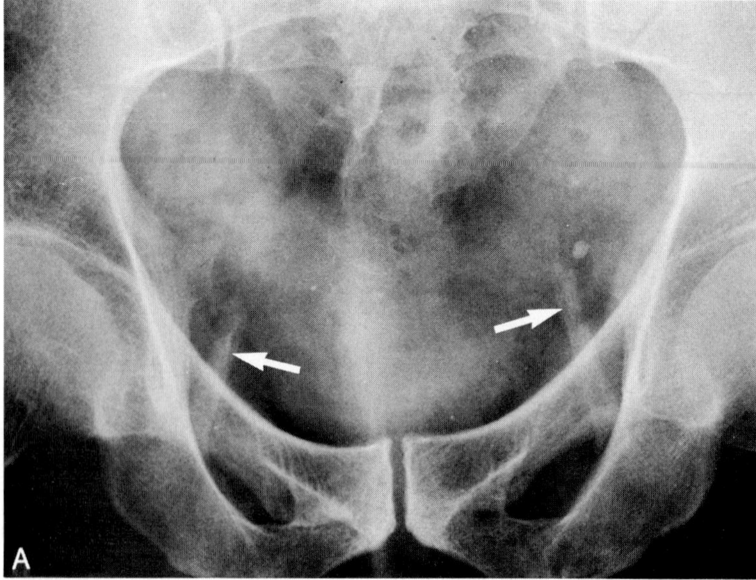

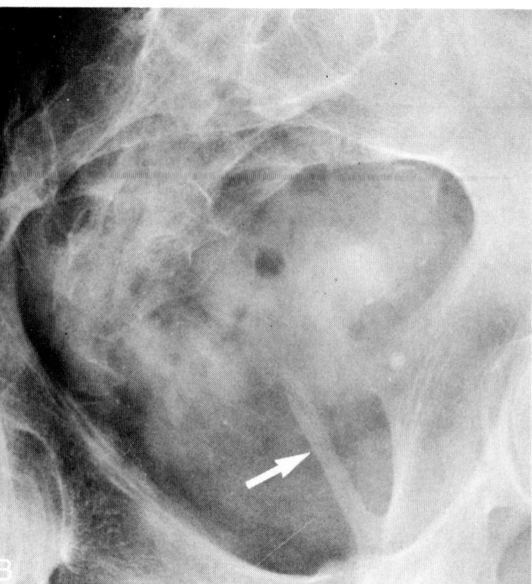

Figure 98–21. Sacrotuberous ligament calcification. *A*, Calcification in the sacrotuberous ligaments is present (*arrows*). *B*, Oblique view of the pelvis reveals that there is a trabecular pattern within the calcification (*arrow*), indicating that this is really ligamentous ossification.

in the fetal skeleton manifest as dense metaphyseal lines. In the adult, bismuth intoxication may simulate osteonecrosis.

FLUOROSIS

Fluoride, when present in a concentration greater than four parts per million in water, may produce skeletal changes. Fluorosis is endemic in India. The average American has become aware of fluoride because of its reported value in the prevention of tooth decay and periodontal disease. Unfortunately, at the concentration of two parts per million, dental fluorosis may occur, with the development of pits of variable size and discoloration of the teeth. At the concentration of 100 parts per million, renal failure and death have been reported.

The diagnosis of skeletal fluorosis should be considered when there is a constellation of findings including osteosclerosis, osteophytosis, ligamentous calcification, periostitis, and osseous excrescences. Taken separately, each finding carries its own differential diagnosis. Skeletal fluorosis is seen most commonly in the ribs, spine, and pelvis. In adults, the most common presentation is osteosclerosis. In children, osteopenia has been reported to occur initially before increased density in the bones occurs. In addition to the increased density of the bone, vertebral osteophytosis may produce symptoms due to nerve root compression. Calcification of the paraspinal, sacrotuberous (Fig. 98–21), and iliolumbar ligaments as well as ligamentous attachments to the iliac crest, ischial tuberosity, and ribs has been described.

POLYVINYL CHLORIDE

In 1950, Hannasch reported shortened, thickened fingers with a widespread dermatologic abnormality in the form of eczema presenting in a blacksmith who worked with oil. Ten years later, the association between the vinyl chloride monomer and acro-osteolysis was made. In addition, the patient may have other constitutional symptoms, including fatigue, asthma, nervousness, and insomnia. Raynaud's phenomenon–like digital pain may occur. The classic physical findings are those of drumstick fingers with watchglass nails. These patients may develop hepatic fibrosis or tumor. Radiographically, the common finding is osteolysis of the terminal phalanges. There may be a lucent band across the midshaft of one or more of the terminal phalanges. The thumb is the digit most commonly involved.

DRUG-INDUCED DISORDERS

LEE D. KATZ

The skeleton is a dynamic system in which bone is broken down and rebuilt daily. With this continual turnover of bone, it should not be surprising that some medicines, which for the most part are voluntarily swallowed, affect normal bone development and growth. What is actually surprising is that there are not more bone abnormalities seen with the tremendous number of pharmacotherapies available today, both over the counter and by prescription.

ALCOHOL

With respect to the developing fetus, alcohol is the single most preventable cause of congenital bone anomalies. If a child is born to a woman suffering from alcoholism, the child may show signs of fetal alcohol syndrome and may go through alcohol withdrawal after delivery. Aside from growth disturbances, other anomalies associated with alcohol include clinodactyly, camptodactyly, and congenital dislocation of the hip. In the adult, the effects of alcohol on bone are mainly those of complications secondary to trauma, malnutrition, and anemia. These are manifested as fracture and osteopenia.

CORTICOSTEROIDS

The role of steroid therapy in medicine at the end of the twentieth century is beyond comment. It is used widely in almost every subspecialty of internal medicine. Although its anti-inflammatory effects can be lifesaving, its effects on bone can be devastating. The most common complications from long-term corticosteroid therapy include osteoporosis, osteonecrosis, and osteomyelitis. In addition, there may be evidence of neuropathy-like articular destruction. Corticosteroids also have dramatic effects on tendons and the soft tissues that surround and support bone.

PHENYTOIN

Phenytoin is a common drug used to treat seizures. When it is given to an expectant mother, it can produce the fetal phenytoin syndrome, which is associated with a peculiar facies, cleft palate, digitate thumb, and hypoplasia of the distal phalanges. Chronic phenytoin administration to growing children may produce thickening of the bony calvarium.

THALIDOMIDE

Thalidomide is a tranquilizer used to induce sleep. If taken between the fifth and tenth weeks of gestation, it produces devastating bone deformities. The effects range from dysplasia of the thumb to four-limb amelia. In addition, other congenital anomalies of the heart and GI tract have been noted.

Bibliography

Osteoporosis

Horsman A, Jones M, Francis R, Nordin C: The effect of estrogen dose on postmenopausal bone loss. N Engl J Med 309:1405–1407, 1983.
Kimmel PL, and the Health and Public Policy Committee of the American College of Physicians: Radiologic methods to evaluate bone mineral content. Ann Intern Med 100:908–911, 1984.
Lang R: Osteoporosis. In Bollet AJ (ed): Harrison's Principles of Internal Medicine, Vol II. New York, McGraw-Hill, 1984.
Seeman E, Melton LJ, O'Fallon WM, Riggs BL: Risk factors for spinal osteoporosis in men. Am J Med 75:977–983, 1983.
Singer FR: Metabolic bone disease. In Felig P, Baxter JD, Broadus AE, Frohman LA (eds): Endocrinology and Metabolism. New York, McGraw-Hill Book Company, 1981.
Whyte MP, Bergfeld MA, Murphy WA, et al: Postmenopausal osteoporosis: A heterogeneous disorder as assessed by histomorphometric analysis of iliac crest bone from untreated patients. Am J Med 72:193–201, 1982.

Osteomalacia and Rickets

Dent CE, Stamp TCB: Vitamin D, rickets, and osteomalacia. In Avioli LV, Krane SM (eds): Metabolic Bone Disease, Vol 1. New York, Academic Press, 1977, p 237.
Frame B, Potts JT Jr (eds): Clinical Disorders of Bone and Mineral Metabolism. Amsterdam, Excerpta Medica, 1983.
Goldring SR, Krane SM: Disorders of calcification: Osteomalacia and rickets. In DeGroot LJ (ed): Endocrinology, Vol 2. New York, Grune and Stratton, 1979, p 853.
Mankin HJ: Rickets, osteomalacia and renal osteodystrophy. J Bone Joint Surg 56A:101, 1974.
Rasmussen H, Bordier P: The Physiological and Cellular Basis of Metabolic Disease. Baltimore, Williams and Wilkins, 1974.

Hypervitaminoses and Hypovitaminoses; Heavy Metal and Chemical Exposures; Drug-Induced Disorders

Garn SM, Silverman FN, Hertzog KP, Rohmann CG: Lines and bands of increased density. Their implication for growth and development. Med Radiogr Photogr 44:58, 1968.
Greengard J: Lead poisoning in childhood: Signs, symptoms, current therapy, clinical expression. Clin Pediatr 5:269, 1966.
Jaffe HL: Metabolic, Degenerative and Inflammatory Diseases of Bones and Joints. Philadelphia, Lea and Febiger, 1972.
Siffert RS: The growth plate and its affections. J Bone Joint Surg 48A:546, 1966.

99 Neurologic and Vascular Disorders

Pamela S. Jensen

The relationship between the nervous and vascular systems and their impact upon the musculoskeletal system are only partially understood. Defective development of these systems during fetal life can have a major impact upon the developing skeleton, leading to a variety of anomalies. For example, the administration of the drug thalidomide during the first trimester of pregnancy causes a decrease in the number and diameter of some of the sensory nerves that serve the extremities. This, in turn, leads to incomplete development or the complete absence of the skeletal elements that these sensory nerves would have innervated. Evidence indicates that a substantial number of skeletal changes are neurovascular in origin; however, it is often difficult to determine the respective contributions of the nervous and vascular systems or the temporal sequence that leads to the skeletal abnormalities. Because the specific etiology and pathogenesis of the conditions described in this chapter are not fully understood, the disorders are organized by their major radiographic manifestations, namely osteoporosis, bone destruction, and increased bone production.

CONDITIONS ASSOCIATED WITH OSTEOPOROSIS

Neuromuscular Diseases

Osteoporosis is a major feature of neuromuscular disorders that involve paralysis, immobilization, or disuse. Changes in the blood flow to the bone may stimulate osteoclastic activity, leading to increased bone resorption. Cortical and trabecular bone are both affected. The extent of bone loss may be so great that spontaneous fracturing occurs. The subsequent healing of the fracture may be accompanied by exuberant callus formation. Soft-tissue atrophy is usually present. Heterotopic ossification is also seen in association with central nervous system and spinal cord injuries, and in particular, with paraplegia. The hip, knee, and shoulder are the sites most commonly affected. The ossifications typically begin in the periarticular area and increase in size, often ultimately surrounding the joint and leading to significant reduction or loss of joint mobility. Local factors such as decubitus ulcers or hemorrhage into the tissues in conjunction with vigorous physiotherapy may play a role in some cases. However, the ossifications can occur in areas not subject to trauma or ulceration. Heterotopic ossification can also be seen in the tissues damaged by electrical and thermal burns. Joint changes associated with neuromuscular disorders include cartilage loss, synovial hypertrophy, and, in some cases, joint destruction. In children, altered muscular activity, immobility, and the lack of weight bearing can lead to abnormal modeling of the bone, joint deformities, premature closure of the growth plates, and neuropathic changes.

Reflex Sympathetic Dystrophy

Reflex sympathetic dystrophy (RSD), also called Sudeck's atrophy, is a disorder characterized by the development of pain, soft-tissue swelling, and regional osteoporosis (Fig. 99–1). The shoulder and hand are most commonly affected. Associated conditions are varied and include trauma, surgery, neoplasia, infection, vasculitis, and myocardial infarction. In some cases no antecedent event can be identified, or the associated condition may be of little consequence when compared with the subsequent symptoms associated with RSD. Overactivity of the sympathetic nervous system, leading to increased blood flow, has been implicated. Extensive bone loss involving the endosteal and periosteal cortical surfaces, intracortical resorption, and trabecular loss, particularly evident in the subarticular and periarticular areas, can occur very rapidly. Joint space preservation helps distinguish RSD from primary joint disease. The increased blood flow results in increased radionuclide uptake about the joints on bone scans. Edema of the bone marrow may be demonstrated by magnetic resonance imaging (MRI) in RSD.

Migratory Osteoporosis

Pain and swelling, most often affecting the lower extremity, are the common features of regional migratory osteoporosis. Characteristically several episodes involving various bones of the extremities occur over a number of years. Radiographs reveal substantial osteoporosis of the affected area. Joint spaces are preserved. Increased uptake of radionuclide on the bone scan also occurs. The pathogenesis is unknown, but evidence suggests that ischemia of the small vessels that supply the proximal nerve roots is associated with a local inflammatory process affecting the nerve endings.

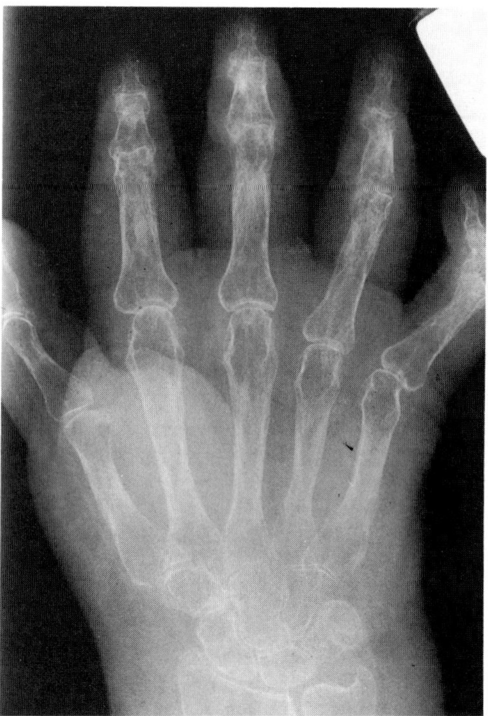

Figure 99–1. Reflex sympathetic dystrophy. Soft-tissue swelling, cortical bone loss, and patchy trabecular loss are characteristic. This 54-year-old woman fell three months earlier, injuring but not fracturing her shoulder.

Transient Osteoporosis of the Hip

Initially described in pregnant women, transient osteoporosis of the hip has now been identified in nonpregnant women and men. Hip pain with no antecedent trauma is present, and the pain is often aggravated by weight bearing, leading to a limp. Radiographs demonstrate osteoporosis of the femoral head and to a lesser degree, of the femoral neck and acetabulum. The joint space is spared. The bone scan is positive before there is radiographic evidence of osteoporosis. Bone marrow edema can be demonstrated by MRI. The affected hip characteristically demonstrates abnormally low signal intensity on T_1 spin-echo images and high signal intensity on T_2 spin-echo images. These MRI findings plus the increased uptake on radionuclide bone scan differentiate transient edema from early osteonecrosis, in which the bone scan demonstrates decreased radionuclide uptake. With transient osteoporosis of the hip, the process usually remits spontaneously within six months and the bone remineralizes. In contrast, osteonecrosis progresses to subcortical bone loss with fracturing and collapse of the femoral head; patchy sclerosis and cyst formation also occur. The pathogenesis of transient osteoporosis of the hip is unknown, but a neurovascular etiology is suspected.

CONDITIONS ASSOCIATED WITH BONE DESTRUCTION

Neuropathic Joint Disease (Charcot's Joint)

Destruction of the bone and cartilage of a joint, usually occurring in conjunction with a neurologic disorder, is termed a neuropathic or Charcot's joint. Neurologic disorders more commonly associated

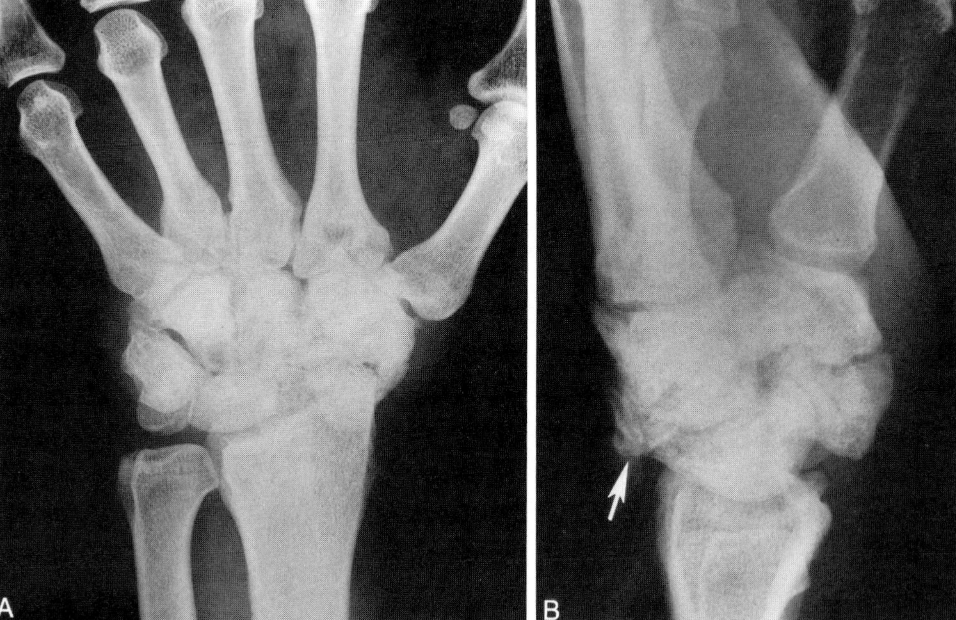

Figure 99–2. Neuropathic joint. *A,* A 26-year-old man with syringomyelia and loss of sensation in his upper extremity. Destruction of the scaphoid and trophic changes of the trapezium and capitate are present. Bone density and cortical thickness are preserved. *B,* Fragmentation (bony shards) from the capitate (*arrow*) and scaphoid are evident on the lateral view of the wrist.

with the development of a neuroarthropathy include syphilis (tabes dorsalis), syringomyelia, meningomyelocele, spinal cord injuries, and peripheral neuropathies, including those associated with diabetes mellitus and alcoholism. Controversy surrounds the pathogenesis of the disorder. Traditionally, the joint changes are thought to be the result of loss of the protective sensations of pain and proprioception, leading to instability of the joint. Repeated trauma then leads to malalignment, fracturing, and ultimate destruction. Others cite evidence supporting a neurovascular cause in which a neurally mediated vascular reflex leads to increased blood flow and increased osteoclastic activity, which, in turn, results in increased bone resorption and osteoporosis. Should this demineralized bone be subjected to trauma, pathologic fracturing and subsequent repair would then be a secondary process, not the initiating one.

The bone and joint changes of neuropathic joint disease can be very dramatic. Gross disorganization of the joint with subluxation or dislocation, fractures, osseous fragments (bony shards) in the surrounding tissues, osteosclerosis, periosteal new bone formation, and marked malalignment are all characteristic radiographic features. The articular ends of the bone lose their articular cartilage, which is replaced by fibrocartilage. The ends of the bones may be resorbed, but the surfaces appear sharp. This feature is helpful in identifying the presence of osteomyelitis; with infection, the edges of bones are often indistinct or fuzzy. Marginal exostoses form and can become quite large in neuropathic disease. They may break off and contribute to the bony shards present about the joint. Again, the cortical margins are typically sharp and well defined.

The joints most commonly affected are generally determined by the underlying disease. With syringomyelia (Fig. 99–2), the joints of the upper extremity and spine are affected. In tabes dorsalis (syphilis), the large joints of the lower extremity (Fig. 99–3) and the spine (Fig. 99–4) are involved. Disorders affecting the peripheral nervous system such as diabetes mellitus and alcoholism exhibit changes more commonly in the tarsal, metatarsal, and interphalangeal joints of the feet (Fig. 99–5). With congenital insensitivity to pain, the joints of the lower extremity are more often affected; acro-osteolysis of the terminal digits of the hands also occurs in this disorder (Fig. 99–6).

In advanced cases, the radiographic changes are so characteristic that confusion with other disorders is unlikely. In earlier stages, neuroarthropathy must be distinguished from osteoarthritis, calcium pyrophosphate dihydrate deposition (CPPD) disease, osteonecrosis, and chronic infection.

Osteonecrosis

Osteonecrosis, also known as avascular, ischemic, or aseptic necrosis of bone, is due to a decrease or cessation of blood flow to the affected area. Many causes can lead to this final outcome: disruption of the vessels (trauma, fracture, irradiation); external compression upon the vessels; internal obstruction due to thrombo-

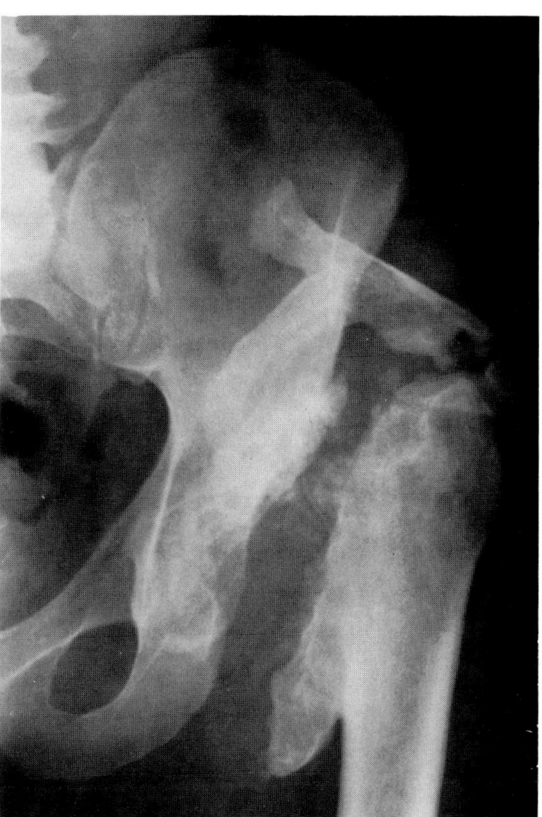

Figure 99–3. Neuropathic joint. Complete destruction of the femoral head and neck with bony shards and new bone formation are present. The ends of the bones are sharply marginated. The cortical thickness of the femoral shaft is preserved.

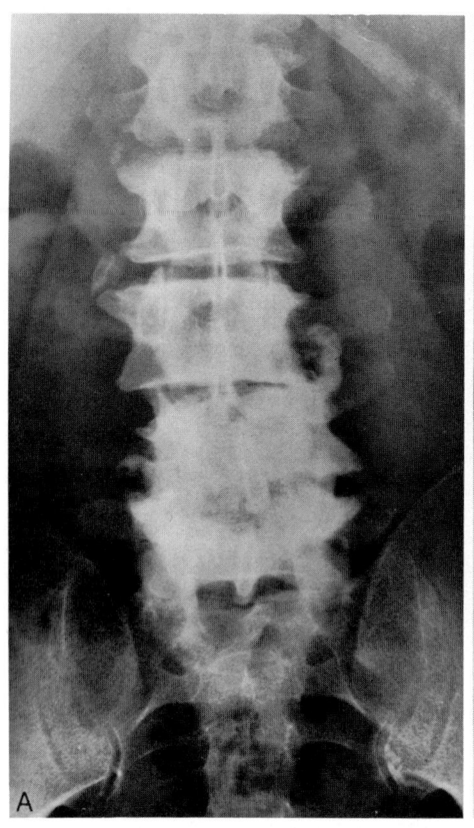

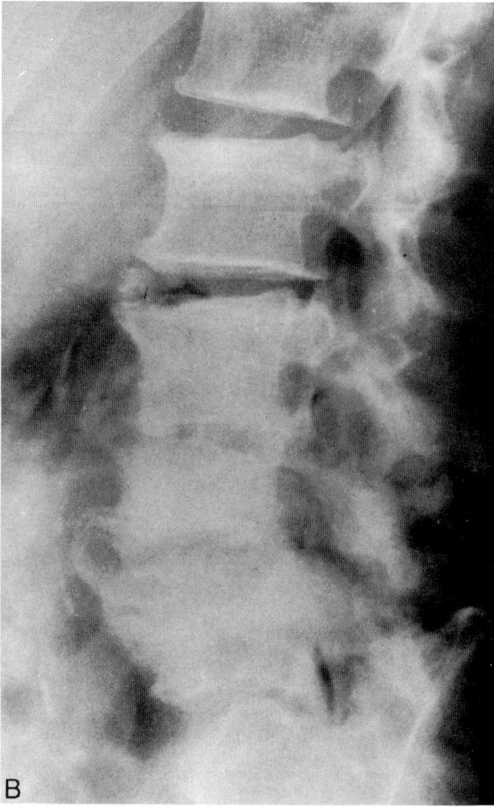

Figure 99–4. Neuropathic joint. *A,* There is subluxation at L3-L4 and L4-L5, trophic bone formation in addition to degenerative osteophytes, and disc narrowing of the lumbar spine in this 52-year-old man with tertiary syphilis. *B,* Lateral view of the lumbar spine also reveals destructive changes of the posterior elements and sclerosis of the involved vertebrae.

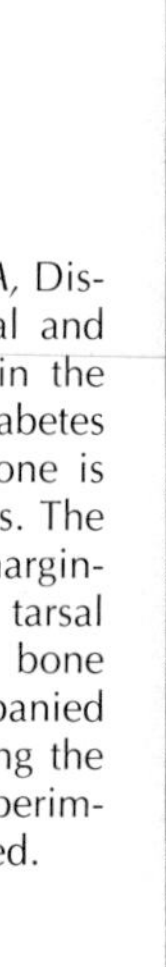

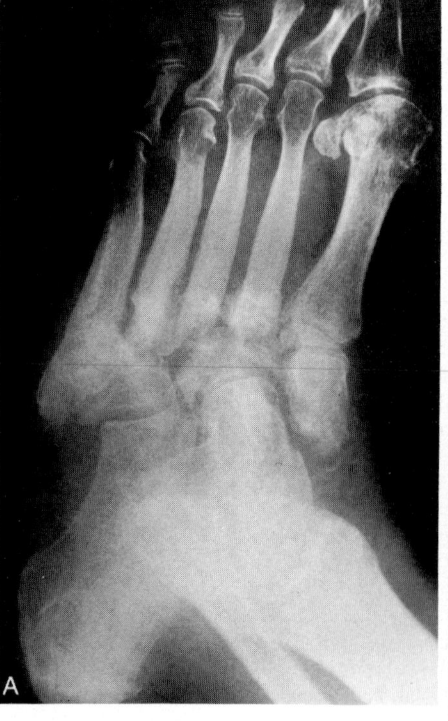

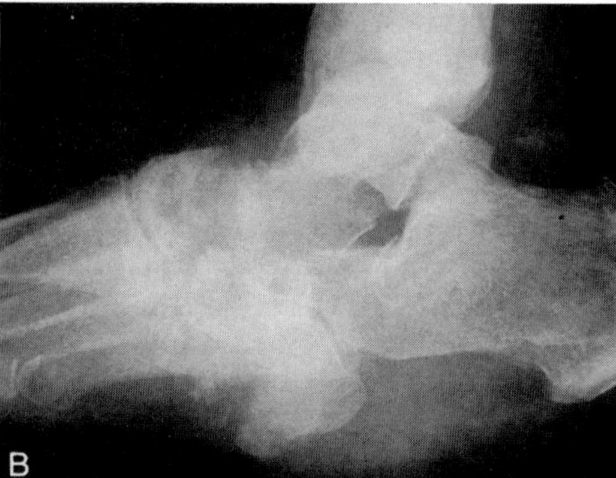

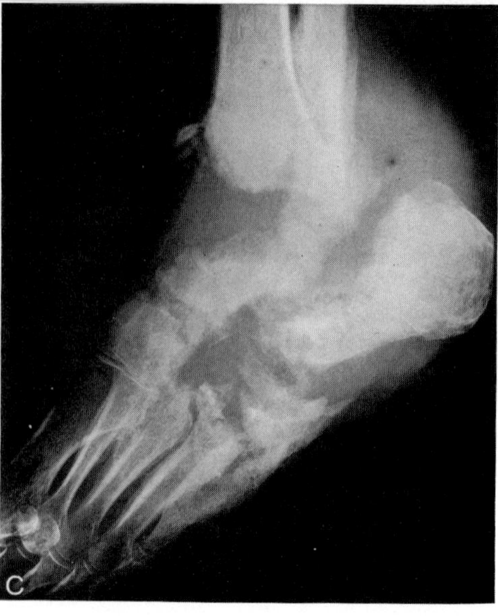

Figure 99–5. Neuropathic joint. *A,* Dislocation of some of the midtarsal and tarsometatarsal joints is present in the foot of this 45-year-old with diabetes mellitus. Thick periosteal new bone is present along the metatarsal shafts. The ends of the bones are sharply marginated. *B,* Lateral view confirms the tarsal dislocation. *C,* More advanced bone loss in another diabetic is accompanied by periosteal bone formation along the tibia, fibula, and metatarsals. Superimposed infection cannot be excluded.

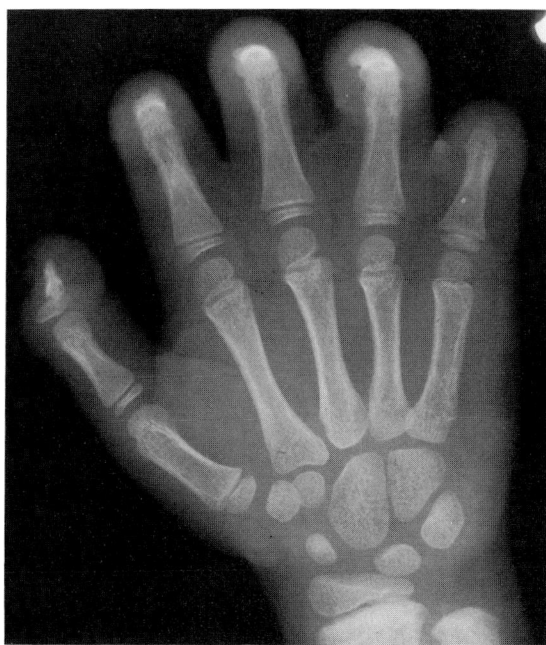

Figure 99–6. Congenital insensitivity to pain. There is loss of the distal and major portions of the middle phalanges and soft tissues of the digits in this eight-year-old girl. Foreshortening of the distal phalanx of the thumb is evident. Extensive soft-tissue swelling and cartilage loss were also present in the right knee.

embolism, fat emboli (alcoholism), nitrogen emboli (dysbaric or caisson disease), and aggregations of cells (sickle cell disease, Gaucher's disease); vasospasm; vasculitis (collagen vascular diseases); and increased intraosseous marrow pressure (steroids). In the relatively closed spaces of the femoral, humeral, and mandibular heads, steroid-induced hypertrophy of fat cells can lead to increased internal marrow pressure. Surgical decompression can reduce this pressure and, if performed early in the course, can in some cases prevent the late consequences of osteonecrosis. Other bones subjected to post-traumatic osteonecrosis because of the nature of their vascular supply include the talus and the scaphoid of the wrist.

The pathogenesis of osteonecrosis involves a number of stages. Following the initiating insult in a bone such as the femoral head, the initial changes (death of the cells) are microscopic. Restoration begins with development of hyperemia of the surrounding bone, which leads to decreased radiodensity; the normal density of the necrotic segment remains unchanged, but relative to the surrounding demineralized bone it appears more dense (Fig. 99–7). Infiltration of the edges of the infarcted area and subsequent remodeling of the trabecular bone lead to further bone loss around the necrotic segment. If the bone becomes sufficiently weakened due to this remodeling process, the subchondral area, which is subjected to weight-bearing forces, fractures, producing a crescent sign (Fig. 99–8) and subsequent collapse of the articular surface that can be detected by radiography or MRI (Fig. 99–9). Following the collapse of the femoral head and disruption of the articular cartilage, changes of osteoarthrosis with joint narrowing, cyst formation, and sclerosis occur (Fig. 99–10). When the infarction occurs in the diametaphyseal shaft of a tubular bone, disruption of the articular surface is not a factor. The edges of the infarct slowly calcify, and residual deformity does not occur (Fig. 99–11).

The MRI pattern reflects the evolving histologic changes through which osteonecrosis passes. Bone marrow edema (low signal intensity on T_1 images and high signal intensity on T_2 images) and the presence of a joint effusion may be the first changes detected. With hemorrhage and formation of necrotic bone the MRI pattern changes. Hemorrhage is characterized by high signal intensity on both T_1 and T_2 images. A peripheral band of low signal intensity characteristically surrounds the area of necrosis in more advanced stages. This corresponds to a margin of reactive bone between viable and necrotic bone.

The plain film radiographic findings appear late in the course of development of osteonecrosis. The earliest changes can be detected by radionuclide bone scanning and MRI. Both methods are sensitive, but it appears that MRI may be somewhat more sensitive because the method does not require comparing one side with the other as does bone scanning. Because osteonecrosis can be bilateral, false negatives can occur with bone scanning. Inasmuch as early surgical intervention provides the best hope for a good outcome, detection of the process should ideally be made before changes are present on plain film radiography.

"Osteochondritis"

In the past, a series of "bone inflammations" was described and collectively called osteochondritis. Pain with an accompanying ab-

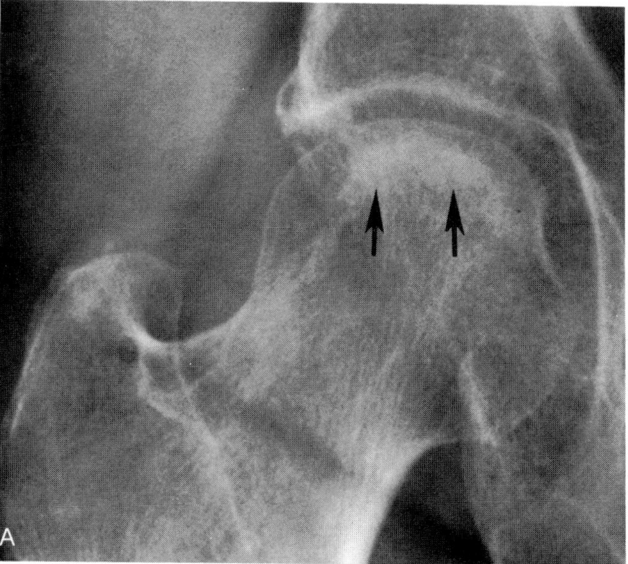

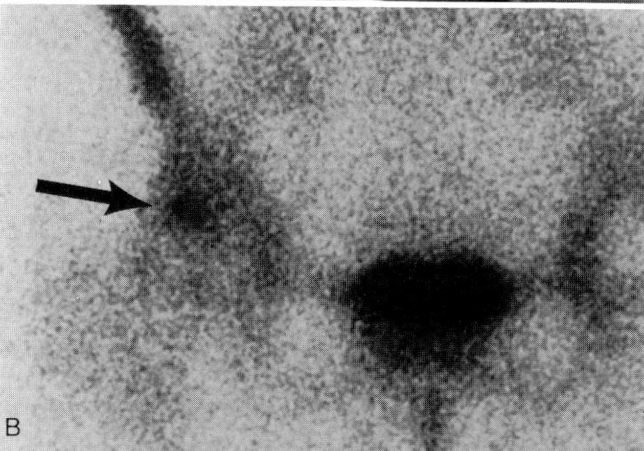

Figure 99–7. Osteonecrosis. *A,* Decreased density of the subarticular bone of the femoral head and increased density of the adjacent underlying bone (*arrows*) are present. The femoral head has retained its normal spherical contour. *B,* ^{99m}Tc bone scan demonstrates an area of increased uptake in the right femoral head (*arrow*) corresponding to the area of change noted on the radiograph. Note the complete absence of radionuclide uptake in the left femoral head and midportion of the neck and shaft due to the presence of a metallic femoral hip prosthesis.

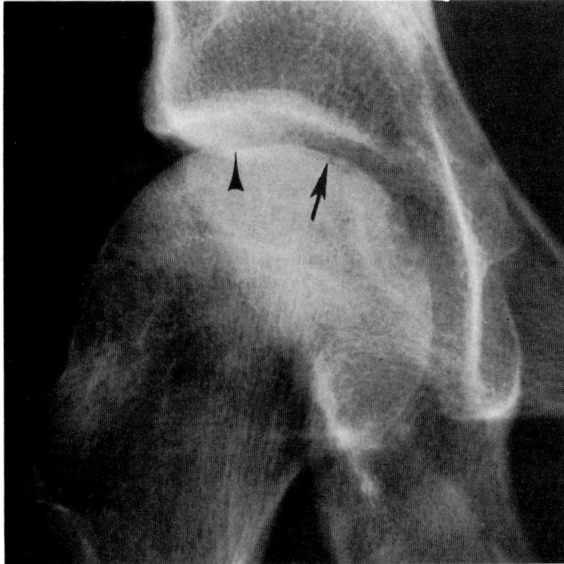

Figure 99–8. Osteonecrosis. Subarticular fracture causing a crescent sign (*arrow*) and early collapse of the femoral head (*arrowhead*) are evident on the frontal projection of the right hip.

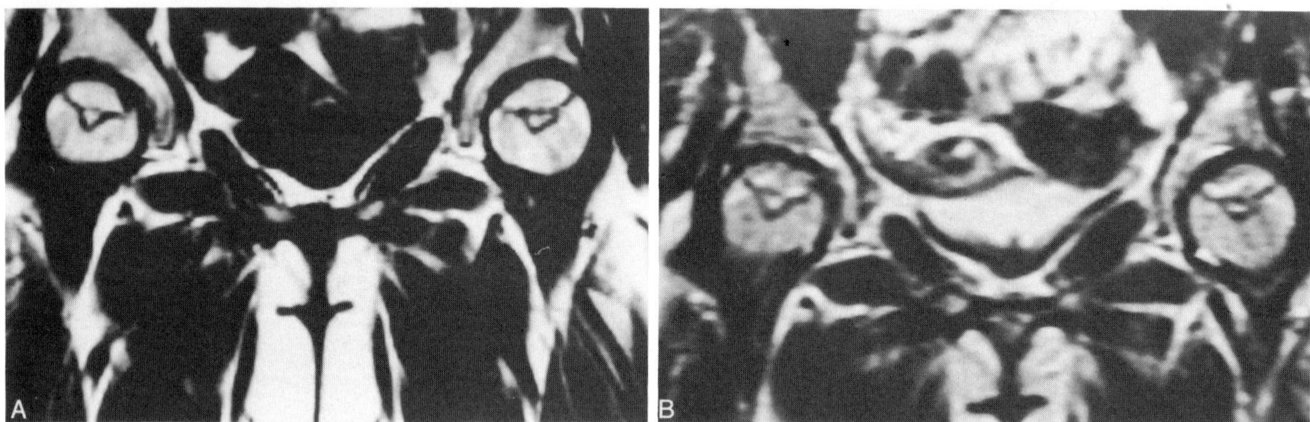

Figure 99–9. MRI of **osteonecrosis of both femoral heads.** *A,* T_1-weighting, coronal plane. *B,* T_2-weighting, coronal plane. MRI is the most accurate diagnostic imaging tool for early osteonecrosis, when available therapies have the greatest chance of preserving joint function. MRI can reliably determine the extent and stage of the disease. The MRI appearance of osteonecrosis is that of a peripheral low-signal intensity rim on T_1- and T_2-weighting, felt to represent sclerosis from reinforcement of existing trabeculae. With T_2-weighting, an inner border of increased signal is seen adjacent to the low-signal rim, consistent with a reactive interface of inflammation, resorption, and granulation. MRI classification of osteonecrosis is based on the central signal within the reactive interface. This example depicts a class A lesion with the central signal isointense to fat in both T_1- and T_2-weighting.

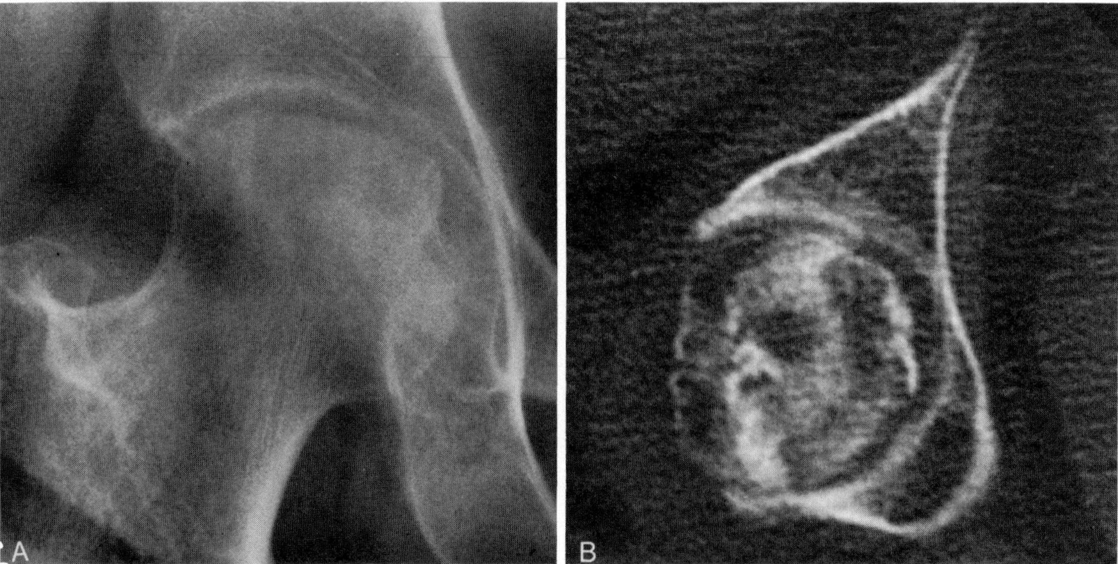

Figure 99–10. Osteonecrosis. *A,* More advanced changes of osteonecrosis are present, with considerable collapse and deformity of the femoral head and cystic changes with adjacent areas of sclerosis. *B,* CT scan reveals cartilage space loss in addition to the osteonecrotic changes demonstrated on the radiograph.

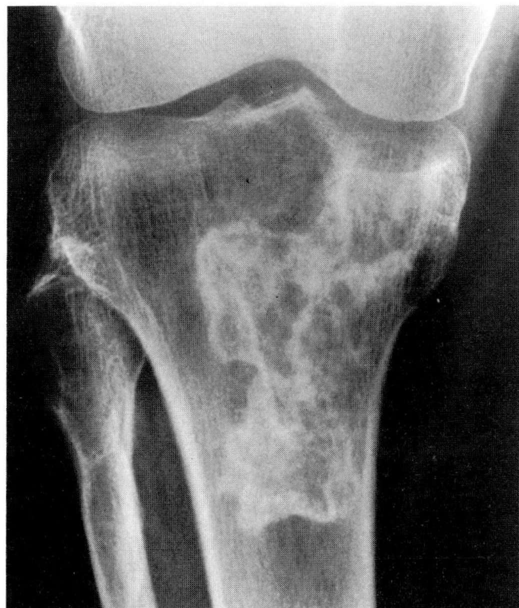

Figure 99–11. Ischemic infarction. Sharply marginated, partially calcified infarct is present in the diametaphyseal area of the right proximal tibia. This infarct followed a medial tibial plateau fracture. Healed fracture of the fibula is also evident.

normal radiographic appearance (sclerosis, fragmentation of epiphyses, and collapse) was the characteristic feature. Eponyms were given to each of the affected anatomic sites. It is now recognized that this is a heterogeneous group of disorders with varying etiologies.

Increased density of the calcaneal apophysis (Sever's disease) is a normal variant. Osgood-Schlatter (tibial tuberosity) and Blount's (proximal tibial epiphysis) diseases (Fig. 99–12) are the result of trauma without evidence of osteonecrosis. Osteonecrosis following trauma characterizes Freiberg's (second metatarsal) (Fig. 99–13), Kienböck's (carpal lunate), and possibly Köhler's (tarsal navicular) diseases (Fig. 99–14). Legg-Calvé-Perthes disease, which is osteonecrosis of the capital femoral epiphysis, occurs in children between the ages of four and eight when the vascular supply to the epiphysis is most vulnerable. Minor trauma leading to synovitis, joint effusion, and increased intra-articular pressure can lead to vascular compression and infarction.

Calvé's disease of the spine (vertebra plana) is now believed to be due almost exclusively to eosinophilic granuloma. Scheuermann's disease, characterized as irregularity of the end-plates of the thoracic spine in the adolescent, represents the herniation of disc material through a weakened end-plate in conjunction with trauma or stress. There is a familial occurrence, suggesting that genetic factors may lead to weakness of the vertebral bodies.

Osteolysis

Post-traumatic osteolysis, due to vascular compromise following fracturing, can occur at a number of anatomic sites and should not be confused with metabolic, arthritic, or neoplastic processes. Fractures of the distal end of the clavicle can progress to non-union with subsequent resorption of the distal fracture fragment, resulting in a widened acromioclavicular junction. The same phenomenon can occur with fractures adjacent to the pubic symphysis involving the pubic and ischial rami. Other bones that can undergo osteolysis following fracture include the distal ulna and radius, the carpal bones, and the femoral neck.

Vanishing bone disease of Gorham is a process of unknown etiology. Extensive osteoporosis and collapse involving multiple bones, usually in a regional distribution, can progress over time. The histologic appearance of the bone is that of extensive vascularity or hemangioma formation.

Acro-osteolysis

Resorption of the distal ends of the digits occurs in many conditions owing to a variety of causes. Vascular insufficiency is a major factor in the development of skeletal changes associated with frostbite. Radiographic manifestations vary with the length of exposure to the freezing temperature and the age of the patient. Soft-tissue loss, resorption of the distal ends of the phalanges, and joint changes resembling osteoarthrosis can occur. The thumb is sometimes spared if it is held inside a clenched fist. In children, destruction of the epiphyses and premature closure of the growth plate leading to brachydactyly are noted.

CONDITIONS ASSOCIATED WITH BONE PRODUCTION

Melorheostosis

The radiographic features of melorheostosis are characteristic (Fig. 99–15). Cortical bone formation (hyperostosis) affects one or more bones of an extremity, with the lower limb being more commonly affected. This new bone formation has the appearance of

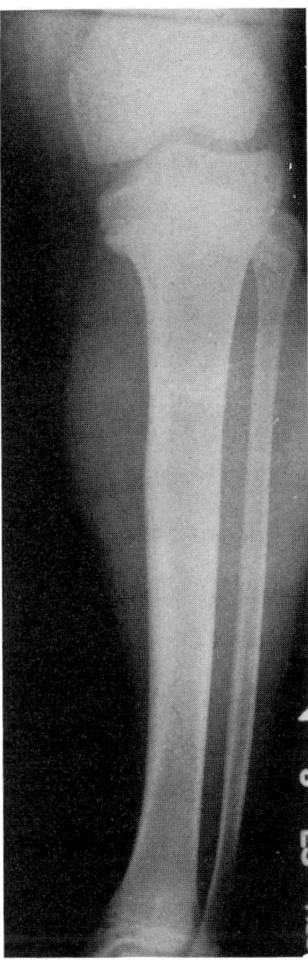

Figure 99–12. Blount's disease. Deformity of the medial tibial plateau (tibia vara) occurring in an adolescent is probably the result of arrest of epiphyseal growth medially following trauma. In this age group, the process is usually unilateral. In the infantile form, the changes are typically bilateral.

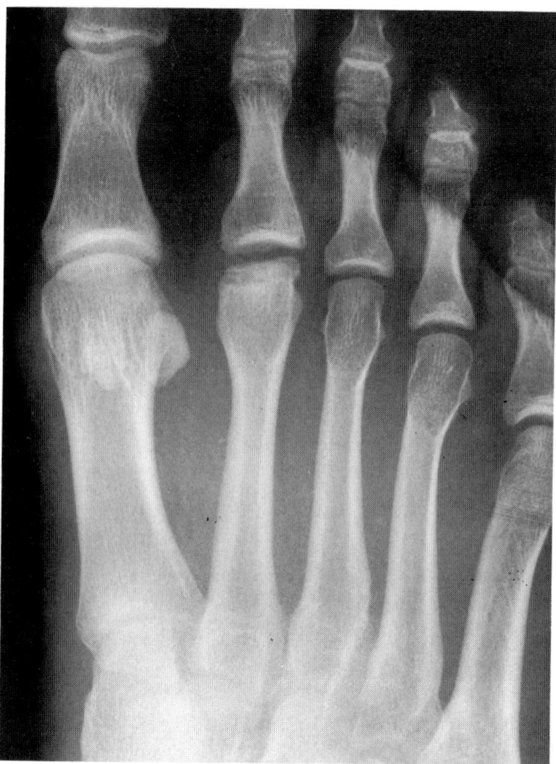

Figure 99–13. Freiberg's infarction. Deformity of the right second metatarsal head with flattening of the articular surface, widening of the head, patchy sclerosis, and thickening of the cortex of the metatarsal shaft are characteristic.

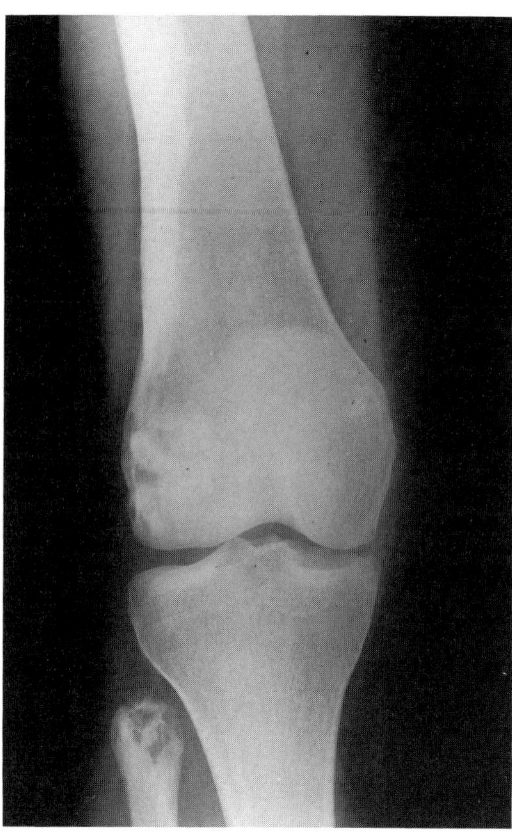

Figure 99–15. Melorheostosis. Cortical thickening involving the lateral aspect of the right femur has a sharply defined, wavy border. The proximal fibula is also involved.

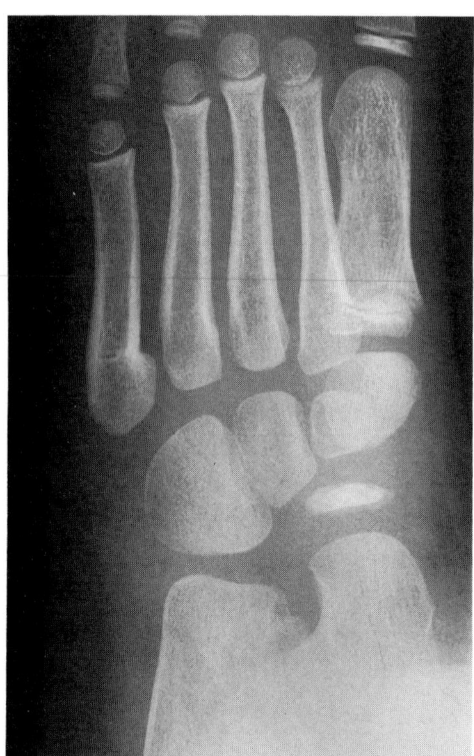

Figure 99–14. Köhler's disease. Flattening and increased density of the tarsal navicular with preservation of the joint spaces are present. Unilateral involvement occurring between the ages of three and seven years is typical.

candle wax dripping down the shaft of the bone. New bone formation can also occur along the endosteal surface of the cortex, leading to narrowing of the medullary cavity. The radionuclide bone scan is positive; thus the distinction between melorheostosis and Paget's disease must be made. Differentiation is based on the anatomic distribution of the lesions and the nature of the bone production. The distribution of melorheostosis follows that of the sclerotomes, which are zones of the skeleton supplied by individual spinal sensory nerves.

Hypertrophic Osteoarthropathy

Primary hypertrophic osteoarthropathy (Fig. 99–16), also known as pachydermoperiostitis, is an uncommon disease transmitted as an autosomal dominant disorder. Clubbing of the digits, painful swollen joints, thickened skin, and bone proliferation in the form of periostitis characterize this disease. The bones most commonly affected are the tubular bones of the extremities, although the smaller bones of the hands and feet, the pelvis, and the skull can also be affected. In contrast to secondary hypertrophic osteoarthropathy, the periosteal new bone extends to the epiphyseal region, and prominent nonlinear outgrowths are typically present.

Secondary hypertrophic osteoarthropathy (Fig. 99–17) is associated with a variety of conditions, including those that are pulmonary in nature (particularly bronchogenic carcinoma), mesothelioma, cyanotic cardiovascular disease, and liver and gastrointestinal disease (Crohn's disease and ulcerative colitis). Periosteal new bone formation, typically linear in nature, is seen along the tibia, fibula, radius, and ulna and is usually bilaterally symmetrical. With progression, other tubular bones are involved. An overgrowth of vascular connective tissue in the affected limbs seems to precede the

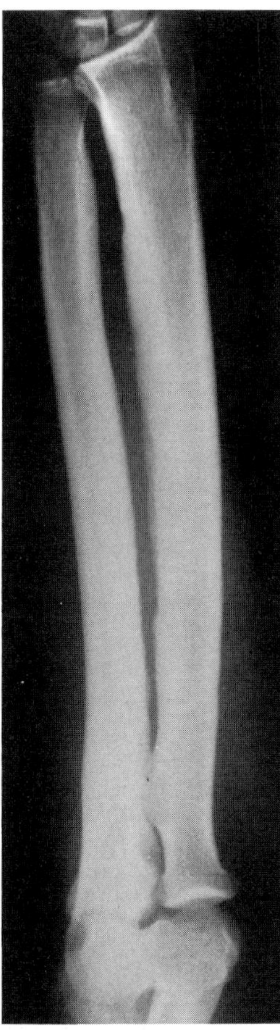

Figure 99–16. Primary hypertrophic osteoarthropathy. Marked thickening of the cortical bone of the radius and ulna is present in this patient with pachydermoperiostitis. The new bone is solid and dense, indicating it is long-standing in nature.

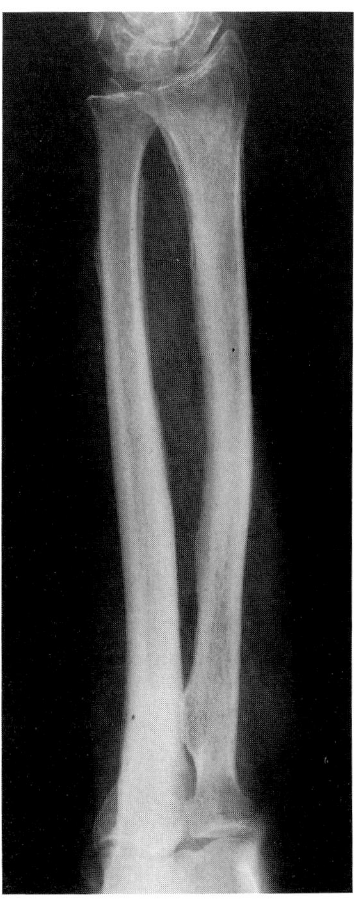

Figure 99–17. Secondary hypertrophic osteoarthropathy. Periosteal elevation along the shafts of the radius and ulna is linear and is not fully ossified in this patient with carcinoma of the lung. The epiphyses are spared.

periosteal new bone formation. Often, radionuclide bone scanning demonstrates increased uptake before there are any radiographic changes. The etiology of the vascular proliferation is unclear; however, disruption of the vagus nerve can lead to decrease in the hypervascularity.

Vascular Insufficiency

Periosteal new bone formation, particularly in the lower extremities, can occur with venous insufficiency and stasis. Soft-tissue edema and calcification of the vessels are often accompanying features.

Bibliography

Brower AC, Allman RM: Pathogenesis of the neurotrophic joint: Neurotraumatic vs neurovascular. Radiology 136:349–354, 1981.

Goergan TG, Resnick D, Riley RR: Post-traumatic abnormalities of the pubic bone simulating malignancy. Radiology 126:85, 1978.

Mankin HJ: Current concepts: Non-traumatic necrosis of bone (osteonecrosis). N Engl J Med 326:1473–1479, 1992.

Murray RO, McCredie J: Melorheostosis and the sclerotomes: A radiologic correlation. Skel Radiol 4:57, 1979.

Sweet DE, Madewell JE: Pathogenesis of osteonecrosis. In Resnick D, Niwayama G: Diagnosis of Bone and Joint Disorders. Philadelphia, WB Saunders Company, 1981, pp 2780–2831.

Thickman D, Axel L, Kressel HY, et al: Magnetic resonance imaging of avascular necrosis. Skel Radiol 15:133–140, 1986.

100 Tumor and Tumor-Like Conditions: Musculoskeletal Tumor Imaging

B. J. Manaster

Musculoskeletal tumor imaging and diagnosis seems somewhat daunting to clinicians and radiologists alike. An introductory textbook such as this should include an overview of the common musculoskeletal lesions; however, uncommon lesions or unusual appearances of common lesions deserve a place only in more specialized texts and therefore will not be included with these discussions.

Perhaps even more important than being able to identify the precise histologic type of a tumor is the radiologist's ability to properly approach the discussion of the lesion. This first section is geared toward introducing the reader to the goals of a proper workup, and to the tools that we have available to meet those goals. The first goal of radiologists is to arrive at a reasonable differential diagnosis or at least categorize a musculoskeletal lesion as to degree of its aggressiveness. If the lesion is aggressive, radiologists should feel comfortable in guiding the clinician in staging, biopsy, and resection of the lesion. Knowledgeable and responsible radiologists will help avoid overly extensive (and therefore overly expensive) staging of nonaggressive lesions. They should help avoid overly aggressive surgery on low-grade lesions, but perhaps most importantly help avoid irreversible undertreatment of aggressive lesions. Finally, radiologists should play an important role in knowledgeable post-treatment follow-up of musculoskeletal tumors.

PLAIN FILM EVALUATION OF A MUSCULOSKELETAL LESION

The approach recommended by the author is to identify a lesion as belonging to one of the following categories:

1. A benign, ''leave me alone'' asymptomatic lesion.
2. An almost certainly benign asymptomatic lesion.
3. A benign symptomatic lesion that may need nothing further than plain filming.
4. A lesion of uncertain diagnosis regarding its benign or malignant status (a good radiologist will have the tools to keep this group small).
5. A clearly malignant lesion.

In this day and age of sophisticated imaging, it is important to remember that, for an osseous lesion, plain films remain the most reliable imaging method for assessment of biologic activity and probable histologic diagnosis. Several parameters or determinants have been found to be useful in plain film assessment of an osseous lesion. The determinants that the author finds to be most useful are:

1. Age of the patient. This can be an extremely important determinant in some lesions in which the age of occurrence may be quite narrow. Furthermore, the age itself may lead to a suggested diagnosis even when the tumor is radiographically atypical. The age ranges of the more common tumors are listed in Table 100–1.
2. Soft-tissue involvement. Cortical breakthrough of an osseous lesion to create a soft-tissue mass should generally suggest an aggressive lesion. It is interesting that tumor mass often distorts muscle planes but otherwise leaves them intact. However, a soft-tissue mass due to infection more commonly obliterates muscle planes, leaving a ''smudgy'' appearance. This plain film finding may help differentiate tumor from infection, either of which can appear extremely aggressive with osseous destruction.
3. Pattern of bone destruction. Commonly accepted terminology for bone destruction includes the terms *geographic, moth-eaten,* and *permeative.* A geographic lesion is one that is so well-circumscribed that the lesion and its extent are immediately obvious (likened to an outline of a country on a map). An example of a geographic lesion is seen in Figure 100–1*A*. On the other hand, a permeative lesion is one in which the destructive pattern is extremely subtle by plain film. Although trabecular destruction is widespread, it may not yet be readily apparent radiographically, and one may even depend on other factors such as host reaction to alert one to the presence of the lesion (Fig. 100–1*B*). This is an extremely aggressive pattern of bone destruction. The moth-eaten appearance has been described as larger, more distinct lytic lesions in an otherwise permeative pattern. The need for this distinction is not clear because this also represents an aggressive pattern of bone destruction.
4. Size of lesion. It is generally true that a larger lesion is more likely to be malignant or aggressive. However, there are many exceptions to this adage (see Fig. 100–1*A,* where this large lesion is in fact a benign nonaggressive tumor), and other determinants are usually more important than size alone.
5. Location. Location is divided into three subsections, and each contribute to one of the most important determinants that we have.
   a. The first type of location might refer to which particular bone harbors the lesion, or whether the bone is a flat or tubular one or axial vs appendicular. Some lesions are noted particularly for localizing in one particular bone (for example, adamantinoma or ossifying fibroma in the tibia). Other lesions are found commonly in flat bones (for example, chondrosarcoma or the older age group of Ewing's sarcoma). Other groups of lesions are found more commonly in the axial skeleton than the appendicular skeleton (for example, chordoma or osteoblastoma). On the other hand, the favorite location of the majority of bone tumors is either the distal femur or the proximal tibia. Thus, this particular location of the tumor may not be of great help.
   b. The second type of location is that on the long axis of a tubular bone. Thus, it is important to determine whether the

TABLE 100–1. AGE RANGES FOR COMMON TUMORS

Age	Tumor
<1	Metastatic neuroblastoma
1–10	Ewing's sarcoma (usually tubular bones)
5–25	Osteosarcoma, solitary bone cyst
10–30	Ewing's sarcoma (tubular and flat bones), chondroblastoma, aneurysmal bone cyst
20–50	Giant cell tumors, parosteal osteosarcoma
30–60	Lymphoma, fibrosarcoma, chondrosarcoma, malignant fibrous histiocytoma
50–80	Metastatic, multiple myeloma
60–80	Osteosarcoma (second peak)

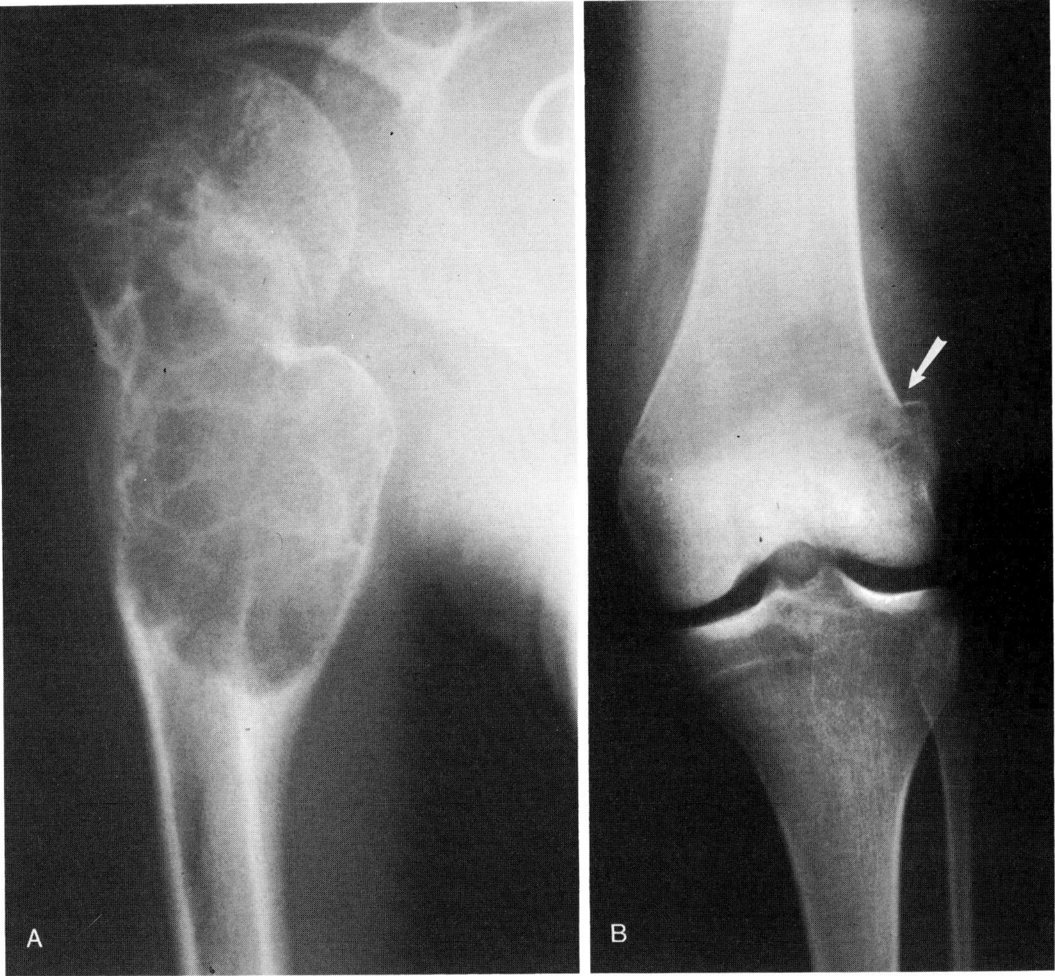

Figure 100–1. Patterns of osseous destruction. *A* demonstrates a geographic pattern. This is a large lesion that happens to be an aneurysmal bone cyst. The radiographic pattern is seen to be that of a very distinct lesion that is clearly separated and different from the underlying normal bone. Despite the large size of this lesion, its geographic nature suggests that it is nonaggressive. *B* contrasts with the appearance shown in *A* and represents a permeative pattern. There is only a slight hint of decreased density in a distal femoral metaphysis. Without the soft-tissue mass and pathologic fracture in the lateral metaphyseal region *(arrow),* it is possible that the underlying lesion (which turned out to be an osteosarcoma) might have been missed. This subtle permeative change is typical of highly aggressive lesions. (*B* reprinted with permission from the ACR Learning File, Musculoskeletal Videodisc, Case 113.)

lesion arises in the epiphysis, metaphysis, or diaphysis. Very few primary bone tumors arise in the epiphysis (chondroblastoma is far and away the most common). Most tumors arise in the metaphysis, or growth center of the bone. On the other hand, fewer lesions arise in the diaphysis (these usually are the round cell lesions, including Ewing's sarcoma and lymphoma).

c. The final location determinant is the location of the lesion along the transverse axis of a tubular bone. This refers to whether the epicenter of the lesion is spaced centrally, eccentrically, or cortically. Examples of central lesions include solitary bone cyst, fibrous dysplasia, Ewing's sarcoma, lymphoma, and a central chondrosarcoma. Many lesions, including osteosarcoma, fibrosarcoma, aneurysmal bone cyst, and giant cell tumor are eccentrically based. Finally, a few lesions, including nonossifying fibroma and benign fibrous cortical defect, are truly cortically based.

6. The zone of transition is an important determinant. Generally, a wide zone of transition from abnormal to normal bone indicates an aggressive lesion.
7. Margination of the lesion. A sclerotic margin usually indicates a nonaggressive lesion. It is generally true that the determinants ''narrow zone of transition'' and ''sclerotic margin'' occur together in a lesion and suggest that it is nonaggressive Fig. 100–2*A*). It is also logical and usually the case that the determinants ''wide zone of transition'' and ''nonsclerotic margin'' occur together in a lesion, suggesting that it is aggressive (Fig. 100–2*B*). However, the utility of using both these determinants becomes clear with the recognition that occasionally one sees the lesion with a narrow zone of transition but no sclerotic margin (Fig. 100–2*C*). This unusual combination of determinants is found most commonly in giant cell tumor and less commonly in plasmacytoma.
8. Tumor matrix. Not only the presence of tumor matrix but its character should be described. Tumor matrix may be tumor-specific, or at least will allow categorization of a lesion as bone-producing or cartilage-producing. Aggressive bone-forming tumors produce amorphous osteoid, which is often less dense and certainly less organized than normal bone (Fig. 100–3*A*). On the other hand, less aggressive bone-forming tumors produce better-organized, denser bone (Fig. 100–3*B*). Finally, the matrix of cartilage-producing tumors is usually stippled (some have described this as C- or J-shaped spicules) and denser than normal bone (Fig. 100–3*C*).

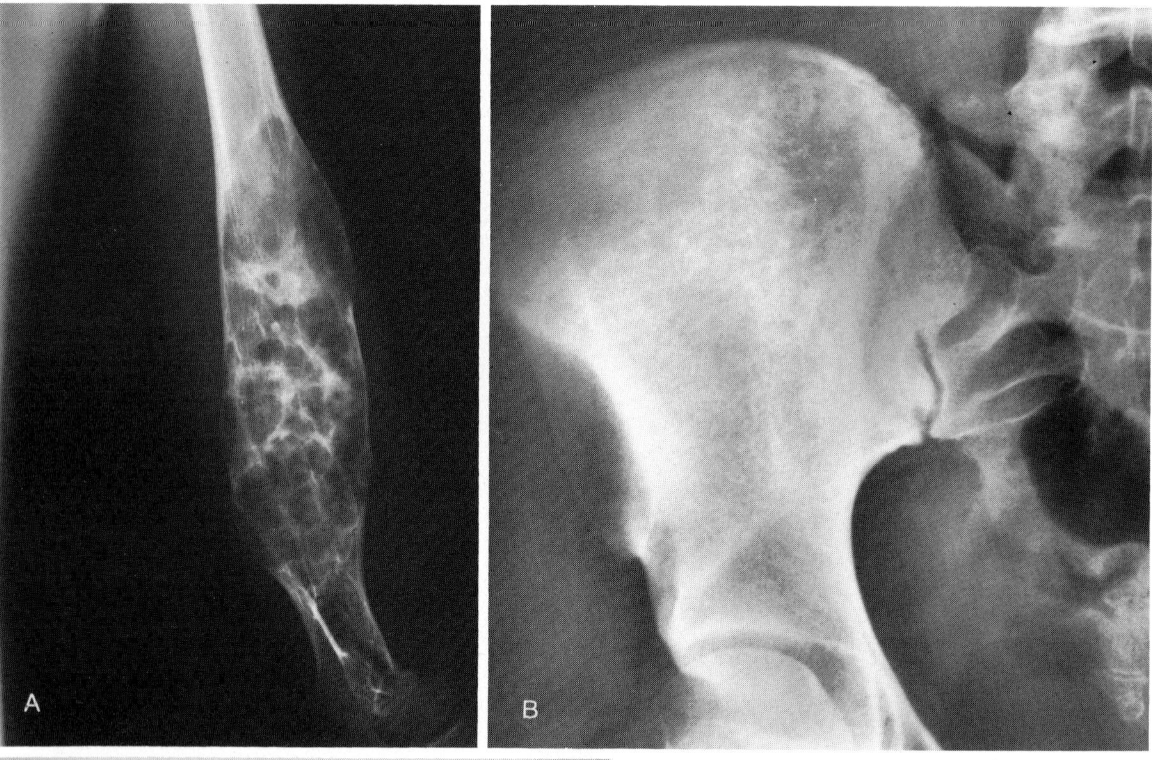

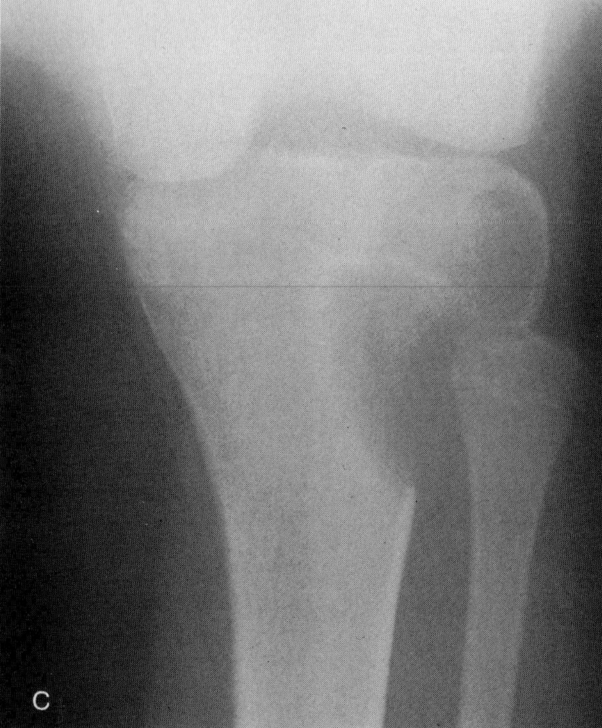

Figure 100–2. Determinants zone of transition and margination. *A,* A large geographic lesion demonstrates a narrow zone of transition and a sclerotic margin. This large lesion is a nonossifying fibroma, and despite its size its benign nature is suggested by the other determinants. *B,* on the other hand, demonstrates a sclerotic permeative lesion in the iliac wing. This lesion has a wide zone of transition and no sclerotic margin. The combination suggests an aggressive lesion, and the matrix makes the diagnosis of chondrosarcoma. *C* demonstrates the unusual combination of a lesion that has a narrow zone of transition but nonsclerotic margination. This combination almost always is seen in giant cell tumor. (*C* from Manaster BJ, et al: Giant cell tumor of bone. Radiol Clin North Am 31(2):303, 1993.)

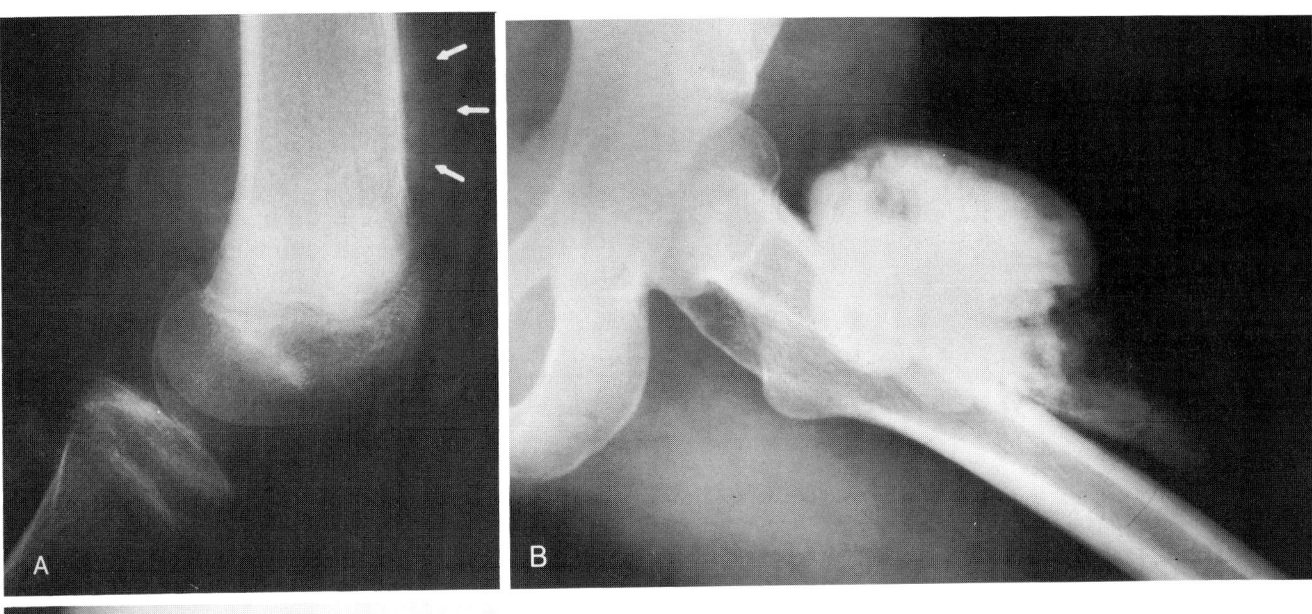

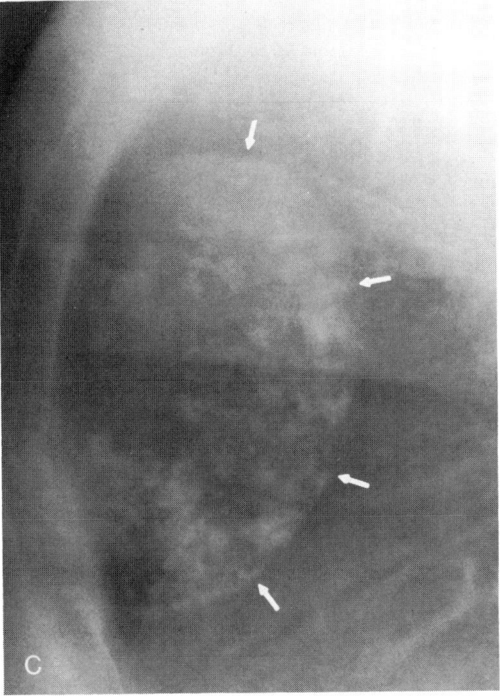

Figure 100–3. Tumor matrix. *A* demonstrates the amorphous tumor osteoid formation *(arrows)* in this patient with osteosarcoma. Aggressive osteosarcomas such as this produce osteoid that is not organized into normal-appearing bone and that is of less density than normal bone. *B,* on the other hand, demonstrates very dense and well-organized bone formation. This is the kind of tumor bone produced by a parosteal osteosarcoma, a less aggressive variety of the osteosarcoma family. *C* demonstrates nicely the characteristic stippling pattern *(arrows)* seen in cartilage-producing tumors. The density produced is often greater than the underlying normal bone. Thus, tumor matrix is often tumor-specific in its roentgenographic appearance.

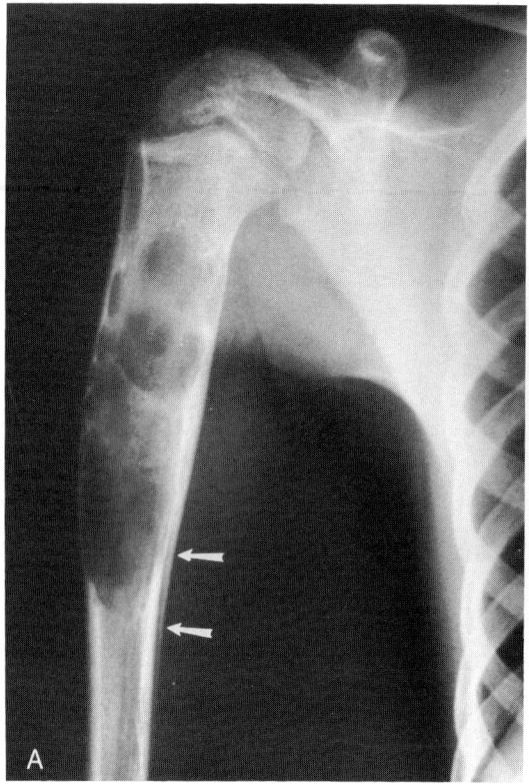

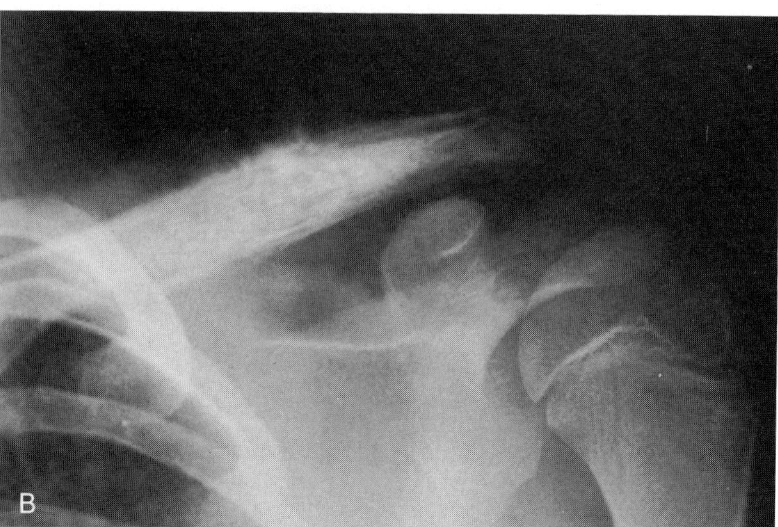

Figure 100–4. Periosteal reaction. Periosteal reaction can either be very linear, thin, and subtle, as shown in *A,* in which the pathologic fracture through the solitary bone cyst has resulted in periosteal reaction *(arrows);* or may be highly visible and aggressive-appearing, as shown in *B,* arising from a Ewing sarcoma of the clavicle. Although one sometimes can determine the aggressiveness of the underlying lesion based on the type of periosteal reaction, this is not uniformly possible because there is fairly wide variability. (*A* reprinted with permission from the ACR Learning File, Musculoskeletal Videodisc, Case 155.)

9. Host reaction. In general, the character of periosteal reaction is not a reliable sign as to malignancy or benignancy of a lesion. However, thin linear periosteal reaction is usually seen in less aggressive lesions whereas ''sunburst'' reaction is clearly more aggressive (Fig. 100–4).

After evaluating these determinants in an osseous lesion, one can often make the diagnosis. However, it is not infrequently the case that the diagnosis cannot be made definitively. In this case, one should conclude with the observation that the lesion appears overall to be either aggressive or nonaggressive. One should specifically avoid stating whether the lesion is benign or malignant. The reason for this avoidance is that malignant lesions may appear nonaggressive (for example, low-grade chondrosarcoma or telangiectatic osteosarcoma), whereas several benign lesions may appear highly aggressive (eosinophilic granuloma or infection).

IMAGING WORK-UP OF AGGRESSIVE OSSEOUS LESIONS

Once the assessment of the plain film has been carefully made, one should be able to categorize the lesion into one of the five categories listed initially in this discussion. If the lesion is aggressive (falling into categories 4 or 5) by plain film, further work-up is required. A cost-effective algorithm is presented in Fig. 100–5. Note that the next step in the algorithm is a radionuclide bone scan. This bone scan is used primarily to determine whether or not a lesion is polyostotic. It should be remembered that in general the degree of uptake on bone scan does not correlate with the grade of the lesion. Furthermore, tumor extent as seen on bone scan is not reliable. Why is it important to determine early in the work-up whether a lesion is polyostotic? If an aggressive lesion is polyostotic, the differential diagnosis is significantly reduced. This differential would include osseous metastases, multiple myeloma, primary bone tumor with osseous metastases (most commonly osteosarcoma, Ewing's sarcoma, or malignant fibrous histiocytoma), an aggressive phase of Paget's disease, multifocal osteomyelitis, histiocytosis, and multifocal vascular bone tumors.

Now look at the right arm of the algorithm. If the bone scan is polyostotic, the next step is to obtain plain films of the other lesions. This will often confirm the diagnosis as one of the above listed entities. The work-up may stop at this point if the films are sufficiently diagnostic, or may continue directly to biopsy of whichever site is most easily needled. Thus, if a lesion is polyostotic, we can often avoid other imaging studies such as CT or MRI scanning.

If the bone scan shows a monostotic lesion, one follows the left arm of the algorithm. This is the point at which plain films and CT of the chest should be obtained to evaluate for metastatic disease and to have as a baseline for follow-up. If the chest examinations demonstrate lung metastases, the work-up may be modified for palliation rather than resection for cure of the primary lesion. The exception to this may be osteosarcoma, where lung lesions can be successfully resected. If on the other hand there are no lung metastases by CT, the lesion should be staged by either MRI or CT. A carefully considered choice of one of these modalities should be made because both should not be required except under exceptional circumstances.

IMAGING WORK-UP OF SOFT-TISSUE LESIONS

Note how far along we are in the algorithm for work-up of osseous lesions before cross-sectional imaging is appropriate. This is not the case for soft-tissue lesions. When a soft-tissue lesion is detected clinically, plain films should be obtained to evaluate for any calcification or osseous involvement or findings that would suggest an unequivocal lipoma. Furthermore, clinical examination and plain film findings rarely (with the exception of lipoma) are

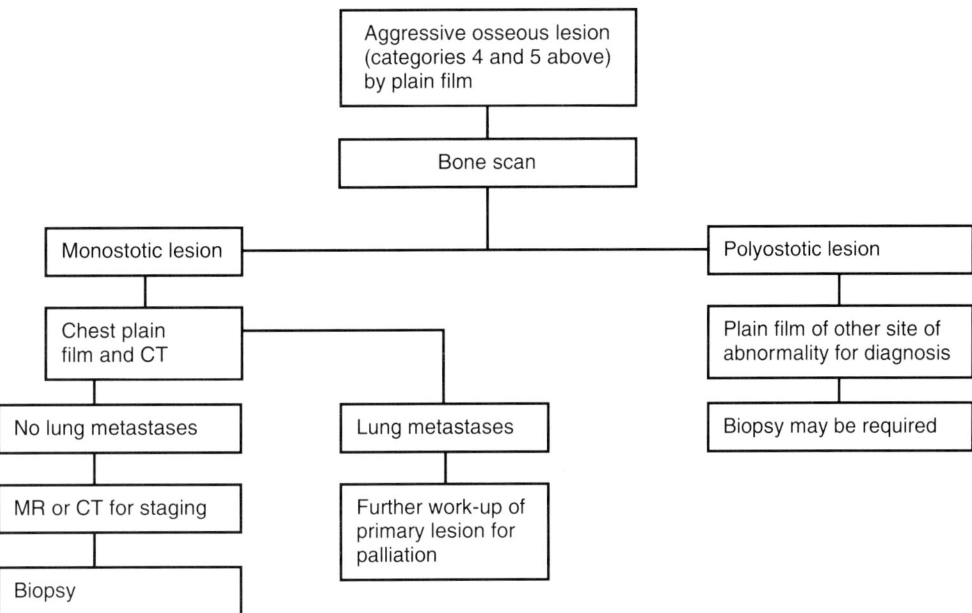

Figure 100–5. Algorithm for work-up of **osseous lesions.** (Reprinted with permission from the ACR Learning File, Musculoskeletal Videodisc, Case 100.)

able to characterize soft-tissue lesions as to their benignancy or malignancy. There is no place for radionuclide scanning in evaluation of soft-tissue lesions. MRI should be obtained very early in the algorithm (Fig. 100–6) for staging of the lesion, planning of biopsy, and therapeutic planning. MRI should then be followed by biopsy. As will be discussed later, MRI does not reliably differentiate between benign and malignant soft-tissue tumors. Therefore, biopsy should be obtained prior to work-up for metastatic lung lesions, with the latter instituted only in the event of biopsy-proven malignant lesions.

SURGICAL TREATMENT OPTIONS FOR MUSCULOSKELETAL LESIONS

Radiologists should be aware of surgical treatment options for musculoskeletal lesions. These are as follows:

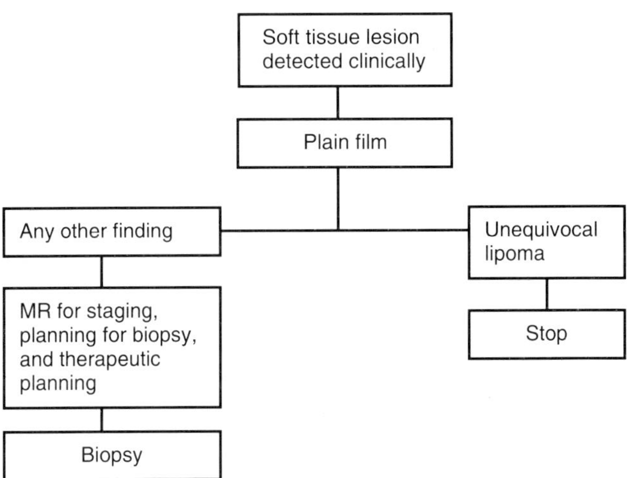

Figure 100–6. Algorithm for work-up of **soft-tissue lesions.** (Reprinted with permission from the ACR Learning File, Musculoskeletal Videodisc, Case 100.)

1. Intralesional excision (curettage), in which tumor remains at the margin of the lesion.
2. Marginal excision, in which the plane of excision passes through reactive but not tumor tissue.
3. Wide excision, in which there is removal of the lesion with intact cuff of surrounding normal tissue. The plane of resection, however, passes through the compartment in which the lesion is located (compartments being defined as bone, muscle, parosteal, skin, and neurovascular).
4. Radical resection, which requires removal of the lesion along with the entire involved compartment. Thus, for example, a wide resection of a tumor of the distal tibia could be accomplished either by en bloc removal of the tumor and several centimeters of normal bone and soft tissue surrounding it or by below-knee amputation. A radical resection requires disarticulation at the knee or above-knee amputation.

The term *limb salvage* has also been used. A limb salvage can be performed using any of the treatment options. Limb salvage thus does not refer to a classification of resection, but refers to surgery that leaves a functional limb. To plan for limb salvage surgery, the surgeon must know the proximal, distal, and transverse extent of osseous and soft-tissue abnormality. The neurovascular bundle's proximity to the lesion must be assessed. Joint involvement is an important part of the assessment. Epiphyseal involvement should be evaluated (an elegant limb salvage procedure in a young child may not be worthwhile if the epiphyseal plate must be sacrificed and the limb cannot grow appropriately). Because a limb salvage should be attempted only if a functional result is likely, it is clear that the radiologist and quality of the CT or MRI play an important role in this decision making.

STAGING OF MUSCULOSKELETAL LESIONS

The surgical staging system for musculoskeletal lesions is useful for both prognosis and treatment planning. The system is based on (a) histologic grade of lesion, (b) presence of metastases (determined by bone scan and chest CT), and (c) evaluation of the site of lesion. This last parameter is used to determine whether the lesion is encapsulated, extracapsular but intracompartmental, or extracapsular and extracompartmental (this last category obviously relating to a higher degree of aggressiveness and a more difficult resection). Conscientiously performed MRI or CT is a requirement for adequate evaluation of site and therefore proper staging of a musculoskeletal lesion.

SITE EVALUATION WITH MRI AND CT

In general, MRI is the preferable modality for staging over CT. However, CT does have a few advantages (Fig. 100–7*B*). Although one can identify tumor matrix and see cortical bone abnormalities with MRI, these are seen to much better advantage with CT. Furthermore, a thin cortical rim can be identified with CT when it may not be seen by either plain film or MRI. Therefore, if one specifically wishes to evaluate these aspects of an osseous lesion, CT may be preferable to MRI (Fig. 100–7). If one chooses CT, how reliable is this modality in evaluation of the extent of lesion? Using Hounsfield unit measurements and comparing with the opposite normal bone, one can evaluate the intraosseous extent of lesion in the diaphysis of tubular bones. Intraosseous extent cannot be as accurately evaluated in the metaphysis of the long bones. Similarly, CT may show soft-tissue involvement as well in regions of the body where there are abundant fat planes, especially if intravenous contrast is used (such as in the pelvis). However, other areas of the body such as the lower leg and forearm can be much more difficult localities for evaluation of soft-tissue extent.

MRI has several obvious advantages in the evaluation of the site of the lesion. The intraosseous extent is highly accurately observed, not only in the diaphysis but also in the metaphysis and epiphysis (Figs. 100–7*C* and 100–8*B*). Joint involvement is much more easily assessed owing to the multiplanar imaging capabilities (Fig. 100–8). Soft-tissue involvement is uniformly easily evaluated with MRI, as is neurovascular involvement. Overall, with the multiplanar imaging, site evaluation of musculoskeletal tumors is often more accurate with MRI than with CT; beyond this, the conclusions are almost invariably reached with greater confidence.

With all the imaging planes and sequences available, what are the optimal imaging sequences for MRI of musculoskeletal lesions? Generally, spin-echo or fast spin-echo sequences should be considered standard. According to the site of the lesion, one coronal (or occasionally sagittal) sequence should be obtained, using T_1-weighting if it is an osseous lesion or T_2-weighting if it is a soft-tissue lesion. Following that, axial T_1- and axial T_2-weighted sequences must be obtained to include the entire lesion and reactive tissue. If the entire lesion is not included, the examination is not complete. Generally, the use of gadolinium, fat suppression techniques, or other sequences should not be required except to answer specific questions or concerns.

A radiologist must be aware of two conditions that may result in overestimation of tumor extent in the soft tissues: hematoma and edema. Either of these processes can have signal intensity identical to tumor. They may also, at least initially, present with a mass-like morphology (Fig. 100–9). Thus, exact site and size of tumor may not be accurately assessed by MRI in the presence of edema or hematoma. Although relatively acute hematomas may have characteristic signal, older hematomas are inhomogeneous, with areas of both high and low signal intensity. They may incite large areas of reactive edema, often crossing compartments and appearing extremely aggressive (Fig. 100–10). However, this is usually a moot point because a wide resection of an aggressive lesion requires removal of reactive tissue as well as the tumor.

HISTOLOGIC SPECIFICITY OF MRI

MRI generally does not reliably add information for histologic diagnosis (either by signal intensity, dynamic studies, or spectroscopy). There are a few exceptions to this statement. Soft-tissue lipomas follow the signal intensity of subcutaneous fat in all sequences (Fig. 100–11*A*). Benign fibrous lesions with abundant collagen and hypocellularity tend to have decreased signal intensity on both T_1 and T_2 sequences (Fig. 100–11*B*). Intermuscular hemangiomas tend to be isointense with muscle on T_1, high signal intensity on T_2, but with lacy areas surrounding and interdigitating the lesion that have the intensity of subcutaneous fat (Fig. 100–11*C*). However, it is worth remembering that up to 20 per cent of benign fibrous lesions and hemangiomas may not have these classic features and may be indistinguishable from other tumors.

Not only does MRI generally not help make a histologic diagnosis, but it also does not reliably differentiate benign from malignant lesions. Use of the signal intensity to try to differentiate lesions is unreliable, even when used in conjunction with gadolinium and dynamic scanning, owing to significant overlap between benign and malignant lesions. Morphologic characteristics of the lesion are generally more useful. As a generalization, malignant lesions tend to be large and inhomogeneous, and to appear infiltrative. Benign lesions tend to be smaller and homogeneous, and to appear encapsulated (Fig. 100–12). There are, however, important exceptions for these generalizations. Malignant lesions may acquire a pseudocapsule of reactive tissue that gives a false appearance of containing the tumor both on MRI and at surgery. Synovial sarcoma is notorious for appearing homogeneous and nonaggressive, but other lesions may give this appearance as well (Fig. 100–13*A*). Conversely, many benign lesions are inhomogeneous, locally aggressive, and infiltrative, giving by MRI an extremely aggressive appearance. The most notorious of these are desmoid tumors, hematomas, and infection (Fig. 100–13*B*). Remember that, because MRI does not reliably give histologic diagnosis, does not differentiate reliably between tumor and edema or hematoma, and does not reliably differentiate between benign and malignant lesions, a combination of clinical information, morphology of the lesion, and a healthy dose of suspicion will be useful in evaluating individual cases.

BIOPSY OF THE LESION

Planning the site of either open or percutaneous biopsy is an important role played by the radiologist. MRI is extremely useful in helping to avoid necrotic or reactive areas and find a representative sample site. Some lesions are particularly amenable to percutaneous biopsy. Metastatic lesions or multiple myeloma need only very small sample sizes for diagnosis. Primary malignant osseous or soft-tissue lesions similarly require relatively small cores of tissue, whereas benign osseous lesions often require larger amounts of tissue for diagnosis than are obtained in needle biopsy specimens. Percutaneous biopsy of cartilage lesions should be avoided because sampling error is especially notorious in these lesions. The pathologists generally require an entire lesion before they will commit themselves to grading a cartilage lesion or even determining whether it is malignant.

The site of biopsy is crucial. The surgeons should be consulted as to preference for biopsy approach because the needle tract must be removed as part of the resection of an aggressive lesion. Biopsy must be carefully planned to avoid crossing more than one compartment and to avoid violating neurovascular compartments. The importance of careful planning for open or percutaneous biopsies is illustrated by a study conducted by the Musculoskeletal Tumor Society (see Enneking, Skeletal Radiology 13:183–194). At 16 in-

Text continued on page 1513

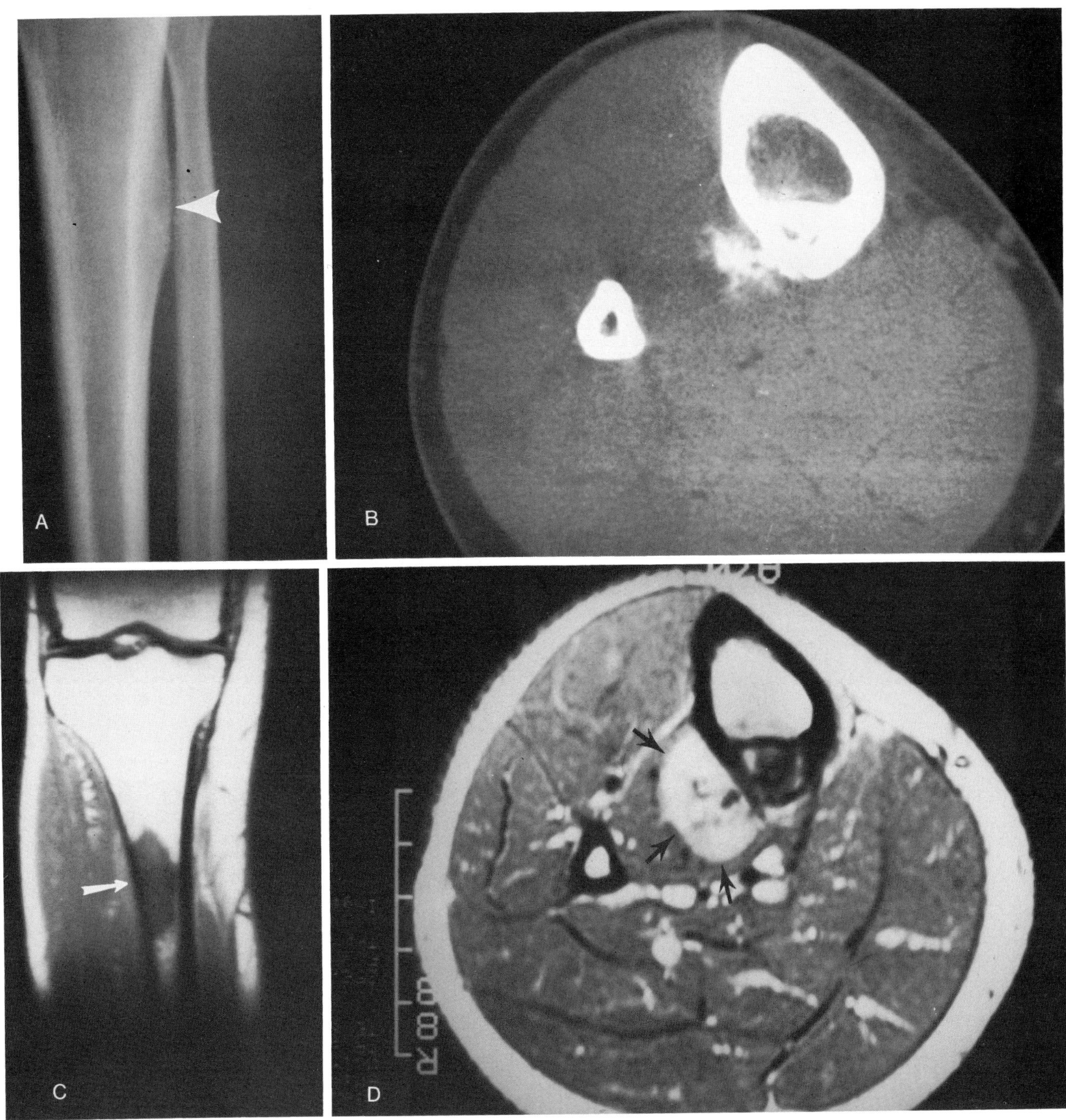

Figure 100–7. Relative advantages of cross-sectional imaging modalities. *A* demonstrates a lesion causing expansion of the posterior cortex of the proximal tibial diaphysis *(arrow head)*. No further feature was discernible by plain film; therefore, computed tomography (CT) was performed. CT *(B)* demonstrates not only the expanded posterior tibial cortex, but also tumor bone formation within the posterior compartment, as well as increased density in the medullary space of the tibia. These features make the diagnosis of parosteal osteosarcoma, but the extent of the lesion is not determined by CT. Magnetic resonance imaging (MRI), however, demonstrates nicely the intraosseous extent on the T_1 sequence *(C)*. The low signal intensity demonstrates marrow replacement *(white arrow)* while the high signal intensity shows the soft-tissue extent *(black arrows)* on the axial T_2 sequence *(D)*. In the final analysis, this patient was an excellent candidate for limb salvage surgery. (*A* to *D* reprinted with permission from the ACR Learning File, Musculoskeletal Videodisc, Case 115.)

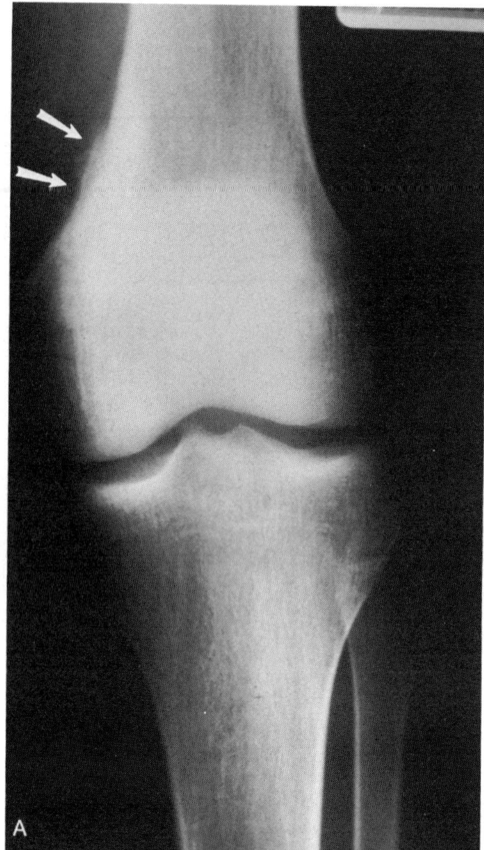

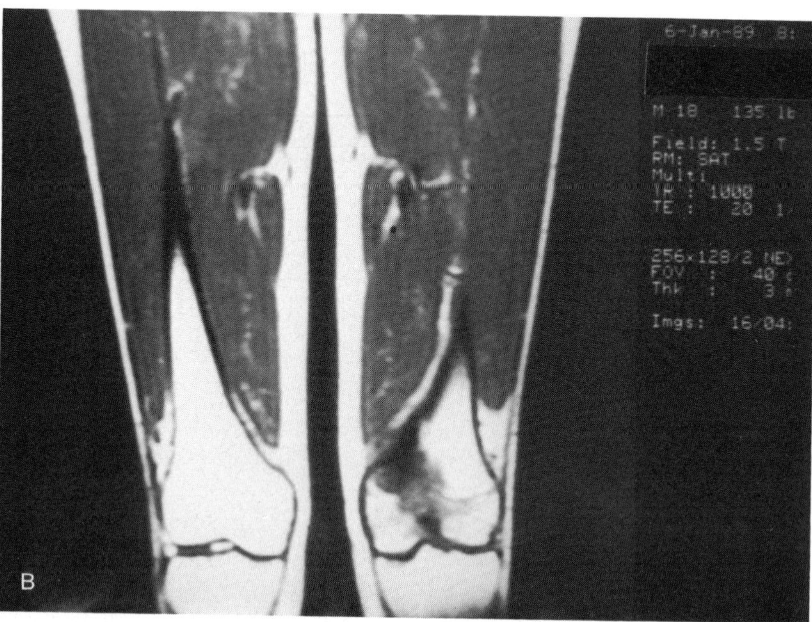

Figure 100–8. *A* demonstrates an early osteosarcoma in this teenaged patient, with tumor bone formation in both the medial metaphysis of the distal femur and the adjacent soft tissues *(arrows)*. Since this was an early lesion, limb salvage surgery was anticipated. It would be vastly preferable to resect the lesion leaving the epiphysis intact so that a cadaver graft could be placed in the defect with the patient retaining his own articular surface. The alternative, if the epiphysis shows tumor involvement, is resection of the distal femur with placement of a custom prosthesis for the knee. *B,* MRI demonstrates very nicely that in fact not only the metaphysis but also the epiphysis is involved with tumor. Therefore, the custom prosthesis was planned for and placed. (*A* and *B* reprinted with permission from the ACR Learning File, Musculoskeletal Videodisc, Case 112.)

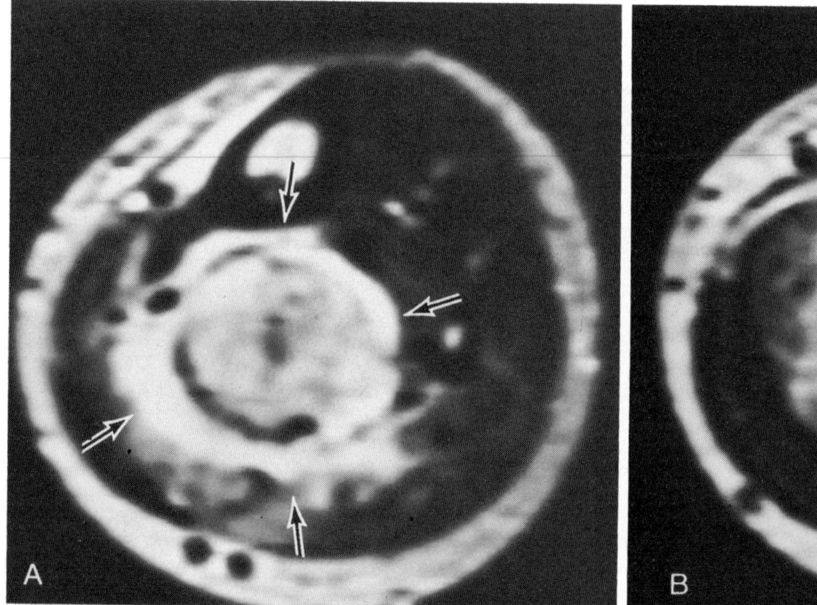

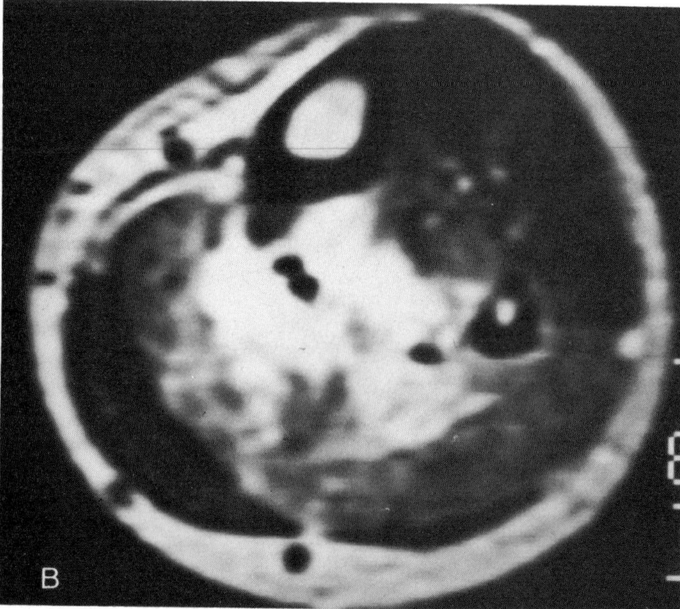

Figure 100–9. MRI does not reliably differentiate tumor from edema. *A,* A T_2 image of a sarcoma of neural origin. The high signal mass *(arrows)* in the posterior compartment is heterogeneous. There is no delineation between apparent tumor and soft-tissue reaction. *B,* More proximally in the leg, there seems to be a "veiling" or less strong signal intensity surrounding a more central high signal intensity. This is a more typical appearance of edema surrounding tumor. However, analysis of the specimen at both of these regions shows the entire area of abnormality in *B* to be reactive edema, and all but a 1-cm diameter central tumor mass in *A* was edema.

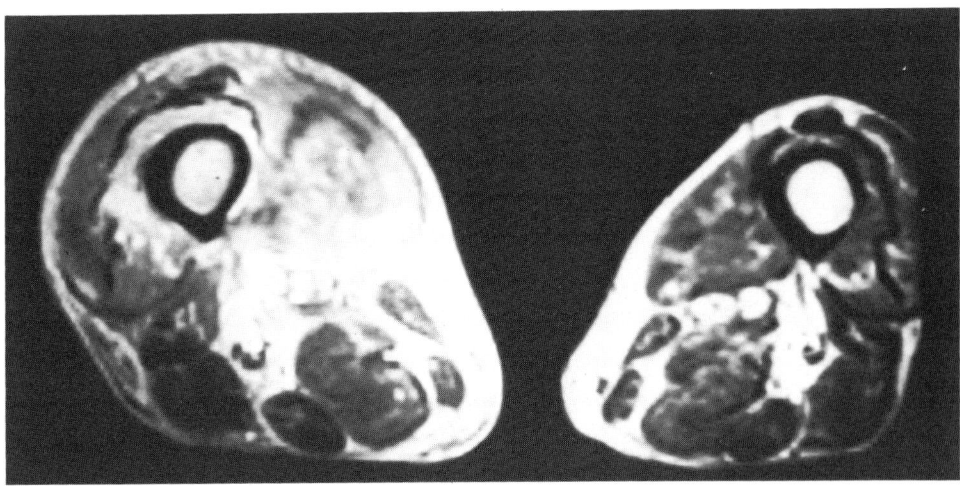

Figure 100–10. This patient has a very large, extremely heterogeneous high signal mass involving all of the vastus muscles of the right thigh. This appears to be an extremely aggressive and invasive lesion. Biopsy specimen demonstrates only hematoma and muscle necrosis in this patient, who did have a history of trauma. Old hematoma thus can quite strongly resemble tumor.

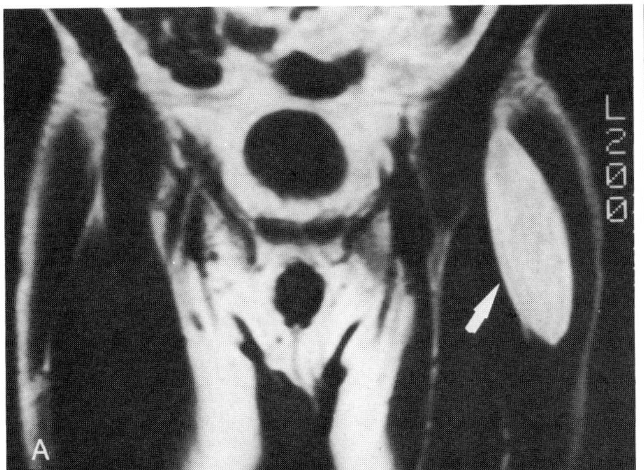

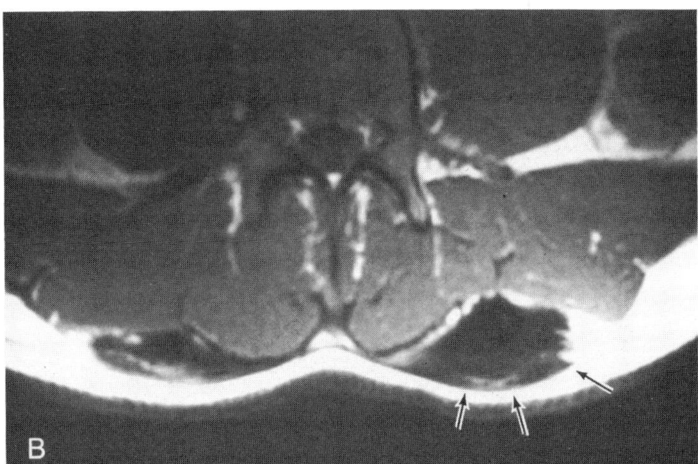

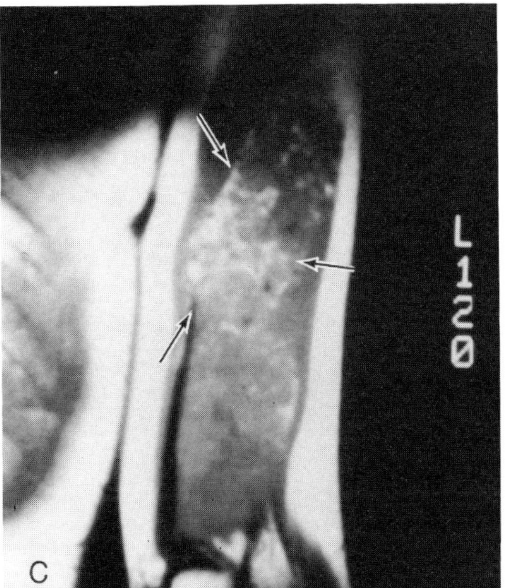

Figure 100–11. MRI characteristics can suggest histology in a very limited number of lesions. Among them are lipoma *(A),* in which the signal of the mass *(arrow)* follows the signal of subcutaneous fat in all sequences. *B* demonstrates a subcutaneous fibromatosis *(arrows),* which was of low signal intensity in all sequences. *C* demonstrates a hemangioma of the arm, in a T_1 coronal sequence, showing the slightly higher than muscle signal intensity mass with interdigitating fat signal *(arrows).* (*A* reprinted with permission from the ACR Learning File, Musculoskeletal Videodisc, Case 147.)

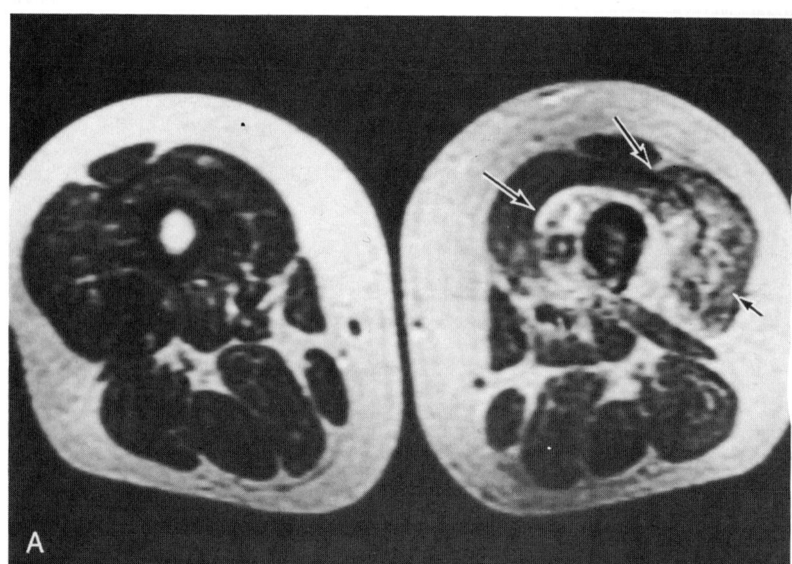

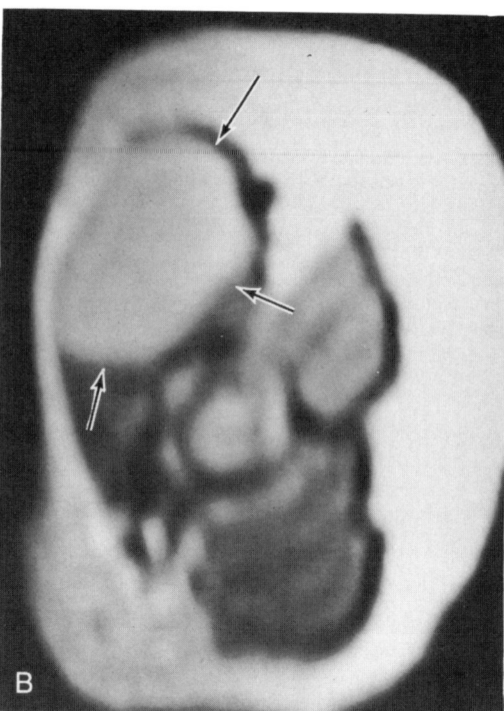

Figure 100–12. *A* demonstrates a typical appearance of a highly aggressive and malignant lesion. There are marrow replacement and cortical destruction in the femur. The soft-tissue mass *(arrows)* is large, inhomogeneous, and infiltrative. This is an osteosarcoma, displaying the typical appearance of an malignant aggressive lesion. For interest, however, you might compare the appearance of this soft-tissue mass with Figure 100–10, which shows a similarly appearing aggressive soft-tissue mass that simply represented hematoma. *B* demonstrates an axial T_2 image of the arm of a child in which the soft-tissue mass *(arrows)* is completely homogeneous and appears encapsulated. This happens to be a rare lesion, a soft-tissue eosinophilic granuloma, which follows the "rules" of appearance for a benign soft-tissue lesion.

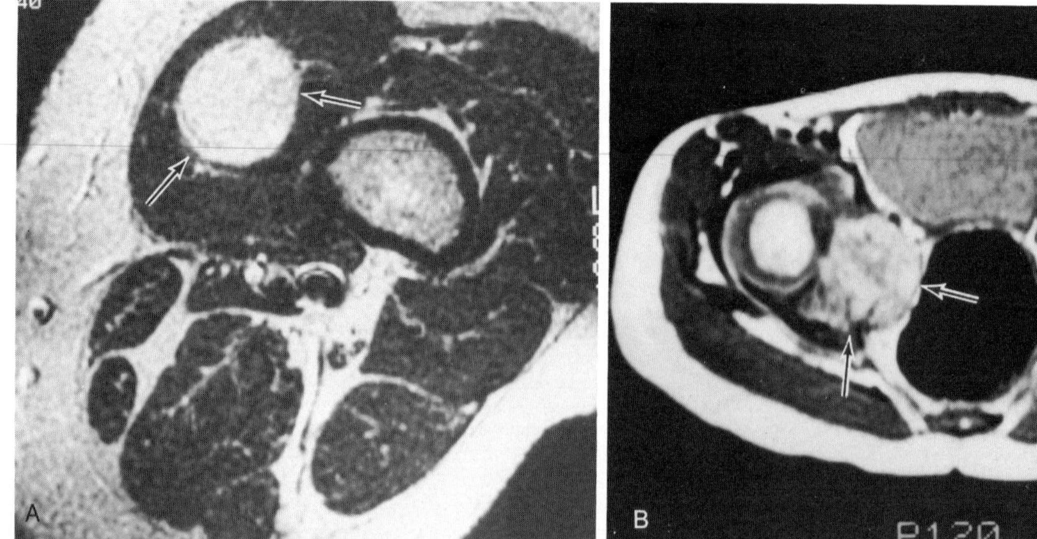

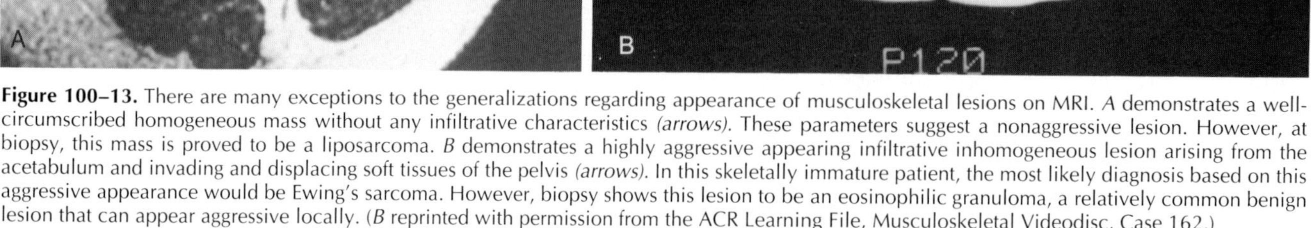

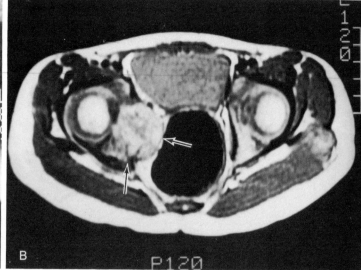

Figure 100–13. There are many exceptions to the generalizations regarding appearance of musculoskeletal lesions on MRI. *A* demonstrates a well-circumscribed homogeneous mass without any infiltrative characteristics *(arrows)*. These parameters suggest a nonaggressive lesion. However, at biopsy, this mass is proved to be a liposarcoma. *B* demonstrates a highly aggressive appearing infiltrative inhomogeneous lesion arising from the acetabulum and invading and displacing soft tissues of the pelvis *(arrows)*. In this skeletally immature patient, the most likely diagnosis based on this aggressive appearance would be Ewing's sarcoma. However, biopsy shows this lesion to be an eosinophilic granuloma, a relatively common benign lesion that can appear aggressive locally. (*B* reprinted with permission from the ACR Learning File, Musculoskeletal Videodisc, Case 162.)

stitutions, 329 consecutive tumors were evaluated. Fifteen per cent of cases had major diagnostic errors related to the biopsy. Ten per cent of the biopsies were either not representative or technically poor. Seventeen per cent had complications resulting from the biopsy, and 18 per cent required alteration of the optimum therapy plan because of the biopsy site (with 4.5 per cent having a limb salvage converted to an amputation). The study also noted that biopsy-related problems occurred three to five times more frequently when the biopsies were performed at a referring institution rather than at the major definitive tumor treatment center. These findings confirm the importance of careful biopsy planning, and strongly suggest that biopsy should be performed only at the treatment center, and planned in conjunction with the treating surgeon.

FOLLOW-UP IMAGING FOR MUSCULOSKELETAL LESIONS

Post-treatment follow-up of musculoskeletal lesions is the least-defined aspect of the radiologist's role in musculoskeletal tumor imaging. Patients with a large amount of orthopedic hardware are generally monitored for local recurrence by plain film because the hardware results in significant CT and MRI artifact. As more titanium hardware is made available, this may allow accurate MRI and follow-up of the primary lesion. Plain film and CT are used for evaluation for lung metastases. MRI is generally used for post-therapeutic evaluation of soft-tissue lesions. MRI does provide a reasonable evaluation of tumor volume, but does not provide accurate evaluation of tumor necrosis at this time. Generally, with a favorable response to therapy, soft-tissue T_2 signal intensity decreases. The time required for this decrease in signal intensity, however, is highly variable, and there is overlap in signal intensity of recurrent/residual tumor and benign post-therapeutic change (Fig. 100–14). Thus, morphology again is a more important determinant than signal intensity. Serial MRI scanning can be useful, however, and baseline follow-up MRI is recommended three months after therapy. Subsequent scanning should be dictated by the nature of the lesion and its hazard rate for developing recurrent or metastatic disease.

BONE-FORMING TUMORS

B. J. Manaster

Benign Bone-Forming Tumors

OSTEOMA AND ENOSTOSIS

The least worrisome benign bone-forming tumors are osteomas and enostoses (bone islands). Both of these represent hamartomatous processes, with histologically normal dense bone formation and no host reaction. Osteomas occur predominantly in membranous bone, being seen most commonly in the outer table of the calvarium or the paranasal sinuses. The osteoma usually has a typical appearance (Fig. 100–15) and should be easily differentiated from an osteoblastic metastasis or a meningioma, which arises on the inner table of the skull.

Enostoses or bone islands may be found in the medullary space of any bone. The entire lesion is homogeneously sclerotic. Although at first glance it appears to be geographic in nature, it actually blends into the surrounding normal bone, and a careful look may reveal several small spiculations extending into the surrounding normal bone. This common lesion may be polyostotic and is never symptomatic. Because it may show additional uptake by bone scan, it at times may need to be differentiated from an osteoblastic metastasis. A solitary bone island may need to be distinguished from a very dense osteoid osteoma (see next section). If the lesion is typical radiographically (Fig. 100–16) and asymptomatic, it should be considered a "leave me alone" lesion.

OSTEOID OSTEOMA

An osteoid osteoma is a painful, small (less than 2 cm) lytic lesion. This lytic nidus may or may not contain calcification. The nidus is surrounded by dense reactive bone in nearly all cases. The nidus has a highly vascular stroma, and therefore shows intense uptake on bone scan.

This lesion is seen most commonly in the second and third decades and in many cases presents with clinical features of aching pain that is worse at night, relieved with aspirin, and dramatically relieved by excision. The lesion can have three fairly distinct appearances depending on its location. One of the common locations is within the cortex in tubular bones. This lesion may be surrounded by such dense reactive sclerosis that the lucent nidus may actually be masked (Fig. 100–17*A*). In this case the differential diagnosis would include Brodie's abscess, and a subacute stress fracture with healing reaction. Osteoid osteomas can also be located at an intracapsular site. The most common example of this location is in the medial femoral neck. Interestingly, these lesions may elicit a sclerotic host reaction that is located at a considerable distance from the nidus. Prominent calcar buttressing may occur as a host reaction as well. Additionally, the patient may develop a sympathetic hip effusion, resulting in significant growth deformities (overgrowth and valgus angulation of the femoral neck, and widened tear drop [Fig. 100–17*D*]). This appearance can certainly mask the underlying small lesion, leading to a misdiagnosis of an arthritic process or dysplasia.

A third common location for osteoid osteoma is the posterior elements of the spine (Fig. 100–18). This lesion typically causes a painful scoliosis that is concave on the side of the lesion. The underlying lesion can be difficult to find, and the reactive density may be misdiagnosed as metastatic disease or bony reaction to another process such as spondylolysis. A fourth location of osteoid osteoma, subperiosteal, is sufficiently rare and difficult to diagnose that it will not be discussed further in this chapter.

Treatment of osteoid osteoma requires resection of the entire lytic nidus. However, none of the reactive bone need be resected. Ideally, this should lead to a very small resection that does not compromise the mechanical integrity of the bone. However, it can be quite difficult for the surgeon to locate the nidus with all of the heaped-up reactive bone around it. Therefore, CT imaging has been found to be extremely useful, giving a precise location of the small nidus (see Fig. 100–17*C*). Methylene blue dye can be used to mark the site of the nidus, or a detachable wire can be placed at the site for even more precise localization. Some investigators are now attempting percutaneous removal of the nidus under CT guidance.

OSTEOBLASTOMA

This rare lesion is histologically similar to osteoid osteoma but radiographically quite distinct. It is geographic, expansile, and usually nonaggressive in appearance. Interestingly, although it is a bone-forming tumor, it may present as a blastic, lytic, or mixed-density lesion. Location can be quite helpful in the diagnosis; 42 per cent of osteoblastomas occur in the posterior elements of the spine (Fig. 100–19). The remainder arise in the long bones. If the lesion appears somewhat aggressive, the differential diagnosis would include a malignant bone-forming tumor, osteosarcoma. If the lesion is lytic, a spinal location may suggest a differential diagnosis of aneurysmal bone cyst or giant cell tumor. Treatment is usually curettage with bone grafting, and the prognosis is excellent.

Text continued on page 1518

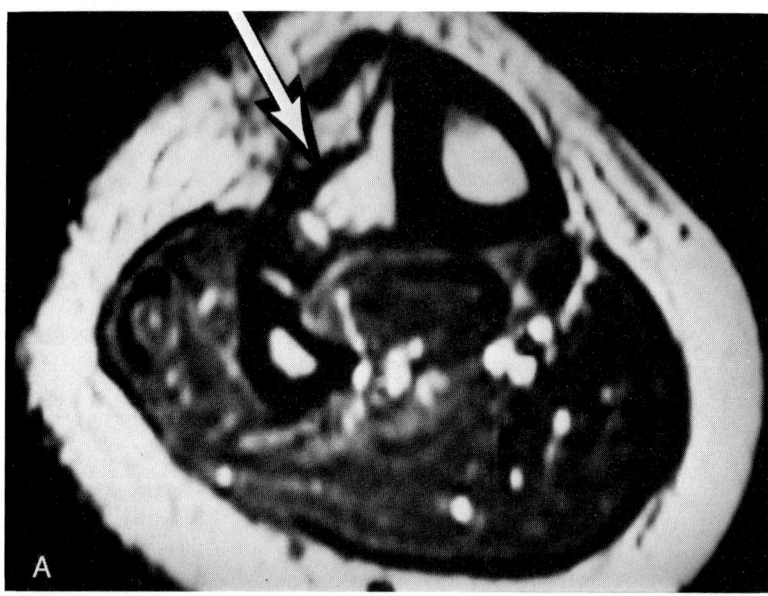

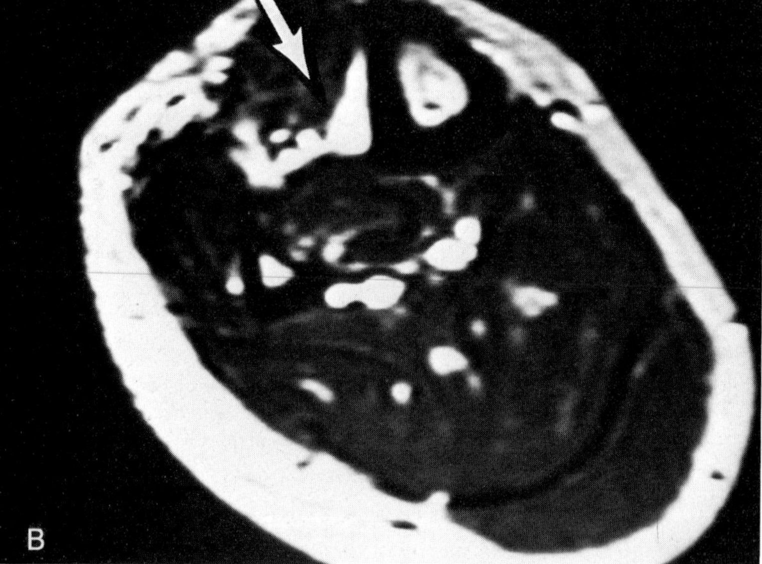

Figure 100–14. Post-therapeutic MRI can be difficult to evaluate. *A* demonstrates a T_2 axial image of the leg in a patient six months after surgery and radiation therapy of a malignant hemangiopericytoma. There is a residual high-signal lesion *(arrow)* that has a convex border, suggesting a mass-like morphology. At biopsy, this represented only fibrotic material. Six months later *(B),* the region still shows high signal intensity *(arrow).* However, the mass-like character is resolving and one can feel more comfortable with a presumption of resolving post-therapeutic fibrosis. (*A* and *B* reprinted with permission from the ACR Learning File, Musculoskeletal Videodisc, Case 106.)

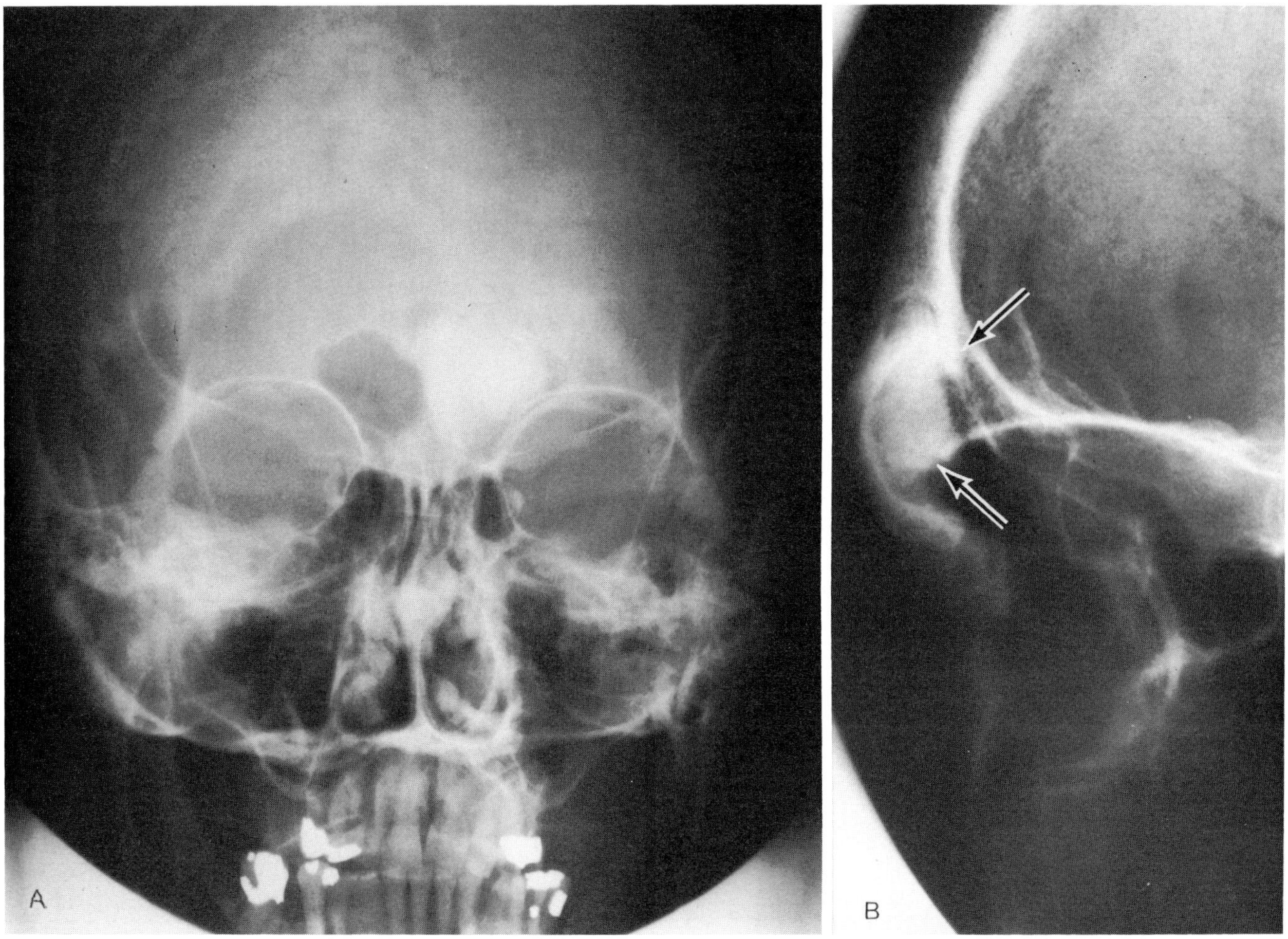

Figure 100–15. *A* and *B,* Round, dense, homogeneous lesion *(arrows in B)* is seen to be located in the frontal sinus on this AP and lateral film. The appearance and location are classic for osteoma.

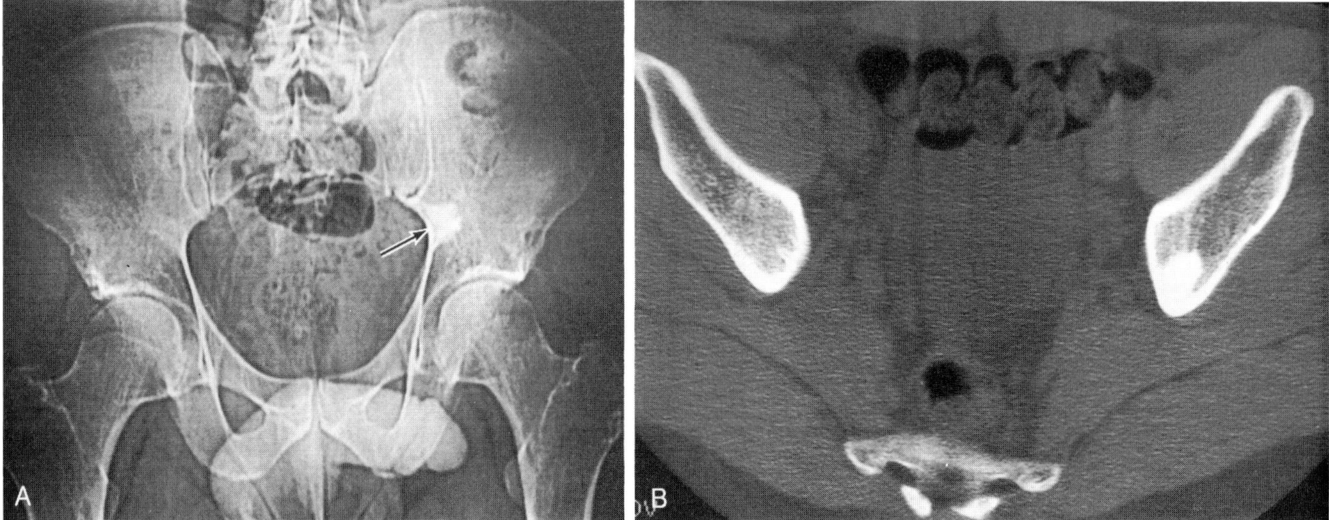

Figure 100–16. The scanogram *(A)* and axial CT scan *(B)* demonstrate the typical features of a bone island or enostosis. This dense hamartomatous bone production occupies medullary space without eliciting host reaction. It blends into the surrounding normal bone with very small spicules.

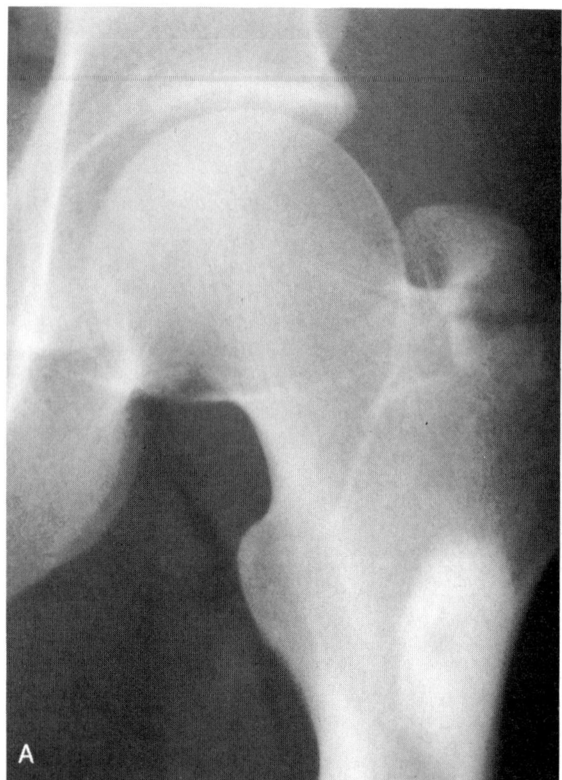

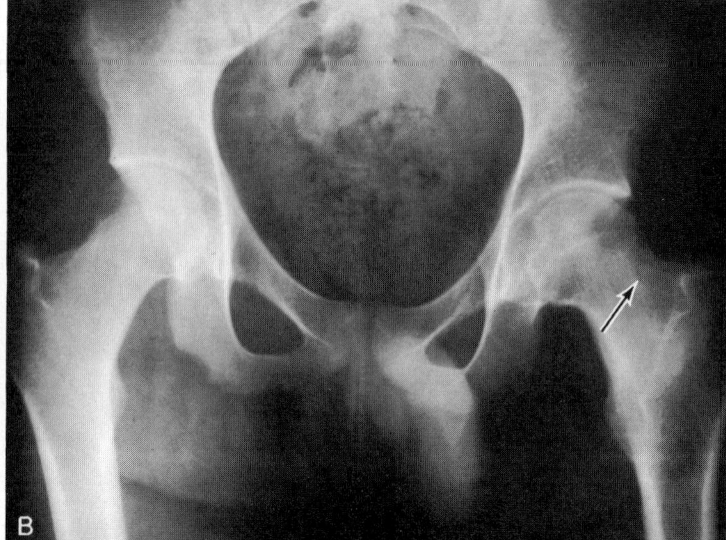

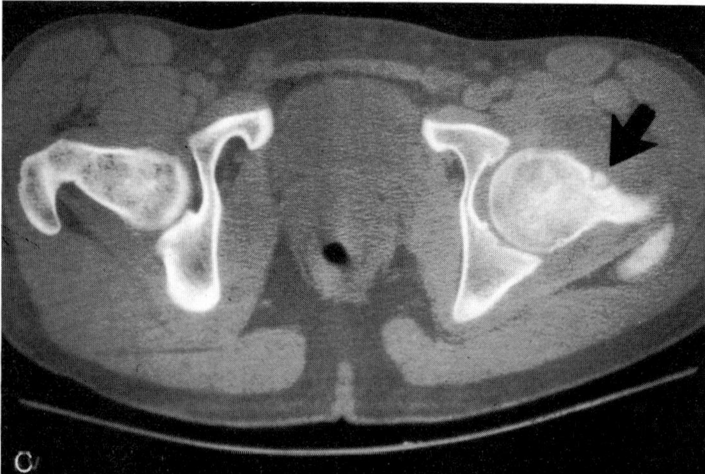

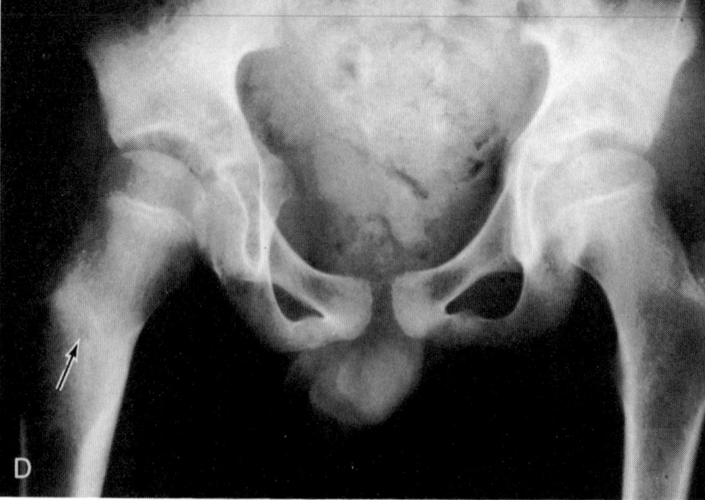

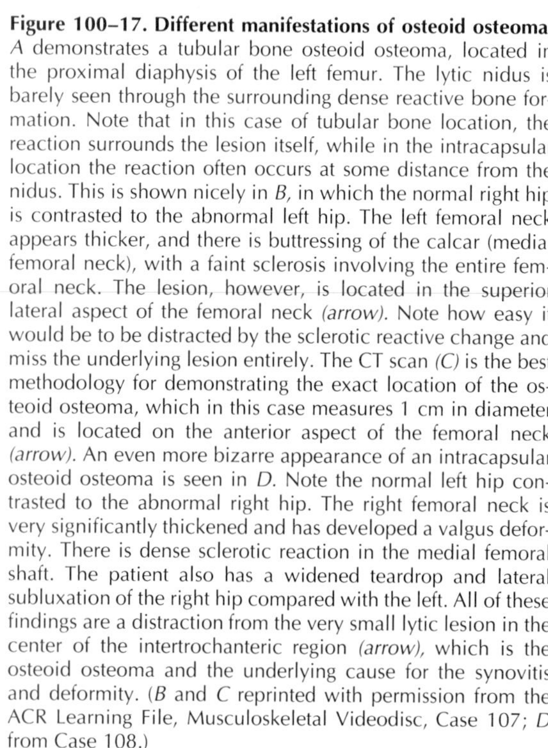

Figure 100–17. Different manifestations of osteoid osteoma. *A* demonstrates a tubular bone osteoid osteoma, located in the proximal diaphysis of the left femur. The lytic nidus is barely seen through the surrounding dense reactive bone formation. Note that in this case of tubular bone location, the reaction surrounds the lesion itself, while in the intracapsular location the reaction often occurs at some distance from the nidus. This is shown nicely in *B,* in which the normal right hip is contrasted to the abnormal left hip. The left femoral neck appears thicker, and there is buttressing of the calcar (medial femoral neck), with a faint sclerosis involving the entire femoral neck. The lesion, however, is located in the superior lateral aspect of the femoral neck *(arrow).* Note how easy it would be to be distracted by the sclerotic reactive change and miss the underlying lesion entirely. The CT scan *(C)* is the best methodology for demonstrating the exact location of the osteoid osteoma, which in this case measures 1 cm in diameter and is located on the anterior aspect of the femoral neck *(arrow).* An even more bizarre appearance of an intracapsular osteoid osteoma is seen in *D.* Note the normal left hip contrasted to the abnormal right hip. The right femoral neck is very significantly thickened and has developed a valgus deformity. There is dense sclerotic reaction in the medial femoral shaft. The patient also has a widened teardrop and lateral subluxation of the right hip compared with the left. All of these findings are a distraction from the very small lytic lesion in the center of the intertrochanteric region *(arrow),* which is the osteoid osteoma and the underlying cause for the synovitis and deformity. (*B* and *C* reprinted with permission from the ACR Learning File, Musculoskeletal Videodisc, Case 107; *D* from Case 108.)

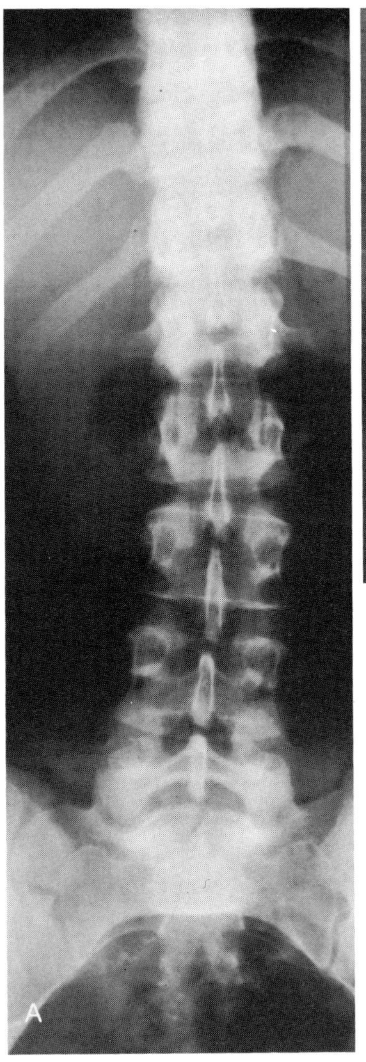

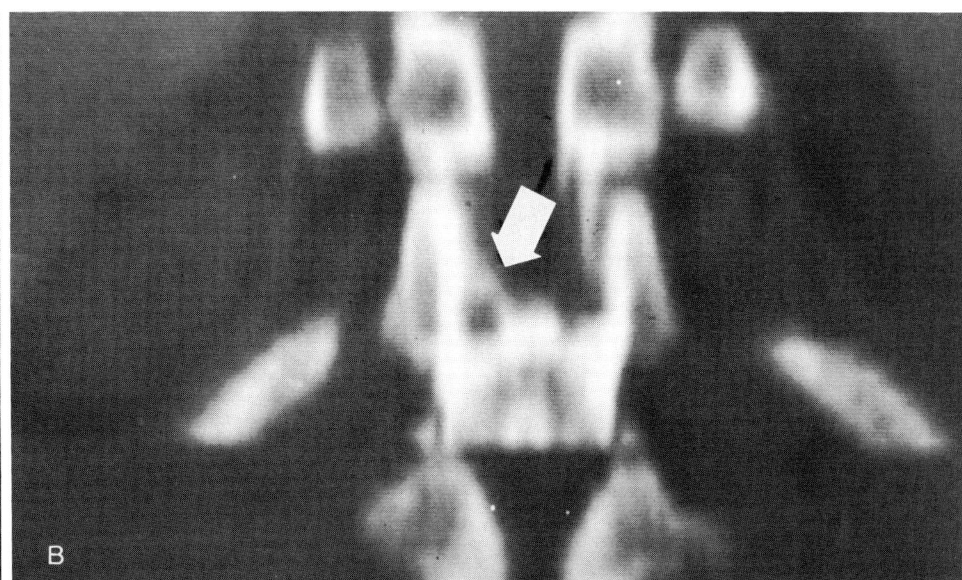

Figure 100–18. Osteoid osteoma of the spine. This is a classic case of spinal location of an osteoid osteoma. The plain film demonstrates a long scoliosis without a rotatory component. An osteoid osteoma is usually located in the apex in the curve of the concave side. No definite diagnosis can be made on the basis of the plain film *(A)*, but bone scan (not shown) demonstrated increased uptake in the posterior elements of T12. CT with reconstruction *(B)* demonstrates very nicely that there is a lytic lesion involving the laminae of T12 *(arrow)*. Resection of this lytic nidus left the patient pain-free. (*A* and *B* reprinted with permission from the ACR Learning File, Musculoskeletal Videodisc, Case 109.)

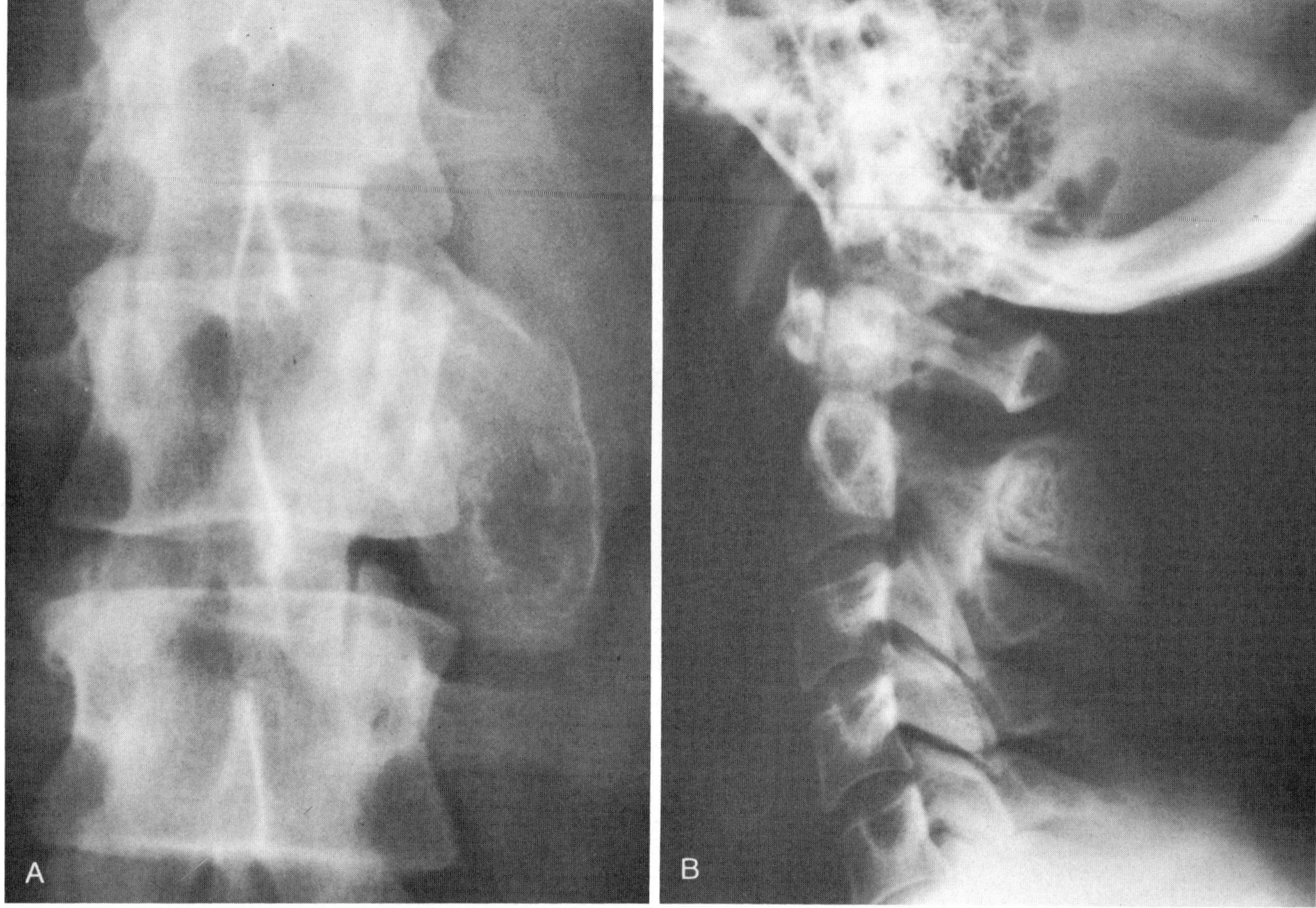

Figure 100–19. Osteoblastoma. *A* demonstrates a prominent expansion of the left posterior elements of L2. The pedicle as well as the transverse process is involved, but there is no other destructive process. The matrix is not prominent but might be described as mixed density. *B* demonstrates a lateral film with a very sclerotic lesion and an expanded spinous process at C2 in a different patient. Both of these findings are typical of osteoblastoma. (*A* reprinted with permission from the ACR Learning File, Musculoskeletal Videodisc, Case 110.)

Malignant Bone-Forming Tumors: Osteosarcoma

CONVENTIONAL OSTEOSARCOMA

Osteosarcoma is one of the more common bone tumors, comprising 20 per cent of all primary bone tumors that are biopsied. It most commonly occurs in the 10- to 25-year age range, with a second peak in the elderly population. Unless specified otherwise, this discussion will be confined to the more common younger age group.

Osteosarcomas are highly aggressive and elicit a host reaction. They most commonly are found in the metaphyses (90 per cent) but can extend to the metadiaphyseal region. Osteosarcomas usually arise in an eccentric location, but with increasing size can appear to be central. There is almost invariably cortical breakthrough and soft-tissue mass.

These lesions all produce tumor osteoid, and bone tumor matrix will be radiographically visible in approximately 90 per cent of cases, but it varies significantly in density. Thus, the tumor matrix can be intensely sclerotic (Fig. 100–20*A*), moderately sclerotic (see Fig. 100–8*A*), have a very mild amorphous density (see Fig. 100–3*A*, seen both in the bone and soft tissues), or be permeative without discernible matrix (see Figs. 100–1*B* and 100–20*B*). This variability in radiographic tumor matrix density is somewhat mirrored by the histology of the lesions. Although all osteosarcomas produce tumor osteoid, 50 per cent produce predominantly osteoid. These are the osteoblastic lesions. Twenty-five per cent of osteosarcomas produce more chondroid matrix than osteoid and may be variably dense, whereas the last 25 per cent of osteosarcomas produce predominantly spindle cells and tend to be the less dense variety.

The prognosis for conventional osteosarcoma is relatively poor, with common hematogenous spread to lung and other bones as well as local lymphatic spread. The primary bone itself may contain intramedullary "skip" lesions. The radiologic work-up is therefore crucial, including bone scan to evaluate for bone metastases, lung CT to evaluate for pulmonary metastases, and MRI to evaluate for intramedullary skip lesions and local involvement at the primary site. MRI shows no features specific for this lesion (see Fig. 100–12*A*); the diagnosis is usually made by plain film. Overall five-year survival is 60 to 70 per cent. If the patient presents with lung metastases, there is a 10 to 20 per cent five-year survival. Resection of limited lung metastases is often attempted. The patients are treated with preoperative induction chemotherapy, which serves to control micrometastases and often produces a shrinkage of the mass, making resection easier. This also helps to assess efficacy of the chemotherapeutic regimen at the time of surgery. Surgical therapy requires a wide resection, and the patient receives adjuvant chemotherapy post-surgically.

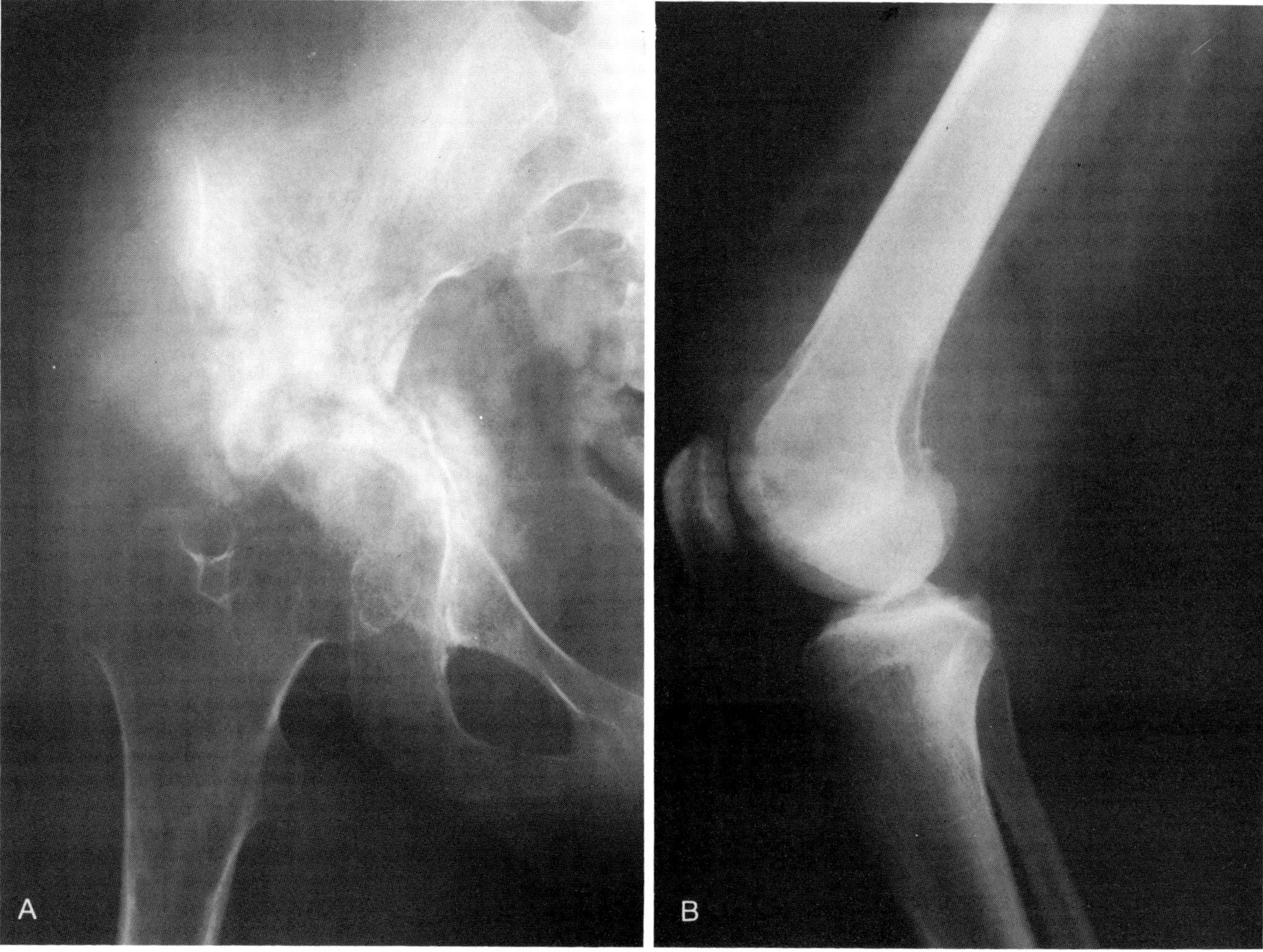

Figure 100–20. Spectrum of matrix density in conventional osteosarcoma. *A* demonstrates the densely sclerotic osteoid formation that can be seen in a classic osteosarcoma. Note that this dense matrix is seen not only within the osseous structures but also within the soft-tissue mass. You might also note that the osteoid is not as well-organized as in parosteal osteosarcoma (see Fig. 100–22). *B* demonstrates an entirely lytic osteosarcoma. The distal femoral metaphysis shows a permeative pattern but no matrix. There is a very large soft-tissue mass both anterior and posterior to the distal femoral metaphysis. No matrix is seen within this soft-tissue mass either. (The AP film of this patient is seen in Fig. 100–1*B*.) In conventional osteosarcomas, the amount of mineralization of the matrix has no prognostic significance. (*B* reprinted with permission from the ACR Learning File, Musculoskeletal Videodisc, Case 113.)

TELANGIECTATIC OSTEOSARCOMA

This is a rare variant of osteosarcoma in which the diagnosis can be extremely difficult. Telangiectatic osteosarcomas arise in the same age range as conventional osteosarcoma and unfortunately have the same dismal prognosis. They present radiographically as a large, round, lytic lesion. The lesion is usually rather geographic in nature, with a fairly narrow zone of transition. This appearance, unfortunately, is one of a less aggressive tumor (Fig. 100–21), and the lesion is often radiographically misdiagnosed as an aneurysmal bone cyst, giant cell tumor, or nonossifying fibroma. At surgery, the lesion predominantly consists of large pools of blood. Tumor is often found only at the periphery. Thus, the surgeon and pathologist can be misled as well. The radiologist therefore needs to be aware of the existence of this lesion and should suggest the diagnosis if an otherwise nonaggressive metaphyseal lesion has some features suggesting an underlying aggressive lesion.

PAROSTEAL OSTEOSARCOMA

This is the second most common variant of osteosarcoma. It is differentiated from conventional osteosarcoma by several features, including patient age, radiographic appearance of the lesion, and prognosis. Parosteal sarcoma is a well-differentiated osteosarcoma. It is located in a metaphyseal site, but rather than being eccentric within the bone, has its epicenter near the periosteum. Thus, dense well-organized bone appears to "wrap around" the underlying bone (Fig. 100–22; see Fig. 100–3*B*). With the newer imaging modalities, we now recognize that there usually is some involvement of the underlying bone (see Fig. 100–7) and this lesion must be evaluated by MRI or CT in addition to plain film. The radiographic appearance is quite typical, varying only with the size of the lesion as shown in the previous examples. The location is typical as well, with 60 per cent of parosteal osteosarcomas arising in the distal femur and most of the remainder arising in the proximal tibia, proximal humerus, and proximal femur.

A relatively early parosteal osteosarcoma might be confused with myositis ossificans (see Chapter 101). However, a zoning pattern distinguishes parosteal osteosarcoma from myositis; parosteal osteosarcoma demonstrates a dense central mass, with less mature bone located peripherally, whereas the opposite zoning occurs in myositis. CT can be useful in further defining this zoning phenomenon in an individual case.

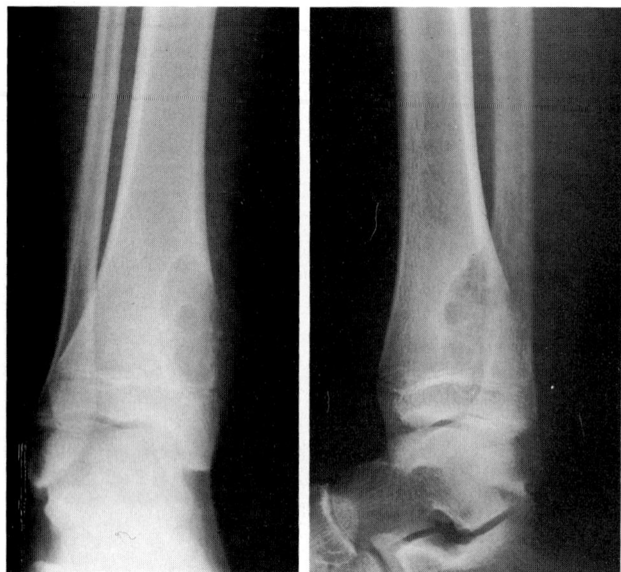

Figure 100–21. Telangiectatic osteosarcoma. This case represents a diagnostic dilemma. The patient has a lytic lesion eccentrically located in the metaphysis of the distal tibia. The lesion has a narrow zone of transition and is rather well-marginated. These features are suggestive of giant cell tumor or chondromyxoid fibroma. However, note that there is medial cortical breakthrough with a small soft-tissue mass. This should raise the possibility of a more aggressive lesion, such as telangiectatic osteosarcoma. (Reprinted with permission from the ACR Learning File, Musculoskeletal Videodisc, Case 114.)

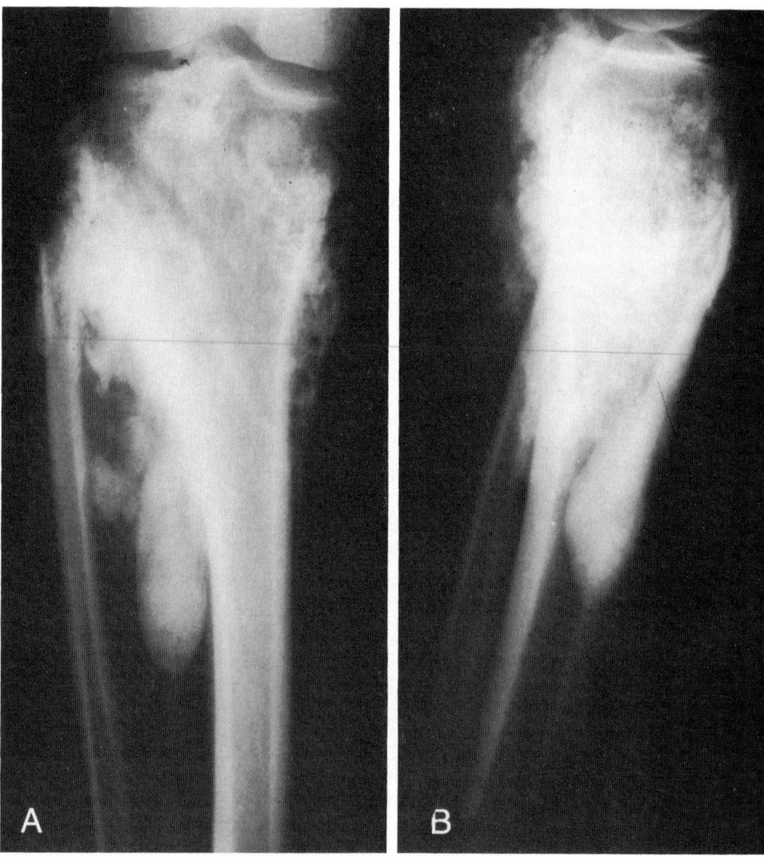

Figure 100–22. Parosteal osteosarcoma. The AP *(A)* and lateral *(B)* films demonstrate a well-differentiated dense matrix in this tumor bone, which is "wrapping around" the proximal tibia. The underlying bone, to the extent that it can be seen, appears normal. This is a typical appearance for parosteal osteosarcoma. It is interesting that five years earlier, this lesion was biopsied and said to be benign and it has been growing slowly ever since. Sampling error can be significant, especially in slow-growing lesions such as this one. (*A* and *B* reprinted with permission from the ACR Learning File, Musculoskeletal Videodisc, Case 115.)

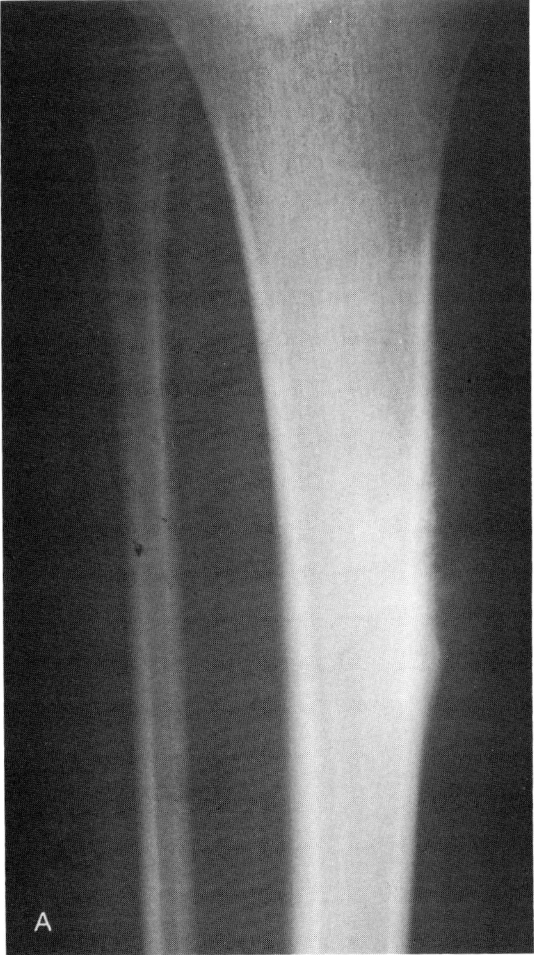

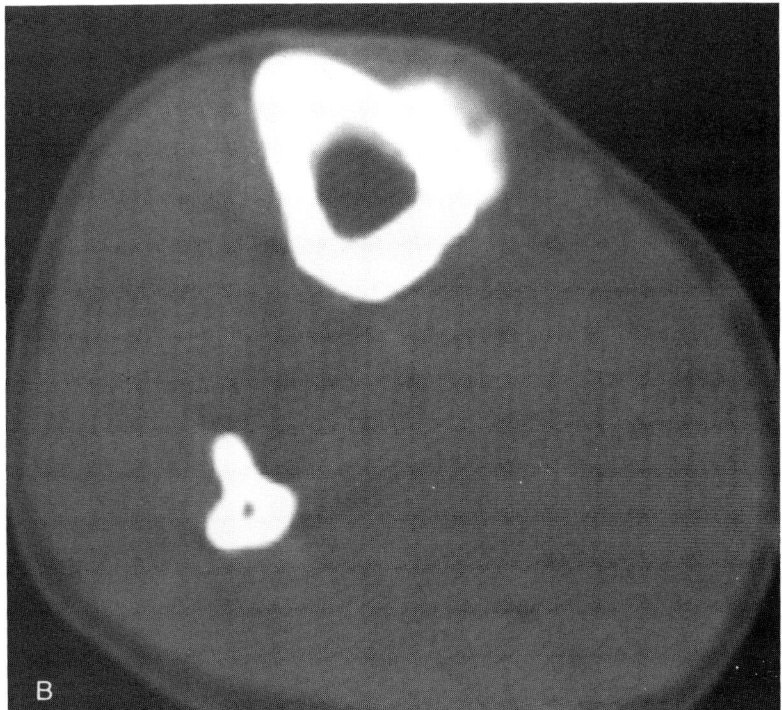

Figure 100–23. Periosteal osteosarcoma. This is a surface lesion in the diaphyseal region of the proximal tibia. There is obvious osteoid matrix in the soft tissue causing slight scalloping of the underlying bone *(A)*. No host reaction is seen. This appearance is typical for but not pathognomonic of periosteal osteosarcoma. CT scan *(B)* confirms the surface location of the tumor bone, and the normal underlying marrow.

Eighty per cent of parosteal osteosarcomas fall in the 20- to 50-year age range, considerably older than the conventional osteosarcomas. The prognosis is significantly better than that of conventional osteosarcoma, with approximately 90 per cent five-year survival. Metastases to the lungs can occur infrequently, but these are generally late. Treatment of parosteal osteosarcoma is wide resection. These patients are often ideal candidates for limb salvage procedures. Radiation and chemotherapy are not a part of the routine treatment of this lesion.

PERIOSTEAL OSTEOSARCOMA

This extremely rare variety of osteosarcoma is usually included in textbooks, although the nonsubspecialized radiologist should not expect to see it in a clinical practice. This is a "surface" osteosarcoma that has no intermedullary involvement. The underlying cortex may be either thickened or saucerized. The lesion presents as a soft-tissue mass that may have either bone spicules within it or an amorphous calcific density (Fig. 100–23). These lesions are of interest because their differential diagnosis includes aggressive malignant lesions (high-grade surface osteosarcoma) and benign lesions (juxtacortical chondroma). They are also of interest because they arise in a slightly older age range of patients than conventional osteosarcomas (second through fourth decade) and have an excellent prognosis (80 per cent five-year survival).

INTRAOSSEOUS LOW-GRADE OSTEOSARCOMA

This extremely rare lesion is entirely intraosseous, without cortical breakthrough or host reaction. It may appear variably aggressive, and the differential diagnosis depends on the degree of permeative change (ranging from fibrous dysplasia or infection to Ewing's sarcoma or fibrosarcoma). This arises in the same age population as conventional osteosarcoma. If the lesion is recognized early and a wide resection achieved, the prognosis is excellent, with an 80 to 90 per cent five-year survival.

MULTICENTRIC OSTEOSARCOMA (OSTEOSARCOMATOSIS)

This is another extremely rare variant of osteosarcoma in which there is synchronous appearance at multiple sites of typical osteoblastic sarcomatous lesions. The lesions are often symmetrical. The similar size of the lesions serves to distinguish multicentric osteosarcoma from a primary osteosarcoma with osseous metastases. The lesions are rapidly progressive and prognosis is dismal.

OSTEOSARCOMA IN THE ELDERLY PATIENT

The elderly patient represents the second peak of osteosarcomas in the patient population. They are distinct from conventional osteosarcomas in many respects other than age of occurrence. The radiographic appearance, although quite aggressive, is very often lytic, without evidence of matrix production (80 per cent). The location of several of these osteosarcomas is distinct, with 27 per cent in the axial skeleton, 13 per cent in the craniofacial bones, and 11 per cent in the soft tissues. These osteosarcomas are also distinct in that 56 per cent arise in pre-existing lesions. These include Paget's disease (approximately 1 per cent of the Paget's population is at risk for developing osteosarcoma) (Fig. 100–24). Bone that has been pre-

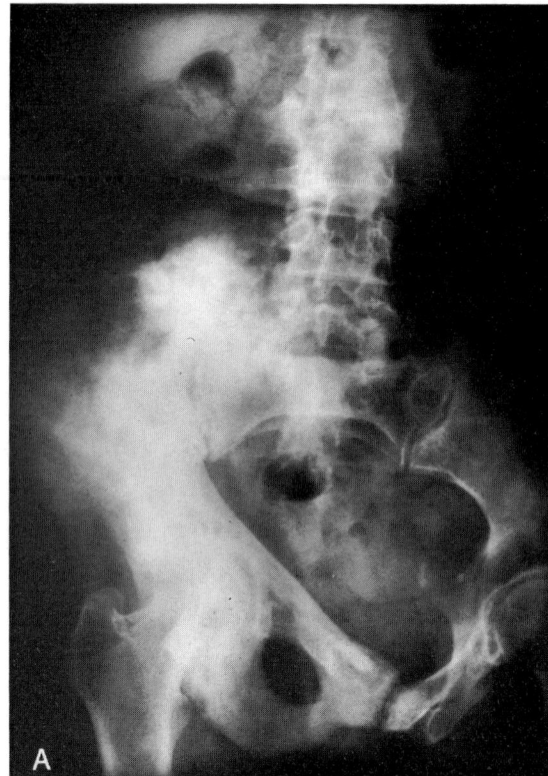

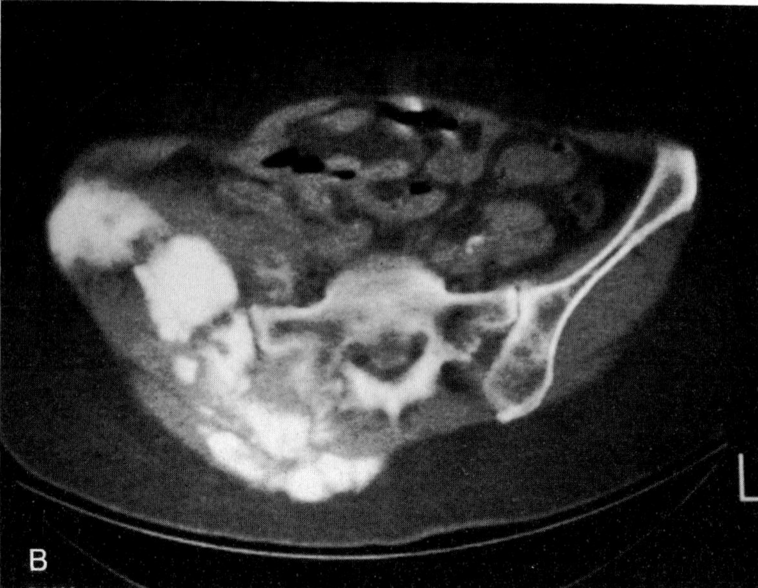

Figure 100–24. *A,* This patient with underlying Paget's disease has developed a large aggressive osteosarcoma of the right iliac wing. The diagnosis of Paget's disease is made by the thickened cortex and expansion of the right hemipelvis. However, the obvious osteoid matrix is not a feature of Paget's and represents secondary development of osteosarcoma. You might also note the widening and destructive change in the body of L2. This is a second focus of Paget's disease. *B,* The CT scan shows to better advantage the bone-forming large soft-tissue mass.

viously radiated is at risk for developing osteosarcoma (with an average 14-year span since the radiation, but much wider range). Chondrosarcomas can dedifferentiate, occasionally into a highly aggressive osteosarcoma. The prognosis of an osteosarcoma arising in the elderly patient is worse than that of conventional osteosarcoma, with a 37 per cent survival in a de novo lesion and 7.5 per cent survival if the osteosarcoma arises in a pre-existing lesion.

CARTILAGE-FORMING TUMORS

B. J. Manaster

Benign Cartilage-Forming Tumors

ENCHONDROMA

Enchondromas are benign cartilaginous neoplasms that are asymptomatic in the absence of pathologic fracture or malignant degeneration and are most often discovered incidentally in the third or fourth decades. These are central metaphyseal lesions which usually present with a geographic pattern. Although the lesion is lobulated, the zone of transition is usually narrow and there may or may not be a fine sclerotic margin present. It is an indolent lesion and usually does not elicit a host response. The lesion does produce chondroid, but radiographically may appear either to have typical cartilaginous stippled dense matrix or to be completely lytic (Fig. 100–25).

Fifty per cent of enchondromas are distributed in the metaphyses of the long tubular bones (especially the humerus, femur, and tibia). These are usually monostotic and easily diagnosed by plain film. The most common differential consideration of an enchondroma that contains matrix is a bone infarct in which the pattern of dystrophic calcification may be quite similar. Most of these lesions remain asymptomatic throughout their lifespan. Thus, if an enchondroma is found incidentally, treatment most often is to watch the lesion for clinical signs of change. Occasionally enchondromas will undergo malignant degeneration to chondrosarcoma. Proximal lesions, particularly in the pelvis or shoulder girdle, have the highest incidence of malignant change. Clinicians must be aware that early malignant degeneration may not be detectable radiographically. Even serial plain films, bone scans, and CT or MRI scans may show no interval change early in the course of degeneration. The diagnosis of malignant degeneration therefore may be based solely on local pain, and appropriate treatment should be instituted on a painful enchondroma in the absence of pathologic fracture. Histology in early malignant degeneration most commonly shows either low-grade chondrosarcoma or an atypical enchondroma.

The other 50 per cent of enchondromas arise in tubular bones of the hand or feet. These lesions often have a different appearance, with significant expansion of the bone, and usually an absence of matrix. Differential diagnosis includes giant cell tumor, aneurysmal bone cyst, and solitary bone cyst, but these last three lesions are less commonly found in this acral distribution than is enchondroma. Although enchondromas in the hands and feet can appear radiographically aggressive and even histologically aggressive, they almost universally behave in a benign manner (Fig. 100–26). Although enchondromas in long tubular bones are usually monostotic, there may be several enchondromas in the hands or feet without raising the specter of multiple enchondromatosis (see next section).

MULTIPLE ENCHONDROMATOSIS (OLLIER'S DISEASE)

Ollier's disease is a rare developmental abnormality characterized by the presence of enchondromas in the metaphyses of multiple

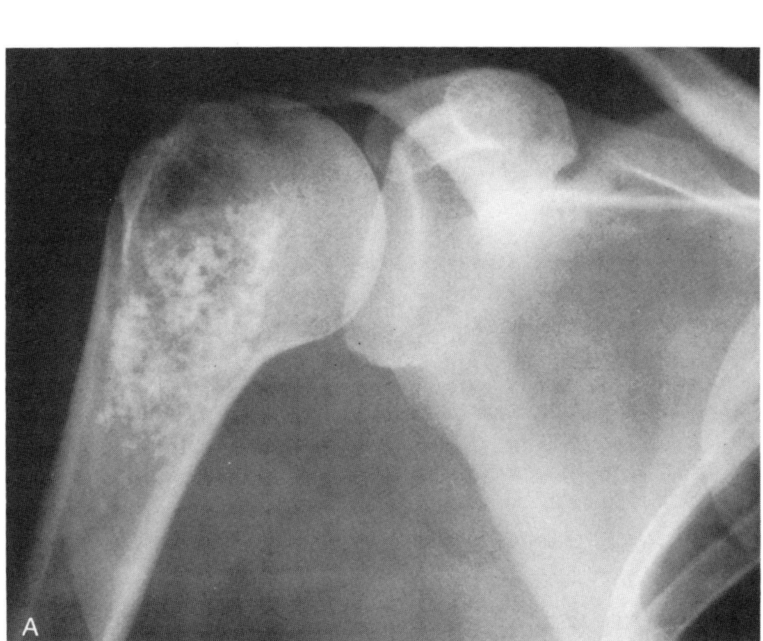

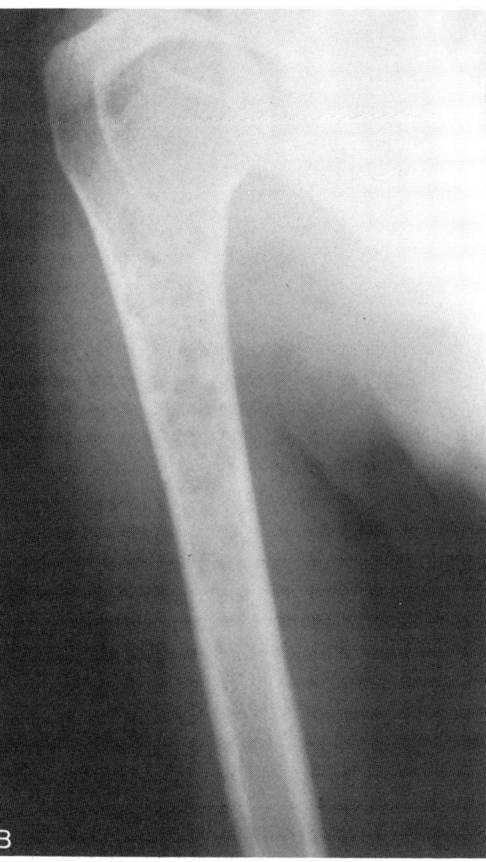

Figure 100–25. Enchondroma. *A* shows a classic enchondroma of the humerus. The radiographic features include dense calcific matrix in a metadiaphyseal lesion. The lesion causes mild scalloping of the cortex, and there is absolutely no host bone reaction. There is a narrow zone of transition, but no true margination of the lesion is seen. A little more difficult lesion to diagnose is shown in *B*. The film demonstrates the central lesion located in the metadiaphysis of the proximal humerus. The lesion is rather large but does appear to have a narrow zone of transition. There is no margination of the lesion. It is completely lytic and causes scalloping of the endosteum with absolutely no host reaction. Occasionally enchondromas such as this occur that do not have calcific matrix. With all the other features pointing toward enchondroma, this diagnosis can be made in this asymptomatic lesion. (*A* reprinted with permission from the ACR Learning File, Musculoskeletal Videodisc, Case 116; *B* from Case 117.)

bones. It is felt to represent a dysplasia rather than a true tumor and is not hereditary or familial. The lesions tend to be unilateral and may be localized to a single extremity. The lesions occasionally appear radiographically like typical enchondromas. However, they may appear much more bizarre, with a striated appearance (Fig. 100–27). This dysplasia causes significant limb shortening and growth deformity. It also carries a risk of malignant transformation to chondrosarcoma in the range of 10 to 30 per cent. Another variant of Ollier's disease, Maffucci's syndrome, consists of enchondromatosis combined with soft-tissue hemangiomas. This syndrome has a much higher malignant degeneration potential than enchondromatosis alone, up to 100 per cent.

OSTEOCHONDROMA (EXOSTOSES)

An exostosis is a very common benign neoplasm that results from growth plate cartilage displaced to the metaphyseal region. Once this mechanism is understood, the radiographic appearance is easily understood as well. The underlying bone is completely normal, and normal bone grows as an excrescence from the underlying metaphysis. There is continuity of the periosteum, cortices, and bone marrow of the exostoses and host bone. As with other growth plates, an exostosis may be expected to continue growth as long as the patient has not reached skeletal maturity. Because of this growth pattern, the mass is usually discovered in the first or second decade. An exostosis may achieve a very large size prior to cessation of growth (Fig. 100–28). When the exostosis has this cauliflower-like appearance, the diagnosis is relatively easy, with only parosteal osteosarcoma or possibly myositis ossificans as a reasonable differential diagnosis. However, exostoses can also appear much more broad-based and sessile. These are more commonly seen when a patient has multiple exostoses and may be confused with a metaphyseal dysplasia.

Although exostoses have the appearance of normal bone, it should be remembered that their growth occurs from a cartilaginous cap. Cartilaginous matrix may occasionally be seen in the cartilaginous cap.

Most (90 per cent) exostoses are solitary. These stop growing with skeletal maturation, but may occasionally be the source of mechanical irritation, sometimes with bursitis developing over them. Solitary osteochondromas that are incidentally found do not require treatment, whereas mechanically painful osteochondromas may be locally excised. Fewer than 1 per cent of solitary exostoses undergo malignant degeneration to chondrosarcoma. Such degeneration may occasionally be detected radiographically with new mineral deposition beyond previously documented contours, or very rarely destructive changes of the neck or base of the exostosis. More commonly, there is no radiographic change, but the patient complains of pain or growth of the exostosis after closure of the epiphyses. In the absence of mechanical reasons for pain or the formation of a bursa simulating the growth of the exostosis, such clinical symptoms indicate malignant degeneration until proven otherwise. These should be worked up and treated as a chondrosarcoma.

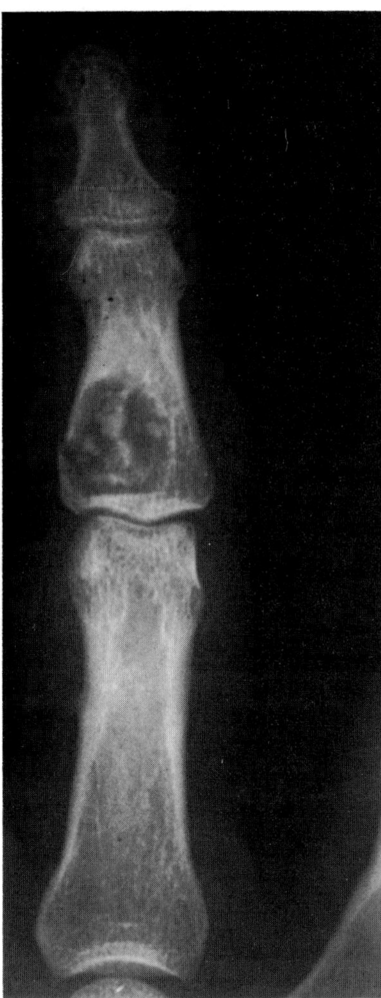

Figure 100–26. Enchondroma of phalanx. There is a pathologic fracture of a round lesion involving the proximal diaphysis of the middle phalanx. The lesion is eccentric and slightly bows the cortex. It uniformly thins the cortex and contains matrix calcification. The most common lesion of the phalanx is enchondroma, and the presence of cartilaginous calcification in this case is confirmation of this diagnosis.

Multiple hereditary exostosis represents an autosomal dominant disorder resulting in the development of multiple osteochondromas. Although some of these exostoses may appear stalk-like, most are broad based in the metaphysis and result in the appearance of a greater circumference of this portion of the bone. This often simulates a dysplasia, and the true nature of the disease process may go unrecognized (Fig. 100–29). The disorder may result in limb shortening and deformity. Even more importantly, these patients have a relatively high incidence of sarcomatous degeneration within the exostoses (10 to 20 per cent), especially the more proximal lesions. These patients therefore should be followed up carefully for degeneration to chondrosarcoma.

CHONDROBLASTOMA

Chondroblastoma is a fairly rare benign cartilaginous lesion that has the radiographic distinction of being located almost exclusively in the epiphysis. It usually arises before epiphyseal closure, most commonly in the second decade. The lesion is geographic, with a sclerotic border (Fig. 100–30). It may be eccentric. The most commonly involved bone is the proximal humerus, but the lesion is also often seen in the proximal femur or around the knee. Chondroblastomas most commonly appear lytic, but may contain small amounts of cartilaginous calcification in up to 50 per cent of cases. Interestingly, these very benign-appearing lesions not infrequently elicit periosteal reaction. With an otherwise classic-appearing chondroblastoma, this periosteal reaction should not mislead the radiologist into consideration of a more aggressive lesion.

The differential diagnosis should not be difficult. Articular lesions with large cysts such as pigmented villonodular synovitis might be considered. Occasionally, a giant cell tumor is also considered. However, it should be remembered that the epicenter for giant cell tumor is metaphyseal whereas the epicenter of chondroblastoma is epiphyseal (Fig. 100–31). Furthermore, the sclerotic margin is much more prominent in chondroblastoma.

This lesion is diagnosed by plain film and only rarely needs additional radiographic work-up. Chondroblastoma can be painful and treatment is curettage with bone grafting. The recurrence rate is relatively low, at 15 per cent.

CHONDROMYXOID FIBROMA

Chondromyxoid fibroma is a very rare benign cartilaginous lesion that finds itself in many differential diagnoses, but rarely actually

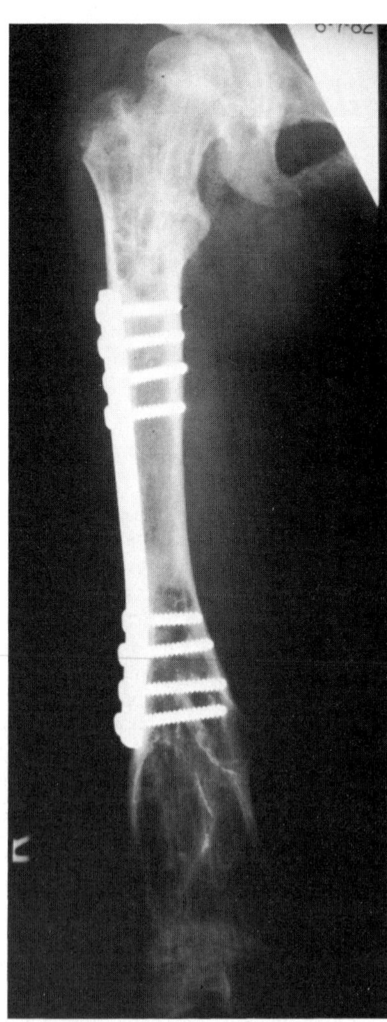

Figure 100–27. Multiple enchondromatosis. This patient had polyostotic metaphyseal lesions involving the right lower extremity only. The metaphyseal lesions appear quite bizarre, with lytic expansion containing streaky or striated calcification. The metaphyses are slightly deformed. The plate along the diaphysis is from a leg-lengthening procedure; not only were the metaphyses deformed, but also the leg was extremely short. This combination of features is descriptive of Ollier's disease, or multiple enchondromatosis. (Reprinted with permission from the ACR Learning File, Musculoskeletal Videodisc, Case 118.)

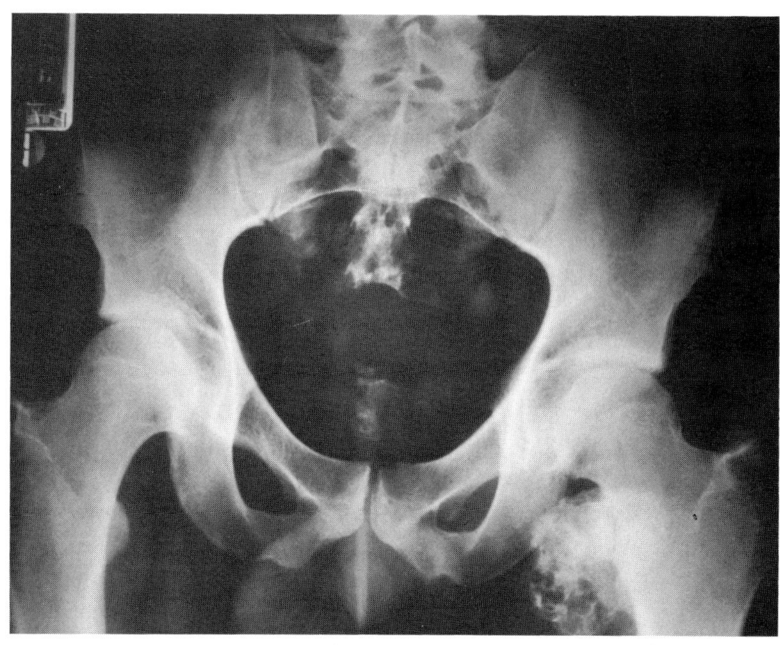

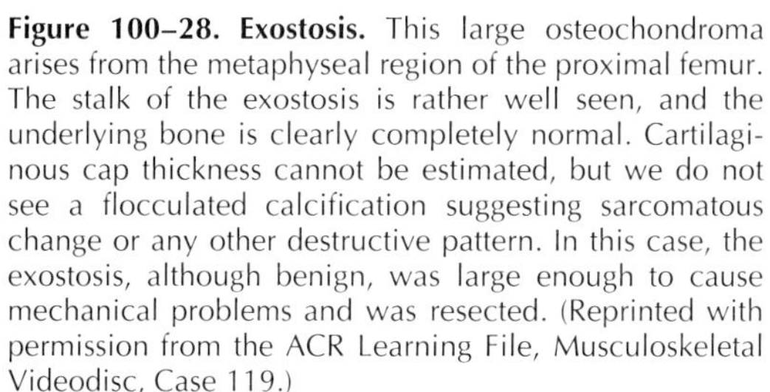

Figure 100–28. Exostosis. This large osteochondroma arises from the metaphyseal region of the proximal femur. The stalk of the exostosis is rather well seen, and the underlying bone is clearly completely normal. Cartilaginous cap thickness cannot be estimated, but we do not see a flocculated calcification suggesting sarcomatous change or any other destructive pattern. In this case, the exostosis, although benign, was large enough to cause mechanical problems and was resected. (Reprinted with permission from the ACR Learning File, Musculoskeletal Videodisc, Case 119.)

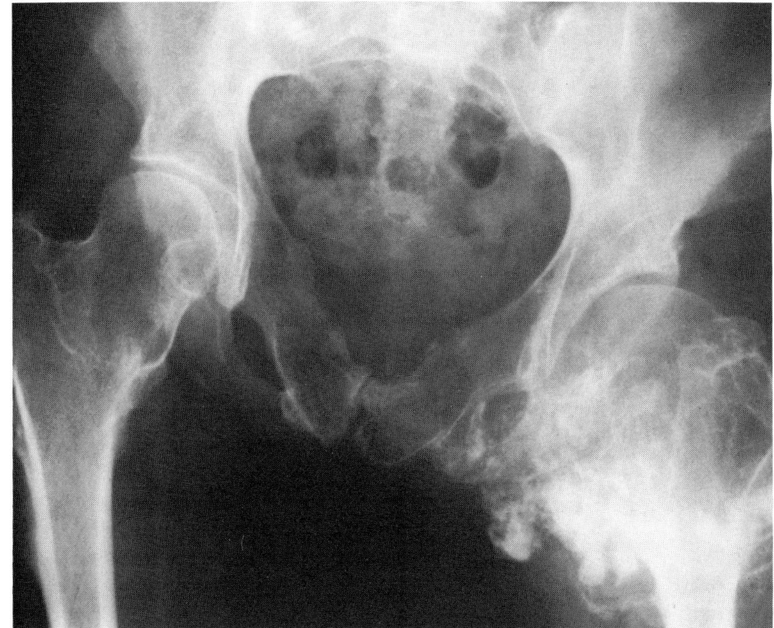

Figure 100–29. Multiple familial exostoses. Both the exophytic variety (left proximal femur) and sessile variety of exostoses are demonstrated. The cauliflower-like exostosis arises from a stalk and leaves the underlying bone completely normal. The left femoral lesion has evidently been this large size and shape for a considerable period of time, since one notes that the femoral head has been subluxated and the head and the acetabulum have remodeled to accommodate this exostosis. Although this lesion is very large, it does not show destructive changes. The broad-based sessile exostoses are seen involving the right femoral metaphyseal region as well as both pubic rami. It is not surprising that this appearance is often mistaken for a metaphyseal dysplasia if there is no cauliflower-like exostosis present to make the diagnosis easy. (Reprinted with permission from the ACR Learning File, Musculoskeletal Videodisc, Case 120.)

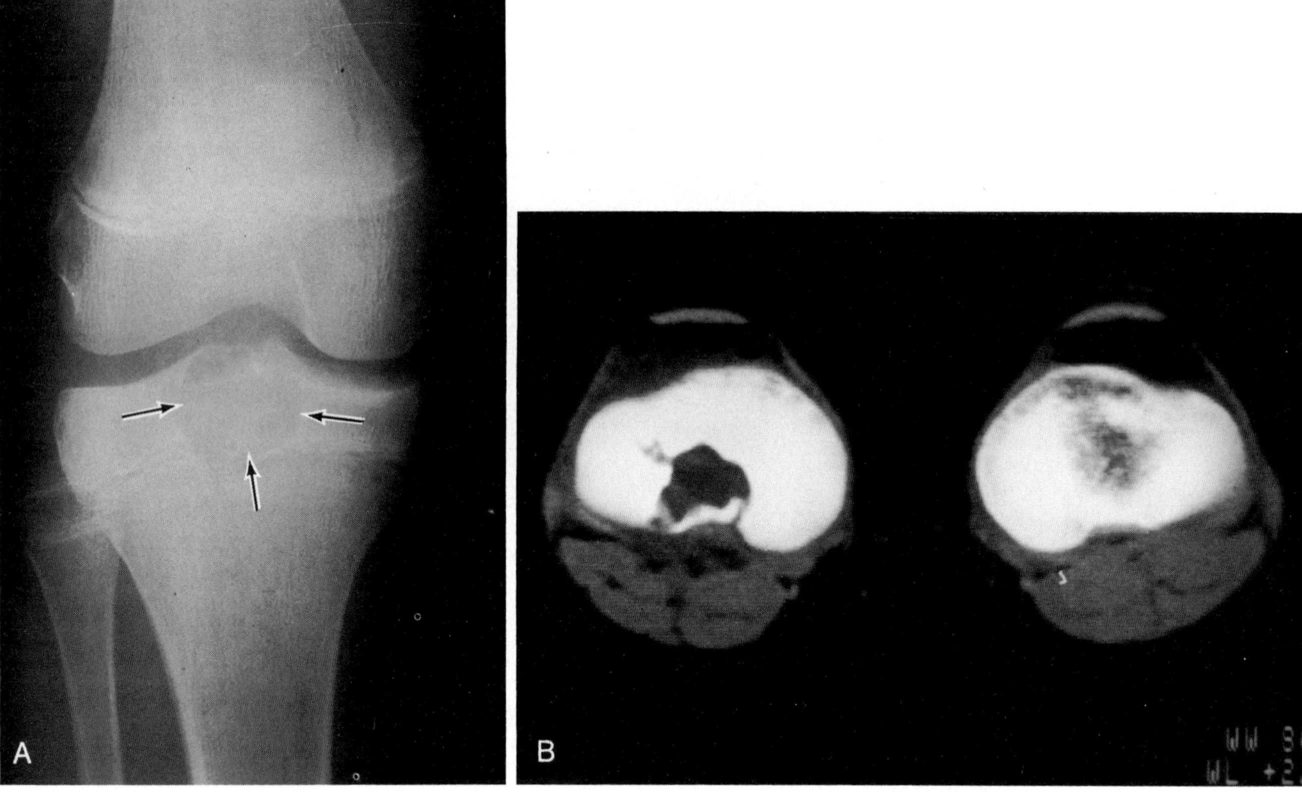

Figure 100–30. Chondroblastoma. The plain film *(A)* demonstrates a lytic lesion located entirely within the epiphysis of the proximal tibia. There is a mildly sclerotic border *(arrows)*. In a skeletally immature patient, this appearance represents chondroblastoma until proven otherwise. The CT scan *(B)* confirms the lytic nature of the lesion. It is interesting that the CT scan demonstrates an extension of the lesion from the rounded epicenter. This suggests that a more extensive curettage than usual would be required in this case to prevent recurrence. (*A* and *B* reprinted with permission from the ACR Learning File, Musculoskeletal Videodisc, Case 121.)

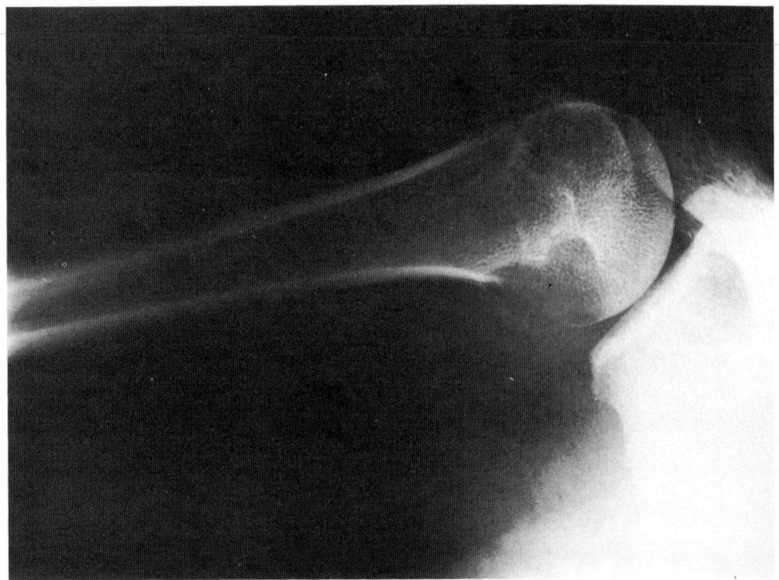

Figure 100–31. This eccentric, well-marginated lesion has its epicenter within the epiphysis, although, as this patient is becoming skeletally mature, the lesion extends into the metaphysis. It might be difficult to differentiate between chondroblastoma and giant cell tumor in this patient. However, the fact that the lesion arises in the proximal humerus and that the origin of the lesion seems to be epiphyseal suggests chondroblastoma more strongly. This diagnosis was confirmed at biopsy. (From Manaster BJ, et al: Giant cell tumor of bone. Radiol Clin North Am 31(2):303, 1993.)

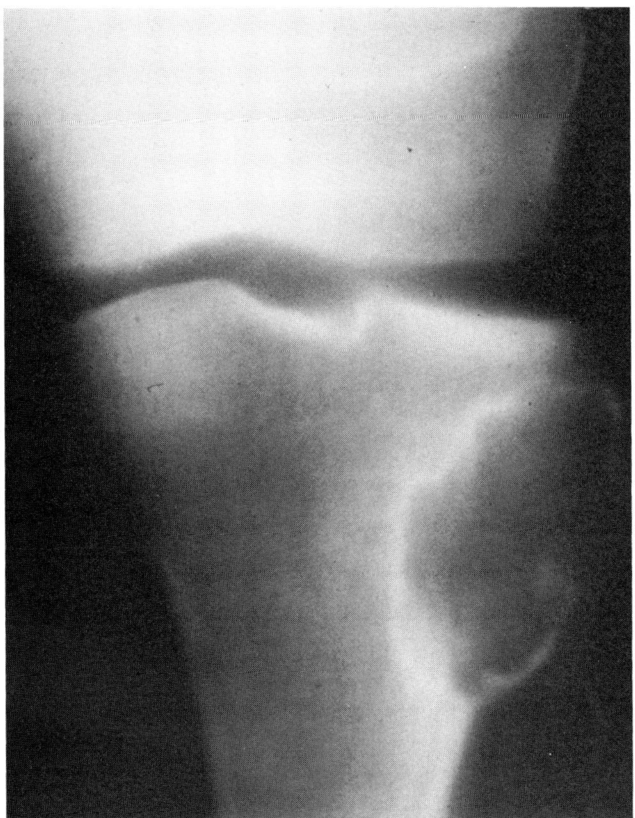

Figure 100–32. Chondromyxoid fibroma. This tomogram shows a lytic lesion located at the proximal tibial metaphysis that is eccentrically placed, slightly bubbly and expansile, and has a strongly sclerotic margin. This is typical of chondromyxoid fibroma. A diagnosis of nonossifying fibroma might also be considered in this case, but the latter lesion tends to be more longitudinally oriented in tubular bones. (Reprinted with permission from the ACR Learning File, Musculoskeletal Videodisc, Case 122.)

occurs. The lesion most commonly occurs in the proximal tibia and is geographic, often appearing lobulated. Like many other lesions, it is found eccentrically in the metaphysis and has a thick sclerotic margin (Fig. 100–32). Although it is a cartilage-producing tumor, calcification is only rarely seen (2 per cent). Host reaction is rare. The differential diagnosis includes other metaphyseal geographic lesions: nonossifying fibromas, aneurysmal bone cyst, chondroblastoma (if the epicenter is in the epiphysis), and giant cell tumor (although the latter generally does not have a sclerotic margin). The diagnosis is suggested by plain film and proven by biopsy; additional imaging generally is not useful. The lesion can be painful, and is treated by curettage and bone grafting initially. There may be a high recurrence rate (25 per cent) owing to the lobulated nature of the lesion.

Malignant Cartilage-Forming Tumors

CENTRAL (MEDULLARY) CHONDROSARCOMA

Chondrosarcomas are the third most common primary malignant bone tumor (following osteosarcoma and multiple myeloma). Unfortunately, these sarcomas are often asymptomatic or only mildly symptomatic, leading to large tumors with late diagnosis. Because they often appear rather indolent, errors in diagnosis are also common, again leading to a delay in appropriate treatment.

Central chondrosarcomas may be either primary or secondary to degeneration of enchondromas. They are most commonly located in the central metaphyseal ends of long bones, or the pelvis and shoulder girdle. Because the lesions are often of low grade and therefore slow growing, large portions of the tumor may appear geographic, with a narrow zone of transition. However, other portions may appear permeative with a less distinct zone of transition or margin. There may or may not be cortical breakthrough soft-tissue invasion. Therefore periosteal reaction is variable. The endosteum may either be thinned and expanded or may show thickening in an effort to contain the tumor.

As is the case with enchondromas, central chondrosarcomas range from being lytic, to lytic with a few flecks of calcification, to dense aggregates of annular calcification (Fig. 100–33).

The above description characterizes the 90 per cent of central chondrosarcomas that are low grade. As described, they appear to be only a moderately aggressive lesion. The astute radiologist will remember that chondrosarcomas are common lesions and therefore, if a central lesion in a patient in the right age group appears slightly to moderately aggressive, subtle calcification should be sought and a diagnosis of chondrosarcoma should be offered, whether or not cartilaginous calcification is found. Central chondrosarcoma is very commonly underdiagnosed because it so often appears rather benign; this underdiagnosis results in undertreatment.

Although chondrosarcomas are often low-grade lesions, they have the disadvantage of very easily seeding surrounding tissue following biopsy or resection. Thus, local recurrence is more common than is metastatic disease. If metastasis occurs, it involves the lung. This can occur quite late in the disease process. The five-year survival with adequate therapy (wide resection) is 75 per cent. Except in a high-grade lesion, radiation and chemotherapy are not a part of the treatment regimen.

PERIPHERAL (EXOSTOTIC) CHONDROSARCOMA

Peripheral chondrosarcomas may arise either primarily or secondarily owing to degeneration of an exostosis. The age range of 30 to 60 years is similar to that of central chondrosarcomas. The tumor often has a large soft-tissue mass (Fig. 100–34). A cartilage cap greater than 1 cm in thickness on an exostosis suggests malignant change to chondrosarcoma, but this may be difficult to detect and quantify. The degenerating cartilage cap may also become densely calcified with a ''snowstorm'' pattern, which helps suggest degeneration to chondrosarcoma. However, degeneration of an exostosis to chondrosarcoma may produce no clear-cut radiographic signs. Therefore, clinical signs of growth and pain in an exostosis after epiphyseal closure should be considered of primary importance in making the diagnosis of peripheral chondrosarcoma. Radiographic workup should include MRI. There is no distinct MRI appearance of chondrosarcomas, but the lobulated nature that is characteristic of cartilage is often seen (Fig. 100–35). Although MRI may not distinctly show the extent of the cartilaginous cap, it will outline the soft-tissue mass. Work-up and treatment are similar to that for central chondrosarcoma.

DEDIFFERENTIATED CHONDROSARCOMA

Chondrosarcomas, either central or peripheral, may degenerate from a typically indolent chondrosarcoma into a highly aggressive lesion. Degeneration may occur to fibrosarcoma, malignant fibrous histiocytoma, high-grade chondrosarcoma, osteosarcoma, or a lesion that has several elements. Ten per cent of chondrosarcomas may dedifferentiate. Furthermore, the original chondrosarcoma and the dedifferentiated elements coexist (Fig. 100–36). Therefore the biopsy site must be chosen to include the more aggressive lesion. MRI can be extremely useful in choosing appropriate and representative biopsy sites in these lesions.

Prognosis for dedifferentiated chondrosarcomas is poor (20 per cent five-year survival rate), and lung metastases are common. Treatment is wide or radical excision and chemotherapy.

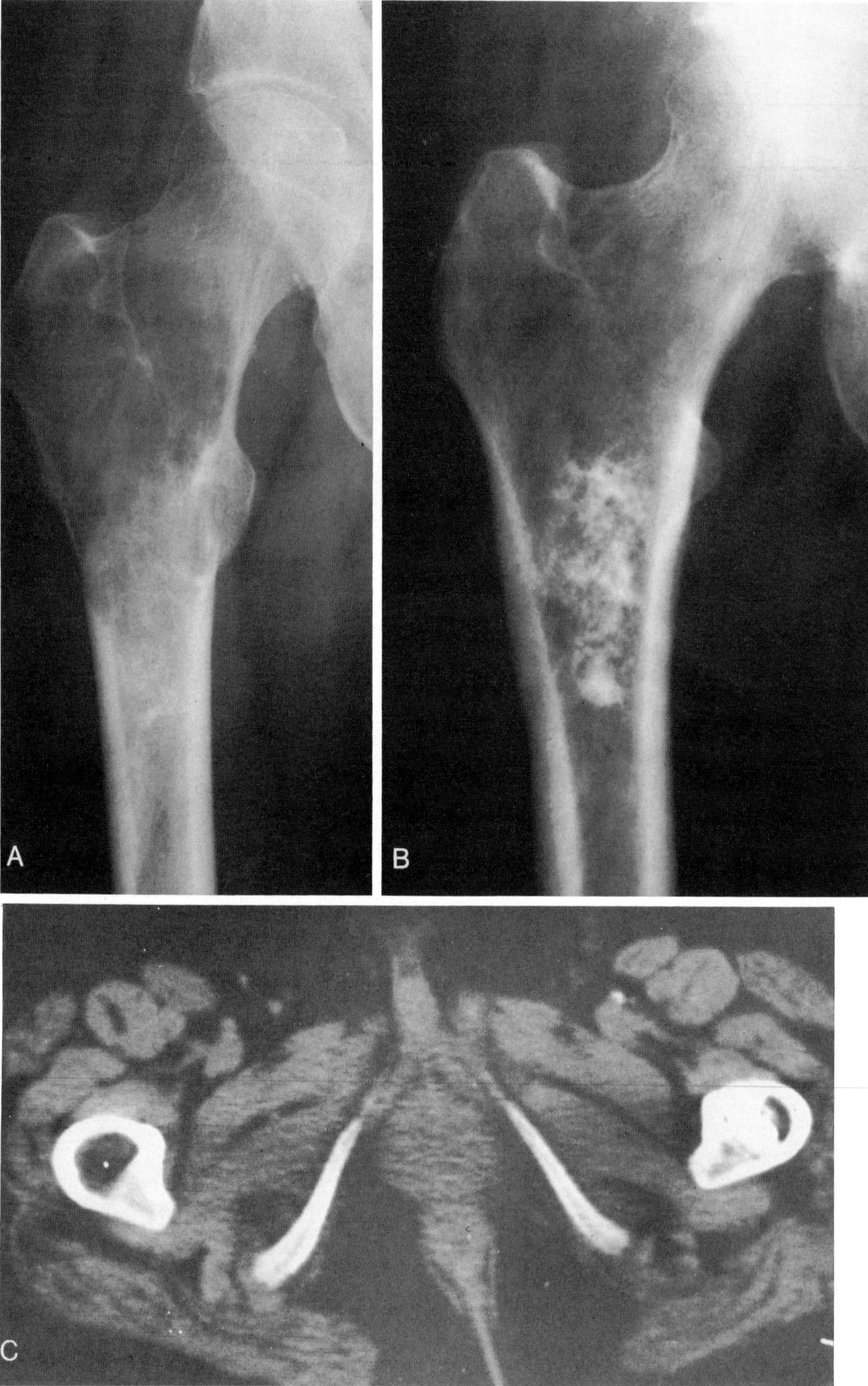

Figure 100–33. Intermedullary chondrosarcoma. *A* demonstrates a typical case of a lytic intermedullary chondrosarcoma. The lesion is in the metaphyseal region of the femur and is only moderately aggressive, being large and having a moderately wide zone of transition and no distinctly sclerotic margin. The lesion is expansile. In this 53-year-old patient, this moderately aggressive central lesion is quite typical for intermedullary chondrosarcoma. Note that the cartilaginous nature of the lesion is confirmed by the subtle calcification seen more distally. *B* demonstrates a densely calcified intermedullary chondrosarcoma. This lesion has the typical appearance of an enchondroma, with typical stippled dense calcifications in the metadiaphyseal region in a geographic and nonaggressive-appearing lesion. The CT scan *(C)* similarly demonstrated no suggestion of aggressive nature, with an intact cortex and no soft-tissue mass. Despite this rather typical appearance of enchondroma, the patient complained of pain localized to this site. The clinical history is therefore suggestive of degeneration to chondrosarcoma, and treatment for this lesion is indicated.

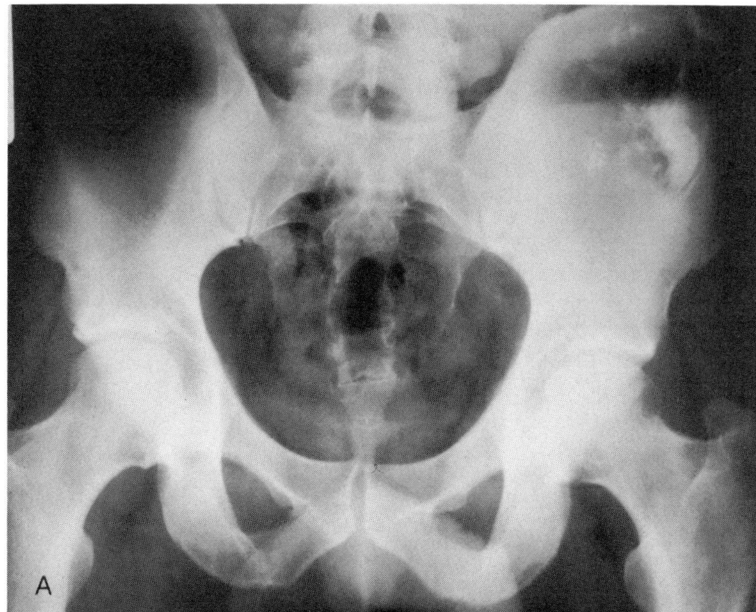

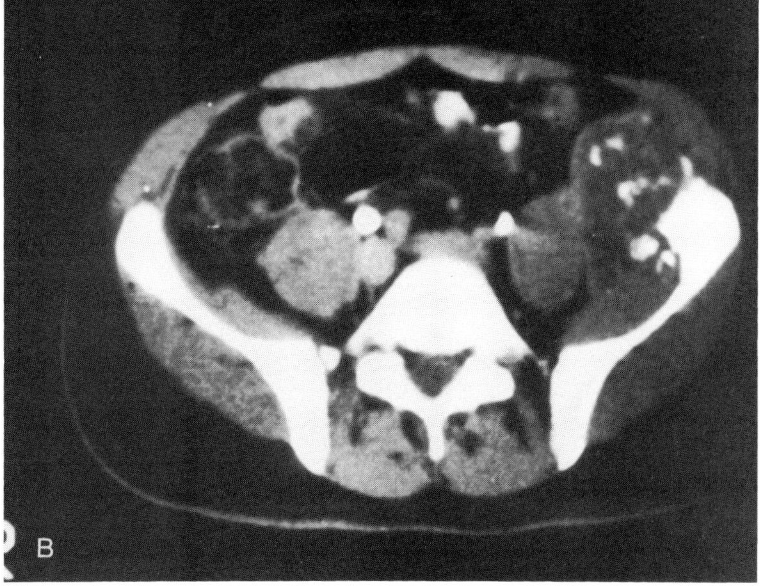

Figure 100–34. Exostotic chondrosarcoma. The plain film *(A)* demonstrates a lytic lesion with dense flocculated cartilage calcification arising in the left iliac wing. This is a very typical location and appearance for chondrosarcoma in this 35-year-old male. The CT scan *(B)* demonstrates that the lesion originated as an exostosis arising from the anterior portion of the iliac wing. The CT scan confirms a large soft-tissue mass and delineates nicely the tumor extent as is required for resection of this chondrosarcoma. (*A* and *B* reprinted with permission from the ACR Learning File, Musculoskeletal Videodisc, Case 123.)

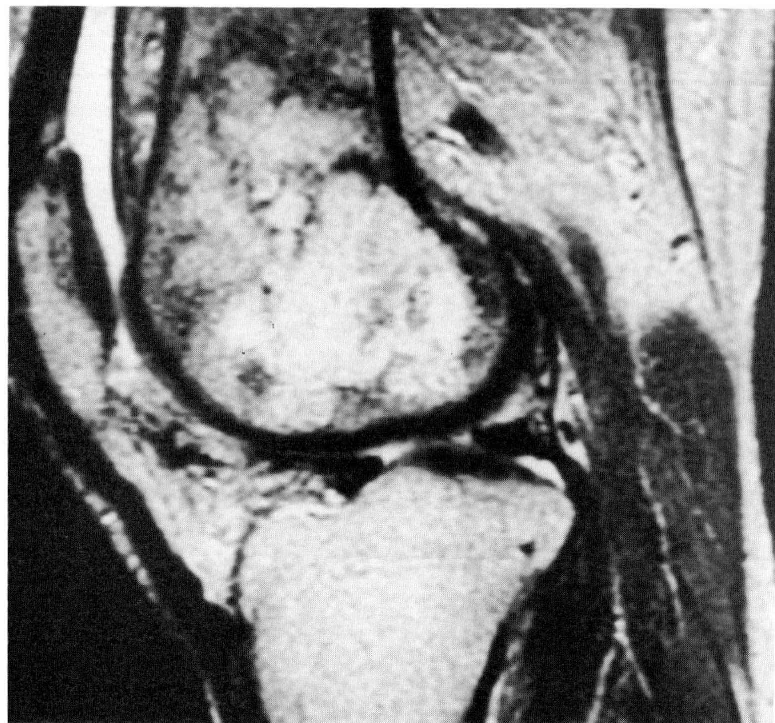

Figure 100–35. MRI of chondrosarcoma. This T_2 sequence demonstrates an intermedullary chondrosarcoma in the distal femur. The signal intensity of the lesion is higher than that of normal intermedullary bone; this is typical of most tumors. However, the MRI also demonstrates the lobulated character of the tumor, which is quite characteristic of cartilaginous lesions. A higher-grade chondrosarcoma need not have this lobulated appearance.

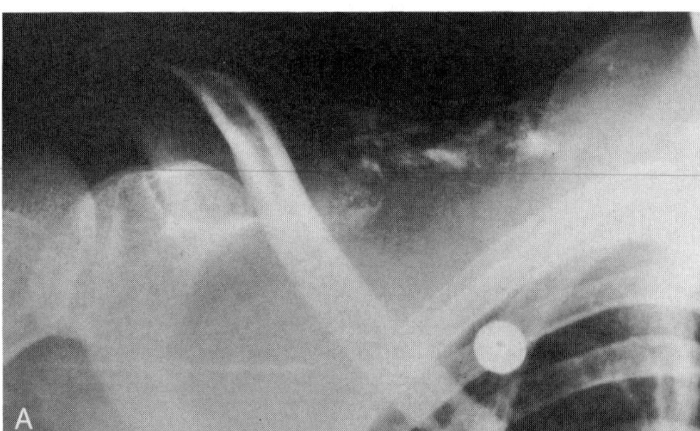

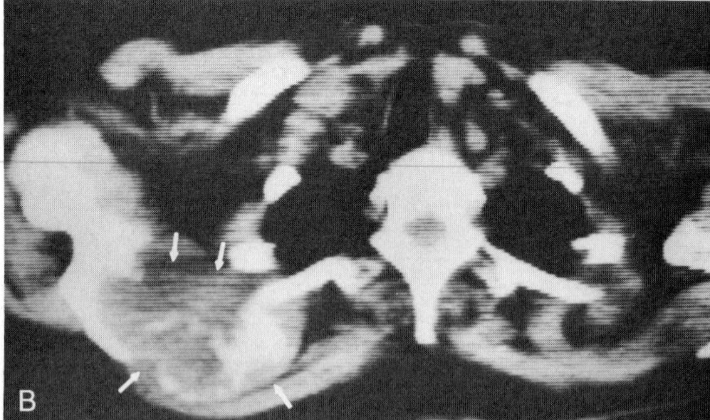

Figure 100–36. Dedifferentiated chondrosarcoma. The plain film *(A)* demonstrates typical cartilaginous calcification in the superior portion of the scapula. It extends beyond the borders of the scapula and, associated with destructive changes in the superspinous fossa, is typical of an exostotic chondrosarcoma. However, the extent of the lesion is not appreciated by plain film. CT scan demonstrates the cartilaginous calcification proximally. However, axial cuts more distally *(B)* show a very large soft-tissue mass that destroys the scapular wing *(arrows)*. These findings are typical of at least a very high grade chondrosarcoma, but dedifferentiation might be expected given the very different appearance of the distal portion of the scapula compared with the proximal. At biopsy, the calcified region demonstrated a typical low-grade chondrosarcoma, while the large soft-tissue mass showed elements of osteosarcoma and fibrosarcoma present along with Grade 4 chondrosarcoma. This specimen therefore represents a dedifferentiated chondrosarcoma and is a more representative tissue sample. (*A* and *B* reprinted with permission from the ACR Learning File, Musculoskeletal Videodisc, Case 127.)

MARROW TUMORS

B. J. Manaster

The group of marrow tumors has always been called the "round cell" tumors. It is useful, however, to remember that round cell lesions include not only primary tumors (Ewing's sarcoma, lymphoma, and multiple myeloma) but also metastatic neuroblastoma, histiocytosis, and infection. With the exception of multiple myeloma, these lesions are often not easily distinguished radiographically. Thus, the differential diagnosis for an aggressive-appearing round cell lesion ranges from completely benign treatable lesions to very malignant lesions.

Ewing's Sarcoma

Ewing's sarcoma is a highly malignant marrow cell tumor found commonly in children (second most common primary bone tumor in children, after osteosarcoma). The age range is 4 to 30 years. Interestingly, the younger patients tend to have the tumor arise in tubular bones whereas the older patients tend to have the tumor located in the axial skeleton, pelvis, and shoulder girdle. The lesion is highly aggressive, with a permeative pattern that destroys rather than expands bone. A soft-tissue mass is almost invariably present. The lesion is located centrally and is most commonly diaphyseal, although a diametaphyseal epicenter is not uncommon. Aggressive periosteal host response is the rule. However, the host also responds in other manners, including rarely developing thick reactive endosteal bone. Sclerotic reactive bone formation can even be seen within the medullary canal. It is not always easy to differentiate this sclerotic reactive bone from tumor osteoid matrix as would be seen in an osteosarcoma. Thus, although approximately 60 per cent of Ewing's sarcomas are completely lytic, 25 per cent have at least minimal reactive bone formation and 15 per cent have marked sclerotic reactive bone (Fig. 100–37). One factor that helps differentiate these patients from osteosarcoma patients is the fact that reactive bone, although being found within the medullary canal, is not found in the soft-tissue mass.

There are some distinct clinical features often found in patients with Ewing's sarcoma. One third of these patients present with fever, leukocytosis, and an elevated erythrocyte sedimentation rate. The overlying skin may be warm and red. Clinical findings and laboratory findings thus may strongly suggest infection; as indicated earlier, the radiographic features may suggest infection as well. It may also be of interest that Ewing's sarcoma is extremely rare in black patients.

Prognosis in this lesion is poor, with a 50 per cent five-year survival. Between 15 and 30 per cent of patients have metastases at the time of diagnosis; metastases affect lung and bone with equal frequency. Central and larger lesions have a worse prognosis than more distal ones. The radiographic work-up should follow that described in the algorithm for aggressive lesions (see Fig. 100–5). Treatment of the primary lesion routinely consists of radiation and chemotherapy. Some protocols call for resection of the primary site after the initial radiation therapy if the primary tumor is in an accessible site. It might be noted that because large radiation doses are used in relatively young patients, the complication rate of the radiation itself is not insignificant. If the patients survive their primary tumor, they can develop radiation-induced sarcomas at a later time. Growth deformities are also not uncommon (see Radiation Changes, later in this chapter).

Primary Lymphoma of Bone

Primary lymphoma uncommonly arises initially in bone. The most common age group affected is 30 to 60 years. Like Ewing's sarcoma, the lesion is large, lytic, and permeative, with cortical breakthrough and a large soft-tissue mass (Fig. 100–38). Occasionally reactive sclerosis may be seen and the patients often have periosteal reaction. Central appendicular sites (femur, pelvis, humerus, and scapula) represent the most common locations.

The major differential diagnoses includes the other aggressive bone tumors that arise in this age group: malignant fibrous-histiocytoma, fibrosarcoma, and chondrosarcoma. Five-year survival approximates 55 per cent. Unlike the other sarcomas, this lesion metastasizes most commonly to local lymph nodes. Occasionally bone and lung metastases are found. Work-up is that for aggressive osseous lesions, and treatment is whole bone radiation with chemotherapy for disseminated disease.

Hodgkin's Disease

Hodgkin's disease of bone is almost always secondary to a primary lymph node lesion. Although 20 per cent of patients with Hodgkin's disease have radiographic evidence of bone involvement, it is extremely rare as a primary bone tumor. Since it is usually a secondary process, polyostotic involvement is common. The axial skeleton represents the most common location (77 per cent), with the vertebral bodies being the prime site. Sclerotic reactive bone formation is often seen, with the classic manifestations of Hodgkin's disease being the ivory vertebra (Fig. 100–39). The major differential diagnosis is metastatic disease.

Multiple Myeloma

Multiple myeloma is a neoplastic proliferation of plasma cells and represents the most common primary bone tumor. The clinical presentation is usually of back pain and anemia in a patient over the age of 40 years. Myeloma has three major patterns of presentation. The majority (70 per cent) are multifocal lesions with a moth-eaten pattern of small discrete punched-out lytic lesions (Fig. 100–40). Multiple myeloma originates in the red marrow but progresses to the cortex and other areas. Thus the most common sites of involvement of multifocal multiple myeloma include the skull, vertebral bodies, ribs, and the proximal appendicular skeleton.

Thirty per cent of myeloma patients present with a solitary plasmacytoma. Plasmacytomas do not have the usual focal punched-out appearance, but are large expanded cystic-appearing lesions that may have permeative components (Fig. 100–41). Plasmacytoma progresses to multifocal disease.

Perhaps the most difficult form of multiple myeloma to diagnose radiographically is the small percentage of patients that present with generalized infiltration but no focal lesions. These patients appear to have only a generalized osteopenia. It is useful to remember that multiple myeloma can present in this manner, especially when one has a relatively young male patient who does not have other reasons for senile osteoporosis. Other unusual presentations include sclerosing myeloma in which there is either a sclerotic margin around the lesion or else entirely sclerotic lesions. This form of myeloma is associated with a syndrome that carries the acronym POEMS (polyneuropathy, organomegaly, endocrinopathy, myeloma, skin changes). Finally, 10 to 15 per cent of patients with myeloma have associated amyloidosis. If amyloid infiltrates the synovium, it may simulate rheumatoid arthritis.

The radiographic work-up of multiple myeloma is controversial, but it seems that skeletal surveys and bone scans are complementary. Technetium bone scan is positive in only 25 to 40 per cent of myeloma lesions, but has been shown to be more sensitive than plain film in 18 per cent of lesions. On the other hand, plain film has been shown to be more sensitive than technetium bone scanning in a different 38 per cent of lesions. Skeletal surveys are also useful in evaluating for the presence of lesions that are at risk for patho-

Text continued on page 1537

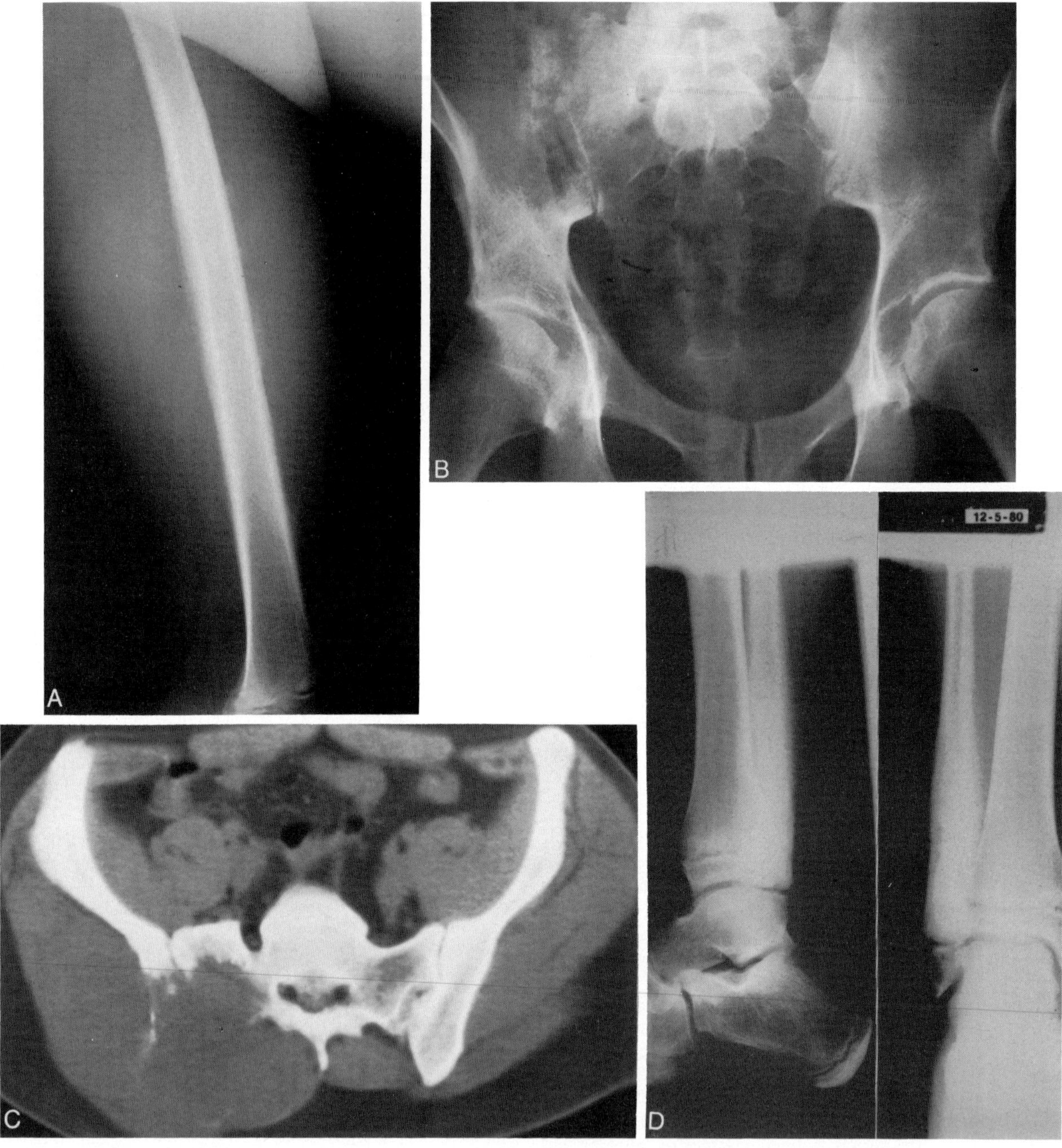

Figure 100–37. Ewing's sarcoma. *A* demonstrates the most classic Ewing's sarcoma you will ever see. It is arising in the diaphysis of a tubular bone in a 10-year-old. There is an obvious large soft-tissue mass that distorts the tissue planes. The osseous lesion is permeative and located centrally. It has a very wide zone of transition and has elicited prominent periosteal reaction. The lesion shown in *B* is another Ewing's sarcoma, which is a diagnostic challenge since it is easy to overlook the lytic destructive lesion in the posterior right iliac wing on the plain film. No other characterization is made on this plain film. However, the CT scan *(C)* demonstrates a very large soft-tissue mass involving the gluteal muscles, with destruction of the posterior right iliac wing as well as adjacent destruction of the right sacral ala. This lytic destructive lesion in a flat bone of a 24-year-old patient is highly characteristic of Ewing's sarcoma. *D* demonstrates a more difficult diagnostic challenge. It shows an aggressive permeative metadiaphyseal lesion that has elicited a sunburst type of periosteal reaction. It does have a soft-tissue mass, not seen on this film. The lesion is extremely dense, but no tumor bone formation is seen in the soft-tissue mass. This is a Ewing's sarcoma with tremendous reactive bone formation, which at times can appear as dense as a blastic osteosarcoma. (*D* reprinted with permission from the ACR Learning File, Musculoskeletal Videodisc, Case 112.)

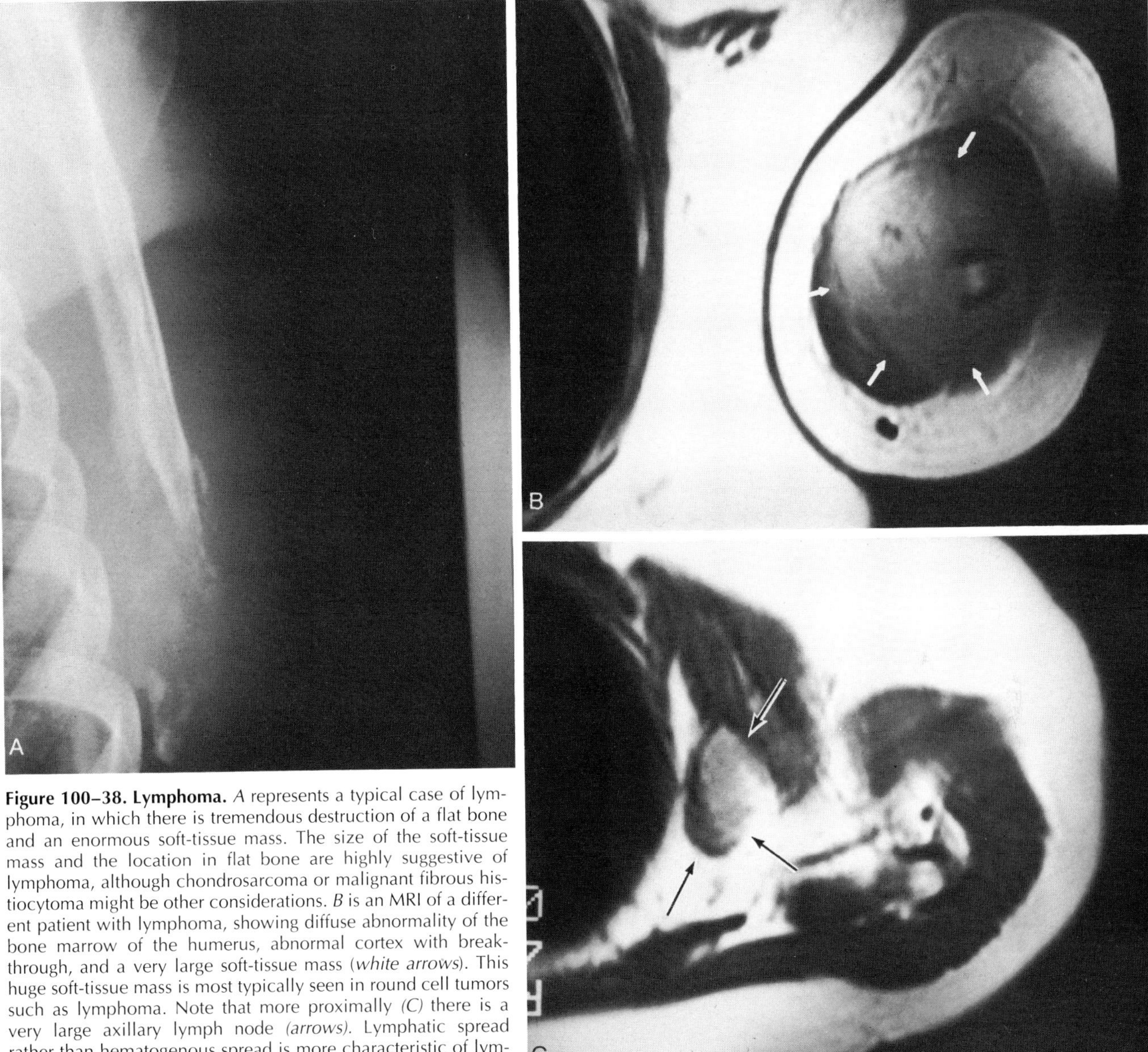

Figure 100–38. Lymphoma. *A* represents a typical case of lymphoma, in which there is tremendous destruction of a flat bone and an enormous soft-tissue mass. The size of the soft-tissue mass and the location in flat bone are highly suggestive of lymphoma, although chondrosarcoma or malignant fibrous histiocytoma might be other considerations. *B* is an MRI of a different patient with lymphoma, showing diffuse abnormality of the bone marrow of the humerus, abnormal cortex with breakthrough, and a very large soft-tissue mass (*white arrows*). This huge soft-tissue mass is most typically seen in round cell tumors such as lymphoma. Note that more proximally *(C)* there is a very large axillary lymph node *(arrows)*. Lymphatic spread rather than hematogenous spread is more characteristic of lymphoma than the other sarcomas. (*A* to *C* reprinted with permission from the ACR Learning File, Musculoskeletal Videodisc Case 133.)

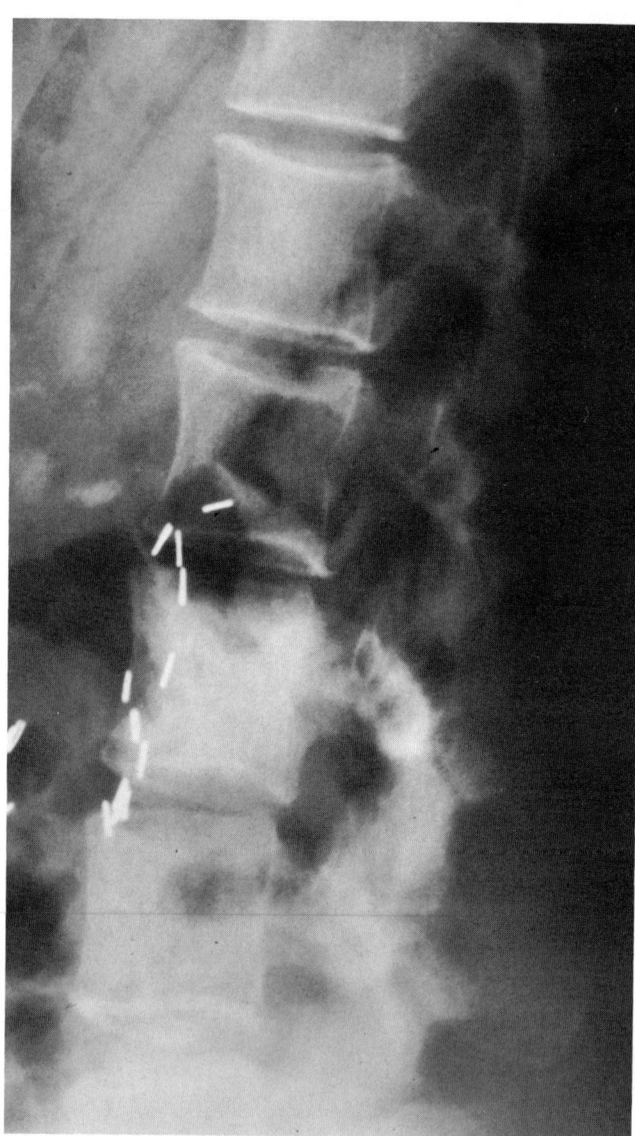

Figure 100–39. Hodgkin's disease. The dense but otherwise normal-appearing L3 vertebral body is typical of the "ivory body" that is characteristic of metastatic Hodgkin's disease. This patient is 29 years old. In an older patient, differential diagnosis of this ivory vertebral body would have included Paget's disease, breast or prostate carcinoma, carcinoid, and sarcoid. (Reprinted with permission from the ACR Learning File, Musculoskeletal Videodisc, Case 136.)

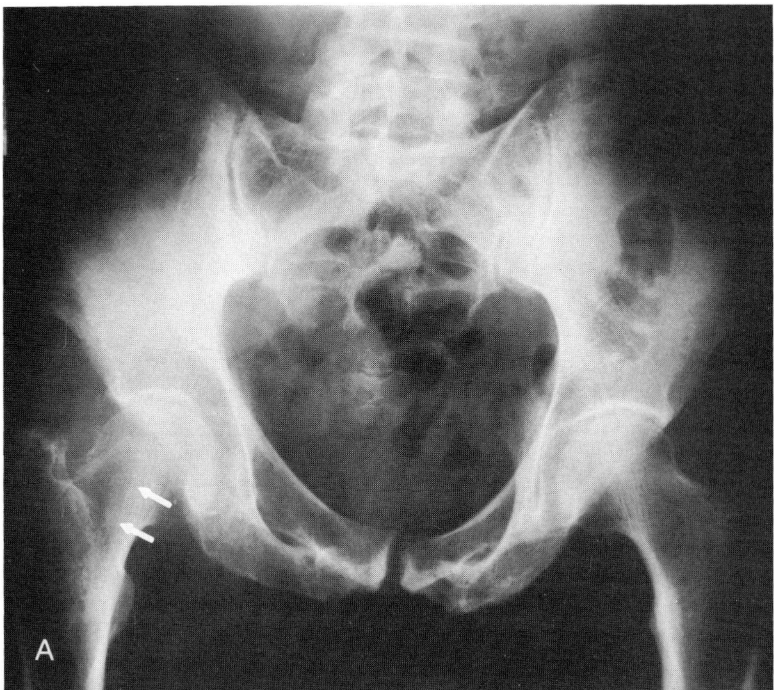

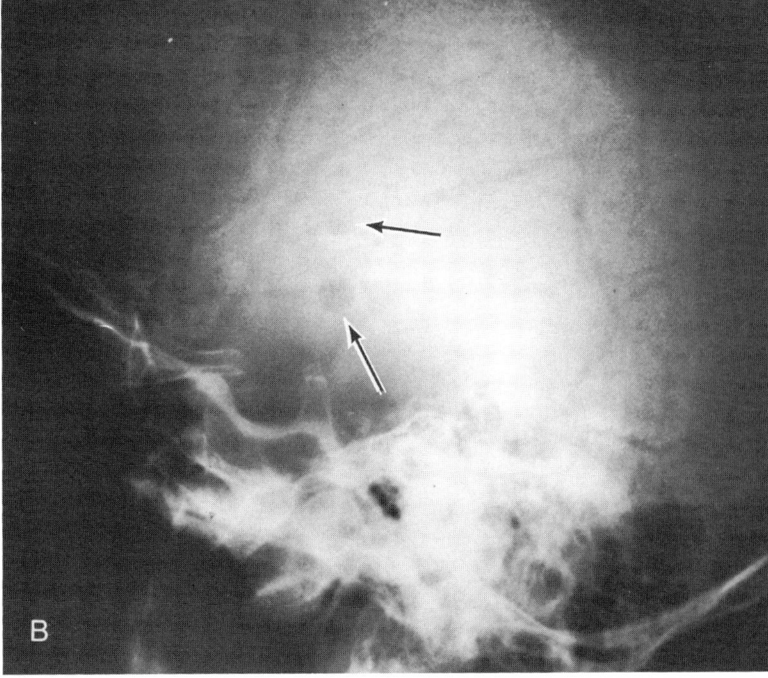

Figure 100–40. Multiple myeloma. The pelvis film *(A)* demonstrates a characteristic of multiple myeloma that can make it quite difficult to diagnose. The film very nearly appears normal. However, there are several areas in which we see fewer trabeculae than would be expected (right femoral neck [*arrows*] and right trochanteric region as well as the right sacral ala). Multiple myeloma can present as an osteopenic skeleton without clearly defined lytic lesions as in this case. However, the skull film *(B)* is much more typical of multiple myeloma, with the classic punched-out lytic lesions *(arrows)*. (*A* and *B* reprinted with permission from the ACR Learning File, Musculoskeletal Videodisc, Case 137.)

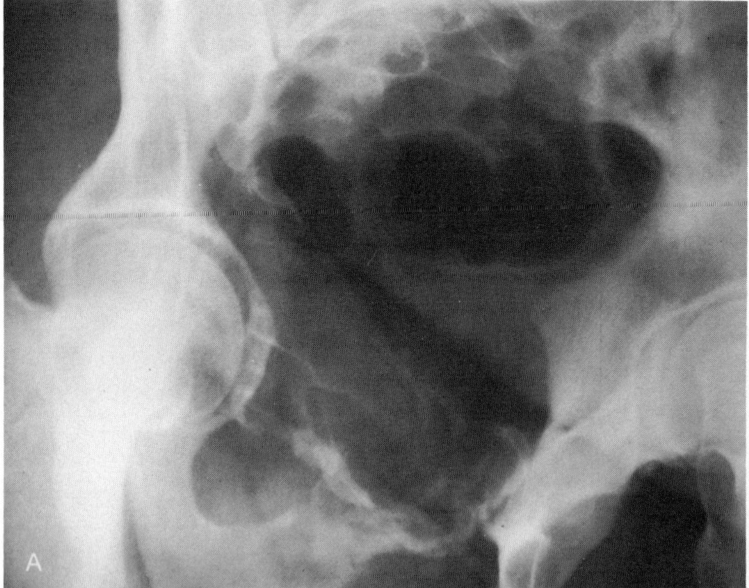

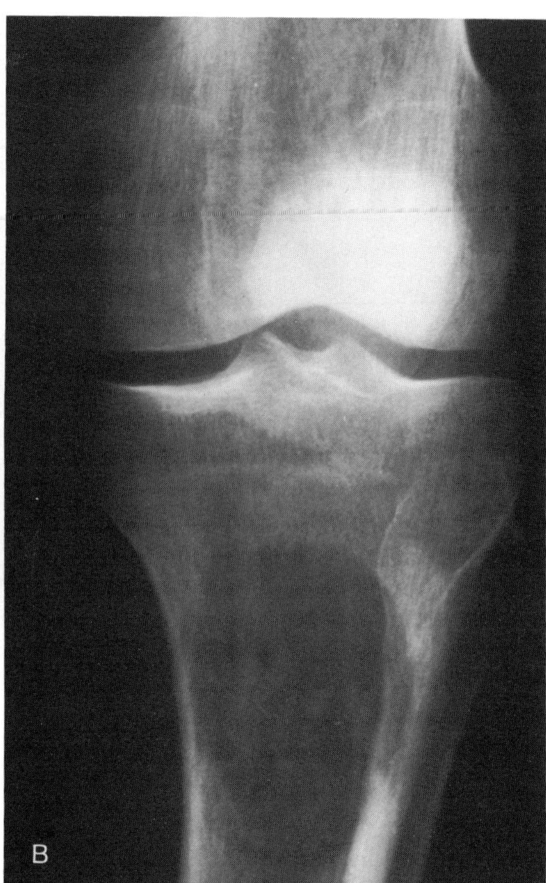

Figure 100–41. Plasmacytoma. *A* demonstrates a bubbly lesion involving both the ilium and superior pubic ramus. The lesion is expansile but does not show cortical breakthrough or a large soft-tissue mass. It is rather geographic. In this 32-year-old patient, plasmacytoma should be high on the differential list. Other moderately aggressive lesions might be considered, including low-grade chondrosarcoma or chondromyxofibroma. *B* demonstrates a different patient in which a large central metaphyseal lytic lesion is seen. The lesion is not well-marginated but has a narrow zone of transition. Plasmacytoma is a better choice in this case than giant cell tumor, since the epicenter is more metadiaphyseal than metaphyseal and the lesion does not approach the subarticular surface. (*A* reprinted with permission from the ACR Learning File, Musculoskeletal Videodisc, Case 138.)

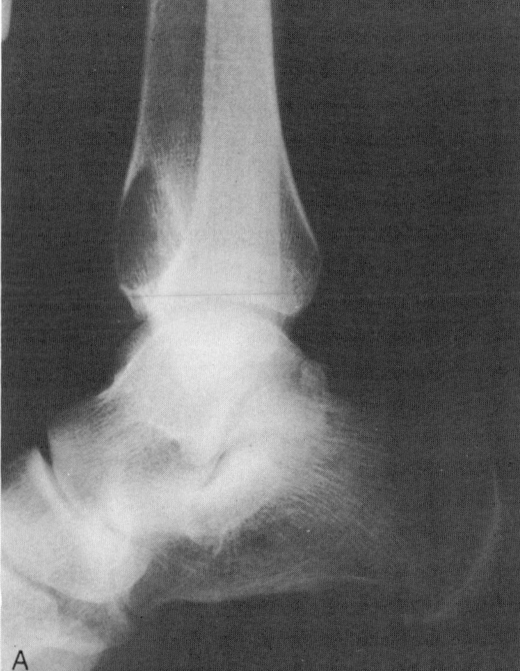

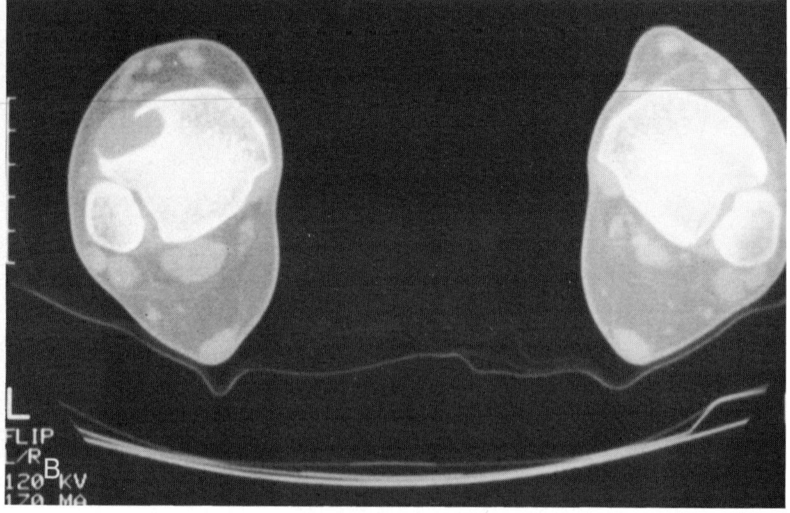

Figure 100–42. The plain film *(A)* demonstrates a classic giant cell tumor. The lesion is located in the distal tibial metaphysis of a patient who is just barely skeletally mature. Although it is metaphyseally based, it has now reached the subarticular region. The lesion is eccentrically located and is completely lytic. Although the zone of transition is narrow, there is no sclerotic margin. This unusual combination of characteristics is extremely helpful in diagnosing giant cell tumor since it occurs in almost no other lesion. The CT scan *(B)* confirms the relatively nonaggressive features of the lesion and the fact that it is not permeative. There is no soft-tissue mass beyond the faintly seen cortical rim. Note that the above-described features of giant cell tumor are quite characteristic by comparing them with the giant cell tumor seen in Figure 100–2*C*. (*A* and *B* reprinted with permission from the ACR Learning File, Musculoskeletal Videodisc, Case 128.)

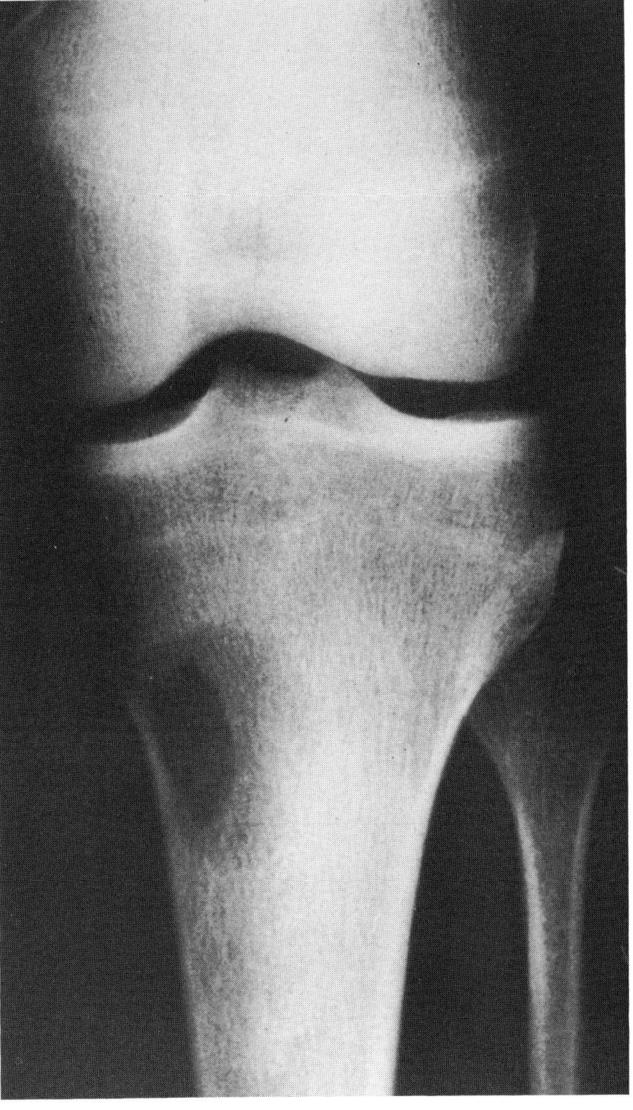

Figure 100–43. Giant cell tumor. This lytic lesion is located entirely within the metaphysis of the proximal tibia. It has a narrow zone of transition and no sclerotic margin. These features should lead us to the diagnosis of giant cell tumor. However, the lesion does not extend to the subarticular surface. This case underscores the fact that giant cell tumors arise in the metaphysis and then extend toward the subarticular region. The subarticular location therefore is a less important parameter than the others in diagnosing a giant cell tumor. (Reprinted with permission from the ACR Learning File, Musculoskeletal Videodisc, Case 129.)

logic fracture and may require palliative or preventative treatment. MRI is quite sensitive and may be helpful when one must resolve a discrepancy between bone scan and plain film results.

The prognosis for this disease process is poor, with a five-year survival rate of 10 per cent for multiple myeloma. Most patients with plasmacytoma go on to multifocal or generalized disease and have a five-year survival of 40 per cent. Chemotherapy and radiation therapy are the treatment modalities.

GIANT CELL TUMORS

B. J. Manaster

This lesion comprises 5 per cent of primary bone tumors and is very distinct radiographically. The most important determinants in this distinct appearance include age, location, and the pattern of zone of transition/margination. The lesion nearly always occurs after epiphyseal fusion, and most (70 per cent) fall between 20 and 40 years of age. Giant cell tumor is a geographic expanding lesion that arises eccentrically in the metaphysis of tubular bones. With growth, it extends to the subarticular end of the bone, involving the epiphysis as well as the metaphysis. The most commonly involved bones include the distal femur, proximal tibia, and distal radius (accounting for 65 per cent of cases). Although giant cell tumor does not commonly involve the spine, when it does the sacrum is the most commonly involved site and the body rather than the posterior elements is preferentially involved. Aside from age and location, the final important determinant in diagnosing giant cell tumor is the fact that these lesions usually have a narrow zone of transition but no sclerotic margin (Figs. 100–42 and 100–43; see Fig. 100–2*C*).

The initial diagnosis of giant cell tumor thus is usually easily made by plain film analysis. However, giant cell tumor can have a wide variety of behavior. Most of these lesions act as a mildly aggressive local tumor that has a high recurrence rate (50 to 60 per cent) when treated with curettage and bone graft (Fig. 100–44). However, giant cell tumors occasionally demonstrate a greater morbidity, and metastasize to the lung. These metastases very often show the same low-grade histologic pattern as the original lesion. Giant cell tumor may also occasionally become malignant, either primarily or secondarily (usually in lesions previously treated by radiation). Unfortunately, much of the literature demonstrates that one cannot reliably differentiate benign from malignant giant cell tumor or those lesions that will metastasize to the lung by either radiographic or histologic features alone. However, it might be noted that some giant cell tumors have clearly more locally aggres-

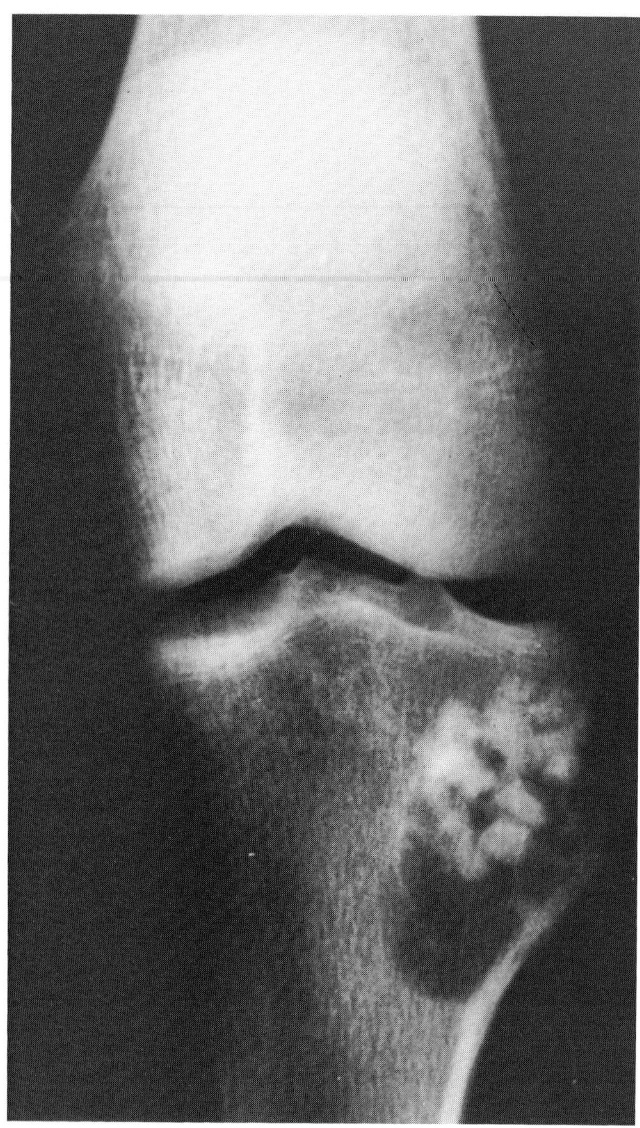

Figure 100–44. Recurrent giant cell tumor. Bone chips are seen in a lytic lesion located eccentrically in the proximal tibial metaphysis. The lesion has a narrow zone of transition and no sclerotic margin. It represents a recurrence of a typical giant cell tumor that had previously been curetted and bone-grafted. This treatment of giant cell tumors results in recurrence 50 to 60 per cent of the time.

sive features than others, including cortical breakthrough and soft-tissue mass (Fig. 100–45). There are now some authors who believe that these radiographic features, in conjunction with histologic features using the musculoskeletal tumor staging system, can predict the tumor's ultimate behavior and suggest appropriate treatment.

The above considerations suggest that curative treatments of giant cell tumor would be to regard each lesion as a low-grade malignant neoplasm and treat it with wide resection. This results in a lower recurrence rate (10 per cent). However, the subarticular nature of the lesion often would require resection of the joint to achieve a wide margin. This would require placement of a long-stemmed custom prosthesis or else fusion of the joint for limb salvage. Either of these procedures produces considerable morbidity in these relatively young patients. The currently accepted compromise in treating these patients is initial treatment with curettage and cryosurgery if wide resection is unacceptable because of subarticular location. With the use of cryosurgery and bone grafting, recurrence may be lower than the 55 per cent expected following simple curettage and bone graft. Radiation therapy is generally avoided because some series have demonstrated a higher-than-expected rate of radiation-induced sarcoma in giant cell tumor patients, thus implicating the lesion with being particularly susceptible to sarcomatous change following radiation.

OTHER TUMORS

B. J. Manaster

Vascular Tumors: Benign

HEMANGIOMA

Hemangiomas are the common benign vascular tumors that can be found in either soft tissues or bone. Hemangiomas are hamartomatous lesions composed of vascular channels. Soft-tissue hemangiomas are characterized on plain film by a mass and may contain calcified phleboliths (Fig. 100–46). By CT, a soft-tissue hemangioma is best seen with contrast enhancement and may have a characteristic "can of worms" appearance due to the tortuous dilated vessels. By MRI, the soft-tissue mass usually shows the slightly higher than muscle signal intensity on T_1 and hyperintense T_2 signal of most tumors. However, interdigitating lacy high signal characteristic of fat density is also seen in a high percentage of soft-tissue hemangiomas (Fig. 100–46). Although the underlying osseous structures are usually normal, soft-tissue hemangiomas may invade bone, giving an extrinsic scalloped appearance.

Intraosseous hemangiomas have a very characteristic location,

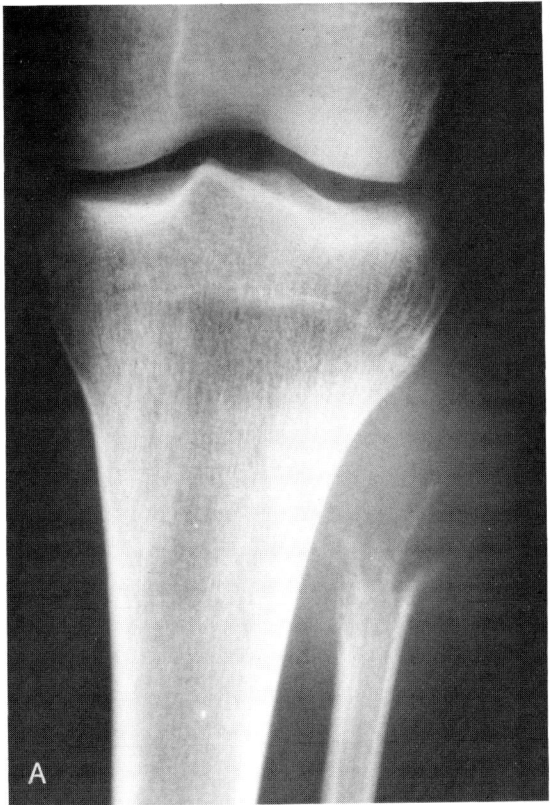

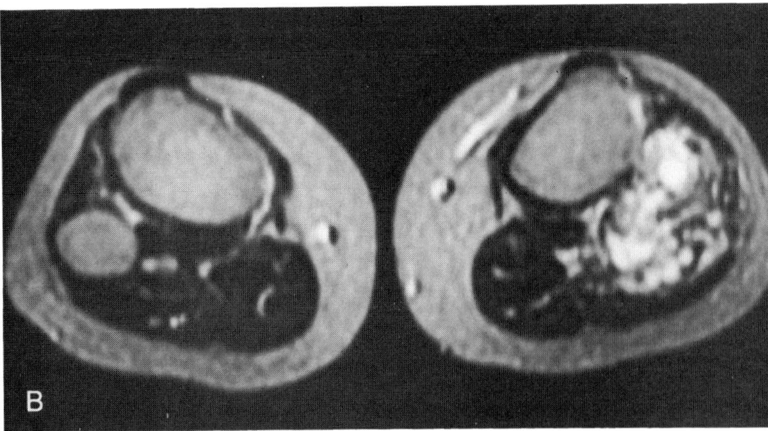

Figure 100–45. Aggressive giant cell tumor. The plain film *(A)* demonstrates a tremendously expanded lesion of the proximal fibula. The lesion extends all the way to the subarticular surface but has a fairly narrow zone of transition and no sclerotic margin. The T_2-weighted MRI *(B)* suggests that the lesion is more aggressive than the usual giant cell tumor, demonstrating highly abnormal osseous tissues as well as what appears to be a large soft-tissue mass surrounding the fibula. Reactive changes extend into both the anterior and posterior compartments. Although this appears to be a highly aggressive giant cell tumor radiographically, it was benign at pathology. The case serves as a nice reminder that giant cell tumors may behave somewhat independent of either their histologic or radiographic appearance. Because of the radiographically aggressive appearance and the fibular location, wide resection rather than curettage was elected. (From Manaster BJ, et al: Giant cell tumor of bone. Radiol Clin North Am 31(2):303, 1993.)

with the vast majority located in vertebral bodies, and most others in the skull and facial bones. In addition to the location, the radiographic appearance is usually characteristic as well. In the vertebral bodies there is a coarsened vertical trabecular pattern that develops without collapse (Fig. 100–47). In the skull there are also coarsened trabeculae but they radiate in a sunburst pattern from a normal inner table to an expanded outer table of the cranium. Occasionally an epidural soft-tissue mass may develop in a vertebral body lesion. MRI is characteristic, with a high signal intensity in T_1- as well as T_2-weighted images, and defines the epidural extent well.

OTHER BENIGN ANGIOMATOUS LESIONS

Lymphangiomas represent hamartomatous lesions consisting of dilated lymphatic vessels. These intraosseous lesions may be geographic or moth-eaten and do not have other characteristic appearances. Lymphangiomatosis is a form of lymphangioma with multiple skeletal lesions, lymphedema, and a chylous pleural effusion. Cystic angiomatosis is a rare, more aggressive lesion of multicentric hemangiomatosis or lymphangiomatosis, often with severe visceral involvement. Multiple expanded aggressive-appearing lesions, associated with phleboliths in the soft tissues, will suggest this diagnosis. Another extremely aggressive form of angiomatosis is seen with massive osteolysis or Gorham's disease. These patients usually give a history of trauma and radiographically demonstrate rapid dissolution of bone, spreading contiguously across joints.

Vascular Tumors: Malignant

The most common malignant vascular tumor is angiosarcoma. The lesion has a radiographically aggressive appearance, with permeative osseous destruction. It is usually found in a metaphyseal location. One characteristic that may help suggest the lesion is that approximately 40 percent of angiosarcomas are polyostotic. Furthermore, the polyostotic lesions may be regional in distribution (Fig. 100–48). Angiosarcomas are highly malignant, with five-year survival ranging from 30 to 50 percent, and metastasize to the lungs or skeleton. Interestingly, the prognosis appears to be slightly better if the lesion is multifocal at presentation.

Hemangiopericytomas and hemangioendotheliomas are vascular lesions that may be either benign or low-grade malignant lesions. As with the other vascular lesions, they may arise in either the soft tissues or skeleton. They may be multicentric, often within a single extremity. No other distinctive radiographic features apply.

Other Connective Tissue Tumors: Benign

FIBROMATOSES

The fibromatoses are a heterogeneous group of lesions that have been described with a variety of terms and classifications but are characterized by a similar histology. Fibromatosis is usually a soft-tissue lesion. One of the more radiographically distinct types is the juvenile aponeurotic fibroma. This is a slowly infiltrative lesion that arises in the aponeurotic tissue of the hands (palm), wrist, and feet (plantar aspect). The lesion is slowly but relentlessly locally infiltrative. It may deform the osseous structures, and calcifications may be seen in the interosseous membrane (Fig. 100–49). As with all fibromatoses, recurrence after resection is common.

The most common type of fibromatosis is the desmoid tumor, also termed *aggressive fibromatosis.* Although benign, this lesion shows aggressive local infiltration of adjacent compartments, muscles, vessels, nerves, and tendons. No pseudocapsule is formed; therefore, these lesions can present an even more aggressive and infiltrative appearance on imaging studies than most malignant tumors (Fig. 100–49). Because of this characteristic, it should not be surprising that the post-resection recurrence rate of aggressive fibromatosis is very high (65 to 75 per cent). Osseous involvement with aggressive fibromatosis is rare, but pressure erosion of the cortex may be seen (Fig. 100–49), and very impressive spiculated periosteal reaction has been described.

Text continued on page 1544

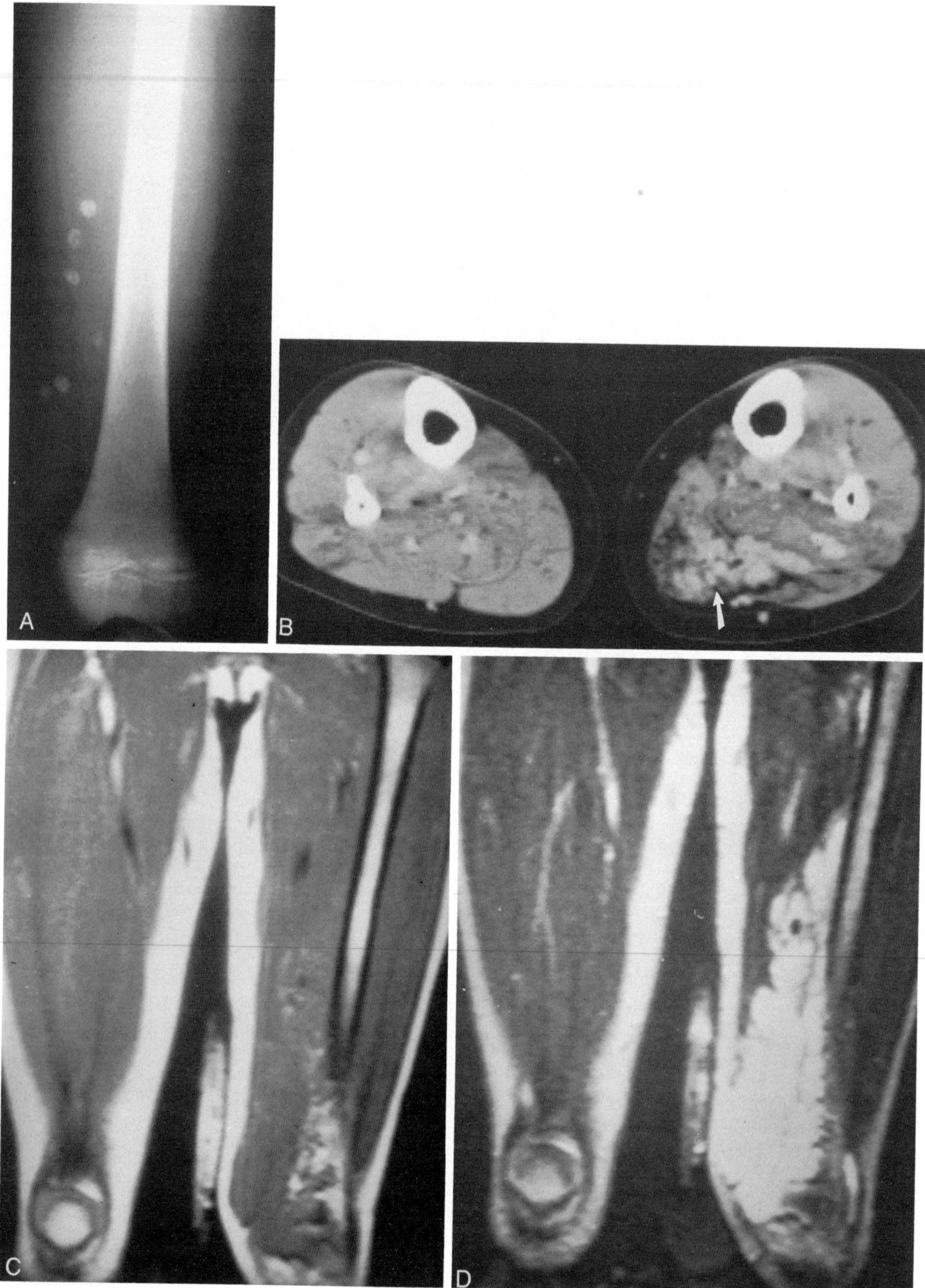

Figure 100–46. Soft-tissue hemangioma. *A* demonstrates a soft-tissue mass in the thigh of a skeletally immature patient. The mass has dense calcifications within it. The calcifications are round, and some have a central lucency. These are characteristic of phleboliths and help make the diagnosis of hemangioma. In this case, there is no involvement with the underlying bone. *B* is a CT scan of a soft-tissue hemangioma in a different patient. Intravenous contrast outlines nicely the tubular structures with the "can of worms" appearance within the medial head of the gastrocnemius muscle *(arrows)*. This is a characteristic CT appearance. *C* and *D* are the T_1 and T_2 coronal MR images, respectively, of the hemangioma shown by plain film in 46*A*. The T_1 image demonstrates the bulk of the mass to be isointense with the surrounding muscle, but the lesion is of high signal on T_2 imaging. However, note the interdigitating lacy pattern that follows fat signal that can be so characteristic of hemangiomas. This is, of course, best seen on the T_1 image. (*A, C,* and *D* courtesy of Mark Kransdorf, M.D., AFIP; reprinted with permission from the ACR Learning File, Musculoskeletal Videodisc, Case 140.)

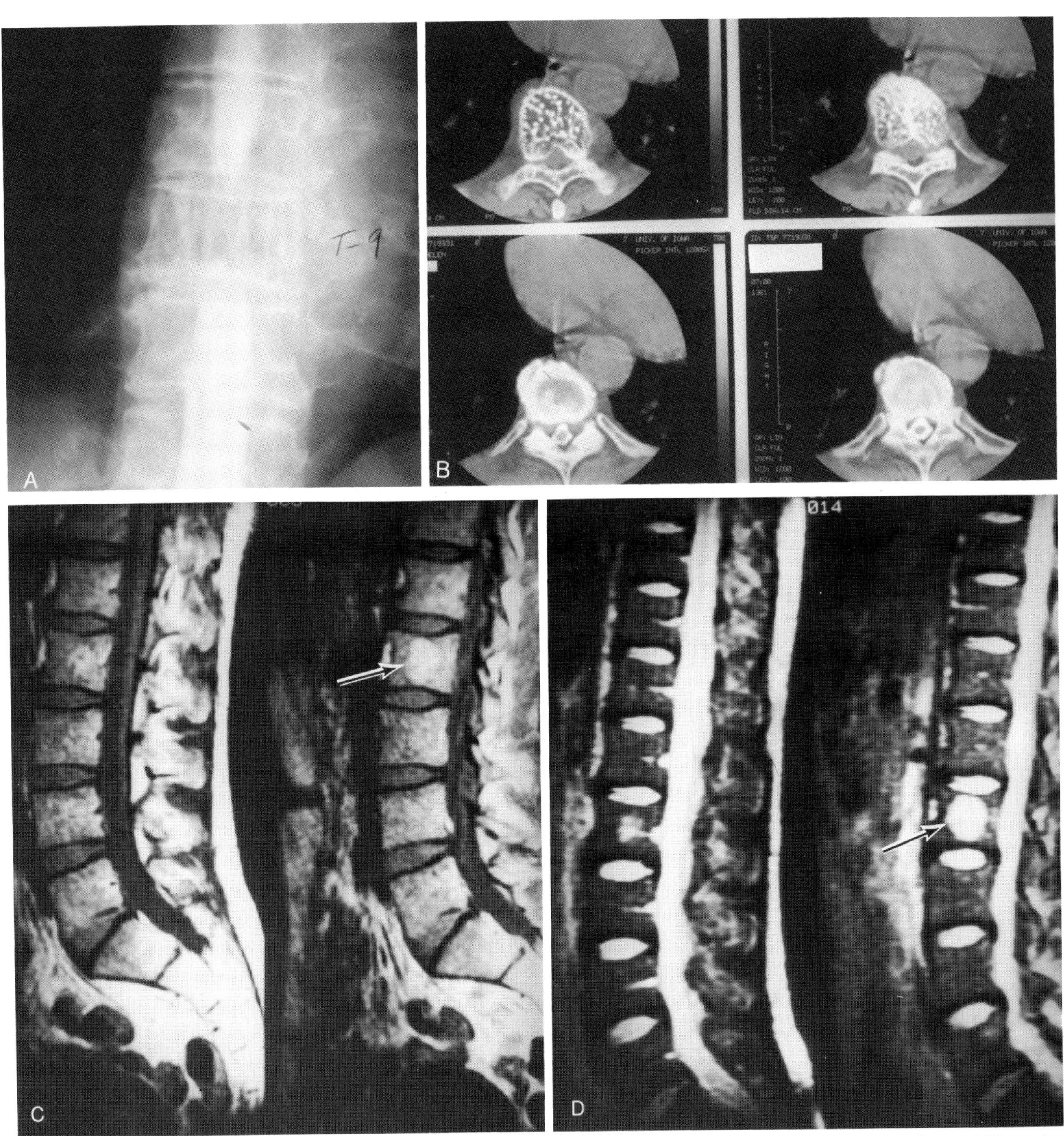

Figure 100–47. Vertebral body hemangioma. *A* is a plain film in a patient who has had a myelogram. It demonstrates an abnormal T9 vertebral body with coarse vertical striations throughout. This is a typical plain film appearance of hemangioma. Additionally, there is an incomplete block of metrizamide at this level. The CT myelogram *(B)* redemonstrates the coarsened trabeculae of the vertebral body. In addition, there is an epidural mass present that is not well-defined since the metrizamide has not surrounded the cord at this level. You might compare the abnormal vertebral body appearance with the normal at the next level *(lower right hand image)*. *C* and *D* are T_1 and T_2 images, respectively, of a different patient. They demonstrate a typical hemangioma in the body of L2 that is of higher signal intensity than the surrounding bone on both T_1 and T_2 imaging *(arrows)*. These characteristics are unlike most other osseous lesions. In this case, the hemangioma was an incidental finding, since the patient did not experience pain at this site and there is no evidence of epidural extension. (Case loaned by Wendy RK Smoker, M.D.; reprinted with permission from the ACR Learning File, Musculoskeletal Videodisc, Case 139.)

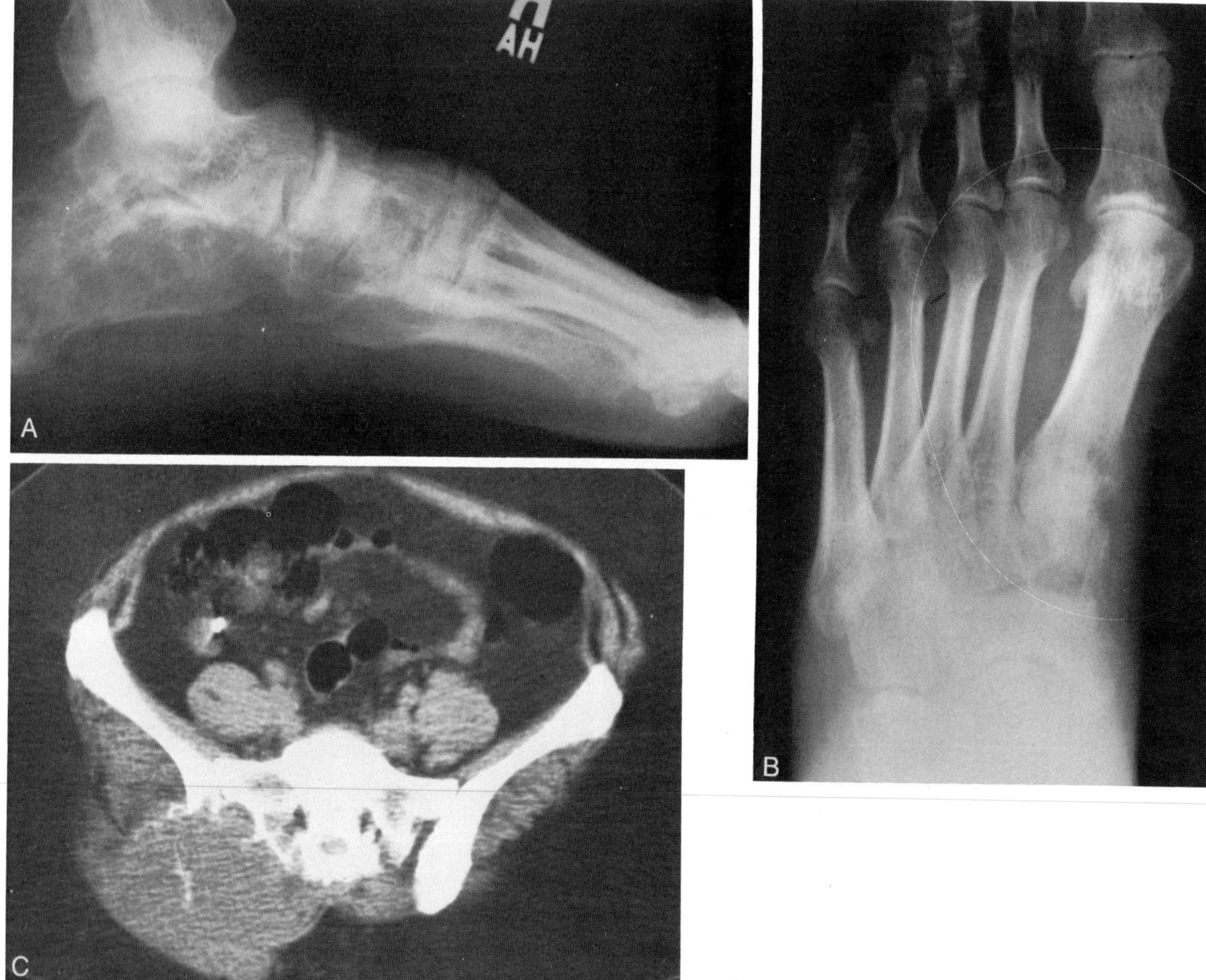

Figure 100–48. Angiosarcoma. *A* and *B* demonstrate the lateral and AP films, respectively, of the involved foot. There is a truly moth-eaten pattern involving the calcaneus, talus, cuboid, and medial cuneiform. It might be tempting to suggest that this represents disuse osteoporosis! However, note that the metatarsals are of normal density and therefore that diagnosis cannot be supported. This is a polyostotic vascular lesion, which is more commonly seen in the lower limb than elsewhere in the body. *C* is a CT scan of a different patient with a solitary angiosarcoma. This large destructive lesion originated in the posterior aspect of the right iliac wing and involves the sacrum by contiguous extent. The density within the mass is residual bone from the destroyed iliac wing and does not represent a calcific matrix. There are no specific findings to help identify this highly destructive lesion as an angiosarcoma.

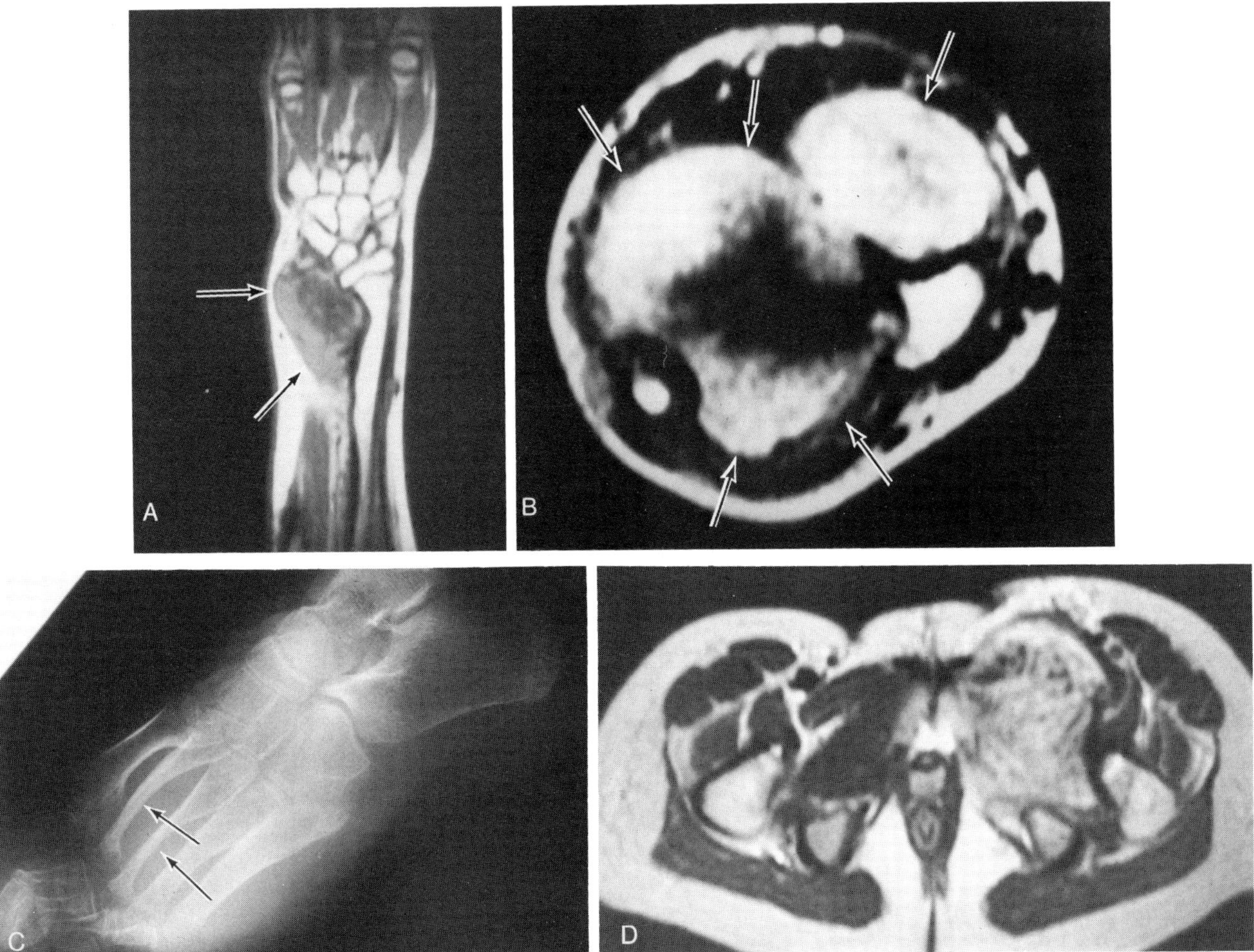

Figure 100–49. Fibromatosis. *A* and *B* demonstrate an MRI of juvenile aponeurotic fibromatosis. The coronal T_1 view nicely demonstrates the large inhomogeneous mass in the interosseous membrane *(arrows)*. The axial T_2 view demonstrates the tremendous size of the mass *(arrows)*, which pushes the flexor and extensor tendons away without apparent involvement. The mass is quite inhomogeneous, a feature that has been suggested to relate to malignancy. However, fibromatosis is well known to produce such an aggressive, large, inhomogeneous appearance. Note that the osseous structures are scalloped and deformed rather than destroyed. This gives a nice hint that the lesion is in fact somewhat slow-growing and only locally aggressive. *C* shows a different patient with aggressive fibromatosis (desmoid tumor). There is an extremely large soft-tissue mass of the foot that has caused extensive scalloping of metatarsals two, three, and four *(arrows)*. This patient has already had multiple soft-tissue tumor resections and has now developed another recurrence. Finally, *D* demonstrates another patient with aggressive fibromatosis. This large inhomogeneous mass arises in the adductor muscle but extends into the obturator muscles through the obturator foramen. Such spread across compartments is highly typical of this kind of desmoid tumor, as is the extremely high recurrence rate. (*A* and *B* reprinted with permission from the ACR Learning File, Musculoskeletal Videodisc, Case 144; *D* from Case 143.)

Desmoplastic fibroma is a very rare form of fibromatosis that is intraosseous. The lesions are usually central and metaphyseal and may present as either mildly or moderately aggressive osseous lesions. They may be difficult to differentiate both radiographically and histologically from a well-differentiated fibrosarcoma.

LIPOMA

Soft-tissue lipomas are extremely common tumors arising from fatty tissues. Most are subcutaneous and easily palpable, but some may be inter- or intramuscular, presenting a greater clinical diagnostic challenge. By plain film or CT, soft-tissue lipomas are radiolucent (fat tissue density) and well-defined. MRI characteristically shows a sharply bordered lesion with signal intensity mirroring that of subcutaneous fat (Fig. 100–50).

Osseous lipomas are rare, but very characteristic. They present as a lytic lesion with a distinct, fine sclerotic margin and no host reaction. They are usually of fat density by CT or MRI, and often have a central calcified nidus (Fig. 100–51). They are metaphyseal lesions, and are most commonly seen in the proximal femur or the calcaneus.

Other Connective Tissue Tumors: Malignant

MALIGNANT FIBROUS HISTIOCYTOMA (MFH)/FIBROSARCOMA

Although fibrosarcoma and MFH usually can be distinguished histologically, there are no distinctive radiographic features. They will be described together. Either MFH or fibrosarcoma may originate in the skeleton, producing usually an aggressive sarcoma, or in the soft tissues, where it may be either low grade or highly aggressive. MFH is the most common soft-tissue sarcoma in adults. It may have a deceptively benign appearance because like many soft-tissue sarcomas it may develop a reactive pseudocapsule that makes it appear encapsulated on CT, MRI, and at surgery (Fig. 100–52*A*). It is important to remember this characteristic, and not be misled into interpreting or treating the lesion as a nonaggressive one: Tumor cells invariably are found outside the margin of the reactive pseudocapsule. MFH follows the typical tumor signal intensity on MRI, and does not have distinguishing features other than its common occurrence.

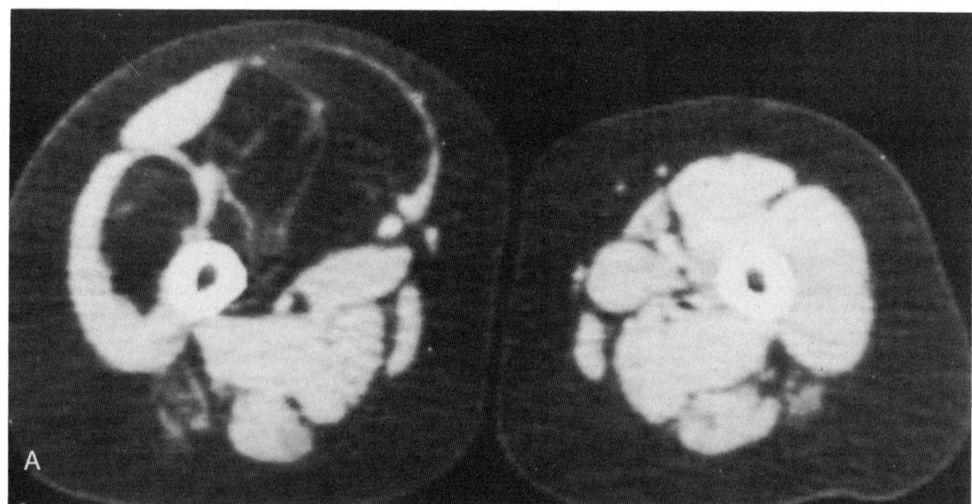

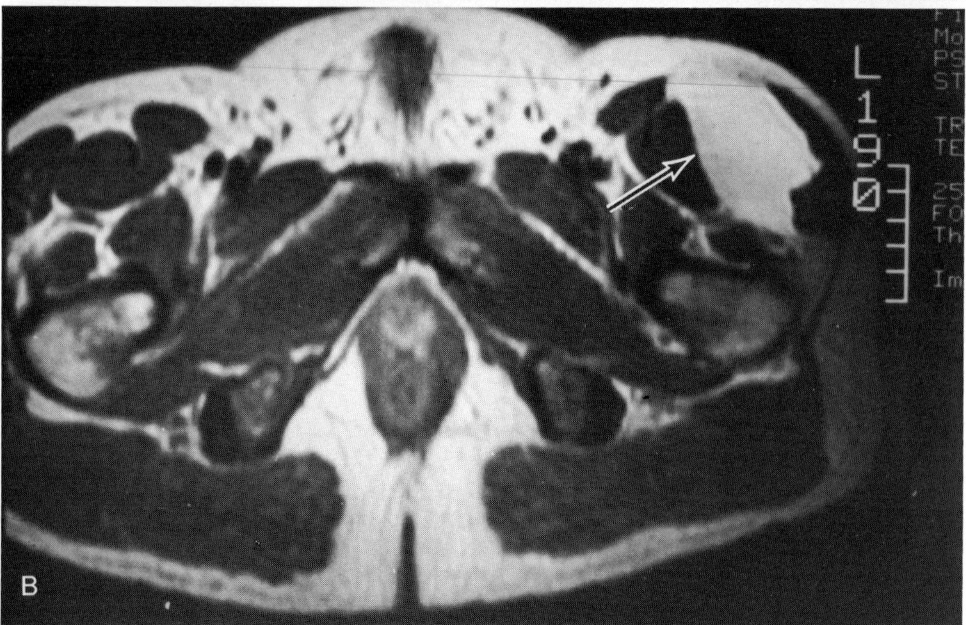

Figure 100–50. Lipoma. *A* is a CT scan of a large intermuscular lipoma that involves the vastus medialis, vastus lateralis, and vastus intermedius. There is obvious fat density (mirroring that of the subcutaneous fat). No cellular areas are seen within it to suggest that a portion might represent liposarcoma. *B* also demonstrates an intermuscular lipoma *(arrow)*. This is just one of the several sequences that showed this anterior thigh lesion following the signal intensity of subcutaneous fat. It is entirely homogeneous, and there is no question that it represents anything other than lipoma. (*B* reprinted with permission from the ACR Learning File, Musculoskeletal Videodisc, Case 147.)

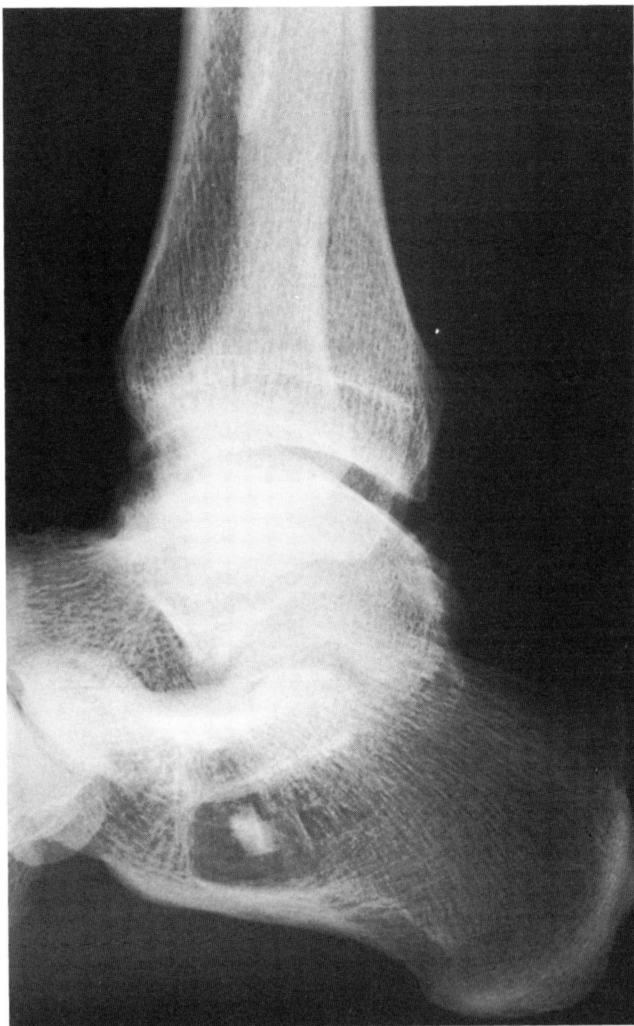

Figure 100–51. Intraosseous lipoma. This is a classic appearance for intraosseous lipoma, with a lytic lesion involving the neck of the calcaneus. Within this lesion, there is a calcific density. Both the location and the appearance are typical for intraosseous lipoma. CT would show fat density within the lesion.

Osseous fibrosarcomas and MFH may be primary bone tumors or may arise secondarily. The secondary lesions may result from previous radiation, Paget's disease degeneration, or dedifferentiation from a chondrosarcoma. MFH may, in addition, arise in a bone infarct. Osseous MFH/fibrosarcomas present as a permeative diametaphyseal lesion, usually in the long tubular bones. Dystrophic calcification may be present, as may serpiginous calcification from residual portions of bone infarcts that have degenerated to MFH (Fig. 100–52*B*). No other distinguishing characteristics are seen in this aggressive osseous lesion. These lesions occur most commonly in the 30- to 60-year age range, and the reasonable differential diagnosis includes chondrosarcoma and lymphoma, representing the other aggressive lesions usually seen in this age range. Five-year survival is poor (25 to 50 per cent if the lesion is high grade), and metastatic lesions are found predominantly in the lung parenchyma and in bone.

LIPOSARCOMA

Soft-tissue liposarcoma is the second most common soft-tissue sarcoma. It may either be well-differentiated or high grade. Consequently, on CT or MRI, it may have fat density of signal intensity if the lesion is well-differentiated. However, a higher grade lesion is more cellular and more often of nonspecific soft-tissue density or signal intensity (Fig. 100–53). Thus a liposarcoma most commonly does not have distinguishing characteristics radiographically. Like soft-tissue MFH, liposarcomas often elicit reactive pseudocapsule formation. This is easily misinterpreted as true encapsulation. If the lesion is "shelled out," there is invariably residual tumor at the margins; recurrence with this marginal type of excision is common and prognosis is poor, with metastatic disease to the lungs and viscera.

Liposarcomas most commonly occur in the buttocks, thigh, and lower leg. The common occurrence of liposarcoma and MFH in the soft tissues of adults should be appreciated and these lesions should be strongly considered when a soft-tissue mass in the extremities is encountered.

Synovial Cell Sarcoma

Synovial cell sarcoma is a soft-tissue sarcoma of synovial origin. However, it need not occur in a joint capsule because it may arise in synovial tissues associated with tendons, tendon sheaths, and bursi. Synovial sarcomas occur most commonly in the age range of 15 to 35 years and are most commonly located in the lower extremity, especially about the knee. Like other soft-tissue sarcomas, the radiographic appearance is not specific, especially since a misleading pseudocapsule may be seen. Besides the characteristic age and location of the lesion, these sarcomas are characterized by the presence of dystrophic calcification (20 to 30 per cent) (Fig. 100–54). Dystrophic calcification may be seen in the other soft-tissue sarcomas but at a much less significant rate.

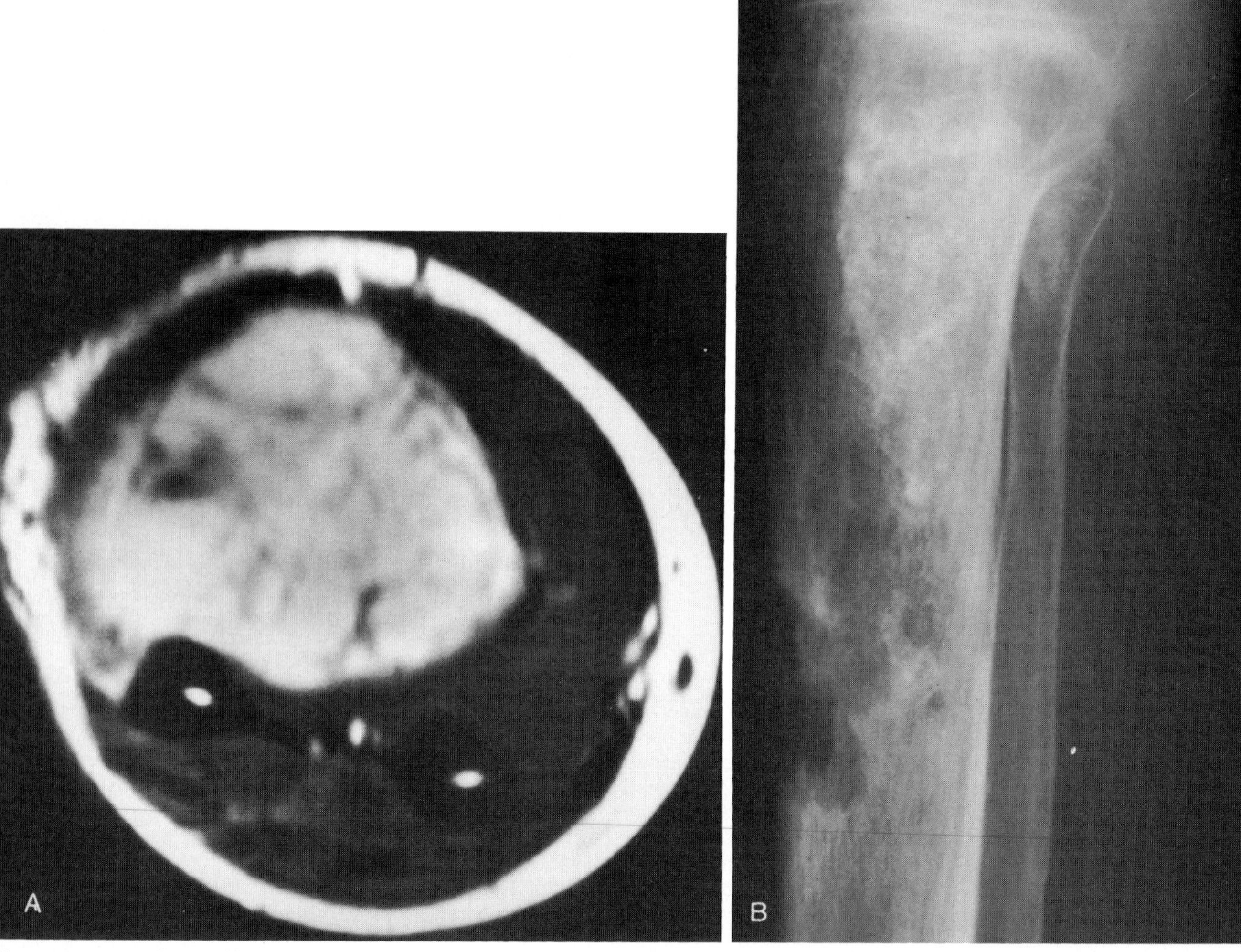

Figure 100–52. Malignant fibrous histiocytoma (MFH). Soft-tissue MFH is the most common sarcoma in the adult population. *A* demonstrates a typical soft-tissue MFH, with a large mass in the volar aspect of the forearm. There is high signal intensity on T_2-weighting, and the mass is rather inhomogeneous. Although it does appear in some areas to have a pseudocapsule, in others it appears more locally aggressive. Although there are no definite characteristics to help suggest the diagnosis, the statistical likelihood of either MFH or liposarcoma is high. *B* demonstrates an osseous MFH. The plain film shows an extremely destructive lytic lesion in the proximal diaphysis of the tibia. This lesion is associated with a small soft-tissue mass. More interestingly, it appears contiguous with a less aggressive lesion that contains a serpiginous cartilaginous calcification. Thus, this lesion should represent either a chondrosarcoma arising from an enchondroma or MFH arising in an infarct. Biopsy proved the latter diagnosis. (*A* reprinted with permission from the ACR Learning File, Musculoskeletal Videodisc, Case 152; *B* from Case 150.)

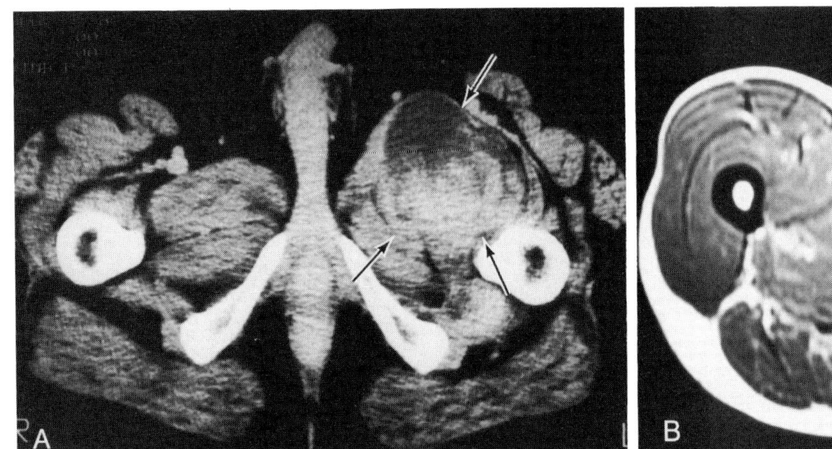

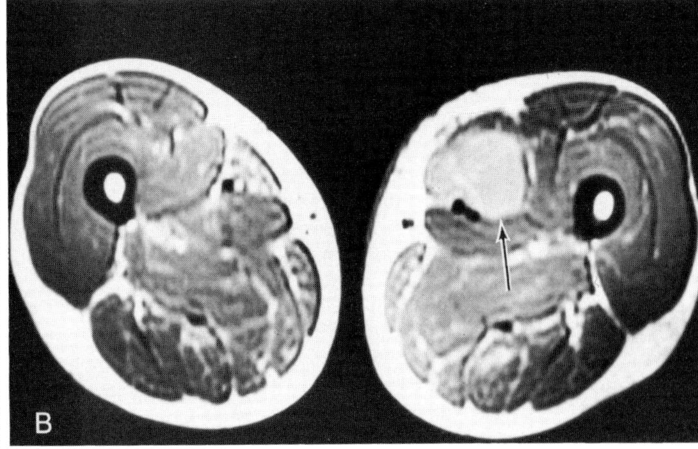

Figure 100–53. Liposarcoma. *A* is a CT of a liposarcoma involving the left adductor muscles. There is inhomogeneous contrast enhancement within the mass *(arrows)*. Although there is some low signal intensity within the mass, this is not sufficient to suggest a fatty tumor, as other sarcomas can contain necrotic areas. This was a high-grade liposarcoma and contains too many cellular areas to demonstrate the differentiated fat tissue that might be seen in lower-grade lesions. *B* is an MRI of a different patient with a liposarcoma of the thigh *(arrow)*. Again, fat signal is not a characteristic of liposarcoma. The lesion is a common one and therefore should be readily suspected when a soft-tissue mass is discovered, especially in the thigh and buttocks area. (*A* reprinted with permission from the ACR Learning File, Musculoskeletal Videodisc, Case 148.)

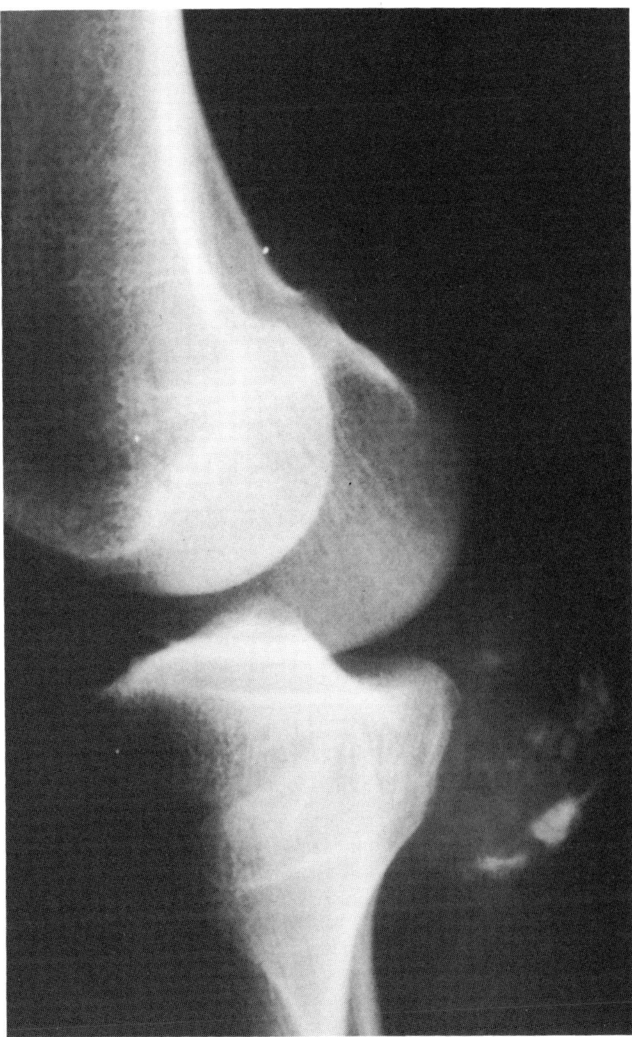

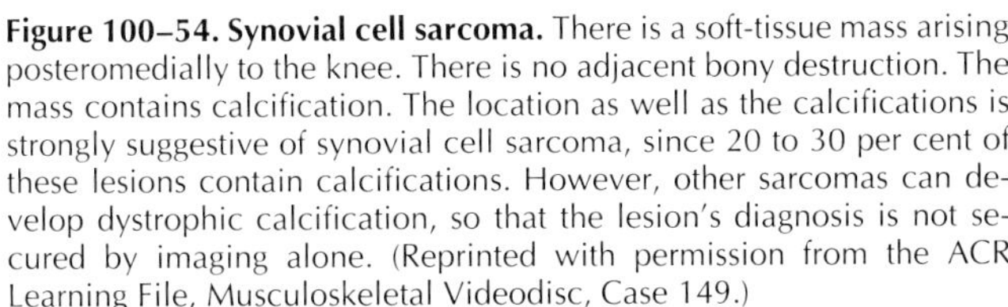
Figure 100–54. Synovial cell sarcoma. There is a soft-tissue mass arising posteromedially to the knee. There is no adjacent bony destruction. The mass contains calcification. The location as well as the calcifications is strongly suggestive of synovial cell sarcoma, since 20 to 30 per cent of these lesions contain calcifications. However, other sarcomas can develop dystrophic calcification, so that the lesion's diagnosis is not secured by imaging alone. (Reprinted with permission from the ACR Learning File, Musculoskeletal Videodisc, Case 149.)

Chordoma

Chordoma is a low-grade malignant neuroplasm that arises from notochordal remnants. Because of its tissue of origin, it is found only in the spine. Fifty per cent of chordomas are found in the sacrum (conversely, 30 per cent of sacral tumors are chordomas). Thirty-five per cent of chordomas are located in the clivus. The remaining 25 per cent are located in the spine. Within these structures, the epicenter of a chordoma is found in the posterior portion of the body rather than the posterior elements, again relating to the position of the notochord.

Chordomas are locally aggressive lesions. However, although extensive local bone destruction and soft-tissue mass are seen, the time course is often so slow that the lesion acquires a sclerotic rim and has a narrow zone of transition, making it appear radiographically less aggressive. The soft-tissue mass may be large, extending anteriorly into the pelvis from the sacrum or posteriorly from a vertebral body with epidural compression (Fig. 100–55).

Because of the location in the posterior vertebral bodies, differential diagnosis includes multiple myeloma and metastatic disease. If a chordoma does not appear terribly aggressive, giant cell tumor might also be considered in the differential diagnosis.

Twenty-five per cent of chordomas develop metastases to the lung, but these often occur very late in the disease process. More commonly, the patient has significant morbidity and mortality from local recurrence (80 per cent if only marginal resection is accomplished) and associated complications.

TUMOR-LIKE LESIONS

Carol L. Andrews

A number of bony lesions may be mistaken for primary tumors of bone even though they are not true neoplasms. By following the

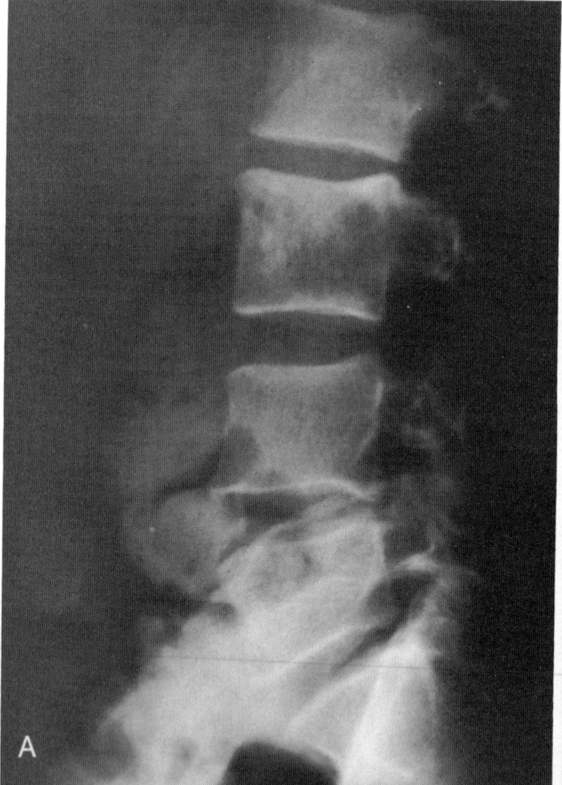

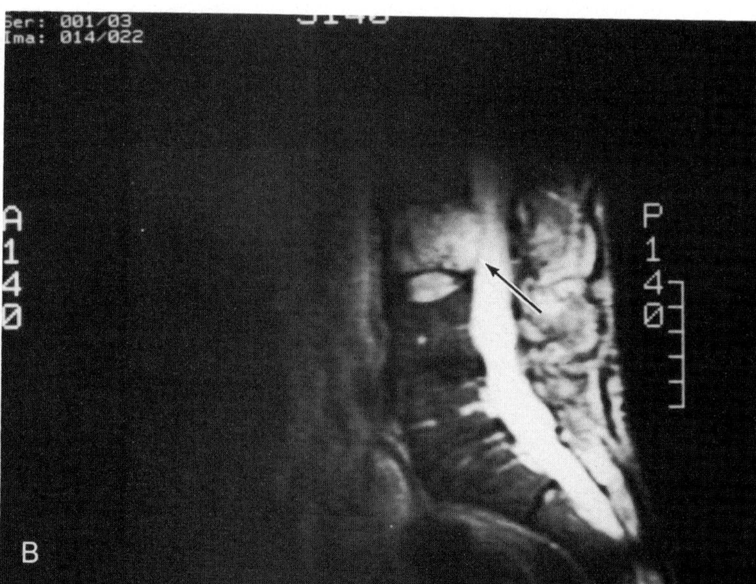

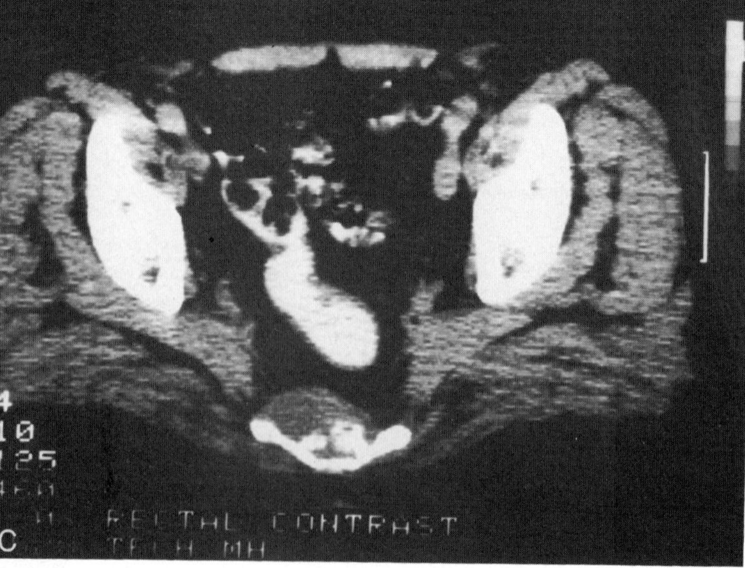

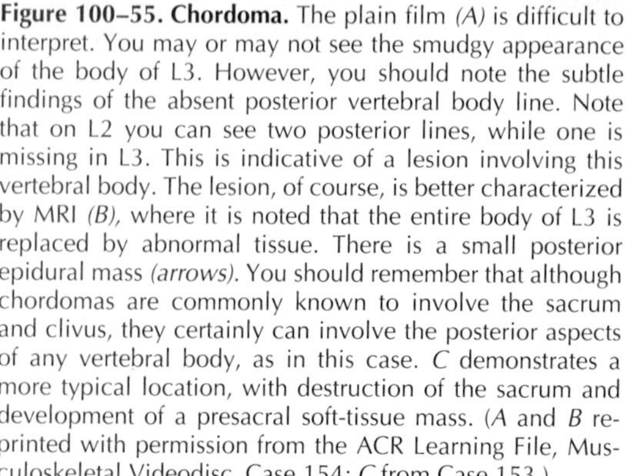

Figure 100–55. Chordoma. The plain film *(A)* is difficult to interpret. You may or may not see the smudgy appearance of the body of L3. However, you should note the subtle findings of the absent posterior vertebral body line. Note that on L2 you can see two posterior lines, while one is missing in L3. This is indicative of a lesion involving this vertebral body. The lesion, of course, is better characterized by MRI *(B),* where it is noted that the entire body of L3 is replaced by abnormal tissue. There is a small posterior epidural mass *(arrows).* You should remember that although chordomas are commonly known to involve the sacrum and clivus, they certainly can involve the posterior aspects of any vertebral body, as in this case. *C* demonstrates a more typical location, with destruction of the sacrum and development of a presacral soft-tissue mass. (*A* and *B* reprinted with permission from the ACR Learning File, Musculoskeletal Videodisc, Case 154; *C* from Case 153.)

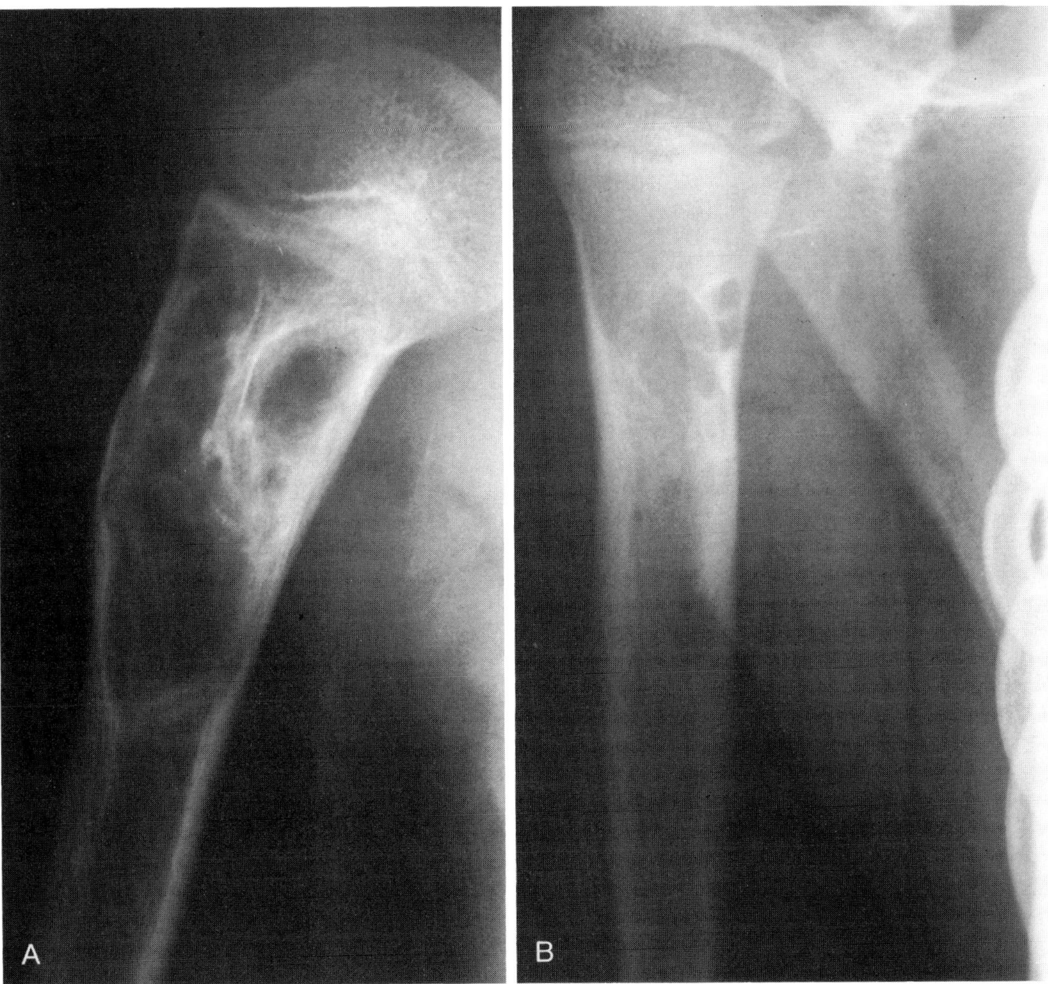

Figure 100–56. *A,* Classic findings of a solitary bone cyst (SBC) are well-demonstrated on a plain film of this lytic, metaphyseal humerus lesion, which is mildly expansile. A pathologic fracture disrupts the cortex in the mid-lateral portion of the lesion. *B,* A film, taken nine months later, demonstrates healing of the proximal portion of the SBC with "migration" of the lesion away from the metaphysis, indicating that the lesion is no longer active and normal bone growth is continuing.

standard format presented in the first section of this chapter, one may effectively identify the characteristics of these lesions and characterize them as nonaggressive or aggressive.

Solitary Bone Cyst

The solitary bone cyst (SBC) is a common benign cystic lesion of childhood, occurring most commonly between ages 3 and 19 (approximately 85 per cent of all SBCs). This well-circumscribed, fusiform, central geographic lesion is also known as a simple or unicameral bone cyst and may be clinically identified when a pathologic fracture occurs, resulting in sudden onset of pain. The unilocular cavity, lined with fibrous tissue, is filled with a serous to serosanguineous fluid unless a recent fracture has occurred, resulting in hemorrhage into the cystic cavity.

The SBC, which usually is 5 cm or greater, is found most commonly in the metaphysis of long bones including the proximal humerus (60 per cent) and the proximal femur (25 per cent). The lesion arises adjacent to the growth plate (Fig. 100–56) and may appear to migrate into the diaphysis during the patient's continued growth. Such "migration" represents normal growth away from a usually inactive lesion. SBCs are mildly expansile with variable cortical thinning. However, the cortex remains intact without evidence of host reaction unless a fracture is sustained. Periosteal reaction, appropriate to fracture healing, will then be identifiable (see Fig. 100–4*A*). A fragment of the cortex may (rarely) be identified within the lesion after a fracture and represents the "fallen fragment" sign—a fracture fragment having "fallen" to the bottom of the cavity.

Surgical treatment of SBCs with curettage and bone graft has a recurrence rate of 35 to 50 per cent. Recurrence is twice as likely in a patient younger than 10 years of age than in an older patient. Intralesional injection of steroids has shown about the same results. A significant proportion of SBCs will spontaneously heal, especially following pathologic fractures. It should be noted that surgery performed close to an open growth plate risks acceleration or arrest of growth.

Aneurysmal Bone Cyst

Up to 50 per cent of aneurysmal bone cysts (ABCs) are believed to be a reparative effort related to some bony lesion, such as trauma or an underlying neoplastic process (e.g., chondroblastoma, fibrous dysplasia, osteosarcoma), that has gone awry, resulting in an osseous vascular malformation. This rapidly expansile lesion histologically resembles a sponge with a fibrous or fibro-osseous latticework and blood-filled interstices.

Occurring most commonly in patients younger than 20 years of age (over 85 per cent of the time), ABCs involve long bones (50 per cent) and posterior spine elements (15 per cent). They range in size from 2 to 25 cm with an average size of 5 to 10 cm. In long bones, the lesion is metaphyseal and eccentrically located. Patients will frequently present with pain and/or swelling related to the lesion itself or an associated pathologic fracture. In the spine, it involves the posterior elements (Fig. 100–57) much more frequently than vertebral bodies. Clinically, these patients may present with neurologic complaints as nerve roots are compressed.

This geographic, lytic lesion has a narrow zone of transition and no tumor matrix. It may appear multilocular or "bubbly." A fine sclerotic rim is present but may not be readily apparent without CT examination. Fluid-fluid levels may be identified on CT or MRI (Fig. 100–58). In its early phase, an ABC may appear permeative.

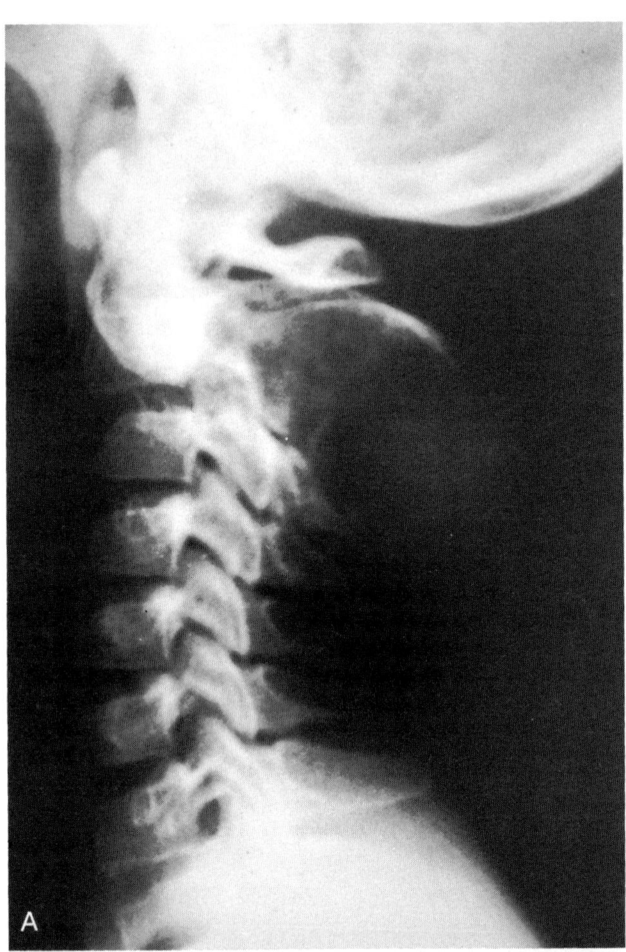

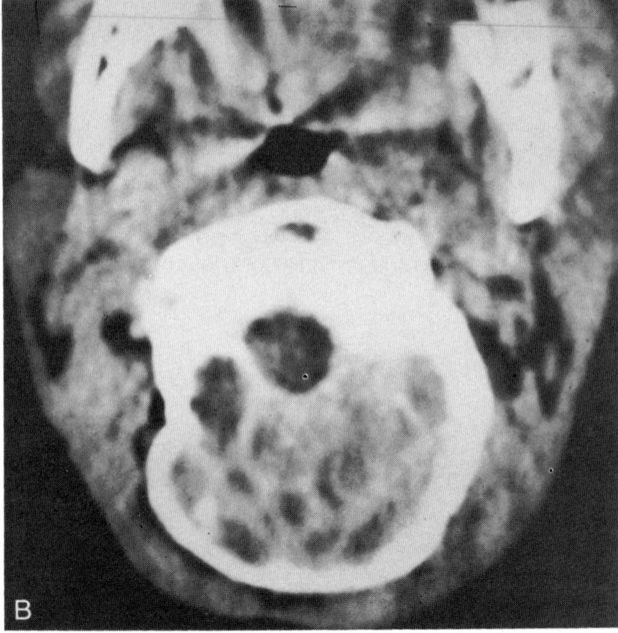

Figure 100–57. A lateral plain film of the cervical spine demonstrates an expansile lytic lesion of C2 posterior elements *(A)* in this nine-year-old female. This aneurysmal bone cyst demonstrates no cortical disruption or associated soft-tissue mass on axial CT scan obtained at the mid-level of this lesion *(B)*. (*A* and *B* reprinted with permission from the ACR Learning File, Musculoskeletal Videodisc, Case 110.)

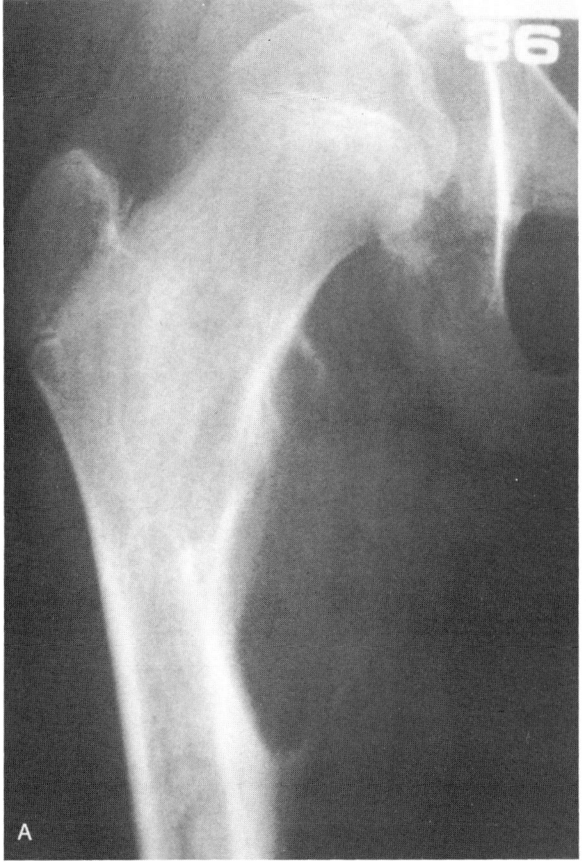

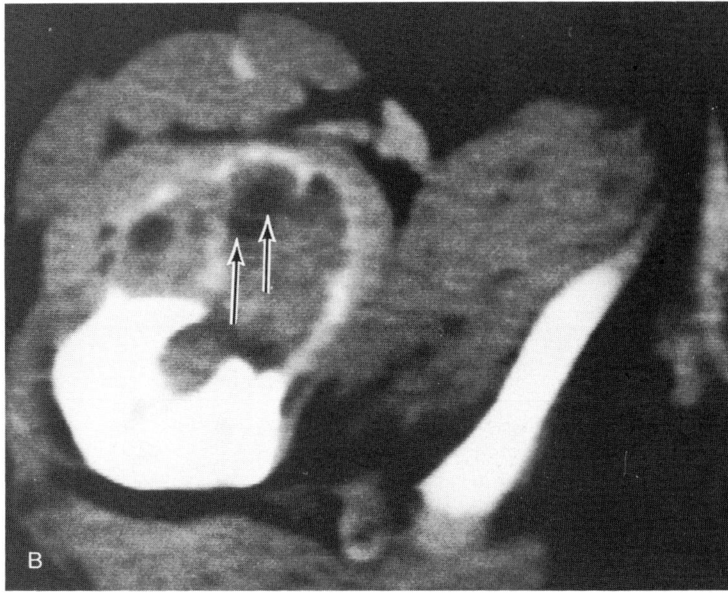

Figure 100–58. *A,* This eccentric metaphyseal lytic lesion in the proximal femur of a 12-year-old female demonstrates marked medial expansion. The cortical rim appears to be intact on plain film. *B,* CT scan confirms the presence of an intact cortical rim in this aneurysmal bone cyst. No associated soft-tissue mass is present, but the normal soft-tissue planes are displaced by the medial expansion of the bony lesion. Fluid-fluid levels can be identified *(arrows).* (Case loaned by Mark Kransdorf, M.D., AFIP; reprinted with permission from the ACR Learning File, Musculoskeletal Videodisc, Case 157.)

As it aggressively expands, it incites a marked host response, resulting in the development of Codman's triangle or periosteal reaction. It may obliterate the underlying osseous lesion responsible for the initial development of the ABC.

Differential diagnostic considerations for ABCs during various stages of evolution include nonossifying fibroma, fibrous dysplasia, and osteoblastoma. Curettage, cryotherapy, and low-dose radiation therapy have each had varying success, with recurrence of up to 50 per cent.

Benign Fibrous Cortical Defect/Nonossifying Fibroma

Benign fibrous cortical defects (BFCDs) and nonossifying fibromas (NOFs) are histologically identical lesions comprised of fibrous tissue. The BFCD is a transitory lesion seen in 30 to 40 per cent of children older than 2 years of age but seen infrequently in adults (suggesting that the lesions heal spontaneously). NOFs occur in the first or second decade, with 95 per cent in patients younger than 20 years of age.

These geographic, lytic lesions are rimmed with sclerosis and have a narrow zone of transition (see Fig. 100–2*A*). BFCDs usually measure less than 2 cm and NOFs greater than 2 cm (it can be enormous). NOFs tend to be expansile with no host reaction or matrix. Both occur in the metaphyseal portion of lower extremity long bones (55 per cent around the knee—distal femur, proximal tibia, and fibula). Both are cortically based except in smaller tubular bones (Fig. 100–59). The NOF may enlarge and encroach upon the intramedullary space, but the BFCD does not (Fig. 100–60).

As noted above, the BFCD heals spontaneously. The NOF may also heal spontaneously, appearing to migrate away from the metaphysis (Fig. 100–61) as the child grows. It may transiently become sclerotic as ossification and remodeling occurs. Large NOFs may require curettage with bone chip packing, especially if the patient is symptomatic secondary to mass effect or pathologic fracture.

Differential diagnostic considerations for the nonossifying fibroma include chondromyxoid fibroma and aneurysmal bone cyst as well as brown tumor of hyperparathyroidism.

Fibrous Dysplasia

Fibrous dysplasia (FD) is a hamartomatous fibro-osseous metaplasia characterized by islands of osteoid and woven bone that arises from the medullary space of the affected bone and may be monostotic or polyostotic (3:1). A wide age range is seen, varying from 1 to 75 years, with the majority of cases (75 per cent) identified by age 20.

This geographic lesion may demonstrate expansion with cortical thinning and varies in size from 1 to 30 cm. Surrounding bony sclerosis is present but not prominent, and other host response such as periosteal reaction is rare in the absence of pathologic fractures. Soft tissues are displaced by expansion of the underlying osseous lesion but are otherwise uninvolved.

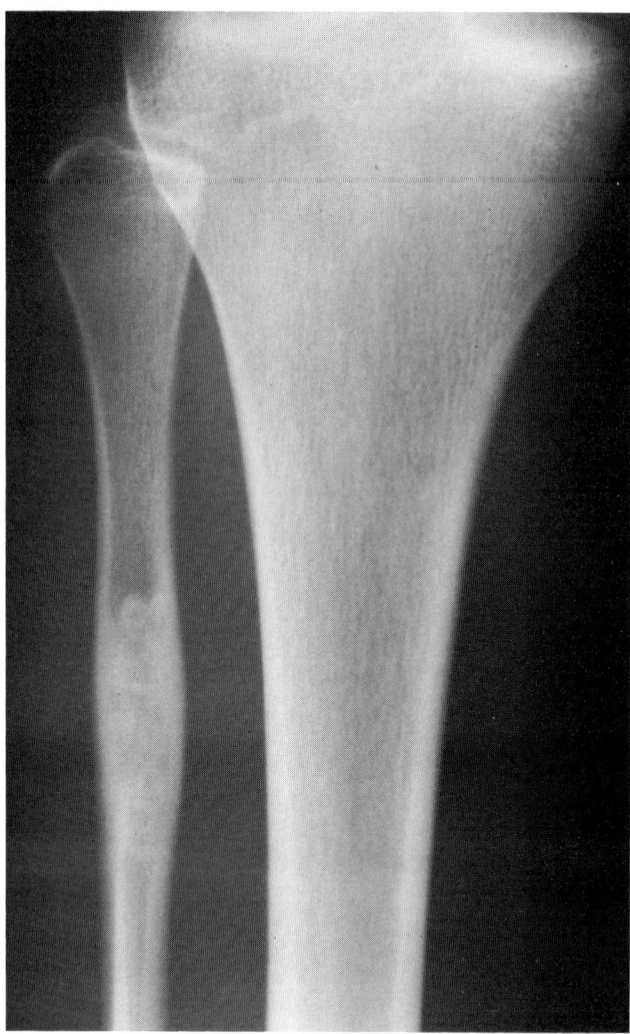

Figure 100–59. This small diaphyseal fibular lesion, incidentally noted on a plain film, is geographic with a narrow zone of transition. This nonossifying fibroma is sclerotic, consistent with expected appearance in the healing phase. Though nonossifying fibromas are most commonly eccentric in location, they may appear central in very thin bones such as the fibula or ulna. This healing fibroma, like an inactive solitary bone cyst, has "migrated" from the metaphysis as normal bone growth has continued.

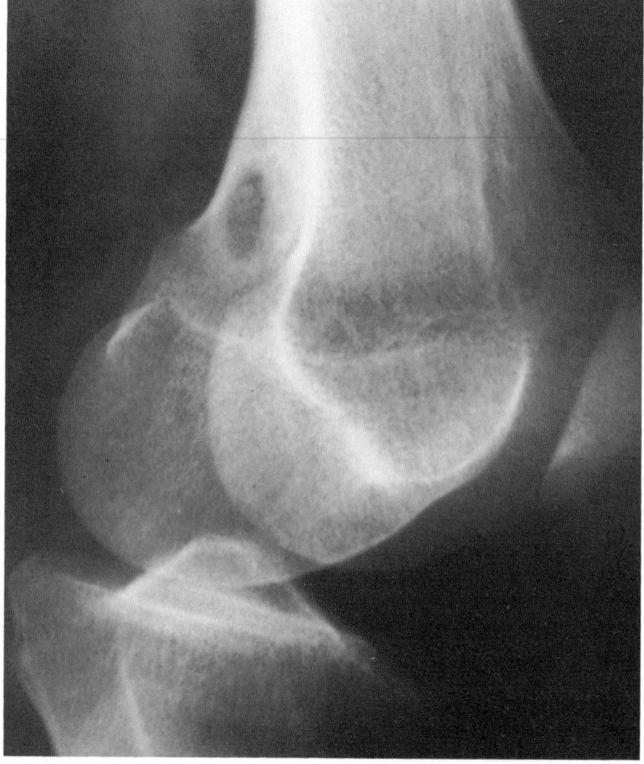

Figure 100–60. This small metaphyseal, cortically based, geographic lesion in the distal femur of an 18-year-old male demonstrates the classic appearance of a benign fibrous cortical defect. It has a narrow zone of transition and a sclerotic margin.

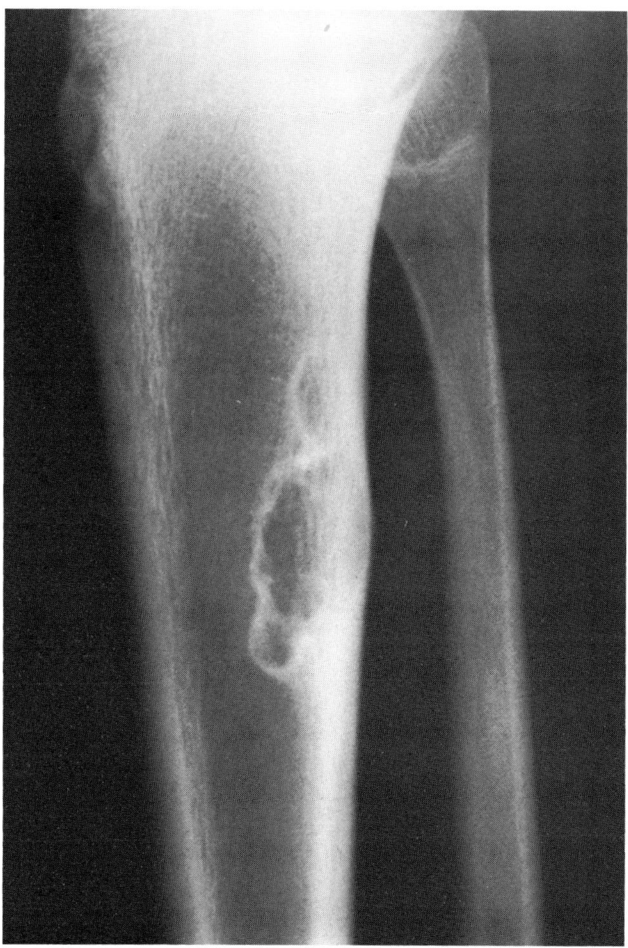

Figure 100–61. This nonossifying fibroma in the proximal tibia is an incidental finding in a 14-year-old male. The cortically based lesion demonstrates a sclerotic margin with a narrow zone of transition. The metadiaphyseal location of this lesion demonstrates the "migration" from the metaphysis as the lesion becomes quiescent in the growing child.

This process is usually central but may be eccentric. Metaphyseal involvement of long bones such as the femur and tibia is common but the metaplasia may involve any bone and the disease often affects the skull, ribs, and pelvis. The polyostotic form of FD tends to affect multiple bones on one side of the body—90 per cent of patients with polyostotic presentation have a unilateral distribution of lesions.

Location of the lesion appears to dictate its density and overall appearance. Thus, tubular bony lesions tend to be mildly expansile, with density ranging from lytic to slightly opaque. The opaque, homogeneous quality results from the presence of osteoid or woven bone in increasing amounts and is known as "ground glass" appearance (Fig. 100–62). Skull lesions are usually densely sclerotic with enlargement of the involved bone (Fig. 100–63). Pelvic lesions are distinct as well, often appearing lytic and "bubbly" (Fig. 100–64).

Albright's syndrome comprises a triad that includes the classic FD bony lesions in polyostotic form, precocious puberty, and cutaneous pigmentation located on the same side as the polyostotic lesions. This rare syndrome is seen in 3 per cent of patients with FD.

Fractures are a common complication of FD. The "shepherd's crook" deformity results from repetitive microfractures of the proximal femur with poor healing (especially poor remodeling) and a subsequent coxa vara angulation. This is considered a hallmark of FD in the femur (Fig. 100–65). Leg length discrepancy secondary to long bone enlargement and bowing may also be seen. Expansile lesions of the paranasal sinuses and mandible can produce a facial deformity termed *cherubism*.

Treatment is directed toward care of fractures and maintenance of function of affected part. Although radiation therapy was once attempted, results were poor and were felt to increase the likelihood of sarcomatous degeneration, which is otherwise rare.

Differential diagnosis includes solitary bone cyst for a monostotic tubular bony lesion and eosinophilic granuloma, Ewing's sarcoma, or metastases for rib lesions. For polyostotic lesions, Ollier's disease or metastases should be considered but easily differentiated. Paget's disease or en plaque meningioma should be considered for base of skull lesions.

Histiocytosis X

Eosinophilic granuloma (EG), Hand-Schüller-Christian disease, and Letterer-Siwe disease are histologically similar diseases, with

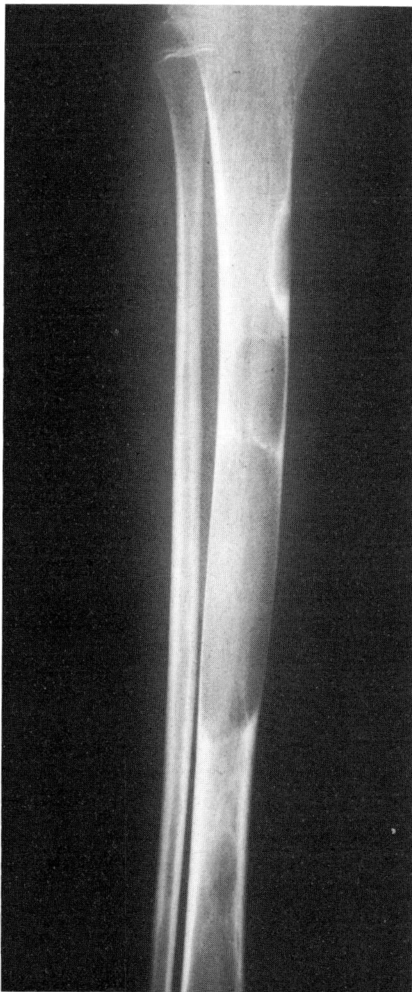

Figure 100–62. Multiple lesions in the tibia of this 10-year-old female are located centrally in the diaphysis. These lytic lesions have caused thinning and slight expansion of the bone. The slight opacity of the lesions represents the classic "ground glass" appearance of fibrous dysplasia. Similar lesions were found in the femur on the same side. The opposite lower extremity demonstrated no abnormality.

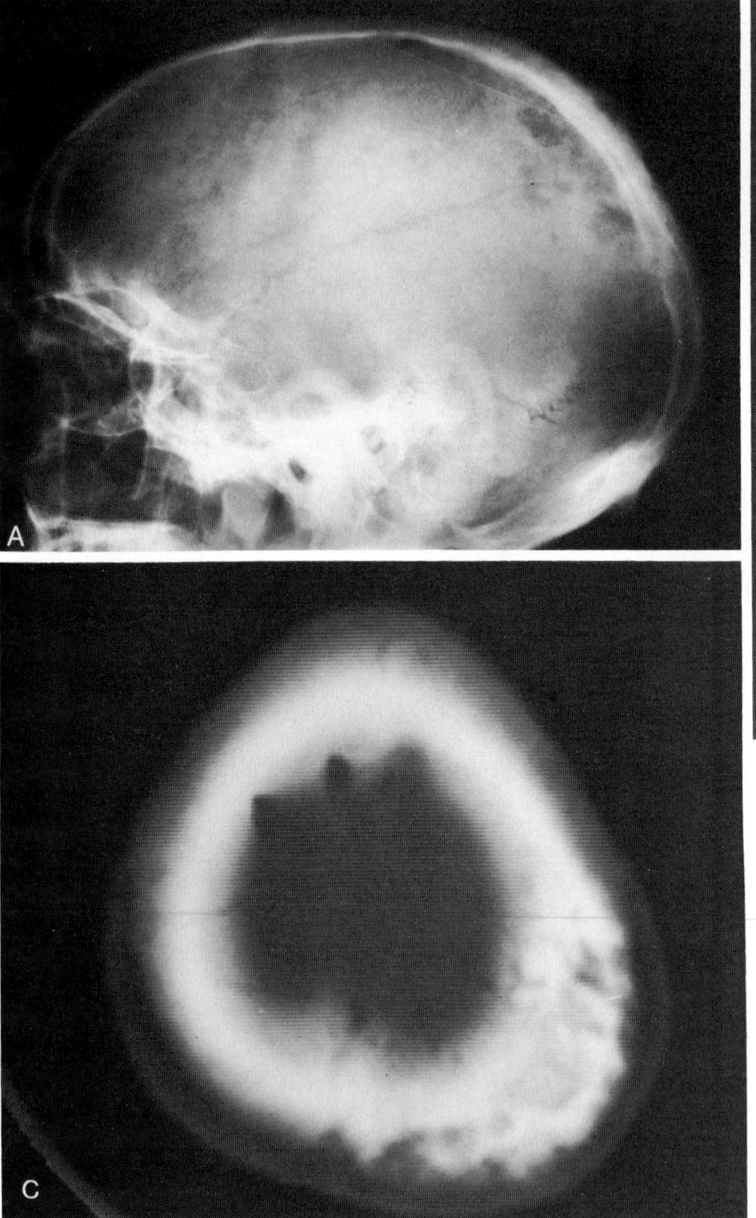

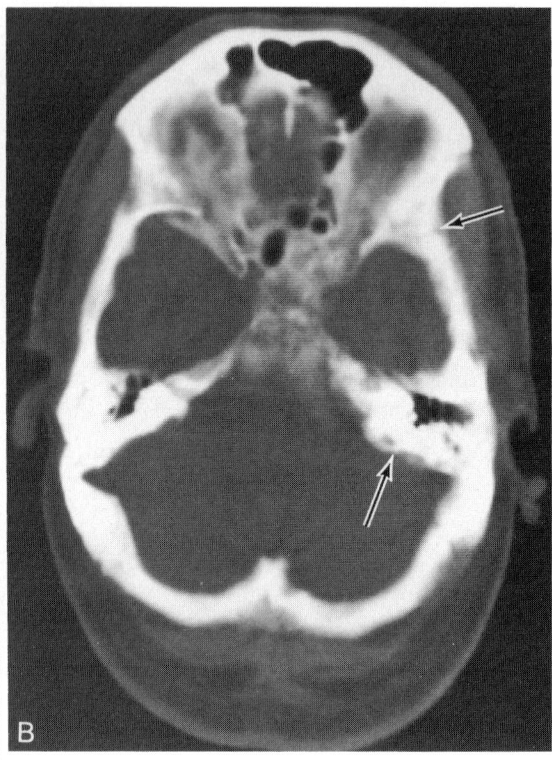

Figure 100–63. *A,* Lateral skull film demonstrates cystic, expansile lesions involving the cranium and skull base. These are lesions of fibrous dysplasia, though somewhat more cystic than the densely sclerotic lesions classically described. *B,* CT scan demonstrates the marked expansion of the skull base *(arrows)* with cystic changes, but sclerosis is also readily apparent. *C,* A slightly higher plane of section emphasizes the expansile nature of these areas of fibrous dysplasia.

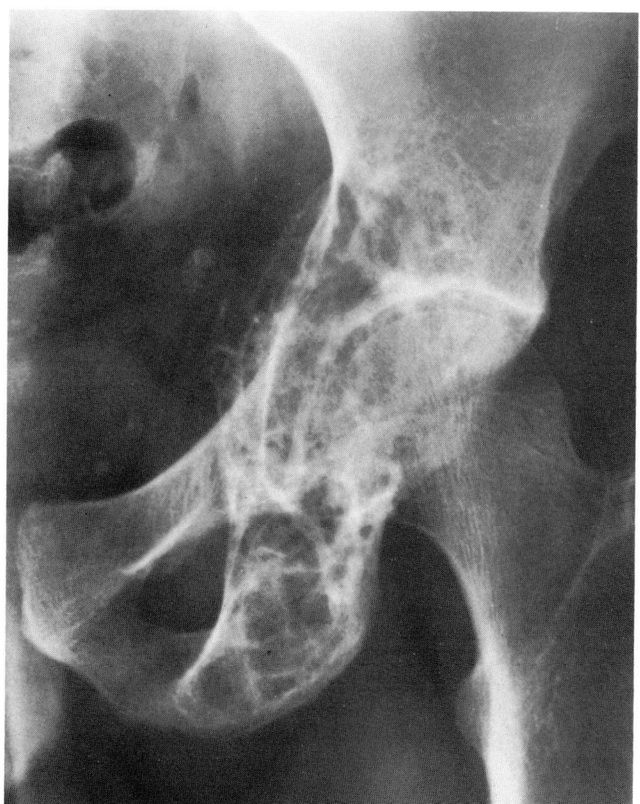

Figure 100–64. This "bubbly" lytic lesion found in a 29-year-old male includes the ischium and neck of the ileum. It has no cortical breakthrough or soft-tissue mass and demonstrates the classic appearance of pelvic lesions in fibrous dysplasia.

varying clinical presentations, known collectively as histiocytosis X. All have histiocytic/eosinophilic infiltration of involved tissues and aggressive bone lesions.

Eosinophilic granuloma is the mildest and most common (60 to 80 per cent) form and is localized to bone or lung. Ninety per cent of patients with this form are between 5 and 15 years of age. The disease course is usually benign. Hand-Schüller-Christian disease is the chronic disseminated form and involves not only the skeleton but other reticuloendothelial system (RES) organs such as the liver, spleen, and lymph nodes. It occurs in patients younger than 15 years, with 66 per cent identified at younger than 5 years of age. Prognosis is variable, with a high morbidity and a 10 per cent mortality. Letterer-Siwe disease is the acute fulminant form of the disease and is seen before age 2. Organ systems involved include not only the RES but skin as well. Mortality is extremely high in this rare form of histiocytosis X.

Eosinophilic granuloma presents with pain and may simulate an infectious process with fever and an elevated sedimentation rate. It has great variability in appearance depending on its phase and bony location. It may appear highly aggressive with a moth-eaten or permeative pattern and a wide zone of transition (Fig. 100–66), no sclerotic margin, and marked periosteal reaction. On the other hand, the skull lesions may have a more discrete appearance, often with the typical "beveled edge" indicating different rates of involvement of the inner and outer skull tables. Soft-tissue masses are often seen.

Approximately 70 per cent of lesions are found in the flat bones of the skull, jaw, ribs, and pelvis (Fig. 100–67) as well as the vertebral bodies. EG is the most common cause, in children, of vertebra plana, which is characterized by the remarkable flattening of the vertebral body, whereas the posterior elements and disk spaces remain intact (Fig. 100–68). Sclerosis develops as the lesions evolve and resolve.

In the long bones, the lesions are diaphyseal 60 per cent of the time, respecting the joint space and growth plate even in the most aggressive growth phase. Although there is no tumor matrix, rapid evolution of the lesions may result in a central fragment of bone being "left behind." This is known as a "button sequestrum." Sclerosis develops as the lesions evolve and resolve.

Treatment of the mild form may include simple curettage, steroid injection, wide excision, low-dose radiation, or no therapy, all with similar rates of recurrence. Therapy is usually directed only toward the symptomatic lesions.

In evaluating this aggressive lesion, one must always consider round cell lesions such as Ewing's sarcoma and lymphoma. Infection and metastatic disease (especially neuroblastoma) might also be considered and may be indistinguishable. A bone scan is helpful in identifying and evaluating polyostotic disease. However, all the lesions in the differential diagnosis may be polyostotic as well.

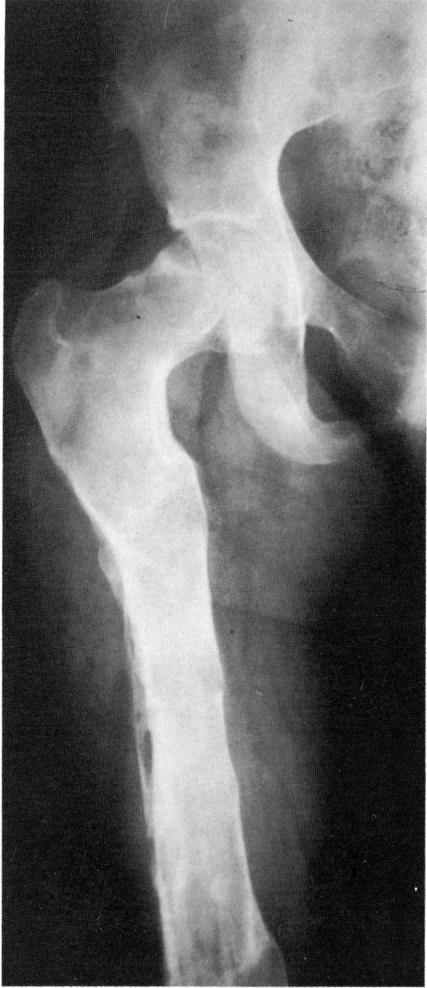

Figure 100–65. Plain film of the proximal femur demonstrates a typical "shepherd's crook" deformity in the femoral neck of this 18-year-old female with fibrous dysplasia. The diffuse ground glass appearance of the femur and hemipelvis represents the abnormal osteoid/woven bone. The linear region of bone formation in the lateral femoral diaphysis represents new bone growth associated with a stabilization plate previously placed and subsequently removed. (Reprinted with permission from the ACR Learning File, Musculoskeletal Videodisc, Case 165.)

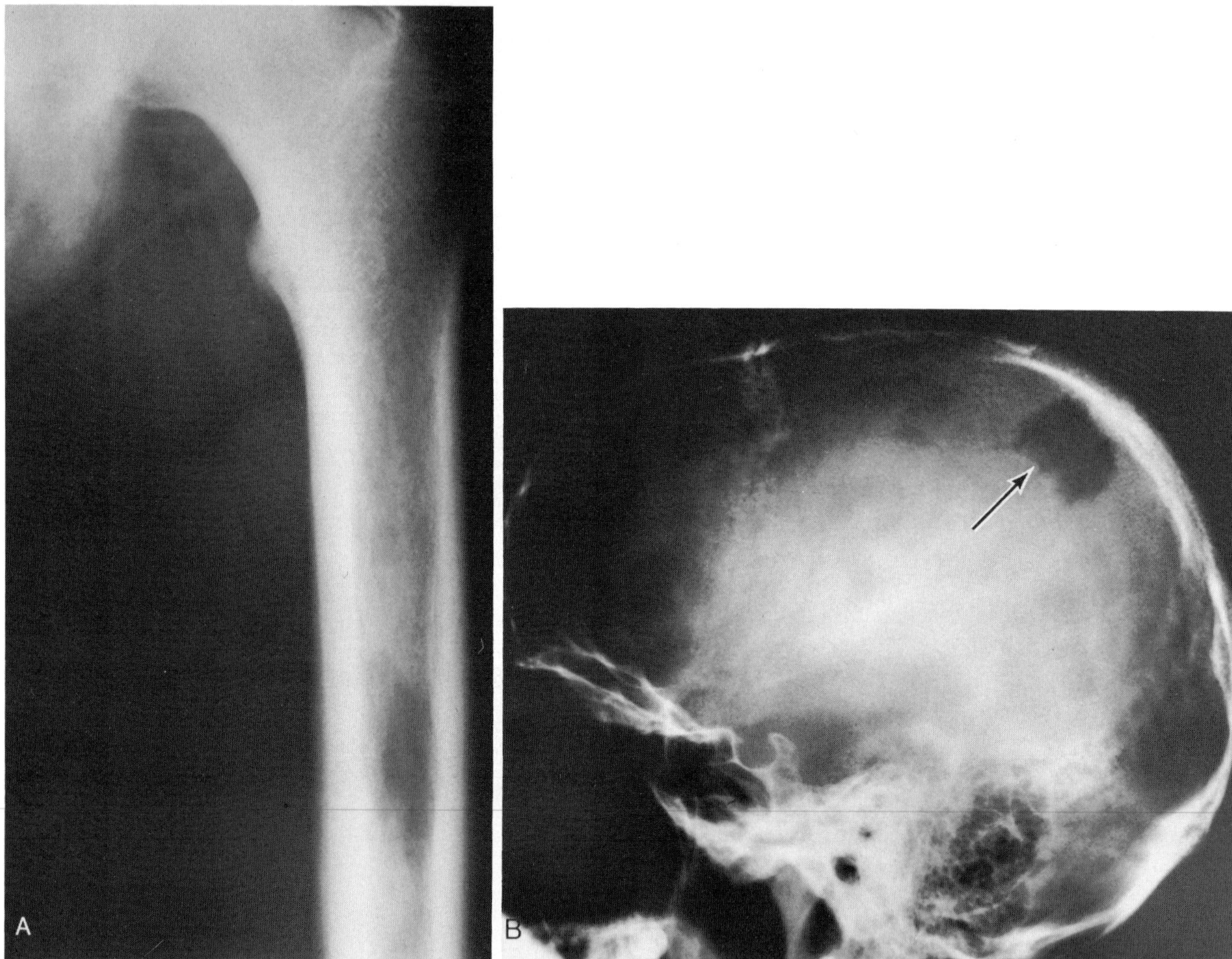

Figure 100–66. A permeative lesion of the femoral diaphysis with adjacent periosteal reaction was identified on plain film *(A)* when this 15-year-old male presented with a complaint of thigh pain. A bone scan was obtained, which revealed increased uptake in the skull. Plain film of the skull *(B)* demonstrates the classic "beveled edge" appearance of eosinophilic granuloma *(arrow)*, which results from differing rates of involvement of the inner and outer tables of the skull. (*A* and *B* reprinted with permission from the ACR Learning File, Musculoskeletal Videodisc, Case 163.)

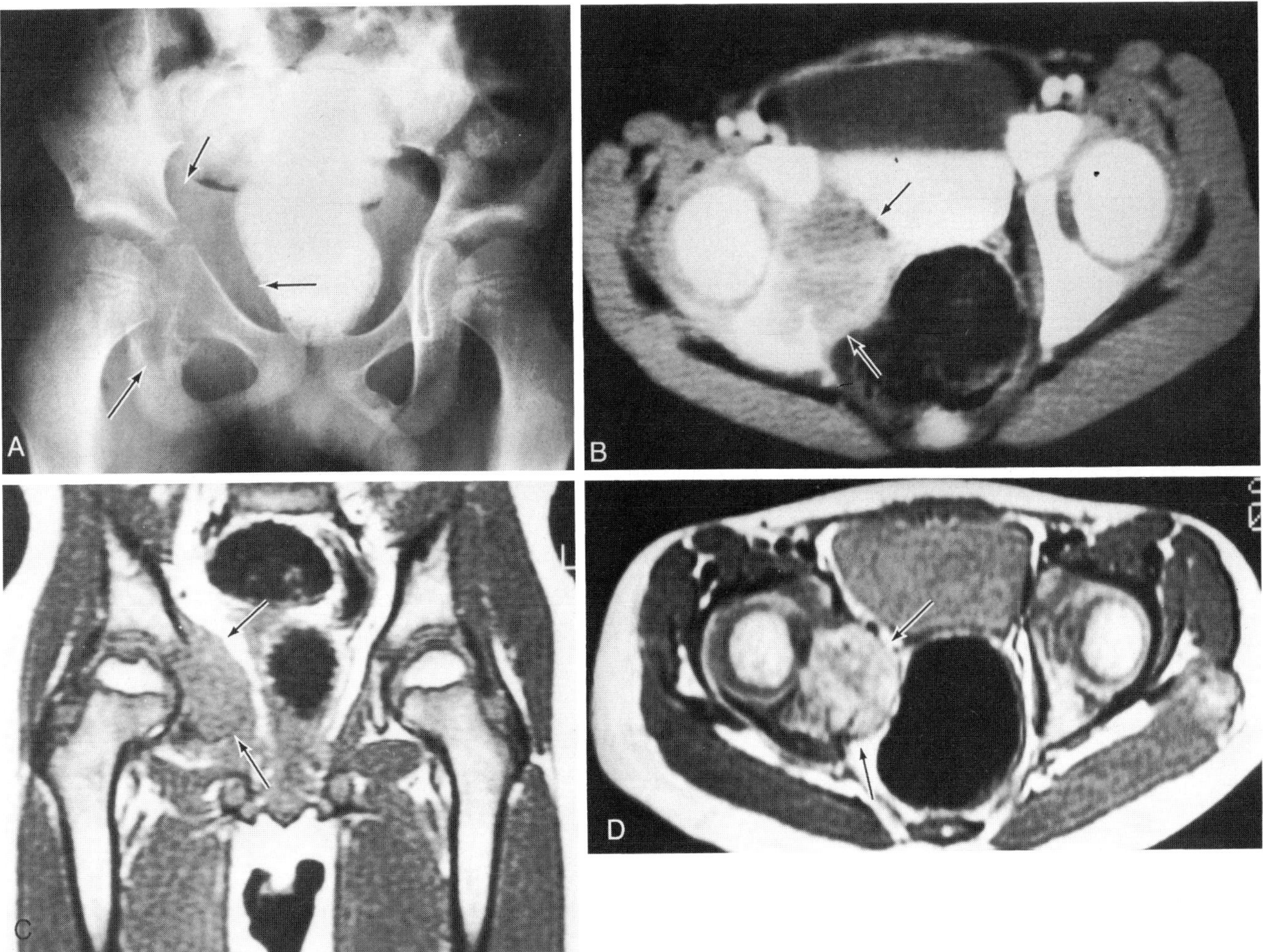

Figure 100–67. *A,* A plain film of the pelvis in this 6-year-old male demonstrates an aggressive lesion of the right acetabulum and ischium with a wide zone of transition and permeative appearance. There is suggestion of a soft-tissue mass. *B,* CT scan reveals a destructive lesion of the medial acetabular wall without a remnant of residual bone. An associated soft-tissue mass displaces the bladder and rectum *(arrows). C,* Coronal T_1-weighted MRI demonstrates the extent of bony disruption of the acetabulum with preservation of normal signal in the adjacent femoral head. Soft-tissue mass with displacement of the pelvic structures is again seen *(arrows). D,* The signal on T_2-weighted imaging is slightly heterogeneous. The soft-tissue component exerts mass effect against the normal pelvic structures, but soft-tissue planes are intact without obvious invasion of surrounding structures *(arrows).* This lesion proved to be eosinophilic granuloma at biopsy. (*A* to *D* reprinted with permission from the ACR Learning File, Musculoskeletal Videodisc, Case 162.)

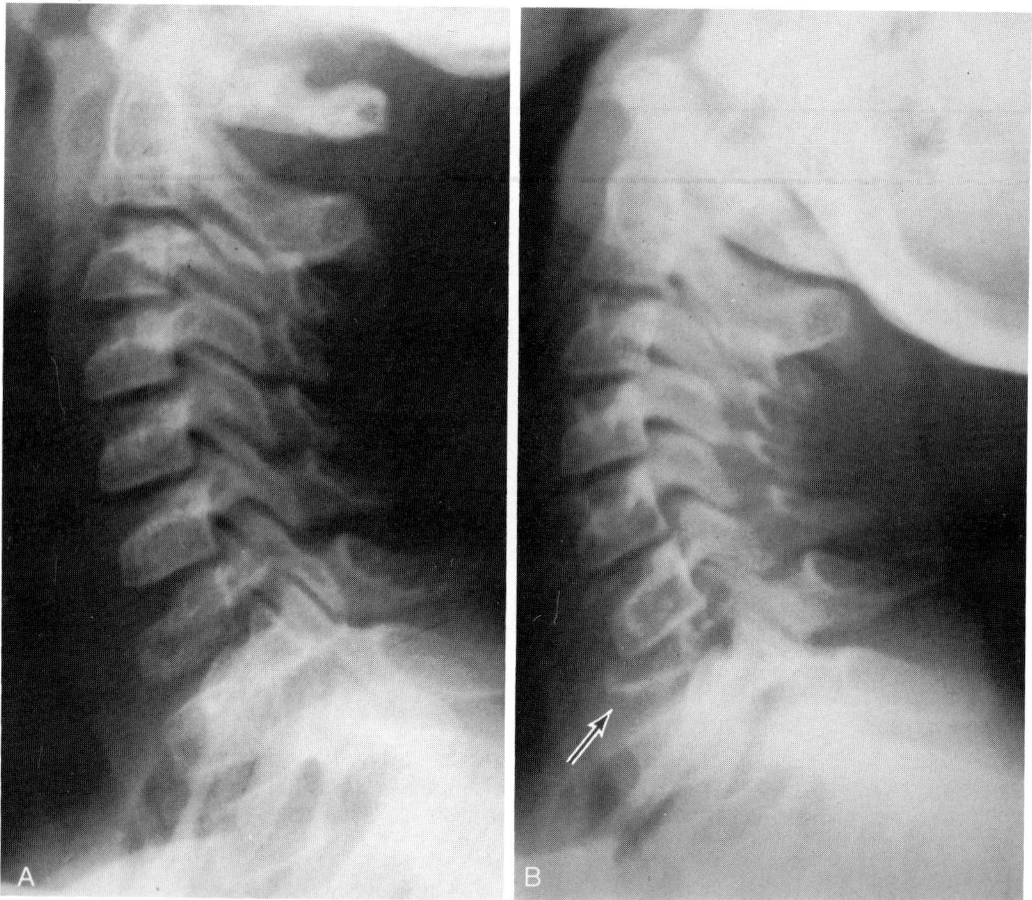

Figure 100–68. *A,* Slight flattening of the C7 vertebral body is identified in this 4-year-old female with known eosinophilic granuloma. Note that the posterior elements are intact. *B,* Within one month, the lesion has progressed to a complete vertebra plana of C7 *(arrow)*. The posterior elements are unaffected, but a slight soft-tissue mass surrounds the abnormal vertebral body. The patient responded well to low-dose radiation with partial restoration of the vertebral body height.

METASTATIC DISEASE AND OTHER CONSIDERATIONS

B. J. Manaster

Metastatic Disease

Metastatic disease to bone is a common occurrence, eventually being found in 20 to 35 per cent of extraskeletal malignancies. To keep the relative importance of primary bone tumors in proper perspective, one should remember that metastases to bone occur 25 times more frequently than do primary bone tumors. Furthermore, establishing a reasonable differential diagnosis for the site of primary disease in patients with metastatic bone lesions is not difficult because 80 per cent of bone metastases arise from four major primary locations (breast, prostate, lung, or kidney). Other common primary sites include gastrointestinal, thyroid, and round cell (lymphoma or neuroblastoma).

Metastases generally have a moth-eaten pattern with an ill-defined zone of transition, no sclerotic margin, and with a variable host reaction. Soft-tissue masses tend to be smaller than in the usual bone sarcoma. Thus, metastatic disease may be moderately to highly aggressive. Metastases usually involve marrow spaces centrally, although a cortical location is not terribly unusual in a patient with widespread metastases. Because metastases to the bone are blood-borne, the most common sites are in the red marrow. Thus, 80 per cent of metastases are located in the axial skeleton and proximal large bones (ribs, pelvis, vertebra, skull, proximal humerus, and proximal femur). Acral lesions are distinctly uncommon. As stated above, metastases involving the spine are very common, found in 38 per cent of malignancies at autopsies (although fewer are detected radiographically). Vertebral metastases may appear either as focal lesions or as nonspecific compression fractures. The epicenter of vertebral metastatic lesions is usually the posterior body, but involvement of pedicles is a commonly noted feature by plain film. Distinguishing tumor from senile osteoporosis or infection as a cause of vertebral body collapse can be difficult. Focal destruction, focal soft-tissue mass, and intact disc spaces are features that are suggestive of metastatic disease.

A few features may be helpful in suggesting the primary lesion. Although most metastases are moth-eaten or permeative in appearance, occasionally metastases present as geographic, bubbly, and expansile. The primary in these cases is usually kidney or thyroid (Fig. 100–69). Furthermore, although most metastatic lesions are polyostotic, kidney or thyroid metastases are often solitary. The density of metastases is variable. In descending order of frequency, purely lytic metastases include lung, kidney, breast, thyroid, gastrointestinal, and neuroblastoma. Purely blastic metastases include prostate, breast, bladder, gastrointestinal (stomach or carcinoid), lung (small cell), and medulloblastoma. Several of these lesions (breast, lung, prostate, bladder, and neuroblastoma) may present as mixed lytic and blastic metastases. Furthermore, a given patient may demonstrate changing patterns of density of the lesions, reflecting healing due to therapy, progressive destruction, or occasionally radiation osteonecrosis.

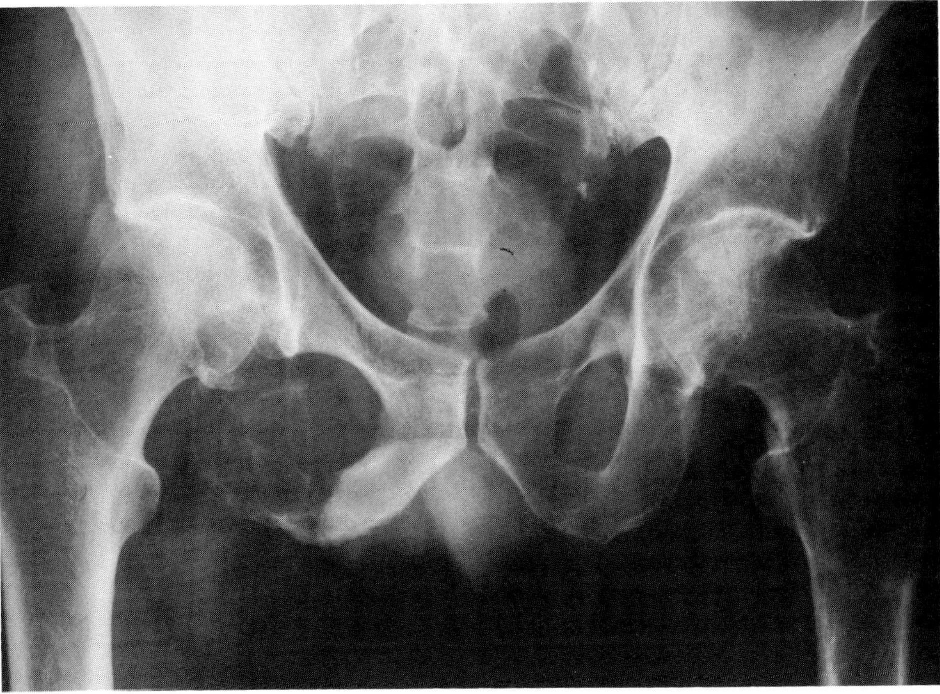

Figure 100–69. Bubbly metastatic lesion. The expansile nature of the right ischial lesion is certainly suggestive of either hypernephroma or thyroid metastatic disease. Note the second lesion involving the left subtrochanteric region. The diagnosis was thyroid in this case.

The most commonly used imaging modalities for detection of metastatic lesions are plain film and radionuclide bone scan. These modalities have complementary roles. Bone scans are highly sensitive compared with plain films. Figures ranging from 10 to 40 per cent have been given of metastatic lesions that are found to be abnormal on bone scan but normal by plain film. On the other hand, fewer than 5 per cent of metastatic lesions are normal on bone scan but abnormal by plain radiography. Radionuclide abnormality can be surprisingly subtle in a few cases with widespread metastatic lesions. Patients who present with diffuse breast or prostate metastases may yield a "superscan" pattern of radionuclide uptake (Fig. 100–70), where the bones appear unusually and uniformly distinct. The key to this diagnosis is the lack of kidney uptake of the radionuclide.

While bone scans are highly sensitive, their specificity is very poor. Abnormalities on radionuclide scan may be due to tumor, trauma, arthritis, or infection. Plain film is more specific and differentiates among these possibilities. Plain radiographs are also used to assess therapeutic success. They are also important in evaluation for signs of impending pathologic fracture. Lesions that are 2.5 cm or larger in diameter, or that involve 50 per cent of cortical width, are at risk for pathologic fracture and should be identified for prophylactic therapy.

It of course must be remembered that not all polyostotic disease represents metastatic lesions. Other possibilities include multiple myeloma, radiation osteonecrosis, sclerosing dysplasias, Paget's disease (which can have aggressive phases), histiocytosis, or fibrous dysplasia. One particular site of abnormality that can cause confusion in the elderly osteoporotic patient is the pubic bones. Stress fractures and post-traumatic osteolysis of the pubis may simulate aggressive metastatic disease. The trauma may be remote and forgotten but the attempts at fracture healing in a bone that continues to bear weight can result in a destructive-appearing lesion (Fig. 100–71). One should remember to consider trauma as an etiology for a lesion with this appearance at this site. If one performs a biopsy on the lesion, the histologic appearance may be aggressive owing to fracture healing, causing further confusion.

Some fracture sites and patterns should make one suspicious of metastatic disease. For example, an isolated fracture of a lesser tuberosity rarely occurs as the result of trauma and should be investigated for the possibility of metastatic disease. Furthermore, a transverse fracture of any long bone in the absence of substantial trauma is suspicious for underlying pathology. Transverse fractures occur in the traumatic setting only with great force, with the more common fractures being oblique or spiral. Therefore, a transverse fracture occurring with minimal force is seen only in situations of either insufficient bone or pathologic bone (Fig. 100–72). In such cases, metastatic disease should be strongly considered.

Although bone scan and plain film remain the major imaging modalities, CT and MRI can demonstrate marrow infiltration and destruction. They are, however, usually nonspecific and rarely cost-effective diagnostic modalities for metastatic disease. Thus, MRI is usually called upon when other modalities present a confusing picture and it is important to evaluate a potential metastatic site.

Radiation Changes

Bone can respond in several different ways to radiation therapy, and can yield a potentially confusing picture. Skeletally immature patients may demonstrate early fusion and growth abnormalities resulting from a radiation-induced vasculitis at the epiphyseal plates (Fig. 100–73). A less common occurrence in the skeletally immature patient who is irradiated is the development of a radiation-induced osteochondroma (Fig. 100–73). These may enlarge quite rapidly.

Radiation osteonecrosis may occur, generally in the 7- to 10-year range following therapy. The osteonecrosis appears as a mixed lytic and blastic destructive change seen in bones restricted to the radiation port. Although the lesions often appear aggressive and result in pathologic fracture (Fig. 100–74), the restriction of the abnormality to a square or oblong radiation port helps to differentiate this change from tumor recurrence. Bones with radiation osteonecrosis have an increased susceptibility to infection, so this diagnosis must also be considered in these patients. If the femoral head is included in the radiation port, it may undergo avascular necrosis as well.

Finally, a sarcoma may arise in previously irradiated bone. These radiation-induced sarcomas most commonly arise in the 4- to 20-year range following therapy. The cell type of sarcoma is usually osteosarcoma, MFH, fibrosarcoma, or chondrosarcoma, or may con-

Text continued on page 1564

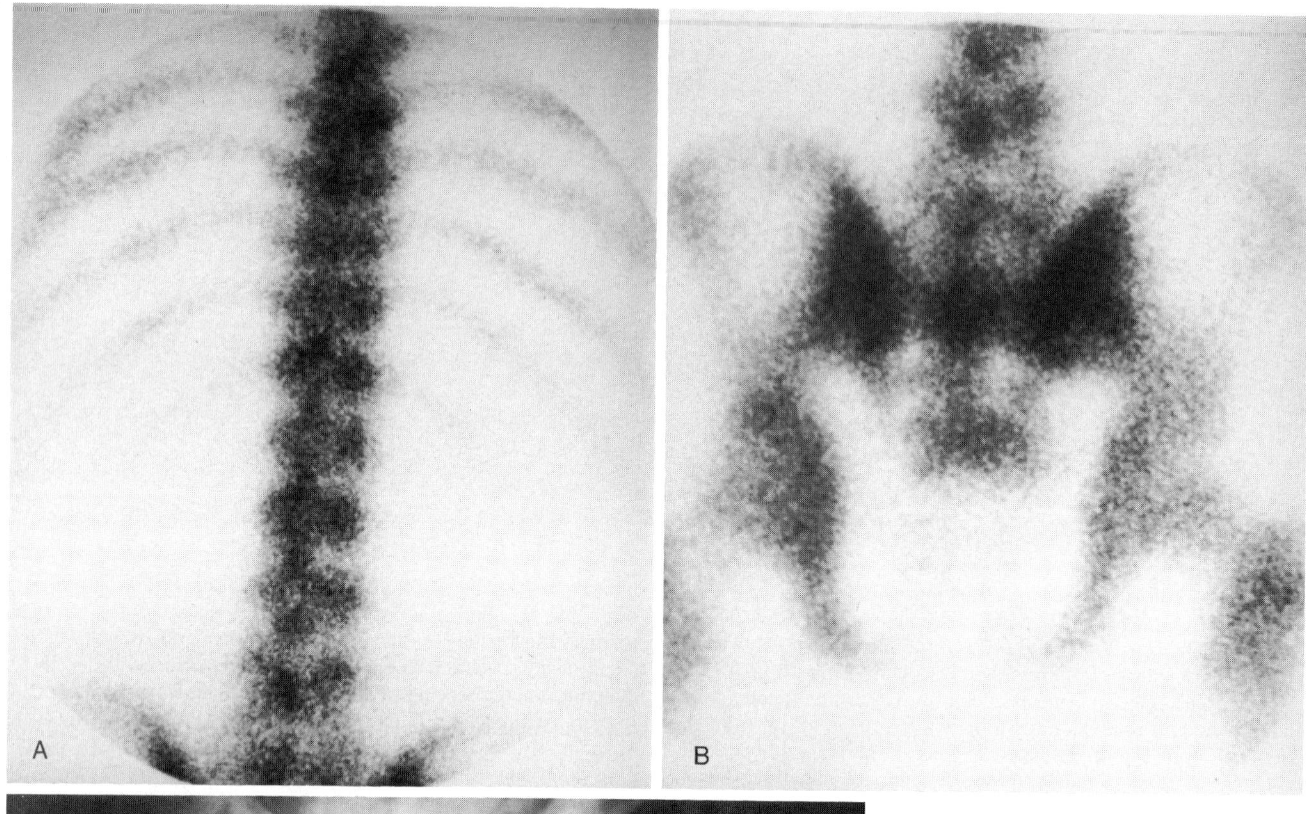

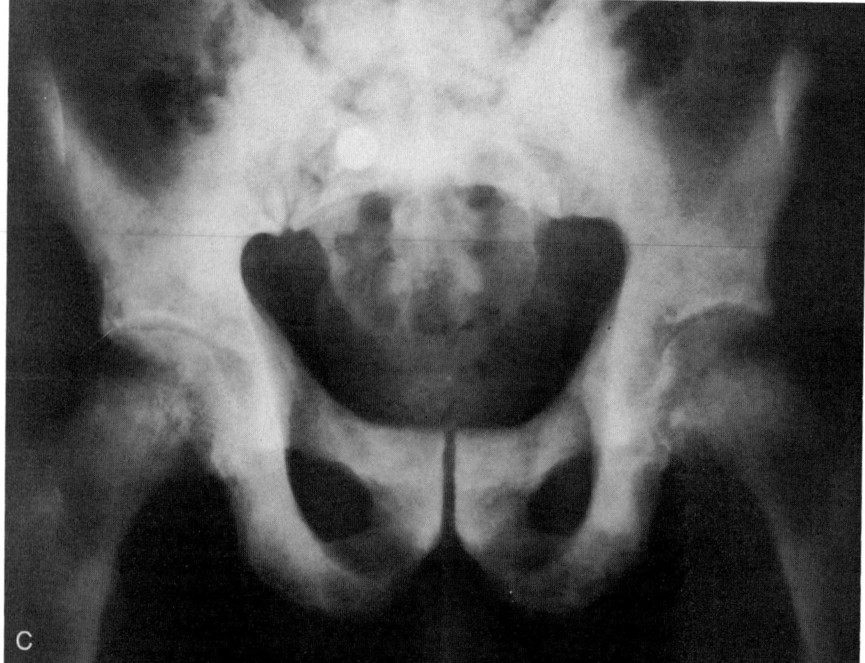

Figure 100–70. Superscan in prostate cancer. *A* and *B* demonstrate a part of the superscan, in which the osseous structures are particularly clearly seen. The uptake is fairly symmetrical in all the bones. The hallmark of the superscan is the lack of uptake by the kidneys. The plain film *(C)* demonstrates the widespread sclerotic lesions of metastatic prostate cancer.

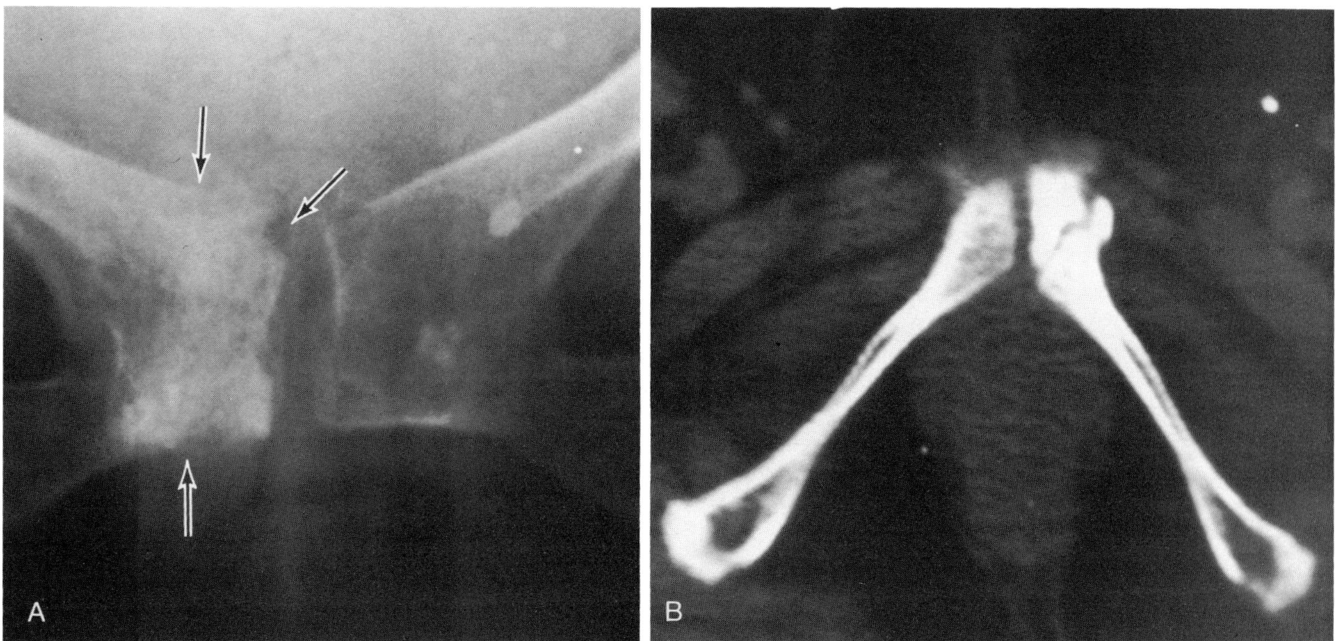

Figure 100–71. Pseudometastasis. The plain film *(A)* shows a fairly aggressive appearing lesion involving the pubic ramus *(arrows)*. The CT scan *(B)* demonstrates the nature of the lesion, which is an insufficiency fracture attempting to heal in a patient who is continuing to bear weight. This appearance is a common source of confusion in the elderly patient suspected of having metastatic disease.

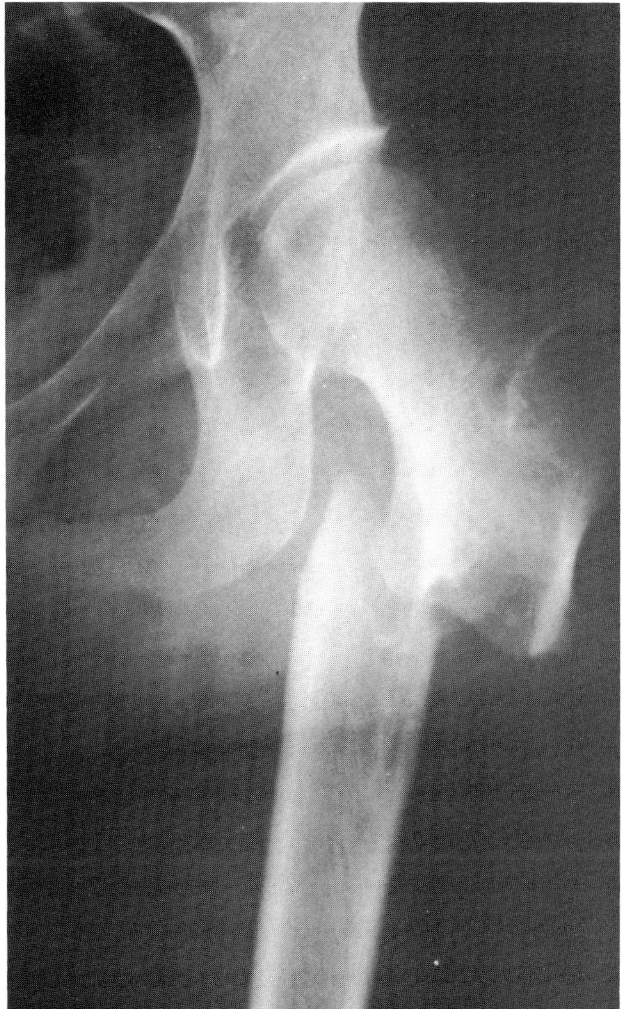

Figure 100–72. Solitary metastasis. This patient demonstrates a transverse fracture in the subtrochanteric region of the left femur. The patient had not experienced significant trauma. This history strongly suggests that the patient has a pathologic or stress fracture. In this case, there simply is not enough bone present and the patient does have a lytic lesion through which the fracture occurred. Primary was breast cancer.

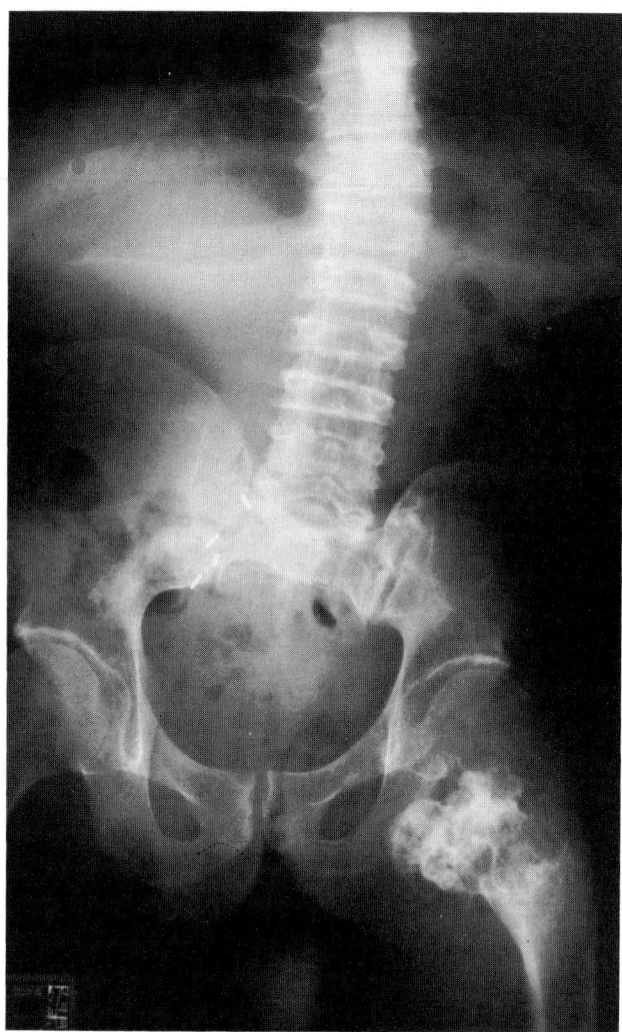

Figure 100–73. Growth abnormalities related to radiation. This plain film shows hypoplasia of the lumbar vertebral bodies, more pronounced on the left than on the right. The sacrum is hypoplastic, again more pronounced on the left than on the right. The left iliac wing is severely hypoplastic when compared with the normal right side. These findings of growth arrest in a port-like configuration are typical of radiation therapy in a skeletally immature patient. This patient was indeed irradiated for a Wilms' tumor on the left side several years earlier. Note also the presence of an exostosis arising from the left femoral neck. Exostoses are uncommon developments related to radiation in the skeletally immature patient. (Reprinted with permission from the ACR Learning File, Musculoskeletal Videodisc, Case 604.)

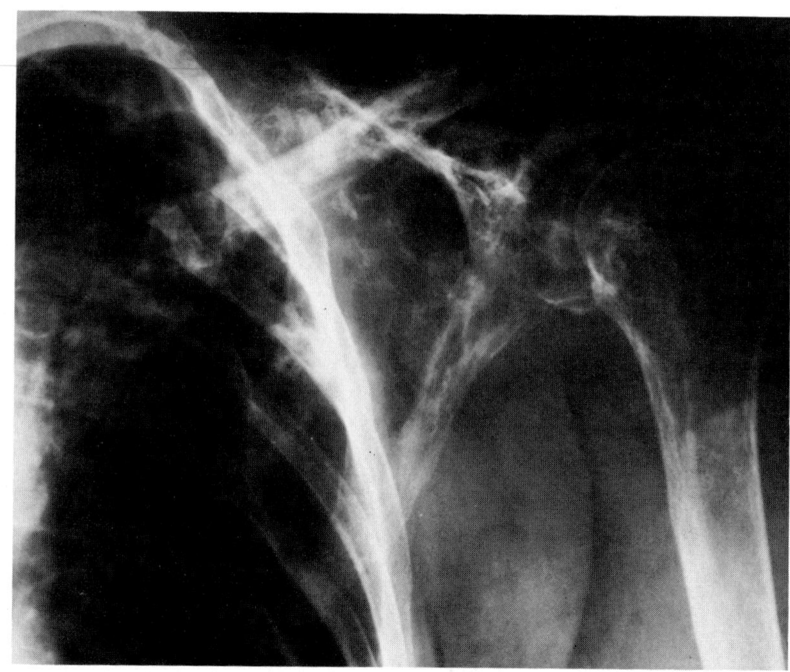

Figure 100–74. Radiation osteonecrosis. This film demonstrates lytic and sclerotic change involving the upper ribs, clavicle, and scapula, as well as proximal humerus. This could easily represent metastatic breast cancer. However, the entire chest film would make the nature of the lesion more readily diagnosed. It would demonstrate the mastectomy, and the port-like distribution of these abnormalities with the remainder of bones appearing normal. This appearance and distribution are typical of radiation osteonecrosis. (Reprinted with permission from the ACR Learning File, Musculoskeletal Videodisc, Case 605.)

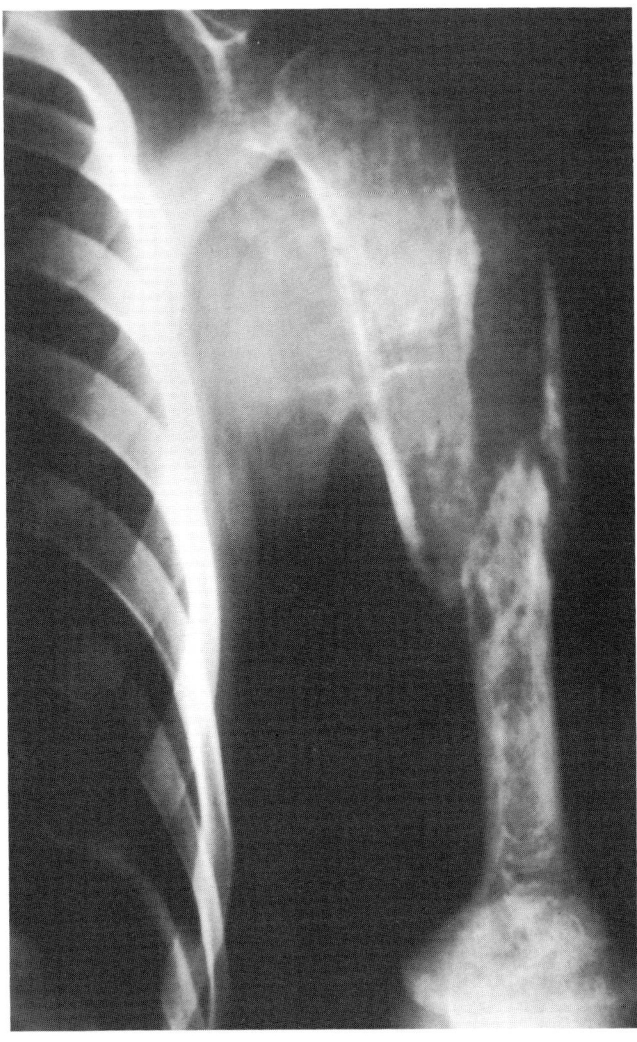

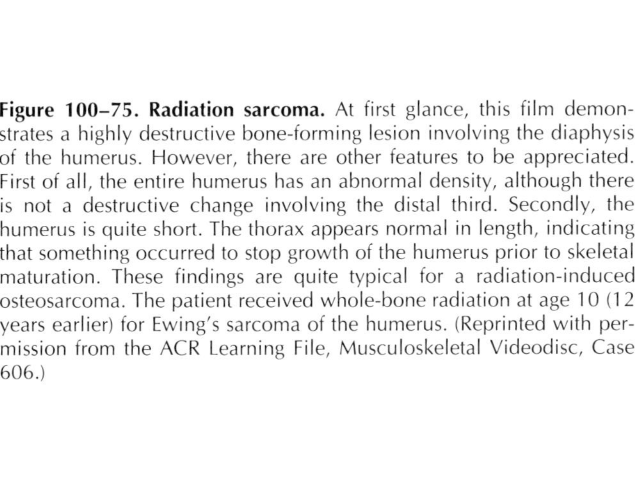

Figure 100–75. Radiation sarcoma. At first glance, this film demonstrates a highly destructive bone-forming lesion involving the diaphysis of the humerus. However, there are other features to be appreciated. First of all, the entire humerus has an abnormal density, although there is not a destructive change involving the distal third. Secondly, the humerus is quite short. The thorax appears normal in length, indicating that something occurred to stop growth of the humerus prior to skeletal maturation. These findings are quite typical for a radiation-induced osteosarcoma. The patient received whole-bone radiation at age 10 (12 years earlier) for Ewing's sarcoma of the humerus. (Reprinted with permission from the ACR Learning File, Musculoskeletal Videodisc, Case 606.)

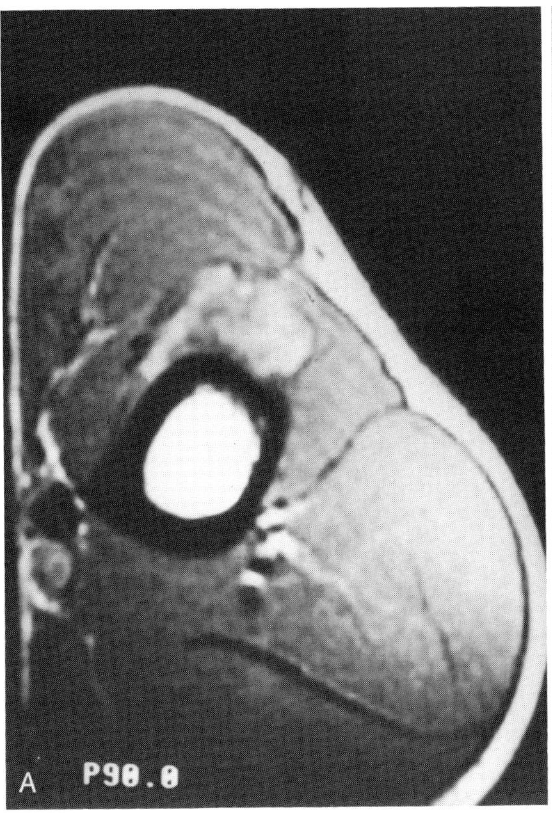

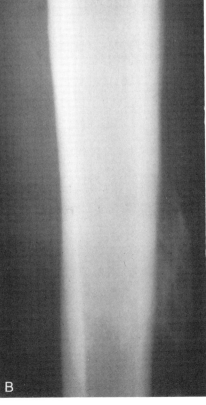

Figure 100–76. Myositis ossificans simulating tumor. *A* is an MRI obtained in this 17-year-old patient when a lump was discovered on his arm. The MRI demonstrates high signal intensity within the mass lesion, as well as abnormal cortex of the bone immediately adjacent to this soft-tissue mass. These findings are alarming but nonspecific. The plain film *(B)* gives the answer. It demonstrates the osseous nature of the soft-tissue mass. This is quite clearly bone matrix, well-differentiated into trabeculae. There is mild adjacent cortical thickening, which is a host reaction to the process of myositis ossificans. It is this reactive change that appeared somewhat aggressive by MRI. When the MRI and plain films are interpreted together, the patient can be safely advised of the diagnosis and can be followed clinically. (*A* and *B* reprinted with permission from the ACR Learning File, Musculoskeletal Videodisc, Case 311.)

tain elements of several of these. These sarcomas may be difficult to differentiate from radiation osteonecrosis or from recurrent tumor (Fig. 100–75). Their aggressive nature is soon demonstrated, and the prognosis is very poor.

Myositis Ossificans

Myositis represents a post-traumatic formation of bone that, in the early stages, may appear as amorphous bone formation, simulating osteosarcoma. Furthermore, if the myositis arises adjacent to underlying bone, it may elicit a periosteal reaction and even cortical response. Thus the lesion can appear quite aggressive (Fig. 100–76). A strong clinical suspicion, combined with understanding of the timing of radiographic changes in myositis, helps the radiologist distinguish this lesion from osteosarcoma.

The early lesion (week one to three following trauma) is a soft-tissue mass that is clinically painful and warm. By week three or four after trauma, flocculated amorphous densities are seen within the mass. Periosteal reaction in the underlying bone may be seen. It is at this stage where myositis ossificans is most commonly mistaken for an early osteosarcoma. By weeks six to eight, the peripheral portion of the lesion demonstrates well-organized cortical bone. This surrounds a lacy pattern of less-organized bone. Maturation proceeds centrifugally. This zoning phenomenon is the opposite of that seen in parosteal osteosarcoma. Finally, after several months, the mature lesion usually reduces in size and occasionally disappears altogether. There is very often a radiolucent zone that separates the lesion from the underlying bone cortex. It can thus be seen that history and timing are crucial in supporting the early diagnosis of myositis ossificans. With good correlation of this information and the radiographic findings, early and potentially confusing biopsies can often be avoided.

Bibliography

Enneking W: Musculoskeletal Tumor Staging, Vols I and II. New York, Churchill-Livingstone, 1983.

Enneking WF: Staging of musculoskeletal neoplasms. Skeletal Radiology 13:183–194, 1985.

Hudson T: Radiologic-Pathologic Correlation of Musculoskeletal Lesions. Baltimore, Williams and Wilkins, 1987.

Manaster BJ: Handbook for Skeletal Radiology. Year Book Medical Publishers, 1989.

Manaster BJ, Ensign MF: Imaging of musculoskeletal tumors. Semin Oncol 18:140–149, 1991.

Mankin HJ, Lang TA, Spanier SS: The hazards of biopsy in patients with malignant primary bone and soft tissue tumors. J Bone Joint Surg 64(8):1121–1127, 1982.

Mirra J: Bone Tumors: Diagnosis and Treatment, 2nd ed. Philadelphia, JB Lippincott, 1980.

Pettersson H, Gillespy T, Hamlin D, et al: Primary musculoskeletal tumors: Examination with MR imaging compared with conventional modality. Radiology 164:237, 1987.

101 Musculoskeletal Trauma

Anthony J. Doyle and B. J. Manaster

INTRODUCTION

Anthony J. Doyle

Imaging of musculoskeletal trauma involves the demonstration and description of fractures, dislocations, and associated soft-tissue injuries. The mainstay of this process is plain film radiography, supplemented by tomography, computed tomography (CT), magnetic resonance imaging (MRI), and nuclear isotope studies. This chapter covers the principal areas of the body commonly involved in trauma and their most common injuries. It is designed as an overview; for more detailed discussion of fracture patterns, the reader is referred to Lee Rogers' text *Radiology of Skeletal Trauma* and other references cited at the end of this chapter. This chapter is divided by anatomic regions with a short passage at the beginning of each covering the normal variants in that region which can mimic trauma. For more detail on normal variants, the reader is referred to Theodore Keats' *Atlas of Normal Roentgen Variants That May Simulate Disease*. Most pediatric trauma is covered in the respective sections with a separate section devoted to nonaccidental injury and the classification of childhood fractures.

Fractures and Their Terminology

A fracture involves the complete or partial disruption of a bone or cartilage by the application of force. When force is applied to a bone, it initially responds by elastic deformation; that is, when the force is removed, the bone returns to its original shape. Further application of force leads to plastic deformation with permanent distortion of the bone—this happens more often in children than in adults. After more force is applied, beyond the "fracture threshold" of a bone, the bone fractures. The break may be complete or incomplete—incomplete fractures are more common in children (Fig. 101–1) and in bones that are abnormally soft due to osteomalacia, Paget's disease, or some other metabolic bone disease. Bony rings, as found in the pelvis, vertebrae and forearm, almost always break in two places, and the second site of disruption should be deliberately looked for if it is not obvious.

Stress, Insufficiency, and Pathologic Fractures

A stress fracture occurs when abnormal stress of a repetitive nature is applied to a normal bone. Repetitive stress lowers the fracture threshold of a bone, just as repeated bending of a piece of metal eventually results in fracture of the metal. Common sites of stress fractures include the metatarsal shafts (especially the second, Fig. 101–2), the calcaneus, tibia, fibula, proximal femur, and pubic rami. They may be very subtle in the early stages and require delayed films, nuclear medicine scan, or MRI for detection (Fig. 101–3). Insufficiency fractures occur when bone weakened by osteoporosis, hyperparathyroidism, or similar metabolic bone disease

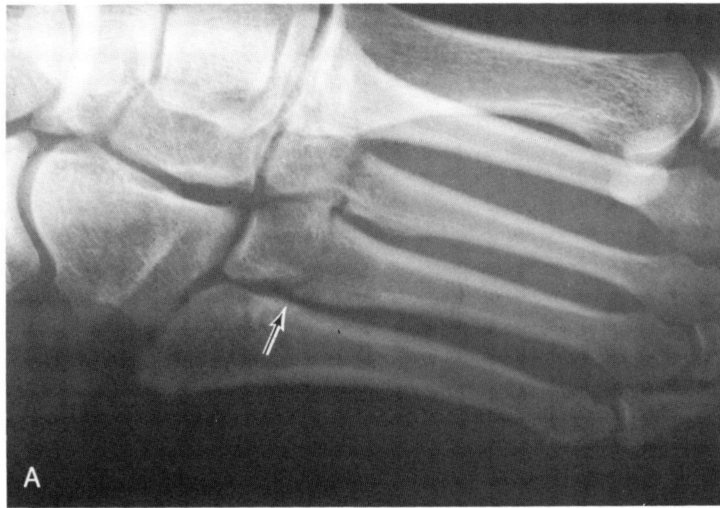
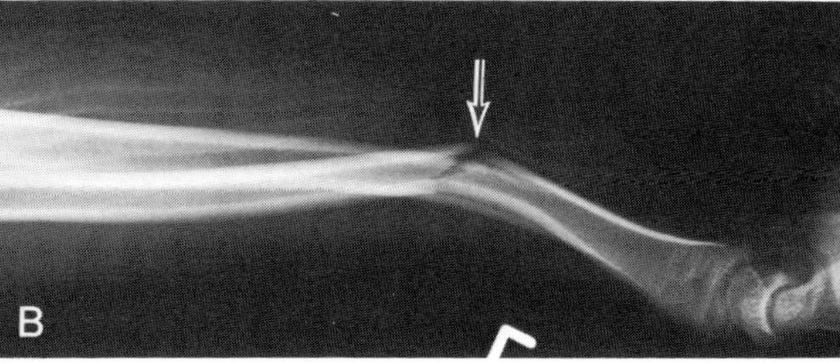

Figure 101–1. *A*, **Complete fractures *(arrow)*** through both cortices of the third and fourth metatarsal bases are seen. *B*, **Plastic bowing and an incomplete fracture** in an adolescent. There is an obvious break in the volar cortex of the radius (*arrow*), but the dorsal cortex is not completely fractured, with the fragments held together by the strong periosteum. This is a greenstick fracture. Note how the ulna at this point has a smooth curve in it with no break in the cortex. This is plastic bowing.

is placed under normal stress (Fig. 101–4). A pathologic fracture occurs when normal stress is placed on bone that is weakened by tumor involvement, either primary (Fig. 101–5) or metastatic. In the large long bones such as the femur, a transverse diaphyseal fracture in the absence of major trauma should raise the suspicion of a pathologic fracture.

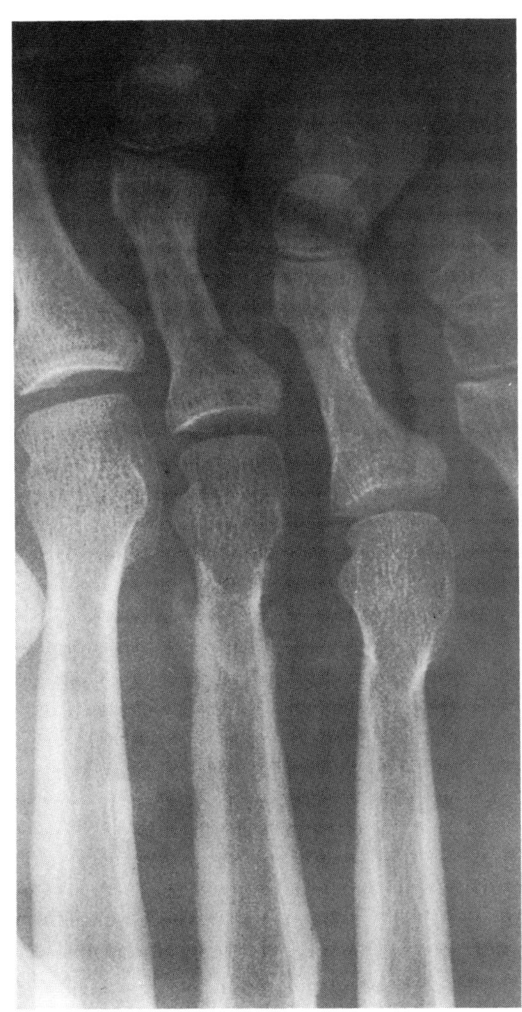

Figure 101–2. Stress fracture of the neck of the third metatarsal in an army recruit. Note the almost invisible lucent fracture line but quite easily appreciated fluffy periosteal new bone on this radiograph taken one week after the onset of pain.

Fracture Detection

Detection of fractures is usually accomplished by plain film radiography using at least two orthogonal views. Subtle nondisplaced fractures may show up only on delayed films after a week to 10 days when early healing has occurred with bone resorption around the fracture site. Alternatively, these fractures may be sought using more sophisticated imaging; MRI and nuclear isotope studies are both more sensitive than plain films for subtle fractures (Fig. 101–6), but they are much more expensive and should be used only when necessary. Both plain and computed tomography can be very useful for demonstrating fractures in complicated areas such as the spine and pelvis.

The importance of clinical correlation in fracture detection cannot be overemphasized; several studies show that an adequate history makes a significant difference to the ability to detect fractures, especially in the extremities. If no history is given, the radiologist is well advised to ask the patient where the pain is or get the technician taking the film to do so. The mechanism of injury can also make a difference in what types of fractures are expected and should be looked for.

Terminology

Precision of terminology is important in describing fractures because this has implications for treatment and prognosis. Fractures are described in terms of the site and direction of the fracture line, the degree of comminution, angulation, the apposition of the fragments, rotation and whether or not the fracture is open. To describe the site, the bone itself is identified as well as the particular part of the bone. By convention, long bones are divided into proximal, middle, and distal thirds and their individual features referred to by name when used as fracture landmarks (e.g., the greater tuberosity of the humerus). Other bones are described in terms of their anatomic features (e.g., the distal pole of the scaphoid). Joint involvement or lack of it is specifically referred to where relevant.

The fracture line is described as transverse, oblique, longitudinal, spiral, or complex and whether or not it is complete. The fracture is described as comminuted if it has two or more fragments. Some comminuted fractures have special names, e.g. the "pilon" fracture in the ankle. These particular subsets of comminuted fractures carry implications for treatment and healing that differ from other frac-

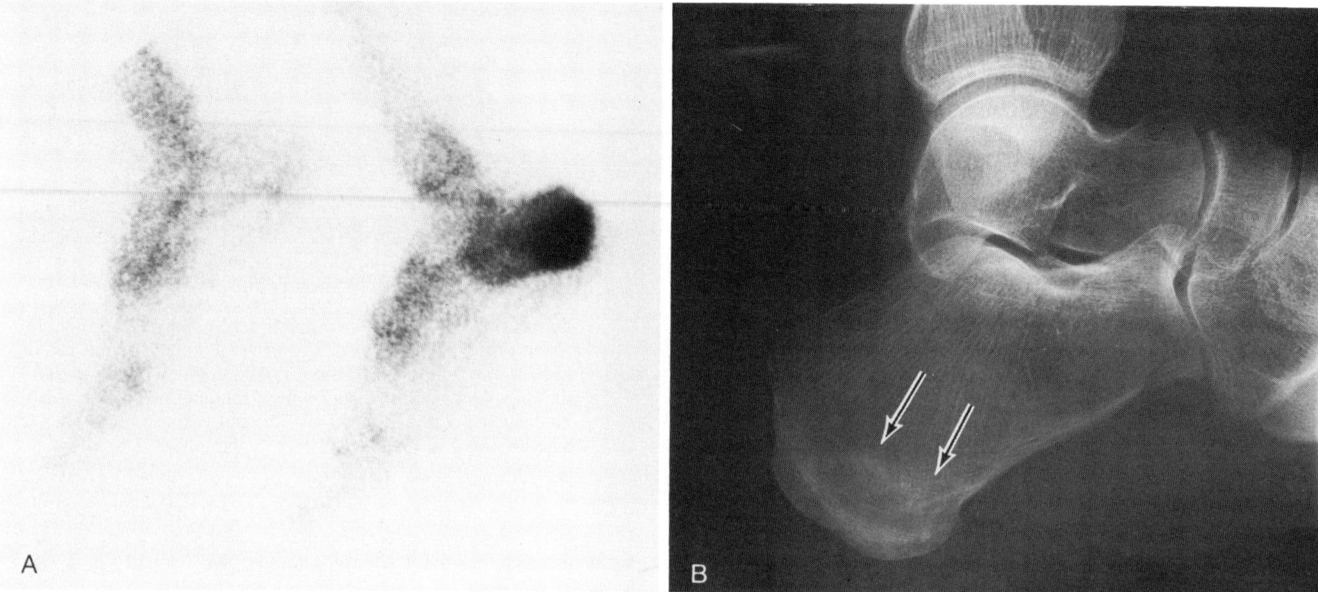

Figure 101–3. Stress fracture of the calcaneus. Initial radiographs in this middle-aged woman with heel pain were normal. The medial view on a bone scan performed after two days (*A*) shows intense increased uptake in the left calcaneus. A lateral radiograph one month later (*B*) shows a faint band of sclerosis (*arrows*), confirming the stress fracture.

tures in the same sites. A triangular fragment along one cortex of a long bone fracture is termed a *butterfly fragment* (Fig. 101–7*A*), whereas a portion of a long bone with a fracture at each end is termed a *segment*.

Apposition refers to the degree of contact of the bone ends. The fragments may be distracted, in which case the gap is measured in centimeters (Fig. 101–7*B*). Distraction may be due to excessive traction, interposed soft tissues, post-traumatic resorption of bone, or bone lysis secondary to infection. Impaction occurs when the fragments are driven into each other, usually producing increased density. Bayonetting refers to overlap of the fragments without angulation (Fig. 101–7*C*), and telescoping refers to the sliding of one fragment into the other fragment (usually when the latter is somewhat splayed open or there is a large displaced butterfly fragment). Displacement is described in terms of proportion of shaft width and direction of shift of the distal fragment with respect to the proximal (e.g., 60 per cent shaft width posterior displacement of the distal fragment, Fig. 101–7*D*) Angulation can be described in two ways. The direction in which the apex of the fracture is pointing can be described (e.g., ''apex medial,'' Fig. 101–7*E*), or the angulation of the distal fragment with respect to the proximal can be described (e.g., ''lateral angulation of the distal fragment''). The former is more concise and favored by many orthopedists, but either is acceptable provided the description is precise. The amount of angulation is referred to in degrees.

Rotation can be very important in long bones and should be specifically looked for. If both ends of the bone are included on the film, as they should be whenever possible, this is easy (Fig. 101–7*F*). When both ends are not included, changes in the size and shape of the bone at the fracture site as well as specific features

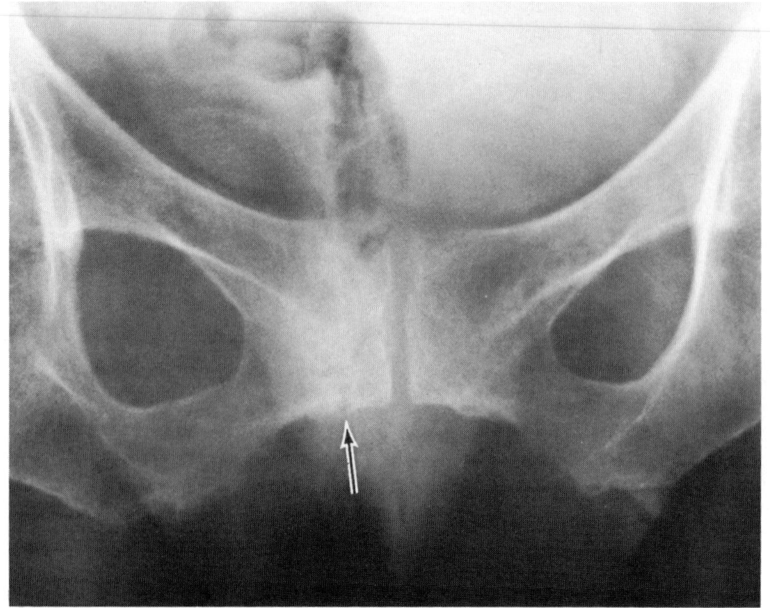

Figure 101–4. Insufficiency fracture of the right pubic bone is shown in an elderly osteoporotic woman who presented with right hip pain. The arrow indicates the fracture line with some surrounding sclerosis.

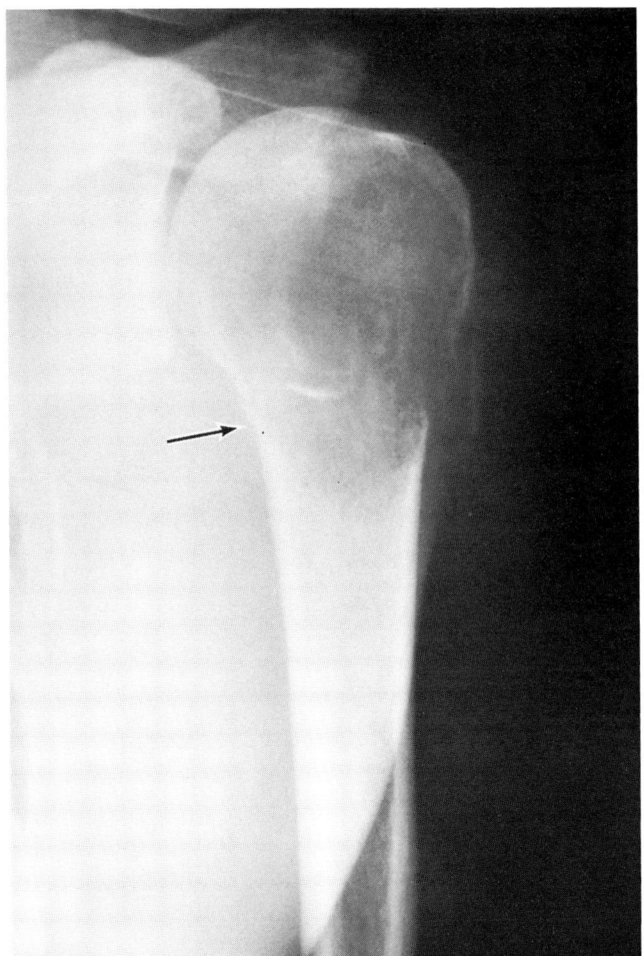

Figure 101–5. Pathologic fracture has occurred through a giant cell tumor in the proximal humerus of this 30-year-old patient. The lateral cortex is disrupted with a fragment displaced laterally, and there is a faint fracture line extending through the medial cortex *(arrow)*. (From Manaster BJ, et al: Giant cell tumor of bone. Radiol Clin North Am 31(2):303, 1993.)

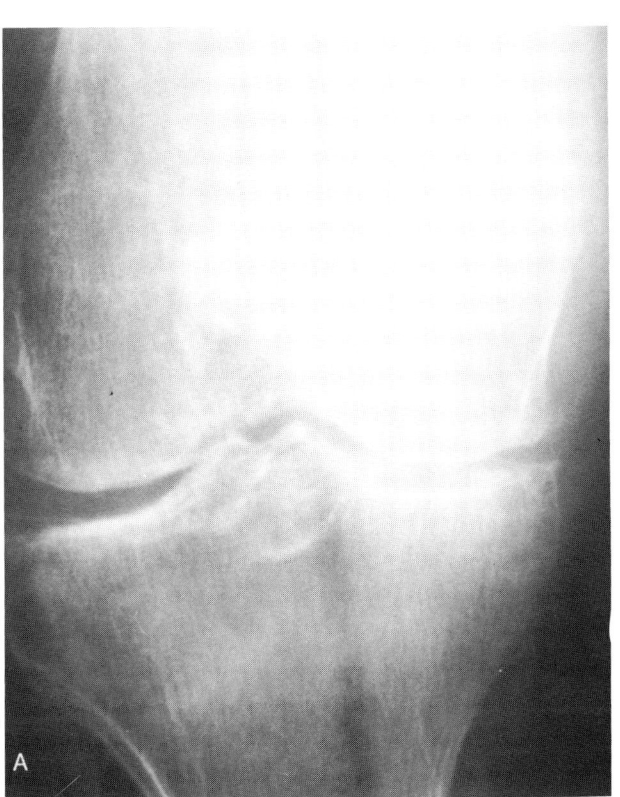

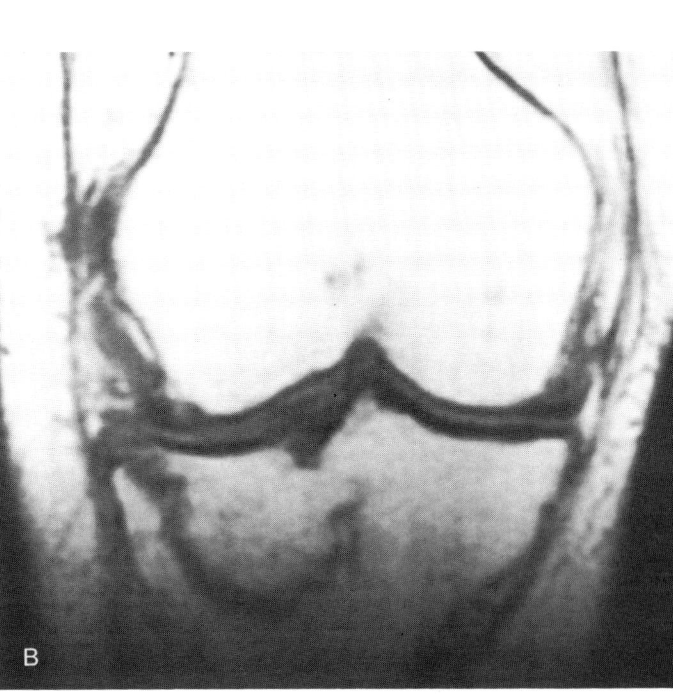

Figure 101–6. *A*, In an osteoporotic elderly woman, the AP view of the tibia shows only a **questionable line of sclerosis** in the proximal lateral aspect. *B*, The coronal T_1-weighted MRI shows very clearly the **low-intensity curvilinear fracture** through the lateral plateau.

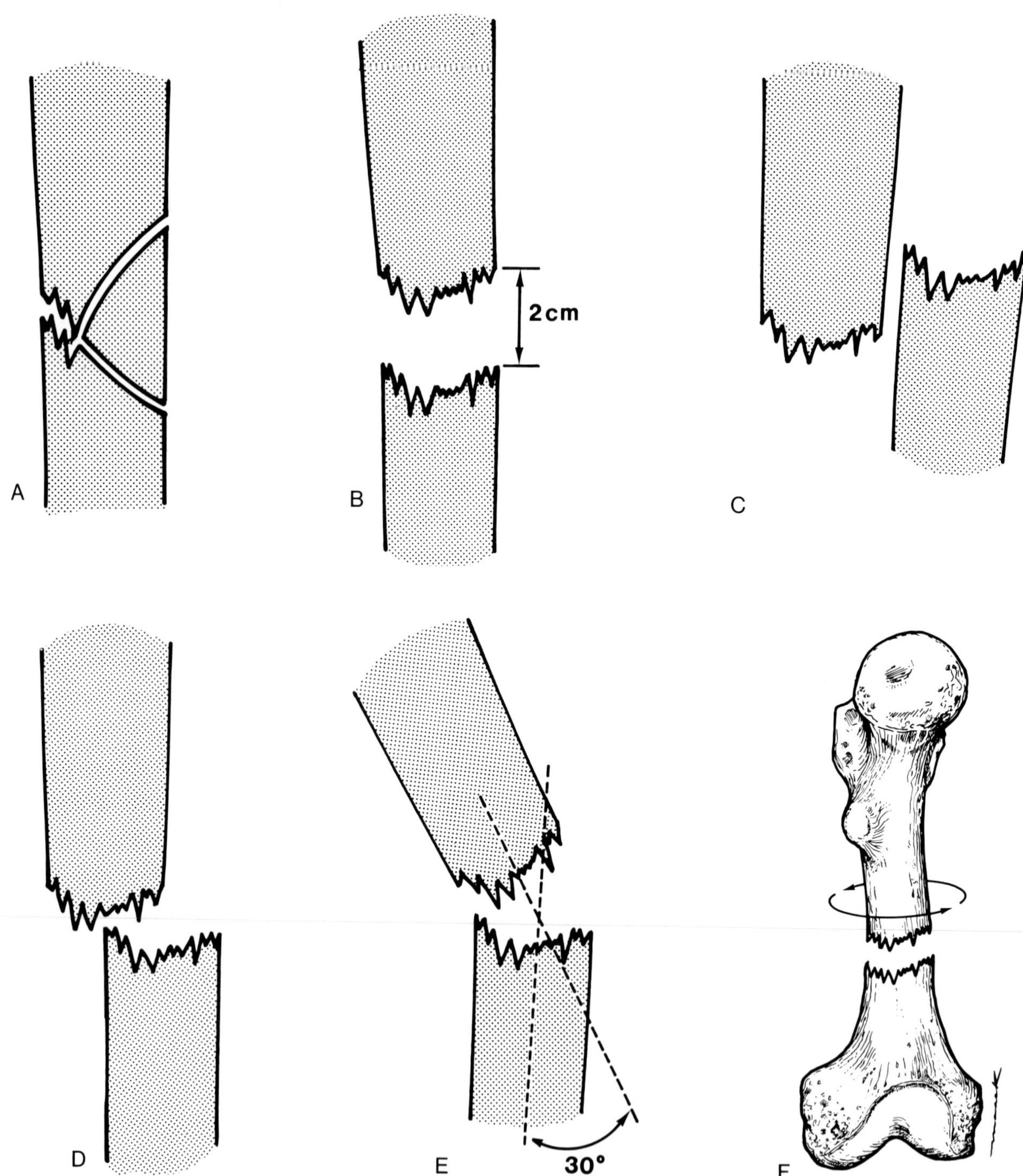

Figure 101–7. *A,* Diagram of a **nondisplaced comminuted fracture with a butterfly fragment** (the triangular fragment on one side of the fracture). *B,* A **simple transverse fracture** that shows **2-cm separation** of the bone ends. *C,* A simple transverse fracture with 100 per cent shaft width displacement and 2-cm **bayonet apposition** of the fragments. *D,* A simple transverse fracture showing **50 per cent shaft width displacement** of the distal fragment. *E,* A simple transverse fracture with **30-degree apex medial angulation** but no displacement. *F,* A foreshortened diagram of the femur showing a simple transverse fracture of the shaft with no displacement but with **90-degree external rotation** of the proximal fragment.

such as the continuity of the linea aspera of the femur should be assessed. Open fractures are often clinically obvious, but puncture wounds may be very difficult to see, with radiographic evidence of communication the only clue. The presence of gas or foreign material at the fracture site or in an adjacent joint alerts the radiologist that there may be communication of the fracture with the outside. This predisposes to infection and is important to detect.

Terms such as "good" or "bad" fracture alignment should be avoided as imprecise and containing value judgements. If alignment is normal, "anatomic" or "near-anatomic" alignment can be used. Many fracture eponyms exist and although they are of historic interest, they are often imprecise and confusing; a concise description of the fracture is usually more useful. There are, however, a few eponyms used very commonly, and these are included in the relevant sections.

Fracture Treatment and Healing

Some fractures heal by themselves without any further intervention (e.g., the common clavicle fracture). Others require casting in a plaster or fiberglass cast, whereas still others need operative reduction and/or fixation with orthopedic hardware. The rate of healing of a fracture depends on the bone in which it occurs; a simple clavicle fracture will heal in a few weeks, whereas a tibial fracture may take months to unite. The presence of infection, ischemia, foreign material (including hardware), interposed soft tissues, and excessive movement at the site all slow the rate of healing.

The first step in healing is resorption of bone around the fracture site leading to fuzziness of the margins and increased visibility of the fracture. This is usually maximal at around 10 days. Following this, woven bone is laid down, forming a callus, and this eventually is replaced with cortical or cancellous bone depending on the site. Remodeling of the fracture occurs to a variable degree depending on the bone involved and the age of the patient; young children can completely remodel the bone so that the fracture becomes indiscernible, but this is rare in adults.

Fracture healing may be abnormal in a number of ways. The bone may unite well but in an abnormal position—this is called a *malunion* (Fig. 101–8). Some joints cannot tolerate even a slight degree of malunion (e.g., the ankle, where malunion leads to early degenerative changes), whereas others can compensate for considerable deformity (e.g., the humerus). A fracture may heal slowly, termed a *delayed union*. This is not a radiographic diagnosis; the rate of healing depends on patient age, soft-tissue injury, and other factors not amenable to radiographic analysis. Finally, a fracture may not heal at all; this is a non-union. There are two types of non-union, one in which no new bone forms around the fracture (the atrophic non-union, Fig. 101–9) and one in which excess bone forms but does not bridge the fracture (the hypertrophic non-union; see Fig. 101–8), in which the fracture line is still visible with dense callus on either side of it. The radiographic hallmark of non-union is the rounded and sclerotic appearance of the bone ends at the fracture site.

Dislocation and Subluxation

This occurs when the surfaces of a joint are displaced with respect to each other. In a dislocation, the surfaces are no longer in contact (Fig. 101–10). A subluxation is a less severe displacement in which the surfaces are still partially in contact. Dislocation and subluxation are described in terms of the displacement of the distal fragment, e.g., anterior, lateral, etc. The presence of a dislocation implies damage to the ligaments and joint capsule contributing to the stability of the joint in question—the extent of this can only be inferred from plain films but can be directly imaged with MRI. There is frequently an associated effusion, and this may be the only

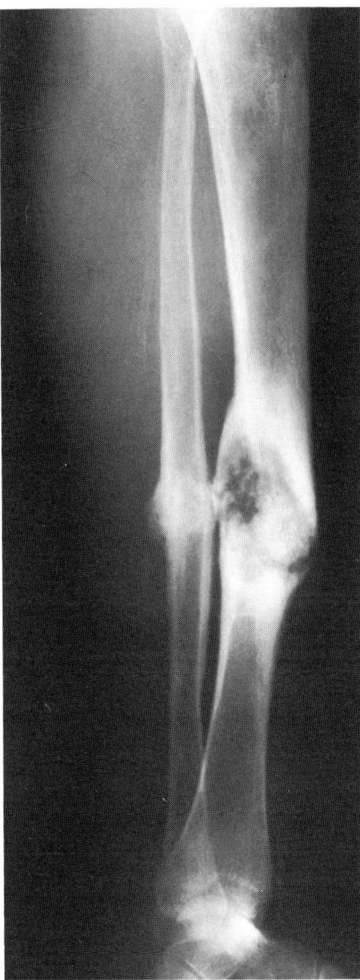

Figure 101–8. Malunion and hypertrophic nonunion are both demonstrated in this tibial fracture. Note the apex anterior angulation, which would result in significant malunion if healing continued. More prominent, however, is the dense callus on either side of the fracture line but without bony bridging. The rounded high-density bony ends are typical of hypertrophic nonunion.

sign of a subluxation that has then reduced, e.g. the lateral subluxation of the patella in the knee. There are often associated fractures and these should be sought.

Soft-Tissue Injuries

These may or may not be imaged radiographically, and can be seen directly only by MRI. The significance of soft-tissue injury is variable; it may be the most important component of the injury, as can happen in the cervical spine, with very little bony injury present but sufficient damage to result in quadriplegia (Fig. 101–11). Alternatively, a soft-tissue abnormality may be unimportant in itself but alert the radiologist to the presence of a bony injury, as in the elbow where the presence of an effusion may lead to the discovery of a subtle radial head fracture through obtaining additional views. Observation of a fat-fluid level in a joint is a sign of an intra-articular fracture that has resulted in fatty bone marrow leaking into the joint. This is observed most commonly in the knee and shoulder and is seen only on a horizontal-beam radiograph.

In some joints, it may be useful to obtain stress views to show that there is ligamentous laxity. In others, this is not important. MRI is the most effective technique and may be very useful to show

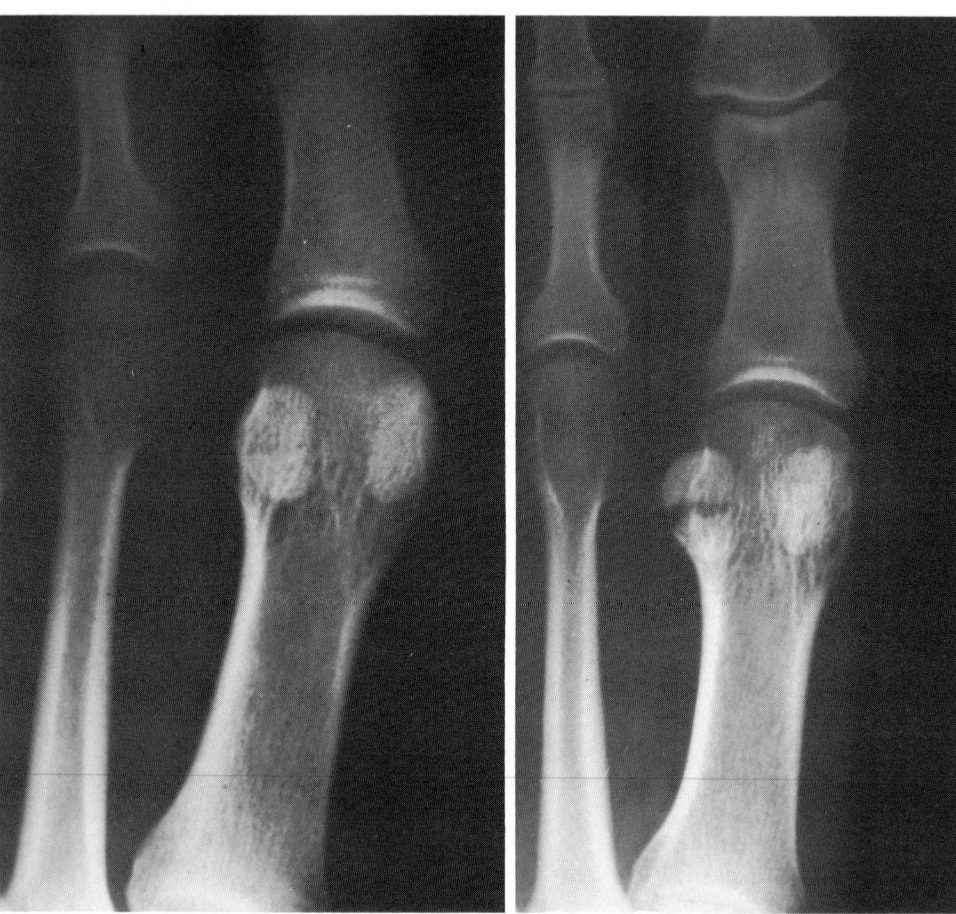

Figure 101–9. Atrophic nonunion of a sesamoid fracture is seen. The initial radiograph (*A*) shows a faint transverse fracture. Six months later (*B*), the fragments have failed to unite and have separated slightly with no callus formation visible.

Figure 101–10. Dislocation of the interphalangeal joints is common, as seen in this example. The articular surfaces are no longer in contact. Tiny bone fragments indicate an associated fracture, which is a common finding.

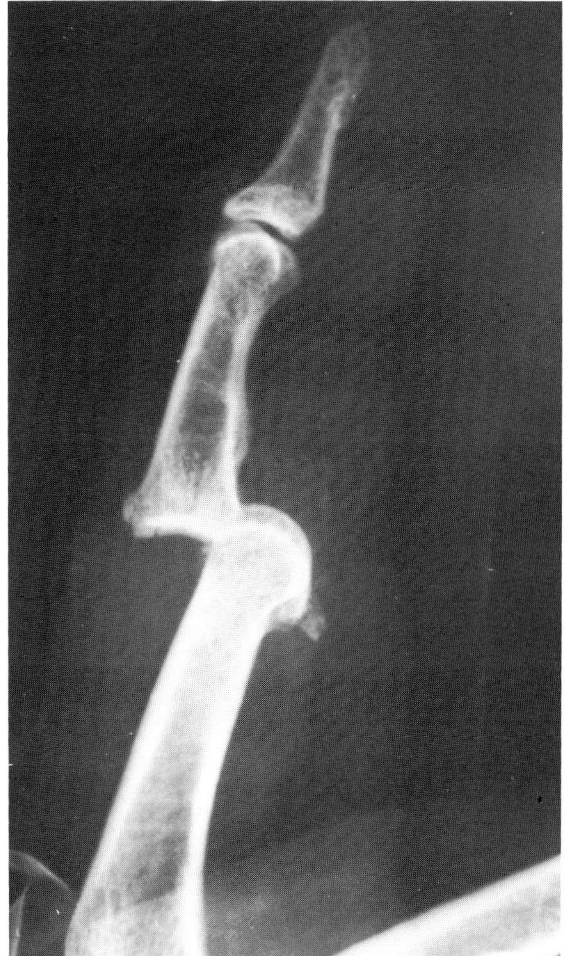

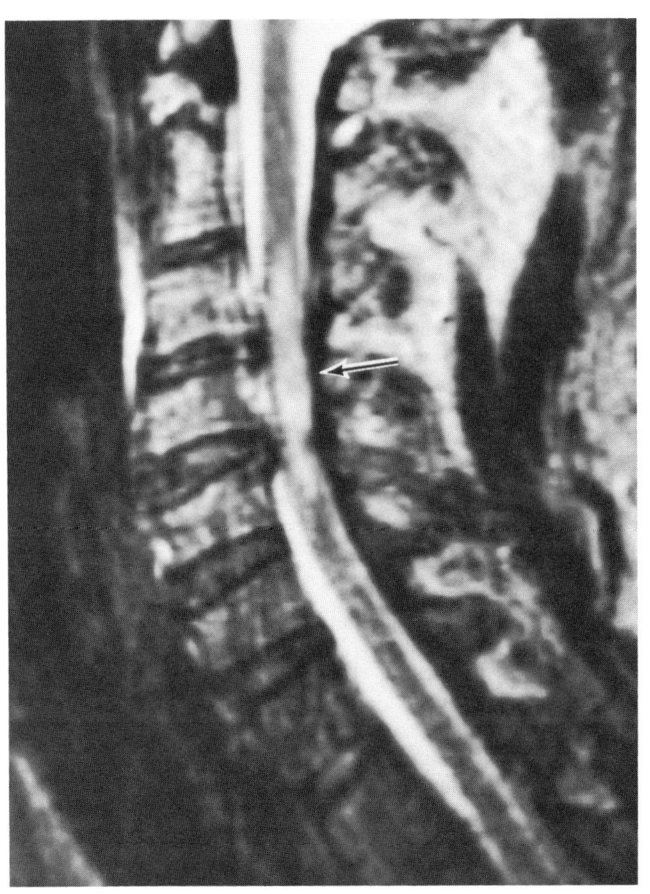

Figure 101–11. Spinal cord edema is seen in this 50-year-old man who suffered a flexion injury in a motor vehicle accident and was immediately rendered quadriplegic. On the sagittal T_2-weighted MRI, note the area of high signal *(arrow)* within the spinal cord. The bony canal is narrowed by osteophytes anteriorly, but no fracture was ever identified. (Reprinted with permission from the ACR Learning File, Skeletal Videodisc [1993], Case 443.)

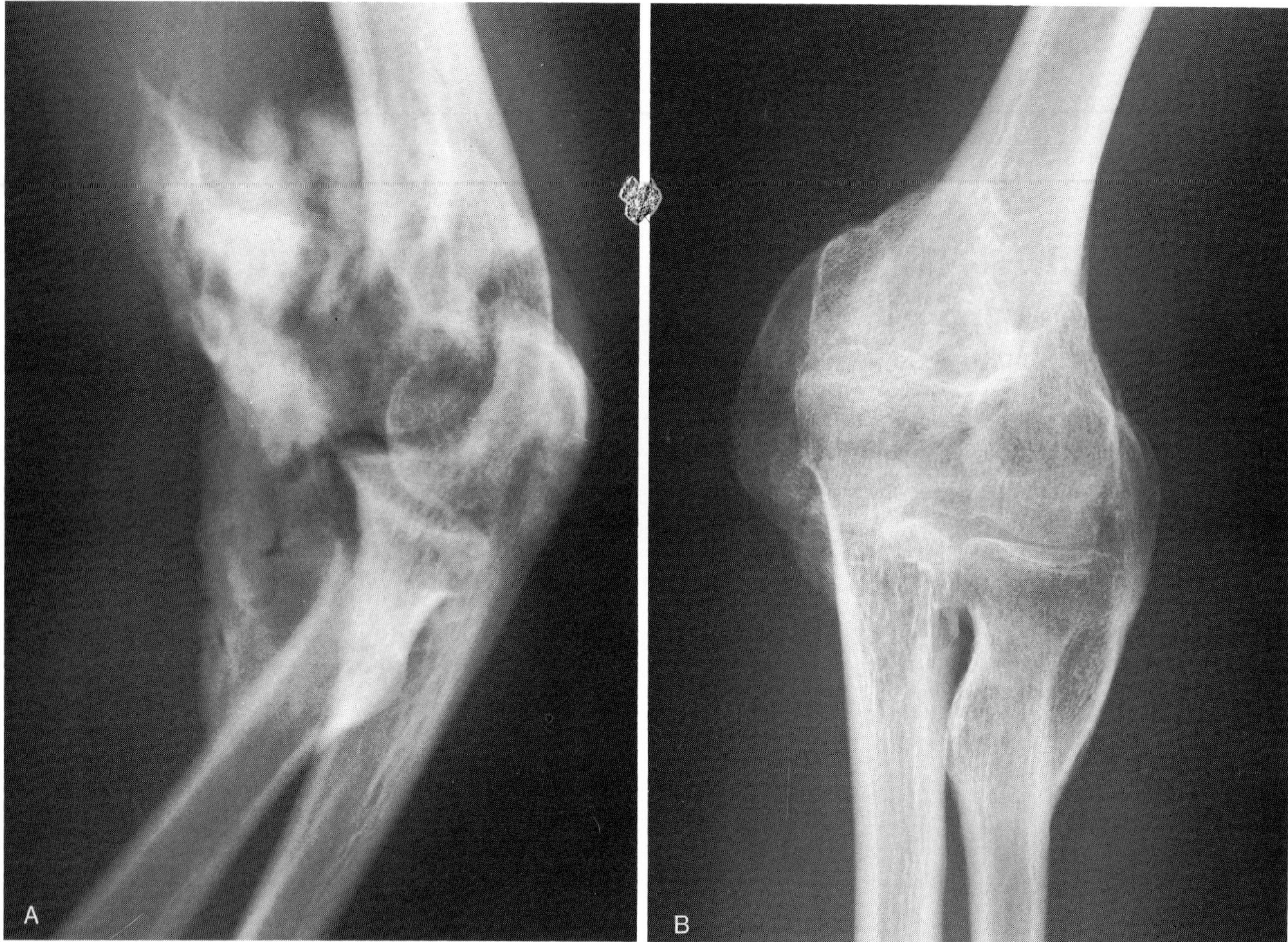

Figure 101–12. Myositis ossificans following an elbow dislocation is shown in a 22-year-old man. There is cloud-like calcification (*A*) forming six weeks after the injury. An AP view taken one year later (*B*) shows consolidation into a bony mass with clearly defined trabeculae within it.

ligament injury and injuries to other soft-tissue structures such as the menisci of the knee. Arthrography has only a minor role to play in acute trauma.

Myositis ossificans is an uncommon but characteristic complication of trauma, seen most frequently in adolescents and young adults. The most common sites are the elbow, the thigh, the gluteal muscles, the shoulder, and the leg. Periosteal reaction and a soft-tissue mass appear around the trauma site followed by cloud-like calcifications between 11 days and 6 weeks post trauma. The mass calcifies in an eggshell fashion with peripheral calcification around a soft-tissue core (Fig. 101–12). This is well demonstrated by CT and it is very characteristic of myositis ossificans. Periosteal reaction may be quite prominent. The calcified mass is initially separated from the underlying bone by a lucent gap in most cases but may fuse with the bone later on. These two features and a history of trauma help differentiate myositis ossificans from other bone-producing lesions such as parosteal osteosarcoma, osteochondroma, and extraskeletal osteosarcoma. It helps to know that the cellular center of myositis ossificans contains rapidly proliferating cells that on biopsy may cause pathologic confusion with an osteosarcoma. The outer ossifying layer of the lesion reflects its true nature and biopsy should be guided to include this if it is performed. A bone scan is usually performed prior to attempted surgical excision to ensure that the lesion is mature; excision of active myositis ossificans can lead to further bone production and actually worsen the condition.

Pediatrics

GENERAL CONSIDERATIONS AND NONACCIDENTAL INJURY

Children's bones differ considerably from adults in that the bones themselves are more resilient and deformable. Furthermore, each bone has a secondary growth center at one or both ends, separated from the rest of the bone by a cartilaginous growth plate in which much of the bone growth occurs. There are two principal types of secondary growth centers: the epiphyses, which are under compression; and the apophyses, which are subject to tension by tendons and ligaments. The weakest areas in the pediatric skeleton are the growth plates, followed by the bones themselves, and then the ligaments. Consequently, ligamentous sprains are uncommon in children whereas growth plate injuries and fractures are relatively more common.

Growth plate fractures are generally grouped by the Salter-Harris classification. Type I is simple separation of the epiphysis, common in infants and toddlers. Type II is the commonest, where the growth plate fractures and takes with it a small part of the metaphysis. Type III is a fracture through the epiphysis with the fracture extending at right angles through the growth plate. Type IV is a fracture through the epiphysis, growth plate, and a portion of the metaphysis. Type V is a crush injury of the epiphysis and is rare. Any injury to the growth plate can lead to premature closure of all or part of it and resultant growth disturbance. Traditionally this complication is said to be maximal in type IV and V fractures and not so common in type I and II. However, this depends on the site and severity of the injury and the type of management employed (Fig. 101–13).

The periosteum in children is thick and tends to hold stray fragments in place, resulting in nondisplaced fractures. The common greenstick fracture involves a complete break in one cortex with an intact cortex and periosteum on the other side acting as a hinge (see Fig. 101–1*B*). Torus fractures are also common in childhood; they result from impaction and are seen as a small buckle usually in one cortex (Fig. 101–14). Children's bones are also more subject than adults' to plastic bowing (see Fig. 101–1*B*), which does not remodel well and can cause growth disturbance.

NONACCIDENTAL INJURY

This is a potentially lethal condition, with up to 5 per cent mortality if the child is returned home with the condition unrecognized. Most victims are younger than three years old with a second peak in incidence at between 11 and 17 years. First-born and premature children, stepchildren, and the handicapped are most at risk. Those inflicting the trauma often include boyfriends, relatives, siblings, babysitters, and stepparents.

Certain fractures are highly specific for nonaccidental injury. These include metaphyseal, posterior rib, scapula, spinous process, and sternal fracture. Eighty per cent of femoral fractures in children younger than two years of age are due to nonaccidental injury (Fig. 101–15). Of medium specificity are multiple or bilateral fractures (Fig. 101–16), fractures of differing ages, epiphyseal separations, vertebral body fractures, digital fractures, and complex skull fractures. Low-specificity fractures are those of the clavicle and long bone shafts and linear skull fractures (but only in the context of an adequate history of trauma). It should be noted that intracranial injuries may occur in the absence of skull trauma and are best demonstrated by CT or MRI. The presence of bilateral subdural hematomas, especially of differing ages, is suggestive of nonaccidental injury.

Although skeletal survey in suspected cases has a fairly low yield, it is generally viewed as worthwhile. Nuclear medicine bone scan can be useful in detecting rib fractures and differentiating fractures from unusual normal variants. Particular findings to look for are metaphyseal corner or "bucket handle" fractures, especially of the long bones of the limbs, which are nearly pathognomonic of nonaccidental injury (Fig. 101–17). They represent Salter II fractures of the growth plates caused while the child is being shaken forcefully. They are present, however, in less than a third of cases. Shaking may also cause periosteal reaction around the shaft of the long bone where the child has been gripped tightly and the periosteum stripped off. Various processes can mimic this, including scurvy, syphilis, Caffey's disease, septic arthritis, rickets, leukemia, and physiologic periostitis. Multiple fractures in various stages of healing can also be seen in osteogenesis imperfecta but this is usually easily distinguished from nonaccidental injury (Fig. 101–18).

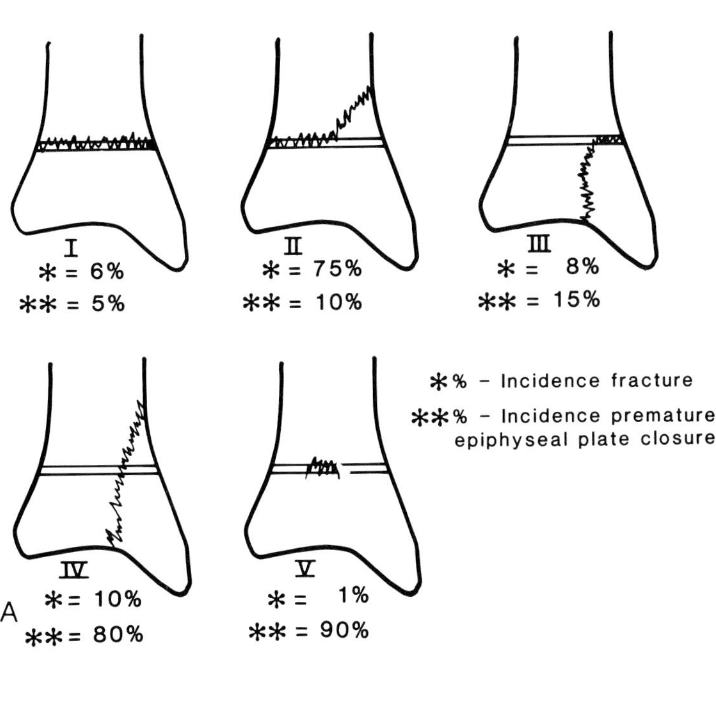

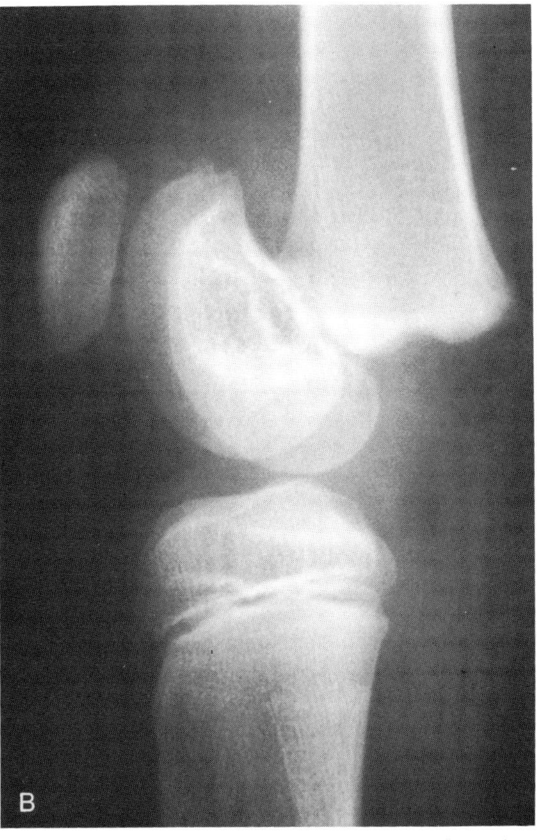

Figure 101–13. Salter-Harris classification of childhood fractures. *A,* Each type of fracture is shown diagrammatically, with both its overall incidence and the evidence of premature growth plate closure associated with it shown below it. *B,* A **type I fracture** of the distal femur is demonstrated. The semicircular distal femur epiphysis has separated from the metaphysis and is displaced anteriorly. The anterior periosteum is intact. (*B* courtesy of Paula Shultz, M.D., Salt Lake City, UT.) *C,* A **type II fracture** is seen on a lateral view of the ankle. The fracture line passes vertically through the posterior tibial metaphysis and then horizontally through the anterior half of the growth plate. The epiphysis and its attached metaphyseal fragment are displaced posteriorly. There is also a fibular fracture.

Illustration continued on following page

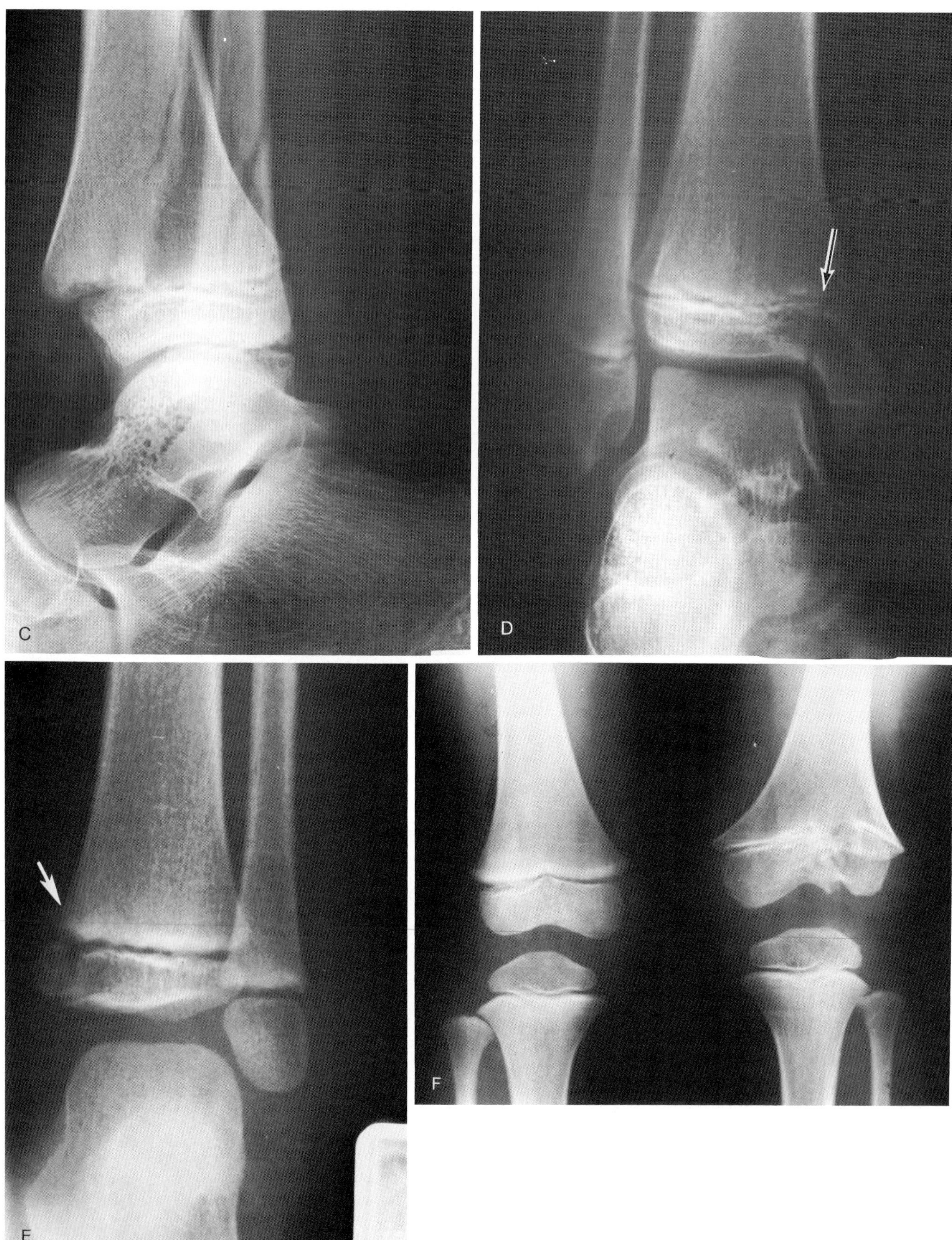

Figure 101–13 *Continued D,* A **type III fracture,** in which the fracture line extends through the medial growth plate and then vertically through the epiphysis *(arrow). E,* A **Salter IV fracture** of the distal tibia. A tiny fracture through the metaphysis *(arrow)* continues through the growth plate and the adjacent epiphysis, with slight displacement. These fractures frequently give rise to growth disturbance. *(E* courtesy of Paula Shultz, M.D., Salt Lake City, UT.) *F,* A **Salter type V fracture** has occurred previously in the left femur. As is often the case, the initial fracture was not detected and here are seen the sequelae in the form of premature fusion of the middle of the left distal femoral growth plate and consequent shortening of the left lower limb. Note that the margins of the distal femoral growth plate remain open and horizontal growth has not been affected, leading to a flared appearance.

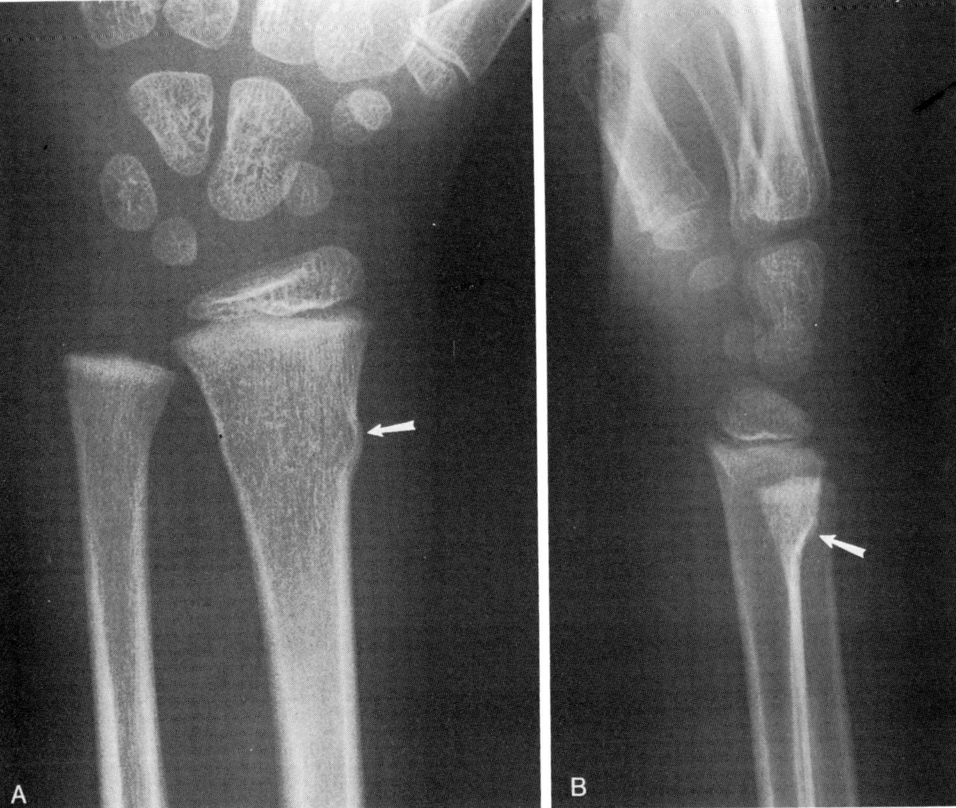

Figure 101–14. Torus fracture of the distal forearm in an eight-year-old patient. Note the buckle of the distal radius, which is most prominent on the radial and dorsal aspect (*arrows*) on the AP and lateral films (*A* and *B*, respectively). A much more subtle buckle fracture is seen on the ulna, better seen on the lateral than on the AP film. These incomplete fractures are typical of a fall on the outstretched arm in this patient age group.

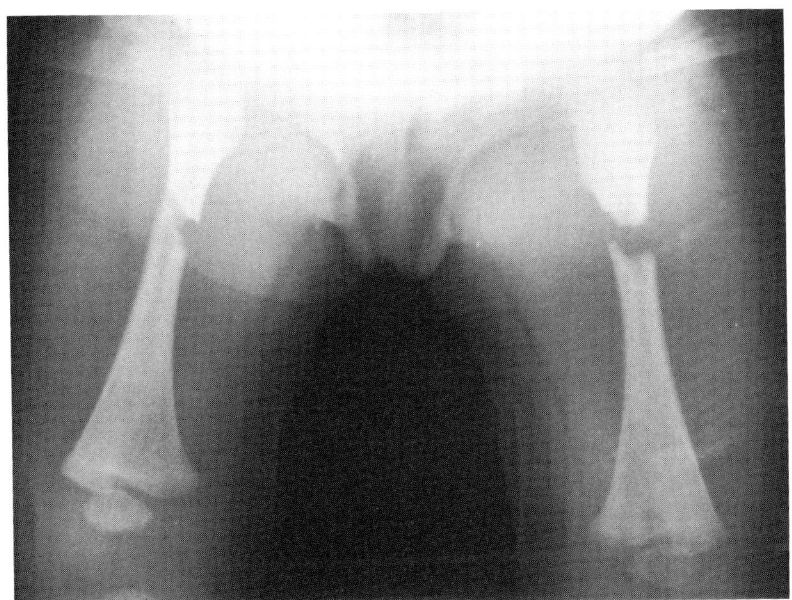

Figure 101–15. Bilateral femoral fractures in this two-month-old girl are typical of nonaccidental injury. The proffered history was that of "falling off a table," a totally inadequate explanation for these fractures.

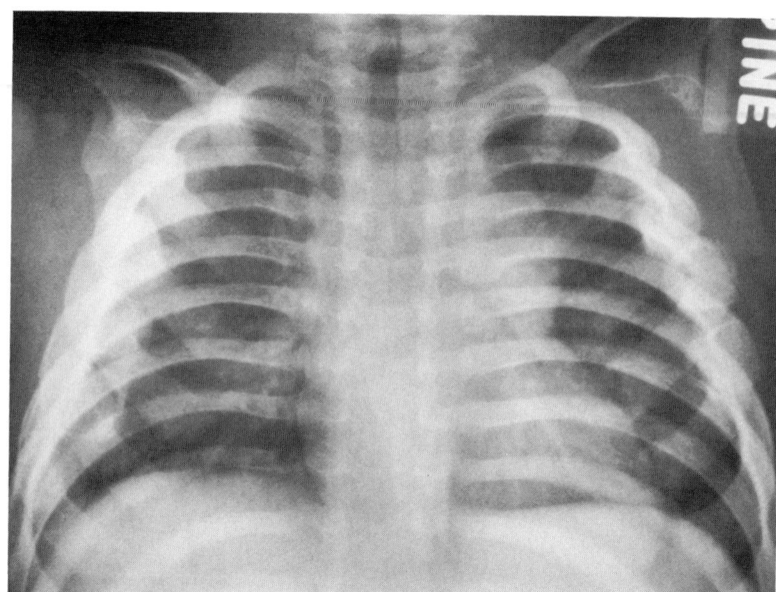

Figure 101–16. Bilateral rib fractures of varying ages are very typical of nonaccidental injury, as seen in this infant.

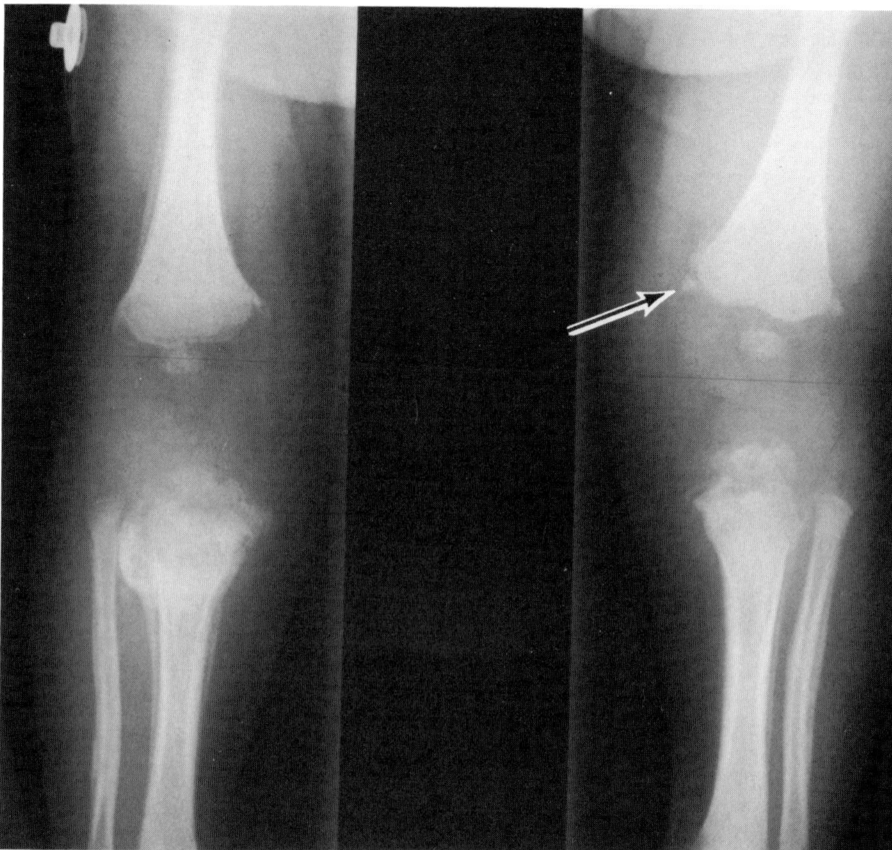

Figure 101–17. Bilateral metaphyseal corner fractures (*arrow*) and extensive periosteal new bone around the femora, tibias, and fibulas are effectively pathognomonic of nonaccidental injury.

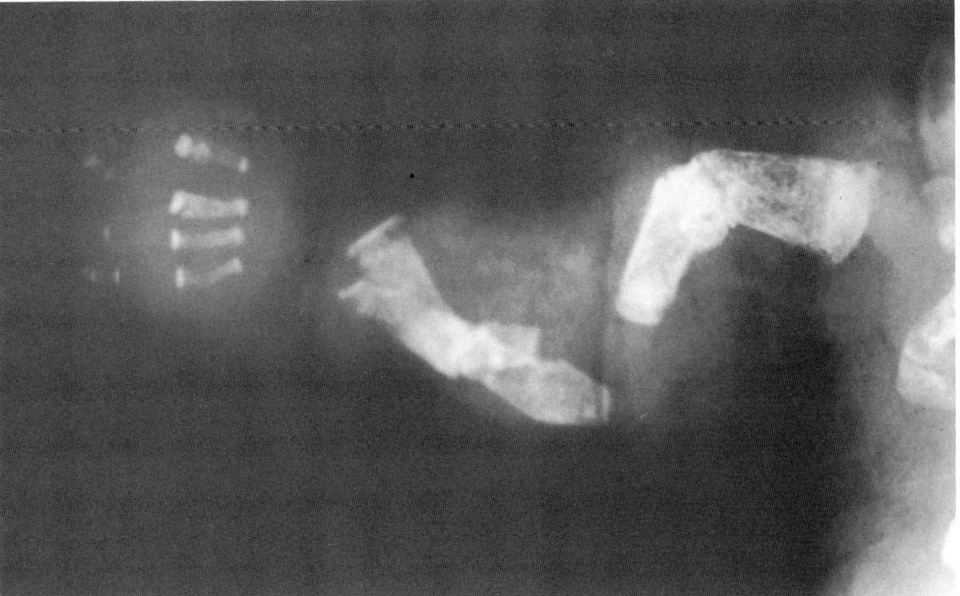

Figure 101–18. Osteogenesis imperfecta of the congenital form has led to multiple fractures and callus formation in the upper limb of this neonate. The abnormally thin cortices, osteopenia, and fractures throughout the skeleton distinguish this from nonaccidental injury.

THE CERVICAL SPINE

Anthony J. Doyle

The function of the cervical spine as a supporting column for the exposed and relatively heavy head makes it vulnerable to injury from accelerating or decelerating forces, direct flexion or extension, rotation, and compression. It may sustain fracture of the bony elements or damage to the ligaments, intervertebral discs, and other soft tissues alone but most frequently there is a combination of such injuries. Involvement of the spinal cord varies with the site and mechanism of injury; where the canal is wide or there is a fracture leading to widening of the canal, the cord may be unaffected. On the other hand, there may be severe cord trauma without much osseous damage, as can happen from severe flexion in a spine with a narrow bony canal (see Fig. 101–11).

Assessment depends strongly on the clinical history. If there is severe trauma, the initial film will be a cross-table lateral view. This is inadequate up to 25 percent of the time owing to lack of visualization of the cervicothoracic junction, rotation, or obscuration of soft-tissue swelling by nasogastric or other tubes. In mobile patients with a low suspicion of injury, a three-view study can be done immediately and may be all that is needed. Frontal and lateral films may be supplemented by swimmer's views, obliques, tomography, CT, or MRI as needed. Whatever is done, the entire cervical spine from the skull base to the top of T1 must be seen in two projections for adequate evaluation. When there is a question of ligament injury raised by the observation of soft-tissue swelling without bony abnormality, gapping of the spinous processes, focal kyphosis or lordosis, or mild subluxation, or change in the intervertebral space, dynamic assessment using flexion and extension views to exclude ligamentous injury may be necessary (on cooperative patients only!).

Care is necessary when moving patients with suspected spine trauma to avoid neurologic damage. If in doubt about the wisdom of moving such patients to get a particular view, consult with the clinical service taking care of them. It is often possible to use an alternative view or procedure to get the desired information.

Initial Assessment

The lateral view provides the most information and should be looked at systematically. Firstly, the prevertebral soft tissues should measure no more than about 7 mm in the upper spine and 21 mm below the level of the larynx, without any focal bulges. Secondly, the anterior and posterior vertebral body lines should form a smooth continuous curve. Thirdly, the spinolaminar lines should align perfectly to the level of C2 with an anterior step to C1 of no more than 2 mm. Fourthly, the spinous processes should form a smooth curve. Finally, the atlanto-axial gap should be less than 3 mm (Fig. 101–19) and the atlas, dens, vertebral bodies, facets, spinous processes, and disc spaces inspected on all views.

Normal Variants

Some common normal appearances may mimic trauma in the cervical spine. A fine black line across the base of the odontoid is often seen on the open-mouth AP odontoid view. This is a Mach effect produced by the arch of the atlas or the teeth overlying the dens (Fig. 101–20). It may be produced by the retina of the eye wherever there is an abrupt step-off in density and can be seen elsewhere (e.g., next to the heart border on the chest radiograph). Repeating the view in a slightly different obliquity can resolve this issue if there is any doubt.

In children, there is a normal slight anterior displacement of C2 on C3 and sometimes of C3 on C4. This physiologic subluxation (Fig. 101–21) decreases with age and should be minimal by adolescence. Under the age of eight years, the arch of the atlas may rest above the dens, especially in extension. The apical apophysis of the odontoid (the os terminale) appears at age 2 and fuses at age 12 or so; it should not be mistaken for a fracture of the tip of the dens, an entity that is virtually unknown in childhood. The spinous processes of the cervical vertebrae are often bifid and should not be mistaken for a fracture on the AP view.

In many normal individuals there is a slight wedged appearance to the bodies of C5 and C6 that can be mistaken for a compression fracture. In older people there may be osteophytes that can produce lucencies overlying the vertebrae (Fig. 101–22) or may be "floating" anteriorly and simulate small avulsion fractures. Correlation with symptoms, lack of soft-tissue swelling, or use of flexion/extension views can aid in recognizing these normal variants.

Pediatrics

Injuries to the cervical spine in childhood are uncommon. They can be divided into infantile (until head control is gained), young

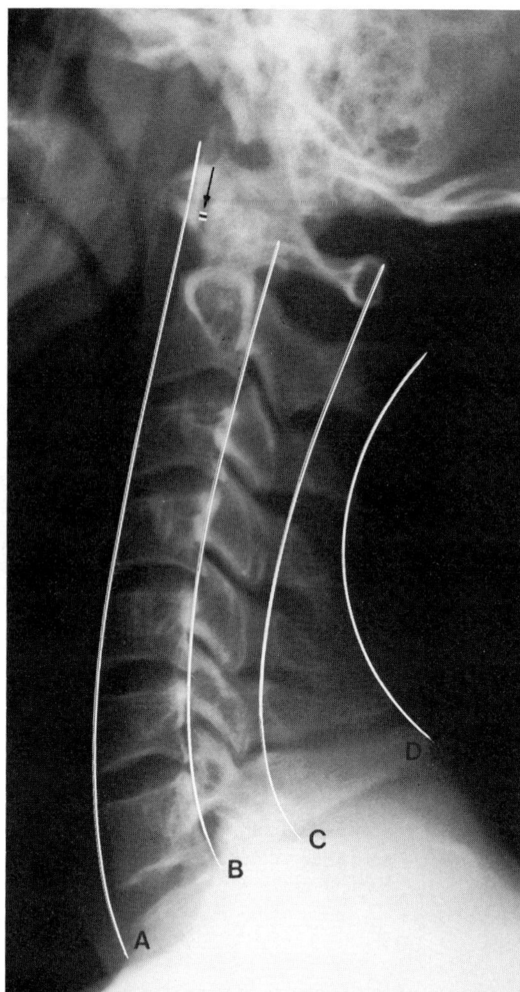

Figure 101–19. Normal cervical spine alignment on the lateral is described by four continuous curves: *A*, Anterior margins of the vertebral bodies. *B*, Posterior margins of the vertebral bodies. *C*, Spinolaminar lines. *D*, Spinous processes. The arrow indicates the atlanto-axial gap measurement. (Courtesy of B. J. Manaster, M.D., Ph.D.)

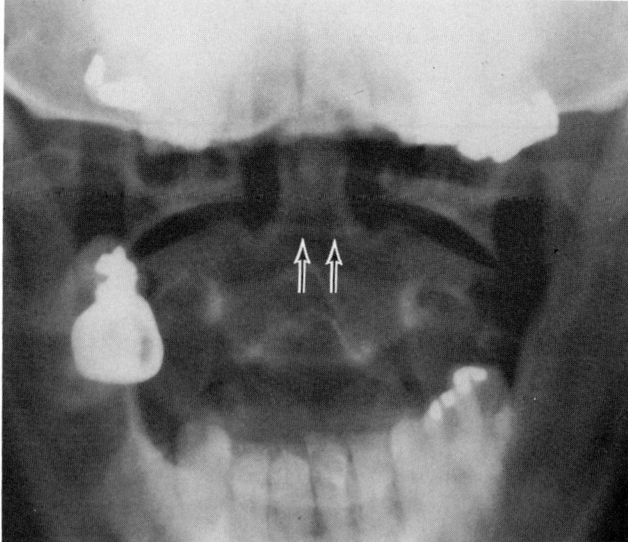

Figure 101–20. A Mach effect simulating a fracture is produced by the posterior arch of the atlas overlying the base of the dens (*arrows*). Note a similar effect produced by the incisors and the anterior arch of the atlas overlying the tip of the dens. (Courtesy of B. J. Manaster, M.D., Ph.D.)

juvenile (up to 7 to 9 years), and juvenile types. The juvenile injuries are essentially the same as those of adults.

In the infant, spinal cord damage may occur during birth or from later trauma, accidental or not. The spine is very elastic and even shaking may cause cord damage. There is usually no radiographic abnormality except on MRI.

In the young juvenile, injuries are most common in the upper cervical spine. Burst fracture of the atlas, fracture through the subdental synchrondrosis, and rotary atlanto-axial subluxation are the most common (although the last more often is not due to trauma).

Pathologic subluxation in the upper cervical spine in this age group is extremely uncommon, as are injuries below the level of C3. Care should be taken not to mistake normal synchondroses for fractures (Fig. 101–23).

Specific Injuries in Adults

Although these are often classified by the mechanism of action, we will approach them here by anatomic region because this is simpler and often more clinically relevant. Most cervical spine injuries occur at C5-C6, with a smaller concentration at C1-C2. Some injuries are regarded as "stable" in that the vertebrae are unlikely to move and compromise the spinal cord, whereas others

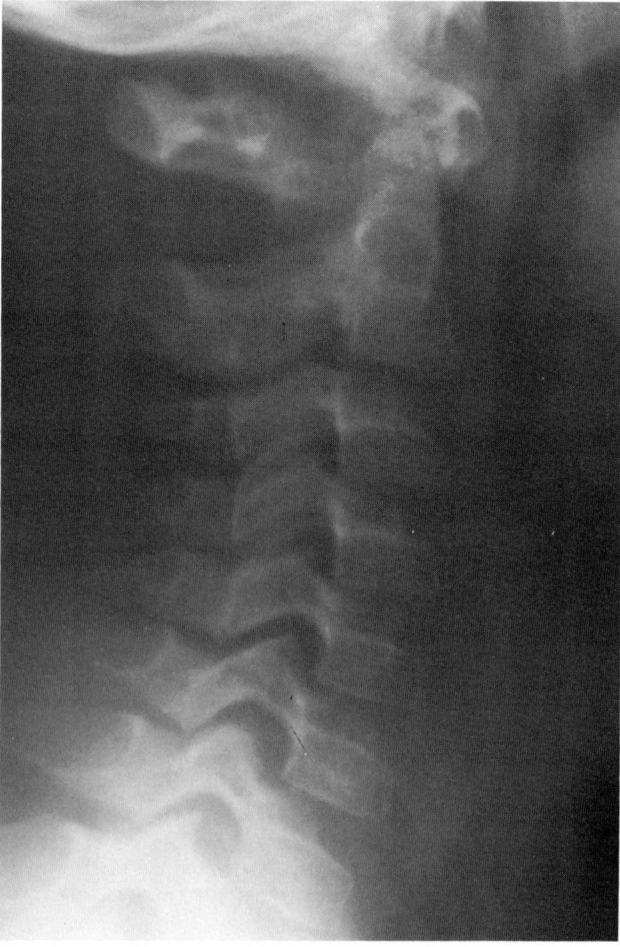

Figure 101–21. Physiologic subluxation of C2 and C3 is common in children. Note also the slight wedge-shaped appearance of the vertebral bodies. This is normal, due to unossified ring apophyses, and may persist into adult life. (Courtesy of B. J. Manaster, M.D., Ph.D.)

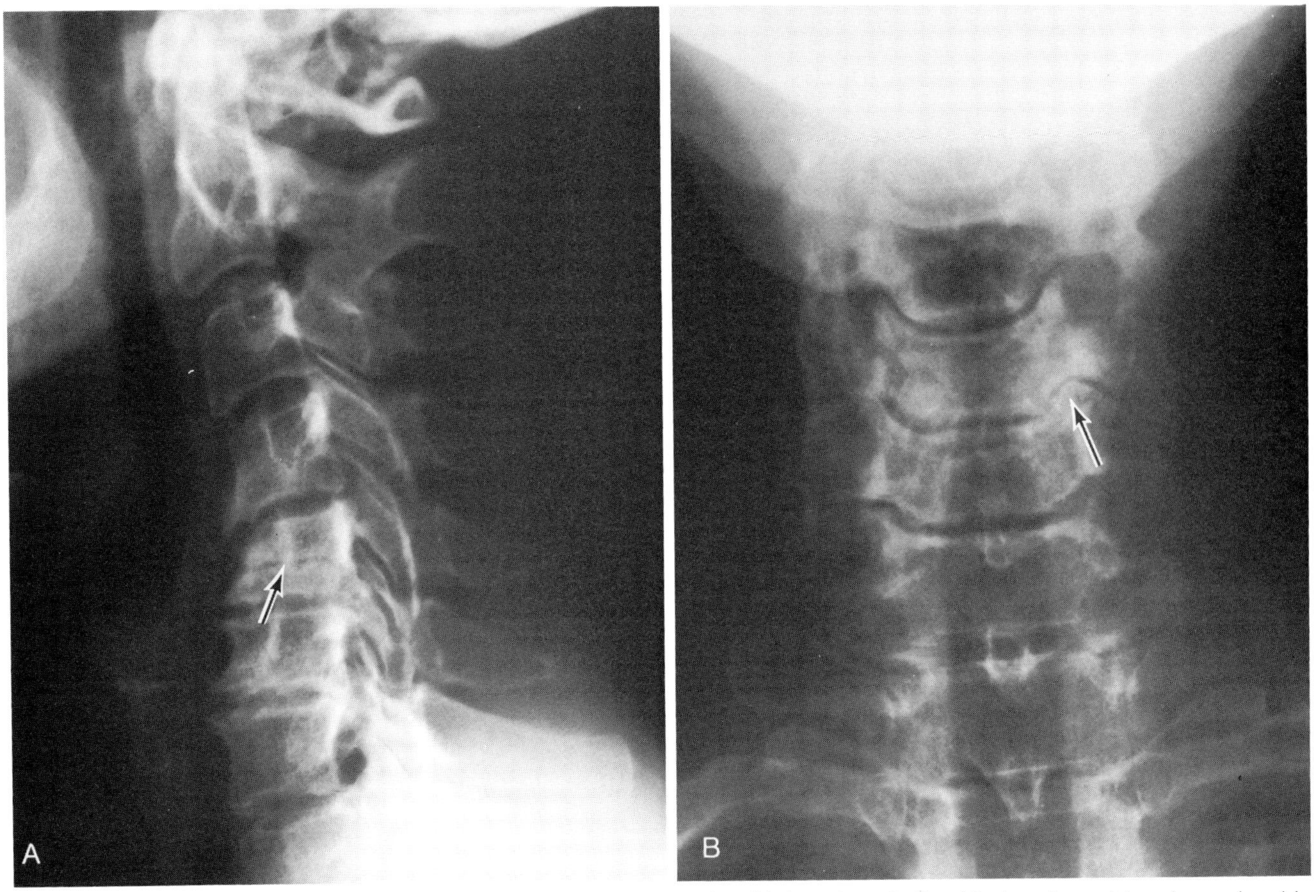

Figure 101–22. *A*, A **lucency overlying C5** (*arrow*) simulates a fracture in this elderly patient. *B*, The AP view shows this to be produced by degenerative changes in the uncovertebral joint (*arrow*). (Courtesy of B. J. Manaster, M.D., Ph.D.)

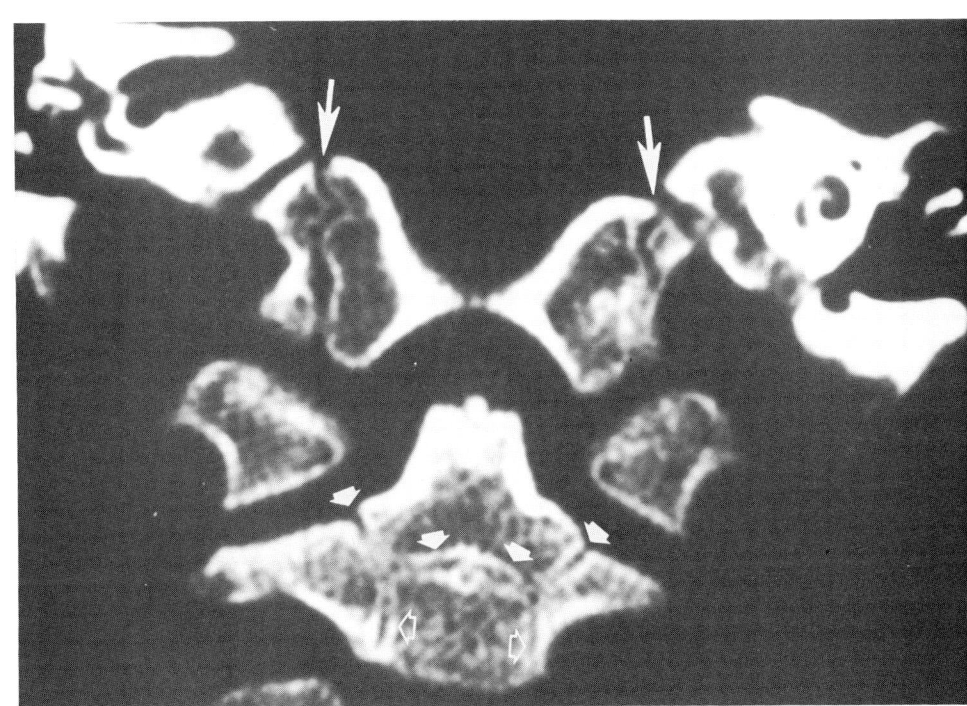

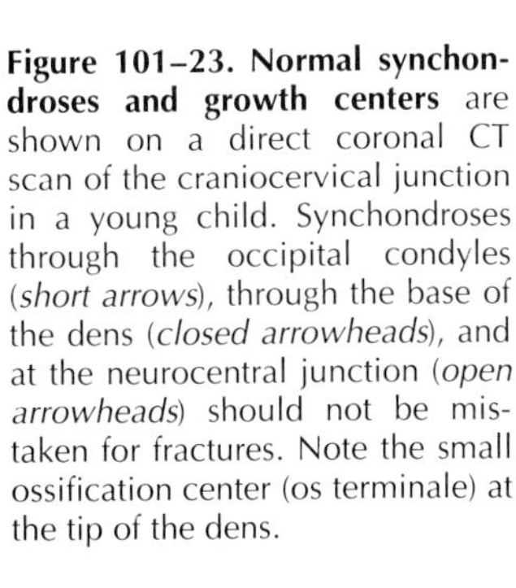

Figure 101–23. Normal synchondroses and growth centers are shown on a direct coronal CT scan of the craniocervical junction in a young child. Synchondroses through the occipital condyles (*short arrows*), through the base of the dens (*closed arrowheads*), and at the neurocentral junction (*open arrowheads*) should not be mistaken for fractures. Note the small ossification center (os terminale) at the tip of the dens.

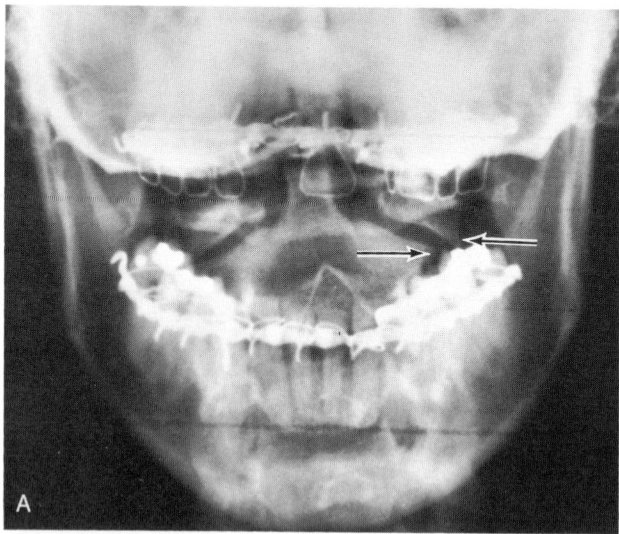

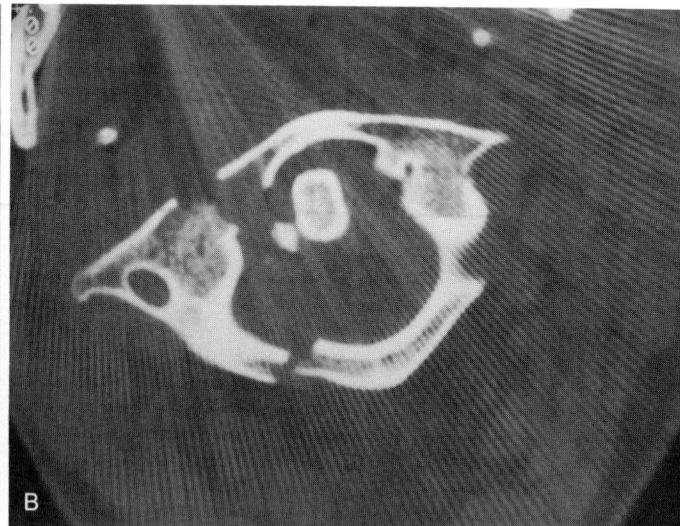

Figure 101–24. *A*, **Jefferson fracture**. The open-mouth odontoid view shows lateral displacement of both articular masses of C1 with lack of congruence of the atlanto-axial joint surfaces (*arrows*). *B*, Thin-section CT scan through the atlas clearly shows the fracture of both anterior and posterior portions of the bony ring. The atlanto-axial joint is also widened.

are "unstable" and extra care must be taken to protect the spinal cord. The division between stable and unstable depends largely on the amount of ligamentous and other soft-tissue damage involved.

As in the lumbar spine, the cervical spine is often thought of as consisting of three columns. The anterior column comprises the anterior longitudinal ligament and anterior half of the vertebral body and intervertebral disc. The middle column includes the posterior half of the vertebral body and disc with the uncovertebral joints (joints of Luschka). The posterior column contains the facet joints and their capsules, neural arch, and the interspinous ligaments and ligamenta flava. Generally speaking, spinal fractures are considered unstable if two or more columns are disrupted.

THE UPPER SPINE

Atlanto-occipital dislocation is uncommon; extreme force is required and it is usually fatal, secondary to transection of the spinal cord at the spinomedullary junction. Other injuries at the atlanto-occipital junction are uncommon and often best looked for with CT because many overlapping shadows make plain film interpretation difficult.

The atlas itself undergoes two common types of injury—fracture of the posterior arch by hyperextension of the neck, crushing the arch between the occiput and the arch of C2 (a stable fracture), and axial loading producing a wedging action of the facet joints, forcing the articular masses of the atlas laterally and bursting the bony ring (the Jefferson fracture, unstable because the transverse ligament of the atlas is torn, Fig. 101–24). These should be initially detected on lateral and odontoid views respectively and are both well seen by CT.

Atlanto-axial subluxation is not uncommon and often appears as a widening of the atlanto-axial distance and/or a larger than usual step-off in the spinolaminar line at C1-C2 posteriorly on the lateral radiograph, sometimes seen only on the flexion view. It implies disruption of the transverse ligament of the atlas, disruption of the bony ring, or a displaced odontoid fracture, and is usually unstable.

Fracture of the odontoid (dens) of the axis may occur through the dens itself (Fig. 101–25) or through the base into the body of the axis (termed types II and III respectively —type I, fracture of the tip of the dens, is very rare). Both types II and III are unstable. Type II fractures tend to go on to non-union because of their high content of cortical bone.

The axis itself may fracture through the posterior arch (traumatic spondylolysis or hangman's fracture, unstable although rarely associated with cord damage because the canal at this point is wide, Fig. 101–26) or suffer avulsion of the inferior corner by the anterior longitudinal ligament (extension teardrop fracture, stable).

THE MID-CERVICAL SPINE

Injuries in this region are commonly caused by flexion, extension, rotation, or a combination of these forces.

The mildest flexion injury is the sprain, in which the ligaments are stretched without fracture or dislocation. More severe flexion

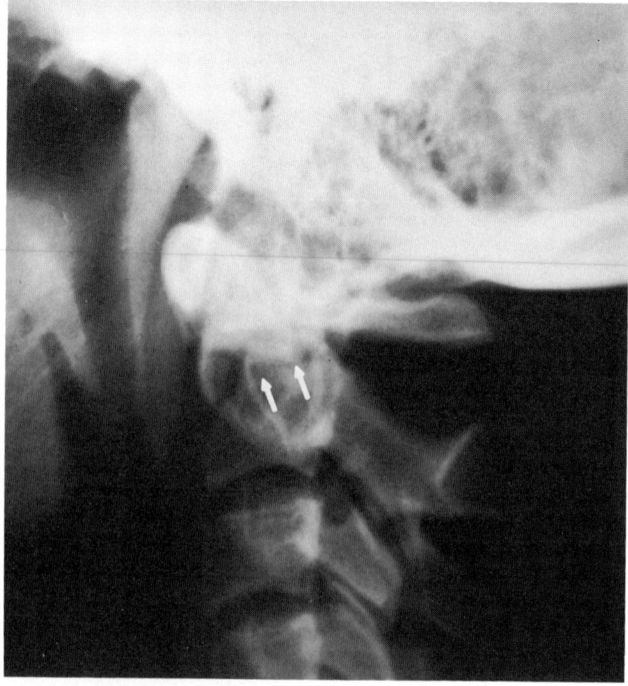

Figure 101–25. There is soft-tissue swelling anterior to C2. Furthermore, the posterior arch of the atlas is anterior from its normal position, and if one follows the anterior and posterior borders of C2 upward, they are not in continuity with the odontoid. A fracture line (*arrows*) is seen obliquely through the base of the odontoid, confirming the **type II fracture of the odontoid.**

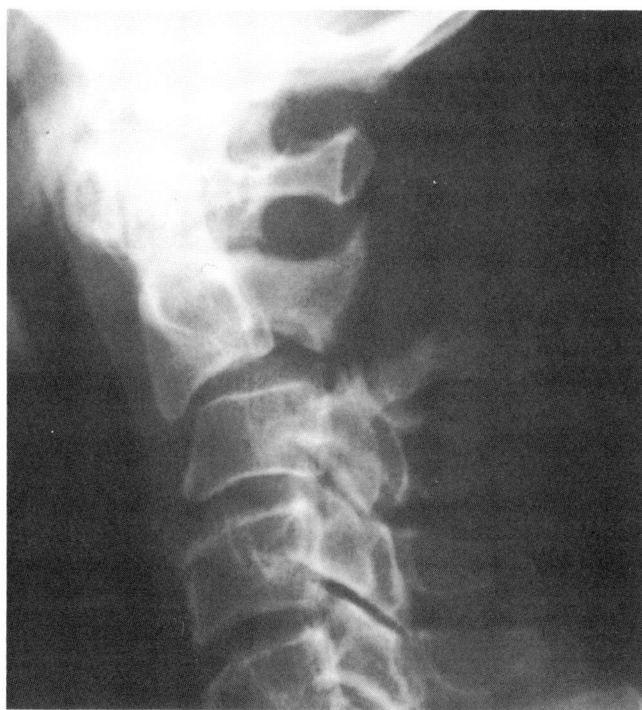

Figure 101–26. This **hangman's fracture** was overlooked on CT because the plane of the slices was parallel to the plane of the fracture. It is very obvious and quite alarming on the lateral flexion view, although the patient had been walking around with it for two weeks. Note that the severe subluxation does not compromise the canal since the neural arch remains posterior.

may lead to complete disruption of the posterior ligaments and facet joint capsules; this may be radiographically occult except with the use of flexion/extension views (Fig. 101–27) and is potentially unstable, leading to progressive kyphosis if untreated.

Vertebral body compression fracture results from moderate flexion forces disrupting the vertebral endplate without other bony or ligamentous injury and is a stable fracture. A combination of flexion and axial loading may cause a "burst" fracture of the vertebral body where there is comminution and widening of the body (Fig. 101–28). Depending on the ligaments involved, these may be stable or unstable. Severe flexion can produce bilateral "facet lock" in which the inferior facets of the upper vertebra ride forward over the superior facets of the lower vertebra and lock anterior to them in a ratchet fashion. This involves disruption of the middle and posterior columns and so is unstable. It is easily seen on the lateral radiograph (Fig. 101–29), with the upper vertebra moving forward half its width or more and the spinolaminar line disrupted. On CT, the "naked facet" sign is seen.

The most severe flexion injury is the "flexion teardrop," in which severe flexion and axial loading crush one vertebral body to produce a small anterior "teardrop" fragment and a larger posterior fragment. The posterior ligaments are disrupted and the entire upper spine dislocates back into the canal, causing severe spinal cord damage (Fig. 101–30).

Rotation combined with flexion may lead to a range of subluxation of the vertebrae of which the end result may be a unilateral facet lock, as opposed to the bilateral facet lock seen on pure flexion and discussed above. This may be recognized on the radiograph by an abrupt change in rotation of the spine at a single interspace, a sudden decrease in the laminar space, or a "bow-tie" appearance of the facets on the lateral view (Fig. 101–31) or an abrupt shift in the spinous processes as seen on the frontal view. There may not be significant listhesis of the vertebral bodies. As an isolated injury this is stable.

Hyperextension injuries may be radiographically subtle or occult yet produce severe neurologic damage. This damage is produced by impingement of the spinal cord between the ligamenta flava posteriorly and the vertebral body anteriorly. Plain film manifestations may include prevertebral soft-tissue swelling, anterior widening of the disc space, compression of the facets, vacuum phenomenon in the disc or annulus, or a small avulsion fragment from the inferior anterior corner of the vertebral body (an injury known as the "hyperextension teardrop," a very different fracture from the flexion teardrop). If there are no plain film findings but there is a neurologic deficit and a suspicion of a hyperextension mechanism of injury (such as the presence of facial fractures), MRI is the method of choice for evaluating the spinal cord.

THE LOWER CERVICAL SPINE

The patterns of injury in this region are influenced by the sudden transition from the flexible cervical spine to the more rigid thoracic spine. There is a tendency toward fracture or dislocation of the C6 and C7 vertebrae, hence the need to image the cervicothoracic junction in trauma, especially because many of these are unstable. More minor injuries that can occur at this level include the avulsion fracture of the spinous process (the "clay-shoveler's" fracture) caused by the pull of the ligamentum nuchae (Fig. 101–32). Occasionally these are associated with significant ligamentous damage and may result in a listhesis and instability.

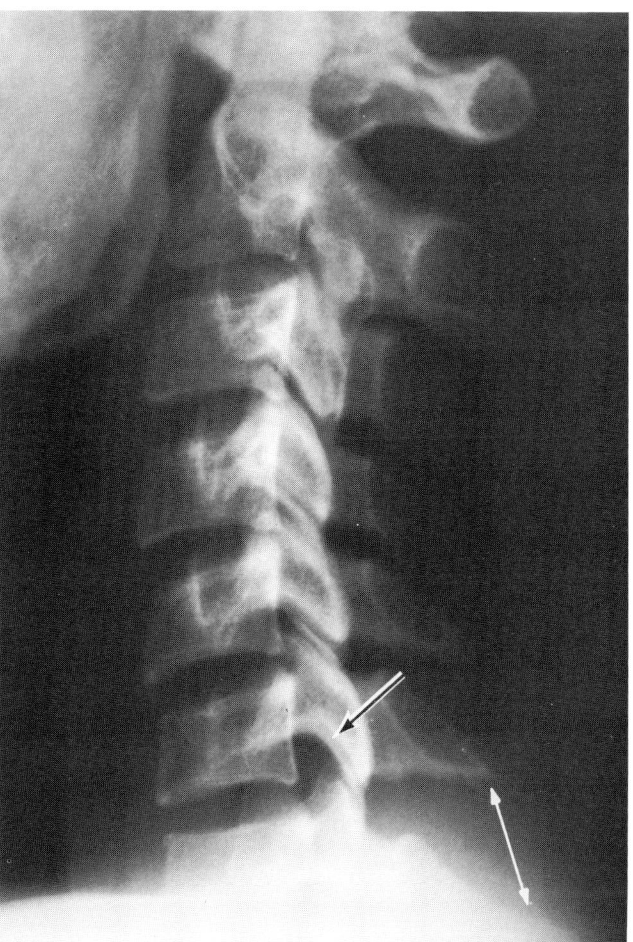

Figure 101–27. A flexion sprain is demonstrated at C6-C7. There is gapping of the spinous processes (*double-ended arrow*) and nearly 50 per cent subluxation of the C6 inferior facets on the superior C7 facets (*arrow*). Significantly, these were visible only on the flexion view.

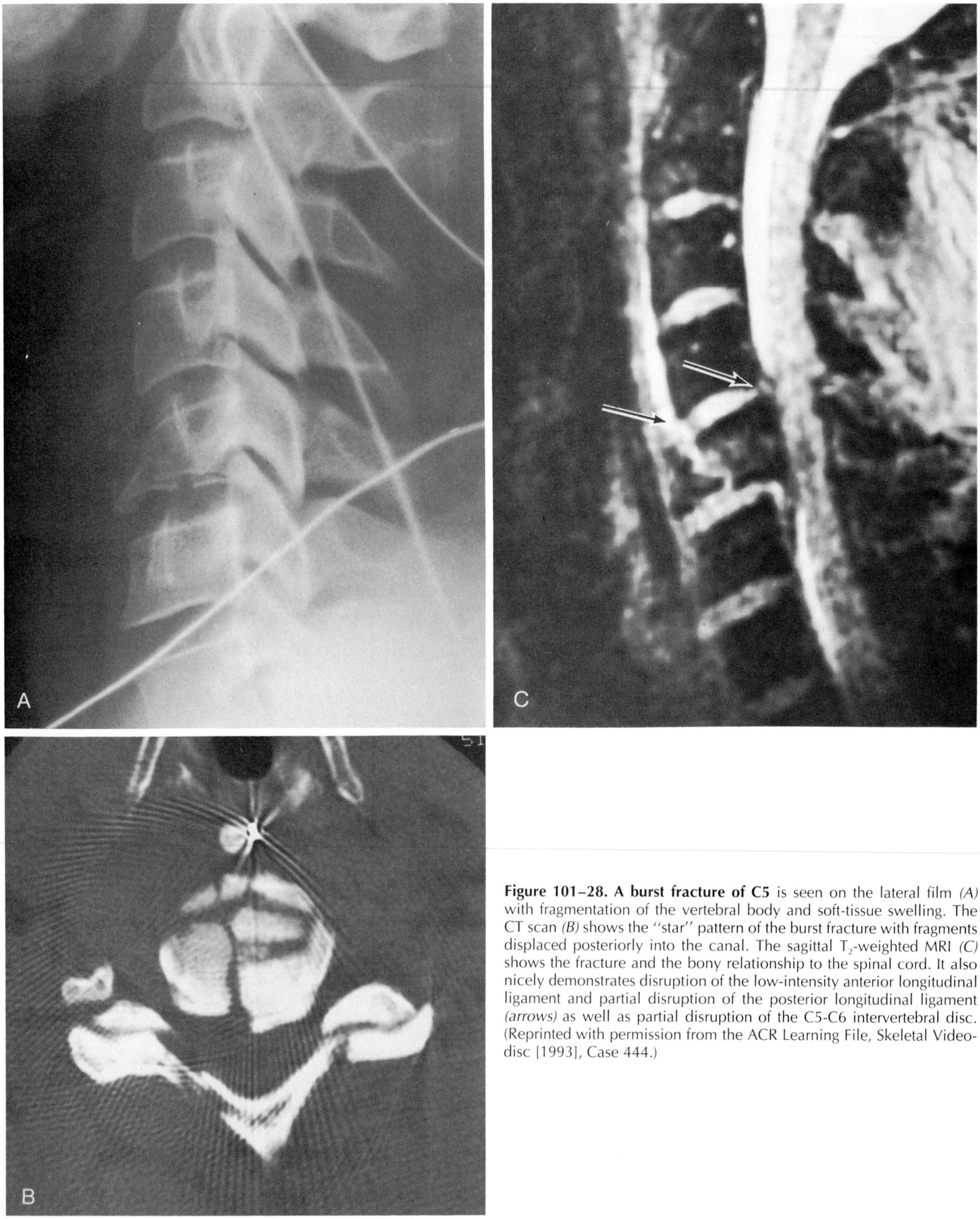

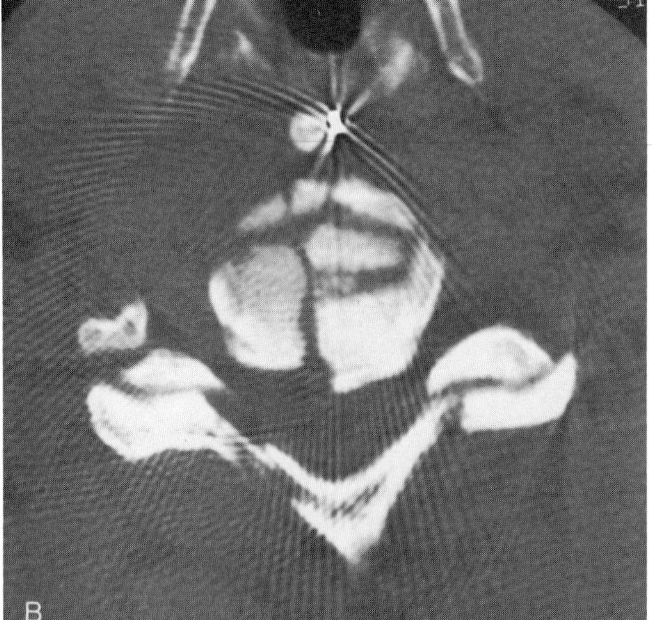

Figure 101–28. A burst fracture of C5 is seen on the lateral film *(A)* with fragmentation of the vertebral body and soft-tissue swelling. The CT scan *(B)* shows the "star" pattern of the burst fracture with fragments displaced posteriorly into the canal. The sagittal T_2-weighted MRI *(C)* shows the fracture and the bony relationship to the spinal cord. It also nicely demonstrates disruption of the low-intensity anterior longitudinal ligament and partial disruption of the posterior longitudinal ligament *(arrows)* as well as partial disruption of the C5-C6 intervertebral disc. (Reprinted with permission from the ACR Learning File, Skeletal Videodisc [1993], Case 444.)

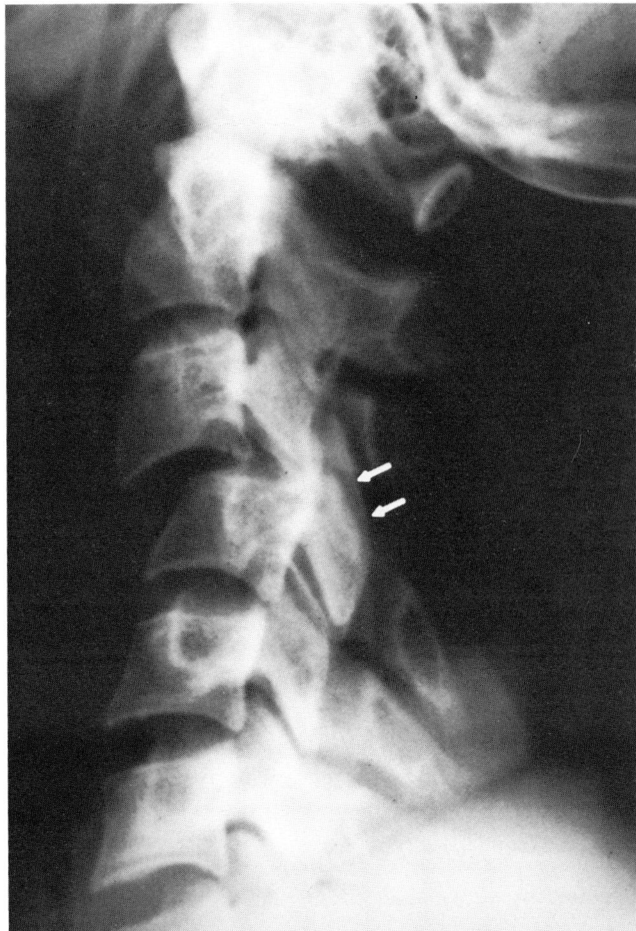

Figure 101–29. A lateral view shows bilateral locked facets at C3-C4. Note the 60 per cent anterolisthesis of C3 on C4 and the inferior facets of C3 locked in front of the superior facets of C4. These facets are uncovered (*arrows*), and there is interspinous widening also. The spinal canal is narrowed to half its normal width.

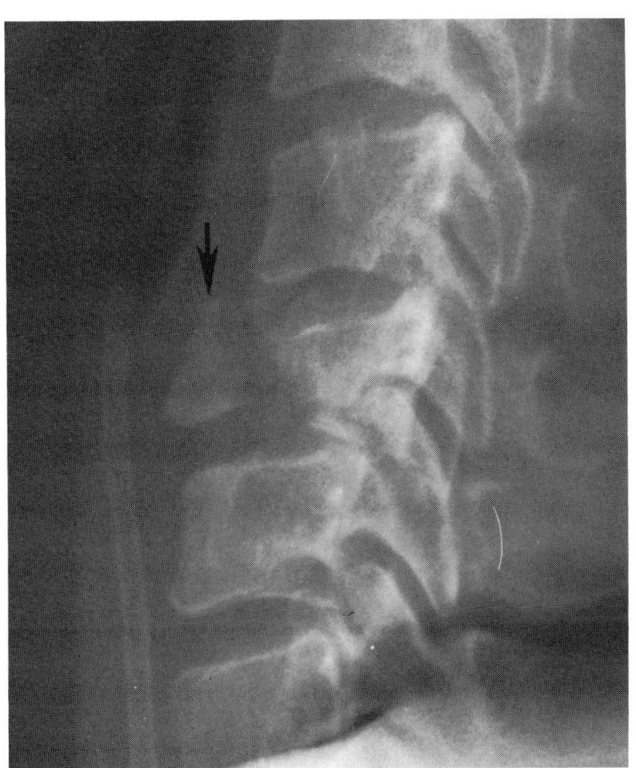

Figure 101–30. Flexion teardrop fracture of C5 showing typical findings. The "teardrop" anteriorly (*arrow*) is separated from the posterior part of the body, which has subluxed posteriorly, narrowing the canal to half its normal width. Severe ligamentous and spinal cord injury is inevitable.

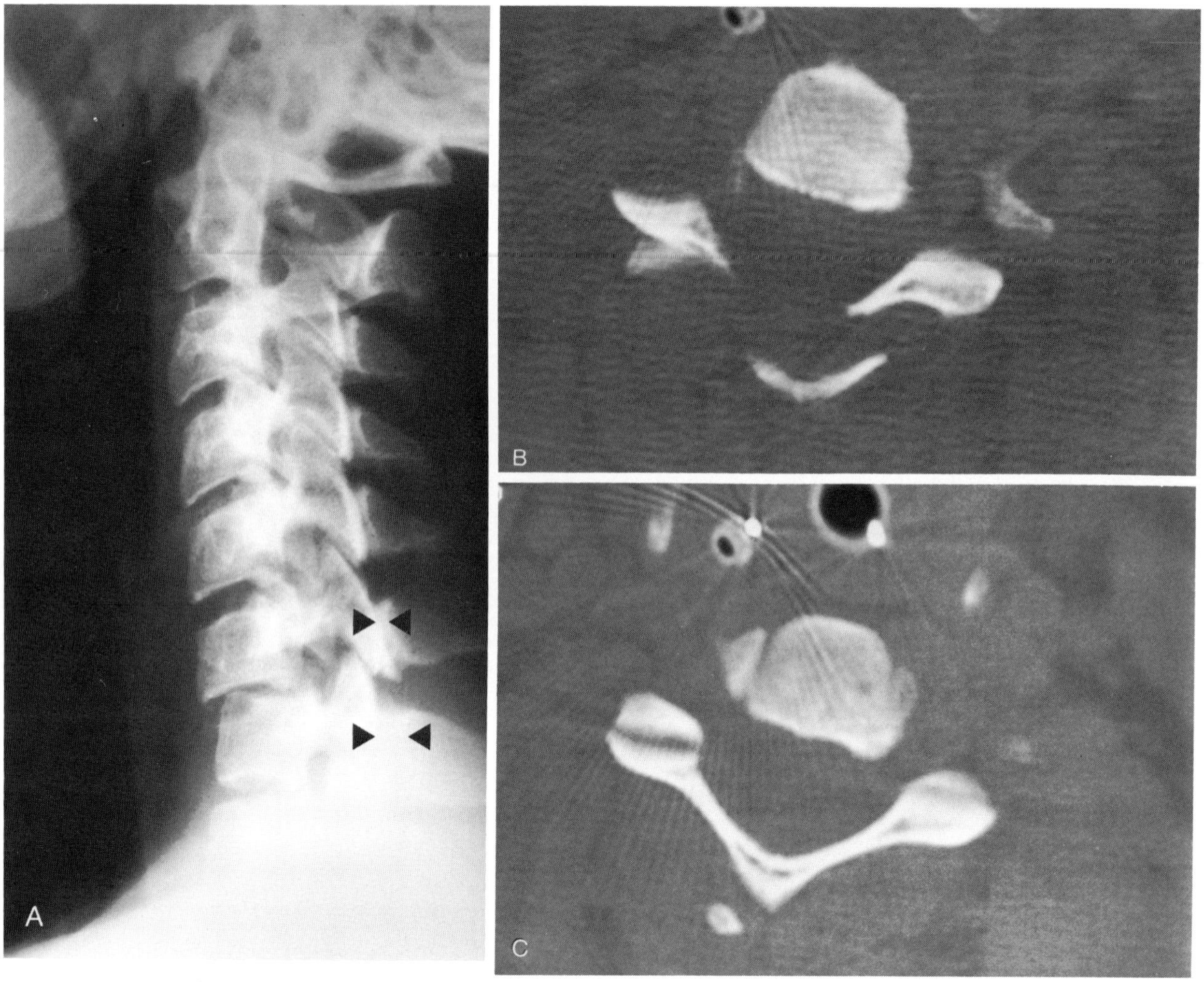

Figure 101–31. *A,* The **unilateral locked facet at C6-C7** is indicated by both the "bow-tie" appearance of the facets from C6 upward and by the sudden decrease of the laminar space (*arrowheads*) between the posterior aspect of the facets and the spinolaminar line at C6 compared with C7. There is only slight subluxation of C6 on C7. *B,* CT scan shows unilateral facet lock on the right where the inferior facet of the upper vertebra is anterior to the superior facet of the lower vertebra (almost like the wings of a bird). *C,* A normal level in which the inferior facet of the upper vertebra is in its normal place posterior to the superior facet of the lower vertebra; this is the "praying hands" appearance (or, more prosaically, the "hamburger").

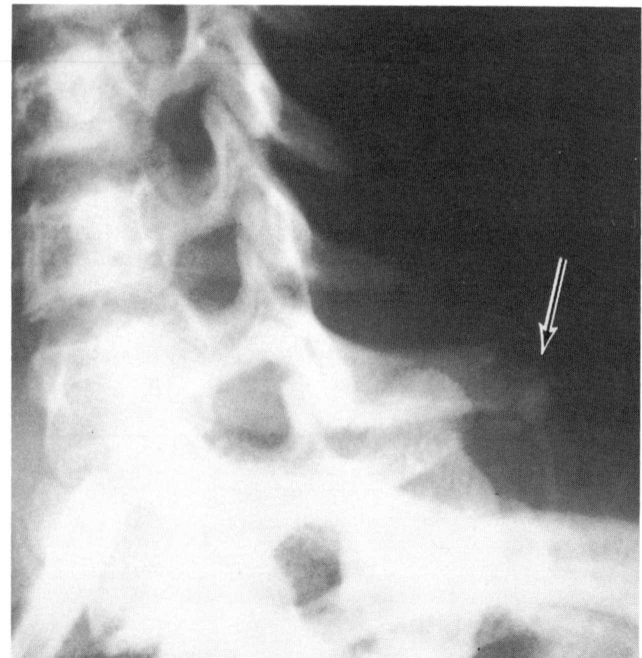

Figure 101–32. The typical clay-shoveler's fracture is a stable injury in which only the very tip of the spinous process (*arrow*) is avulsed by the ligamentum nuchae.

THORACOLUMBAR SPINE

B. J. Manaster

The thoracic spine is conventionally filmed in the AP and lateral positions. On the AP film, attention should be paid to the interpediculate distance, which should gradually increase from the upper to the lower thoracic bodies. A sudden increase in interpediculate width suggests a burst fracture (Fig. 101–33). Similarly, the paravertebral tissues should be inspected for evidence of hematoma. On the high-kV chest films initially obtained in trauma situations, this paraspinous fullness may simulate either adenopathy or large vessel bleed. Remember that it can be simply secondary to hematoma from a thoracic spine fracture.

Vertebral body height and compression fractures should not be evaluated on the AP film of the thoracic spine. Owing to the normal kyphosis of the thoracic spine, these features are often somewhat distorted. Furthermore, the manubrium is normally superimposed on T4 or T5. This may give the impression of a vertebral endplate fracture on the AP view.

The lateral thoracic spine film is usually obtained with a long-exposure breathing technique that blurs the overlying lung structures. A swimmer's view is necessary for viewing the upper thoracic spine (see Cervical Spine section). The vertebral body height should remain uniform over the length of the thoracic spine. The exception to this is a normal slight anterior wedging in the T11, T12, L1 region, the site of transition from the kyphotic to lordotic curve of the lumbar spine. The normal expected kyphosis of the thoracic spine ranges from 20 to 40 degrees, as measured from T4 to T12. On the lateral view, occasional superimposition of the tip of the scapula or of the glenoid fossa on the swimmer's view may simulate thoracic vertebral fracture.

The thoracic spine is an unusual site of fracture except for the stable flexion anterior compression type injury. Even the occasional burst type of fracture in the thoracic spine is often stable owing to the support from the thoracic cage and the orientation of the facet joints. Instability is more likely to occur in the presence of multiple rib fractures or a sternal fracture; these associated injuries must be sought in the rare case of a thoracic vertebral body burst fracture.

Standard lumbar spine films include AP, lateral, and oblique. On the AP film, the interpediculate distance is expected to gradually widen from L1 to L5. Spina bifida occulta, failure of the posterior normal arch to fuse, is a common variant at L5. The psoas muscle, arising from the transverse processes of the lumbar spine, gradually widens from the upper to the lower lumbar spine. On the lateral film, the disc spaces gradually increase in size from L1-L2 to L4-L5; the L5-S1 disc space may be slightly narrower than L4-L5 normally. The vertebral bodies normally have a slight concavity both anteriorly and posteriorly. The pars interarticularis and facet joints are seen; the spinous processes are viewed well with the aid of a bright light. Skeletally immature patients demonstrate their normal growth centers (ring apophyses, Fig. 101–34). The limbus vertebra is an unfused ring apophysis, developed secondary to anterior disc herniation between the apophysis and vertebral body; this could simulate a fracture (Fig. 101–35).

The anatomy as demonstrated on the oblique film is detailed in Fig. 101–36. The pars intra-articularis, the site for spondylolysis, is especially well seen on this view. Spondylolysis is a defect in the pars intra-articularis, seen most commonly at L5. The defect is more prevalent in males than females and in whites than other races. The etiology of spondylolysis is uncertain, but it is felt that it may

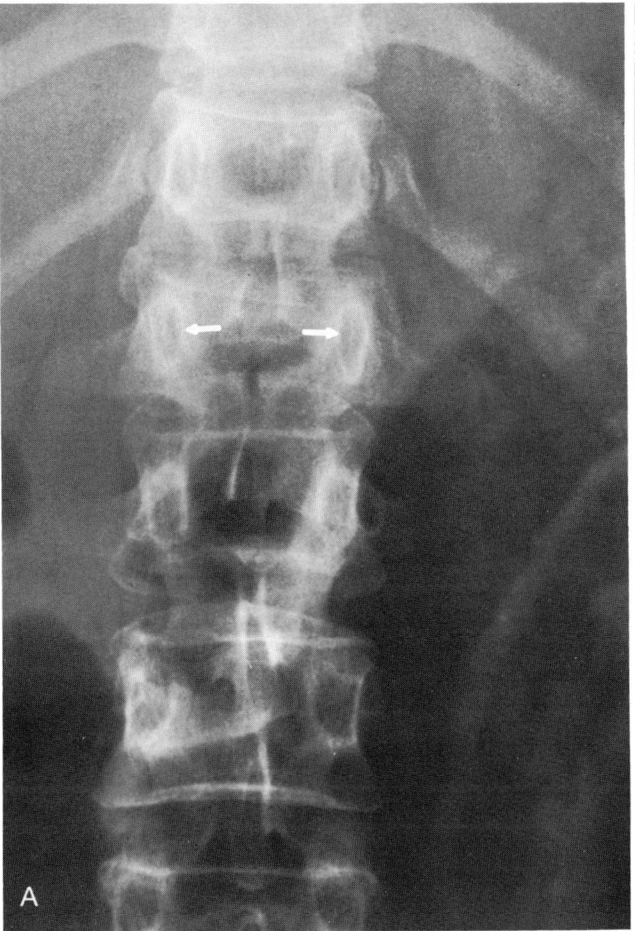

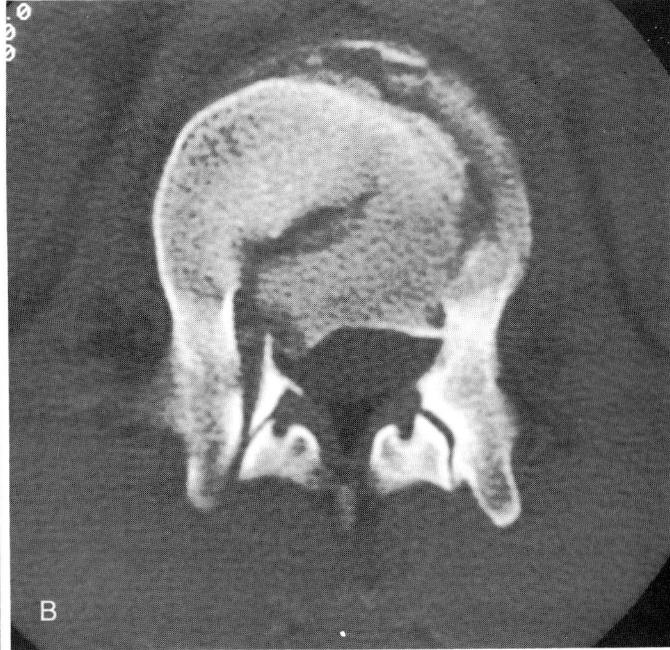

Figure 101–33. *A,* Note the **widening of the interpediculate distance** on this AP film at L1 *(arrows).* The interpediculate distance should normally gradually widen from T12 distally. With a sudden increase in distance as in this case, one must make diagnosis of a **burst fracture**. *B,* The corresponding CT scan, with the comminuted fracture of the body of L1 seen in association with the widened pedicles. There is retropulsion of a large body fragment, which narrows the canal by 50 per cent.

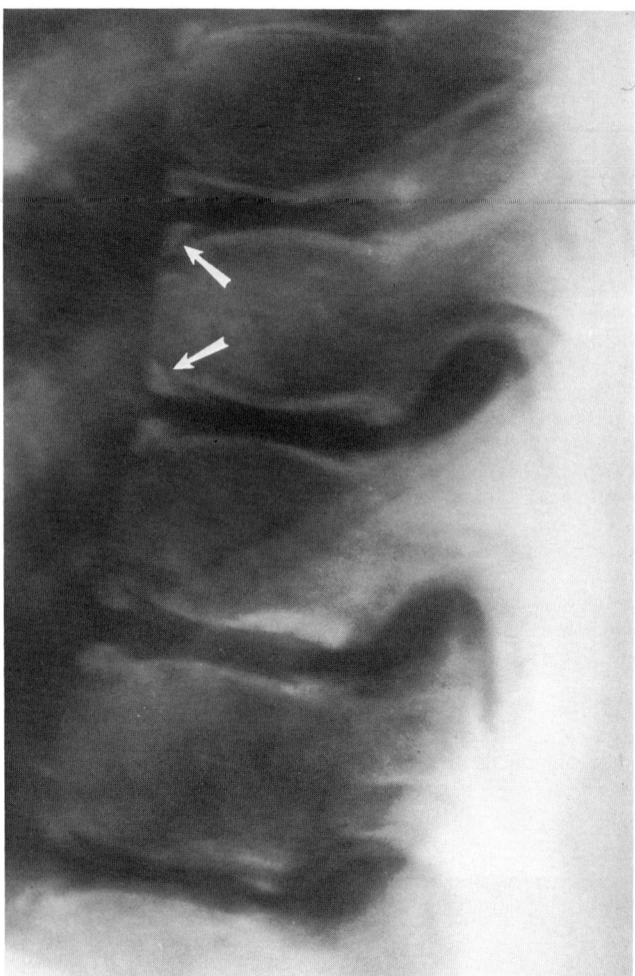

Figure 101–34. Multiple ring apophyses *(arrow)* are seen in the thoracic spine in this skeletally immature patient. These are the growth centers for the vertebral body and should not be mistaken for fractures. They are seen at all levels of the spine.

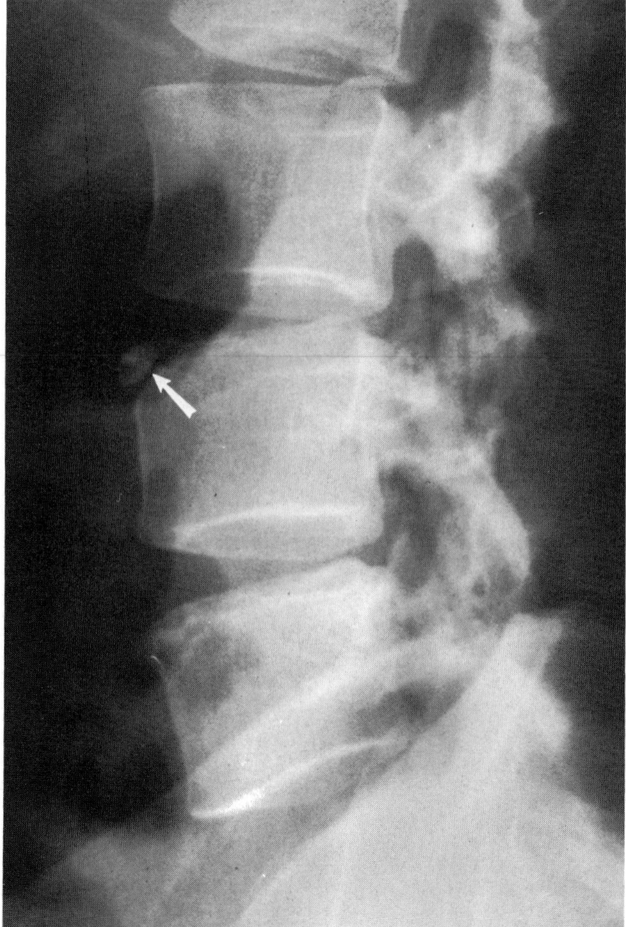

Figure 101–35. Limbus vertebra (*arrow*) where the patient has developed an anterior disc herniation through the ring apophysis. This is a relatively common finding and should not be mistaken for a fracture. Note the sclerotic margins, indicating that this is a long-term finding.

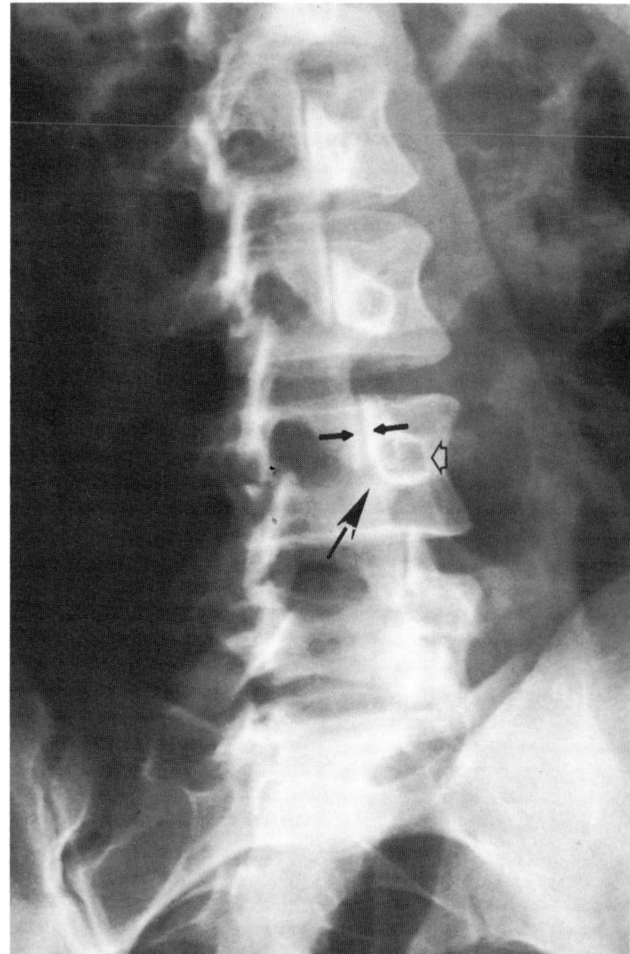

Figure 101–36. This figure details the **normal anatomy of the lumbar spine on the oblique view.** Shown to best advantage on this view are the superior and inferior facets (*short arrows*), pedicle (*open arrow*), and pars intra-articularis (*long arrow*). This view is particularly helpful for evaluating not only degenerative change of the facets, but also integrity of the pedicles and the pars intra-articularis. If there is a lucency through the pars, this represents a spondylolysis.

represent a stress fracture from repeated normal trauma, perhaps aggravated by dysplasia or hypoplasia of the pars. It is usually diagnosed in the second or third decade. Spondylolysis may be unilateral or bilateral. If it is bilateral, an associated spondylolisthesis may develop (Fig. 101–37). If it is unilateral, there is no listhesis, but reactive hyperplasia and sclerosis of the contralateral facet may develop, which can simulate metastatic disease or other disease processes.

There are very specific patterns of injury involving the thoracolumbar spine that have both diagnostic and therapeutic implications. First of all, most of the injuries occur in the transition zone between the thoracic and lumbar spine. Sixty per cent of thoracolumbar fractures are found to involve T12, L1, or L2; 90 per cent are found in the T11-L4 region.

Seventy-five per cent of thoracolumbar fractures are the compression variety, with anterior wedging or depression of the superior end-plate and intact posterior elements. These are diagnosed by plain film, and intact elements are confirmed by the presence of a normal interpediculate width and lack of interspinous process gapping on the AP film. Generally, no further work-up is required and therapy is conservative.

Twenty to twenty-five per cent of thoracolumbar spine fractures are fracture-dislocations, involving the posterior elements as well as the body. Plain film findings indicating this more serious variety of injury include interpediculate widening, gapping of the spinous processes, translation of vertebral bodies in either the AP or mediolateral plane, and posterior element fractures or dislocations. Many of these features are better evaluated by CT than plain film. CT allows evaluation of the integrity of the spinal canal, disc herniation or fragmentation, and the facets. The facets may be fractured, subluxed, perched, dislocated, or locked, and these situations are not always obvious on CT unless the anatomy is understood (Fig. 101–38). Lumbar facets are identified by their orientation with respect to the vertebral body (superior facets are directed posteromedially and inferior facets are directed anterolaterally) as well as the shape of the intra-articular surface (superior facet articular surface is concave, inferior articular surface is flat or convex) as demonstrated in Fig. 101–39. Using these guidelines, facet dislocation will not be missed on CT; subluxation of the facets can be seen well with sagittal CT reconstruction.

Not all burst fractures are unstable. To assess stability, one generally divides the spine into three columns. The anterior column consists of the anterior vertebral body, anterior longitudinal ligament, and the anterior portion of the annulus fibrosus. The middle column consists of the posterior half of the vertebral body, the posterior longitudinal ligament, and the posterior half of the annulus fibrosus. The posterior column consists of the posterior elements, facet capsules, and intraspinous ligaments. In general, two of these three columns must be intact for intrinsic stability. Thus you should not be surprised to see some "burst" fractures treated conservatively because it may be determined that they are nonetheless intrinsically stable. One "named" fracture that is generally fairly extensive but nonetheless stable is the Chance fracture. The pattern for this fracture consists of a transverse fracture through the vertebral body (or with the line of stress going through the disc space) and continuing with transverse fractures through the posterior elements (Fig. 101–40). Any of the posterior elements may be involved, including the pedicles, facets, transverse processes, and spinous process. Lap type seat belts in a sudden deceleration accident are the most common culprit in a Chance fracture, acting as a fulcrum

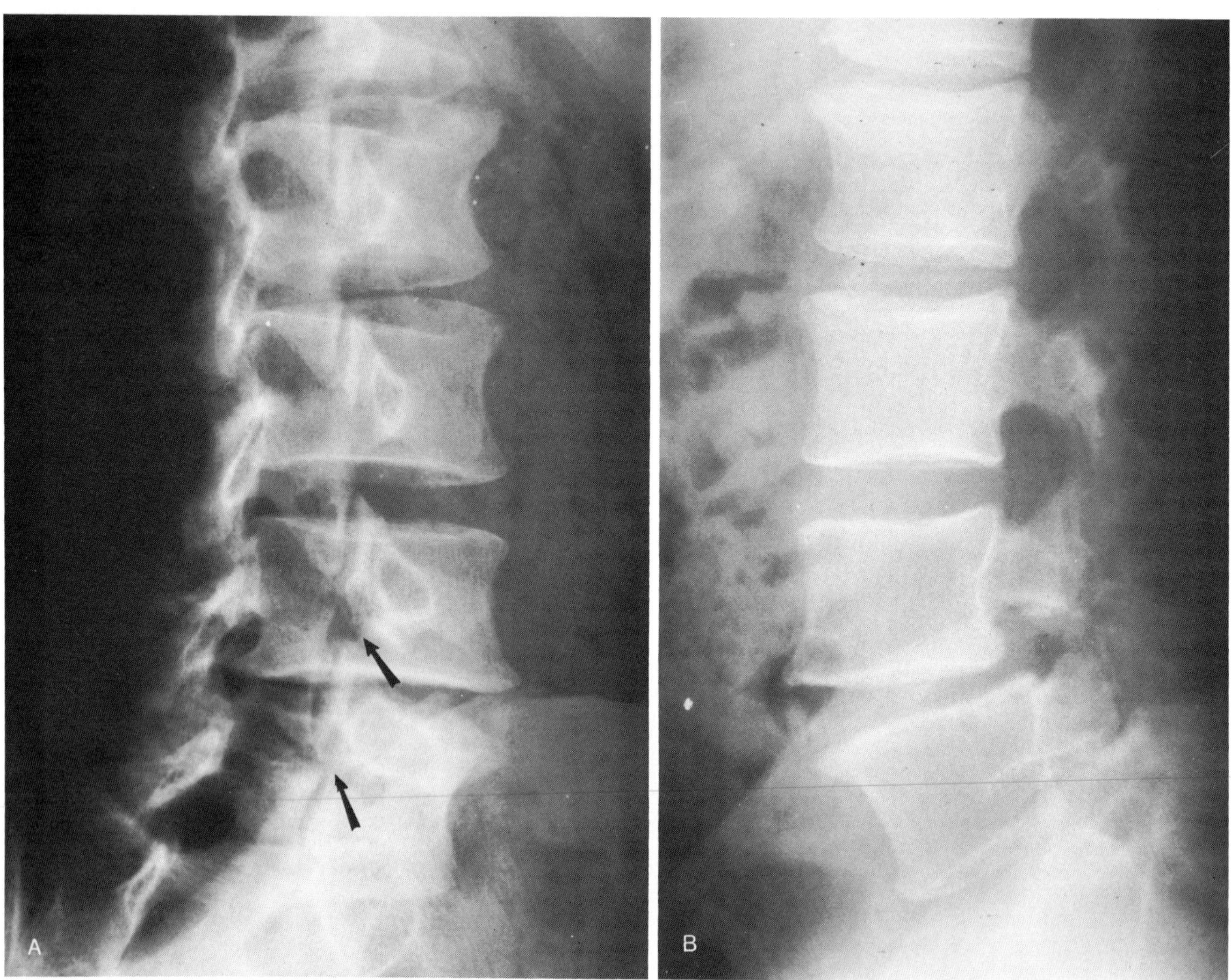

Figure 101–37. *A*, **Spondylolysis** (lysis at the pars intra-articularis) of both L4 and L5 (*arrows*). For comparison, note the intact pars intra-articularis at other levels in this spine. Only one side is shown on the oblique films, but the opposite side was identical. This patient therefore has bilateral spondylolysis of both L4 and L5. The lateral film (*B*) shows **mild spondylolisthesis or anterolisthesis** of L4 on L5. L5 has not moved with respect to S1, despite the presence of bilateral pars defects.

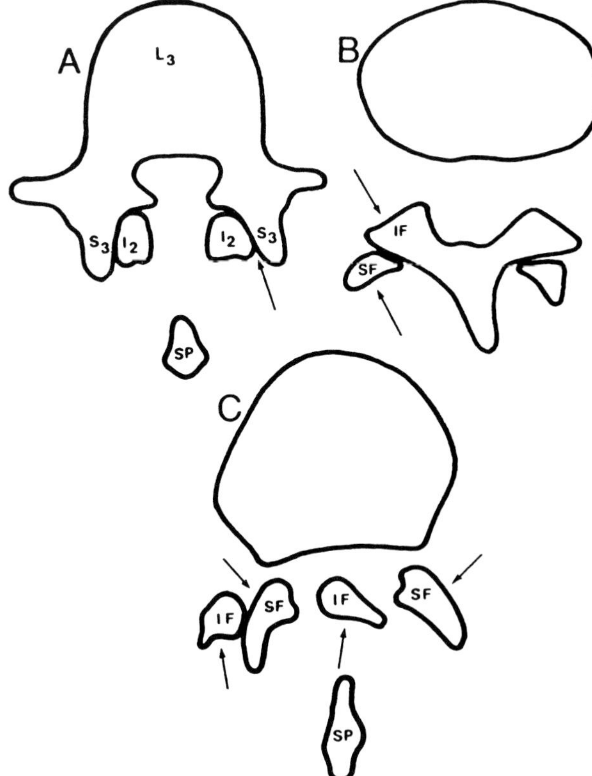

Figure 101–38. CT appearance of facets in lumbar spine. *A*, Normal. *B*, Anterior lock. *C*, Lateral lock. (SF = superior facet; IF = inferior facet; SP = spinous process; *arrows* = articular surface.) (From Manaster BJ: Handbooks in Radiology: Skeletal Radiology. Chicago, Year Book Medical Publishers, 1989.)

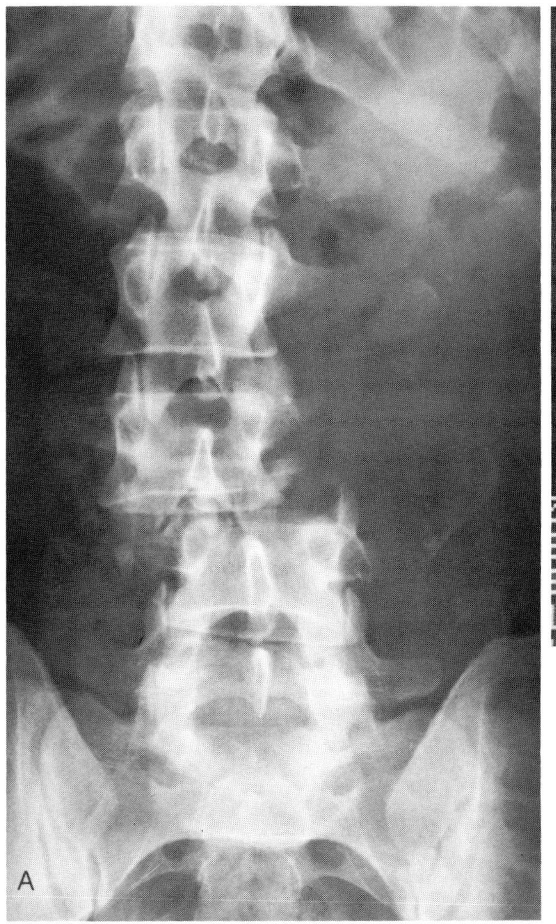

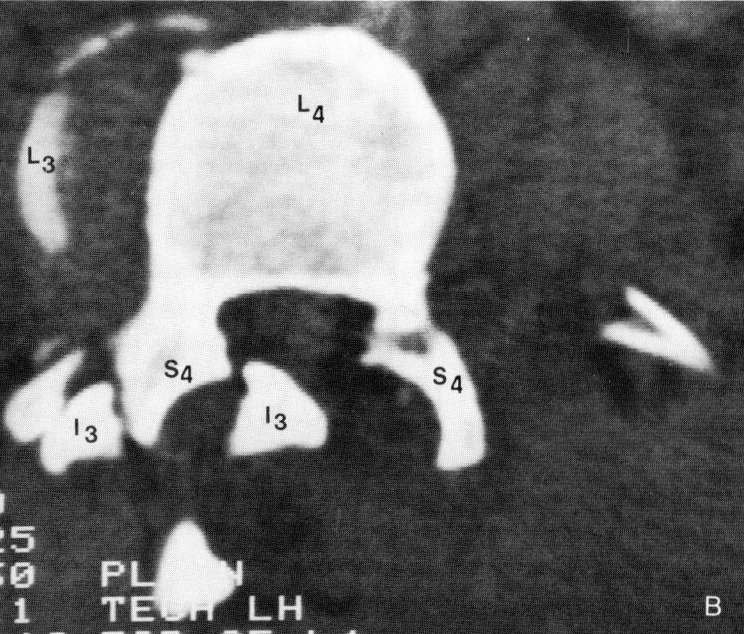

Figure 101–39. Complex fracture-dislocation. The plain film (*A*) demonstrates a lateral translation of L3 on L4. There are clearly fractured facets, but also there is a strong possibility of locked facets. The CT scan (*B*) demonstrates to much better advantage the pattern of the posterior element fracture-dislocation. Note that the diagram in Figure 101–38*C* is of this CT scan. Here one sees that the inferior facets (I3) of lumbar vertebra 3 are laterally dislocated, with the right inferior facet locked laterally on the right superior facet of L4. Both superior facets are "naked." Additionally, one sees a portion of the body of L3 laterally translated with respect to L4.

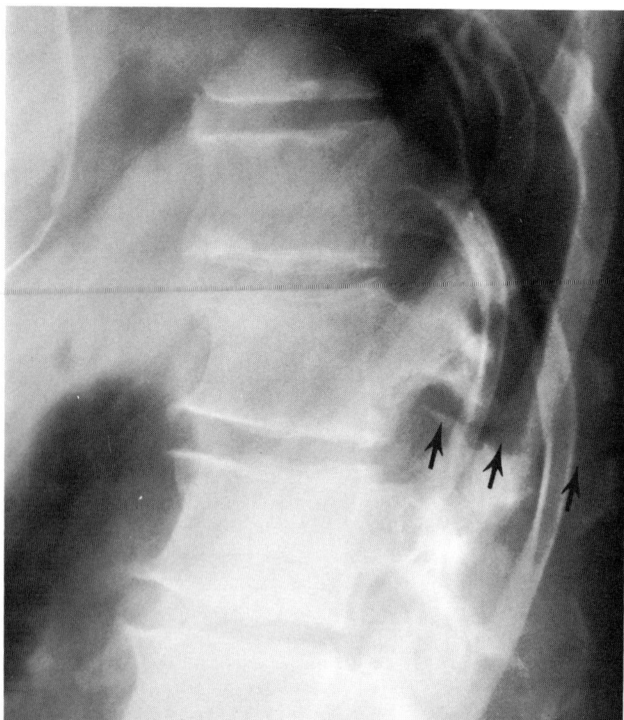

Figure 101–40. This plain film demonstrates a slight wedge compression fracture of L1 with a small anterior superior corner fracture of L2. These findings suggest a flexion mechanism. Note also, however, that the patient has a fracture through the inferior articular facet of L1 that extends posteriorly through the spinous process (*arrows*). These findings are very typical of a **Chance fracture**. This is often a stable fracture, which in this case was treated with a brace.

at L1 or L2. The tensile stress in hyperflexion causes the usual transverse fracture. There need be little or no vertebral body compression. Abdominal injury is often associated, and should be sought.

THE SHOULDER AND HUMERUS

Anthony J. Doyle

This region includes the clavicle and sternoclavicular joints as part of the shoulder girdle. Dislocations and fracture-dislocations are common around the shoulder.

Normal Variants

In the newborn, the clavicle may be foreshortened on a chest radiograph and simulate a fracture, or the nutrient foramen may project so as to appear as a cortical break (Fig. 101–41). This appearance can usually be remedied by repositioning. A common source of overreading on the adult chest radiograph is that of calling the glenohumeral joint dislocated when in fact the relationship is simply distorted by the projection used.

Several ossification centers around the shoulder may be confusing. The ossification center for the tip of the acromion may never fuse, forming an "os acromiale" that is bilateral in 60 percent. The center at the tip of the coracoid process may also be mistaken for a fracture. The proximal humeral physis has a complex shape and may be mistaken for a fracture at first glance (Fig. 101–42). The small flake-like epiphysis at the medial end of the clavicle is last in the body to fuse, in the early twenties. These growth centers are distinguished from fractures by their corticated margins.

PEDIATRICS

Fracture of the clavicle is not uncommon in the neonate, from birth trauma, and is also frequent in childhood, from direct trauma. Most of these fractures are in the mid-clavicle and heal rapidly without any sequelae.

The proximal humerus may be fractured by direct trauma (including birth trauma in the neonate, usually Salter type I) or indirectly, as in Little League pitchers, usually Salter type II. Fractures through the proximal diaphysis are often pathologic, most commonly secondary to an underlying asymptomatic simple bone cyst. The mid-humerus may fracture from a direct blow or from angulation and twisting forces.

ADULTS

Sternoclavicular Joints

Dislocation of the sternoclavicular joint is uncommon, and usually requires considerable force. The most common direction of dislocation is anterior, usually easy to diagnose clinically. The more dangerous dislocation is posterior, where the clavicular head may damage or compress major structures such as the large vessels in the thoracic area or the trachea. Both types of dislocation may be difficult to detect radiographically. Widening of the sternoclavicular joint may be visible. Special views such as a 40-degree cephalad angled AP (the "serendipity" view) can be helpful, but the best way to assess the sternoclavicular joints is undoubtedly CT. The dislocation, any associated fractures, and the adjacent soft-tissue structures are well shown by a limited thin-section CT through the joints.

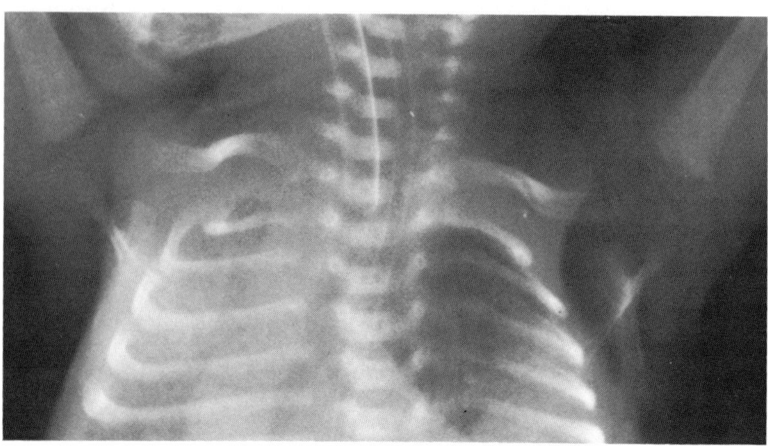

Figure 101–41. AP chest film on a neonate shows **angulation of the right clavicle and lucency in the left clavicle, both of which could be mistaken for fracture**. The angle on the right is due to rotation; the lucency on the left is the normal nutrient foramen.

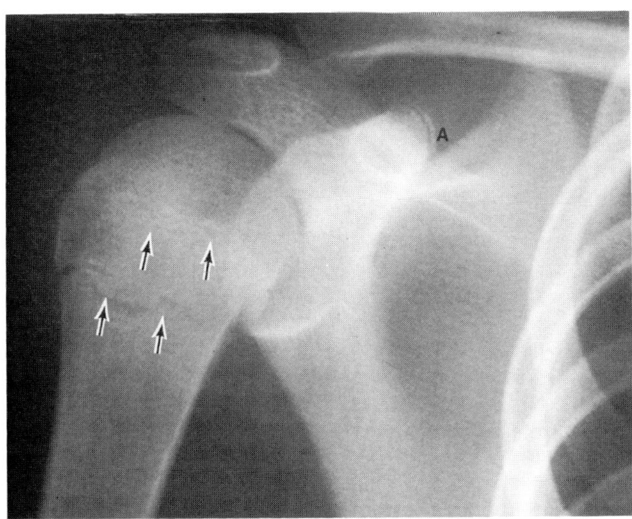

Figure 101–42. Normal undulating epiphyseal line, simulating a fracture (***arrows***). Similarly, the apophysis of the coracoid process (A) should not be mistaken for an avulsion injury in this skeletally immature patient.

Clavicle

This is the most commonly fractured bone of all and has been written about since 2000 B.C. Fractures of the clavicle are commonly classified as group I, II, and III, referring to fractures of the middle third (80 per cent, Fig. 101–43), distal third (15 per cent), and proximal third (5 per cent) respectively. AP and 45-degree cephalad angled views usually provide sufficient assessment. The mechanism of injury is usually a fall on the point of the shoulder. Associated rib fractures and pneumothorax (in up to 3 per cent) should be looked for. Both proximal and distal clavicle fractures may be unstable if the sternoclavicular or coracoclavicular ligaments are disrupted. This is sometimes assessed with stress views.

Healing is usually rapid and uncomplicated. Distal fractures are somewhat more prone to non-union and, although acute neurovascular injury is rare, abundant callus may impinge on the brachial plexus or subclavian vessel. In this case, MRI can be usefully employed to show the impingement.

The Acromioclavicular Joints

The acromioclavicular (AC) joints are also injured by falls on the shoulder. The injuries are usually divided into grade I (slight ligamentous stretching), grade II (slight elevation of the distal clavicle), grade III (disruption of the coracoclavicular and acromioclavicular ligaments with elevation of the distal clavicle), and grade IV (posterior dislocation of the distal clavicle, Fig. 101–44). There may be an associated distal clavicle fracture. Assessment is usually with an AP view angled 15 degrees cephalad (including the opposite AC joint for comparison) and an axillary lateral view to detect posterior dislocation. Some orthopedists favor stress views of the AC joints whereas others find them unnecessary.

Scapula

Fractures of the scapula are most commonly located in the body, with fractures of the neck slightly less common and intra-articular fractures distinctly uncommon. They are associated with other major injuries in up to 90 per cent, including fractured ribs, lung contusion, brachial plexus injuries, pneumothorax, and trauma elsewhere (Fig. 101–45). They are frequently overlooked on portable chest x-rays taken for trauma. Assessment is best made with AP and transscapular lateral views but still may be difficult. CT is often helpful.

Fractures through the body and neck of the scapula may be unstable if the clavicle is fractured or the coracoclavicular ligament is disrupted. Fractures through the glenoid itself may require operative treatment depending on the size and position of the fragments. Fractures of the acromion or coracoid are uncommon although a stress fracture of the coracoid is sometimes seen in trap shooters. Rarely, the scapula may be dislocated into the chest or avulsed from the chest wall. This requires severe trauma.

Glenohumeral Dislocation

This is the most common joint dislocation, making up 50 per cent of all dislocations. Ninety-five per cent are anterior, with the head of the humerus in an anteromedial subcoracoid position (Fig. 101–46). They are usually secondary to a fall on an abducted arm. The uncommon posterior dislocation is frequently secondary to muscle spasm from electric shock or convulsion and is easily overlooked radiographically because the head dislocates directly posteriorly without any superior or inferior displacement. Radiographic

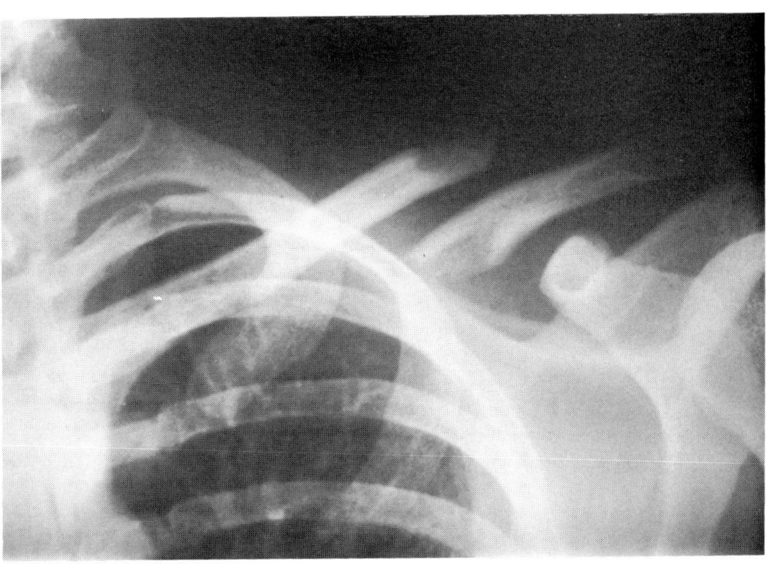

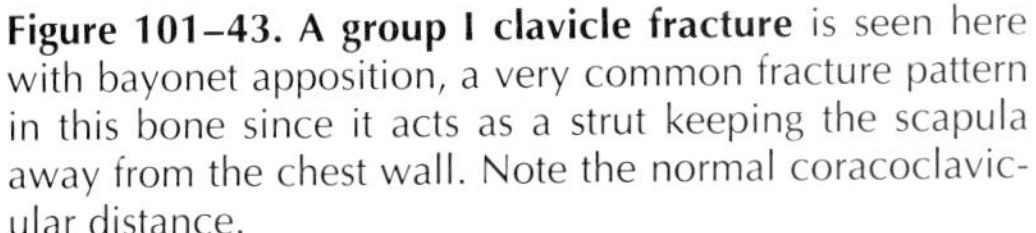

Figure 101–43. A group I clavicle fracture is seen here with bayonet apposition, a very common fracture pattern in this bone since it acts as a strut keeping the scapula away from the chest wall. Note the normal coracoclavicular distance.

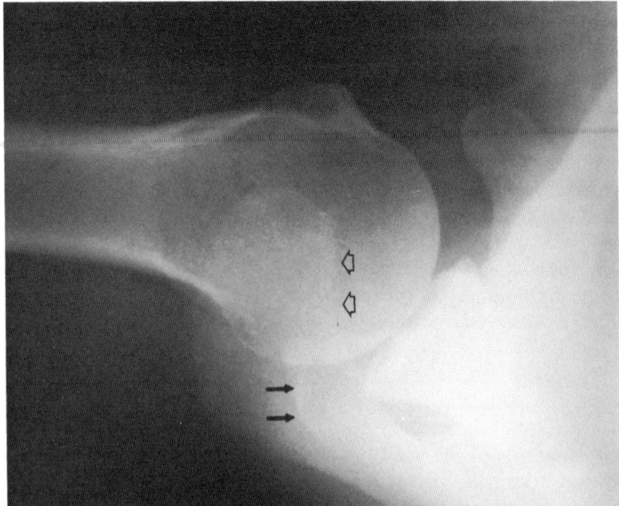

Figure 101–44. Grade IV acromionavicular dislocation is uncommon. This axillary lateral view shows a naked facet on the acromium (*open arrowheads*) where the clavicle should be. The clavicle head is posterior (*arrows*), having rotated about the coracoclavicular ligaments. The associated proximal clavicle fracture is not shown.

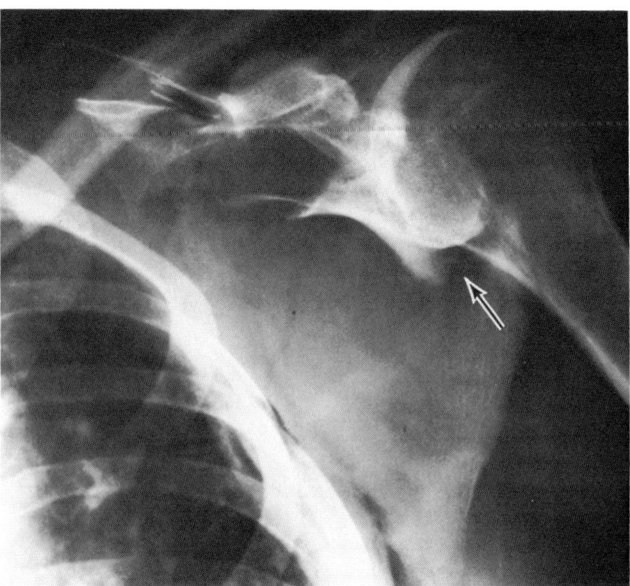

Figure 101–45. Fractures of the body and neck of the scapula are seen on an AP view. The fracture through the neck (*arrow*) is displaced, but the glenoid itself is not involved. Associated rib fractures and subcutaneous air from a treated pneumothorax are seen.

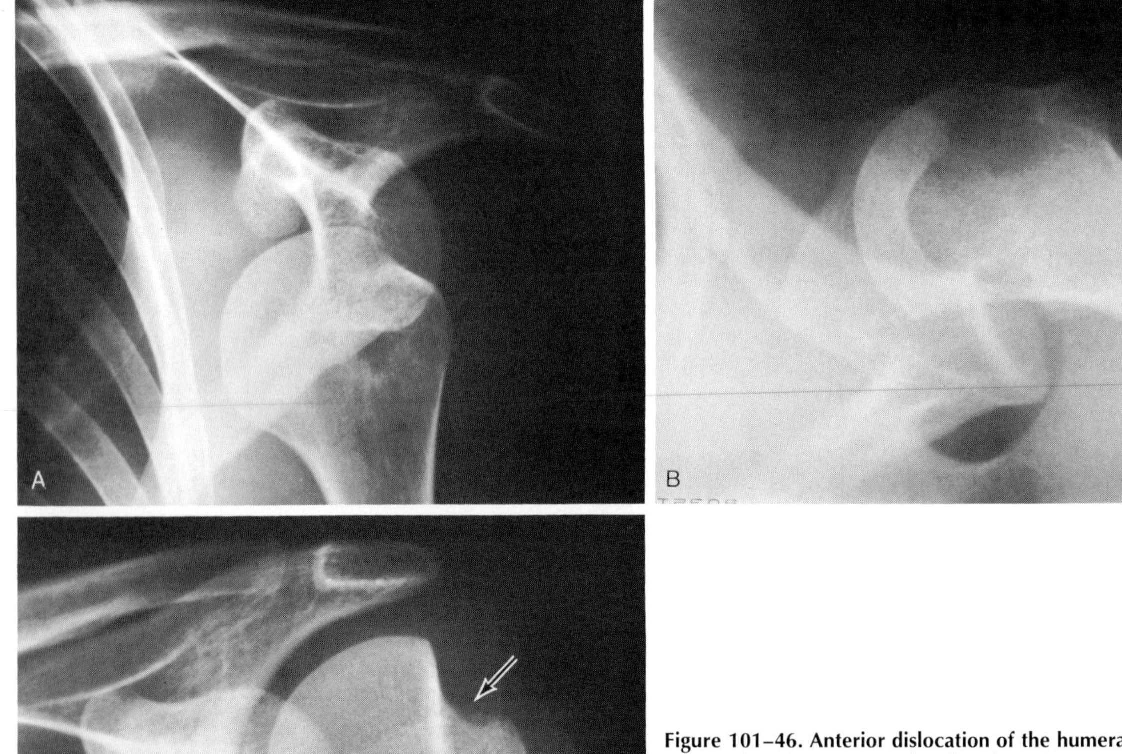

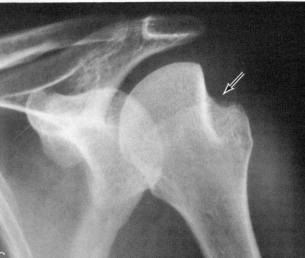

Figure 101–46. Anterior dislocation of the humeral head is well-demonstrated on the AP (*A*) and axillary lateral (*B*) views. Note the subcoracoid position of the humeral head. After reduction, the internal rotation view (*C*) shows the very large Hill-Sachs defect (*arrow*) in the anatomic neck of the humerus.

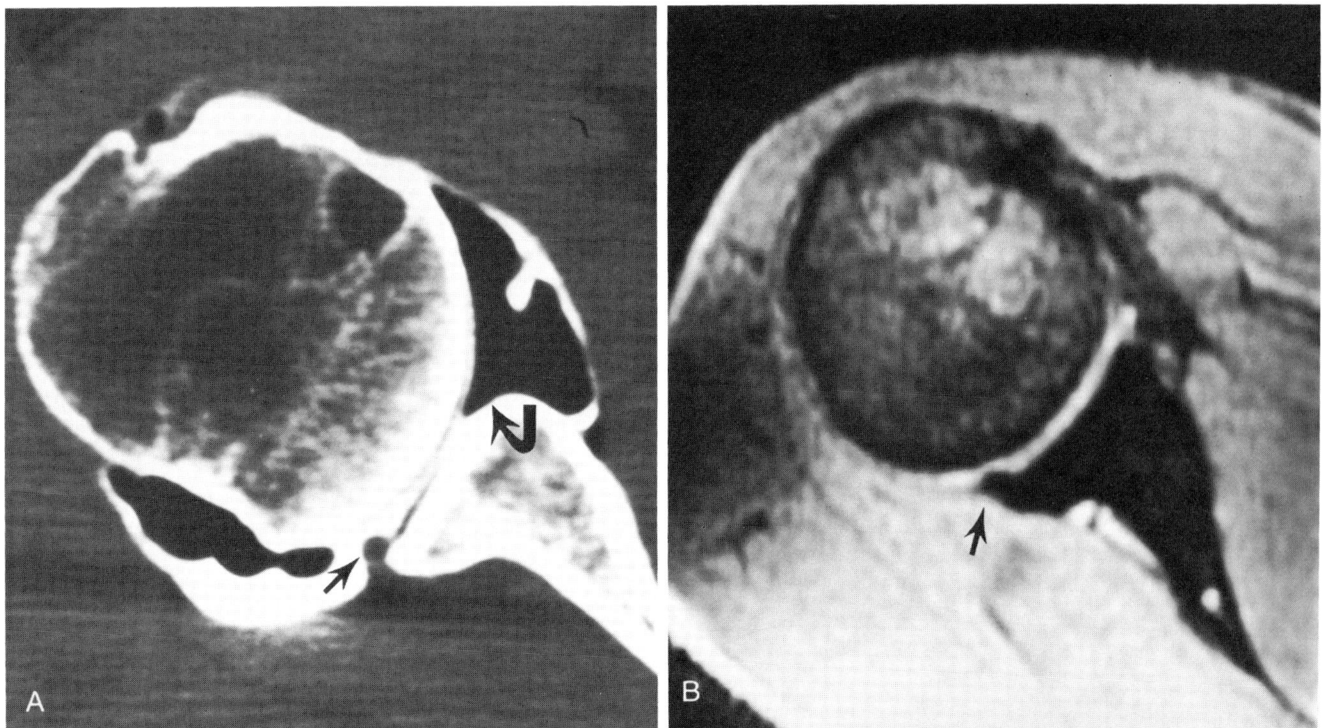

Figure 101–47. *A,* **Complete deficiency of the anterior glenoid labrum** is demonstrated on double-contrast CT arthrography. The posterior labrum (*arrow*) is present and normal. The anterior labrum, however, is missing altogether and there is only a bare bone surface remaining (*curved arrow*). *B,* Anterior labral deficiency is shown on an axial MRI (gradient-recalled acquisition). The intact posterior labrum (*arrow*) contrasts with the absence of a visible labrum on the anterior glenoid. Both these patients were young males with recurrent anterior shoulder dislocation.

assessment is best made with AP and true lateral views in the plane of the scapula (i.e., to profile the glenohumeral joint on the AP and to get the "Y" or "Mercedes Benz" view of the scapula on the lateral) rather than the outdated anatomic AP and lateral views. An axillary lateral should also be obtained if at all possible. There may be associated fractures, in particular fracture of the greater tuberosity.

Anterior dislocation frequently results in an impaction fracture on the posterolateral portion of the head of the humerus (the Hill-Sachs lesion). This is best seen on the internal rotation AP view (Fig. 101–46). Conversely, a fragment of cartilage and/or bone may be broken off the anterior glenoid lip (the Bankart lesion). Reverse Hill-Sachs and Bankart lesions may be seen on posterior dislocations. Shoulders with recurrent subluxation/dislocation may require CT arthrography or MRI to determine whether a glenoid labrum injury is the source of instability (Fig. 101–47).

Rotator Cuff Tears

Although small tears in the rotator cuff may occur as the result of degenerative changes, large tears are frequently associated with acute trauma. There is usually a background of rotator cuff degeneration from impingement by the acromium and acromioclavicular joints in older people or from glenohumeral instability in younger, more athletic patients. The most common site of rotator cuff tear is in the lateral "critical zone" of the supraspinatus tendon just before its insertion onto the greater tuberosity. A complete tear of the rotator cuff is readily diagnosed by arthrography. Contrast is injected into the glenohumeral joint capsule and the tear diagnosed on the basis of contrast leaking through the defect into the subacromial and/or subdeltoid bursae (Fig. 101–48*A*). Complete or partial tears can also be demonstrated by MRI (Fig. 101–48*B* to *D*).

Proximal Humerus Fractures

These are usually secondary to a fall on the outstretched hand and are related to osteoporosis, being more common in the elderly, with a female to male ratio of 2:1. They are usually classified by the Neer classification, in which the humeral head, greater tuberosity, lesser tuberosity, and shaft are regarded as separate parts. A part is regarded as displaced if it is separated from the others by more than 1 cm or angulated by more than 45 degrees. About 80 per cent of proximal humerus fractures are nondisplaced (Fig. 101–49). The rest are two-, three-, or four-part fractures depending on how many parts are displaced. Four-part fractures carry a high risk of avascular necrosis of the humeral head (because the blood supply is via the tuberosities) and are usually treated by hemiarthroplasty. Nondisplaced fractures are treated nonoperatively and treatment of two- or three-part fractures depends on the severity. There may be an associated dislocation. Occasionally there is simply an impaction fracture of the articular surface or a linear split through the humeral head.

Humeral Shaft

Because fracture of the humeral shaft is often secondary to a direct blow, open fractures are common. Fractures above the deltoid insertion lead to outward displacement of the distal fragment whereas fractures below the deltoid insertion lead to upward displacement of the distal fragment because of the differing pull of the muscles. Radiographs must include both ends of the humerus to check for rotation. The radial nerve may be affected, especially in spiral fractures of the distal third. Healing with conservative treatment is usually fairly rapid.

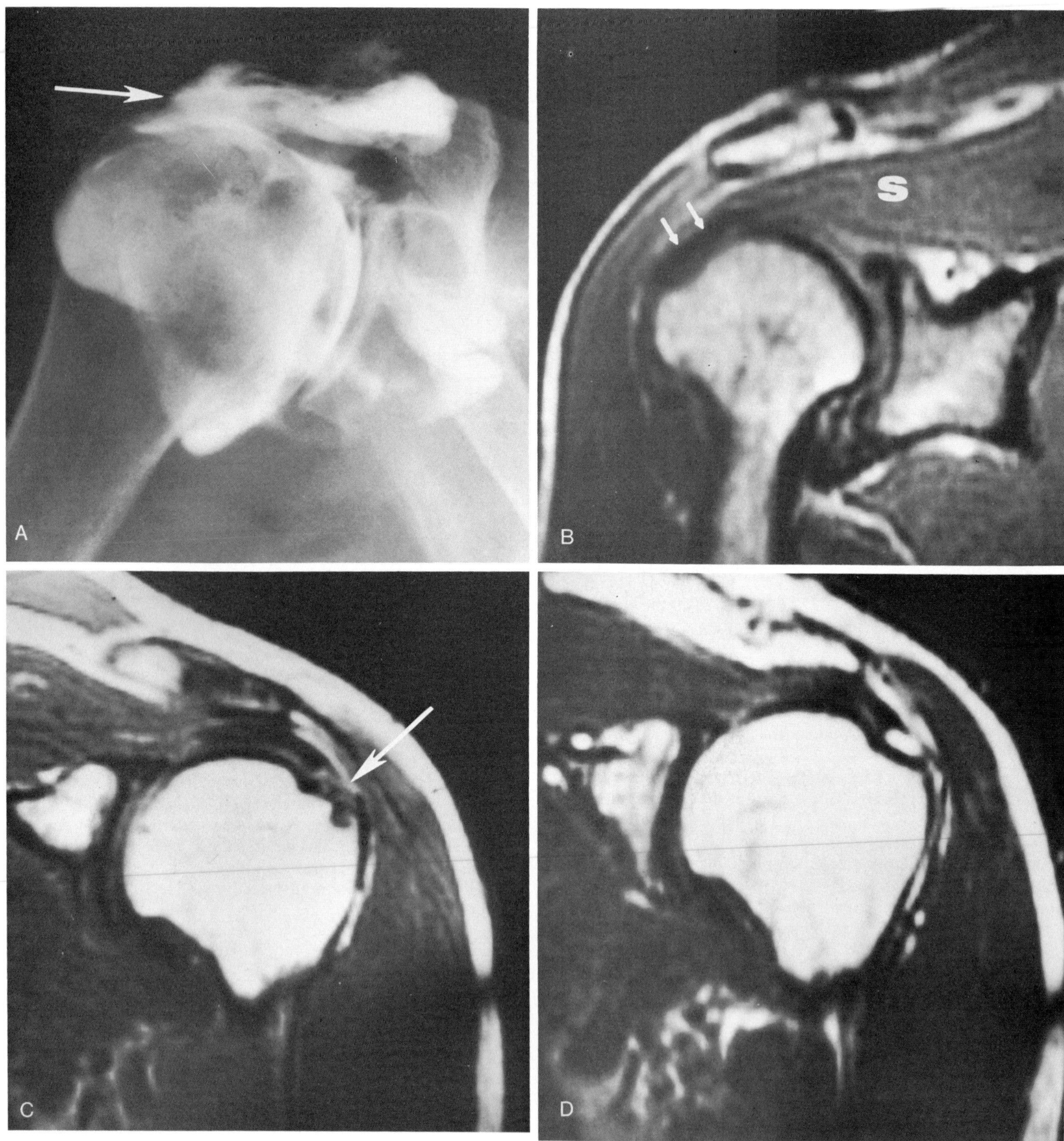

Figure 101–48. Complete tear of the rotator cuff is shown by single-contrast arthrography *(A)*. Contrast outlines the joint capsule, with a thin line of contrast overlying the humeral articular cartilage in a normal manner superolaterally. However, there is a large amount of contrast in the subacromial bursa between the humeral head and the acromion *(arrow)*, establishing the presence of a complete tear. The normal rotator cuff is seen on MRI *(B)* as a low signal band *(arrows)* connecting the supraspinatus muscle (S) to the greater tuberosity of the humerus. A tear is shown by increased signal in this tendon, indicated by the arrow in *C*, and confirmed by brightening of this signal on the T_2-weighted image *(D)*.

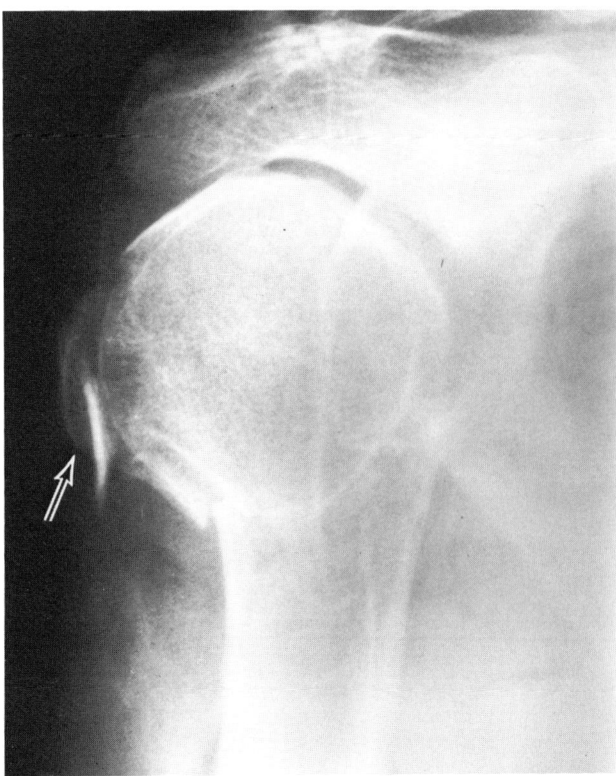

Figure 101–49. A nondisplaced humeral neck fracture is shown in internal rotation. The greater tuberosity fragment (*arrow*) is less than 1 cm displaced. The age of the patient (75 years) is typical.

THE ELBOW AND FOREARM

Anthony J. Doyle

Pediatrics

The elbow in children can be challenging because of the large number of ossification centers. It is important to know the order of ossification of these centers; one easy way to remember this is the mnemonic CRITOE (Capitellum at 1 year, Radius at 3+ years, Internal epicondyle at 5+ years, Trochlea at 10 years, Olecranon at 6 to 10 years, and External epicondyle at 10 + years, Fig. 101–50). Remembering this sequence will avoid the pitfall of overlooking a medial epicondylar avulsion. This injury is secondary to the pull of the common flexor tendon (Little League pitchers again) and often occurs in young patients with ossification of only the capitellum, radial head, and medial epicondyle. The pull of the flexor tendon may result in displacement of the medial epicondylar fragment into the medial elbow joint. There it may mimic a trochlear ossification center (Fig. 101–51). This mistake is avoided by recognizing that the presence of an ossified trochlear center implies that there must be an ossified medial epicondyle center present, and if this is not in its usual place, it is probably displaced into the joint. If in doubt, comparison with the other side is helpful, as in other childhood trauma.

Secondary signs of trauma in the elbow in children are important. The "fat pad sign" consisting of a visible posterior fat pad or (less reliably) a perpendicular, elevated anterior fat pad indicates a fracture in up to 90 per cent of cases in children. Alignment is also important, as indicated by the anterior humeral line and the radiocapitellar line. The anterior humeral line should pass through the middle third of the capitellum; in a supracondylar fracture it will pass through the anterior third (Fig. 101–52) or even in front of the capitellum altogether because the fracture fragment is posteriorly angulated. Supracondylar fractures may be otherwise occult because they are angulated but generally not displaced. A line along the axis of the radius (the radiocapitellar line) should similarly pass through the capitellum in all projections; failure to do so indicates dislocation of the radial head, as in a "Monteggia" fracture, where the proximal ulna is fractured and the radial head dislocation is the other break in the bony ring formed by the radius and ulna.

The most common fracture around the elbow in children is in fact the supracondylar fracture (60 per cent), with lateral condyle fracture next (15 per cent) followed by medial epicondyle separation (10 per cent). The supracondylar fracture is greenstick in nature in 25 per cent, with the fracture line often not visible, hence the importance of detecting the posterior angulation of the condyles, the usual direction of angulation. Severe angulation or displacement of the distal fragment may lead to impingement on the brachial artery and median nerve, which if untreated can go on to permanent contracture of the flexors of the forearm. Fracture of the lateral condyle is a Salter type IV injury in which the fracture line extends through the metaphysis, along the growth plate, and then between the capitellar and trochlear ossification centers. The pull of the common extensors often results in displacement of the fragment, which contains the capitellum and a flake of metaphysis (Fig. 101–53). These almost always require fixation but produce little growth disturbance because the fracture line passes between the trochlear and capitellar growth centers rather than through the capitellar center. For this reason some authorities regard these as Salter type II lesions. Separation of the medial condyle, to which the common flexors are attached, is discussed above. Rarely, the entire distal humeral epiphysis may separate.

The radial head epiphysis may suffer a Salter II fracture; this may be nondisplaced, in which case the metaphyseal fracture leads to the diagnosis. The radial head may be dislocated (almost always anterior) in the Monteggia fracture as described above. The "nursemaid's elbow" or "pulled elbow" results from a sudden pull on the arm in a toddler and is common. It shows no radiographic abnormality but is very easily reduced by gentle supination and often reduces during positioning for the radiograph.

Distal to the elbow, fractures of the forearm bones are common in children, often from falls. Most frequently both bones are broken

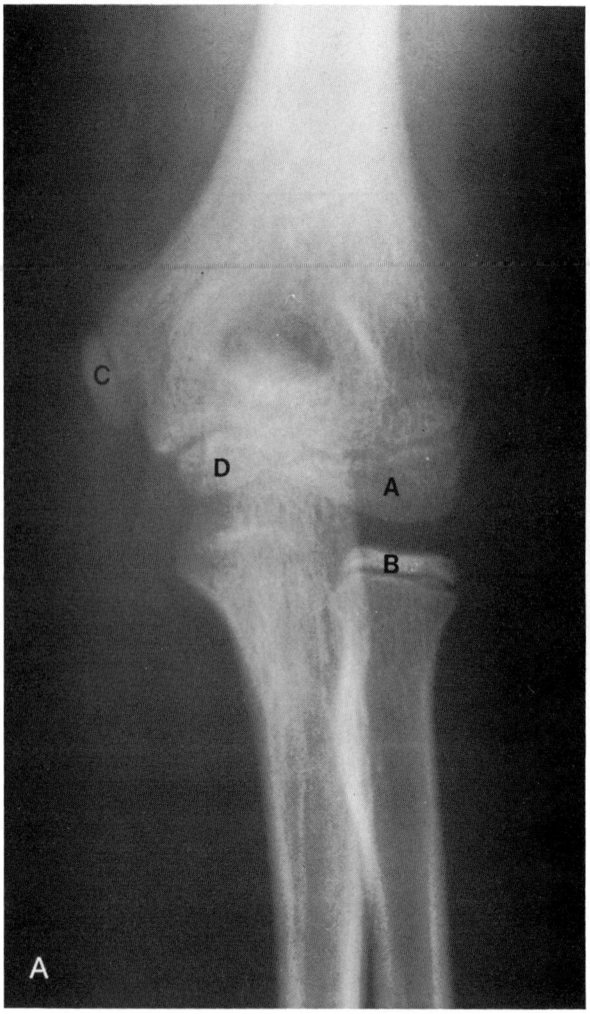

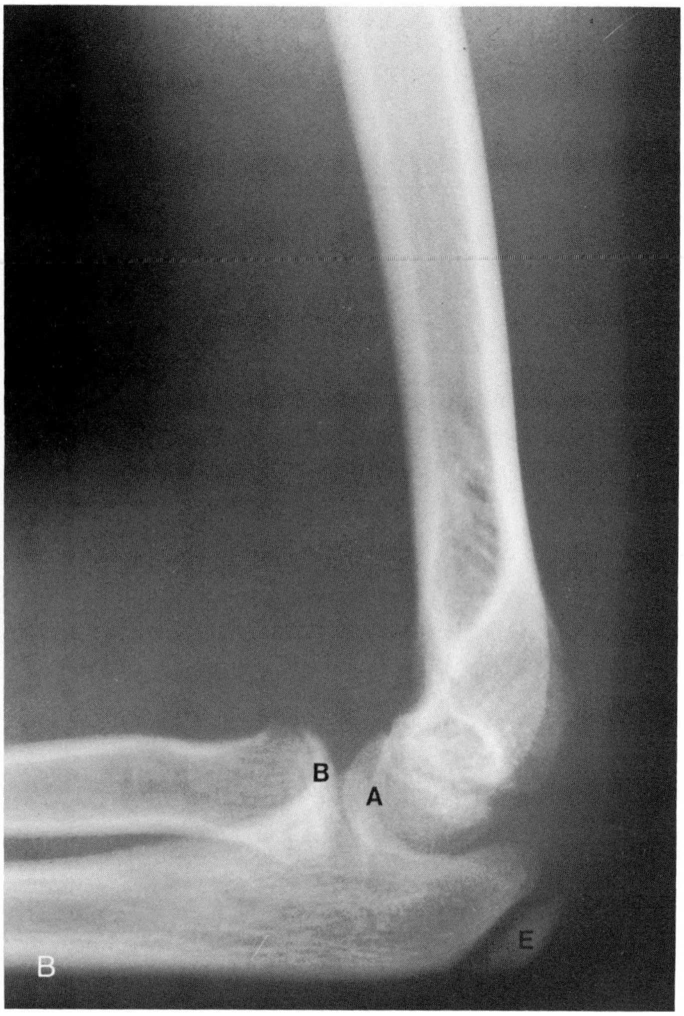

Figure 101–50. *A* and *B*, **Ossification centers of the elbow** are shown in chronologic order: capitellum (A), radial head (B), medial epicondyle (C), trochlea (D), olecranon (E), and lateral epicondyle (not yet ossified in this patient). (Courtesy of B. J. Manaster, M.D., Ph.D.)

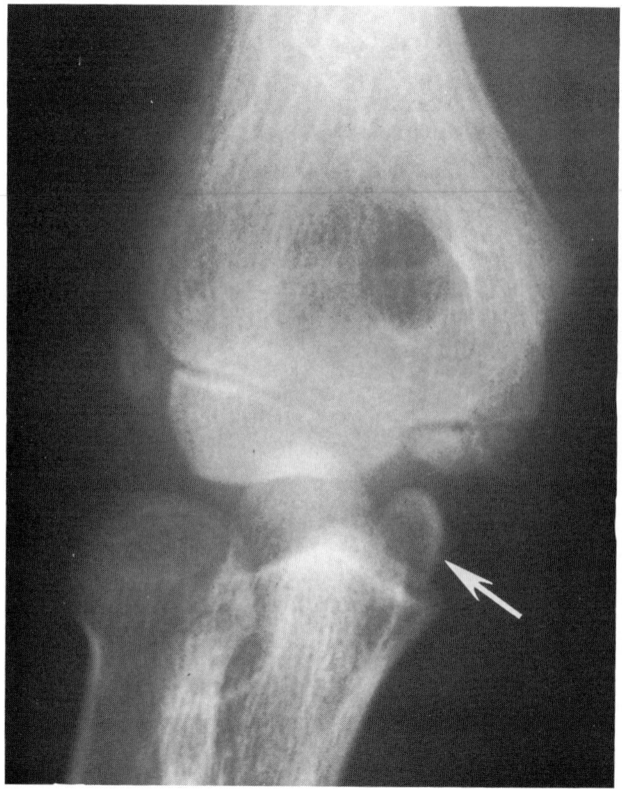

Figure 101–51. The medial epicondyle has been avulsed in this child. Going through the CRITOE sequence shows that the capitellum and radius are present but the internal epicondyle is displaced into the joint (*arrow*). In a younger child, it may simulate the center for the trochlea in this position. (Courtesy of Paula Shultz, M.D., Salt Lake City, UT.)

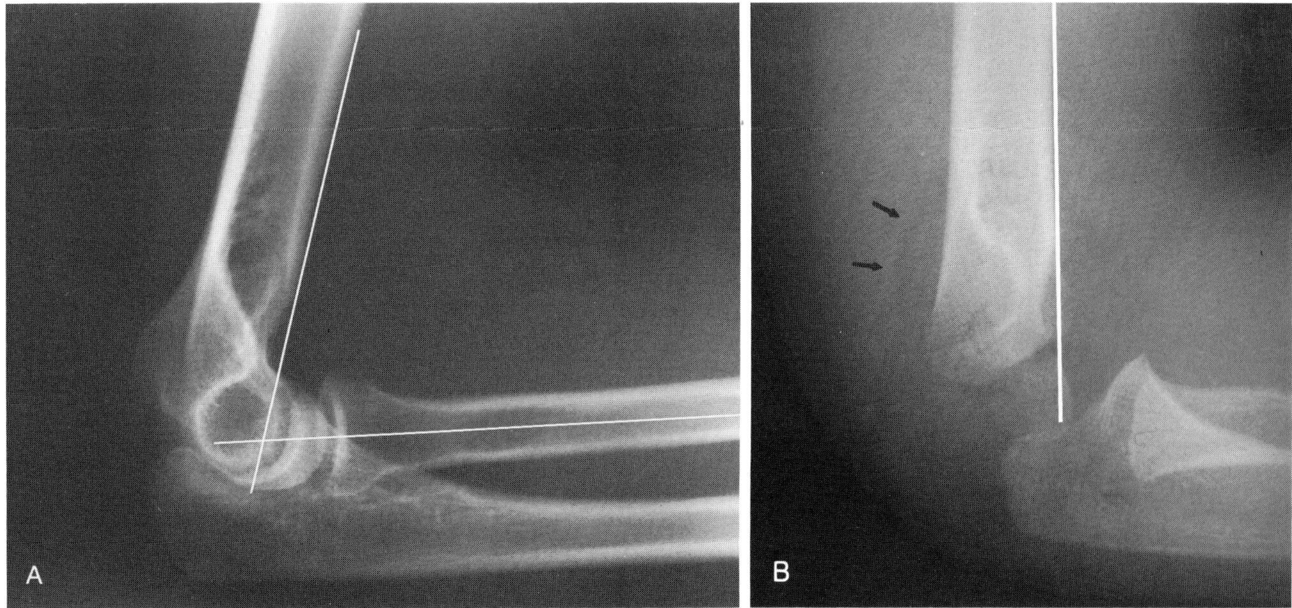

Figure 101–52. *A*, The **anterior humeral line** passing along the anterior cortex and intersecting the middle third of the capitellum is seen on the lateral radiograph, as well as the **radiocapitellar line**, passing along the axis of the radius and intersecting the middle of the capitellum. *B*, Both the **"fat pad sign" and the anterior humeral line** are seen in this supracondylar fracture. Note the faint semicircular lucency of the displaced posterior fat pad (*arrows*) indicating an effusion. The anterior humeral line (*white line*) intersects the anterior capitellum rather than the middle, indicating posterior displacement. Although no fracture line is visible, the appearance of periosteal new bone 10 days later confirmed a supracondylar fracture.

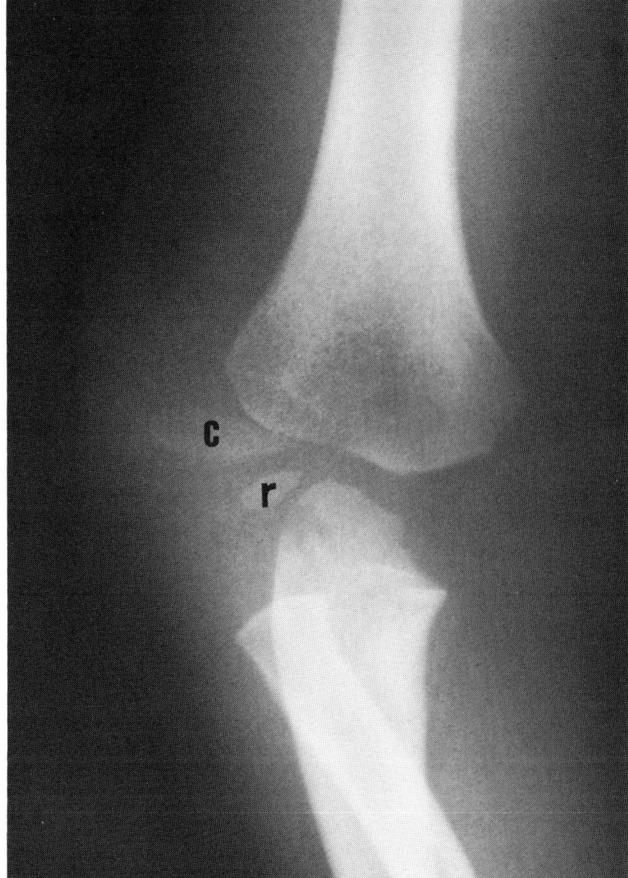

Figure 101–53. A fracture of the lateral humeral epicondyle is demonstrated in this three-year-old. The capitellum (C) is displaced laterally with the radial head epiphysis (r) following it. The expected fleck of metaphysis is nonossified so not visible. The ulna is in normal position, but there is a nondisplaced olecranon fracture.

and, depending on the age of the child, site of the fracture, and degree of angulation, may need reduction to preserve function. One or both distal forearm fractures are often incomplete, presenting as torus or greenstick fractures. This is also the most common site for plastic bowing to occur (see Fig. 101–1), usually in the radius in association with an ulnar fracture. Plastic bowing does not remodel well and operative reduction is often necessary.

Adults

ELBOW

Supracondylar fractures in adults usually result from a fall with hyperextension and similar considerations apply as in children. Another common distal humeral fracture is the intercondylar T or Y fracture. This is probably secondary to ulnar impaction, driving the fragments apart. These consequently are frequently comminuted and displaced and may require tomography or CT for full evaluation. They are often classified as types I to IV and usually treated with open reduction and internal fixation.

Condylar fractures usually involve the lateral condyle rather than the medial. If the fracture line passes outside the lateral trochlear ridge it is stable, but if it passes medial to this ridge it is unstable (Fig. 101–54). The capitellum may be fractured by force transmitted through the radial head, frequently resulting in an osteochondral fracture. Isolated fractures of the trochlea and epicondyles are unusual in the adult.

Overt dislocation is reasonably common, especially in the 10- to 20-year age group. Most involve posterior displacement of the ulna with respect to the humerus (Fig. 101–55). Isolated dislocation of the ulna is uncommon and of the radius, rare. Associated fractures are often present; avulsion of the medial epicondyle of the humerus (which may become entrapped) is more common than fracture of the coronoid process of the ulna. A common post-reduction complication is heterotopic ossification, myositis ossificans, or ossification of the capsule and ligaments (see Fig. 101–12).

The olecranon process may be fractured by a direct blow, sudden triceps contraction in a fall, or both. A good true lateral and AP are necessary to diagnose nondisplaced fractures and the occasional hairline sagittal fracture. The triceps insertion may be avulsed, the fracture may be comminuted, or there may be an associated dislocation. Depending on the size of the fragment, these are often open-reduced and internally fixed with a wire tension band.

Fracture of the radial head is the most common fracture in the adult elbow. In nondisplaced fractures, the fracture line may be difficult to see. An effusion as shown by the presence of elevated fat pads should lead to a search for occult radial head fracture with oblique views or cephalad angled views (Fig. 101–56). Severely comminuted radial head fractures may be associated with disruption of the interosseous membrane and distal radio-ulnar joint (acute longitudinal radio-ulnar dissociation or ''Essex-Lopresti'' fracture), which may be radiographically occult.

FOREARM

Fractures of both forearm bones may result from many different mechanisms. Accurate reduction is of crucial importance because malalignment, especially loss of the normal radial bowing, leads to impaired pronation and supination. Very little remodeling occurs in the adult, unlike in the child. Consequently, good radiographs are essential. The elbow and wrist must be included in two views at right angles. Most two-bone fractures of the forearm are treated operatively to achieve anatomic alignment. Comminuted fractures may be treated with an external fixator. Malunion, non-union or delayed union may occur. Post-traumatic synostosis is uncommon (3 per cent).

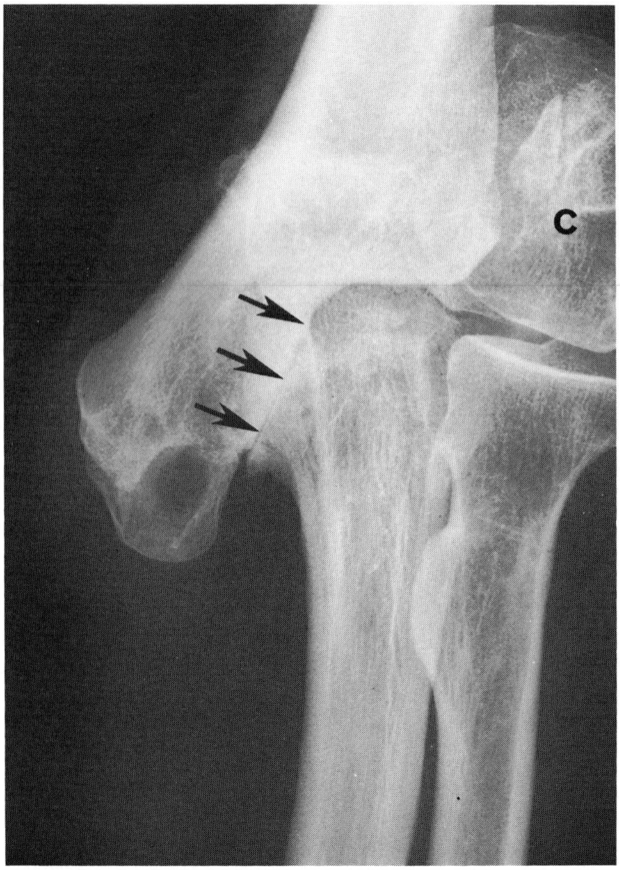

Figure 101–54. Unstable lateral condyle fracture with nonunion. The old fracture line (*arrows*) passed medial to the trochlear ridge and was unstable. The condylar/capitellar fragment (C) did not reunite and has migrated proximally, taking both radius and ulna with it, so that there is now a pseudarthrosis along the old fracture line.

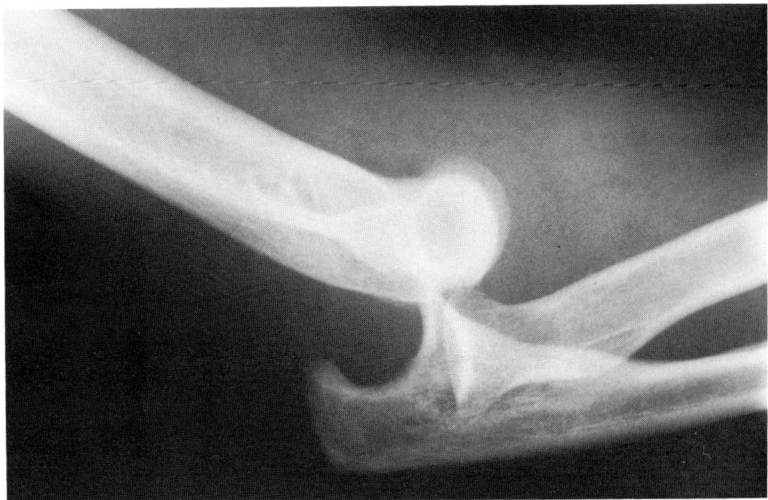

Figure 101–55. Complete posterior dislocation of both the radius and ulna is seen on the lateral projection. The coronoid process of the ulna is at risk of avulsion fracture by the biceps brachii tendon, which inserts at this point.

Fractures of a single forearm bone usually fall into one of three patterns. The "night stick" fracture of the ulna is caused by a direct blow to the ulna that is subcutaneous for much of its length. Associated injuries are uncommon. The other two injury patterns, however, involve significant dislocations. Fracture of the proximal ulna usually is apex anterior. An associated anterior dislocation of the radial head must be looked for on the elbow films. This can be subtle (a survey in 1940 showed that 52 per cent of these were missed initially) and requires observation of the radio-capitellar line (Fig. 101–57). This fracture-dislocation is known as the Monteggia complex after the Italian who described it in 1814. The other and somewhat more common fracture-dislocation is the Galeazzi lesion, in which there is a fracture of the distal radius with dislocation at the distal radio-ulnar joint. The dislocation must be carefully looked for in a good lateral (Fig. 101–58) film and is sometimes better demonstrated by CT. Both of these are treated by open reduction and internal fixation.

WRIST TRAUMA

B. J. Manaster

Because the natural tendency is to break the force of any fall by reaching out with the hand, a "fall on the outstretched hand" or FOOSH is a very common mechanism of injury to the wrist. Although fracture of the wrist is extremely common, dislocations and instability patterns are often seen as well. These can be quite subtle injuries, and one must be familiar with normal anatomy in order to

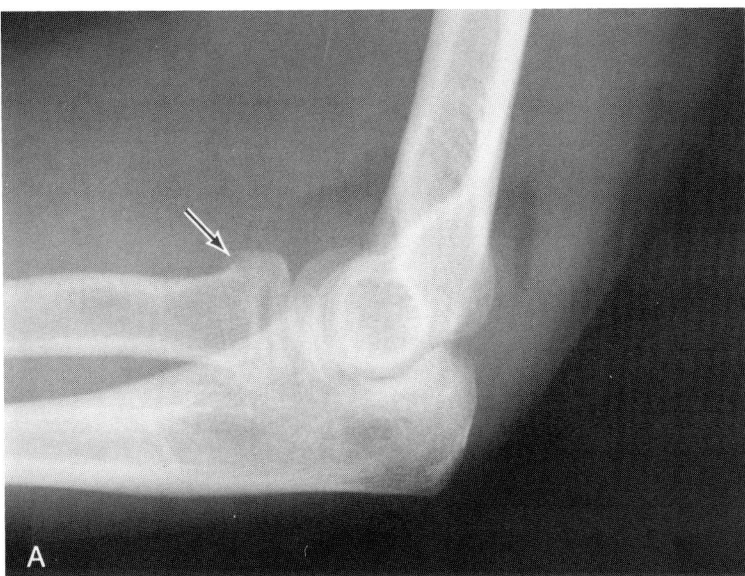

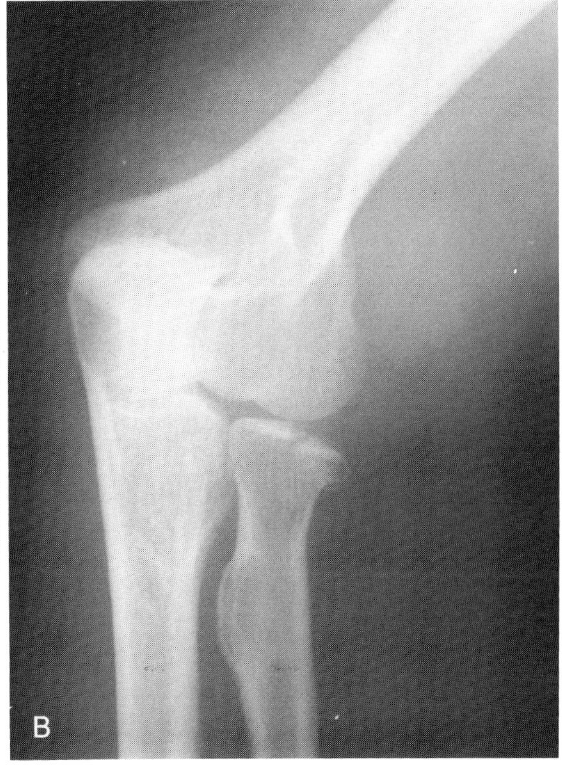

Figure 101–56. *A,* The **fat pad sign** is easily seen on this lateral elbow, indicating an effusion. The underlying radial head fracture (*arrow*) is subtle. *B,* An oblique view shows the radial head fracture much more clearly.

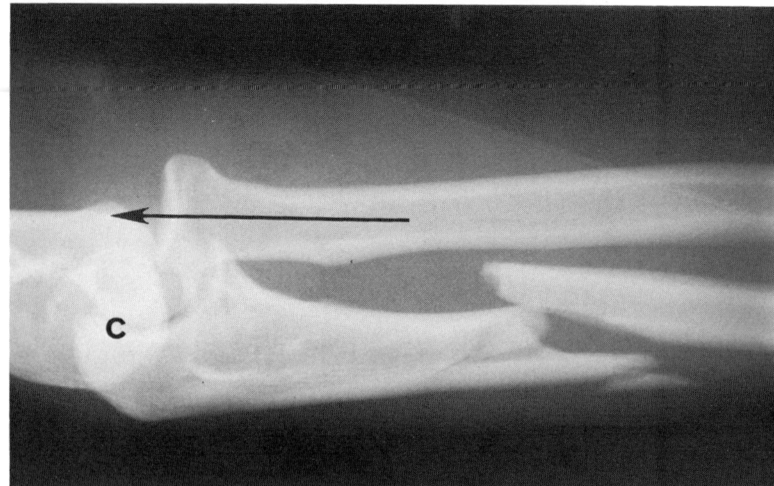

Figure 101–57. This **Monteggia fracture-dislocation** could be overlooked if one were not careful to assess the radiocapitellar line. The ulnar fracture is obvious; more subtle is the complete anterior dislocation of the radius with its axis (*arrow*) well anterior to the rounded capitellum (C). Diagnosis is not helped by the fact that the elbow film is not a true lateral, but trauma films are not always perfect!

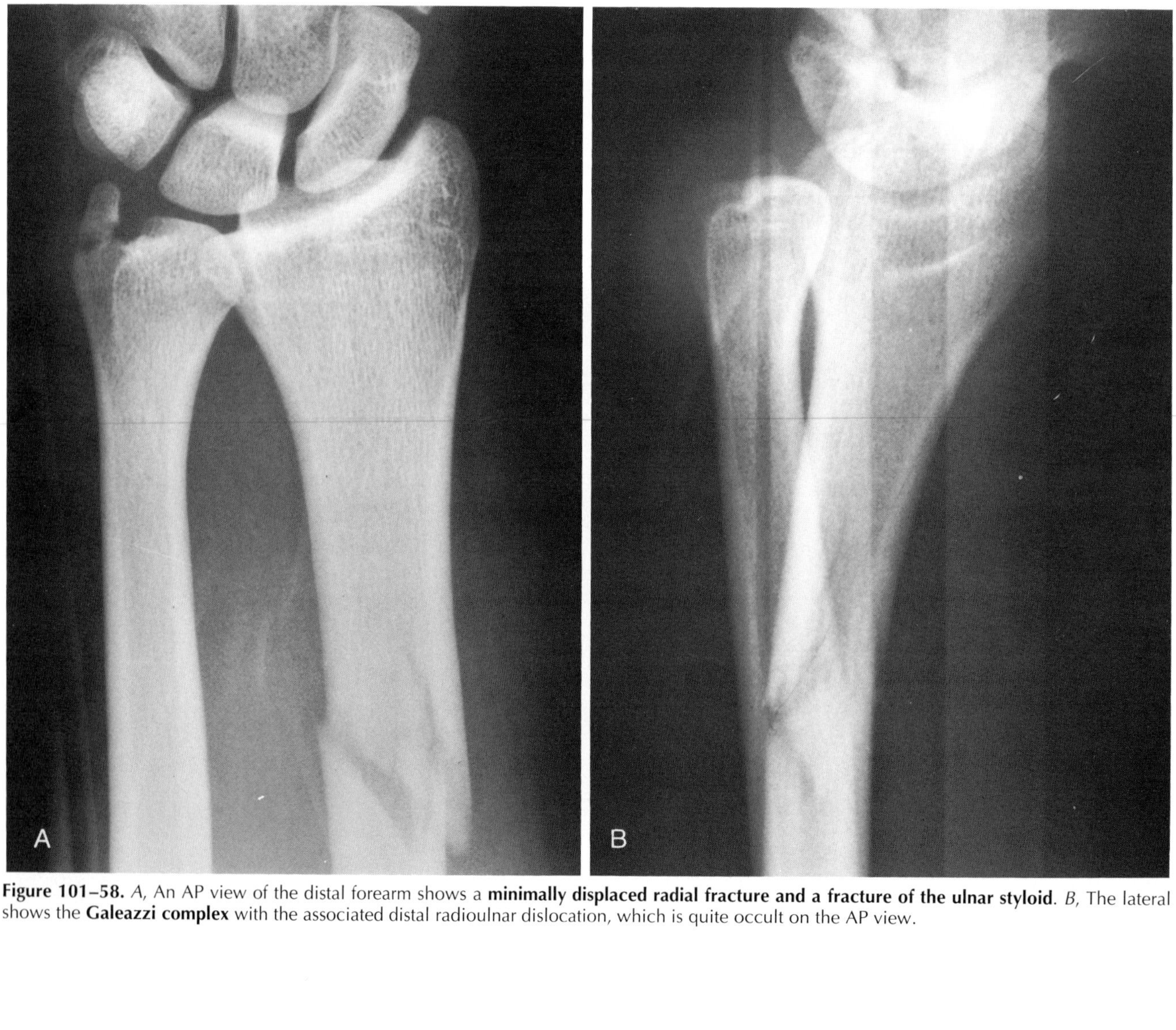

Figure 101–58. *A*, An AP view of the distal forearm shows a **minimally displaced radial fracture and a fracture of the ulnar styloid**. *B*, The lateral shows the **Galeazzi complex** with the associated distal radioulnar dislocation, which is quite occult on the AP view.

reliably diagnose these abnormalities. Knowledge of normal anatomy is also useful in assessing post-reduction alignment of fractures and dislocations.

Distal Forearm

The distal forearm must be evaluated separately from the carpus. The normal anatomy is outlined in diagram form in Fig. 101–59*A*. The distal radial articular surface is seen to tilt normally 17 degrees towards the ulna on the PA film. Medially, the radius articulates with the head of the ulna at the ulnar notch. The head of the ulna is usually 1 to 2 mm shorter than the radius (although it may be slightly longer or shorter, representing an ulnar plus or ulnar minus variant, respectively). The head of the ulna generally touches or slightly overlaps the radius at the distal radial ulnar joint on the PA view. The triangular fibrocartilage, seen only by arthrography or MRI, extends from the medial radial surface to insert at the base of the ulnar styloid, helping to maintain the integrity of the distal radial ulnar joint.

On the lateral film (Fig. 101–59*B*), the distal radial articular surface is angled 10 to 15 degrees volarly (palmarly). On a true lateral film, the dorsal surface of the distal ulna lies 1 to 3 mm posterior to the dorsal surface of the radius. The pronator quadratus muscle is located across the volar aspect of the digital radius and ulna; the fat overlying the pronator quadratus is seen on the lateral film as a flat lucent line, and it may be a clue to soft-tissue injury if it is seen to bulge volarly.

The most common injury of the skeletal system is a fracture of the distal forearm. As stated earlier, most result from a fall on the outstretched hand. Interestingly, age alone is a very good predictor of the type of FOOSH injury. The young patient (4 to 10 years of age) will most commonly demonstrate a transverse fracture in the metaphyseal region of both forearm bones. This fracture may be complete or incomplete, with the latter seen as either a greenstick or torus variety (see Fig. 101–14). The patient in the 11- to 16-year age range is much more likely to suffer a Salter II fracture of the distal radial epiphysis. Epiphyseal plate injuries are especially common in this age range, and the Salter II variety is the most frequently seen. Because the etiology is again a fall on the outstretched forearm, the Salter II fracture is usually manifest as an epiphyseal plate separation with a small dorsal metaphyseal fragment. Because there is usually little displacement, the Salter II injury of the distal forearm may be convincingly demonstrated only on the lateral film (Fig. 101–60).

The young adult patient (17 to 40 years) is most likely to suffer a scaphoid fracture with a fall on the outstretched arm (Fig. 101–61). Seventy per cent of scaphoid fractures are at the waist, and nondisplaced. They therefore may be radiographically occult at the time of acute injury. Bulging of the navicular fat pad may serve as a clue. Specially angulated scaphoid views may also be useful. If a scaphoid fracture is clinically suspected but not seen, films may be repeated in 7 to 10 days, when sclerosis or resorption about the fracture line may be seen. If it is essential to make the diagnosis acutely, bone scan, CT, or MRI will demonstrate the abnormality. The proximal half of the scaphoid has a tenuous arterial supply. Thus, with a waist of scaphoid or proximal scaphoid fracture, the patient is at risk for development of either avascular necrosis of the proximal pole or non-union. The importance of diagnosis of this sometimes subtle fracture is thus emphasized.

Finally, a fall on the outstretched arm in the more elderly osteoporotic patient results most commonly in a Colles fracture (Fig. 101–62). A Colles fracture is a fracture of the distal radius that results in apex volar angulation with dorsal impaction. There may or may not be an intra-articular component, and there may or may not be an associated ulnar styloid fracture.

Other fractures of the distal forearm are quite infrequent, but should be recognized as distinct from those that have previously been described. Not all distal radial fractures are Colles' fractures! Those that are not Colles' fractures have different treatments and prognoses, and must be recognized. Some of these fractures are quite unstable, including the Barton and reverse Barton fractures, in which the carpus usually stays with a dorsal or volar fragment rather than with a normal alignment of the forearm.

Other distal forearm injuries are rare. These include distal radioulnar subluxation. This diagnosis may be suggested by an abnormal position of the head of the ulna in the ulnar notch. However, the diagnosis can be quite subtle and is usually best made by CT axial images through the distal radio-ulnar joint.

The triangular fibrocartilage may be ruptured, either as an aging phenomenon, or from a traumatic etiology. Rupture of this ligament is diagnosed either by MRI or arthrography (Fig. 101–63).

Carpus

Carpal injuries are relatively infrequent compared with forearm injuries (1 to 10). Furthermore, carpal injuries are rare in patients under the age of 12. Finally, of all carpal injuries, 60 to 70 per cent are scaphoid fractures, discussed earlier in this chapter. The remaining carpal injuries can be quite subtle or may have no findings on plain films. As always, it is crucial to understand the normal anatomy.

On the PA film, one can see that there are proximal and distal rows of the carpus that are bridged by the scaphoid. The width of the intercarpal joints is uniform, approximating 2 mm. However, intercarpal width can easily be obscured by slight obliquity of the wrist on the radiograph. Three parallel arcs have been described by Gilula to aid in evaluation of the carpus (Fig. 101–64). The first arc is a smooth curve along the proximal articular margins of the proximal carpal row, the second is the curve along the distal articular margins of the proximal carpal row, and the third is the curve

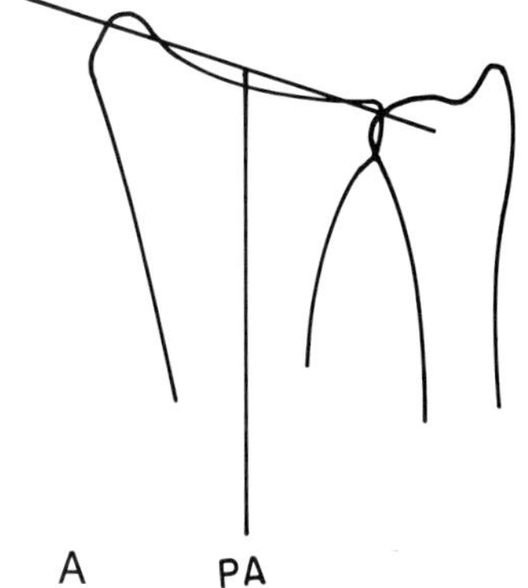

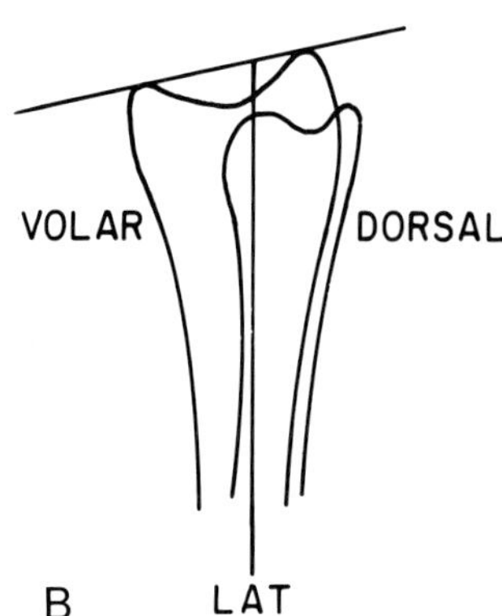

Figure 101–59. *A*, **Normal ulnar tilt** of the distal radial articular surface on the PA film. *B*, **normal volar tilt** of the distal radial articular surface on the lateral film. Note that the distal ulna is slightly shorter and posteriorly placed with respect to the radial articular surface on a well-positioned lateral film. (LAT = lateral.) (From Manaster BJ: Handbooks in Radiology: Skeletal Radiology. Chicago, Year Book Medical Publishers, 1989.)

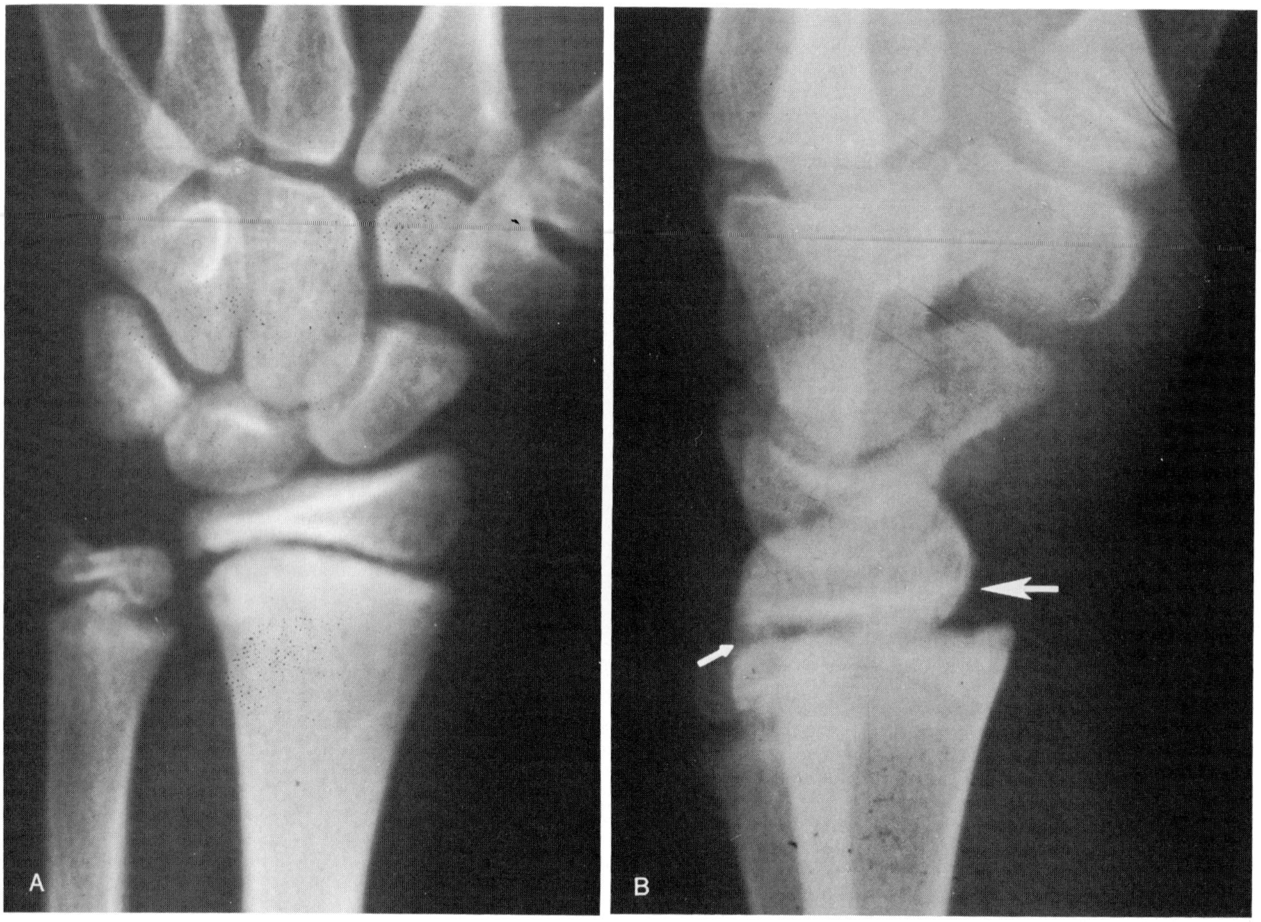

Figure 101–60. AP (*A*) and lateral (*B*) films of a **Salter II fracture** in a 13-year-old patient. Note that the fracture is extremely difficult to detect on the AP view. However, on the lateral view the hints consist of dorsal displacement of the radial epiphysis (*long arrow*) and the small dorsal metaphyseal fragment (*short arrow*).

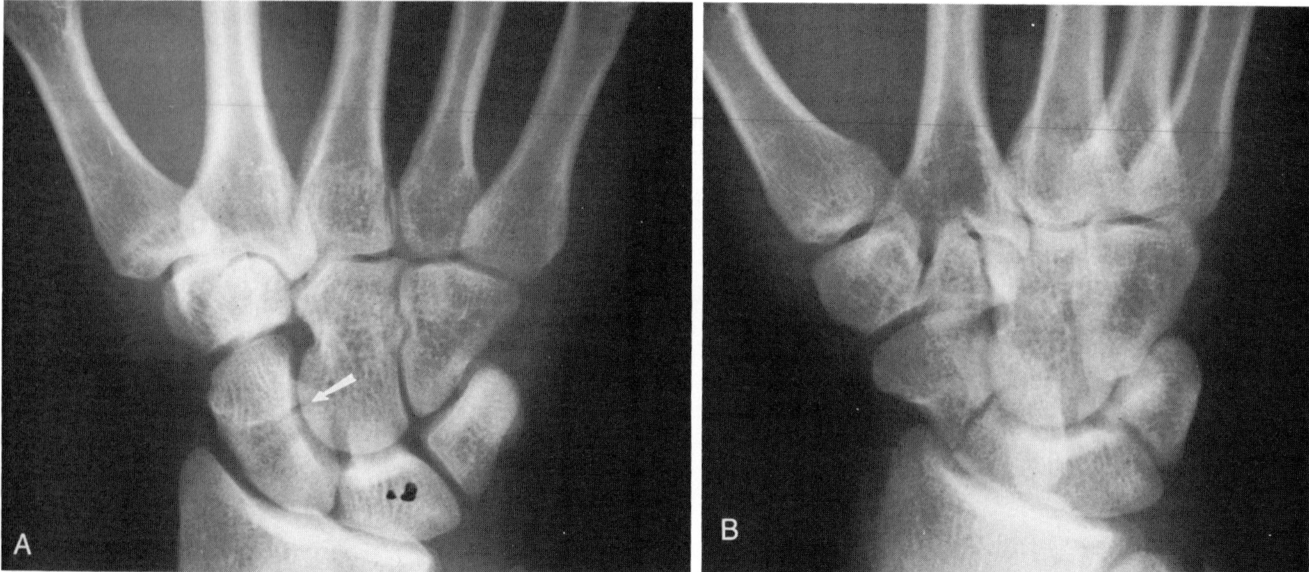

Figure 101–61. Twenty-year-old male with **waist of scaphoid fracture** from a fall on the outstretched hand. The fracture is difficult to detect on the PA film (*arrow in A*), but is easily seen on the oblique film (*B*). Occasionally other, more highly angulated films are needed for diagnosis.

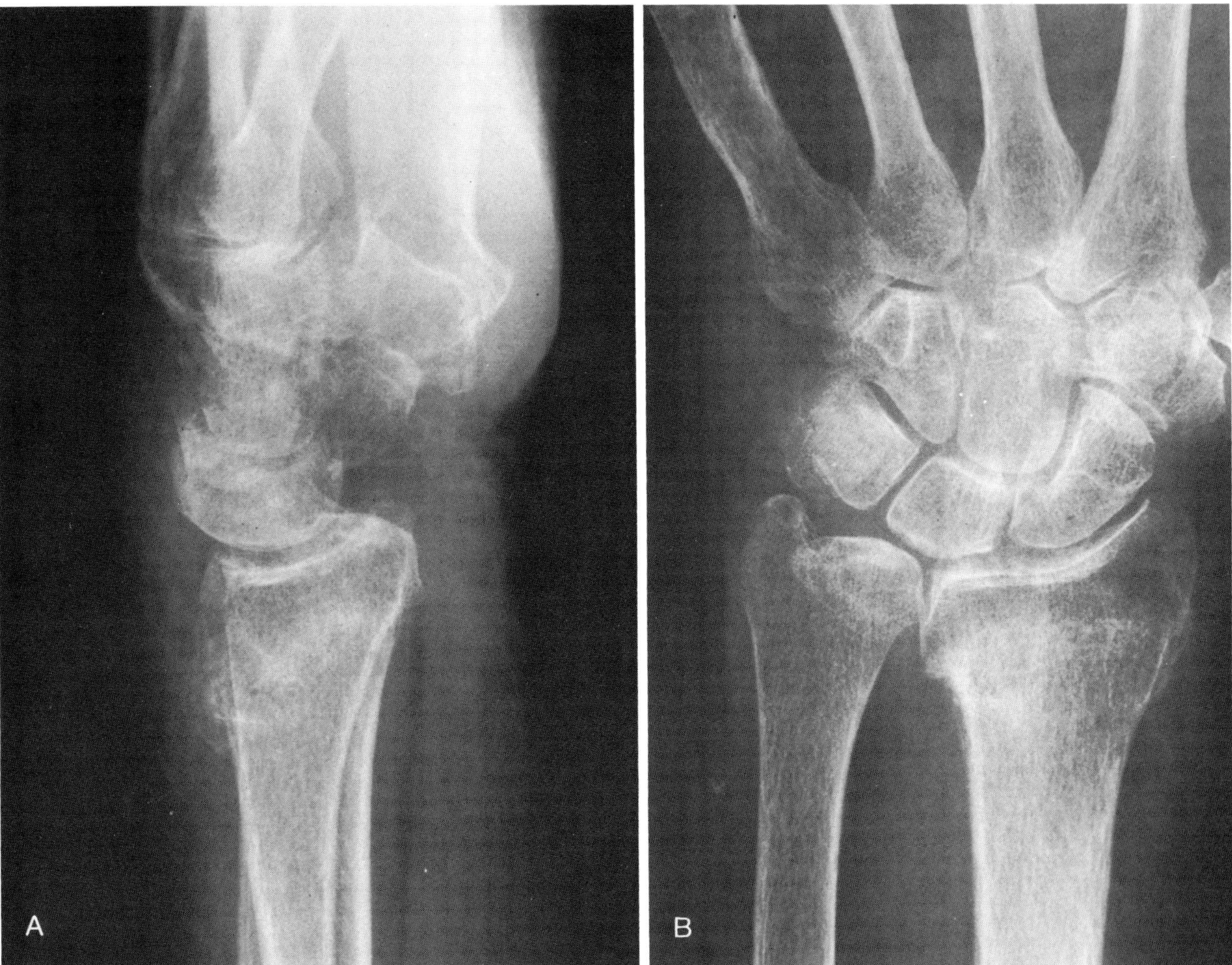

Figure 101–62. Example of a **Colles fracture**. In this case there is a transverse fracture through the distal radius with impaction. Note that the normal volar tilt of the radial articular surface has been reversed (lateral, *A*), resulting from the apex volar angulation at the fracture site. There is also decrease in the length of radius (AP, *B*), as is typically seen in this patient. There is no intra-articular extension and no ulnar styloid process fracture, but these need not be components of a Colles fracture. Note the osteopenia consistent with the patient's age of 70.

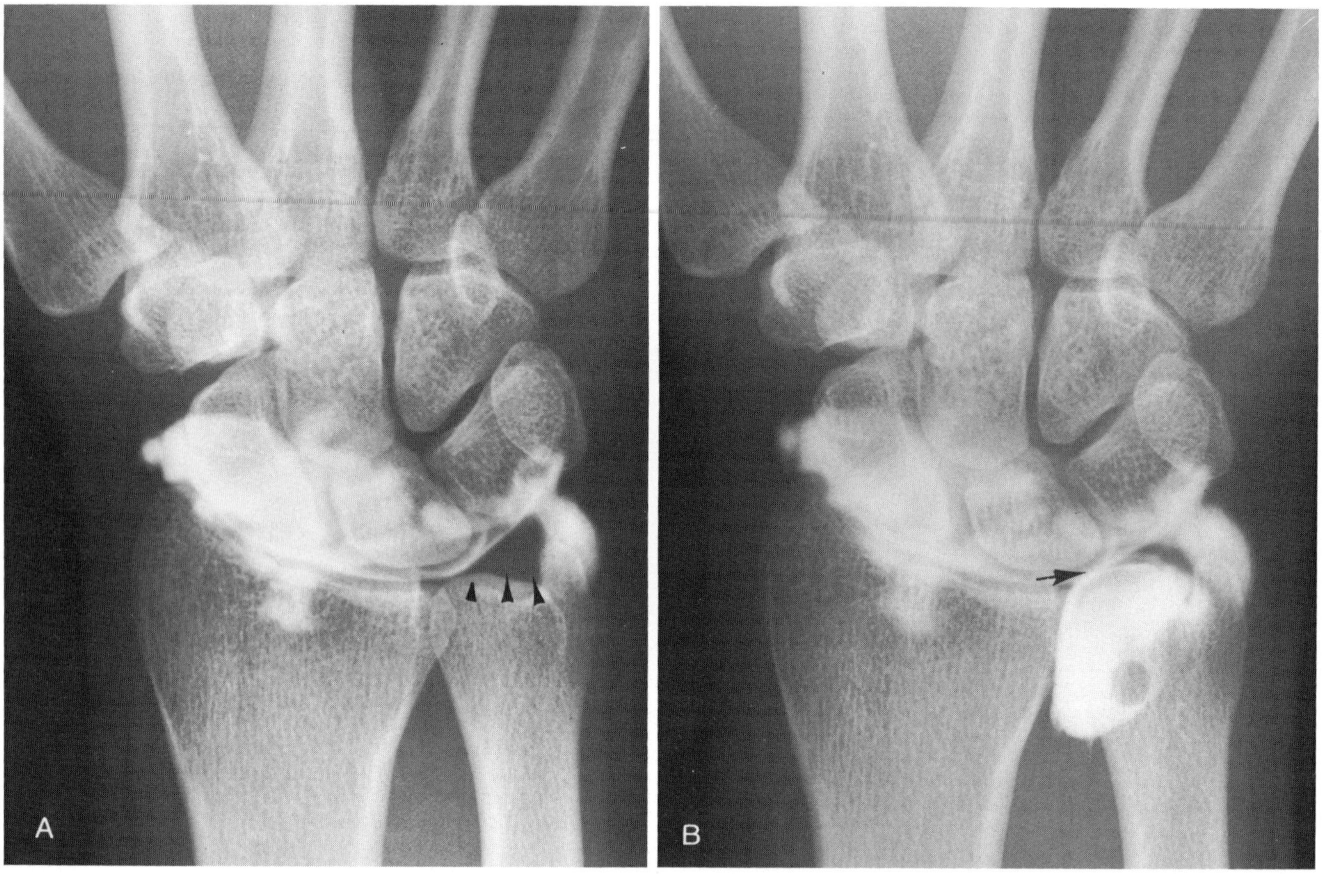

Figure 101–63. *A*, A **normal arthrographic injection** of the radiocarpal joint. The contrast is restricted from entering the distal radioulnar joint by an intact triangular fibrocartilage complex (soft-tissue structure not seen, but location outlined by *arrow*) that stretches between the lateral radius and the ulnar styloid. *B*, A similar radiocarpal injection in which the contrast flowed not only into the radiocarpal joint, but also through a tear in the triangular fibrocartilage complex to fill the distal radioulnar joint (*arrow*). This arthrographic result is diagnostic of a **triangular fibrocartilage complex tear.**

along the proximal articular margins of the capitate and hamate. Disruption of any of these gentle curves implies subluxation or dislocation of the carpus. Another hint suggesting carpal abnormality is the shape of the lunate. This bone is normally trapezoidal on the PA film. If the lunate is abnormally rotated as in a subluxation or dislocation, it becomes triangular in shape. However, poor positioning with wrist held in either dorsi or palmar flexion will also make the lunate appear triangular in shape, thus simulating an abnormality.

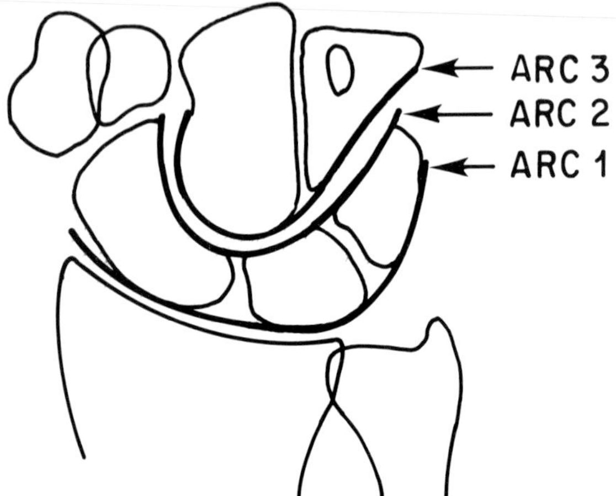

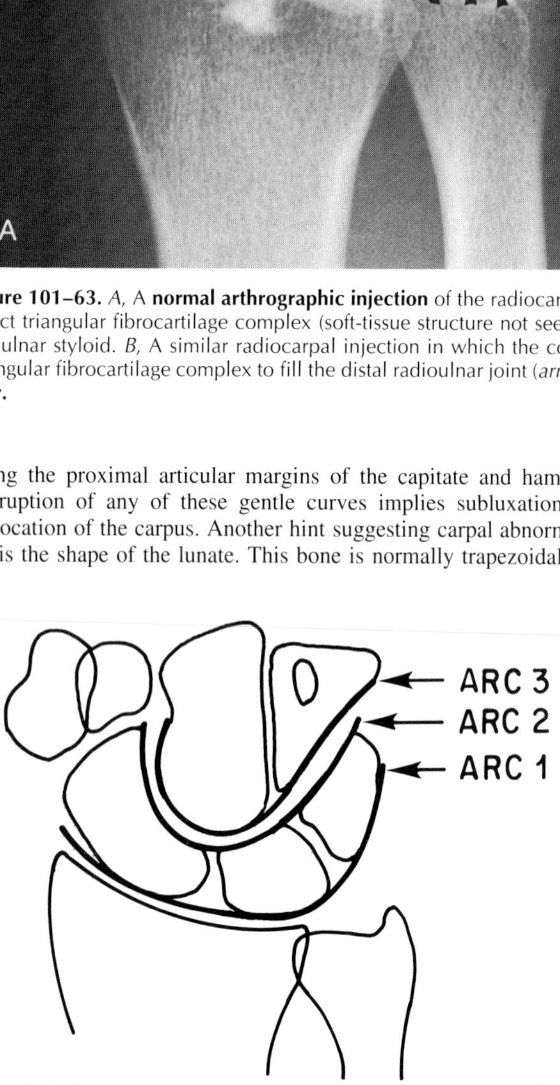

Figure 101–64. Normal PA carpal view demonstrating particularly the normal shapes of the scaphoid and lunate as well as the three continuous arcs of the proximal and distal carpal rows. Continuity of these arcs ensures carpal row integrity. (From Manaster BJ: Handbooks in Radiology: Skeletal Radiology. Chicago, Year Book Medical Publishers, 1989.)

In neutral position on the PA film, 50 per cent or more of the lunate articulates with the radius. With ulnar deviation of the hand, the scaphoid appears elongated and the entire lunate articulates with the radius (Fig. 101–65*A*). In radial deviation, only 25 per cent of the lunate articulates with the radius and the scaphoid appears foreshortened and distorted. This foreshortening of the scaphoid owing to poor positioning may simulate a "ring sign," suggesting abnormal rotation of the scaphoid, which can be seen in ligamentous injuries. More importantly, it also may obscure a waist of scaphoid fracture. Furthermore, patients with painful wrists normally hold the hand in radial deviation. With this positioning, scaphoid fractures may easily be missed (Fig. 101–65*B*).

Several normal variants may be observed on the PA view of the wrist. A number of accessory ossicles occur, which may be confused with fracture. The accessory ossicles are outlined in Theodore Keats' *Atlas of Normal Roentgen Variants That May Simulate Disease*. Use of this reference is recommended. Additionally, accessory ossicles are generally smoothly rounded and well corticated, and therefore usually distinguishable from acute fracture.

The lateral film of the carpus presents a confusing overlap (Fig. 101–66), but the coaxial relationship among the articular surfaces of the radius, lunate, capitate, and third metacarpal *must* be picked out. An exact linear relationship among these bones is uncommon,

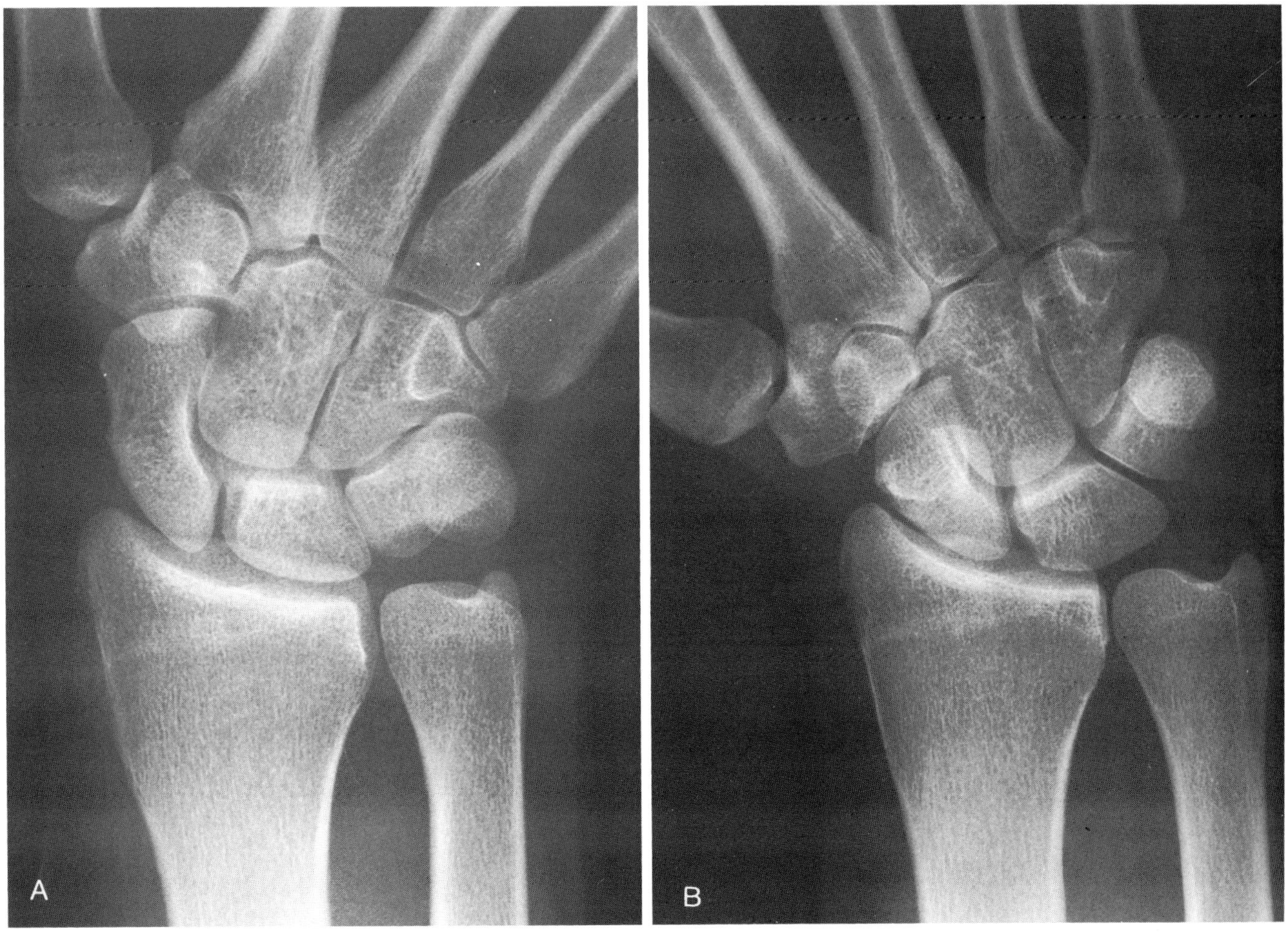

Figure 101–65. *A*, In **ulnar deviation**, note the elongation of the scaphoid, which is extremely well seen. Confirmation of this positioning is made by noting that the lunate completely articulates with the radius. *B*, The wrist is held in **radial deviation**. The scaphoid is foreshortened, with a "ring sign," making evaluation of waist area extremely difficult. Confirmation of positioning is made by the fact that less than 50 per cent of the lunate is covered by the radius.

but the coaxial relationship must be demonstrated in order to rule out subluxation or dislocation.

Most fracture dislocations of the carpus follow the vulnerable zone outlined by Yeager: The inner arc roughly outlines the disrupted ligaments around the lunate, as seen in a pure dislocation, whereas the outer arc outlines the fractures commonly associated with carpal fracture dislocation (radial styloid, waist of scaphoid, proximal capitate, base of hamate, lunar surface of the triquetrum, and ulnar styloid). It is interesting to note that with progression from the radial to the ulnar side of the arc, the severity of the injury increases (for example, a scapholunate dissociation is less severe than a perilunate dislocation, which in turn is less severe than a lunate dislocation). Additionally, with progression from the radial to ulnar side, the frequency of the injury decreases (for example, a scapholunate dissociation may be a less severe injury than a perilunate dislocation, but it is also much more common; perilunate dislocations are more common than lunate dislocations). The radiographic analysis of carpal dislocations is not difficult if the rules are followed. On the PA film, Gilula's first and second arcs are disrupted. On the lateral film, the coaxial radius-lunate-capitate arrangement is disrupted. The PA film is not reliably useful for diagnosing the type of dislocation. This information is found entirely on

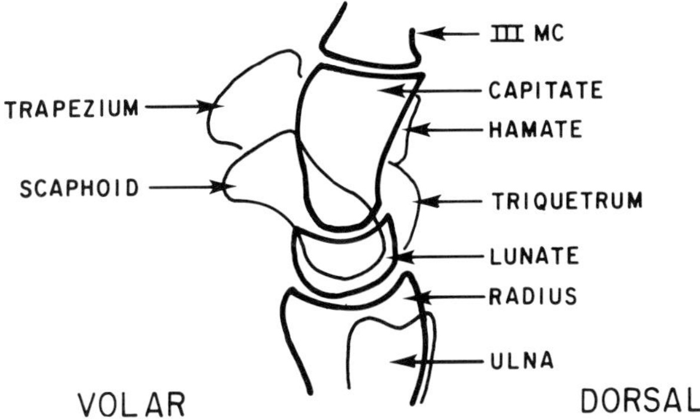

Figure 101–66. Normal lateral carpal view, in which one must pick out the articulating distal radius, lunate, capitate, and third metacarpal (*bold outline*). (From Manaster BJ: Handbooks in Radiology: Skeletal Radiology. Chicago, Year Book Medical Publishers, 1989.)

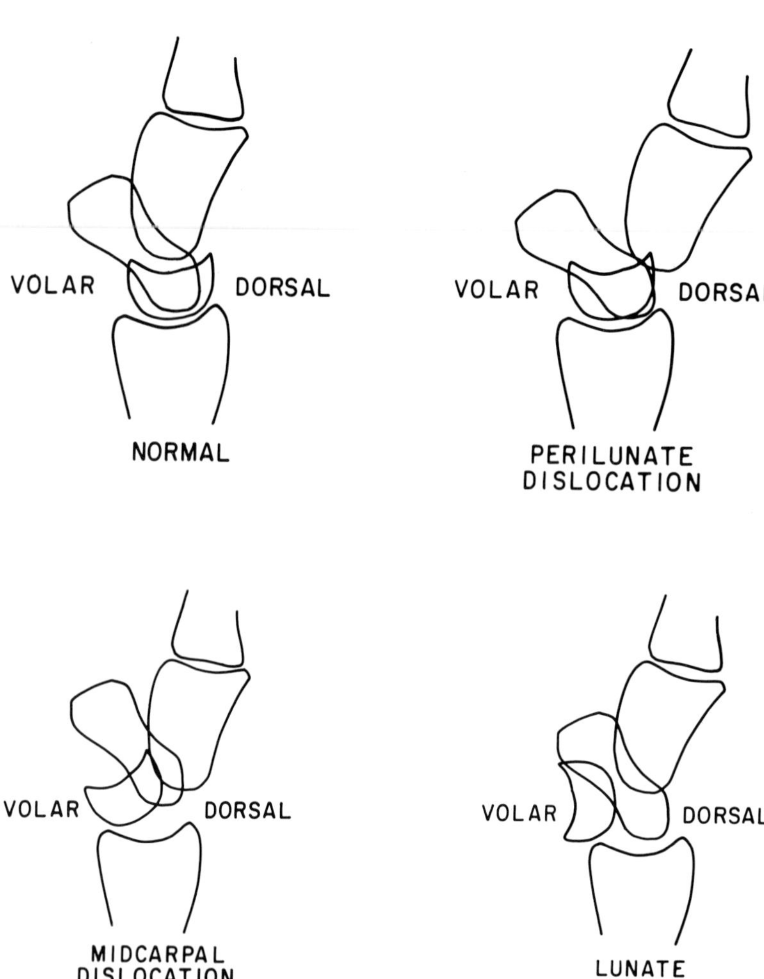

Figure 101–67. Carpal dislocation patterns as seen on the lateral film. The progression from normal (*A*) to perilunate (loss of articulation of the capitate with the lunate) (*B*) through midcarpal (dislocation of the capitate from the lunate, and subluxation but not dislocation of the lunate from the radius) (*C*) to lunate (dislocation of the capitate from the lunate and of the lunate from the radius) (*D*) demonstrates increasing severity of injury as well as the possible sequence of injury patterns in a single person. A patient who presents initially with a perilunate dislocation may go on to a midcarpal dislocation, and convert to a lunate dislocation if there is sufficient ligamentous disruption. (From Manaster BJ: Handbooks in Radiology: Skeletal Radiology. Chicago, Year Book Medical Publishers, 1989.)

the lateral film (Fig. 101–67). In a perilunate dislocation, the capitate articular surface is dislocated from the lunate, almost invariably dorsally. The lunate maintains its normal articulation with the radius. In a mid-carpal dislocation, the capitate is dislocated from the lunate (as in a perilunate dislocation), and the lunate tilts volarly but is not dislocated from the radius (Fig. 101–68). This may represent a carpus in transition from a perilunate to a lunate dislocation. Finally, in a lunate dislocation, the lunate loses its articulation with both the capitate and the radius and is displaced volarly with 90 degrees of rotation (Fig. 101–69). The capitate remains aligned with the radius but sinks proximally towards it.

Fractures of the carpus, with the exception of the scaphoid, are quite rare. It is unusual to see an acute lunate fracture, but the lunate is vulnerable to avascular necrosis, usually secondary to microtrauma, so collapse and increased density may be seen (Kienböck's disease or lunatomalacia, Fig. 101–70). Dorsal chip fractures of the triquetrum are seen only on the lateral film and are not treated. Capitate fractures are extremely rare, except as a part of a complex fracture dislocation. The same is true of proximal pole fractures of the hamate. Hook of hamate fractures are less rare and are best detected on PA films by the absence of the hook and then confirmed on CT.

Collapse between the proximal and distal carpal rows is normally prevented by the rigid scaphoid link as well as strong ligamentous attachments. Loss of these mechanisms leads to zig-zag collapse deformities, termed carpal instabilities. These are diagnosed radiographically by a change in alignment of the capitate, lunate, radius, and scaphoid as seen on the lateral film (Fig. 101–71). The most common instability pattern is scapholunate dissociation, in which the gap at the scapholunate joint is greater than 2 mm on the PA films. These patients may or may not have associated scaphoid rotation, which is best evaluated on lateral film (Fig. 101–71*B*).

Dorsiflexion carpal instability (dorsal intercalated segmental instability [DISI]) most commonly results from a traumatic episode. This instability is diagnosed on the lateral film by an increased dorsiflexion of the lunate, with a consequent increase in lunate capitate angle. There is usually associated volar flexion of the scaphoid, with a consequent increase in the scapholunate angle on the lateral film (Fig. 101–71*C*). Finally, volar flexion carpal instability (volar intercalated segmental instability [VISI]) is seen most commonly in patients with rheumatoid arthritis and subsequent ligamentous laxity. It is diagnosed by detection of a volar flexion of the lunate and dorsiflexion of the capitate, giving a zig-zag deformity and abnormally large lunate capitate angle on the lateral film (Figs. 101–71*D* and 101–72). Often, but not invariably, there is a decrease in the scapholunate angle as well.

Ligamentous injury can also result in nondissociative instability patterns that are not readily apparent by plain film. These are sometimes seen transiently under fluoroscopy (recommended particularly when a patient has a reproducible painful click of the wrist). Stress views may also elicit these nondissociative patterns. Finally, wrist arthrography and/or MRI examination may be required to evaluate the integrity of the intraosseous ligaments. The accuracy of arthrography and MRI is equivalent for evaluation of the triangular fibrocartilage complex. Arthrography is generally felt to be equal or superior in accuracy in evaluation of the intraosseous ligaments (Fig. 101–73). Both examinations are highly dependent on technical expertise and careful examination technique.

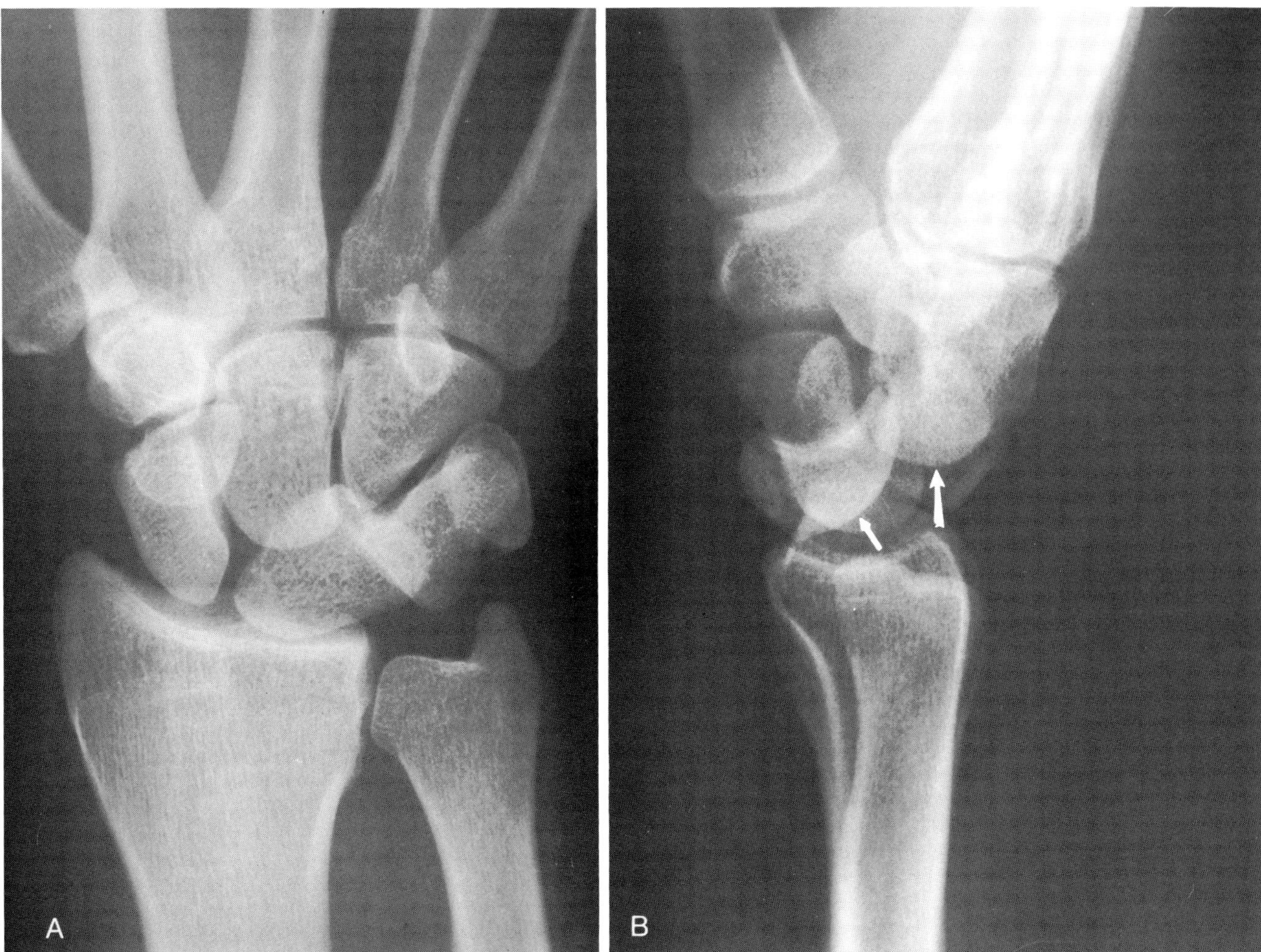

Figure 101–68. The PA film (*A*) demonstrates **interruption of arcs 1 and 2**. The lunate is also abnormally shaped, appearing somewhat triangular. The lateral film (*B*) confirms that there is a dislocation. The capitate (*long arrow*) is completely dislocated from the lunate (*short arrow*) in a dorsal direction. This is typical for a perilunate dislocation. However, note that the capitate is nudging the lunate into more of a volar position, so that, although the lunate still articulates with the radius, it is not sitting concentrically within this articulation. Therefore, this perilunate dislocation is converting to a midcarpal dislocation and perhaps will continue to convert, resulting in a lunate dislocation pattern.

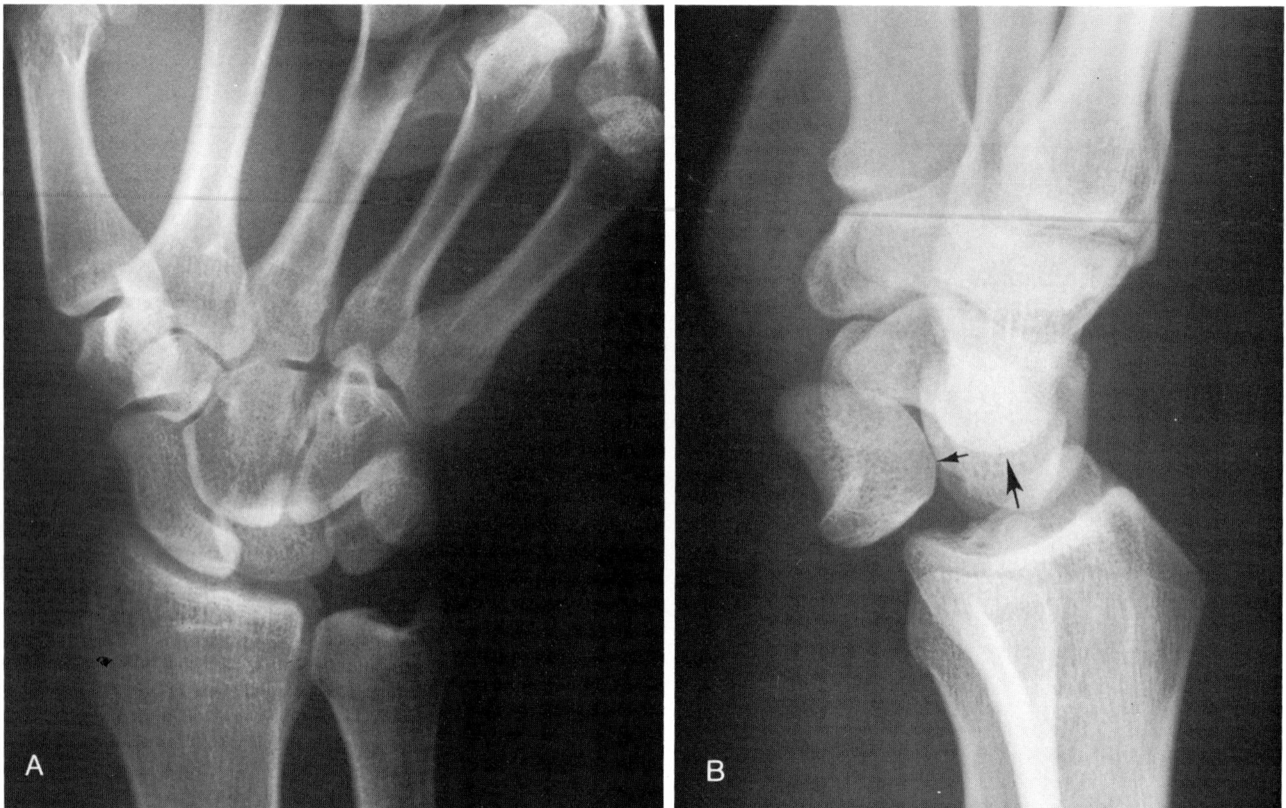

Figure 101–69. These films are classic for lunate dislocation. On the PA view (*A*) there is disruption of arcs 1 and 2 with a triangular-shaped lunate. The lateral film (*B*) demonstrates complete dislocation of the capitate (*long arrow*) from its articulation with the lunate (*short arrow*). In addition, there is dislocation of the articular surface of the lunate with the radius. The lunate is rotated 90 degrees and has been pushed out volarly.

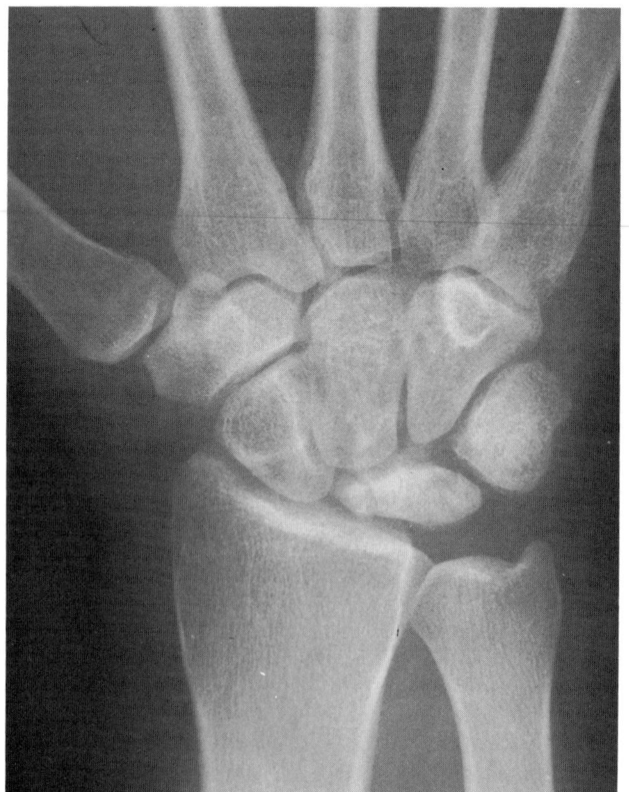

Figure 101–70. This film demonstrates **Kienböck's disease or lunate malacia**. The findings are of increased density, collapse of the lunate with normal cartilage, and otherwise normal bone.

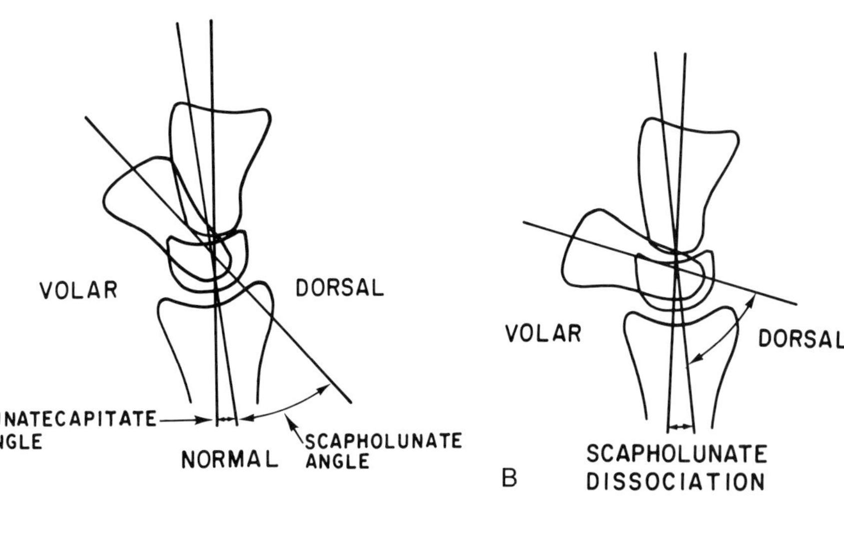

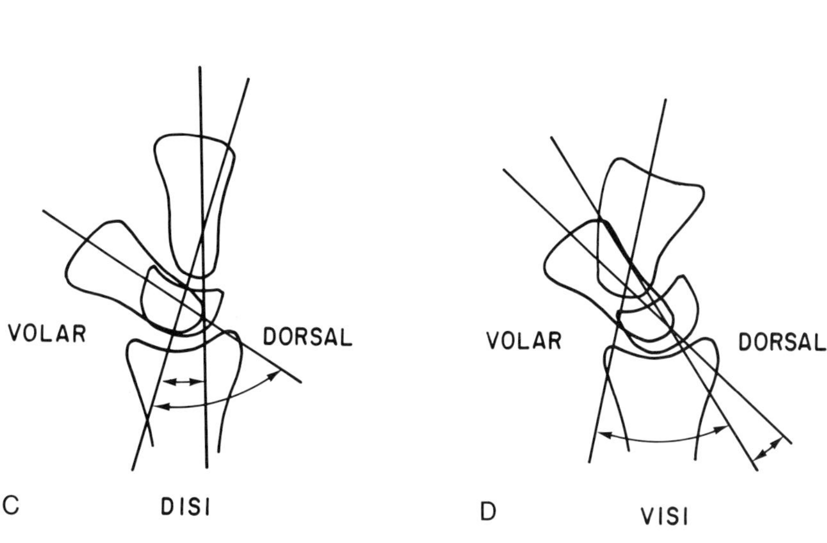

Figure 101–71. Carpal instability patterns. *A*, Normal, with lunate-capitate angle less than 20 degrees and scapholunate angle of 30 to 60 degrees. *B*, Scapholunate dissociation, with rotary subluxation of the scaphoid (normal lunate-capitate angle, abnormally large scapholunate angle). *C*, Dorsiflexion carpal instability pattern, with increased lunate-capitate angle, increased scapholunate angle, and dorsiflexion of the lunate. *D*, Volar flexion carpal instability, with increased lunate-capitate angle, often decreased scapholunate angle, and volar flexion of the lunate. (From Manaster BJ: Handbooks in Radiology: Skeletal Radiology. Chicago, Year Book Medical Publishers, 1989.)

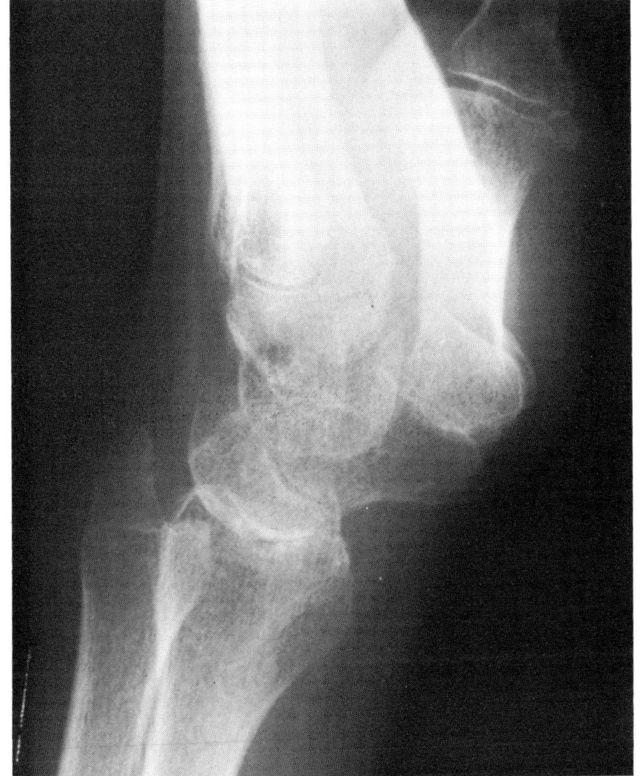

Figure 101–72. Example of a **volar flexion carpal instability pattern (VISI)**. One sees severe volar tilt of the lunate that has resulted in an increased lunate-capitate angle (approximating 90 degrees here) and a significantly decreased scapholunate angle (approximately 10 degrees). (For confirmation, compare this example with the diagram in Fig. 101–71*D*.) The combination of these findings makes the diagnosis of VISI.

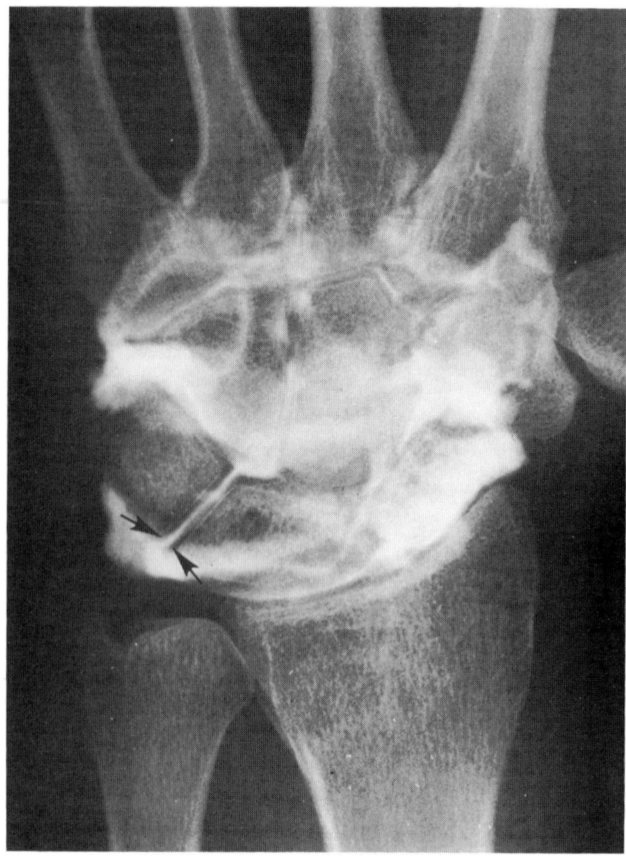

Figure 101–73. This arthrogram was produced by a single radiocarpal joint injection. The radiocarpal joint fills normally (compare with Fig. 101–63*A*). There is no evidence of a triangular fibrocartilage complex tear (compare with Fig. 101–63*B*). However, it is seen that there is flow from the radiocarpal joint into the midcarpal joints. The source of flow from one compartment to another is through a **perforation in the lunate triquetral interosseous ligament** (*arrow*).

PELVIS

Anthony J. Doyle

The bony pelvis is most often fractured in young adults by high energy trauma such as motor vehicle accidents. In the elderly, much less trauma may be required. An AP pelvis film should be obtained in most people with high-speed trauma and the following normal bony structures carefully inspected: the iliopectineal line, the ilioischial line, the sacroiliac joints, pubic symphysis, and the sacral foramina (Fig. 101–74).

Normal Variants

In children around the age of six or seven there is very commonly a prominent bony mass at the ischiopubic growth plate. This may be asymmetrical and therefore mistaken for a healing fracture or tumor by the unwary (Fig. 101–75). The apophysis along the iliac crest and the Y-shaped acetabular cartilage should not be mistaken for fractures. The nutrient foramen of the iliac wing may sometimes appear like a linear fracture but has a sclerotic margin and disappears on oblique projections. Widening of the symphysis may rarely be secondary to exstrophy of the bladder or cleidocranial dysostosis rather than trauma.

Pediatrics

The child's pelvis is deformable, with more elastic bones and ligaments than the adult; consequently, bony fractures imply severe trauma, with bladder and bowel injuries commonly associated. Associated fractures elsewhere in the body occur in up to 45 per cent of childhood pelvic fractures owing to the severity of the trauma involved. In the infant, nonaccidental injury should be suspected if there is not a strong history of trauma to account for pelvic fracture. In adolescents, avulsion injuries of apophyses are common, mostly related to sports. The anterior-superior iliac spine may be avulsed

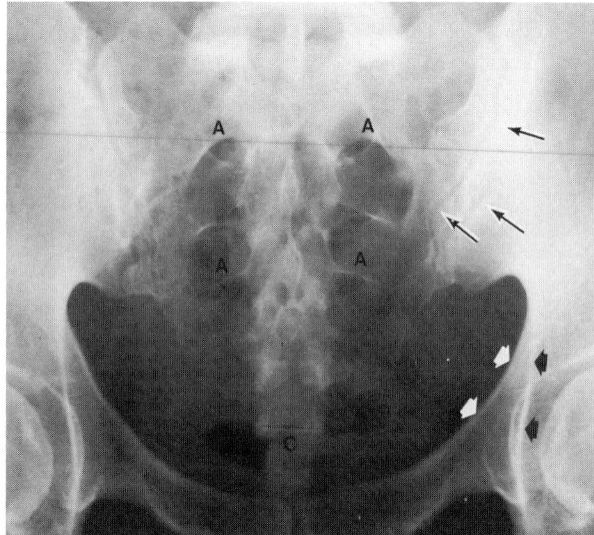

Figure 101–74. The sacral foramina and their arches (A) are indicated and should be almost perfectly symmetrical. The undulating sacroiliac joints (*arrows*) should also be symmetrical. The ilioischial (*black arrowheads*) and iliopectineal lines (*white arrowheads*) should be smooth and continuous. The coccyx (C) lines up with the symphysis pubis in a true AP projection. (Courtesy of B. J. Manaster, M.D., Ph.D.)

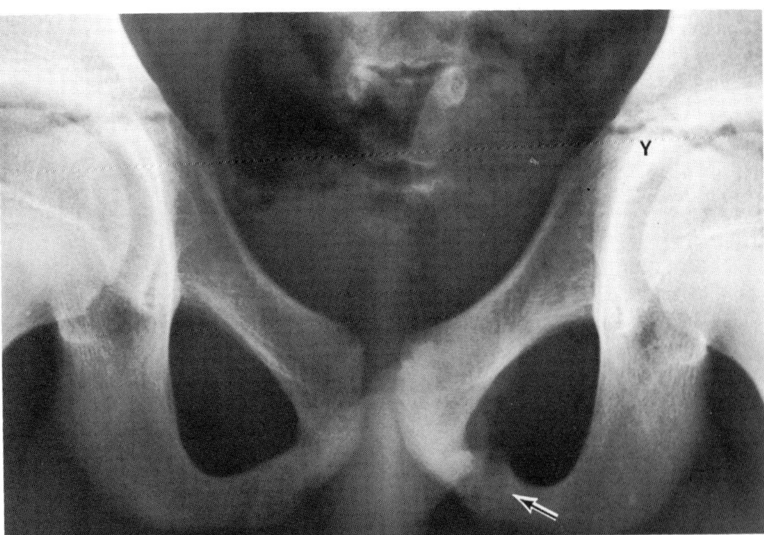

Figure 101–75. The prominent fusing pubic synchondrosis (*arrow*) and the slightly irregular lucency of the Y cartilage (Y) are normal appearances in this adolescent. (Courtesy of B. J. Manaster, M.D., Ph.D.)

by the sartorius and the anterior-inferior iliac spine by the rectus femoris in kicking type activities. The ischial tuberosity apophysis may be avulsed by the hamstrings during gymnastics. These injuries can lead to exuberant callus formation that can be painful and, with the appropriate history, should not be mistaken for a tumor (Fig. 101–76). The callus may impinge on nerves and require excision, however. Stress fractures of the pelvis are uncommon in children. Acetabular fractures in children are rare but may damage the triradiate Y cartilage and cause growth arrest with consequent acetabular dysplasia.

Adults

Because it is a bony ring, the pelvis usually is injured in two places. Lateral compression may produce pubic ramus fracture, sacral compression fracture, iliac wing fracture (Fig. 101–77) or an ''open book'' injury where the sacroiliac joint is widened and the ilium rotated to a more ''open'' position. Anteroposterior compression tends to produce widening of the symphysis pubis and/or sacroiliac joint; if severe, the sacroiliac, sacrotuberous and sacrospinous ligaments may be damaged with complete disruption of the symphysis. Vertical shear forces produce fracture or joint disruption

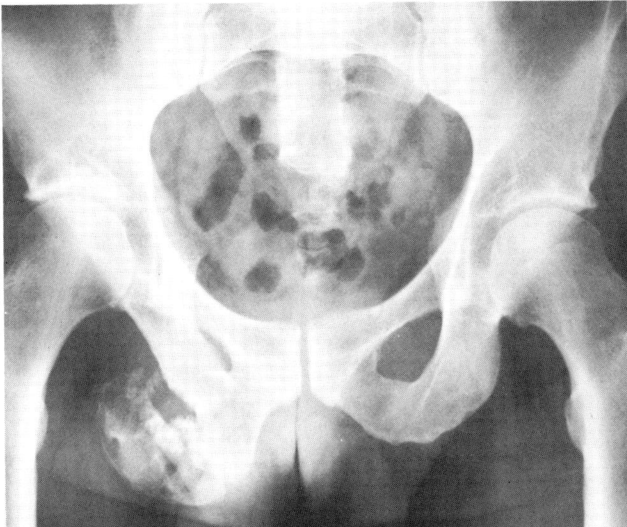

Figure 101–76. This young man had experienced a water skiing injury with forceful abduction of the right leg some years ago followed by progressive swelling and discomfort in the right buttock. The AP film clearly shows a healed avulsion of the ischial tuberosity caused by the pull of the hamstring and adductor tendons. This had compressed the sciatic nerve and was symptomatic enough to require removal of the callus.

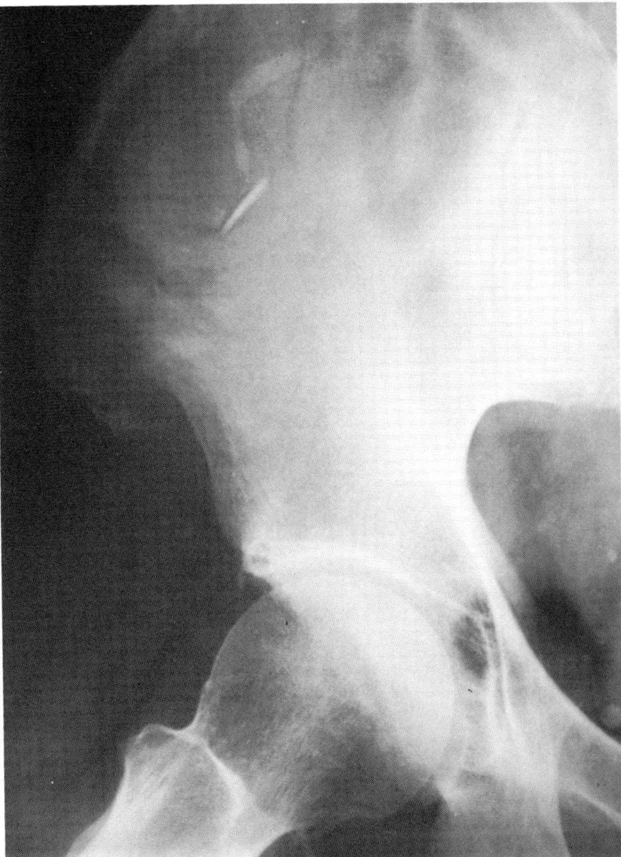

Figure 101–77. Fracture of the iliac wing was caused by a direct blow in this case. Note that part of the fracture is lucent, whereas in other places the fracture is manifested as linear densities due to overlapping bony edges.

through the anterior and posterior parts of the bony ring, usually on one side, with vertical displacement of part of the pelvis (the Malgaigne fracture, Fig. 101–78). In severe trauma there may be a combination of these fracture patterns. Although understanding the patterns of injury can aid in detecting fractures, it is more important to accurately define all the injuries that are present than to attempt to pigeonhole the injury into a rigid classification system.

Because the plane of the pelvis is not vertical, inlet/outlet views (i.e., with cranial or caudal angulation) are useful adjuncts to the straight AP film. Obliques at 45 degrees (Judet views, Fig. 101–79) and CT are also very helpful, especially where complex mechanisms leading to multiple fractures are involved. Sacral fractures can be especially difficult to diagnose. CT is very helpful for these (Fig. 101–80), and MRI can be useful, especially if nerve involvement is suspected. Fractures of the coccyx can occur secondary to a direct blow from falling upon one's posterior and are better diagnosed clinically than radiographically. The "solitary" fracture of the pubic ramus almost always has an associated posterior sacroiliac or sacral injury that may be subtle and detected only by CT. The exception to this generalization is found in the elderly or osteoporotic patient who suffers an insufficiency fracture of the pubis (see Fig. 101–4).

Double breaks in the bony ring are unstable, may require fixation, and often have associated soft-tissue injuries. The "straddle" fracture where the pubic rami are broken bilaterally is notoriously associated with urethral injuries in young people. In the elderly, however, it may result from a low-energy injury secondary to a straddling fall such as on the edge of the bathtub.

Acetabular fractures in adults may be associated with a more generalized injury to the pelvis or may be isolated, secondary to impaction of the femur into the acetabulum or femoral head dislocation (Fig. 101–81*A*). When part of a general pelvic injury, the fracture is usually severe and often requires fixation or joint replacement. Isolated acetabular fractures may involve the anterior column (i.e., the anterior acetabulum formed by the ilium and pubic ramus), the posterior column (i.e., the posterior acetabulum formed by the ilium and the ischium, Fig. 101–81*B*), the dome of the acetabulum, or the medial wall. Many classifications exist and again it is more important to describe accurately the fracture than to assign a classification. Fragments may enter the hip joint, preventing reduction of

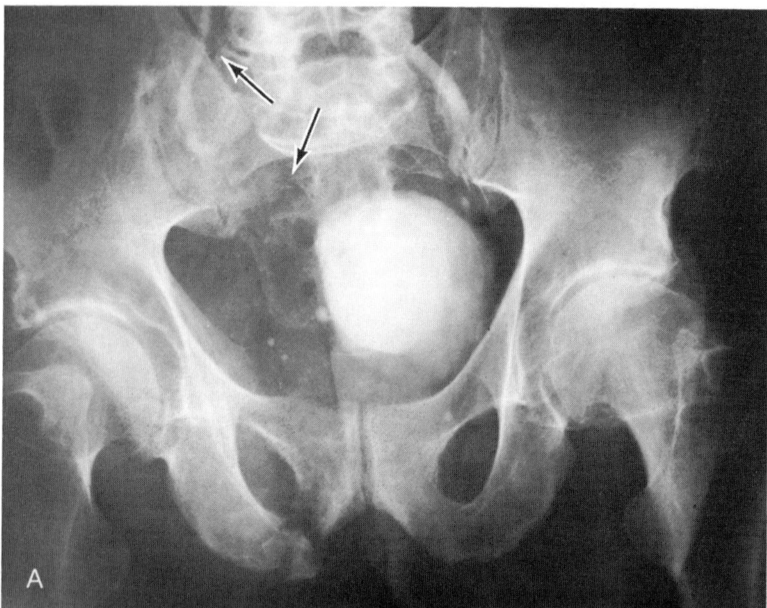

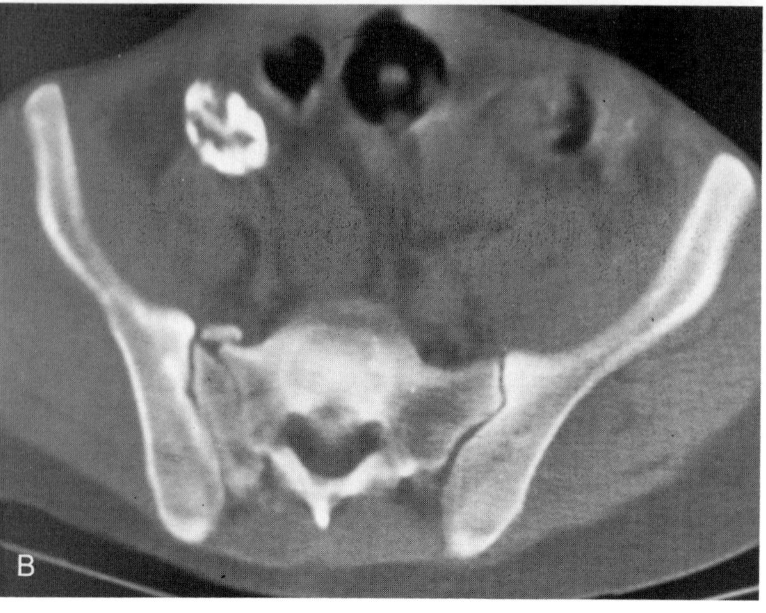

Figure 101–78. *A*, **Malgaigne fracture** showing several interesting findings. First, note the displacement of the contrast-filled bladder to the left by a large hematoma occupying the right hemipelvis. Second, note the right superior and inferior pubic ramus fractures, which are fairly obvious. Much less obvious is the **right sacral fracture**, best appreciated by noting the asymmetry of the right second sacral arch compared with the left and the discontinuity of the superior margin of the right sacral ala (*arrows*). *B*, The sacral fracture is easier to see by CT. The degree of displacement and the small anterior fragment are very difficult to appreciate on the plain film.

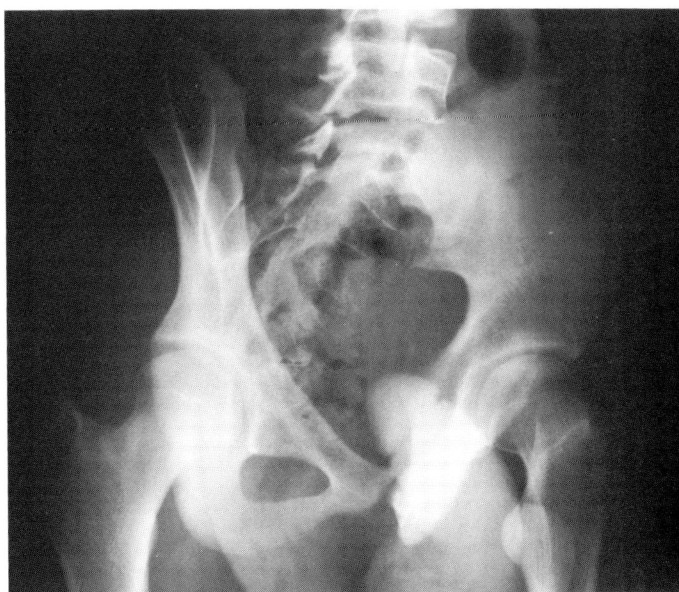

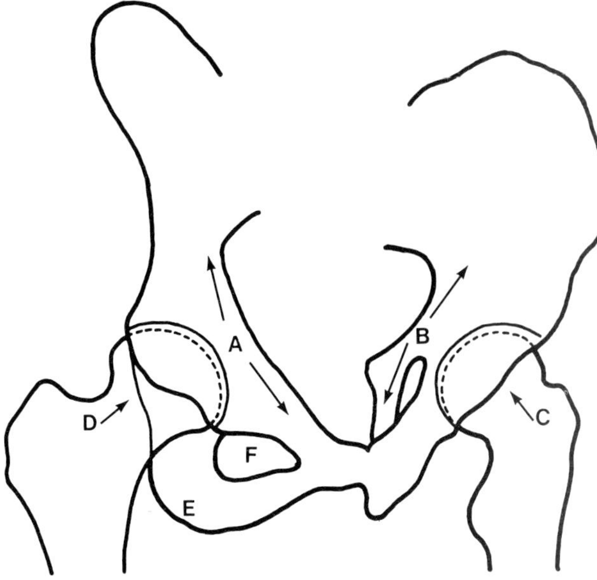

Figure 101–79. Judet (45-degree olique) view of the pelvis. Note that the anterior column (A) and posterior column (B) are seen much more completely than on the AP view. The anterior (C) and posterior (D) rims of the acetabula are also seen to much better advantage. (E = ischial tuberosity; F = obturator foramen.) (Courtesy of B. J. Manaster, M.D., Ph.D.)

Figure 101–80. A subtle right sacral fracture *(arrow)* demonstrated on CT was invisible on plain film. Note also very slight left sacroiliac joint distraction. Note the improved image quality compared with that of Figure 101–78*B* with the use of 5-mm sections and bone algorithm reconstruction.

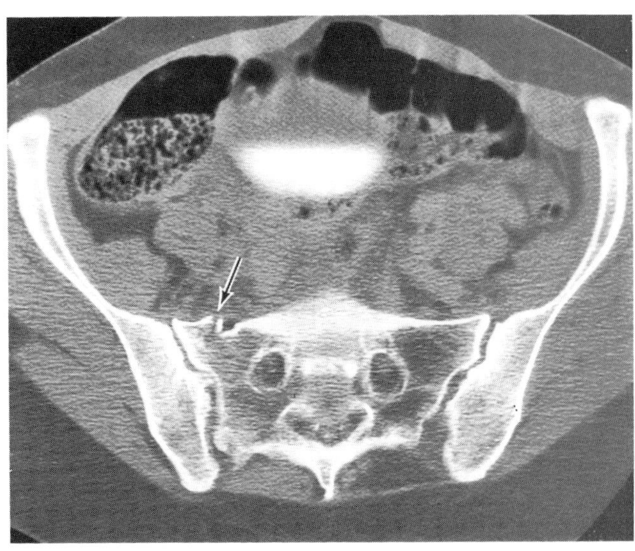

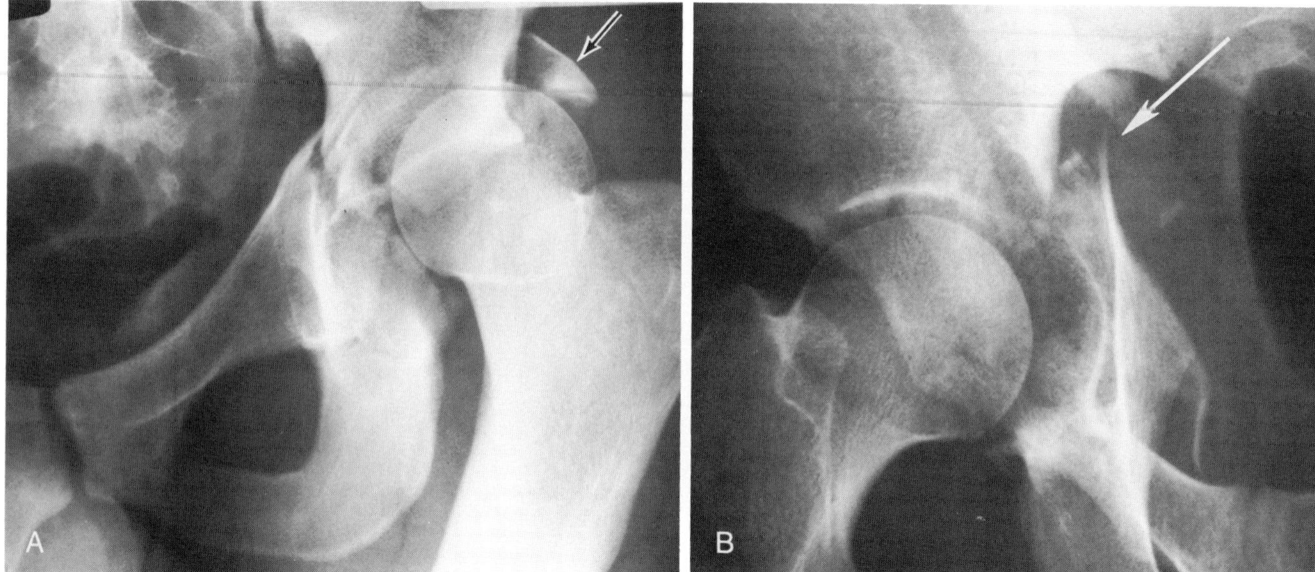

Figure 101–81. *A,* This **acetabular fracture** extends through the anterior column (well seen on this oblique view), the medial wall of the acetabulum, and into the posterior column. There is associated posterior dislocation of the femoral head that has caused a fracture of the posterior acetabular rim (*arrow*). *B,* **Fracture through the posterior column** in a different patient (*arrow*) is well shown on a right oblique Judet view. Note also the vertical component of the fracture extending into the ilium.

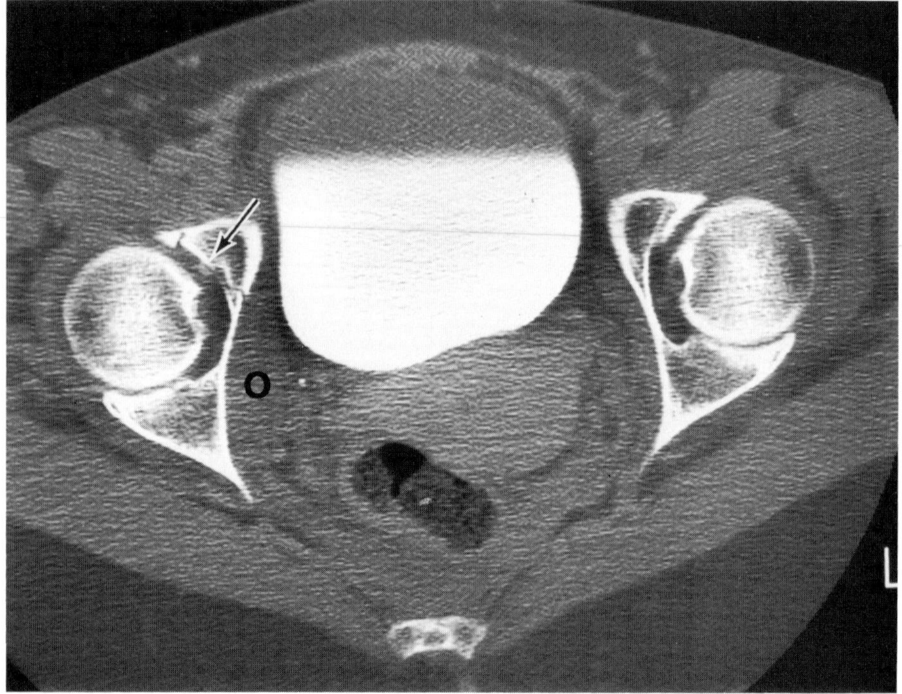

Figure 101–82. Anterior column fracture on the right is nicely shown on CT. Note the subtle widening of the right anterior joint space with a tiny fragment trapped within the joint (*arrow*). Slight thickening of the obturator internus muscle (O) on the right secondary to hematoma is present.

the hip, and are well detected by CT (Fig. 101–82) or seen as widening of the teardrop distance and/or lack of concentricity of the femoral head with the acetabulum on plain film. Hip dislocation is seven times more common in the posterior than anterior direction and may lead to fracture of the lip of the acetabulum and/or impaction fracture of the femoral head. AP and lateral or slightly oblique lateral views usually show the dislocation and fragments well. Hip dislocation is an orthopedic emergency because it compromises the blood supply to the femoral head. Post-reduction films should show concentric reduction of the head.

HIP AND FEMUR

Anthony J. Doyle

Fracture patterns in the hip vary markedly with age.

Normal Variants

In the elderly, a rim of osteophytes around the femoral head may overlap the neck and give a spurious appearance of impacted femoral neck fracture (Fig. 101–83). Occasionally in the same age group, prominent soft-tissue shadows may produce lucencies overlying the proximal femur, mimicking fracture.

Pediatrics

Hip fractures are rare in children. Dislocation is more common, especially in the 12- to 15-year age group. Fractures of the femoral neck in childhood are usually Salter type II, with Salter type I less common. Complications are common with avascular necrosis (Fig. 101–84) developing in up to 40 per cent. Coxa vara, non-union, and premature epiphyseal closure may also occur. Most are secondary to severe trauma, either from a direct vehicle impact or from non-accidental injury.

Femoral shaft fractures in children are often nondisplaced owing to the thick periosteum holding the fragments in place. Open fractures are rare. Birth trauma may uncommonly cause femoral shaft fracture especially in breech delivery; other abnormalities such as osteogenesis imperfecta (see Fig. 101–18) should be looked for. In infancy, nonaccidental injury is the most common cause of femoral fracture (see Fig. 101–15). Radiographs should include the hip and knee, and shielding should be supplied for the gonads.

SLIPPING OF THE CAPITAL FEMORAL EPIPHYSIS

Slipping of the capital femoral epiphysis is usually not related to one specific episode of trauma. It most commonly occurs in obese adolescents between the ages of 10 and 16 and more frequently in males. There is a slightly higher incidence in African-Americans than in other racial groups. The process may be bilateral in 20 per cent.

During the adolescent "growth spurt," the cartilage of the growth plate is relatively weak. The femoral neck changes configuration from valgus to varus at this time, introducing a shear force that predisposes to slipping of the capital epiphysis. The radiographic appearance may be quite subtle but is characteristic (Fig. 101–85). Movement of the epiphysis posteromedially leads to foreshortening of the epiphysis on the AP view and "widening" of the growth plate. A line drawn along the lateral femoral neck fails to intersect the epiphysis. The frog-leg lateral shows the displacement more strikingly, an appearance likened to a melting ice-cream cone. Treatment consists of pinning and leads to a short broad femoral

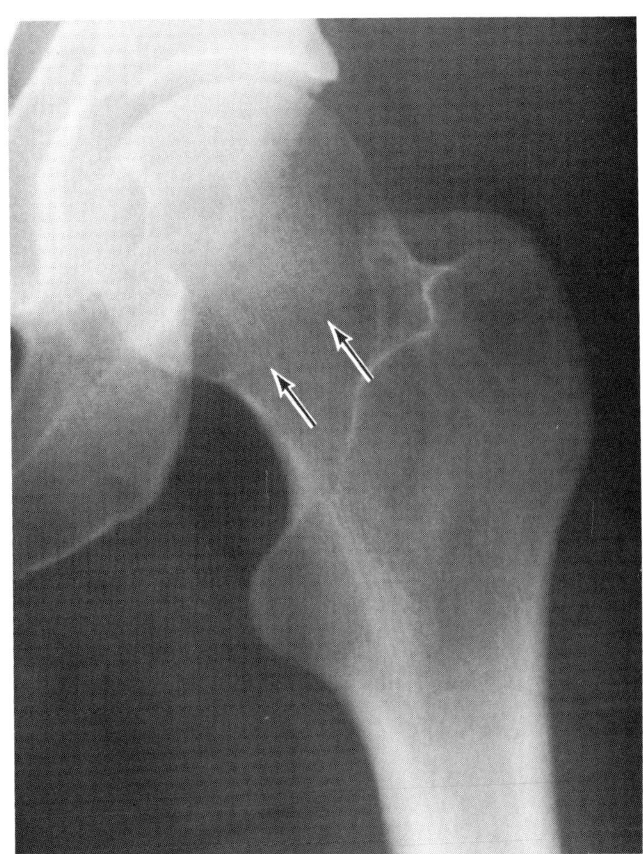

Figure 101–83. Simulated fracture of the femoral neck is seen in the form of a fine white line overlying the neck (*arrows*). This is due to the margin of the femoral head accentuated by small osteophytes and most obvious in external rotation, as in this case. (Courtesy of B. J. Manaster, M.D., Ph.D.)

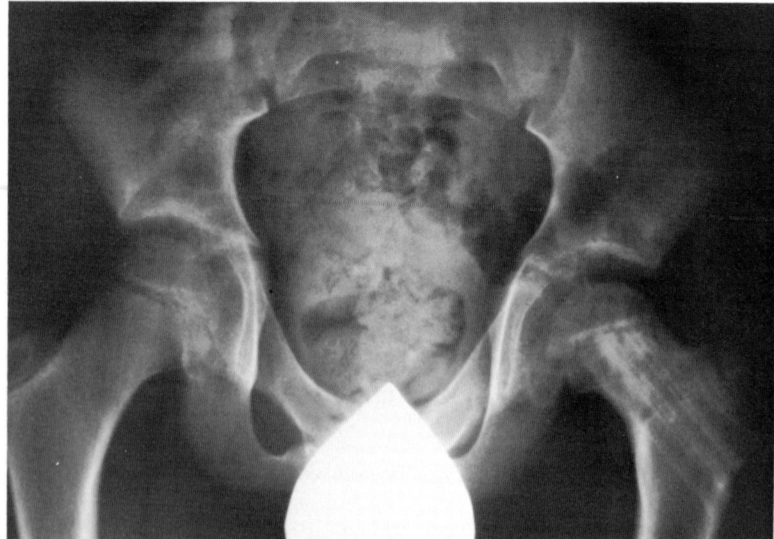

Figure 101–84. Post-traumatic avascular necrosis has developed in the left femoral capital epiphysis. The epiphysis is flattened and irregular. The pintracks and residual deformity of the femoral neck from the previously treated femoral neck fracture are still visible.

neck. Degenerative changes are a late complication occurring up to 30 years or so later. Avascular necrosis may occur in around 10 per cent and is related to the severity of the slip and difficulty in repositioning. Chondrolysis (spontaneous resorption of articular cartilage) may occur as a complication but is fairly uncommon and infection must be considered in the differential diagnosis of cartilage loss seen radiographically.

Adult

Proximal femoral fractures are very common in the elderly on the basis of osteoporosis, but occur infrequently in groups where osteoporosis is uncommon. In the osteoporotic patient the fracture often occurs with trivial trauma. AP and groin lateral films usually show the fracture, but it can be subtle on a background of osteoporosis. Limited coronal T_1-weighted MRI is a very effective way of diagnosing these occult fractures (Fig. 101–86). Delayed films, tomograms (Fig. 101–87) or radioisotope bone scans may also be helpful. Many orthopedists use the Garden classification for subcapital fractures, in which I is incomplete/impacted, II is complete nondisplaced, III is slightly displaced, and IV is separated. Grade III and IV fractures (Fig. 101–88) often require arthroplasty. In younger adults, stress fractures from unusual or repetitive activity may occur in the femoral neck. Other femoral neck fractures in the young adult require significant force; the subcapital fracture is, as in any patient, at risk for developing avascular necrosis.

Intertrochanteric fractures are also common in the elderly. They occur about a decade later in life than femoral neck fractures and are associated with falls. An AP and groin lateral are essential to show the degree of comminution and position of the fragments. The fracture usually runs obliquely distally and medially. Fractures with reverse obliquity, badly comminuted fractures with a loss of contact between the proximal and distal fragments, and fractures in which

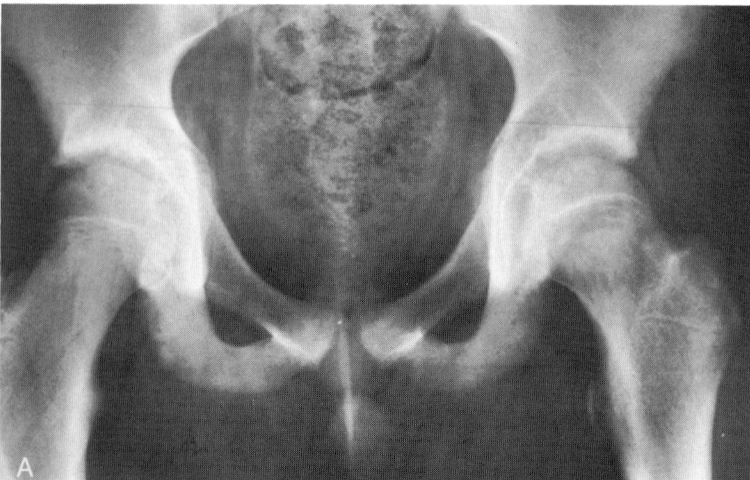

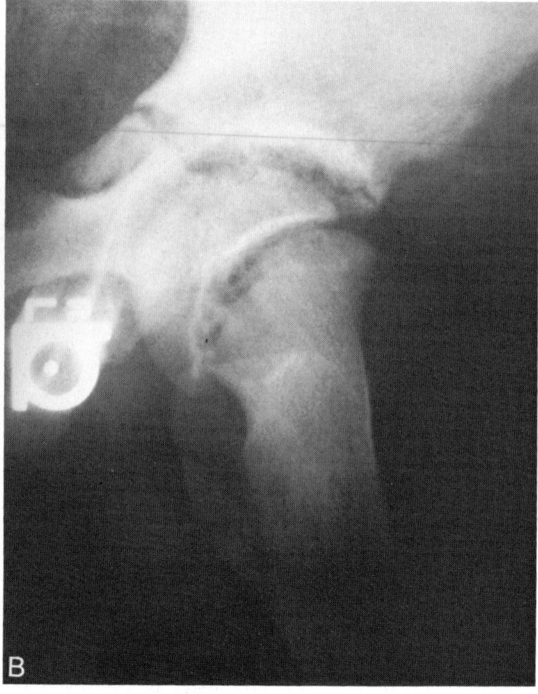

Figure 101–85. *A*, **Slipping of the left femoral capital epiphysis** in this obese 14-year-old boy is manifested on the AP view by asymmetrical placement of the left epiphysis with respect to the right. A line drawn along the lateral femoral neck and metaphysis does not intersect the epiphysis. Compare with the normal right side the slight widening of the left growth plate. *B*, The frog-leg lateral clearly shows the posterior displacement of the epiphysis, which should sit perfectly on the end of the femoral neck.

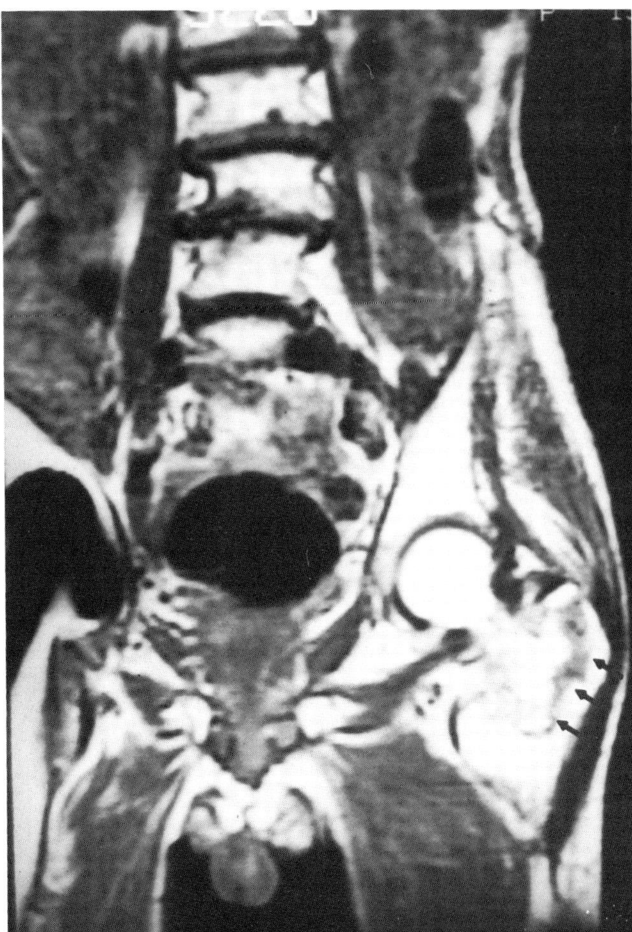

Figure 101–86. Coronal T_1-weighted MRI shows an **intertrochanteric fracture** in an elderly man who had hip pain. The plain radiographs were negative even in retrospect. The small black arrows indicate the low signal intensity fracture line extending through the intertrochanteric region of the femur.

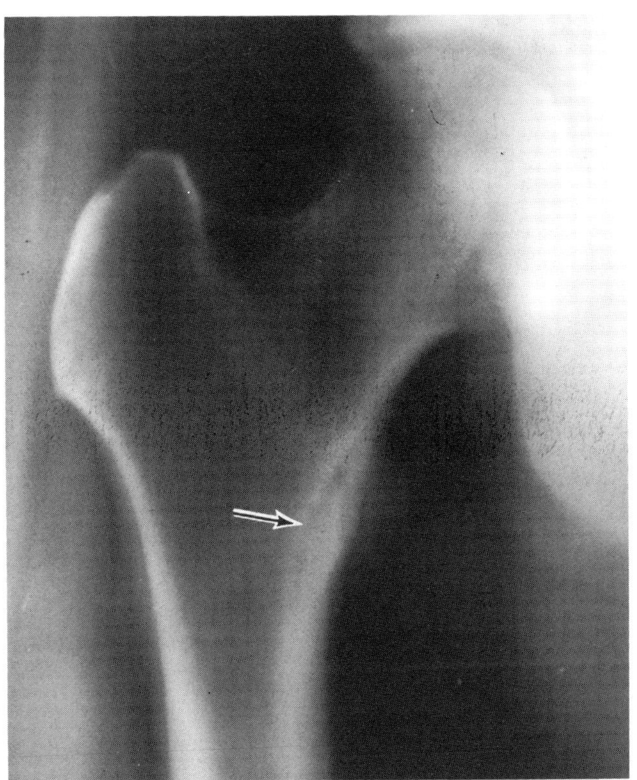

Figure 101–87. Coronal polydirectional tomography shows a **curvilinear nondisplaced fracture** (*arrow*) **through the medial femoral cortex**. This somewhat unusual fracture in a middle-aged woman was occult on the initial radiographs.

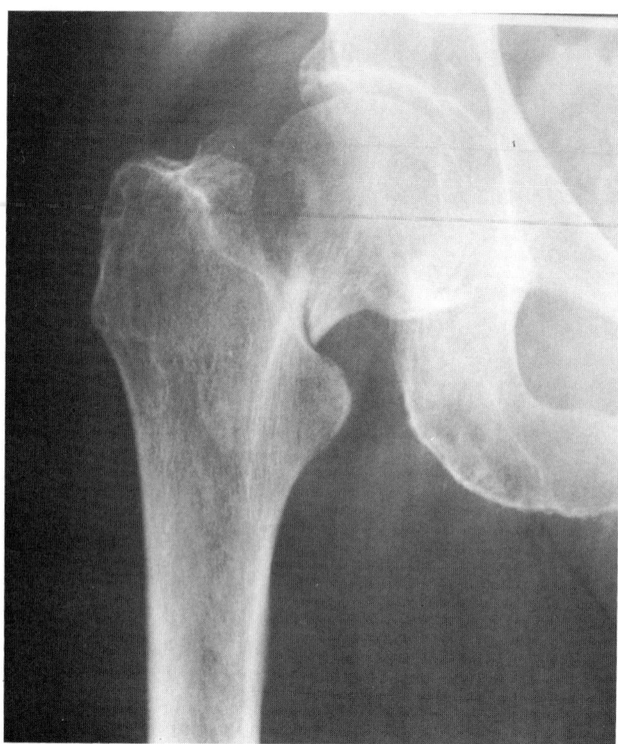

Figure 101–88. An obvious Garden grade IV femoral neck fracture is seen in this 75-year-old osteoporotic woman. Note the significant displacement. There is a high risk of avascular necrosis, so the patient was treated with a bipolar arthroplasty.

the lesser trochanter is avulsed with loss of the posterior cortex are often unstable (Fig. 101–89). Instability is present in up to 60 per cent of intertrochanteric fractures and influences the operative technique. Subtrochanteric fractures are uncommon and pathologic fracture should be strongly suspected in the absence of the history of severe trauma. Trochanter avulsions do occur in adults but are also uncommon and often pathologic.

Fractures of the femoral shaft usually require violent force. The AP films should include the hip and knee, and the lateral include the knee to look for associated fractures or dislocations and malalignment. Ipsilateral femoral neck fractures or head dislocations occur in up to 5 per cent of femoral shaft fractures. The films must be adequate to show fine linear extensions of the fracture and any signs of pathologic fracture such as endosteal scalloping or soft-

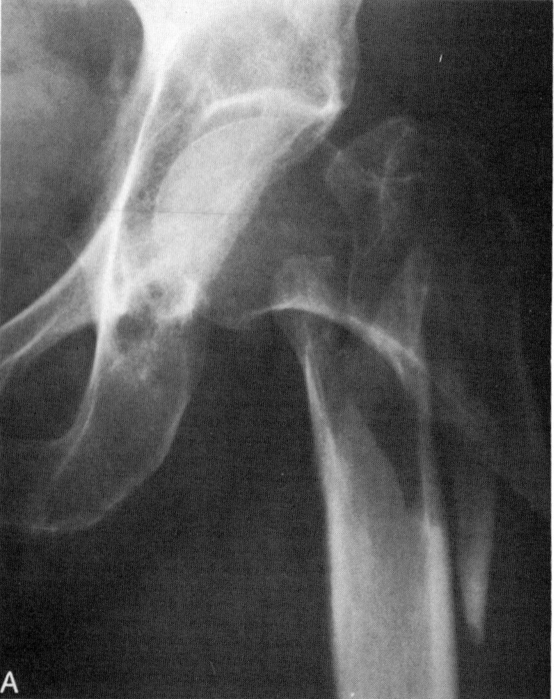

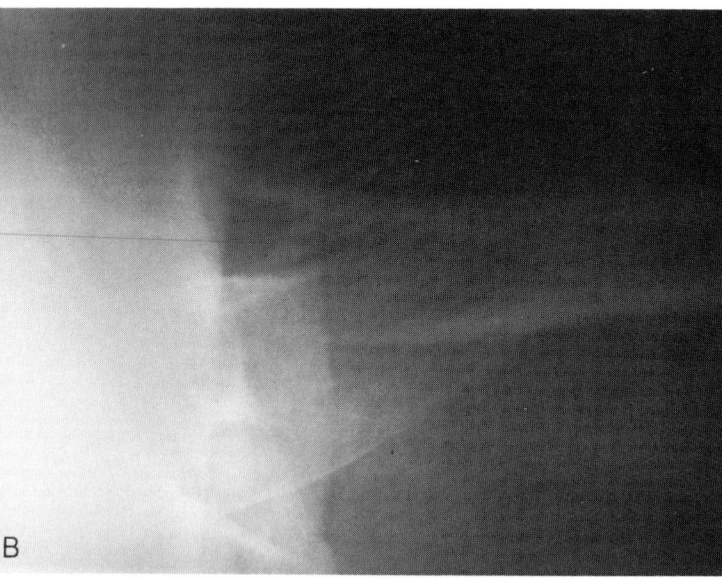

Figure 101–89. A comminuted intertrochanteric fracture is well shown on AP (*A*) and lateral (*B*) radiographs. The loss of contact of the cortical margins and difficulty of closed reduction can be appreciated from the films. Operative fixation of the medial fragment with the attached lesser trochanter was in fact necessary in this case.

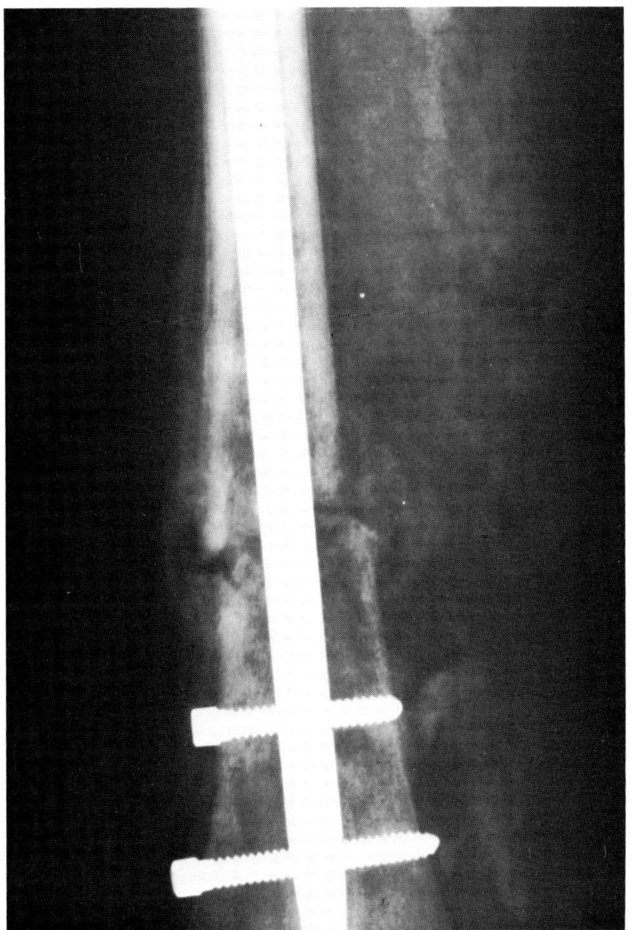

Figure 101–90. This **pathologic fracture of the femur** went unrecognized initially. The patient, a well-built 14-year-old male, had been playing basketball and fractured the femur upon turning, a totally inadequate explanation for a femoral fracture in normal bone. Six weeks after placement of the intermedullary rod seen here, a soft-tissue mass was noted and this proved to be a highly aggressive osteosarcoma. All of the soft-tissue ossification and periosteal new bone seen here are secondary to the tumor, not a manifestation of fracture healing.

tissue calcification. It is again emphasized that, in a young person, a femoral fracture should be assumed to be pathologic if there is not a history of severe trauma (Fig. 101–90). Pathologic fractures are often transverse or short oblique in nature. Femoral shaft fractures are usually fixed with an intermedullary rod; this may have interlocking nails at one or both ends, and both projections should be scrutinized on the postoperative films to ensure that the nails do in fact pass through the holes in the rod.

THE KNEE

Anthony J. Doyle

This complex joint is frequently subject to excessive twisting, hyperextension, or valgus and varus strains. Impaction forces through the tibia are a less common cause of injury, whereas direct blows usually affect only the patella and sometimes the head of the fibula. Soft-tissue injuries are frequent. Indirect signs of trauma are important, and effusion or a fat-fluid level are best seen in the suprapatellar pouch on the cross-table lateral view (Fig. 101–91)

Normal Variants

The distal femoral epiphyses are often irregular in late childhood, simulating osteochondritis dissecans (Fig. 101–92). The lateral femoral condyles in adults frequently have an indentation anteriorly that may be mistaken for an osteochondral fracture. The patella frequently ossifies in an irregular fashion and the bipartite patella is common; the secondary center is usually in the upper outer aspect of the patella (Fig. 101–93), although it can occur elsewhere. The margins are rounded and sclerotic, thus differentiating it from a fracture. Occasionally, there may be small accessory ossicles in the intercondylar notch related to the tibial spines. On the lateral film, overlap of the posterior margins of the tibial plateau may simulate a fracture; improved positioning should make this obvious. In adolescents, the growth plate for the tibial tubercle seen en face may simulate a fracture (Fig. 101–94), and the tubercle itself often has multiple ossification centers.

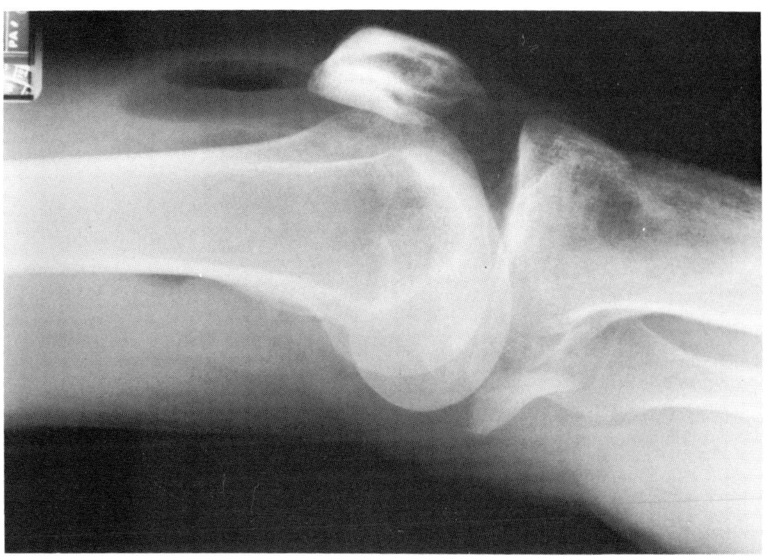

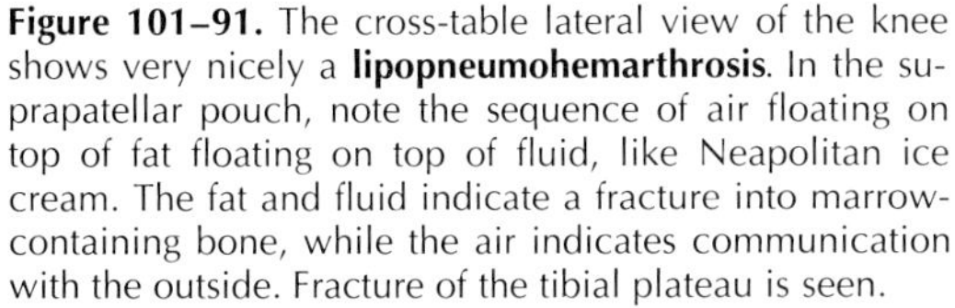

Figure 101–91. The cross-table lateral view of the knee shows very nicely a **lipopneumohemarthrosis**. In the suprapatellar pouch, note the sequence of air floating on top of fat floating on top of fluid, like Neapolitan ice cream. The fat and fluid indicate a fracture into marrow-containing bone, while the air indicates communication with the outside. Fracture of the tibial plateau is seen.

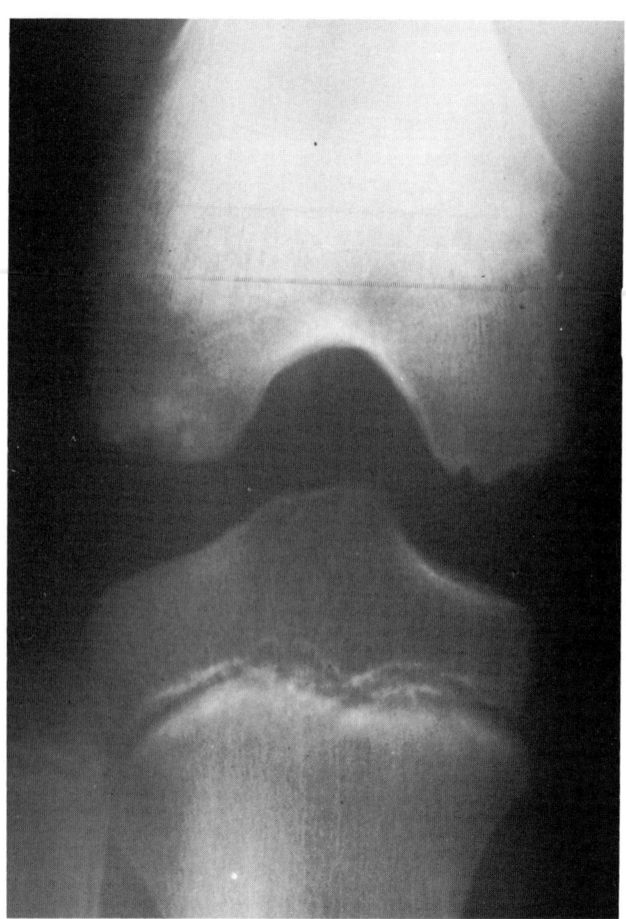

Figure 101–92. Normal irregularities in the distal femoral epiphysis are seen in this skeletally immature patient. Note that these irregularities are better seen on this notch view than on a true AP because of their relatively posterior position.

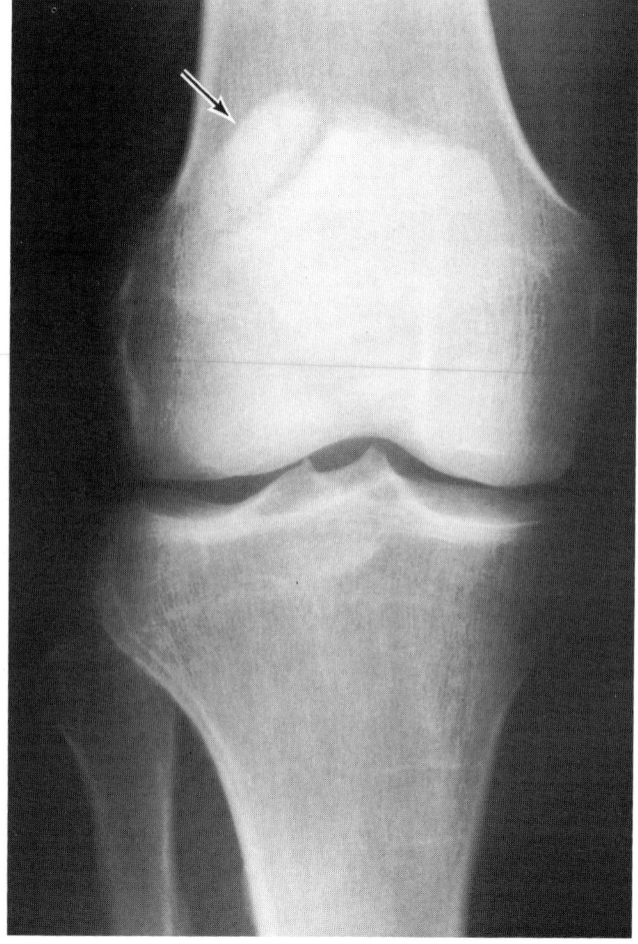

Figure 101–93. A typical bipartite patella is seen here with the secondary center in the upper outer aspect (***arrow***). Note that the margins are more rounded and sclerotic than in a fracture.

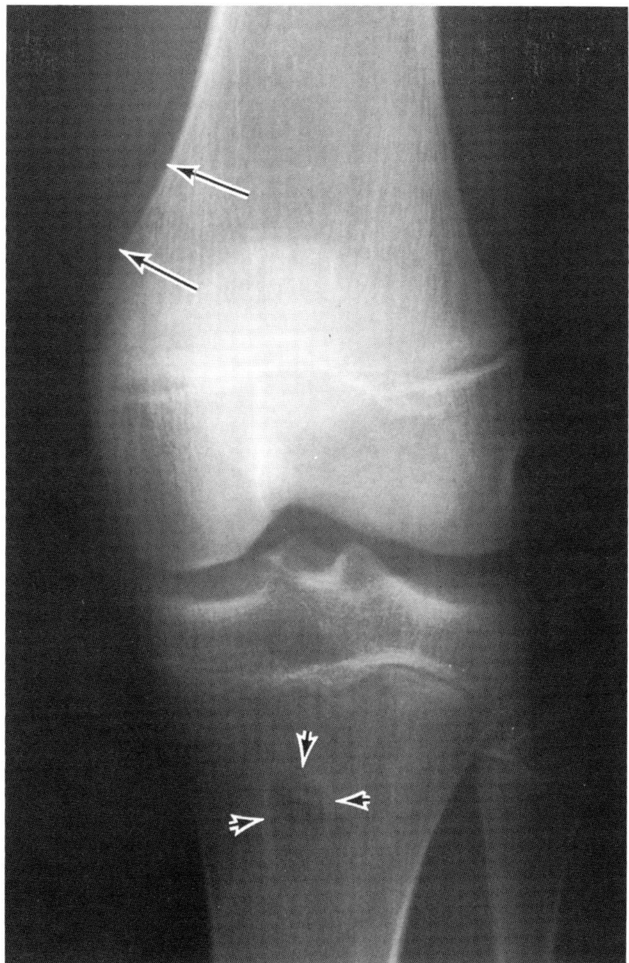

Figure 101–94. The **normal tibial tubercle** seen on the AP film creates a lucent area (*arrowheads*). A normal slight irregularity in the medial distal femur (*arrows*) is not periosteal new bone.

Pediatrics

Fractures of the distal femoral growth plate are common, although less so than those of the distal radius or tibia. Adolescents make up two thirds of the affected population, and the injury is usually due to indirect trauma. In infants, it may be secondary to birth trauma or nonaccidental injury. Salter type II fractures are the most common, with type I (see Fig. 101–13*B*) the next most common. Although in many other locations growth is not affected by such injuries, in the distal femur there is frequently either early fusion or partial bony bridging of the growth plate secondary to these fractures, causing limb length discrepancy or distal femoral deformity (see Fig. 101–13*F*). The fracture itself may be occult and be shown only by close comparison with the opposite side, stress views, or MRI. There is often associated ligamentous damage. If the epiphysis is severely displaced anteriorly, the metaphysis may impinge on vascular structures.

Fracture and displacement of the proximal tibial growth plate is rare and often subtle but if severe can also cause vascular injury (Fig. 101–95). Acute fracture of the tibial tubercle is often related to sports involving jumping and should be distinguished from the more chronic apophysitis seen in Osgood-Schlatter disease. It may present as a small avulsion fracture or as a larger injury involving a Salter type III fracture of the tibial epiphysis (Fig. 101–95). The patella may be elevated compared with the opposite side. Fracture of the tibial spine is occasionally seen; because the anterior cruciate ligament is stronger than the adjacent bone in children, avulsion fracture rather than ligament tear tends to occur.

Fracture of the patella is uncommon in childhood. It is often, however, hypoplastic, bipartite (Fig. 101–93), or even absent. One of the poles may be avulsed, especially the lower pole. In the "sleeve" fracture there is a very small bone fragment but quite a large cartilage fragment (best seen by MRI) avulsed from the lower pole that if undetected may lead to lengthening of the patella and disordered mechanics. Occasionally, the patella may fracture but the posterior cartilage remain intact so that the patella "books" open anteriorly. Patellar dislocation laterally is not uncommon. There may be small osteochondral fractures from the medial patellar facet or lateral femoral condyle; these are best detected on axial views of the patella, arthrography, or MRI, which may also show acute changes in the medial patellar retinaculum. Fifteen per cent of those with acute dislocation go on to develop recurrent dislocation. In many of these patients the quadriceps tendon makes an angle with the patellar tendon (the Q angle) that predisposes to lateral displacement. Defining which patients are at risk for patellar dislocation is controversial, but lateral patellar tilt or displacement as seen on the sunrise view are associated with lateral dislocation.

Although ligamentous injuries are uncommon in children, they do occur. The medial collateral and the cruciate ligaments are the most commonly affected, with the lateral collateral ligaments seldom affected. Stress views or MRI can detect these. The menisci can be damaged also, especially in adolescents. A discoid meniscus (Fig. 101–96) is one in which the meniscus substance is discoid rather than semicircular in shape and continuous across the entire compartment of the knee. It is more common laterally and frequently gives rise to symptoms because it is prone to injury. It is easily detected on MRI.

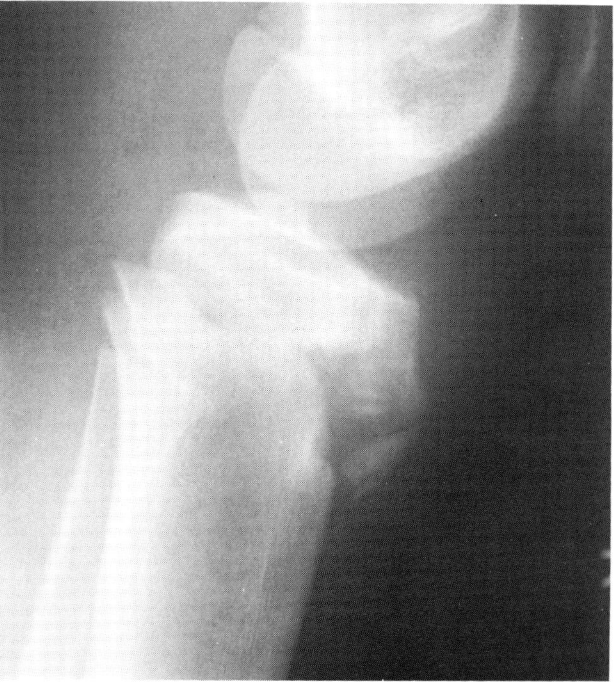

Figure 101–95. A complex fracture of the proximal tibial growth plate is present in this 16-year-old who was in a motor vehicle accident. Note that the proximal tibial epiphysis is displaced anteriorly with a fracture extending vertically through its anterior portion. The tibial tubercle is also separated from the tibial metaphysis. This is effectively a Salter type III injury. At this point, the fracture has been partly reduced. Posterior displacement of the sharp margin of the tibial metaphysis had already caused a laceration of the popliteal artery.

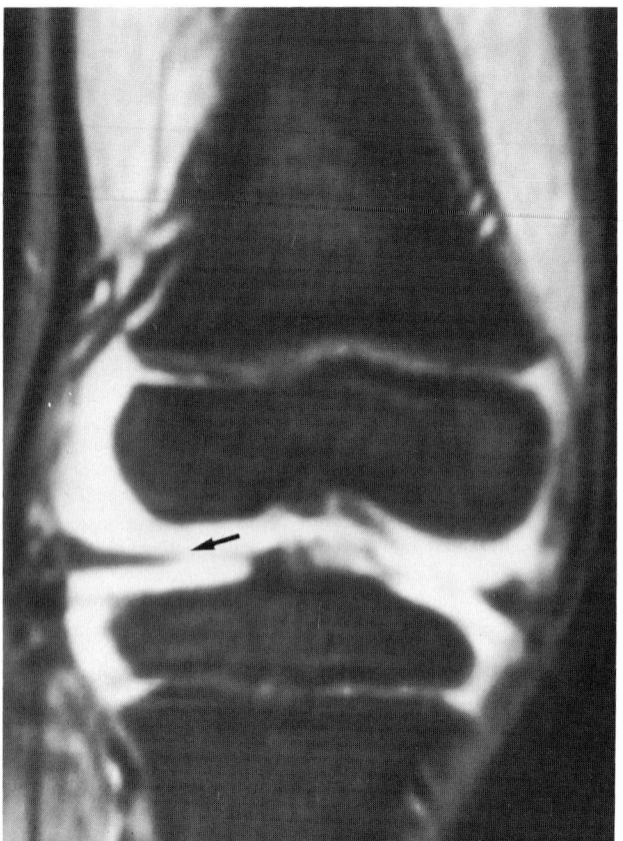

Figure 101–96. A discoid lateral meniscus (*arrow*) is readily seen on this coronal T_2-weighted MRI. Compare the plate-like shape of the lateral meniscus with the triangular medial meniscus. The open growth plates are visible. (From Manaster BJ: MRI of the knee. Semin US CT MRI 11(4):307–326, 1990.)

Adult

Supracondylar fractures of the distal femur in young adults require high-energy trauma (Fig. 101–97), usually involving axial loading, varus or valgus force, and rotation, whereas in the elderly they may be secondary to minor trauma. There are many classification systems in use. They are usually treated operatively with blade or buttress plating or similar hardware. Osteochondral fractures of the femoral condyles are not uncommon. Osteochondritis dissecans, affecting the lateral aspect of the medial femoral condyle, is probably such a lesion and is found mostly in young males.

The tibial plateau is a common site of fracture, especially in the elderly. The lateral plateau is more commonly fractured than the medial or both combined. Classically, plateau fractures are secondary to motor vehicle vs pedestrian accidents causing a valgus or varus force (the so-called fender fracture). The opposite collateral ligament acts as a hinge and is usually intact but may be disrupted in up to 20 per cent. Most plateau fractures involve simple depression of the surface or an oblique split through the proximal tibia. There may be a combination of both of these findings and a variable degree of comminution and displacement. These fractures are regarded as minimally displaced if there is less than 4 mm depression or displacement. The degree and direction of displacement are important for operative planning and may be best shown by tomography, CT, or MRI. The fracture itself may be difficult to detect and seen best with oblique or tangential views (Fig. 101–98), or MRI (see Fig. 101–6).

Fractures of the tibial spines and intercondylar eminence are often isolated, but this area is also involved in about 15 per cent of tibial plateau fractures. If the origins of the cruciate ligaments are involved (Fig. 101–99), the knee may be unstable or may heal with reduced motion. Hyperextension, flexion, varus/valgus and twisting forces may cause these injuries. Often the tunnel view (between the femoral condyles in flexion) shows these avulsions best. They are often graded according to degree of separation of the fragment. Fracture of the tibial tubercle is uncommon except in association with proximal tibial fracture, which is also uncommon. The same applies to fracture of the proximal fibula. Either may have associated neurovascular injury.

Patellar fractures are mostly secondary to a direct blow. Males in the 20- to 50-year age group are most commonly affected. The fracture is transverse in 50 per cent, involving the central to lower patella. These fractures are usually fixed operatively, frequently with a tension band wire. Stellate (Fig. 101–100), longitudinal (marginal), and osteochondral fractures are less common. AP and lateral films and the "sunrise" view in which the x-ray beam is directed along the patellofemoral joint are useful. Arthrography or MRI may be useful for identifying small osteochondral fragments. Patellar dislocation is discussed above.

Ligament and tendon injuries are common around the knee. The quadriceps may rupture, usually involving the muscle, and may manifest as a low-riding patella. The patellar tendon itself may rupture and can lead to a high-riding patella. Both these injuries are

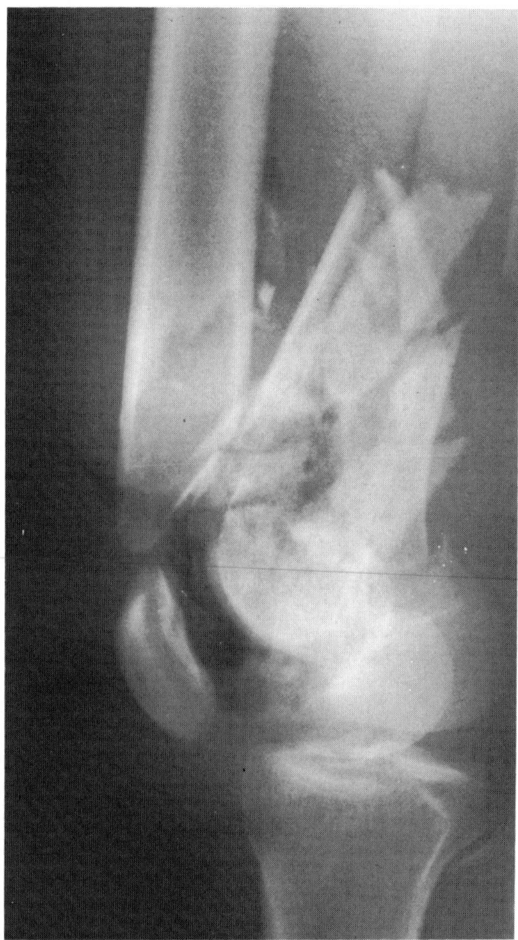

Figure 101–97. A highly comminuted supracondylar fracture of the femur is seen in this young adult involved in a motor vehicle accident. The posterior displacement and bayonet apposition of the highly fragmented distal femur and condyles are seen with the patella displaced almost behind the proximal shaft fragment. Gas within the joint indicates an open fracture. A similarly highly comminuted appearance may be seen in the pilon fracture of the distal tibia.

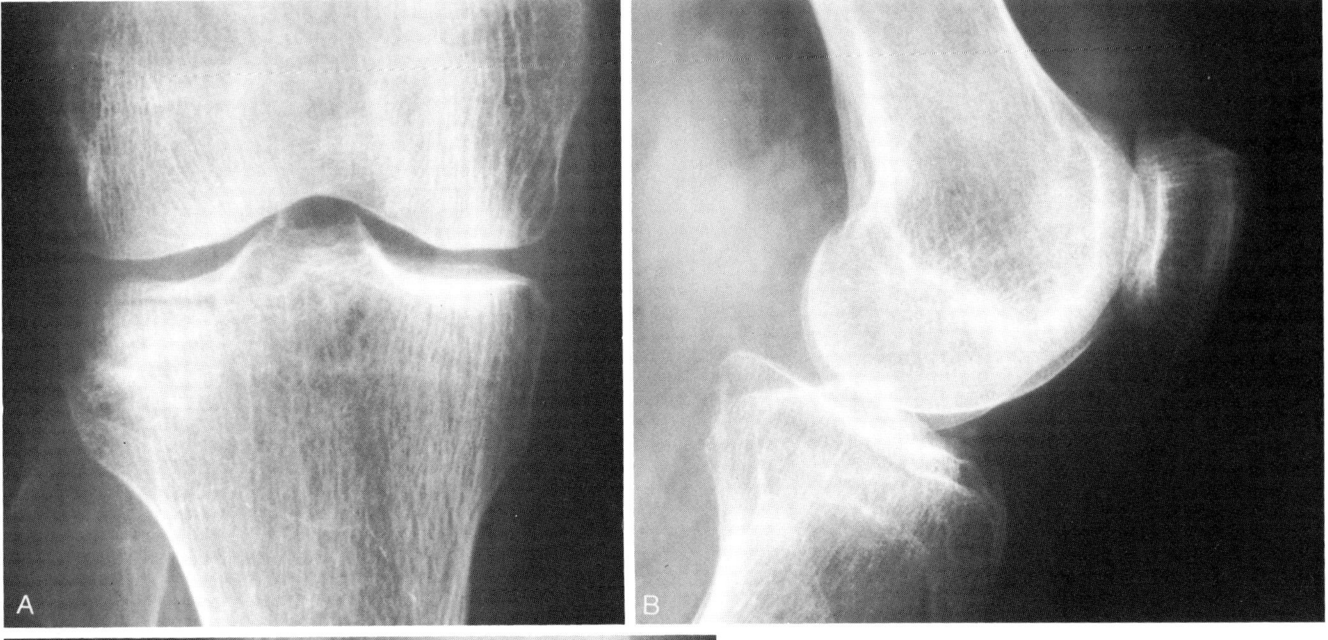

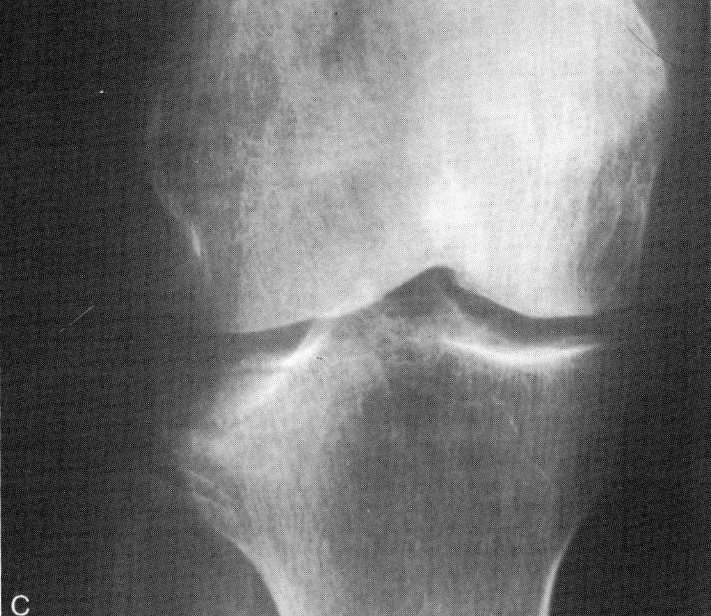

Figure 101–98. AP (*A*) and lateral (*B*) radiographs show a joint effusion and slight increased density in the lateral tibial plateau. More subtle is the loss of the smooth white line of subchondral bone in the lateral plateau on both AP and lateral films. An oblique film (*C*) very clearly shows the **depressed lateral tibial plateau fracture** in this osteoporotic elderly woman.

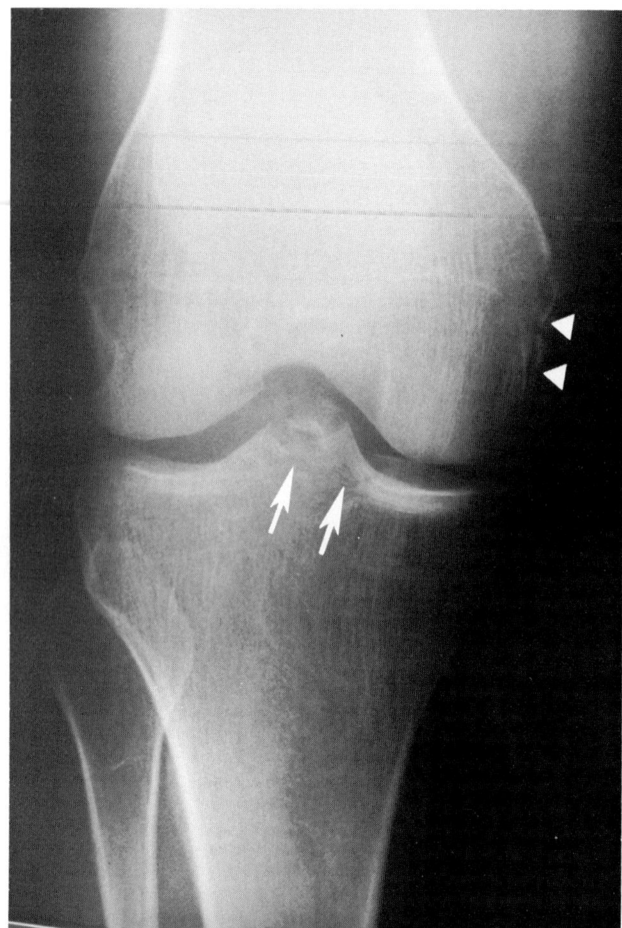

Figure 101–99. Fracture of the medial tibial spine is demonstrated (***arrows***) with a fragment at the origin of the anterior cruciate ligament between the spines situated slightly more superiorly. Also note the linear ossific density adjacent to the medial condyle (*arrowheads*) consistent with prior trauma to the origin of the medial collateral ligament.

secondary to quadriceps contraction during applied stretching and are both well visualized by MRI (Fig. 101–101).

Injury to the collateral ligaments due to varus/valgus and rotation forces is also well seen on MRI as loss of continuity of the normal low-signal ligament (Fig. 101–102) and increased signal in the ligament on T_2-weighted MRI. Occasionally, avulsion from the lateral tibial plateau by the lateral capsular ligament may be seen (the Segond fracture, Fig. 101–103); this has an association with anterior cruciate ligament injury. The anterior cruciate ligament itself is commonly disrupted by a combination of twisting and deceleration forces, often with external rotation. It is well seen on MRI, especially on thin-section sagittal images (Fig. 101–104). With good technique, one can attain greater than 90 per cent accuracy. The posterior cruciate is much less commonly injured, usually by a posteriorly directed force applied to the tibia. It is also well seen on MRI (Fig. 101–105). Because the posterior cruciate is much stronger than the anterior, small bony avulsions are more frequently seen with posterior cruciate injuries, located at the posterior margin of the tibial plateau (Fig. 101–106).

The menisci may be torn by a twisting injury, which may also affect the collateral and cruciate ligaments. The "terrible triad" recognized by O'Donoghue is one such association involving the anterior cruciate and medial collateral ligaments and medial meniscus. The pattern of meniscal tear may be "bucket handle" with a fragment displaced into the middle of the joint, horizontal cleavage tear, a radial tear, or a more complex degenerative tear. These are well seen on MRI, as are associated bone lesions that may be radiographically occult (Fig. 101–107).

Dislocation of the knee is uncommon. The tibia most often dislocates anteriorly and the popliteal artery is at risk. Arteriography may be required if this cannot be assessed clinically. Dislocation of the proximal tibio-fibular joint is rare and may be subtle (Fig. 101–108), requiring close comparison with the opposite side.

THE LEG AND ANKLE

Anthony J. Doyle

Fractures of the tibia are almost ten times as common as fractures of the femur. Fibular fractures are almost always associated with tibial fractures but may be secondary to disruption of the ankle, and plastic bowing of the fibula may occur with a tibial fracture (Fig. 101–109). Ligamentous injuries, fractures, and dislocations of the ankle are quite common, with the type of injury being related to the age of the patient, the bone quality, and the direction, magnitude, and rate of application of the loading force.

Text continued on page 1629

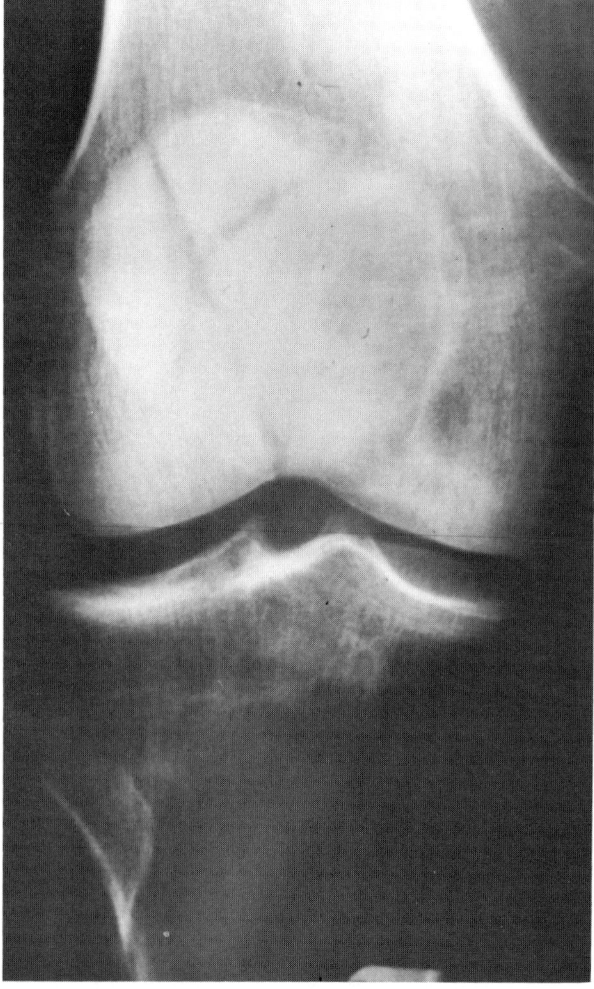

Figure 101–100. A stellate fracture of the patella is seen in this young male. Compare the sharply defined fracture lines with the rounded sclerotic borders seen in the bipartite patella in Figure 101–93.

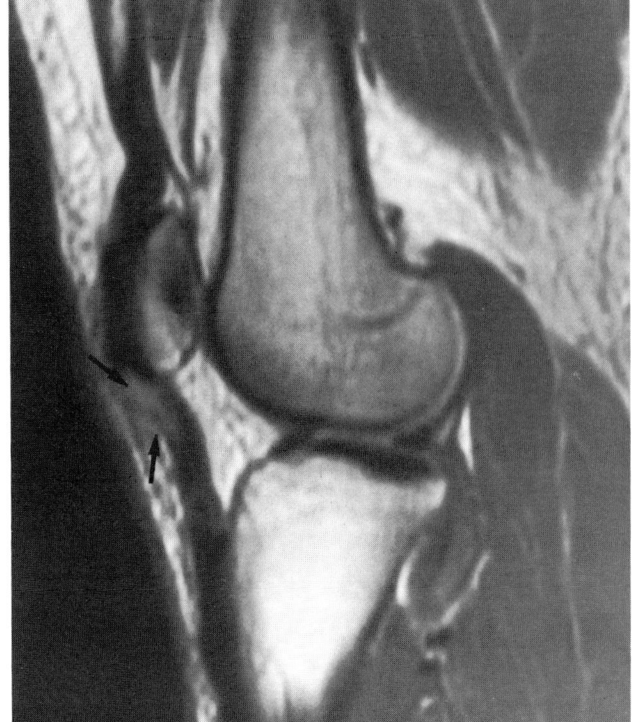

Figure 101–101. Partial tear of the patellar tendon near its origin on the patella is easily seen on this sagittal T_1-weighted MRI. Increased signal in the anterior tendon (*arrows*) is present, but there are some intact low-signal fibers posteriorly. (From Manaster BJ: MRI of the knee. Semin US CT MRI 11(4):307–326, 1990.)

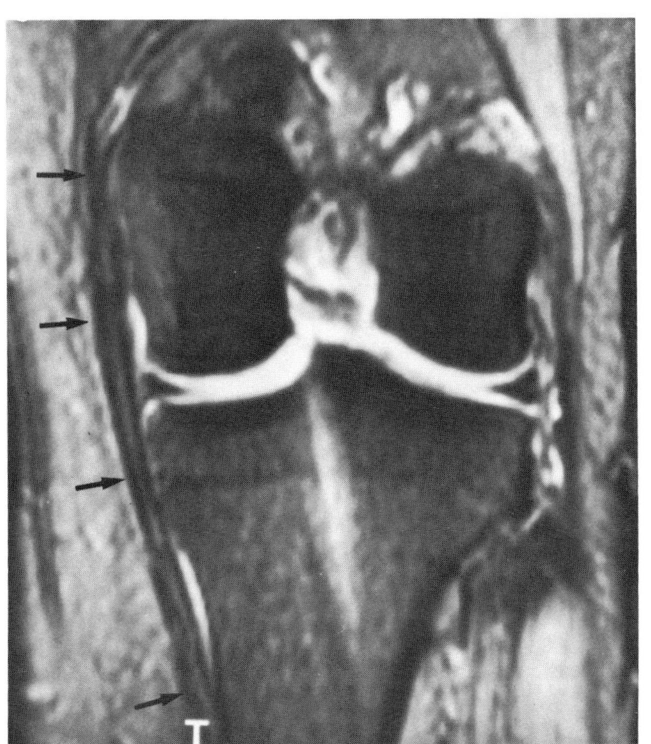

Figure 101–102. The normal medial collateral ligament (*arrows*) is beautifully seen on this coronal T_2-weighted MRI. Note that it is in two parts, with the deep portion separated from the superficial by a slightly higher signal line of fat. Increased signal in or around the ligament and/or discontinuity of the low-intensity ligament itself indicates trauma. (From Manaster BJ: MRI of the knee. Semin US CT MRI 11(4):307–326, 1990.)

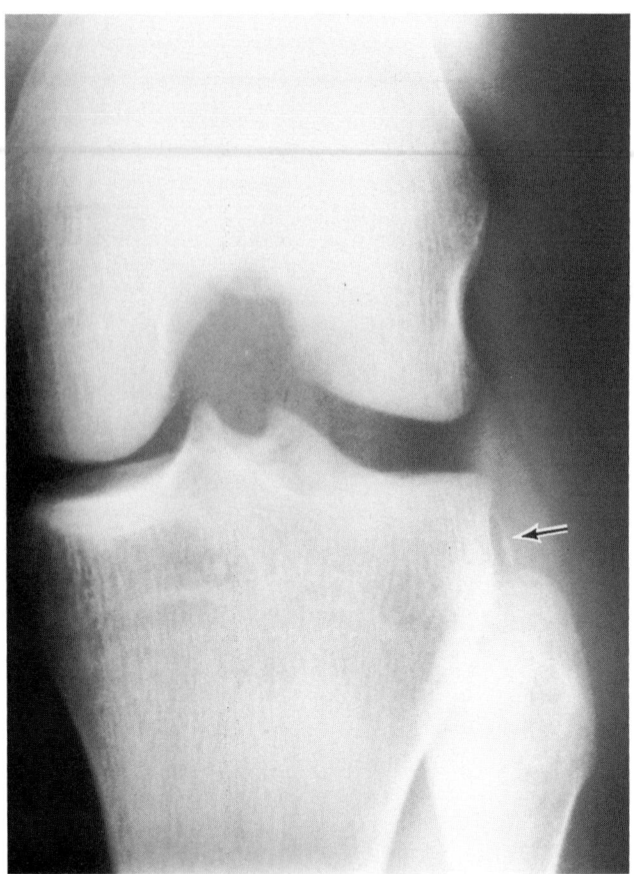

Figure 101–103. The lateral capsular insertion (Segond) fracture seen on this notch view is a small avulsion fracture from the tibial plateau (*arrow*). Its significance is the association with anterior cruciate and other ligamentous injuries.

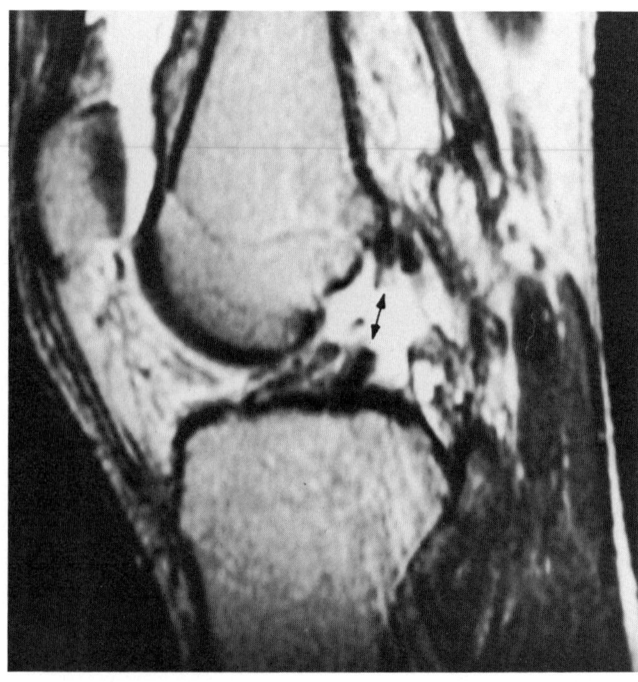

Figure 101–104. A complete tear of the anterior cruciate ligament is seen on this sagittal T_2-weighted MRI. The low-signal ends of the ligament (*double-ended arrow*) are separated by high-signal fluid. Sometimes, the ligament fragments are not identified and abnormal signal in the location of the anterior cruciate ligament is the major clue to the diagnosis.

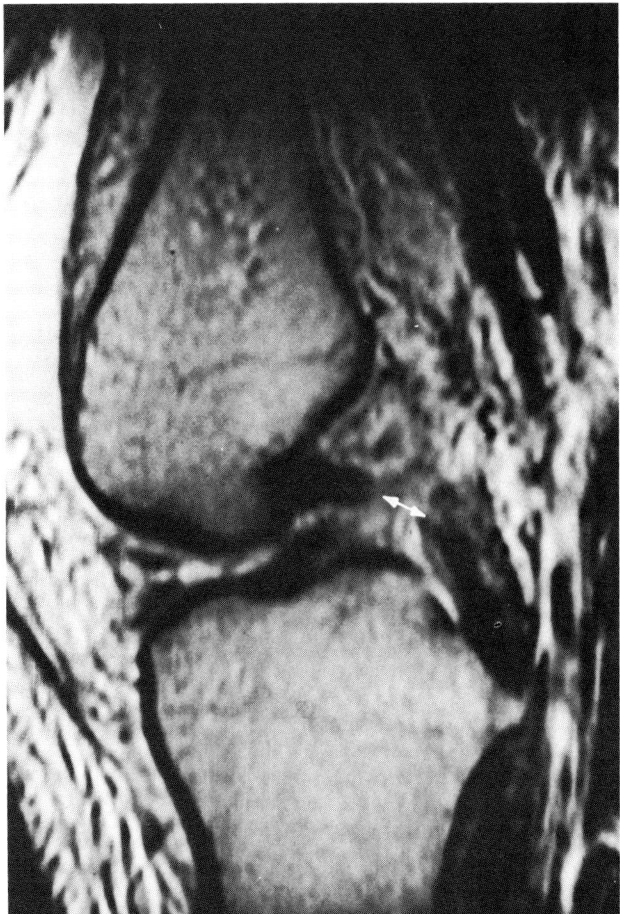

Figure 101–105. Complete disruption of the posterior cruciate ligament is shown on this sagittal T_2-weighted MRI. The gap between the ends of the low-signal ligament is easily seen (*double-ended arrow*). Compare with Figure 101–104 to see how much larger the posterior cruciate is than the anterior cruciate.

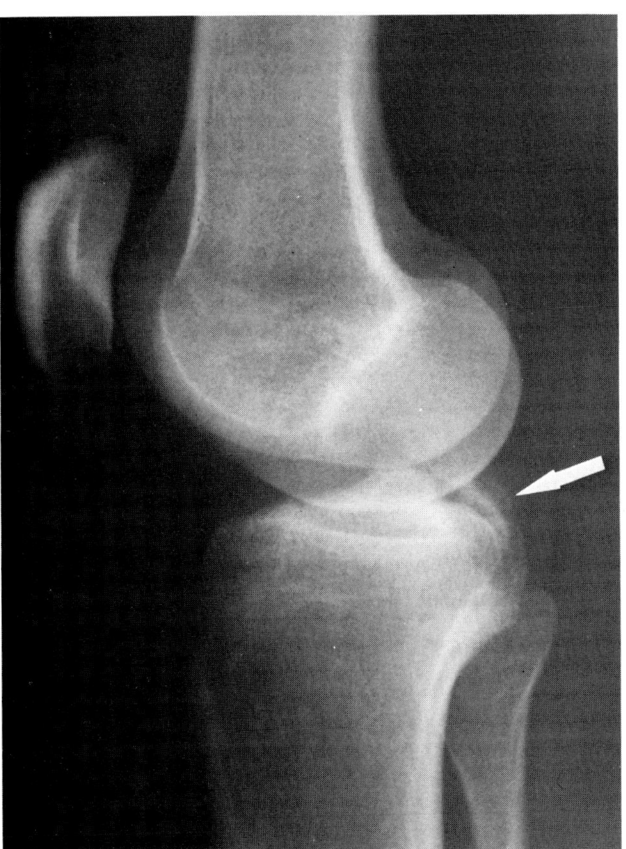

Figure 101–106. Avulsion of a piece of bone is more common with posterior cruciate than with anterior cruciate injuries due to the greater strength of the ligament. Such an avulsion is visible here at the origin of the posterior cruciate from the posterior tibial plateau (*arrow*).

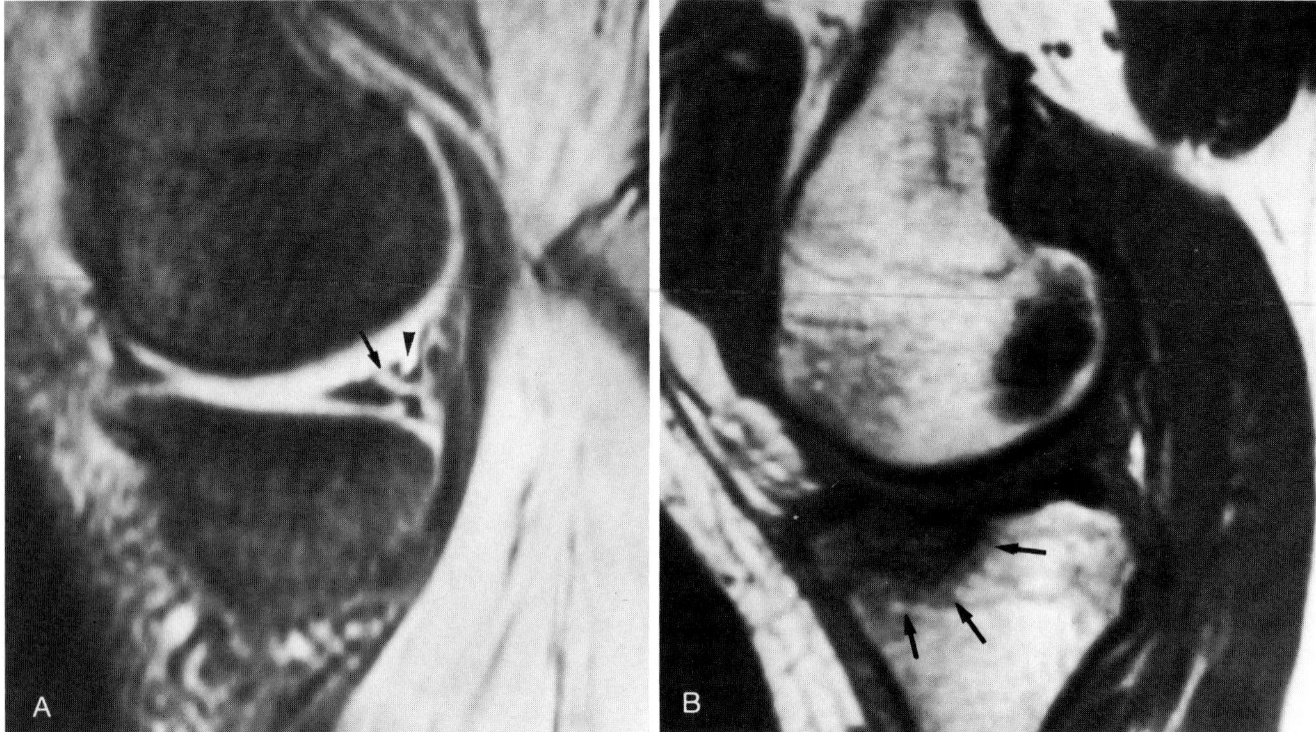

Figure 101–107. *A*, **Tear of the posterior medial horn of the meniscus** (***arrow***) is shown on this sagittal T_2-weighted image by high signal extending through the surface of the meniscus. The normal posterior sulcus at the base of the meniscus (*arrowhead*) should not be mistaken for a tear. *B*, An associated radiographically occult fracture of the tibial plateau (*arrows*) is shown on this sagittal T_1-weighted MRI. Here, there is both low signal in the marrow containing cancellous bone and discontinuity of the cortex. More minor injuries may produce merely decreased signal in the marrow, which may be quite subtle. (From Manaster BJ: MRI of the knee. Semin US CT MRI 11(4):307–326, 1990.)

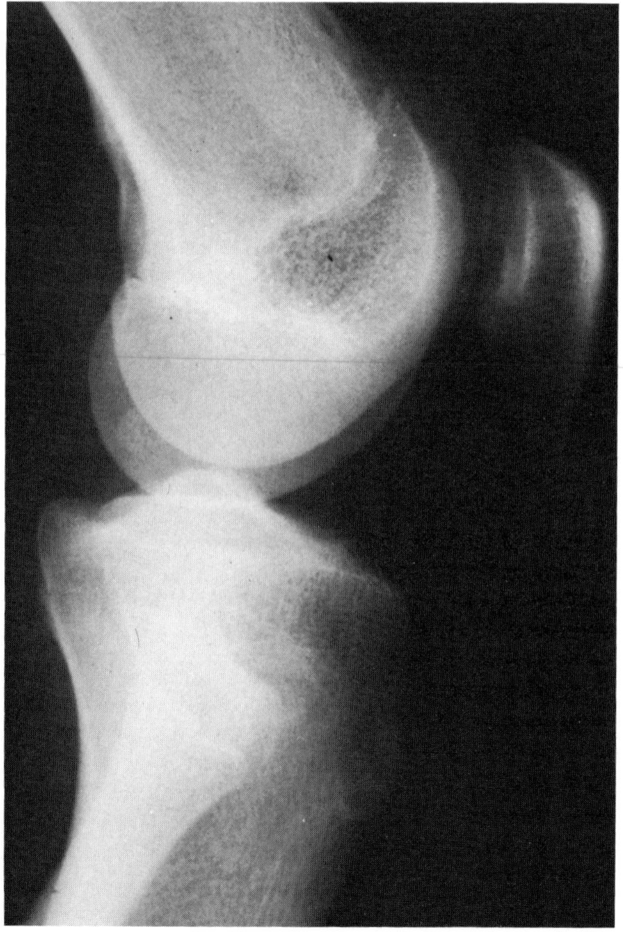

Figure 101–108. Anterior dislocation of the fibular head is seen on this lateral radiograph. The fibular head is almost a full shaft width anterior to its normal position (compare with Figs. 101–91 and 101–106).

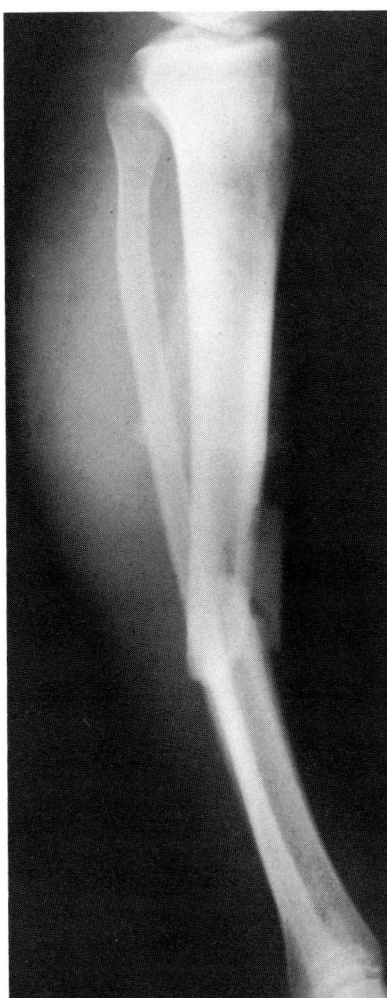

Figure 101–109. A midshaft tibial fracture with an anterior butterfly fragment is seen on this lateral radiograph. The fibula has not fractured but has undergone plastic bowing and has a smooth curve that is convex-posterior. This is important to detect, since it may seriously affect reduction of the tibial fracture.

Normal Variants

The nutrient artery of the tibia piercing the posterior cortex and heading away from the knee joint can be quite prominent and mistaken for a fracture. Distally, irregularities in the fibula may simulate a fracture, and the overlapping cortices of the tibia and fibula may do the same. There are frequently small accessory ossicles subjacent to the medial and lateral malleoli, distinguished from avulsion fractures by their smooth borders and well-corticated margins.

Pediatrics

Tibial fractures in children are common and heal well, in contrast to those in adults. They are frequently greenstick or nondisplaced and may be difficult to see on the initial radiographs, especially if these are taken using a low-dose high-speed film/screen combination with relatively low spatial resolution (Fig. 101–110). Radiographs should include the knee and ankle to assess rotation, and CT is sometimes useful to evaluate this also. The "toddler fracture" is found up to six years of age. It is a spiral fracture produced by torsion of the tibia without a fibular fracture (Fig. 101–110). An AP with internal rotation may show the fracture best or it may be detected on delayed films. Bicycle spoke injury in children is common and may produce a distal tibial fracture.

Stress fractures of the tibia in children are almost always in the upper third of the bone. As in adults, they may not show up on plain films but are well seen by bone scan or MRI. In paraplegics, minor trauma may lead to fractures producing massive callus formation that can be mistaken for an osteogenic tumor. Pathologic fractures through a nonossifying fibroma, simple bone cyst, or other benign process are not uncommon. Fractures of the distal metaphysis are frequently greenstick fractures.

Ankle fractures in children, as in adults, are usually due to rotation of the leg on top of the fixed foot (see discussion below). The ankle ligaments are attached to the epiphyses so growth plate injury is frequent, usually a Salter type I or II fracture (see Fig. 101–13*C*). These may or may not lead to growth disturbance, whereas Salter III and IV fractures in this location frequently do. Supination/inversion injuries are most common, causing avulsion of the fibular tip (a Salter type I fracture) and in more severe cases causing a Salter type III or IV medial tibial injury that frequently leads to medial growth arrest. Other common injury patterns are supination/external rotation leading to a tibial Salter type II fracture and pronation/eversion/external rotation leading to a Salter type II fracture of the tibia with a fibular shaft fracture that may be quite proximal.

The "juvenile Tillaux" fracture is a Salter type III avulsion of the lateral portion of the tibial epiphysis by the anterior tibio-fibular ligament. It occurs in skeletally maturing patients; the medial portion of the distal tibial growth plate fuses early, leaving the lateral portion at risk for a Salter fracture. Tomography or CT may be useful in demonstrating this fracture, which can be subtle on plain film.

The triplane fracture also occurs in the adolescent patient. The three fracture planes are (1) coronally through the posterior metaphysis, (2) horizontally through the growth plate, and (3) sagittally through the epiphysis. There are usually two fragments: the anterolateral epiphysis attached to the metaphysis and the fibula, and the remainder of the epiphysis attached to the posterior portion of the metaphysis (Fig. 101–111). Variations may have three or four fragments, depending on whether the epiphyseal fragments remain attached to their respective portions of metaphysis. Tomograms, CT, and 3-D reconstruction can be useful in this complex fracture.

Focal soft-tissue swelling around the ankle may be a pointer to a nondisplaced type I or II fracture that may be very subtle and detected only on stress views. In young children, type I fractures of the distal tibial physis may be overlooked until the interosseous membrane shows calcification (indicating a membrane tear) three weeks or so afterwards.

Adults

Tibial fractures are frequently due to motor vehicle accidents, penetrating trauma, or indirect twisting forces such as in skiing accidents and falls with a fixed foot. The fibula is usually also fractured. Spiral fractures commonly are caused by twisting forces, with oblique, transverse, and segmental fractures appearing in direct trauma with varying degrees of comminution. It is uncommon for the fracture to extend to the tibial plafond (the distal articular surface of the tibia), except in falls from a height (Fig. 101–112). There are several different orthopedic classifications in use. One distinctive and difficult to treat fracture pattern is the "pilon fracture" of the distal tibia. This is caused by axial compression and torsion especially in osteoporotic bones. It results in severe comminution of the distal tibia (cf Fig. 101–97) with intra-articular involvement and many variably displaced fragments. Pathologic fractures of the tibia are uncommon.

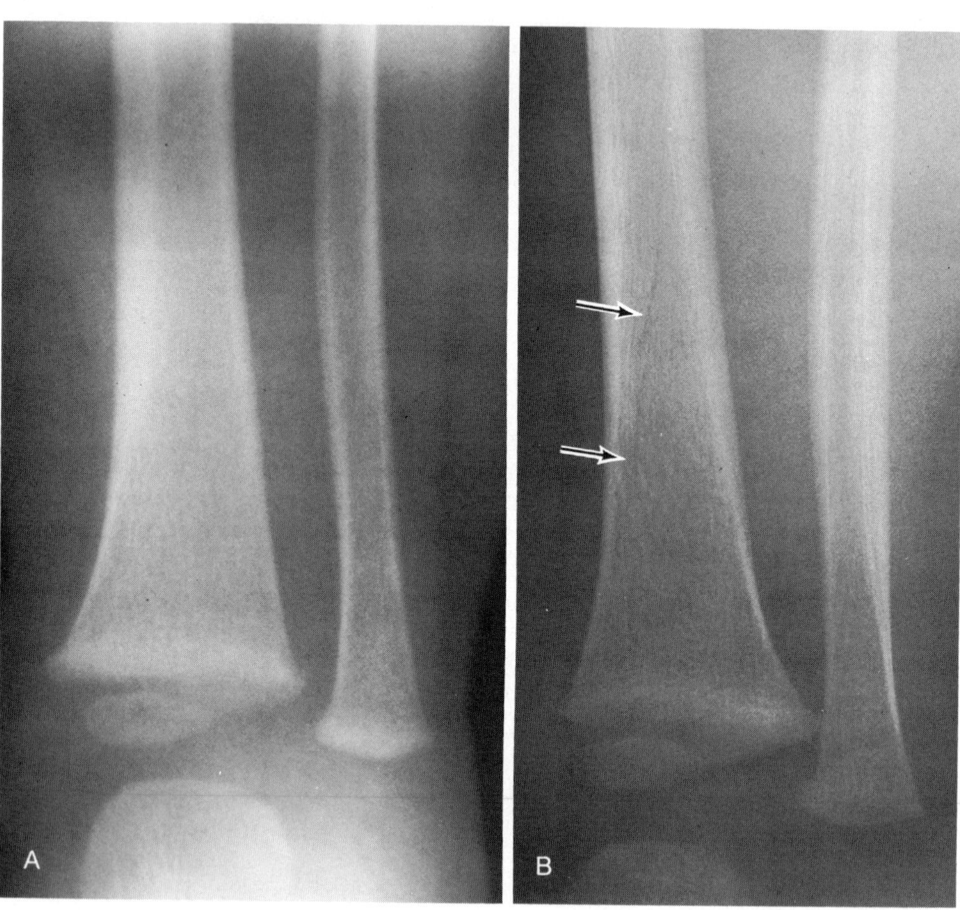

Figure 101–110. This **toddler fracture of the distal tibia** was not seen on the initial low-dose radiograph (*A*). A repeat examination on high-detail film two days later (*B*) shows the nondisplaced spiral fracture well (*arrows*).

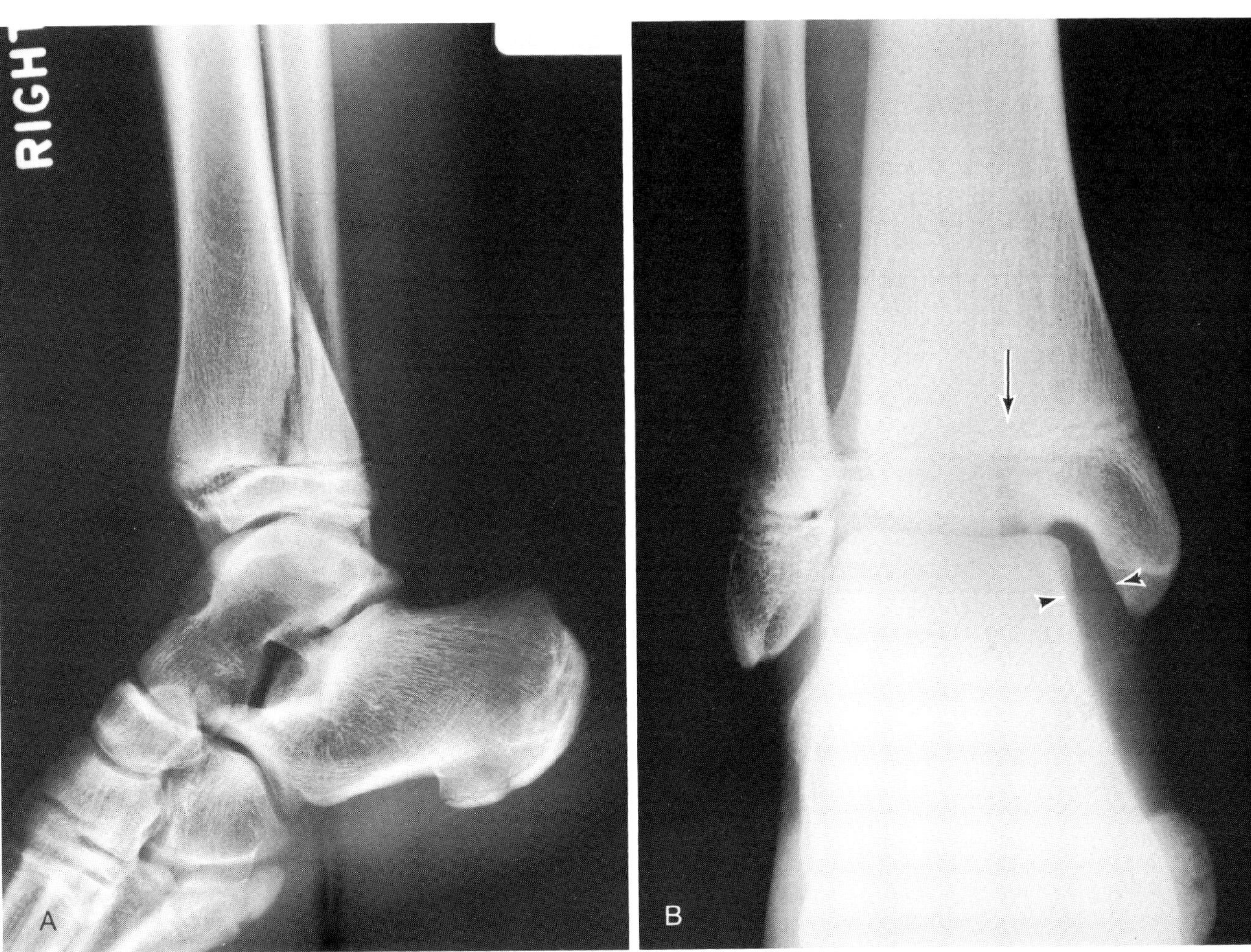

Figure 101–111. Triplane fracture of the distal tibia. On the lateral view (*A*), note the vertical metaphyseal and horizontal growth plate fracture much like a Salter II injury. However, the AP view (*B*) shows a vertical fracture through the epiphysis (*arrow*) allowing the lateral portion of the epiphysis to stay attached to the tibia and fibula. Consequently, there is no fibular fracture. The medial widening of the mortise (*arrowheads*) indicates the instability of this fracture.

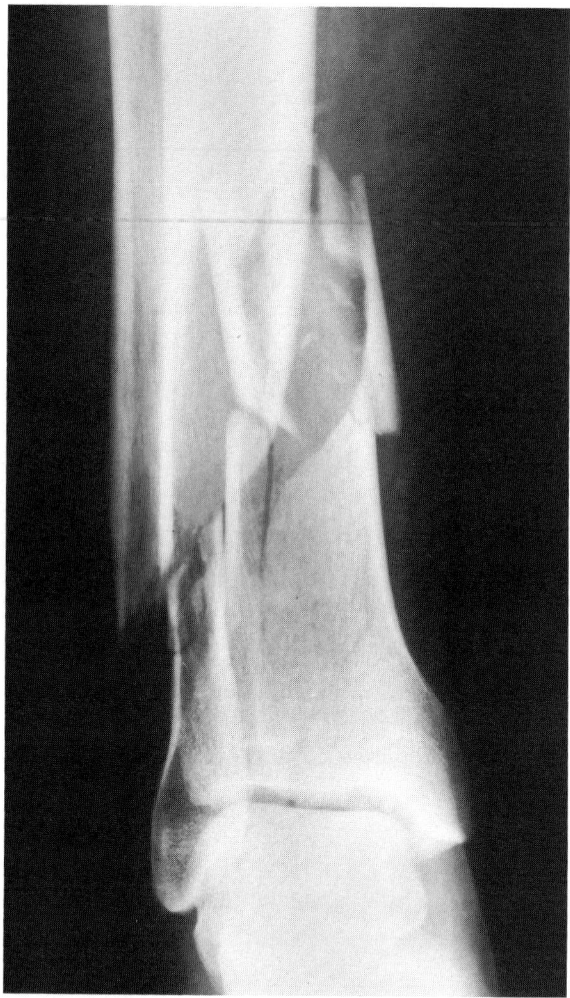

Figure 101–112. Comminuted fractures of both the tibia and fibula are visible. The basic fracture is spiral-oblique, with medial displacement of the distal fragment and slight bayoneting. Note that the tibial fracture extends down to the joint surface, an important consideration in planning treatment. The ankle mortise itself is not disrupted.

Radiographic assessment with plain films should include the knee and the ankle. Complications consisting of delayed union or non-union, infection, and disuse osteoporosis are relatively common owing to the lack of muscle mass on the anterior tibia. These fractures are often treated with an intramedullary nail. A plate may also be used, and if there is a large bony defect, bone graft may be inserted.

Stress fractures may have no plain film manifestations or may manifest as an area of sclerosis with or without a lucency. In military recruits they tend to affect the upper third of the tibia, in ballet dancers the mid third, in gymnasts the lower third, and in runners the distal fibula. They are easily detected by bone scan or MRI.

The Ankle

The basic ankle radiographs are the AP, the lateral and the mortise view (in which the ankle is internally rotated 20 degrees to have the intermalleolar line parallel with the film). The tibio-fibular clear space, tibio-fibular overlap, medial clear space, and talar tilt should be assessed. A line drawn through the tibio-talar joint and going down along the fibulo-talar joint (the tibio-fibular line) should follow a smooth curve. Stress views may be useful to show ligamentous disruption. Tomography, CT, arthrography and MRI all have a place in assessing complex fractures. Reduction at the ankle must be to within 1–2 mm to avoid postoperative degenerative arthritis, which occurs in 10 per cent of well-reduced fractures but 85 per cent of poorly reduced fractures.

Fractures of the ankle are commonly due to rotation of the leg upon a fixed foot. The work of Lauge-Hansen on cadavers showed the importance of the position of the foot and talus in determining the pattern of fracture. The ankle ligaments, including the anterior and posterior tibio-fibular, the talo-fibular, the calcaneo-fibular, and the deltoid ligaments, influence the fracture pattern either by avulsion of portions of bone or by providing a hinge around which the bones rotate. Impaction of the talus on the medial or lateral malleoli secondary to inversion/eversion or rotation is the other principal factor determining the fracture pattern. Avulsion fractures tend to be transverse or in the form of tiny fragments, whereas impaction causes a vertical or spiral/oblique fracture. The simplest classification and one that is frequently used is the Weber system, which relies on the position of the fibular fracture. The Weber A fracture is an avulsion fracture of the tip of the lateral malleolus by the lateral talo-fibular and calcaneo-fibular ligaments or, in its more severe form, this plus an oblique vertical fracture of the medial malleolus produced by impaction of the talus on the malleolus (Fig. 101–113*A*). This corresponds to the Lauge-Hansen supination adduction injury. The Weber B is oblique or spiral with the fracture line entering the joint at the level of the syndesmosis (in which the anterior tibio-fibular ligament is torn in more than 50 per cent) with, in the more severe form, a medial or posterior malleolar fracture (Fig. 101–113*B*). This corresponds to a Lauge-Hansen supination-eversion injury. The Weber type C has a fibular fracture above the tibio-fibular syndesmosis, which is disrupted, and a medial injury (Fig. 101–113*C* and D). The fracture may be in the distal fibula or may be in the proximal fibula, even up to the neck of the fibula (the "Maisonneuve" injury in which the whole interosseous membrane is disrupted, Fig. 101–114). Simple Weber A and B fractures may be stable and may not need operative treatment, whereas Weber C fractures inevitably have disruption of the ankle mortise and require operative reduction and fixation. It should be remembered that fractures occur in sequence, so that seeing the later stage of a fracture implies that the earlier stages are necessarily present.

More minor ankle injuries include small avulsed fragments from the distal fibula, lateral process of the talus or neck of the calcaneus

Figure 101–113. *A,* **Weber A fracture of the ankle** is seen with a transverse avulsion fracture of the distal fibula. Inversion and rotation of the talus have also produced a vertical fracture of the medial malleolus from impaction of the talus against it. Furthermore, there is an impaction fracture of the tibial articular surface just medial to this (*arrow*), also caused by impaction of the talus. *B,* **Weber B fracture of the ankle** is diagnosed on the basis of the fibular fracture at the level of the plafond. In this case, the fibular fracture is caused by impaction of the rotating talus against the fibular tip. The distal tibiofibular syndesmosis is intact. The mortise is widened, however, secondary to an avulsion injury of the medial malleolus caused by the pull of the deltoid ligament. This is shown by the small bony fragments on the medial side (*arrow*). *C,* This **Weber C fracture** probably resulted from external rotation of the foot in a pronated position. The AP view shows the fibular fracture caused by impaction of the talus on the distal fibula disrupting the tibiofibular ligament and interosseous membrane along with the medial widening secondary to deltoid ligament injury. *D,* The lateral view shows the posterior malleolar fracture (*arrow*) produced by the rotating talus impacting on the distal tibia.

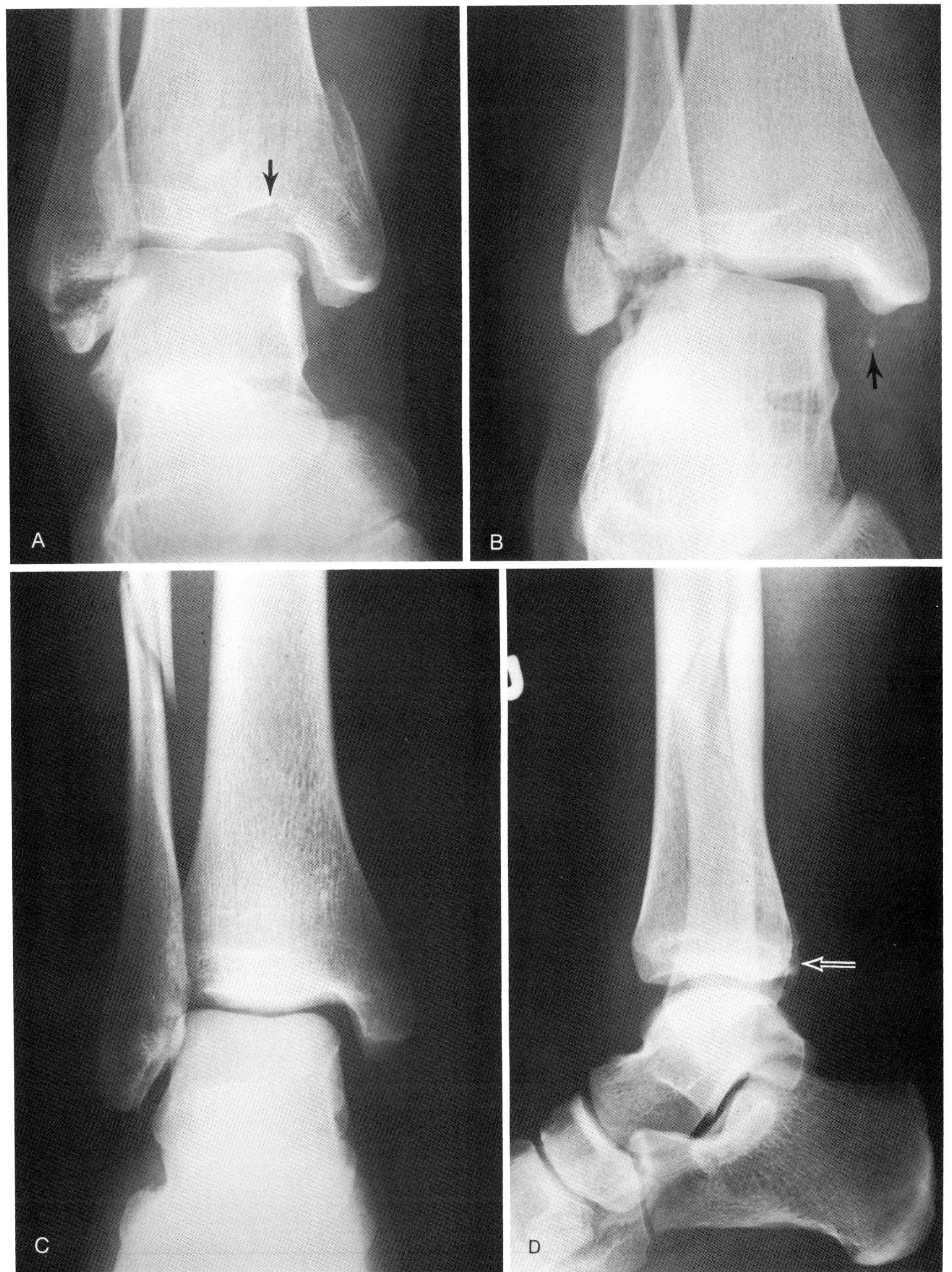

Figure 101–113 *See legend on opposite page*

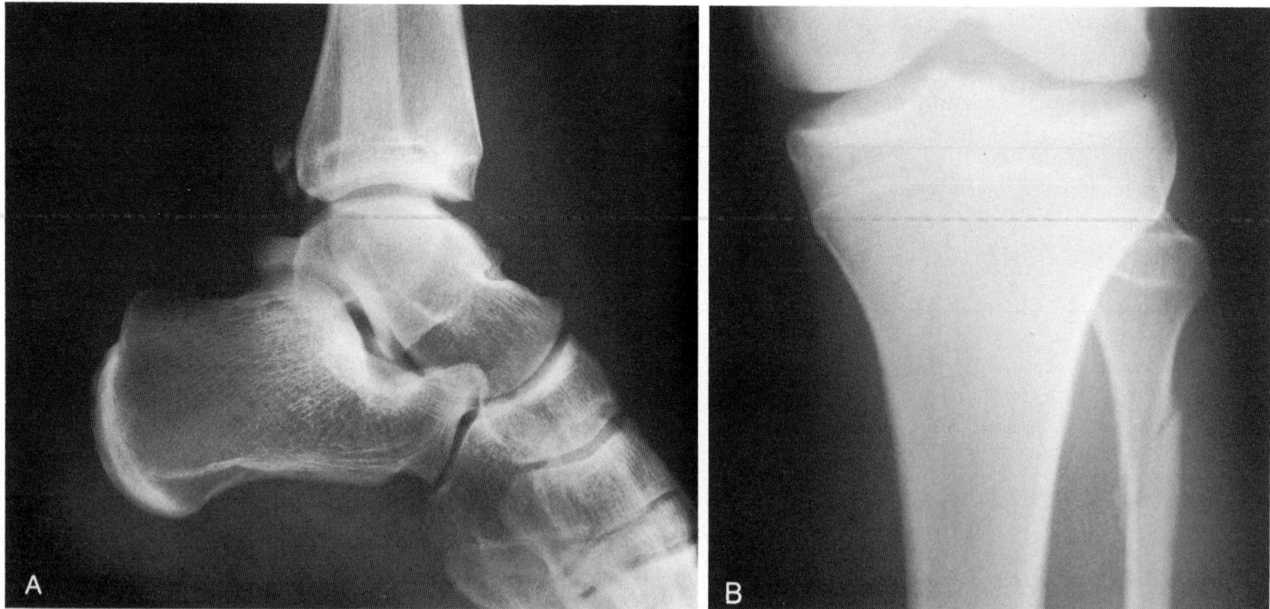

Figure 101–114. Maisonneuve fracture. The fracture of the posterior malleolus seen on lateral view (*A*) indicates considerable movement and rotation of the talus with probable disruption of the distal tibiofibular joint. No fracture was found distally, but the proximal fibula is fractured (*B*), indicating disruption of the interosseous membrane up to this level.

at the origin of the extensor digitorum brevis, all of which are seen with the common inversion injuries of the ankle. Soft-tissue swelling is important to assess. If there is less than 1 cm soft-tissue swelling, the chances of bony injury are less than 5 per cent. Osteochondral fractures are fairly common, especially in the talus; these may be best seen by tomography or by MRI, which can also sometimes assess whether the fragment is partially or completely loose. Impaction fractures on the medial corner of the plafond by the talus should be looked for and sometimes are manifest only by subtle increased density at this point (Fig. 101–115). Reflex sym-

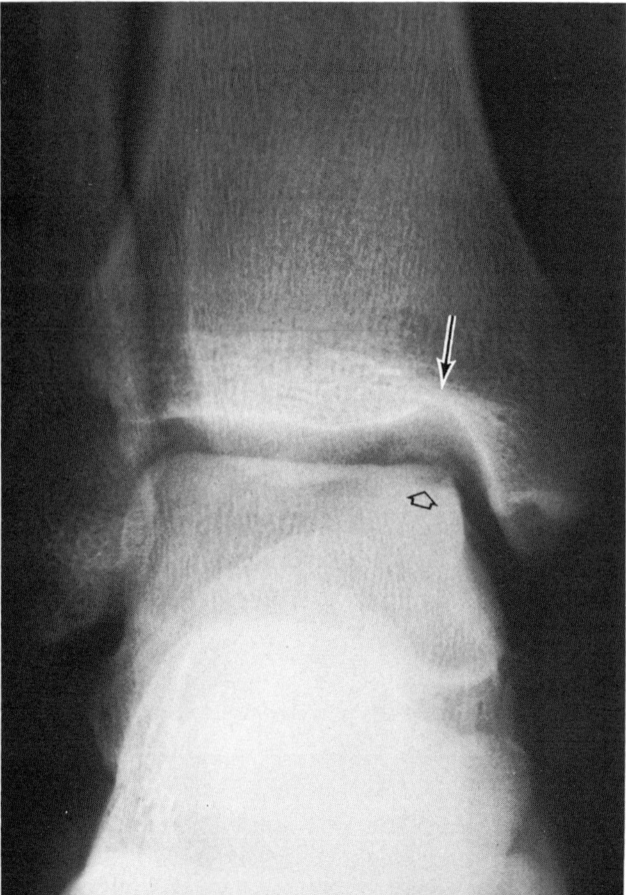

Figure 101–115. Both an **impaction fracture of the medial plafond** (***arrow***) **and an osteochondral fracture of the margin of the talus** (***open arrowhead***) are seen in this man who suffered a supination injury to the ankle.

pathetic dystrophy sometimes occurs, and a synostosis between the distal tibia and fibula may occur in severe trauma. Dislocation of the ankle is extremely uncommon as an isolated injury, as is fracture of the posterior malleolus. If the latter is observed, evidence of interosseous membrane separation and a proximal fibula fracture should be sought (see Fig. 101–114).

THE FOOT

Anthony J. Doyle

For diagnostic purposes the foot is divided into the hindfoot, consisting of the calcaneus and talus; the midfoot, consisting of the navicular, cuboid, and cuneiforms; and the forefoot, which contains the metatarsals and phalanges. Generally speaking, fractures of the foot can be divided into those that involve joints and those that do not. The latter have a considerably better prognosis. Because many of the bones in the foot overlap on straight AP and lateral views (especially the bases of the mesatarsals and the cuneiforms), AP, lateral, and medial oblique views are usually taken to evaluate the foot. Special views such as the lateral oblique, weight-bearing views, stress views, or tangential views of various joints and bones may also be useful in addition to tomograms, CT, MRI, and bone scan.

Normal Variants

There are numerous accessory bones in the foot, seen in up to 30 per cent of normal adults. Some of the most common are the os trigonum (at the posterior margin of the talus), the os tibiale externum (at the tubercle of the navicular), the os peroneum (in the peroneus longus tendon as it crosses the cuboid), and the os vesalianum (at the base of the fifth metatarsal) (Fig. 101–116). Numerous sesamoid bones are also present. It should be remarked that these are frequently not symmetrical from one foot to the other and are often bipartite or fragmented, thus leading to confusion with fractures. However, true fractures of the sesamoids are usually transverse and sharply marginated. Numerous secondary ossification centers appear in adolescents. In addition, there are normal clefts in the epiphyses of the phalanges in particular that can simulate fractures. The complex anatomy of the midfoot with many overlapping cortices can lead to simulated lucencies that are usually readily evaluated with oblique views.

Pediatrics

Significant fractures of the foot are unusual in children owing to the pliability of the foot. Fractures that do occur are similar to those in adults.

Adults

The calcaneus is the most frequently fractured foot bone. The usual mechanism is a fall from a height. The fractures are intra-articular in 75 per cent. Associated injuries of the spine and lower extremities are present in up to 60 per cent. The most common fracture passes obliquely through the calcaneus (Fig. 101–117*B* and *C*), separating it into an anteromedial and a posterolateral fragment. The posterior subtalar joint is usually involved. Boehler's angle (the angle subtended by a line drawn from the anterior process of the calcaneus to the subtalar joint and a line drawn across the subtalar

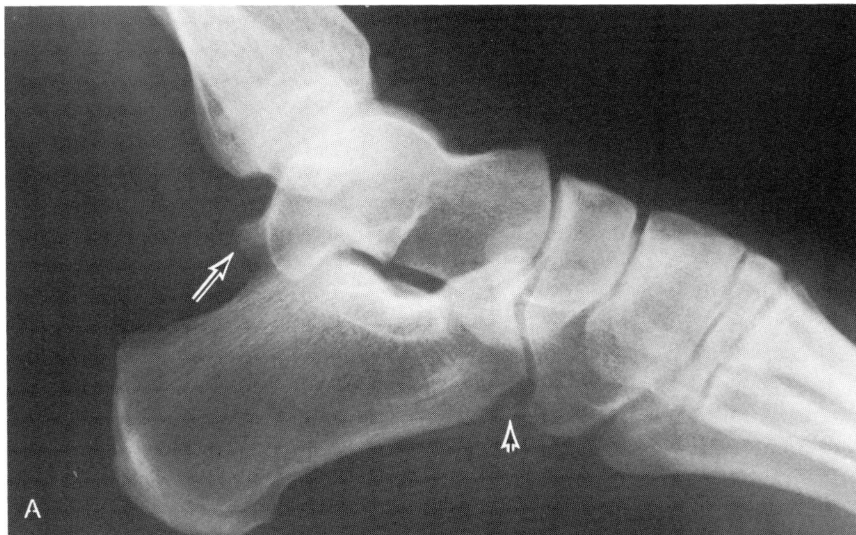

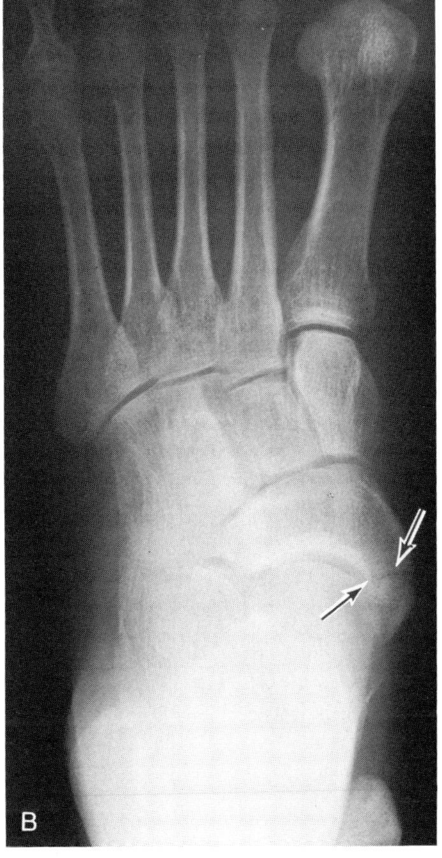

Figure 101–116. *A,* The **os trigonum** (***arrow***) is seen at the posterior margin of the talus and the **os peroneum** (***arrowhead***) near the inferolateral margin of the cuboid. *B,* On the medial side, the **os tibiale externum** (***arrows***) is seen at the tubercle of the navicular. These are normal variants.

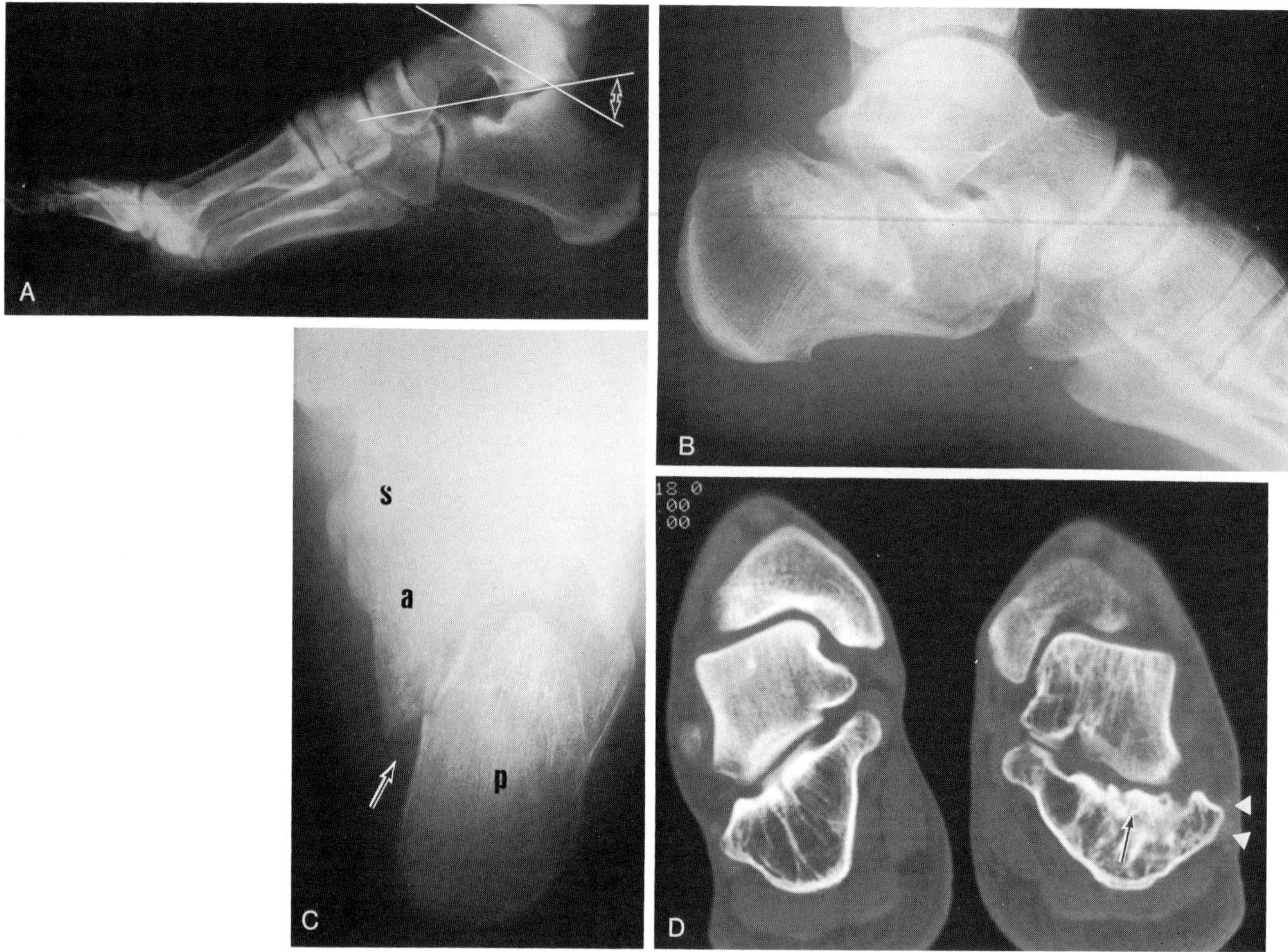

Figure 101–117. *A,* **Boehler's angle** is indicated by the double-ended arrow and is normally between 28 and 42 degrees. *B,* There is an **oblique comminuted fracture** through the body and neck of the calcaneus extending into the subtalar joint posteriorly and effectively reducing Boehler's angle to zero. *C,* Axial view showing the fracture (*arrow*) passing obliquely through the subtalar joint and separating the smaller enteromedial fragment (a) from the larger posterolateral fragment (p). The sustentaculum tali (s) is part of fragment (a). *D,* CT scan through the subtalar joint three months post-injury shows irregularity of the posterior calcaneal facet (*arrow*) predisposing to degenerative changes. Laterally, note the spike of bone adjacent to the peroneal tendons (*arrowheads*), which can be quite irregular and produce fraying or entrapment of these tendons.

joint and the Achilles bursal eminence) is flattened from its normal value of between 28 and 42 degrees (Fig. 101–117*A*). The fragments are best seen with CT performed in the coronal plane (Fig. 101–117*D*). This will show the degree of override of the medial on the lateral fragment, the number of fragments, and the degree of impingement on the peroneal tendons and other structures. The second most common fracture of the calcaneus is avulsion of the anterior process by the bifurcate ligament while the foot is in adduction and plantar flexion, best shown on the lateral oblique film. Compression fractures of the anterior calcaneus, fracture of the sustentaculum tali, and fracture of the tuberosity near the Achilles tendon insertion are less common fractures. Dislocation of the calcaneus is very rare.

The talus is second to the calcaneus in frequency of fracture. Because this bone is three fifths covered in cartilage it is susceptible to avascular necrosis, especially if the vessels entering inferiorly through the talar neck are disrupted. The usual mechanism of talar neck fracture (Fig. 101–118) is hyperdorsiflexion such as occurs as when the foot is jammed against the floor of a car or the rudder bar of an airplane (hence the old term "aviator's astragalus"). The fracture may not be obvious and CT, tomography, or MRI may be needed to show it. Evidence of an intact blood supply is shown by decreased density of the body and dome of the talus from disuse osteoporosis about three weeks postinjury (Hawkins' sign). Persistent normal density of the talar dome (which stands out against the surrounding osteoporosis) indicates avascular necrosis (Fig. 101–119), which can also be diagnosed by MRI. Small chip fractures from the talus are common and are secondary to avulsion by ligaments, usually the talofibular ligament laterally. Fractures of the talar head and body are uncommon as are fractures of the lateral process (although many of these are simply overlooked). The posterior process is also uncommonly fractured; the acute irregular sharp fracture line should be distinguished from the smooth borders associated with a normal os trigonum (Fig. 101–120). Subtalar dislocation is not uncommon. Talo-navicular alignment should be carefully assessed on both the AP and lateral views. Complete dislocation of the talus is a rare but devastating injury with a high incidence of AVN.

The mid-tarsal (Chopart) joint may be subject to medial, longitudinal, or lateral carpal stress and crush injury in descending order of frequency. This gives rise to various subluxation and fracture patterns. In lateral stress, the cuboid may be fractured (the "nutcracker" fracture).

The navicular may suffer avulsion of the dorsal surface by the insertion of the talo-navicular capsule and portions of the deltoid ligament. Less commonly, the posterior tuberosity may be avulsed by the tibialis posterior tendon. This fracture should be distinguished from the fairly common accessory ossicle at this point by the smooth corticated margin of the latter (Fig. 101–121). The body of the navicular is usually fractured in association with other bones.

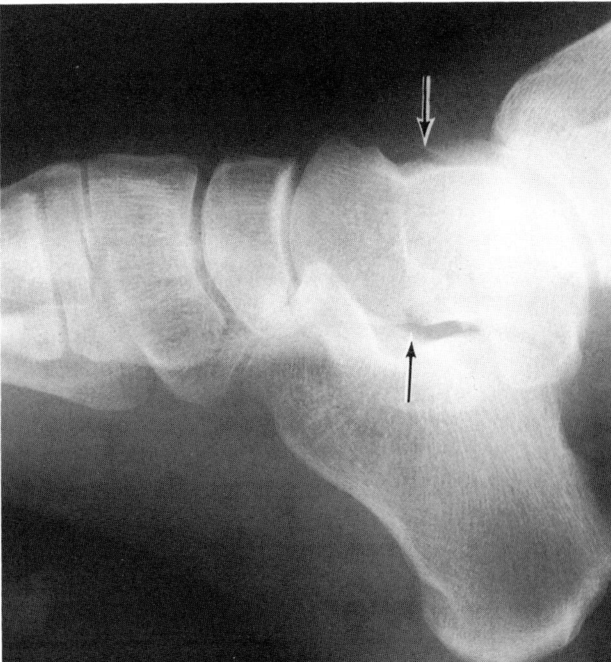

Figure 101–118. Talar neck fracture is seen here in a typical location (*arrows*) and is nondisplaced.

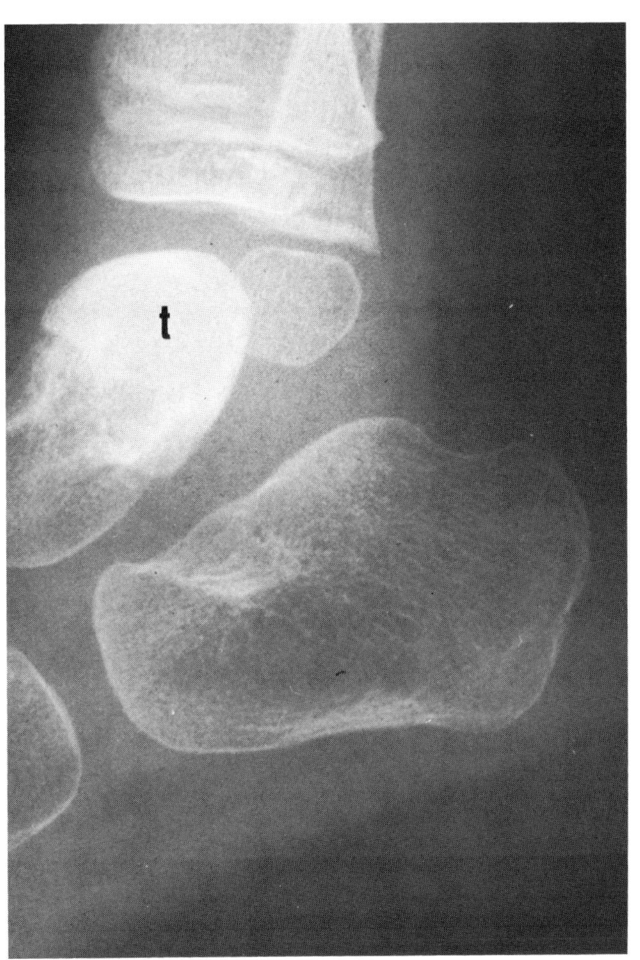

Figure 101–119. Avascular necrosis of the body and dome of the talus is seen in a two-year-old child with a healing talar neck fracture. The avascular talar dome (t) remains of high density, while the surrounding bones are more lucent due to subacute osteoporosis from hyperemia associated with the fracture healing.

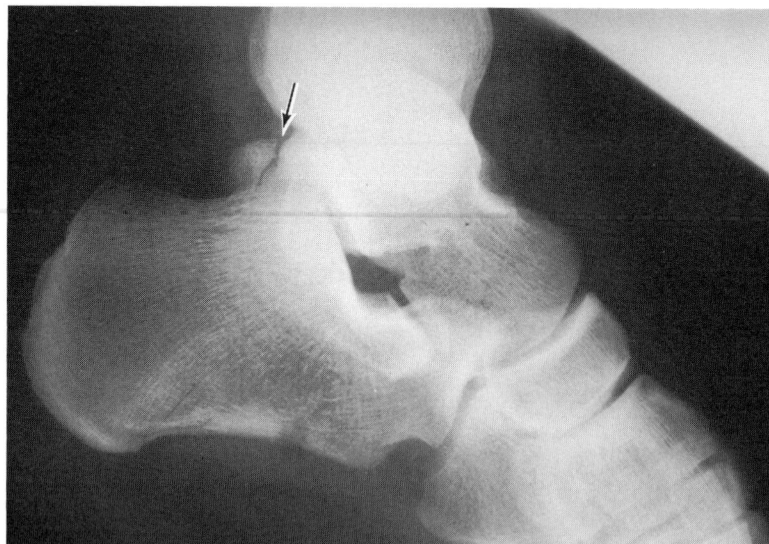

Figure 101–120. Fracture of the os trigonum is seen with the sharp fracture line (*arrows*) having a different appearance from the normal rounded borders of the os trigonum. This uncommon fracture may also be manifested by pain on flexion of the great toe, since the flexor hallucis longus runs around this point.

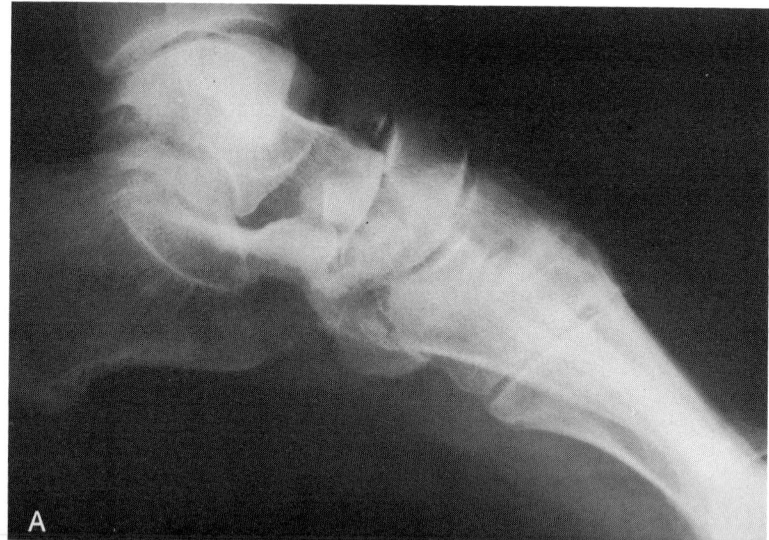

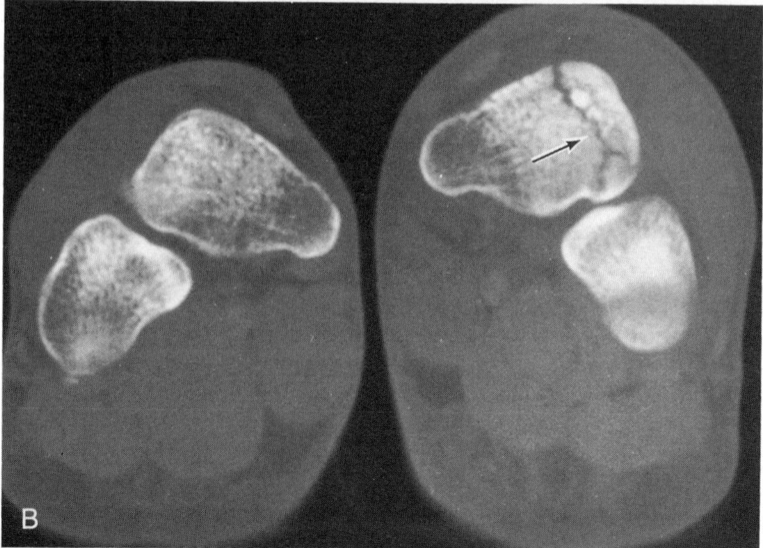

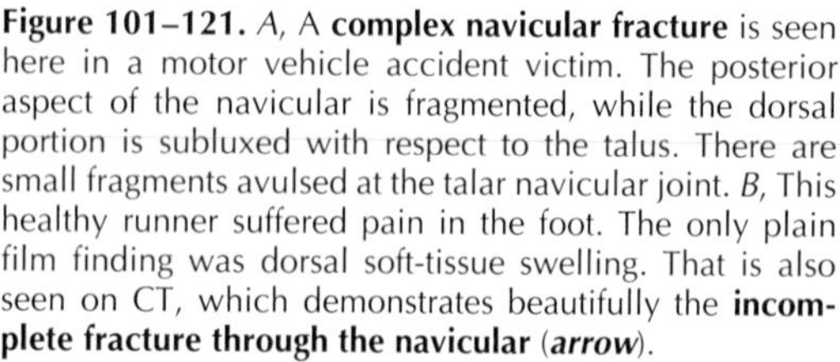

Figure 101–121. *A,* A **complex navicular fracture** is seen here in a motor vehicle accident victim. The posterior aspect of the navicular is fragmented, while the dorsal portion is subluxed with respect to the talus. There are small fragments avulsed at the talar navicular joint. *B,* This healthy runner suffered pain in the foot. The only plain film finding was dorsal soft-tissue swelling. That is also seen on CT, which demonstrates beautifully the **incomplete fracture through the navicular** (*arrow*).

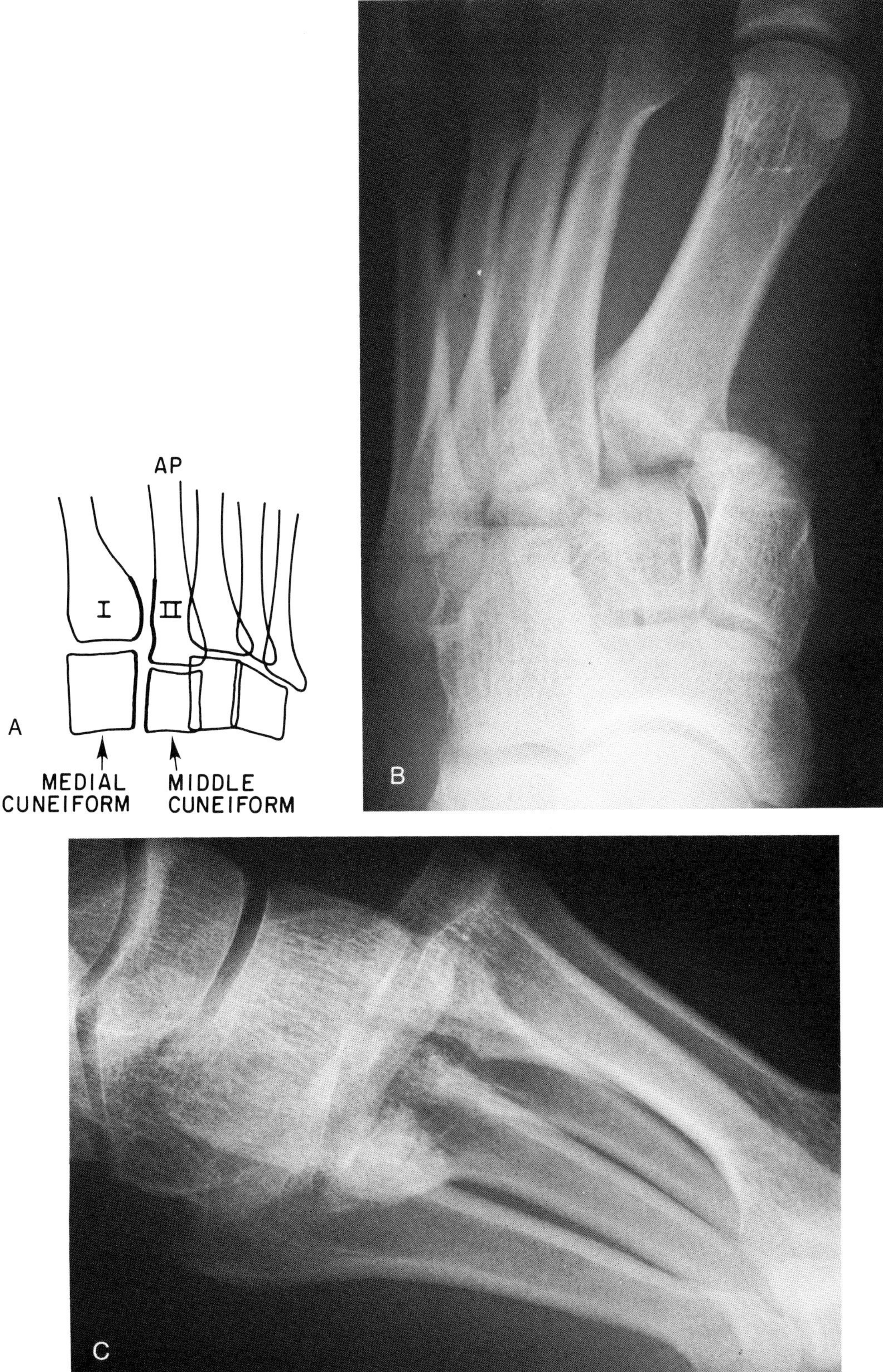

Figure 101–122. *A*, Diagrammatically, the **normal perfect alignment of the adjacent surfaces of the first and second metatarsals and their respective cuneiforms** is shown by the heavy black lines. (*A* from Manaster BJ: Handbooks in Radiology: Skeletal Radiology. Chicago, Year Book Medical Publishers, 1989.) *B* and *C*, A very obvious homolateral **Lisfranc fracture-dislocation**. It is visible on both AP and lateral views. The first through third metatarsals are dislocated dorsolaterally. Note the small bony fragments adjacent to the medial cuneiform.

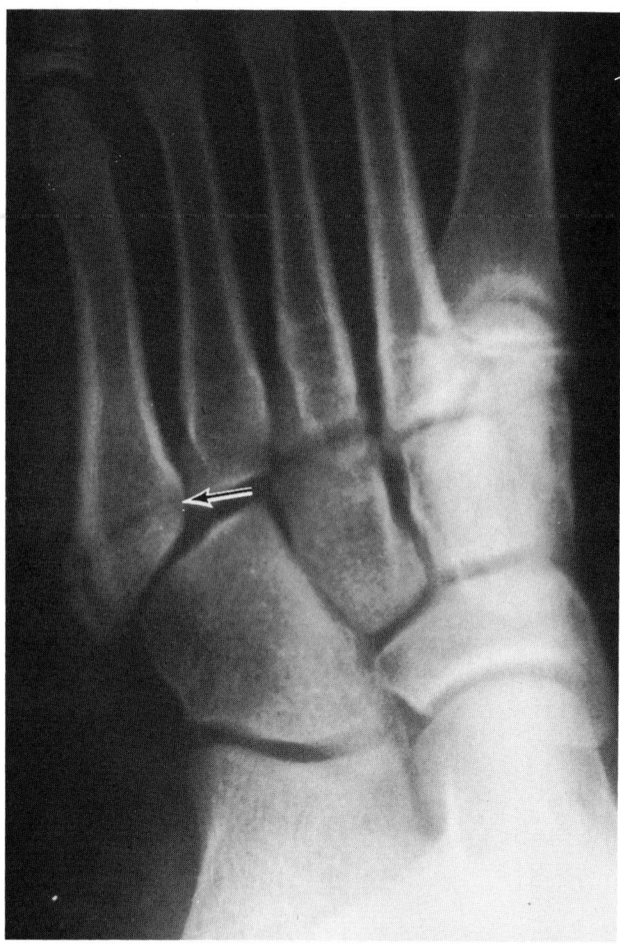

Figure 101–123. This adolescent has a **transverse avulsion fracture of the base of the fifth metatarsal** (***arrow***). Note also the longitudinally oriented apophysis at this site, a normal finding.

Stress fractures may occur and can be difficult to see; they are easily demonstrated on CT or MRI (Fig. 101–121*B*). The cuneiforms fracture uncommonly, usually in association with other bones.

The tarsometatarsal (Lisfranc) joint is injured by a variety of mechanisms mostly involving load along the axis of the foot and ranging from stepping off a curb to severe trauma. It frequently occurs in patients with diminished sensation, especially diabetics, patients with tabes dorsalis, and those with subacute combined degeneration of the spinal cord. There is usually a combination of dislocation and tiny fracture fragments. Normally, the medial aspect of the second metatarsal lines up perfectly with the middle cuneiform, the lateral aspect of the first metatarsal lines up with the medial cuneiform and the third metatarsal lines up nearly perfectly with the lateral cuneiform. Any deviation from this raises the suspicion of a Lisfranc dislocation (Fig. 101–122). The injury may be homolateral (where the metatarsals are all displaced the same way), isolated (in which one or two bones are displaced away from the others), or divergent (where the bones are displaced away from the midline of the foot).

The metatarsals frequently are fractured by direct load such as a heavy weight landing on them. Stress fractures may affect any of them but particularly the second, third, and fifth. The lateral films should be carefully inspected for sagittal displacement; this requires reduction—otherwise the function of the foot is affected. There is a common avulsion fracture of the base of the fifth metatarsal (Fig. 101–123) from the pull of either the peroneus brevis or abductor digiti minimi quinti tendon. The fracture line is transverse in contradistinction to the physis at this site, which is longitudinal. Although often called a Jones fracture, this is not accurate; Robert Jones described a fracture in the diaphysis of the metatarsal that he suffered in 1902 while dancing, a stress fracture that heals much more slowly than the typical base of metatarsal avulsion fracture.

The toes may be injured by the foot striking a solid object or having something dropped on them. Dislocations are common except at the first metatarsophalangeal joint, which has strong ligaments. Complete reduction should be checked for because occasionally a small bone fragment or a sesamoid bone can be trapped in the joint and prevent reduction. The sesamoids themselves rarely fracture (see Fig. 101–9); multipartite sesamoids are more common.

Bibliography

Dunn A: Fractures and dislocations of the carpus. Surg Clin North Am 52:1513, 1972.

Gilula L: Carpal injuries: Analytic approach and case exercises. AJR 133:503, 1979.

Harris JH: The Radiology of Acute Cervical Spine Trauma, 2nd ed. Baltimore, Williams and Wilkins, 1987.

Keats T: Atlas of Normal Roentgen Variants That May Simulate Disease, 3rd ed. Chicago, Year Book Medical Publishers, 1984.

Manaster B: Digital arthrography of the wrist. AJR 147:563–566, 1986.

Manaster BJ: Skeletal Radiology (Handbooks in Radiology). Chicago, Year Book Medical Publishers, 1989.

Martire JR, Levinsohn EM: Imaging of Athletic Injuries, A Multimodality Approach. New York, McGraw-Hill, 1992.

Reicher MA, Kellerhouse LE (eds): MRI of the Wrist and Hand. New York, Raven, 1990.

Rockwood CA, Green DP, Bucholz RW: Rockwood and Green's Fractures in Adults, 3rd ed. Philadelphia, JB Lippincott, 1991.

Rockwood CA, Green DP, Bucholz RW. Rockwood and Green's Fractures in Children, 3rd ed. Philadelphia, JB Lippincott, 1991.

Rogers LF: Radiology of Skeletal Trauma. New York, Churchill-Livingstone, 1982.

Stark DD, Bradley WG: Magnetic Resonance Imaging, 2nd ed. St. Louis, Mosby Year Book, 1992.

Yeager B, Dalinka M: Radiology of trauma to the wrist: Dislocations, fracture dislocations, and instability patterns. Skel Radiol 13:120–130, 1985.

CARDIOVASCULAR SYSTEM

Cardiovascular disease continues to be the principal cause of mortality and morbidity in the United States. The need for improved diagnosis and therapy continues. In the diagnosis of cardiovascular disease, imaging modalities are used to establish the presence or absence of disease and to help accurately define the abnormality and its severity. The time-honored components of the cardiovascular work-up—the history, the physical examination, and the electrocardiogram—have been supplemented in most cases with the imaging data from chest radiographs, echocardiograms, Doppler ultrasound studies, radionuclide studies, computed tomography, cardiac catheterization, and angiography. Positron emission tomography and magnetic resonance imaging offer unique insights into cardiovascular diagnosis. These imaging modalities play a central role in the diagnosis of cardiovascular disease and aid in quantifying the severity of disease. Data accumulated from these techniques can help determine the most appropriate course of treatment, whether it is surgery or some other therapeutic interventional option such as angioplasty, thrombolytic therapy, or embolotherapy.

Hence, the four major tasks for the clinician confronted with a patient suspected of having cardiovascular disease are:

1. To establish the presence or absence of cardiovascular disease.
2. To define the specific anatomic and/or physiologic abnormality, its etiology, and its severity.
3. To determine the appropriate treatment plan.
4. To accomplish the above three with as little risk and expense to the patient as possible.

In the following chapters, currently available imaging modalities used in the evaluation of cardiovascular disease will be reviewed. First, an attempt will be made to describe specific techniques: their indications, performance, risks, and cost. Subsequent chapters will deal with disease states affecting the cardiovascular system and certain percutaneous techniques used to treat these conditions.

MICHAEL J. KELLEY

Cardiovascular Anatomy and Imaging Techniques

102 Cardiovascular Anatomy and Function

Michael J. Kelley

The cardiovascular system is a complex, regulated system, capable of wide variations in performance. In employing the many imaging techniques used to study it, one should be aware of the factors that underlie the image, whether one is dealing with the normal state, the compensated state, or the failing cardiovascular system.

FUNCTIONAL ANATOMY

The normal adult heart weighs approximately 300 g. The thin-walled atria act as reservoirs for collecting systemic and pulmonary venous blood when the atrioventricular valves are closed (ventricular systole). In mid-diastole, when the AV valves open, the atria serve as conduits from the veins to the ventricles. Near the end of diastole, the atria contract and eject a small amount of blood into the ventricles prior to ventricular contraction.

The right ventricle consists of a relatively thin-walled (0.4 cm) concave free wall and a convex septum. Ejection of blood occurs as the free wall shortens and moves toward the interventricular septum. This ventricle has a low filling pressure (approximately 5 mm Hg) and ejects blood into the low-pressure (20 mm Hg) pulmonary artery.

The left ventricle is a relatively thick-walled (0.9 cm) conical pump from which blood is ejected by a process of constriction. The thickness of the ventricular wall is dependent on wall stress (which is relatively constant), intraventricular pressure, and the radius of wall curvature. Normal cardiovascular pressure and volume measurements are given in Table 102–1.

CARDIAC PERFORMANCE

Cardiac performance is primarily determined by four factors:

1. PRELOAD. This refers to the initial stretching force prior to muscular contraction. Preload is generally estimated by measuring the end-diastolic volume or pressure of the ventricle. In patients, preload is reflected in the filling pressures (atrial pressures) of the

TABLE 102–1. NORMAL CARDIOVASCULAR PRESSURE AND VOLUME MEASUREMENTS

PRESSURES
1. Left atrium—normal mean = 12 mm Hg
2. Left ventricle
   a. Peak systolic pressure = 100–150 mm Hg (adults)
   b. End-diastolic pressure = 12 mm Hg
3. Aorta
   a. Systolic pressure = 100–150 mm Hg (adults)
   b. Diastolic pressure = 60–90 mm Hg (adults)
4. Right atrium—normal mean = 6 mm Hg
5. Pulmonary artery
   a. Systolic pressure = 15–30 mm Hg
   b. Diastolic pressure = 4–12 m Hg

VOLUMES
1. Left ventricular end-diastolic volume (EDV) = 70–100 cc/sq m
2. Left ventricular end systolic volume = 25–35 cc/sq m
3. Stroke volume (SV) = 40–70 cc/sq m
4. Ejection fraction (SV/EDV) = 0.55–0.80

OTHER MEASUREMENTS
1. Heart rate = 60–100 beats/min
2. Cardiac index = 2.8–4.2 liters/min/sq m
3. Systemic vascular resistance = 770–1500 dynes · sec · cm^{-5}
4. Pulmonary vascular resistance = 20–120 dynes · sec · cm^{-5}

ventricles. In general, increasing the preload (end-diastolic pressure or volume) increases cardiac performance. The normal left atrial pressure is 12 mm Hg. The optimal left atrial pressure in critically ill patients is 15 to 20 mm Hg. In this situation, the elevated atrial pressure (increased preload) will optimize left ventricular filling pressure and maximize stroke volume.

2. AFTERLOAD. This refers to the load against which the heart must contract. In patients, afterload is approximated from the arterial pressure against which the heart must work. As arterial pressure is increased, the stroke volume decreases because the ventricle must eject blood against a higher load. If arterial pressure and systemic vascular resistance are reduced, the forward stroke volume and cardiac output will increase. Changes in preload and afterload are closely related. Thus, if arterial pressure (afterload) is raised, the ventricle has greater difficulty ejecting blood and more end-diastolic volume is retained. This increases preload. These changes can be followed in the clinical setting by monitoring arterial and left atrial (pulmonary capillary wedge) pressures.

3. CONTRACTILITY. The vigor of heart muscle contraction is measured in the isolated heart as an increase in velocity of shortening of the heart muscle at a given load. Positive inotropic agents such as catecholamines and digitalis increase contractility, whereas ischemia, acidosis, and beta-adrenergic blocking agents reduce contractility. In the face of reduced coronary blood flow secondary to coronary artery disease, increase in contractility caused by a positive inotropic agent or exercise may increase myocardial oxygen demand beyond the ability of the arteries to deliver oxygen and lead to further ischemia.

4. HEART RATE. The heart rate is determined by the frequency of the sinoatrial node impulses and is markedly affected by the autonomic nervous system (primarily the parasympathetic system through the vagus nerve). Factors that influence heart rate include emotions, changes in arterial pressure (baroreceptors), and carotid body stimulation. Cardiac performance is directly affected by heart rate in that it enables the heart to increase cardiac output by the following relationship:

$$\text{Cardiac output} = \text{stroke volume} \times \text{heart rate}$$

This may be seen in the patient with acute heart failure and reduced stroke volume, in whom the heart rate is increased to maintain the cardiac output.

PERIPHERAL VASCULAR SYSTEM

Blood pressure in the arterial system is maintained at a constant range until the level of the terminal arterioles is reached. There is an 80 per cent drop in pressure across the arterioles. This is the site responsible for the regulation of peripheral vascular resistance. The large cross-sectional area of the capillaries results in a large drop in the velocity of blood in the aorta, from 50 cm/second to 0.05 cm/second. The main factor that keeps fluid from leaving the capillaries is the osmotic pressure of the plasma proteins. The Starling hypothesis states that hydrostatic forces are primarily responsible for fluid movement out of capillaries, whereas oncotic pressure is primarily responsible for fluid movement into capillaries. An imbalance between these forces results in edema, either peripheral or pulmonary, when there is a substantial increase in venous pressure, either systemic or pulmonary. Hydrostatic pressure exceeds oncotic pressure, and fluid moves from the capillaries into the interstitial space. In the lungs, it may eventually move into the alveoli.

Approximately 75 per cent of the total blood volume is present in the venous system. These vessels play an important role in regulating shifts in blood volume between the peripheral and central circulation.

The kidney receives approximately 20 per cent of cardiac output, and reductions in cardiac output can have a detrimental effect on renal function. Certain "regional circulations" such as the cerebral and coronary circulations and the skin and splanchnic bed are affected by autoregulatory mechanisms that can maintain or reduce blood flow during reductions in arterial pressure. The amount of oxygen delivered to the body by the heart is a product of the cardiac output and the arterial-venous oxygen difference. The kidneys have a relatively low demand for oxygen, so that the arterial-venous oxygen difference is less than for the rest of the body. In contrast, the heart extracts oxygen nearly completely from the coronary arteries. Therefore, in order to deliver increased oxygen to the myocardium, coronary blood flow must be increased.

CARDIAC OUTPUT

Under normal resting conditions in the healthy individual, cardiac output is related to the peripheral requirements of the body and is determined by venous return to the heart. The heart itself becomes the limiting factor in regulating cardiac output when it begins to fail. A state of heart failure exists when the diseased heart is unable to pump all the blood that has returned to it and is therefore unable to supply sufficient blood for the metabolic demands of the body.

HEART FAILURE

Heart failure may be caused by a number of factors, including loss of heart muscle (myocardial infarction), abnormal valve function, failure of the myocardium (cardiomyopathy), and mechanical defects that place excess stress on the heart (ventricular septal defect). As myocardial failure occurs, there is a reduction in contractility and cardiac output. As cardiac output is decreased, preload increases owing to the reduced ability of the heart to eject blood (reduced ejection fraction) and to an increase in circulating blood volume (secondary to increased retention of salt and water and edema formation). This reduction in cardiac output leads to an increase in peripheral vascular resistance (an attempt to maintain arterial blood pressure). The ensuing increase in resistance to ejection of blood by the heart leads to a further reduction in cardiac output, and a vicious circle is created.

In the presence of heart failure, certain compensatory mechanisms occur in an attempt to maintain cardiovascular compensation. These include increased venoconstriction and increased heart rate. Arterial pressure tends to be lower as the ventricle loses its capacity to generate a normal pressure.

The various therapeutic interventions employed to deal with heart failure are geared to altering three of the four factors that control cardiac performance—namely preload, contractility, and afterload. Thus, diuretics and salt restriction are used to reduce intravascular volume and preload; digitalis is employed to improve contractility of the failing myocardium; arterial dilators are used to reduce systemic resistance; and venodilators are used to redistribute blood away from the central circulation and reduce the pulmonary capillary wedge pressure.

Bibliography

Braunwald E (ed): Heart Disease: A Textbook of Cardiovascular Medicine, 3rd ed. Philadelphia, WB Saunders Company, 1987.

103 Chest Radiography and Cardiac Fluoroscopy

James T. T. Chen

In the age of high technology, conventional radiologic methods are often overlooked in favor of newer imaging modalities in the diagnosis of cardiovascular disease. This is unfortunate, since more often than not, a problem can be quickly solved and costly workups avoided by first making full use of the standard chest radiograph and cardiac fluoroscopy.

The main purpose of chest radiography is to provide anatomic details by filming with short exposure time that stops motion. Cardiac fluoroscopy, on the other hand, primarily deals with dynamic alterations or small calcifications in the heart that are discernible only in motion.

Whether by filming or fluoroscoping, the patient should be examined in at least two (posteroanterior and lateral) views and preferably four views for the first time as well as in any subsequent study called for by a new development.

CARDIAC SERIES AND ANATOMY

The standard views are (1) posteroanterior (PA) view with barium (Fig. 103–1), (2) left lateral (lateral) view with barium (Fig. 103–2), (3) right anterior oblique (RAO) view at 45 degrees with barium (Fig. 103–3), and (4) left anterior oblique (LAO) view at 60 degrees without barium (Fig. 103–4).

The obvious reason for choosing the posteroanterior and left lateral views is to minimize magnification of the image by putting the heart close to the x-ray film (or the image intensifier). The barium in the esophagus helps in the detection of certain vascular abnormalities and left atrial enlargement.

PA View

This view (Fig. 103–1) is best suited for assessment of the pulmonary vascularity and cardiac size. From top to bottom, the right cardiac border is formed by the superior vena cava, the right atrium, and occasionally the inferior vena cava. On the left side, the structures visualized are, from top to bottom, the aortic arch, the pulmonary trunk, the left atrial appendage, and the left ventricle. Normally, the inferior vena cava image is faint and is frequently obscured by the fat pad in the right cardiophrenic sulcus. The left atrial appendage merges imperceptibly with the left ventricle and cannot be recognized as a separate structure. The barium-filled esophagus descends through the mediastinum in a straight course except for a slight rightward deviation produced by the aortic arch.

In the presence of cardiomegaly, each cardiac chamber expands in a specific direction in each view. In the PA view, the right atrium dilates to the right side, as do the venae cavae (see Figs. 103–10 and 103–16*A*). The azygos vein expands rightward and superiorly (see Fig. 103–9*A*). The right ventricle expands leftward and superiorly, displacing the left-sided cardiac chambers, displacing the left-sided cardiac chambers, forming a convexity along the left cardiac border from below the pulmonary trunk to the cardiac apex. This is why isolated right ventricular enlargement causes an upturned appearance of the left ventricular apex (see Figs. 103–9*A*, 103–12, 103–16*A*, and 103–19*A*). The pulmonary trunk, when dilated, also bulges in a superolateral direction to the left (see Figs. 103–11 and 103–12).

The aorta dilates laterally and superiorly, perpendicular to its long axis. For instance, the ascending aorta bulges to the right side, the aortic arch superiorly and to the left, and the descending aorta to the left (see Figs. 103–13, 103–14*A*, 103–15*A*, 103–21, and 103–22*B*). Left atrial enlargement displaces the esophagus to the right side and the descending aorta to the left. The left ventricle enlarges leftward and inferiorly (see Figs. 103–13, 103–14*A*, 103–15*A*, and 103–22).

Lateral View

This view (Fig. 103–2) is best suited for detection of pericardial disease and cardiovascular calcifications.

The anterior contour of the cardiovascular silhouette is formed by the ascending aorta and the pulmonary trunk above and the right ventricle below. In the uppermost area, the faint images of the left

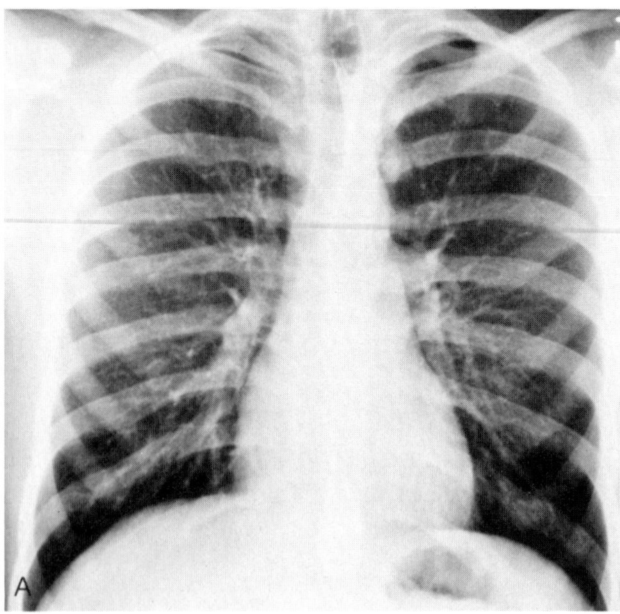

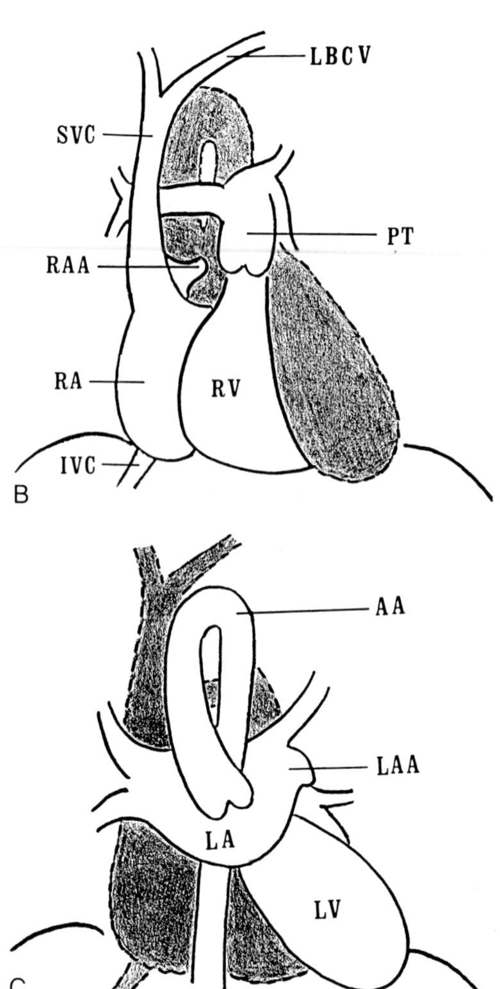

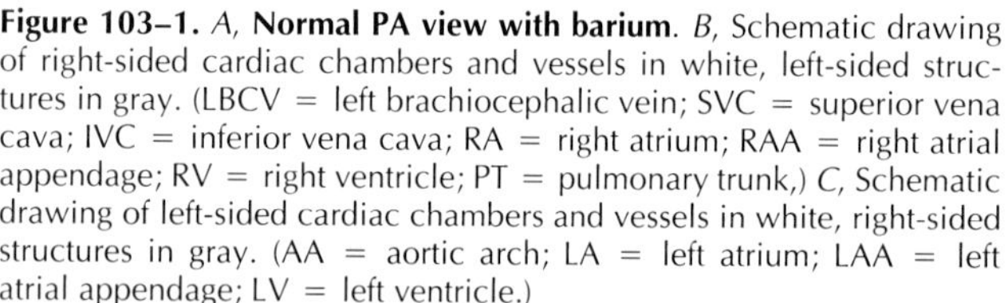

Figure 103–1. *A,* **Normal PA view with barium.** *B,* Schematic drawing of right-sided cardiac chambers and vessels in white, left-sided structures in gray. (LBCV = left brachiocephalic vein; SVC = superior vena cava; IVC = inferior vena cava; RA = right atrium; RAA = right atrial appendage; RV = right ventricle; PT = pulmonary trunk,) *C,* Schematic drawing of left-sided cardiac chambers and vessels in white, right-sided structures in gray. (AA = aortic arch; LA = left atrium; LAA = left atrial appendage; LV = left ventricle.)

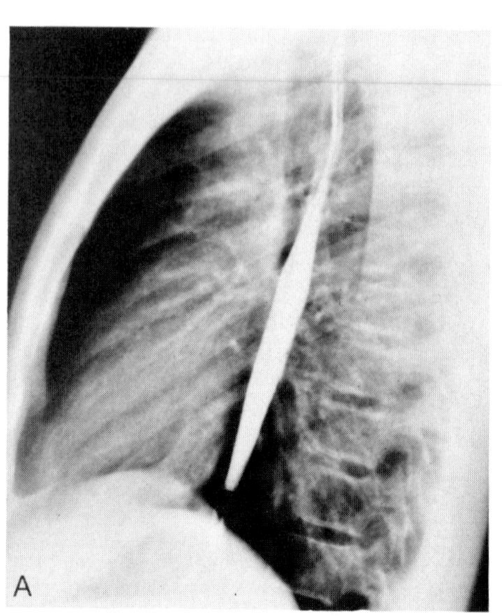

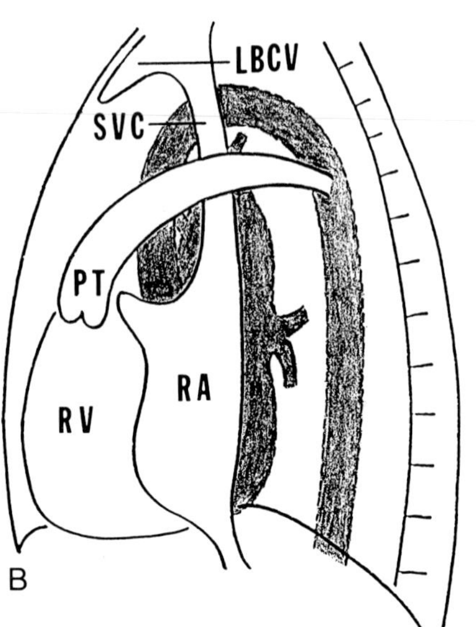

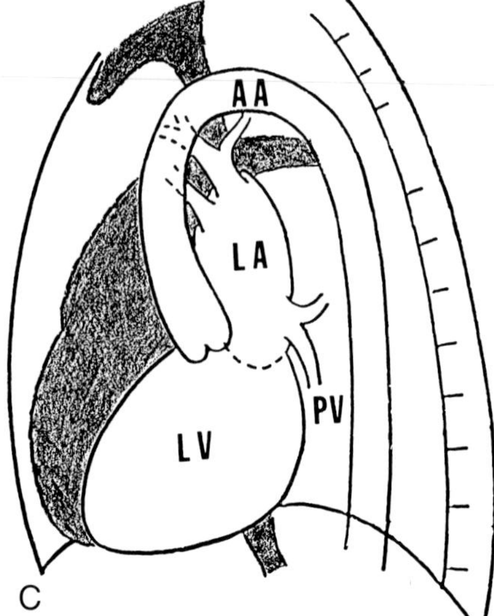

Figure 103–2. *A,* **Normal lateral view with barium.** *B,* Schematic drawing of right-sided cardiac chambers and vessels in white, left-sided structures in gray. (Abbreviations as in Figure 103–1.) *C,* Schematic drawing of left-sided cardiac chambers and vessels in white, right-sided structures in gray. (PV = pulmonary vein. Other abbreviations as in Figure 103–1.)

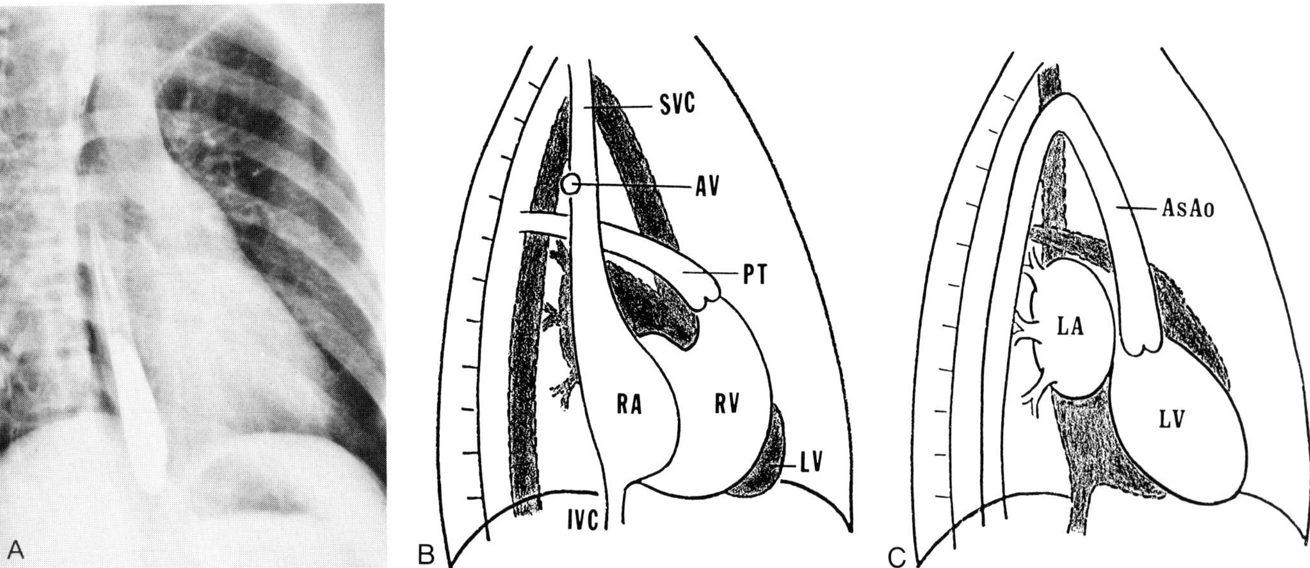

Figure 103–3. *A,* **Normal RAO view at 45 degrees with barium.** *B,* Schematic drawing of right-sided cardiac chambers in white, left-sided structures in gray. (AV = azygos vein. Other abbreviations as in Figure 103–1.) *C,* Schematic drawing of left-sided cardiac chambers and vessels in white, right-sided structures in gray. (AsAo = ascending aorta. Other abbreviations as in Figure 103–1.)

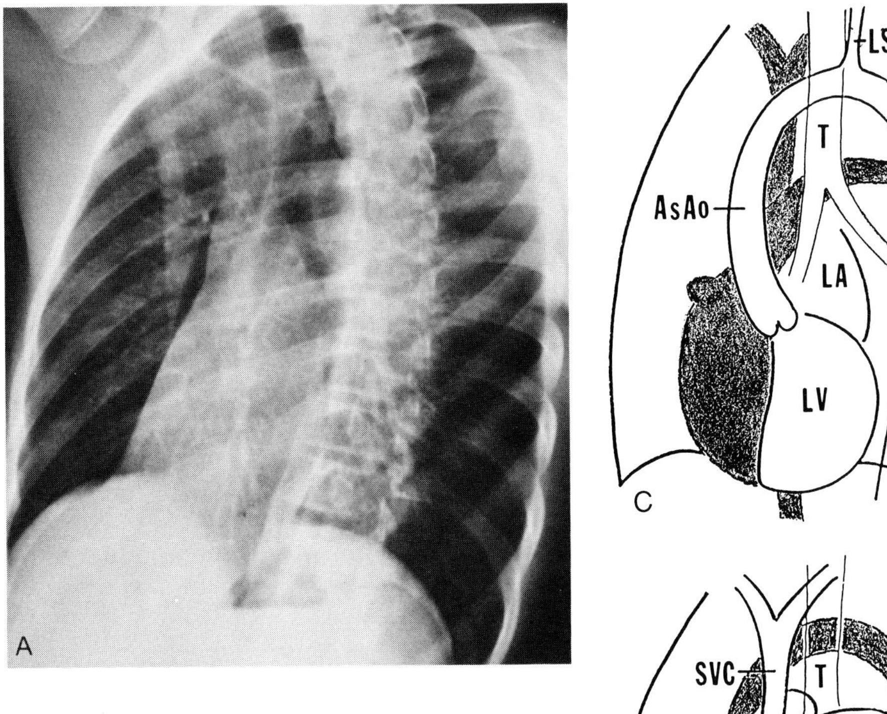

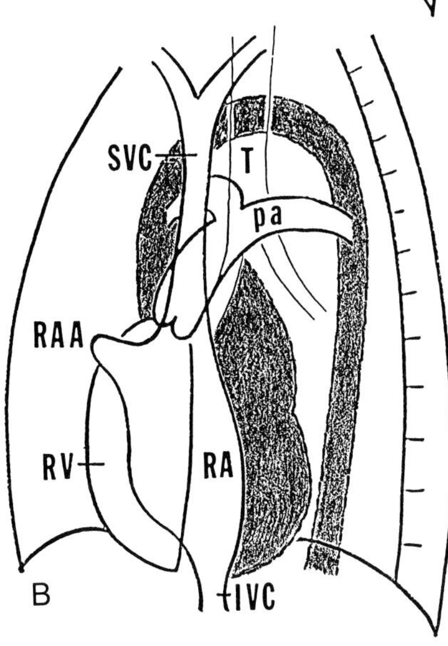

Figure 103–4. *A,* **LAO view at 60 degrees without barium.** *B,* Schematic drawing of right-sided structures in white, left-sided structures in gray. (pa = left pulmonary artery; T = trachea. Other abbreviations as in Figure 103–1.) *C,* Schematic drawing of left-sided structures in white, right-sided structures in gray. (LSA = left subclavian artery. Other abbreviations as in Figure 103–1.)

brachiocephalic vein and superior vena cava are occasionally visualized. The right ventricle abuts the sternum for a distance approximately one third of that from the diaphragm to the angle of Louis (the sternal angle). The posterior contour of the silhouette is formed, from top to bottom, by the aortic arch and the left pulmonary artery above, the left atrium and the lower lobe pulmonary veins in the middle, and the left ventricle and the inferior vena cava below. The esophagus courses behind the heart in a straight line, deviated slightly posteriorly by the aortic arch (Fig. 103–2).

The enlarged right atrium casts a double density in the lateral view that merges with the dilated inferior vena cava (see Fig. 103–16*B*). The dilated superior vena cava produces a band-like density in front of the trachea. The dilated azygos vein may show a distinct arcade below the aortic arch, obscuring the image of the left pulmonary artery (see Fig. 103–9*B*). The right ventricle enlarges anteriorly and superiorly, usually associated with a dilated pulmonary trunk that courses posteriorly and superiorly. The left atrium enlarges posteriorly below the carina, deviating the esophagus in the same direction (see Fig. 103–16*B*). Before entering the lower portion of the left atrium, the lower pulmonary veins may form a large confluence. The left ventricle enlarges posteriorly and inferiorly (see Fig. 103–14*B*).

RAO View

The RAO view at 45 degrees is a four-chamber view (Fig. 103–3). In this projection, each atrium is separate from its corresponding ventricle. The two ventricles are divided along the anterior cardiac border. The posterior (right) border of the cardiovascular silhouette is formed, from top to bottom, by the superior vena cava, the aortic arch, the azygos vein at the right tracheobronchial junction, and the left and right atria. The anterior (left) border of the silhouette is outlined, from top to bottom, by the ascending aorta, the pulmonary trunk, and the right and left ventricles. The barium-filled esophagus runs straight behind the cardiovascular silhouette, indented slightly by the aortic arch to the right side and posteriorly. The aorta for the most part folds on itself and is difficult to evaluate in this view.

As the right atrium and the inferior vena cava enlarge, they cast a triangular opacity behind the barium column without deviating its course (see Fig. 103–5*A*). This opacity is below the level of the left atrium. The dilated superior vena cava and its azygos vein bulge posteriorly and to the right side from the right border of the tracheobronchial tree. The right ventricle and its pulmonary trunk enlarge to the left side and superiorly, forming a bulge along the upper two thirds of the anterior cardiac border (see Fig. 103–5*A*). The left atrium enlarges immediately below the carina in a rightward and superior direction, deviating the esophagus and splaying the two main bronchi (see Figs. 103–5*A* and 103–6). The left ventricle enlarges in a leftward and downward direction, tending to obliterate the left costophrenic sulcus and depressing the gastric air bubble (see Fig. 103–6). Tortuosity and dilatation of the aorta cause only mild dilatation of the superior mediastinum in this projection.

LAO View

This view (Fig. 103–4) is ideal for evaluating the aorta in its entirety as well as for detecting left coronary artery calcification and for distinguishing right from left ventricular enlargement.

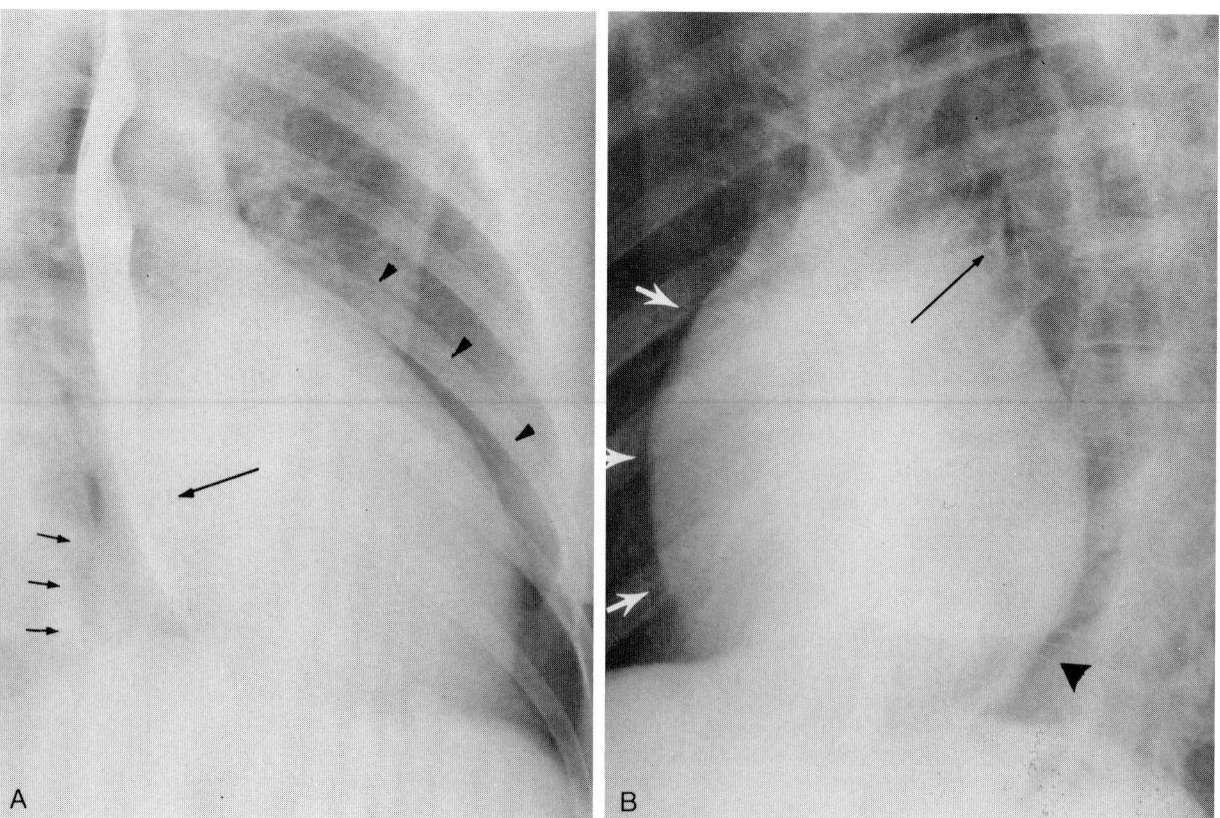

Figure 103–5. A 38-year-old woman with **severe tricuspid stenosis and moderate mitral stenosis.** *A*, RAO view shows a triangular opacity (*arrows*) behind the barium-filled esophagus representing the enlarged right atrium and inferior vena cava. Also noted is a bulge along the upper two thirds of the anterior cardiac border (*arrowheads*) representing the enlarged right ventricle and pulmonary trunk. Note that the left ventricle is normal and the left costophrenic sulcus is clear. *B*, LAO view shows bulging of the anterior cardiac border (*arrows*) representing the enlarged right heart. The left ventricle is displaced posteriorly and upward by the enlarged right ventricle, with a notch (*arrowheads*) between the two ventricles representing the lower end of the posteriorly displaced interventricular septum. The left mainstem bronchus is elevated (*long arrow*) by the enlarged left atrium.

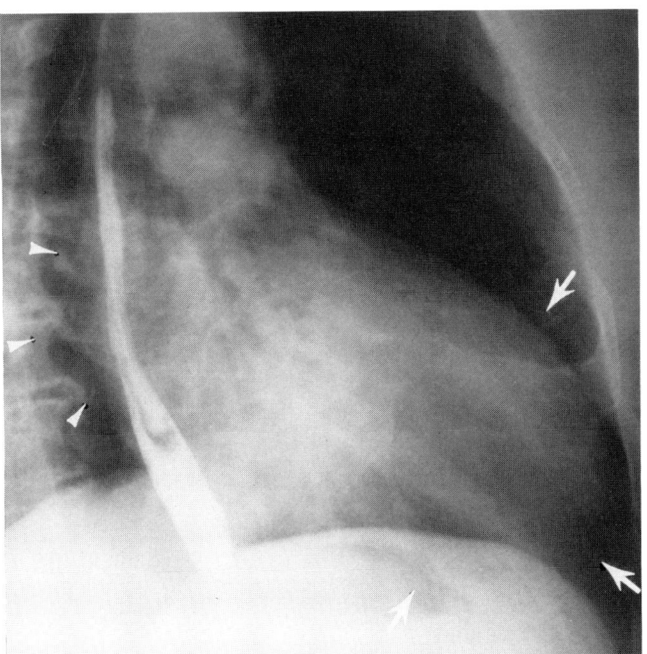

Figure 103–6. A man with **calcific aortic stenosis**. In the RAO view, the left ventricle enlarges inferiorly and leftward, obliterating the left costophrenic sulcus (*arrows*). The upper portion of the anterior cardiac border remains flat and normal in the absence of right-sided cardiomegaly. The left atrium (*arrowheads*) is mildly enlarged, splaying the two main bronchi and deviating the esophagus.

The anterior (right) contour of the cardiovascular silhouette is formed, from top to bottom, by the right brachiocephalic vein, the superior vena cava, the ascending aorta, the right atrial appendage, and the right ventricle. The posterior (left) contour of the silhouette is formed, in the same downward order, by the left subclavian artery, the aortic arch, the left pulmonary artery, the left atrium, and the left ventricle. A barium meal is usually omitted in the LAO view so that the left atrial border can be clearly seen through the aortic window. The aortic window is a clear space below the aortic arch with the tracheal bifurcation astride the left atrium. When the aorta is being evaluated, however, barium should be given to outline the aortic arch and the anteromedial border of the descending aorta.

Although the LAO view is of limited value in evaluating right atrial enlargement because this chamber is almost completely hidden in the middle of the cardiac silhouette, in general, conditions that enlarge the right atrium also enlarge the right ventricle. The right ventricle enlarges anteriorly while the left ventricle protrudes posteriorly (Fig. 103–5*B*). The left atrium expands posteriorly and superiorly, displacing and compressing the left main bronchus in that direction (Fig. 103–5*B*). The aorta is spread out in this view, so that any deviation from the norm in any segment of the organ can be clearly delineated (Fig. 103–7).

CHEST RADIOGRAPHY

Good working habits in analyzing the chest radiograph are of prime importance. The film must be examined in an orderly fashion so that no important information will be overlooked.

An Overview

The first step is to survey the radiograph, providing an overview of the entire situation. At this time, one should search briefly for noncardiac conditions and for abnormalities not directly related to the cardiovascular system that may reflect heart disease. For example, rib notching is an important clue to the diagnosis of coarctation of the aorta (Fig. 103–8). A right-sided stomach in the absence of the inferior vena cava may provide a logical explanation for an enlarged azygos vein (interruption of the inferior vena cava with azygos continuation) (Fig. 103–9).

The Lung and Its Vasculature

The lung can be likened to a mirror faithfully reflecting the underlying pathophysiology of the heart. Failure of the right side of the heart is manifested by scanty flow, small vessels, and unusually radiolucent lungs (Fig. 103–10). Failure on the left side, on the other hand, is characterized by cephalad flow and pulmonary edema. When cephalization (''redistribution'') of the pulmonary vascularity is encountered (Fig. 103–11), simple left-to-right shunts are practically excluded in favor of lesions associated with pulmonary venous hypertension. When striking cephalization of the pulmonary flow is associated with well-delineated septal lines (Kerley's B lines) in mitral stenosis (Fig. 103–11), the mitral valve area is almost always smaller than 1.3 cm^3, the mean pressure of the pulmonary artery higher than 30 mm Hg, and the pulmonary capillary wedge vein pressure higher than 20 mm Hg. A uniform increase in pulmonary vascularity (Fig. 103–12), on the other hand, suggests an uncomplicated left-to-right shunt.

Cardiac Size

Radiographic assessment of cardiac size is extremely important in the diagnosis of heart disease. The simplest way to accomplish this task is by measuring the cardiothoracic ratio. In adults, the

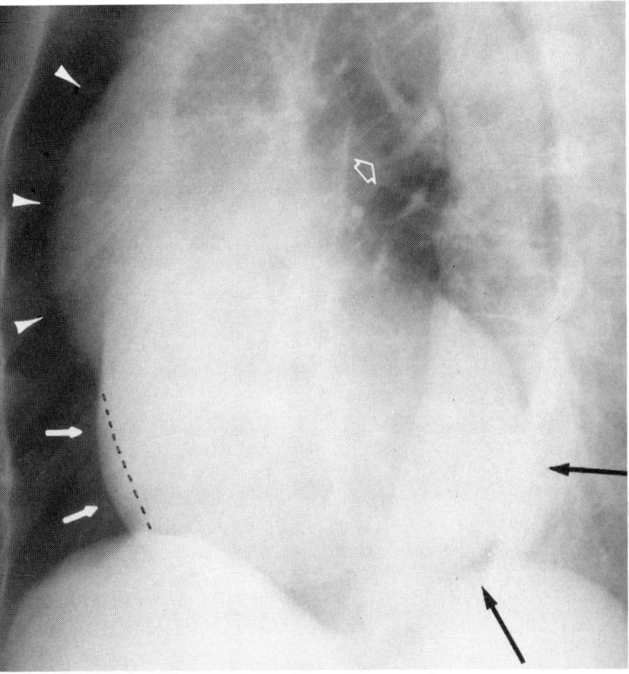

Figure 103–7. A woman with **calcific aortic stenosis**. In the LAO view, the left ventricle enlarges posteriorly and inferiorly (*long arrows*). The post-stenotic dilatation of the ascending aorta (*arrowheads*) is striking. The normal right ventricle forms a flat anterior border (*dashed line*). The breast shadow (*short arrows*) should not be confused with the right ventricular border. The left mainstem bronchus (*open arrow*) is not elevated in the absence of left atrial enlargement.

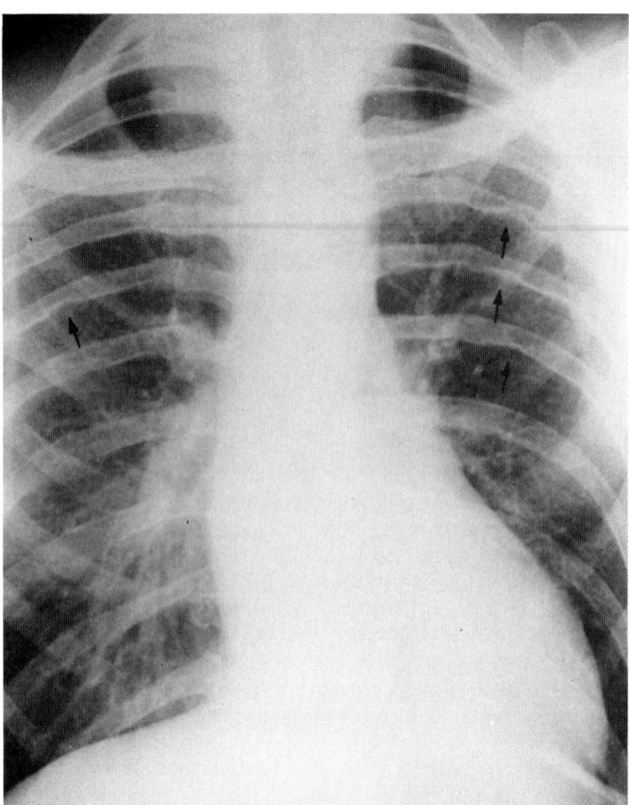

Figure 103–8. PA view of a patient with **coarctation of the aorta** showing notching of the ribs bilaterally (*arrows*).

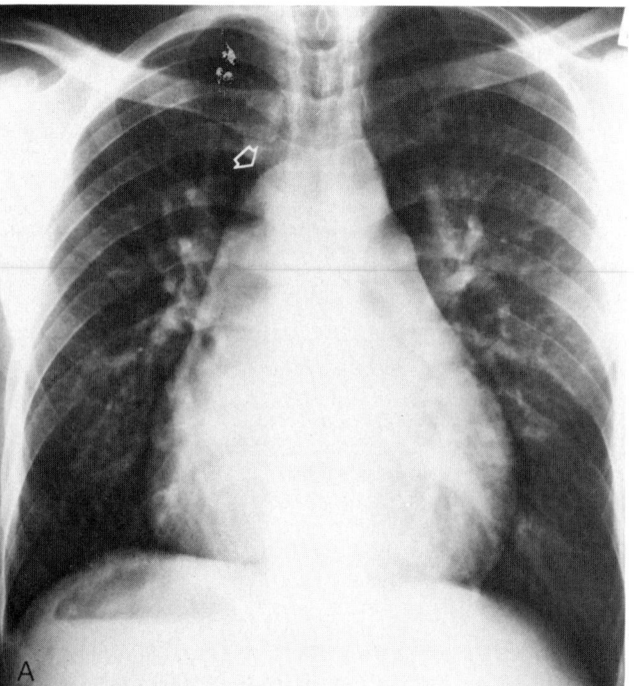

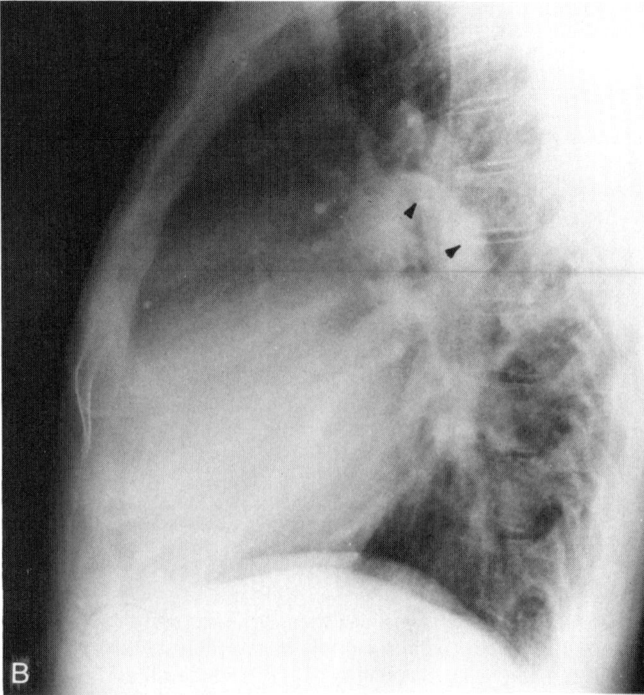

Figure 103–9. *A*, Patient with **situs ambiguus**. In the PA view, the gastric air bubble is on the right side and the aorta and cardiac apex are on the left. The azygos vein is markedly dilated (*arrow*) as a result of congenital interruption of the inferior vena cava. The pulmonary vascularity is increased because of coexisting endocardial cushion defect and a left-to-right shunt. Both the right atrium and the right ventricle are enlarged. *B*, In the lateral view, the density of the inferior vena cava is absent. The azygos arch (*arrowheads*) is huge. The pulmonary trunk and the right ventricle bulge anteriorly. (From Chen JTT: The plain radiograph in the diagnosis of cardiovascular disease. Radiol Clin North Am 21:609, 1983.)

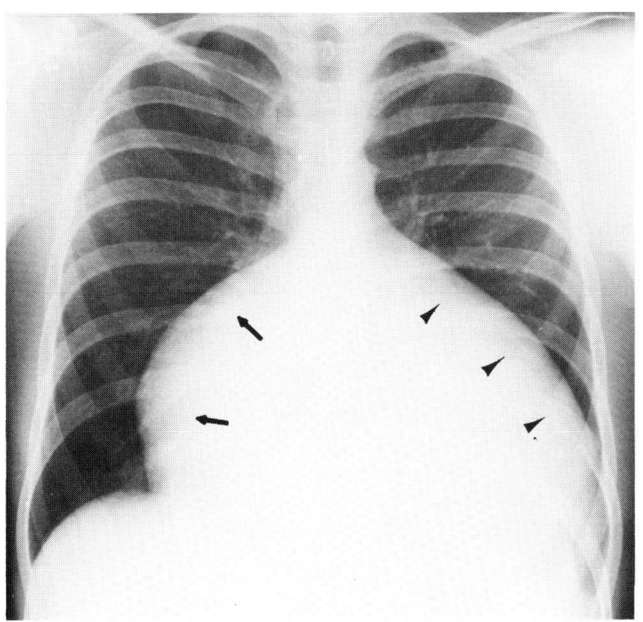

Figure 103–10. Patient with **Ebstein's anomaly**. Note the enormous dimensions of both right atrium (*arrows*) and right ventricle (*arrowheads*). The left-sided chambers are displaced posteriorly and hidden in the PA view. The pulmonary vessels are very small, and the lungs appear "hyperlucent" owing to decreased pulmonary blood flow. (From Chen JTT: The plain radiograph in the diagnosis of cardiovascular disease. Radiol Clin North Am 21:609, 1983.)

average normal value of the ratio is 0.50. In general, all enlarged hearts are abnormal hearts; when the cardiac size is within normal limits, the heart may or may not be normal. The diagnosis of an abnormally small heart (as seen in Addison's disease) often requires a retrospective observation when the heart has come back to its normal capacity after successful therapy (steroids in this case).

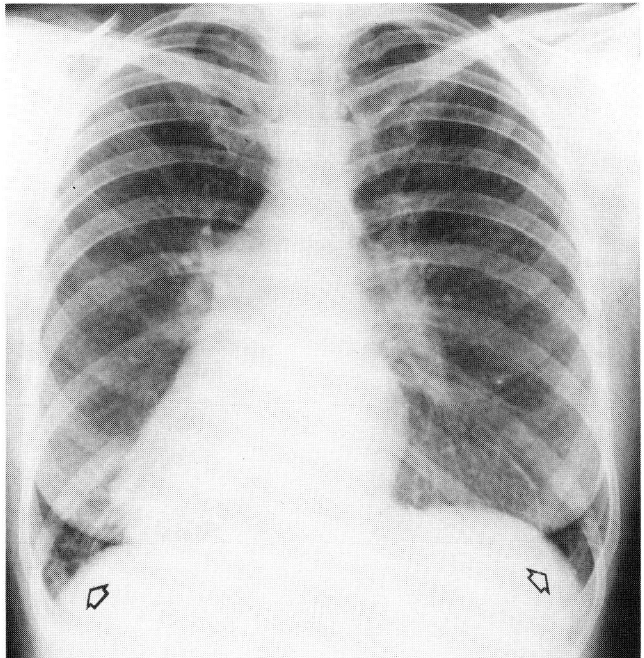

Figure 103–11. Patient with **severe rheumatic mitral stenosis**. Note the dilated upper vessels and the constricted lower vessels and Kerley B lines (*arrows*) in the costophrenic sulci. The pulmonary trunk is prominent, and the aorta is inconspicuous. (From Chen JTT: The plain radiograph in the diagnosis of cardiovascular disease. Radiol Clin North Am 21:609, 1983.)

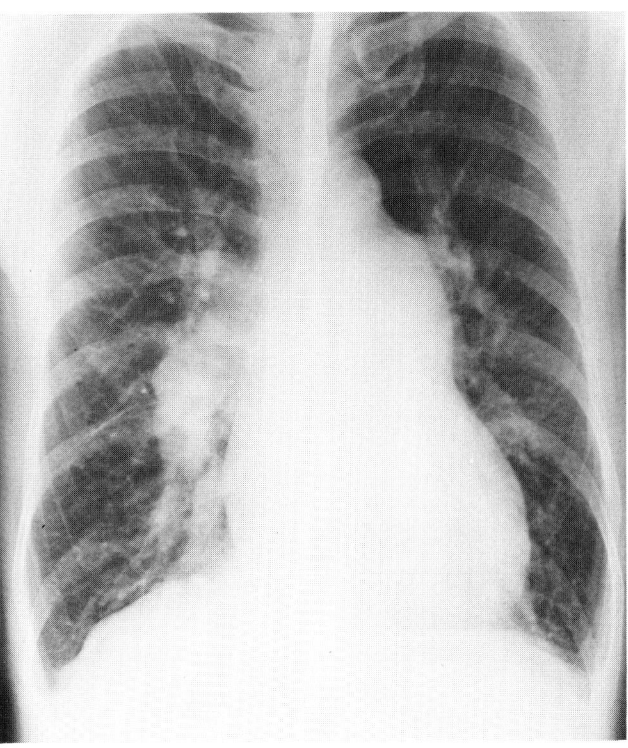

Figure 103–12. Patient with a large **secundum atrial septal defect**. Note the diffuse increase in pulmonary vascularity; cardiomegaly with rounded, upturned apex (right ventricular enlargement); small aorta; and large pulmonary trunk. (From Chen JTT: The plain radiograph in the diagnosis of cardiovascular disease. Radiol Clin North Am 21:609, 1983.)

Gross cardiomegaly without signs of congestive heart failure suggests a problem of volume overload. This could be the result of valvular regurgitation, hyperkinetic state, or severe bradycardia with prolonged filling time (Fig. 103–13). At this stage, the left ventricle is significantly dilated with excessive volume. Pressure abnormalities are not reflected in the pulmonary vascular bed until there is cardiac decompensation. On the other hand, mild cardiomegaly frequently results from lesions associated with pressure overload states. This is exemplified by a patient with a severe aortic stenosis prior to congestive heart failure (Fig. 103–14). At this point, the left ventricle is operating against high pressure but with normal or reduced volume. The pulmonary vascularity remains normal. The heart is only mildly enlarged, with a cardiothoracic ratio slightly greater than 0.50. The convexity of the left lower cardiac border is increased, and the Hoffman-Rigler sign of left ventricular enlargement is positive. All these findings are in keeping with left ventricular pressure overload without dilatation. As soon as the left ventricle fails, however, the heart begins to dilate and the lungs become congested with edema.

The diagnosis of a volume overload lesion such as aortic regurgitation is preferred to that of a pressure overload lesion (e.g., aortic stenosis) when gross left ventricular enlargement is associated with normal pulmonary vascularity. In aortic stenosis or other entities causing pressure overload of the left ventricle (e.g., hypertrophic cardiomyopathy, systemic hypertension), the heart almost never reaches such a magnitude without some radiographic evidence of pulmonary venous hypertension. When pressure alone is at fault, significant cardiomegaly is usually associated with cardiac decompensation and congestive heart failure.

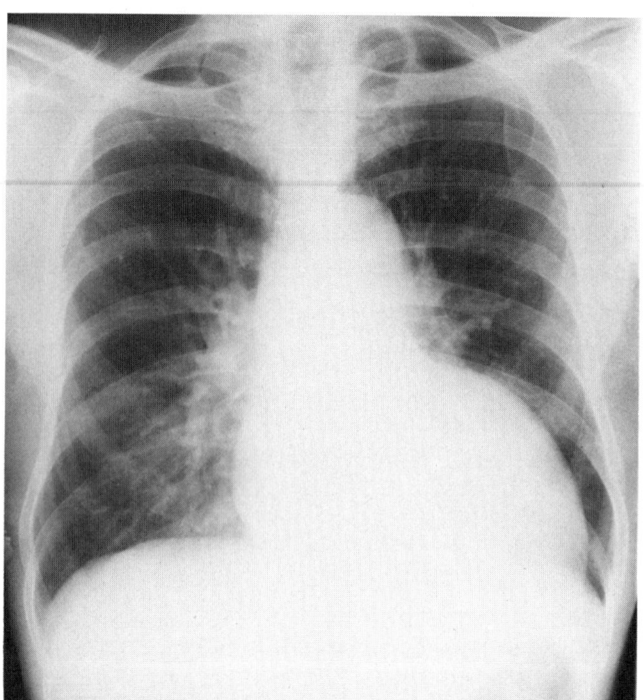

Figure 103–13. Patient with **severe aortic regurgitation**. The pulmonary vascularity is normal. Note the marked enlargement of the left ventricle and diffuse dilatation of the aorta due to volume overload. The cardiothoracic ratio is 0.60. Lateral view (not shown) gave a Hoffman-Rigler measurement of 3.8 cm (normal < 1.8 cm). (From Chen JTT: The plain radiograph in the diagnosis of cardiovascular disease. Radiol Clin North Am 21:609, 1983.)

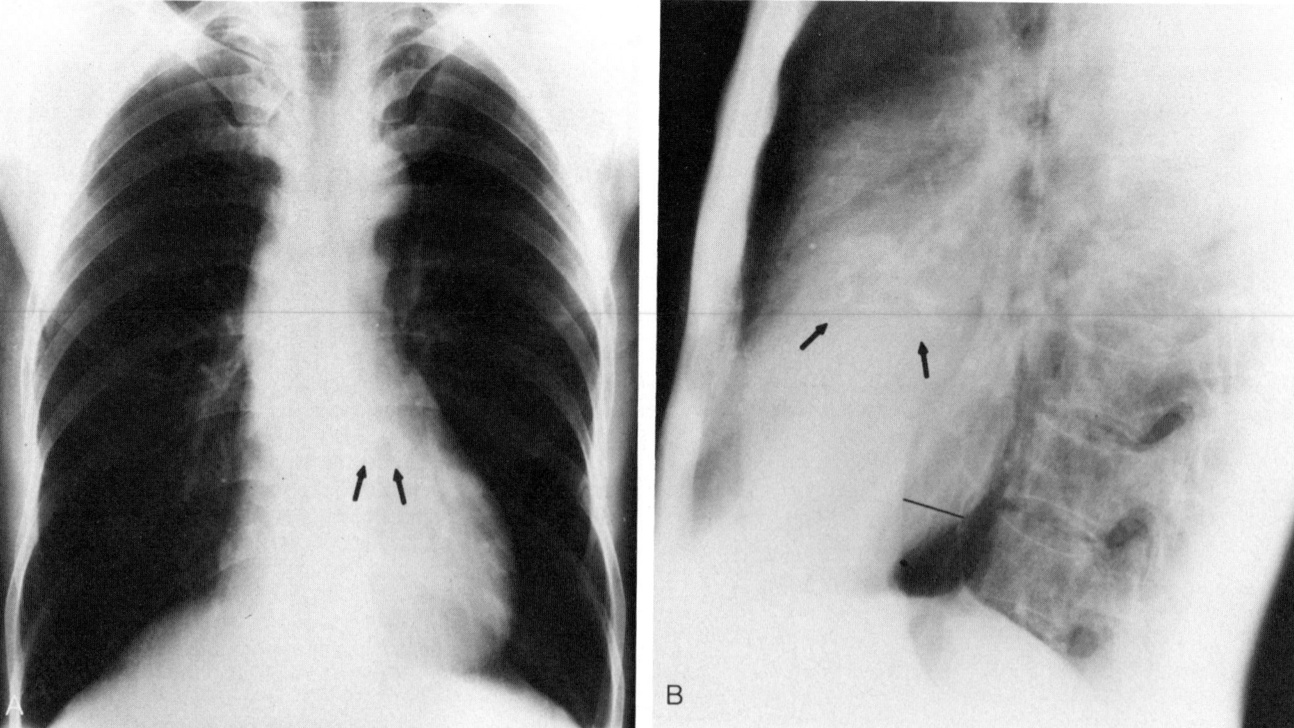

Figure 103–14. *A*, Patient with **severe aortic stenosis**. The pulmonary vascularity is normal and the heart is only mildly enlarged, with a cardiothoracic ratio of 0.50. *B*, Hoffman-Rigler measurement of 2.2 cm (normal < 1.8 cm) is present (*horizontal line*) on lateral view. Note the dilated ascending aorta and the calcified aortic valve (*arrows*). (From Chen JTT: The plain radiograph in the diagnosis of cardiovascular disease. Radiol Clin North Am 21:609, 1983.)

Cardiac Contour

The radiologist must become familiar with the normal contour of the heart and great vessels in each view, must learn the various conditions that may cause an odd shape of the heart, and finally must remember the pathologic anatomy associated with a variety of cardiac conditions.

In Figure 103–15*A*, a bulge is found along the left lower cardiac border in the PA view. In the lateral view (Fig. 103–15*B*), the density is situated anteriorly. There are sharply demarcated borders laterally, anteriorly, and superiorly. The pulmonary vascularity appears within normal limits, as do other cardiopulmonary structures. Here, the most essential radiologic assessment of the problem lies in the analysis of the unusual cardiac contour. First, the anterior location of the bulge seems to suggest a right ventricular problem. However, the sharp anterosuperior margins of the opacity suggest a lesion separated from the right ventricle by the air-filled lung. Furthermore, the site of the lesion is too low for the right ventricle. This favors its being in the region of the left ventricle. In the PA view, the lesion is inseparable from the image of the left ventricle. At this point, the most likely diagnosis is a left ventricular aneurysm. This argument is further strengthened by the location of most ventricular aneurysms in the anterolateral and apical segments of the left ventricle.

Abnormal Opacities

An enlarged left atrium creates a "double density" in the PA view. A similar double opacity is cast by an enlarged right atrium in the lateral view (Fig. 103–16*B*). One must also search diligently for intracardiac calcifications, which are always clinically significant. Any radiographic evidence of cardiac valve calcification is diagnostic of stenosis of that valve with or without associated regurgitation. The heavier the calcium is, the narrower the valve becomes regardless of other signs. Calcification of the coronary artery indicates the presence of advanced atherosclerosis. When chest pain is associated with such a calcification (Fig. 103–17), over 94 per cent of the patients will have angiographic evidence of occlusive coronary disease.

Abnormal Lucencies

Abnormal lucencies in and around the heart are seen in a variety of conditions. The tracheobronchial tree may be displaced by enlarged cardiovascular structures and become conspicuous. For example, a right-sided aortic arch with aberrant left subclavian artery may cause marked leftward and anterior displacement of the trachea, which reflects the underlying arch anomaly. A huge left atrium almost always displaces the major bronchi. The presence of pericardial effusion, thickening, or both, often provides a background of water density, which is outlined by the subepicardial fat stripe and the apical fat pad (Fig. 103–18).

Great Vessels

Examination of the great vessels is an integral part of the radiographic diagnosis of heart disease. General dilatation of the aorta (see Fig. 103–13) with increased pulsation is the hallmark of severe aortic regurgitation. Selective enlargement of the ascending aorta, on the other hand, is suggestive of aortic stenosis (see Fig. 103–14). The position of the aortic arch may strongly suggest or militate against congenital cardiac defects (Figs. 103–19 and 103–20). A "snowman" cardiovascular configuration (in the case of total anomalous pulmonary venous connection) is formed, in part, by the dilated systemic veins in the mediastinum. The "figure 3" sign of the descending aorta and the "reversed 3" sign on the barium-filled esophagus (Fig. 103–21) not only diagnose but also pinpoint the site of coarctation of the aorta.

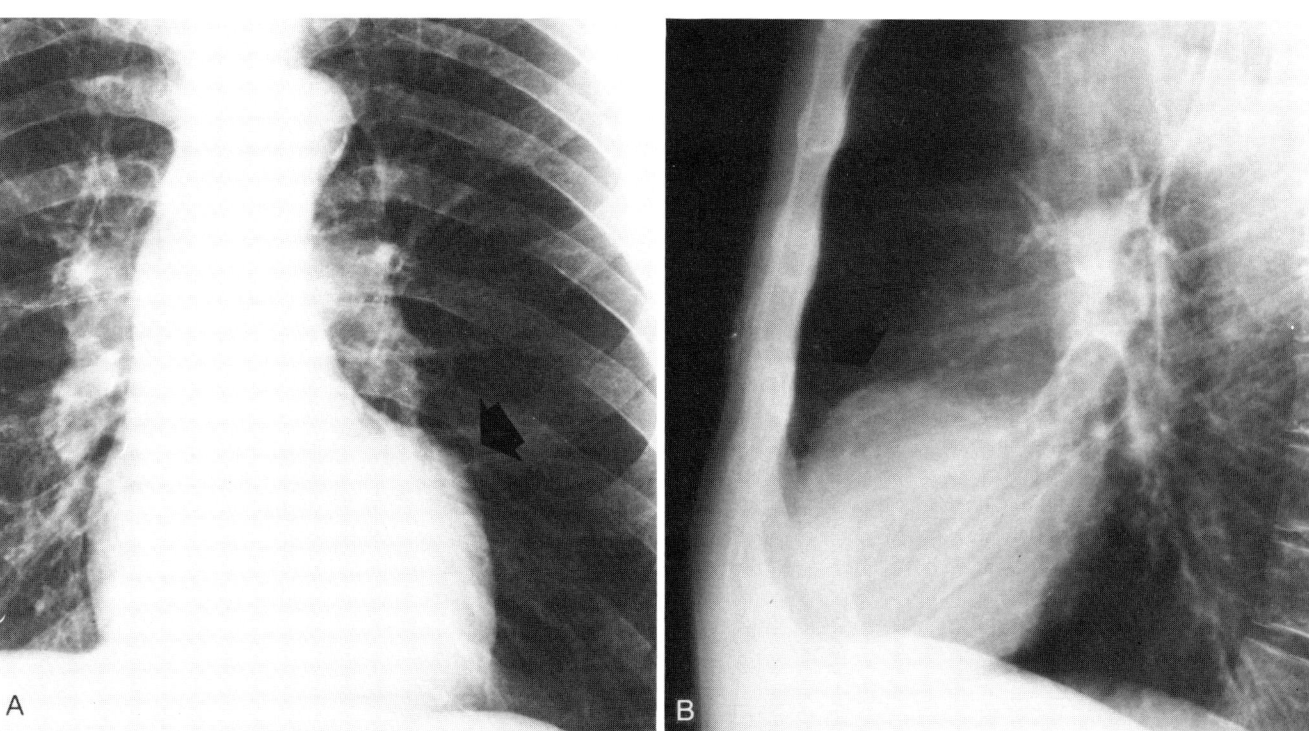

Figure 103–15. *A*, PA view. Patient with a **large left ventricular aneurysm of the anterolateral wall**. A bulge (*arrow*) is noted to arise from the left cardiac border and protrude anteriorly and to the left. Note the sharply demarcated borders anteriorly, superiorly, and on the left, representing a continuous air-water interface separated from the right ventricle. *B*, Lateral view. The aneurysm casts a double density shadow on the right ventricle in the lateral view. (From Chen JTT: The plain radiograph in the diagnosis of cardiovascular disease. Radiol Clin North Am 21:609, 1983.)

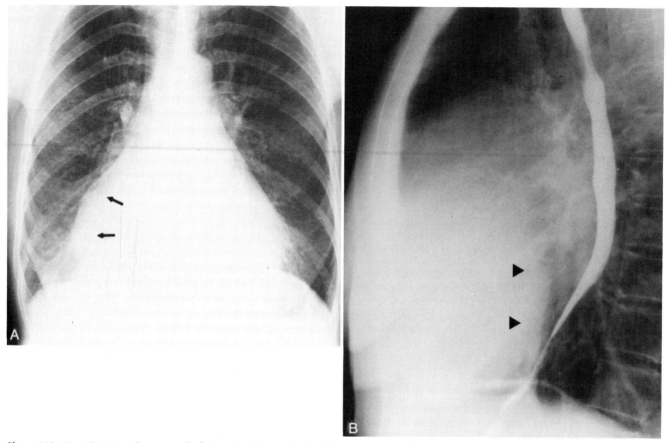

Figure 103–16. *A*, Patient with **severe mitral stenosis**, right ventricular failure, and tricuspid regurgitation. Note the large right atrium (*arrows*) in the PA view. *B*, A double density (*arrowheads*) is present in the lateral view and represents the dilated right atrium. (From Chen JTT: The plain radiograph in the diagnosis of cardiovascular disease. Radiol Clin North Am 21:609, 1983.)

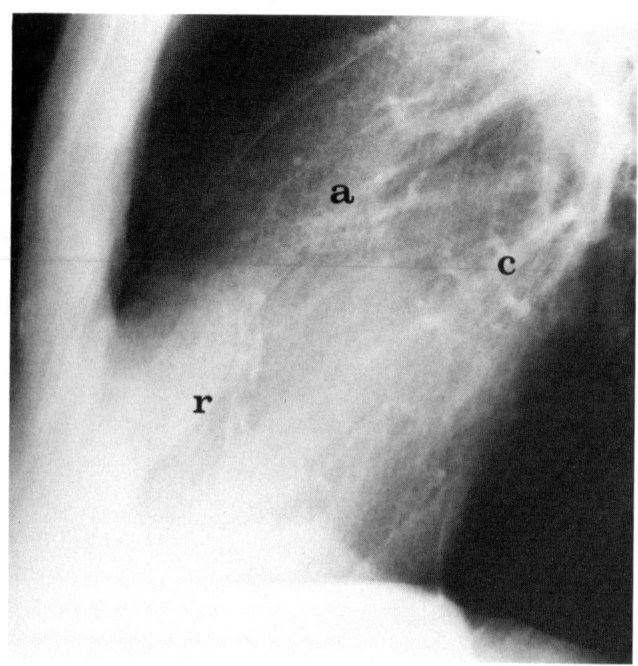

Figure 103–17. Patient with **angina pectoris**. Note the calcified coronary arteries. (a = anterior descending artery; c = circumflex artery; r = right coronary artery.) This patient had angiographic evidence of subtotal obstruction of all three vessels. (From Chen JTT: The plain radiograph in the diagnosis of cardiovascular disease. Radiol Clin North Am 21:609, 1983.)

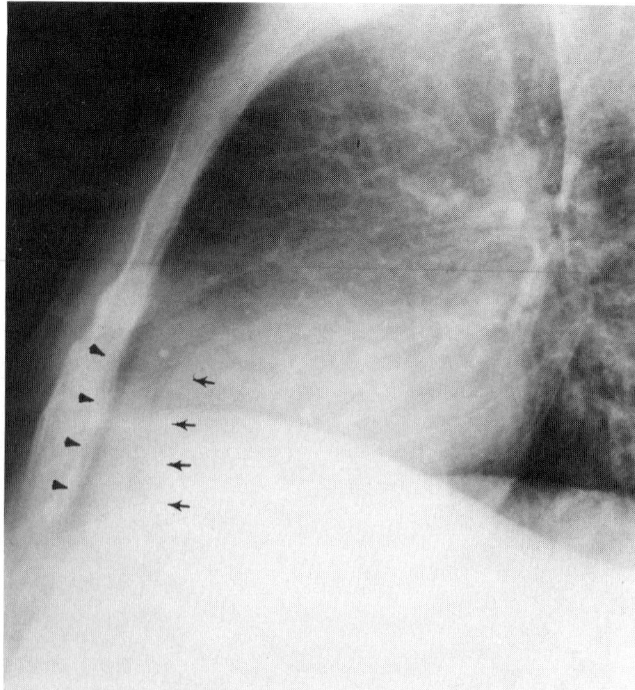

Figure 103–18. Patient with **pericardial effusion** showing widening of the pericardial density sandwiched between the subepicardial fat stripe (*arrows*) and apical fat pad (*arrowheads*) in the lateral view. (From Chen JTT: The plain radiograph in the diagnosis of cardiovascular disease. Radiol Clin North Am 21:609, 1983.)

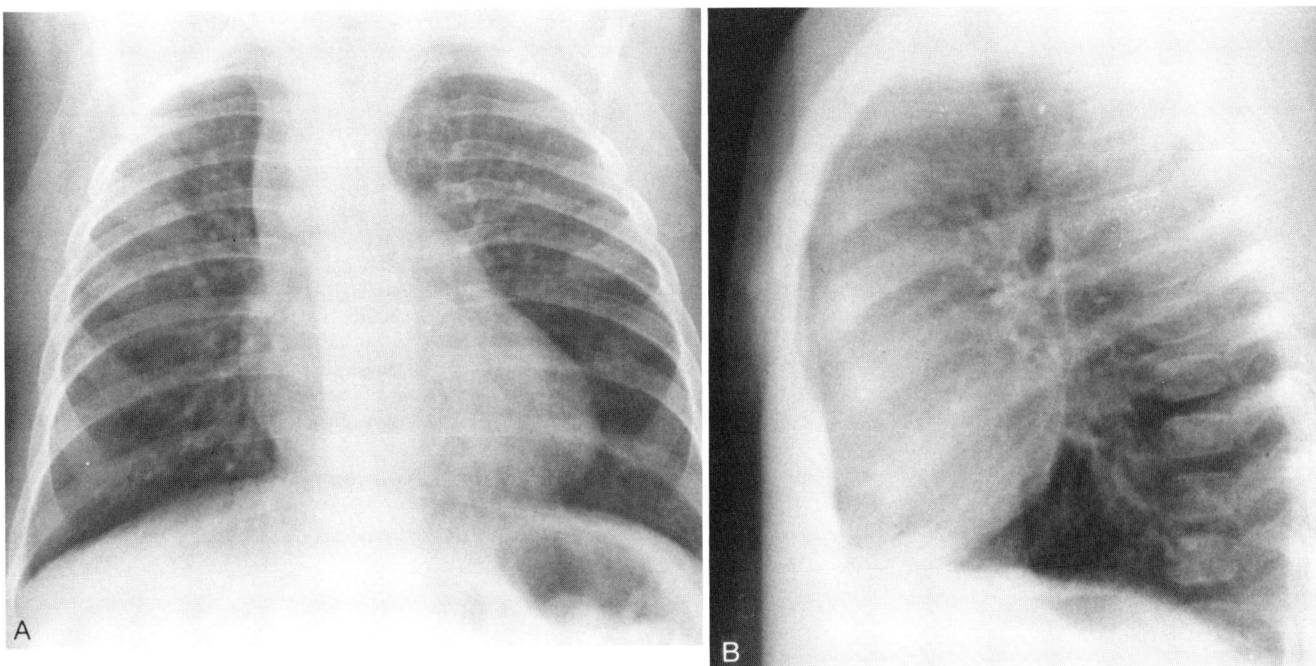

Figure 103–19. *A,* PA view. Patient with **a right-sided aortic arch with mirror image branching**. The trachea is deviated to the left and posteriorly. Note the decreased pulmonary vascularity in this infant with tetralogy of Fallot. *B,* Lateral view. (From Chen JTT: The plain radiograph in the diagnosis of cardiovascular disease. Radiol Clin North Am 21:609, 1983.)

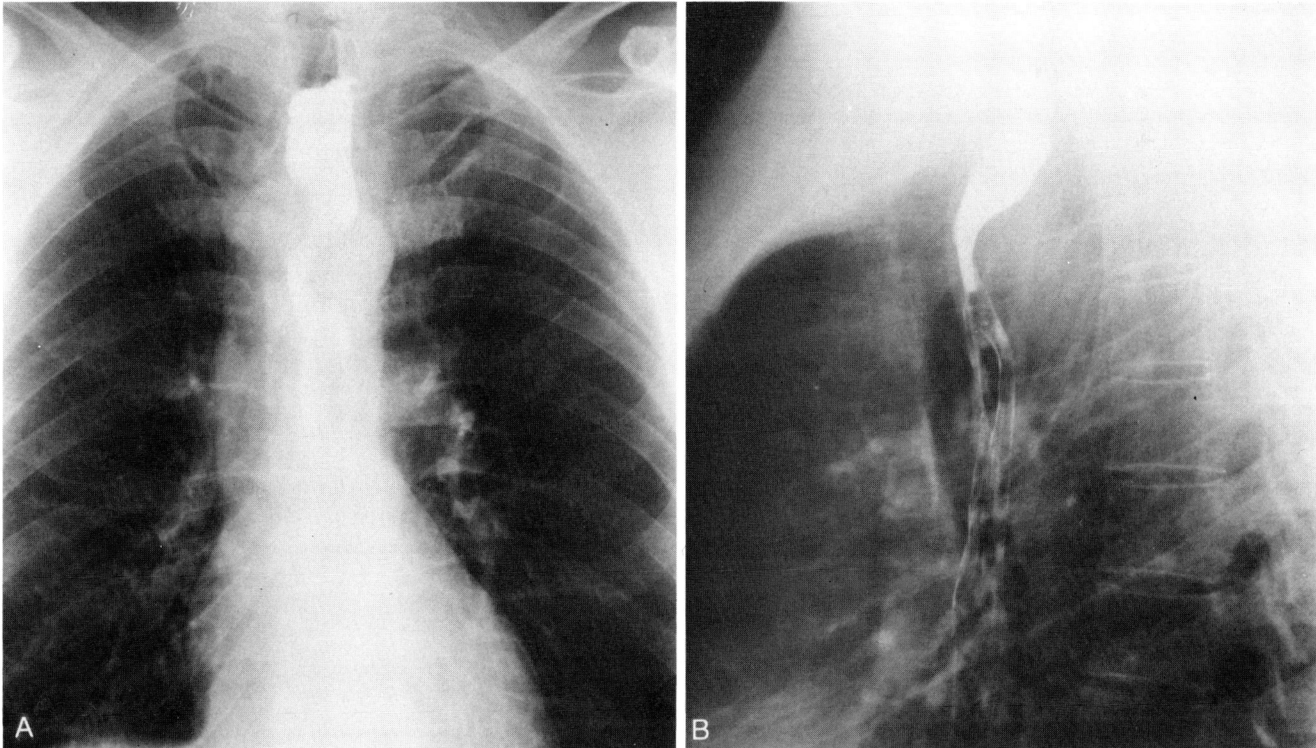

Figure 103–20. *A,* Patient with **a double aortic arch**. Note the bilateral indentation on the esophagus on the PA view. *B,* Posterior indentation on the esophagus and anterior indentation on the trachea are demonstrated on the lateral view. The patient's heart is entirely normal, however. (From Chen JTT: The plain radiograph in the diagnosis of cardiovascular disease. Radiol Clin North Am 21:609, 1983.)

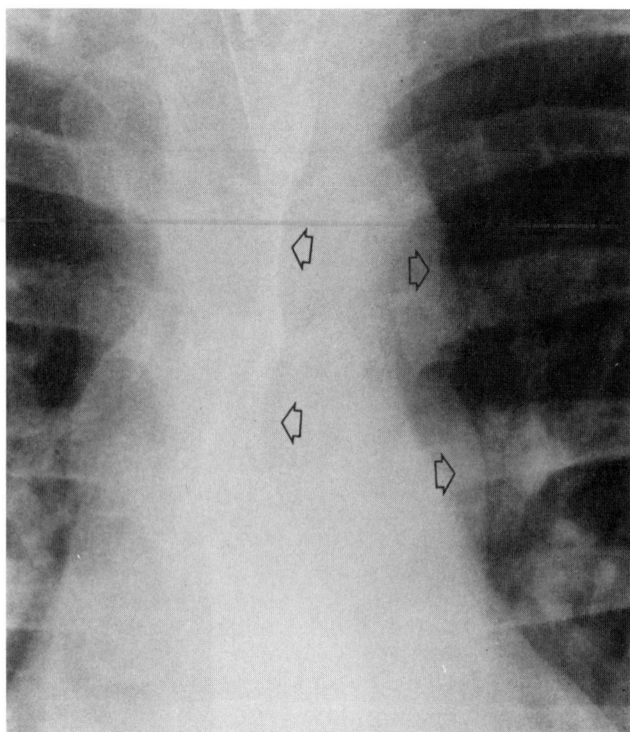

Figure 103–21. Patient with **coarctation of the aorta**. Note the "3" sign (*right arrows*) on the descending aorta and the "reversed 3" sign, or "E" sign (*left arrows*), on the barium-filled esophagus. (From Chen JTT: The plain radiograph in the diagnosis of cardiovascular disease. Radiol Clin North Am 21:609, 1983.)

Pleura

Failure of the left side of the heart is typically associated with a right-sided pleural effusion. Bilateral pleural effusion is suggestive of biventricular heart failure. Unilateral left-sided effusion is suggestive of a noncardiac problem. An interlobar collection of pleural fluid ("pseudotumor," or "vanishing tumor") is an unusual manifestation of congestive heart failure.

Statistical Guidance

Some radiographic findings are by themselves diagnostic of a disease because they directly disclose the underlying pathoanatomy and pathophysiology. Other signs are indirectly suggestive of the diagnosis on statistical grounds alone. However, the latter can have such a high predictive value of disease that they should be used routinely in clinical medicine. For instance, the incidence of congenital heart disease is 100-fold greater than normal when a right aortic arch with mirror-image branching is present. Ninety per cent of the congenital defects found in this setting are tetralogy of Fallot (see Fig. 103–19). Therefore, all patients with such an arch anomaly should be scrutinized for the overwhelming probability of having cyanotic heart disease. Double aortic arch typically compresses both the esophagus and the trachea (see Fig. 103–20) but only rarely coexists with intracardiac defects.

Clinical Correlation

When the objective analysis of the radiograph is completed, one should correlate the radiographic signs with the clinical, hemodynamic, and other measures before drawing the final conclusion. At this point, re-examination of the radiograph, the patient, or both may be necessary. After detailed roentgen analysis of some finer points, a correct diagnosis may be strengthened or a wrong impression corrected.

To avoid bias, it is desirable to first interpret the radiograph without prior clinical knowledge. Both the clinical and the radiologic diagnoses may be correct but not consistent. For example, the clinical manifestations of a ventricular septal defect may be convincing, but the roentgen signs may be within normal limits. This is explained by the fact that a left-to-right shunt with a pulmonary-to-systemic flow ratio less than 2-to-1 is very difficult, if not impossible, to detect radiographically. On the other hand, a large secundum atrial septal defect may occasionally be misdiagnosed as mitral stenosis because of similar physical findings. The radiographic features are, however, characteristic for atrial septal defect (see Fig. 103–12) and essentially rule out mitral stenosis (see Fig. 103–11).

CARDIAC FLUOROSCOPY

Indications

Cardiac fluoroscopy is indicated for the following reasons: (1) to evaluate cardiovascular dynamics; (2) to detect cardiovascular calcification; (3) to help visualize delicate fat stripes; (4) to differentiate cardiac from noncardiac diseases; (5) to evaluate cardiac pacemakers, valve prostheses, and radiopaque foreign bodies; and (6) to assist cardiac catheterization and angiocardiography.

Methodology

There are four basic positions in which fluoroscopy of heart disease is accomplished: the PA view, the lateral view, the RAO view, and the LAO view. The degree of rotation for oblique views varies between 20 and 70 degrees, depending on what particular structures one is trying to visualize. For instance, to see calcified left coronary arteries, a shallow LAO view at 25 to 35 degrees is optimal. On the other hand, to see a calcified aortic valve, a 60-degree LAO view is usually required. A 45-degree RAO view is ideal for evaluating right atrial size but unsuitable for the aortic valve, which is more clearly seen with a shallower RAO view. Barium meal is used only after a thorough search for cardiovascular calcifications has been completed.

The x-ray exposure should be adjusted for each view, depending on the body thickness in that view. Therefore, relatively speaking, the least exposure is needed for the PA view and the most for the lateral view. The proper exposures for the oblique views fall somewhere in between according to the obliquity actually chosen. As a rule, the kilovoltage ranges from 75 to 120, and the milliamperage varies between 1.5 and 3.5. Excessive milliamperage produces an undesirable glow, blurring off the interfaces between structures. Too high a kilovoltage reduces the contrast of the image. The shortest fluoroscopic time and the smallest shutter opening are recommended to reduce radiation exposure to the patient. The average time for fluoroscopic examination by this author is about three minutes.

The patient is usually examined in the erect position. A recumbent position is preferred, however, under special conditions, such as (1) extreme obesity, (2) very small calcifications, and (3) equivocal cardiac asynergy. When an obese patient is recumbent, the thick layers of soft tissue are compressed and pushed aside, thereby improving the fluoroscopic image. For an obese or slim patient, the cardiac output increases and the heart rate decreases in nearly all patients as soon as they lie down. Furthermore, the heart seems to be more "relaxed" and less affected by gravity when the patient is in the recumbent position. All these factors, physiologic or mechanical, tend to bring about a truer and more representative picture of cardiac contractility. For the same reasons, smaller calcific foci are more likely to be seen in this position.

Patients should hold their breath during cardiac fluoroscopy, but this is not absolutely necessary. Suspension of respiration after taking a small breath is ideal. Holding too big a breath, particularly if associated with an involuntary Valsalva maneuver, tends to produce a false-positive asynergy of the left ventricle. Hyperventilation or prolonged breath-holding may provoke premature ventricular contractions or fainting spells. Short and easy suspension of respiration, on the other hand, helps eliminate all motion except the rhythmic movements from the cardiovascular system. If the patient cannot hold his or her breath, a slow, quiet breathing pattern should be encouraged.

Evaluation of Cardiovascular Dynamics

Fluoroscopy is particularly suited to the evaluation of cardiovascular dynamics. It provides a continuous vision of the moving organs throughout the cardiac cycle. By noting the strength, character, and rhythm of the heart and great vessels, the radiologist can frequently infer underlying pathophysiology. For example, vigorous pulsations of the entire thoracic aorta (see Fig. 103–22*B*) are the hallmark of aortic regurgitation, while increased pulsations are confined to the ascending aorta in aortic stenosis. Standard chest radiographs obtained at random most frequently provide a diastolic image of the heart. Fluoroscopic observation, on the other hand, encompasses all images from systole to diastole. Since many cardiac lesions manifest their abnormalities only in systole, the diagnosis can easily be missed if fluoroscopy is not used. Young adults and children with severe aortic regurgitation may not show an enlarged aorta radiographically (Fig. 103–22*A*) as expected. The striking systolic expansion of the whole aorta, however, is readily appreciated fluoroscopically and is diagnostic of the disease (Fig. 103–22*B*).

In mitral regurgitation, there may not be any radiographic evidence of left atrial enlargement, but fluoroscopically, the exaggerated systolic expansion of the left atrium is typical for mitral regurgitation. The enlarging left atrium in systole can wedge between the barium-filled esophagus and the descending aorta, pushing them apart. This phenomenon has been termed "the posterior wedging sign of mitral insufficiency" (Fig. 103–23). Sometimes intermittent left atrial enlargement is noted in patients with a large atrial myxoma. Since this tumor may move to and fro across the mitral valve on a long pedicle, the volume of the left atrium increases only during systole when the mass is within the chamber. A similar phenomenon is also observed in patients with severe prolapse of the mitral valve with or without mitral insufficiency. This sign is more easily appreciated when the esophagus is filled with barium paste.

In a large left-to-right shunt, there is a uniform increase in pulmonary blood flow. The caliber and length of all pulmonary vessels increase throughout both lungs. The dynamic aspect of these changes is represented by the increased amplitude of pulsation of all the vessels. When discrepancy in size and pulsation gradually develops between the central and the peripheral vessels, one should be alerted to the possibility of Eisenmenger's syndrome.

In valvular pulmonary stenosis with an intact ventricular septum, there is an uneven distribution of pulmonary blood flow with more blood circulating to the left lung at the expense of the right. The dynamic expression of this pathophysiology includes (1) a striking increase in the pulsation of the dilated pulmonary trunk and the left pulmonary artery, and (2) a decrease in the pulsation of the smaller right pulmonary artery.

Detection of Small Cardiovascular Calcifications

One of the most useful functions of fluoroscopy is its ability to detect and localize small cardiovascular calcifications. Even a tiny

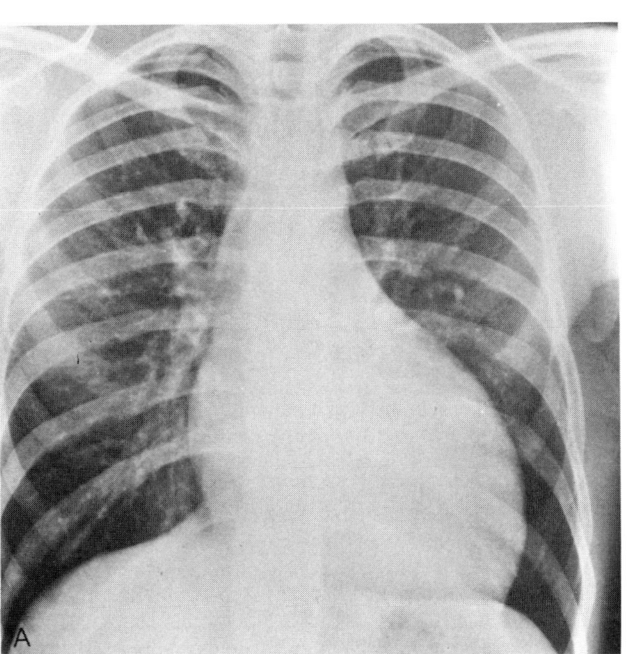

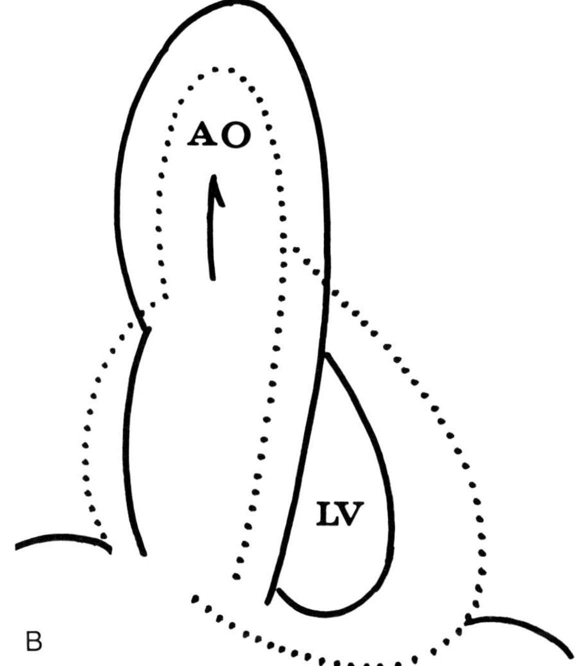

Figure 103–22. 20-year-old patient with **severe aortic regurgitation**. *A*, Posteroanterior radiograph shows a large left ventricle with normal pulmonary vascularity and normal aorta. *B*, A schematic drawing of the patient's fluoroscopic findings: The dotted lines depict the diastolic status of the heart and the aorta, the solid lines the systolic. Note the normal aorta (AO) and the dilated left ventricle (LV) in diastole, and the dilated aorta and a smaller left ventricle in systole. (From Chen JTT: Cardiac fluoroscopy. Cardiol Clin North Am 1:565, 1983.)

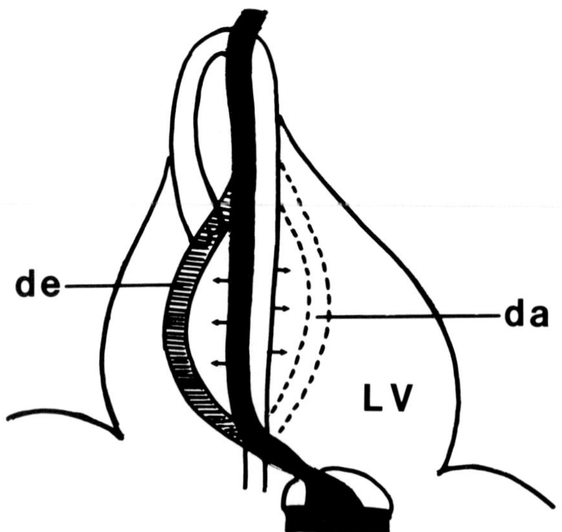

Figure 103–23. Schematic drawing depicting **posterior wedging sign of mitral insufficiency**. The aorta *(white)* and the esophagus *(black)* are together in diastole. They are separated by the enlarging left atrium in systole. (de = laterally displaced esophagus; da = laterally displaced aorta. Arrows point to the direction of displacement of the respective organs. LV = left ventricle.) (From Chen JTT: Cardiac fluoroscopy. Cardiol Clin North Am 1:565, 1983.)

fleck of calcium in the wall of the coronary artery can be clearly seen fluoroscopically by virtue of its vigorous rhythmic movement. On the contrary, such small calcifications are frequently fuzzed out by motion on the standard chest radiograph. Large calcifications (a calcified aortic valve or extensive pericardial calcifications) can be seen in certain views of the chest radiograph (see Fig. 103–14). At times, even large cardiac calcifications require fluoroscopy for their clarification and confirmation.

Diagnosing and localizing cardiac calcifications are of major clinical importance. In the adult population, the presence of calcium in the mitral valve almost always indicates rheumatic mitral stenosis. Calcification of the left atrial wall is associated with severe rheumatic mitral stenosis with a high incidence of mural thrombi and arterial embolization. The degree of calcification of a cardiac valve is proportional to the severity of stenosis of that valve.

The significance of coronary artery calcification has been reemphasized in the literature. The combination of chest pain and any fluoroscopically detected coronary calcification constitutes a firm diagnosis of major vessel stenosis 94 per cent of the time. In most of the patients (91 per cent), the site of the calcification coincides with the site of the stenosis of the vessel. The frequency of the coronary calcification increases with more advanced coronary disease detected angiographically. Also, the severity of the coronary disease increases progressively with the extent of coronary calcification. In a series of 800 patients with coronary artery disease, calcification of the coronary artery was found to reflect a poorer prognosis than in patients without coronary calcification.

In an asymptomatic population, cardiac fluoroscopy followed by exercise electrocardiography has been used to detect possible latent ischemic heart disease. Of 108 middle-aged asymptomatic male office workers, 37 (34 per cent) had coronary artery calcification. Of these 37 men, 13 (35 per cent) had a positive exercise test. Only 3 of 71 men (4 per cent) without coronary calcification had a positive exercise test. Conversely, of the 16 men with a positive exercise test, 13 (81 per cent) had calcium in their coronary artery (or arteries), implying a ninefold increased risk of a positive exercise test for those with coronary artery calcification. Twelve of the 13 patients (92 per cent) who had both coronary calcification and a positive exercise test were subsequently found to have stenosis greater than 50 per cent in at least one major coronary artery.

Detection of Delicate Fat Stripes

Subepicardial fat stripes are an important landmark separating the myocardium from the pericardium. Their visualization is of major importance in the diagnosis of heart disease. The fat stripes are usually small, delicate, and highly mobile. They are not seen on chest radiographs except retrosternally in the lateral view. Fluoroscopically, however, the fat stripes can be seen as pulsating linear lucencies against the opaque shadow of the myocardium.

Since the coronary arteries are embedded in the subepicardial fat stripes, between the cardiac chambers, the latter can be used to identify the calcified coronary arteries. If the calcified artery (dark line) coincides with the fat stripe (bright line) within the left atrioventricular groove, it represents the circumflex coronary artery. The anterior descending artery moves synchronously with the fat stripe within the anterior interventricular groove. The right coronary artery runs in the right atrioventricular groove, as does the posterior descending artery in the posterior interventricular groove (Figs. 103–17 and 103–24).

The subepicardial fat stripe separates the myocardium from the pericardium. Identification of the subepicardial fat stripes helps detect pericardial disease. Normally, fat stripes are difficult to see because of the adjacent similar radiolucency of the lung. The in-between, delicate, hairline density of the normal pericardium is not visualized except retrosternally in the lateral view. In the presence of pericardial thickening or effusion, however, the subepicardial fat stripes become readily discernible because of the added background of water density (see Fig. 103–18).

In the case of pericardial effusion, the vigorously pulsating fat stripe is in bold contrast to the immobile band of pericardial fluid. Pulsation of the outer border of the heart is absent. In pericardial thickening, the thickened pericardium pulsates synchronously with the subepicardial fat stripe. Therefore, pulsation of the outer border of the heart is present. In either case, amplitude of excursion of the fat stripe represents the contractility of myocardium. A diminished excursion of the fat stripe suggests the presence of cardiac tamponade or pericardial constriction, depending on the presence of effusion or thickening. Since the advent of echocardiography, cardiac fluoroscopy has been used less frequently for the diagnosis of pericardial disease. When not clinically suspected, however, a pericardial effusion may first be detected by fluoroscopy, making other procedures unnecessary. For the assessment of a small anterior pericardial effusion, cardiac fluoroscopy is superior to echocardiography. Fluoroscopy is particularly helpful when special conditions make echocardiography technically difficult to perform for the detection of pericardial disease. These conditions include patients with severe emphysema, extreme obesity, marked chest deformity, and inability to cooperate.

Differentiation Between Cardiac and Noncardiac Diseases

With suspension of respiration, any moving structures are likely to be cardiovascular. Conversely, noncardiac structures are immobile. A pulmonary varix or an azygos vein collapses on Valsalva maneuver with rebound pulsation upon release of the breath. An enlarged mediastinal lymph node, on the other hand, does not change either in size or in contour with the Valsalva maneuver. However, it is not always possible to differentiate an aortic aneurysm from a mediastinal mass by fluoroscopy alone. A clot-filled aneurysm may fail to pulsate. A tumor adherent to the aorta may transmit the aortic pulsation and therefore mimic an aneurysm. If there is any doubt about the exact nature of the lesion, more sophisticated modalities, such as computed tomography with enhancement, radionuclide imaging, or angiocardiography, should be used for clarification.

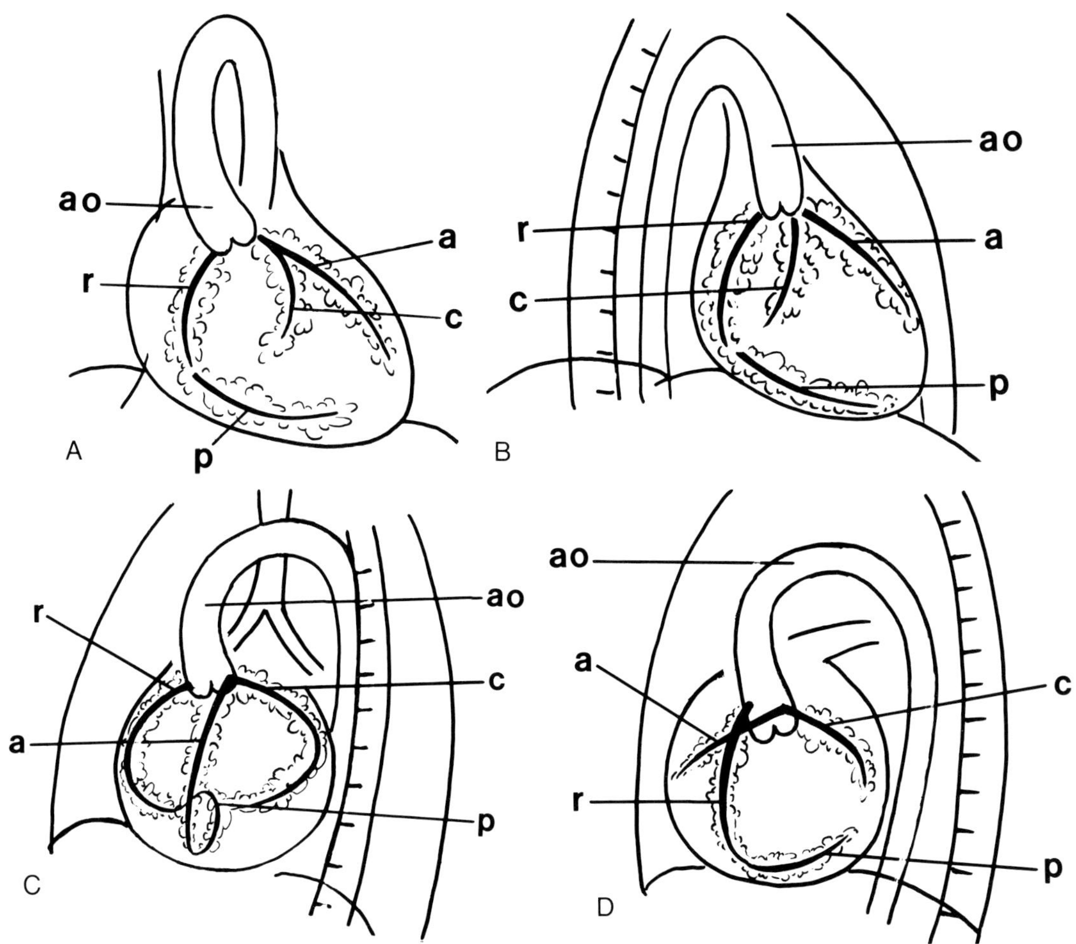

Figure 103–24. Schematic drawing depicts the **subepicardial fat stripes** in relation to the coronary arteries in four views. *A*, Posteroanterior view. *B*, Right anterior oblique view. *C*, Left anterior oblique view. *D*, Left lateral view. (ao = aorta; r = right coronary artery, which is embedded in the right atrioventricular groove; p = posterior descending coronary artery, which is embedded in the posterior interventricular groove; a = anterior descending coronary artery, which is embedded in the anterior interventricular groove; c = circumflex coronary artery, which is embedded in the left atrioventricular groove.) (From Chen JTT: Cardiac fluoroscopy. Cardiol Clin North Am 1:565, 1983.)

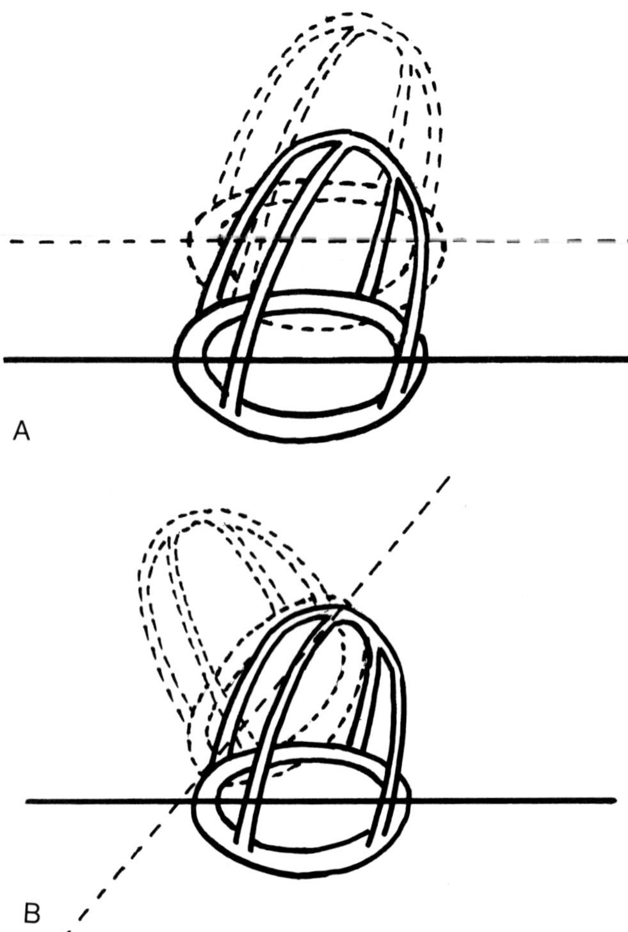

Figure 103–25. Schematic drawings depicting **normal and abnormal movements of a prosthetic valve.** *A,* Normal movement. Note that the base of the valve between the two phases of the cardiac cycle remains parallel. *B,* Abnormal movement. Note that the base forms an angle greater than 12 degrees between end-systole and end-diastole. (From Chen JTT: Cardiac fluoroscopy. Cardiol Clin North Am 1:565, 1983.)

Evaluation of Cardiac Pacemakers and Prosthetic Valves

Atrial pacing via the coronary sinus or right atrial appendage has become increasingly popular, as has atrioventricular sequential pacing. The position of a variety of pacing catheters can be determined promptly by fluoroscopy if not detected by radiography.

When confronted with a malfunctioning valve prosthesis, the radiologist can use fluoroscopy to quickly assess the stability of the prosthesis by measuring the degree of valve tilt. A tilt of more than 12 degrees between the phases of the cardiac cycle is considered significant instability (Fig. 103–25). This would imply loosening of surgical sutures at the base of the prosthesis associated with valvular regurgitation. A metallic foreign body in the heart is easily detected by its rhythmic motion, in contrast to an immobile foreign body in the chest wall when respiration is suspended. The exact location of the foreign body in the heart can then be determined by its relation to the subepicardial fat stripes.

Assistance to Cardiac Catheterization and Angiocardiography

The advent of image intensification fluoroscopy has greatly facilitated cardiac catheterization. The precise placement of a catheter in the heart and great vessels ensures the accuracy of blood sampling, pressure measurement, and pacemaker function and unobstructed views of angiocardiography.

Bibliography

Bartel AG, Chen JTT, Peter RH, et al: The significance of coronary calcification detected by fluoroscopy. A report of 360 patients. Circulation 49:1247, 1974.

Chen JTT: Radiologic demonstration of anomalous pulmonary venous connection and its clinical significance. CRC Crit Rev Diagn Imaging 11:383, 1979.

Chen JTT: Cardiac fluoroscopy. Cardiol Clin North Am 1:565, 1983.

Chen JTT: The chest roentgenogram. *In* Hurst JW (ed): The Heart, 6th ed. New York, McGraw-Hill, 1985.

Chen JTT: The plain radiograph in the diagnosis of cardiovascular disease. Radiol Clin North Am 21:609, 1983.

Chen JTT, Behar VS, Morris JJ, et al: Correlation of roentgen findings with hemodynamic data in pure mitral stenosis. AJR 102:280, 1968.

Chen JTT, Capp MP, Johnsrude IS, et al: Roentgen appearance of pulmonary vascularity in the diagnosis of heart disease. AJR 112:559, 1971.

Chen JTT, Lester RG, Peter RG: Posterior wedging sign of mitral insufficiency. Radiology 113:451, 1974.

Eddleman EE Jr, Frommeyer WB Jr, Lyle DP, et al: Critical analysis of clinical factors in estimating severity of aortic valve disease. Am J Cardiol 31:687, 1973.

Elkin M: President's address. Issues in radiology related to the new technologies. Radiology 143:1–6, 1982.

Green CE, Kelley MJ: A renewed role for fluoroscopy in the evaluation of cardiac disease. Radiol Clin North Am 18:345, 1980.

Hewitt MJ, Chen JTT, Ravin CE, Gallagher JJ: Coronary sinus atrial pacing: Radiographic considerations. AJR 136:323, 1981.

Hoffman RB, Rigler LG: Evaluation of left ventricular enlargement in the lateral projection of the chest. Radiology 85:93, 1965.

Kelley MJ, Huang EK, Langou RA: Correlation of fluoroscopically detected coronary artery calcification with exercise testing in asymptomatic men. Radiology 129:1, 1978.

Kelley MJ, Jaffe CC, Kleinman CS: Cardiac Imaging in Infants and Children. Philadelphia, WB Saunders Company, 1982, pp 251–252.

Lachman AS, Roberts WC: Calcific deposits in stenotic mitral valves. Circulation 57:808, 1978.

Langou RA, Kelley MJ, Huang EK, et al: Predictive accuracy of coronary artery calcification and positive exercise test in asymptomatic non-hyperlipidemic men for coronary artery disease. Am J Cardiol 45:400, 1980.

Margolis JR, Chen JTT, Kong YL, et al: The diagnostic and prognostic significance of coronary calcification. A report of 800 patients. Radiology 137:609, 1980.

Torrance DJ: Demonstration of subepicardial fat as an aid in the diagnosis of pericardial effusion or thickening. AJR 74:850, 1955.

104 Echocardiography

C. Carl Jaffe

As an imaging technology for visualizing the heart and great vessels, ultrasound has a number of very significant advantages: (1) since its mechanism of imaging uses acoustic waves, it has virtually negligible biologic effect, and therefore imaging can be repeated at frequent intervals on the same patient, making it an excellent means of monitoring; (2) since blood is hypoechogenic compared with tissue, cardiac images show excellent contrast at the endocardial-blood boundary and valve structures; (3) using different imaging windows between the ribs of the chest, sequential multiple planar views are obtainable, which permit visualization of virtually all portions of the myocardium at real-time imaging rates (greater than 30 images per second); and (4) Doppler assessment of local blood velocities using a sample position guided by the two-dimensional image or whole-image color-encoded Doppler imaging permits accurate characterization of the direction and pattern of blood flow. The combination of structural and flow information allowed by the technology offers nearly complete definition of a variety of cardiac abnormalities.

INSTRUMENTATION

Ultrasound creates its image by emitting high-frequency acoustic pulses from a piezoelectric crystal transducer and allowing the sonic pulses to travel through soft tissue. Because tissues of various types possess different acoustic properties, each interface causes a small portion of the pulse energy to be reflected as an echo. The return of these echoes to the transducer generates a small voltage signal. Using knowledge of the speed of sound in the tissue (approximately 1540 m/sec in soft tissue), timing of the return echoes permits estimation of the distance of the tissue plane from which the echoes arose. As the original pulse travels through tissue, it undergoes continued attenuation at each interface until the return echo is too weak to record. The amplitude of these echoes varies from very strong (arising from sharp boundaries [specular reflectors] such as found at blood-valve interfaces) to very weak (arising from the internal structure of organs that generate low-level backscatter echoes from structures such as myocardium).

The mechanism by which the acoustic impulses are generated is known as the piezoelectric effect. When polarized by a brief high electric voltage, crystals of certain compositions physically vibrate. If the crystal is directly coupled to tissue by a fluid gel, the acoustic pulse will be transmitted to the tissue. The frequencies employed are in the megahertz range (well above audible, which is limited to 20,000 hertz). The most useful frequencies for imaging purposes lie between 2.5 and 7.5 mHz. The physics equation relating the various acoustic properties is written as $V = f \times \lambda$, where V is the velocity of sound in tissue, f is the frequency, and λ (lambda) is the wavelength. This implies that for a sound velocity of 1540 meters per second, the wave length of a 5 -mHz pulse is 0.3 mm. Since the total length of the acoustic pulse is only a few wave cycles (the voltage pulse driving the transducer lasts a few microseconds), the instrument is able to resolve structures that are less than a millimeter thick. Because of the high velocity with which the sound travels through tissue, all of the echoes occurring from a tissue depth of 10 cm have arrived back at the transducer within slightly more than 100 microseconds. By rapidly pulsing the transducer while sweeping the beam through slight increments in angle over approximately 90 degrees, a wedge-shaped planar image can be generated, forming new images at a rate of up to 60 per second. This image rate permits favorable capture of rapidly moving cardiac structures, which can be recorded on video tape and played back by the viewer either in real time or in slow motion for more careful analysis.

The most significant enhancement of ultrasound technology occurring in the last few years has been the opportunity to use the two-dimensional image to direct the position from which range-gated echoes can be examined for their Doppler shift information. The Doppler equation notes that as sound with a known original frequency interacts with structures in motion, a frequency shift is generated that if measured allows the observer to extract the velocity of motion of the object imposing the shift. Using electronics that rapidly switch from generating an image to monitoring the Doppler shift of an echo pulse arising from a designated time range gate, one can extract information representing both the velocity and direction of blood flow within a specified region of the heart (see Figs. 104–9 and 104–10).

ECHOCARDIOGRAPHIC IMAGING

Current instrumentation permits even the relatively inexperienced user to easily produce useful diagnostic images. The narrow transducer head (usually less than 20 mm wide) and triangular image format are designed to take advantage of the narrow acoustic window that occurs between the rib spaces. Obstruction of the acoustic pulse occurs when the sound must pass through either rib or lung, and therefore an effort is made to view the heart where it is in contact with the chest wall. By convention, this implies that the most favorable access windows are in the parasternal, apical, or subxiphoid positions. Although useful information can be generated from any view, it is conventional to generate images from at least a few standard planes. An image accessible from the left parasternal position, usually at the fourth or fifth intercostal space, defines the well-known long axis of the heart with the aorta located superiorly (Fig. 104–1). Because of the relative hypoechogenicity of blood,

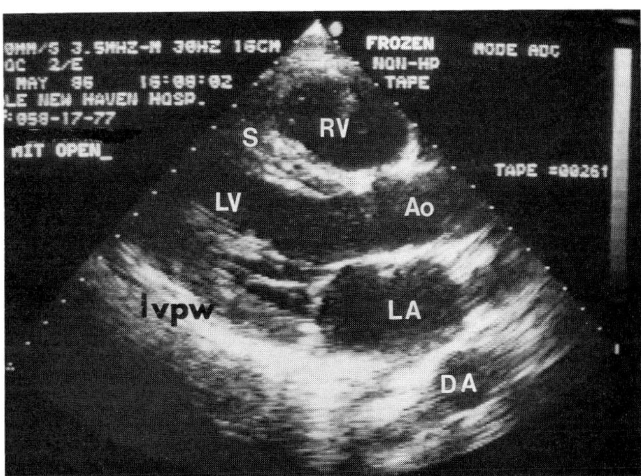

Figure 104–1. Parasternal long-axis view of the left ventricle with the apex at image left. The left and right ventricles (LV, RV), aorta (Ao), left atrium (LA), septum (S), descending aorta (DA), and left ventricular posterior wall (lvpw) are all well-imaged.

the myocardium and valve structures are sharply defined, although the still frame photograph shown (Fig. 104–1) does not do full justice to the rich dynamic information that can be extracted from the original real-time video. From this viewing angle the first intracardiac structure visible (at the apex of the sector—closest to the transducer) is the right ventricular anterior wall, below which is the cavity of the right ventricle. Continuity of the intraventricular septum with the anterior aortic root can easily be determined. Additionally, the motion and thickening of the septum during systole provide highly useful diagnostic information. The left ventricle, because it represents the high-pressure chamber, is a bullet-shaped cavity that undergoes the most visible change in volume and configuration during ventricular systole. The structural attachments of the mitral valve chordae to the papillary muscles are readily defined, and the characteristic flapping motion of the mitral valve provides information about its flexibility. The mitral valve opening motion is normally double-phased, demonstrating a rapid opening during early diastole-followed by a gradual closure as the left ventricle fills with blood. This is followed by a second rapid opening, which is due to the onset of atrial contraction. During ventricular systole, the mitral valve remains closed, and its configuration is readjusted to conform to the smaller volume of blood remaining in the chamber. The aortic valve undergoes an opening and closing cycle complementary to that of the mitral valve. In this plane, only two valve leaflets are visible, consisting of the right and noncoronary cusps. Behind the left ventricular outflow tract and aortic root lies the left atrium and behind it a cross-section of the descending aorta. All instruments provide depth markers that allow measurement of the various structures, but the experienced observer usually develops a sense of proportionality between structures that allows a rapid assessment of normal or abnormal configuration. The instruments provide a variety of techniques for enhancing the detailed visualization of specific structures of interest. Narrow-angle viewing (Fig. 104–2) and use of higher frequency transducers, which permit improved structural resolution along the axis of the beam, offer an opportunity for detailed evaluation of structures of specific interest.

With the transducer lying in the same position along the left parasternal border, rotation of the imaging plane creates a short-axis view at the level of the great vessels (Fig. 104–3). The view is looking upward through the apex of the left ventricle with the three leaflets of the aortic valve seen directly en face. Superiorly lies the right ventricular outflow tract, which connects on the patient's left with the pulmonary valve. Posterior to the aortic valve is the left atrium and (somewhat medially) the interatrial septum. The dynamics of valve opening are clearly evident as one follows the cardiac cycle in real time. The three leaflets of the aortic valve peel back as if they were wedges and display the full opening extent of the valve orifice (Fig. 104–4). Returning to the long-axis plane by rotating the transducer 90 degrees but now tilting under the sternum reveals a long-axis view of the right ventricle and right atrium and a sharp definition of two of the tricuspid valve leaflets (Fig. 104–5).

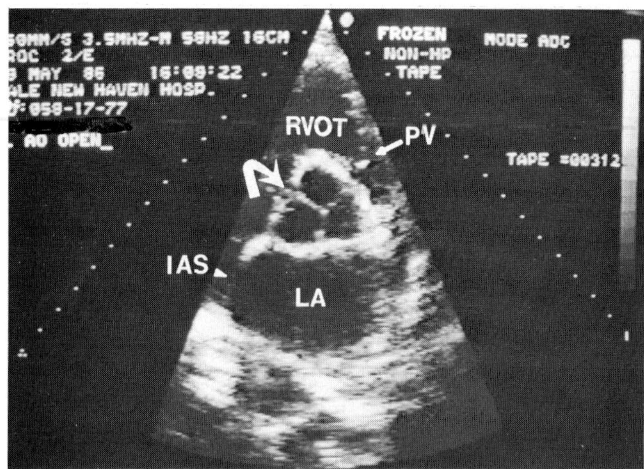

Figure 104–3. Parasternal short-axis view at the level of the aortic root with the three cusps of the aortic valve in the center of the image (*curved arrow*). Anterior to the aorta is the right ventricular outflow tract (RVOT), and to the patient's left is the pulmonary valve (PV). The intra-atrial septum (IAS) is medial to the left atrium (LA).

The full dynamics of left ventricular contraction and the reduction in volume that occurs during the cardiac cycle are often best displayed by remaining in the long-axis view but moving the transducer until it lies at the ventricular apex (Fig. 104–6). This view is particularly helpful for defining the full extent of the endocardial border and for making decisions concerning segmental wall motion abnormalities. This view is one of the most favorable for separating the regional myocardial distributions served by the right and left coronary arteries. The septum and apex are supplied by the left anterior descending artery and the posterior wall by the posterior descending artery, which in the majority of individuals arises from the right coronary artery. The shortening of the endocardial circumference during systole is easily visible (Fig. 104–7), but it is also

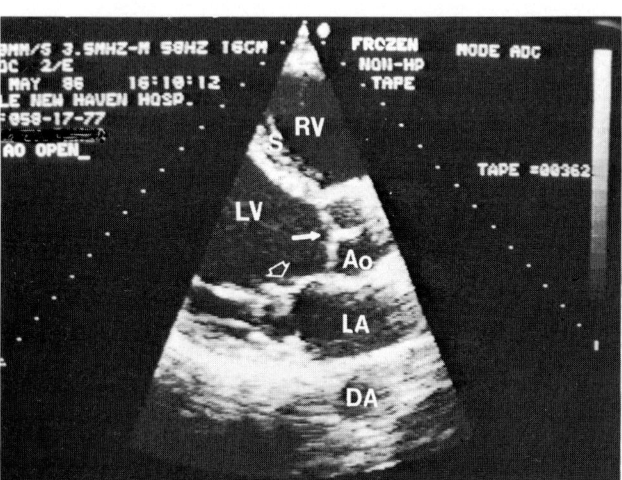

Figure 104–2. Parasternal long-axis narrow-angle view of the **aortic valve** (*closed arrow*) and **mitral valve** (*open arrow*). Labels as in Figure 104–1.

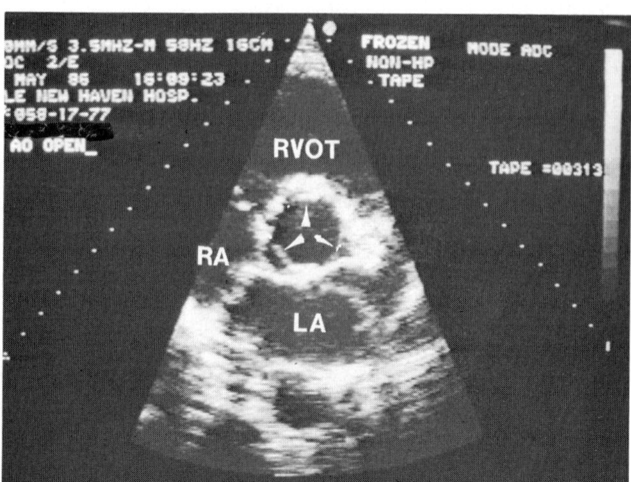

Figure 104–4. Parasternal short-axis view as in Figure 104–3, showing **the opening pattern of the aortic valve leaflets** (*arrowheads*), which peel open in a triangular manner. Labels as in Figure 104–3. (RA = right atrium.)

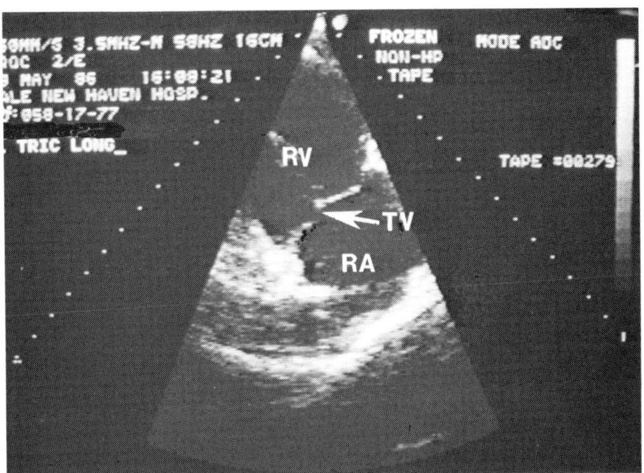

Figure 104–5. Parasternal long-axis view of the right ventricle (apex to viewer's left) displaying a section of the tricuspid valve (TV), which separates the right ventricle (RV) from the right atrium (RA).

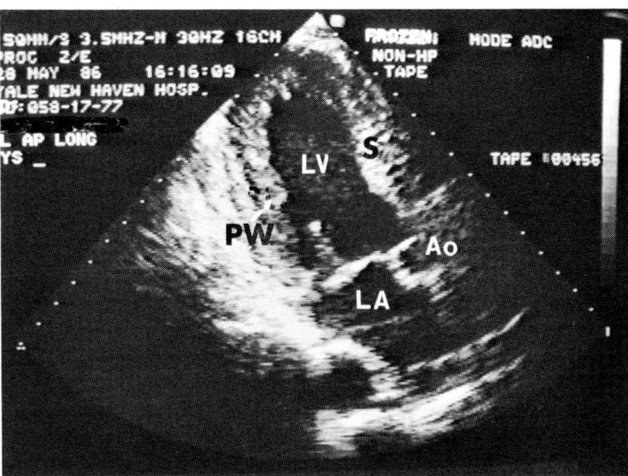

Figure 104–7. Same view as Figure 104–6 but at **end-systole** when the left ventricle (LV) has its smallest area. Note increase in wall thickness of the septum (S) and posterior wall (PW). Other labels as in Figure 104–6.

important to note the thickening of the myocardium as a further indicator of proper contractile function. This view and a closely related one (the two-chamber apical view) parallel the silhouette configuration derived during the RAO left ventricular angiogram at catheterization. Investigators have shown that quantitative area-length methods for estimating ventricular volume and function show comparable results between the two techniques.

At the apex, the transducer can be rotated 90 degrees to obtain a four-chamber view of the heart (Fig. 104–8). The septal tissue between the ventricles and atria falls into a vertical line, and it is perpendicularly transected by the atrioventricular groove aligning the tricuspid and mitral valves. The structures are easily differentiated in motion, with the septum contracting toward the left ventricular cavity and the left atrium showing orifices of the draining pulmonary veins.

The four-chamber view is the most useful for directed Doppler recordings to define the blood velocity patterns entering the ventricles, since it allows sampling axially along the blood flow (Fig. 104–9). Most instruments time-share between generating the two-dimensional image, from which the position of the Doppler sample can be directed. The Doppler signal is presented as a linear graphic display that scrolls horizontally along a time axis. The direction of blood velocity is assigned as positive relative to zero if the blood is flowing toward the transducer and negative when flowing away (Fig. 104–10). For example, the blood velocities flowing through the mitral annulus during diastole normally create an M-shaped pattern with an early rapid rise in velocity as the mitral valve opens, followed by a rapid descent as the left ventricular cavity is filled to capacity (Fig. 104–10). By directing the Doppler sample to other areas of the cardiac image, it is possible to characterize blood flow patterns throughout the cardiac cycle. Valvar regurgitation is detected as a distinct turbulent signal appearing at a place and time inappropriate for normal flow. Moreover, valvar stenoses can be detected by the abnormal high-velocity jets that their narrow orifices generate. Quantitation of the degrees of stenosis and regurgitation has become a vital role that Doppler echocardiography effectively serves.

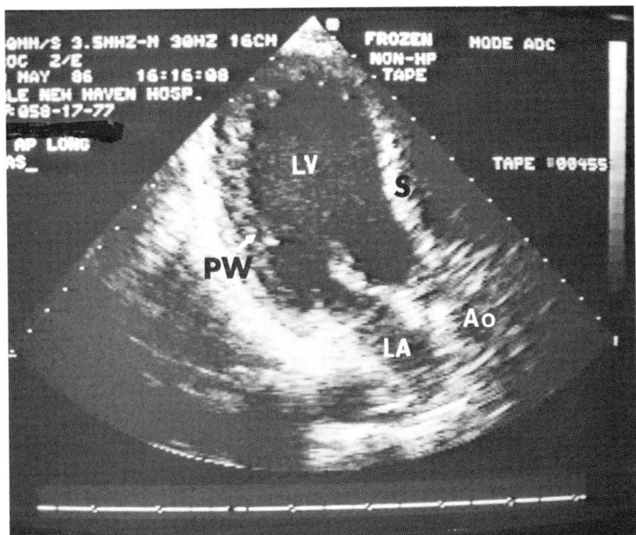

Figure 104–6. Long-axis view of the left ventricle from the apex during diastole. The septum (S) and posterior wall (PW) show the thickness that occurs during myocardial relaxation. The left ventricle (LV) encompasses its largest area. (LA = left atrium; Ao = aorta.)

Although cardiac structures represent the region of greatest clinical interest, ultrasound is capable of providing an image of any portion of the chest that is accessible by an acoustic window free of interference by air-containing lung. In patients without chronic pul-

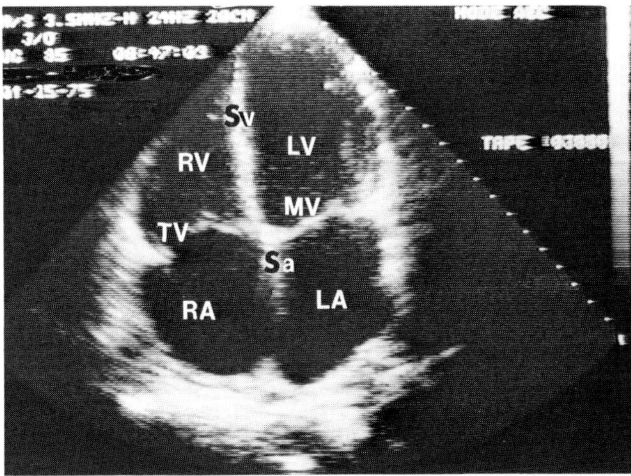

Figure 104–8. Four-chamber apical view of ventricles (RV, LV) **and atria** (RA, LA) forming a cross-configuration with the septa (Sv, Sa) and atrioventricular valves (TV, MV).

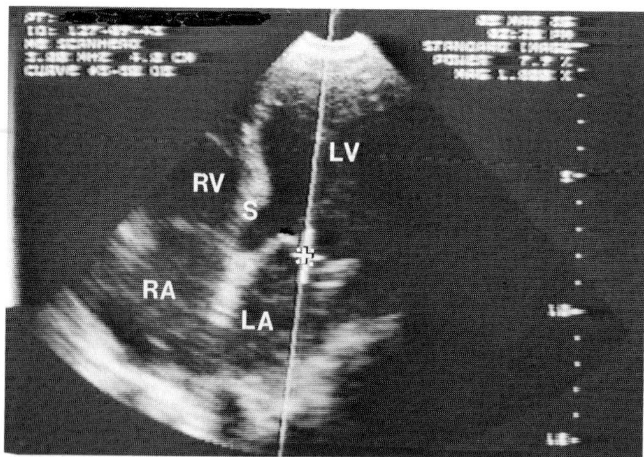

Figure 104–9. Pulsed Doppler sampling at the orifice of the mitral valve (*asterisk*). Four-chamber apical view as in Figure 104–8.

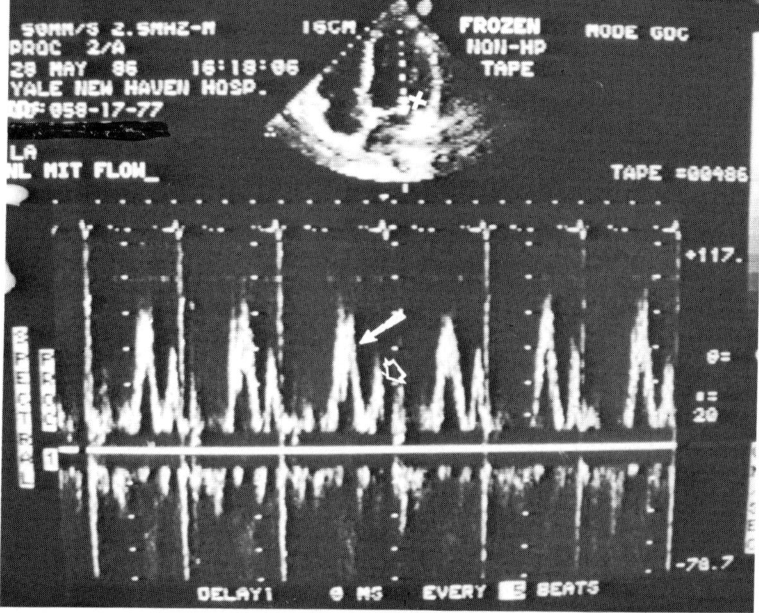

Figure 104–10. Pulsed Doppler pattern at the mitral orifice from the apical four-chamber view (X). The flow pattern during diastole shows blood velocity toward the apex that is most rapid in early diastole (*solid arrow*), decreasing and then followed by a rapid late diastolic filling due to atrial contraction (*open arrow*).

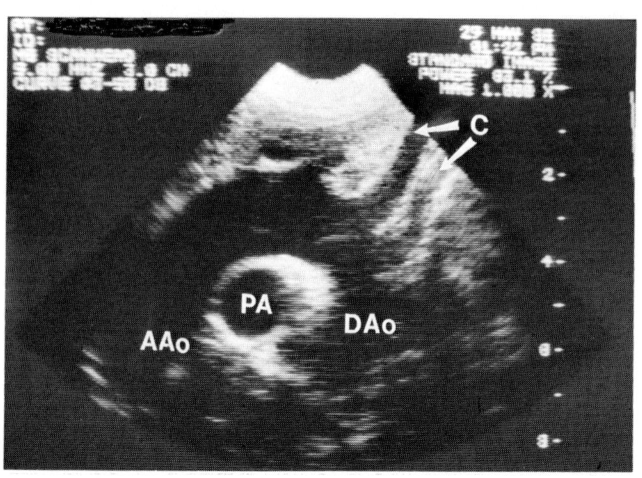

Figure 104–11. Longitudinal view of the aortic arch from the suprasternal notch. The ascending (AAo) and descending aorta (DAo) arch around the right pulmonary artery (PA). The take-off points of the cephalic vessels (C) are well-visualized.

monary disease, a suprasternal window is usually available for viewing a cross-sectional plane of the aortic arch (Fig. 104–11). This access not only allows remarkable definition of the origins of the cephalic vessels but also permits Doppler samples to be directed into the ascending or descending aorta. Noninvasive detection of patent ductus arteriosus and coarctation of the aorta is now possible with a high degree of sensitivity and specificity.

The gradual evolution of improvements in image quality and the major contribution that Doppler imaging has made to accurate, noninvasive assessment of valvar disease have placed ultrasonography in the forefront of cardiac diagnosis. It can be expected that much wider dissemination of the technology is inevitable as electronic miniaturization continues and the cost of equipment falls. Ultimately, it is more than likely that it will take a diagnostic position comparable to, and directly competitive with, the stethoscope.

Bibliography

Baker DW, Rubenstein SA, Lorch GS: Pulsed Doppler echocardiography: Principles and applications. Am J Med 63:69, 1977.

Edwards WD, Tajik AJ, Seward JB: Standardized nomenclature and anatomic basis for regional tomographic analysis of the heart. Mayo Clin Proc 56:479, 1981.

Feigenbaum H: Echocardiography, 4th ed. Philadelphia, Lea and Febiger, 1986.

Griffith JM, Henry WL: A sector scanner for real time two-dimensional echocardiography. Circulation 49:1147, 1974.

Hatle L, Angelsen B: Doppler Ultrasound in Cardiology: Physical Principles and Clinical Applications, 2nd ed. Philadelphia, Lea and Febiger, 1984.

Henry WL, DeMaria A, Gramiak R, et al: Report of the American Society of Echocardiography Committee on Nomenclature and Standards in Two-Dimensional Echocardiography. Circulation 62:212, 1980.

Kalmanson D, Veyrat C, Bouchareine F, Degroote A: A non-invasive recording of mitral valve flow velocity patterns using pulsed Doppler echocardiography. Application to diagnosis and evaluation of mitral valve disease. Br Heart J 39:517, 1977.

King DL: Cardiac ultrasonography: Cross-sectional ultrasonic imaging of the heart. Circulation 47:843, 1973.

Popp RL, Fowles R, Coltart J, Martin RP: Cardiac anatomy viewed systematically with two-dimensional echocardiography. Chest 75:579, 1979.

Salcedo E: Atlas of Echocardiography, 2nd ed. Philadelphia, WB Saunders Company, 1985.

Schmittger I, Gordon EP, Fitzgerald PJ, Popp RL: Standardized intracardiac measurements of two dimensional echocardiography. J Am Cardiol 2:934, 1983.

Stewart HD, Stewart HF, Moore RM, Garry J: Compilation of reported biologic effects data and ultrasound exposure levels. J Clin Ultrasound 13:167, 1985.

Tajik AJ, Seward JB, Hagler DJ, et al: Two dimensional real-time ultrasonic imaging of the heart and great vessels. Technic, image orientation, structure identification, and validation. Mayo Clin Proc 53:271, 1978.

Wells PNT: Absorption and dispersion of ultrasound in biological tissue. Ultrasound Med Biol 1:369, 1975.

Wells PNT: Biomedical Ultrasonics. London, Academic Press, 1977.

Weyman AE: Cross-Sectional Echocardiography. Philadelphia, Lea and Febiger, 1982.

105 Radionuclide Cardiac Imaging

Michael W. Hanson and R. Edward Coleman

The first application of radioactive tracers in cardiovascular studies was done in 1927 by Herman Blumgart and Soma Weiss. They studied the time of blood circulation by injecting an aqueous solution of radon intravenously into one arm, and, using a cloud chamber, detecting the arrival of the radon in the other arm. Although several cardiac studies were performed with radioisotopes in the 1950s and 1960s, radionuclide cardiac imaging did not become widely available clinically until the 1970s. Imaging of myocardial infarction with technetium-99m (^{99m}Tc) pyrophosphate was the first cardiac imaging technique to be used in a large number of hospitals. The information provided by infarct imaging demonstrated that unique information, important for patient management, could be obtained from cardiac imaging studies. Subsequently, other techniques for cardiovascular nuclear imaging became available and are now widely utilized. The primary techniques currently in use include first-pass radionuclide angiography (RNA), gated blood pool imaging (multigated radionuclide angiogram [MUGA]), and imaging of myocardial perfusion. These studies are readily available in most institutions for the evaluation of patients with known or suspected cardiovascular disease.

FIRST-PASS RADIONUCLIDE ANGIOGRAPHY (RNA)

Radiopharmaceuticals

The first-pass RNA study can be performed with one of several radiopharmaceuticals. The agent chosen for the study must have enough radioactivity in the single bolus injection to generate an adequate count rate to produce an interpretable image as it traverses the ventricles during its first pass through the heart and lungs.

Technetium-99m pertechnetate is a commonly used radiopharmaceutical for first-pass RNA studies; it is the eluate from the ^{99}Mo-^{99m}Tc generator and thus requires no further preparation. The usual administered dose is 10 to 15 mCi (370 to 555 MBq) per injection, with a maximum of 30 mCi (1110 MBq). If a rest and maximum exercise study is planned, two 15-mCi (555 MBq) doses are used. If a rest, intermediate level, and maximum exercise study is planned, three 10-mCi (370 MBq) doses are used. Other radiopharmaceuticals, such as ^{99m}Tc diethylenetriamine penta-acetic acid (DTPA) or ^{99m}Tc sulfur colloid, can be used for first-pass RNA studies. When ^{99m}Tc sestamibi or ^{99m}Tc teboroxime are used for evaluation of myocardial perfusion, a first-pass RNA study can be obtained at the time of injection of either of these radiopharmaceuticals. Because the clearance of each of these ^{99m}Tc-labeled agents is not the same, the patient will receive different radiation absorbed doses (rad) from these radiopharmaceuticals.

Radioactive gold (^{195m}Au) is a generator-produced radionuclide that has also been used for performing first-pass RNA studies. It is the daughter of ^{195m}Hg, a cyclotron-produced radionuclide with a half life of 41.6 hours. Owing to the short half life of ^{195m}Au (30.5 seconds), large amounts of radioactivity (30 to 50 mCi [1110 to 1850 MBq]) can be administered with significantly less radiation dose to the patient than would be received using ^{99m}Tc pertechnetate. Although ^{195m}Au has been used for routine clinical studies in Europe, and for research studies in the United States, the cost-effectiveness factor for the manufacture of the generator will likely prohibit its availability for routine clinical studies in the United States.

Imaging Technique

It is essential that the tracer for first-pass RNA studies be delivered by rapid bolus injection. A slow non-bolus infusion results in erroneous data. To optimize the likelihood for a good bolus injection, an external jugular vein is the preferable site for injection of the first-pass RNA tracers.

The first-pass RNA can be performed with either a single-crystal or a multi-crystal camera. The multi-crystal camera is specially designed for high count-rate first-pass studies; however, the newer single-crystal digital cameras also have high count-rate capabilities without significant dead-time loss. Because the first-pass technique evaluates the transit of a bolus of radioactivity through the heart, high temporal resolution is required, and 25 to 50 msec framing rates are needed. After identification of the left ventricle, one determines time activity curves of the transit and background. A single representative cardiac cycle is then generated from the left ventricular phase of the study.

If a rest-exercise study is to be performed in which only the first-pass RNA is to be acquired, the patient is positioned in a seated position on an upright bicycle in an anterior or RAO position. The anterior position is preferred because it facilitates patient positioning. After the rest study is done, exercise is started. Blood pressure, heart rate, and an electrocardiogram (EKG) are monitored. Bicycle ergometry with progressive multi-staged exercise is used, beginning at 100 to 300 kilopound-meter (kpm) per minute, and is increased 100 to 200 kpm per minute at each stage, depending on the study protocol. Exercise is continued until the patient is limited by symptoms or reaches a predetermined target heart rate (85 per cent of the age-predicted maximum heart rate, which can be calculated by subtracting the patient's age in years from 220). The exercise is considered to demonstrate an adequate heart rate if the patient attains his or her predetermined target rate. The second injection is given at maximum exercise, and the patient continues to exercise during the data acquisition. If maximum exercise is not maintained during the second study, rapid changes in the data can occur that will compromise the accuracy of the study.

If a rest-exercise first-pass study is done in conjunction with perfusion imaging (using ^{99m}Tc sestamibi), the resting study is performed in an anterior position with the patient standing. About one hour after the resting first-pass study is completed, the patient has perfusion images of the myocardium obtained. When the perfusion images are completed, the patient returns for the exercise first-pass RNA. The patient is placed on a treadmill, and exercise is started. Blood pressure, heart rate, and an EKG are monitored. Although any exercise protocol can be used, the most commonly used protocol for exercise is the standard Bruce protocol, which provides multi-level exercise. The treadmill starts at a speed of 1.7 mph and an incline, or grade, of 10 per cent. The speed and incline of the treadmill progressively increase by predetermined amounts every three minutes. As with bicycle exercise, the second injection of tracer is given when the patient reaches maximum exercise (either symptom-limited or target heart rate). With the gamma camera in front of the patient, he or she continues to walk on the treadmill during the data acquisition. Patient motion at peak exercise presents somewhat more of a problem with treadmill exercise than with bicycle exercise, but motion correction programs can be used to assist with analysis of the data.

Image Interpretation

Various measurements can be derived from the first-pass data, including global and/or regional ventricular ejection fractions, wall motion, and left ventricular end-systolic and end-diastolic volumes. The anterior projection allows for segmental wall motion analysis of the anterior and inferior walls and the apex of the left ventricle (Fig. 105–1). The rest-exercise studies can be viewed simultaneously to evaluate for changes that may occur in any of these parameters. The walls are determined to be normal, hypokinetic (motion less than normal), akinetic (portion of the wall has no motion), or dyskinetic (portion of the wall moves outward during systole).

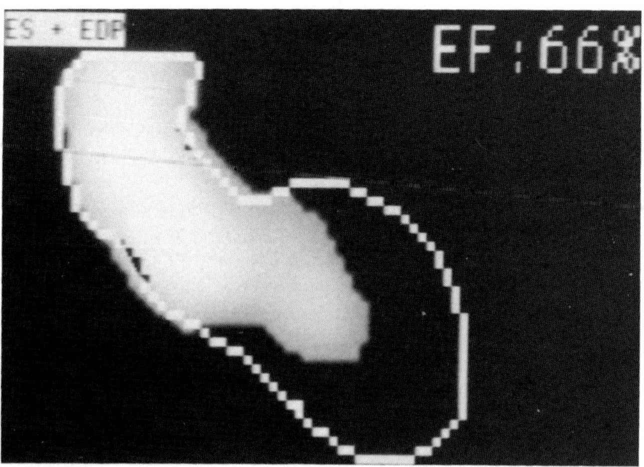

Figure 105–1. A normal first-pass RNA study acquired in the anterior projection demonstrating the anterior wall, apex, and inferior wall of the left ventricle. The single perimeter line represents the profile of the left ventricle at end-diastole, while the end-systolic image is represented by the gray-scale inner image. The left ventricle demonstrates normal wall motion and a normal ejection fraction of 66 per cent.

GATED BLOOD POOL STUDIES (MUGA)

Radiopharmaceuticals

The single-image first-pass RNA study requires that radioactivity remain in the blood pool only during its first transit through the heart and is acquired in a matter of seconds. The acquisition time for a multiple-view gated blood pool study, however, is longer, and therefore the radioactivity must remain constant within the blood pool during the entire period of acquisition during rest and/or exercise. Good labeling of the blood pool is necessary to optimize the heart-to-background ratio for these studies. The definition of the cardiac chambers is more difficult if there is radioactivity outside of the blood pool. The initial radiopharmaceutical used for these studies was ^{99m}Tc human serum albumin, but this agent has been almost completely replaced by ^{99m}Tc-labeled autologous red blood cells. Labeled human serum albumin has considerable accumulation in the liver and a faster clearance from the blood than labeled red blood cells.

Red blood cells are labeled by the in vivo, in vitro, or modified in vitro technique. The in vivo technique is most widely used owing to its simplicity and satisfactory labeling. The in vivo technique consists of administering 5 to 15 mg of stannous pyrophosphate that contains 1 to 2 mg of tin for an average adult dose. The stannous pyrophosphate is commercially available in a kit, and provides a convenient method of administering the stannous ion, which is a reducing agent that can cross the red cell membrane. Approximately 20 to 30 minutes after the administration of the stannous pyrophosphate, 20 to 30 mCi (740 to 1110 MBq) of ^{99m}Tc pertechnetate are given. The ^{99m}Tc pertechnetate crosses the red cell membrane, is reduced inside the red cell by the stannous ion, and labels hemoglobin. The labeling occurs in the intravascular space. The stannous pyrophosphate and ^{99m}Tc pertechnetate should be injected directly into a peripheral vein; administration of either agent through an indwelling intravenous line may result in poor labeling efficiency because they bind to the surface of the intravenous line.

The in vitro technique requires blood to be drawn and the labeling process to be done externally in a sterile vial. The blood is mixed with stannous ion and the pertechnetate is added to the vial. Red blood cell labeling with commercial kits provides a high labeling efficiency and excellent images.

The modified in vitro technique requires the administration of stannous pyrophosphate intravenously. The red blood cell labeling is then performed in a closed system attached to the patient. Venous access is obtained with a butterfly needle attached to extension tubing with a three-way stopcock. One outlet of the stopcock is attached to a shielded syringe containing the ^{99m}Tc pertechnetate, and the other outlet contains a syringe with heparinized saline. Fifteen minutes after stannous pyrophosphate administration, the line is flushed with heparinized saline, and approximately 10 ml of blood are withdrawn into the syringe containing radioactivity. The shielded syringe is gently agitated for approximately 15 minutes to permit red cell labeling, and the red cells are then reinjected into the patient. The modified in vitro technique has a labeling efficiency of 95 per cent, similar to that of the in vitro technique and higher than the 85 to 90 per cent reported with the in vivo technique.

Imaging Technique

Gated blood pool studies use a dedicated computer and special software for data processing. The blood pool data are collected in synchrony with the EKG. Thus, a good EKG signal is important to obtain a good study. The R-wave of the EKG is used to start framing intervals for the acquisition. If a good R-wave is not present, if other waves of the EKG signal are of similar height, or if artifacts are present on the EKG, gating problems that allow random framing of the data will occur and degrade the study. The R-R interval is usually divided into 16 to 24 equal time frames. The radiotracer counts during consecutive time intervals are sorted into the frames, and the temporal sequence is determined by the time since the previous R-wave. A single representative cardiac cycle is produced and is composed of data from several hundred individual beats. The EKG and gamma camera data can be obtained in a list mode, which requires a large amount of disk space for storage. The list mode acquisition permits cardiac cycles of a specified, uniform duration to be selected retrospectively. Thus, if a patient has multiple ventricular premature contractions, they can be excluded using this type of acquisition. Although most dedicated computer systems have list mode acquisitions available, it is rarely used for clinical studies. Most patients are able to be evaluated adequately by the frame mode acquisition. It is not clear that patients with inadequate frame mode studies have adequate list mode studies. Most patients with atrial fibrillation and ventricular premature contractions can be adequately evaluated by frame mode gated blood pool studies.

Rest studies are performed in the supine position with a high resolution collimator. The images are acquired until at least 200,000 to 250,000 counts per frame are obtained. The rest acquisition generally requires 7 to 10 minutes per view. Rest images include a 45-degree LAO (best septal), 70-degree LAO, and an anterior or 20-degree RAO image. These views permit analysis of all chambers and calculation of the ejection fraction. The best septal (approximately 45-degree LAO) view gives the best separation of the two ventricles and frequently requires approximately a 10-degree tilt of the detector toward the feet. This caudal tilt helps to minimize left atrial radioactivity overlapping into the left ventricular region of interest. The septal, inferoapical and posterolateral walls of the left ventricle are evaluated on the best septal view. The 70-degree LAO view is used to evaluate the posterior and inferior walls. The anterior or 20-degree RAO view is used to evaluate the anterior and apical walls.

A left ventricular time-activity curve is generated from the best septal view for the calculation of the left ventricular ejection fraction because it is the only view in which the left ventricle is separated from the other cardiac chambers. Radioactive counts from the left ventricular region of interest include photon emissions from overlying structures such as chest wall, lungs, and atria. Scattered radiation from adjacent structures, such as the spleen and right ventricle, is also included in a left ventricular region of interest. The normal left atrium does not contribute much to the left ventricular count because the atrium is further from the detector and above the left ventricle. In left atrial enlargement, the left atrium can contribute significantly to the count and falsely lower the left ventricular ejection fraction.

The left ventricular ejection fraction calculation uses counts instead of volumes. Because attenuation remains relatively constant during the cardiac cycle, counts are proportional to volume. Background correction is necessary because many of the counts in the left ventricular region of interest are from structures around the ventricle.

Most dedicated computers use a semi-automatic technique for calculating the left ventricular ejection fraction. After the left ventricle is identified by a rectangular box or circle, an automated program is used to define the left ventricular edges. This program is interactive, and the operator can adjust the calculated edge if it does not correspond to the visual determination of the edge. This edge detection program goes through each of the frames constituting the gated blood pool study. The background region of interest is automatically selected adjacent to the posterolateral wall of the left ventricle in the end systolic frame. If this automated selection is not appropriate because of incorporation of the spleen, aorta, or other high- or low-count structures, a background region of interest is generated manually. The background counts per pixel are recorded for evaluating quality of studies and are especially important in the quality control of sequential studies.

The ejection fraction is calculated from the difference between the end-diastolic and systolic counts divided by the end-diastolic counts, with the counts corrected for background. Various methods have been suggested for determining left ventricular volume. Geometric methods have been used, but have the limitation of assuming that all ventricles conform to a certain shape. Count-based methods, with attenuation correction, are used more widely for volume determination. These methods require determination of the ventricular depth, the amount of attenuating material, and the counts per ml of blood. The measurements of the ventricular depth and amount of attenuating material are not simple, and volume calculations are not performed routinely with gated blood pool studies in most laboratories.

Rest-exercise studies are performed with an all-purpose or high-sensitivity collimator to obtain more counts in a shorter period, although with some loss in resolution. The counts per frame are also reduced to 150,000. These changes permit a study to be acquired in approximately two minutes, an acceptable length of time for exercise acquisition. The patient is positioned in the best septal view for the exercise study, which can be performed in either the supine or the upright position. After the rest data are obtained, multi-stage exercise is started. Three-minute stages are used, with data collection during the last two minutes of each stage. Although the rest and maximal exercise stages are generally the stages used for interpretation, the other stages may provide useful information. Because ejection fraction increases rapidly with small decreases in workload, the maximal exercise data must be acquired at a constant level of exercise.

Image Interpretation

Left ventricular wall motion is evaluated from a cinematic display. The location and extent of any abnormality are recorded for each view. As with first-pass RNA studies, the walls are determined to be normal, hypokinetic, akinetic, or dyskinetic.

Various quantitative methods have been proposed to determine regional function. Although the methods have demonstrated utility in numerous studies, the amount of information that these methods provide, in addition to the ejection fraction and regional wall motion determination, is not clear. These quantitative techniques include regional ejection fraction and stroke volume images, phase analysis, amplitude analysis, etc. They are useful to inexperienced observers, but seem to provide little, if any, additional information to the experienced observer of these studies.

MYOCARDIAL PERFUSION IMAGING

Planar and SPECT Imaging Modalities

In contrast to the first-pass RNA and the MUGA study, in which cardiac wall motion is assessed by imaging activity within the blood pool, myocardial perfusion studies acquire images of radioactive tracer that is distributed and accumulated within the myocardium relative to coronary artery blood flow. These static images can be acquired and displayed either as planar images or as single photon emission computed tomographic (SPECT) images. With either technique, images should be obtained in a standardized manner so that stress and rest images can be compared.

With planar imaging, a minimum of three views is obtained. A 45-degree LAO view, or the oblique view that best demonstrates a circle or ellipse, is the first view obtained. The other two views should be an anterior view (or 45 degrees to the right of the first view) and a 70-degree LAO view (or 25 degrees to the left of the first view) (Fig. 105–2). Planar imaging is technically less demanding than SPECT imaging. Generally, there is less image contrast with a lesser target-to-background ratio on planar images when compared with SPECT studies. Planar images may be interpreted directly or with the assistance of a semi-quantitative computer analysis program, which is available in standard software on most nuclear medicine computers for thallium-201 (^{201}Tl). These methods are well suited for comparing the exercise and redistribution studies. The most widely used analysis is a circumferential profile of activity in the left ventricle. After performing a background subtraction, one plots the maximum counts along six-degree radii from the center of the left ventricle. The counts are plotted in relation to angular location and are displayed as a curve for analysis. Wash-out circumferential profiles can be calculated as per cent wash-out from the stress circumferential profiles to the four-hour delayed profiles if ^{201}Tl is not reinjected at redistribution. Normal profiles are established for the initial distribution, delayed distribution, and wash-out in normal subjects (healthy individuals with a very low probability of coronary disease). Other semi-quantitative techniques are also used, but the circumferential profile appears to have the widest use. These semi-quantitative techniques have improved the sensitivity of ^{201}Tl imaging for detecting significant coronary artery disease and recognition of multi-vessel disease. The ability to detect intermediate (50 to 70 per cent) levels of stenosis and isolated single-vessel disease is also improved with semi-quantitative analysis.

SPECT imaging produces images without the superimposition of activity that occurs in planar imaging. SPECT is a volume imaging modality that gathers data from the whole organ from a circumferential perspective. Data is collected from multiple projections around the patient. The SPECT camera is designed with one to four rotating gamma camera heads. The more heads there are in a SPECT camera, the less time is needed to acquire the data or the greater the counts per slice that can be acquired per time; however, the cost of the camera increases significantly with the addition of each individual head. The basic principle is to acquire data from multiple lines of response that can be reconstructed into tomographic planes representing a three-dimensional structure.

A single-headed camera rotates from the 30-degree RAO position to the 150-degree LPO position when acquiring data for a 180-degree acquisition (Fig. 105–3). Some studies have suggested that a 180-degree data collection is superior to a complete 360-degree collection. Other studies, however, have identified artifacts in 180-degree acquisition that are not present on the 360-degree acquisition. Furthermore, attenuation correction is not as well documented with the 180-degree data collection as it is with the 360-degree collection. There are ongoing efforts to resolve these issues. The myocardial images can be acquired with the rotating camera collecting data continuously as it rotates, or with the camera stopping at selected points for a predetermined length of time at each stop. With a single-headed gamma camera, using a 180-degree rotation with 32 stops at 40 seconds each, a typical SPECT scan can be acquired in approximately 20 minutes. The SPECT images, which can be oriented to any plane, are most commonly displayed in the short axis, vertical long axis, and horizontal long axis planes (Fig. 105–4).

Semi-quantitative computer programs are also available for analysis of SPECT myocardial images. A program available on some nuclear medicine computers is the bull's-eye display and analysis. This program takes each of the short axis images from the apex to the base of the heart and displays them as progressively enlarging concentric circles into a single image. This program displays the extent of any defect, relative to the entire ventricle, and is helpful in determining the percentage of abnormal myocardium.

THALLIUM-201

Radiopharmaceutical

Thallium-201, a cyclotron-produced radionuclide, is a potassium analog and the first commercially produced myocardial perfusion imaging agent; it is administered in the form of thallous chloride. Thallium-201 has a half-life of 73 hours and decays by electron capture to mercury-201. During this decay process, characteristic x-rays, which are 90 per cent abundant, are given off with photon energies of 69 to 83 keV. It is these characteristic x-rays that are primarily imaged for the thallium data acquisition. Gamma-rays of 135 keV and 167 keV are also emitted by ^{201}Tl in 2.7 per cent and 10 per cent abundance, respectively.

Thallium-201 is distributed to all organs proportional to blood flow. The blood-brain barrier prevents accumulation in the brain. Because 3 to 5 per cent of the cardiac output goes to the myocardium, 3 to 5 per cent of the administered dose of ^{201}Tl accumulates in the myocardium. The amount of ^{201}Tl in the myocardium depends on blood flow, extraction, and wash-out. The accumulation of ^{201}Tl is linearly related to myocardial blood flow over a wide range of flow rates. Thallium-201 has a high extraction fraction during its first pass through the myocardium. The mechanism of extraction of the thallous ion is not well understood. The intracellular localization of ^{201}Tl was originally thought to be related to the ATPase-dependent sodium-potassium pump. Subsequent studies have suggested that the accumulation is passive and relates to the concentration difference across the cell membrane.

Because the ^{201}Tl is highly extracted during its first pass, its blood level decreases rapidly. The gradient across the myocardial cell membrane then favors clearance of the ^{201}Tl from the cell into the blood. Experimental studies have demonstrated that reactive hyperemia is associated with an absolute increase in myocardial ischemia with an absolute decrease in ^{201}Tl accumulation, compared with normal myocardium. The half-clearance time is 3.4 hours, 5.3 hours, and 11.0 hours in the hyperemic, normal, and ischemic areas,

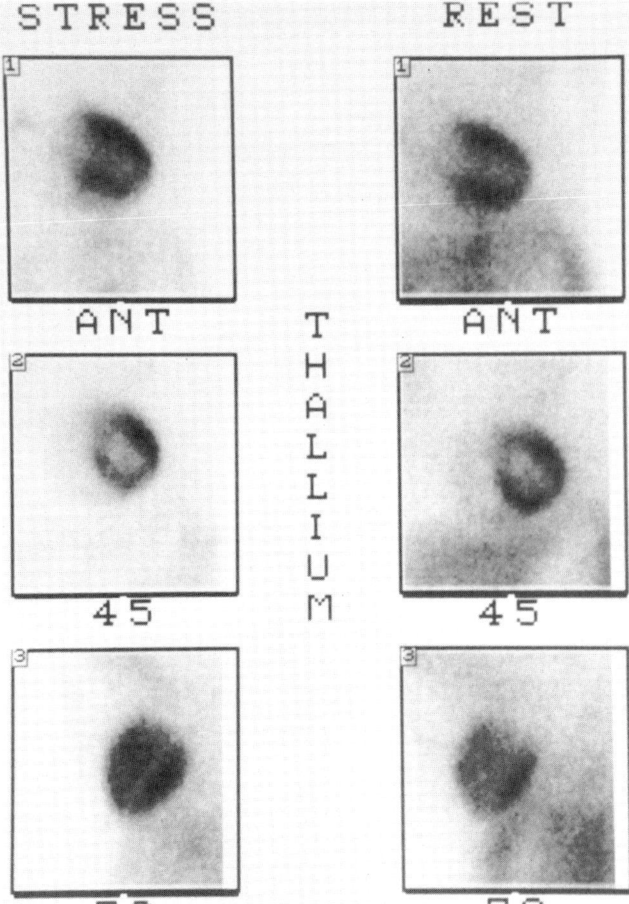

Figure 105–2. A normal planar thallium-201 imaging study obtained in three standard views.

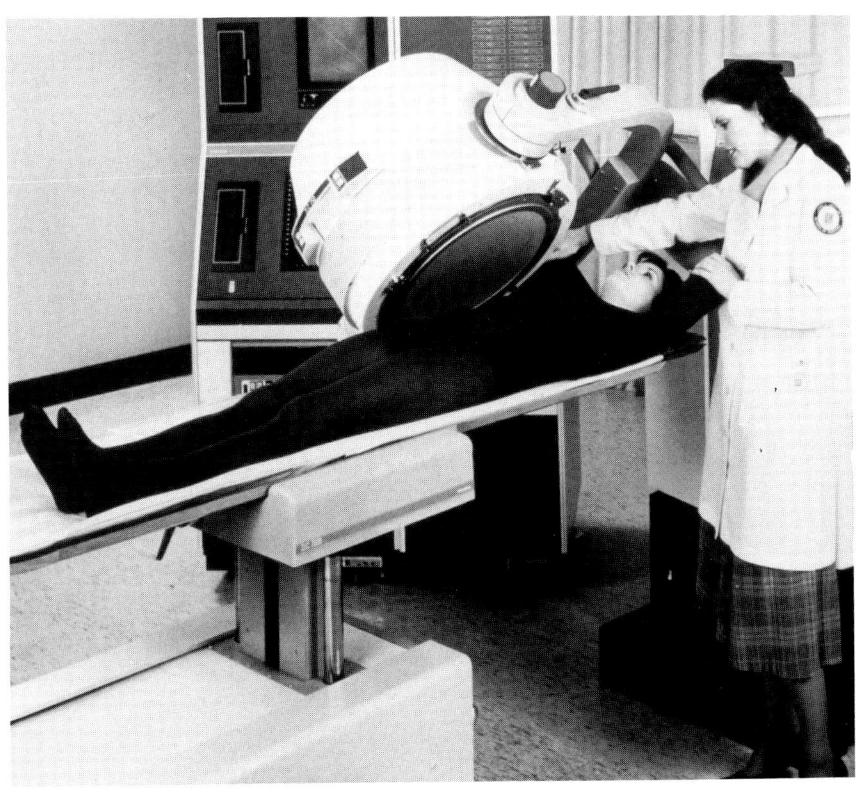

Figure 105–3. A rotating single-head gamma camera SPECT system demonstrating patient positioning.

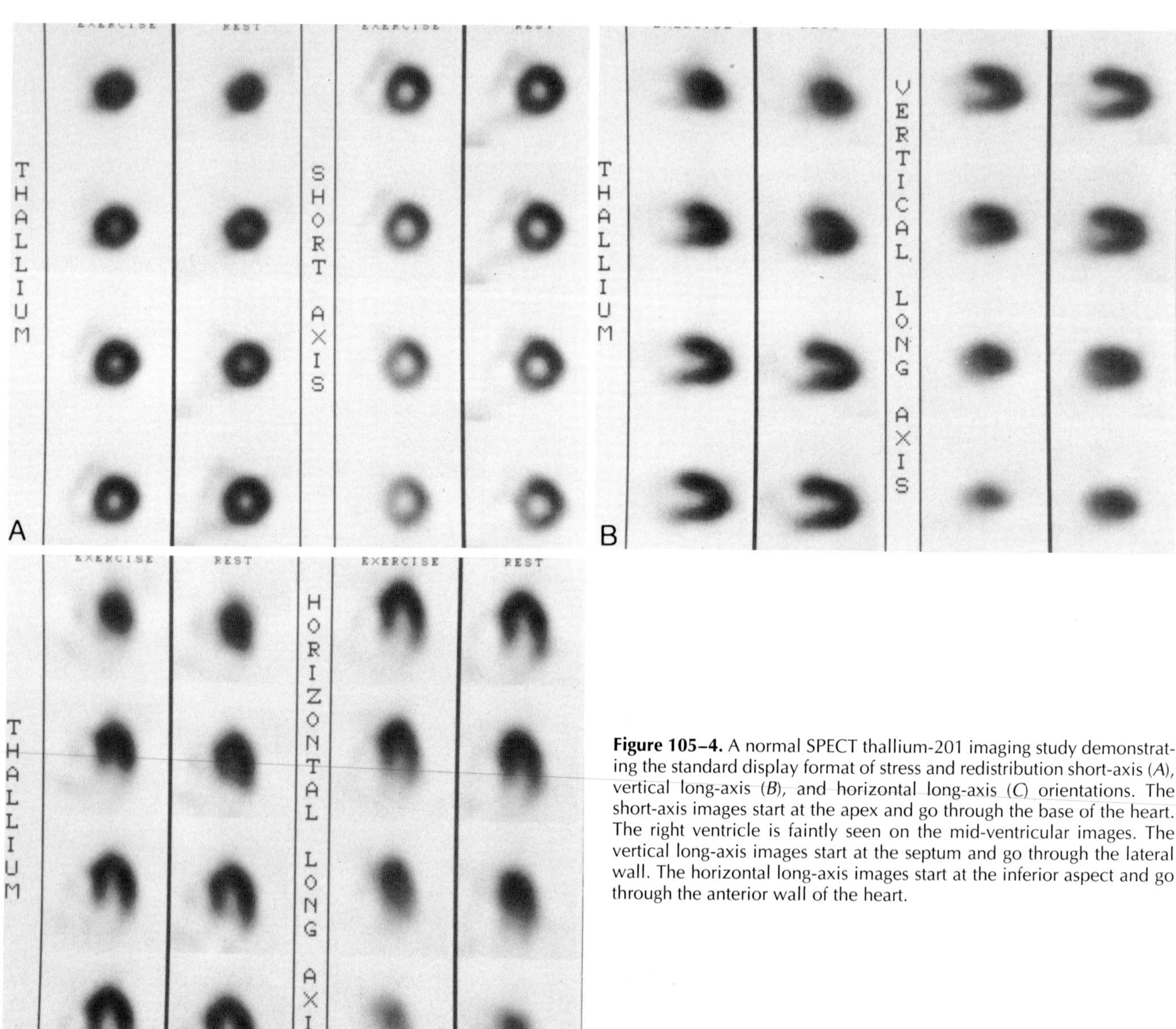

Figure 105–4. A normal SPECT thallium-201 imaging study demonstrating the standard display format of stress and redistribution short-axis (*A*), vertical long-axis (*B*), and horizontal long-axis (*C*) orientations. The short-axis images start at the apex and go through the base of the heart. The right ventricle is faintly seen on the mid-ventricular images. The vertical long-axis images start at the septum and go through the lateral wall. The horizontal long-axis images start at the inferior aspect and go through the anterior wall of the heart.

respectively. The redistribution phenomenon, thus, relates to the initial differential accumulation and the differential clearance. There may be an absolute increase in the ischemic zone early in the redistribution phase.

Imaging Technique

The protocol for stress-redistribution studies includes having the patient fasting and establishing an intravenous line for the administration of ^{201}Tl. The patient undergoes a standard exercise treadmill test with 3 mCi (111 MBq) of ^{201}Tl injected at peak exercise. The patient continues to exercise for an additional minute to keep myocardial blood flow constant while the ^{201}Tl is being extracted. The patient is monitored for three to six minutes following exercise, and imaging is begun 10 minutes after exercise. Redistribution images are obtained three to four hours after injection. Caloric intake should be minimized between the exercise and redistribution studies. Approximately 10 minutes before the redistribution image is started, the patient is injected with an additional 1 mCi (37 MBq) of ^{201}Tl. This re-injection technique has improved the ability of ^{201}Tl imaging to identify regions of reversible ischemia (thus, viable myocardium) that may have otherwise appeared to be irreversible (thus, nonviable myocardium). Acquiring the redistribution image at 24 hours has also been proposed as another technique to improve the accuracy of ^{201}Tl imaging for identifying viable myocardium. However, this technique is often not practical and produces marginal redistribution image quality.

High-resolution instrumentation is necessary for ^{201}Tl imaging. A current generation gamma camera with a 0.25-inch thick crystal and at least 37 photomultiplier tubes should be used. The thin crystal provides better spatial resolution with minimal loss of efficiency for the low photon energy. A window is used to include the 69 to 83 keV characteristic x-rays of mercury-201. Cameras with multiple photo peaks may include the 10 per cent abundant 167 keV photopeak. Images may be acquired in either the planar or SPECT mode.

Image Interpretation

The interpretation of ^{201}Tl images utilizes the wash-in and wash-out properties of the radiopharmaceutical. Homogeneous tracer accumulation in the myocardium at stress indicates no significant differences in coronary artery blood flow (see Fig. 105–2). With equivalent wash-out throughout the myocardium, the redistribution image will also be homogeneous. On the stress image, an area of diminished perfusion can be due to infarct, ischemia, or a region of combined infarct and ischemia, which can be determined by the redistribution image. Regions of stress-induced ischemia become homogeneous with normal myocardium on the redistribution image (Fig. 105–5), whereas a region of infarct at stress shows a persistent defect at redistribution (Fig. 105–6). Regions of perfusion defect at stress that show some improvement, but do not become completely homogeneous with normal myocardium, are considered to be segments that have a combination of infarcted and ischemic myocardium. Caution must be taken when interpreting the apical segment of the left ventricle where thinning of the normal myocardium can mimic an infarct. Likewise, normal drop-out of activity near the base of the heart in the membranous septum and at the valve plane along the upper posterolateral wall can mimic a myocardial infarction.

TECHNETIUM-99M LABELED PERFUSION AGENTS

Several new ^{99m}Tc myocardial perfusion imaging radiopharmaceuticals are being evaluated. Two agents have been approved by the Food and Drug Administration (FDA) for perfusion imaging (^{99m}Tc sestamibi and ^{99m}Tc teboroxime). A ^{99m}Tc-labeled perfusion agent offers several potential advantages over ^{201}Tl. The physical characteristics for imaging are better for ^{99m}Tc than for ^{201}Tl. Larger amounts of radioactivity can be administered with ^{99m}Tc radiopharmaceuticals than with ^{201}Tl. Thus, better imaging statistics can be obtained. Because of the larger amounts of administered activity, first-pass studies can be performed to give functional information, in addition to the perfusion study (Fig. 105–7). A ^{99m}Tc agent can be prepared on site, whereas ^{201}Tl must be delivered from the production site. Thus, ^{99m}Tc is more readily available to a larger number of centers.

Technetium-99m Sestamibi

Technetium-99m sestamibi (methoxyisobutylisonitrile) is accumulated within the myocardium in proportion to regional myocardial blood flow. The uptake is by passive diffusion and is linear up to 2.5 times normal flow rates. The myocardial extraction fraction of sestamibi at resting coronary blood flow is less than that of ^{201}Tl (66 per cent versus 82 per cent, respectively). Sestamibi undergoes rapid clearance from the blood. Over 90 per cent of the initial activity is cleared in less than five minutes. Sestamibi is excreted intact by the kidneys, and the hepatobiliary system and shows no evidence of in vivo metabolism. Unlike ^{201}Tl, there is no significant redistribution of sestamibi within the myocardium, and, thus, the initial uptake pattern remains relatively fixed with a half-life for myocardial clearance of approximately seven hours. Because there is no wash-out of tracer from the myocardium, two separate injections of sestamibi must be given for a rest and stress evaluation of myocardial perfusion. These injections could be given on separate days, but this approach is often not practical. Therefore, protocols have been developed to complete the study in one day, using two separate doses with the dose of radiopharmaceutical for the stress study being approximately three times the dose for the rest study. If a first-pass RNA is to be performed, the patient is given an 8-mCi (296 MBq) bolus injection of sestamibi through an intravenous line in the external jugular vein with acquisition of a first-pass RNA during the injection. The patient then waits 45 to 60 minutes prior to myocardial perfusion imaging. During this time, a small amount of food and/or liquid is given to help clear some of the hepatobiliary and intestinal tracer. After completing the resting perfusion images, the patient is exercised in a standard manner. At peak exercise, a 24-mCi (888 MBq) bolus injection is given in the external jugular line, and a first-pass RNA is repeated. After a briefer, 30-minute, interval, the stress perfusion image is acquired (see Fig. 105–7). The first-pass study and the perfusion images are analyzed for evidence of ischemia or infarct. Thus, this agent allows for simultaneous analysis of left ventricular function and perfusion. The first-pass RNA studies are analyzed for changes in ejection fraction and segmental wall motion. Patterns of perfusion abnormalities are analyzed similarly to ^{201}Tl images for analysis of ischemia and/or infarct (Fig. 105–8).

Technetium-99m Teboroxime

Technetium-99m teboroxime, a neutral lipophilic compound derived from a boronic acid adduct of technetium oxime, is taken up by the myocardium proportional to regional myocardial blood flow. Myocardial uptake occurs by passive diffusion with an extraction fraction of greater than 90 per cent. After uptake, however, the tracer clears the myocardium rapidly with a bi-exponential pattern of wash-out with effective half-lives of six minutes (66 per cent of myocardial activity) and four hours (33 per cent of myocardial activity). Thus, the first half-life for the myocardium is between 10 and 15 minutes. Teboroxime is excreted through the liver, where peak uptake occurs at approximately six minutes.

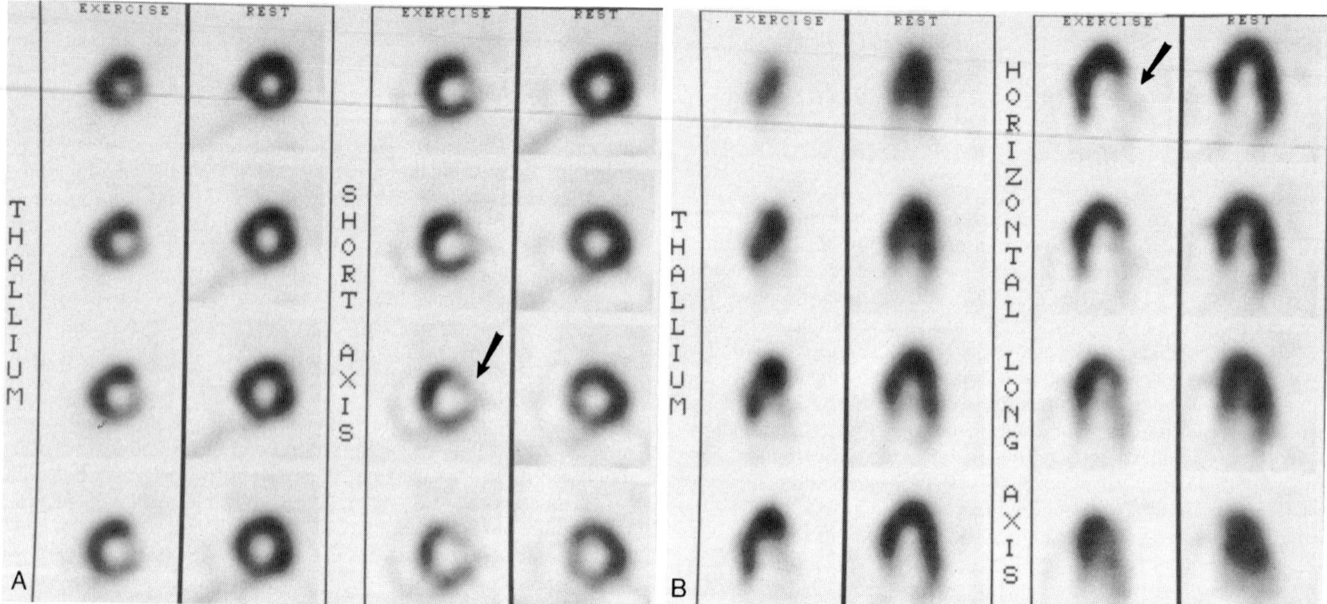

Figure 105–5. Short-axis (*A*) and horizontal long-axis (*B*) SPECT images of thallium-201 in a patient with coronary artery disease. The stress images demonstrate a perfusion defect in the lateral wall of the left ventricle (*arrows*) in *A* and *B* that shows complete reversibility on the redistribution images. These findings demonstrate exercise-induced myocardial ischemia.

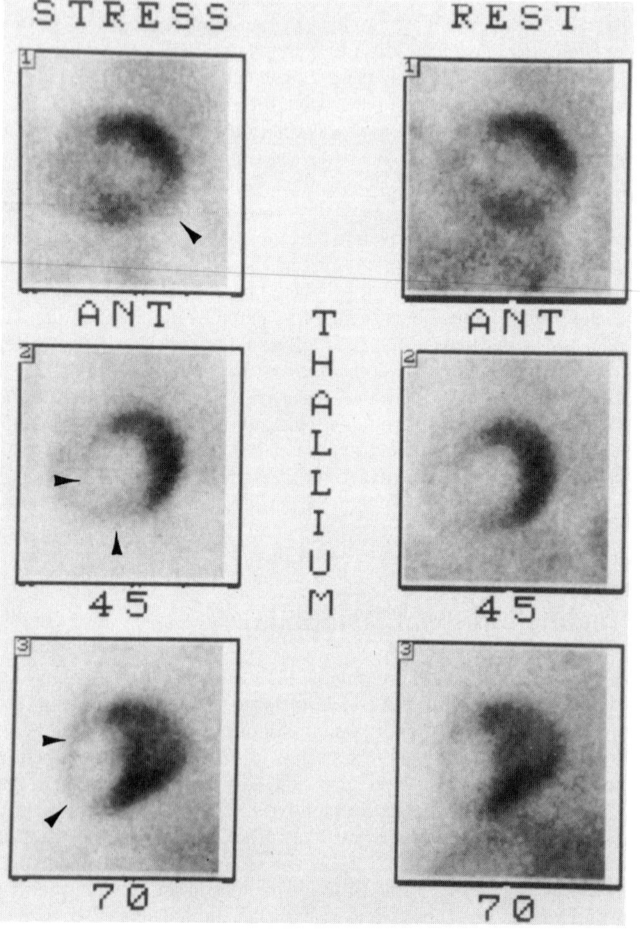

Figure 105–6. Thallium-201 planar images in a patient with coronary artery disease. There are extensive perfusion defects on the stress images in the interventricular septum and infero-apex (*arrows*: 45-degree LAO view) and the anterior wall and apex of the left ventricle (*arrows*: 70-degree LAO and anterior view). These defects show no improvement at redistribution. These findings demonstrate prior myocardial infarction.

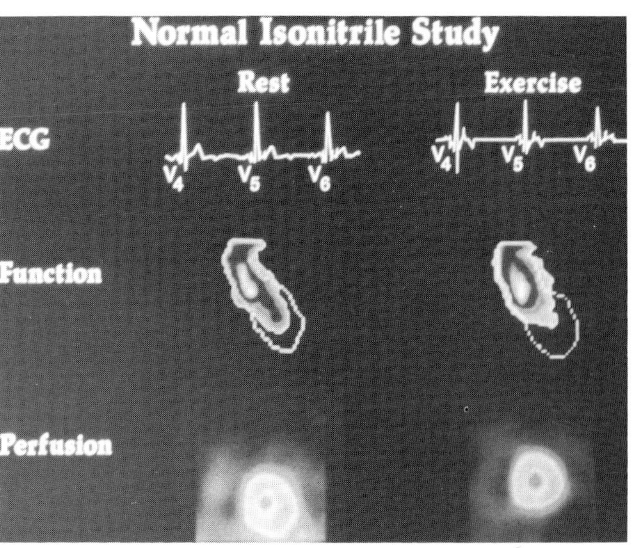

Figure 105–7. A combined myocardial functional study and myocardial perfusion study (short-axis projection) performed as a one-day protocol with ^{99m}Tc sestamibi in a normal volunteer. The EKG has no ST-segment changes with exercise. The ejection fraction, wall motion, and myocardial perfusion are normal at rest. With exercise, there is some ventricular dilatation. Myocardial contractility increases with exercise with no segmental wall motion abnormalities. The exercise ejection fraction is increased over the resting study. The exercise short-axis SPECT perfusion images demonstrate homogeneous tracer accumulation throughout the myocardium.

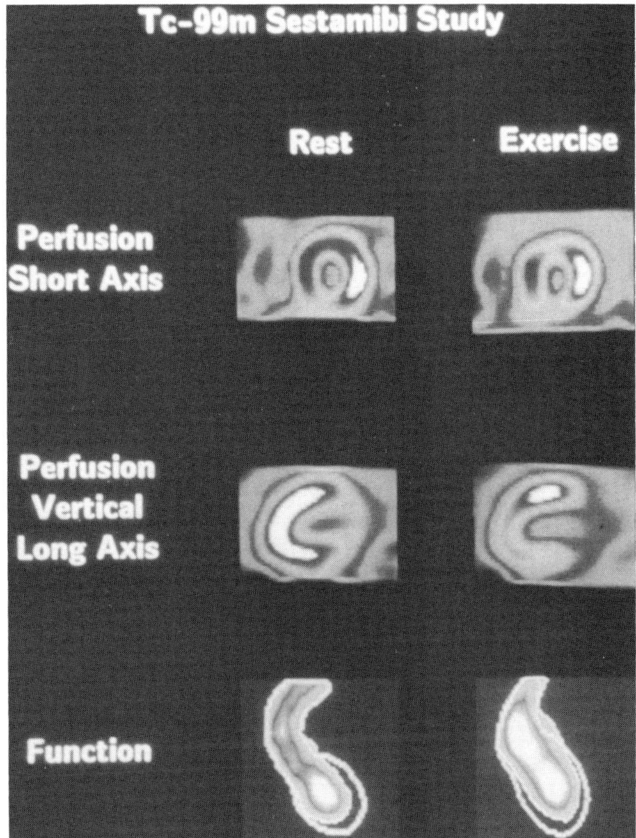

Figure 105–8. A combined myocardial functional study and myocardial perfusion study done as a one-day protocol with ^{99m}Tc sestamibi in a patient with coronary artery disease. There is a perfusion defect in the inferior wall of the left ventricle on the resting perfusion study and hypokinesis of the inferior wall on the resting first-pass RNA study. At exercise, the inferior wall perfusion defect persists, and there is also a new anterior wall and apical perfusion defect noted. The stress first-pass RNA study demonstrates slight improvement in the inferior wall contractility, while the anterior wall and apex become hypokinetic with a decrease in ejection fraction. These findings demonstrate a prior inferior wall myocardial infarction and exercise-induced ischemia in the anterior wall and apex of the left ventricle.

With the rapid clearance of this tracer from the myocardium, imaging must begin immediately after injection. Two separate injections are required for a stress and rest perfusion study. Unlike ^{201}Tl and ^{99m}Tc sestamibi, in which exercise is continued for an additional minute after injection, with teboroxime, exercise is stopped at the time of injection and imaging is started within two minutes. Although there is rapid clearance, successful planar and SPECT imaging has been done with this agent. The average dose of teboroxime for the rest or stress images is 15 to 25 mCi (555 to 925 MBq). With the rapid clearance of tracer from the myocardium, the stress and rest studies can generally be completed in about two hours. The ability to use high doses of activity allows for a first-pass RNA study to also be done with this agent, similar to sestamibi. Thus, teboroxime also allows for simultaneous left ventricular functional and perfusion analysis.

PHARMACOLOGIC STRESS TESTING

Many patients cannot exercise to their target heart rate (85 per cent of maximum predicted) owing to a variety of diseases, poor physical condition, or to medication, such as beta blockers, that limit heart rate response to exercise. The inability to achieve the target heart rate is an important factor in determining the significance of the results of the perfusion imaging study. Inadequate exercise does not create the desired differential in blood flow through altered coronary arteries. Thus, the perfusion images more closely reflect a basal coronary flow state that may be relatively similar in each of the vessels, in spite of the presence of stenosis in some. Therefore, inadequate exercise may result in a false-negative perfusion scan. Several alternatives to treadmill or bicycle exercise have been proposed, including hand-grip exercise, arm ergometer exercise, isometric exercise, rapid atrial pacing, and pharmacologic cardiac stress. Currently, the most accepted alternative to standard exercise is pharmacologic stress agents.

Dipyridamole (Persantine), a potent, indirect coronary vasodilator, is the only drug currently approved by the FDA for use as a pharmacologic cardiac stress agent. Dipyridamole increases myocardial blood flow to areas supplied by normal coronary arteries (by as much as three to four times normal resting flow), but it does not increase myocardial blood flow to the same extent, if at all, to areas supplied by stenosed coronary arteries. Dipyridamole acts by blocking the uptake of endogenous adenosine. The increased extracellular level of adenosine then interacts with the adenosine A-2 receptor in the wall of the endothelial cells that subsequently results in coronary vasodilation. Dipyridamole is administered intravenously in a dose of 142 μg/kg/min for four minutes. Heart rate, blood pressure, and an EKG are monitored. An increase in heart rate of 10 beats per minute and a decrease in blood pressure of 10 mm of mercury are expected after the intravenous infusion. The perfusion tracer (most often ^{201}Tl) is injected at three to five minutes after completion of the dipyridamole infusion, when blood levels are their highest. Acquisition of the stress image is started within five to six minutes of the ^{201}Tl injection and redistribution images are acquired at three to four hours after the stress images. A re-injection technique can also be used for redistribution, as is done with standard exercise studies. The diagnostic accuracy of intravenous dipyridamole ^{201}Tl perfusion imaging has been found to be similar to exercise studies in the diagnosis of coronary artery disease. Side effects from dipyridamole have been observed in 30 to 50 per cent of patients. Chest pain occurs frequently. Other reported side effects include headache, flushing, dizziness, and nausea. In some patients, typical angina may occur with ischemic ST segment changes on the EKG. In many, however, the chest pain is atypical, and the presence of chest pain is not diagnostic of coronary artery disease because this symptom has been reported in many normal subjects. Serious side effects are not common, but there have been reports of lethal ventricular arrhythmias, bronchospasm with respiratory failure, myocardial infarction, and death. Thus, precautions must be taken to exclude some patients from the study, such as patients with a history of asthma or wheezing at the time of the study or patients with hypertension or congestive heart failure. Aminophylline is a pharmacologic antagonist of dipyridamole and brings about rapid reversal of symptoms caused by the administration of the dipyridamole. Patients taking theophylline drugs must have these medications withheld prior to the performance of the study. The experience to date with dipyridamole demonstrates that it is an acceptable alternative to exercise testing in patients unable to exercise adequately.

Adenosine can be administered directly by intravenous infusion, which results in increased levels of available extracellular adenosine, while bypassing the need for a drug to increase levels of endogenous adenosine. The current commercially available form of adenosine has been approved by the FDA for the treatment of supraventricular tachycardia, but has not been approved as an adjunct for myocardial perfusion imaging. Adenosine can be administered as a six-minute continuous infusion at a rate of 140 μg/kg/min, with the perfusion tracer (usually ^{201}Tl) injected at three minutes into the infusion. At this dose, maximum coronary vasodilation occurs in most patients. Stress thallium images are obtained about five minutes after the termination of the infusion and redistribution images are acquired three to four hours later. Side effects are frequent with intravenous adenosine, occurring in approximately 80 per cent of patients. Chest pain occurs in 30 to 50 per cent of patients. Like dipyridamole, the chest pain may be typical of angina, but more often is atypical and does not correlate with the presence of coronary artery disease. First-degree heart block may be seen in approximately 10 per cent of patients whereas second-degree heart block is seen in about 4 per cent, and third-degree heart block in about 1 per cent of patients. The A-V conduction delay is due to the direct effect of adenosine on the conducting system. The side effects of adenosine are very similar to dipyridamole. The accuracy of adenosine in diagnosing coronary artery disease is similar to dipyridamole stress imaging and standard exercise imaging. The same precautions and contraindications apply to adenosine as with dipyridamole. Aminophylline can also be used to reverse the effects of adenosine, but is rarely needed due to the ultra-short half-life of intravenous adenosine of less than 10 seconds, which is a main advantage of this agent for pharmacologic stress perfusion imaging.

Whereas dipyridamole and adenosine are primarily vasodilators, dobutamine, a synthetic catecholamine, increases heart rate, myocardial contractility, and myocardial oxygen demand, thus mimicking exercise better than any other pharmacologic stress agent. Thus, at high levels of dobutamine infusion, regional coronary blood flow increases in normal vessels, but not in stenotic vessels; therefore, the differential in blood flow in this setting can be demonstrated with the injection of perfusion tracers at peak infusion. Dobutamine is given as a progressive infusion starting at 5 μg/kg/min and increasing at three-minute intervals to a maximum of 40 μg/kg/min or to patient tolerance. Patients with significant ventricular arrhythmias or hypertension should not be considered for this study. Fewer scintigraphic studies have been done with dobutamine than with either of the vasodilator perfusion agents, but preliminary data are encouraging that this study can be done safely with accuracy comparable to other pharmacologic and exercise stress studies for the diagnosis of coronary artery disease.

MYOCARDIAL INFARCT IMAGING

^{99m}Tc Stannous Pyrophosphate

Several radiopharmaceuticals have been demonstrated to localize in areas of acute myocardial infarction. Mercury-203 chlormerodrin was the first agent used to localize in acute infarction; subsequently, radiolabeled tetracycline, mercury fluorescein, and glucoheptonate have demonstrated localization. All of these agents, however, have limitations in their usefulness. The first agent to gain widespread use was ^{99m}Tc pyrophosphate. Although other bone-seeking radiotracers also accumulate in acute myocardial infarctions, ^{99m}Tc pyrophosphate is the agent of choice of this group of radiopharmaceuticals because it provides images superior to those of other tracers. The mechanism of tracer accumulation of this agent in myocardial infarctions relates to the deposition of calcium in necrosing myocardium. The original studies suggested that deposition occurs in the mitochondria of irreversibly damaged myocardial cells. For the scan to be abnormal, some residual collateral blood flow to the damaged myocardium must be present. The study will be negative for the first 24 hours after infarction, and becomes maximally abnormal at two to three days after the myocardial infarction has occurred. The usual dose of ^{99m}Tc pyrophosphate to be injected for this study is 15 to 20 mCi (555 to 740 MBq). Because ^{99m}Tc pyrophosphate is also taken up in bone as well as the infarcted myocardium, overlying rib activity can interfere with abnormalities of uptake into the myocardium, especially on planar imaging. SPECT imaging improves the detection of abnormal localization of ^{99m}Tc pyrophosphate in regions of infarcted myocardium. Because SPECT provides three-dimensional information and improves image contrast, a better definition of abnormal localization is realized. Although SPECT has been able to quantitate infarct size in animal models, its ability to accurately quantitate infarct size in human patients has not been documented.

The use of ^{99m}Tc pyrophosphate is not indicated in the routine evaluation of a patient who has a known myocardial infarction documented by either electrocardiography or characteristic cardiac isoenzyme changes. The study may be helpful, however, in patients who present late after the onset of symptomatology and the rise and fall of the cardiac isoenzymes may have already occurred. Because the ^{99m}Tc pyrophosphate scan may be abnormal for as long as 14 days following the acute event, an abnormal study would confirm the occurrence of a recent myocardial infarction.

Indium-111 Antimyosin

Antimyosin is a murine-produced monoclonal antibody that is directed against heavy-chain myosin. Binding of this monoclonal antibody with myosin occurs only when the myocyte membrane is disrupted and there is irreversible cell damage. Thus, the binding of this monoclonal antibody is specific for myocyte necrosis. The F(ab')$_2$ fragment of antimyosin is a fairly large protein molecule with relatively slow clearance from the blood pool. Therefore, to visualize the distribution of this monoclonal antibody, radionuclides with longer half-lives have been used to label the monoclonal antibody for imaging at 24 to 48 hours after administration. Most of the imaging studies with this monoclonal antibody have used indium-111 (^{111}In). This radionuclide (half-life of 67 hours) has been linked to the antimyosin molecule via the chelating agent, DTPA. Using planar imaging, investigators have shown that this radiopharmaceutical demonstrates a high sensitivity and specificity in the detection and localization of acute myocardial infarctions. This agent has also been shown to assist in the diagnosis and assessment of prognosis in cardiac transplant rejection and myocarditis. To evaluate patients who are at potential risk for future myocardial ischemic events, antimyosin has been used in conjunction with ^{201}Tl myocardial perfusion tracer to simultaneously evaluate regions of abnormal myocardial perfusion as compared with the region of myocardial necrosis.

The typical planar antimyosin scan is acquired at 24 to 48 hours after the injection of 0.5 mg of antimyosin labeled with 2 mCi (74 MBq) of ^{111}In. Images are acquired in the standard anterior, 45-degree LAO and 70-degree LAO projections, with each image being acquired for 7 minutes (300,000 to 500,000 counts). Both photopeaks of ^{111}In (174 and 247 keV) are imaged, using a medium-energy general purpose collimator.

The interpretation of myocardial images with antimyosin is similar to that with ^{99m}Tc pyrophosphate. On a 48-hour delayed image, the target-to-background ratio is greater with ^{111}In antimyosin than what is seen on the typical ^{99m}Tc pyrophosphate scan. A more diffuse pattern of uptake would be expected in the evaluation of myocarditis, whereas a more focal, segmental region of abnormality would be seen in areas of myocardial infarction. Currently, most of these studies are being done as research. However, some of these applications may soon be useful in the clinical evaluation of these patients.

CARDIAC IMAGING BY POSITRON EMISSION TOMOGRAPHY

Positron emission tomography (PET) has been available for more than 15 years, but has only recently emerged as a clinical diagnostic option for the evaluation of myocardial ischemia and viability. PET offers selected advantages over either planar or tomographic imaging of ^{201}Tl- or ^{99m}Tc-labeled agents. The inability to correct for attenuation in either planar or SPECT imaging can affect the accurate interpretation of myocardial perfusion studies. In contrast, PET can accurately correct for attenuation. PET can accurately assess myocardial perfusion and metabolism, which is important in the evaluation of viability. PET measures the concentration of radioactivity in a given volume of tissue, and it is the only modality currently available that can provide quantitative measurements of in vivo biochemistry. The high-resolution images of PET can be analyzed qualitatively, semi-quantitatively, or quantitatively.

Evaluation of Myocardial Perfusion

The most commonly used tracers in PET for evaluating myocardial perfusion are rubidium-82 and nitrogen-13 ammonia.

Rubidium-82 (^{82}Rb) is similar to ^{201}Tl in that it acts as a potassium analog. Being a generator-produced radionuclide, an on-site cyclotron and radiopharmacy are not needed for its use, thus making it more readily and widely available. Rubidium-82 is FDA-approved for myocardial perfusion imaging. The very short physical half-life of this radionuclide (76 seconds) allows rapid imaging and allows for serial studies to be done easily. The extraction fraction of ^{82}Rb is approximately 65 per cent at normal resting myocardial blood flow and is nonlinear at higher flow rates. Several studies have reported myocardial perfusion imaging with ^{82}Rb to have sensitivities of 90 to 95 per cent and specificities of 75 to 95 per cent for the detection of coronary artery disease.

In centers that have an on-site cyclotron, nitrogen-13 (^{13}N) ammonia is the predominant tracer used in the evaluation of myocardial perfusion. Ammonia, labeled with ^{13}N (half-life of 10 minutes) has an extraction fraction of approximately 90 per cent at normal resting myocardial blood flow, which exceeds that of both ^{201}Tl and ^{82}Rb. The extraction of ^{13}N ammonia is not linear at higher flow rates. It clears rapidly from the blood pool, enters the extravascular space, and is converted in the myocardium to ^{13}N glutamine. Because the clearance of ^{13}N from the myocardium is slow, images with high contrast between the myocardium and blood pool are produced. Thus, image quality is excellent. Although pulmonary accumulation of ^{13}N ammonia occurs in smokers and in patients with congestive heart failure, the tomographic technique of PET produces good-quality images of the myocardium in those instances. Studies have reported sensitivities and specificities for the diagnosis of coronary artery disease with ^{13}N ammonia comparable to those with ^{82}Rb.

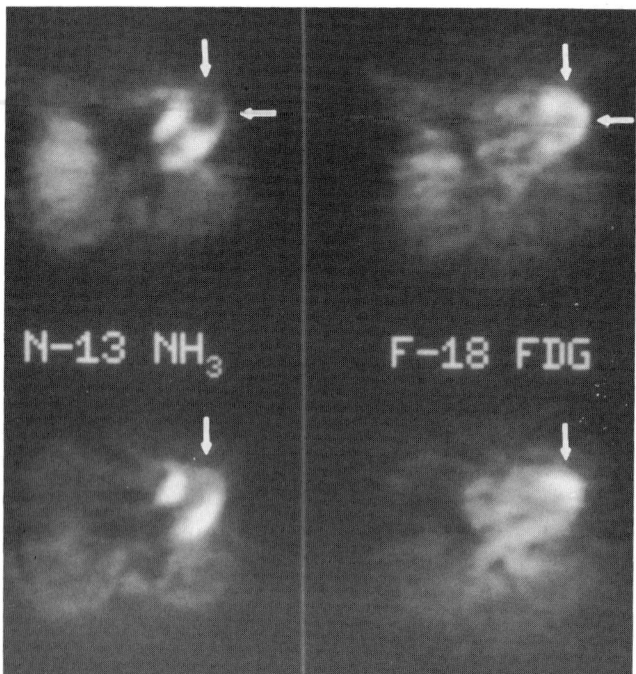

Figure 105–9. Transaxial ^{13}N ammonia and ^{18}F FDG-PET images in a patient with coronary artery disease. The ^{13}N ammonia images demonstrate an extensive perfusion abnormality in the anterior and anterolateral segments of the left ventricle (*arrows*). The corresponding planes of the ^{18}F FDG images, acquired in the fasting state, demonstrate moderate accumulation of ^{18}F FDG in the same regions where perfusion is diminished (*arrows*) and little, if any, FDG accumulation in the rest of the myocardium. These findings demonstrate viable, ischemic myocardium in the anterior and anterolateral regions of the left ventricle.

Owing to the technical requirements for PET imaging, standard treadmill or upright bicycle exercise in the PET facility is not practical. Supine bicycle exercise is feasible, but difficult and cumbersome to perform. Thus, the various pharmacologic stress agents for evaluation of myocardial ischemia offer an alternative that is more suitable for use with PET imaging than either treadmill or bicycle exercise.

Evaluation of Myocardial Viability

With the increasing resources and capabilities of performing coronary artery bypass graft surgery and percutaneous transluminal coronary angioplasty in patients with coronary artery disease, the question of tissue viability becomes increasingly important. These patients generally have a history of prior myocardial infarction and have wall motion abnormalities. The ability to distinguish viable from nonviable myocardium can dramatically alter clinical decisions whether to treat a patient medically or to proceed to surgery, angioplasty, or cardiac transplantation.

Wall motion analysis by contrast ventriculography, echocardiography, or multi-gated acquisition studies cannot accurately distinguish a region of ischemic viable myocardium from a region of infarcted nonviable myocardium. Even with re-injection and/or 24-hour delayed redistribution imaging techniques, ^{201}Tl scintigraphy can overestimate nonviable myocardium in these patients. Thus, there is a need to develop better noninvasive methods for identifying and distinguishing viable from nonviable myocardium.

One method for assessing myocardial viability using PET is by evaluating myocardial intermediary metabolism with ^{18}F fluorodeoxyglucose (^{18}F FDG). In ischemic, but viable, myocardium, metabolism is shifted to anaerobic glycolysis, which results in a greater uptake of glucose (thus, FDG) into those segments, relative to the surrounding normal myocardium. Thus, this characteristic allows identification of ischemic, viable myocardium because nonviable myocardium will not accumulate FDG. The finding of maintained or increased FDG accumulation, relative to coronary artery blood flow, assessed with ^{13}N ammonia, can identify regions of ischemia with preserved ischemic viable myocardium (Fig. 105–9). The combination of ^{13}N ammonia and ^{18}F FDG has been reported to have a positive predictive accuracy of 78 to 85 per cent in the identification of viable myocardium and a negative predictive accuracy of 78 to 92 per cent. If these studies are done in the fasting state, the unpredictability of FDG uptake results in as many as 30 per cent of the studies being uninterpretable. Therefore, to assist in a more reliable uptake, patients are usually given 50 g of oral glucose approximately 30 minutes prior to the injection of FDG for these studies.

In spite of some of the benefits of myocardial PET imaging, the cost of cardiac PET and the lack of reimbursement policies for these procedures by third-party payers remain major obstacles in the further development and widespread use of these techniques at this time. Most third-party payers are reimbursing for the studies, but only a few have policies for reimbursement. The advantages of PET must be shown to result not only in improved accuracy in the diagnosis of coronary artery disease, as compared with existing modalities, but also to be cost-effective in the management of these patients. This challenge will determine the future role of cardiac PET in the overall management of patients with ischemic heart disease.

Bibliography

Bonow RO, Berman DS, Gibbons RJ, et al: Cardiac positron emission tomography—a report for health professionals from the Committee on Advanced Cardiac Imaging and Technology of the Council on Clinical Cardiology, American Heart Association. Circulation 84(1):447–454, 1991.

Bonow RO, Dilsizian V, Cuocolo A, Bacharach SL: Identification of viable myocardium in patients with chronic coronary artery disease and left ventricular dysfunction: Comparison of thallium scintigraphy with reinjection and PET imaging with 18F-fluorodeoxyglucose. Circulation 83:26–37, 1991.

Borges-Neto S, Coleman RE, Potts JM, Jones RH: Combined exercise radionuclide angiography and single photon emission computed tomography perfusion studies for assessment of coronary artery disease. Semin Nucl Med 21:223–229, 1991.

Johnson LL: Monoclonal Fab antimyosin in cardiac imaging. Clin Cardiol 15: 145–153, 1992.

Kahn JK, McGhie I, Akers MS, et al: Quantitative rotational tomography with Tl-201 and Tc-99m 2-methoxy-isobutyl-isonitrile: A direct comparison in normal individuals and patients with coronary artery disease. Circulation 79:1282–1293, 1989.

Leppo JA, De Puey EG, Johnson LL: A review of cardiac imaging with sestamibi and teboroxime. J Nucl Med 32(10):2012–2022, 1991.

Levison JR, Boucher CA, Coley CM, et al: Usefulness of semiquantitative analysis of dipyridamole thallium-201 redistribution for improving risk stratification before vascular surgery. Am J Cardiol 66:406–410, 1990.

Verani MS, Mahmarian JJ, Hixon JB, et al: Diagnosis of coronary artery disease by controlled coronary vasodilation with adenosine thallium-201 scintigraphy in patients unable to exercise. Circulation 82(1):80–87, 1990.

106 Conventional and Digital Angiography of the Heart

Julius H. Grollman, Jr.

TECHNICAL FACTORS NEEDED TO GENERATE THE IMAGE

Cine radiography is the preferred recording medium for cardiac and coronary anatomy, although large film serialography and small format (70 to 105 mm) photofluorography are useful imaging modalities. Similar factors apply to whatever technique is being used. The peak kilovoltage (kVp) should be approximately 70 to take advantage of iodinated contrast medium. Short exposure times of 4 to 10 msec are mandatory to eliminate motion unsharpness due to cardiac movement. The shorter times are required for cine, with up to 10 msec being necessary for large film serialography. The amperage levels depend on the modality used: 800 to 1200 mA for large films and 200 to 500 mA for cine.

Large Film Serialography

Large film serialography with conventional film-screen combinations requires relatively high kVp levels, especially for large adults, for whom 100 kVp or more is needed to maintain short exposure times. Although rare-earth screens have helped considerably in reducing the kVp, careful coning to just cover the heart and the use of 10:1 or 12:1 grids are imperative to reduce scatter and to produce high-quality studies even with a high kVp. Conventional cine and/or digital angiography has replaced large film serialography in the study of the heart and has the potential to replace it in the study of the great vessels.

Cine and Photofluorography

Rapid development in cesium iodide image amplifier technology has resulted in tubes with resolution of the output phosphor approaching that of large films, that is, 5 to 7 line-pairs/mm. Because of the greater efficiency of conversion of x-ray to light with high gain, short exposure times are obtainable. An exposure time of 4 msec is optimal to eliminate motion, although frequently in the right anterior oblique (RAO) projection, vessels in the atrioventricular grooves (right coronary and circumflex arteries) are blurred in patients with tachycardia. Although some cine systems allow exposures up to 10 msec, motion unsharpness on the film during coronary angiography eliminates any benefit from kVp reduction. In visualization of the cardiac chambers, however, motion unsharpness is much less critical, and longer exposure times are more acceptable. Although it is desirable to maintain kVp around 70, larger patients require higher kVp to allow adequate penetration, especially when the angled projections are used. Close coning to the area of interest is imperative to obtain a high quality image. A grid ratio of 8 to 10:1 is generally recommended. The focal spot size of the x-ray tube should be between 0.6 and 0.8 mm for coronary arteriography. Larger focal spots are acceptable for contrast studies of the chambers and great vessels.

Since image amplifiers are of variable quality, care must be taken in their selection. One looks for the "ideal" combination of gain, noise, and contrast, realizing that noise increases with gain. Since the highest gain will be found on the largest mode of a dual- or triple-mode amplifier, the choice should depend on the case selection in the laboratory. The 15 to 17 cm (6 to 7 inch) image amplifier is optimal for the study of adults with ischemic coronary disease. However, more and more patients are being studied with significant cardiac enlargement, necessitating larger 22 to 25 cm (9 to 10 inch) multiple mode image amplifiers to cover the heart. Patients with congenital heart disease in whom simultaneous visualization of the chambers and great vessels is important are also more suitably studied on the larger image amplifiers. With the larger intensifiers, the overall quality of coronary imaging is somewhat reduced owing to the higher kVp needed in the smaller 15 to 17 cm mode, as there is a loss in gain proportional to the square of the change of field size. For example, the decrease in gain from the 22-cm field to the 15-cm field in the same intensifier is $15^2/22^2 = 0.46$. However, the compromise of a larger format image amplifier is acceptable, and even larger 30-cm (12-inch) amplifiers are now being used in laboratories in which noncardiac procedures are also performed.

A physicist will be helpful in evaluating the intensifier tube, but the experienced angiographer may also evaluate these factors by viewing the cine films, realizing that choice of cine film and processing are equally important in the chain leading to the final image. It should be remembered that the image amplifier has a life expectancy limited to only a few years. Occasional re-evaluation is important to detect decreasing contrast and gain.

The cine camera should be capable of 60 frames per second. Using 30 frames per second reduces radiation demands on the x-ray tube by 50 per cent and still yields adequate information on coronary anatomy. Higher frame rates allow easier chamber motion analysis and are helpful in children or adults with rapid heart rates.

The lens in the camera is selected according to the degree of overframing desired on the cine film. Exact framing refers to including the entire circular image on the rectangular cine film. Any exclusion of the image on the film results in overframing. Moderate overframing is preferred in most laboratories, with the degree of overframing being dependent on the image amplifier output phosphor diameter and objective lens focal length as well as lens size. Lenses of 85 and 100 mm are usually recommended.

Television monitors in conjunction with magnetic videotape and/or disc recorders are used for visualizing the progress of the examination. Until recently, 525-line television systems, as used commercially, were used. With the currently available higher line scan of above 1000, greater vertical resolution is obtained, with improvement in diagnostic information from the television monitor and much easier visualization of the fine wires and catheters used in coronary angioplasty. Digital fluoroscopy with 512^2 matrix and high line display of greater than 1000 lines are available and are further improving the fluoroscopic image.

Initially, cine imaging was adapted to gastrointestinal fluoroscopic rooms. Special procedure rooms were then designed with floating table tops to which a rotational cradle was added to allow rapid change to oblique projections. With the current additional need to image the coronary arteries with cranial and caudal angulation, multiangular C and U arms with x-ray tube and image intensifier are now widely used to maintain the patient in a relatively isocentric plane. The functions of a cardiac laboratory are different from those of a vascular laboratory. In spite of similarities between vascular and cardiac imaging techniques, laboratory design is significantly different between the two facilities to encourage separate facilities when the caseload is adequate.

Photofluorography may be used as an adjunct to cardiac and coronary angiography when static images are desired. The same technical factors apply as noted with cine radiography, except that slightly longer exposure times are usually necessary. Since fewer exposures at slower rates are made, higher x-ray tube loads are possible, allowing more radiation to produce a less noisy image. Because resolution has improved so much with the most recent image intensifiers, most angiographers are content with the high-quality images available on cine.

Cine and photofluorographic film selected for angiographic studies should have a wide latitude with low base fog. The use of a very high contrast film will limit recording of the necessary wide range of anatomic information from the spine to the lungs. A professional film processor is needed for proper processing. Frequent quality control with daily determination of base fog and gamma are necessary to prevent variations from processor malfunction and solution deterioration or contamination. A high-quality cine projector is necessary to display the images accurately. Considerably more detailed information on equipment, film, and processing is available in the "ACC/AHA Guidelines for Cardiac Catheterization and Cardiac Catheterization Laboratories" (Pepine et al., 1991).

Digital Cardiac Angiography

Digital subtraction angiocardiography is difficult to apply to cardiac imaging. Although digital subtraction angiography is an established modality for relatively static vascular imaging, cardiac motion presents significant problems and limitations in the use of this technique. The conventional mask-mode technique in which a selected single mask is used for subtraction from subsequent images has not been as successful as with conventional digital subtraction because of rapid cardiac motion. Considerable improvement in subtraction of the moving heart has been obtained by averaging or summing several preinjection images into one mask. Other techniques have been tried, such as constantly updating the mask to allow "panning" of the image intensifier, electrocardiographic (ECG) gating, functional subtraction (end systolic image minus end diastolic image), and dual energy subtraction, but have not been generally accepted.

On the other hand, digital cine angiography without subtraction in 512^2 matrix at 30 frames per second has been very successful in cardiac and coronary angiography and in some laboratories has replaced conventional cine angiography as the images approach the older technique in resolution and equal the quality because of improved contrast. There are significant advantages of digital angiocardiography such as instant or real-time processing and viewing of the study, avoiding the 15 to 30 minute delay needed to process cine film. Film and film-processing costs are significantly reduced. Computer software programs have been developed that allow rapid chamber volumetric and ejection fraction measurements with segmental wall motion analysis using computer edge recognition and stenosis measurement both geometrically and densitometrically.

There are significant problems with the integration of digital imaging into a cardiac catheterization laboratory. The accuracy of digital coronary arteriography as compared with conventional cine coronary arteriography awaits clinical validation. However, digital angiography with 1024^2 matrix at 30 frames per second is now becoming available and may significantly improve resolution, but there are major problems because of the increase in radiation dose and storage needed. There is also an increase of close to 50 per cent in the total cost of this addition to the laboratory, without a major improvement in imaging quality over conventional cine technique except in contrast. If conventional cine is eliminated, the total cost decreases about 10 per cent. Permanent recording and easy access storage of the images present a major problem in dealing with motion studies. Memory requirements are immense, although they can be handled by hard discs with gigabyte storage capacity, optical discs, and digital videotape. Until an industrial standard is decided on, digitally recorded images are not transferrable from one institution to another for consultation unless similar equipment is available. Converting the image to conventional television recording medium such as VHS is not adequate to allow primary diagnosis because of image degradation.

Intravenous digital coronary angiography and angiocardiography, although theoretic possibilities, have the same limitations as conventional cine radiography in which intravenous injections have been tried and abandoned. The problems are overlap by unwanted moving contrast-filled vascular structures and the increased volume of contrast medium needed for the study.

PERFORMANCE OF THE EXAMINATION

Right Heart

RIGHT ATRIUM. Positive contrast angiograms of the right atrium are now used primarily for the diagnosis of right heart masses and certain congenital cardiac anomalies. Injection of 0.5 ml/kg body weight of 350 to 370 mg I/ml contrast medium in 1 to 1.5 seconds through a closed-end (N.I.H.) or pigtail catheter is usually performed in the posteroanterior (PA) or shallow RAO projection so that the right atrium and right ventricle are not superimposed (Figs. 106–1 and 106–2). The PA projection projects the spine over the middle of the heart, necessitating increasing the radiation exposure and thereby causing difficulty in detecting the lateral borders of the chambers. Digital angiocardiography requires similar contrast flow rates and volumes. Digital subtraction angiocardiography, because of the contrast enhancement resulting from the subtraction technique, allows a reduced contrast amount to be used. The reduction is better obtained through dilution of the contrast medium (about one half) rather than through a reduced flow rate so that proper mixing of the contrast agent used with the blood is obtained.

RIGHT VENTRICLE. In the adult population with acquired heart disease, the major indication for right ventriculography is the assessment of tricuspid regurgitation. Closed-end N.I.H., tip-occluded, or pigtail catheters are usually used. Steaming a 90-degree bend in the catheter 6 to 10 cm from the tip permits more exact positioning toward the right ventricular apex rather than the infundibulum. End- and side-hole Gensini-type catheters should be tip occluded to avoid myocardial perforation by the jet of contrast from the catheter tip. N.I.H. catheters are more likely to perforate the right ventricular myocardium than are pigtail catheters. Although the pigtail is more likely associated with thromboembolic complications, this risk is almost totally eliminated by the use of systemic heparinization during the procedure. Volumes and flow rates of contrast medium are similar to those used for right atrial injections; however, if maintenance of a sinus rhythmn is desired, a slower flow rate is necessary. In adults, 12 to 15 ml/sec usually suffices.

PULMONARY ARTERY. In pulmonary angiography, as in right ventriculography, N.I.H. and pigtail catheters are preferred over end- and side-hole catheters, with pigtail catheters having the best safety record. A 90-degree angle placed 3 to 6 cm from the pigtail or even the more gentle N.I.H. curve facilitates catheterization of the pulmonary artery, with many variations having been described in the literature (Fig. 106–3). When the right atrium is dilated, making pulmonary artery catheterization more difficult, use of a gentle reverse primary curve prior to the shorter more acute secondary curve is of help.

In contrast with studies of the cardiac chambers and coronary

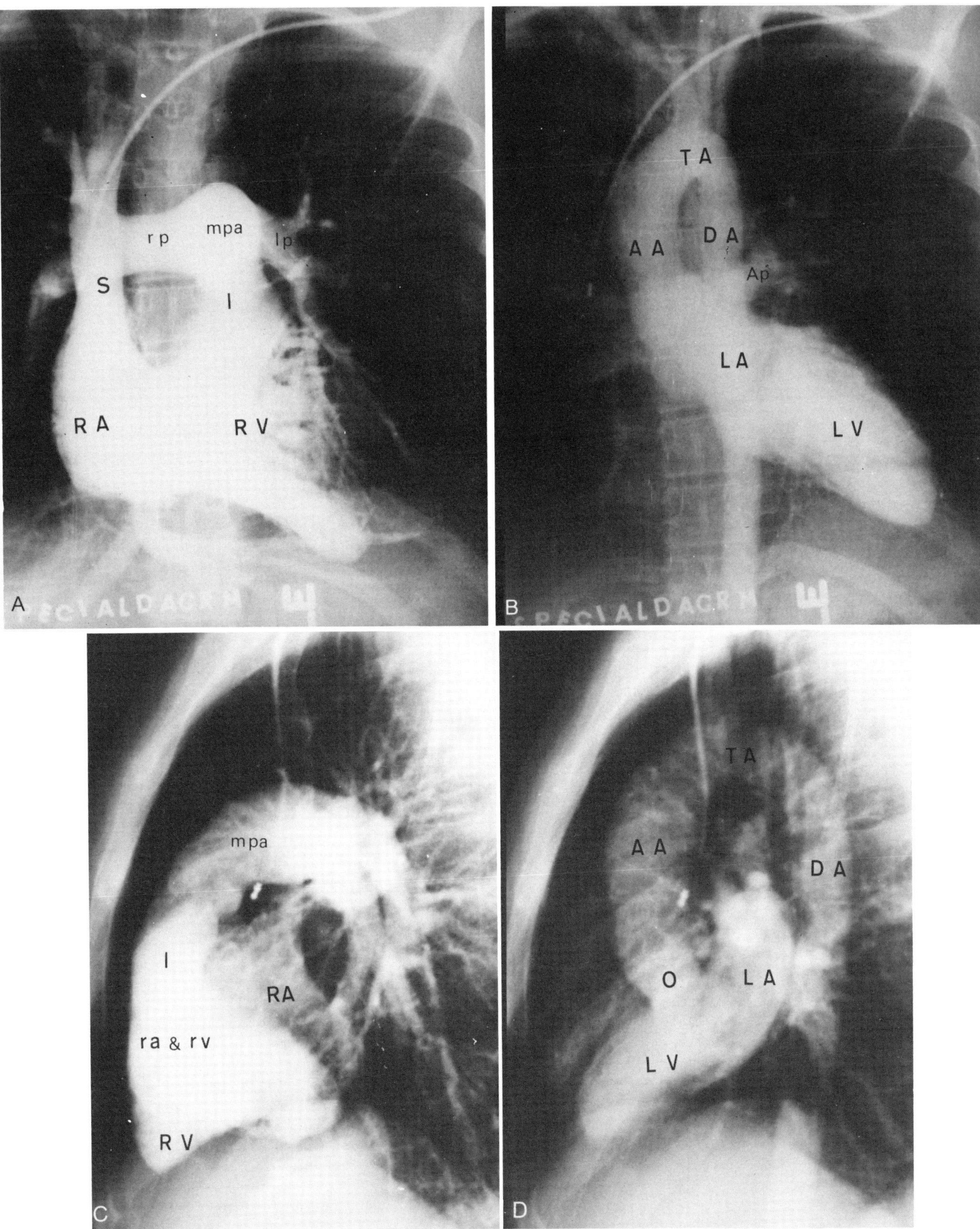

Figure 106–1. Anteroposterior (*A* ***and*** *B*), **and lateral** (*C* ***and*** *D*) **right and left angiocardiograms** performed by injecting contrast into the superior vena cava (S) through a closed-end and side-hole N.I.H. catheter. The lateral view superimposes major portions of the right atrium and ventricle (ra and rv) and shows the short left ventricular outflow (O) formed anteriorly by the septum and posteriorly by the anterior leaflet of the mitral valve (see also Figure 106–8). (AA = ascending thoracic aorta; Ap = left atrial appendage; DA = descending thoracic aorta; I = infundibulum; LA = left atrium; lp = left pulmonary artery; LV = left ventricle; mpa = main pulmonary artery; RA = right atrium; rp = right pulmonary artery; RV = right ventricle; TA = transverse arch.)

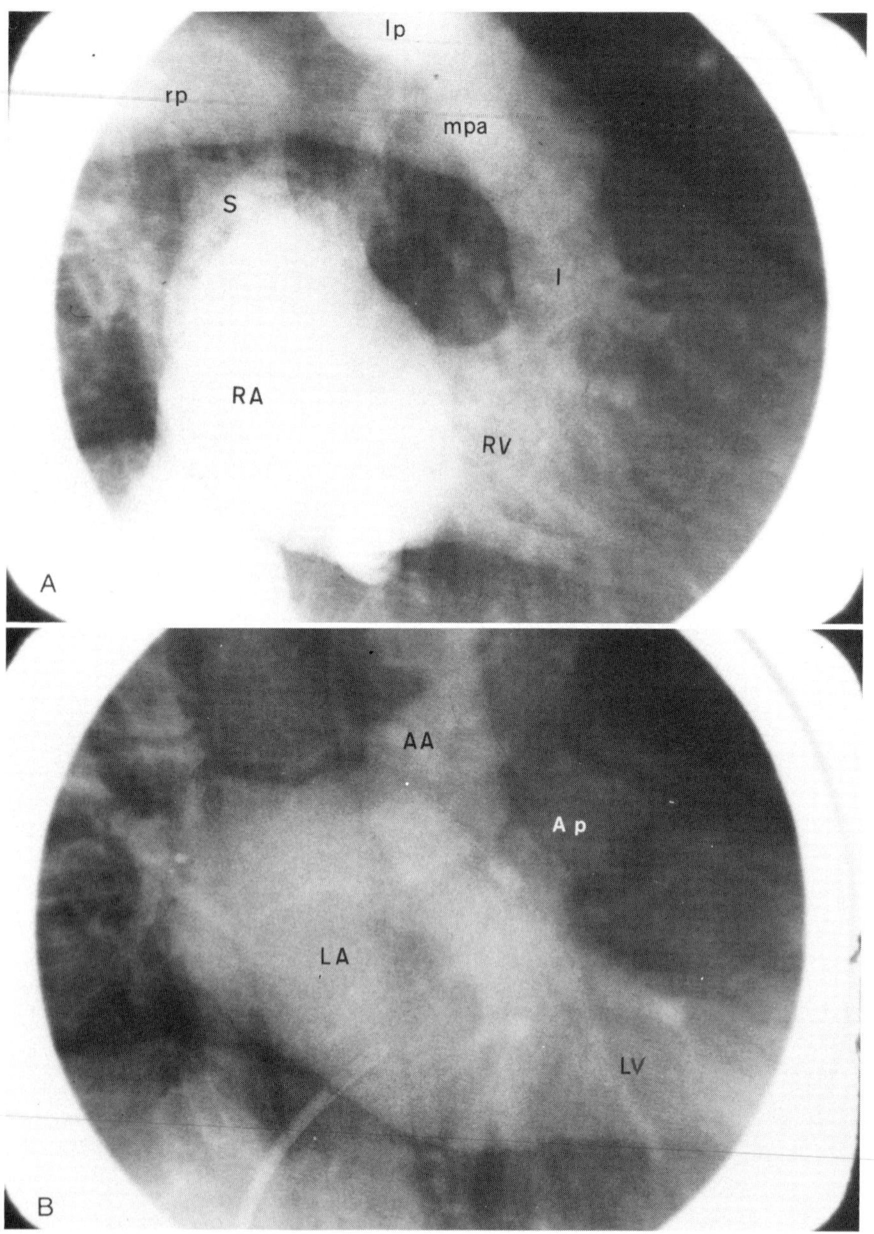

Figure 106–2. Right anterior oblique right atrial (*A*) **and levoangiocardiograms** (*B*). (S = Superior vena cava. Other labels as in Figure 106–1.)

arteries, for which cine radiography is preferred, large film serialography has been the recording technique of choice in the diagnosis of pulmonary embolism because of the large field of view needed. A contrast volume of approximately 0.7 ml/kg body weight delivered in 1.5 seconds is necessary for satisfactory opacification of the entire pulmonary arterial tree, regardless of whether conventional or digital (nonsubtracted) radiographic imaging is used. For selective right and left pulmonary artery injections, the flow rate is reduced by one half for 1.5 to 2 seconds. Digital angiography with large format 30 to 40 cm (14 to 16 inch) image amplifiers is beginning to supplant large film serialography since imaging processing is real-time with almost immediate recall of the study for review, allowing the elimination of film processing time. In addition, digital cine pulmonary angiography surpasses large film serialography in visualizing small pulmonary thrombi in moving vascular structures, particularly in sick patients.

Other adjuncts such as cine and photofluorography are suitable adjunctive imaging modalities in limited circumstances, depending on the size of the image amplifier used. Most cardiac catheterization laboratories have small image tubes designed for angiocardiography and coronary arteriography, and although they can be used for pulmonary arteriography, they are not ideal because of the limited field coverage. Cine fluorography, because of its rapid frame rates and short exposure time, is especially helpful in patients with tachycardia and those who cannot hold their breath during filming (digital cine pulmonary arteriography has the same advantage). Digital subtraction angiography has only limited application as it is more difficult because of the normal "vasomotion" of the pulmonary arterial tree as well as transmitted motion from the heart. However, it may be useful in situations where the effect of cardiac motion is minor, such as when visualizing very peripheral thrombi, and it allows use of dilute contrast (discussed in **Digital Cardiac Angiography**). Magnification arteriography also may be useful in similar circumstances.

Left Heart

Left Atrium. Although the left atrium can be catheterized in a retrograde fashion from the left ventricle by placing an acute

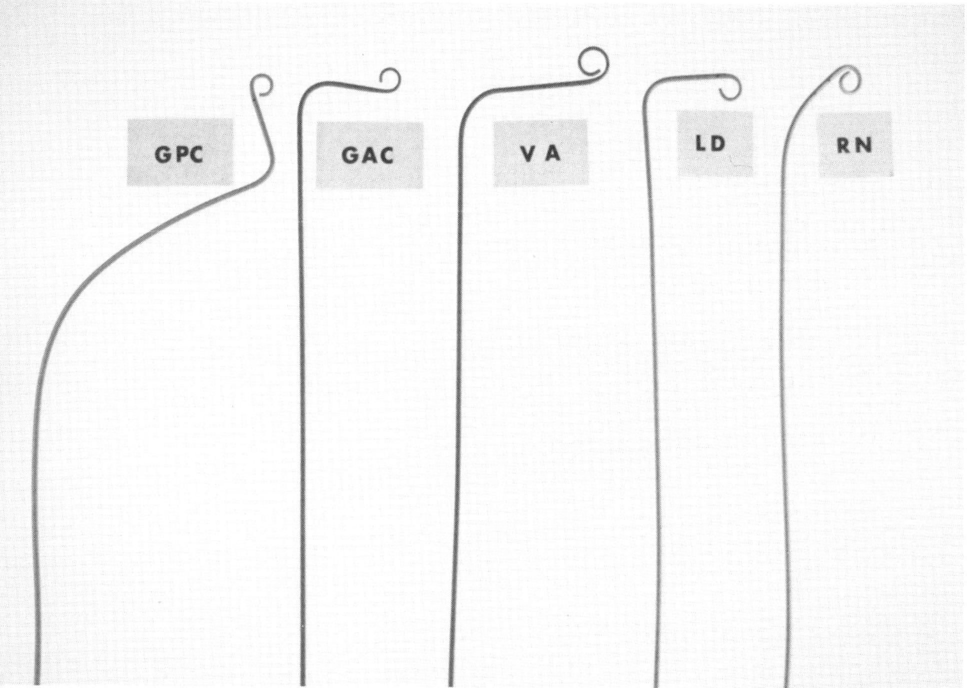

Figure 106–3. Five pigtail catheters out of many suitable for pulmonary angiography. (GPC = reverse primary curve, which tends to seek out the pulmonary artery [should be used only from the femoral approach]; GAC = modified version of the GPC, with a simple 90-degree angle useful for most cases; VA = Van Aman, with elongated distal segment; LD = Ledor, with downward turning pigtail; RN = Renner, with an N.I.H.-like distal curve.) (Reproduced with permission of Springer International from Grollman JH Jr: Pulmonary angiography. Cardiovasc Interv Radiol 15:166–170, 1992.)

angle 3 to 4 cm from the tip of the catheter, this technique is rarely used. The major means of opacifying the left atrium is with an injection of contrast (1 to 1.2 ml/kg in 2 seconds) into either the right atrium or the main pulmonary artery. The 30 to 45 degree RAO projection is ideal, because it reduces overlap with the left ventricle (see Fig. 106–2). If another approximately 90-degree view is needed, a lateral or cranially angled left anterior oblique (LAO) projection is helpful, especially for localization of masses. The standard LAO projection results in superimposition of the left atrium and ventricle, especially in patients with a horizontally positioned heart. Cine and digital angiocardiography are the preferred recording techniques, although large film serialography and photofluorography are acceptable.

Left Ventricle. Assessment of the left heart with a right heart contrast injection is only rarely performed because large volumes of contrast are necessary (1 to 1.2 ml/kg in 2 seconds) and because of the safety of left heart catheterization and angiocardiography with the techniques now available. The principal indication for this technique is visualization of suspected masses such as thrombus or tumor; a less common indication is assessment of wall motion. Wall motion studies performed by either conventional or digital cine radiography after right heart contrast medium injections are more accurate than the radionuclide techniques, owing to better edge detection, but they are more invasive because catheter techniques are necessary to allow adequate contrast medium delivery. Other noninvasive imaging techniques including echocardiography, computed tomography, and magnetic resonance imaging have become the primary diagnostic media in the diagnosis of cardiac masses.

Direct catheterization and opacification of the left ventricle are desirable, especially when evaluation of wall motion abnormalities and mitral regurgitation is desired. It is preferable to maintain sinus rhythm during these studies. The preferred method is to position a pigtail catheter toward the midportion of the left ventricle. A relatively slow flow rate of contrast media of 9 to 14 ml per second for 3 to 4 seconds should be used to prevent significant arrhythmias and to allow an adequate number of cardiac cycles for evaluation. Phased diastolic injections of contrast will help reduce contrast volume and arrhythmias but are successful only with relatively slow heart rates of no more than 70 to 80 beats per minute and preferably less. The Sones catheter, developed for transbrachial coronary arteriography, and the all-purpose transfemoral catheter are frequently used for left ventriculography by those experienced with their use. Owing to the long taper and limited effectiveness of the side holes in these catheters, there is considerable recoil during left ventricular injection, resulting in a high incidence of multiple ectopic beats.

The RAO view is the best single projection for evaluating the left ventricle including segmental wall motion and calculating the ejection fraction (Fig. 106–4). For evaluation of the septum and posterolateral wall as well as the anterior mitral leaflet, the cranially angled LAO view is optimal (Fig. 106–5).

Coronary Arteries. Visualization of the coronary arteries is performed selectively. The Sones catheter placed via a brachial artery cutdown is manipulated off the coronary cusps into the coronary arteries. It has only a minimal curve at the distal tip and does not seek out the coronary arteries directly. Considerable skill by the angiographer is necessary to catheterize the coronary arteries selectively, and frequent performance is necessary to maintain this skill. Proponents of this approach indicate that one catheter may be used to perform the entire study (left ventriculography and selective coronary arteriography) and that bed rest following the study is not necessary as it is with the transfemoral technique, more readily permitting outpatient coronary angiography. This technique has been simplified by using a percutaneous transbrachial or transaxillary approach with preformed Amplatz catheters from the right arm and Judkins catheters from the left arm.

Selective coronary arteriography with preformed catheters placed by the percutaneous transfemoral approach is relatively easily learned by even inexperienced angiographers. The right Judkins (see Fig. 106–14) and Amplatz catheters (Fig. 106–6) are similar in use for right coronary arteriography in that rotation of the catheter from a point just above the right coronary ostium will usually allow entrance into this artery. The Amplatz right coronary catheter enters the artery more deeply and is usually more stable. The Judkins left coronary catheter is supported by the ascending aortic wall with direction of its tip into the left coronary artery, whereas the Amplatz catheter is displaced off the left coronary cusp into the sinus and then into the left coronary artery, similar to the Sones technique (Fig. 106–7). Various sizes of both Amplatz and Judkins catheters are available to fit the aortic configuration. Similar techniques using

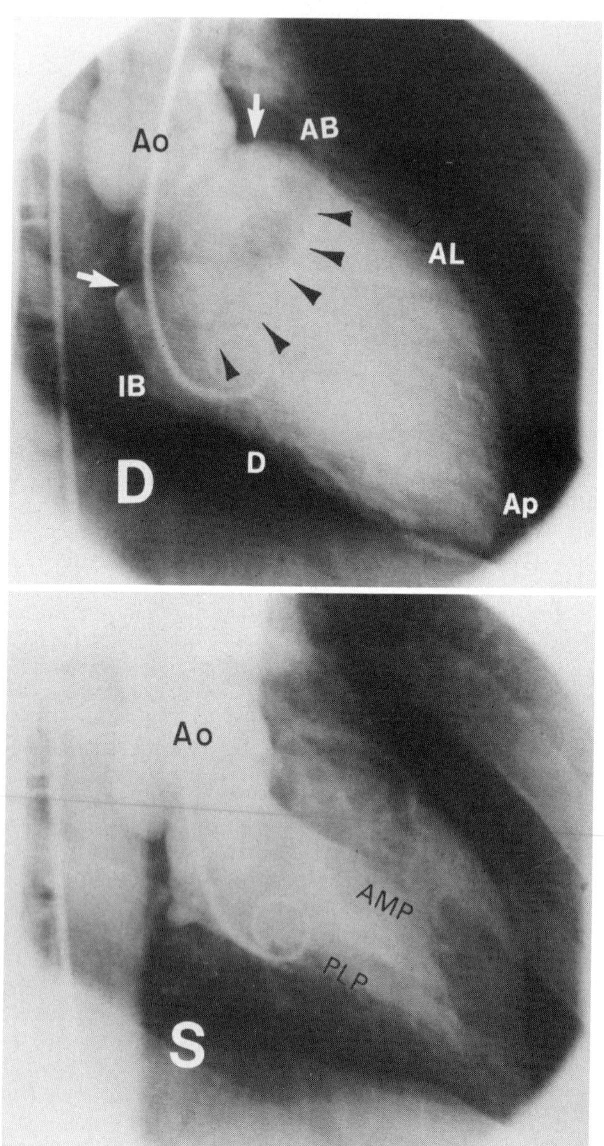

Figure 106–4. Right anterior oblique end diastolic (*D*) and end systolic (*S*) left ventriculograms performed with pigtail catheter. *White arrows* indicate the anterior and posterior commissure of the mitral valve ring. *Black arrowheads* indicate the broad wave of unopacified blood entering the left ventricle from the left atrium (mitral valve has opened). (AB = anterobasal segment; AL = anterolateral segment; AMP = anteromedial papillary muscle; Ao = aorta; AP = apical segment; D = diaphragmatic segment; IB = inferobasal segment; PLP = posterolateral papillary muscle.)

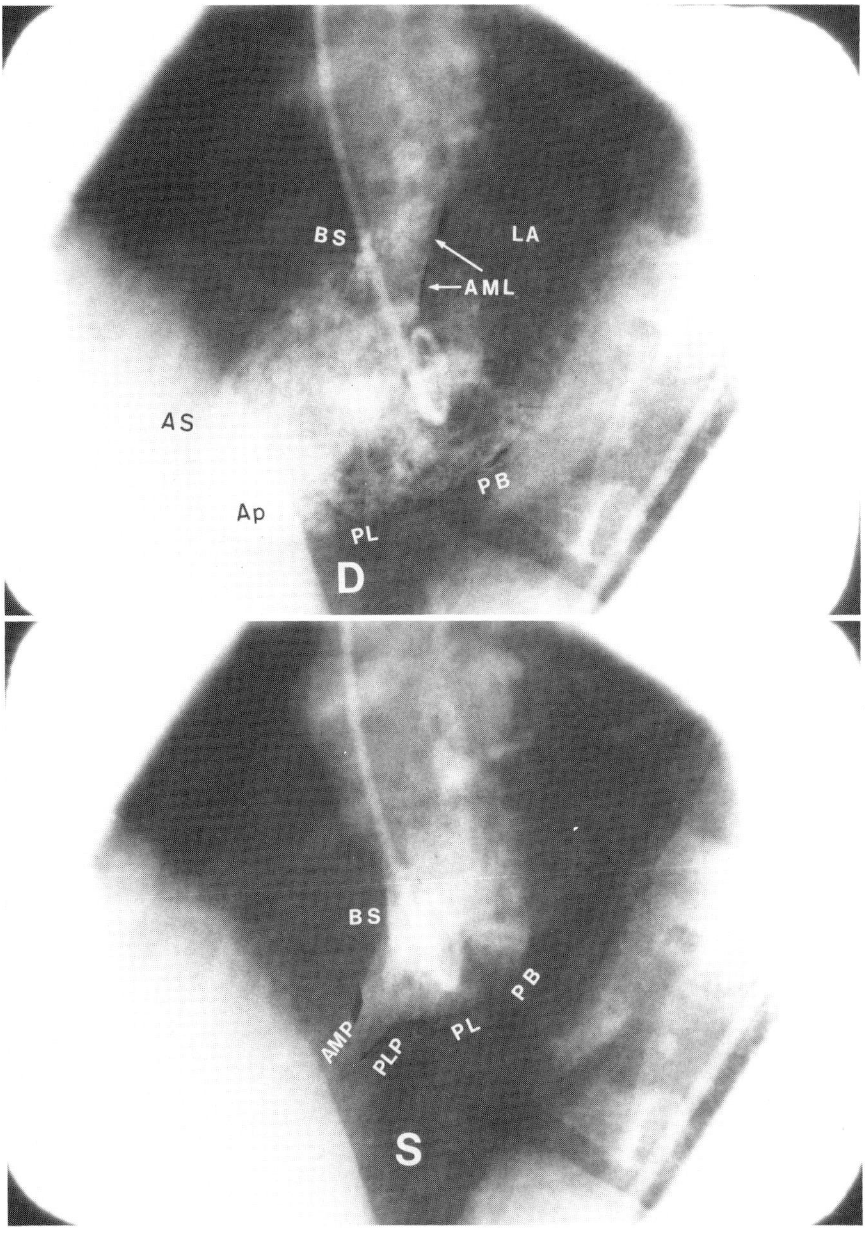

Figure 106–5. Cranially angled left anterior oblique end diastolic (*D*) and end-systolic (*S*) left ventriculograms. (AML = anterior mitral leaflet; AS = apical septum; BS = basal septum; LA = left atrium; PB = posterobasal segment; PL = posterolateral segment. Other labels as in Figure 106–4.)

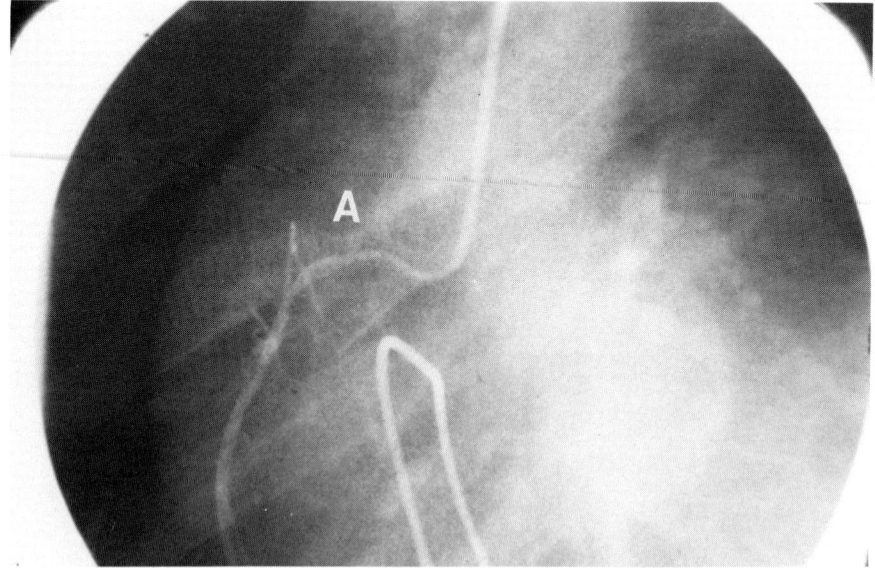

Figure 106–6. Right Amplatz *(A)* **catheter** in left anterior oblique projection of right coronary artery.

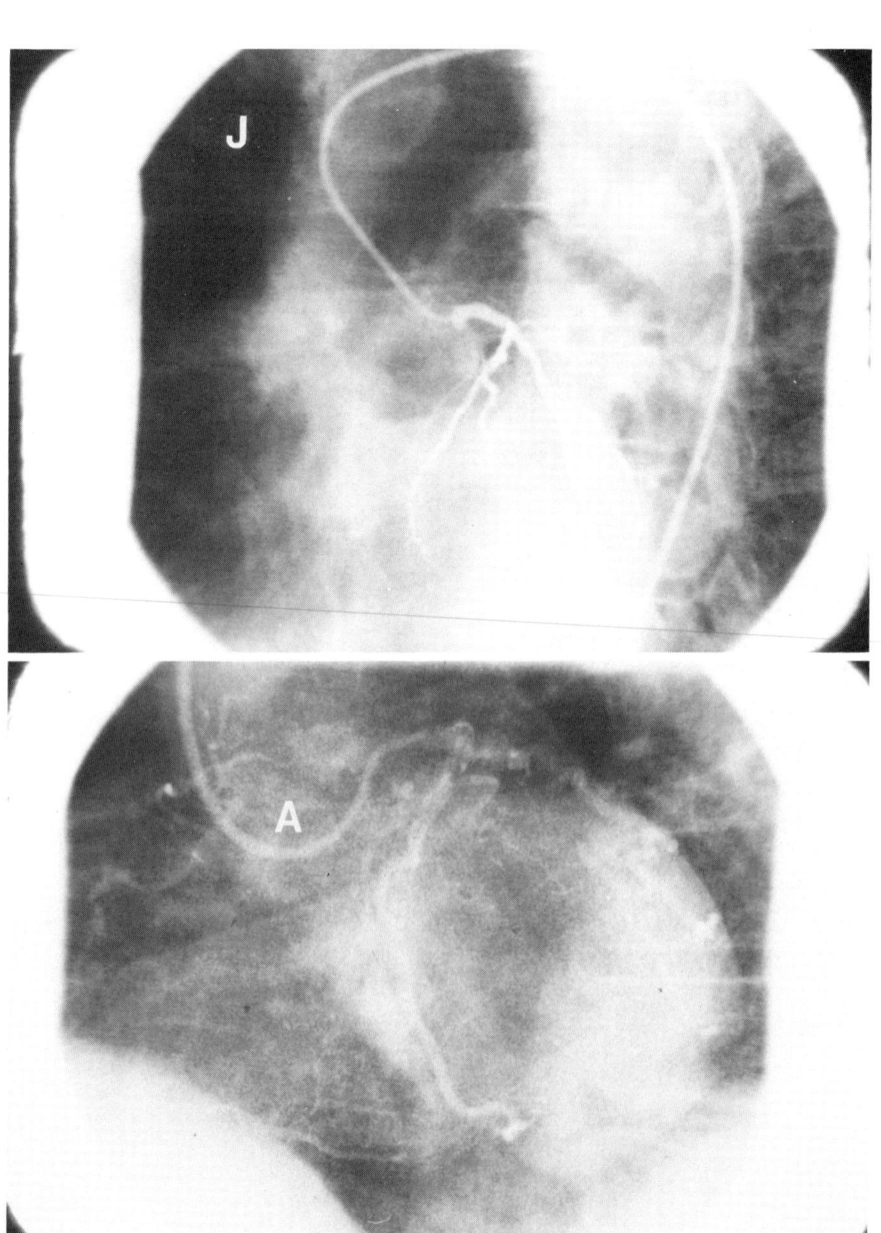

Figure 106–7. Left Judkins (J) and left Amplatz (A) catheters in left anterior oblique projections during contrast injections of left coronary artery.

other catheters have been described but have not received wide recognition.

Injection of contrast medium is generally by hand, using 6 to 8 ml in 1.5 to 2 seconds for the left coronary artery and 3 to 6 ml for the right, depending on the size and distribution of these arteries. Large film serialography is not used now, the imaging modality of choice being conventional and digital cineangiography. ECG monitoring and pressure measurements at the catheter tip are mandatory in all forms of cardiac and coronary angiography because of the arrhythmias and pressure changes frequently associated with contrast injections. Multiple projections are necessary to localize and quantitate the obstructive process because of frequent eccentricity of the stenotic lesions and overlap by adjacent branches.

NORMAL ANATOMY AND PROJECTIONS

Cardiac Chambers

Angiocardiographic anatomy is easily correlated with gross anatomy, and therefore the cardiac angiographer needs a firm basis in the anatomy of the heart and blood vessels. With this knowledge, it is relatively easy to evaluate angiocardiograms in any projection. The normal frontal and lateral angiocardiographic anatomy of the cardiac chambers may be found in Fig. 106–1. It is seen that the RAO (see Fig. 106–2) and PA projections of the right and left heart are somewhat similar. The 30-degree RAO projection is used for single-plane studies of the left heart (see Figs. 106–2 and 106–4). In this view the largest number of segments of the left ventricle in reference to coronary blood supply are seen. In addition, this view reduces superimposition of the left atrium and left ventricle. Angling the x-ray beam in these projections is rarely of value in adult acquired heart disease.

The lateral (see Fig. 106–1) and LAO (see Fig. 106–5) views of the left ventricle are somewhat similar and may be necessary if a projection 90 degrees to the RAO or frontal view is needed. For the right heart, the direct lateral projection is usually used. The LAO with cranial angulation is helpful in the evaluation of intracardiac masses involving the right atrium or right ventricle.

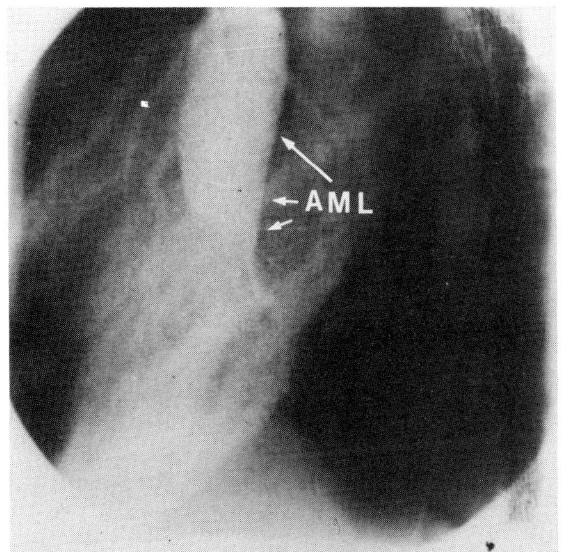

Figure 106–8. Lateral left ventriculogram showing the **anterior leaflet of the mitral valve** (AML). Cine studies will best show its anterior and posterior motion.

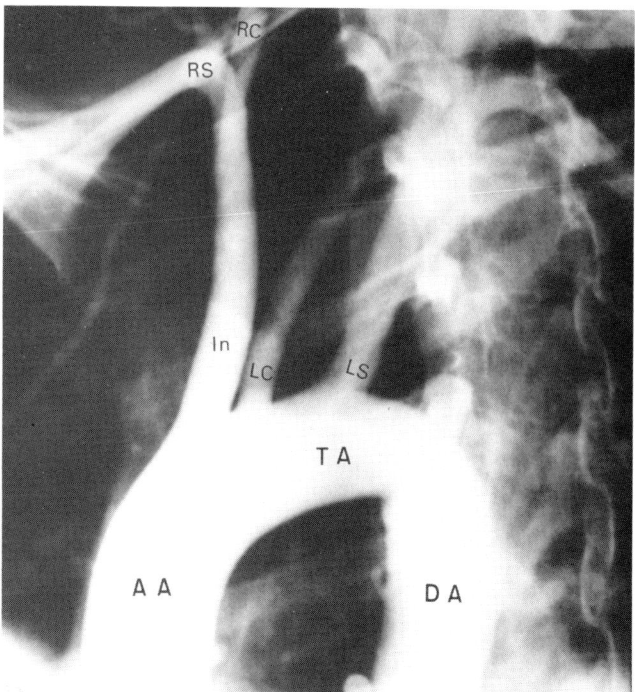

Figure 106–9. Left anterior oblique thoracic aortogram including the proximal brachiocephalic arteries. (AA = ascending aorta; DA = descending aorta; In = innominate artery; LC = left common carotid artery; LS = left subclavian artery; RC = right common carotid artery; RS = right subclavian artery; TA = transverse aorta.)

The standard LAO projection of the left heart is suboptimal because the left atrium and left ventricle are usually superimposed, especially when the heart has a horizontal orientation. A cranially angled LAO projection of the left ventricle (see Fig. 106–5) is ideal for evaluation of the septum and posterolateral wall, because the base and apex of the left ventricle are displaced away from each other and the left atrium is displaced away from the left ventricle. Care must be taken in setting up this view so that the right hemidiaphragm is not excessively superimposed over the left ventricle. It may be necessary to modify the angles (40 to 60 degrees LAO with cranial angulation of 15 to 20 degrees) to obtain the best compromise. A slow, constant inspiration by the patient is helpful in lowering the diaphragm and preventing a Valsalva maneuver. Both the cranial LAO and the lateral projection are beneficial for evaluating the anterior leaflet of the mitral valve and the left ventricular outflow tract (Fig. 106–8).

Great Vessels

The thoracic aorta is best imaged in a steep LAO projection (Fig. 106–9) or, if two planes are needed, frontal and lateral. The RAO projection superimposes the ascending and descending thoracic aorta on each other and therefore should not generally be used. The normal aortic valve anatomy is seen in Fig. 106–10. The pulmonary artery is best evaluated in the frontal projection if both branches are imaged with a main pulmonary artery contrast injection. Appropriate oblique and lateral projections are helpful with selective injections, depending on which branches are being studied.

Coronary Arteries

Although the coronary arteries have classically been studied in oblique projections, overlapping vessels make multiple projections

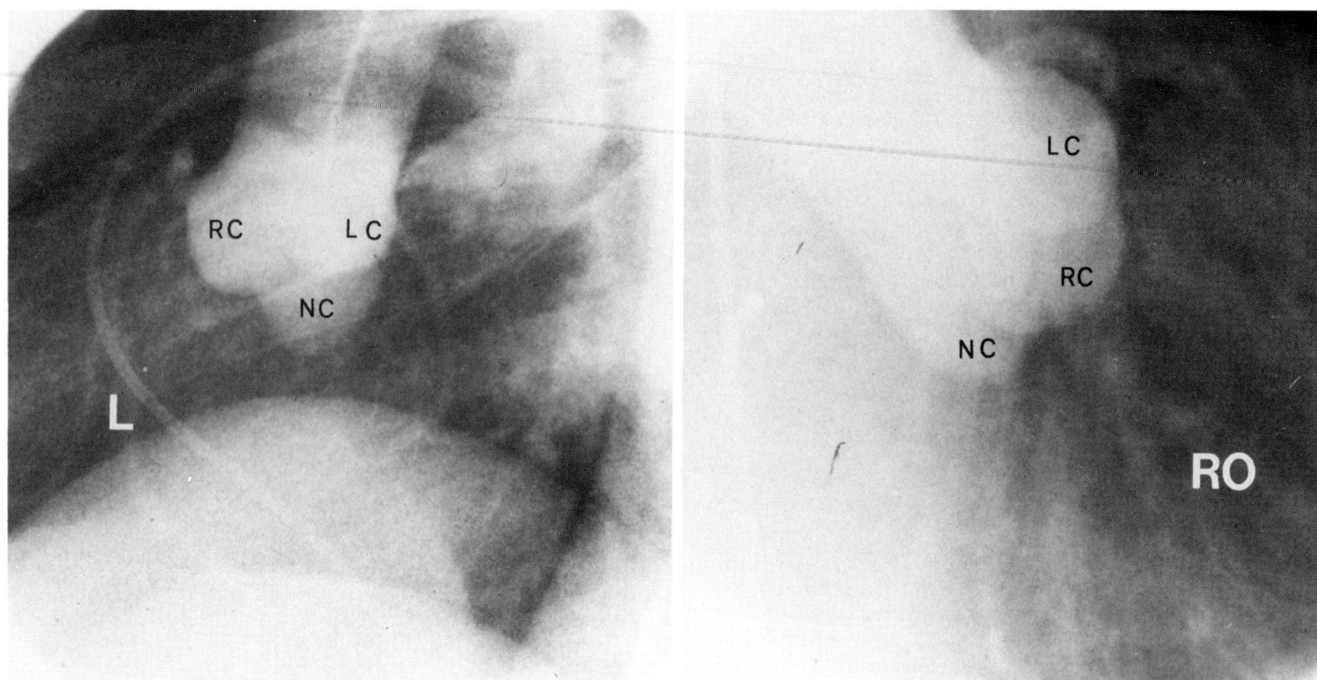

Figure 106–10. Lateral (L) and right anterior oblique (RO) ascending thoracic aortograms. (RC = right coronary sinus; LC = left coronary sinus; NC = noncoronary sinus.)

including frontal, lateral, and oblique views with various degrees of cranial and caudal angulation necessary in the evaluation of coronary artery obstructive disease. Accurate assessment is particularly imperative when consideration is being given to coronary bypass surgery or percutaneous transluminal coronary angioplasty. Anatomically, the coronary arteries may be divided according to their location into four major segments: (1) anterior interventricular groove–anterior descending artery, (2) posterior interventricular groove–posterior descending artery, (3) anterior atrioventricular groove–right coronary artery, and (4) posterior atrioventricular groove–circumflex artery. The anterior descending and circumflex arteries normally originate from the left coronary sinus as a short common trunk, properly called the left coronary artery but often referred to as the "left main coronary artery." This artery is of variable length and may be looked on as a fifth segment, its importance being emphasized because of the high morbidity and mortality associated with left main coronary artery obstructive disease. The right coronary artery and circumflex arteries coursing in their respective atrioventricular grooves form a nearly complete circle. The anterior and posterior descending arteries coursing in their respective interventricular grooves toward the apex form a loop.

There is considerable variation in the nomenclature used for the coronary arteries and branches. This is unfortunate, since institutions may not use the same terminology, particularly with regard to the branches of the major coronary arteries. The cardiac radiologist and angiographer must be aware of this variability in interacting with their colleagues from other institutions.

Left Coronary Artery (Fig. 106–11). This vessel usually arises from the left coronary sinus, passing between the pulmonary artery and left atrium to the junction of the anterior interventricular and posterior atrioventricular grooves under the left atrial appendage. It is of variable length before dividing into the anterior descending and circumflex arteries. Occasionally this segment is absent, with the anterior descending and circumflex arteries arising separately from the left coronary sinus. Less frequently, the left coronary artery arises from above the sinus, making catheterization more difficult. Rarely it may arise from the right coronary artery or right coronary sinus and course anterior to the pulmonary artery, between the pulmonary artery and aorta, through the crista supraventricularis, or posterior to the aorta.

Anterior Descending Artery (Fig. 106–11). This artery, usually referred to as the left anterior descending artery (LAD), courses in the anterior interventricular groove, giving off as its major branches the diagonal and septal arteries. The septal arteries perforate somewhat perpendicularly into the septum and are frequently referred to as "perforators." Diagonal arteries course from the anterior descending artery to the anterior and sometimes anterolateral free wall of the left ventricle and may be numbered as first, second, third, etc. diagonals. Proximally they frequently give off septal arteries. Occasionally, small arteries to the right ventricle and conus can be identified arising from the anterior descending artery.

Circumflex Artery (Fig. 106–11). The circumflex artery by definition courses in the posterior atrioventricular groove. A relatively frequent variation (0.7 per cent) is anomalous origin in the right coronary artery or sinus, passing posterior to the aorta to the posterior atrioventricular groove. The angiographer must be alert to this variation by noting the absence of an artery supplying the posterolateral left ventricular wall. The anomalous circumflex artery frequently is not initially visualized because the right coronary catheter tip is beyond its origin.

When the circumflex artery leaves the groove, it is usually referred to as a marginal artery. When one artery dominates, it is referred to as the obtuse marginal artery, because it courses to the obtuse margin of the heart, as seen in the LAO projection. Usually, there are several marginal branches and it is best to describe them by their distribution to the lateral, posterolateral, and posterior wall of the left ventricle, although many angiographers and surgeons prefer to number them. If the circumflex artery has an inferior emphasis (discussed in Right Coronary Artery), it will give off the posterior descending artery as well as the artery to the atrioventricular node (Fig. 106–12). Frequently, an artery arises from the bifurcation of the left coronary artery, resulting in a trifurcation (see Fig.

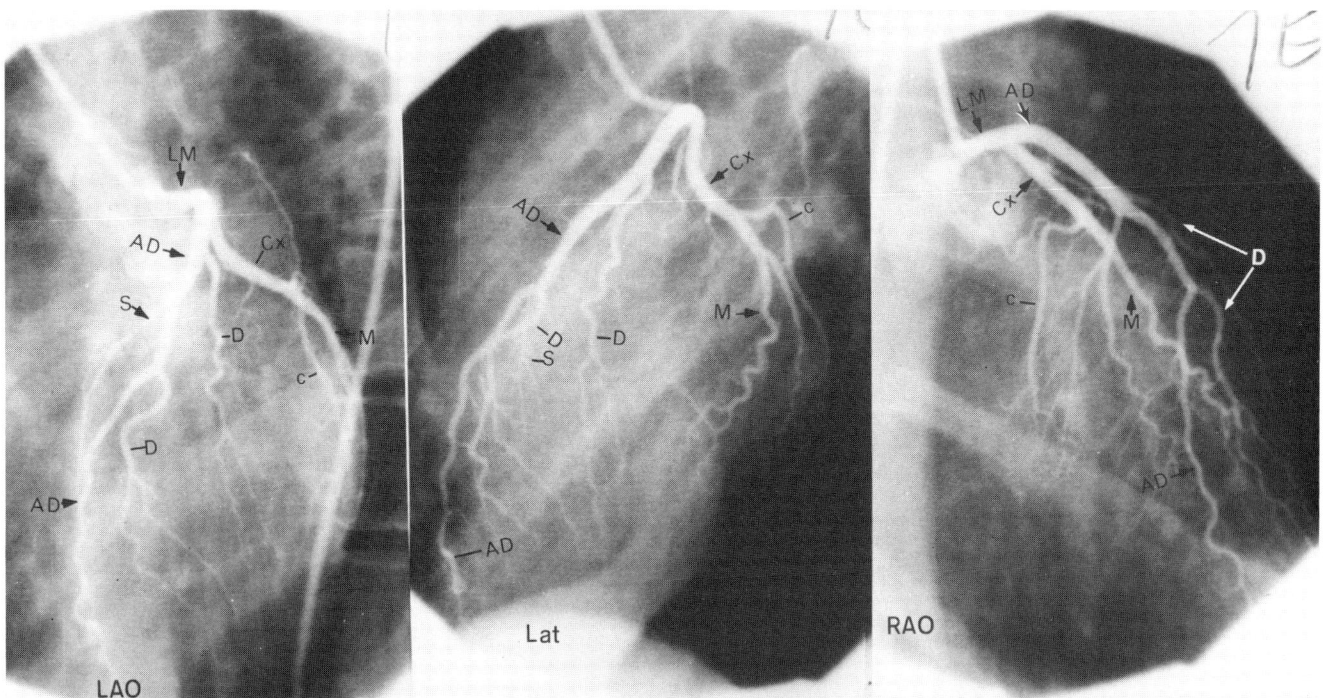

Figure 106–11. Left coronary arteriograms in left anterior oblique (LAO), lateral (Lat), and right anterior oblique (RAO) projections. (AD = anterior descending artery; c = distal circumflex artery; Cx = circumflex artery; D = diagonal branch; M = marginal artery [lateral distribution in this case]; LM = left main coronary artery; S = septal branch.)

106–20). This artery is referred to as a median ramus (or ramus medianus) branch and usually has a lateral distribution halfway between the diagonal and marginal arteries.

Atrial branches can be seen arising from the circumflex artery and can be best recognized in the RAO projection coursing posteriorly over the left atrium. In a large number of patients, a proximally arising atrial branch courses posteriorly around the left atrium to the right atrium to eventually supply the sinoatrial node (Fig. 106–13).

Right Coronary Artery (Fig. 106–14). The right coronary artery usually arises from the right coronary sinus, but not infrequently it arises above the sinus and less commonly it arises anteriorly and more toward the left coronary sinus. Then the right coronary artery courses in the anterior atrioventricular groove proximally, giving off branches to the pulmonary conus and the sinoatrial node (Fig. 106–15). In roughly one third of patients, the conus artery has a separate ostium from the right coronary sinus, usually a few millimeters anterior to the origin of the main right coronary

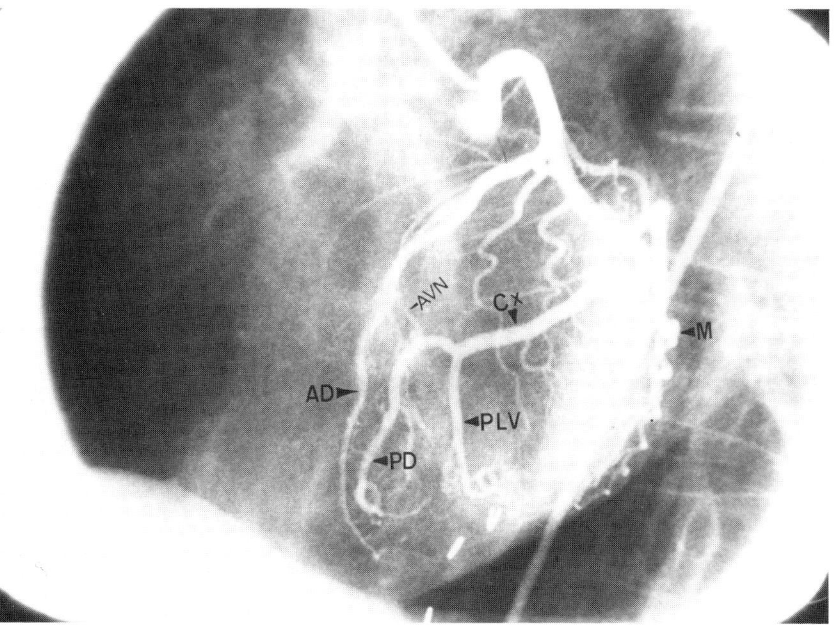

Figure 106–12. Left coronary artery in cranial left anterior oblique projection with circumflex having an inferior emphasis. (AVN = atrioventricular node artery; PD = posterior descending artery; PLV = posterior left ventricular branch [posterior marginal]. Other labels as in Figure 106–11.)

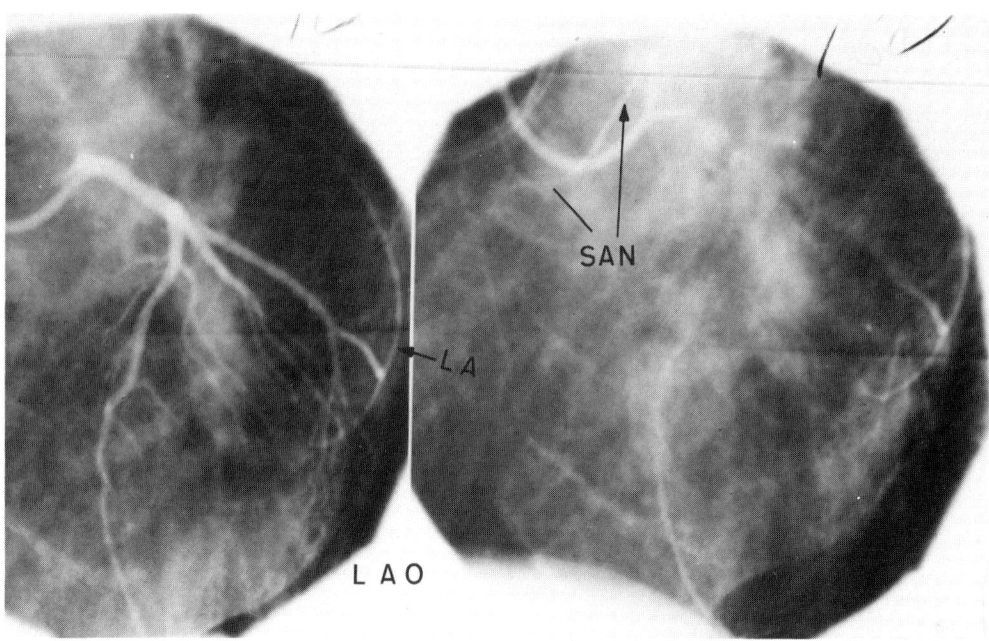

Figure 106–13. Left coronary arteriogram in cranial left anterior oblique projection showing left atrial branch (LA) coursing in back of the left atrium to supply the sinoatrial node (SAN). The right coronary arteriogram showed absence of this artery.

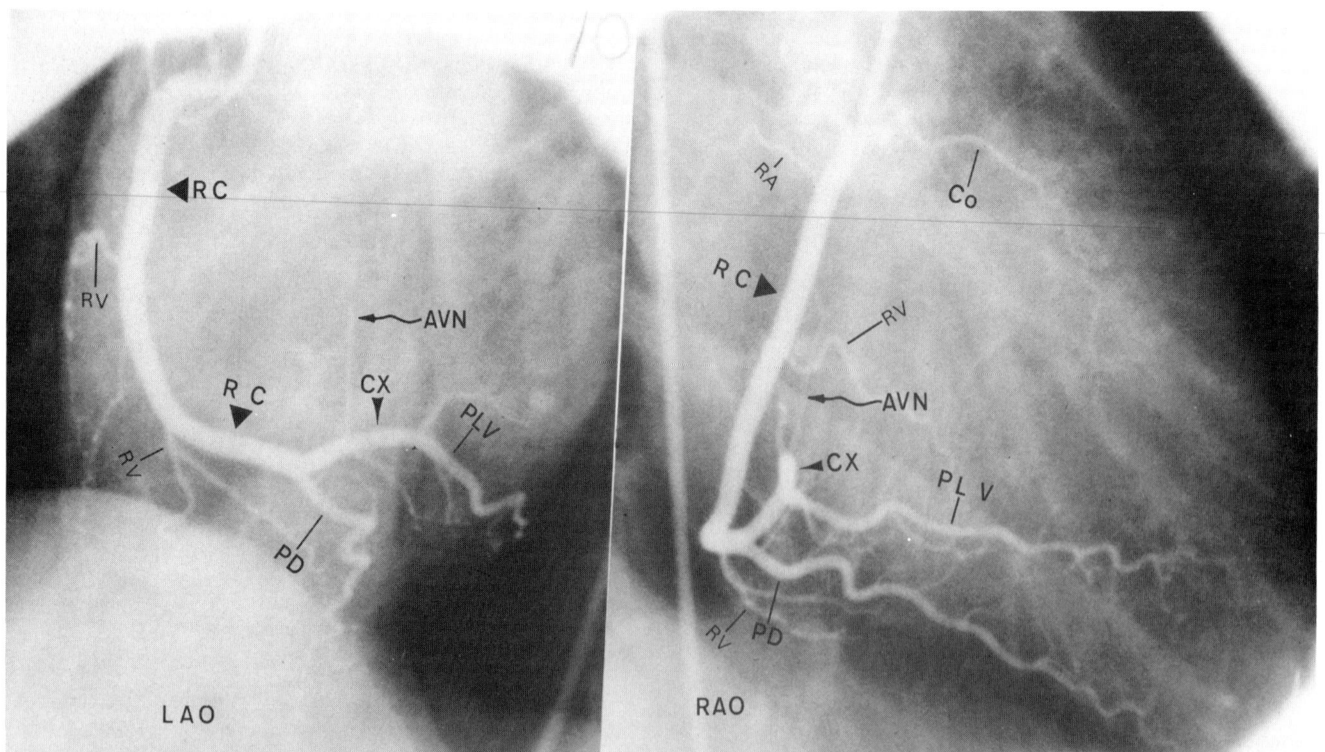

Figure 106–14. Right coronary (RC) arteriogram in left (LAO) and right (RAO) anterior oblique. Note the inverted U shape of the vessel at the crux (CX). (AVN = atrioventricular node artery; Co = conus artery; PD = posterior descending artery; PLV = posterior left ventricular branch; RA = right atrial branch; RV = right ventricular branch.)

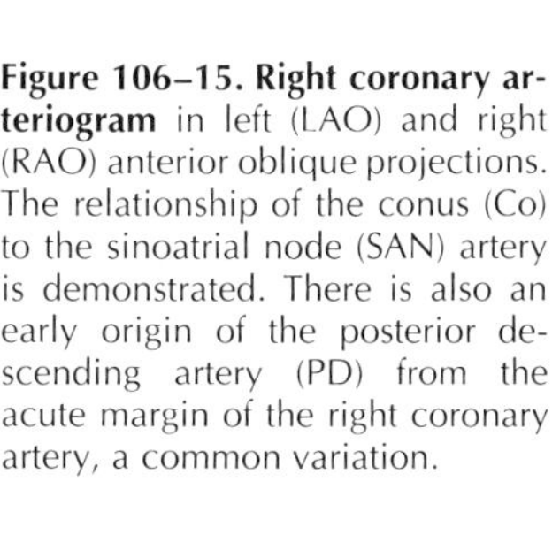

Figure 106–15. Right coronary arteriogram in left (LAO) and right (RAO) anterior oblique projections. The relationship of the conus (Co) to the sinoatrial node (SAN) artery is demonstrated. There is also an early origin of the posterior descending artery (PD) from the acute margin of the right coronary artery, a common variation.

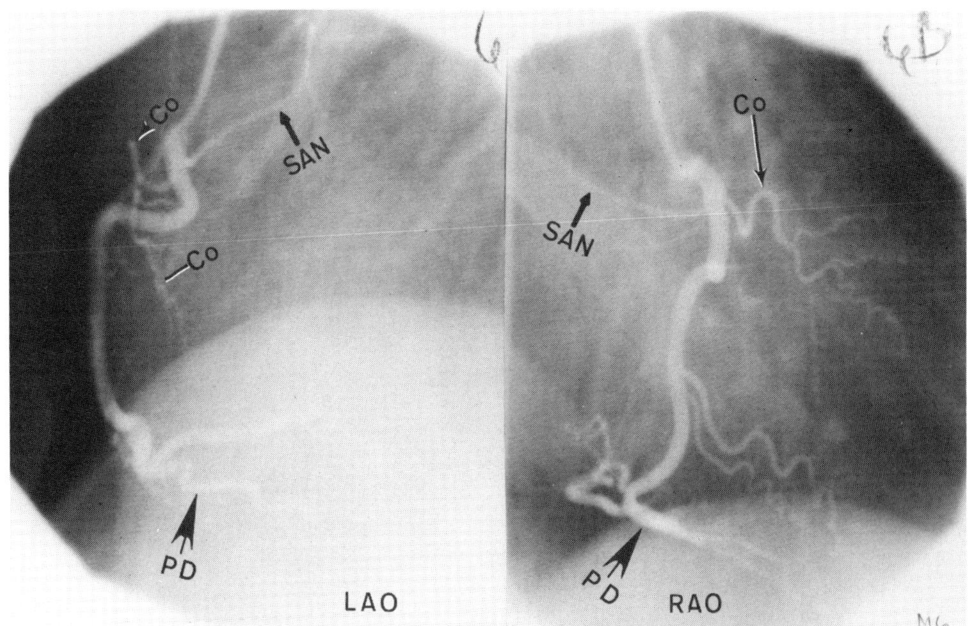

artery. The next major branches of the right coronary artery supply the right ventricle. The dominating artery has been referred to as the acute marginal artery because it courses to the acute margin of the heart, as seen in the LAO projection. Most angiographers just use the term *right ventricular branch* for all the right ventricular arteries.

As the right coronary artery courses to the diaphragmatic surface of the heart, it traverses the acute margin and usually (approximately 90 per cent of patients) gives off the posterior descending artery a variable distance before the crux (the junction of the intersection of the anterior and posterior atrioventricular grooves with the posterior interventricular groove). Occasionally, the posterior descending artery arises from the right coronary artery at or proximal to the acute margin of the heart, and this is referred to as early origin of the posterior descending artery (see Fig. 106–15). As the right coronary artery continues to the crux, it may occasionally give off a second smaller posterior descending artery. When these anatomic situations occur, the right coronary artery is referred as the "dominant" artery. On the other hand, in approximately 10 per cent of the normal population, the posterior descending artery arises from the circumflex artery; this is known as left coronary "dominance." It has been suggested that a more appropriate term would be circumflex or right coronary "emphasis" to the inferior left ventricle. More simply, it can be noted whether either the circumflex or right coronary artery has an inferior dominance or emphasis. Infrequently, mixed dominance can occur, with both the circumflex and right coronary arteries terminating as posterior descending branches.

At the crux, a characteristic inverted U-shaped course of the right coronary artery is seen as it passes over the coronary sinus and continues in the posterior atrioventricular groove to send branches to the posterior wall of the left ventricle (see Fig. 106–14). Beyond the crux, the right coronary artery sends a branch to the atrioventricular node as well as major branches to the posterior left ventricular wall. There is considerable variation in the degree of supply to the posterior left ventricle by either the right coronary or circumflex artery, with either or both sending branches to this region. Rarely, a right coronary artery will be so dominant that it sends branches to the posterolateral and lateral left ventricular wall (Fig. 106–16). This variability can also be considered a form of emphasis to a given area. In a nondominant right coronary artery, the vessel terminates as small right ventricular and atrial branches (Fig. 106–17).

The concept of dominance also applies to other areas of the heart where there may be variable supply to one region of the myocardium, such as the apex of the left ventricle, which is normally supplied by the anterior descending artery but occasionally may be

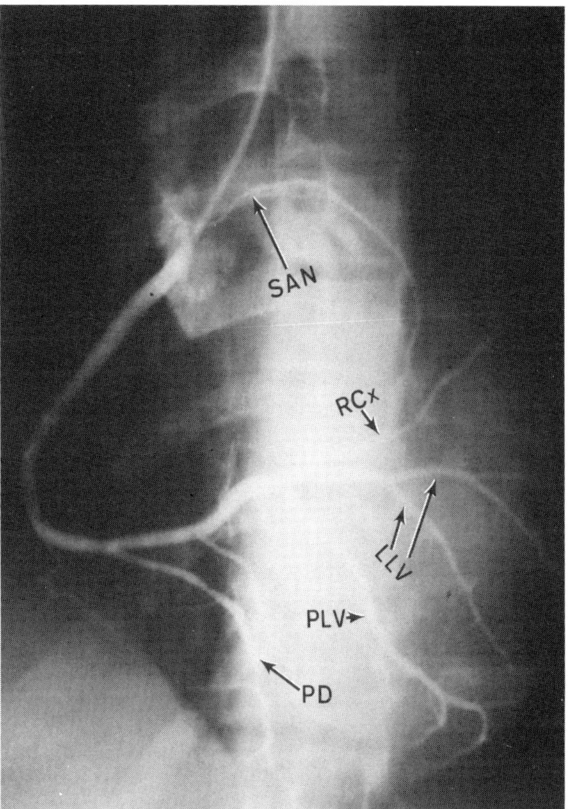

Figure 106–16. Unusually dominant right coronary artery in cranial left anterior oblique projection. The right circumflex artery (RCx) courses in the posterior atrioventricular groove to give off a left atrial branch that supplies the sinoatrial node (SAN). (LLV = lateral left ventricular branch; PLV = posterior left ventricular branch; PD = posterior descending artery.)

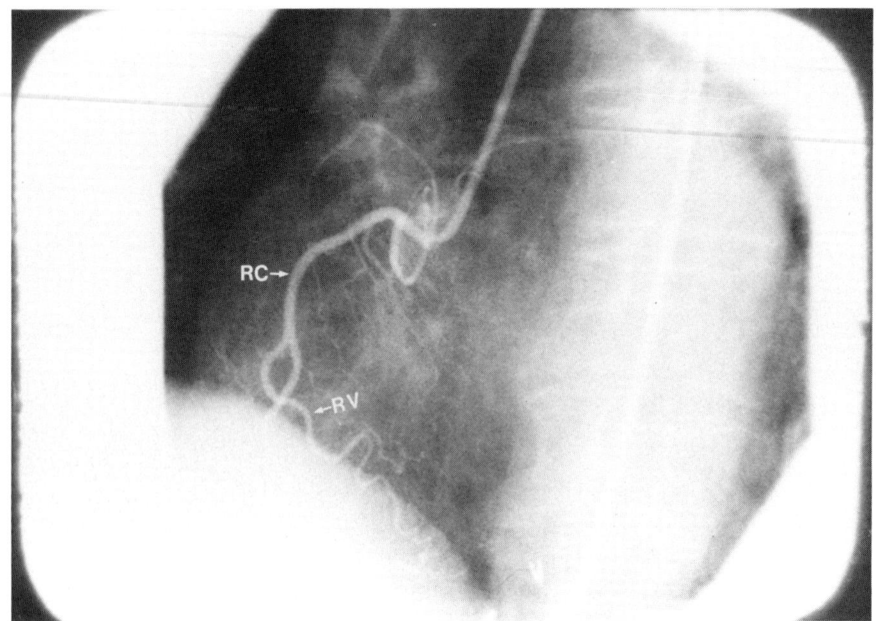

Figure 106–17. "Nondominant" right coronary artery in left anterior oblique projection. (RC = right coronary artery; RV = right ventricular branch.)

supplied by the posterior descending artery. The exact distribution, origin, and size of the branches are extremely important in the preoperative assessment for surgical bypass or angioplasty.

Coronary Artery Views. The left main coronary artery is best evaluated with a very shallow LAO projection for the proximal segment and the PA or slightly RAO projection for the distal segment.

For the left coronary artery, in addition to the conventional LAO and RAO and lateral projections (see Fig. 106–11), angled projections are imperative to evaluate the vessels fully. This is especially true in the proximal portion, where the anterior descending artery and circumflex branches have a more horizontal course and there is considerable overlap of these branches. Although these views may be obtained by sitting the patient up or elevating the hips, it is preferable and easier to obtain them by angulating the x-ray tube–image amplifier axis. This is most often done with a variation of a C-arm mount. Cranial angulation refers to shifting the overpatient image amplifier toward the head, whereas caudal angulation refers to shifting the image amplifier toward the feet. The cranially angled LAO projection is now considered mandatory (Fig. 106–18), and supplemental PA cranial and RAO cranial views may be extremely valuable, the latter being particularly important in horizontally positioned hearts. Caudal angulation in both the LAO and RAO projections (Figs. 106–19 and 106–20) is especially valuable in evaluating the left main coronary artery bifurcation or if there is a trifurcation.

The right coronary artery can be studied with fewer views because there is less problem of overlap. LAO and RAO projections are standard (see Fig. 106–14). The lateral projection is helpful in visualizing the origin of the right coronary artery as well as the posterior descending artery as it courses toward the apex. This view also helps to distinguish the posterior descending artery from the posterior left ventricular branches. The cranially angled LAO projection is helpful in evaluating the proximal posterior descending artery and crux (see Fig. 106–16), because in the standard LAO projection these vessels tend to be markedly foreshortened, especially in patients with horizontally positioned hearts. A very shallow RAO cranially angled projection can also be helpful in certain instances when further evaluation of the crux and proximal posterior left ventricular branches is necessary. A standard 30 to 45 degree cranially angled RAO projection results in superimposition of the proximal and distal crux vessels on themselves, defeating the value of this view. Rarely caudal projections may be of value if in this view the lesion to be evaluated is oriented perpendicularly to the x-ray beam.

RISKS OF PROCEDURE

Complications of cardiac catheterization and angiography may be classified either symptomatically or etiologically. Symptomatic complications include death, acute myocardial infarction, cerebral vascular accident, arrhythmias, local vascular problems (thrombosis, hemorrhage, and false aneursym), pericardial tamponade, hypotension, congestive heart failure, and renal failure. It is important to understand the etiology of these complications to reduce their incidence (Table 106–1). Although most coronary angiographers prefer systemic heparinization to prevent thromboembolic complications, meticulous technique is equally important.

The frequency of these complications varies with the experience of the cardiac laboratory. It is appropriate to consider the incidence of these complications in the light of experience at the largest laboratories, where in stable patients the rate of mortality is approximately 0.1 per cent, the rate of acute mycardial infarction is 0.3 per cent, the rate of stroke is 0.1 per cent, and the total of these three severe complications is no greater than 0.4 per cent. Higher rates may be seen in infants and elderly patients. Laboratories not performing procedures at these levels of safety should re-examine their techniques. The increased mortality and morbidity in less frequently used laboratories is undoubtedly related to the experience of the angiographer, the laboratory, and its personnel. A minimum caseload of 300 per year is recommended for adult laboratories, and a caseload of 150 per year is recommended for pediatric laboratories to maintain a satisfactory level of activity for efficiency and safety.

The stability and severity of the patient's cardiac and medical condition also affect the complication rate. Increased risk is found in patients with significant left main coronary artery disease, severe triple vessel disease, unstable angina, congestive heart failure, multiple premature ventricular contractions, and systemic hypertension. Ostial left main coronary artery stenoses are particularly dangerous, because the trauma from the catheter entering the stenosis may increase the degree of narrowing, precipitating cardiac arrest. When a significant ostial lesion is found, views should be limited to the key angles necessary for showing the appropriate target vessels and urgent surgical bypass should be considered.

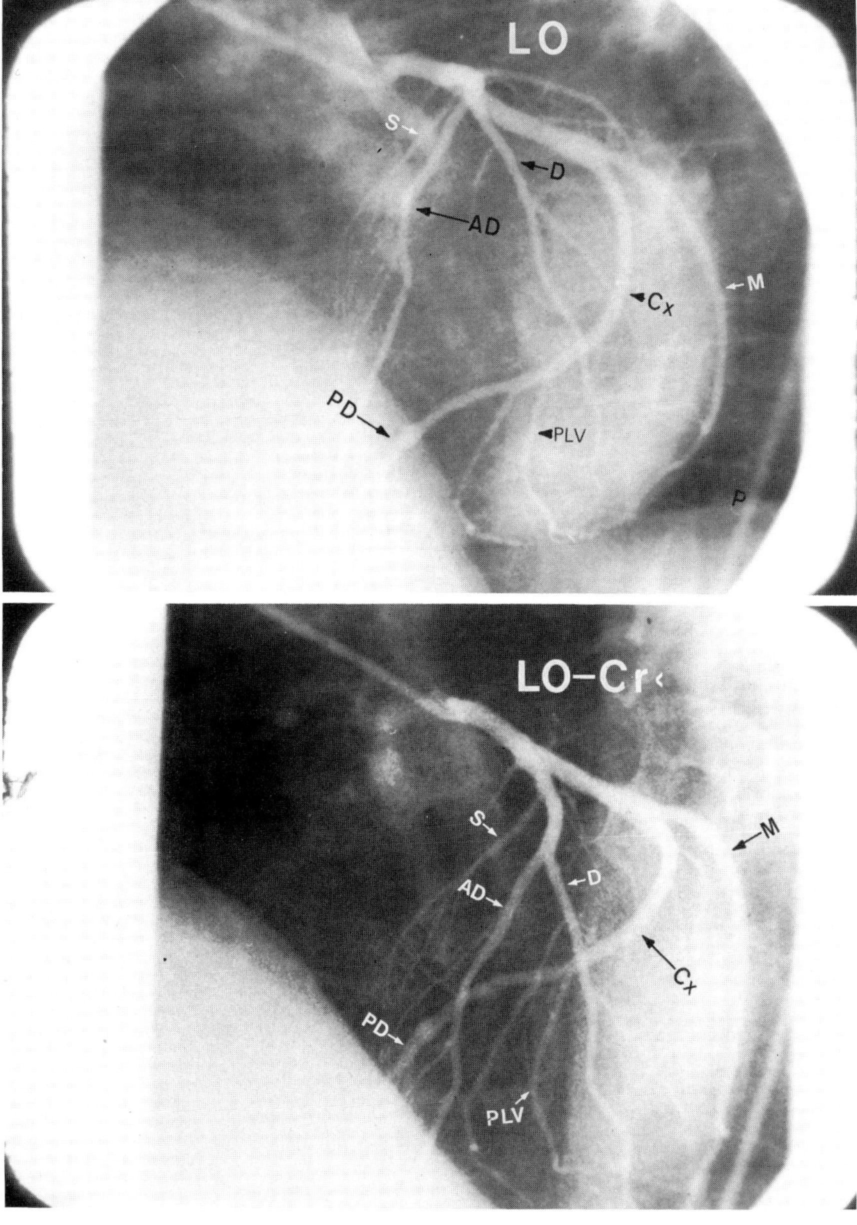

Figure 106–18. Routine (LO) and cranially angled (LO-Cr<) left anterior oblique **left coronary arteriograms**. Note improved depiction of the proximal anterior descending artery (AD) as well as the origin of the diagonal branch (D) from the anterior descending artery. The circumflex artery (Cx) has an inferior emphasis ("dominant"). (M = marginal artery; S = septal branch; PD = posterior descending artery; PLV = posterior left ventricular branch.)

TABLE 106–1. ETIOLOGY OF MAJOR COMPLICATIONS OF CARDIAC ANGIOGRAPHY

I. Contrast Media
- A. Arrhythmias
  1. Ventricular fibrillation and/or tachycardia
  2. Prolonged asystole
  3. Others—supraventricular arrhythmias, heart blocks, bigeminy
- B. Reactions
  1. Allergic
  2. Hypertension
  3. Hypotension
- C. Congestive heart failure
- D. Renal failure

II. Catheterization Technique
- A. Thromboembolic
  1. Cause
     a. Thrombus
     b. Air
     c. Particulate
        1) Catheter or guidewire fragment
        2) Contaminant
  2. Effect
     a. Acute myocardial infarction
     b. Cerebral vascular accident
     c. Renal infarction
     d. Extremity ischemia
- B. Improper catheter or guidewire passage
  1. Dissection
  2. Perforation
- C. Local
  1. Thrombus
  2. Dissection
  3. False aneurysm
- D. Inadequate or incomplete examination requiring repeat study or leading to improper treatment

The choice of contrast medium affects morbidity. Most angiographers prefer contrast with 350 or 370 mg I/ml for angiocardiography and selective coronary arteriography. Although low-osmolality contrast agents, particularly nonionic ones, have been shown to be safer in cardiac and coronary studies, their cost (20 times that of high-osmolality agents) restricts their general use. At a minimum, low-osmolality agents should be used in high-risk patients such as those with unstable angina, congestive heart failure, or cardiogenic shock and those over 60. Since nonionic agents have a decreased anticoagulant effect compared with ionic media, with a possible association with thromboembolic complications, systemic heparinization is recommended and good technique must be emphasized, including not allowing the blood to be withdrawn in the manifold and tubes connected to the catheter. When ionic high-osmolar contrast medium is used, 100 per cent meglumine agents must be avoided because of their high incidence of ventricular fibrillation associated with selective coronary angiography. Agents that contain a small amount of sodium salt and do not contain calcium-binding additives should be selected because of the reduced incidence of cardiac arrythmias.

Previously there was controversy regarding the relative safety of the brachial and femoral artery approach for coronary angiography. Reports have established that the key is *experience* and that both methods are acceptably safe. It has been shown that laboratories that only occasionally perform a transbrachial (cut-down) approach have a significantly higher complication rate than those that use this technique routinely. An alternative is the percutaneous brachial approach, using 5 and 6 Fr preformed catheters through a vascular access sheath.

Special mention should be made of pulmonary angiography. Although it is a remarkably safe procedure, the risk is significantly elevated in patients with severe pulmonary arterial hypertension. The use of nonionic contrast medium significantly reduces but does not completely eliminate this problem, and caution in these patients is advisable, entailing the use of superselective injections of small amounts of the contrast agent.

COSTS OF PROCEDURES

Cardiac catheterization laboratories frequently have more complicated x-ray and physiological equipment and require more personnel to scrub, circulate, and run the equipment than do noncardiac laboratories. At a minimum, a registered nurse, radiologic technologist, and cardiopulmonary technologist should be present in a dedicated cardiac laboratory. The time required to perform the procedure depends on the needed information. A routine left heart catheterization, left ventriculogram, and selective coronary angiogram should be accomplished in about 30 minutes skin to skin. Even a simple right heart catheterization should add only a few more minutes. However, coronary angioplasty adds significantly to the time burden in cardiac catheterization laboratories. The study of patients with valvular or congenital heart disease requires considerably more time, depending on the complexity of the condition. The experienced catheterizing physician will be able to perform the study efficiently in the minimum necessary time. It is necessary that the catheterizing physician be familiar with the patient's condition so that a complete but not superfluous study will be obtained.

The costs vary considerably across the United States but may be significantly reduced by increasing volume, because the federal government is encouraging regionalization as well as packaging with cardiac surgery or angioplasty to reduce this significant burden on our health care costs. It is projected that the total cost both technical and professional of the diagnosis and therapy of a patient with coronary heart disease can be reduced from a high of more than $40,000 to about $25,000, the diagnostic catheterization and angiographic study costing about 10 to 15 per cent of the total.

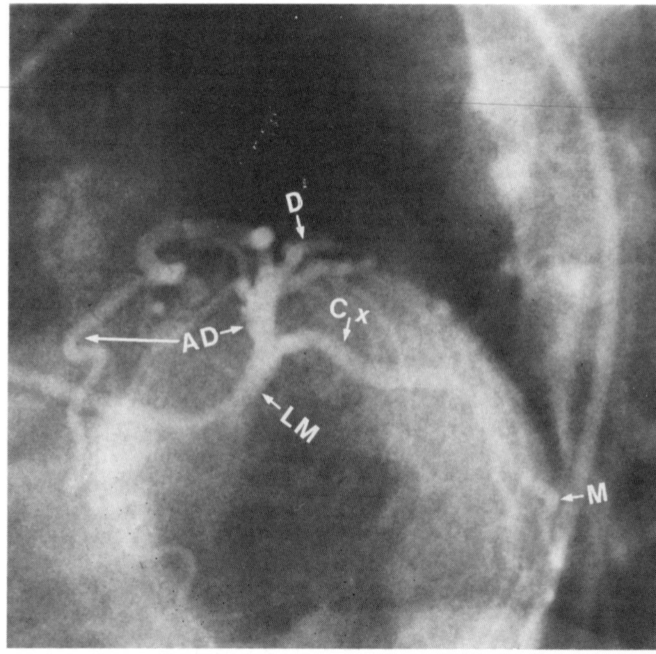

Figure 106–19. Caudally angled **left anterior oblique left coronary arteriogram** ("spider view"). (AD = anterior descending artery; D = diagonal branch; Cx = circumflex artery; M = marginal artery; LM = left main coronary artery.)

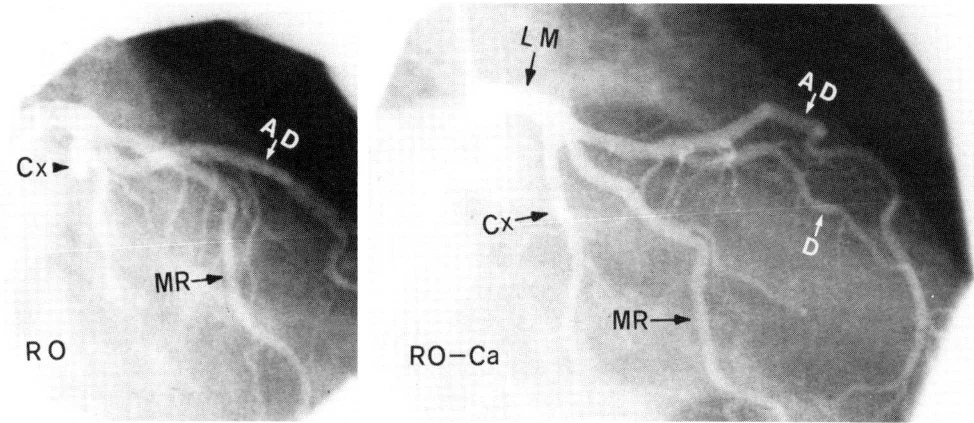

Figure 106–20. Routine (RO) and caudally angled (RO-Ca) **right anterior oblique left coronary arteriograms**. A trifurcation of the left coronary artery is seen (a common variation). The central vessel is the median ramus branch (MR) with its origin best seen on the caudally angled view. (AD = anterior descending artery; Cx = circumflex artery; D = diagonal branch; LM = left main coronary artery.)

Bibliography

Adams DF, Abrams HL: Complications of coronary arteriography: A follow up report. Cardiovasc Radiol 2:89–96, 1979.

Amplatz K, Formanek G, Stanger P, Wilson W: Mechanics of selective coronary artery catheterization via femoral approach. Radiology 89:1040–1047, 1967.

Bettmann MA, Bourdillon PD, Barry WH, et al: Contrast agents for cardiac angiography: Effects of a nonionic agent vs a standard ionic agent. Radiology 153:583–587, 1984.

Daves ML: Cardiac roentgenology. The loop and circle approach. Radiology 95:157–160, 1970.

Davis K, Kennedy JW, Kemp HG, et al: Complications of coronary arteriography from the Collaborative Study of Coronary Artery Surgery (CASS). Circulation 59:1105–1112, 1979.

Engel HJ, Torres C, Page HL: Major variations in anatomical origin of the coronary arteries: Angiographic observations in 4,250 patients with associated congenital heart disease. Cathet Cardiovasc Diagn 1:157–169, 1975.

Pepine CJ, Allen HD, Bashore TM, et al: ACC/AHA Guidelines for cardiac catheterization and cardiac catheterization laboratories. J Am Coll Cardiol 18:1149–1182, 1991.

Grollman JH Jr: Pigtail catheters in pulmonary angiography. Cathet Cardiovasc Diagn 10:389–391, 1984.

Grollman JH Jr: Pulmonary angiography. Cardiovasc Interv Radiol 15:166–170, 1992.

Gurley JC, Nissen SE, Booth DC, et al: Comparison of simultaneously performed digital and film-based angiography in assessment of coronary artery disease. Circulation 78:1411–1420, 1988.

Holmes DR Jr, Wondrow MA, Gray JE: Isn't it time to abandon cine film? Cathet Cardiovasc Diagn 20:1–4, 1990.

James TN: Anatomy of the coronary arteries in health and disease. Circulation 32:1020–1033, 1965.

Judkins MP: Percutaneous transfemoral selective coronary arteriography. Radiol Clin North Am 6:467–492, 1968.

Kennedy JW: Complications associated with cardiac catheterization and angiography. Cathet Cardiovasc Diagn 8:5–11, 1982.

Mills SR, Jackson DC, Older RA, et al: The incidence, etiologies and avoidance of complications of pulmonary angiography in a large series. Radiology 136:295–299, 1980.

Newell JD II, Kelley MJ, Ovitt TW: Digital cardiac radiology. Radiol Clin North Am 23:261–273, 1985.

O'Reilly RJ: Coronary angiographic nomenclature. Current status and a plea for standardization. Radiology 115:229–232, 1975.

Schoonmaker FW, King SB: Coronary arteriography by the single catheter percutaneous femoral technique. Experience in 6,800 cases. Circulation 50:735–740, 1974.

Sones FM Jr, Shirey EK: Cine coronary arteriography. Mod Concepts Cardiovasc Dis 31:735–738, 1962.

Steinberg EP, Moore RD, Powe NR, et al: Safety and cost effectiveness of high-osmolality as compared with low-osmolality contrast material in patients undergoing cardiac angiography. N Engl J Med 326:425–430, 1992.

107 Conventional and Digital Angiography of the Peripheral Vascular System

Antoinette S. Gomes, Robert J. Cassling, and Julius H. Grollman, Jr.

EQUIPMENT NEEDED TO GENERATE THE EXAMINATION

Angiography of the peripheral vascular system should be performed in a dedicated room with adequate fluoroscopic, digital, and rapid filming capabilities. The generator should be at least three-phase and preferably constant-potential, with a minimum output of 100 kw and 1000 MA. Radiographic technique should use high milliamperage with peak kilovoltage around 70 and a reasonably short exposure time of 100 msec or less to minimize patient and vessel motion artifacts. At least a dual–focal spot x-ray tube should be available, with focal spots of approximately 0.6 and 1.0 to 1.2 mm. Larger 2-mm focal spots result in too much geometric unsharpness because there is always a moderate degree (1.2 to 1.3 times) of magnification in most angiographic systems. Greater magnifications of 1.5 to 2 times with a 0.3-mm focal spot tube are occasionally helpful. Stationary fine-line grids (100 lines per inch) with a ratio of 12:1 are important. A high-speed film and screen combination is preferable, but it should not be too fast or the resulting noisy image will degrade resolution. Scatter radiation, which degrades the image, can be reduced by tight collimation of the x-ray beam to the field of interest.

Image recording should be appropriate to the organ or region being studied. Catheter manipulation with 15 to 25 cm (6 to 10 inch) diameter image intensifiers is acceptable, but imaging with this size is limited, especially in the extremities. Image intensifiers with resolution approaching standard film-screen techniques have allowed the development of fluoroscopic imaging. Large format image intensifiers of 30 to 40 cm (12 to 16 inch) are now preferred for peripheral angiography because much of the filming is now imaged from the output phosphor rather than a large film changer. Photofluorography with a spot film camera mounted on the intensifier has been used, but this is being supplanted by digital imaging. Cine fluorography at 15 to 60 frames per second is useful when rapid flow is encountered, such as with arteriovenous malformations, but it *should not* be relied on as the only means of recording the image.

Large film seriography is the standard for peripheral arteriography against which other techniques are compared (Figs. 107–1 and 107–2). Rapid film changers with up to four frames per second are preferable. The latest versions have a low profile, allowing a mounting directly on the image intensifier housing, facilitating change from fluoroscopic to film changer imaging. Most changers are 36 × 36 cm (14 × 14 inches), although actual coverage is less, as is the case with image intensifiers.

Peripheral runoff angiography is best handled by either a moving tabletop or a long-leg film changer. The latter has the advantage of ease of timing since the entire pelvis and lower extremities are included on a single film—the commonly used changers allow four or five exposures at variable time intervals. The disadvantage of the long-leg film changer is that an entire separate x-ray system is needed in addition to the standard film changer and its x-ray tube, because a ceiling mount tube is necessary to allow enough beam divergence to cover the entire long-film cassette. This addition also requires extra space and a means of moving the patient from the fluoroscopic table to the film changer. On the other hand, using a moving tabletop over a standard film changer requires only an inexpensive addition to the angiographic laboratory (see Fig. 107–1). An adequate diagnostic study however, requires accurate timing and judgment, in spite of which 20 to 40 per cent of cases need some repetition because of inadequate visualization of segments of the peripheral circulation.

Digital subtraction angiography (DSA) is now a mandatory adjunct to a complete angiographic facility, and digital angiography without subtraction (DA) has become a primary diagnostic technique. DSA is an angiographic image processing technique that digitizes the sequential photofluoroscopic images, allowing real-time subtraction and display of these images (Fig. 107–3). DA is simply the same process without subtraction—the simultaneous acquisition and display of digitally enhanced images with instant replay of the same quality images.

Intravenous DSA (IV-DSA), with intravenous injection of contrast medium in the peripheral veins, superior vena cava, or right atrium and recording of the image during the arterial phase, is now rarely used. Patient motion, low cardiac output, and the need for large volumes of contrast medium have resulted in its being supplanted by intra-arterial DSA (IA-DSA), which has all the advantages of conventional angiography, the only disadvantage being the invasive transarterial approach.

Overall, digital studies have lower resolution than conventional film-screen arteriography, and there can be a significant problem with field size, which is limited by the diameter of the image intensifier. Newer large format image intensifiers of 30 to 40 cm have helped, but there is a tradeoff in terms of loss of gain and resolution. Recording the image with a 1024^2 matrix is of particular value with these larger intensifiers (the older matrix standard was 512^2). The resolution for peripheral vascular obstructive disease is generally adequate. The reduced film and processing costs help to justify the extra expense of the added equipment. The immediate display and instant replay of the study shorten the time of the examination, allowing greater efficiency and scheduling of more cases and especially facilitating interventional procedures. Other benefits include postprocessing techniques that improve the quality of the study, road mapping, and quantitative techniques such as diameter and densitometric stenosis measurement.

Digital imaging for lower extremity vascular disease is usually used as an adjunct to standard large film seriography, especially to facilitate the oblique studies of the pelvis and the femoral and popliteal bifurcation. Primary imaging with digital recording presents special problems in studying the lower extremities. DSA is difficult because following a bolus of contrast from the pelvis to the feet with one injection requires acquiring a mask for each level as a separate run immediately before or after the injection; however, it is not impossible. DA is more commonly used, and the bolus of contrast is visually followed as it flows down the lower extremities by moving the image intensifier or tabletop (Fig. 107–4). Unfortunately, the round field cuts off portions of the legs even with the largest intensifiers, making simultaneous bilateral lower extremity studies difficult, especially in large patients. In addition, resolution

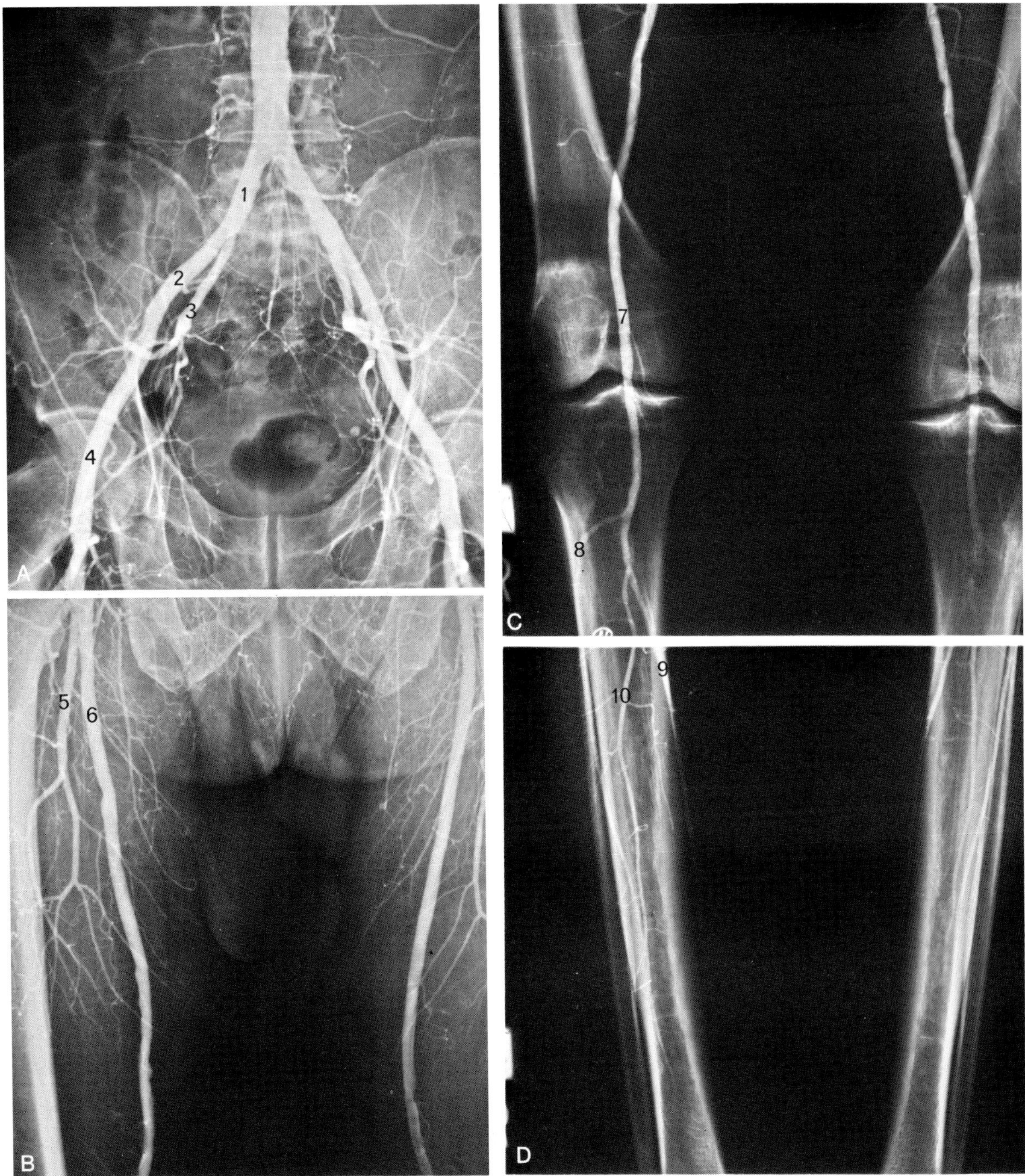

Figure 107–1. Normal arterial runoff examination. *A,* Pelvic level showing pelvic vessels: common iliac artery (1), external iliac artery (2), internal iliac artery (3), and common femoral artery (4). *B* , Thigh level showing profunda femoral artery (5) and superficial artery (6). *C,* Knee level demonstrating popliteal artery (7) and anterior tibial artery (8). *D,* Lower leg runoff showing posterior tibial artery (9) and peroneal artery (10).

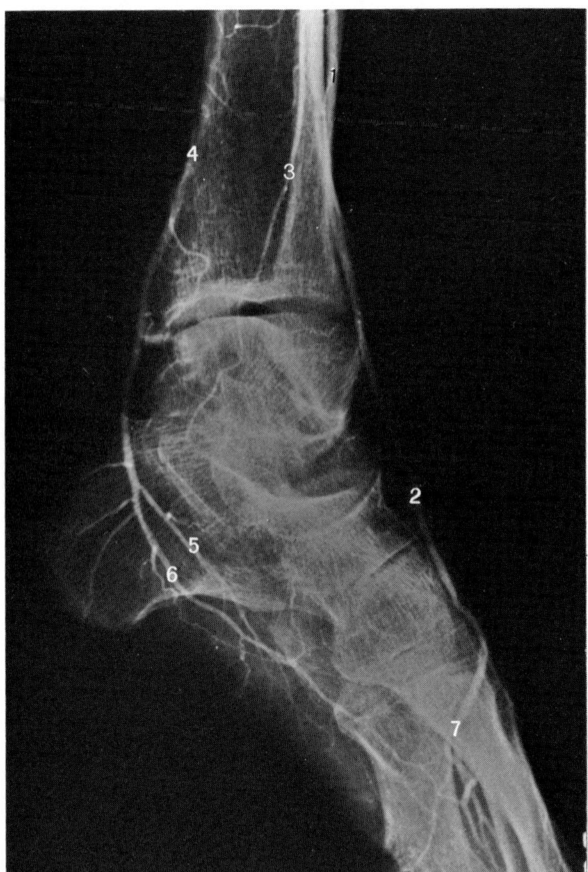

Figure 107–2. Arterial anatomy of the foot. Steep oblique view from a study using a conventional bilateral large film seriography over a stepping table shows anterior tibial artery (1), dorsal pedal artery (2), peroneal artery (3), posterior tibial artery (4), medial plantar artery (5), lateral plantar artery (6), and deep plantar branch artery (7).

drops off toward the periphery of the field. Bolusing of the region between and around the legs presents a special problem, because the unfiltered beam results in halation (bright spots in the image). Bolusing may be accomplished externally by water bags, Play-Doh, etc, and internally by filters in the x-ray tube housing and an electronic thresholding technique. These problems are not as severe with unilateral lower extremity peripheral angiography. Digital imaging is more suitable to upper extremity peripheral angiography because it is always unilateral.

Performing the DA study in the anteroposterior plane with the image intensifier under the table ensures more uniform magnification from level to level and results in less magnification than is found with posteroanterior imaging, where the abdomen and feet prevent close approximation of the image tube. It is important to remember, however, that fluoroscopy in the anteroposterior plane results in considerably more radiation exposure to the angiographer. Oblique unilateral studies may be performed quite easily with a posteroanterior x-ray beam without as much varying magnification because the abdomen and feet do not prevent lowering the image intensifier close to the patient.

Physiologic recording equipment must be available to ensure adequate diagnostic studies in peripheral angiography as well as safety. Routine intra-arterial monitoring of blood pressure allows ready access to measuring gradients across borderline stenotic lesions, especially in the aortoiliac vessels, where the diameter of the vessel being studied and the catheter used (4 and 5 Fr) generally allow accurate pressure determinations. Although two pressure channels are ideal, a single channel will suffice. If direct intra-arterial pressures are not monitored, automatic frequent arm cuff pressures are mandatory. Routine electrocardiographic monitoring is also mandatory, especially since these patients usually have concomitant coronary artery disease. A pulse oximeter mounted on an appropriate digit is also recommended. An emergency cart and oxygen supply should be in or readily available to the angiography suite.

PERFORMANCE OF THE EXAMINATION

With small-diameter, 4 and 5 Fr, high-flow catheters, most diagnostic arteriography is performed on an outpatient basis followed by a four to six hour observation period prior to discharge from an outpatient surgery or angiography recovery unit. Angiography is generally performed on an inpatient basis only when the patient has to be hospitalized for other medical problems or immediate intervention is planned. Use of the Seldinger technique modified by advances in catheter and guidewire technology has rendered percutaneous vascular access a remarkably safe procedure.

Approaches

Because of its ease and safety, the most common route of entry into the arterial system is percutaneous puncture of the common femoral artery below the inguinal ligament. Following careful aseptic preparation of the skin and adequate local anesthesia, the anterior arterial wall is punctured with the ''one-wall'' technique, using a beveled needle without an obturator (alternatively, both walls may be punctured with a double- or triple-component needle, with the pulsatile blood return being obtained during slow withdrawal of the needle with the obturator removed). The needle hub should be slightly depressed and a guidewire gently fed through the needle into the artery. If resistance is felt, minimal further withdrawal of the needle may free the tip from the posterior wall. After the guidewire has been advanced to its proper destination with fluoroscopic guidance, the needle is withdrawn, hemostasis is maintained by digital compression at the puncture site, and a catheter is inserted over the guidewire to the desired area.

When severe iliofemoral disease precludes catheter introduction into either femoral artery, alternate routes are available. Many angiographers' first choice is the axillary or brachial arterial puncture. Either of these approaches is more difficult than the femoral because of the mobility of the vessels and their smaller caliber. The axillary artery is larger in diameter but is more prone to neurologic complications than the brachial artery (see Risks of Procedure). The brachial artery may be approached at multiple sites. The high brachial artery is large and relatively fixed. The midbrachial artery is fairly large but is deep and mobile. The brachial artery at the antecubital fossa is more superficial and easier to puncture, but its smaller size makes it more susceptible to spasm and thrombosis. With the antecubital approach, a small 4 Fr catheter is advisable, and if selective studies are planned, a vascular access sheath is recommended. Systemic heparinization should be used when the approach is at the antecubital fossa, with reversal by protamine sulfate only after removal of the catheter. Compression is applied only to the point of maintaining hemostasis while still allowing distal flow controlled by monitoring the radial pulse.

Direct puncture of the aorta via a translumbar approach is an alternative used in many institutions. This procedure carries less morbidity than the transaxillary approach but probably not less than the brachial approach. If not properly performed, it can be quite uncomfortable to the patient. Careful preliminary injection of local anesthetic through a 22-gauge Chiba needle along the expected soft

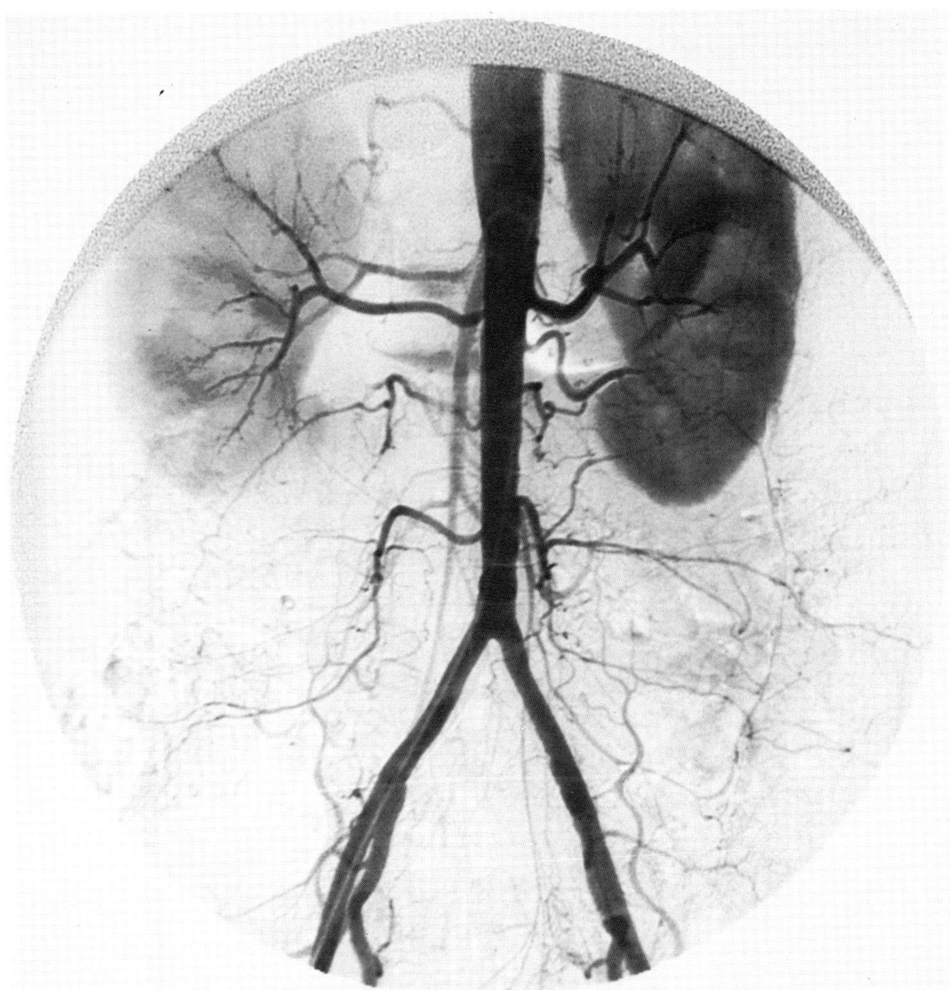

Figure 107–3. Intra-arterial digital subtraction aortogram (DSA) of the abdominal aorta and its branches on a 36-cm image intensifier using a 1024^2-pixel matrix. There is excellent central resolution but decreased resolution peripherally. Note the cutoff at the corners because of the circular field and the preferential filling of the posteriorly arising arteries. The superior and inferior mesenteric arteries and superior right renal artery are faintly filled because the contrast medium, which is heavier than blood, is settling posteriorly due to the relatively slow injection rates used for DSA, in this case 12 ml/sec for 1 and 1½ seconds. The image has been manipulated by edge enhancement and the "peak pixel" mode in which all images during the arterial phase have been summed, allowing depiction of the entire abdominal aorta and branches on this single film in spite of the relatively short injection.

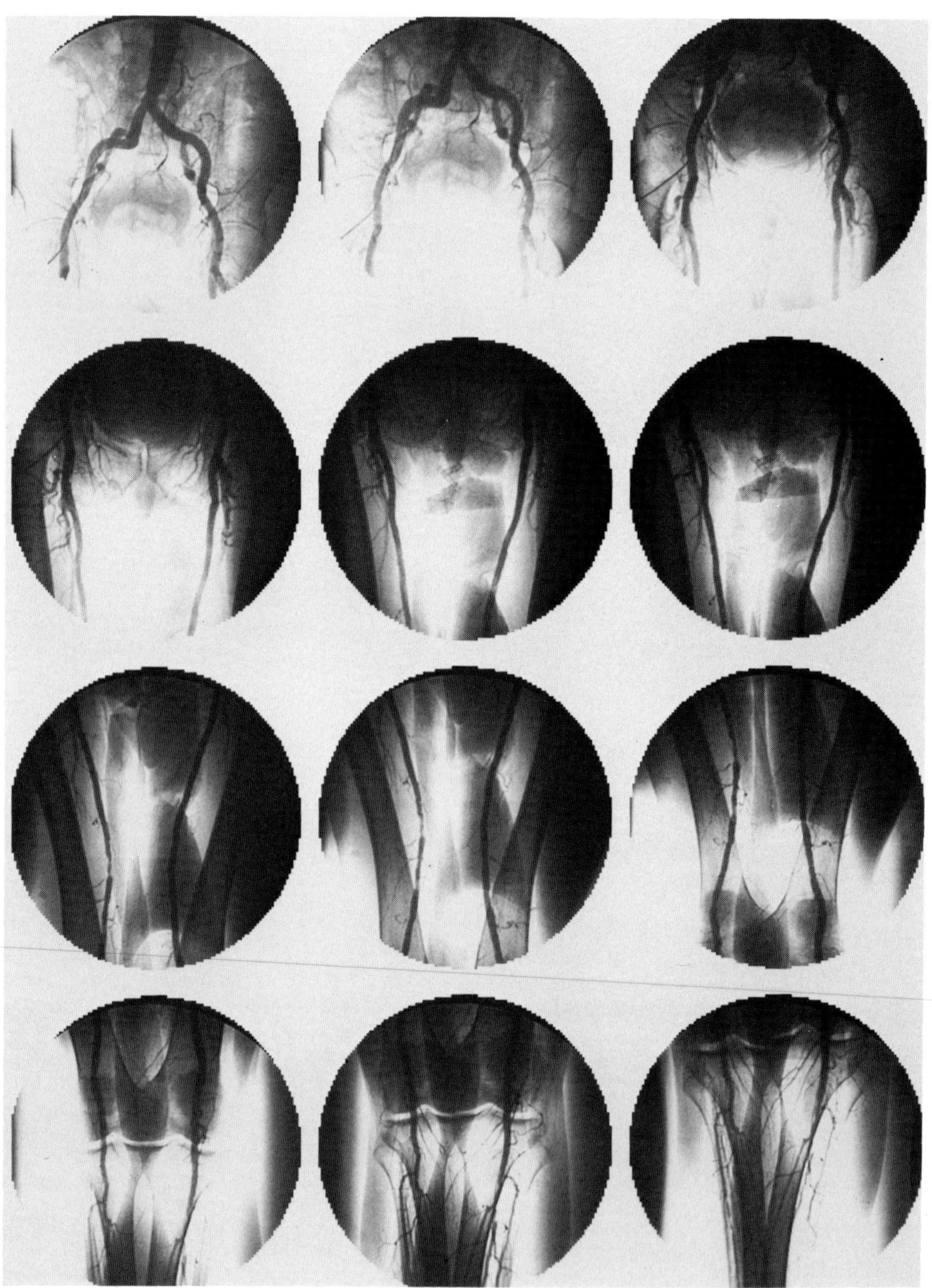

Figure 107–4. Anteroposterior bolus chase digital peripheral angiogram (DA) performed on a 36-cm image intensifier injecting 60 ml of non-ionic contrast medium 370 mg I/ml contrast medium at a rate of 10 ml/sec. The contrast bolus has been followed by stepping the table using visual monitoring. Note the cutoff at the corners and marginal field coverage on this standard-sized adult, requiring multiple images instead of the four or five stations used with large film seriography. The ankles have been crossed to decrease the distance between the knees and to reduce halation. In spite of these problems, the study is diagnostic.

tissue approach will relieve much of the discomfort. This approach has a relative contraindication in patients with abdominal aortic aneurysms, bleeding disorders, aortic grafts, or severe hypertension.

Either a suprarenal T12 or infrarenal approach may be used. The infrarenal puncture is suitable only in the absence of significant aortic occlusive disease. A conventional T12 puncture site results in injection of contrast into the thoracic aorta, as is appropriate when there is significant aortic obstruction. It results in filling of the intercostal arteries, which are the major collateral pathway. Because the internal mammary arteries also supply collaterals, an ascending thoracic aortic injection may result in the best opacification of the femoral arteries. If an infrarenal delivery of contrast is needed, a translumbar catheter with a short distal 90-degree angle may be used to direct the catheter over a guidewire into the distal aorta after a T12 puncture. In this situation, a tip occluder should be used to prevent the catheter tip from injecting into the aortic wall.

If peripheral access is unavailable because of arterial outflow obstruction in all four extremities, the translumbar approach becomes the technique of choice and may be used safely for thoracic aortography as well as selective upper extremity, carotid, vertebral, and coronary arteriography. Introduction of a long vascular access sheath is imperative so that catheter exchanges can be accomplished without retroperitoneal bleeding.

Lower Extremity Arteriography

A standard lower extremity arteriogram for occlusive disease includes opacification of the vascular system from the aortic bifurcation down to the feet. As part of this assessment, visualization of the abdominal aorta at least in the frontal projection is routinely included to assess the aortic bifurcation and renal artery origins. A lateral view may be necessary to evaluate the extent and severity of aneurysmal and obstructive disease, as well as the origins of the visceral branches. Using the usual common femoral artery approach, an end- and multiside-hole catheter, either straight or in a pigtail or other loop configuration, is passed into the abdominal aorta to the level of the renal arteries or celiac axis, depending on the extent of visualization needed. For standard film or DA angiography, 30 to 50 ml of 350 to 370 mg I/ml contrast is injected over 1.5 to 2 seconds, depending on the size of the patient and aorta being studied. The angiographer should know the variable flow rate limitations of the individual catheters. For DSA, half-strength contrast will frequently suffice, depending on the characteristics of the digital system being used, but the flow rate should not be reduced too much, or adequate mixing with blood will not be obtained (see Fig. 107–3). Abdominal compression or intravenous glucagon (0.5 to 1.0 mg) may be use to improve the quality of DSA studies by reducing bowel motion artifacts.

The catheter is positioned just above the aortic bifurcation for the peripheral angiogram. Prior to filming, a test injection of contrast medium under fluoroscopy should be made to estimate the transit time to the knees, which will help the angiographer select a proper combination of contrast volume, flow rate, and filming sequence. When distal flow is slow, reactive hyperemia may be used to improve visualization. Reactive hyperemia is induced by the application of tourniquets to the thigh, occluding flow bilaterally for 5 to 7 minutes with release immediately before the contrast injection. As an alternative, intra-aortic tolazoline in doses of 35 to 50 mg may be used. Although tolazoline is not as effective as reactive hyperemia, it produces less patient discomfort. In the event of a marked disparity between the lower extremities, such as with a unilateral iliac or femoral occlusion, it can be helpful to induce a hyperemic state on the affected side only. Inflation of the thigh cuff for only 2 to 3 minutes will be adequate to equalize the flow rates in both extremities in most patients.

Although sequential runs may be made for the various segments of the lower extremities, a better quality study will be obtained with a net lower total volume of contrast by injecting a large bolus of contrast relatively slowly using either a long-leg film changer or a stepping tabletop. Depending on the patient's size and distal flow, 60 to 100 ml of 300 or 320 mg I/ml contrast is injected over a 10 to 14 second interval; for patients with slower distal flow, a longer injection is required to obtain good distal visualization. The long column of contrast in the distal vessels at each instant increases the likelihood of proper visualization during the filming sequence, despite differences in blood flow from one extremity to the other. During this period, the angiographic table is moved in steps to cover the pelvis, thighs, knees, ankles, and feet (see Figs. 107–1 and 107–2). Filming is usually extended to 14 to 16 seconds and sometimes longer. A long-film changer will require less total volume since timing is not so critical.

If a single extremity is to be evaluated, the femoral artery on the ipsilateral side may be punctured and contrast injected through a catheter in the ipsilateral common or external iliac artery. Alternately, the other femoral artery may be punctured and the iliac artery on the side of interest may be catheterized using a catheter with a short distal curve passed over a floppy or hydrophilic guidewire. If the aortic bifurcation is very acute, a pigtail or sidewinder shape facilitates the catheterization. If one is studying the entire extremity with one injection, half the volume and flow rate recommended for bilateral studies will suffice.

Overlap of the superficial and profunda femoral and the external and internal iliac arteries in the frontal projections may mask a significant lesion. Oblique pelvic views are necessary to visualize both these areas (Figs. 107–5 and 107–6). A right anterior oblique (left posterior oblique) projection typically opens up the right common femoral and the left common iliac bifurcation, and the left anterior oblique (right posterior oblique) conversely opens up the left common femoral and right common iliac bifurcations. DSA using dilute contrast is particularly useful in obtaining these and all ancillary views. Single-station pelvic arteriography requires 30 to 45 ml of contrast over 2 to 3 seconds for large film studies, with DSA again requiring considerably less and more dilute media. Single-station unilateral studies need approximately half these amounts.

However, since orthogonal views that reliably evaluate a lesion are not always obtainable because of overlap or lesion eccentricity, pressure measurements above and below the lesion will be helpful. A systolic gradient of greater than 10 mm Hg is regarded as significant in the aortoiliac arteries. If a hemodynamically significant gradient is not measured at rest, a hyperemic state should be induced, because this may unmask a lesion significant under stress. In hyperemic states induced pharmacologically by vasodilators such as tolazoline or papaverine or by reactive hyperemia, a gradient of 15 to 20 mm Hg or more is considered significant. These measurements are particularly important in assessing the significance of aortoiliac stenoses; these measurements may be obtained by simple withdrawal of the catheter across an ipsilateral lesion. Contralateral catheterization is more difficult, but it should be performed when there are questionable lesions (40 to 60 per cent by diameter) whose significance will influence the therapeutic course of action. This technique is acceptably safe in patients without severe ulcerative aortoiliac disease and aortic aneurysms containing mural thrombus. The use of 4 or 5 Fr catheters yields valid pressure measurements in most external and common iliac arteries with diameters of 6 to 12 mm. If contralateral catheterization is contraindicated or impossible because of the acuteness of the angle of the aortoiliac bifurcation, catheterization of the opposite common femoral artery with comparison between the pressure in the side of interest through a needle, small catheter, or vascular dilator and the aortic pressure will yield the necessary information.

Beyond their origins, the superficial femoral and profunda femoral arteries are typically only imaged in the frontal projection because overlap is usually not a problem. However, lateral views may

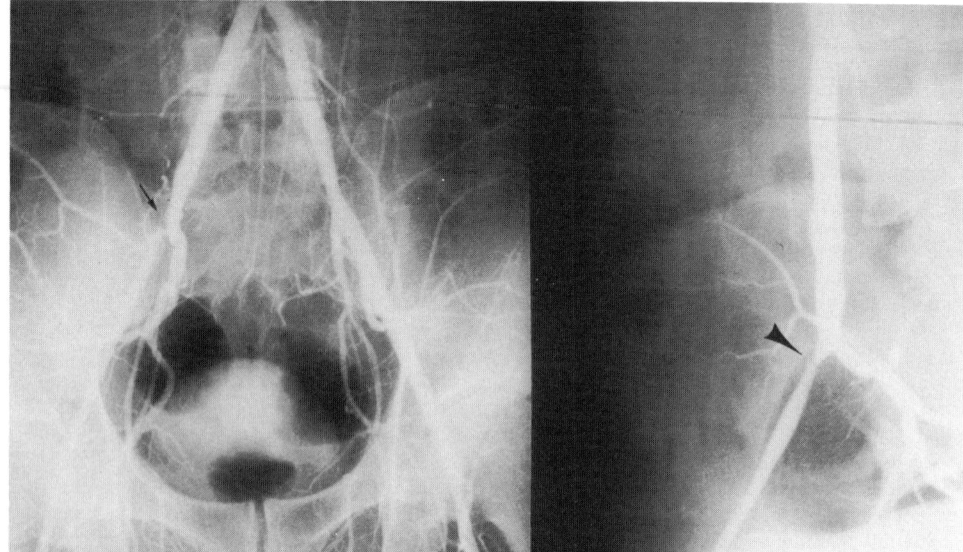

Figure 107–5. *Left,* **Anteroposterior pelvic arteriogram showing a lesion** *(arrow)* **in the very proximal right external iliac artery** that is impossible to quantify due to overlap with the hypogastric artery. *Right,* A right posterior oblique selective iliac arteriogram was then performed, clearly demonstrating a high-grade stenosis *(arrowhead).*

be important for the full assessment of a borderline stenosis (Fig. 107–7). Equally important may be orthogonal views of the popliteal bifurcation and the tibial and peroneal arteries. Visualization of the feet is important, especially when there is infrapopliteal disease (a single lateral or oblique view is usually sufficient).

Hemodynamic evaluation of infrainguinal lesions is more difficult because of the distance of the contralateral lesions from the puncture site and may be impossible when the lesion in question is ipsilateral to the puncture site. The distal vessels are relatively small in relation to the catheter diameter. Familiarity with the clinical situation via pertinent history, complete assessment of all peripheral pulses, and knowledge of the findings of noninvasive vascular tests facilitates the selection of the important additional views (see Fig. 107–7). Contrast medium limitations will prevent routinely obtaining orthogonal views of the entire lower extremities.

In the evaluation of angiographic studies, it is important to indicate whether a stenosis is described by diameter or area per cent reduction: A 50 per cent diameter and a 75 per cent cross-sectional area reduction are equivalent and considered the borderline of significance (Table 107–1). The angiographer should be careful in relying on cross-section area analysis unless two orthogonal views are available, because arteriosclerotic lesions are typically eccentric. When orthogonal views are available, it is not accurate to rate eccentric stenoses as the severest diameter of the two views; instead, it is preferable to indicate the equivalent cross-section area reduction if possible. For example, a 60 × 40 per cent lesion is approx-

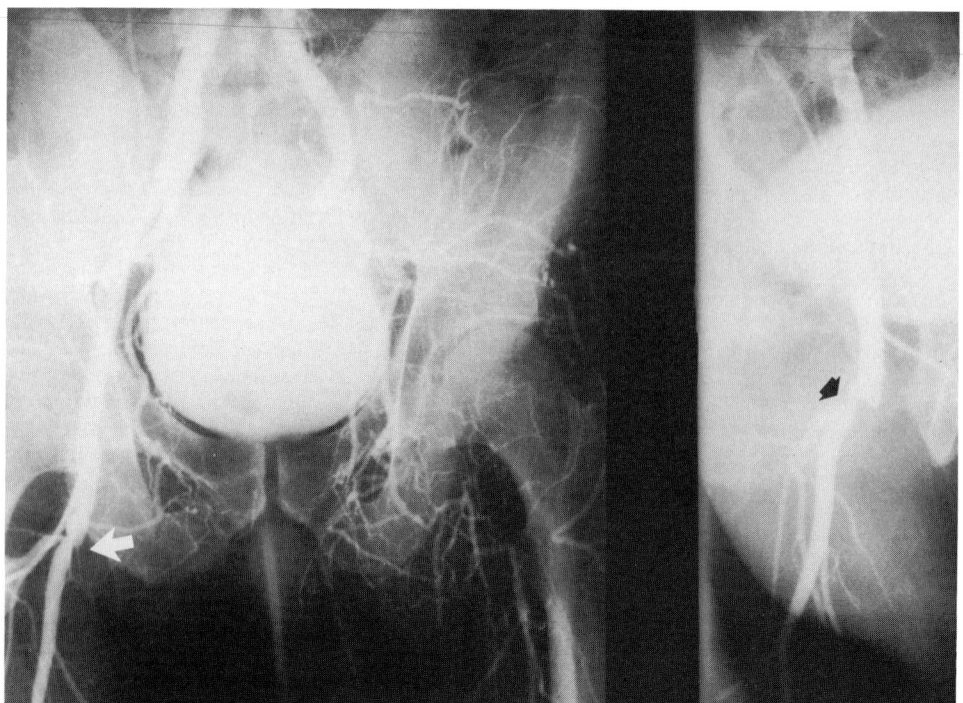

Figure 107–6. *Left,* **Anteroposterior pelvic arteriogram showing an occluded superficial femoral artery** with a patent profunda femoral artery *(arrow). Right,* A left anterior oblique selective iliac arteriogram unmasks a hidden significant origin profunda femoral artery stenosis *(arrow).*

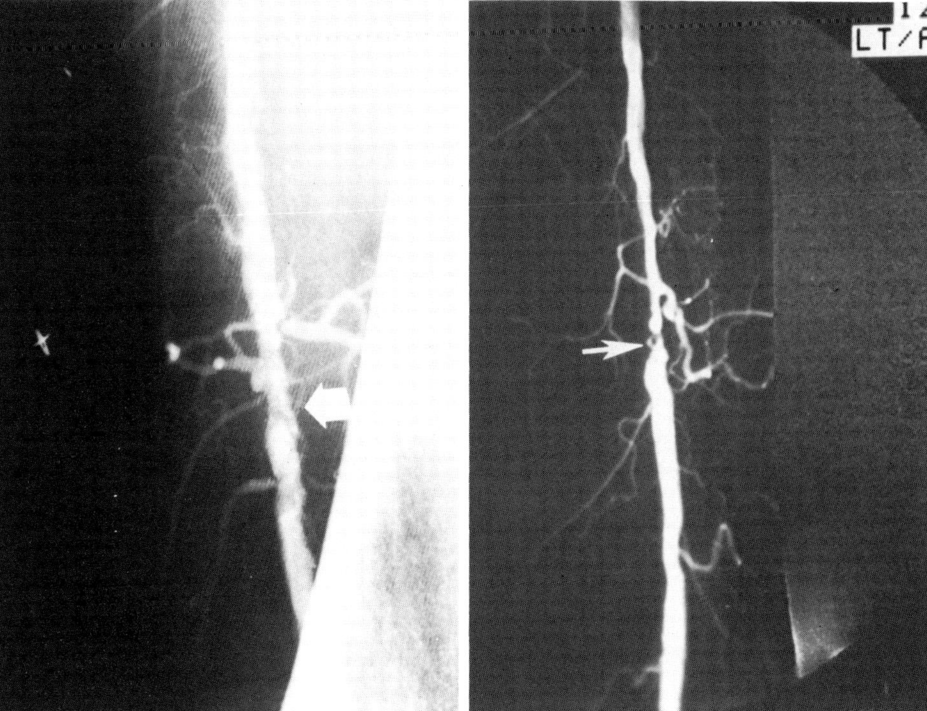

Figure 107–7. *Left,* **Significant stenosis at the adductor hiatus** obscured on the anteroposterior view because of eccentricity *(arrow). Right,* A lateral view was obtained because of decreased popliteal and pedal pulses showing a significant stenosis *(arrow).*

imately equivalent to a 50 per cent concentric diameter stenosis and a 75 per cent area stenosis.

Upper Extremity Arteriography

Although large film serialography previously was used for aortic arch aortography and brachiocephalic arteriography, many centers with adequate equipment now rely almost solely on DSA. Conventional aortic arch aortography performed to study extracranial occlusive disease requires rapid flow rates of at least 30 to 45 ml/sec of 350 or 370 mg I/ml contrast medium for 1 to 1.5 seconds to opacify these vessels adequately in patients with normal cardiac output. Short injections through 6 to 8 Fr high-flow end- and side-hole or pigtail catheters with rapid 3 or 4/sec filming frame rates during the arterial phase result in diagnostic studies in most patients. On the other hand, flow rates of 15 to 25 ml/sec of 300 mg I/ml contrast medium injected for 1 to 1.5 seconds through 4 and 5 Fr high-flow catheters are adequate for DSA.

Many variations of selective catheters are available for selective brachiocephalic arteriography, most of which have a "reverse" primary curve to be chosen by the angiographer to fit the configuration of the transverse thoracic aorta and the origins of the brachiocephalic arteries. The selective catheter is carefully advanced over a guidewire to the point of interest. Again, imaging may be accomplished by large film serialography and/or DA.

Subclavian and common carotid arteriography is best accomplished with flow rates of 5 to 8 ml/sec of 300 or 320 mg I/ml contrast medium over 2 to 3 seconds. A flow rate of 4 to 5 ml/sec suffices for vertebral arteriography. Reduced volumes and slightly reduced flow rates are adequate for DSA.

Arm, forearm, and hand arteriography require lower flow rates of 3 to 4 ml/sec. Somewhat longer injection times of 4 or 5 seconds are helpful in studying the more distal arterial tree. It is generally not useful to place the catheter any farther than the brachial artery, even when studying the hand, because it is imperative to fill both the radial and ulnar arteries. A high bifurcation of the brachial artery may result in too distal an injection.

The study of obstructive arterial problems in the hand is particularly difficult because of the very slow flow rates encountered. Enhancing the flow rate pharmacologically with tolazoline or other techniques is imperative for visualizing the small distal digital arteries. Immersing the hand in warm water for about 5 minutes just before the arterial contrast injection is particularly of value. Magnification to bring out fine arterial changes is often helpful.

TABLE 107–1. DIAMETER VERSUS CROSS-SECTION AREA STENOSIS

Diameter		Area
30%	=	51%
40%	=	64%
50%	=	75%
60%	=	84%
70%	=	91%
80%	=	96%
90%	=	99%
95%	=	99+%

Venography

Pelvis and Lower Extremity Veins. The technique of lower extremity venography is described in Chapter 45. It is the most common form of contrast venographic examination, and it may be modified by using digital imaging if a large image intensifier is available.

Selective visualization of the iliac veins and inferior vena cava is occasionally necessary and is most commonly performed by percutaneous catheterization of the femoral vein at the groin, with selective injections into the ipsilateral and contralateral iliac veins or inferior vena cava. Transpopliteal venous access to the femoral and pelvic veins is a rare but safely used technique if the femoral vein is inaccessible due to thrombosis or tumor. The catheter configurations used tend to be simple because vessel tortuosity is generally not a problem. The contrast medium flow rates and volumes used are similar to those used for the adjacent arteries. DSA and DA are very useful in these studies.

SUPERIOR VENA CAVA AND BRACHIOCEPHALIC VEINS. Superior vena cavagrams are most commonly performed using bilateral antecubital vein access with small catheters placed in both basilic veins. Hand injection of 30 to 40 ml of contrast medium bilaterally with or without tourniquets is performed with conventional serial radiography or DA or DSA. A transfemoral or transjugular (internal or external) approach may also be used. Rare alternative sites include the axillary and subclavian veins. Catheter designs again are simple, and contrast medium flow rates and volumes are similar to those for the adjacent arteries. Hand injection of contrast into veins of the hands and wrist is suitable for forearm and arm venography. These peripheral sites may be used for subclavian, innominate, and superior vena caval visualization when swelling or anatomy precludes the use of the basilic vein. In these incidences a tourniquet should be applied to the forearm and released midway through the injection. Simultaneous elevation of the arms facilitates visualization of the more central veins.

NORMAL ANATOMY

Arterial Anatomy

PELVIS AND LOWER EXTREMITIES. The common iliac arteries arise at the aortic bifurcation, at the level of the fourth lumbar vertebral body, and extend a variable length (usually about 5 to 8 cm) anterolaterally until they divide into the external and internal iliac arteries (see Fig. 107–1*A*). The internal iliac (hypogastric) artery passes posteromedially into the true pelvis and supplies blood to the pelvic structures via two major trunks. The posterior division becomes the superior gluteal artery, which courses through the greater sciatic foramen to supply the musculature of the buttocks. Also arising from the posterior division are the iliolumbar, lateral sacral, and inferior gluteal arteries. The anterior division of the internal iliac artery divides into the obturator and the internal pudendal arteries.

The external iliac artery is a direct continuation of the common iliac artery and extends to the inguinal ligament. The inferior epigastric artery (supplying the anterior abdominal wall) and deep circumflex iliac artery (supplying the lateral pelvis and hip) are its major branches. The external iliac artery continues as the common femoral artery beyond the inguinal ligament. The common femoral artery then bifurcates into the superficial and deep femoral arteries (see Fig. 107–1*B*). The deep (profunda) femoral artery is the major supplier of blood to the hip and thigh region via the medial and lateral femoral circumflex arteries. The superficial femoral artery sends off multiple small muscular branches to the thigh while coursing to the popliteal fossa, where it becomes the popliteal artery. The popliteal artery begins at the distal aspect of the adductor canal (adductor hiatus) and sends off multiple geniculate branches (see Fig. 107–1*C*). Beyond the knee joint, the popliteal artery bifurcates into the anterior tibial and tibioperoneal arteries.

The anterior tibial artery runs anterolaterally along the fibula and crosses the ankle to become the dorsalis pedis artery in the foot (see Figs. 107–1*D* and 107–2). The tibioperoneal artery divides into the posterior tibial and peroneal arteries. The posterior tibial artery courses medially to supply the posterior calf and crosses the ankle, where it becomes the medial and lateral plantar arteries of the foot. The lateral plantar and dorsal pedal arteries form the plantar arch of the foot. The peroneal artery travels posterior to the interosseous membrane to the lateral malleolus.

Clinically significant anomalies of the arteries of the lower extremities are rare, although minor variations are common. In the pelvis variable levels of bifurcation of the common iliac and femoral arteries are frequent, the latter being of clinical importance because a high bifurcation close to the inguinal ligament complicates antegrade puncture of the common femoral artery. Very rarely the external iliac artery is hypoplastic, continuing into the proximal thigh as the deep femoral artery. The major supplier of blood to the lower extremity in this situation is the inferior gluteal branch of the hypogastric artery, which is a persistent umbilical artery and is referred to as the ''primitive sciatic artery.'' This artery courses through the greater sciatic notch, continues into the thigh, and eventually becomes the popliteal artery. Another unusual but clinically significant anomaly is entrapment of the popliteal artery by the medial head of the gastrocnemius muscle, resulting in transitory muscular obstruction of the artery during exercise, a surgically remedial condition. Variations in the origins of the tibial and peroneal arteries are relatively common. The most common variation of the popliteal artery is high bifurcation near or above the level of the knee joint. Occasionally, the peroneal artery arises from the anterior tibial artery.

BRACHIOCEPHALIC AND UPPER EXTREMITY ARTERIES. The thoracic aorta and proximal brachiocephalic arterial anatomy is described in Chapter 116. The subclavian artery becomes the axillary artery after it crosses the first rib and becomes the brachial artery at the distal border of the teres major muscle normally near the anterior axillary fold. The brachial artery continues to the distal forearm, where it divides into the the radial and ulnar arteries, with an interosseous branch typically arising from the proximal ulnar artery. The radial and ulnar arteries continue to the hand with considerable variation in dominance of these arteries as they form the deep and superficial palmar arches. The metacarpal and digital arteries arise from the palmar arches.

Venous Anatomy

LOWER EXTREMITIES. The veins of the calf are typically paired and accompany the tibial and peroneal arteries. Into these veins drain muscular veins, the largest of which are the soleal and gastrocnemius veins, which empty respectively into the posterior tibial and popliteal veins. The tibial veins converge just below the knee to become the popliteal vein. The short saphenous vein, which drains the superficial system of the posterior calf, empties into the popliteal vein at about the level of the knee.

At the adductor hiatus the popliteal vein becomes the *femoral* vein, both of which can be duplicated. Although the femoral vein accompanies the superficial femoral artery, it is preferable not to call it the superficial femoral vein because it is not part of the superficial system. On the other hand, the deep veins, that drain the thigh musculature are referred to as deep femoral veins and converge with the femoral vein to become the common femoral vein. The greater saphenous vein (the large superficial vein that courses up the medial lower leg and thigh) enters the common femoral vein, which in turn becomes the external iliac vein at the inguinal ligament.

The names of the pelvic veins correspond to the names of their arterial counterparts. The confluence of the common iliac veins is different in that the left iliac vein has a more horizontal course than its accompanying artery, resulting in a more obtuse angle as it enters the inferior vena cava. Significant congenital variations of the pelvic venous system are rare. Fibrous bands, probably congenital, may compress the left common iliac vein just before its confluence with the right common iliac vein. This compression is seen more commonly in females and may be associated with significant obstruction, perhaps accounting for the higher incidence of deep venous thrombosis in the left lower extremity.

Upper Extremities. Similar to the lower extremities, there are deep and superficial networks of veins in the upper extremities. In the hands there are dorsal digital and metacarpal veins, which drain laterally into the cephalic veins and medially into the basilic veins of the forearm, which are part of the superficial system. The median cubital vein connects these two superficial networks, which are larger than the deep veins. These veins eventually drain into the axillary vein. The size and dominance of these various superficial veins are extremely variable.

The deep veins of the hand, forearm, and arm are generally smaller than the superficial veins. In the hand, the superficial and deep palmar veins drain into the radial, ulnar, and interosseous veins of the forearm, which are usually paired and follow their similarly named arteries, continuing in the arm as the brachial vein. The axillary vein is the continuation of the brachial, cephalic, and basilic veins and accompanies the axillary artery. The axillary vein becomes the subclavian vein and then the innominate or brachiocephalic vein, the latter joining with the opposite brachiocephalic vein to become the superior vena cava.

RISKS OF PROCEDURE

Bleeding

The most common angiographic complication is hematoma formation at the arterial puncture site due to too high or low a puncture site, inadequate compression after catheter removal, excessive movement or Valsalva by the patient, poor wall structure, or bleeding diathesis. Fortunately, most hematomas are self-limited and resolve spontaneously, rarely requiring transfusion or operative intervention. Arterial puncture above the inguinal ligament is particularly likely to lead to hemorrhage into both the anterior abdominal wall and retroperitoneum. After compression is completed, hemostasis is still tenuous, probably because of reduced secondary soft tissue compression in this region. Puncture too low and distal to the common femoral bifurcation may lead to significant bleeding into the thigh, particularly medially. The inguinal crease is frequently not a good landmark for the inguinal ligament, especially in obese patients. If there is any question, it is advisable to guide the puncture fluoroscopically using the midfemoral head as the level of entry.

Occlusion

Loss of the pulse at the puncture site may result from vessel spasm, local intimal dissection, or thrombosis, the last possibly contributed to by excessively heavy postprocedural compression (Fig. 107–8). After catheter removal, compression should be forceful only initially and just enough to maintain hemostasis. After about one minute, compression should be reduced just enough to allow distal flow without bleeding. Spasm and intimal dissection tend to be self-limited unless thrombosis ensues. Persistent loss of the pulse with or without rest symptoms presumes thrombosis, whatever the cause, and requires intervention by surgical thrombectomy or, rarely, by selective thrombolysis. Distal embolization of thrombus or atheromatous plaque may occur during the procedure and may also require intervention, depending on the clinical severity of ischemia of the distal limb (Fig. 107–9).

Arteriovenous Fistulas

Postcatheterization arteriovenous fistulas are uncommon complications of both transfemoral and transbrachial approaches. In the former situation, fistula is associated with a low puncture below the common femoral artery. False aneurysm is also an unusual complication seen most often with larger catheters and extensive manipulation. False aneurysms of the common femoral artery may be closed nonsurgically by prolonged mechanical compression with ultrasound control.

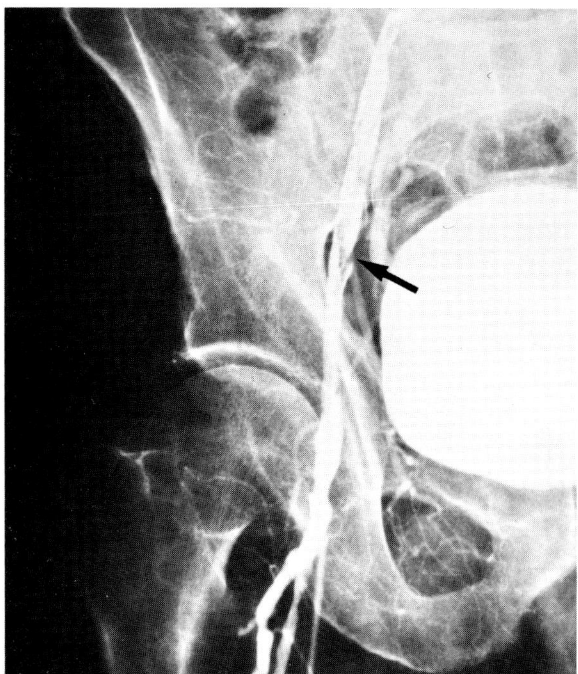

Figure 107–8. Traumatic catheter dissection of the external iliac and common femoral arteries in a patient with severe obstructive atherosclerotic disease.

Neurologic Complications

Neurologic complications due to pressure on adjacent nerves by hematoma or needle trauma may be seen with any of the approaches. They are uncommon but are most significant with transaxillary catheterization (in the range of 0.05 to 0.1 per cent). Brachial plexus injury from compression of the nerves in the axillary sheath by even a small hematoma may have disastrous results. Brachial artery catheterization in the antecubital fossa is associated with fewer and less severe neurologic complications, but since the vessel is smaller there is a higher incidence of brachial thrombosis (0.5 to 2 or 3 per cent, depending on the catheter size and amount of manipulation involved), a surgically remedial complication. High brachial artery catheterization is probably associated with fewer neurologic complications than is the axillary approach.

Any motor deficit following a transaxillary or transbrachial study requires urgent surgical incision of the neurovascular sheath to release the pressure of the hematoma, regardless of whether the hematoma is palpable. Otherwise, permanent brachial plexus injury in the distribution of the median and ulnar nerves will result with paresis and causalgia, an incapacitating condition. Paresthesias without motor deficit may be observed and will eventually resolve but sometimes require several months. Paresthesias in the lower extremities due to compression of branches of the femoral nerve in the femoral triangle can also occur, especially in the medial cutaneous nerve, resulting in numbness and pain along the medial thigh.

Toxicity of Contrast Medium

The iodinated contrast material injected to visualize the vascular system has associated risks. Formerly the most widely used agents

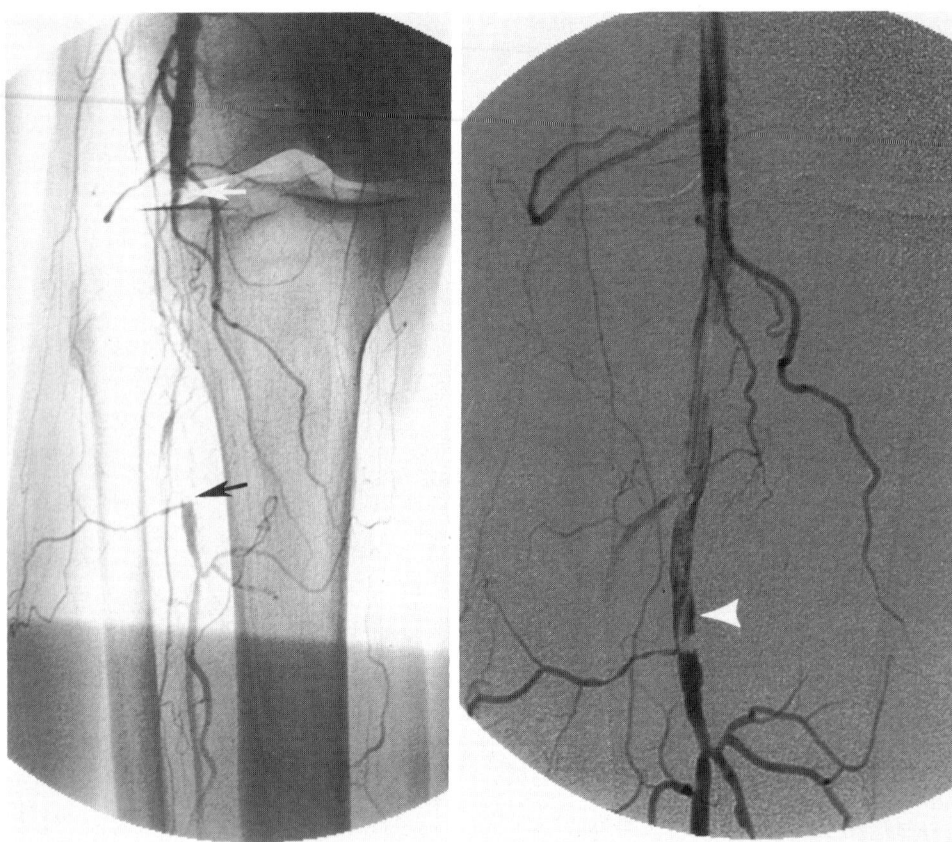

Figure 107–9. Thromboembolic complication of arteriography angiographically shown by a popliteal arteriogram. *Left,* There is total occlusion of the middle and distal popliteal artery. Note the meniscus effect at the beginning *(white arrow)* and the end *(black arrow)* of the occlusion characteristic of an occluding thrombus. *Right,* The embolic clot was treated by direct infusion of urokinase into the clot with the first follow-up study showing partial lysis. Note the wormlike filling defect *(arrowhead)* also typical of thrombus.

were sodium and meglumine salts of tri-iodobenzoic acid. The osmolality of these agents is higher than that of blood, causing a severe sensation of heat and pain. Symptoms are also related to the quantity and rapidity of the injection. Newer contrast agents with lower osmolality are associated with less sensation of heat and pain. Contrast media may induce acute renal dysfunction. They are excreted by glomerular filtration and produce a transient decrease in renal blood flow. In addition, they may cause acute renal dysfunction via a direct nephrotoxic effect even in patients without a history of renal disease. However, patients with prior renal disease, proteinuria, diabetes, and dehydration are at a higher risk for renal dysfunction. The degree of renal damage is usually relatively mild, often resolving spontaneously within several days. But it can progress to severe renal failure. The clinician and angiographer should be aware of high-risk patient groups to minimize potential problems. The examination should be tailored to decrease the amount of contrast material used. Adequate hydration via clear liquids by mouth and intravenous administration of fluids prior to angiography is the single most important factor in lowering the risk of renal insufficiency. Intravenous mannitol or furosemide infusion before and during angiography may also reduce this risk.

Contrast agents may precipitate an allergic-like reaction. Hives most commonly occur and often require no treatment. However, for relief of itching, intravenous diphenhydramine may be administered. Anaphylactoid reactions, characterized by severe periorbital edema, bronchial spasm, and hypotension, are uncommon. Immediate therapy is mandatory and entails intravenous epinephrine, steroids, and antihistamines—sometimes both H_1 (diphenhydramine) and H_2 (cimetidine) blockers are required if immediate results are not apparent. Patients with a history of serious contrast reaction should have their indications for angiography carefully evaluated. Pretreatment with steroids at least 18 hours prior to the study plus antihistamines immediately prior to the study has been found to block the recurrence of the severe reactions in a high percentage of patients.

Bibliography

Fester A, Hildner FJ: Cross sectional coronary artery stenosis. Cathet Cardiovasc Diagn 3:107–110, 1977.

Gomes AS, Baker JD, Martin-Paredero V, et al: Acute renal dysfunction following major arteriography. AJR 145:1249–1253, 1985.

Grollman JH Jr, Marcus R: Antegrade translumbar aortography. Radiology 153:249–250, 1984.

Grollman JH Jr, Marcus R, Averbook BD, Fiaschetti FL: Bilateral aortoiliac pressure measurements from a single puncture site. Cardiovasc Intervent Radiol 13:367–371, 1990.

Hessel SJ, Adams DF, Abrams HL: Complications of angiography. Radiology 138:273–281, 1981.

Johnsrude IS, Jackson PC: A Practical Approach to Angiography. Boston, Little, Brown, 1979.

Kim D, Orron DE, Skillman JJ: Surgical significance of popliteal arterial variants. A unified angiographic classification. Ann Surg 210:776–781, 1989.

Lasser EC, Berry CC, Talner LB, et al: Pretreatment with corticosteroids to alleviate reactions to intravenous contrast material. N Engl J Med 317:845–849, 1987.

May AG, Van de Berg L, DeWeese JA, Rob CG: Critical arterial stenosis. Surgery 54:250–258, 1963.

Negus D, Fletcher EWL, Cockett FB, Thomas ML: Compression and band formation at the mouth of the left common iliac vein. Br J Surg 55:369–375, 1968.

Picus D, Hicks ME, Darcy MD, Kleinhoffer MA: Comparison of nonsubtracted digital angiography and conventional screen-film angiography for the evaluation of patients with peripheral vascular disease. JVIR 2:359–364, 1991.

Sherwood T, Laverde JD: Does renal flow rise or fall in response to diatrizoate? Invest Radiol 4:327–328, 1969.

Smith DC, Mitchell DA, Peterson GW, et al: Medial brachial fascial compartment syndrome: Anatomic basis of neuropathy after transaxillary arteriography. Radiology 173:149–154, 1989.

108 Interventional Techniques for Coronary Artery Disease

Lowell F. Satler and Curtis E. Green

The last 15 years have witnessed research focused on the treatment of patients presenting with acute and chronic myocardial ischemia. As experience with medical and surgical therapy in the management of angina and acute infarction has developed, it has become apparent that improvement in morbidity and mortality requires early definition of the coronary anatomy. With coronary angiography, the pathophysiology of ischemic syndromes can be identified as being due to atherosclerosis, coronary spasm, or coronary thrombosis. After determination of the etiology of the ischemia, coronary flow can usually be improved by coronary angioplasty, thrombolytic therapy, coronary bypass surgery, or intensification of anti-ischemic pharmacologic therapy. The focus of this chapter is on the non-surgical techniques for improvement of coronary flow, that is, percutaneous transluminal coronary angioplasty (PTCA) and thrombolytic therapy, and their role in the treatment of stable and unstable angina and acute myocardial infarction.

PERCUTANEOUS TRANSLUMINAL CORONARY ANGIOPLASTY

Indications

The range of patients who may ultimately be candidates for PTCA has not yet been established. Initially, the ideal candidate was one with single-vessel coronary artery disease and a discrete, noncalcified proximal stenosis, preferably less than 1 cm in length. With recent advances in angioplasty equipment design, particularly the development of steerable systems, and newer techniques such as directional atherectomy, rotational atherectomy, and laser angioplasty, more complex lesions are amenable to the technique. Even calcified lesions, although more difficult to cross and dilate, can now be dilated. Patients now considered for PTCA include those with previous coronary artery bypass grafting, multivessel disease, sequential lesions, and totally occluded vessels.

PTCA after Coronary Bypass Surgery. Despite the well-defined merits of coronary bypass surgery, progression of disease in the native vessels or stenosis of the grafts can lead to recurrent symptoms. In some of these patients, PTCA represents a reasonable alternative to an often technically difficult and higher risk second surgical bypass procedure. Angioplasty can be performed at several different sites, including vessels not previously bypassed, lesions distal to the implanted grafts, stenoses of the body of the graft, and stenosis at the distal anastomosis (Fig. 108–1). Ostial lesions (aorta-to-vein graft anastomosis) are associated with more technical difficulty and a higher recurrence rate.

Multivessel Disease. The state of the art of coronary angioplasty now permits inclusion of many patients with multivessel (most frequently double-vessel) disease as candidates. The most significant lesion is usually dilated first, after which the procedure should be continued only if the first dilatation is successful (Fig. 108–2). Unfortunately, restenosis rates are higher with multivessel PTCA than with single-vessel PTCA.

Sequential Lesions. Multiple lesions in the same vessel can also frequently be dilated, particularly if they are relatively discrete (Fig. 108–3). If the lesions are of relatively the same severity, the most proximal one is dilated first. The more distal lesion is then approached if the first dilatation is successful.

Coronary Occlusion. Recently, experience has been gained in recanalizing chronically occluded vessels. Although recurrence rates have not been well-defined, the preliminary success rate is about 50 per cent. Clinical and angiographic considerations

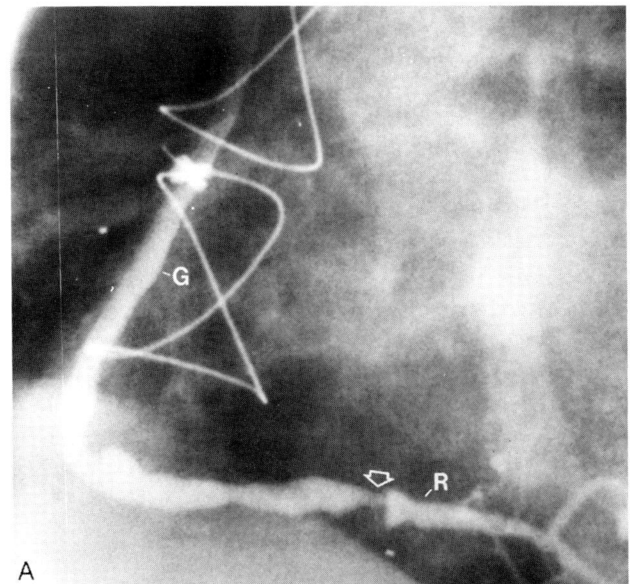

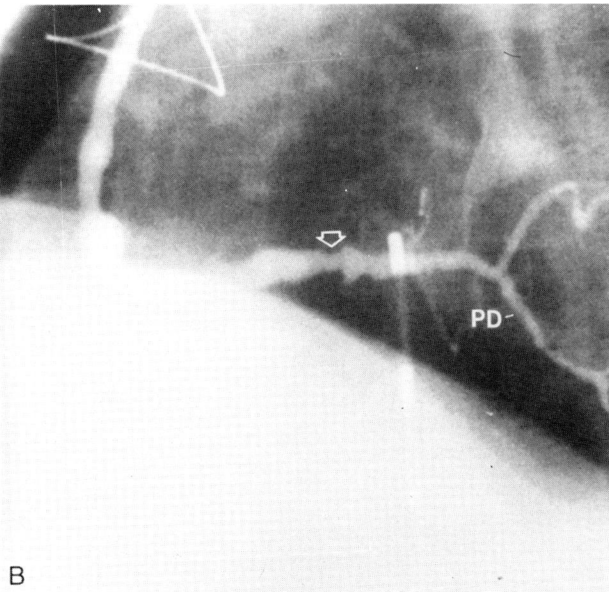

Figure 108–1. Lateral anterior oblique views before (A) and after (B) angioplasty of a stenosis at the distal anastomosis of a saphenous vein graft (G) to the distal right coronary artery (R). The degree of narrowing is reduced from approximately 75 per cent to 40 per cent (arrows). (PD = posterior descending artery.)

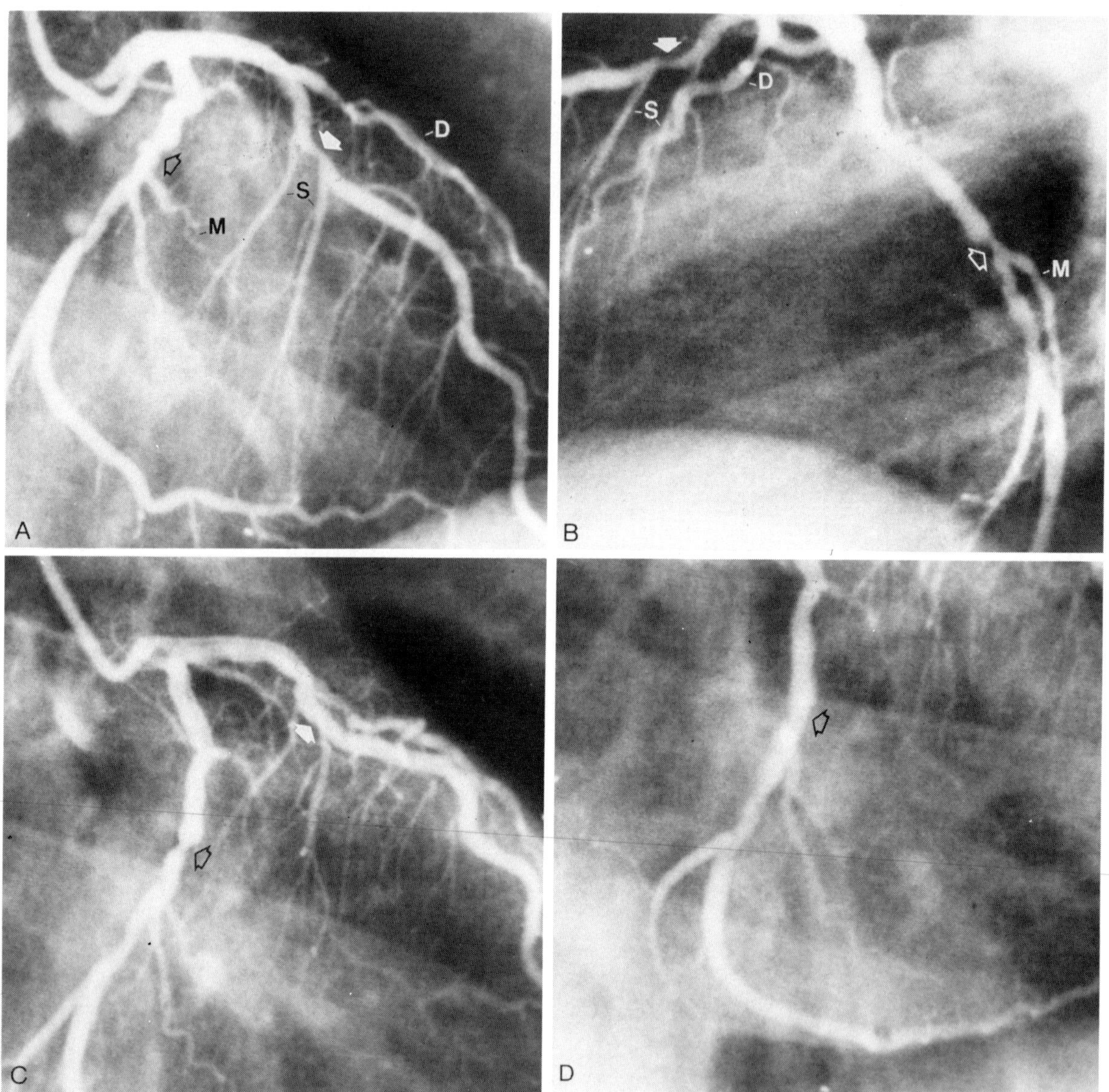

Figure 108–2. Multivessel angioplasty. *A,* Right anterior oblique view demonstrates a 60 per cent stenosis of the left anterior descending artery (LAD) (*closed arrow*) between two septal branches (S). A stenosis of the left circumflex artery (LCx) (*open arrow*) is obscured in this view owing to foreshortening. (D = first diagonal; M = second obtuse marginal.) *B,* Lateral view demonstrates both stenoses (*open and closed arrows*). *C,* After angioplasty of the LAD, there is no apparent residual narrowing (*closed arrow*). The 75 per cent stenosis of the LCx is much better seen in this caudal right anterior oblique view. *D,* Following angioplasty of the LCx, there is less than 20 per cent residual stenosis.

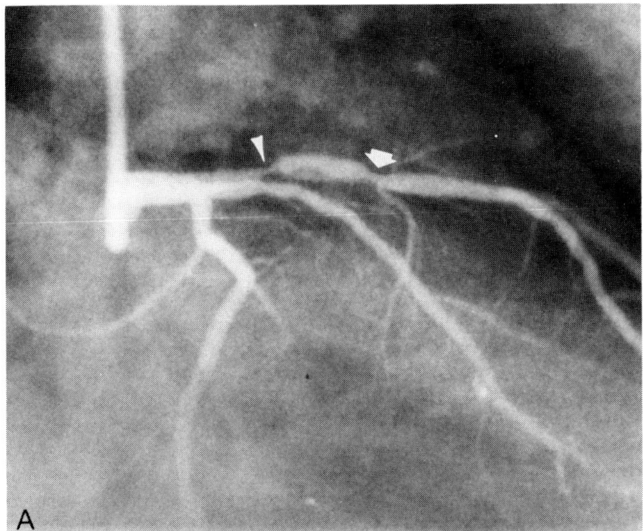

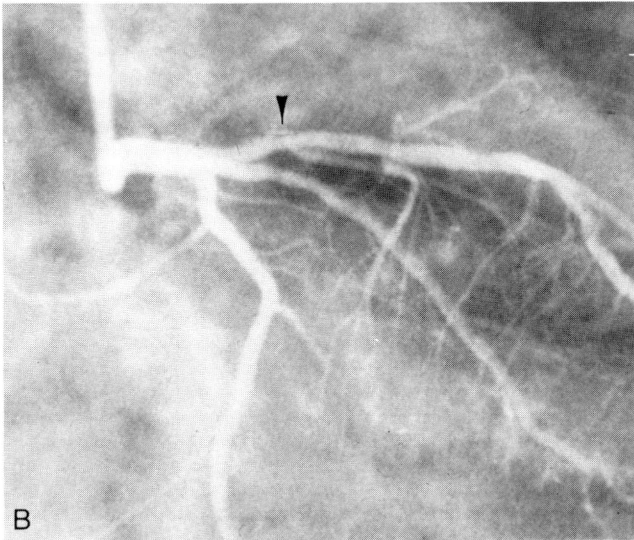

Figure 108–3. Sequential angioplasty. *A,* Right anterior oblique view of the left coronary artery shows sequential 90 per cent (*arrowhead*) and 50 per cent (*arrow*) stenoses of the proximal left anterior descending artery. *B,* After dilatation of both lesions there is less than 20 per cent narrowing of the distal lesion and 30 per cent stenosis of the proximal one. A small dissection is present at the proximal site (*arrowhead*).

for attempted recanalization of chronically occluded vessels include (1) persistent ischemic symptoms despite therapy, (2) duration of suspected occlusion less than six months, (3) viable myocardium subtended by the occluded vessel, (4) good visualization of the distal vessel, and (5) a short occluded segment (<15 mm). The presence of a funnel-shaped "entrance port" proximal to the occlusion may help to channel the guidewire into the area of the true lumen (Fig. 108–4). Laser PTCA may be of some value in total occlusions.

Contraindications

Certain types of stenoses carry an increased risk of failure or complication. Left main coronary artery stenoses represent one absolute contraindication to angioplasty, owing to the life-threatening hazard presented by the possibility of dissection and the disappointing long-term survival rates. Other sites associated with an increased risk are sharply angulated portions of a vessel and hyperkinetic segments of arteries situated in the atrioventricular groove (right coronary artery, left circumflex artery). Ostial stenoses deserve particular mention as poor sites for angioplasty, since they are characteristically resistant to dilatation and are associated with a high recurrence rate, apparently owing to the inherent resilience of the aortic wall. Finally, the angiographic appearance of the stenotic segment affects the selection process. Lesions of borderline significance should probably be avoided, since the benefit is unclear and there is risk of accelerating the disease process. Alternatively, extremely severe stenoses are associated with an increased risk of dissection, particularly if they are long and/or eccentric. If there is good collateral flow to the distal vessel, however, dilatation can be attempted with less trepidation.

Angioplasty Technique

There are several different manufacturers of angioplasty equipment. Although balloon constructions are dissimilar, allowing for different deflated profiles, peak inflation sizes are similar, ranging from 2.0 to 4.0 mm. Commonly used guidewires range from 0.010 to 0.018 inch. Various types of guidewire tip configurations are available to aid in negotiating bends in the coronary arteries.

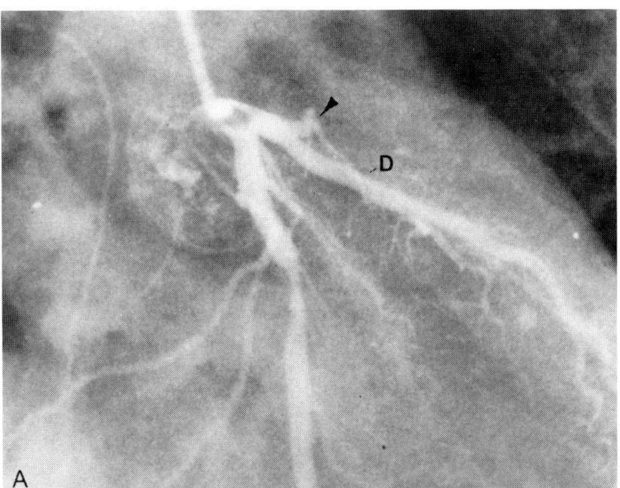

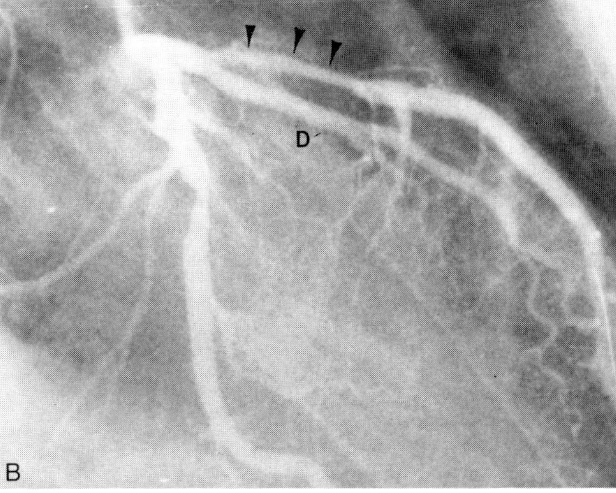

Figure 108–4. *A,* **Right anterior oblique views of the left coronary artery showing successful angioplasty of an occluded left anterior descending artery** (LAD). Before dilatation, the LAD is occluded (*arrowhead*) just after the first diagonal (D). The mid and distal LAD was visualized by collaterals from the right coronary artery. *B,* After angioplasty there is recanalization of the LAD with a long, residual 40 per cent stenosis (*arrowheads*).

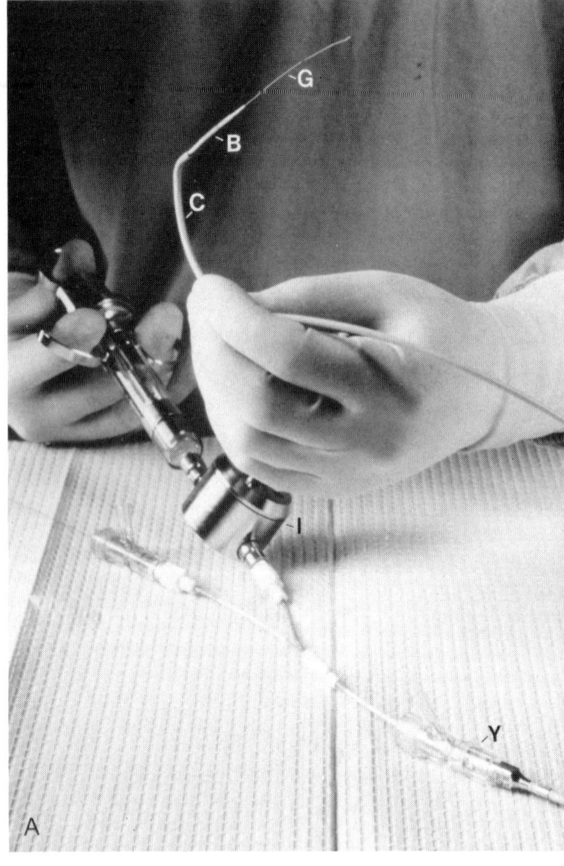

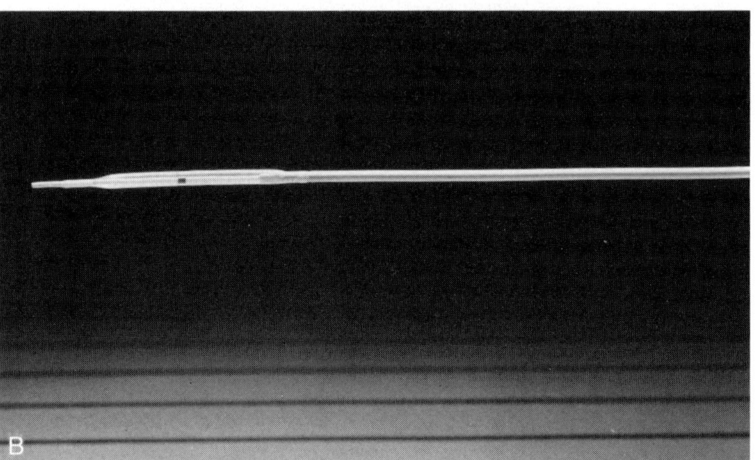

Figure 108–5. Typical coronary angioplasty system. *A*, The major components are the guidewire (G), balloon catheter (B), guiding catheter (C), Y connector (Y), and inflation device (I). *B*, Close-up of a coronary angioplasty catheter with balloon deflated.

The equipment used in a typical system is shown in Figure 108–5. The essential components are the guiding catheter, angioplasty balloon catheter, guidewire, Y-connector allowing for balloon entry and simultaneous pressure monitoring, and manifold. In addition, a torquing control is usually present at the end of the guidewire, to aid in manipulation of the flexible wire.

Prior to angiography, patients are usually premedicated with a calcium channel blocker and withdrawn from beta-blockers. Initial angiograms can be taken with a guiding catheter, but because it tends to be less flexible, angiography is probably more safely obtained with a standard angiographic catheter. For the right coronary artery (RCA), several views are completed, with a final guiding picture in the 30-degree left anterior oblique (LAO) view. If the stenosis is overlying the diaphragm, slight caudal angulation usually depresses the diaphragm sufficiently to allow for better visualization of the distal RCA. For the left coronary artery (LCA), standard views are usually obtained, with a final view of the left system obtained in the 30-degree right anterior oblique (RAO) view. If the lesion is in the proximal left circumflex (LCx) artery, caudal angulation may allow better visualization of the stenosis. It is useful to record the optimal LAO and RAO views on a video recorder or digital subtraction system. These "fixed" images may be used to assist the angiographer in properly positioning the balloon catheter prior to dilatation.

After the angiograms are obtained, the guiding catheter is placed in the coronary ostium, and the guidewire and balloon are placed into the guiding catheter and advanced to the top of the aortic arch. The balloon is left near the top of the arch while the guiding wire is advanced into the coronary ostium. The guidewire is then slowly advanced down the coronary artery. For the RCA, this can generally be accomplished using only the 30-degree LAO view (Fig. 108–6*A*). In the LCA, biplane fluoroscopy is extremely helpful in negotiating the proximal left anterior descending (LAD) and LCx. In addition, in the RAO view it may be difficult to determine whether the wire is in the LAD, a diagonal, or a ramus medianus branch. A shallow cranial LAO view (30-degree cranial, 30-degree LAO) will usually show whether the guidewire is in the LAD, a diagonal, or a septal branch. Reference may also be made to "fixed" video or digital subtraction images to check guidewire location within the coronary system.

The guidewire is then carefully negotiated through the stenosis and as far out into the distal vessel as possible (Fig. 108–6*B*). This stabilizes the dilatation system and allows more pressure to be applied to push the balloon through the stenosis without disengaging the guiding catheter. Once this has been achieved and the balloon is maximally deflated with a mechanical inflation-deflation device (see Fig. 108–5*A*), it is slowly advanced over the guidewire and manipulated carefully through the stenosis. Test injections of contrast material are used to demonstrate proper balloon placement. After measurement of the trans-stenotic gradient, the balloon is inflated to 2 atmospheres of pressure. Indentation of the balloon at this stage indicates that proper orientation of the balloon in relation to the plaque has been achieved (Fig. 108–6*C*). Pressures are increased as necessary to a maximum of 10 to 12 atmospheres if indentation is present at the lower pressure. The balloon is then inflated to at least 1 to 2 atmospheres above the indentation point (Fig. 108–6*D*). Inflation is maintained for an average of 60 to 180 seconds or until the development of chest pain. This procedure may be repeated up to three times, with the last inflation being slightly less than that required for peak inflation. Multiple inflations are thought to be important for molding of the plaque to help ensure long-term patency. After the inflations are completed, the balloon is pulled back, with the wire left in place, and repeat angiography is performed to determine whether any significant irregularity or dissection is present, in which case the balloon is placed again across the stenosis and inflated several more times to lessen the chance of

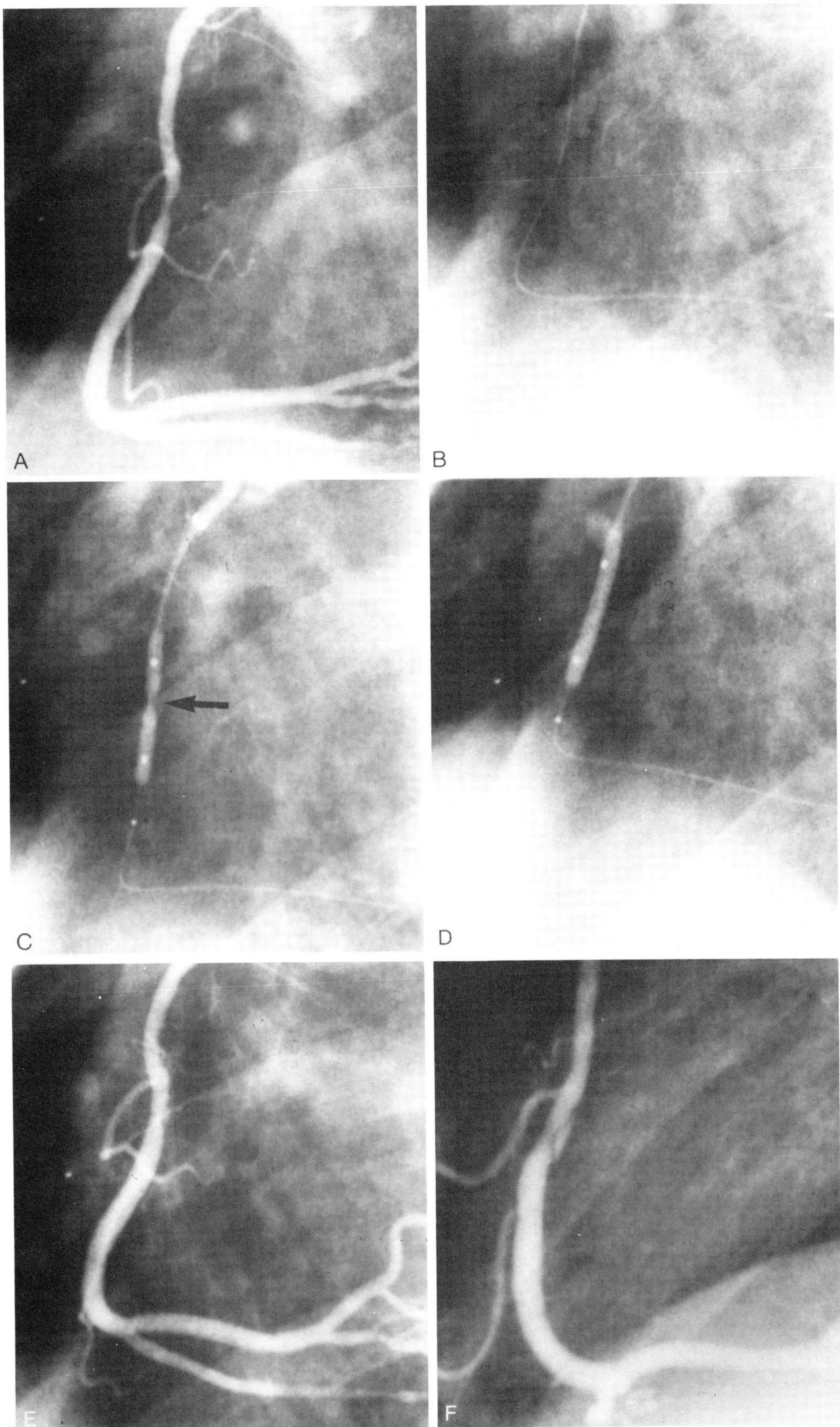

Figure 108–6. *A*, **Left anterior oblique view of the right coronary artery before, during, and after angioplasty** of a 70 per cent stenosis of the mid-portion of the vessel. Although the vessel proximal to the anastomosis is narrowed, the lesion appears fairly discrete. *B*, The guidewire has been placed far out into the posterior descending artery. *C*, Initial inflation shows indentation of the balloon (*arrow*). *D*, On a later inflation at high pressure there is no indentation. *E*, Following angioplasty there is 40 per cent stenosis with a small dissection of the medial wall. *F*, Lateral view shows the dissection to be somewhat larger than suspected on the left anterior oblique.

reocclusion of the vessel. After adequate vessel patency has been established, the balloon and wire are removed and final angiographic pictures are obtained (Fig. 108–6*E* and *F*). Perfusion balloons, which allow blood to flow to the distal vessel, can be used for prolonged inflations when dissection compromises the lumen.

Radiographic Findings

Following successful dilatation, a variety of angiographic findings can be seen. Most commonly, haziness is seen in the area of the dilatation, resulting from fracturing of the plaque. This results in a considerable amount of absorption unsharpness, which often makes delineation of the edges of the vessel difficult. As with any coronary artery stenosis, it is important to obtain more than one view of the dilatation site, since, just as with any stenotic lesion, the residual stenosis may be eccentric. Small dissections are very common and are usually of no significance (see Figs. 108–3*B* and 108–6*E* and *F*). Sometimes, marked dissection is present which may resolve with time; however, if patency of the vessel is compromised, emergency coronary bypass may be required even in the absence of complete occlusion. Dissection can also occur distal to the dilatation site. This is usually caused by the tip of the guidewire. One should also pay close attention to the status of large branch vessels near the dilatation site. These may become occluded during dilatation and result in ischemia or infarction. If unsuccessful, angioplasty can result in either no visible change in the angiographic appearance of the stenosis, a more severe stenosis, or occlusion. The hemodynamic effects of occlusion depend to a large extent on the adequacy of collateral blood flow to the occluded vessel (Fig. 108–7).

Postangioplasty Care

The major function of postangioplasty care is to monitor the patient for ischemia. Upon the patient's arrival in the coronary care unit, a 12-lead electrocardiogram is obtained and blood is drawn for determination of creatinine phosphokinase level, after which telemetry is begun. Routine medications in the immediate postangioplasty period include 75 mg aspirin per day, dipyridamole 75 mg tid, and calcium channel blockers. The patient is generally allowed to ambulate at will the morning after the procedure and usually undergoes an exercise test prior to discharge. If there is a significant dissection, heparin is continued overnight.

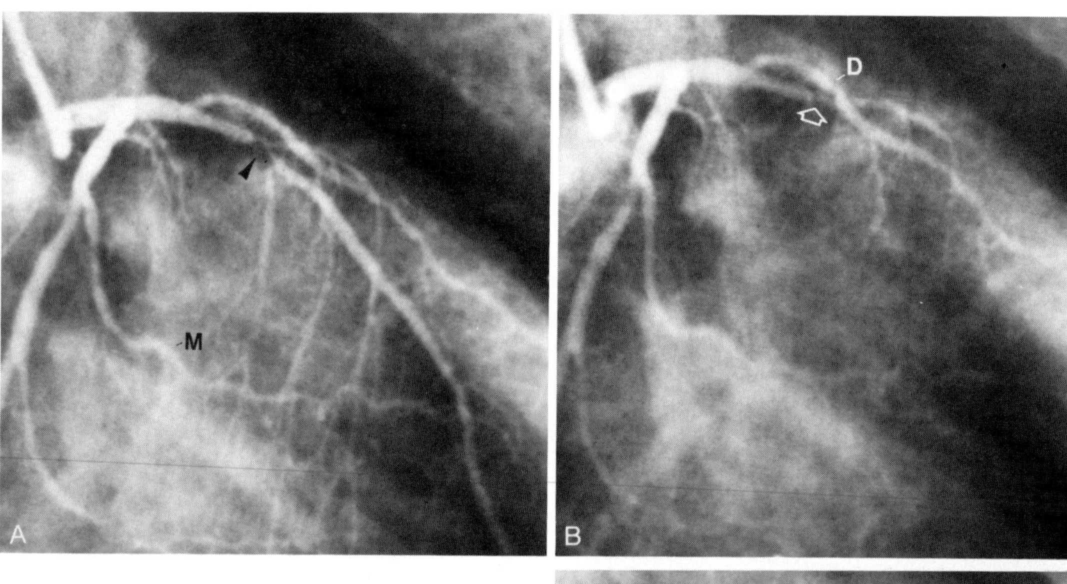

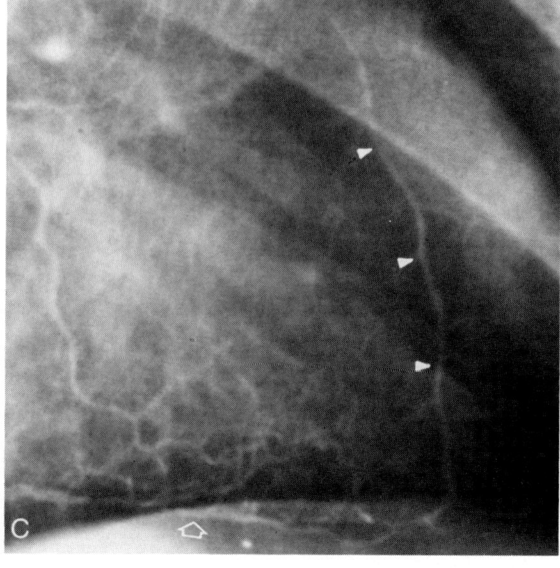

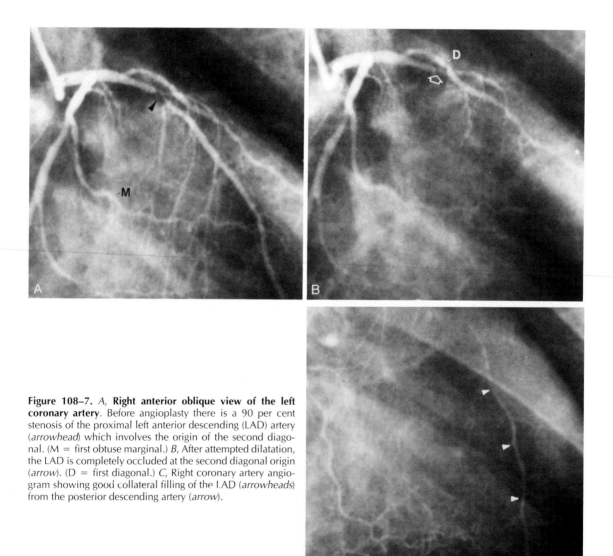

Figure 108–7. *A*, **Right anterior oblique view of the left coronary artery**. Before angioplasty there is a 90 per cent stenosis of the proximal left anterior descending (LAD) artery (*arrowhead*) which involves the origin of the second diagonal. (M = first obtuse marginal.) *B*, After attempted dilatation, the LAD is completely occluded at the second diagonal origin (*arrow*). (D = first diagonal.) *C*, Right coronary artery angiogram showing good collateral filling of the LAD (*arrowheads*) from the posterior descending artery (*arrow*).

Complications

In terms of likelihood and clinical impact, the most common major complication of coronary dilatation is an acute reduction of regional coronary flow. This occurs in approximately 3 per cent of patients. It can often be treated with the placement of a metallic coronary stent. If stent placement is not possible, coronary bypass surgery is recommended. Overall mortality is 1 per cent or less.

Results and Long-Term Follow-up

Since coronary dilatation was first performed in 1977, it has been shown that the majority of individuals maintain angiographic and clinical improvement. Some patients will, however, develop restenosis. Clinical manifestations of restenosis usually occur within the first six months after the procedure, most often as recurrent angina. Infarction seems to be an uncommon presentation of recurrent stenosis. Initially, angiography was performed routinely in these patients at six months. Now it is recognized that restenosis is usually heralded either by the development of chest pain or by an abnormal exercise stress test. Should either of these be present, repeat angiography with possible angioplasty is then planned. In patients with recurrent chest pain, it has been found that approximately two thirds will have evidence of recurrent stenosis. In the remainder, angiography demonstrates either progression of disease in another vessel or a different part of the same vessel, or a widely patent dilated lesion (possibly indicating coronary spasm or noncardiac chest pain).

THROMBOLYTIC THERAPY

Initial efforts at coronary thrombolysis involved intracoronary administration of a thrombolytic agent, usually streptokinase (Fig. 108–8). There was an obligatory time delay in getting the agent to the patient because of the necessity for cardiac catheterization. As a

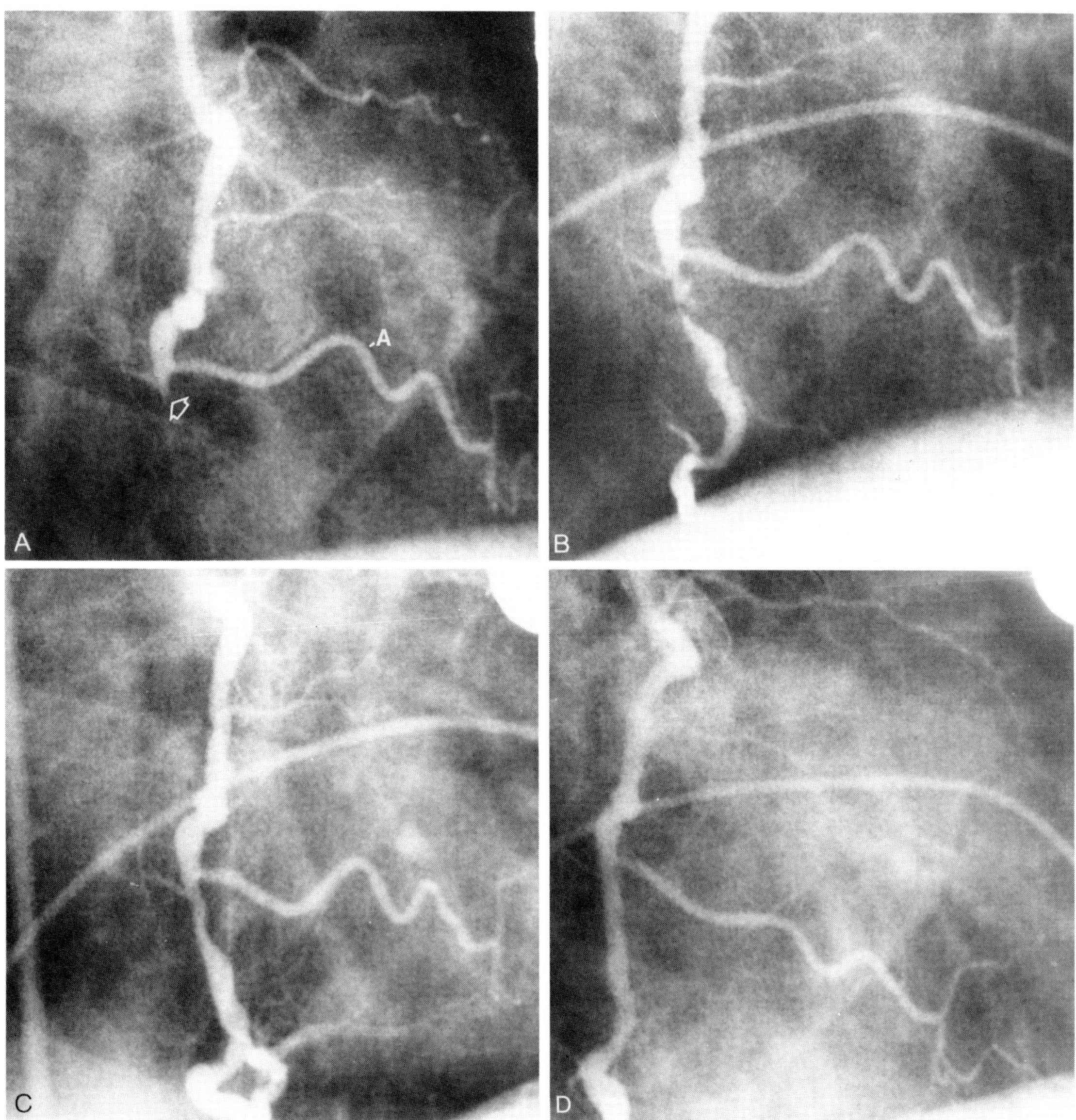

Figure 108–8. *A*, **Right anterior oblique view of the right coronary artery** (RCA) in a patient with acute myocardial infarction. The distal RCA is occluded (*arrow*) just distal to a large acute marginal branch (A). *B*, After intracoronary administration of 100,000 units of streptokinase, there is reperfusion. *C*, A residual 70 per cent stenosis is present after 250,000 units. *D*, Angioplasty resulted in no apparent residual stenosis. Note the haziness of the border of the vessel.

result, intravenous therapy has become the standard and has been shown to reduce mortality from acute myocardial infarction. Benefit appears to be greatest if therapy is begun within 6 hours after the onset of pain, but may be effective up to 24 hours after onset in patients with so-called stuttering infarction. Currently used agents include streptokinase, tissue plasminogen activator (tPA), urokinase, and an isolated plasminogen–streptokinase activator complex. In a recent randomized trial (GUSTO), tPA appeared superior to streptokinase.

When the lytic agent is unsuccessful or if there is a contraindication to thrombolysis, emergency angioplasty offers an immediate means of mechanical revascularization to salvage myocardium.

NEW CORONARY DEVICES

Standard PTCA has certain limitations in addressing specific anatomic, pathologic, and clinical problems, including total coronary occlusions, intracoronary thrombi, diffuse disease, ostial disease, large proximal lesions, saphenous vein graft disease, restenotic lesions, eccentric lesions, heavily calcified lesions, and nondilatable fibrotic lesions. A variety of new transcatheter techniques have been developed to address these limitations of angioplasty and to permit safer, more successful revascularization.

The introduction of coronary laser angioplasty using a pulsed 308-nm excimer source with variously sized over-the-wire multiple fiber catheters allows ablation of approximately 50 μm of atherosclerotic plaque per pulse (1 mm per second) with minimal thermal effects. Anatomic lesions most amenable to this technique include diffuse disease and total occlusions.

Directional atherectomy utilizes a catheter with a side window and a rotating cutter cup. An inflatable balloon pressures the side window against the plaque, and the cutter is driven by a motor at 2000 rpm. As the rotating blade is advanced manually, atheromatous material is shaved, collected, and then stored in the distal nose cone. Rotating the catheter permits directional repositioning, allowing removal of the core of plaque in multiple directions. This technique appears most effective in ablating large, proximal (including ostial and/or eccentric) lesions in native vessels. It has also been used to salvage an unsuccessful or uncomplicated balloon angioplasty by removing a focal, occlusive coronary dissection flap.

Rotational atherectomy employs a high-speed (180,000 rpm), rotating, over-the-wire, granular diamond-chipped burr to pulverize plaque into microparticles. These particles are usually less than 5 to 10 μm in size and pass innocuously through the coronary microcirculation. This system is most effective in treating patients with heavily calcified lesions, nondilatable fibrotic lesions, restenotic lesions, ostial lesions, and lesions in tortuous vessels.

Finally, the deployment of metallic intracoronary stents, which exert a scaffolding force to tack down intimal flaps and prevent elastic recoil, can optimize coronary arterial lumen patency and potentially improve suboptimal angioplasty results. Preliminary data regarding the efficacy of stents in enhancing the results of vein graft angioplasty have been encouraging.

Bibliography

Anderson JL, Marshall HW, Bray BE, et al: A randomized trial of intracoronary streptokinase in the treatment of acute myocardial infarction. N Engl J Med 308:1312–1318, 1983.

Braunwald E, Kloner RA: The stunned myocardium: Prolonged, postischemic ventricular dysfunction. Circulation 66:1146–1149, 1982.

Campeau L, Enjalbert M, Lesperance J, et al: The relation of risk factors to the development of atherosclerosis in saphenous-vein bypass grafts and the progression of disease in the native circulation. A study 10 years after aortocoronary bypass surgery. N Engl J Med 211:1329–1332, 1984.

DeWood MA, Spores J, Notske MD, et al: Prevalence of total coronary occlusion during the early hours of transmural myocardial infarction. N Engl J Med 303:897–902, 1980.

Dorros G, Cowley MJ, Simpson J, et al: Percutaneous transluminal coronary angioplasty: Report of complications from the National Heart, Lung and Blood Institute PTCA Registry. Circulation 67:723–730, 1983.

Dorros G, Johnson WD, Tector AJ, et al: Percutaneous transluminal coronary angioplasty in patients with prior coronary artery bypass grafting. J Thorac Cardiovasc Surg 87:17–26, 1984.

Dorros G, Stertzer SH, Cowley MJ, Myler RK: Complex coronary angioplasty: Multiple coronary dilatations. Am J Cardiol 53:126C–130C, 1984.

Gruentzig AR, Meier B: Current status of dilation catheters and guiding systems. Am J Cardiol 53:92C, 1984.

The GUSTO Investigators: An international randomized trial comparing four thrombolytic strategies for acute myocardial infarction. N Engl J Med 329:673–682, 1993.

Hall DP, Gruentzig AR: Percutaneous transluminal coronary angioplasty. Current procedure and future directions. AJR 142:13, 1984.

Hartzler GO, Rutherford BD, McConahay DR, et al: PTCA: Application for AMI. Am J Cardiol 53:117C, 1984.

Holmes DR, Vliestra RE, Mock MB, et al: Angiographic changes produced by percutaneous transluminal coronary angioplasty. Am J Cardiol 51:673–683, 1983.

Holmes DR, Vliestra RE, Reeder GS, et al: Angioplasty in total coronary occlusion. J Am Coll Cardiol 3:845–849, 1984.

Ischinger T, Gruentzig AR, Hollman J, et al: Should coronary arteries with less than 60% diameter stenosis be treated by angioplasty? Circulation 68:149–154, 1983.

Kennedy JW, Ritchie JL, Davis KB, Fritz JK: Western Washington randomized trial of intracoronary streptokinase in acute myocardial infarction. N Engl J Med 309:1477–1482, 1983.

Kennedy JW, Ritchie JL, Davis KB, et al: The Western Washington randomized trial of intracoronary streptokinase in acute myocardial infarction. A 12 month follow-up report. N Engl J Med 312:1073–1078, 1985.

Kent KM, Bentivoglio LG, Block PC, et al: Percutaneous transluminal coronary angioplasty: Report from the Registry of the National Heart, Lung and Blood Institute. Am J Cardiol 49:2011–2019, 1982.

Kereiakes DJ, Selmon MR, McAuley BJ, et al: Angioplasty in total coronary occlusion: Experience in 76 consecutive patients. J Am Coll Cardiol 6:526–533, 1985.

Khaja F, Walton JA, Brymer JF, et al: Intracoronary fibrinolytic therapy in acute myocardial infarction. Report of a prospective randomized trial. N Engl J Med 308:1305–1314, 1983.

Laffel GL, Braunwald E: Thrombolytic therapy. A new strategy for the treatment of acute myocardial infarction. N Engl J Med 311:710–716, 1984.

Leiboff RH, Katz RJ, Wasserman AG, et al: A randomized, angiographically controlled trial of intracoronary streptokinase in acute myocardial infarction. Am J Cardiol 53:404–407, 1984.

Levine S, Ewels CJ, Rosing DR, Kent KM: Coronary angioplasty: Clinical and angiographic follow-up. Am J Cardiol 55:673–678, 1985.

Satler LF, Levine S, Kent KM, et al: Aortic dissection masquerading as acute myocardial infarction: Implication for thrombolytic therapy without cardiac catheterization. Am J Cardiol 54:1134–1135, 1984.

Thornton MA, Gruentzig AR, Hollman J, et al: Coumadin and aspirin in the prevention of recurrence after transluminal coronary angioplasty. Circulation 69:721–727, 1984.

109 Vascular Interventional Techniques in the Abdominal Aorta and Its Pelvic and Peripheral Branches

Michael J. Kelley, Arl Van Moore, and Mark H. LeQuire

In considering vascular interventional techniques for diseases affecting the abdominal aorta and its pelvic and peripheral branches, one is dealing primarily with three disease states: acute and chronic peripheral arterial disease, trauma to the abdominal aorta and its pelvic and peripheral arterial branches, and acquired and congenital arteriovenous malformations.

This chapter discusses the use of certain accepted methods of vascular intervention as applied to these disease states. After presenting an overview of arteriosclerotic peripheral vascular disease, we focus on three therapeutic modalities: (1) angioplasty, atherectomy, and intravascular stents; (2) thrombolytic therapy; and (3) embolotherapy.

ATHEROSCLEROTIC PERIPHERAL VASCULAR DISEASE

The Abdominal Aorta

Abdominal aortic aneurysms, the vast majority of which are atherosclerotic in origin and distal to the renal arteries, are presently treated by surgical means. Percutaneously placed endovascular stents appear to be a promising alternative to surgical grafting, especially in patients with abdominal aortic dissection. The role of stents in this setting awaits controlled, randomized trials comparing stents with surgery.

Peripheral Arterial Disease

When considering interventional therapy for the management of peripheral arterial disease, one should be familiar with the prevalence of peripheral arterial disease, its clinical presentation, and possible differential diagnoses.

Several studies have determined the approximate prevalence of intermittent claudication: 1.8 per cent in patients younger than 60 years; 3.7 per cent in patients 60 to 70 years; and 5.2 per cent in patients older than 70 years. Approximately two thirds of patients older than 40 years have femoropopliteal disease. More than half of patients younger than 40 years have isolated aortoiliac disease. Intermittent claudication is five times more prevalent in diabetics than in nondiabetics.

On the basis of symptoms at presentation, approximately 75 per cent of patients with peripheral arterial disease present with intermittent claudication, whereas 25 per cent present with a threatened limb (ischemic ulcer, rest pain, or gangrene).

Certain differential diagnoses should be considered in patients with possible peripheral arterial disease. These include spinal stenosis, osteoarthritis, neuritis, and gout. True rest pain should be associated with specific physical signs, including atrophy and coolness as well as color changes in the dependent extremity.

Noninvasive Vascular Laboratory

The noninvasive vascular laboratory is invaluable in screening patients with suspected peripheral arterial disease. One study reported that 44 per cent of positive histories for peripheral arterial disease were false-positive and 19 per cent were false-negative. At minimum, these laboratories should include Doppler waveforms of the common femoral arteries, segmental Doppler limb pressures, and bilateral segmental pulse volume recordings (Fig. 109–1). Repeat ankle pressures should be obtained after exercise or hyperemic stress. Color flow Doppler imaging may also be helpful, often confirming suspected occlusions or stenoses (see Fig. 109–1). The

TABLE 109–1. CRITERIA FOR CATEGORIZING PATIENTS WITH CHRONIC LOWER EXTREMITY ISCHEMIA

Grade	Category	Description	Objective Criteria
0		Asymptomatic	Normal treadmill or stress test
I	1	Mild	Patient completes treadmill; post-exercise ankle pressure > 50 mm Hg but > 25 mm Hg below normal
	2	Moderate IC	Between categories 1 and 3
	3	Severe IC	Patient cannot complete treadmill; post-exercise ankle pressure < 50 mm Hg
II	4	Rest pain	Resting ankle pressure ≤ 40 mm Hg; toe pressure ≤ 30 mm Hg; PVR flat or barely pulsatile
III	5	Minor tissue loss—nonhealing ulcer, focal gangrene	Ankle pressure ≤ 60 mm Hg; ankle or metatarsal PVR flat or barely pulsatile
	6	Major tissue loss—extending above tarsal-metatarsal level, functional foot no longer salvageable	Same as category 5

IC = intermittent claudication; PVR = pulse volume recordings.

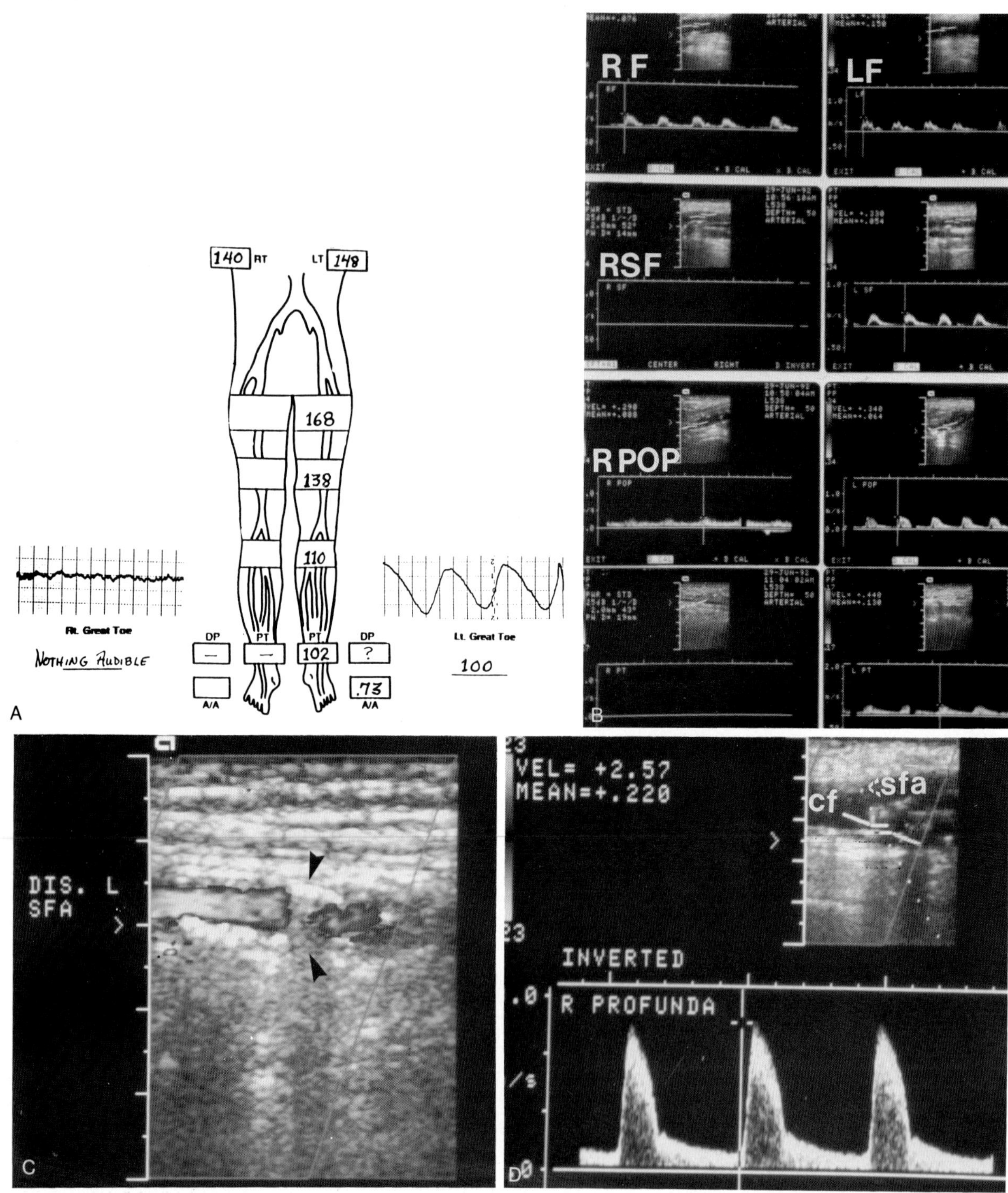

Figure 109–1. Noninvasive lower extremity Doppler arterial evaluation in a man with severe right leg claudication. *A,* Segmental Doppler leg pressures demonstrate a 58-mm gradient between the left thigh and left knee (168 minus 110) and no recordable pressures in the right leg or right great toe. The left ankle arm index (A/A) is reduced at .73. *B,* Doppler velocity waveforms reveal bilateral common femoral (RF and LF) flow with relatively low velocity. Although there is no flow recorded in the right superficial femoral (RSF), low amplitude right popliteal (RPOP) arterial flow is recorded. *C,* Color-flow Doppler recording of the distal left superficial femoral artery (DIS.L SFA) reveals turbulence and a calcified plaque (*arrowheads*). *D,* Color-flow Doppler recording of the right common femoral artery (cf) shows occlusion of the proximal superficial femoral artery (*arrowhead,* sfa) with vigorous Doppler flow in the right profunda femoris artery (R PROFUNDA). (See Fig. 109–2 for angiographic correlation.)

noninvasive vascular laboratory is essential for planning diagnostic and therapeutic procedures; for assessing pre- and post-therapeutic results; and for conducting long-term follow-up of patients who have undergone vascular interventional therapy.

Staging and Prognosis in Peripheral Arterial Disease

Table 109–1 presents criteria that have been accepted by both vascular surgeons and interventional radiologists for categorizing patients with chronic lower extremity ischemia. A summary by Hertzer of several long-term follow-up studies of approximately 6000 patients with intermittent claudication included several important findings. First, the stability of claudication versus progressive claudication was not a good predictor of an individual's likelihood of developing severe ischemia. Both groups had a 21 to 27 per cent likelihood of such deterioration. Second, the amputation rate in a follow-up period greater than five years was approximately 6 per cent for all patients with peripheral arterial disease. The amputation rate for smokers was 11 per cent, and that for diabetics was 21 per cent. A third observation was that the risk of acute, severe deterioration was less in patients with aortoiliac disease (14 per cent) but greater in smokers (31 per cent) and diabetics (35 per cent).

If one considers all patients with lower extremity ischemia, the five-year mortality rate is 30 per cent. Most deaths are due to coronary artery disease. Such deaths are twice as likely in male claudicants than they are in the general male population. The rate of coronary deaths in female claudicants is five times that in the general female population. Correction of underlying coronary artery disease can improve survival in patients with peripheral arterial disease. Since coronary comorbidity is such an important factor in determining survival in these individuals, it is recommended that patients being considered for therapy of peripheral vascular disease have their coronary artery status assessed with a history, a physical examination, an electrocardiogram (EKG), and noninvasive testing.

VASCULAR INTERVENTION FOR CHRONIC PERIPHERAL ARTERIAL DISEASE

Arteriographic/Hemodynamic Work-up

Once the clinical diagnosis of peripheral arterial disease is made, arteriography is reserved for patients in whom percutaneous or surgical intervention is contemplated. Arteriography, then, is performed primarily for preoperative or preinterventional staging rather than for diagnosis. It should be used to define the anatomy; evaluate the severity and extent of disease; assess collateral flow and patency of distal vessels; and identify unsuspected lesions such as emboli, aneurysms, or dissections. High-quality arteriography of the abdominal aorta, iliac arteries, femoral arteries, and peripheral arteries to the feet is required (Fig. 109–2).

The hemodynamic significance of an arterial stenosis should be correlated with the patient's symptomatology, the degree of stenosis as a percentage of the normal luminal diameter, and the pressure gradient across the lesion (Fig. 109–3). The arterial diameter ($2r$) must be decreased by 50 per cent to produce the 75 per cent decrease in a cross-sectional area (πr^2) of the lumen necessary to significantly reduce blood flow. A pressure gradient of 20 mm Hg or greater at rest across a stenosis indicates a significant lesion. Hyperemia, induced by the administration of 30 mg of papaverine intra-arterially to simulate physical exertion, may uncover a significant gradient across a stenosis. Pressures should also be obtained across multiple subcritical stenoses in series. The presence of collateral vessels around a stenosis offers indirect information on its hemodynamic significance. Once the hemodynamic severity of a lesion is determined, a decision regarding appropriate surgical or nonsurgical management can be made.

Treatment Choices for Peripheral Arterial Disease

The treatment of chronic peripheral arterial disease depends on the level and extent of disease. Treatment options for aortoiliac disease include angioplasty and surgery. Focal stenoses or short (<3 cm) occlusions are treated with angioplasty, whereas long stenoses or occlusions are usually considered surgical, unless the patient is not a surgical candidate. Surgical inflow procedures include aortic bifurcation grafts (aortobi-iliac and aortobifemoral), axillofemoral grafts, and femoral-femoral grafts. If both inflow and outflow disease exists, consideration is given to correction of inflow first. The patient may then be followed to determine whether outflow repair is also needed.

Femoropopliteal and/or tibial peroneal occlusive disease carries a less favorable outcome than aortofemoral disease. Angioplasty of focal stenoses or short (<4 cm) segment occlusions is a consideration. Long segment occlusions or severe diffuse lesions do not respond well, and surgical grafting is usually the treatment of choice. Autologous saphenous vein graft is the material of choice because synthetic grafts such as Gore-Tex have poorer patency rates.

Percutaneous Transluminal Angioplasty

The primary pathophysiologic event that occurs during percutaneous transluminal angioplasty (PTA) has been described as a "controlled vessel injury." As the balloon expands, there is rupture of the atherosclerotic arterial intima and separation (dehiscence) from the media. This intima-media dehiscence is seen as an extraluminal collection of contrast on post-PTA angiograms (see Fig. 109–3). The media then stretches and is kept distended by the blood pressure. This fracture and separation of the atheromatous intima allow the media to distend and increase the luminal diameter. This explains the continued improvement in vessel diameter seen on follow-up angiograms after PTA. Within 24 hours of dilatation, medial architecture degenerates, macrophages clear away the debris, and fibroblasts proliferate to repair the "damaged" artery. This repair process takes four to six weeks.

INDICATIONS FOR ANGIOPLASTY IN PERIPHERAL ARTERIAL DISEASE

The indications for PTA are similar to those for surgery and thus should be limited to symptomatic patients. The following are the generally accepted indications for PTA:

1. All anatomically and hemodynamically significant lesions that produce intermittent claudication adversely affecting the patient's lifestyle.*
2. Rest pain.
3. Ischemic ulceration or poor wound healing.
4. Impending or overt gangrene.

PTA may be considered as an adjunct to surgery in the following situations:

*Note that patients at high risk for surgery because of age or other health problems are not excluded as candidates for PTA.

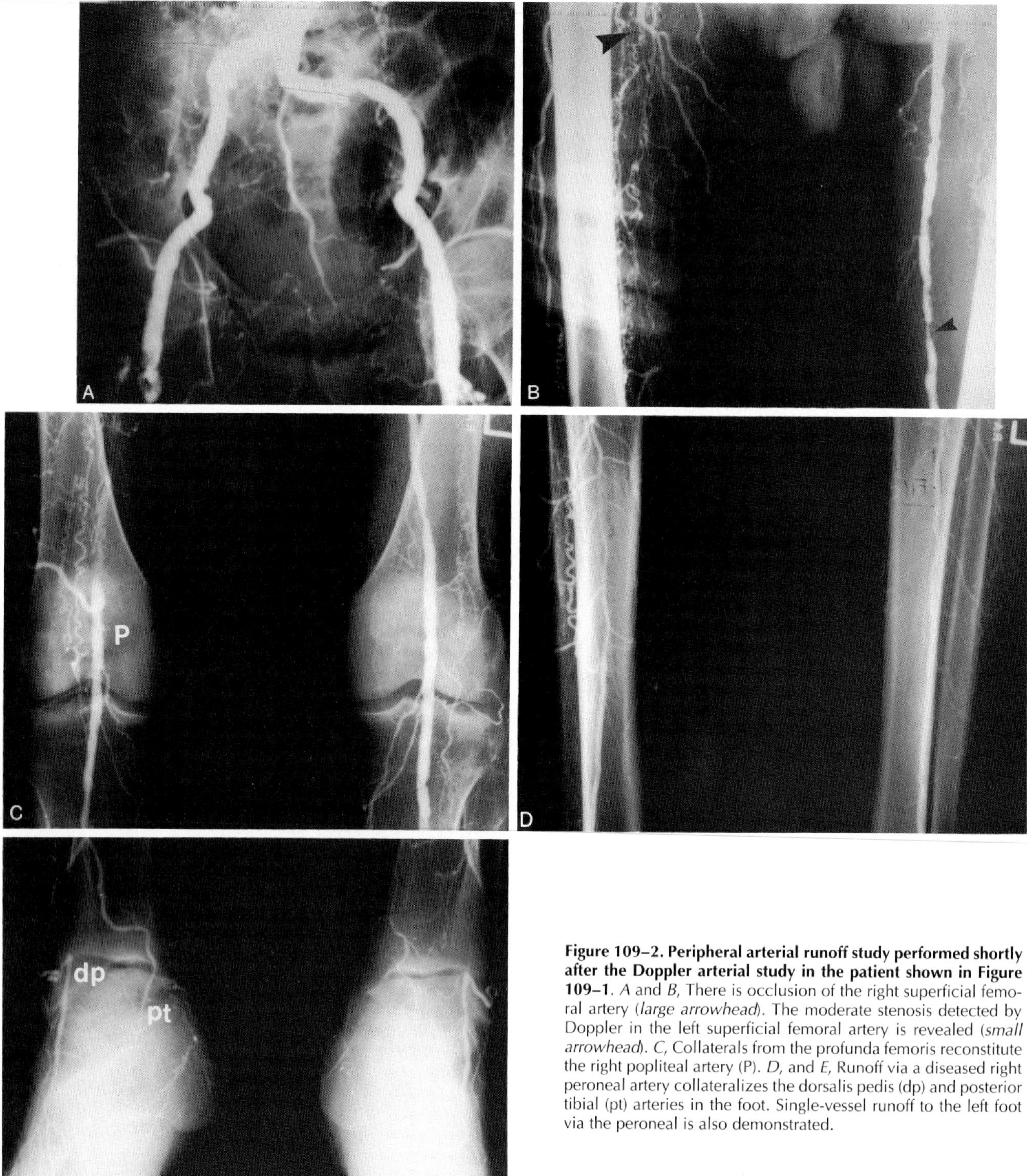

Figure 109–2. Peripheral arterial runoff study performed shortly after the Doppler arterial study in the patient shown in Figure 109–1. *A* and *B*, There is occlusion of the right superficial femoral artery (*large arrowhead*). The moderate stenosis detected by Doppler in the left superficial femoral artery is revealed (*small arrowhead*). *C*, Collaterals from the profunda femoris reconstitute the right popliteal artery (P). *D*, and *E*, Runoff via a diseased right peroneal artery collateralizes the dorsalis pedis (dp) and posterior tibial (pt) arteries in the foot. Single-vessel runoff to the left foot via the peroneal is also demonstrated.

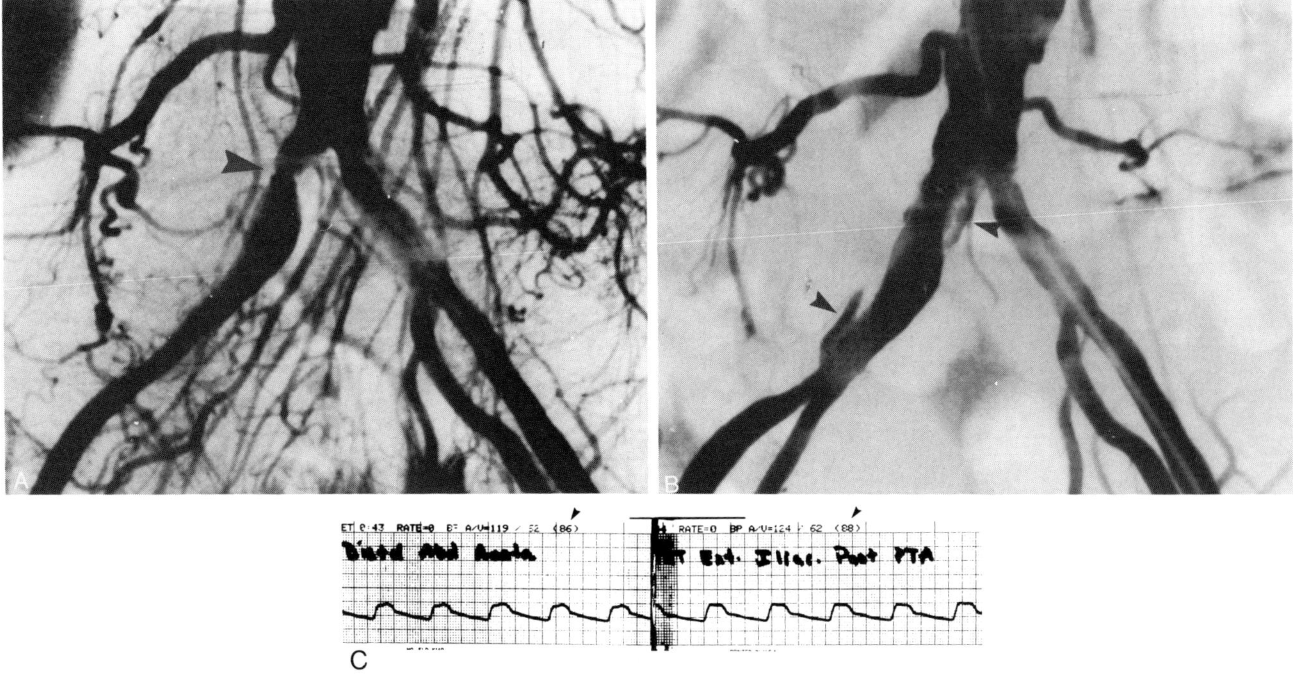

Figure 109–3. Pelvic arteriograms (subtracted) in a patient with right hip and leg claudication. *A,* The pressure gradient across the 70 per cent stenosis (*arrowhead*) in the right common iliac artery was 30 mm Hg. Note occlusion of the right internal iliac artery. *B,* After percutaneous transluminal angioplasty (PTA) there is a good angiographic result with typical separation of the intima from the media and an extraluminal collection of contrast in two locations (*arrowheads*). Note that the previously occluded right internal iliac artery is now patent. *C,* Pullback pressure recording from the distal abdominal aorta to the right external iliac artery following PTA in Figure 109–2B demonstrates no systolic or mean (86 to 88 arrowheads) arterial gradient.

1. Correction of significant iliac stenosis to improve flow prior to femoropopliteal bypass surgery.
2. Correction of native stenosis threatening the patency of a previously placed bypass graft.
3. Correction of anastomotic site stenoses in bypass grafts, especially in threatened limbs.

Certain anatomic considerations are important in the proper selection of patients for PTA. Ideal lesions include:

The aortoiliac junction: short (<3 cm) stenoses.
The iliac arteries: single or multiple discrete stenoses and short (<3 cm) occlusions.
The femoral arteries: stenoses and occlusions.
The superficial femoral arteries: single stenoses, multiple short stenoses, occlusions less than 10 cm.
The popliteal arteries: stenoses and short occlusions.
The infrapopliteal arteries: single or multiple focal stenoses and short (<4 cm) occlusions.

Patients with any of the above amenable lesions who have poor distal runoff will have poorer long-term results than patients with good distal runoff.

CONTRAINDICATIONS FOR ANGIOPLASTY IN PERIPHERAL ARTERIAL DISEASE

The clinical situation should dictate whether angioplasty is indicated or not. A good result may be less likely in the following circumstances:

1. Patients with blue-toe syndrome who have an ulcerated plaque in the aorta or iliac arteries.
2. Patients with long (>10 cm) occlusions in the iliac or superficial femoral arteries.
3. Patients with embolic occlusions.
4. Patients whose clinical history indicates recent complete occlusion. In these patients, thrombolytic therapy may precede angioplasty.

PERCUTANEOUS TRANSLUMINAL ANGIOPLASTY: TECHNIQUE

In patients in whom the diagnostic angiogram is to be coupled with possible intravascular intervention, multiple views may be needed to determine the location and extent of disease. In general, the least symptomatic side is chosen so that the symptomatic side may be approached with either a retrograde or antegrade puncture. Vascular access for typical lesions includes:

1. Unilateral iliac stenosis: Retrograde (contralateral—"around the horn"—or ipsilateral) femoral approach (see Figs. 109–3, 109–6, and 109–9).
2. Bilateral iliac stenoses: Unilateral femoral (less stenotic side) or bilateral femoral ("kissing balloon"—see Fig. 109–4) approach.
3. Common femoral stenosis: Retrograde (contralateral) femoral approach.
4. Multiple iliac/femoral lesions: Retrograde (contralateral) femoral; dilate distal contralateral lesion first.
5. Proximal superficial femoral or profunda stenoses: Retrograde (contralateral) femoral approach.
6. Distal superficial femoral, popliteal, and infrapopliteal stenoses: antegrade femoral approach (see Fig. 109–8).

Transaxillary or transbrachial techniques are not recommended for angioplasty of iliac or femoral lesions, since the size of the balloon catheter predisposes the patient to possible complications, including hematoma and thrombosis, at the puncture site.

The size of the angioplasty balloon (Fig. 109–5) used is deter-

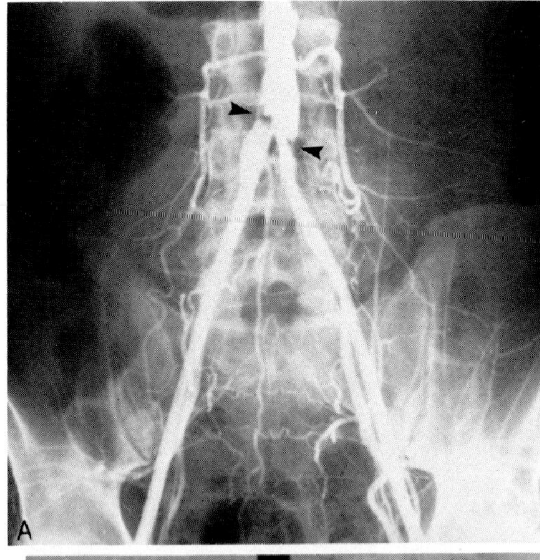

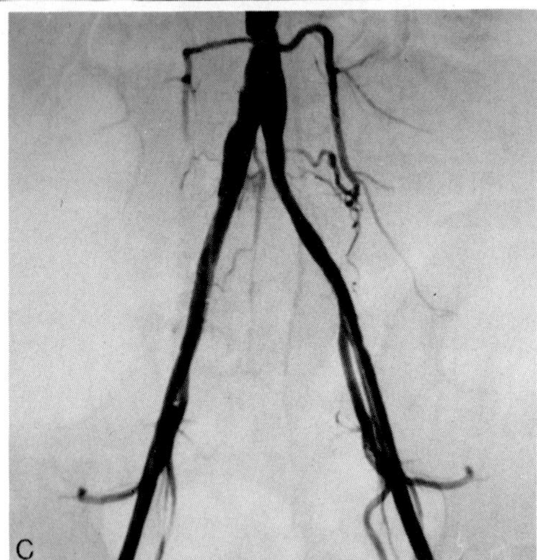

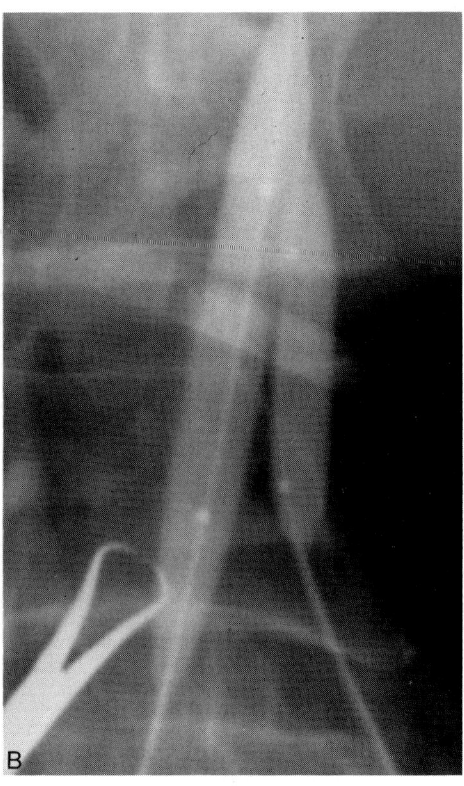

Figure 109–4. *A,* **Pelvic arteriogram demonstrates bilateral iliac stenoses** (*arrowheads*) **in a patient with bilateral hip claudication**. *B,* Patient shown in A after retrograde femoral placement of two angioplasty balloons. With balloons centered on iliac stenosis, simultaneous inflation of each balloon is accomplished—the "kissing balloon" technique. *C,* Substraction arteriogram shows good angiographic result.

Figure 109–5. Balloon angioplasty catheter with balloon inflated.

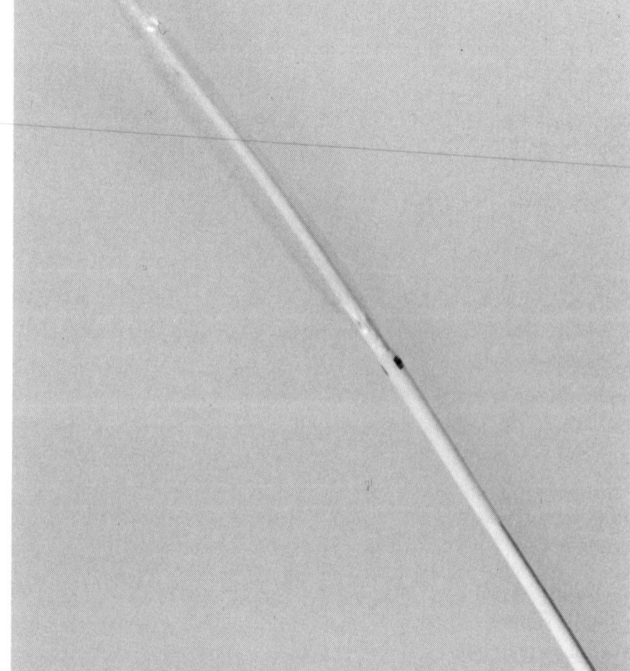

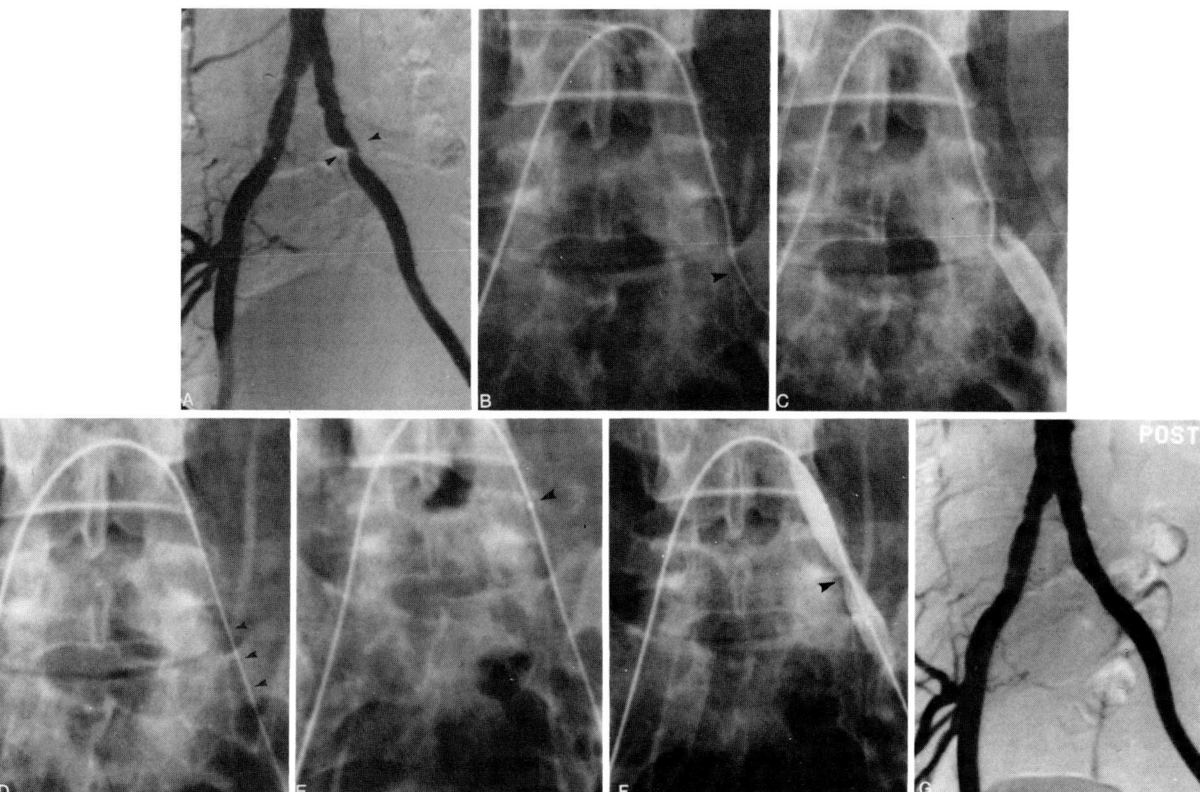

Figure 109–6. Sequential films taken during percutaneous angioplasty of left common iliac artery stenosis. *A*, Focal 80 per cent stenosis is demonstrated (*arrowheads*). *B*, Contralateral right femoral approach is used. Multipurpose catheter has been advanced into left common iliac artery, and flexible guidewire (*arrowhead*) has been used to cross the lesion. *C*, Contrast is injected, and pressures are obtained beyond stenosis. *D*, Heavy-duty .038-inch guidewire (*arrowheads*) is introduced to facilitate balloon catheter placement. *E*, Balloon catheter with radiopaque marker (*arrowhead*) is passed around the iliac bifurcation and centered on lesion. *F*, Initial balloon dilatation results in an "hourglass" deformity (*arrowhead*) as the balloon is centered on the lesion. *G*, Postprocedure arteriogram shows excellent result.

mined by a direct measurement of the normal lumen adjacent to the stenosis on the cut film angiogram. These films are usually magnified approximately 20 per cent, so that lesions in the periphery are generally "overdilated."

A typical percutaneous angioplasty of an 80 per cent left iliac stenosis is described and illustrated in Figure 109–6. This lesion could be approached either from a retrograde left femoral approach or, as in this case, from a contralateral right femoral approach (Fig. 109-6*A*). Arterial access is obtained in the usual way. The left common iliac artery is selected with a 5 Fr multipurpose or curved visceral catheter. Pressure is recorded. The catheter is advanced just proximal to the lesion. An angiogram is performed and recorded on 105-mm spot film or digital format. Lesion landmarks are noted or external markers are placed on the patient. The lesion is crossed with a flexible (floppy) straight or 1.5-mm J guidewire to decrease the incidence of subintimal dissection. The multipurpose or curved visceral catheter can be used to direct the guidewire through the eccentric lumen (Fig. 109–6*B*). Once the guidewire and catheter have crossed the lesion, an angiogram and pressure measurements are made (Fig. 109–6*C*). The patient is given intravenous heparin (5000 units) to inhibit thrombus formation. Procardia (10 mg sublingual) may be administered to prevent vascular spasm. This is mandatory in the smaller peripheral vessels. A standard 0.035-inch guidewire should be exchanged for a sturdier 0.038-inch guidewire prior to balloon catheter placement (Fig. 109–6*D*). This is especially true when contralateral iliac stenoses are to be crossed. The balloon catheter is placed over the wire and centered on the lesion previously marked (Fig. 109–6*E*). The balloon is inflated to approximately 5 atmospheres with a 10-ml syringe or inflation device containing dilute contrast material. With the initial dilatation, an hourglass deformity is seen (Fig. 109–6*F*). The balloon gradually assumes a cylindrical shape. Inflation should be maintained from 20 to 60 seconds. The balloon is then rapidly deflated using a larger (60-ml) syringe. Inflations are repeated until the pressure gradient has been abolished or decreased to less than 10 mm Hg. A postprocedure angiogram and pressure measurements proximal and distal to the lesion are then obtained (Fig. 109–6*G*). The catheter is removed and hemostasis achieved. The effects of heparin may be reversed with protamine sulfate immediately or if bleeding at the puncture site does not stop after 45 minutes of compression.

COMPLICATIONS OF ANGIOPLASTY

The complication rate for peripheral angioplasty ranges from 1 to 20 per cent. Most complications are minor and resolve with conservative therapy. Surgical management may be required in 2 to 3 per cent of cases. Complications of PTA may occur at the puncture site, at the site of angioplasty, or in the periphery. A hematoma develops at the puncture site in 5 to 6 per cent of patients. A high puncture (above the inguinal ligament) that cannot be compressed will lead to a retroperitoneal bleed. Hypotension and tachycardia following a PTA should raise the suspicion of this complication. The diagnosis can be confirmed with a computed tomographic scan.

There is a risk of subintimal dissection by the guidewire at the site of stenosis. Longitudinal dissection with thrombosis and occlusion occurs in 3 to 4 per cent of patients. Percutaneous placement of vascular stents offers a remedy for this complication. Severe pain that occurs during balloon dilatation and persists during deflation may indicate an arterial rupture. If this rare complication occurs, the balloon should be inflated across the rupture site to seal it and the patient should be taken to surgery.

Distal embolization of blood clot or atheromatous material is uncommon. Those events requiring surgical intervention occur in approximately 2 per cent of patients. Catheter- or guidewire-induced arterial spasm is not uncommon, especially in smaller distal arteries. This can be prevented by pretreatment with calcium channel blockers and procedural use of intra-arterial nitroglycerine.

RESULTS OF ANGIOPLASTY IN PERIPHERAL ARTERIAL DISEASE

In general, the three-year patency rate for PTA taken from several series is as follows:

	PERCENTAGE
Common iliac artery	85 to 95
External iliac artery	75 to 90
Superficial femoral artery (stenosis)	75 to 80
Superficial femoral artery (occlusion)	60 to 75
Infrapopliteal (two years)	70 to 88

These rates compare favorably with five-year surgical success rates for aortofemoral bypass grafts of 90 to 95 per cent; for femoropopliteal above the knee bypass grafts of 50 to 70 per cent; and for below the knee bypass grafts of 50 to 70 per cent.

Other Techniques for Endovascular Recanalization

The significant drawbacks to current endovascular therapy using PTA include:

1. Unsuitability of some lesions for therapy.
2. Acute failures following PTA.
3. Late failures due to restenosis and/or progressive disease.

Several different strategies have been or are being used to solve one or more of these problems. These include technical, pharmacologic, and even genetic approaches. It is beyond the scope of this chapter to delve into the history or current research of these myriad technologies and methods. Two technologies, directional atherectomy and intravascular stents, are discussed briefly.

DIRECTIONAL ATHERECTOMY

Atherectomy is the process of physically removing an obstructing atheroma. Extirpative atherectomy involves shaving or cutting of the atheroma and retrieving the debris. The Simpson or directional atherectomy device has enjoyed the widest clinical application (Fig. 109–7). The device employs a soft balloon to press a compact cutting chamber against the protruding atheroma. The atheroma is then shaved off by a rotating cutter. Debris is accumulated in the collection chamber, and when the chamber is full the entire catheter is removed and the debris is flushed clean from the chamber. Multiple overlapping cuts (8 to 10) are usually required (Fig. 109–8).

Directional atherectomy devices are much larger than angioplasty balloons, requiring a 9 Fr arteriotomy to produce a 7-mm lumen. The results obtained with atherectomy can be achieved with a 5 Fr balloon catheter. Atherectomy devices are expensive, approximately two to three times the cost of a balloon catheter. Finally, the atherectomy catheter is not time-efficient, especially for long-segment stenoses. The directional atherectomy catheter has been used in an attempt to debulk atheromatous lesions and leave a smoother surface. This approach was directed at preventing intimal fibrous proliferation and reducing the 20 to 30 per cent restenosis rate associated with PTA.

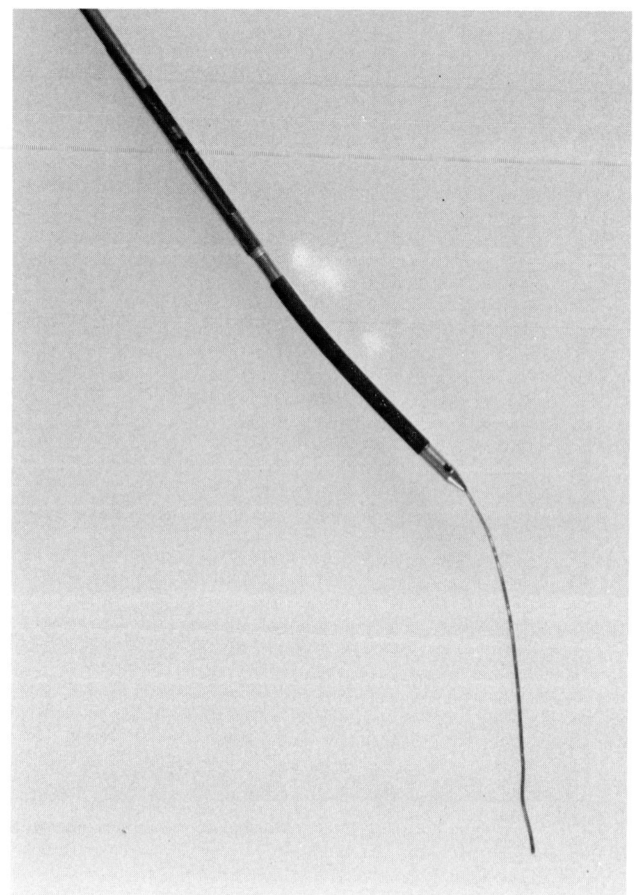

Figure 109–7. Simpson directional atherectomy device.

The effectiveness of this therapeutic modality is now becoming evident. Unfortunately, the restenosis rate in patients treated with directional atherectomy is essentially identical to that in patients treated with simple balloon angioplasty. Although the device may be used to resect obstructing intimal flaps following conventional PTA, there is currently little support for its widespread application for the treatment of lesions amenable to PTA.

INTRAVASCULAR STENTS

Expandable metallic stents are one of the most important developments in interventional radiology. Beginning in the 1980s, several types of stents were introduced, initially in the laboratory and then in various clinical settings. Expandable metallic stents are being used for treatment of obstructions in arteries, veins, biliary ducts, the esophagus, the trachea, and bronchi. Clinical experience obtained in the past five years has shown that balloon expandable stents have performed well in the aortoiliac junction and in the iliac arteries (Fig. 109–9). The current recommendation is that stainless steel iliac stents of the Palmaz type be placed when there is an inadequate post-angioplasty response, an intimal dissection, a persistent gradient of 5 mm Hg, or a persistent stenosis greater than 30 per cent (see Fig. 109–9).

Other indications for stent placement are restenosis after previous iliac balloon angioplasty and total iliac artery occlusion. Contraindications for stent placement include (1) extravasation of contrast material after PTA; (2) markedly tortuous iliac vessels; and (3) dense, extensive arterial calcification. Recent studies comparing

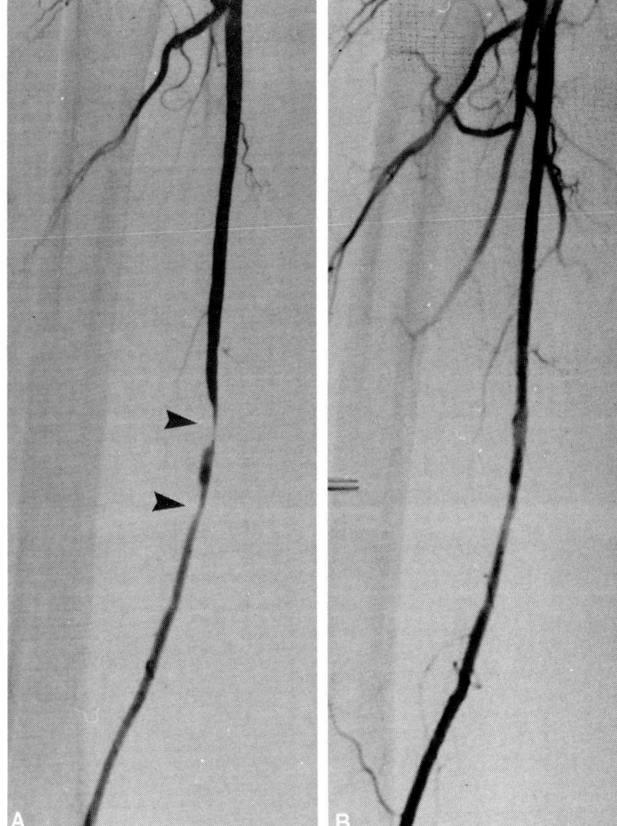

Figure 109–8. Antegrade right superficial femoral arteriogram. *A*, There is subtotal occlusion followed by 80 per cent stenosis of the mid-superficial femoral artery (*arrowheads*). *B*, Following multiple overlapping cuts with atherectomy device, excellent angiographic result is seen.

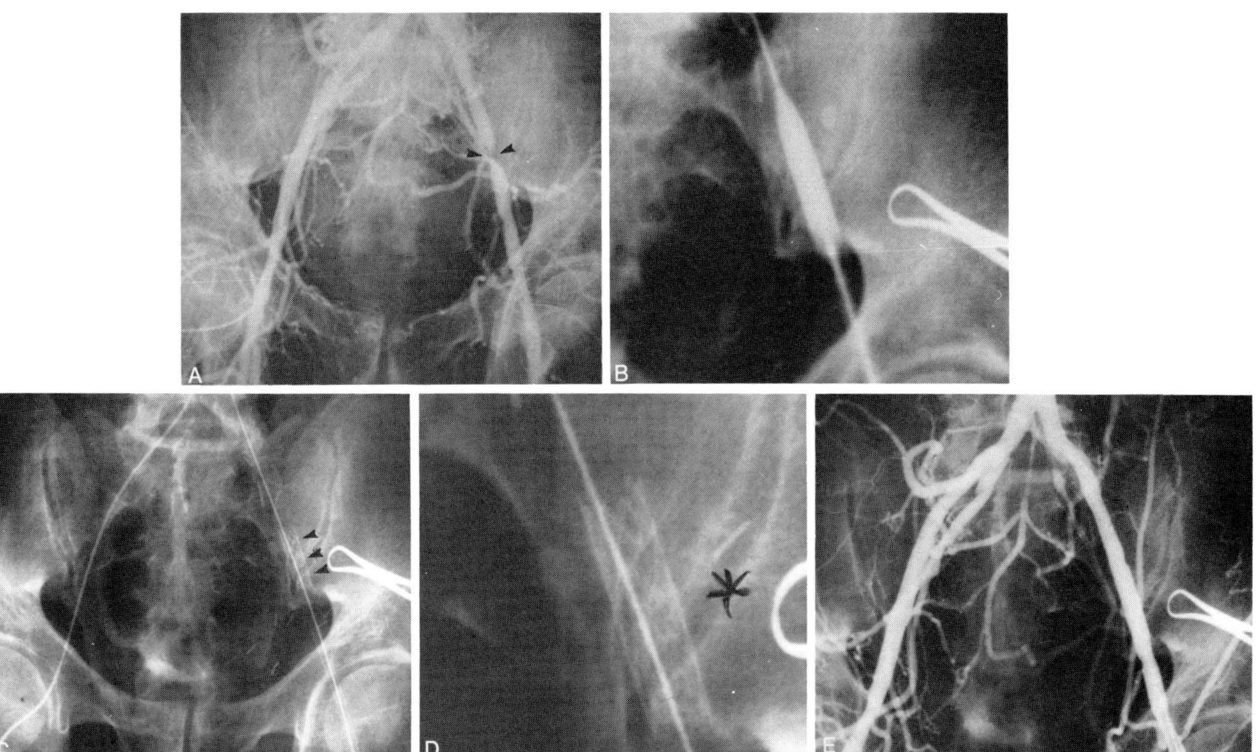

Figure 109–9. Expandable arterial stent placement. *A*, Pelvic arteriogram with subtotal occlusion of left external iliac artery (*arrowheads*). Routine PTA produced a poor angiographic and hemodynamic result. *B*, Balloon catheter carrying expandable stent is inflated across lesion. *C*, Metallic stent is fully deployed across the lesion (*arrowheads*), and balloon catheter is removed. *D*, Close-up of expanded metallic stent. *E*, Postprocedure arteriogram shows excellent angiographic result.

PTA with balloon expandable stent placement (Palmaz type) indicate a two-year success rate of 96 per cent after stent placement versus a 72 per cent two-year success rate after PTA. This improved result is thought to be due to the better morphologic restoration of lumen patency achieved with stents (see Fig. 109–9).

As with any new device, only controlled clinical trials with long-term follow-up can establish efficacy of stents and determine their limitations in different situations. Comparison of stents with both balloon angioplasty and with surgery should provide the answers.

THROMBOLYTIC THERAPY IN THE PERIPHERAL ARTERIAL SYSTEM

Since 1974, when Dotter's landmark article initially described the technique of intrathrombus administration of a thrombolytic agent as an alternative to the intravenous route, the literature has become replete with descriptions of lytic agents and techniques. As a result, thrombolytic therapy has become a mainstay for treatment of atherosclerotic occlusions, graft thromboses, and post-angioplasty thrombosis. Efforts continue to define the ideal delivery system and therapeutic dosage. In this section, we review available thrombolytic agents, patient selection, technique, complications, the predictors of successful therapy, and the success rate for thrombolytic therapy in the peripheral arterial system.

Available Agents

Dotter's initial series presented 17 patients treated with an intra-arterial regimen of streptokinase delivered either directly into the thrombus or proximal to it. This technique remained dormant until 1981 when Katzen and van Breda reported their series of 12 patients treated in a similar fashion. In 1985, McNamara and Fischer focused attention on urokinase as an intrathrombus thrombolytic agent. Since then, in a search for the ideal thrombolytic agent, pro-urokinase, acylated streptokinase-plasminogen activator complex (APSAC), tissue-plasminogen activator (t-PA), recombinant tissue-plasminogen activator (rt-PA) and recombinant single-chain urokinase plasminogen activator (SCU-PA) have all been investigated. Only streptokinase and urokinase are presently in use for thrombolysis in the peripheral arterial system.

Streptokinase is produced from cultures of group C beta-hemolytic streptococci. Therefore, the agent is antigenic and may cause serious allergic reactions. In addition, patients with previous streptococcal infections or recent streptokinase therapy have circulating antibodies. The streptokinase can effectively be neutralized by these antibodies, and large loading doses may be required to overcome them. Streptokinase acts on plasminogen in a two-step process. It first forms a 1:1 equimolar complex with plasminogen, resulting in an intermediate complex. This complex then converts nonbound molecules of plasminogen to plasmin to initiate fibrinolysis. It can cause systemic fibrinolytic activation and has minimal fibrin specificity. It has a half-life of 83 minutes.

In contrast, urokinase is a natural protein obtained from tissue cultures of human renal tubular cells and is therefore nonantigenic. Allergic reactions do not occur, and previous exposure is not an issue. Therefore, retreatment can be performed as soon as needed. Urokinase is a direct activator of plasminogen, converting it to its active form, plasmin. Although urokinase can cause systemic fibrinolytic activation, it has a greater affinity for fibrin-bound plasminogen than does streptokinase, and therefore it is less likely to cause systemic fibrinolysis and subsequent hemorrhagic complications. Its fibrin specificity is moderate. It has a half-life of 16 minutes.

Urokinase has a higher incidence of clot lysis with shorter infusion times than does streptokinase. The rate of hemorrhagic complications with urokinase is also lower. Given its more predictable response, safer profile, and nonantigenicity, it is the agent of choice in the periphery.

Patient Selection

Thrombolytic therapy has been shown to be effective in lysing clots within both arteries and surgical grafts. The decision to select thrombolysis as a treatment for a patient is complex and multifactorial. Unquestionably, the primary criterion for selection is the degree of underlying ischemia. Restoration of flow to an ischemic limb arrests major tissue damage, but it can result in the reperfusion syndrome, which can cause acute tubular necrosis, adult respiratory distress syndrome, disseminated intravascular coagulation, lactic acidosis, hyperkalemia, compartment syndrome, or death.

In considering a patient for thrombolytic therapy, a distinction should be made between time to restoration of blood flow and the time of complete clot lysis. Restoration of flow decreases the risk of ischemic damage and is accomplished in a shorter time period than the complete clot lysis that is considered the end point of thrombolytic therapy. Because the presence of a thrombus is itself a thrombogenic stimulus, the clot must be completely lysed to reduce the risk of rethrombosis after therapy is discontinued.

The average time until complete clot lysis varies between 6 and 18 hours, and therefore patients with intolerable ischemia and cadaveric limbs should be excluded from therapy. Signs of intolerable ischemia include markedly diminished sensation and motor deficits, such as difficulty in flexing the ankle. In addition to irreversible or intolerable ischemia, active internal bleeding; recent intracranial, intraspinal, or intraocular surgery; and recent cerebrovascular accident or transient ischemic attack are absolute contraindications. Recent major surgery, previous biopsy of organs with noncompressible arteries, and conditions that might cause serious bleeding, severe hypertension, or recent trauma are relative contraindications.

Otherwise, patients with acute, subacute, or even chronic occlusions of native arteries and grafts or thrombosis post-angioplasty may be ideal candidates for lytic therapy. Patients with embolic occlusions or emboli post-angioplasty may also be suitable, although less than ideal, candidates.

Technique

The initial studies on the use of thrombolysis in peripheral vascular thromboembolic disease used a relatively high-dose intravenous regimen of streptokinase. These studies were associated with an unacceptably high rate of bleeding secondary to systemic fibrinolysis. Dotter was one of the first to consider intrathrombus administration of streptokinase. He used much smaller doses, avoided systemic fibrinolysis, and subsequently reduced the rate of complications to a more acceptable level. Subsequent researchers continued to deliver the lytic agent locally, within the thrombus. Due to its lack of antigenicity, its more predictable response, its higher incidence of thrombolysis success, and its lower complication rate, urokinase has supplanted streptokinase as the agent of choice in the periphery.

McNamara and Fischer significantly altered the technical approach beyond simple implantation of the catheter within the clot. A guidewire traversal test was described as a predictor of successful lysis. An angiographic guidewire was passed through the clotted segment. If the guidewire passed through the clot entirely, results of lytic therapy were uniformly successful. If not, success occurred in only 10 per cent of the cases. If the guidewire passed only partially though an occlusion, an eccentric underlying stenosis or atherosclerotic occlusion was likely present and a therapeutic trial of thrombolysis for four to six hours was found to be of benefit. If

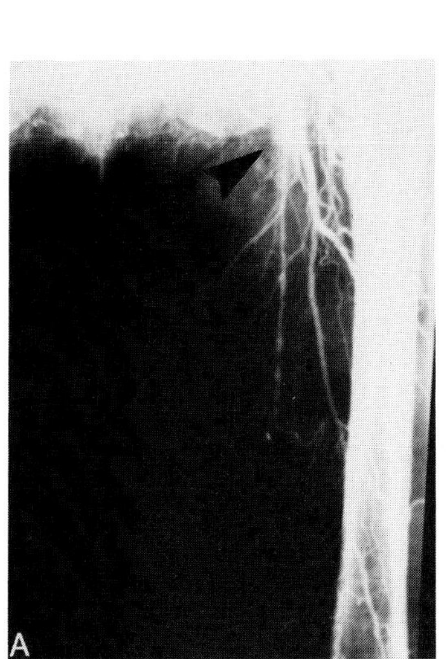

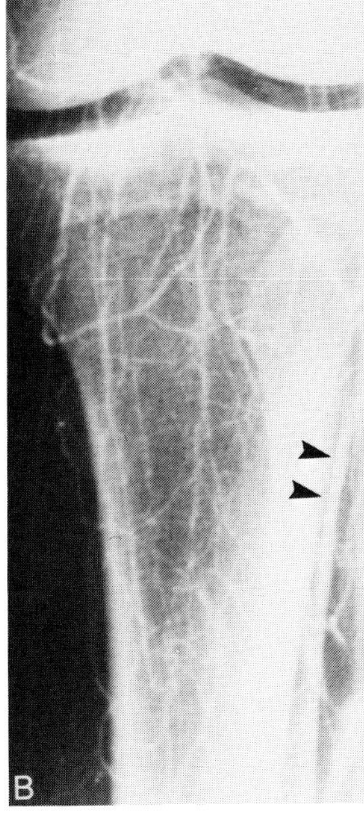

Figure 109–10. Patient who 3 months previously had a left composite, Gore-Tex/reversed saphenous vein femorotibial bypass graft placed. Patient presented with a cold, pulseless left foot. *A,* Origin of composite femorotibial bypass graft is occluded (*arrowhead*). *B,* Reconstitution of the proximal anterior tibial artery is seen distally (*arrowheads*).

flow was restored or a channel created through the thrombus in this time period, therapy was continued and was likely to be successful. In addition, a high-dose infusion protocol was proposed that had a higher rate of complete clot lysis, faster recanalization times, and fewer complications than previously described with the low-dose streptokinase regimens. With this protocol, an overall success rate of 83 per cent was established.

An initial diagnostic arteriogram must be performed prior to the institution of thrombolytic therapy (Fig. 109–10). Also, if a previous surgical graft has been placed for revascularization, knowledge of its location and extent is extremely beneficial. It is important to know from the diagnostic study and the surgical history the proximal origin point of occlusion and the point where reconstitution of flow occurs before initiating therapy (see Fig. 109–10). Recanalization of the entire thrombosed segment with a guidewire is essential for successful therapy and must be attempted (Fig. 109–11). Once recanalization has been performed with the guidewire, the next therapeutic goal is the rapid reinstitution of flow through the thrombosed segment to assist thrombolysis further and prevent rethrombosis. Both high- and low-dose regimens exist to re-establish flow.

Indications for high-dose therapy include an acutely ischemic limb, a thrombus of unknown age, and the desire to avoid overnight infusions in patients who present earlier in the day. Most regimens use doses up to 250,000 units of urokinase per hour over the first four hours. Doses are then tapered to more standard low-dose regimens (60,000 units/hour).

Indications for low-dose therapy include nonacute ischemia or situations where overnight infusions are unavoidable, such as a patient who presents later in the day. Infusion rates range between 40,000 and 80,000 units of urokinase per hour.

The final therapeutic goal of the infusion is to determine the cause of the thrombosis (Fig. 109–12). Long-term patency rates are significantly affected by the demonstration and correction of underlying causes for the thrombosis. Flow-limiting lesions in either the inflow or outflow of the thrombosed arterial segment or graft must be diligently sought out. If a graft has been placed, the proximal and distal anastomoses should be carefully studied for stenoses (see Fig. 109–12). Oblique angiographic views are almost always needed. If a flow-limiting lesion amenable to angioplasty is found, this procedure should be considered. If not, surgical intervention or revision of the graft should be considered. Failure to correct an underlying flow-limiting lesion or the absence of an identifiable lesion speaks poorly for long-term patency.

Systemic anticoagulation with heparin is advocated by most authors. Heparinization prevents pericatheter thrombus formation and prevents rethrombosis as thrombolysis progresses. Heparin is usually initiated at a rate of 1000 units/hour intravenously to maintain a partial thromboplastin time (PTT) of 80 to 150 seconds or a ratio 2.5 to 3.5 times normal. If heparin is used, intramuscular injections should be avoided and the catheter site monitored closely.

Appropriate baseline laboratory studies include hemoglobin, hematocrit, platelets, fibrinogen, PTT, and serum creatinine. The PTT should be monitored as the heparin is adjusted. A serum fibrinogen level less than 100 mg/dl correlates with a significantly increased bleeding risk. The time at which these parameters should be reassessed is quite variable among authors.

Additional variations in technique have been described that have shortened clot lysis times, resulting in continued, improved success and fewer complications. Coaxial catheter techniques with split dosing have been described to improve delivery over longer segments of occlusion. Injection of high doses of an intrathrombus bolus of urokinase ("lacing") has been shown to shorten clot lysis times significantly. A pulsed-spray method has been developed that, when combined with a positive guidewire traversal test, has a reported success rate as high as 98 per cent. Multiport catheters and guidewires have been recently released that allow the frequent delivery of small volumes of concentrated lytic agent over long infusion lengths. As a result of these additional variations, success rates have improved and clot lysis times have been shortened even further.

Complications

Unfortunately, the complication rates during thrombolytic therapy remain high, especially when compared with rates associated with other interventional procedures such as angioplasty. Fortunately, most of these complications are rarely associated with serious, long-term clinical sequelae. The rate of complications has been found to be directly proportional to the length of the procedure. Complication rates range between 15 and 25 per cent, 4 to 12 per cent of which are hemorrhagic. Overall, rates of hemorrhagic complications are higher for streptokinase (48 per cent) than urokinase (25 per cent). Complications from streptokinase are believed to be related to its more profound systemic fibrinolysis and those of urokinase to the technical aspects of catheter manipulation. Hemorrhagic complications can be managed by attempting as atraumatic an initial puncture and catheter placement as possible, placing an arterial sheath to minimize catheter exchanges, reducing the heparin dosage, or discontinuing the infusion if necessary.

Additional complications include pericatheter thrombus formation, distal clot embolization, contrast-induced acute renal failure, and the reperfusion syndrome. The chances of pericatheter thrombus can be reduced with systemic anticoagulation and avoidance of catheter placement across flow-limiting lesions. Distal embolization of clot has been reported in 8 per cent of cases. It may be manifested as acute worsening of the patient's ischemic symptoms. Therapy should be continued because the majority of these emboli will lyse with continuation of the infusion. Many patients present acutely and have not had preprocedural hydration. Therefore, contrast volumes should be closely monitored to prevent contrast-induced acute renal failure. Serum creatinine should be followed, and injections should be limited to those absolutely necessary to document the progression of treatment and determine adjustments in the

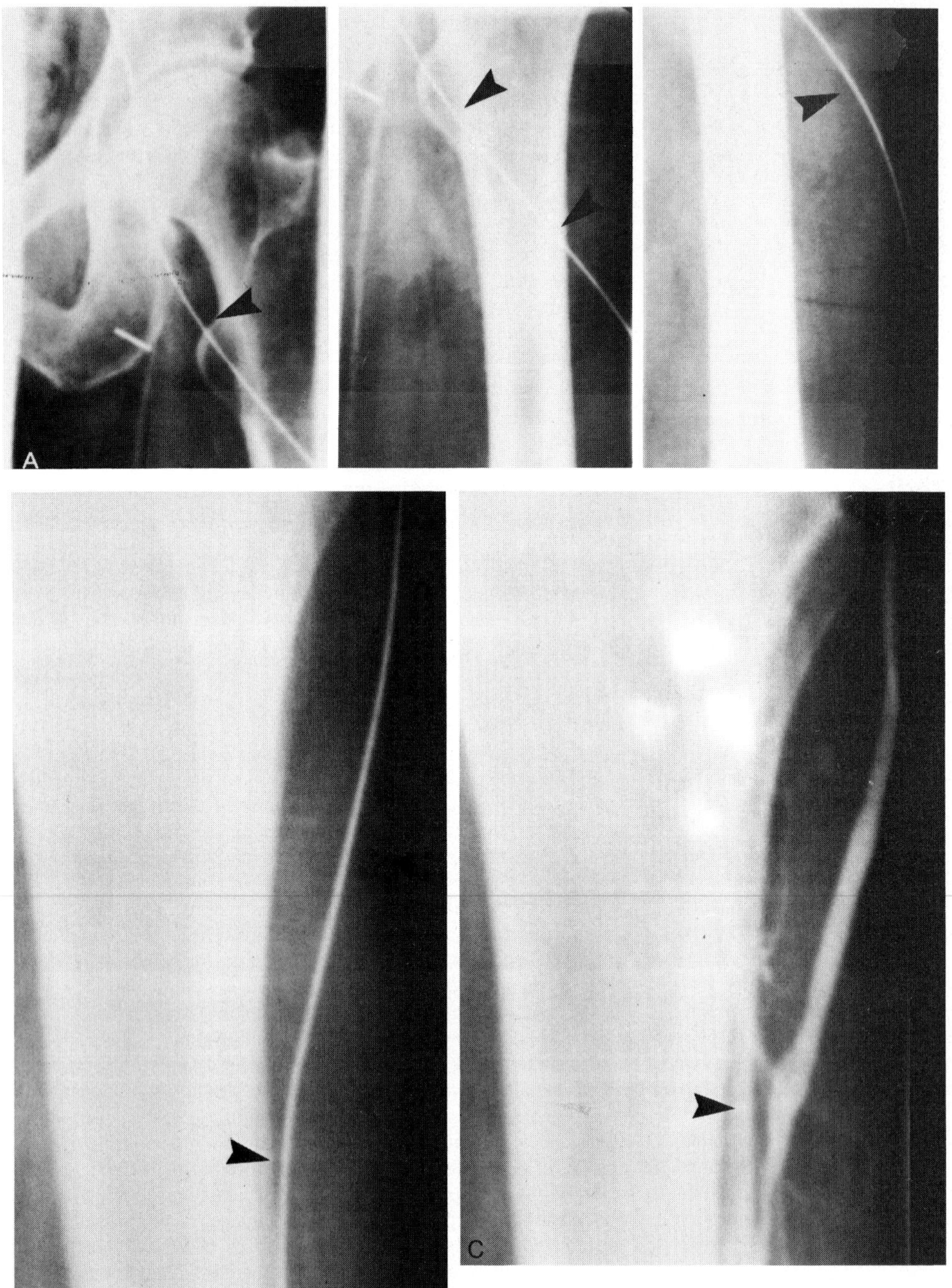

Figure 109–11. Same patient as shown in Figure 109–10. *A,* A guidewire is passed across the graft occlusion from its point of occlusion distally (*arrowheads*). *B,* Complete recanalization with the guidewire through the entirety of the graft across the distal anastomosis (*arrowhead*) is ideal. *C,* Limited contrast injection after guidewire passage confirms recanalization through the distal anastomosis (*arrowhead*).

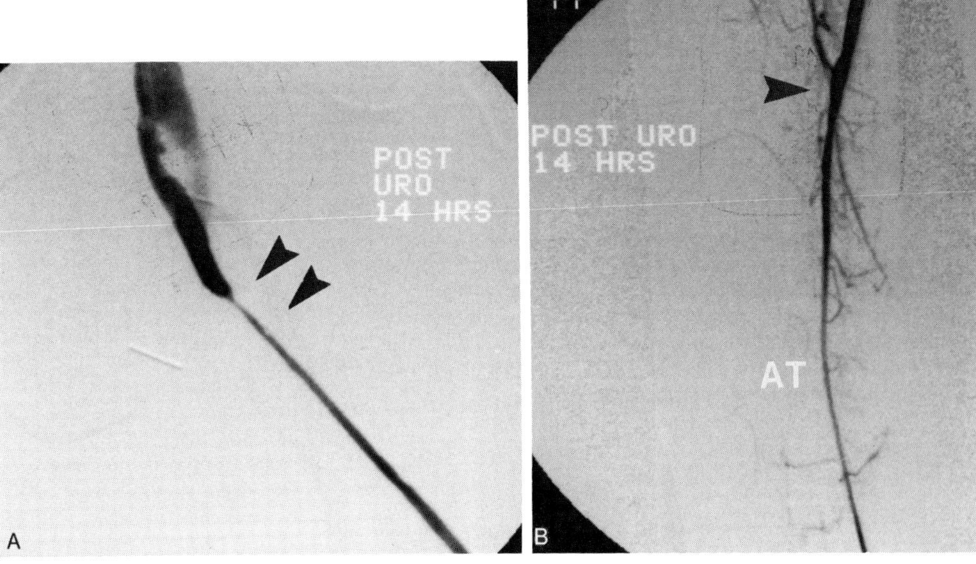

Figure 109–12. Digital subtraction angiograms obtained following 14 hours of urokinase infusion in patient shown in Figure 109–10. *A,* Common femoral angiogram demonstrates stretching of the vein graft at the composite anastomosis as the cause of thrombosis (*arrowheads*). *B,* Distal anastomosis (*arrowhead*) and anterior tibial artery (AT) are widely patent following thrombolysis. The intervening segment of graft (not shown) was also patent. This patient had surgical revision of his graft.

therapy. The reperfusion syndrome can be avoided by not attempting thrombolysis in cadaveric limbs.

Predictors of Successful Therapy

Many factors can affect success. These include acuity of the thrombosis, the location of the occlusion, and whether a native artery or a graft is affected. Once therapy is instituted, technical factors including the result of the guidewire traversal test, rapidity of reinstitution of flow, and the type and mode of administration of the lytic agent may determine outcome.

Acute thrombus lyses better than chronic thrombus. In thrombus less than three days old, overall success rates as high as 97 per cent have been reported; in clot older than three weeks, success rates as high as 70 to 75 per cent have been reported. Although statistically significant differences exist in clot lysis times, some authors suggest that this is of no clinical significance.

The incidence of complete clot lysis is associated with vessel location. The likelihood of successful clot lysis decreases as the location becomes more peripheral. Whether native artery or graft, suprainguinal locations have success rates of about 90 per cent, and infrainguinal locations have an approximately 70 per cent success rate.

No significant difference in initial success rates has been reported between artery and graft. Patency rates, however, are better for arteries than for grafts. At six months, the overall patency rate for recanalized arteries is 71 per cent and that for recanalized grafts is 41 per cent.

The guidewire traversal test is the single best predictor of the likelihood of recanalizing a given occlusion and obtaining clot lysis. Complete passage of the wire virtually ensures success. As a corollary, if recanalization is evident at two hours with reinstitution of flow, there is a 100 per cent likelihood of success if therapy can be completed.

Most authors agree that urokinase is more effective. In native arteries, the success rates for urokinase and streptokinase have been reported to be 75 per cent and 45 per cent, respectively. In grafts, the respective success rates of 84 per cent and 48 per cent have been reported.

High-dose therapy, intrathrombus bolus of urokinase, and the pulsed-spray method have all been shown to improve success as well.

Success and Patency Rates

Success can be defined as complete or virtually complete clot lysis with the return of antegrade flow. Overall success rates between 77 and 80 per cent have been reported. In acute thromboses, success rates as high as 90 to 97 per cent have been reported. Chronic thromboses may be successfully lysed 70 to 75 per cent of the time. Success in suprainguinal arteries and grafts is 90 per cent, and that in infrainguinal arteries and grafts is 70 per cent.

Patency can be defined as the time between the end of the infusion and the occurrence of reocclusion. The primary determinant of long-term patency is the presence or absence of an underlying, correctable lesion. Slow flow secondary to poor runoff in the periphery or hemodynamically significant residual stenoses also affect long-term patency. If at the completion of lysis and after the correction of an underlying lesion no residual stenosis is evident above, within, or below the previously occluded segment, six-month patency is 85 per cent.

If a flow-limiting lesion is present and left untreated, six-month patency is only 8 per cent. Occlusions above the inguinal ligament do better than those below it and are reported at 86 per cent vs 38 per cent at six months. Six-month patency of arteries exceeds that of grafts, regardless of location, at 71 per cent vs 41 per cent.

Thrombolytic therapy has been established as an effective way to manage thromboembolic occlusions of peripheral arteries, occluded surgical bypass grafts, and thrombosis post-angioplasty. Except for those patients with intolerable limb ischemia, lysis is successful in most acute and the majority of chronic occlusions. If a guidewire will completely traverse an occlusion and clot lysis is performed quickly with rapid reinstitution of antegrade flow, success rates will generally be high and complication rates low. Patency rates will be greater if an underlying correctable cause or lesion is identified and treated.

EMBOLOTHERAPY

Embolotherapy is a percutaneous catheter technique that has applications not only in the periphery, but in other parts of the arterial and venous systems as well. The purpose of this section is to provide a broad overview of the basics of embolotherapy: We review the indications for embolotherapy, discuss the more common materials and equipment used in the procedure, and review some of the common clinical applications of embolotherapy.

Indications

HEMORRHAGE

A majority of patients who undergo embolotherapy are treated because of uncontrollable arterial or venous hemorrhage. Penetrating or blunt trauma is a frequent cause of arterial injury resulting in uncontrollable bleeding. Gastrointestinal tract bleeding may result from mucosal laceration, gastritis, or variceal bleeding secondary to portal hypertension. In the tracheobronchial tree cystic fibrosis and other chronic inflammatory diseases such as tuberculosis may result in bronchial artery hemorrhage. In each of these situations, embolotherapy may play an important role in controlling the bleeding.

TUMOR DEVASCULARIZATION

In certain settings, embolotherapy plays an important role in tumor dearterialization and infarction. Indications include tumor devascularization prior to surgical removal to minimize intraoperative blood loss, in situ tumor infarction for pain palliation, or control of intermittent bleeding produced by primary and metastatic tumors.

VASCULAR MALFORMATIONS

Vascular malformations have unique characteristics that make them amenable to embolotherapy. They respond favorably to arterial occlusion. The intent is to obliterate or devascularize significantly the arteriovenous fistulas or arteriovenous malformations by eliminating the abnormal arterial communication(s). Testicular varicoceles and other venous malformations may also respond to embolotherapy.

Materials

There are three broad categories of occlusive material and delivery systems: short-term reversible; intermediate-term, potentially reversible; and permanent occlusive materials.

SHORT-TERM REVERSIBLE

Reversible, short-term occlusion devices are limited to occlusion balloons. These devices are inflated in the primary feeding vessel and occlude blood flow until a surgical repair can be effected. The advantages of these devices are that they can be inserted rapidly and used to occlude both large and small vessels. The occlusion can be rapidly reversed. The balloon may also act as a palpable landmark for the surgeon, facilitating identification of the involved vessel. These balloons can be used in the acute trauma setting; for example, in the case of a lacerated aorta, the balloon can help stabilize the patient until the injury can be repaired.

Balloons can be used in the nonacute setting as well. Reversible occlusion of carotid arteries prior to surgery can be used as a provocative test to determine whether carotid ligation can be accomplished safely. When ethanol is used as the infarction agent, balloons are useful in maintaining the ethanol in a closed space, preventing seepage into nontarget vessels.

INTERMEDIATE-TERM, POTENTIALLY REVERSIBLE

The object of intermediate-term occlusion is to produce an occlusion that will be effective for a few days to weeks. The purpose is to occlude the vessel for a period of time long enough to produce the desired therapeutic effect. For example, therapeutic occlusion of a gastric or duodenal artery to control bleeding resulting from a mucosal ulcer need not be permanent. Once acute bleeding from the ulcer has resolved, the vessel no longer needs to be occluded. Material that is gradually absorbed by the body is ideal for this clinical application. Autologous clot; patient tissue (fat, muscle, dura, or fascia); and Gelfoam, Avitene, Oxycel, and Angiostat all produce temporary vascular occlusion. The duration of the occlusion varies, depending on the material used.

AUTOLOGOUS CLOT. A patient's own blood is readily available material that can be used to produce a short-term vascular occlusion. Fresh autologous clot can be difficult to manipulate. In order to improve the handling characteristics, blood may be either mixed with Amicar (epsilon-aminocaproic acid) or heat treated. This produces a more rigid thrombus with more malleable properties. Autologous clot, heat-treated autologous clot, and autologous clot mixed with Amicar have a relatively short duration of occlusion. Untreated clot begins to be resorbed almost immediately, leading to possible recanalization in a matter of a few hours. Embolic occlusion with modified clot produces a more durable occlusion, retarding the intrinsic thrombolytic process for perhaps twice the duration of unadulterated thrombus.

GELFOAM. Gelfoam is a purified gelatin sponge that may be injected by catheter in a number of forms (Figs. 109–13 and 109–14). Powder and small particles can be injected as a "slurry." Larger particles ("torpedoes") may be injected as individual pledgets through the catheter into the target vessel. The particle size is chosen on the basis of the result desired. Gelfoam powder migrates into the capillary bed and has a high incidence of producing target organ infarction. The larger the particle, the more proximal the occlusion and the greater the likelihood that collateral vessels will develop. This lessens the likelihood of infarction. Some believe that a proximal occlusion enhances the prospects for later complete recanalization of the vessel. The particles, 3 to 5 mm × 12 mm strips of Gelfoam, are compressed and then extruded through the smaller caliber catheter, producing a very proximal occlusion. The material re-expands immediately after release, usually occluding the vessel just distal to the catheter tip. The occlusion is very proximal with the Gelfoam torpedo, and this embolus greatly diminishes the pressure downstream to the occlusion. In most cases, this pressure reduction is all that is needed to stop the bleeding.

OTHER OCCLUSIVE MATERIALS. A number of other absorbable occlusive materials are available. Avitene is microfibrillar collagen in powder form and is usually injected as a slurry. Oxycel is oxidized cellulose, similar in form to Gelfoam. Angiostat is highly purified bovine dermal collagen that has been cross-linked with glutaraldehyde. It is sold in premixed syringes. These three materials have more specific embolotherapy applications and are seldom used in current general embolotherapy practice.

PERMANENT OCCLUSION

Permanent occlusion is produced by a variety of embolic materials. The most commonly used device is the stainless steel coil. The original Gianturco coil has been modified in countless ways to adapt to a large variety of delivery systems and applications. Since then a variety of materials have been developed to produce permanent occlusion. Ivalon, silk threads, silicone beads, polystyrene spheres, and detachable balloons are other nonabsorbable materials and devices that produce permanent vessel occlusion. Injection of ethanol and boiling contrast directly into the vessel destroys red cell and endothelial protein on contact, producing a permanent occlusion. Tissue glue (isobutyl-2-cyanoacrylate) injected into the vessel forms a permanent cast of the vessel one or two seconds after injection. This not only occludes the target vessel but also extends into first-, second-, and third-order branches. The extent of the cast and the number of vessels occluded by the cast are varied by altering the

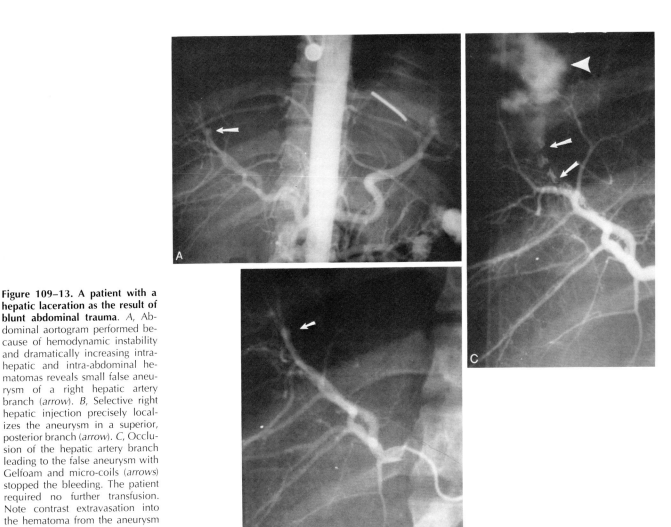

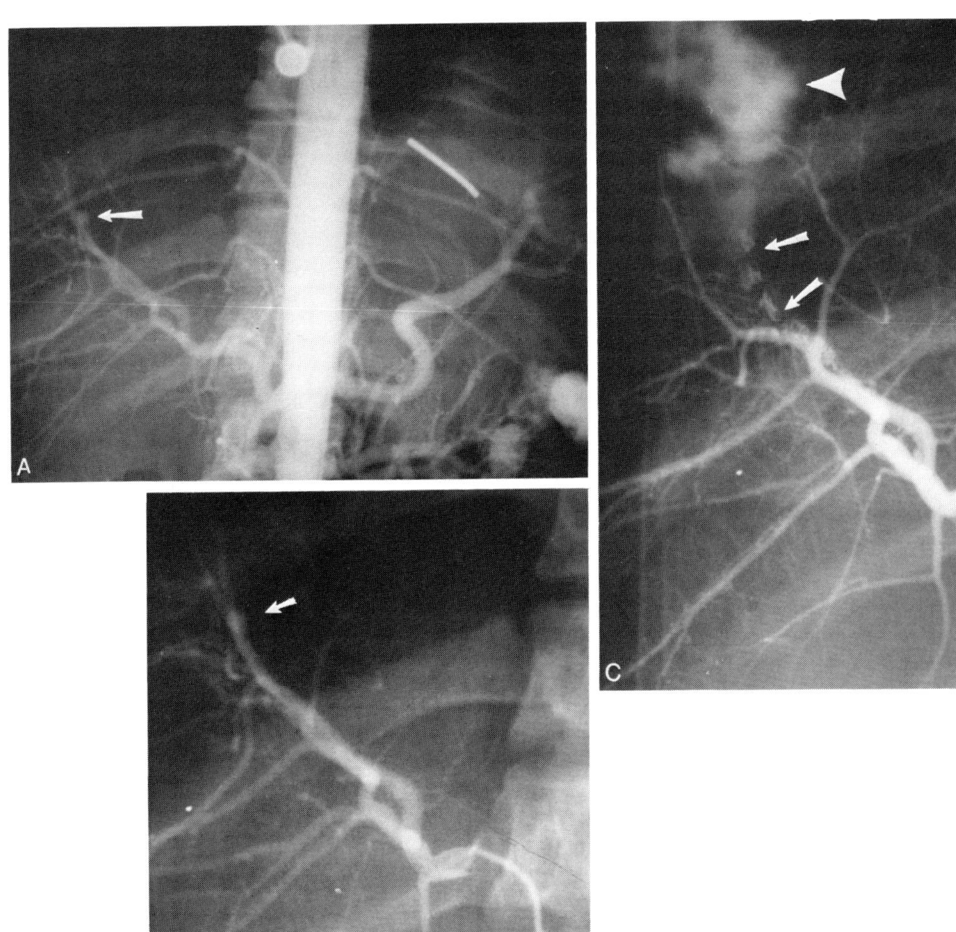

Figure 109–13. A patient with a hepatic laceration as the result of blunt abdominal trauma. *A*, Abdominal aortogram performed because of hemodynamic instability and dramatically increasing intrahepatic and intra-abdominal hematomas reveals small false aneurysm of a right hepatic artery branch (*arrow*). *B*, Selective right hepatic injection precisely localizes the aneurysm in a superior, posterior branch (*arrow*). *C*, Occlusion of the hepatic artery branch leading to the false aneurysm with Gelfoam and micro-coils (*arrows*) stopped the bleeding. The patient required no further transfusion. Note contrast extravasation into the hematoma from the aneurysm (*arrowhead*).

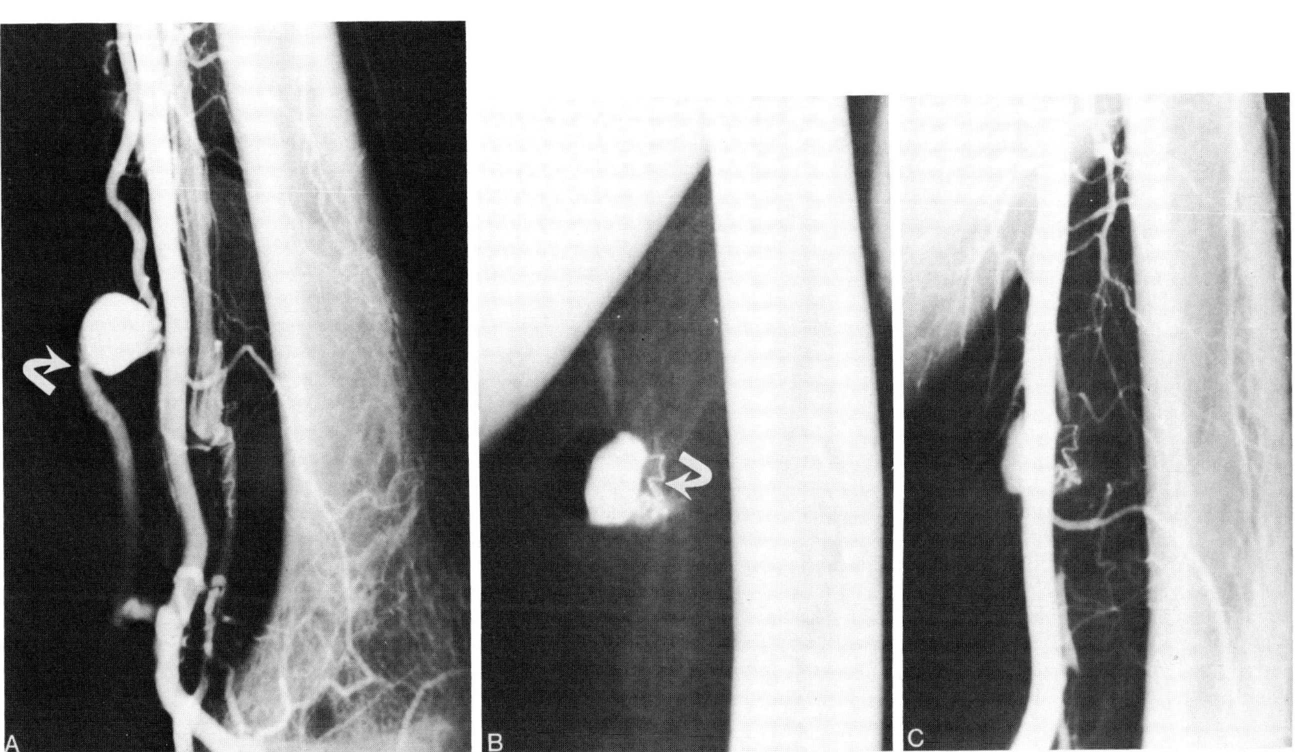

Figure 109–14. Patient who sustained a stab wound to the left arm and in whom a bruit was noted. *A*, A left axillary arteriogram demonstrates a false aneurysm of a profunda brachii branch with fistulous communication to the deep venous system (*arrow*). *B*, Occlusion of the proximal and distal feeding branches to the aneurysm with Gelfoam and micro-coils (*arrow*) isolates the aneurysm. Contrast is static in the aneurysm lumen. *C*, Arteriography following embolotherapy reveals no filling of the arteriovenous fistula.

polymerization time of the glue. Sclerosing agents such as Sotradecol produce endothelial lining irritation and necrosis, which promotes platelet deposition and thrombosis.

STAINLESS STEEL COILS. The ease of use and availability of a broad selection of coil configurations and delivery systems make the coil the most widely used permanent embolic device. Stainless steel spring coils of varying size and configuration usually incorporate a thrombogenic fiber. Dacron fiber is most often used, although wool and silk have been used as well. The coils are advanced out of the catheter tip. Once in the target vessel, they assume their preloaded configuration. Since coils are sized slightly larger than the caliber of the target vessel, the catheter tip must be positioned at the exact location of the desired occlusion. Malposition of a coil may lead to inadvertent occlusion of a nontarget vessel. Undersizing the coil may allow it to migrate distally into a nontarget vessel. Oversizing the coil may result in protrusion of some of the coil into a major vessel. Having the coil or coil fibers exposed in a nontarget feeding vessel can lead to formation of microemboli and subsequent distal emboli in nontarget organs.

Coils can be configured to form cylinders, spirals, helical designs, or other configurations as large as 20 mm in diameter. Thus coils can occlude a vessel many times the diameter of the delivery catheter. Development of sophisticated small catheters such as the Tracker and its microcoil delivery system have broadened the scope of embolotherapy applications (see Figs. 109–13 and 109–14). These catheters can be maneuvered into fourth- and fifth-order branching vessels, allowing precise placement of tiny occlusion coils in the brain, liver, kidney, and extremities.

IVALON. Ivalon (polyvinyl alcohol) is a nonabsorbable material that is injected as a particle suspension or slurry. Because Ivalon is a solid sponge, the particle size can be tightly controlled. This permits the interventionalist to select a particle size commensurate with the size of the artery requiring occlusion. Most particles are sized less than 700 microns, with the 200 to 300 micron and the 300 to 500 micron sizes the most popular. The advantages of Ivalon are that it is a relatively nonreactive material and it can produce a very distal permanent occlusion. This distal occlusion reduces the number of collateral capillary pathways available for revascularization of the target tissue. Although revascularization may occur, the degree of revascularization is significantly reduced. A disadvantage of Ivalon is that it is not very compressible. Attempts to inject too many particles at one time or too large a particle may occlude the catheter, requiring recatheterization of the vessel to complete the procedure.

BALLOONS. The Debrun balloon, now being used on an investigational basis in the treatment and occlusion of cerebral aneurysms and fistulas, has yet to be released for general use.

There is a wide variety of additional permanent occlusive embolic material in addition to the more commonly used material discussed above. These materials are infrequently used and require special skills and training.

Applications

THORAX

HEMOPTYSIS. Uncontrollable massive hemoptysis in patients with severe lung disease such as cystic fibrosis or tuberculosis may require embolization for bleeding control. The bleeding is frequently from the systemic arterial system, usually the bronchial arteries. Pulmonary hypertension is also a factor in this life-threatening setting. Prior to embolization, the source of bleeding should be localized bronchoscopically to either a specific lung segment or a lobe. Angiographic delineation of the bronchial arteries with subsequent embolization of the involved segment or lobe using absorbable material is the procedure of choice in patients who are inoperable. These patients often have compromised pulmonary circulation. Recanalization is desirable to minimize further compromise, and therefore absorbable embolic material is the preferred embolic agent in this patient group.

TRAUMA. Penetrating chest wall trauma may produce severe hemorrhage from either an intercostal artery or a fistula between an artery and the associated intercostal vein. Embolization may play a role in the management of these patients. In the acute setting with hemorrhage into the pleural space, control by embolization of the feeding vessel with absorbable material is an option. Arteriovenous fistulas may be controlled in the elective setting with either permanent or absorbable material. Occlusion of an intercostal artery should not be undertaken without a good deal of deliberation and preparation. Embolization of an intercostal artery or bronchial artery requires identification of the anterior spinal artery (the artery of Adamkiewicz) prior to embolotherapy. Inadvertent occlusion of this artery during embolization may lead to permanent paraplegia.

ABDOMEN

HEPATIC ARTERY. Indications for hepatic artery embolization include uncontrollable acute hemorrhage from blunt or penetrating trauma (see Fig. 109–13); hemobilia as the result of prior penetrating trauma often presenting as a false aneurysm; occlusion of a hepatic artery branch containing a visceral artery aneurysm; a high output state secondary to hepatic hemangioendothelioma in infants; and infarction of intrahepatic metastatic deposits for palliation of pain. Embolization is also used in patients with aberrant hepatic arteries prior to intra-arterial infusion of chemotherapeutic agents. The occlusions redistribute hepatic blood supply in an attempt to ensure that as much hepatic parenchyma as possible is perfused from a single catheter infusion site.

SPLENIC ARTERY. Partial splenic ablation using embolotherapy is directed at elevating the platelet count in patients with thrombocytopenia secondary to splenic platelet sequestration. The embolic material, usually stainless steel coils and Gelfoam, is released in the midportion of the splenic artery. The goal is to starve the spleen of most but not all of its blood supply. The intent is to prevent infarction. The effect is to reduce overall splenic size, diminishing the degree of platelet sequestration. Numerous retroperitoneal collateral vessels continue to feed the spleen through the pancreatic tail and the short gastric arteries. Splenic infarction is no longer being advocated as a means of nonsurgical removal of the spleen because of the high incidence of post-infarction abscess formation.

Pancreatic pseudocyst erosion into the splenic artery or one of its branches can create a false aneurysm of the involved vessel. Occlusion of the artery, placing coils on either side of the aneurysm origin, isolates the neck of the aneurysm. This eliminates the need for surgical exploration, which is associated with high morbidity and mortality.

GASTRIC/GASTRODUODENAL ARTERY. Acute uncontrollable upper gastrointestinal tract hemorrhage secondary to a bleeding peptic ulcer is an indication for embolotherapy. The advent of H_2 receptor blockers and endoscopic cautery techniques has virtually eliminated the need for embolization in this acute setting. If indicated, absorbable material is used so that recanalization may occur once the acute episode is over.

Visceral artery aneurysm formation and pseudoaneurysms from pancreatic pseudocyst erosion into these vessels may also be an indication for transcatheter ligation of the involved vessels in certain clinical settings. The techniques are similar to those used in the splenic artery.

RENAL ARTERY. Trauma and adjuvant therapy in the management of renal neoplasms provide the primary indications for embolotherapy in the kidney. Management of pseudoaneurysms or arteriovenous fistulas resulting from penetrating or blunt trauma currently is the leading indication for renal embolization. The advent of highly steerable guidewires and small, supple catheters that easily follow these newer guidewires permits superselective embolization of third-, fourth-, and fifth-order branching vessels in the renal parenchyma. Small-particle Ivalon and small micro coils allow permanent occlusion of these small vessels, sparing a significant portion of uninvolved renal tissue.

Main renal artery occlusion is effective in the management of hematuria and pain in patients with unresectable renal neoplasms. Preoperative renal artery occlusion to minimize intraoperative blood loss can be effective in tumor management in certain clinical settings.

Renal infarction in the management of uncontrollable hypertension is a more recent indication for renal artery occlusion and renal infarction. Ethanol or Gelfoam powder produces an effective renal infarction. In this setting, patients either are on dialysis or have renal transplants and have native kidneys that secrete renin.

TRANSPLANT RENAL ARTERY. False aneurysms or arteriovenous fistulas in renal transplants as the sequela of renal biopsy, percutaneous nephrostomy, or other invasive procedures are abnormalities that, if asymptomatic, can be managed effectively by renal embolization. Superselective techniques allow the conservative management of these problems with a minimal loss of the uninvolved, functioning transplant parenchyma.

PORTAL VEIN. Variceal bleeding, especially bleeding esophageal varices in patients with portal hypertension, may be controlled with embolotherapy. Access to the portal vein usually requires a transhepatic approach, although access using an umbilical vein approach has been described. The portal vein may also be accessed by means of a transjugular or a transabdominal wall approach. The coronary vein is the major vessel feeding esophageal varices with hepatofugal flow from the portal system. Permanent occlusion with coils and Gelfoam or ethanol is the usual occlusive technique. There is no advantage to temporary occlusion with absorbable material. The portal system has seemingly limitless collateral pathways, and, despite occlusion of the coronary vein or the short gastric veins, varices often reoccur via other pathways.

GONADAL VEIN. Testicular varicocele is a common cause of male infertility and a less frequent cause of chronic scrotal pain. Transcatheter occlusion of the testicular vein is one therapeutic approach to this problem. Permanent occlusion of the gonadal vein may be accomplished with a variety of techniques. Occlusions with detachable balloons, boiling contrast, and tissue adhesives have been described. The preferred choice is the combination of coils and Gelfoam. This combination is easy to use and keeps procedure time and fluoroscopy time to a minimum. In addition, it is highly effective in producing permanent gonadal vein occlusion. Access to the gonadal vein may be achieved from the internal jugular vein or the common femoral vein or from peripheral venous access in the arm. The femoral vein is a popular approach because of the familiarity most angiographers have with the transfemoral approach to most angiographic problems. The transjugular approach, however, allows for greater ease in selecting multiple accessory gonadal veins, as well as the right gonadal vein.

EXTREMITIES

ARTERIAL. Extremity embolotherapy has two primary areas of focus. The first is directed at lesions that result from penetrating and blunt trauma, such as false aneurysm formation and traumatic arteriovenous fistulas. When false aneurysms involve branches of the major vessels of the extremities, they can be isolated with permanent embolic material much as the surgeon would ligate the neck of an aneurysm by isolating both portions of the feeding vessel (see Fig. 109–14). Arteriovenous fistulas in branch vessels may be occluded by direct fistula embolization (see Fig. 109–14). When the major supply vessels in an extremity are involved, such as the superficial femoral artery in the thigh, these lesions are repaired surgically.

Embolotherapy also plays a role in the adjuvant therapy and the management of extremity neoplasms. Preoperative embolization of a primary or metastatic lesion to reduce the blood supply and the number of feeding vessels can diminish the complexity of a surgical procedure. This not only has the advantage of reducing the associated intraoperative blood loss, but also decreases the anesthesia time.

VENOUS. The most common symptomatic venous malformation that does not have direct arterial feeding branches is the venous hemangioma. At this time, transcatheter and transcutaneous approaches to the problem are in the early clinical trial stage.

Embolotherapy in the thorax, abdomen, and periphery is an established modality in the correct clinical setting. Expanded use is anticipated as newer materials become available and innovative techniques are developed.

Bibliography

General Bibliography

Castaneda-Zuniga WR: Transluminal Angioplasty. New York, Thieme-Stratton, 1983.

Johnsrude I, Jackson D, Dunnick N: A Practical Approach to Angiography, 2nd ed. Boston/Toronto, Little, Brown 1987.

Kadir S: Diagnostic Angiography. Philadelphia, WB Saunders Company, 1986.

Tegtmeyer C: Percutaneous transluminal angioplasty. Curr Prob Diagn Radiol, March/April, 1987.

Udoff EJ, Barth KH, Harrington DP, et al: Hemodynamic significance of iliac artery stenosis: Pressure measurements during angiography. Radiology 132:289–293, 1979.

Zwiebel WJ: Introduction to Vascular Ultrasonography, 3rd ed. Philadelphia, WB Saunders Company, 1992.

Vascular Intervention for Chronic Peripheral Arterial Disease

Castaneda-Zuniga WR, Formanek A, Tadavarthy M, et al: The mechanism of balloon angioplasty. Radiology 135:565–571, 1980.

Gunther RW, Vorwerk D, Antonucci F, et al: Iliac artery stenosis or obstruction after successful balloon angioplasty: Treatment with a self-expandable stent. AJR 156:389–393, 1991.

Hertzer NR: The natural history of peripheral vascular disease: Implications for its management. Circulation 83 (Suppl I):I-17–I-19, 1991.

Juergens JL, Barker NW, Hines EA Jr: Arterioscleroses obliterans: Review of 520 cases with special reference to pathogenic and prognostic factors. Circulation 21:118–195, 1960.

Kannel WB, McGee DL: Update on some epidemiologic features of intermittent claudification: The Framingham Study. J Am Geriatr Soc 33:13–18, 1985.

Kim D, Granturco LE, Porter DH, et al: Peripheral directional atherectony: 4-year experience. Radiology 183:778–793, 1992.

Martinelli MR, Beach KW, Glass MJ, et al: Noninvasive testing versus clinical evaluation of arterial disease: A prospective study. JAMA 241:2031–2034, 1979.

McDaniel MD, Cronenwett JL: Basic data related to the natural history of intermittent claudication. Ann Vasc Surg 3:273–277, 1989.

Palmaz JC: Balloon-expandable intravascular stent. AJR 150:1263–1269, 1988.

Palmaz JC, Garcia OH, Schatz RA, et al: Placement of balloon-expandable intraluminal stents in iliac arteries: First 171 procedures. Radiology 174:969–975, 1990.

Richter GM, Noeldge G, Roeren T, et al: First long-term results of a randomized multicenter trial: Iliac balloon expandable stent placement versus percutaneous transluminal angioplasty (abstract). Radiology 177(p):152, 1990.

Rutherford RB: Standards for evaluating and reporting results of interventional therapy for peripheral vascular disease. Circulation 83 (Suppl I):I-6–I-11, 1991.

Simpson JB, Selmon MR, Robertson GC, et al: Transluminal atherectomy for occlusive peripheral vascular disease. Am J Cardiol 61:96G–101G, 1988.

Smith GD, Shipley MJ, Rose G: Intermittent claudication, heart disease risk factors and mortality: The Whitehall Study. Circulation 82:1925–1931, 1990.

Thrombolytic Therapy in the Peripheral Arterial System

Belkin MB, Belkin B, Bucknam CA, et al: Intra-arterial fibrinolytic therapy. Arch Surg 121:769–773, 1986.

Bookstein JJ, Fellmeth B, Roberts A, et al: Pulsed-spray pharmacomechanical thrombolysis: Preliminary clinical results. AJR 15:1097–1100, 1989.

Dotter CT, Rosch J, Seaman AJ: Selective clot lysis with low-dose streptokinase. Radiology 111:31–37, 1974.

Gardiner GA: Thrombolysis of occluded arterial bypass grafts. Cardiovasc Intervent Radiol 11:558–559, 1988.
Gardiner GA, Harrington DP, Koltun W, et al: Salvage of occluded arterial bypass grafts by means of thrombolysis. J Vasc Surg 9:426–431, 1989.
Katzen BT: Technique and results of "low-dose" infusion. Cardiovasc Intervent Radiol 11:541–547, 1988.
Katzen BT, van Breda A: Low-dose streptokinase in the treatment of arterial occlusions. AJR 136:1171–1178, 1981.
Lammer J, Pilger E, Neumayer K, Schreyer H: Intra-arterial fibrinolysis: Long-term results. Radiology 161:159–163, 1986.
McNamara TO: Technique and results of "higher-dose" infusion. Cardiovasc Intervent Radiol 11:548–557, 1988.
McNamara TO, Bomberger RA: Factors affecting initial and six month patency rates after intra-arterial thrombolysis with high-dose urokinase. Am J Surg 152:709–712, 1986.
McNamara TO, Bomberger RA, Merchant RF: Intra-arterial urokinase as the initial therapy for acutely ischemic lower limbs. Circulation 83 (Suppl 1):I-106–I-119, 1991.
McNamara TO, Fischer JR: Thrombolysis of peripheral arterial and graft occlusions: Improved results using high-dose urokinase. AJR 144:769–775, 1985.
Sullivan KL, Gardiner GA, Shapiro MJ, et al: Acceleration of thrombolysis with a high-dose transthrombus bolus technique. Radiology 173:805–808, 1989.
van Breda A, Katzen BT, Deutsch AS: Urokinase versus streptokinase in local thrombolysis. Radiology 165:109–111, 1987.

Embolotherapy

Kadir S, Athanasoulis CA, Ring EJ, et al: Transcatheter embolization of intrahepatic arterial aneurysm. Radiology 128:335–338, 1980.
Levey DS, Teitelbaum GP, Finch EJ, et al: Safety and efficacy of transcatheter embolization of axillary and shoulder arterial injuries. JVIR 2:99–104, 1991.
Panetta T, Sclafani SJA, Goldstein AS, et al: Percutaneous transcatheter embolization for massive bleeding from pelvic fractures. J Trauma 25:1021–1029, 1985.
Sclafani SJA, Cooper R, Shafton GW, et al: Arterial trauma: Diagnostic and therapeutic angiography. Radiology 161:163–172, 1986.
Sclafani SJA, Shafton GW: Transcatheter treatment of injuries to the profunda femoris artery. AJR 138:463–466, 1982.

110 Cardiac MRI

Kerry M. Link, Eric M. Martin, and Stephen P. Loehr

Magnetic resonance imaging (MRI) can provide extremely useful information concerning the cardiovascular system. Spin-echo (SE) MRI provides excellent anatomic images of the heart and great vessels. Pathophysiologic information demonstrating the ramifications of congenital anomalies and acquired diseases is obtainable using gradient echo (cine) and phase (velocity) mapping techniques (VINNIE, FEER). MRI is a noninvasive, nonionizing technique that is essentially a three-dimensional imaging method with excellent contrast resolution. Flowing blood exhibits a dark signal on SE images and a bright signal on cine images, creating excellent contrast demarcation between the blood pool and the endocardium and lumen of vessels.

Its freedom from operator dependence, three-dimensional multiplanar imaging capability, large field of view (FOV), and improved spatial resolution give MRI clear advantages over echocardiography and computed tomography (CT). The ability to image all four cardiac chambers simultaneously, map myocardial contraction dynamics, and calculate velocities and pressures within the heart chambers and great arteries (phase mapping) provides clear advantages over cardiac catheterization and cine angiography.

Magnetic resonance imaging has the capability to revolutionize the way we examine cardiac diseases in a fashion similar to its role in redefining imaging studies of the nervous and musculoskeletal systems. However, despite obvious advantages, the acceptance of magnetic resonance (MR) as a primary imaging technique has been slow. In addition to the natural reluctance of physicians to accept new methods and the competition between subspecialty groups over diagnostic procedures ("turf" battles), some potential drawbacks of MRI are frequently cited. Concern exists over issues such as examination expense, resource availability, the frequent need for patient sedation, and the tendency towards long examination times. Inconsistent MR examination quality and the generally limited knowledge of MR capabilities have also slowed the acceptance of cardiovascular MRI as a valuable technique.

The purpose of this chapter is to address the last point by discussing how to tailor the capabilities of MR to specific indications for cardiovascular imaging. It is our belief that MR will soon play a major role in the examination of patients with cardiovascular disease. Considering that 50 per cent of the American population will die as a result of some form of cardiovascular disease, MR will undoubtedly increase the potential for early diagnosis of treatable conditions. Unfortunately, through the years, the radiologist's role in studying the heart has greatly diminished. Residents and practitioners alike have limited training or experience in this arena. MR can provide an avenue for radiologists to resume their role as cardiac diagnosticians, and therefore, it is important for all radiologists to become aware of the techniques of cardiac MRI, and to gain a greater understanding of cardiac embryology, anatomy, and physiology. We encourage those interested to become familiar with these subjects and basic cardiac MRI protocols, and to learn how to modify a MRI study to suit each and every patient. The interested reader should refer to additional works written by and for radiologists (Link, 1992; Kondo and Higgins, 1992).

SAFETY

Although strong magnetic fields may theoretically affect biological systems, there is no concrete evidence that detrimental effects occur at standard clinical imaging field strengths (0.15 to 1.5 Tesla [T]) (Shellock, 1989).

Perhaps the greatest safety issue for support personnel is the potential for local environmental objects of ferromagnetic composition (metal tools, IV poles, scissors, etc.) to be attracted to the bore of the magnet. This creates a potentially hazardous situation because these objects may become projectiles. Similarly, earrings, hairclips, and jewelry may pull, causing lacerations or injury. From an inconvenience standpoint, the magnet can damage credit cards, watches, and nonshielded monitoring devices. For these reasons, most devices and tools used in an MR facility are nonferromagnetic (MR-compatible) in nature.

In vivo ferromagnetic substances can be similarly affected, and, therefore, a careful patient history is mandatory prior to any MR examination. Older male patients may have shrapnel in their soft tissues, and although the shrapnel is usually "fixed" in scar, it can move and disturb the patient. When one performs rapid gradient echo exams, the shrapnel may serve as a heat depository, which can also cause the patient mild discomfort. We have studied a teenager with magnetic orthodontics who experienced significant pain when placed in the bore of the magnet (unpublished case). We therefore have these devices removed by the patient's orthodontist prior to scanning. Permanent make-up, or tattoos, are generally not a problem; however, when present on the eyelids (permanent eyeliners), any ferromagnetic material within the pigment will be affected and can lead to fairly significant lid swelling. Patients and physicians should be advised of this situation and a risk-benefit analysis discussed with the patient prior to scanning. Orthopedic traction devices are usually stainless steel. We keep a small magnet in the MR suite and simply test these devices prior to scanning. The magnetic field will not adversely move these devices; however, heat may be deposited. In these cases and all the others listed above, the patient should have access to some type of device within the magnet bore (bell, etc.) to notify the technician of any discomfort.

A much more serious problem is the presence of a ferromagnetic clip on a delicate vascular structure, such as an intracranial aneurysm clip. Independent of what part of the body is being studied, any patient with an aneurysm clip must be thoroughly investigated prior to scanning. Currently, most neurosurgeons are aware of the need to clearly document the composition of clips. New non-metallic clips are available that do not cause artifacts on follow-up scans. If there is uncertainty regarding a clip's composition and you know the type of clip, consult the classic article by Shellock and Curtis (1991) regarding biomedical implants, materials, and devices. Remember that otologic implants, bullets, dentures, and any other foreign material may be affected by the magnetic field, as well. Reviewing Shellock and Curtis (1991) prior to undertaking a rotation or career in MRI is strongly recommended.

A careful occupational history of every patient is also important. Sheet metal workers, mechanics, and other patients may have iron filings in their eyes, where heat deposition can cause significant complications. Debate still exists regarding the best way to document metallic foreign bodies. Thus, it is necessary to stay current with the literature for the sake of your patients and from a medical-legal standpoint of view.

With regard to cardiovascular system prosthetics, it is important to realize that the torque and strain induced by normal myocardial contractile forces on prosthetic heart valves exceeds any deflection induced by the magnetic field. The recommendations are that all patients with prosthetic heart valves can be imaged, except patients with Starr-Edwards pre-6000 valves. These patients must not be imaged with a greater than 0.35 T MR system when there is concern regarding valve dehiscence and annular integrity (Shellock and Curtis, 1991). Remember, however, that the metallic component of these prosthetic valves will cause localized signal loss that can interfere with interpretation of the examination, especially if there is suspicion of a valvular abscess. Similarly, patent ductus arteriosus (PDA) clips and sternal wires can also interfere with interpretation. With only limited exceptions, *no one* with a pacemaker or cardiac-assisting electromechanical device should walk into a scanner room, no less undergo an MRI study! The magnetic field and/or gradient switching may cause device malfunction with potentially life-threatening complications.

Although rapid switching of gradient fields at very high ($\geqslant$4 T) magnetic field strengths has been shown to affect the biochemical environment of certain cells, this phenomenon does not seem to occur with standard, clinical high-strength magnetic fields ($\leqslant$1.5 T). However, there have been some reports of patients suffering first-, second-, and third-degree burns because of heat deposition in electrocardiograph (EKG) wires and monitor lines after exposure to rapidly shifting gradient fields. Patients should always be instructed to notify the technician if they have any sensation of "burning." This presents a special problem with children and infants, and frequent inspections of these patients should take place when undertaking gradient echo sequences.

Although considerable evidence supports the safety of limited MRI during pregnancy (Kanal et al, 1990), examination is not advised during the first trimester unless there is no safer alternative. MRI has been effectively used in evaluating morphology and cardiovascular status in utero without adverse affects. Above all, the decision to use MRI must be made with the best interest of mother and fetus in mind, and under the advisement of the referring obstetrician. Although currently, the use of contrast agents in cardiovascular MRI is limited, there is occasionally the need to use contrast in lactating women (for cardiac tumors, myocardial ischemia). These women should be advised to refrain from breast-feeding after contrast injection for 48 hours (>90 per cent gadolinium–diethylenetriamine penta-acetic acid [Gd-DTPA] will have been excreted), during which time they should continue to express milk for discard. Women may manually express milk prior to the study and store it for use during this 48-hour period.

PULSE SEQUENCES

Cardiovascular MRI can be divided into two broad categories, which invariably demonstrate considerable overlap. By chance they are usually discussed in order of their chronological development. The first category involves anatomic or static imaging based on spin-echo (SE) imaging techniques. Spin-echo MRI offers as its greatest asset tremendous contrast resolution. With this technique, flowing fluid (blood, cerebrospinal fluid [CSF], pericardial fluid, etc.) with a velocity of greater than approximately 4 cm/sec produces a dark image, or signal void, that enables depiction of intracardiac structures (moderator band, valve apparatus, etc.) and delineation of the endocardial, myocardial, epicardial, pericardial, and other blood-vessel wall interfaces. This, coupled with its large FOV, multiplanar imaging capability, and excellent spatial resolution, gives MRI obvious advantages over echocardiography, CT, and angiography (Crooks et al, 1984). Although SE MRI is primarily a tool for anatomic diagnosis, observations regarding the pathophysiologic consequences of diseases such as left ventricular hypertrophy can be discerned. When MRI is used in conjunction with contrast agents, functional information can also be ascertained (identification of jeopardized myocardium).

The major criticism of early cardiac MRI was its inability to provide functional information similar to echocardiography and cardiac catheterization. With the advent of dynamic MRI techniques, including gradient recalled echo (GRE or cine MRI), phase or velocity mapping, breath-holding (ultra-fast MRI), and echoplanar imaging (EPI) this criticism is no longer valid. The two most widely available techniques within this second category are cine and phase mapping, both of which image the blood pool as a bright signal. The resulting image is similar to an angiogram with the important exception that the myocardium can be visualized. These techniques have been used to assess wall motion, systolic wall thickening (SWT), myocardial mass, volumetric data, the severity of valvular disease, and myocardial ischemic disease.

SPIN ECHO

The standard magnetic resonance protocol is the spin-echo sequence (Fig. 110–1). A slice is selected by creating a linearly varying gradient field along the z axis and applying a narrow band-

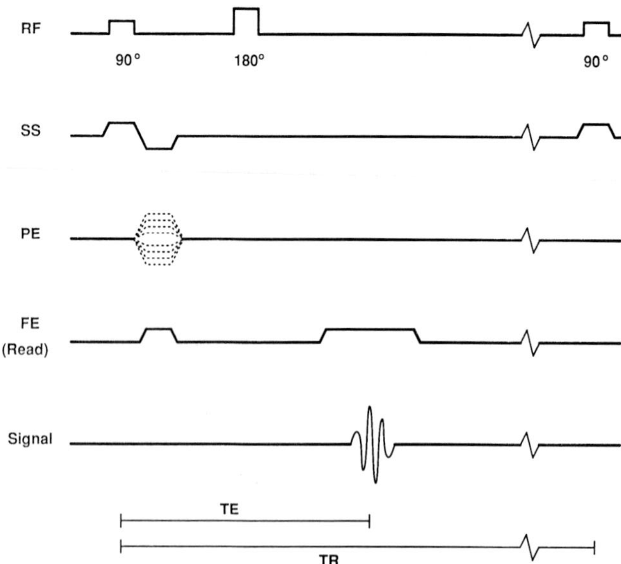

Figure 110–1. Pulse diagram of a spin-echo (SE) sequence. A 90-degree radiowave frequency (RF) pulse applied perpendicular to the z axis is combined with the slice select (SS) gradient applied along the z axis in order to define an anatomic slice for signal acquisition. The subsequent phase encoding (PE) and frequency encoding (FE or Read) gradients spatially localize information from protons within the slice, along the x and y axes, respectively. The MR signal, or echo, occurs at TE (time to echo) after application of a 180-degree, phase refocusing RF pulse at time ½ TE. The interval TR (time to repetition) represents the delay provided for magnetization to relax, or recover, before repetition of the sequence.

width radiofrequency (RF) pulse, matching the RF of the Larmor frequency of protons across a narrow region of the patient. A 90-degree RF pulse tips the net magnetization into the transverse plane and instantaneously produces phase coherence although the phase quickly disperses throughout the xy plane. After a time, ½ TE, a 180-degree RF pulse refocuses the phases back into coherence. At time TE the phases coalesce to produce an MR signal termed an echo. Accordingly, the term *TE* (time to echo) defines the interval between the 90-degree pulse and the echo. Before another 90-degree RF pulse can be generated, the magnetization must at least partially relax back to its initial state, aligned with the z axis. The required delay is termed the repetition time (TR), or the time between 90-degree pulses. This sequence of 90-degree–180-degree pulses is repeated a number of times equal to the number of phase-encoding steps in order to acquire sufficient phase information to fill the data matrix (k-space).

The parameters TE and TR can be manipulated to enhance the tissue contrast created by inherent relaxation properties specific to different tissues. T_1- (short TR, short TE) and T_2- (long TR, long TE) weighting describe sequences that accentuate differences in tissue T_1 and T_2 relaxation times, respectively. A short TR allows tissues with short T_1 to relax to equilibrium to a greater extent than those with long T_1. With cardiac MR, the pulse sequences are timed according to the ECG pattern of the patient, whereby TR is equal to the R-R interval or a multiple thereof. TR is typically on the order of 800 to 1000 msec. It is important to realize that, because TR is equal to the R-R interval, standard SE cardiac studies are not truly T_1-weighted. A short TE minimizes the effects of T_2 relaxation and provides more T_1 weighting. With cardiac MR, TEs are generally on the order of 20 to 30 msec.

On standard cardiac "T_1-weighted" studies (the bread and butter pulse sequence), fat appears with high (bright) signal intensity, the myocardium and fibrous tissues have intermediate (gray) signal intensity; and flowing blood and pericardial fluid have low (black) signal, or signal void. The absence of signal is due to exit effects: Rapidly flowing substances do not remain within the slice long enough to experience both pulses, and therefore, return no signal. By the same reasoning, slow flow may result in the production of regions of high signal within the intravascular pool (Bradley and Waluch, 1985; Waluch and Bradley, 1984). Because this may obscure intracavitary and intravascular structures, presaturation slabs are often used to overcome this phenomenon by limiting the possible signal intensity from slow inflowing spins.

To obtain images at comparable phases of the cardiac cycle, one employs ECG gating techniques. Image acquisition is triggered by the R wave of the ECG tracing. A typical acquisition delay of 40 to 60 msec from the R wave initiates data acquisition during systole, when steady flow velocities produce a more constant signal void.

Multi-slice SE techniques utilize the time normally spent waiting during TR to obtain data from additional slices. This technique is also triggered by the R wave and produces a series of images that usually encompass the entire heart. The advantage is a tremendous saving in overall image acquisition time. The disadvantage is that neighboring slices are obtained at different phases of the cardiac cycle. This must always be remembered when analyzing the images and as a result, this technique cannot be used to calculate volumetric data.

GRADIENT RECALLED ECHO

Gradient recalled echo (GRE) sequences obtain an MR echo signal by using rapidly reversing magnetic field gradients instead of the 180-degree RF pulse used to produce an echo with SE techniques (Fig. 110–2). Gradient echo sequences also differ from SE studies in the fact that they employ a shorter TE and a flip angle (FA) less than 90 degrees. This RF pulse transfers only a fraction of the net magnetization into the xy plane, leaving a greater net magnetization residual along the z axis. The result is more magnetization that can be flipped on the next pass without having to depend on T_1 relaxation processes. The overall effect is to shorten the delay between RF pulses (TR) while maintaining a steady state of net magnetization along the z axis. Acronyms for this technique include GRASS (gradient recall at steady state) and FLASH (fast low angle shot).

With a 1.5-T system, flip angles of 30 degrees are routinely used to obtain a steady state. TE ranges between 6 and 12 msec, depending on gradient capabilities and FOV. Smaller FOVs require longer TE values. TR ranges from 20 to 30 msec, enabling data acquisition from multiple phases of the cardiac cycle during each R-R interval. The sequence is repeated by the number of phase encoding steps to complete the data matrix.

ECG gating techniques are employed to obtain images at comparable points in the cardiac cycle. Since the TR is shorter than the R-R interval, images are post-processed by techniques that retrospectively reference each acquisition to the ECG R wave signal (Crooks et al, 1984). For this reason, GRE techniques are ECG-referenced and not strictly ECG-gated. The first image of the multiphase series of images is obtained 40 to 60 msec after the R wave. Subsequent reordering enables cine display of up to 50 phases of a single cardiac cycle at a single plane, providing temporal resolution equivalent to or better than ventriculography.

Overall tissue contrast in GRE studies is inferior to that demonstrated with SE techniques; however, image acquisition time is substantially shortened. Another important advantage is the bright signal generated by flowing blood (Sechtem et al, 1987). GRE techniques create flow signal enhancement by maximizing entry effects and minimizing exit effects. Entry effects describe how new fully magnetized spins enter an anatomic slice on the time scale of TR, providing for increased magnetization transfer upon the next

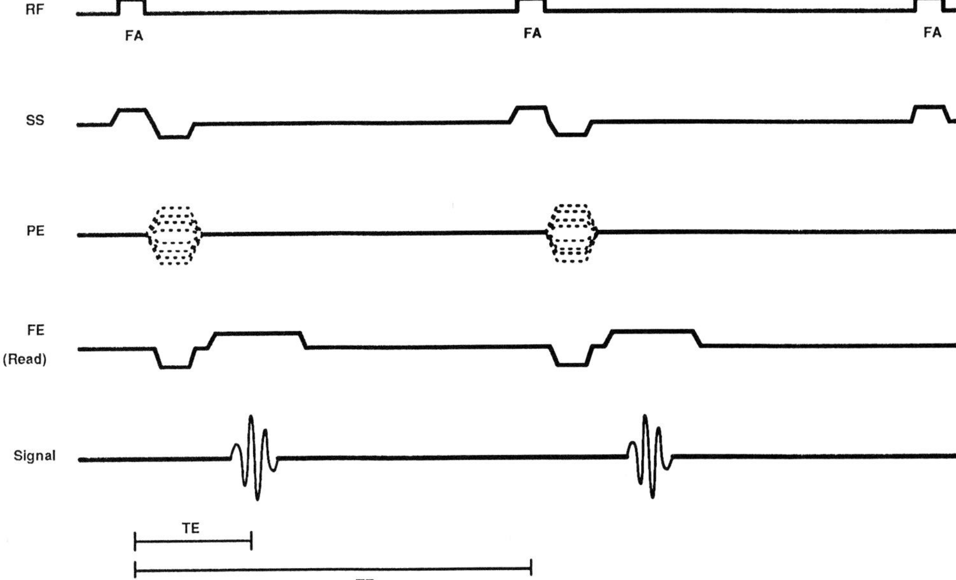

Figure 110–2. Pulse diagram of a gradient recalled echo (GRE) sequence. Information is spatially localized in the same manner as the SE sequence. SS, PE, and FE have their standard meanings. The 90-degree pulse of the SE sequence is replaced by a RF pulse of a lower flip angle (FA). An echo is generated by the reversal of gradients instead of a 180-degree RF pulse. As a result, TR and TE are much shorter than in the corresponding SE values.

RF pulse. A short TE then ensures a high proportion of the spins within a slice are able to return an echo. Signal enhancement is thus proportional to blood velocity and allows qualitative interpretation of flow within cardiac chambers and the great vessels. Excessive flow velocities and turbulent flow lead to loss of signal intensity, which is useful in the detection of valvular disease (Evans et al, 1988). Delineation of both the intrachamber blood pool and myocardium on images from end-diastole and end-systole allows calculation of volumetric data and assessment of ventricular contraction dynamics (Fig. 110–3).

PHASE MAPPING TECHNIQUES

Phase or velocity mapping techniques utilize the phase component of the MR signal to produce images that reflect the movement of protons over time. Spins accumulate phase shifts proportional to their velocity as they flow through a slice during and in the direction of an applied gradient field (Moran, 1982; Bryant et al, 1984). These techniques make use of phase compensation methods such as gradient moment nulling (GMN) to refocus spins initially, and then to adjust spins according to the degree of phase shift experienced after a specified time (Fig. 110–4). The resultant phase shifts are directly proportional to the velocity of spins. To account for bidirectional flow, phases are recorded on a scale from −180 to +180 degrees, with negative phase shifts corresponding to retrograde flow and positive phase shifts corresponding to antegrade flow (Fig. 110–5). Higher velocities correspond to larger phase shifts. The gray scale is also split equally, assigning a phase shift of +180 to the brightest pixel and −180 to black. Phase techniques allow for both qualitative and quantitative information regarding cardiovascular function. Complex flow patterns can impair velocity measurements by enhancing phase dispersion, leading to signal loss and less accurate flow measurements.

To maximize sensitivity to velocity, a range of velocities must be assigned to the spectrum of phase shifts. Phase shifts that exceed prior estimations lead to misregistration effects called aliasing. A high velocity may actually register a +200 degree phase shift, but, limited by the convention, this would correspond to a phase shift of −20 degrees, and therefore, be misrepresented on the final image as retrograde flow by a low (meaning slow) signal intensity. These techniques currently play a role in the quantitative assessment of valvular disease, shunt lesions, and cardiomyopathies (Fig. 110–6) (Underwood et al, 1987).

PRE-EXAMINATION SCREENING

As with all radiographic examinations, patients scheduled to undergo a cardiovascular MR study must be thoroughly screened by the radiologist. In addition to the safety issues discussed above, it is mandatory to review the patient's chart and discuss the case with the referring physician. It must be determined whether or not the patient will require sedation (almost universally needed in patients < 10 years of age). In the usual situation, children can be

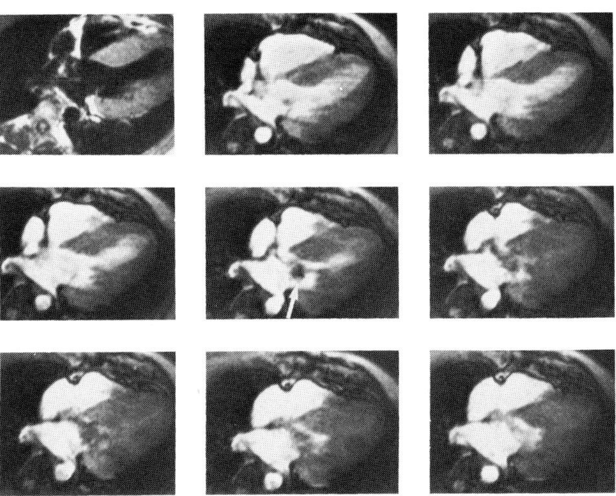

Figure 110–3. *Left,* **ECG-gated horizontal long-axis SE image depicts symmetrical hypertrophic cardiomyopathy, with normal myocardium at the apex.** The remaining images are GRE ECG-referenced images at the same location during multiple phases of the cardiac cycle. Notice the region of turbulent flow *(arrow)* corresponding to valvular regurgitation. At peak systole, there is no demonstrable end-systolic volume, corresponding to an approximate 100 per cent ejection fraction.

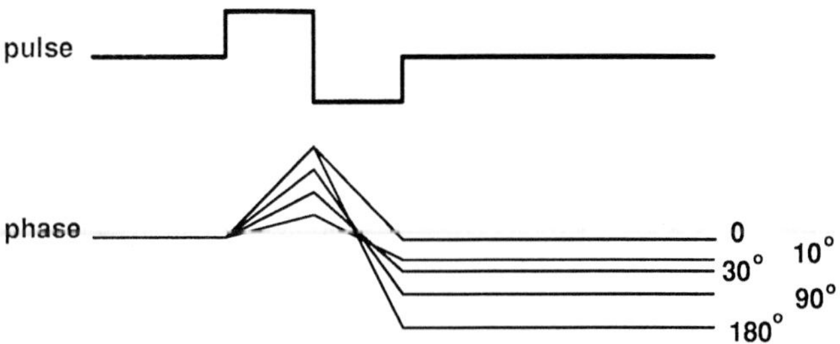

Figure 110–4. Effects of gradients and velocity on phase. Two gradient pulses of equal magnitude and opposite polarity refocus the phases of spins in static tissue back to their initial value. Spins moving along an applied gradient accumulate phase changes at rates proportional to their velocities. The second gradient pulse adjusts the phase shifts experienced after a certain time. The resultant phase changes (10, 30, 90 and 180 degrees) are translated into velocities. Dipolar velocity encoding gradients may be applied in one, two, or three directions, allowing determination of velocity along three dimensions.

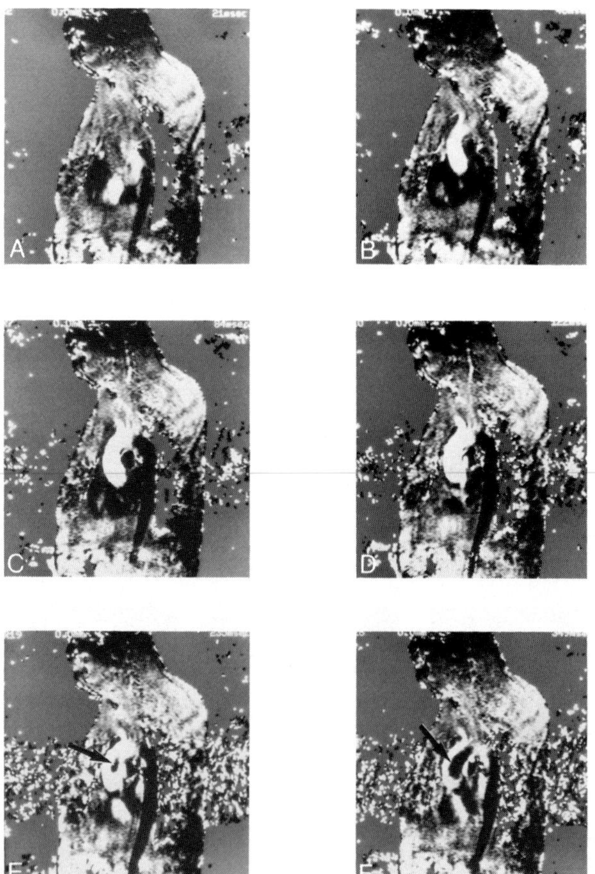

Figure 110–5. *A* to *F*, **Left anterior oblique phase (velocity) mapping images taken at the same plane during different phases of the cardiac cycle demonstrate the directional information obtained from aortic flow with such techniques.** The ascending aortic flow in *B* appears bright, whereas the descending aortic flow appears dark *(C and D).* Retrograde aortic flow *(arrows in E and F)* back into the ascending aorta during early diastole appears dark. This flow will eventually fill the coronary arteries during mid-to-late diastole.

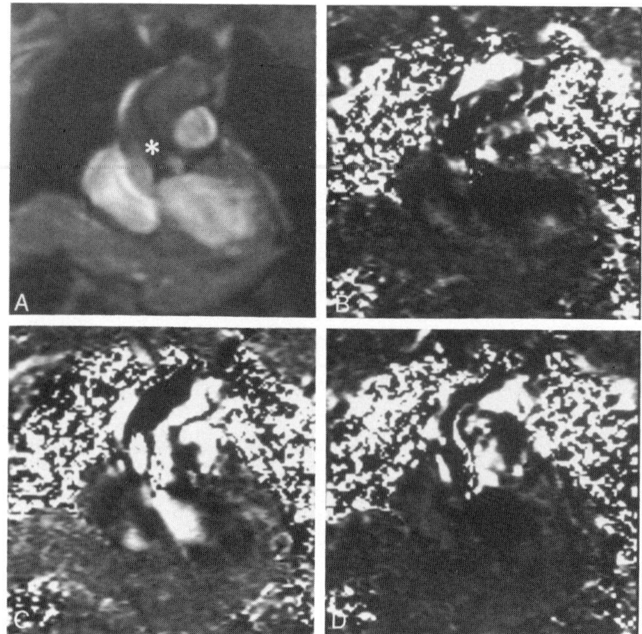

Figure 110–6. Coronal magnitude (*A*) and tridirectional phase mapping (*B* to *D*) images depict aortic valvular stenosis. The post-stenotic flow jet *(asterisk)* appears dark (signal void) and extends distally into the ascending aorta. The phase mapping data correspond to the velocity in the right-to-left, anterior-to-posterior, and superior-to-inferior directions. A composite of the phase images can be generated to compute a final velocity. In this patient, the peak transvalvular flow velocity was 2874 mm/second or 2.87 m/second. Using a modified Bernoulli's equation ($P = 4v^2$), a pressure gradient of 33 mm Hg was obtained.

sedated and monitored by the staff radiologist or MRI nurse. Although there are a number of sedation protocols advocated with children, we prefer to administer pentobarbital (Nembutal), 2 to 6 mg/kg IM, 30 minutes before the examination. For adults, we have found diazepam (Valium), 5 to 10 mg parenterally, to work in most cases.

The cardiopulmonary status must be assessed because this patient population is in general sicker than patients routinely studied with MRI. All cardiac patients require close supervision, and this is especially true in patients with complex congenital heart disease (CHD) and those with ischemic myocardial disease. In most cases, this can be done by the radiologist or MRI nurse. Patients can be monitored using pulse oximetry (units are now made specifically for MR suites) and respiratory bellows. The latter is routinely used to employ respiratory compensation schemes and therefore may already be in place for use as a monitoring device. It is not uncommon to require assistance from an anesthesiologist. This is mandatory with intubated patients.

As discussed below, the magnetic field has a dramatic and deleterious effect on the patient's ECG tracing; thus, only the heart rate can reliably be followed using current ECG gating devices. This becomes a disadvantage when performing dipyridamide stress studies with MRI. Presently several companies are investigating truly MRI-compatible ECG monitoring devices.

ECG GATING

Perhaps the foremost practical limitation of MRI is its sensitivity to motion. Both voluntary and involuntary motion create artifacts that degrade the quality of cardiovascular images. An obvious cause of induced artifact is patient motion, hence the need for sedation in infants, most children, patients in pain, and those suffering from claustrophobia. Perhaps less apparent are motion-induced artifacts caused by eye movement, CSF pulsations, swallowing, peristalsis, respiratory motion, blood flow, and myocardial contraction. Presuming that the patient remains still during the examination, motion degradations from ocular movements, CSF pulsations and swallowing are insignificant when studying the heart. Esophageal peristalsis may interfere when looking for vascular rings or performing MR angiography of the thoracic aorta.

The most obvious and troublesome type of motion is that of the beating heart itself. This problem may be overcome by acquiring data at a consistent specified time within the heart cycle over a series of heart beats. MR systems sequence acquisitions using the patient's R-R cycle as a temporal reference, hence the need for continual ECG monitoring throughout the study. Systems either predetermine exactly when in the cardiac cycle information will be gathered (ECG-gated), or use the cardiac cycle as a reference over which information is post-processed (ECG-referenced). Thus, the single most important means to overcome motion degradation when studying the heart is the use of ECG gating. It is imperative that the radiologist be intimately familiar with the implementation of this technique (Mirowitz et al, 1992).

The ECG is a measurement of electrical potentials of the heart, and is in turn the result of voltages generated from individual cardiac muscle cells. The magnetic field will have an affect on the electrical potentials and therefore on the ECG tracing (distortion). It is not important to interpret the actual tracing (except for in dipyridamole-induced stress MRI), but rather to maintain a point in the cardiac cycle (R-wave) that the scanner can consistently recognize and use as a trigger or reference. As such, certain steps must be taken to maximize the vector sum of myocardial voltages, so as to produce a distinguishable R-wave for proper gating and therefore "motion-free" images.

The first step in setting up the cardiac MRI examination is to review the patient's most recent 12-lead ECG. Patients with dysrhythmias usually are not candidates for ECG-gated MRI. In these cases, a standard SE MRI performed with a high number of averages or excitations (NSA or NEX) will almost always provide better image quality than an ECG-gated study. This is an area where breath-holding techniques and EPI will play an important role.

Recall that ferromagnetic substances placed in a magnetic field will be magnetized (alignment of electrons), and when exposed to cyclic/switching gradients can generate a localized small electric field. Thus, metallic ECG electrodes will adversely affect the tracing and serve as a heat sink that may potentially burn a patient. The electrodes on the ECG patches must be nonferromagnetic (i.e., graphite). Several investigators have found that placing the ECG patches on the patient's chest (as opposed to the extremities) in a tight triangular configuration maximizes the vector sums and produces a more reliable ECG tracing (Fig. 110–7*A*). This also avoids the ECG tracing degradation that occurs when a patient inevitably moves an extremity. In order to minimize tracing degradation due to normal respiratory movement, many advocate lead placement on the patient's back (Fig. 110–7*B*). In our experience, this is uncomfortable to the patient, and a lead invariably becomes dislodged during the course of the study. It is recommended that the patches be placed on the patient prior to administration of sedative medications. Once the patient is asleep, there is a high probability that the patient will awaken during patch placement. This is especially true with children and infants.

When draping the leads over the patient, one should place them across the patient's chest parallel to the z axis (the bore of the magnet). The leads themselves can cause electric flux if they form a loop within the magnetic field. To minimize this phenomenon, braid the leads about one another, thereby negating the flux of each individual lead.

Initially check the ECG tracing with the patient on the gantry outside of the magnetic bore. If necessary, rearrange the leads (at the junction box and not on the patient's chest) to achieve a tall R-wave. Re-evaluate the tracing after the patient is in the magnet because there is invariably distortion of the tracing. Again, if necessary, rearrange the leads to achieve a maximal R-wave. Although this may seem time-consuming, the routine is critical, and otherwise image quality is almost certainly sacrificed. Finally, check the ECG

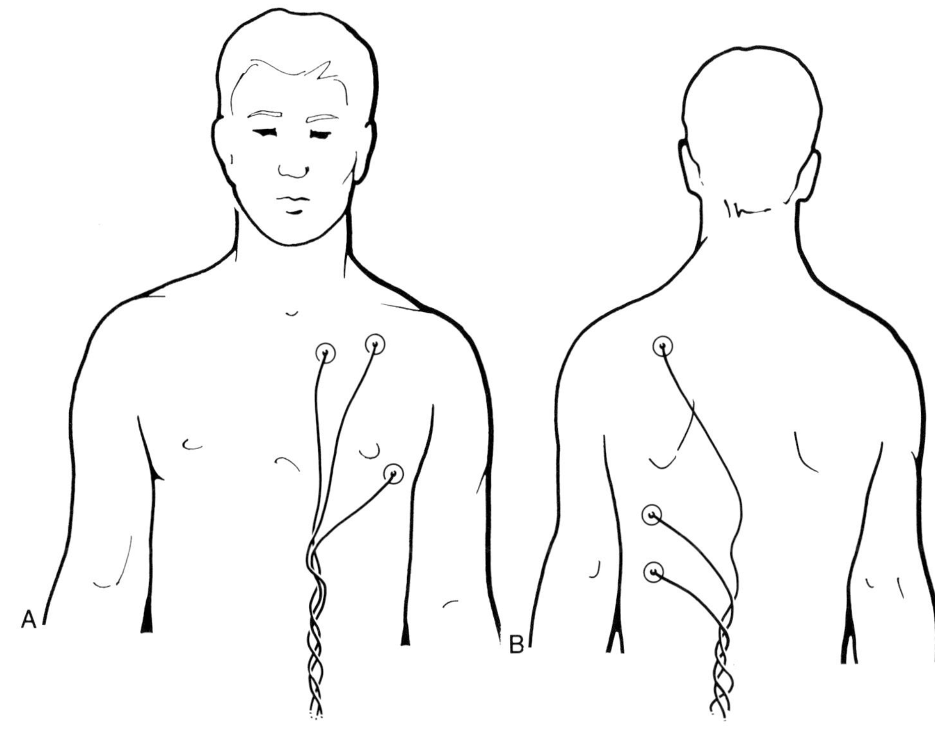

Figure 110–7. *A,* **ECG lead placement on the anterior chest wall.** A triangular configuration with two electrodes forming the base of the triangle just below the left clavicle and the third electrode just below the left nipple maximizes cardiac vector potentials. Braiding the ECG leads negates the electric flux generated by a wire loop in a magnetic field. Although respiratory motion may adversely affect the signal with the anterior placement, there is less tendency for electrode dislodgement than with posterior placement. *B,* **ECG lead placement on the posterior left hemithorax.** The electrodes are placed parallel to the long axis of the scapula. Again, the leads are braided. ECG signal intensity is weaker with the posterior placement secondary to the increased distance from the heart.

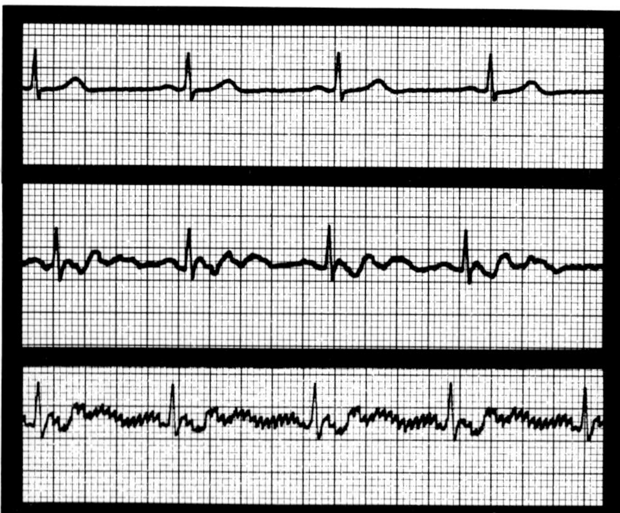

Figure 110–8. Series of ECG tracings from a patient undergoing cardiovascular SE MRI. The top strip was taken with the patient lying on the gantry outside the bore of the magnet. Note the optimally distinct R-waveform. The middle strip is of the same patient after positioning within the bore of the magnet, but prior to initiation of the scan. Notice the distortion caused by the magnetic field, and the still distinct R-waveform. The bottom tracing was obtained during a SE sequence. The multiple small inflections after the R-wave represent the pulsed slice select gradient, and correspond to the number of slices acquired. Despite this additional degradation of the ECG tracing, the R-waveform remains distinct for use as a reference for ECG gating.

tracing during the course of the study to make sure the R-wave is preserved. The applied gradient magnetic fields further distort the ECG tracing (Fig. 110–8).

RESPIRATORY COMPENSATION

Compensation for respiratory motion involves a technique similar to that used for cardiac motion. Data are referenced to specific phases of the respiratory cycle, which is monitored by a bellows apparatus affixed to the chest of the patient. Images are acquired in the normal fashion and then reordered to match the phases of a single inspiratory/expiratory cycle. No increase in scan time results. The technique is called respiratory ordered phase encoding (ROPE) (Bailes et al, 1985). The improvement in image quality is significant, and if available, respiratory motion compensation techniques should be used during all cardiac MRI studies.

IMAGING PARAMETERS

The typical cardiac MRI study starts with a series of SE acquisitions. Because the study is gated, the TR is equal to the patient's heart rate, or the R-R interval of the ECG tracing. Because no patient has a truly regular rate and rhythm, it is advisable to set the TR to 85 per cent of the R-R interval. In this manner, if the patient's heart rate increases (shortening the R-R interval), data acquisition may still take place. Otherwise data acquisition may not occur for several heart beats and the study time will become longer. As a general rule, the TE should be 20 to 30 msec and the FA should remain constant at 90 degrees.

When setting up an MRI study, one must make many decisions regarding several other imaging parameters. These must be balanced against possible trade-offs in signal-to-noise ratio (SNR), spatial resolution, contrast resolution, and total image acquisition time. Contrast resolution is not really a problem when seeking to establish an anatomic diagnosis. Occasionally, a T_2-weighted study is required for evaluation of a myocardial tumor, ischemia, or documentation of the relative age of hemopericardium. This is achieved by making the TR two to three times the R-R interval and increasing the TE to 60 msec.

The challenge of cardiac MR is balancing the length of an individual sequence with the need for spatial resolution and adequate SNR. Although guidelines dictating the specific parameters for the slice thickness, matrix size, and number of signal acquisitions (NSA) are helpful, set protocols may require modification for image optimization, especially with cardiac MRI. Understanding the rationale for selecting values for the various imaging parameters is essential and warrants additional discussion.

A few basic relationships between variable parameters and their effects on scan time, spatial resolution, and SNR must be understood. The relationships are best described as follows:

$$\text{Scanning time} = \text{TR} \times \text{NSA} \times N_x$$

$$\text{Spatial resolution} = \text{FOV}_x/N_x \times \text{FOV}_y/N_y \text{ (for 2-D imaging)}$$

where TR and NSA have their standard meanings, N_x is the number of phase encoding steps (with routine anterior-posterior direction), N_y is the number of frequency encoding steps, and FOV is typically measured in centimeters along both the x and y axes. FOV_x and FOV_y are routinely equivalent in 2-dimensional (2-D) imaging. The dimensions N_x and N_y describe the data matrix.

The SNR is another important measure of image quality. Equations defining SNR are complex, but within the scope of this article, a brief description of how to improve or increase SNR is warranted. A straightforward way to increase SNR is to increase the size of the voxel from which the signal emanates, although this will decrease spatial resolution. Methods to increase voxel size include increasing FOV, increasing slice thickness, and reducing the dimensions of the data matrix by decreasing N_x. All these changes result in a decrease in spatial resolution. Increasing NSA and TR also improve SNR at the cost of increasing scan time. Another method to increase SNR involves increasing the gap between slices in order to exclude cross-talk between neighboring slices. A widened gap, however, may miss anatomic structures or pathology. Review of the above relationships makes it apparent that changing any one parameter usually affects one or more measure of image quality.

Because the TR is set by the R-R interval in ECG-gated SE MR, scanning time can be modified by changing the NSA or number of phase encodings. Shortening the study time by decreasing the NSA decreases SNR. Diminishing the number of phase encoding steps adversely affects spatial resolution. Attempting to increase spatial resolution by decreasing the FOV decreases SNR. Increasing the number of phase encodings to increase spatial resolution increases scan time and also decreases SNR.

Advantages of decreasing sequence acquisition time include decreasing the amount of motion degradation and increasing the number of individual sequences possible during the allotted study time. By increasing spatial resolution the images become less "blurry," allowing visualization of smaller anatomic structures such as valve leaflets and coronary arteries. Increasing SNR makes the image less grainy, giving overall better image quality.

Why are these variables less of an issue with MR of the nervous and musculoskeletal systems? Firstly these studies are not cardiac-gated and are shorter in duration. Secondly and very importantly, there are dedicated coils available for these organ systems. These coils provide a dramatic decrease in FOV while maintaining good SNR, and result in better spatial resolution and image quality. For these reasons, whenever possible, scan infants and small children in a head or knee coil. Work is taking place to develop a dedicated cardiac coil for adults. Our experience with the use of cardiac coils has demonstrated a marked improvement in spatial resolution and image quality.

In summary, the following protocol describes the typical SE cardiac exam:

TR = R-R interval
TE = 20 msec
FOV = 35 to 45 cm (body coil)
16 to 25 cm (dedicated coil)
NSA = 4
Matrix 192 × 256
Slice thickness 8 mm (adults)
4 mm (infants and children)
Interslice gap 2 mm (adults)
1 mm (infants and children)

With GRE and phase mapping sequences, the same fundamental concepts dictate the manipulation of parameters to control scan time, spatial resolution, and SNR. Additional improvements in contrast resolution may result from alteration of the TR, TE, and FA. Similar to SE exams, selecting a shorter TR and TE favors more T_1 weighting, whereas selecting a longer TR and TE favors more T_2* weighting. A larger FA favors T_1 weighting and a smaller FA favors T_2* weighting. Thus, optimal contrast between the blood pool and myocardium on GRE studies results from selection of short TR and TE and a low FA. These parameter settings also favor flow enhancement caused by entry and exit effects. A typical protocol for GRE cardiac imaging on a high-field (1.5-T) scanner may involve:

TR = 20 to 30 msec
TE = 6 to 12 msec
FA = 30 degrees
FOV = 30 to 45 cm (body coil)
16 to 25 cm (dedicated coil)
NSA = 2
Matrix 192 × 256
Slice thickness 8 mm (adults)
4 mm (infants and children)
Interslice gap 2 mm (adults)
1 mm (infants and children)
Cardiac phases 16 to 32

IMAGING PLANES AND CARDIAC ANATOMY

It is probably safe to assume that most radiologists are not as familiar with cardiac anatomy as they are with the rest of the body. Because of the heart's configuration, it is necessary to be familiar not only with transaxial, coronal, and sagittal views but also with the horizontal long- (four-chamber) and short-axis views used with echocardiography. Although it is not our purpose to present an atlas of cardiac anatomy, it is important to discuss certain aspects of anatomy encountered on the more commonly used imaging planes, and indicate which planes are best suited for studying particular aspects of the heart.

The transaxial plane is the bread-and-butter imaging plane in cardiac MRI (Fig. 110–9). It also serves as an excellent starting point for discussions regarding cardiac anatomy. The interventricular septum (IVS) lies at approximately a 45-degree angle in relationship to the patient's back. This oblique orientation is parallel, but slightly anterior, to the oblique angulation of the interatrial septum (IAS). In cases of malrotation and malposition this angulation will be altered. The IVS bows slightly into the right ventricle (RV), reflecting the normally higher pressures within the left ventricle. In cases of Eisenmenger's physiology there will be a straightening or reversal of the IVS configuration. The tricuspid valve apparatus lies closer to the cardiac apex than does the mitral valve apparatus. In the normal anatomic situation, this results in a portion of the IVS (the membranous portion) separating the right atrium (RA) and left ventricle (LV). The muscular portion of the IVS and the LV myocardium average 10 mm in thickness. The RV myocardium and atrial walls are usually 3 mm in thickness. In SE MRI, the flow void of blood is contrasted against the endocardium, allowing visualization of intracavitary structures such as the papillary muscles and the moderator band. The latter, a hallmark of the RV, is helpful in identifying the ventricle in cases of complex congenital heart disease. Typically the anterior and septal leaflets of the tricuspid valve are also demonstrated in this imaging plane. Where the inferior vena cava (IVC) joins the posterolateral aspect of the RA, it is common to see what at first glance looks like an atrial septal defect (ASD). This is in fact the fossa ovalis, a very thin portion of the IAS that is typically volume averaged so as to appear similar to an ASD. This positional relationship of the IVC and fossa ovalis should remind you that oxygenated blood entering the IVC from the placenta is shunted across the fossa ovalis, thereby bypassing the lungs in fetal circulation. It is not uncommon to see a curvilinear structure anterior to the IVC extending into the RA, the eustachian valve, which in utero deflected blood from the IVC across the fossa ovalis.

The transaxial view is also best for identifying the pulmonary veins (all four typically seen in over 90 per cent of studies) and pulmonary arteries. The transverse orientation of the main pulmonary arteries enables studying patients with congenital obstructive lesions of the pulmonary arteries, such as tetralogy of Fallot, and with acquired obstructive lesions such as central pulmonary emboli. The pericardial sac and pericardial fluid demonstrate a dark signal that is contrasted against the white epicardial and pericardial fat. The combination of the pericardial sac and space (filled with fluid) is referred to as the pericardial complex, and is typically 2 mm or less in thickness. A normal thinning of the pericardial fat along the posterolateral aspect of the left ventricle makes it difficult to assess the pericardial complex. Nevertheless, transaxial MRI is the diagnostic imaging modality of choice for studying pericardial disease.

Utilizing a large FOV and the coronal imaging plane (Fig. 110–10), MR becomes an invaluable tool for assessment of patients with mesocardia and dextrocardia. The heart must be evaluated for bulboventricular loop configuration, type of situs (determined by the location of the RA), ventricular inversion (reversal of left-right orientation) and transposition (reversal of the anterior-posterior orientation). The types of atrioventricular and ventriculoarterial connections, and the bronchial and abdominal situs should be evaluated at the same time. The normal right-sided placement of the aorta (d-aorta) in relationship to the pulmonary artery is also nicely depicted in this plane.

Anatomically the coronal imaging plane is very well suited for studying the systemic venous return patterns and the LV outflow tract. Usually the entire length of the SVC can be visualized as it enters the RA. Because of the continuity of the left ventricular outflow tract, aortic annulus, sinuses of Valsalva, and sinotubular junction, this plane is also well suited for studying subaortic, aortic valvular, and supra-aortic stenoses, asymmetrical subaortic hypertrophic cardiomyopathy, and aortic insufficiency with left ventricular dilation. Because of the orientation of the IVS, the septum is seen en face on several adjacent coronal images. The ascending aorta can usually be demonstrated in a single coronal image. For this reason, this is the plane of choice for evaluation of ascending aortic abnormalities, including aneurysms, dissections, and aortic valvular processes. The view is especially informative when using cine and phase mapping techniques.

The horizontal long-axis view (four-chamber view) is a double-oblique view that is very useful for evaluating the myocardium and the mitral and aortic valves, even though it is somewhat time-consuming to perform the two scout views required to establish the proper imaging plane (Fig. 110–11). Because of the spiral nature of the IVS, the transaxial view actually shortens the IVS. The IVS is

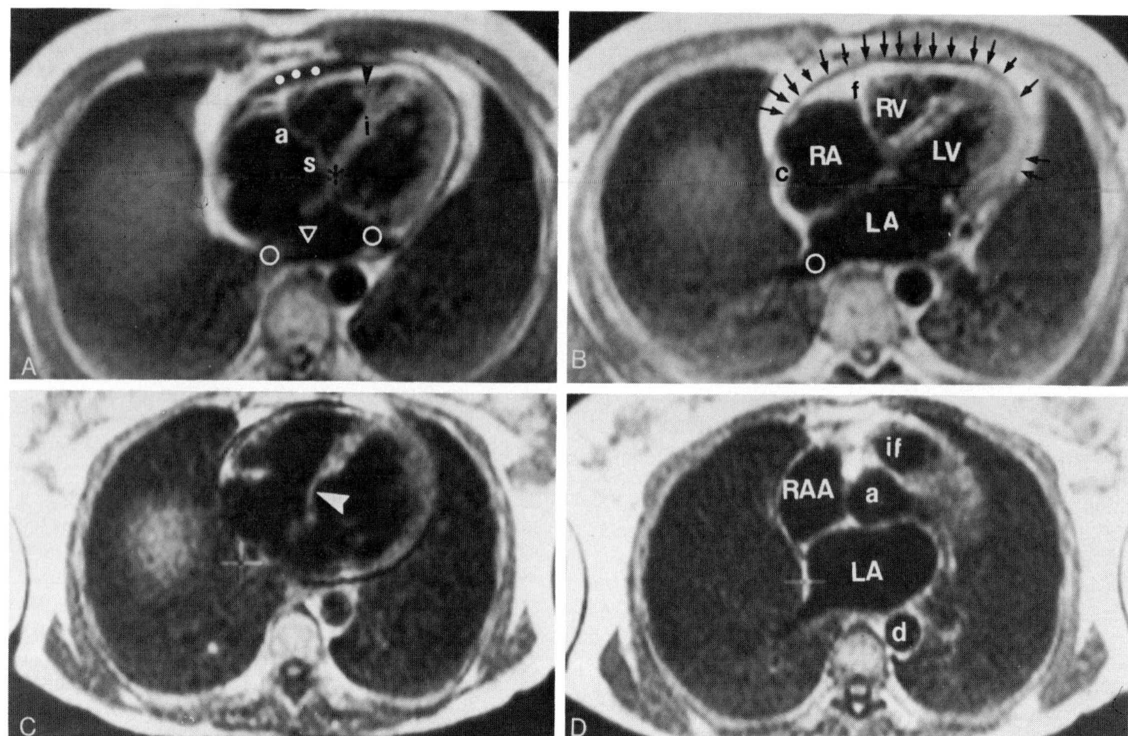

Figure 110–9. Series of transverse images through the heart beginning at the diaphragm (*A*) and extending to the cardiac base (*D*). *A* and *B,* The interventricular septum (IVS) (i) forms approximately a 45-degree angle with the back of the patient. It is parallel, but slightly anterior, to the interatrial septum (IAS). The IVS bows slightly towards the RV, reflecting the increased pressure in the LV. The tricuspid valve apparatus is closer to the cardiac apex than is the mitral valve apparatus. This leaves a portion of the RA separated from the LV by the membranous IVS *(asterisk).* The anterior (a) and septal (s) leaflets of the tricuspid valve are commonly imaged. Also note the moderator band *(arrowhead)* in the RV. The IVC-RA junction is seen on the more inferior images. The IAS in this region is thinned out and mimics an ASD *(open arrowhead).* This represents the region of the fossa ovalis. The pulmonary veins *(open circles)* are best demonstrated on the transverse view. There is high–signal intensity fat (f) in the right atrioventricular (AV) groove, which reflects the normal presence of epicardial fat. The low signal surrounding the heart represents the pericardial complex *(small arrows).* It is difficult to discern the complex along the posterolateral aspect of the LV due to typical absence of epicardial fat in that region. The complex is normally 2 mm thick or less. In this patient, it is 4 mm thick directly behind the sternum, where barely distinguishable fibrous bands are seen *(dots),* indicating localized constrictive pericarditis. The crista terminalis (c) is visible in the posterior aspect of the RA. This ridge along the internal atrial surface corresponds to the junction of the right auricle and sinus venereum. *C and D,* Note the normal thinning of the membranous IVS as it approaches the cardiac base *(arrowhead).* The RV possesses an infundibulum (if) that separates the tricuspid valve from the pulmonary valve. As a result, the pulmonic valve lies anterior and to the left of the normal d-aorta (a). The LA is the most posterior and superior chamber. The RA appendage (RAA) has a broad triangular base. The lumen of the descending aorta (d) is seen along the left paraspinal border.

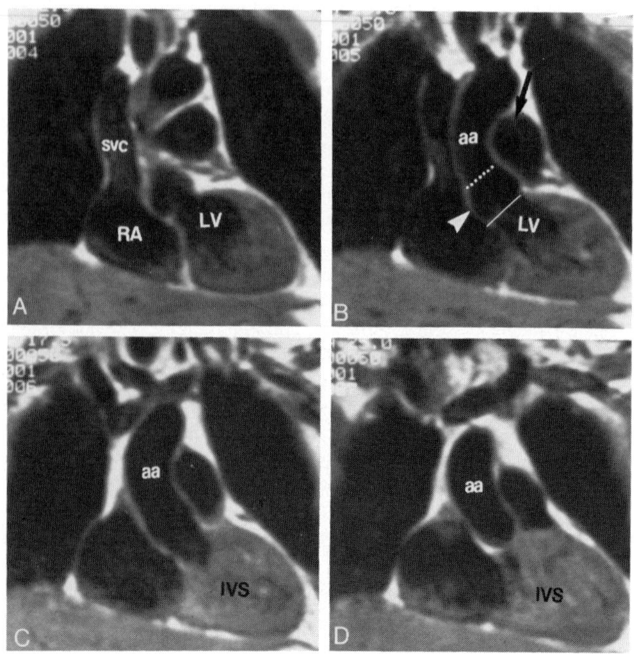

Figure 110–10. Sequential posterior to anterior (*A* to *D*) ECG-gated coronal SE MR images. The continuity of the SVC and RA is beautifully demonstrated in this imaging plane, as is the ascending aorta (aa). The continuity of the LV, aortic annulus *(solid line),* sinus of Valsalva *(arrowhead),* sinotubular junction *(dotted line),* and ascending aorta (aa) are best demonstrated in the coronal plane. This makes this plane ideal for studying aortic valve abnormalities. As we proceed anteriorly, we see the IVS en face. The anteriorly located RV is not demonstrated well with this particular plane. Note that the aortic valve is to the right and is posterior to the pulmonic valve *(arrow),* hence the name dextro- or d-aorta.

Figure 110–11. Method for set-up of the horizontal long-axis (four-chamber) view and the short-axis view. A transaxial scout view is obtained through the mid-aspect of the heart *(A)*. A second scout view *(B)* is obtained by scanning along a line drawn between the apex and the mid-aspect of the LA *(dotted line)*. This second scout view is the longitudinal long-axis view. A set of horizontal long-axis views are obtained by scanning the axis parallel to a line drawn between the apex and LA *(dotted line)*. By scanning perpendicular to this line *(solid line)*, short-axis views are generated.

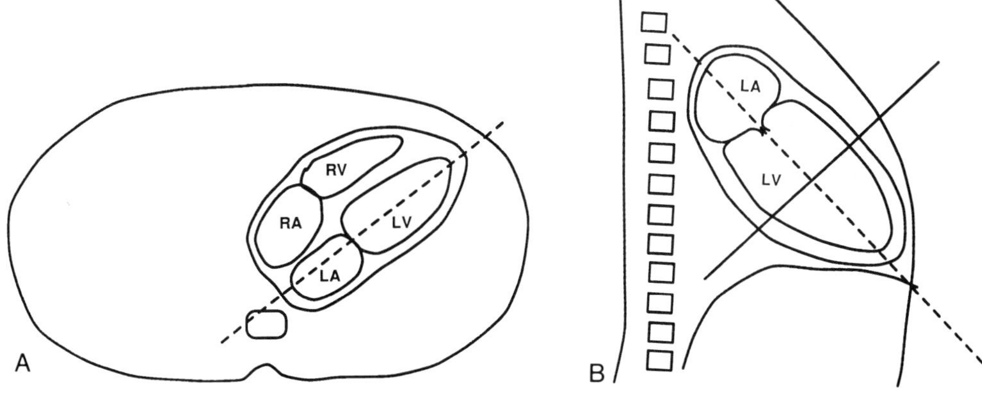

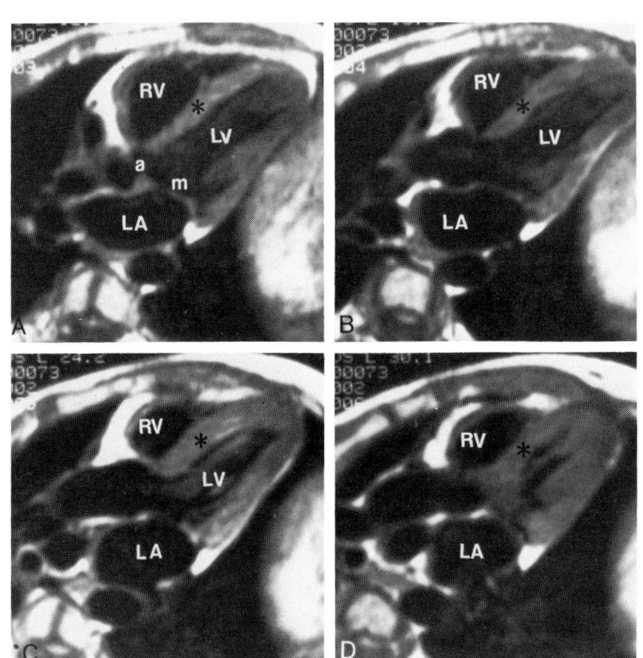

Figure 110–12. Series of horizontal long-axis views starting at the mid-aspect of the heart and extending superiorly (*A* to *D*). Note that the IVS *(asterisk)* is longer than on transaxial views. This is due to the "unraveling" of the spiraled IVS. Also note the graphic demonstration of the continuity of the aortic (a) and mitral (m) valves. This view is ideally suited for studying the hypertrophic cardiomyopathies and their associated mitral leaflet abnormalities (systolic anterior motion). This plane is also used to study aortic valve abnormalities, left ventricular outflow obstruction, and left-to-right shunt lesions.

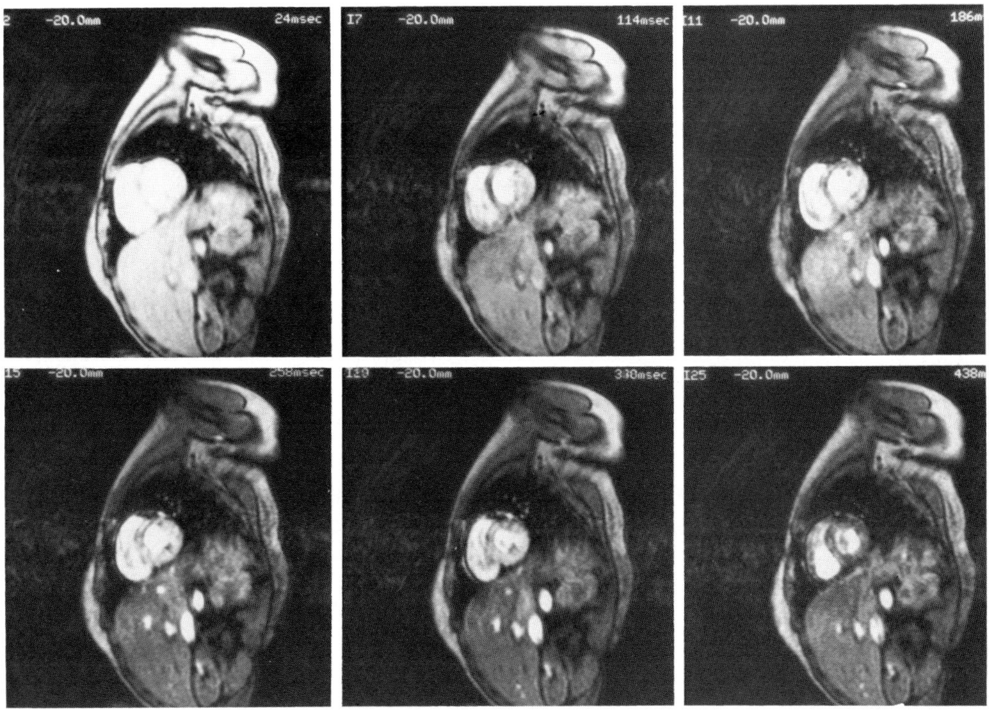

Figure 110–13. Multiple frames from a short-axis view cine study through the mid-aspect of the heart demonstrating **normal and progressive myocardial wall thickening.**

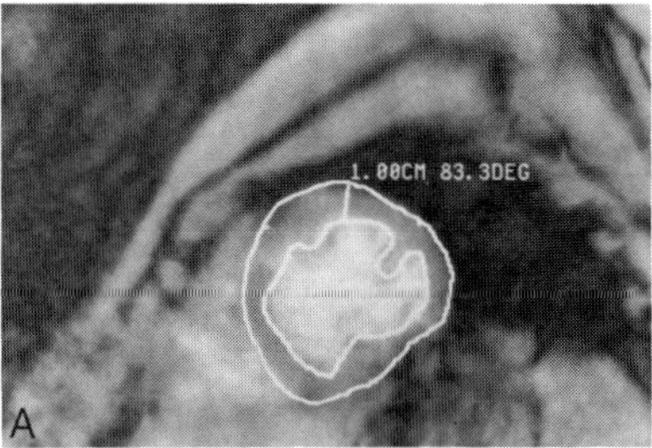

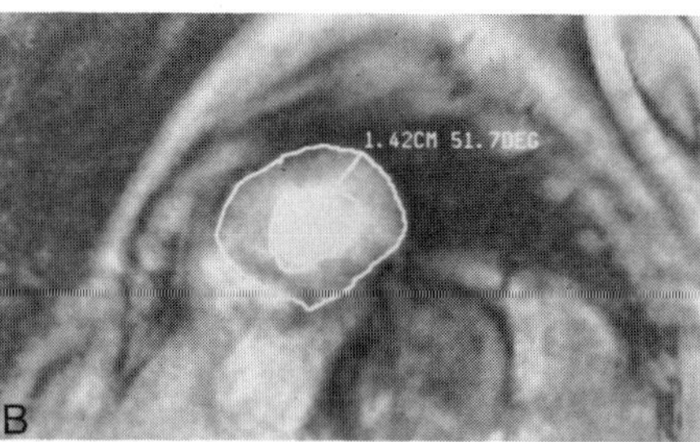

Figure 110–14. Short-axis images in end-diastole (*A*) and end-systole (*B*) through the mid-aspect of the ventricles. These data can be used to calculate cardiac indices such as stroke volume and ejection fraction, as well as assess contraction dynamics.

unfolded, as it were, on the long-axis view (Fig. 110–12). This allows for assessment of the entire IVS as well as the apex and free wall. The view is therefore quite well suited to studying the symmetrical and asymmetrical forms of hypertrophic cardiomyopathy. As with the transaxial view, the moderator band and papillary muscles can be identified. Very importantly, this view demonstrates the continuity of the aortic and mitral values that occurs because of the lack of a left ventricular infundibulum. When this view is used in conjunction with cine or phase mapping techniques, valvular pathology is nicely demonstrated. Using an area-length method, volumetric data may also be generated.

The short-axis view uses a plane that is perpendicular to the long-axis view. The utility of this view lies in the fact that it cross-sections the myocardium for measurement of myocardial wall thickness (Fig. 110–13). When this view is used in conjunction with cine MR, systolic wall thickening (SWT) can be plotted as a function of the cardiac cycle (Fig. 110–14). SWT is a very good indicator in cases of myocardial ischemia. Myocardial mass and volumetric data are easily calculated when cine studies acquire images from adjacent slices through the ventricles. Papillary muscle function can be qualitatively assessed by measurement of the thickness of the muscle at different phases of the cardiac cycle. It must be remembered that during the normal clockwise rotation of the heart (as viewed from the apex looking to the cardiac base), the apex moves 1 to 2 cm toward the cardiac base. As a result, the myocardium visualized at a particular point of the cardiac cycle may move out of the imaging plane during the course of contraction. For this reason care must be taken when assessing SWT.

CONCLUSION

The role of MRI in the evaluation of the cardiovascular system has yet to be defined. It is necessary for radiologists and their referring physicians, both of whom will help define this role, to gain a better understanding of the current capabilities of and indications for cardiovascular MRI. Although there are uncertainties regarding the clinical utility of new hardware and software developments in ultra-fast and echo planar imaging (EPI) techniques, the clinical applications of standard imaging equipment and pulse sequences are supported in the literature. The flexibility and versatility of MR make it ideal for studying both anatomic structure and physiologic function in the cardiovascular system. Realization of the ultimate potential of this imaging modality will require the ability to combine a firm understanding of cardiac embryology, anatomy, and physiology, with a knowledge of the technical aspects unique to MRI. It is hoped that this basic introduction will foster active interest in the rapidly changing field of cardiovascular MRI.

Bibliography

Bailes DR, Gilerdale DJ, Bydder GM, et al: Respiratory ordered phase encoding (ROPE): A method for reducing respiratory motion artifacts in MR imaging. J Comput Assist Tomogr 9(4), 835, 1985.

Bradley WG, Waluch V: Blood flow: Magnetic resonance imaging. Radiology 154:443, 1985.

Bryant DJ, Payne JA, Firmin DN, Longmore DB: Measurement of flow with NMR imaging using a gradient pulse and phase difference technique. J Comput Assist Tomogr 8:588–593, 1984.

Chapman B, Turner R, Ordidge RJ, et al: Real-time movie imaging from a single cardiac cycle by NMR. Magn Reson Med 5:246, 1987.

Crooks LE, Barker B, Change H, et al: Magnetic resonance imaging strategies for heart studies. Radiology 153:459–465, 1984.

Evans A, Blinder A, Herfkens, RJ, et al: Effects of turbulence on signal intensity in gradient-echo images. Invest Radiology 23:512, 1988.

Glover GH, Pelc NJ: A rapid-gated cine MRI technique. In Kressel HY (ed): Magnetic Resonance Annual 1988. New York, Raven, 1988.

Kanal E, Shellock FG, Talagala L: Safety Considerations in MR Imaging. Radiology 176:593–606, 1990.

Kondo C, Higgins C: Congenital heart disease. In Stark DD, Bradley WC (eds): Magnetic Resonance Imaging, 2nd ed. St. Louis, CV Mosby, 1992, pp 1531–1562.

Link KM: Cardiovascular MR imaging: Present status. Radiology Syllabus 1990, pp 123–140.

Link KM: Great vessels. In Stark, Bradley (eds): Magnetic Resonance Imaging, 2nd ed. pp 1490–1530.

Mirowitz SA, Eilenberg SS, White RD: Cardiac MR imaging techniques and strategies in cardiovascular magnetic resonance imaging. St. Louis, Mosby Year Book, 1992, pp 12–25.

Moran PR: A flow velocity zeugmatographic interlace for NMR imaging in humans. Magn Reson Imaging 1:197–203, 1982.

Nayler GL, Firmin DN, Longmore DB: Blood flow imaging by cine magnetic resonance. J Comput Assist Tomogr 10:715–722, 1986.

Sechtem U, Pflugfelder PW, White RD, et al: Cine MR imaging: Potential for the evaluation of cardiovascular function. AJR 148:239–246, 1987.

Shellock FG: Biological effects and safety aspects of magnetic resonance imaging. Magn Reson Quart 5:243, 1989.

Shellock FG, Curtis JS: MR Imaging and biomedical implants, materials and devices: An updated review. Radiology 180:541–550, 1991.

Underwood SR, Firmin DN, Klipstein RH, et al: Magnetic resonance velocity mapping: Clinical application of new technique. Br Heart J 57:404–412, 1987.

Waluch V, Bradley WG: NMR even echo rephasing in slow laminar flow. J Comput Assist Tomogr 8:594, 1984.

Clinical Applications

111 Congenital Cardiovascular Disease

Patricia E. Burrows, Jeffrey F. Smallhorn, and C. A. F. Moes

This chapter outlines an approach to the imaging of congenital heart disease and the basic anatomic defects present in the more common anomalies.

Congenital heart disease involves a huge spectrum of lesions from simple, isolated septal defects to complex primitive anomalies. Many anomalies are rare; the eight defects listed in Table 111–1 include 85 per cent of patients with congenital heart disease. The radiologist must remember that congenital cardiac anomalies are frequently associated with anomalies in other organ systems. Some syndromes that involve the heart are listed in Table 111–2.

The analysis of individual patients with congenital heart disease requires an integrated approach involving physical examination, electrocardiography, plain chest radiographs, and cardiac imaging, which may involve one or a combination of the following modalities: two-dimensional and Doppler echocardiography, nuclear angiography, magnetic resonance imaging (MRI), and finally cardiac catheterization and angiocardiography. Chest radiography, when combined with findings of the initial physical examination, provides information about the physiologic changes caused by the anomaly at that moment in time and also provides a basis for differential diagnosis. Echocardiography displays the intracardiac anatomy and with Doppler techniques can accurately estimate the severity of obstructive or regurgitant lesions. Transesophageal echocardiography is a recent development that allows accurate assessment of atrial septal defects and other intracardiac anatomy, and also permits evaluation of surgical results both during and after surgery. Nuclear cardiac imaging may be used to assess the magnitude of left-to-right shunting, especially in patients with borderline clinical findings, and is also used to assess ventricular function and myocardial ischemia in selected patients. MRI is a superb modality for imaging the heart, and in congenital heart disease it has proved to be most useful in the assessment of anomalies of the thoracic great vessels, and in postoperative evaluations. With the increased accuracy of noninvasive methods, especially echocardiography, cardiac catheterization and cineangiography can be avoided as diagnostic procedures in most patients with isolated atrial septal defects, atrioventricular septal defects, coarctation of the aorta, and patent ductus arteriosus and can be reserved as a single preoperative procedure in many other patients. In patients with surgical congenital heart disease, echocardiography, cardiac catheterization data, and cineangiography are all required for a complete anatomic and physiologic assessment.

TABLE 111–1. INCIDENCE OF CONGENITAL HEART DEFECTS*

Defect	Per Cent
Ventricular septal defect	28.3
Atrial septal defect	10.3
Pulmonary stenosis	9.9
Patent ductus arteriosus	9.8
Tetralogy of Fallot	9.7
Aortic stenosis	7.1
Coarctation of the aorta	5.1
Transposition	4.9
Total	85

*Hospital for Sick Children, Toronto, Ontario, 1950 to 1973, 15,104 cases.

THE SEGMENTAL APPROACH

The segmental approach to congenital heart disease is useful in conveying anatomic information about complex cardiac anomalies. It involves a step-by-step analysis of five cardiac segments: the atria, the atrioventricular valves, the ventricles, the infundibulum, and the great arteries. The atria and ventricles are named according to their morphologic characteristics rather than their location. The

TABLE 111–2. HEREDITARY DISORDERS AND CHROMOSOMAL DEFECTS WITH ASSOCIATED CONGENITAL CARDIAC ANOMALIES

Lesion/Syndrome	Usual Cardiac Defect
Marfan's, Ehlers-Danlos	Valvar regurgitation, aneurysms
Mucopolysaccharidoses	Valvar regurgitation
Osteogenesis imperfecta	Valvar regurgitation
Holt-Oram	Septal defects, TOF
Ellis–van Creveld	Septal defects
Acrocephalosyndactyly	PDA, septal defects
Oculoauriculovertebral dysplasia	Septal defects, TOF
Smith-Lemli-Opitz	Septal defects, TOF
Cornelia de Lange's	Septal defects
Klippel-Feil	Septal defects
Noonan's	Dysplastic pulmonary valve, hypertrophic cardiomyopathy
Turner's	Coarctation of aorta, PDA
Williams'	Supravalvar AS, peripheral PS
Intrauterine rubella	Supravalvar AS, peripheral PS, PDA
Kartagener's	Dextrocardia
Alkaptonuria	Aortic stenosis
Tuberous sclerosis	Rhabdomyomas
Glycogen storage disease	Cardiomyopathy
DiGeorge's	Interrupted aortic arch, complex CHD
Klinefelter's	VSD
Pierre Robin	PDA, septal defects
Trisomy 21	AV septal defects, VSD, PDA, TOF
Trisomy 13–15	Varied
Trisomy 16–18	Varied

AS = aortic stenosis; CHD = congenital heart disease; PDA = patent ductus arteriosus; PS = pulmonary stenosis; TOF = tetralogy of Fallot; VSD = ventricular septal defect.

concepts of *concordance* and *discordance* refer to the connections between the major segments. The atria and ventricles are concordant if the morphologic left atrium is connected to the morphologic left ventricle and the right atrium is connected to the right ventricle. Atrioventricular discordance is present if the morphologic left atrium connects with the morphologic right ventricle. The terms are also useful in describing the ventriculoarterial connections. Concordance indicates that the aorta is connected to the left ventricle and the pulmonary artery to the right ventricle. With ventriculoarterial discordance (e.g., transposition), the aorta connects to the right ventricle and the pulmonary artery to the left ventricle.

The term *situs* refers to the sidedness or lateralization of normally asymmetrical organs within the body and is used to describe the abdominal viscera, atria, and tracheobronchial tree. *Situs solitus* is the normal or usual situation, *situs inversus* is the mirror image of normal, and *situs ambiguus* describes a situation in which lateralization has not occurred. Situs ambiguus often involves organ isomerism—that is, both atria resemble right or left atria, or both lungs are structured as left or right lungs. These anomalies form part of the visceral heterotaxia syndromes, which include asplenia and polysplenia.

The *bulboventricular loop* describes the spatial relationship of the ventricles. During development, the normal primitive heart tube loops to the right (D-loop) before rotating into the left hemithorax so that the morphologic right ventricle is situated to the right of and anterior to the morphologic left ventricle. If the heart tube loops to the left (L-loop), *ventricular inversion* results, with the morphologic right ventricle to the left of the morphologic left ventricle. This is the situation in corrected transposition of the great arteries.

The relationship of the great arteries to each other is described as *N* (normal), *D* (aorta to the right of pulmonary artery), *L* (aorta to the left of pulmonary artery), or *AP* (aorta directly anterior to the pulmonary artery).

A heart with an isolated ventricular septal defect could be described as: ventricular septal defect (S, D, N) (situs solitus, D bulboventricular loop, normally related great arteries). A form of complete transposition is summarized as transposition of the great arteries (S, D, D), or may be further described as having atrioventricular concordance and ventriculoarterial discordance.

THE CHEST RADIOGRAPH

Radiographs of the chest provide information regarding the physiologic effects of the underlying cardiac malformation at a given moment in time. Although a precise diagnosis is frequently not possible, a systematic approach to the analysis of the plain chest film, when combined with clinical data, will help to categorize individual patients into narrow differential diagnoses. The following parameters should be assessed on each chest radiograph:

1. Pulmonary vascular pattern
2. Cardiac size and contour
3. The aorta
4. The pulmonary artery
5. Abdominal visceral situs
6. Cardiac position
7. Pulmonary parenchyma
8. Skeletal anomalies

In most patients, upright posteroanterior (PA) and lateral radiographs are sufficient. Barium esophagography is useful in the investigation of patients with suspected vascular ring.

Chest radiographs of infants and small children exhibit important differences from those of adults. The heart occupies a more horizontal position in infants, and extends more superiorly in the retrosternal space, so assessment of chamber size is difficult. The degree of inspiration is important in the assessment of cardiac size at all ages. Improper x-ray tube centering or arching of the infant's back may result in a lordotic projection, which causes an apparent upturned cardiac apex and increased transverse diameter. The predominance of pulmonary blood flow in the lower lobes compared with the upper lobes seen in upright chest radiographs of adults is not evident in infants and small children. Finally, children of all ages, and especially those younger than six years, may have prominent thymic tissue that obscures mediastinal vascular structures and chamber outlines.

Pulmonary Vascular Pattern

The pulmonary vascularity provides the most useful information about the physiologic effects of the cardiac anomalies. There are five basic patterns of abnormal pulmonary blood flow: (1) shunt vascularity, (2) decreased pulmonary blood flow, (3) precapillary pulmonary hypertension, (4) pulmonary venous hypertension, and (5) systemic collateral flow.

Normally, pulmonary vascular markings branch in an orderly fashion and taper smoothly from hilum to periphery (Fig. 111–1*A*). Only fine markings are seen in the outer portions of the lungs. The right descending pulmonary artery measured just below the hilar angle normally has the same diameter as the trachea. If an adjacent artery and bronchus are seen end-on, they should be equal in size.

Shunt vascularity is characterized by dilated tortuous pulmonary arteries and veins with well-defined margins (Fig. 111–1*B*). Diagnostic features include enlarged vessels in the periphery of the lungs, a larger vessel when an adjacent bronchus and artery are seen end-on, and an interlobar artery larger than the trachea (useful in infants). The central and main pulmonary arteries are enlarged in the presence of a left-to-right shunt, but these features are less specific than the identification of shunt vessels peripherally. An overexposed film can mask the presence of shunt vessels. The lateral view is frequently helpful, as the markings in the perihilar regions appear too prominent and extend into the retrosternal air space. Shunt vasculature is generally not seen until the pulmonary-to-systemic flow ratio is greater than 2:1. The most common lesions associated with shunt vascularity are ventricular septal defects (VSDs), atrial septal defects (ASDs), atrioventricular (AV) septal defects and patent ductus arteriosus in acyanotic patients, and transposition of the great arteries in cyanotic patients.

Decreased pulmonary flow can be diagnosed when the pulmonary vascular markings are abnormally small and the lungs are more radiolucent than normal (Fig. 111–1*C*). The lateral projection is helpful in showing small or absent central pulmonary arteries. Decreased pulmonary blood flow is seen in cyanotic patients with obstruction to pulmonary blood flow plus intracardiac defects that allow right-to-left shunting, most commonly tetralogy of Fallot.

In patients with congenital heart disease, precapillary pulmonary hypertension is usually secondary to a left-to-right shunt that has resulted in an increase in peripheral pulmonary arterial resistance and eventual decrease in the left-to-right shunt followed by right-to-left shunting (pulmonary vaso-occlusive disease, or Eisenmenger's syndrome). The main and central pulmonary arteries are usually dilated out of proportion to the peripheral pulmonary vessels (Fig. 111–2). The heart is frequently normal in size.

Radiographic signs of pulmonary venous hypertension include redistribution of pulmonary blood flow (older children and adults), bronchial wall cuffing, indistinctness of vessel margins, Kerley's lines, and small pleural effusions (Fig. 111–3). Large pleural effusions are infrequently seen in children with congestive heart failure with the exception of volume overload due to renal disease.

The pattern of vascularity seen in patients with systemic collaterals to the lungs is often referred to as bronchial circulation, although the bronchial arteries contribute very little to the radiologic findings. In patients with absence or hypoplasia of the true pulmonary arteries, segments of the lung may be perfused by primitive

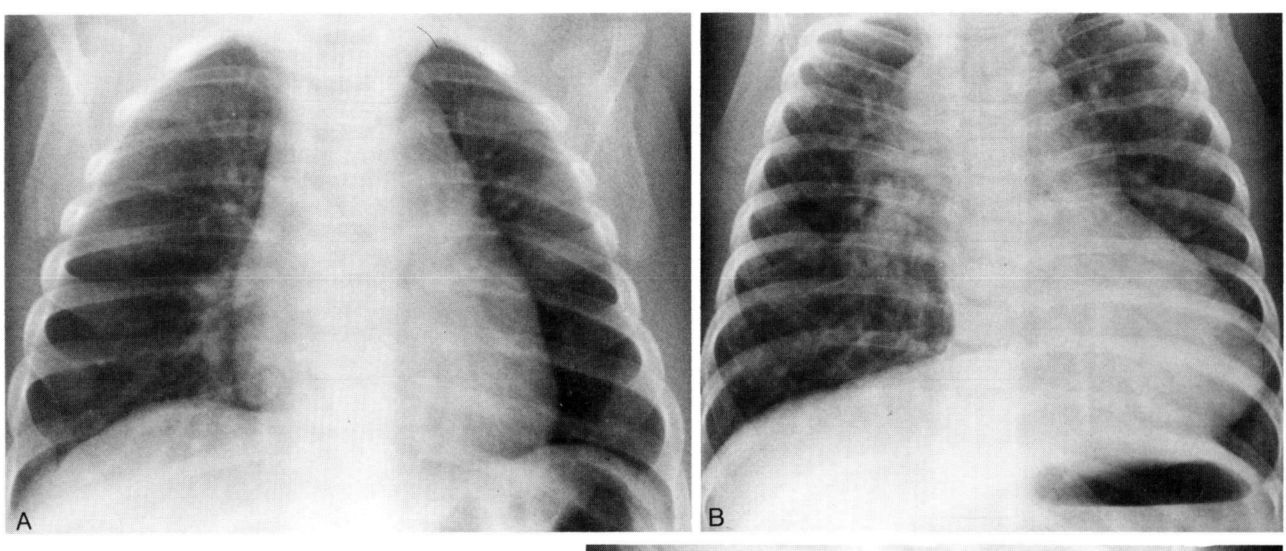

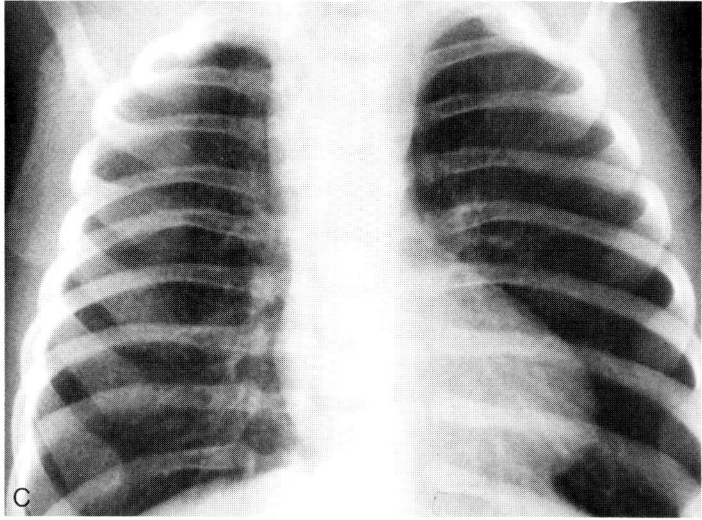

Figure 111–1. Pulmonary vascular patterns. PA projections of three infants with normal vasculature *(A)*, shunt vasculature *(B)*, and decreased pulmonary blood flow *(C)*.

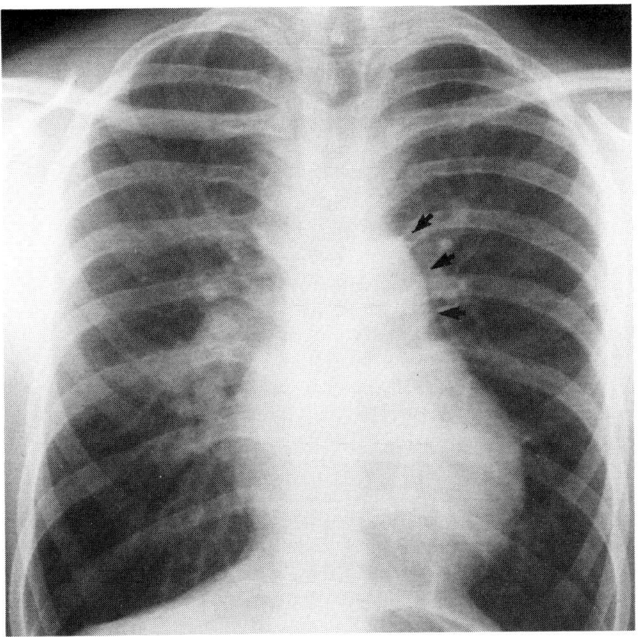

Figure 111–2. Precapillary pulmonary hypertension. The main *(arrows)* and central pulmonary arteries are dilated out of proportion to the peripheral pulmonary vascular markings and heart size in this 15-year-old boy with a large ventricular septal defect (VSD).

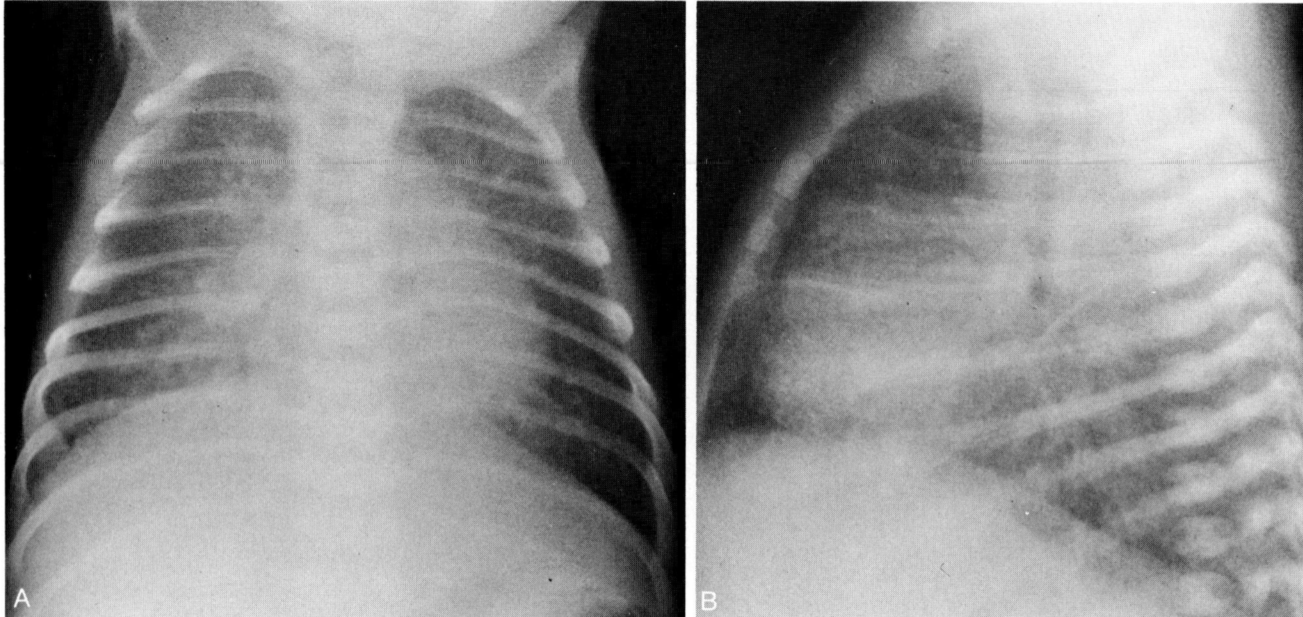

Figure 111–3. Pulmonary venous hypertension with indistinctness of the pulmonary vascular margins, Kerley's lines, thickening of the interlobar fissures, and pulmonary hyperinflation in a newborn boy with obstructed infradiaphragmatic total anomalous pulmonary venous connection. Septal lines are best seen in the right costophrenic angle on the PA film *(A)* and in the retrosternal space in the lateral projection *(B).*

collateral arteries from the aorta and brachiocephalic arteries. As a result, the pulmonary vessels do not converge normally at the hila but have an irregular distribution, with increased markings in some segments and decreased markings in others (Fig. 111–4). Vessels from the chest wall may also supply the lungs via profuse tiny transpleural collaterals, producing a pattern of reticulated vascular markings and sometimes rib notching due to enlargement of the intercostal arteries.

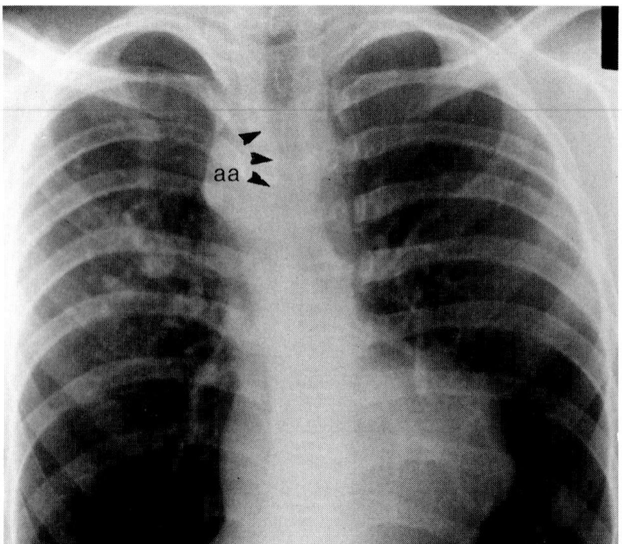

Figure 111–4. Systemic collateral flow is indicated by the uneven size and distribution of the pulmonary vascular markings in this patient with pulmonary atresia and VSD. The largest vessels are seen in the right upper lobe. Notching of the fourth and fifth ribs indicates enlargement of intercostal arteries, which provide transpleural collateral flow. Note the right aortic arch (aa, *arrowheads*), concave main pulmonary artery segment, and upturned cardiac apex.

Cardiac Size and Contour

The assessment of cardiac size is best done with an examination of two views, taking into account the degree of inspiration and the size of the thymus. If measurements are used, the cardiothoracic ratio from a standard PA upright chest radiograph should be less than 50 per cent after the first month of age. A ratio of up to 60 per cent may be normal on portable radiographs of neonates.

In infancy and early childhood, the assessment of specific cardiac chamber enlargement is difficult and is best done with two-dimensional echocardiography. Typical forms of abnormal cardiac contour may be more useful in suggesting some cardiac anomalies.

Ventricular dilatation in patients with congenital cardiac anomalies is caused by volume overload secondary to left-to-right shunting, valvar regurgitation, or myocardial dysfunction. Ventricular outflow obstruction causes myocardial hypertrophy, usually without cardiomegaly. The neonate is an exception to this generalization, as severe obstructive lesions may lead to myocardial ischemia and atrioventricular valve regurgitation, resulting in cardiac enlargement.

The Aorta

The ascending aorta is normally inconspicuous in infants and children and becomes progressively more prominent with age after the third decade. Abnormal prominence may be caused by turbulence due to aortic stenosis; by volume overload secondary to aortic regurgitation, right-to-left intracardiac shunting, aortopulmonary shunting, or arteriovenous shunting; by pressure overload from systemic hypertension; or by intrinsic aortic wall abnormalities as in Marfan's syndrome.

The position of the aortic arch is best determined by the identification of the aortic knob on the PA chest radiograph. When the aortic knob cannot be identified in infants, the position of the descending aorta or the trachea may be helpful (Fig. 111–5*A*). Normally, the trachea is situated slightly to the right of the midline (Fig. 111–5*A*) and buckles to the side opposite the arch on expira-

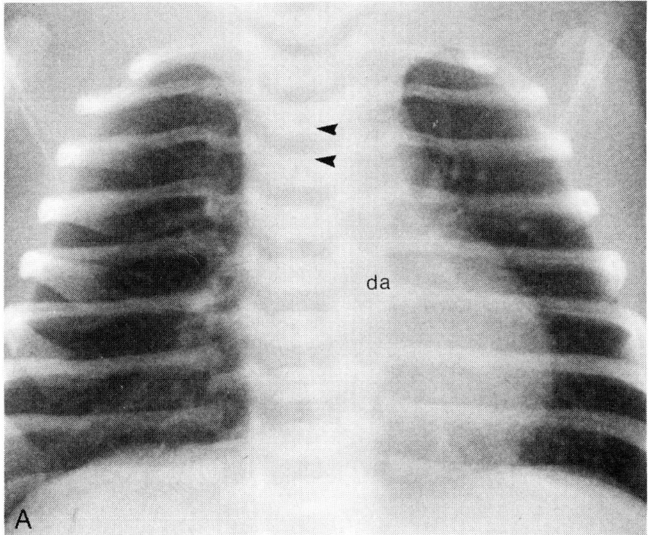

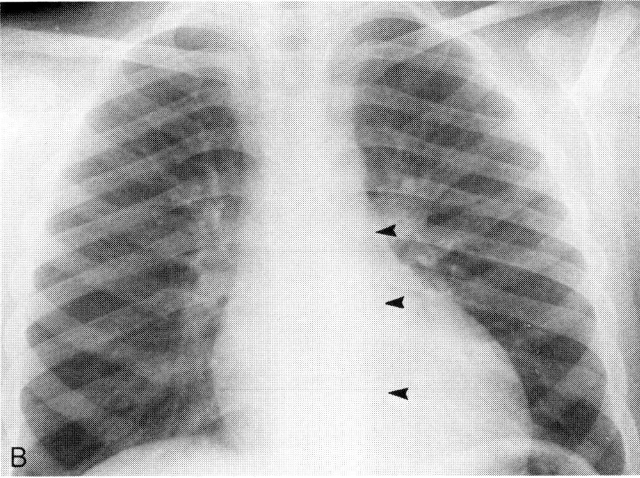

Figure 111–5. *A,* **Normal left aortic arch.** Although the aortic arch is obscured by the thymus, the descending aorta is clearly left-sided, and there is a subtle left-sided indentation in the tracheal air column *(arrowheads).* Compare this appearance with the right aortic arch in Figure 111–4. *B,* **Systemic hypertension.** The aortic arch and descending aorta *(arrowheads)* are dilated and tortuous in this child with systemic hypertension due to chronic renal failure.

tion. In the presence of a right-sided aortic arch, the trachea is *usually* at or to the left of the midline (see Fig. 111–4). The arch also produces a focal indentation in the tracheal air column just above the carina.

A right-sided aortic arch is seen with increased incidence in patients with the following cardiac anomalies: tetralogy of Fallot (30 per cent of patients), pulmonary atresia with VSD (30 per cent), persistent truncus arteriosus (30 per cent), transposition of the great arteries (8 per cent), tricuspid atresia (5 per cent), and VSD (3 per cent).

In the presence of a right aortic arch, the tracheal air column should be carefully examined on the lateral projection to exclude narrowing or displacement by a vascular ring. The right aortic arch in patients with congenital heart disease usually has mirror image branching, with no retroesophageal or retrotracheal branches. The right aortic arch with aberrant retroesophageal left subclavian artery and the double aortic arch are usually isolated anomalies. In all forms of right aortic arch with normal abdominal situs, the descending aorta usually crosses the midline at or above the diaphragm.

Enlargement of the descending aorta is seen in most of the conditions that produce dilatation of the ascending aorta (Fig. 111–5*B*). Inability to define a normally shaped aortic arch in the presence of a well-defined descending aorta suggests coarctation of the descending aorta.

The Pulmonary Artery

Enlargement of the main pulmonary artery is seen with idiopathic dilatation in normal older children and adolescents and in patients with valvar pulmonary stenosis in whom the left pulmonary artery is also dilated, in left-to-right shunts, and in pulmonary hypertension (see Fig. 111–2). Decreased size of the main pulmonary artery segment is seen in patients with tetralogy of Fallot (see Fig. 111–1*C*), pulmonary atresia with VSD (see Fig. 111–4), and transposition of the great arteries, where the aorta and pulmonary artery are anteroposteriorly related. It can be seen, therefore, that the size of the pulmonary trunk usually has meaning only when interpreted in conjunction with the pulmonary vascularity.

Abdominal Visceral (Visceroatrial) Situs

The inferior vena cava, which is on the same side as the dominant lobe of the liver, is essentially always connected to the morphologic right atrium. In abdominal situs solitus, the liver has a triangular shape, with the larger lobe on the right and the gas-filled gastric fundus under the left hemidiaphragm. The opposite is true in patients with abdominal situs inversus. Patients with undetermined situs (ambiguus) often have a horizontal, bilobed liver, and the gastric air bubble may be central, right-sided, or left-sided but is usually displaced inferiorly from the diaphragm (Fig. 111–6*A*). Patients with abdominal situs ambiguus (visceral heterotaxia syndromes) have a high incidence of systemic venous anomalies and complex cardiac anomalies, with ambiguous atrial situs.

Cardiac Position

The heart may be predominantly in the left hemithorax (levocardia), in the midline (mesocardia), or predominantly in the right hemithorax (dextrocardia). Dextrocardia may be further categorized as primary or secondary and congenital or acquired. Thoracic mass lesions, pulmonary hypoplasia, pneumonectomy, and skeletal deformities may cause secondary dextrocardia. The terms *dextroposition* and *dextroversion* are confusing and unnecessary. Scimitar syndrome is a form of secondary dextrocardia, with a hypoplastic right lung and partial anomalous pulmonary venous connection to the inferior vena cava (Fig. 111–6*B*). Kartagener's syndrome includes dextrocardia, bronchiectasis, and immotile cilia. Patients with dextrocardia and abdominal situs inversus (situs inversus totalus) have a low incidence of congenital cardiac defects, whereas patients with dextrocardia and abdominal situs solitus (isolated dextrocardia) or situs ambiguus or with levocardia and abdominal situs inversus (isolated levocardia) usually have cardiac defects and often have complex anomalies such as transposition of the great arteries. Mesocardia is also associated with an increased incidence of congenital heart disease.

Pulmonary Parenchyma

Pneumonia and atelectasis are frequent complications in infants with large left-to-right shunts, especially those with Down's syndrome. Infants with large shunts or pulmonary edema often have pulmonary hyperinflation due to obstruction of the small, relatively soft-walled airways. Focal air trapping in the left lung or left lower

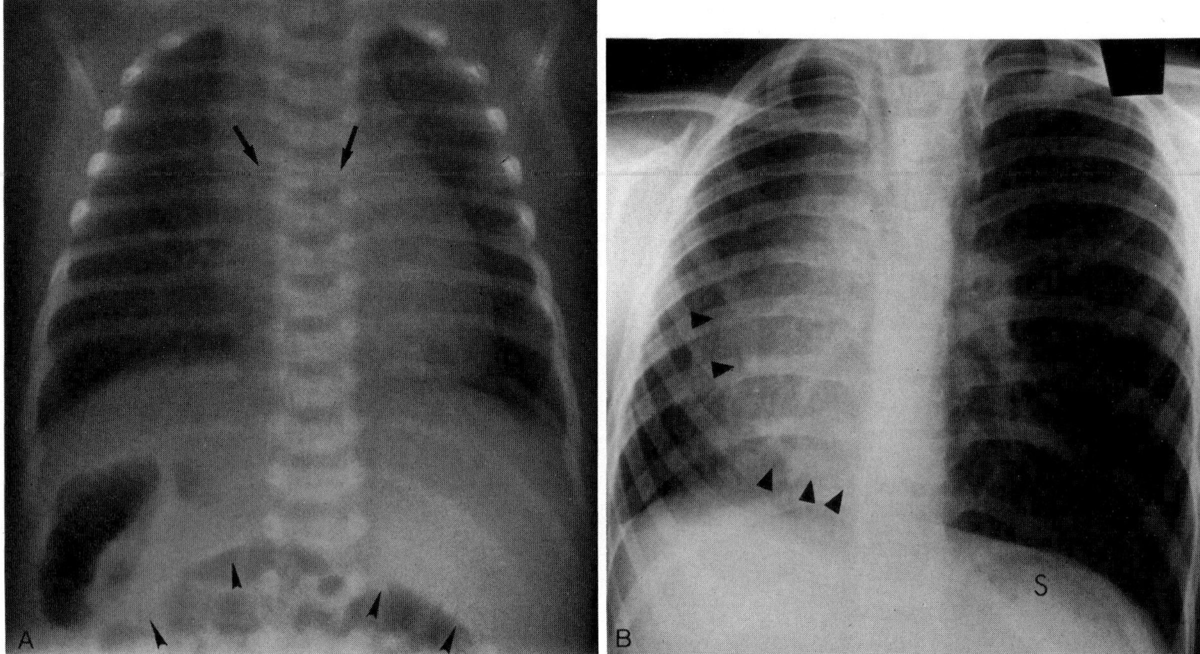

Figure 111–6. *A,* **Abdominal situs ambiguus.** *Arrowheads* indicate the inferior margin of the symmetrical, bilobed liver. The gastric air bubble is difficult to identify. Bilateral eparterial bronchi are present (upper lobe bronchi are indicated by *arrows*) in this infant with asplenia syndrome. *B,* **Secondary congenital dextrocardia in a patient with the scimitar syndrome.** The right lung is hypoplastic, and anomalous pulmonary veins draining toward the inferior vena cava are indicated by *arrowheads.* (S = stomach.)

lobe or collapse of the left lower lobe may be present in infants with moderate or severe cardiomegaly, owing to compression of the left bronchus. Focal air trapping, especially in the right lung, should alert one to the possibility of a vascular ring, such as a pulmonary artery sling. Aneurysmal enlargement of the central pulmonary arteries, seen in absent pulmonary valve syndrome, can also cause central airway compression and aeration abnormalities. Pulmonary hypoplasia should be suspected if one hemithorax is significantly smaller than the other on a nonrotated film and may be secondary to congenital absence of one pulmonary artery, acquired pulmonary artery obstruction (e.g., surgical), or unilateral pulmonary venous obstruction.

Skeletal Anomalies

Twenty-five per cent of infants with congenital cardiac defects have extracardiac anomalies, most often musculoskeletal. Each syndrome listed in Table 111–2 includes skeletal deformities. The most common skeletal anomalies involve the sternum and include early fusion of the sternomanubrial joint and segments of the sternal body, leading to a pectus carinatum deformity. Pectus carinatum is more common with cyanotic than acyanotic forms of congenital heart disease. Segmental anomalies of the spine and ribs are also frequent. Radial ray hypoplasia coexists with cardiac septal defects in the Holt-Oram syndrome, which has an autosomal dominant inheritance (Fig. 111–7).

Acquired bone deformities include rib notching due to enlargement of intercostal arteries in patients with obstructive lesions (coarctation) of the aorta, caval obstruction, cyanotic disease with transpleural collaterals, and those created by Blalock-Taussig shunt procedures. Extramedullary hematopoiesis occurs in severely cyanosed children and may produce expansion of vertebrae or ribs.

Rib deformities may also be secondary to thoracotomy for palliative shunt procedures, atrial septectomy, pulmonary artery banding, ductus ligation, and coarctation repair. Generalized cortical hyperostosis has been noted in infants receiving prostaglandin infusion.

CLINICAL/RADIOLOGIC CORRELATION

A certain amount of clinical information is essential before the findings noted on plain chest radiography can be used in forming a useful differential diagnosis. The most helpful clinical data are the presence or absence of cyanosis and the age at onset of symptoms. Most cyanotic congenital heart diseases are detected shortly after birth, although pulmonary parenchymal disease may be initially considered as a cause of cyanosis. Patients who have lesions with predominant left-to-right shunting typically develop symptoms toward the end of the first month of life after pulmonary vascular resistance falls, although large shunts may become evident earlier. Severe left ventricular outlet obstruction (critical aortic stenosis and hypoplastic left heart syndrome) typically produces symptoms within the first week of life. Coarctation may present in the first week but usually is diagnosed slightly later. Bicuspid aortic valve, coarctation of the aorta, ASDs, small VSDs, and right ventricular outlet obstruction frequently produce no symptoms and may be detected at routine preschool physical examination or during evaluation of an unrelated illness. Table 111–3 lists the most likely diagnoses in four clinical/radiologic categories, combining the clinical picture with the appearance of the pulmonary vascularity.

Table 111–4 lists the causes of pulmonary venous hypertension in infants at different ages. Although primary congenital cardiac lesions are less common than noncardiac lesions in the first week of life, they must be considered, as timely surgical intervention may make a critical difference in the outcome. Lesions that benefit from urgent surgical treatment in the first weeks of life include coarcta-

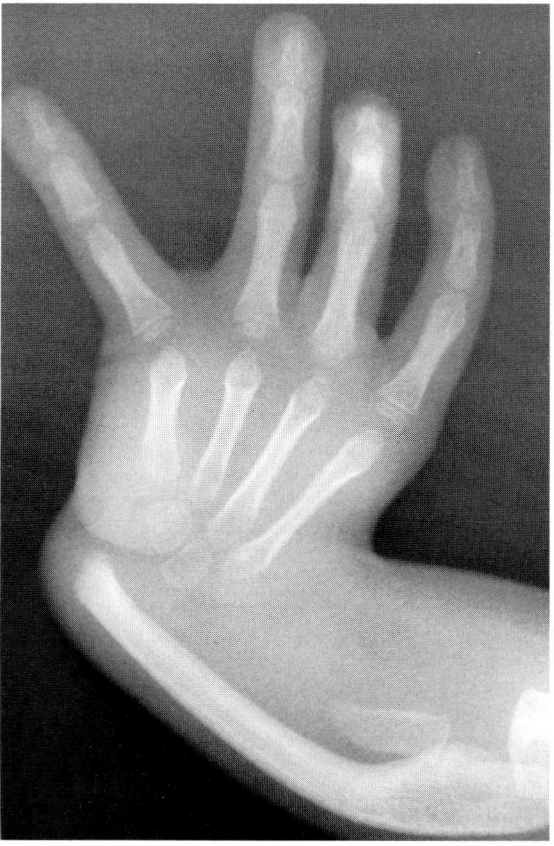

Figure 111–7. Holt-Oram syndrome. Radial clubhand due to hypoplastic radius, with absent first metacarpal, carpal bones, and thumb.

tion of the descending aorta, critical aortic stenosis, total anomalous pulmonary venous connection with obstruction, and hypoplastic left heart syndrome.

ANGIOCARDIOGRAPHY

Accurate demonstration of anatomy in patients with congenital heart disease requires adequate delivery of contrast medium, rapid filming (cine at 60 frames per second), and the use of appropriate projections. Axial projections optimize the demonstration of vascular anatomy by separating the chambers and elongating the ventricular outflow tracts and great arteries. The most commonly used projections are illustrated in Figures 111–8 through 111–10.

1. LONG AXIAL OBLIQUE (60-degree left anterior oblique, 20 to 30 degree cranial) (Fig. 111–8*A*). Used with left ventricular contrast injection, this projection optimally profiles the anterior ventricular septum and elongates the left ventricular outflow tract. It is used for imaging perimembranous and anterior trabecular VSDs; valvar, subvalvar, and supravalvar aortic stenosis; coronary artery abnormalities; and aortic arch anomalies.

2. THIRTY-DEGREE RIGHT ANTERIOR OBLIQUE (Fig. 111–8*B*). This projection is the reciprocal of the long axial oblique view. It optimally demonstrates the mitral valve apparatus, the infundibular septum, and the most anterior part of the ventricular septum anterior to the septal band. The levophase shows the left atrium and shunting at the atrial level. Cranial angulation may be added to elongate the infundibular septum.

3. SITTING-UP PROJECTION (PA, 30 to 45 degree cranial) (Fig. 111–9*A*). With contrast injection in the right ventricle, this projection demonstrates the right ventricular anatomy, the pulmonary valve, and the central pulmonary arteries. It is especially useful in demonstrating main and branch pulmonary artery stenoses. The levophase shows pulmonary venous return and interatrial shunting.

4. LATERAL PROJECTION (Fig. 111–9*B*). As a reciprocal view in right ventriculography, the lateral projection demonstrates the right ventricular infundibulum, infundibular septum, pulmonary valve, and main pulmonary artery to advantage.

5. FOUR-CHAMBER OR HEPATOCLAVICULAR PROJECTION (45-degree left anterior oblique, 30-degree cranial) (Fig. 111–10). This projection is usually used with left ventriculography to profile the posterior ventricular septum (that part between the AV valves) and separate the four chambers. It is the best projection to image AV septal defects, abnormal AV connections, and straddling AV valves; it also demonstrates perimembranous and most trabecular VSDs. Additionally, it is used with contrast injection in the right upper pulmonary vein to demonstrate ASDs.

DIGITAL ANGIOGRAPHY

As the technology for digital acquisition of angiographic data improves, this technology may be useful in image enhancement, computer-facilitated functional analysis and measurement, and, pos-

TABLE 111–3. DIFFERENTIAL DIAGNOSIS BASED ON PULMONARY BLOOD FLOW (CHEST RADIOGRAPH) AND PRESENCE OR ABSENCE OF CYANOSIS

Acyanotic Patient with Shunt Vascularity
VSD
ASD
AV septal defects
Patent ductus arteriosus
Aortopulmonary septal defect (window)
Partial anomalous pulmonary venous connection
Coronary-cameral communication
Ruptured sinus of Valsalva aneurysm
Peripheral or intracranial arteriovenous malformations
Anomalous left coronary artery
Acyanotic Patient with Normal Vasculature or Pulmonary Venous Hypertension
Aortic stenosis (bicuspid aortic valve)
Coarctation of aorta
Pulmonary stenosis
Congenital mitral valve anomalies
Cor triatriatum
Endocardial fibroelastosis
Anomalous left coronary artery
Cardiomyopathies
Corrected transposition of the great arteries
Cyanotic Patient with Shunt Vasculature
Transposition of the great arteries
Double-outlet right ventricle
Single ventricle
Truncus arteriosus
Total anomalous pulmonary venous connection
Tricuspid atresia
Cyanotic Patient with Decreased or Normal Pulmonary Blood Flow
Tetralogy of Fallot
Pulmonary atresia with VSD
Pulmonary atresia with intact ventricular septum
Critical pulmonary stenosis with ASD
Transposition of the great arteries with pulmonary stenosis
Tricuspid atresia with pulmonary stenosis
Double-outlet right ventricle with pulmonary stenosis
Single ventricle with pulmonary stenosis
Ebstein's anomaly

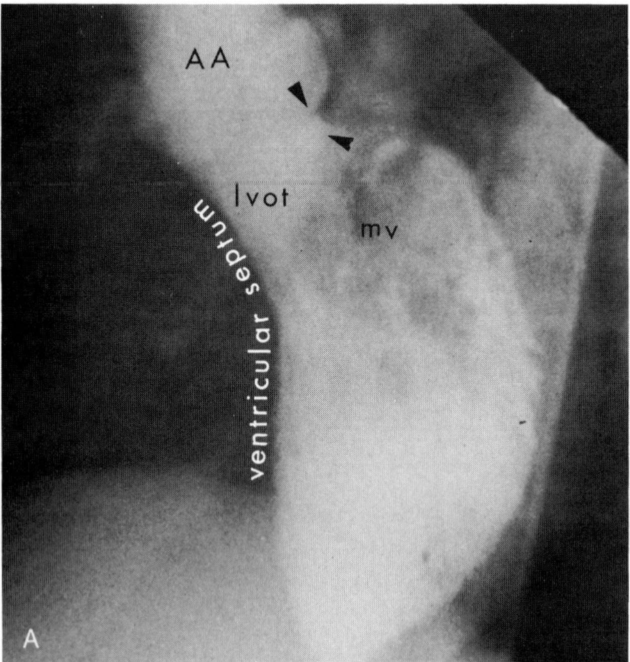

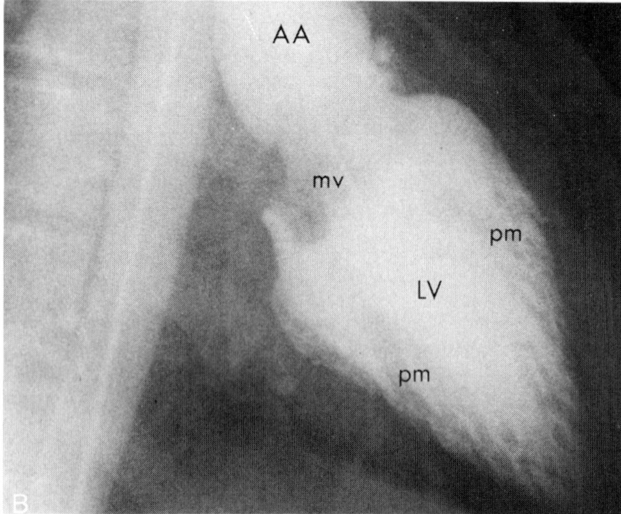

Figure 111–8. *A,* **Normal left ventriculogram.** Long axial oblique projection elongates the left ventricular outflow tract (lvot) and profiles the membranous and anterior trabecular septum. *Arrowheads* indicate aortic-mitral valve continuity. *B,* **Right anterior oblique projection.** (AA = ascending aorta; LV = left ventricle; mv = mitral valve; pm = papillary muscle.)

sibly, ultimate replacement of cine film. Digital subtraction angiography (DSA) is a useful adjunct to cineangiography in imaging the pulmonary arteries, the aorta and its branches, and the pulmonary veins, especially in patients with obstructive lesions (Fig. 111–11). DSA for functional analysis and intravenous DSA for imaging of the thoracic great vessels are used in selected situations but compete with MRI, radionuclide functional analysis, and echocardiography.

MAGNETIC RESONANCE IMAGING

With the advantages of electrocardiographic gating and multiplanar imaging, MRI is a superb modality for imaging the heart and great vessels. MRI can be used to image any cardiac malformation or mass. Currently, its most important role in congenital cardiac disease is in the evaluation of the thoracic great vessels. Anomalies of the aorta, central pulmonary arteries, and systemic and pulmonary veins are accurately demonstrated by MRI. This modality is also indicated in the assessment of cardiac tumors and in the evaluation of postoperative congenital heart disease. Functional analysis and three-dimensional imaging are currently areas of research interest.

TRANSCATHETER INTERVENTIONAL TECHNIQUES

Cardiac catheter intervention is a rapidly developing specialty. Balloon atrial septostomy is still widely used in neonates with transposition of the great arteries. Balloon angioplasty or valvuloplasty is the treatment of choice for coarctation restenosis and valvar pulmonary stenosis. Other common techniques include balloon dilation angioplasty of native coarctation, balloon aortic valvuloplasty, device closure of patent ductus arteriosus and other cardiovascular communications, and stent angioplasty of pulmonary artery stenosis. Device closure of ASDs and VSDs, stenting of aortopulmonary collaterals, and laser valvuloplasty for pulmonary valve atresia are currently investigational techniques.

TABLE 111–4. CAUSES OF PULMONARY VENOUS HYPERTENSION PATTERN IN INFANTS

First Week
Overhydration
Transient tachypnea of the newborn
Asphyxia
Hypoglycemia
Arrhythmia
Persistent fetal circulation
Hypoplastic left heart syndrome
Critical aortic stenosis
Coarctation of aorta
Total anomalous pulmonary venous connection with obstruction
Arteriovenous malformation
Cor triatriatum
Pulmonary vein atresia
Hydrops fetalis
Myocarditis
Second and Third Weeks
Coarctation of aorta
Critical aortic stenosis
Interruption of aortic arch
Endocardial fibroelastosis
Hypertrophic cardiomyopathy
Cor triatriatum
Congenital mitral valve disease
Peripheral arteriovenous malformation
Fourth to Sixth Weeks
Coarctation of aorta
Critical aortic stenosis
Endocardial fibroelastosis
Anomalous origin of left coronary artery
Glycogen storage disease
Hypertrophic cardiomyopathy
Cor triatriatum
Congenital mitral valve disease
Hepatic hemangioma

Modified from Edwards DK, Higgins CB: Radiology of neonatal heart disease. Radiol Clin North Am 18:369–385, 1980.

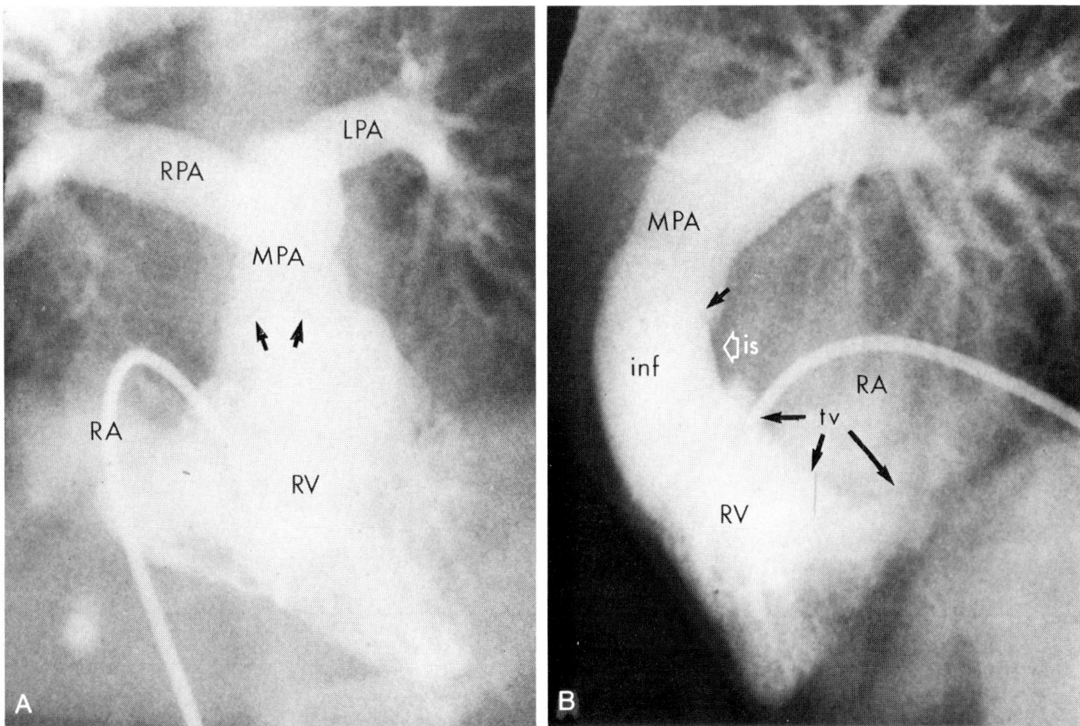

Figure 111–9. *A,* **Normal right ventriculogram.** Axial (cranially) angled PA (sitting up) projection elongates the outflow tract and demonstrates the origins of both pulmonary arteries. *Arrows* indicate the pulmonary valve. *B,* **Lateral projection** shows the infundibular septum (is) separating the pulmonary and tricuspid valves. (inf = infundibulum; LPA = left pulmonary artery; MPA = main pulmonary artery; RA = right atrium; RPA = right pulmonary artery; RV = right ventricle; tv = tricuspid valve.)

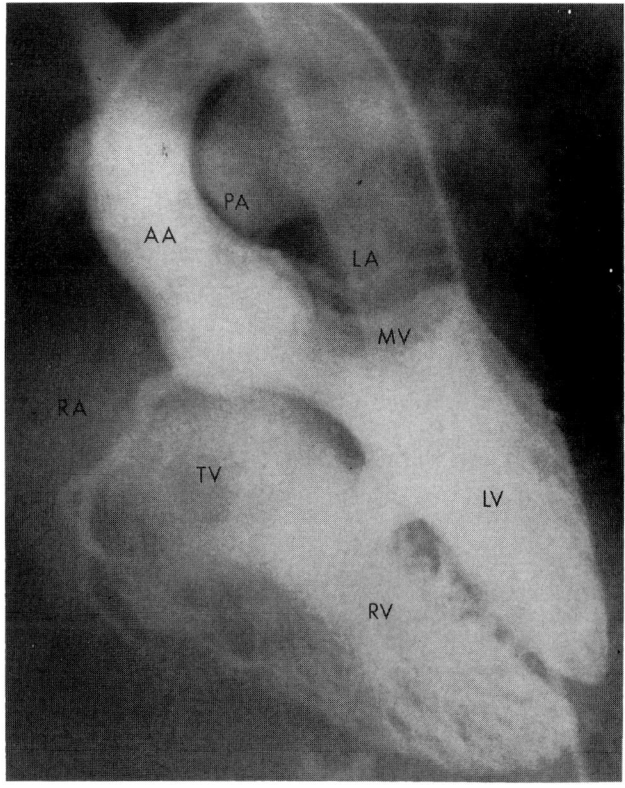

Figure 111–10. Four-chamber projection in a patient with VSDs. This projection profiles the posterior part of the ventricular septum and separates the four chambers. Note the normal orientation of the tricuspid (TV) and mitral (MV) valves. (AA = ascending aorta; LA = left atrium; LV = left ventricle; PA = pulmonary artery; RA = right atrium; RV = right ventricle.)

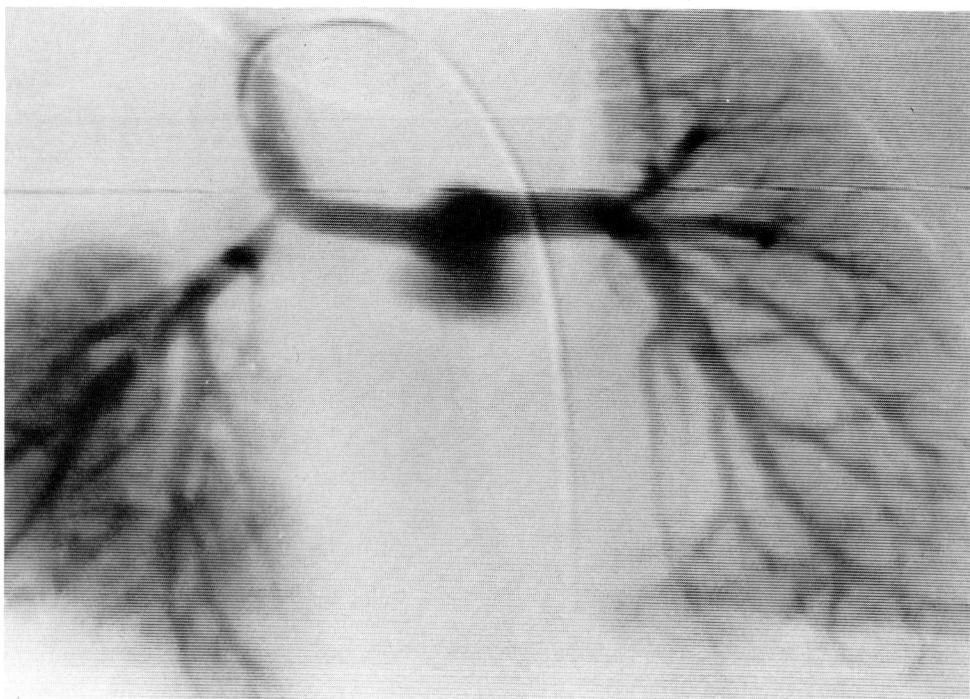

Figure 111–11. Digital subtraction image of the pulmonary arteries in a newborn infant with **right pulmonary artery stenosis secondary to a modified Blalock-Taussig shunt.** The angiogram was made using a 3 Fr catheter and dilute contrast medium.

IMAGING OF SPECIFIC CARDIAC ANOMALIES

Acyanotic Heart Disease

LESIONS WITH LEFT-TO-RIGHT SHUNTS

Ventricular Septal Defects

VSDs are the most common congenital cardiac anomaly with the exception of the bicuspid aortic valve. The defects are classified according to size and location. The locations of different VSDs are illustrated in Figure 111–12.

The ventricular septum is a spiral- or sigmoid-shaped structure consisting of inlet, trabecular, and infundibular or outlet portions, with the membranous septum at the junction. Perimembranous VSDs are the most common, accounting for approximately 70 per cent of all ventricular septal defects and for most of the isolated VSDs. They typically extend from the true membranous septum to the adjacent inlet, trabecular, or infundibular septum. Tricuspid valve tissue is frequently adherent to the margins of perimembranous VSDs and contributes to spontaneous closure and to the angiographic findings of an aneurysm of the membranous septum. Large perimembranous VSDs that extend into the inlet septum adjacent to the tricuspid valve annulus may be associated with a straddling tricuspid valve.

Muscular VSDs may occur in the inlet, trabecular, or infundibular septum. Trabecular VSDs are frequently multiple, and extreme forms are termed "Swiss cheese septum."

Infundibular septal defects may extend to the semilunar valves (subpulmonary, doubly committed subarterial, or supracristal VSD) or may be associated with malalignment of the infundibular septum relative to the septal band, producing subpulmonary or subaortic obstruction. Malalignment VSDs are usually associated with more complex congenital cardiac anomalies, such as tetralogy of Fallot, transposition, and forms of hypoplastic left heart.

High VSDs (perimembranous and subpulmonary) may be associated with prolapse of the right and noncoronary aortic cusps, resulting in aortic regurgitation and a decrease in size of the left-to-right shunt.

The size of the left-to-right shunt associated with a VSD depends upon the size of the defect and the difference in resistance between the systemic and pulmonary circuits. Left-to-right shunting increases after birth as pulmonary vascular resistance decreases and causes increased flow through the pulmonary circuit and volume overload of the left atrium and both ventricles. Infants with large shunts present with symptoms, usually toward the end of the first month of age. Children with small shunts may be entirely asymptomatic. Older patients may develop exercise intolerance and cyanosis due to the presence of pulmonary hypertension and right-to-left shunting caused by the development of pulmonary vaso-occlusive disease (Eisenmenger's syndrome).

CHEST RADIOGRAPHY. Children with small VSDs have normal findings on plain chest radiography. Larger defects are associated with cardiomegaly and shunt vasculature. Left atrial enlargement is best appreciated on the lateral projections. The main pulmonary artery is usually dilated (see Fig. 111–2). Pulmonary edema and pulmonary hyperinflation are often present in infants with large left-to-right shunts. The aortic arch is right-sided in only 3 per cent of patients with isolated VSD.

ANGIOGRAPHY. The locations of various VSDs on right anterior oblique and long axial oblique left ventriculograms are demonstrated diagrammatically in Figure 111–12. The location of a VSD can be determined when the defect is seen in profile in a known projection. Perimembranous (Fig. 111–13*A*) and anterior trabecular VSDs are best profiled in the long axial oblique projection, whereas posterior trabecular (see Fig. 111–10) and AV septal defects are best profiled in the four-chamber view. The right anterior oblique projection profiles VSDs anterior to the septal band and infundibular (subpulmonary) defects. Multiple VSDs require the use of multiple projections. Aortography is necessary in patients with VSD and aortic regurgitation to demonstrate prolapse of the aortic valve.

ECHOCARDIOGRAPHY. Using multiple cross-sectional planes and Doppler interrogation, most VSDs in infants and small children

LOCATION OF VENTRICULAR SEPTAL DEFECTS

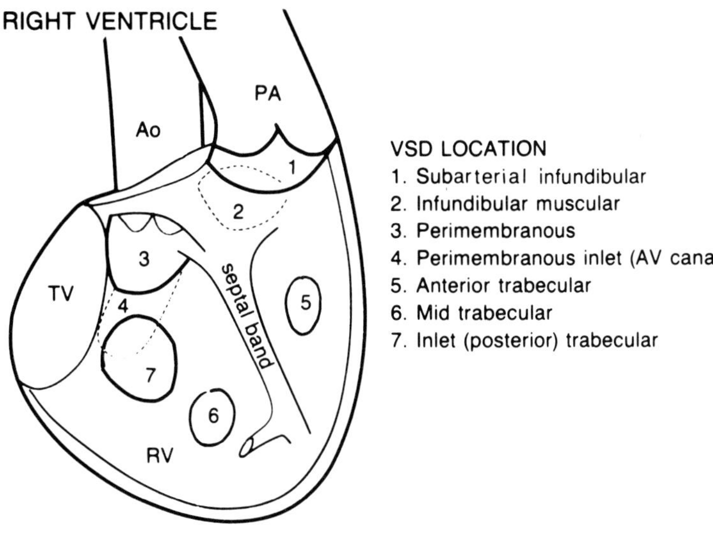

LEFT VENTRICULOGRAPHY

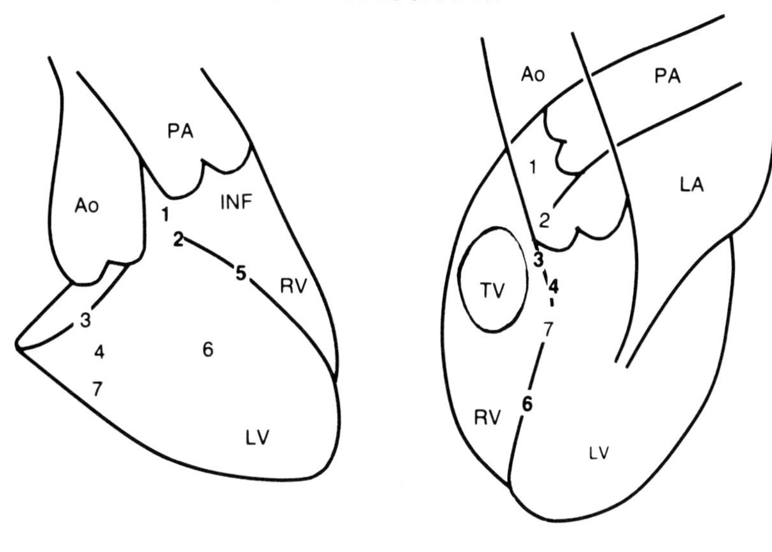

Figure 111–12. The **location of the major types of VSD** as seen from the right ventricle *(top)* and on left ventriculography *(bottom)*. Defects indicated by heavy type numbers are seen in profile in the illustrated projection, while those in lighter type are not. (Ao = aorta; INF = infundibulum; LA = left atrium; LV = left ventricle; PA = pulmonary artery; RV = right ventricle; TV = tricuspid valve.)

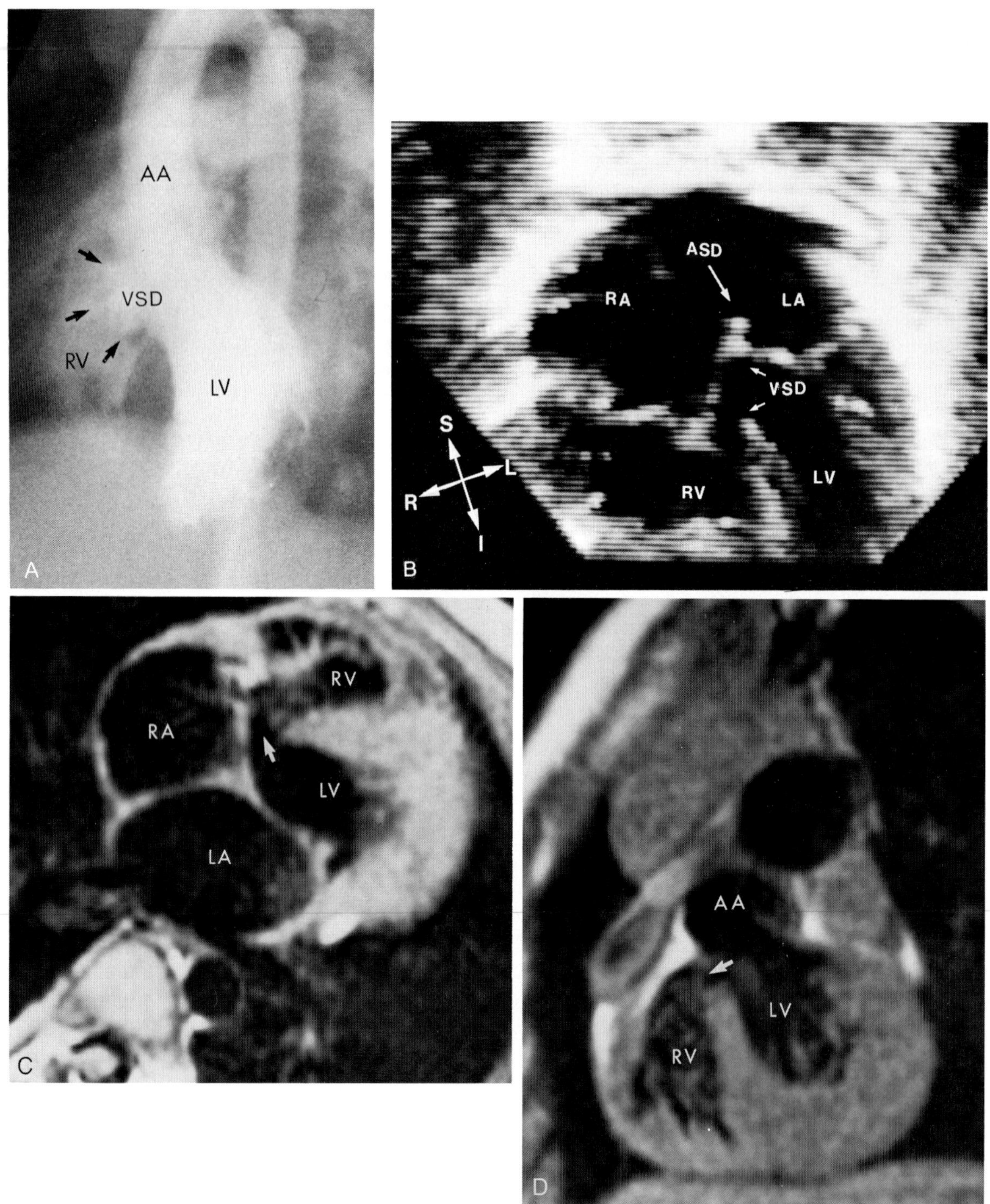

Figure 111–13. *A,* The **perimembranous VSD** is well-profiled under the aortic valve on the long axial oblique projection. The *arrows* indicate tricuspid valve tissue adherent to the margins of the VSD. *B,* A precordial four-chamber echocardiographic image shows the VSD adjacent to the AV valve annuli, under the septal leaflet of the tricuspid valve. The patient also has a secundum atrial septal defect (ASD) *(arrow). C* and *D,* Spin-echo MRIs in transverse axial *(C)* and LAO sagittal *(D)* planes show the relationship between the VSD *(single arrows) (D)* and the tricuspid and aortic valves. (AA = ascending aorta; LA = left atrium; LV = left ventricle; RA = right atrium; RV = right ventricle.)

can be demonstrated and localized with ultrasound (Fig. 111–13*B*). Small muscular defects may be missed.

MRI. VSDs can be imaged with MRI (Fig. 111–13*C* and *D*), especially if an en face plane parallel to the septum is used. MRI is useful in demonstrating the spatial relations between the VSD and the great arteries in complex congenital heart disease such as double-outlet right ventricle.

Atrial Septal Defects

Excluding bicuspid aortic valve, ASD is the second most common congenital cardiac defect and occurs more frequently in females than in males. The five types according to location are (1) ostium secundum defect (secundum type), (2) ostium primum defect (primum type), (3) sinus venosus defect (superior and inferior), (4) coronary sinus—left atrial communication, and (5) common atrium. In addition, the foramen ovale is patent in up to 35 per cent of adult hearts and a higher number of infants and may contribute to atrial shunting, especially in association with other structural defects.

Secundum type defects are the most common and may be associated with pulmonary stenosis, mitral valve prolapse, and aneurysms of the atrial septum. Primum ASDs are usually part of more complex AV septal defects. Sinus venosus ASDs are often associated with partial anomalous pulmonary venous connection to the superior vena cava or right atrium.

Most infants and children with ASD are asymptomatic. Pulmonary artery pressure is usually normal until early adult life in spite of high pulmonary-to-systemic flow ratios. Older adults may have symptoms related to pulmonary hypertension, left ventricular dysfunction, or arrhythmias.

CHEST RADIOGRAPHY. ASD produces volume overload (dilatation) of the right atrium, right ventricle, and pulmonary vessels (Fig. 111–14*A* and *B*). Shunt vascularity is present. The cardiac silhouette is enlarged, with straightening of the left heart border due to dilatation of the outflow portion of the right ventricle. The main pulmonary artery is enlarged. The superior vena caval shadow may be absent on the PA film, presumably owing to rotation of the heart by right-sided enlargement so that the cava is superimposed on the spine. In older children, the retrosternal space may be filled in by the enlarged right ventricular outflow tract and right atrium.

ANGIOGRAPHY. The optimal method to image the atrial septum angiographically is by contrast injection in the right upper pulmonary vein filmed in the four-chamber projection. Secundum type ASDs are seen in the center of the septum, with a rim of septum posteriorly between the superior vena cava and right upper pulmonary vein and anteriorly between the ASD and AV valves (Fig. 111–14*C*). Primum type ASDs are seen anteriorly extending up to the AV valves (Fig. 111–15*A*). The sinus venosus defect (superior vena cava type) is seen postero-superiorly, usually with anterior displacement of the ostium of the right upper pulmonary vein (partial anomalous pulmonary venous connection to the right atrium).

Shunting at the atrial level may also be detected on the levophase of right ventricular or pulmonary artery injection, although the exact location of the defect may be difficult to determine.

ECHOCARDIOGRAPHY. Two-dimensional echocardiography is the modality of choice for imaging the atrial septum. ASDs can be readily identified on the subcostal four-chamber view (see Fig. 111–14*D*). Dropout in the region of the foramen ovale may occur normally in the apical four-chamber view, making it less reliable. The direction of the shunt can be determined with Doppler echocardiography and by observing the direction of bulging of the atrial septum.

MRI. Normal thinning of the atrial septum at the fossa ovalis, seen as signal dropout, must be distinguished from true atrial septal defects. The latter typically have thickening of the margins.

Atrioventricular Septal Defects

The morphology of AV septal defects (also known as AV canal defects and endocardial cushion defects) has been well-described. These complex anomalies involve deficiency of the AV septum and defects or clefts in the septal leaflets of the AV valves. The septal defect involves a varying amount of the anterior atrial septum in the region of the annulus fibrosus of the AV valves and the inlet portion of the ventricular septum, part of which normally separates the right atrium from the left ventricle. AV septal defects are classified in terms of the degree of partitioning of the AV valve as complete, incomplete, and partial.

A complete AV septal defect or AV canal has a primum type ASD, an inlet VSD, and a common or unpartitioned AV valve. The left AV (mitral) valve is cleft; the anterior leaflet is divided into two portions that arise from the crest of the ventricular septum. The superior component of the cleft anterior mitral leaflet is continuous with the anterior leaflet of the tricuspid valve, forming a bridging anterior leaflet. The inferior component forms part of a posterior bridging leaflet.

The heart with a partial AV septal defect has partitioned AV valves (two separate annuli), although the septal defects are in the same location as in complete AV septal defects. The primum type ASD with intact ventricular septum is the most common form of partial AV septal defect and is usually associated with a displaced, cleft mitral valve. Blood that regurgitates through the cleft mitral valve crosses the atrial septal defect to produce a high-pressure left ventricular—right atrial shunt.

Forty per cent of patients with AV septal defects have Down's syndrome, and these patients also have an increased incidence of patent ductus arteriosus and aberrant right subclavian artery. AV septal defects are frequently present in association with primitive complex congenital anomalies such as those seen in asplenia and polysplenia syndromes.

Infants and children with primum type ASD without mitral insufficiency are usually asymptomatic. Those with complete AV septal defects or with severe AV valve regurgitation present in congestive heart failure toward the end of the first month of age.

CHEST RADIOGRAPHY. Chest radiographs demonstrate cardiomegaly with shunt vasculature (Fig. 111–16*A*). The main pulmonary artery is usually dilated, and pulmonary edema with hyperinflated lungs is commonly present in infants. Cardiomegaly out of proportion to the pulmonary blood flow or prominence of the right heart border suggests the presence of AV valve regurgitation. Pulmonary parenchymal disease, including pneumonia and atelectasis, is common, especially in infants with Down's syndrome. Skeletal anomalies including double manubrial ossification centers (Fig. 111–16*B*) and 11 ribs have an increased incidence in patients with Down's syndrome.

ANGIOGRAPHY. Left ventriculography in the frontal projection (PA or RAO) demonstrates the "gooseneck" appearance caused by the deficiency of the inlet septum and displacement of the mitral valve (Fig. 111–17*A*). The cleft in the anterior mitral leaflet appears as a radiolucent notch. The four-chamber view is the preferred projection (Fig. 111–17*B*) and demonstrates the posterior (inlet) VSD, attachments of the AV valves, undercutting of the left ventricular outflow tract, and left ventricular-right atrial shunting. A right upper pulmonary vein injection in the four-chamber projection demonstrates the anterior, primum-type ASD (see Fig. 111–15*A*).

ECHOCARDIOGRAPHY. The morphologic features of AV septal defects are imaged optimally with cross-sectional sonography. Using subcostal and apical four-chamber views, the presence of an atrial and/or ventricular component of the defect and the valve attachments can be assessed (Fig. 111–17*C*). Similar features can be shown by MRI (Fig. 111–7*D*). Doppler echocardiography permits quantitation of AV valve regurgitation.

Text continued on page 1756

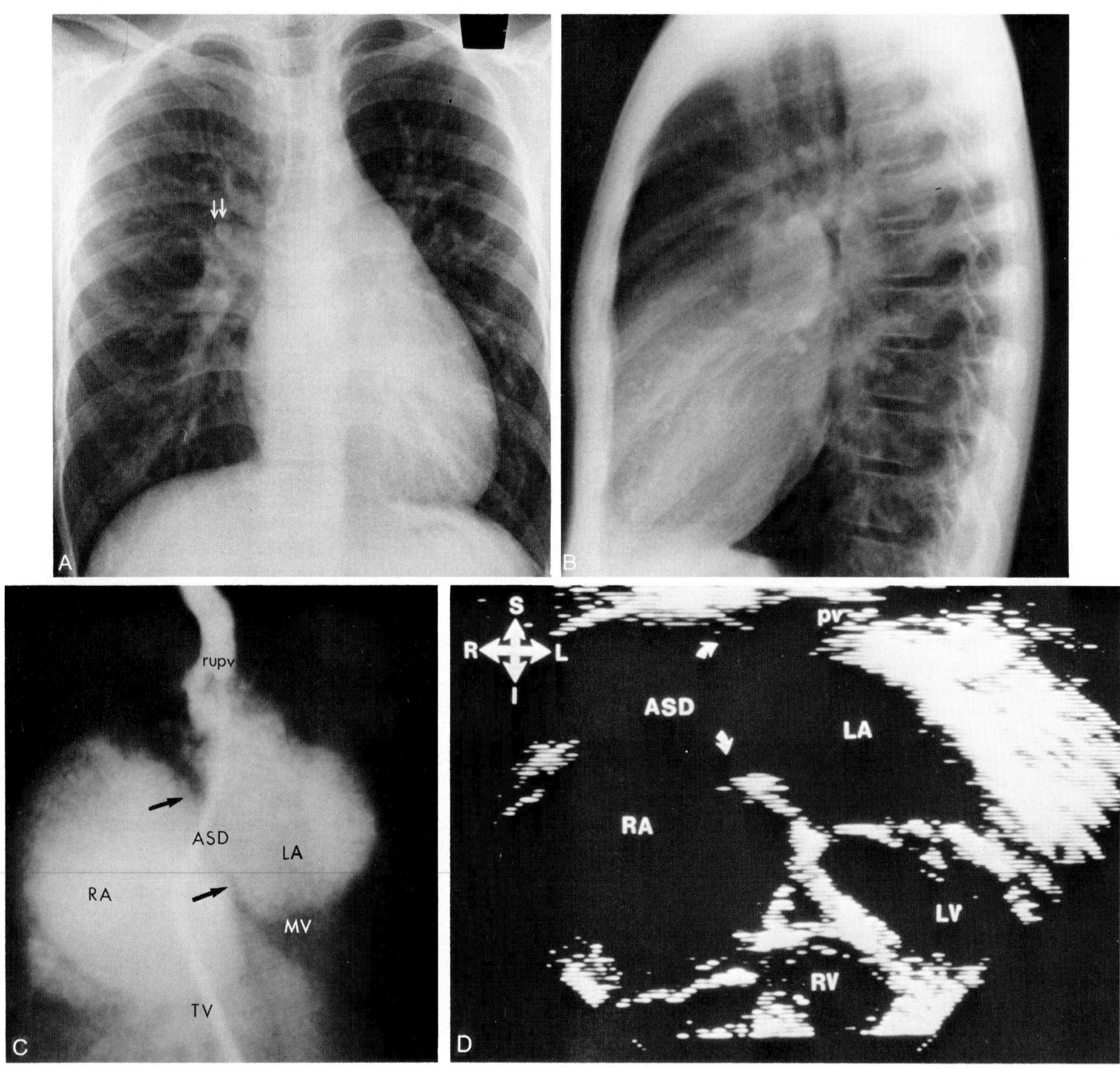

Figure 111–14. Secundum ASD. *A* and *B*, Chest radiographs demonstrate shunt vasculature (note large vessel adjacent to bronchus *[arrows]*), cardiomegaly, straight left heart border, prominent main pulmonary artery, and absent superior vena caval shadow. On the lateral projection *(B)*, the retrosternal space is occupied by the dilated right heart and main pulmonary artery. *C* and *D*, Right upper pulmonary vein (rupv) angiogram, four-chamber projection *(C)*, and subcostal four-chamber echocardiographic image *(D)* show a centrally positioned ASD (*arrows* indicate septal rim), dilated right atrium (RA), and normal offsetting of the AV valves. (LA = left atrium; LV = left ventricle; MV = mitral valve; PV = pulmonary vein; RA = right atrium; RV = right ventricle; TV = tricuspid valve.)

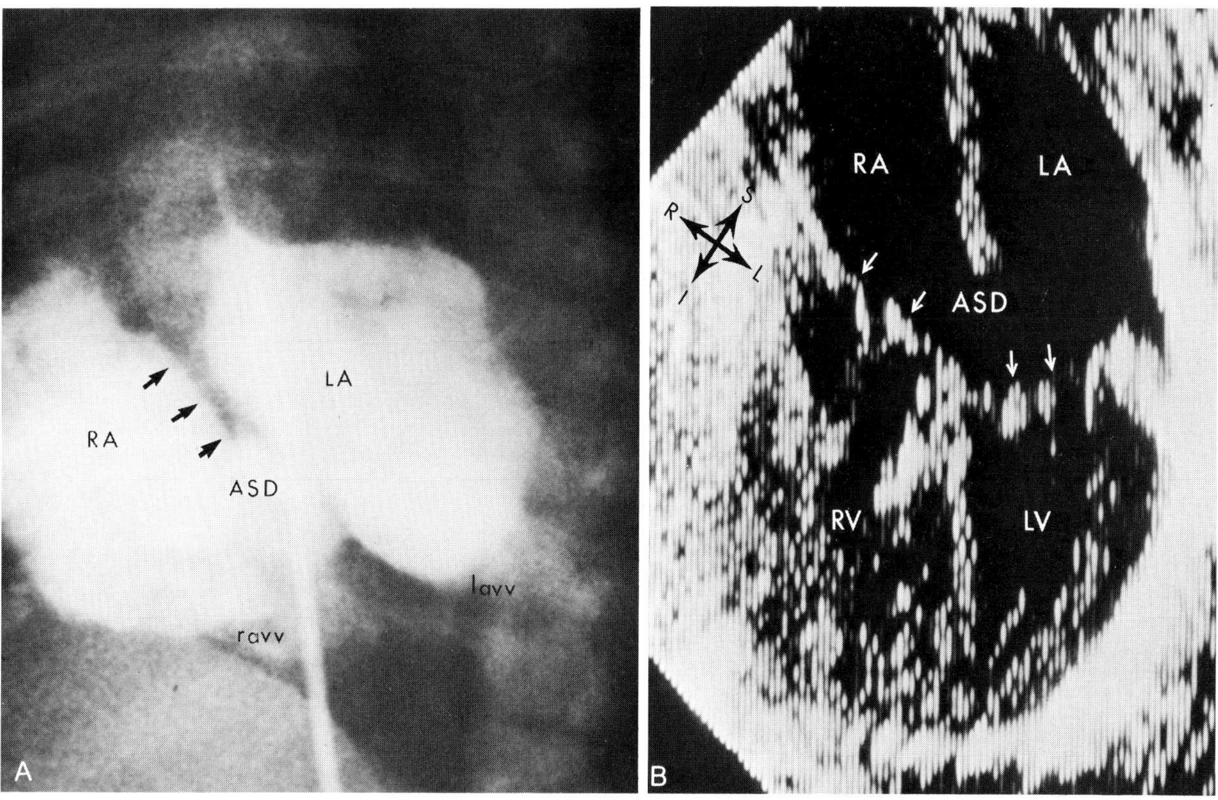

Figure 111–15. Ostium primum ASD. Right upper pulmonary vein angiocardiogram in the four-chamber projection *(A)* and subcostal four-chamber echocardiographic image *(B)* show an anterior ASD that extends to the annuli of the AV valves *(arrows)*. *Arrowheads* indicate the remaining atrial septum. (LA = left atrium; lavv = left AV valve; LV = left ventricle; RA = right atrium; ravv = right AV valve; RV = right ventricle.)

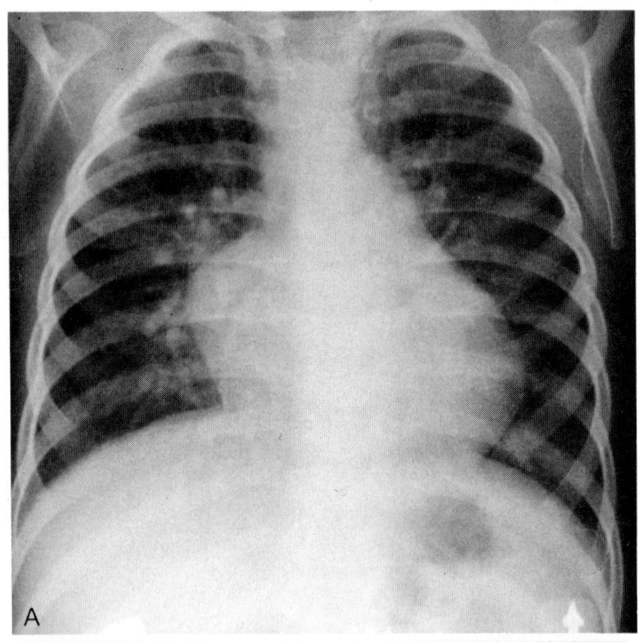

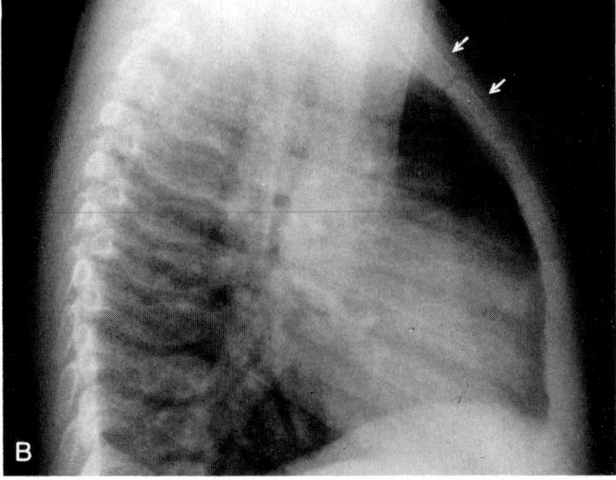

Figure 111–16. AV septal defect. Shunt vasculature is present with cardiomegaly. The right heart border is prominent owing to left ventricular–right atrial shunting *(A)*. *B,* The double manubrial ossification center *(white arrows)* has an increased incidence in patients with Down's syndrome.

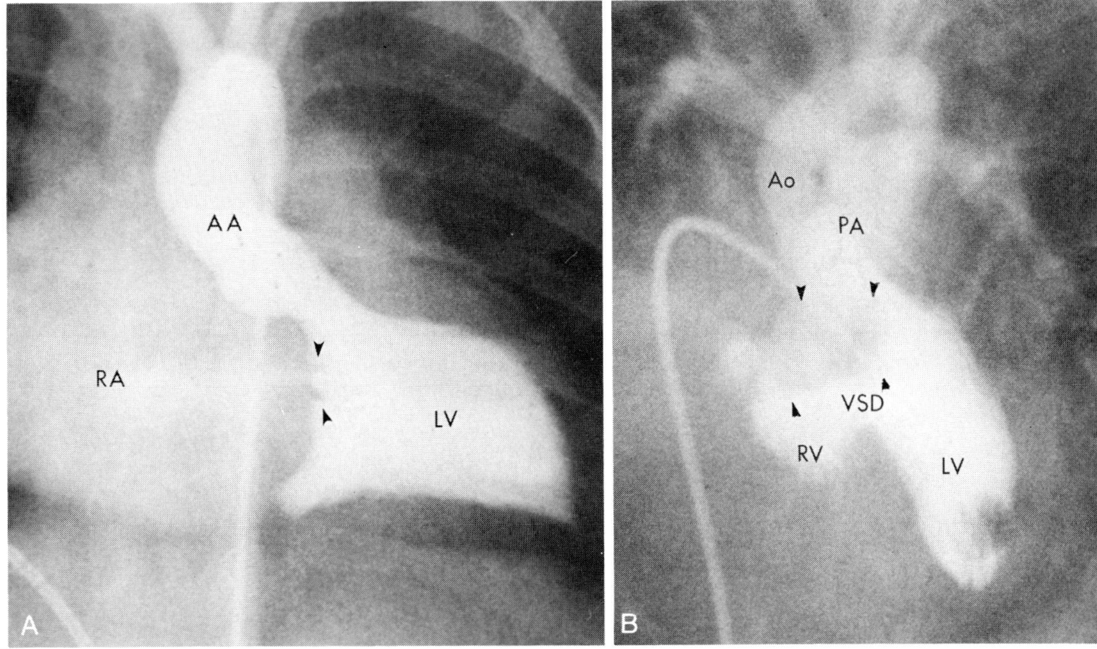

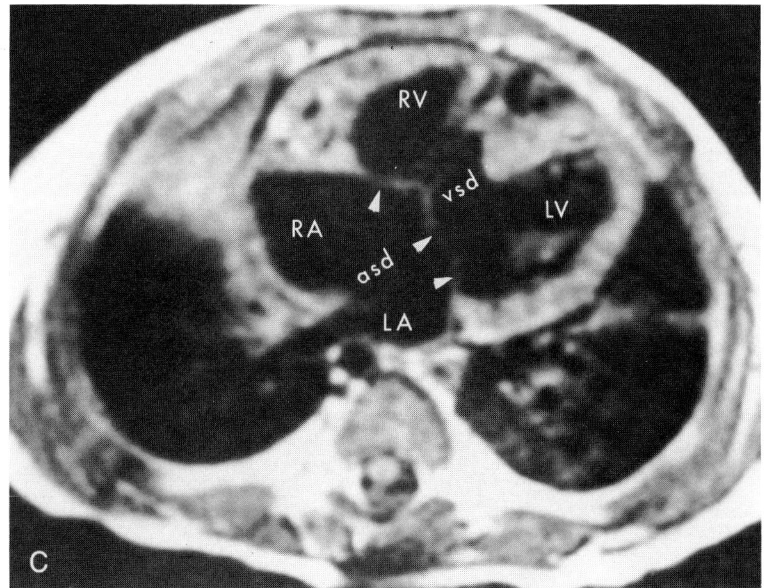

Figure 111–17. *A,* PA projection of left ventriculogram shows **displacement of the mitral valve**, producing a "gooseneck" configuration of the outflow tract. Note the left ventricular (LV)–right atrial (RA) shunt and the cleft in the mitral valve *(arrowheads).* (AA = ascending aorta.) *B,* Left ventriculogram (four-chamber projection) shows a **complete AV septal defect** with an inlet VSD and common AV valve (dark area within *arrowheads*). Note the superior bridging leaflet *(upper arrowheads)* and the inferior bridging leaflet *(lower arrowheads). C,* Axial spin-echo MRI shows the anterior common bridging leaflet *(arrowheads),* the inlet VSD (vsd), and the primum ASD (asd). (Ao = aorta; LV = left ventricle; RV = right ventricle; LA = left atrium; S = septum.)

Patent Ductus Arteriosus

Patent ductus arteriosus (PDA) is the third most common congenital cardiac anomaly (12 per cent), excluding bicuspid aortic valve. Fifteen per cent of premature infants with respiratory distress syndrome have a PDA. Hypoxia associated with immaturity of the ductal tissue is an underlying factor in PDA of the premature. Persistent patency of the ductus arteriosus in full-term infants is felt to be related to a structural abnormality of the ductal wall. As an isolated lesion, the PDA almost always arises from the underside of the proximal descending aorta, distal to the origin of the left subclavian artery, and connects with the pulmonary circuit at the posterior end of the main pulmonary artery or the proximal left pulmonary artery. In the presence of complex congenital heart disease, the ductus may arise from the subclavian or innominate artery and may be bilateral.

Chest Radiography. Chest radiographs of premature neonates with PDA show progressive cardiomegaly and usually hazy central pulmonary densities due to pulmonary edema (Fig. 111–18*A*). Underlying pulmonary disease may complicate radiologic diagnosis. Older infants and children demonstrate cardiomegaly with prominence of the left atrium, main pulmonary artery, and sometimes the aortic arch, associated with shunt vascularity.

Angiography. Cardiac catheterization is rarely needed to diagnose an isolated PDA, as clinical examination and two-dimensional and Doppler echocardiography are accurate, especially in infants. Aortography in the lateral projection is optimal (Fig. 111–18*B*).

Echocardiography. Suprasternal imaging permits demonstration of the ductus along its entire length (Fig. 111–18*C*). Doppler examination confirms patency by detection of continuous flow at the pulmonary artery end of the ductus.

Other Causes of Left-to-Right Shunting

1. Aortopulmonary window (aortopulmonary septal defect)
2. Hemitruncus (origin of one pulmonary artery from the ascending aorta)
3. Coronary-cameral fistula (communication between coronary artery and a cardiac chamber)
4. Aortocameral communications
5. Anomalous origin of the left coronary artery from the pulmonary artery
6. Partial anomalous pulmonary venous return
7. Cerebral or peripheral arteriovenous malformations

LEFT-SIDED OBSTRUCTIVE LESIONS

Aortic Stenosis

Congenital aortic stenosis is present in 7 per cent of patients with congenital cardiac disease and is classified by location as valvar,

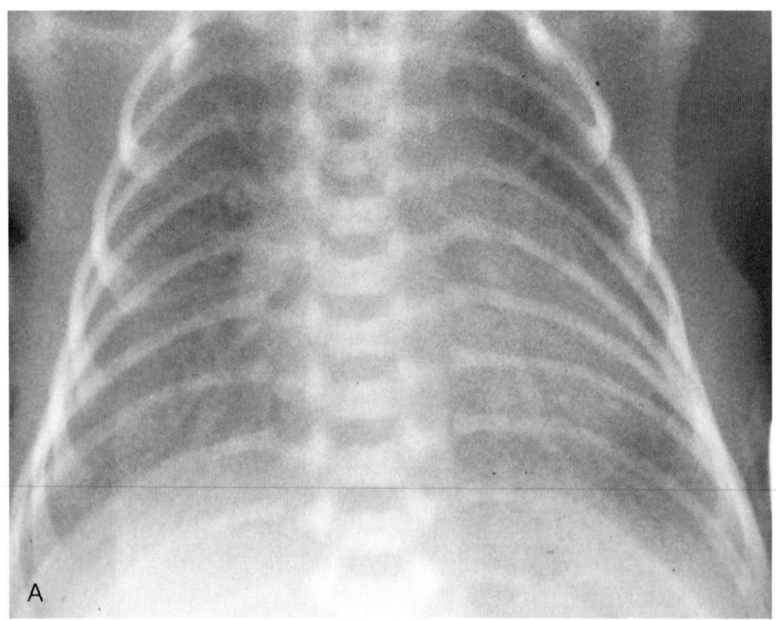

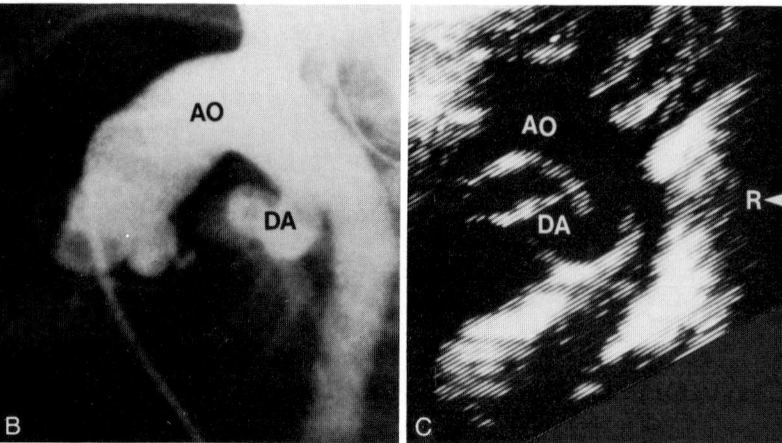

Figure 111–18. *A,* **Patent ductus arteriosus.** This AP chest radiograph of a one-week-old premature infant shows cardiomegaly and haziness of the lungs due to pulmonary edema. *B* and *C,* A patent ductus arteriosus (DA) arising from the undersurface of the aortic arch is shown on a lateral aortogram *(B)* and on a suprasternal echocardiographic image *(C).* (AO = aorta.)

subvalvar, or supravalvar and by the severity of the gradient at cardiac catheterization (30 mm Hg = mild; 30 to 60 mm Hg = moderate; > 60 mm Hg = severe). Obstruction occasionally occurs at more than one site.

VALVAR AORTIC STENOSIS. The abnormal aortic valve may be unicuspid, bicuspid, or tricuspid. The unicuspid aortic valve is uncommon and is usually seen in infants with critical aortic stenosis. The bicuspid aortic valve is the most common anomaly associated with congenital aortic stenosis and is probably the most common congenital cardiac anomaly, present in 1 per cent of the population. The valve anomaly includes varying degrees of abnormal commissure development with thickening and rigidity of the leaflets. Obstruction becomes more severe with time. Calcification of the abnormal leaflets usually occurs in early adulthood. Less frequently, aortic stenosis is caused by a tricuspid valve with commissural fusion. In all forms, the aortic valve annulus may be small.

Twenty per cent of patients with valvar aortic stenosis have other cardiac anomalies. These include mitral valve anomalies, coarctation of the descending aorta, endocardial fibroelastosis, and VSD. Twenty-five per cent of patients have associated aortic regurgitation.

Chest Radiography. Infants with critical aortic stenosis have cardiomegaly with pulmonary venous hypertension. Marked cardiomegaly usually indicates mitral regurgitation due to endocardial fibroelastosis or severe ventricular dysfunction.

Children with isolated aortic stenosis usually have normal heart size and dilatation of the ascending aorta (Fig. 111–19*A*). Serial films showing progressive left ventricular enlargement usually indicate the presence of aortic regurgitation. Valve calcification may be seen in adults, optimally with fluoroscopy.

Angiography. Left ventriculography (RAO and long axial oblique projections) demonstrates left ventricular hypertrophy with increased wall thickness and papillary muscle enlargement.

A supravalvar aortic injection of contrast is made to assess valve competence. The stenotic aortic valve is thickened and domes in systole (Fig. 111–19*B*). Moderate to severe aortic stenosis is usually associated with an eccentric jet (Fig. 111–19*B*) that indicates the size of the valve orifice. The valve annulus may be hypoplastic. A bicuspid aortic valve is easily recognized when only two sinuses of Valsalva are present (Fig. 111–19*C*). In the presence of three sinuses, one, usually the noncoronary sinus, is larger. The ascending aorta is dilated in an eccentric fashion.

Echocardiography. Echocardiography demonstrates thickening and doming and the number of valve leaflets, as well as associated anomalies (Fig. 111–19*D*). Doppler evaluation provides an accurate assessment of stenosis and regurgitation (Fig. 111–19*E*).

SUBAORTIC STENOSIS. Subaortic stenosis is usually caused by one of three morphologic abnormalities: a discrete membrane, a tunnel form of obstruction, and hypertrophic cardiomyopathy.

Discrete and tunnel forms of subaortic stenosis are often associated with other left-sided obstructions such as coarctation, supravalvar aortic stenosis, mitral stenosis, and supravalvar stenosing mitral ring, as well as ventricular septal defects and right ventricular obstructing muscle bundles.

Hypertrophic cardiomyopathy is a hereditary disorder of cardiac muscle that affects both ventricles but with disproportionate thickening of the ventricular septum. Although symptoms usually do not develop until adult years or late childhood, patients may present earlier.

Chest Radiography. Heart size and pulmonary blood flow are usually normal with isolated subaortic obstruction. Approximately 30 per cent of patients have dilatation of the ascending aorta.

Angiography. Left ventriculography in the long axial oblique projections best demonstrates the left ventricular outflow tract. Discrete subaortic stenosis appears as a radiolucent line across the left ventricular outflow tract, a variable distance from the aortic valve. The aortic valve leaflets are thickened, flutter, and may open eccentrically. An aortogram should be performed to demonstrate secondary aortic regurgitation.

Tunnel subaortic stenosis is characterized by a long, tubular, fixed narrowing of the left ventricular outflow tract. In hypertrophic cardiomyopathy, a septal bulge is associated with systolic anterior motion of the anterior mitral leaflet, which may be thickened at the site of impact. Left ventricular hypertrophy is present in all forms of subaortic stenosis.

Echocardiography. Two-dimensional echocardiography reliably demonstrates subaortic obstructions and appears to be more sensitive than angiography in the detection of small subaortic ridges. The long-axis view best shows the obstructing membranes.

SUPRAVALVAR AORTIC STENOSIS. Congenital supravalvar aortic stenosis may occur as a focal ''hourglass'' narrowing (most common), a discrete web, or diffuse narrowing or hypoplasia of the ascending aorta. The hourglass deformity begins at the superior margin of the sinuses of Valsalva. The coronary ostia may be narrowed. This form of obstruction is seen in patients with Williams' syndrome or idiopathic infantile hypercalcemia (elfin facies, mental retardation, and dental anomalies) and intrauterine rubella infection.

Patients with Williams' syndrome and rubella syndrome may also have supravalvar pulmonary stenosis and peripheral pulmonary artery stenoses as well as obstructive lesions in other systemic vessels, including the abdominal aorta and renal arteries.

In the absence of associated lesions, plain chest films are usually normal without post-stenotic dilatation of the aorta.

Hypoplastic Left Heart Syndrome

The term *hypoplastic left heart syndrome* encompasses a spectrum of anomalies associated with severe obstruction, usually at multiple levels, in the systemic cardiac structures. The anomalies account for approximately 7 per cent of congenital cardiac disease.

The most common form includes aortic valve atresia with hypoplastic ascending aorta; tiny, thick-walled left ventricle; and abnormal (stenotic or atretic) mitral valve. Coarctation and interruption of the aortic arch may be present. The ductus arteriosus is patent initially, and an atrial septal defect or patent foramen ovale is usually present.

Forty per cent of infants come to medical attention in the first two days of life, and 95 per cent die in the first month. The usual presentation is that of congestive cardiac failure or vascular collapse.

CHEST RADIOGRAPHY. Plain film findings are variable. Usually the heart is moderately enlarged with a globular configuration, the lungs are overinflated, and vascularity reflects pulmonary venous hypertension with pulmonary edema (Fig. 111–20*A*).

ANGIOGRAPHY. Retrograde aortography demonstrates the severe tubular hypoplasia of the ascending aorta, usually with normal-sized coronary and brachiocephalic arteries and transverse arch and coarctation at the isthmus (Fig. 111–20*B*). Right ventriculography shows enlargement of the right ventricle and pulmonary artery with a large patent ductus arteriosus.

ECHOCARDIOGRAPHY. Cross-sectional echocardiography demonstrates the tiny ascending aorta and left ventricle and associated anomalies (Fig. 111–20*C*). Cardiac catheterization is rarely necessary.

Coarctation of the Descending Aorta

Coarctation of the descending aorta is present in 5 per cent of patients with congenital cardiac disease and occurs in males twice as often as in females. Coarctation usually occurs as a discrete narrowing of the aortic isthmus distal to the origin of the left subclavian artery and near the aortic end of the ductus or ligamen-

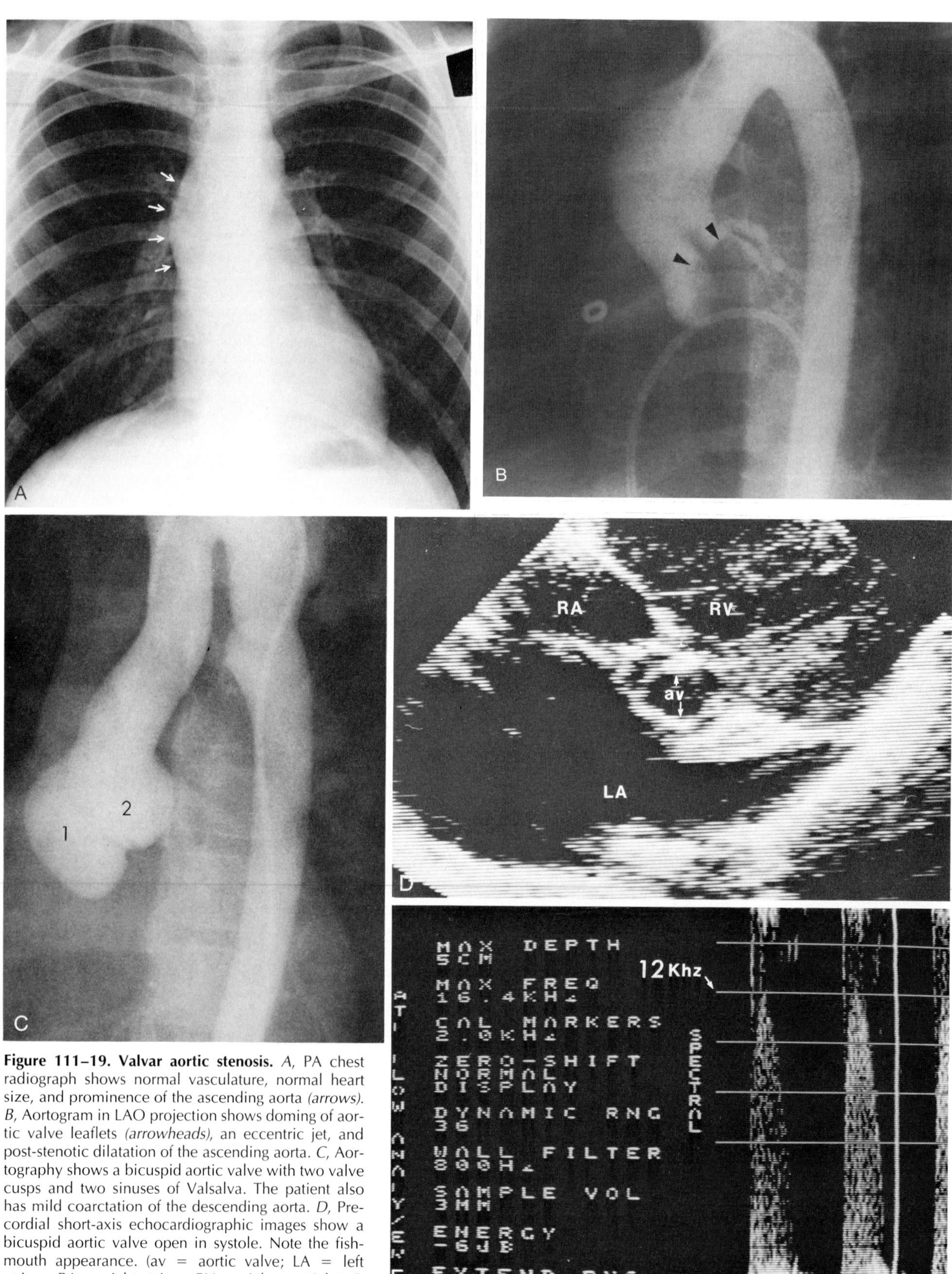

Figure 111–19. Valvar aortic stenosis. *A,* PA chest radiograph shows normal vasculature, normal heart size, and prominence of the ascending aorta *(arrows). B,* Aortogram in LAO projection shows doming of aortic valve leaflets *(arrowheads),* an eccentric jet, and post-stenotic dilatation of the ascending aorta. *C,* Aortography shows a bicuspid aortic valve with two valve cusps and two sinuses of Valsalva. The patient also has mild coarctation of the descending aorta. *D,* Precordial short-axis echocardiographic images show a bicuspid aortic valve open in systole. Note the fish-mouth appearance. (av = aortic valve; LA = left atrium; RA = right atrium; RV = right ventricle.) *E,* Spectral Doppler tracing in a patient with valvar aortic stenosis has a high-velocity turbulent jet (12 kHz).

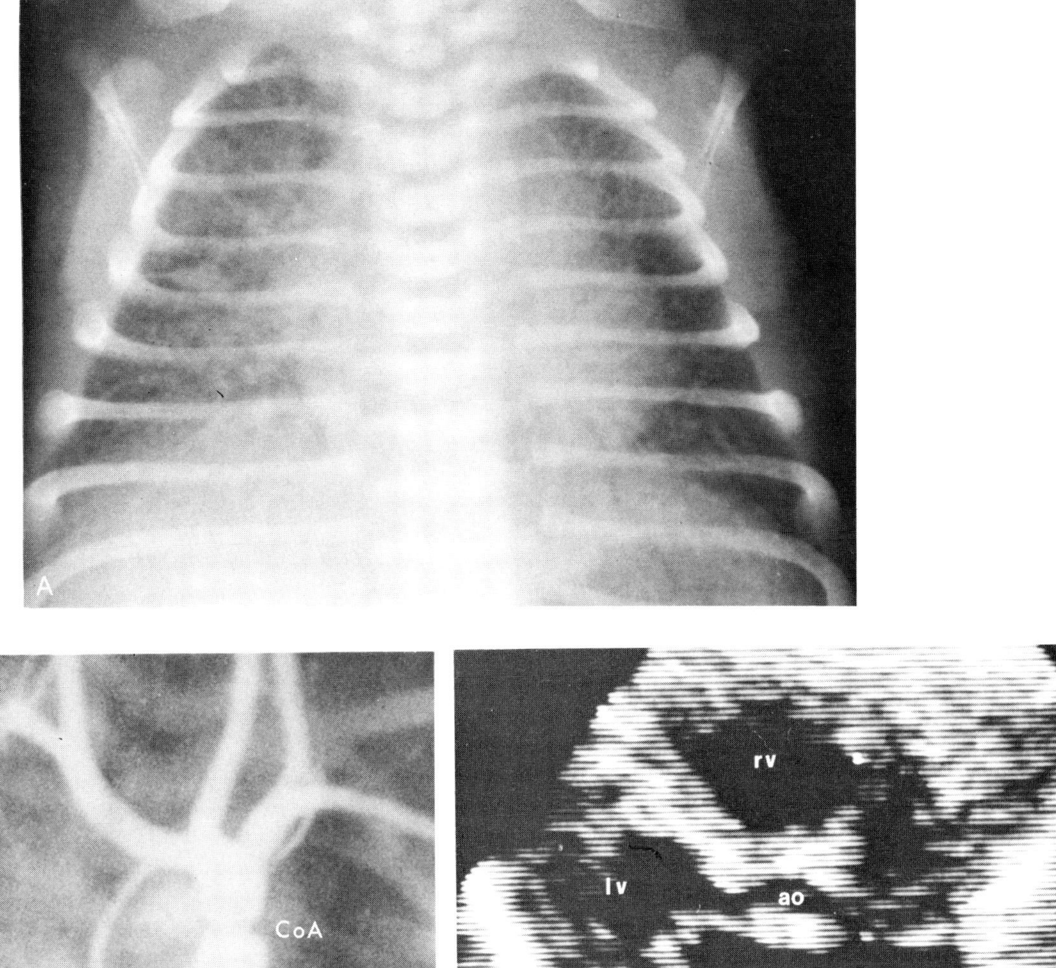

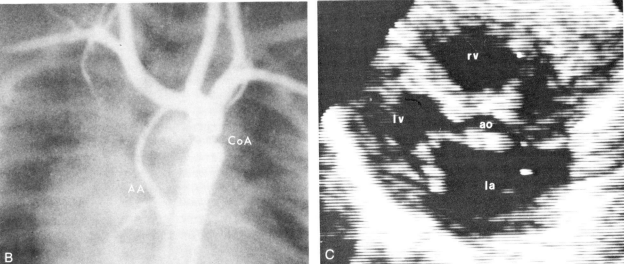

Figure 111–20. Hypoplastic left heart syndrome. *A,* AP chest film shows cardiomegaly and pulmonary venous hypertension. *B,* Contrast injection in the aortic arch fills a tiny ascending aorta (AA) and normal-sized coronary arteries and arch vessels. Note coarctation (CoA) of the descending aorta. *C,* Precordial long-axis cut demonstrates severe hypoplasia of the left ventricle (lv), an abnormal mitral valve, a dilated left atrium (la), a large right ventricle (rv), and a very small ascending aorta (ao).

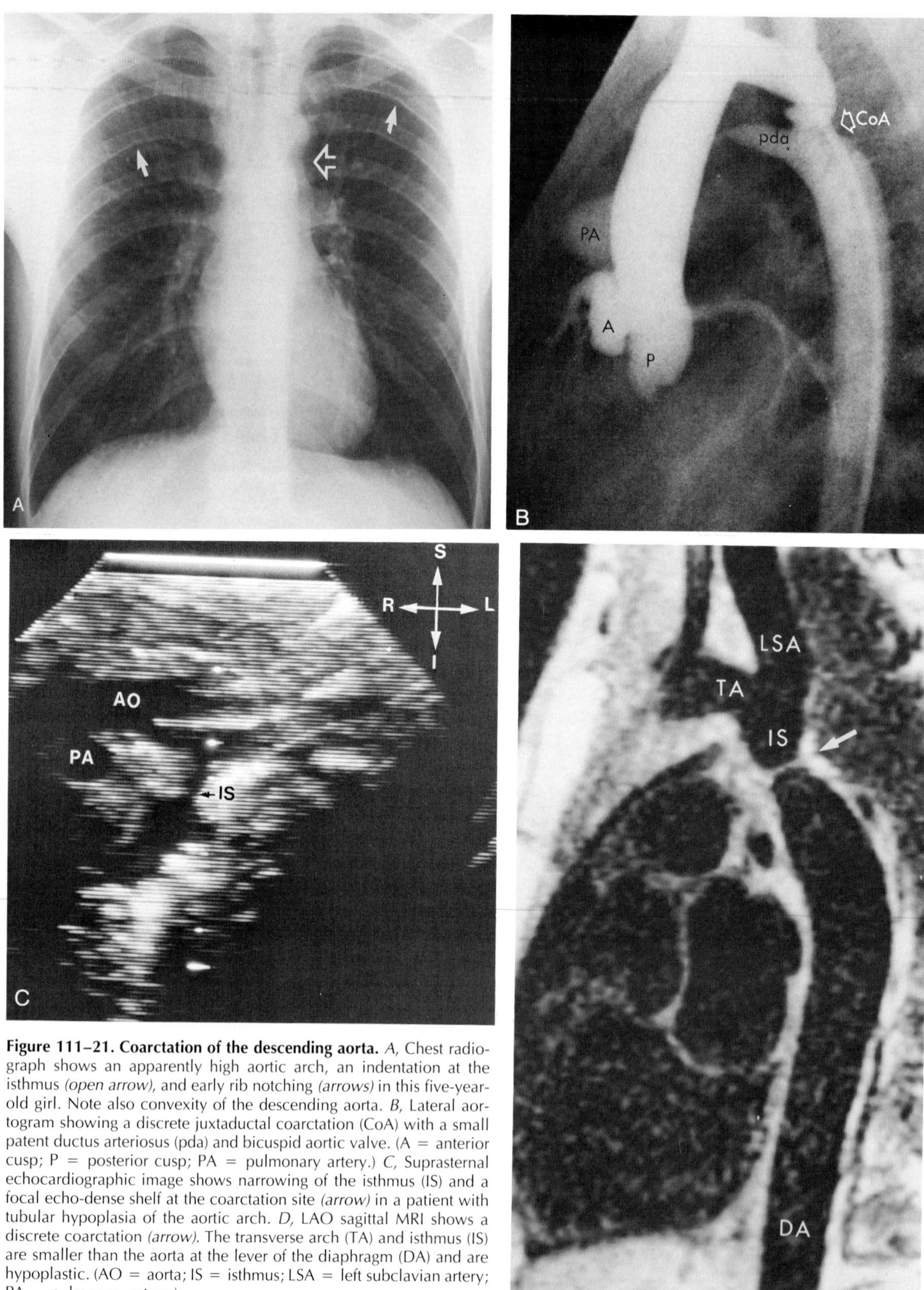

Figure 111–21. Coarctation of the descending aorta. *A,* Chest radiograph shows an apparently high aortic arch, an indentation at the isthmus *(open arrow),* and early rib notching *(arrows)* in this five-year-old girl. Note also convexity of the descending aorta. *B,* Lateral aortogram showing a discrete juxtaductal coarctation (CoA) with a small patent ductus arteriosus (pda) and bicuspid aortic valve. (A = anterior cusp; P = posterior cusp; PA = pulmonary artery.) *C,* Suprasternal echocardiographic image shows narrowing of the isthmus (IS) and a focal echo-dense shelf at the coarctation site *(arrow)* in a patient with tubular hypoplasia of the aortic arch. *D,* LAO sagittal MRI shows a discrete coarctation *(arrow).* The transverse arch (TA) and isthmus (IS) are smaller than the aorta at the lever of the diaphragm (DA) and are hypoplastic. (AO = aorta; IS = isthmus; LSA = left subclavian artery; PA = pulmonary artery.)

tum arteriosus (juxtaductal). Less frequently, the narrowing involves a long segment of transverse aortic arch (tubular hypoplasia), usually also associated with discrete narrowing at the isthmus. When the ductus is patent, it is useful to describe the coarctation as preductal, juxtaductal, or postductal.

Collaterals to the lower body include the following arteries: intercostal, internal mammary, muscular phrenic, superior epigastric, transverse cervical, scapular, lateral thoracic, and anterior spinal. A bicuspid aortic valve is present in a high percentage of patients, with estimates of 30 to 85 per cent. Eighty to 85 per cent of the symptomatic *infants* with coarctation have associated anomalies, especially aortic stenosis, patent ductus arteriosus, and VSD. Symptomatic infants present with signs of congestive heart failure as early as 48 hours of age. Coarctation of the abdominal aorta is much less common and is seen in patients with Williams' syndrome, rubella syndrome, neurofibromatosis, and Takayasu's arteritis. Pseudocoarctation describes elongation of the aorta with kinking at the isthmus, but without dilated collaterals or a gradient.

Interruption of the aortic arch involves absence of a segment of the arch, most often the portion between the left carotid and left subclavian arteries, and is almost always associated with a VSD and subaortic obstruction. The lower body is perfused via a patent ductus arteriosus.

Chest Radiography. Symptomatic infants usually have cardiomegaly and pulmonary venous hypertension. Shunt vascularity is present in those with additional left-to-right shunts. The aortic knob may be difficult to identify in infants, but convexity of the descending aorta is a sign of coarctation. Older children and adults usually have evidence of an abnormal aortic arch contour on the PA radiograph with a normal heart size and pulmonary vascularity (Fig. 111–21*A*). The "3" sign with an indentation at the aortic isthmus and post-stenotic dilatation of the descending aorta are typical findings. Others include a poorly defined aortic arch, "high" aortic arch due to a prominent left subclavian artery, and curvilinear densities superimposed on the isthmus. A barium esophagram is useful in confirming the site of coarctation and shows a reverse 3 sign. The ascending aorta is often dilated, especially in the presence of a bicuspid aortic valve. Notching or sclerosis of the undersurface of ribs, usually the third to eighth ribs bilaterally, and lateral margins of the scapulae is caused by dilated collaterals. These signs are infrequently seen before six years of age (Fig. 111–21*A*).

Angiography. As clinical examination and echocardiography are accurate in the diagnosis of coarctation of the aorta, only patients with atypical findings or additional lesions require angiography or MRI (Fig. 111–21*D*). In discrete coarctation, ascending aortography demonstrates a focal posterolateral shelf-like indentation distal to the origin of the subclavian artery, with post-stenotic dilatation of the descending aorta and dilated collaterals (Fig. 111–21*B*). Variations include left subclavian artery stenosis, aberrant right subclavian artery, aneurysms of the aorta or intercostals, patent ductus arteriosus, bicuspid aortic valve, and additional left-sided obstructions. Hypoplasia of the transverse arch involves segments of variable length and is usually associated with additional discrete isthmic narrowing (Fig. 111–21*C*).

Echocardiography. Suprasternal views demonstrate the site of narrowing with a posterior shelf in infants and small children (Fig. 111–21*C*), and Doppler examination predicts the pressure gradient.

MRI. The optimal imaging plane to evaluate coarctation of the descending aorta is LAO sagittal (Fig. 111–21*D*). Additional planes, such as transverse axial and RAO coronal, are useful to confirm the dimensions. The abdominal aorta at the diaphragm should be smaller than the arch and isthmus and can be used to "normalize" the arch dimensions.

Rare Causes of Left-Sided Obstruction

1. Congenital mitral stenosis
2. Mitral atresia
3. Cor triatriatum
4. Tumors: myxoma, fibroma, rhabdomyoma
5. Congenital pulmonary vein stenosis or atresia
6. Pulmonary veno-occlusive disease

RIGHT-SIDED OBSTRUCTIVE LESIONS

Obstruction to pulmonary blood flow may occur at any level from systemic veins to the peripheral pulmonary arteries. The more common obstructions will be discussed in this section.

Valvar Pulmonary Stenosis

Valvar pulmonary stenosis is present in 10 per cent of patients with congenital heart disease and may be caused by commissural fusion of a tricuspid valve (most common form of isolated pulmonary stenosis), a bicuspid pulmonary valve (usually associated with complex malformations), or a dysplastic pulmonary valve. Patients with Noonan's syndrome and pulmonary stenosis typically have dysplastic pulmonary valves. Secundum type atrial septal defect is often associated with valvar pulmonary stenosis.

Infants and children with severe pulmonary stenosis (peak systolic gradient > 60 mm Hg) may be cyanotic due to right-to-left shunting only in the presence of a patent foramen ovale or atrial septal defect. Those with mild to moderate pulmonary stenosis are usually asymptomatic and are detected because of an ejection systolic murmur and click. Unlike aortic stenosis, valvar pulmonary stenosis is usually nonprogressive.

Chest Radiography. Heart size is usually normal or mildly increased unless severe tricuspid insufficiency is present. Pulmonary blood flow is normal in the absence of a right-to-left shunt, when it may be decreased. The main and left pulmonary arteries are usually dilated, secondary to the jet through the valve orifice (Fig. 111–22*A* and *B*), except in patients with a dysplastic pulmonary valve.

Angiography. Right ventriculography in cranially angled PA and lateral projections shows evidence of right ventricular hypertrophy, often with dynamic subpulmonary narrowing, thickening and systolic doming of the pulmonary valve, and usually post-stenotic dilatation of the main and left pulmonary arteries (Fig. 111–22*C* and *D*). In moderate and severe stenosis, a jet indicates the size of the orifice. Fixed subpulmonary stenosis or hypoplasia of the main branch pulmonary arteries must be ruled out, as these lesions require modification of the surgical approach. The dysplastic valve typically has marked irregular thickening of the cusps, a small annulus, and a small main pulmonary artery.

Echocardiography. Echocardiographic imaging demonstrates the thickened, doming valve and the presence of subvalvar obstruction. Doppler assessment usually accurately predicts the gradient across the stenotic pulmonary valve.

Subpulmonary Obstruction

Subpulmonary fixed obstruction may be caused by hypertrophied, abnormally positioned muscle bundles (anomalous right ventricular muscle bundle, double-chambered right ventricle), deviation of the infundibular septum, discrete membranes, accessory tricuspid valve tissue, and windsock aneurysms of the membranous septum. Obstructing right ventricular muscle bundles are frequently associated with perimembranous VSD and discrete subaortic stenosis.

Supravalvar and Peripheral Pulmonary Stenosis

Stenosis or hypoplasia of the main pulmonary artery, right and left branches, and origins of the segmental or lobar branches may be isolated anomalies or associated with Williams' or rubella syndrome and complex anomalies, especially tetralogy of Fallot. Supra-

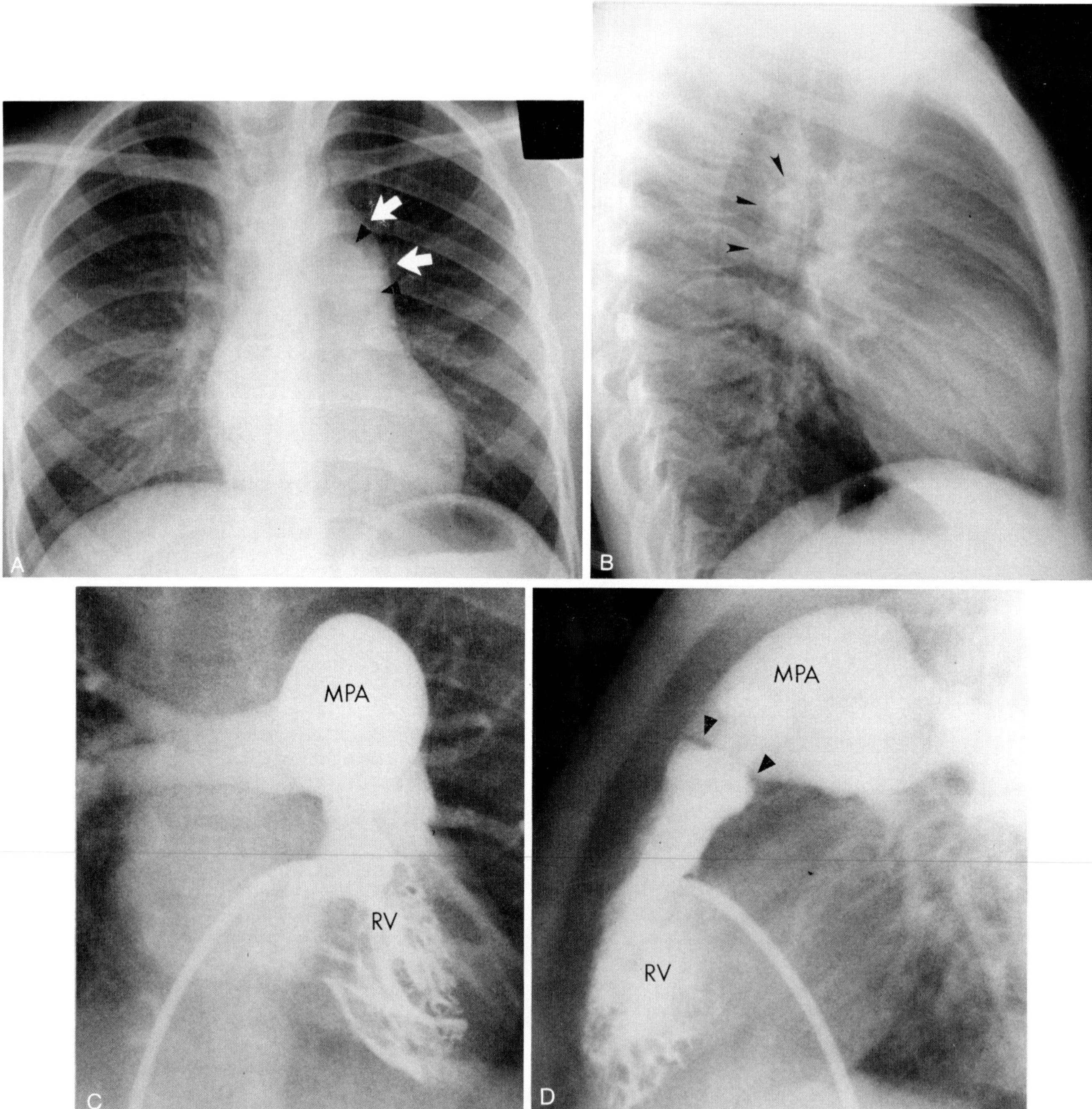

Figure 111–22. Valvar pulmonary stenosis. *A* and *B*, Chest radiographs show normal vascularity, normal heart size, and enlargement of the main *(arrows)* and left *(arrowheads)* pulmonary arteries. *C* and *D*, PA and lateral right ventriculograms demonstrate thickening and doming of the pulmonary valve *(arrowheads)*, an eccentric jet through the orifice, and post-stenotic dilatation of the main pulmonary artery (MPA). (RV = right ventricle.)

valvar pulmonary stenosis is also seen with the dysplastic pulmonary valve. Obstructions are frequently multiple.

Ebstein's Anomaly of the Tricuspid Valve

Ebstein's anomaly is a rare malformation in which the origin or proximal attachments of the tricuspid valve leaflets are displaced into the right ventricular cavity, away from the normal annulus at the AV junction. The anterior leaflet tends to be large and sail-like. The right ventricle is divided by the displaced leaflets into atrialized and functional parts. An atrial septal defect or patent foramen ovale is present in over 50 per cent of patients, and pulmonary stenosis or atresia may be an associated finding. Tricuspid regurgitation with reduced right ventricular function and right-to-left shunting at the atrial level occurs in the more severe forms. Cyanosis may be most pronounced in the neonatal period, whereas patients with milder lesions are acyanotic and asymptomatic until early adult life.

CHEST RADIOGRAPHY. In patients with severe Ebstein's anomaly, the cardiac silhouette is moderately to severely enlarged and pulmonary blood flow is normal or decreased. Typically, the cardiac silhouette is "square," with a prominent right heart border composed of massively dilated right atrium and a prominent left upper heart border formed by a dilated right ventricular outflow tract (Fig. 111–23*A* and *B*).

ANGIOGRAPHY. Contrast injections in the atrialized and functional parts of the right ventricle in PA or RAO projections best demonstrate the anatomy. The expected location of the tricuspid valve annulus can be identified by a notch or indentation in the inferior surface at the atrioventricular junction or by the course of the right coronary artery (Fig. 111–23*C*). The inlet part of the right ventricle is smooth, and the origin of the displaced leaflets produces a second notch, indicating the demarcation between atrialized and functional right ventricle. Tricuspid regurgitation is usually present.

ECHOCARDIOGRAPHY AND MRI. Cross-sectional imaging directly demonstrates the displacement of tricuspid valve leaflets and the degree of valve dysplasia (Fig. 111–23*D* and *E*). Doppler assessment indicates the severity of tricuspid regurgitation.

CYANOTIC CONGENITAL CARDIAC DISEASE

Cyanosis results from obstruction to pulmonary blood flow with right-to-left shunting across a septal defect, or "admixture" of oxygenated and deoxygenated blood when the pulmonary and systemic circulations are not in series. Cyanotic lesions tend to be more complex than acyanotic lesions, often involving malformations of conotruncal development and positional abnormalities of the cardiac chambers or great vessels. Only the most common forms of cyanotic congenital heart disease will be discussed.

Tetralogy of Fallot

Tetralogy or tetrad of Fallot is the most common form of cyanotic congenital heart disease. Traditionally the four components listed as part of the tetrad are pulmonary stenosis, VSD, overriding aorta, and right ventricular hypertrophy. The primary defect is anterior deviation of the infundibular or conal septum, which causes narrowing of the right ventricular outflow tract, the large malalignment VSD, and overriding of the aorta. The pulmonary valve is usually bicuspid and stenotic, and the main pulmonary artery and pulmonary artery branches are hypoplastic to a variable degree. Tetralogy of Fallot may also be associated with atrial septal defects (pentalogy of Fallot), AV septal defects, multiple VSDs, and stenosis or atresia of a pulmonary artery branch (usually the left). Anomalies of coronary artery anatomy are present in 10 per cent of patients. The most important variation is origin of the anterior descending branch from the right coronary artery.

In the most severe form of tetralogy, pulmonary atresia with ventricular septal defect ("pseudotruncus"), the pulmonary valve and proximal main pulmonary artery are atretic (no lumen), so that there is no direct communication between the right ventricle and pulmonary arteries. The lungs are perfused by a ductus or by primitive collateral vessels that arise from the thoracic aorta or brachiocephalic arteries. Central or true pulmonary arteries are usually present but are often tiny. A right aortic arch is present in approximately 30 per cent of patients.

Rarely, the pulmonary valve leaflets may be absent in patients with tetralogy of Fallot. The pulmonary valve annulus is hypoplastic and mildly stenotic. The main and central right and left pulmonary arteries are grossly dilated, forming aneurysms that frequently cause bronchial obstruction.

In all forms of tetralogy of Fallot, the combination of severe pulmonary stenosis and ventricular septal defect leads to right-to-left interventricular shunting and cyanosis. The severity of cyanosis is related to the degree of obstruction to pulmonary blood flow. Infants with mild obstruction may initially be acyanotic with a small left-to-right shunt (pink tetralogy).

CHEST RADIOGRAPHY. The cardiac size is usually normal or mildly increased and pulmonary blood flow is normal to severely diminished, depending upon the severity of pulmonary stenosis (Fig. 111–24*A*). The *coeur-en-sabot,* or boot-shaped heart contour, is typically seen in pulmonary atresia with VSD, with an upturned apex and concave main pulmonary artery segment (Fig. 111–25*A*). The thoracic aorta is often dilated, and a right aortic arch is present in about one third of patients (Fig. 111–24*A*). Segmentation anomalies of the spine and other congenital anomalies are frequent.

ANGIOGRAPHY. Preoperative angiographic assessment of patients with tetralogy of Fallot should include right and left ventriculography and aortography. Right ventriculography in cranially angled frontal and lateral projections demonstrates a large, heavily trabeculated right ventricle, with anterior deviation of the infundibular septum; a horizontal right ventricular outflow tract; valvar, subvalvar, and often supravalvar pulmonary stenosis; and right-to-left shunting across the ventricular defect (see Fig. 111–24*B* and *C*). Left ventriculography in long axial oblique projections typically shows a large subaortic ventricular septal defect with aortic valve override (see Fig. 111–24*D*). The presence of additional septal defects, subaortic stenosis, and other left-sided anomalies occurs rarely and must be ruled out. Aortography is required to delineate the pulmonary blood supply in pulmonary atresia with VSD (Fig. 111–25*B*) and is necessary to delineate the coronary artery anatomy in all forms of tetralogy.

ECHOCARDIOGRAPHY. All of the intracardiac anomalies can be demonstrated with cross-sectional echocardiography. The main and central pulmonary arteries can be imaged, but peripheral pulmonary stenoses, aortopulmonary collaterals, additional septal defects, and coronary artery anomalies require careful angiographic evaluation.

MRI. MRI is useful in evaluating the pulmonary artery stenoses, especially after surgical repair, as well as outflow tract reconstructions and patency of palliative systemic-to-pulmonary shunts.

Tricuspid Atresia

The right AV connection is absent in this anomaly, so that systemic venous blood is shunted across an ASD into the left atrium and then into the left ventricle. Usually the small right ventricle fills through a VSD (Fig. 111–26). The great arteries may be transposed but usually are normally related, with the pulmonary artery arising above the small right ventricle. Pulmonary and subpulmonary stenoses are common. Patients are cyanotic owing to admixture, often with obstructed pulmonary blood flow. Plain chest film findings are variable but in the most common form show normal heart size and

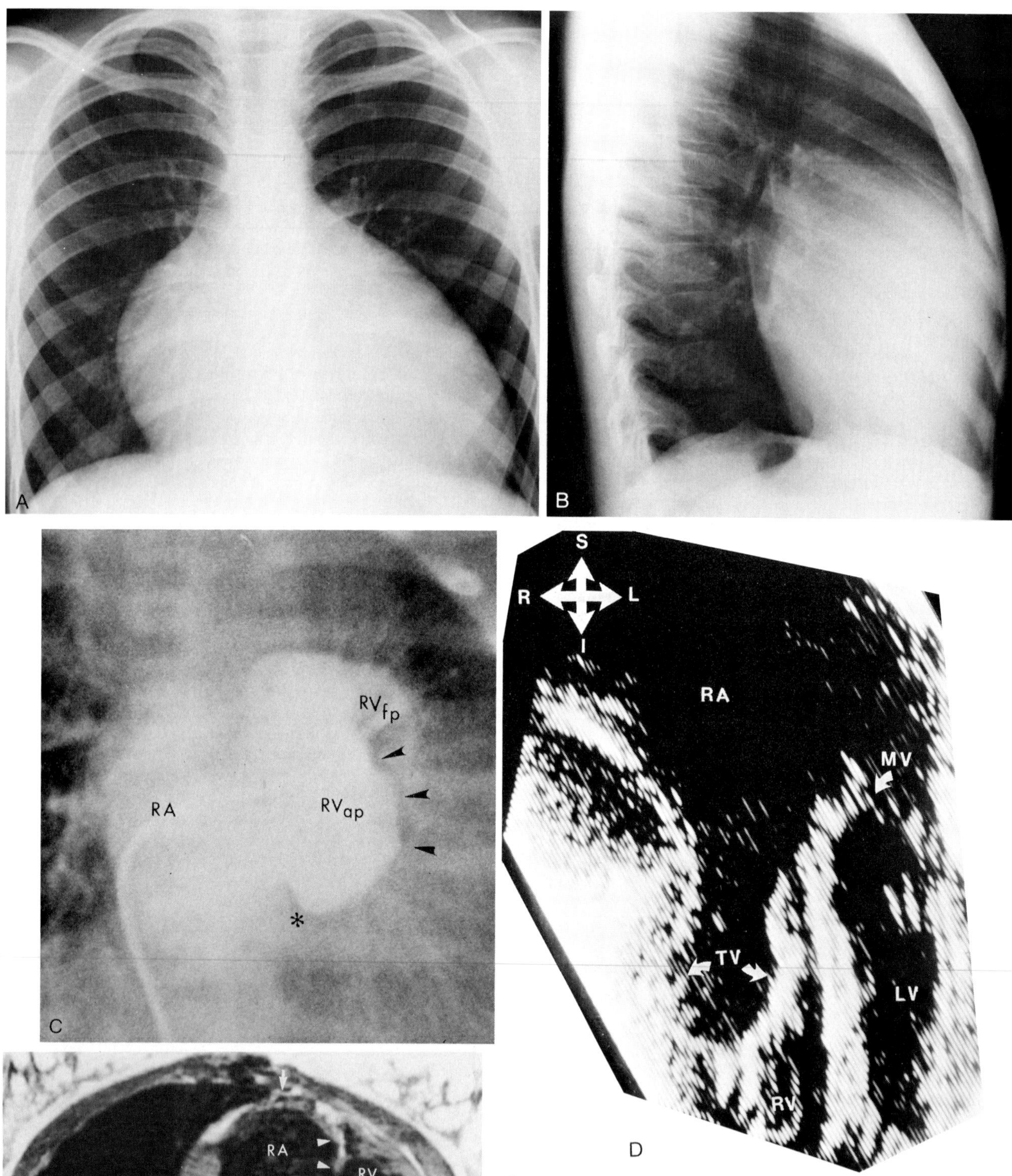

Figure 111–23. Ebstein's anomaly. *A,* PA chest radiograph in a 10-year-old boy shows the typical massive cardiomegaly with a "box-shaped" contour and decreased pulmonary blood flow. *B,* The lateral view demonstrates enlargement of the right heart chambers. *C,* A right ventricular angiogram shows the displacement of the tricuspid valve. The *asterisk* marks the position of the AV groove; the *arrowheads* indicate the displaced valve. (ap = atrialized portion; fp = functional portion.) *D,* Precordial fourth-chamber echocardiographic image demonstrates the large right atrium (RA) and displacement of the tricuspid valve (TV) into the body of the right ventricle (RV). The right ventricular functional cavity is reduced in size. (LA = left atrium; LV = left ventricle; MV = mitral valve.) *E,* Transverse axial MRI demonstrating anterior displacement of the tricuspid valve *(arrowheads)* in Ebstein's anomaly. The right coronary artery *(arrow)* demonstrates the normal location of the atrioventricular junction.

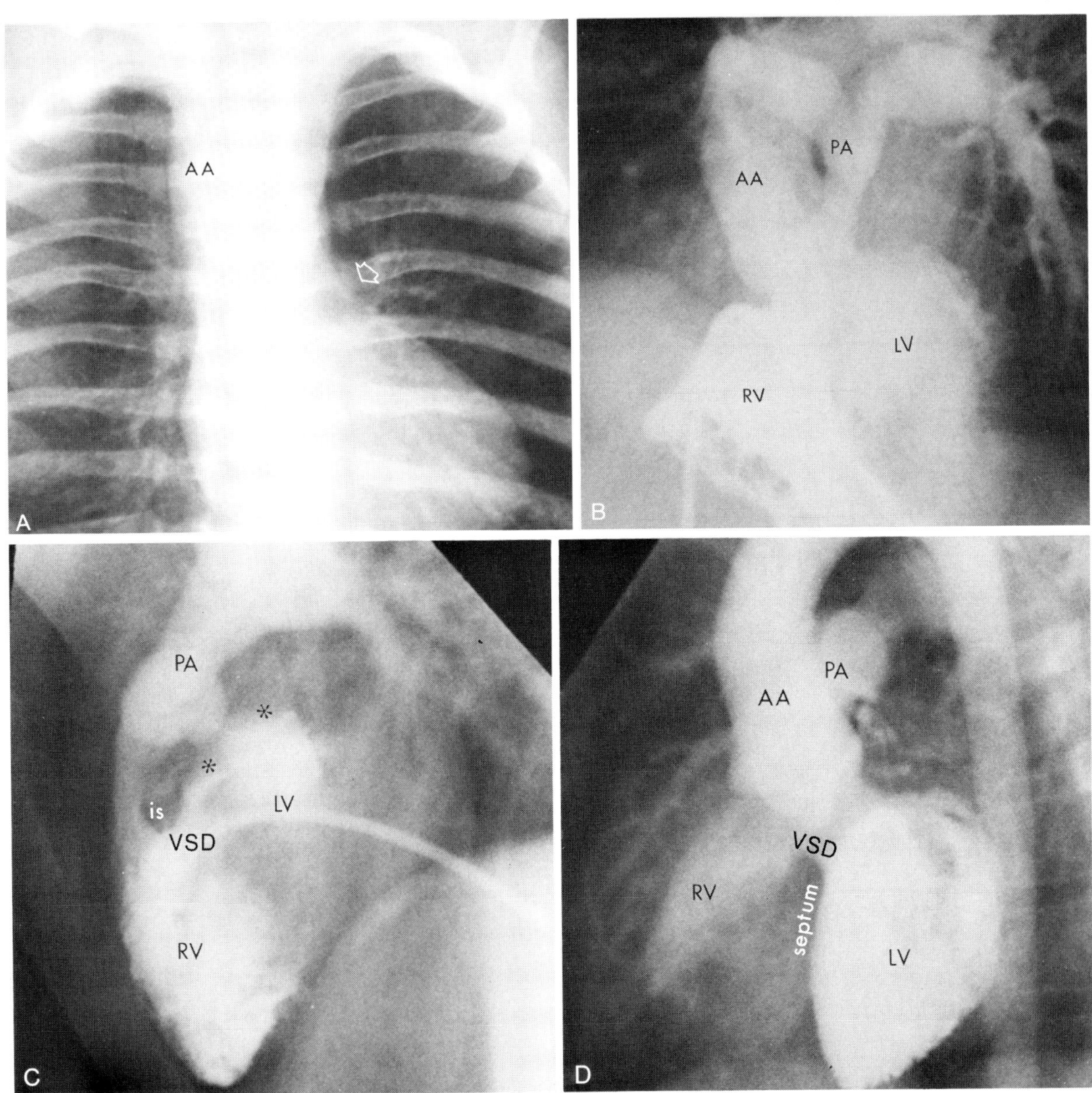

Figure 111–24. Tetralogy of Fallot. *A,* AP chest radiograph demonstrates diminished pulmonary vasculature, a normal heart size, a concave main pulmonary artery segment *(open arrow),* and a right aortic arch (AA). *B,* Cranially angled PA right ventriculogram shows right ventricular (RV) hypertrophy, discrete subpulmonary stenosis at the level of the os infundibulum, and mild hypoplasia of the pulmonary arteries. *C,* The lateral view of the right ventriculogram shows the anterior deviation of the infundibular septum (is) and, immediately below it, the malalignment VSD. The positions of the aortic valve cusps are indicated by *asterisks. D,* The left ventriculogram (long axial oblique projection) shows the large VSD and the overriding aorta.

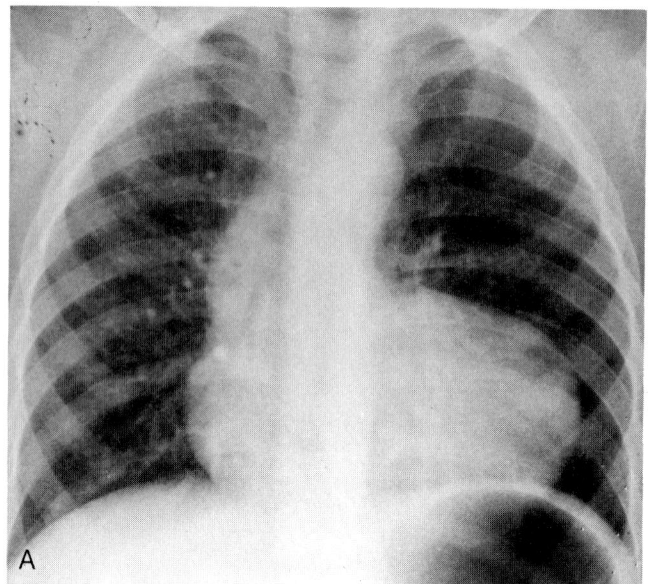

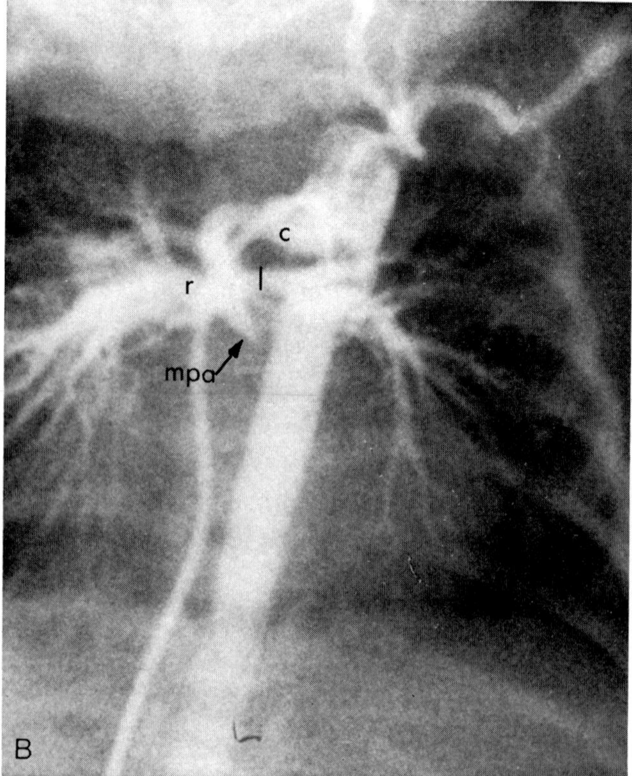

Figure 111–25. Pulmonary atresia with VSD. *A,* PA chest radiograph demonstrates decreased vascularity, marked concavity of the main pulmonary artery segment, a dilated aorta, and *coeur-en-sabot. B,* Antegrade descending aortogram shows a large collateral (c) from the descending aorta to the hilum and retrograde filling of the tiny central pulmonary arteries. (l = left pulmonary artery; mpa = main pulmonary artery; r = right pulmonary artery.)

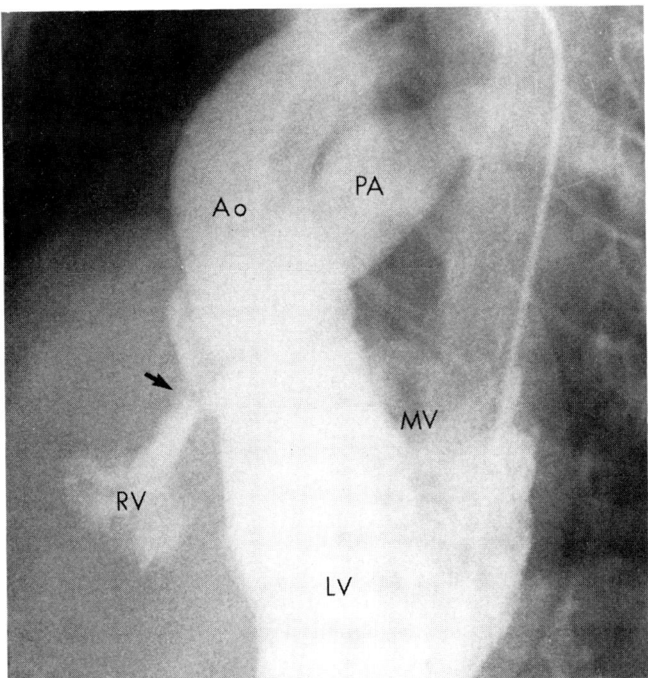

Figure 111–26. Tricuspid atresia. Left ventriculogram, four-chamber projection, shows the large left ventricle (LV), which receives the mitral valve (MV), and filling of a tiny right ventricle (RV) through a VSD. The *arrow* indicates subpulmonary stenosis. (Ao = Aorta; PA = pulmonary artery.)

decreased pulmonary blood flow. Typically the right heart border is flat and the left heart border is more rounded than usual.

Pulmonary Atresia with Intact Ventricular Septum

This uncommon lesion accounts for approximately 1 to 3 per cent of patients with congenital cardiac malformations and has a poor prognosis. The pulmonary valve is atretic, with fusion of the leaflets. The right ventricle is hypoplastic and thick-walled, and the tricuspid valve is dysplastic, with a small annulus and thickened leaflets. Some patients have persistent myocardial sinusoids that allow communication between the right ventricular cavity and the coronary arteries. The coronary arteries in these patients may be stenotic owing to myointimal thickening. The pulmonary circulation is usually perfused by a patent ductus arteriosus. An atrial septal defect or patent foramen ovale must be present to allow right-to-left shunting.

CHEST RADIOGRAPHY. Usually the early films show mild cardiomegaly and normal or decreased pulmonary blood flow, although infants with severe tricuspid insufficiency may have marked cardiac enlargement. The aortic arch is usually left-sided.

ANGIOGRAPHY. Contrast material injected into the right ventricle demonstrates a tiny irregular cavity with contrast filling spaces between prominent trabeculae. The tricuspid valve annulus is small, and the leaflets are thickened. No antegrade flow occurs across the pulmonary valve, so injected contrast material must either reflux into the right atrium or fill coronary arteries via myocardial sinusoids. The pulmonary artery is usually opacified via a patent ductus arteriosus during left ventriculography or aortography.

Transposition of the Great Arteries

By definition, the aorta is supported by the morphologic right ventricle and the pulmonary artery is supported by the morphologic left ventricle (i.e., in transposition of the great arteries, there is ventriculoarterial discordance). The aorta is anterior and usually slightly to the right of the pulmonary artery (D-transposition). As transposition is often associated with complex cardiac malformations, the segmental approach is usually utilized in describing these hearts. For example, a heart associated with normal (solitus) visceroatrial situs, atrioventricular concordance, D-loop ventricles (morphologic right ventricle anterior and to the right of the left ventricle), and ventriculoarterial discordance with the aorta to the right of the pulmonary valve is described as "transposition of the great arteries (SDD)." (SDA and SDL describe similar hearts with "anteroposterior" and "L" (left) related great arteries, respectively.)

About 70 per cent of patients with complete transposition of the great arteries have an intact ventricular septum and unobstructed left ventricular outflow tract. VSDs (usually either perimembranous or infundibular) and left ventricular outflow obstruction are the most common associated anomalies. A right aortic arch is present in up to 8 per cent of patients and has its highest incidence in those with associated anomalies.

The pulmonary and systemic circulations in patients with transposition of the great arteries function in parallel rather than in series, resulting in cyanosis and severe tissue hypoxia. Infants without sufficient intracardiac mixing die within a few days of birth. Those with VSDs have shunting from the systemic to pulmonary circulations, resulting in better oxygenation, but suffer from increased volume overload of the heart and symptoms of congestive heart failure.

CHEST RADIOGRAPHY. In the first few days of life the chest radiograph may appear normal, but with time, the cardiac silhouette enlarges inferiorly and to the left on the frontal projection and pulmonary blood flow increases (Fig. 111–27*A*). The vascular pedicle is narrow, as the aorta and pulmonary artery are anteroposteriorly related, resulting in the typical "egg on its side" appearance of the cardiac contour (Fig. 111–27*A*). A pattern of shunt vascularity plus pulmonary edema is frequently present, especially in those patients with VSD or patent ductus arteriosus.

ANGIOGRAPHY. Right ventriculography is best recorded in frontal and lateral projections and demonstrates a large, heavily trabeculated right ventricle, with the aorta arising above a well-developed infundibulum or conus (Fig. 111–27*B* and *C*). Typically the aortic valve is superior, anterior, and slightly to the right of the pulmonary valve. Left ventriculography should be recorded in axial oblique projections, to assess the ventricular septum, left ventricular outflow tract, and pulmonary valve (Fig. 111–27*D*). Usually, the pulmonary valve is in fibrous continuity with the anterior mitral leaflet owing to absence of subpulmonary infundibulum or conus. The ventricular septum bows toward the left ventricle in most patients, producing dynamic subpulmonary obstruction (Fig. 111–27*D*). Corrective surgery usually consists of the neonatal arterial switch procedure. Accurate angiographic delineation of the coronary arteries is necessary prior to surgery.

ECHOCARDIOGRAPHY. The subcostal long-axis view demonstrates the branching great artery (pulmonary artery) above the morphologic left ventricle and the aorta above the right ventricle (Fig. 111–27*E* and *F*). After the neonatal period, the left ventricle has a banana shape due to leftward bowing of the ventricular septum. Fixed subpulmonary obstruction, the size and position of the VSD, and the size of the ASD are important features that can be determined and followed with echocardiography.

Corrected Transposition of the Great Arteries

Individuals with corrected transposition of the great arteries are not usually cyanotic. As in complete transposition, the aorta arises above the morphologic right ventricle and the pulmonary artery above the morphologic left ventricle—that is, there is ventriculoarterial discordance. The additional anomaly of atrioventricular dis-

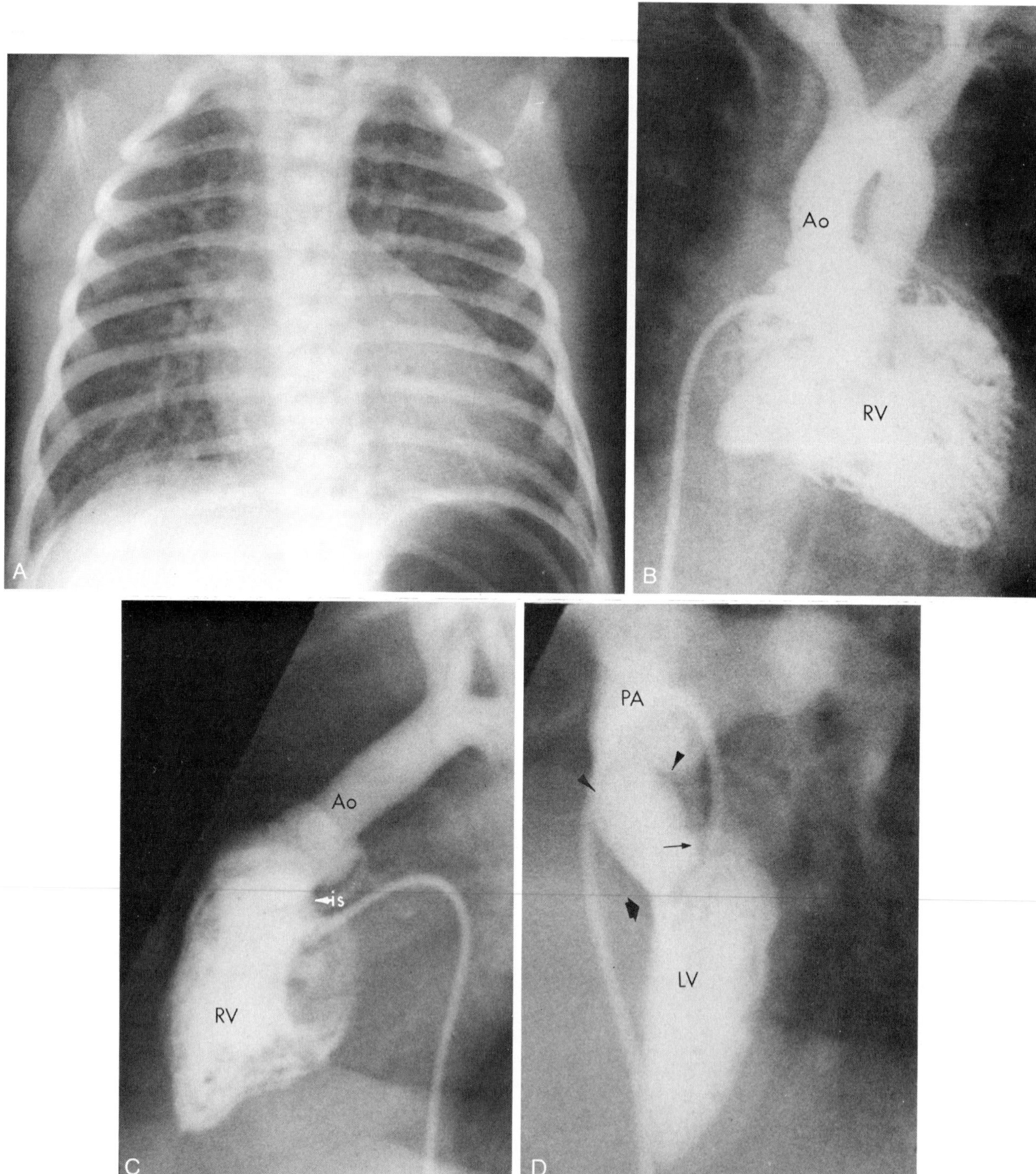

Figure 111–27. Transposition of the great arteries. *A*, AP chest radiograph with "egg on its side" cardiac contour, narrow vascular pedicle, and shunt vascularity. PA *(B)* and lateral *(C)* right ventriculograms show the large morphologic right ventricle (RV) supporting the aorta (Ao). Note the infundibular septum (is), which separates the tricuspid valve from the aortic valve. *D*, Left ventriculogram in long axial oblique view shows the pulmonary artery (PA) arising above the morphologic left ventricle (LV). Note the pulmonary valve *(arrowheads)*–mitral valve *(thin arrow)* continuity and bowing of the ventricular septum toward the left ventricle *(wide arrow)*. Mild pulmonary stenosis is also present.

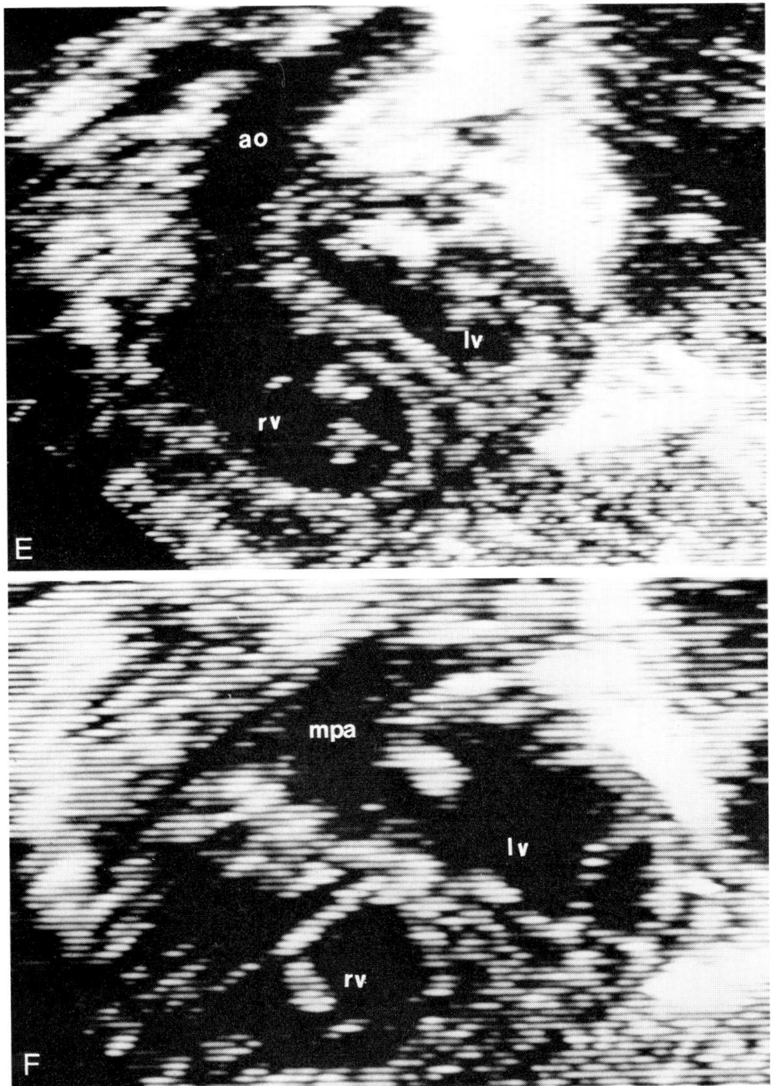

Figure 111–27 *Continued E* and *F*, Subcostal echocardiographic images. By angling the transducer, the examiner can show that the aorta (ao) arises above the morphologic right ventricle (rv) and that the pulmonary artery (mpa), with its typical branching pattern, arises above the morphologic left ventricle (lv).

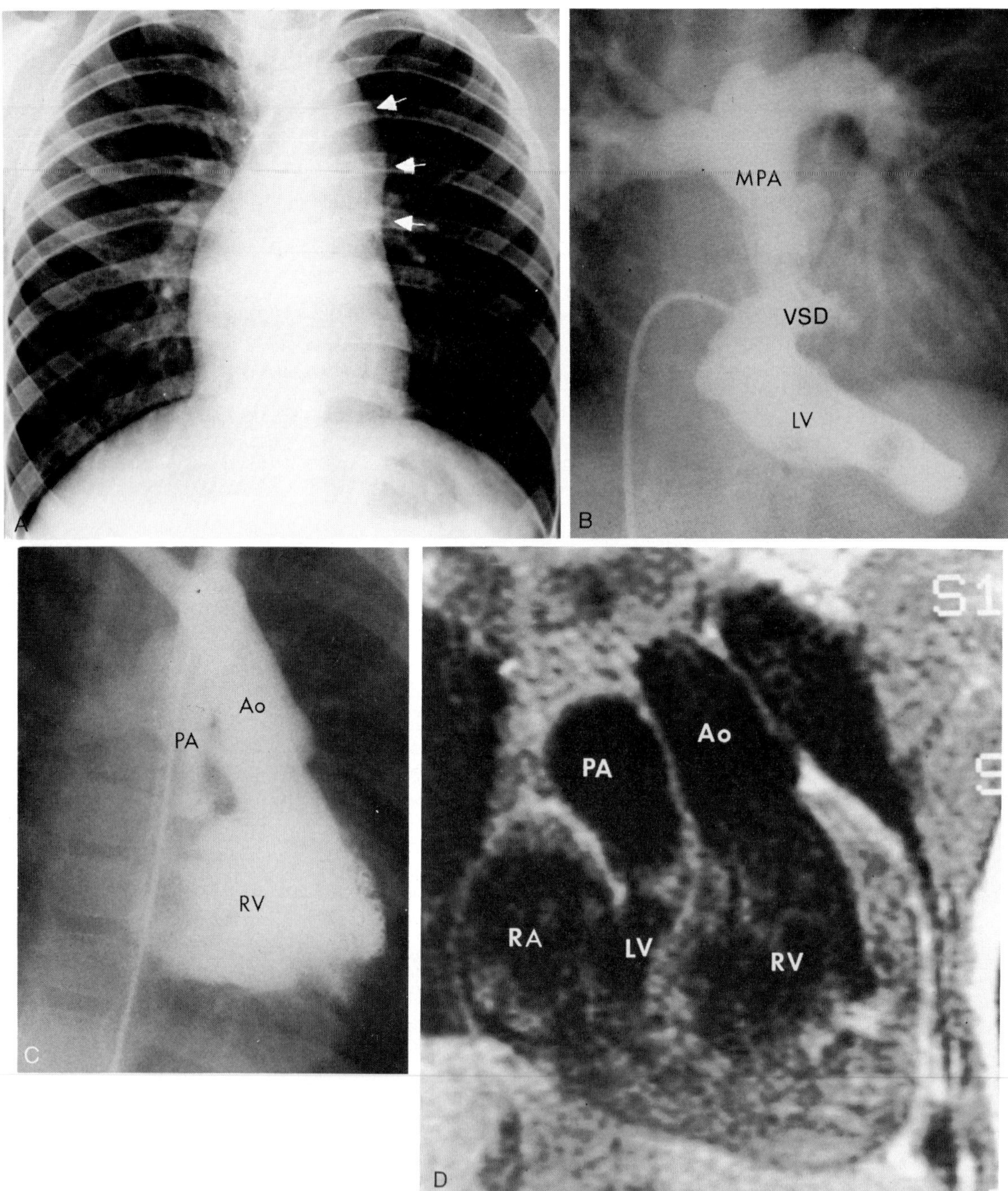

Figure 111–28. Corrected transposition of the great arteries. *A,* Chest radiograph shows the characteristic prominence of the left superior mediastinum *(arrows),* which represents the left-sided ascending aorta. *B* and *C,* Angiography in a patient with corrected transposition of the great arteries (S,L,L) (atrioventricular and ventriculoarterial discordance) reveals that the morphologic left ventricle (LV) is to the right of the morphologic right ventricle (RV) and supports the pulmonary artery (MPA). The catheter position in *B* indicates the presence of atrioventricular discordance (right atrium connects with left ventricle). Note the additional presence of a perimembranous ventricular septal defect (VSD). *D,* Coronal MRI demonstrates anatomy similar to that shown in *B* and *C,* in a postoperative patient who has corrected transposition with VSD and subpulmonary stenosis. (Ao = aorta; LV = left ventricle; PA = pulmonary artery; RA = right atrium; RV = right ventricle.)

cordance (ventricular inversion) causes the circulation to be physiologically corrected. A small percentage of patients have no associated anomalies and live normal lives. Most have associated cardiac lesions that include dysplastic tricuspid valve with tricuspid (systemic AV valve) insufficiency, ventricular septal defect, valvar and subvalvar pulmonary stenosis, and conduction abnormalities with arrhythmias.

Chest Radiography. The findings on chest radiography depend upon the associated anomalies. A characteristic feature is the abnormally prominent left cardiac and superior mediastinal border, caused by the left-sided position of the ascending aorta (Fig. 111–28*A*). Patients with severe tricuspid insufficiency have cardiomegaly with a dilated left atrium and pulmonary venous hypertension.

Angiography. In the patient with levocardia and atrial situs solitus, the right atrium is connected to a right-sided morphologic left ventricle, which supports the pulmonary artery (Fig. 111–28*B*). In the levophase, the pulmonary veins drain into the left atrium; this connects with the left-sided morphologic right ventricle, which supports the aorta (Fig. 111–28*C* and *D*). The ventricular septum has a nearly sagittal orientation. The dysplastic tricuspid valve may be displaced (Ebstein-like malformation) but more frequently appears thickened and regurgitant.

Double-Outlet Right Ventricle

Double-outlet right ventricle includes a spectrum of anomalies in which both, or the greater part of both, great arteries are situated above the right ventricle. Patients are cyanotic owing to admixture and, in some cases, obstruction to pulmonary blood flow. Angiographic and echocardiographic findings also vary, but frequently both great arteries are positioned side by side with infundibulum supporting both semilunar valves and producing semilunar-AV valve discontinuity. A VSD is usually present and is described as subpulmonary, subaortic, double-committed, or uncommitted to the great arteries.

Truncus Arteriosus

In this rare anomaly, the pulmonary arteries, coronary arteries, and ascending aorta arise from a common trunk with a single, usually dysplastic truncal valve. The truncal valve is usually regurgitant and overrides an outlet VSD. Infants are mildly cyanotic and have symptoms of congestive heart failure. Plain chest radiographs show cardiomegaly and shunt vasculature, with a right aortic arch in approximately 30 per cent.

Single Ventricle

Single ventricle or univentricular heart is a complex, primitive cardiac anomaly. The ventricular chamber may resemble a left ventricle or a right ventricle or may be undifferentiated. Subpulmonary or subaortic obstruction is frequently present.

Anomalous Pulmonary Venous Connection

One or more pulmonary veins may connect to the right atrium or its tributaries instead of to the left atrium. Total anomalous pulmonary venous connections (TAPVC) exist when all of the pulmonary veins connect anomalously. The anomalous sites of pulmonary venous connection are classified as follows (incidence figures from Burroughs and Edwards):

Supracardiac	Left innominate vein via left vertical vein	36%
	Right superior vena cava	11%
	Azygos vein	Rare
Cardiac	Coronary sinus	16%
	Right atrium	15%
Infracardiac (subdiaphragmatic)	Portal vein, ductus venosus, inferior vena cava, hepatic vein	13%
Mixed		7%

A patent foramen ovale or ASD is present in all patients. Pulmonary venous flow is often obstructed in the intradiaphragmatic form, owing to focal stenosis of the anomalous vein, increased resistance in the hepatic vessels, or extrinsic pressure at the diaphragm. Infrequently, TAPVC to the left ventricular vein may also be obstructed if the vertical vein passes between the left main bronchus and left pulmonary artery.

The physiology of TAPVC is that of total admixture in the right heart. In the absence of obstructive lesions, pulmonary blood flow is increased and the right atrium and ventricle are dilated. The left atrium and left ventricle are small. In the presence of obstruction to pulmonary venous return, pulmonary blood flow is decreased and the right side of the heart is not dilated.

Patients with TAPVC without obstruction usually develop signs of congestive heart failure toward the end of the first month of life and are usually mildly cyanotic. Infants with obstructed TAPVC are cyanotic and tachypneic from birth. Most die in the first few months of life without surgery.

In partial anomalous pulmonary venous connection (PAPVC), some pulmonary veins connect with the right atrium or its tributaries, whereas others drain into the left atrium. PAPVC is frequently present in association with ASD of the sinus venous type and in scimitar syndrome, which includes dextrocardia, hypoplastic right lung, and anomalous connection of the right pulmonary veins to the inferior vena cava (see Fig. 111–6*B*).

Chest Radiography. In TAPVC without obstruction, the heart is enlarged with shunt vascularity. In the supracardiac forms, the vein that receives the anomalous vein is also dilated, producing the characteristic contour abnormalities. With TAPVC to the left vertical vein, the left vertical vein and superior vena cava are dilated, producing a ''snowman heart,'' although this finding is usually not seen before nine months of age (Fig. 111–29*A*).

In TAPVC with obstruction, especially the infradiaphragmatic form, the cardiac silhouette is small and there is a pattern of diffuse pulmonary edema (see Fig. 111–3). Kerley's lines are very prominent, probably caused partly by distended lymphatics.

Angiography. Each pulmonary vein must be identified angiographically. This may be done using a main pulmonary artery injection (Fig. 111–30*A*), but frequently selective or wedged injections in the right and left pulmonary arteries or retrograde injections in the anomalous veins are required (Fig. 111–29*B*). Left ventriculography is necessary to assess the size of the left ventricle and to rule out additional anomalies.

Echocardiography. In normal infants, using a combination of suprasternal and subcostal views the pulmonary veins can usually be identified and traced to the left atrium. In TAPVC the left atrium is small, with the pulmonary venous confluence lying behind the left atrium (Fig. 111–30*B*). It is important to identify all the veins draining into the confluence and from the confluence to the site of drainage (Fig. 111–30*C*). Doppler echocardiography permits the detection of obstruction and the direction of flow in the venous channels.

Heterotaxia Syndromes

Heterotaxia syndromes are those that lack the normal position of the abdominal and thoracic viscera. The best-defined complexes of anomalies are asplenia and polysplenia syndromes (Fig. 111–31).

Asplenia Syndrome. The atria, liver, and lungs typically show features that suggest bilateral right-sidedness or right isomerism. The liver is usually symmetrically bilobed, frequently with two gallbladders; both atria have appendages resembling right atrial appendages, and the lungs tend to be trilobed with bilateral eparterial bronchi (Fig. 111–31). Nonrotation of the bowel is constant. No splenic tissue is present (Fig. 111–32). Cardiac anomalies are usually complex and primitive and include bilateral superior vena cava, anomalous pulmonary venous connection, pulmonary stenosis or atresia, common atrium, single ventricle, AV septal defects, double-outlet right ventricle, and transposition. Dextrocardia is frequent. Usually, the abdominal aorta and inferior vena cava are on the same side of the spine. Patients with asplenia syndrome are usually cyanotic and have a poor prognosis owing to their cardiac anomalies and immunologic defects.

Polysplenia Syndrome. Abnormalities in the polysplenia syndrome are less constant and usually less severe than in the asplenia syndrome and are suggestive of bilateral left-sidedness. Multiple small splenules are usually present, adjacent to the greater curvature of the stomach (Fig. 111–31). Abdominal situs may be

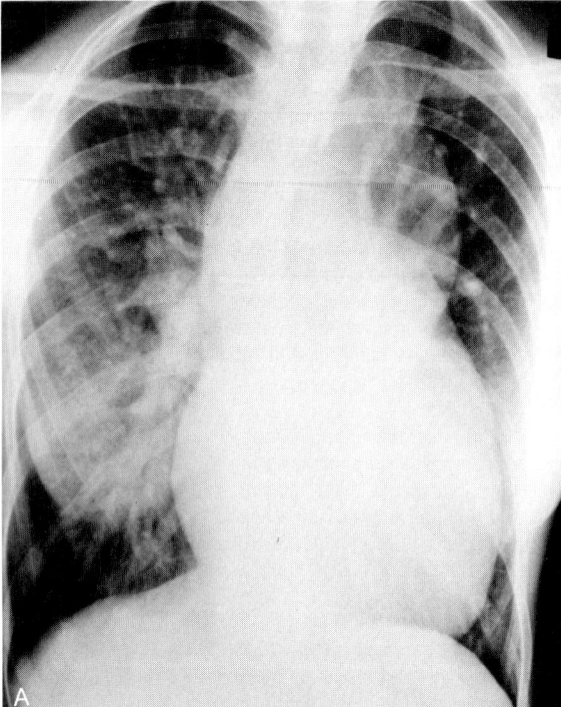

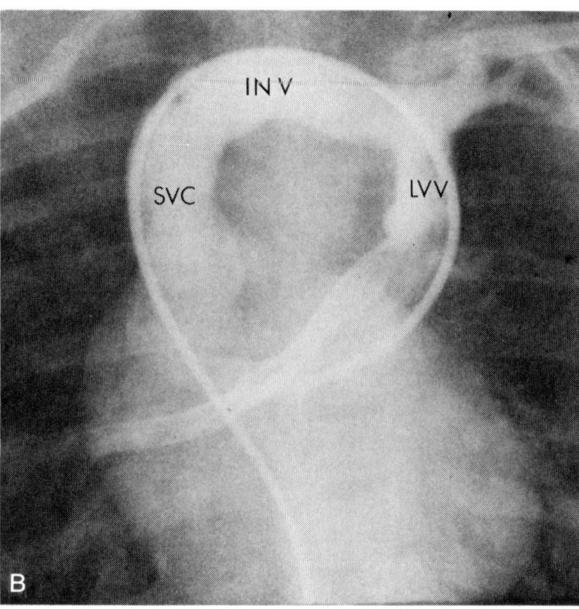

Figure 111–29. Total anomalous pulmonary venous connection to the left vertical vein. *A,* The PA chest radiograph shows shunt vascularity and the characteristic "snowman" cardiac configuration due to enlargement of the left vertical vein in the left superior mediastinum and the superior vena cava on the right. *B,* Retrograde contrast injection in the pulmonary veins shows the veins from both lungs joining to form a confluence before draining into the left vertical vein (LVV). The innominate vein (INV) and superior vena cava (SVC) are dilated.

ambiguous, inverted, or normal. Bowel malrotation is frequent, and biliary atresia or absent gallbladder may occur. Usually, the intrahepatic portion of the inferior vena cava is absent (interrupted) and venous return from the lower body is via the azygos vein. Both atrial appendages may resemble left atrial appendages, and typically but not always both lungs have hyparterial bronchi (Fig. 111–33*A*). Cardiac anomalies encompass a wide spectrum but are usually less severe than those in the asplenia syndrome. Most patients with polysplenia and cardiac anomalies have septal defects with increased pulmonary blood flow and are acyanotic. Dextrocardia is less common than in asplenia.

Radiographic Findings. Although not constant, the presence of abdominal situs ambiguus, decreased pulmonary blood flow, and symmetrical eparterial bronchi is strongly suggestive of asplenia syndrome (see Fig. 111–6*A*). Scintigraphy with ^{99m}Tc sulfur colloid or tagged red blood cells is useful in confirming the absence of splenic tissue (see Fig. 111–32). Ultrasound examination of the abdomen may help define the visceral and vascular anatomy.

Bilateral hyparterial bronchi with any form of abdominal situs suggests the polysplenia syndrome (Fig. 111–33*A*). Interruption of the inferior vena cava with azygous continuation is suggested by the presence of a large azygos vein on the frontal radiograph and absent inferior vena caval shadow on the lateral view. Abdominal ultrasound, computed tomography, and scintigraphy combine to demonstrate the multiple splenules (Fig. 111–33*B*) and vascular anomalies.

CONGENITAL VASCULAR MALFORMATIONS

Aortic Arch Anomalies

Aortic arch anomalies are the result of persistent patency of a vascular segment that normally disappears or the abnormal disappearance of a segment that normally remains patent. These tend to involve either the right or left fourth aortic arch or the right or left aortic root. Aortic arch abnormalities may or may not be associated with a vascular ring encircling the trachea and esophagus. The laterality of the ductus arteriosus (whether patent or represented by a fibrous cord) plays an important role in determining whether or not a vascular ring is present. All possible vascular malformations are illustrated in the hypothetical double aortic arch plan proposed by Edwards (Fig. 111–34).

The left aortic arch with normal brachiocephalic artery branching is formed when there is regression of the right dorsal aortic root (left side of diagram—Fig. 111–34) from the level of the right subclavian artery to the descending aorta. The ductus arteriosus on the right almost always disappears.

A left aortic arch with aberrant right subclavian artery is formed if there is interruption of the right fourth arch between the right common carotid and right subclavian arteries (left side of diagram—Fig. 111–34). The right subclavian artery arises as the fourth branch from the aortic arch distal to the left subclavian artery via the right dorsal aortic root and passes posterior to the esophagus. The ductus arteriosus usually persists on the left, and no vascular ring is present. This anomaly has been reported to occur in 0.5 per cent of individuals.

A *right aortic arch with mirror image branching* of the brachiocephalic arteries is the result of the left dorsal aortic root from the level of the ductus arteriosus to the descending aorta (right side of diagram—Fig. 111–34). The ductus arteriosus on the right usually disappears. No vascular ring is present.

Aortic Arch Anomalies with Airway Obstruction. *A double aortic arch* is formed when the fourth arch and the dorsal aortic root on both sides persist and are patent (top of diagram—Fig. 111–34). A vascular ring is present, since the trachea and esophagus are completely encircled. The ductus arteriosus on the right usually disappears. Separate carotid and subclavian arteries arise from each arch. The arches may be of equal size, although in

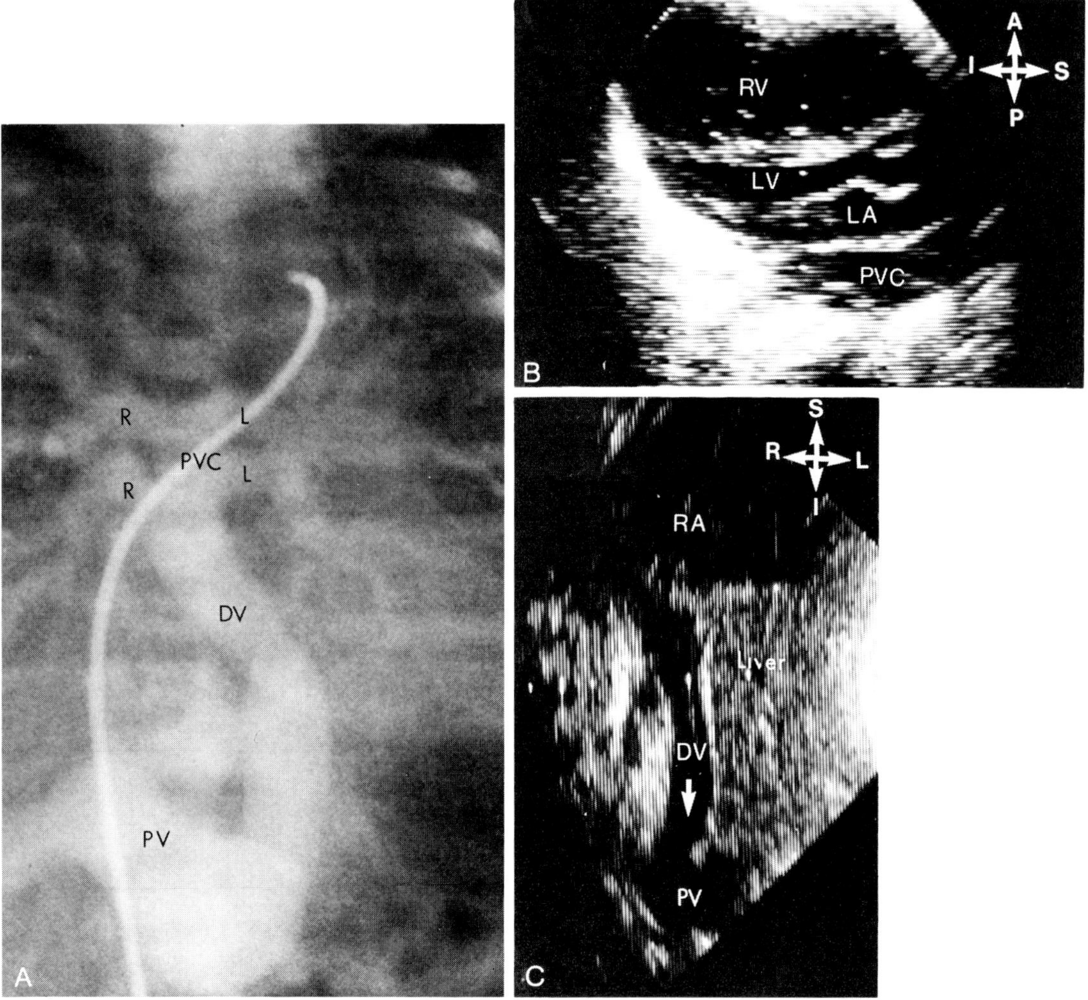

Figure 111–30. Obstructed infradiaphragmatic total anomalous pulmonary venous connection. *A*, The levophase of a pulmonary artery injection shows four pulmonary veins (R and L) entering the pulmonary venous confluence (PVC) and a descending vein (DV), which connects with the portal vein (PV). *B*, Precordial long-axis echocardiographic image shows the pulmonary venous confluence (PVC) posterior to and separate from the left atrium (LA). *C*, Subcostal image shows the descending vein (DV) entering the portal vein (PV) in the liver. (LV = left ventricle; RA = right atrium; RV = right ventricle.)

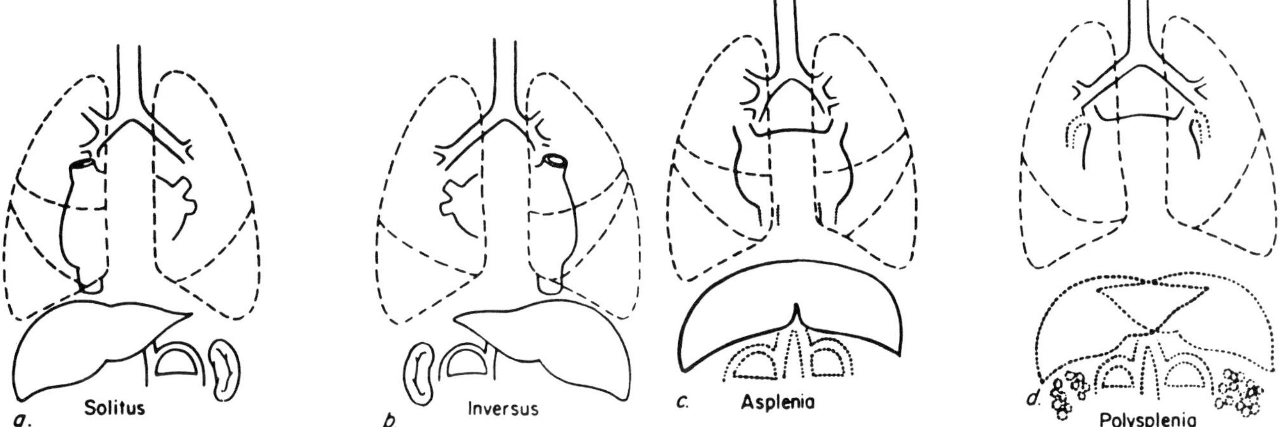

Figure 111–31. Heterotaxia syndromes. (From Stanger P, et al: Cardiac malpositions. An overview based on study of sixty-five necropsy specimens. Circulation 56:160, 1977. Reproduced by permission of the American Heart Association, Inc.)

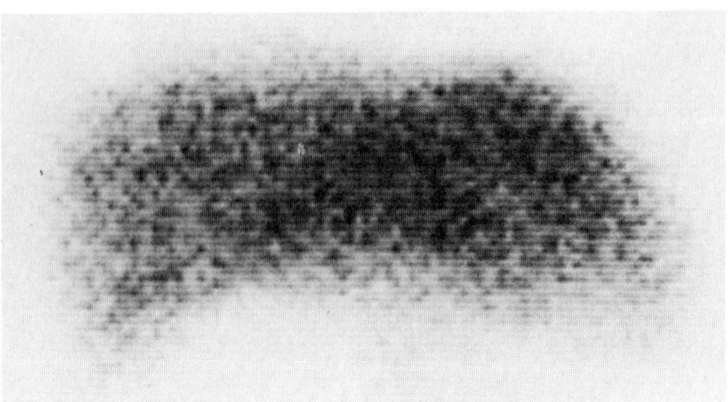

Figure 111–32. Technetium-99m sulfur colloid liver scan shows a symmetrical, bilobed liver with no spleen in a patient with **asplenia syndrome**.

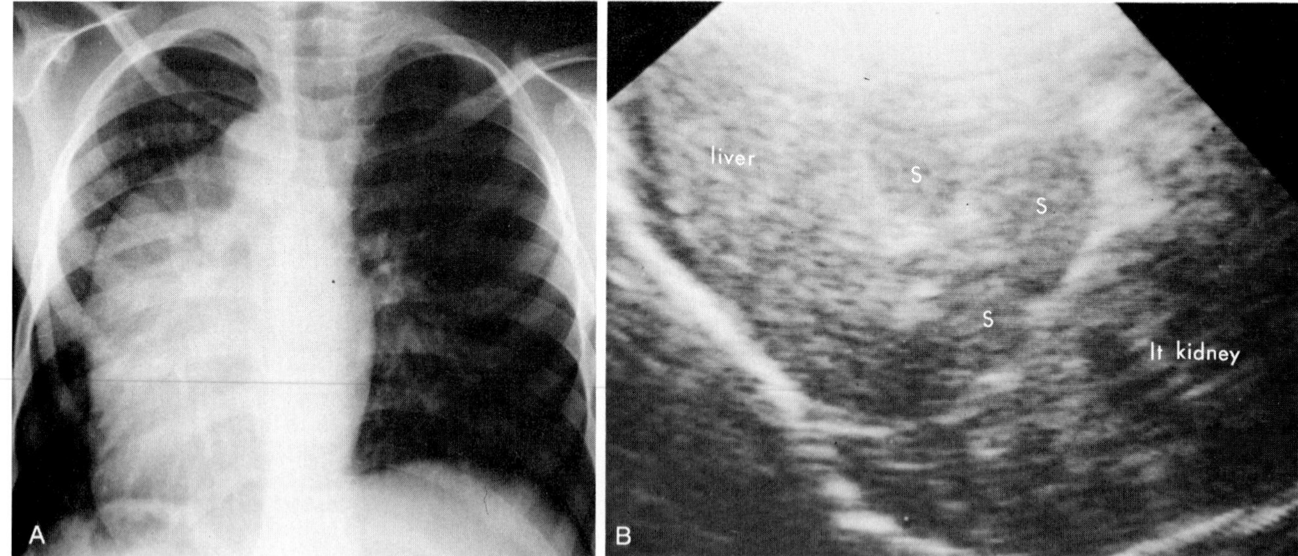

Figure 111–33. Polysplenia syndrome. *A,* PA chest radiograph with bilateral hyparterial bronchi and abdominal situs inversus. *B,* A longitudinal abdominal sonographic image shows multiple small splenules (S) between the left lobe of the liver and the left kidney.

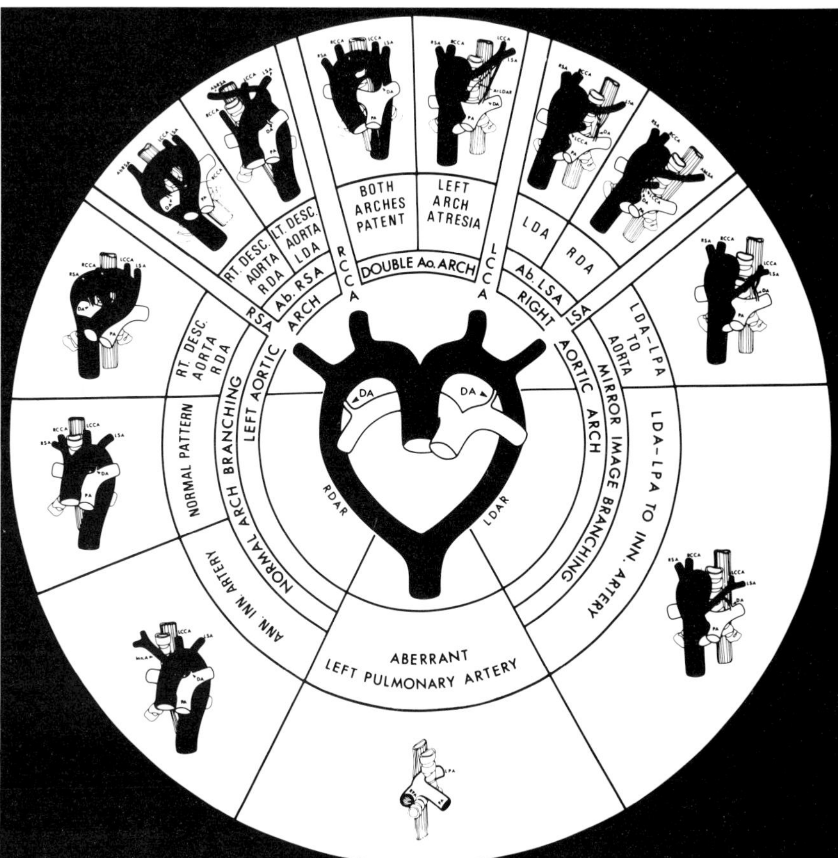

Figure 111–34. Schematic diagram of **aortic arch anomalies** using the hypothetic double aortic arch of Edwards.

approximately 75 per cent the right is the larger vessel. The descending aorta may be on either side of the midline. Typically, the frontal view of the plain chest radiograph shows a midline trachea indented on both sides, and the lateral view shows narrowing and anterior displacement of the trachea. The anterior projection of a barium esophagram (Fig. 111–35*A*) defines an indentation on both sides of the esophagus. On the lateral projection (Fig. 111–35*B*) the esophagus is indented in a deep fashion posteriorly where the two arches unite. The esophagus is frequently flat as it abuts against the trachea anteriorly. Aortography (Fig. 111–35*C*) defines the size of each arch and demonstrates if one arch, usually the left, is actually atretic. This is important information if surgery is contemplated, as the smaller arch should be divided. Currently, patients undergo presurgical evaluation with chest radiographs, contrast esophagography, and echocardiography. If any anatomic questions remain unanswered, MRI in multiple planes (Fig. 111–35*D* to *G*) is capable of demonstrating both the vascular anatomy and the effects on the airways.

A right aortic arch with aberrant left subclavian artery is the result of interruption of the left fourth arch between the left common carotid and subclavian arteries (right side of diagram—Fig. 111–34). The ductus arteriosus usually persists on the left and passes between the aberrant subclavian artery and pulmonary artery. Thus, a vascular ring is present. The origin of the aberrant subclavian artery is often bulbous (as this segment represents the left dorsal aortic root) and is termed the diverticulum of Kommerell. The PA chest radiograph defines the arch to the right of the trachea with mild deviation of the trachea to the left. On the lateral projection the trachea is often bowed anteriorly in its lower third. A frontal esophagram shows an indentation on the right produced by the aortic arch (Fig. 111–36*A*). On the left a small indentation may sometimes be present and is produced by the subclavian artery or ductus arteriosus. The lateral esophagram demonstrates a posterior defect that may be of variable size (Fig. 111–36*B*). A right aortic arch with aberrant left subclavian artery and a double aortic arch may be indistinguishable by plain chest radiography and barium esophagography. On aortography (Fig. 111–36*C*), the first branch to arise from the aortic arch is the left common carotid artery, followed by the right common carotid and subclavian arteries. The aberrant left subclavian artery arises as the fourth branch from the upper descending aorta and proceeds to the left behind the esophagus.

ABERRANT LEFT PULMONARY ARTERY. An aberrant left pulmonary artery (''pulmonary sling'') is characterized by the absence of a normal left pulmonary artery. Embryologically the proximal position of the left sixth arch, which normally forms the left main pulmonary artery, fails to develop or, once formed, becomes obliterated at an early stage. As a result of the lack of arterial supply to a portion of the primitive lung bud, a collateral branch from the pulmonary segment of the right sixth arch extends into the primitive lung tissue. With maturation and separation of the pulmonary tissue into the right and left lungs, the collateral vessel elongates and grows to assume the function of the left pulmonary artery.

The main pulmonary artery gives rise to the right pulmonary artery. The anomalous left pulmonary artery arises from the distal portion of the main pulmonary artery or the right pulmonary artery to the right of the trachea. This branch arches over the right bronchus, then passes to the left between the trachea and the esophagus to enter the left hilum. The ''sling'' that is formed compresses the right bronchus and the distal end of the trachea.

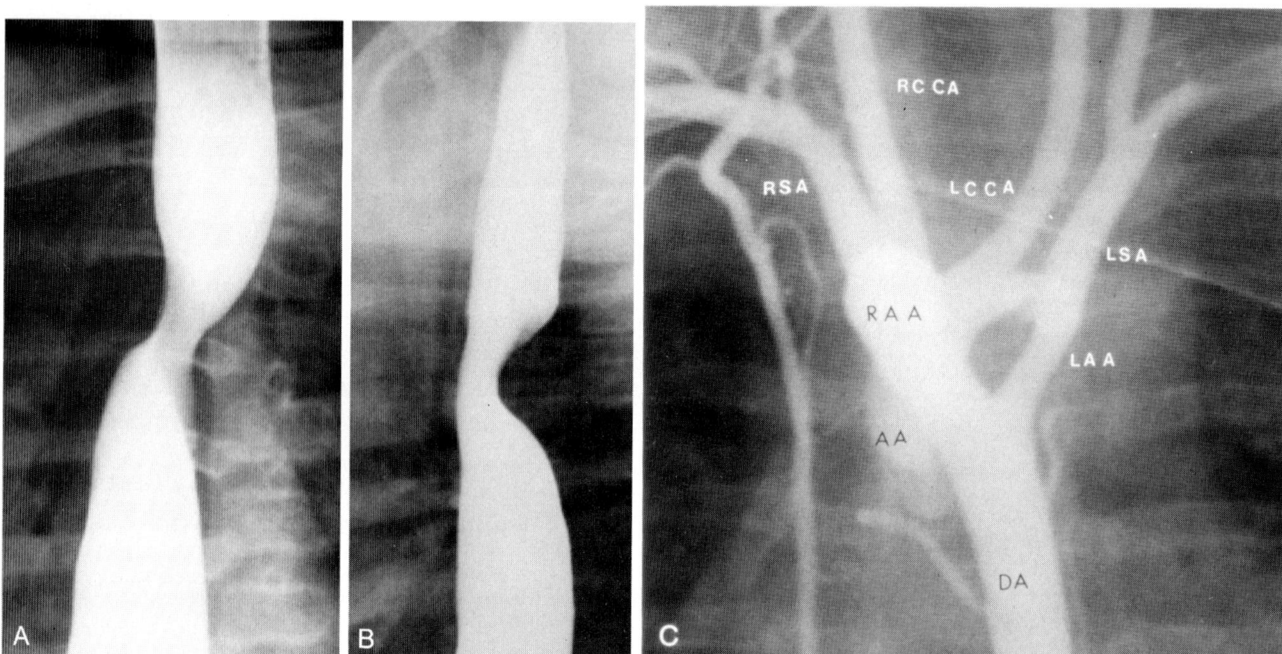

Figure 111–35. Double aortic arch. *A*, Anteroposterior esophagram of a double aortic arch. A bilateral indentation is present. That on the right, representing the right arch, lies at a higher level than the left defect due to the left arch. The lateral view *(B)* shows a deep posterior indentation produced by the united aortic arches. The anterior esophageal outline is flat as it abuts against the trachea, which is narrowed. *C*, Frontal aortogram demonstrates a large right aortic arch (RAA) supporting separate right subclavian (RSA) and right common carotid arteries (RCCA). The smaller left arch (LAA) gives rise to the left common carotid (LCCA) and left subclavian arteries (LSA). The left arch lies anterior to the trachea. The right arch is to the right of the trachea and esophagus, and the left arch is to the left of the trachea and esophagus. The descending portion of the right arch produces the deep indentation seen in *B* as it passes behind the esophagus. (AA = ascending aorta; DA = descending aorta.)

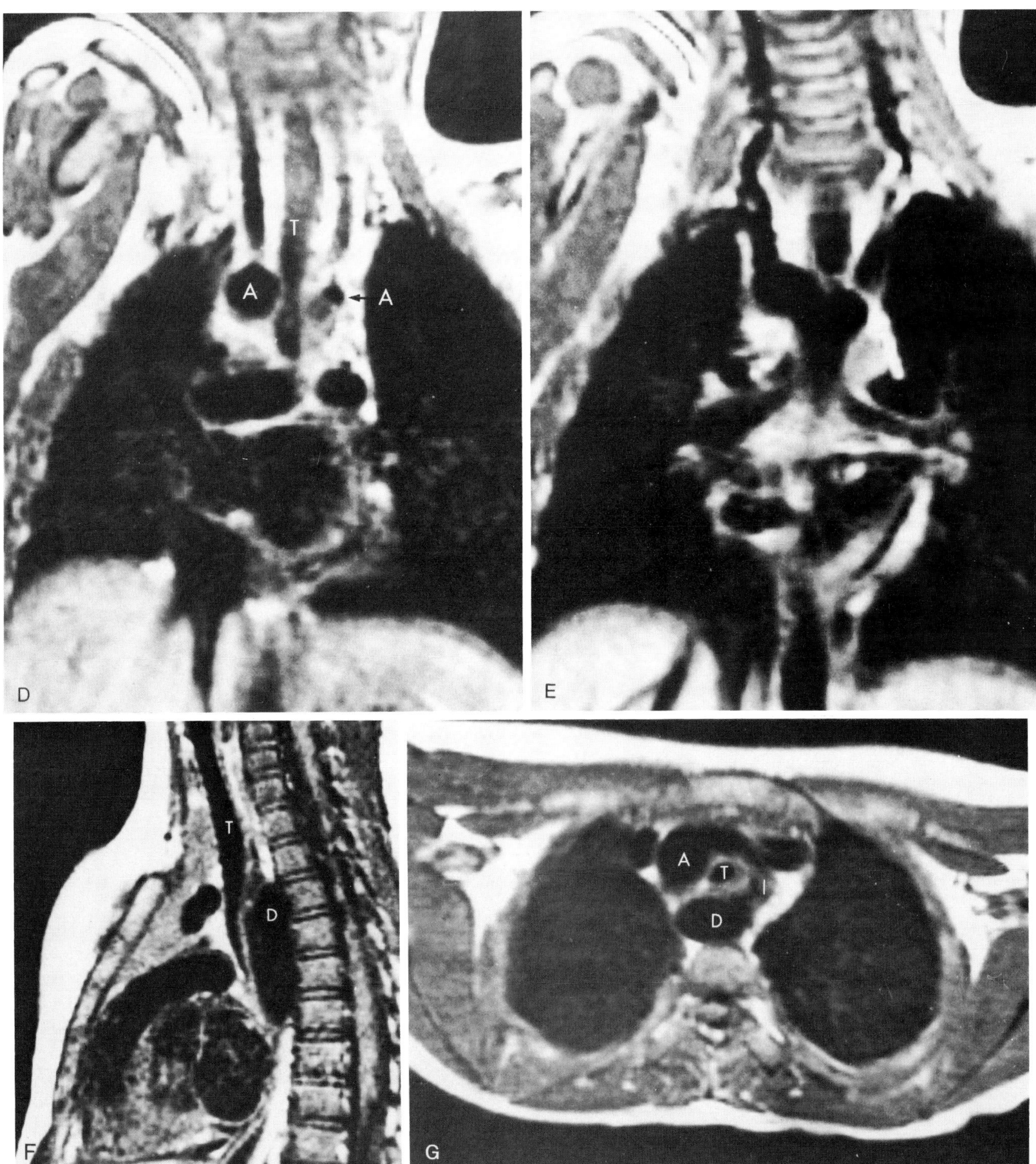

Figure 111–35 *Continued. D,* Coronal MRI at the level of the trachea (T) in another patient with double aortic arch demonstrates the two aortic arches (A); the left one is smaller. *E,* Coronal image posterior to *D* shows the large left dorsal aorta. *F,* Sagittal MRI shows the compression of the distal trachea (T) by the left dorsal aorta (D). *G,* Transverse axial image shows the vascular ring encircling the trachea (T) and esophagus. (A = ascending aorta; D = descending aorta; I = left aortic arch.)

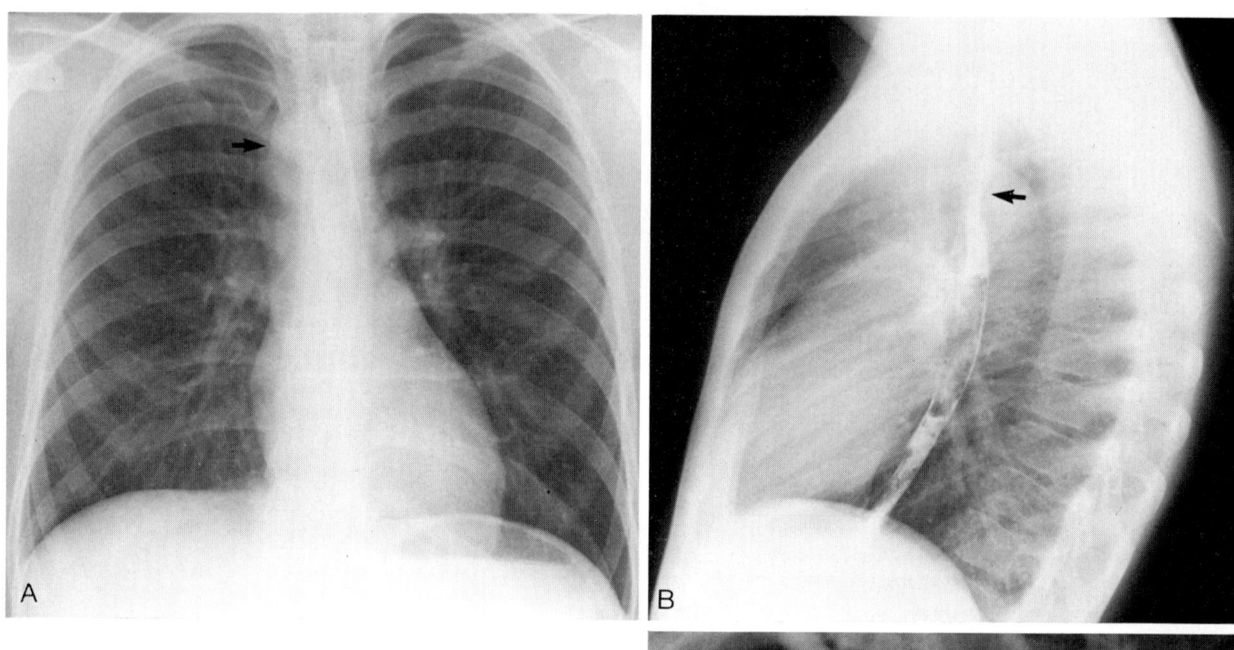

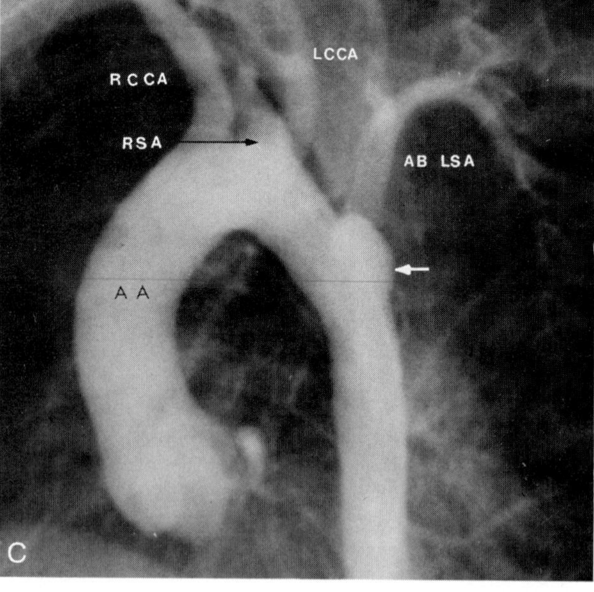

Figure 111–36. Right aortic arch with aberrant left subclavian artery. *A,* PA chest radiograph with esophagram demonstrates a right aortic arch. The barium-filled esophagus and the trachea are both deviated to the left *(arrow). B,* Lateral view with barium in the esophagus demonstrates a posterior indentation *(arrow)* due to the aortic diverticulum and aberrant left subclavian artery. *C,* Left anterior oblique thoracic aortogram demonstrates the aberrant left subclavian artery (AB LSA) arising as the last branch of the aortic arch. The density at the base of the subclavian artery *(arrow)* represents the remnant of the left dorsal aortic root, which appears as a diverticulum. (AA = ascending aorta; LCCA = left common carotid artery; RCCA = right common carotid artery; RSA = right subclavian artery.)

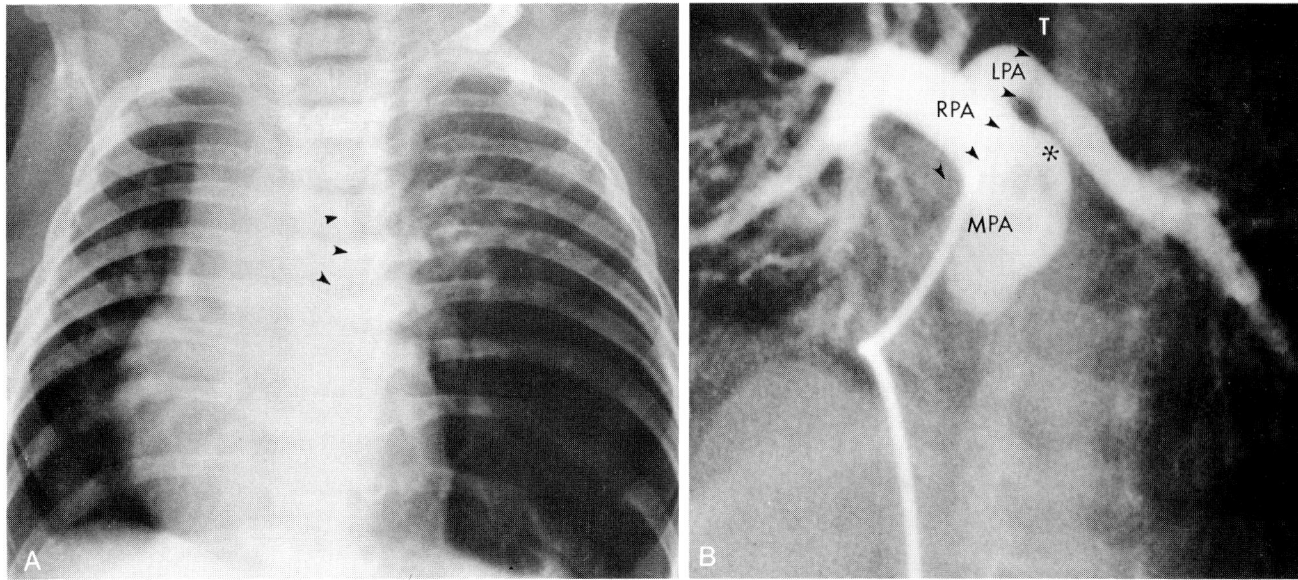

Figure 111–37. Pulmonary artery sling. *A,* A chest radiograph shows extensive pulmonary emphysema, most marked in the left lower lobe, and compression of the trachea and right bronchus *(arrowheads). B,* A pulmonary arteriogram (four-chamber projection) shows the left pulmonary artery (LPA) arising as a branch of the right pulmonary artery (RPA) and passing behind the trachea (T). *Arrowheads* indicate the margin of the trachea and right bronchus. The *asterisk* indicates the expected site of the origin of the left pulmonary artery. MPA = main pulmonary artery. (*A* and *B* courtesy of J. B. Norton, M. D., Arkansas Children's Hospital, Little Rock, Arkansas.)

The chest radiograph may show equally inflated, clear lungs, although obstructive emphysema or atelectasis is often present (Fig. 111–37*A*), usually on the right if compression of the right bronchus is present. Associated tracheal and/or bronchial hypoplasia or stenosis may coexist and may be demonstrated at bronchography or CT. An esophagram will often show an anterior indentation at the level of the tracheal bifurcation, although the study may be normal. Pulmonary angiography, preferably in a cranially angled projection, will define the left pulmonary artery arising from the right and coursing obliquely, inferiorly, and to the left behind the trachea to reach the left hilum (Fig. 111–37*B*).

SURGICAL PROCEDURES FOR CONGENITAL HEART DISEASE

Some commonly used surgical procedures for congenital cardiac lesions are listed in Table 111–5. Palliative procedures are used in children with cardiac anomalies deemed currently inoperable and in symptomatic patients felt to be too small or too young for complete repair. Surgical palliation usually involves increasing (shunt procedures, first four procedures cited in Table 111–5, Fig. 111–38) or decreasing (pulmonary artery banding) the pulmonary blood flow.

TABLE 111–5. SURGICAL PROCEDURES FOR CONGENITAL HEART DISEASE

Procedure	Anatomy	Lesions	Potential Complications
Blalock-Taussig shunt	Subclavian artery to PA	TOF, cyanosis with PBF	CHF, asymmetrical PBF, PPS, thrombosis
Waterston anastomosis	Ascending aorta to PA	TOF, cyanosis with PBF	CHF, pulmonary vaso-occlusive disease, PPS
Potts' procedure	Descending aorta to PA	TOF, cyanosis with PBF	CHF, pulmonary vaso-occlusive disease, PPS
Glenn procedure	SVC to PA	TOF, cyanosis with PBF	Thromboses, pulmonary AV shunting
PA banding	Band around main PA	Left to right shunts	Obstruction or PAS (usually right), migration, perforation
Senning or Mustard procedure	Atrial baffle	TGA	Baffle leak, pulmonary or systemic venous obstruction
Arterial switch procedure	Aorta and PA switched	TGA	CHF, pulmonary or aortic stenosis
Rastelli procedure	LV to aorta baffle	TGA, VSD	Conduit stenosis
	RV to PA conduit	DORV	Subaortic stenosis
Fontan procedure	RA to PA	Tricuspid atresia, single ventricle	CHF, pleural and pericardial effusions
RV outflow patch	Patch RVOT to MPA	TOF	RVOT patch aneurysm if residual PS or VSD
Norwood procedure	Stage 1 Ascending aorta to MPA Shunt to PAs Stage 2 Fontan procedure	Hypoplastic left heart	PA stenosis Residual coarctation

AV = arteriovenous; CHF = congestive heart failure; MPA = main pulmonary artery; PA = pulmonary artery; PAS = pulmonary artery stenosis; PBF = pulmonary blood flow; PPS = peripheral pulmonary stenosis; PS = pulmonary stenosis; RA = right atrium; RV = right ventricle; RVOT = right ventricular outflow tract; LV = left ventricle; DORV = double-outlet right ventricle; SVC = superior vena cava; TOF = tetralogy of Fallot; TGA = transposition of the great arteries; VSD = ventricular septal defect.

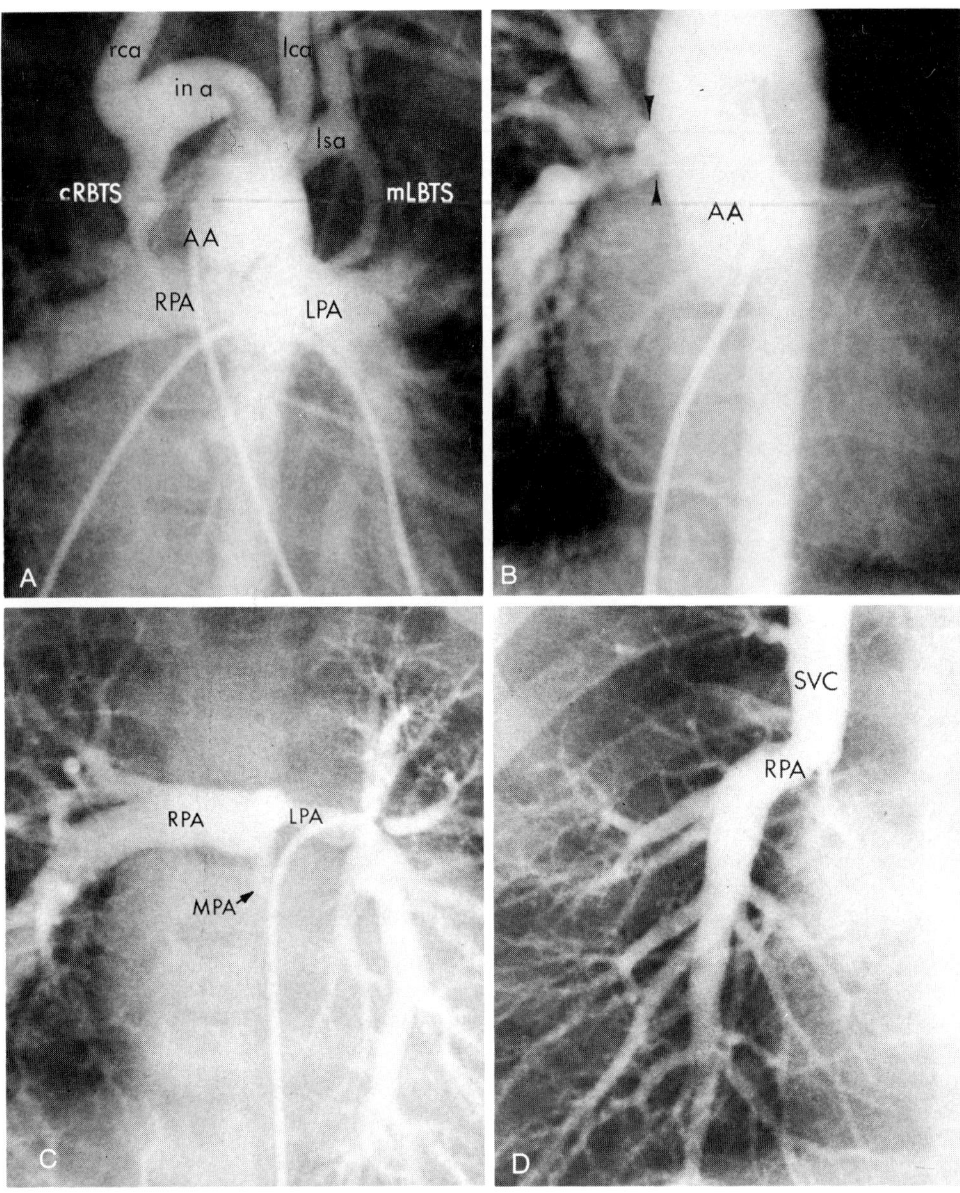

Figure 111–38. Shunt procedures for cyanotic congenital heart disease. *A*, Classic (cRBTS) and modified (mLBTS) Blalock-Taussig shunts. *B*, Waterston anastomosis. *C*, Potts' procedure, with left pulmonary artery stenoses (catheter in the descending aorta has been advanced across the anastomosis). *D*, Glenn procedure. (AA = ascending aorta; ina = innominate artery; lca = left carotid artery; LPA = left pulmonary artery; lsa = left subclavian artery; MPA = main pulmonary artery; rca = right carotid artery; RPA = right pulmonary artery; SVC = superior vena cava.)

Each surgical procedure has its own expected results and complications. After repair of isolated septal defects, heart size and pulmonary vascularity should gradually diminish; failure to do so suggests a residual defect. Following coarctation repair, rib notching usually gradually disappears, but it may reappear with restenosis at the coarctation site.

Bibliography

Adams FH, Emmanoulides GC (eds): Moss' Heart Disease in Infants, Children and Adolescents, 3rd ed. Baltimore, Williams and Wilkins, 1983.

Bargeron LM Jr, Elliott LP, Soto B, et al: Axial cineangiography in congenital heart disease. Section I. Concept, technical and anatomic considerations. Circulation 56:1075–1083, 1977.

Burroughs JR, Edwards JE: Total anomalous pulmonary venous connection. Am Heart J 59:913–931, 1960.

Edwards DK, Higgins CB: Radiology of neonatal heart disease. Radiol Clin North Am 18:369–385, 1980.

Edwards JE: Malformations of the aortic arch system manifested as ''vascular rings.'' Lab Invest 2:56, 1953.

Elliott LP: Cardiac Imaging in Infants, Children and Adults. Philadelphia, JB Lippincott, 1991.

Elliott LP, Bargeron LM, Bream PR, et al: Axial cineangiography in congenital heart disease. Section II. Specific lesions. Circulation 56:1084–1093, 1977.

Elliott LP, Schiebler GL: The X-ray Diagnosis of Congenital Heart Disease in Infants, Children and Adults, 2nd ed. Springfield, IL, Charles C Thomas, 1979.

Fellows KE, Rosenthal A: Extracardiac roentgenographic abnormalities in cyanotic congenital heart disease. AJR 114:371–379, 1972.

Freedom RM, Benson LN, Smallhorn JF (eds): Neonatal Heart Disease. London, Springer-Verlag, 1992.

Freedom RM, Culham JAG, Moes CAF: Angiocardiography of Congenital Heart Disease. New York, MacMillan, 1984.

Gussenhoven EJ, Becker AE: Congenital Heart Disease—Morphologic Echocardiographic Correlations. New York, Churchill Livingstone, 1983.

Higgins CB, Silverman NH, Kersting-Sommerhoff BA, Schmidt K: Congenital Heart Disease: Echocardiography and Magnetic Resonance Imaging. New York, Raven Press, 1990.

Kelley, MJ, Jaffe CC, Kleinman CS: Cardiac Imaging in Infants and Children. Philadelphia, WB Saunders Company, 1982.

Picoli GP, Gerlis LM, Wilkinson JL, et al: Morphology and classification of atrioventricular defects. Br Heart J 42:621–632, 1979.

Picoli GP, Gerlis LM, Wilkinson JL, et al: Morphology and classification of complete atrioventricular defects. Br Heart J 42:633–639, 1979.

Santamonia H, Soto B, Ceballos R, et al: Angiographic differentiation of types of ventricular septal defects. AJR 141:273–281, 1983.

Soto B, Pacifico AD, Cebullos R, et al: Tetralogy of Fallot: An angiographic-pathologic correlative study. Circulation 64:558–566, 1981.

Stanger P, Rudolf AM, Edwards JE: Cardiac malpositions. An overview based on study of sixty-five necropsy specimens. Circulation 56:159–172, 1977.

112 Acquired Valvular Heart Disease

John D. Newell, Jr., Michael J. Kelley, and Randolph S. Pallas

The purpose of this chapter is to give the reader an overview of the assessment of acquired valvular heart disease using modern imaging techniques. The work-up of valvular heart disease begins with a clinical history, physical examination, electrocardiogram, and standard radiographic examination of the thorax. The radiologist is almost always involved at this point in the detection or evaluation of patients with suspected or known acquired valvular heart disease. It is important for the radiologist to know what useful information can be successfully obtained from the plain radiographic examination and what information is better obtained or inferred from more sophisticated imaging techniques such as ultrasound and angiocardiography. The complete imaging evaluation of patients with severe valvular heart disease includes M-mode, two-dimensional, and Doppler echocardiography; hemodynamic assessment of the heart; and angiocardiography. Magnetic resonance imaging (MRI) has been used to assess regurgitant and stenotic valvular cardiac lesions in several research studies. The role of MRI in assessing valvular heart disease is discussed in Chapter 110.

In the following sections of this chapter, we will stress the approach to acquired lesions of the aortic and mitral valves, since these constitute the majority of acquired valvular heart lesions. The features of tricuspid valve disease will be dealt with briefly at the end of the chapter. Essentially, most all pulmonary valvular lesions are congenital in nature and are discussed elsewhere in this textbook.

AORTIC VALVE

Aortic Stenosis

Aortic stenosis develops when the normal diameter of the aortic valve of 2.5 to 3.5 cm^2 decreases to a critical range of 0.5 to 1.0 cm^2. The gradient across the aortic valve is dependent on the cardiac output, which will increase with exercise. Cardiac output generally is normal at rest in patients with critical aortic stenosis until late in the disease. The increased gradient across the valve produces left ventricular hypertrophy and diminished left ventricular compliance. These changes in the left ventricle cause a disproportionate increase in left ventricular pressure and hence pulmonary venous pressure whenever the left ventricular diastolic volume is increased. During the initial compensated period of hypertrophy, end-systolic and end-diastolic dimensions are reduced. This maintains a nearly normal level of wall stress, despite elevated intraventricular pressure. As the disease progresses, the increased muscle mass of the left ventricle may outstrip the coronary blood supply, and subendocardial myocardial ischemia and angina develop.

In the later stages of aortic stenosis, the left ventricle decompensates and its dimensions increase. At this stage of the disease, left ventricular dilatation and pulmonary venous congestion are detected on imaging studies, and there are accompanying clinical findings of heart failure, dyspnea, fatigability, and exertional syncope. Isolated aortic stenosis usually has a nonrheumatic etiology. This disease most frequently develops as a result of degeneration of a congenitally bicuspid aortic valve. This common congenital cardiac malformation occurs in 0.5 to 2 per cent of the population. Less commonly, acquired aortic stenosis is secondary to rheumatic heart disease or degeneration of a tricuspid aortic valve in patients over 65 years of age.

RADIOGRAPHIC FINDINGS

The classic findings of compensated aortic stenosis on the standard frontal and lateral chest radiograph are normal pulmonary vascularity, normal heart size, discrete enlargement of the ascending aorta, and visible calcification of the aortic valve (Figs. 112–1 and 112–2). The cardiac contour usually demonstrates a concavity along its mid-left lateral border and an increased convexity along the lower left lateral border (Figs. 112–1 and 112–2). This has been referred to as the "left ventricular configuration" and may be seen in any condition associated with left ventricular hypertrophy or dilatation. The left atrium and right chambers of the heart are normal in size and contour. The degree of enlargement of the ascending aorta does not correlate with the severity of the aortic stenosis, but the presence of a visibly calcified aortic valve on the radiograph generally indicates a ventricular-to-aortic gradient of greater than 50 mm Hg. The cardiothoracic ratio remains normal (<0.50) or nearly normal (<0.55) in this disease unless the left ventricle begins to dilate and left ventricular failure develops (Fig. 112–3*A*). Cardiac fluoroscopy is most sensitive for detecting aortic valve calcification and should be utilized when the radiographic or clinical features are in doubt. Computed tomography can accurately detect aortic valve calcification (Fig. 112–3*B*).

ECHOCARDIOGRAPHIC FINDINGS

There have been multiple developments in echocardiography over the past 25 years that have increased our ability to diagnose and assess the severity of aortic stenosis. M-mode echocardiography is frequently diagnostic of patients with aortic stenosis (Fig. 112–4). This examination can reveal thickened and eccentric aortic valve leaflets (Fig. 112–4*A*); decreased separation of aortic valve leaflets (Fig. 112–4*B*); increased thickness of the left ventricular walls at end-diastole; and, in well-compensated disease states, hyperdynamic contraction of the left ventricle. The severity of the aortic valve gradient can be assessed using M-mode techniques by computing the left ventricular peak systolic pressure using the following formula:

$$225 \times LVPW_s / LVEDD \quad (1)$$

LVEDD is the left ventricular end-diastolic dimension and $LVPW_s$ is the left ventricular posterior wall thickness at end-systole. The left ventricular pressure value is then compared with the patient's systolic blood pressure to obtain the aortic valve gradient.

Two-dimensional echocardiography has been useful in detecting aortic stenosis (Fig. 112–5), and direct measurement of the aortic valve area (AVA) has been evaluated using this technique. Prior to Doppler echocardiographic techniques, none of the above noninvasive measurements of aortic stenosis were sufficiently accurate to allow quantitation of aortic stenosis in individual patients.

Doppler ultrasound examinations of the heart can now be used to determine the pressure gradient across a stenotic valve and the cross-sectional area of the valve orifice (Fig. 112–6). The pressure gradient across a stenotic valve can be determined by using the following formula:

$$(P_2 - P_1) = 4V^2 \quad (2)$$

The term on the left side of the equation is the pressure gradient across the narrowed valve (e.g., aortic valve), and V is equal to the

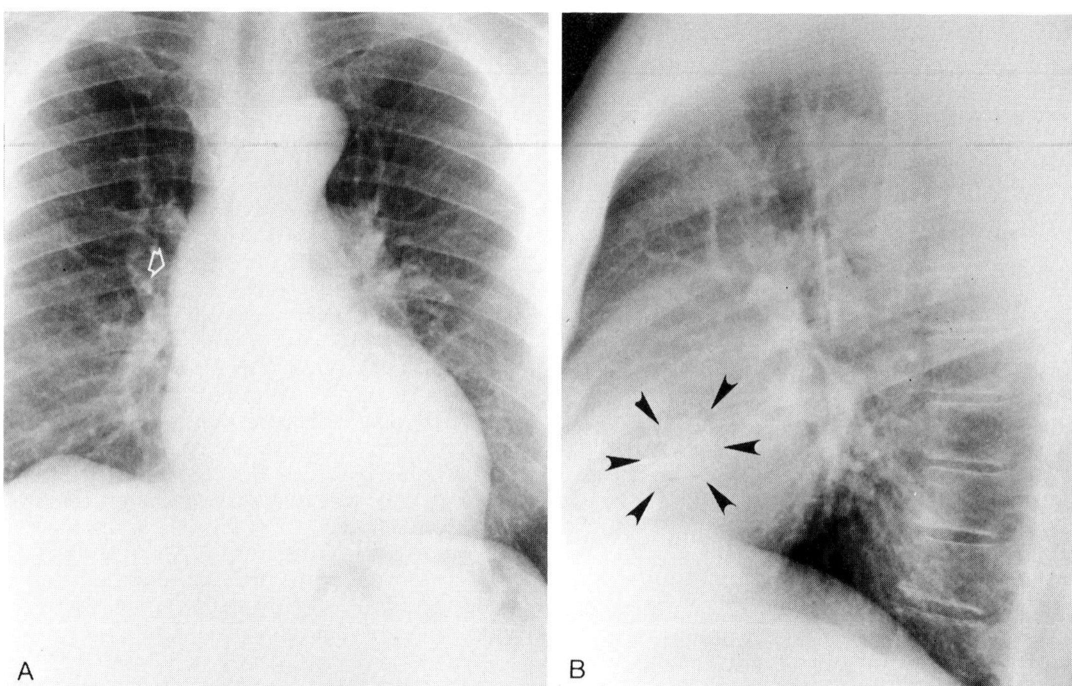

Figure 112–1. Calcific aortic stenosis. *A,* Posteroanterior (PA) and *(B)* lateral chest radiographs in a 45-year-old patient with a systolic murmur. Note the normal pulmonary vascularity and normal heart size with a left ventricular configuration. In the PA view there is prominence of the ascending aorta *(arrow),* and in the lateral projection there is calcification in the region of the aortic valve *(arrowheads).* The latter finding was confirmed at cardiac fluoroscopy.This patient had a bicuspid aortic valve.

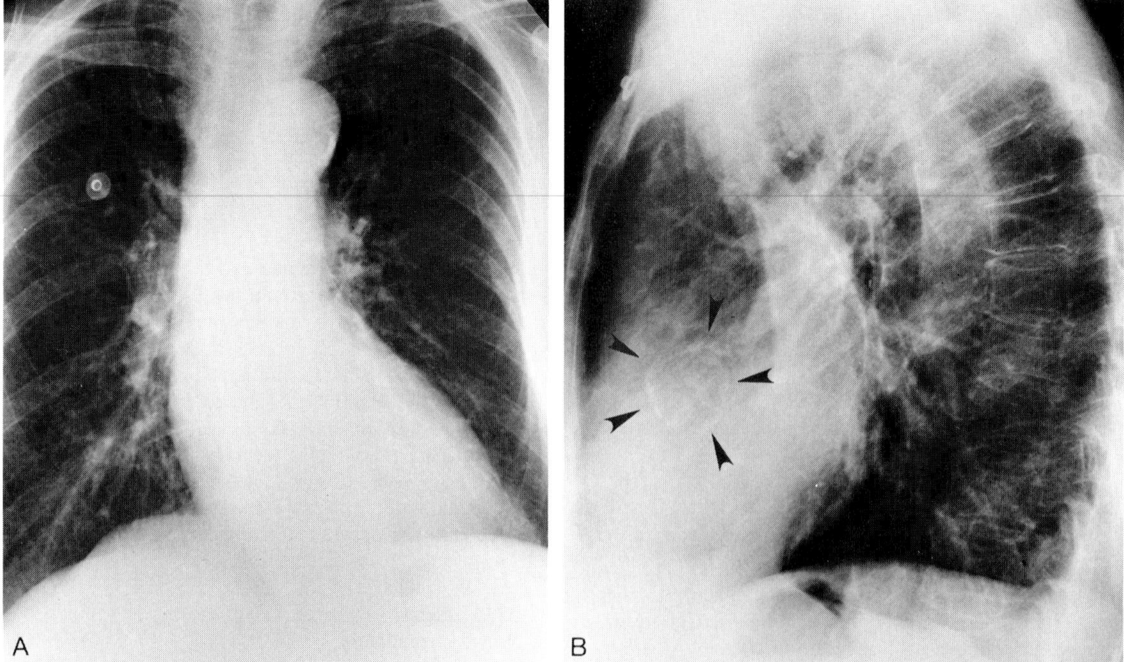

Figure 112–2. Calcific aortic stenosis. PA *(A)* and lateral *(B)* chest radiographs in an 80-year-old patient with a systolic murmur. Normal pulmonary vascularity and normal heart size are noted. Curvilinear calcifications are seen in the region of the aortic valve on the lateral projection *(arrowheads).* At cardiac catheterization, this patient had a tricuspid aortic valve and findings consistent with degenerative calcific aortic stenosis.

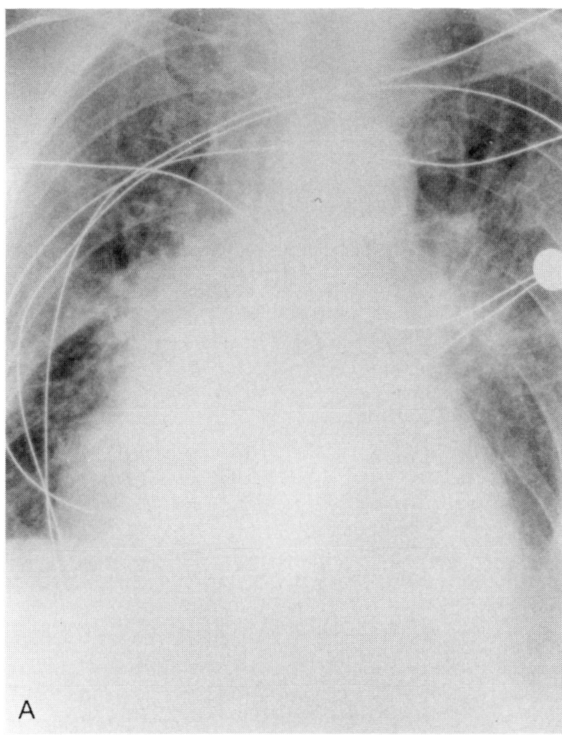

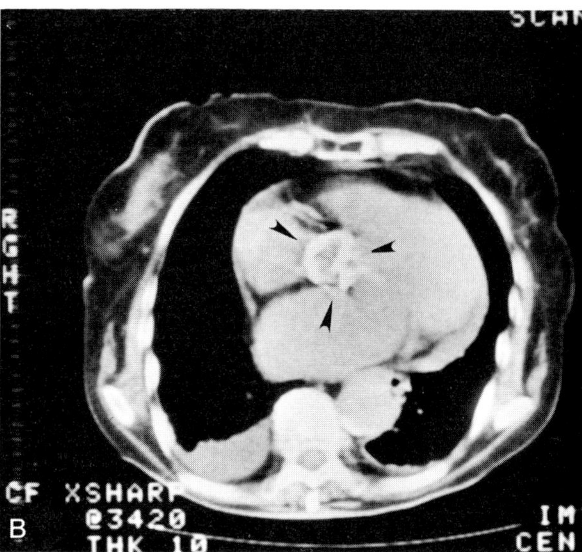

Figure 112–3. Calcific aortic stenosis. *A,* AP portable chest radiograph. *B,* Single slice from a computed tomographic study of the thorax. This patient presented with congestive heart failure of uncertain etiology. The chest film reveals pulmonary edema. The computed tomographic section at the level of the aortic valve reveals dense calcifications in the aortic valve *(arrowheads).* Severe aortic stenosis may present in this fashion with heart murmur inaudible due to congestive failure. Cardiac fluoroscopy or CT scanning may be valuable in assessing aortic valve calcification.

maximum systolic blood flow velocity across the valve. The accurate measurement of the high velocities across the aortic valve requires continuous Doppler recording techniques rather than pulsed Doppler techniques. The aortic valve area can also be determined by means of continuous Doppler recordings using the following equation:

$$AVA = CO/(0.9\ SEP \times V) \quad (3)$$

This is the Gorlin formula from above, the pressure gradient term ($P_2 - P_1$) being replaced with the Doppler-derived term $4V^2$. The aortic valve area has been determined using Doppler techniques without the necessity of performing a left heart catheterization with its recognized morbidity and mortality. In these patients, the cardiac output must be determined by thermodilution techniques in conjunction with right heart catheterization. The SEP and V terms are determined by the Doppler examination. The CO may be determined by Doppler techniques, so that even a right heart catheterization may not be necessary to determine the AVA in a given patient with aortic stenosis.

In the absence of Doppler echocardiography, the majority of adult patients with suspected aortic stenosis undergo left heart catheterization; aortic valve gradients and systolic ejection times are calculated directly from both simultaneous LV and aortic artery pressure recordings. If simultaneous cardiac outputs are determined by standard thermodilution techniques, aortic valve areas can be determined by using the formula of Gorlin and Gorlin:

$$AVA = CO/(44.5\ SEP\ (P_2 - P_1)^{1/2}) \quad (4)$$

AVA is aortic valve area, SEP is systolic ejection time, P_2 is peak left ventricular pressure, P_1 is peak aortic or radial artery pressure, and CO is cardiac output.

ANGIOGRAPHIC FINDINGS

The technique used to evaluate aortic stenosis using angiocardiography usually involves obtaining a standard RAO left ventriculogram and an aortogram using a 40-degree left anterior oblique projection, with 40 degrees of cranial angulation of the x-ray beam relative to the patient. The injection rates and volume of contrast injected must be tailored to the individual patient and the degree of stenosis. In patients with large gradients (>80 mm Hg), the left ventriculogram should be performed with lower volumes of contrast material than for the standard left ventriculogram. Ideally, low-osmolality agents and digital subtraction techniques should be utilized.

When evaluating the angiograms, it is important to keep in mind that acquired aortic valvular stenosis can result from degeneration of a congenitally bicuspid aortic valve, with fibrosis and calcification gradually narrowing the orifice of the valve; or can involve an initially normal tricuspid aortic valve in which commissural fusion, leaflet thickening, and fibrosis have developed. The end stage of any of these processes may be a severely calcified valve, and the etiology may not be recognizable either angiographically or pathologically.

The thoracic aortogram of a congenital bicuspid aortic valve that is stenotic but not calcified reveals thickening with doming of the valve leaflets in systole (Fig. 112–7). A jet of nonopacified blood visible through the stenotic valve may be slightly eccentric in direction but is roughly centered in the middle of the aortic valve annulus (Fig. 112–7). The jet of blood in the supravalvular area may produce post-stenotic dilatation of the ascending aorta in the direction of the jet. The congenital bicuspid aortic valve usually has three sinuses of Valsalva, with one sinus equal in size to the other two sinuses combined (Fig. 112–7). This large sinus is usually the noncoronary sinus. The single commissure of a congenitally bicuspid aortic valve is seen best during systole.

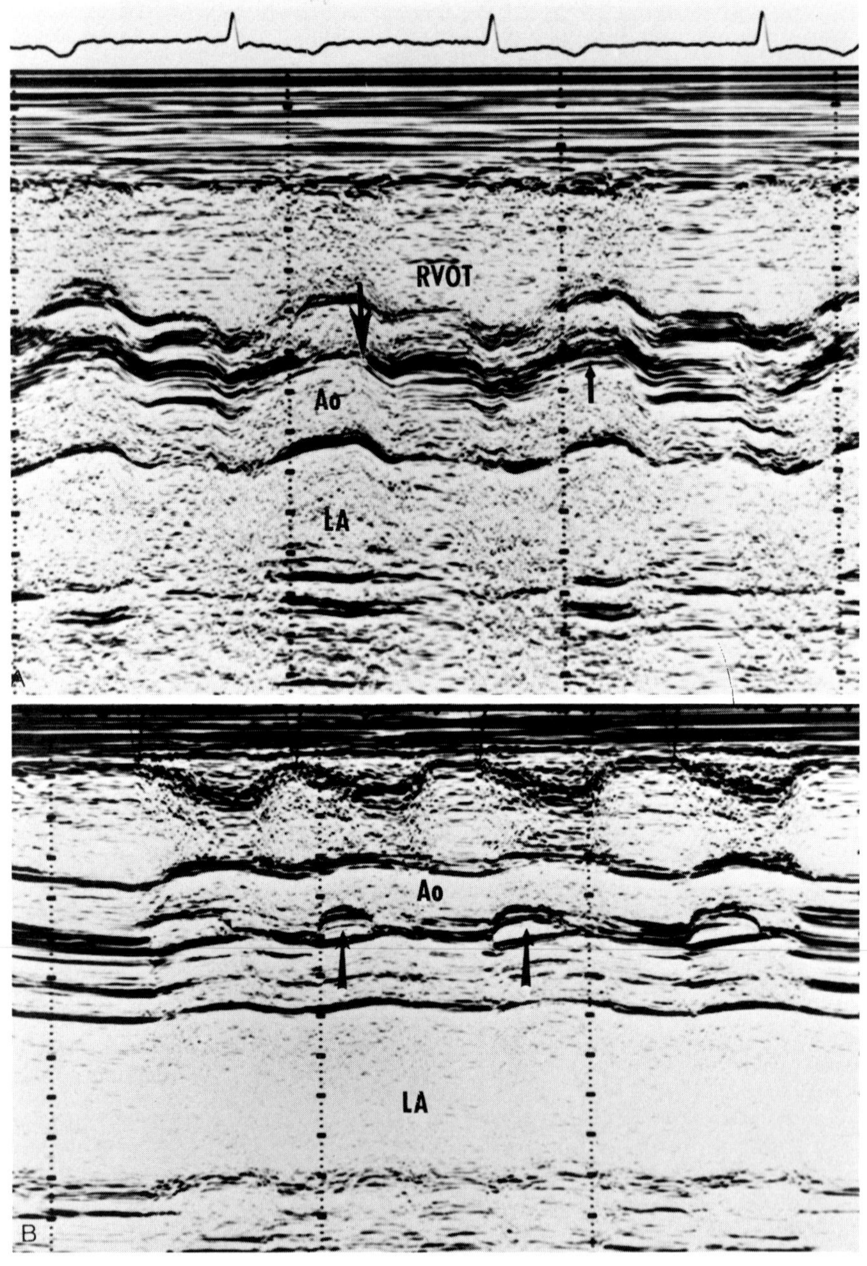

Figure 112–4. Aortic stenosis. *A,* M-mode echocardiographic cut through the RV outflow tract (RVOT), aorta (Ao), and left atrium (LA). The *large arrow* denotes the eccentric closure point of the aortic valve leaflets. No significant aortic valve cusp excursion can be demonstrated *(small arrow). B,* M-mode echocardiographic cut through the aortic valve in a patient with rheumatic aortic stenosis. Note the significantly limited aortic valve cusp excursion *(arrows).*

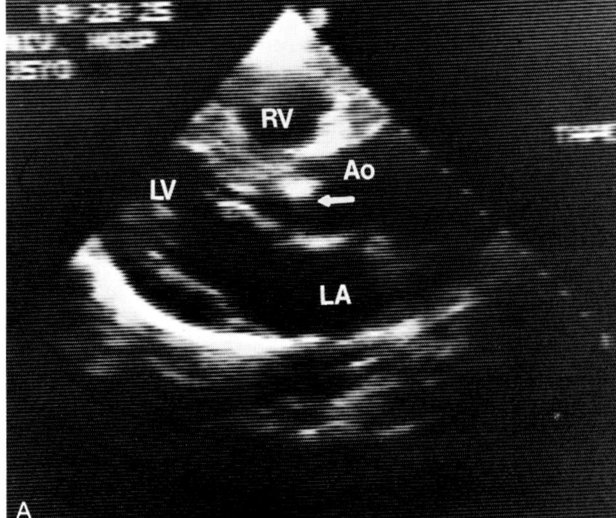

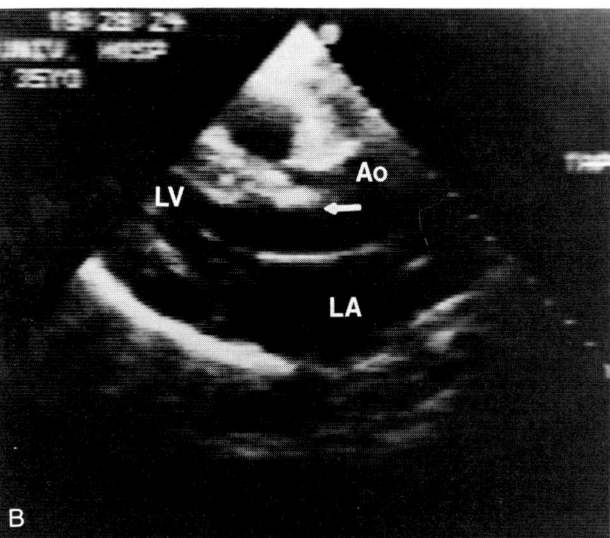

Figure 112–5. Aortic stenosis. *A,* Two-dimensional (2-D) echocardiographic long-axis view in a patient with a bicuspid valve and aortic stenosis. This view demonstrates the right ventricle (RV), the left ventricle (LV), the left atrium (LA), and the aorta (Ao). A calcified aortic valve with the predominant calcification involving the anterior cusp is demonstrated *(arrow).* This still frame is obtained in **diastole** (note the open mitral valve leaflets). *B,* 2-D long-axis echocardiographic view of the left ventricle in the same patient as in *A* in **systole,** demonstrating the predominant calcification involving the anterior leaflet of this bicuspid valve *(arrow).* The patient was a 35-year-old woman with clinically severe aortic stenosis.

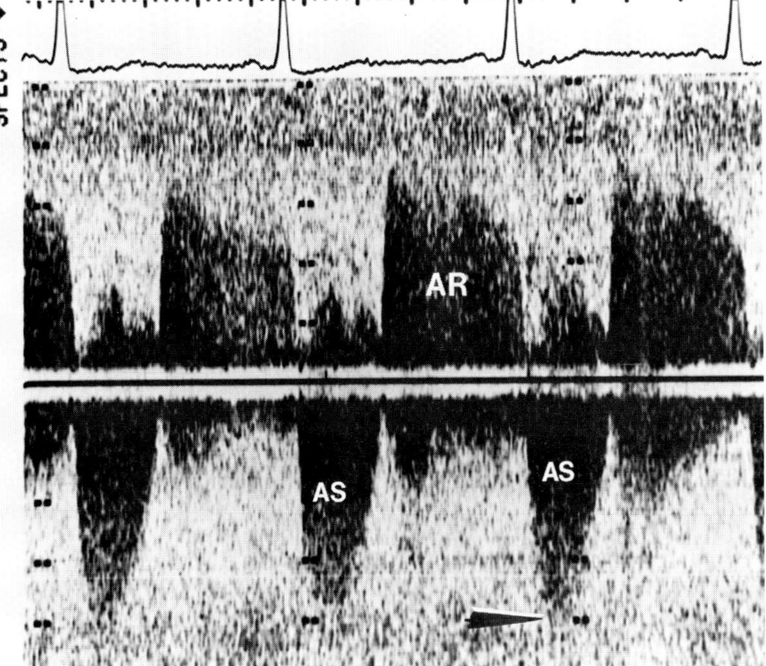

Figure 112–6. Aortic stenosis and aortic regurgitation. Continuous Doppler profile in a patient with a bicuspid aortic valve and aortic stenosis and regurgitation. Imaging is performed from the apex. A high-velocity diastolic flow disturbance is depicted consistent with aortic stenosis (AS). The velocity of this aortic stenosis jet is 4 m/sec *(arrow),* consistent with an instantaneous transaortic valve gradient of 64 mm Hg. A high-velocity diastolic flow disturbance is consistent with aortic regurgitation (AR).

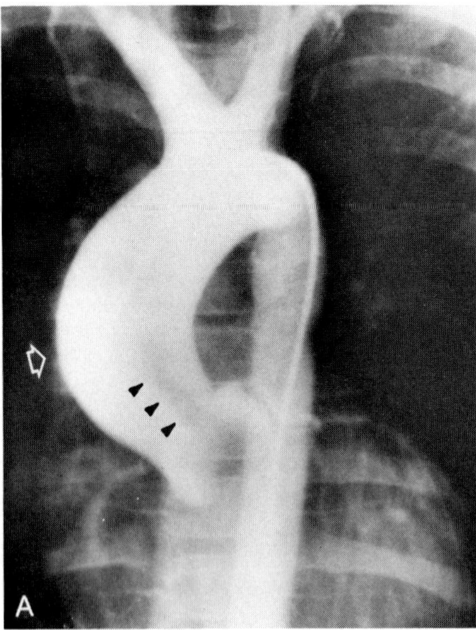

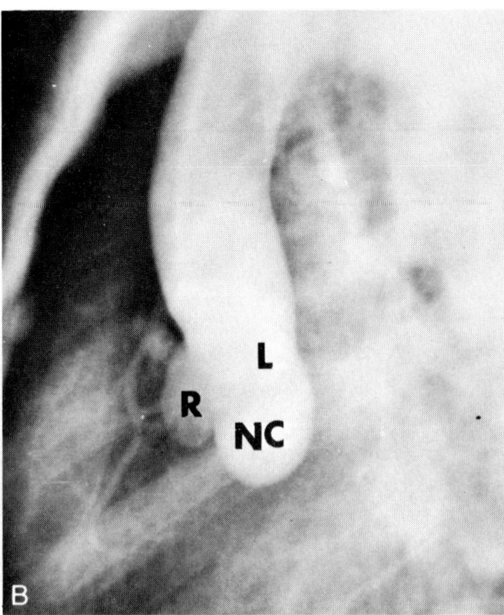

Figure 112–7. Aortic stenosis and bicuspid aortic valve. AP *(A)* and lateral *(B)* ascending aortograms demonstrate dilatation of the ascending aorta *(arrow)* and a nonopacified jet of blood *(arrowheads)* in the systolic AP frame. In the lateral projection, asymmetrical valve cusps are noted. The right (R) and left (L) cusps are small, and the noncoronary (NC) cusp is twice as large. These angiographic features are typical of bicuspid aortic valve with moderate aortic stenosis.

As calcification occurs in the congenital bicuspid aortic valve, the leaflets may not dome during systole, and the jet of blood through the leaflets may not be seen (Fig. 112–8). In order to suggest the most likely etiology of the acquired aortic valve disease when calcification occurs, the age of the patient and certain morphologic features must be taken into consideration. The congenital bicuspid valve begins to calcify in the fourth decade. Rheumatic aortic stenosis also usually begins to calcify in the fourth decade, although it may occur earlier, and "degenerative" aortic stenosis of the elderly is a disease that is seen in patients over the age of 65 years. Fusion of the aortic valve commissures adjacent to the aortic wall occurs typically in patients with rheumatic aortic stenosis, and these patients usually have a tricuspid valve with three equal sinuses of Valsalva (Fig. 112–8*B*). If only one commissure fuses, rheumatic aortic stenosis may closely resemble a calcified congenital bicuspid aortic valve. The patients with rheumatic aortic stenosis may have associated mitral stenosis and/or regurgitation, and there may be evidence of calcification in the mitral valve leaflets as well as thickening of the mitral leaflets. The presence of a calcified mitral valve in association with calcific aortic stenosis makes rheumatic aortic stenosis very likely. Aortic stenosis in the elderly results from thickening and calcification of a tricuspid valve. Coronary and mitral annulus calcification is also frequently present in these patients (Fig. 112–8*C*). The leaflets have clumps of calcium in them, and, in contrast to rheumatic valves, the aortic valve commissures are not fused. If aortography is performed, a narrow jet of blood across the valve is absent, and usually no significant aortic regurgitation is present. The aortic valve leaflets in this form of stenosis have limited mobility.

Aortic Regurgitation

Aortic regurgitation may result from disease of the aortic valve or from conditions primarily affecting the ascending aorta. The most common cause of aortic regurgitation is rheumatic fibrosis. Infective endocarditis is another cause in which regurgitation results from perforation or prolapse of a cusp. The underlying valve is normal in 15 per cent of cases. In the remaining cases the valve may be damaged from a previous condition such as rheumatic fever or a congenital bicuspid valve. Diseases affecting the ascending aorta such as ankylosing spondylitis, rheumatoid arthritis, and cystic medial necrosis can produce aortic regurgitation due to dilatation of the aortic annulus.

The predominant pathophysiologic process in aortic regurgitation is progressive enlargement of both the diastolic and systolic dimensions of the left ventricle. The resultant increase in myocardial fiber length from the dilatation permits an increase in stroke volume (effective systemic forward flow plus regurgitant volume). The compliance of the left ventricle remains normal during the compensated stage of the disease, so that left ventricular diastolic and pulmonary venous pressures remain at or near normal levels. When the length of the myocardial fibers reaches a critical limit, irreversible myocardial failure results. In the late stage of the disease, retrograde flow at the root of the aorta may lead to a relative decrease in coronary blood flow and subendocardial ischemia. In acute aortic regurgitation, the pathologic changes described above may be telescoped in time owing to failure of the normal compensatory mechanisms.

RADIOGRAPHIC FINDINGS

The chest radiograph in compensated aortic regurgitation demonstrates normal pulmonary vascularity and substantial cardiomegaly (cardiothoracic ratio > 0.55) owing to enlargement of the left ventricle (Fig. 112–9). The ascending thoracic aorta and the transverse thoracic aorta are enlarged as well (Fig 112–9). Valvular calcifications are not as common in isolated aortic regurgitation as they are in aortic stenosis. The pulmonary vascularity is normal in the compensated state of the disease (Figs. 112–9 and 112–10). The apparent dichotomy of a large heart with normal pulmonary vascularity may also be seen in patients with congestive cardiomyopathy or pericardial effusion. The clue to radiographic diagnosis in this situation resides in the dilated ascending and descending aorta seen in cases of aortic regurgitation (Fig. 112–10). The presence of pulmonary venous hypertension (usually late in the disease) is a sign of myocardial failure and is associated with a poor prognosis. As the disease progresses and the cardiothoracic ratio exceeds 0.60, the chance of a good postoperative result from aortic valve replace-

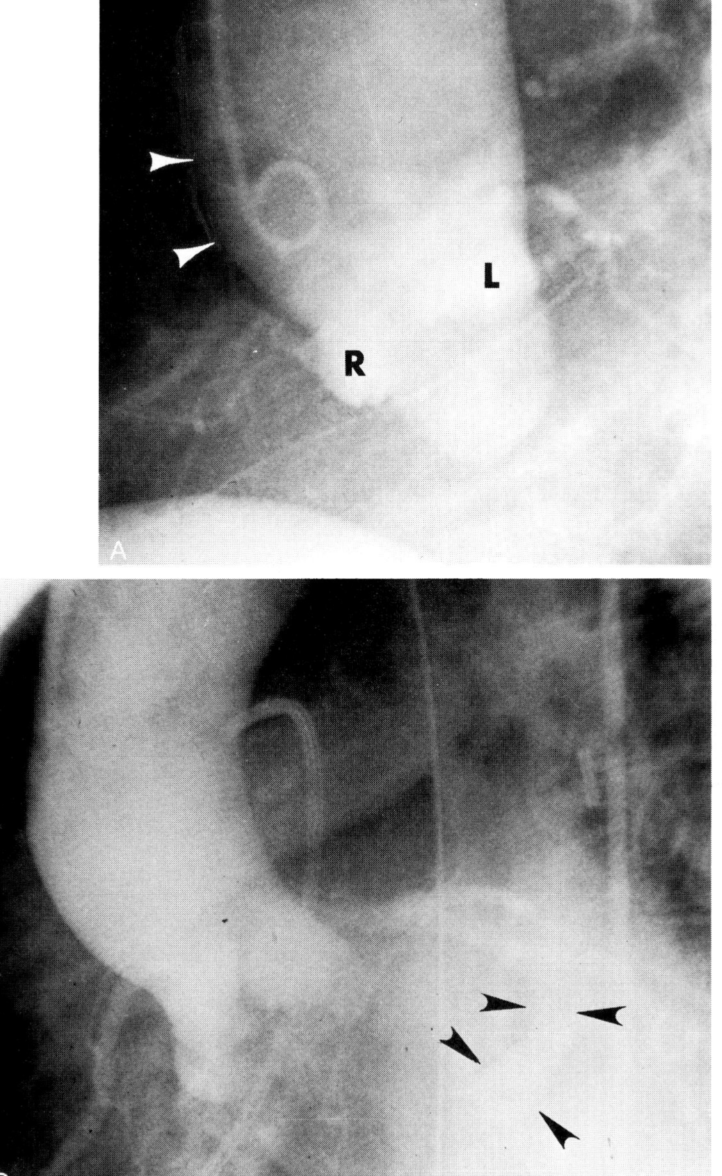

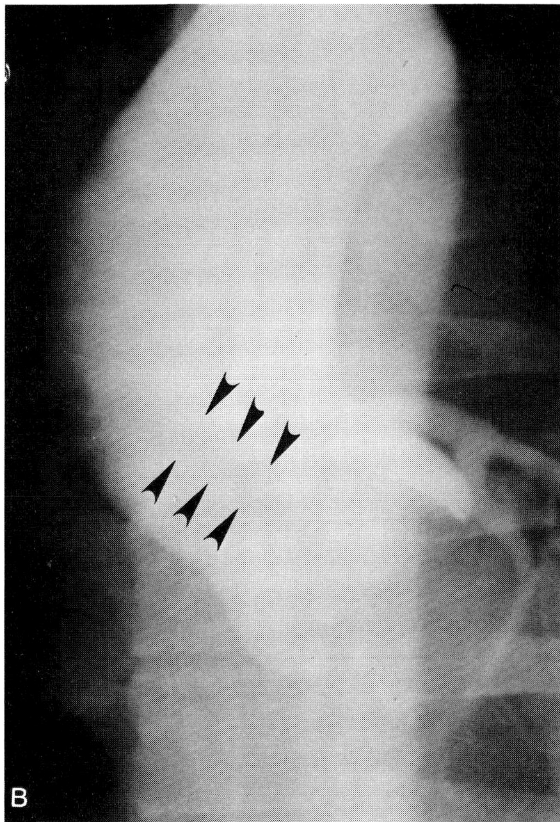

Figure 112–8. Calcific aortic stenosis. *A,* Single LAO cine frame from an ascending aortogram. *B,* AP frame from an ascending aortogram. *C,* Cine frame in LAO projection from an ascending aortogram. In *A,* there is asymmetrical yet small right (R) and left (L) sinuses with a large noncoronary cusp present. There is post-stenotic dilatation *(arrowheads).* This frame is taken in systole; there is minimal doming of the valve, and no jet of nonopacified blood is noted. At surgery, this patient had a congenitally bicuspid aortic valve. In *B,* relatively symmetric cusps are present, and a faint nonopacified jet of blood is noted *(arrowheads).* This patient has rheumatic aortic stenosis with a tricuspid valve. In *C,* this 80-year-old patient has both calcific aortic stenosis with a thickened valve and post-stenotic dilatation of the ascending aorta. Note also the presence of heavy calcification in the mitral annulus *(arrowheads).*

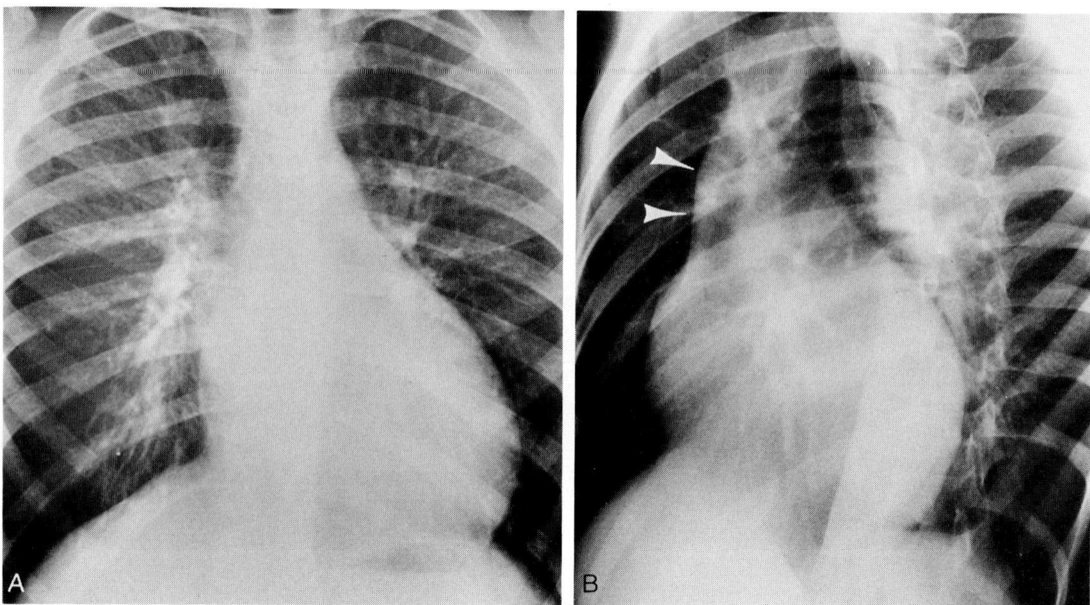

Figure 112–9. Aortic regurgitation. PA *(A)* and LAO *(B)* chest radiographs in a young individual with rheumatic aortic regurgitation. Note the normal pulmonary vascularity and the large cardiothoracic ratio with left ventricular enlargement (best appreciated in the LAO projection). There is prominence of the ascending aorta *(arrowheads)* in the LAO projection. Note the discrepancy between normal pulmonary vascularity and significant cardiomegaly.

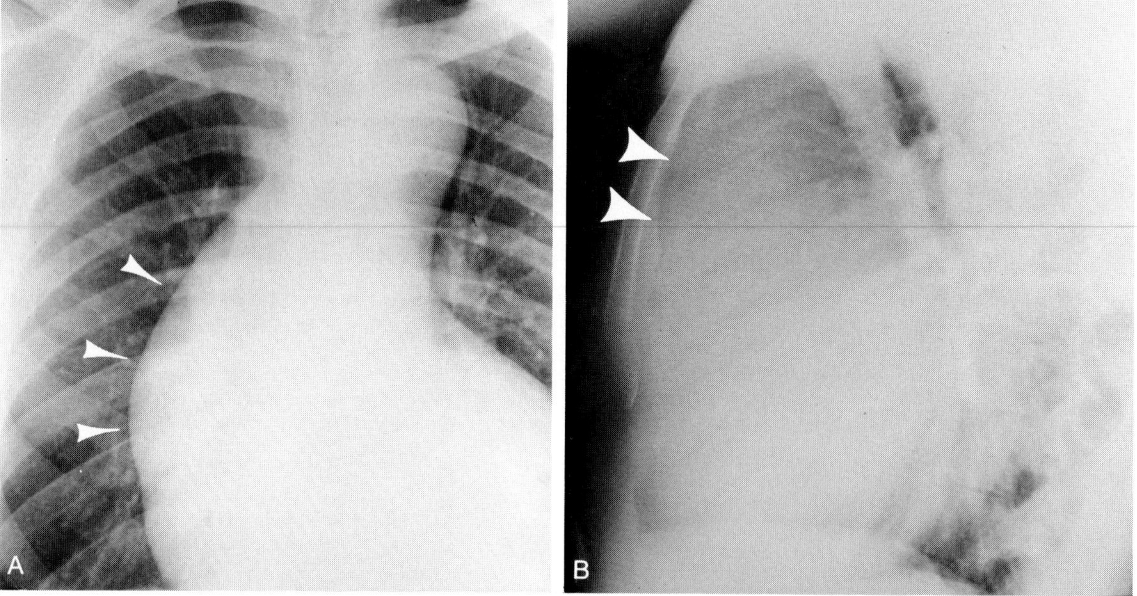

Figure 112–10. Aortic regurgitation. PA *(A)* and lateral *(B)* chest radiographs in a patient with cystic medial necrosis and significant aortic regurgitation. The right lung field is demonstrated on the PA view, showing normal pulmonary vascularity. There is marked left ventricular enlargement and significant enlargement of the ascending aorta on both the PA and lateral projections *(arrowheads)*. On the lateral view, the entire anterior mediastinum is filled in by the dilated ascending aorta *(arrowheads)*.

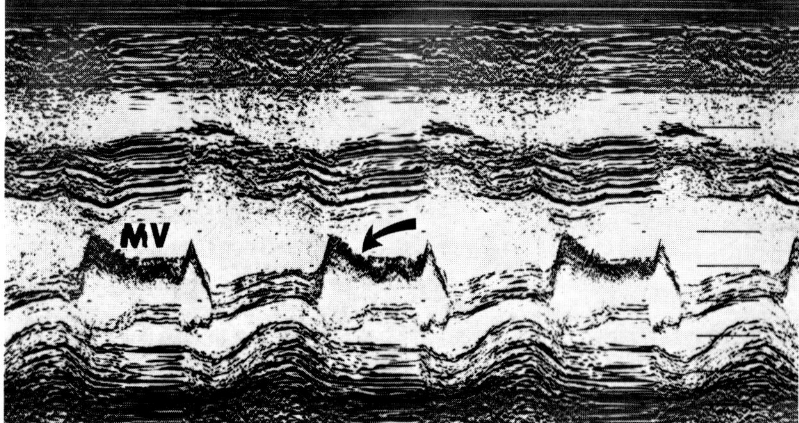

Figure 112–11. Aortic regurgitation. M-mode echocardiogram taken at the level of the mitral valve in a patient with mild rheumatic aortic regurgitation. Although the left ventricular cavity is relatively small, there is diastolic fluttering of the anterior leaflet of the mitral valve (MV—*curved arrow*).

ment decreases, and the five-year survival rate is significantly lowered.

ECHOCARDIOGRAPHIC FINDINGS

The increased dimensions of the aortic root and the left ventricle associated with aortic regurgitation can be assessed on both M-mode and two-dimensional echocardiograms. The extent of contraction or fractional shortening can be assessed as well. Visualization of the anterior leaflet of the mitral valve may demonstrate diastolic fluttering of the leaflet, which represents the echocardiographic equivalent of the Austin Flint murmur (Fig. 112–11). Changes in the geometry of the ventricle may make it difficult to follow the enlargement of the left ventricle accurately with echocardiographic techniques. Pulsed Doppler techniques to quantitate the aortic regurgitation, similar in some respects to the process of quantitating the regurgitation on angiocardiograms of the heart, have been developed and may provide an accurate quantitative method of assessing severity and of following patients with this disease prior to surgical intervention (see Fig. 112–6).

ANGIOCARDIOGRAPHIC FINDINGS

The objectives in assessing aortic regurgitation using angiocardiography are to demonstrate and quantitate the regurgitation and to elucidate the pathology (aortic root vs valve) responsible for the regurgitation (Figs. 112–12 and 112–13). A biplane supravalvular aortogram is usually obtained in both the left and right anterior oblique projections using modern cineangiographic techniques similar to those used in aortic stenosis. The tip of the catheter should be free in the ascending aorta at the sinotubular ridge. Cineangiographic techniques are required if the movement of the aortic cusps is to be assessed accurately. It should be noted that some aortic

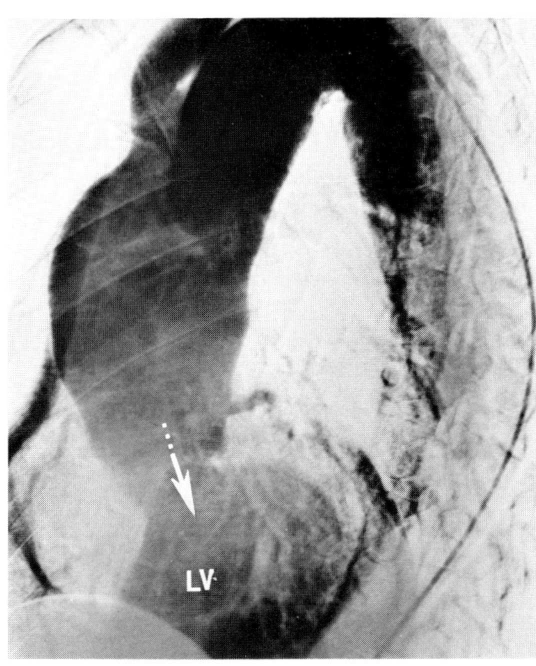

Figure 112–12. Aortic regurgitation. RPO cut film ascending aortogram in an elderly individual with cystic medial necrosis of the ascending aorta. Note the fusiform dilatation of the ascending aorta and the 4+/4+ aortic regurgitation (*arrow*—LV).

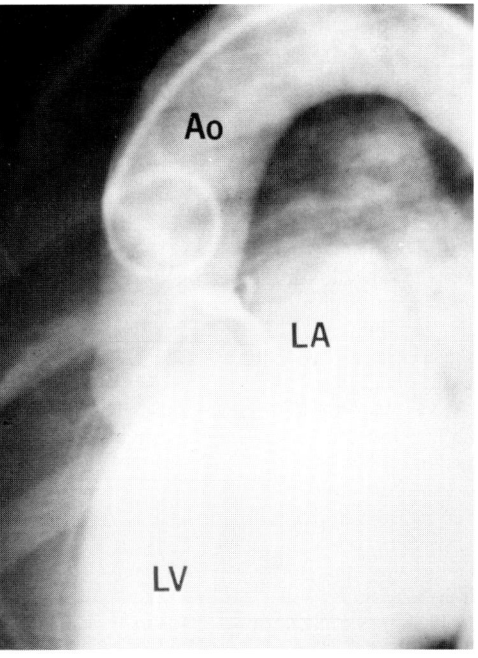

Figure 112–13. Aortic regurgitation and mitral regurgitation. Lateral view of an ascending aortogram. There is 4+/4+ aortic regurgitation and 4+/4+ mitral regurgitation. Note enlargement of the left ventricle (LV) and the left atrium (LA). This young patient had rheumatic valvular heart disease.

regurgitation may be seen in patients who have a normal aortic valve but suffer poor left ventricular contraction or arrhythmia. These may cause erratic opening of the valve. The most accurate way to quantitatively assess aortic regurgitation is to calculate a regurgitant fraction. Subjective assessment using angiocardiography is considerably less accurate. If aortic and mitral regurgitation coexist in a given patient, quantitating the regurgitation using angiocardiography may be useful, since the quantitative technique will not work in the presence of two sequential regurgitant lesions (Fig. 112–13). The following scheme may be used to estimate and grade aortic regurgitation following an ascending aortogram:

Grade 1: Minimal opacification of the ventricle adjacent to the aortic and mitral valves

Grade 2: Faint opacification of the entire left ventricle with subsequent clearing of the left ventricle after one heartbeat

Grade 3: Dense opacification of the left ventricle with subsequent clearing of the left ventricle after two or three beats

Grade 4: Dense opacification of the left ventricle with the density of the left ventricle exceeding that of the aorta and lasting at least four beats after the end of contrast injection

It should be noted that there are several factors that may lead to inaccurate assessment of aortic regurgitation using angiocardiographic grading schemes. These include the position of the catheter, the amount of contrast material injected, the size and contractility of the left ventricle, and the pressure gradient in diastole between the aorta and the left ventricle. If the aortic and left ventricular diastolic pressures become equal, the amount of regurgitation may be severely underestimated.

MITRAL VALVE

Mitral Stenosis

The principal cause of acquired mitral stenosis is rheumatic heart disease. Left atrial myxomas and ball-valve type thrombi of the left atrium will obstruct the passage of blood into the left ventricle and produce similar pathophysiologic states, but they are not, strictly speaking, valvular heart lesions. The pathophysiologic change that occurs in mitral stenosis is increased resistance to emptying of the left atrium, with left atrial pressure and pulmonary vascular pressure rising throughout diastole. In later stages of the disease, medial hypertrophy and intimal sclerosis develop in the pulmonary arterioles, causing an even greater increase in pulmonary arteriolar resistance and pulmonary arterial pressure. The resulting pulmonary arterial hypertension causes right ventricular hypertrophy, dilatation, and eventually right heart failure. The dilatation of the right ventricle may eventually dilate the annulus of the tricuspid valve, so that tricuspid regurgitation develops. If right heart failure develops in a patient with mitral stenosis, the pulmonary vascular abnormalities may resolve, making the diagnosis more difficult. The compensatory mechanism of mitral stenosis is hypertrophy, since this is a lesion that obstructs flow out of the left atrium. However, unlike the hypertrophic response of the left ventricle in aortic stenosis, the thin-walled left atrium will dilate in response to the high pressures that result from obstruction of the mitral valve orifice. In this disease, normal atrial contraction becomes an important mechanism for delivery of blood into the left ventricle. The development of atrial fibrillation therefore has a detrimental effect on cardiac output in these patients.

The changes that occur in the pulmonary vasculature in mitral stenosis are due to the increased pressure in the left atrium that is then transmitted back into the pulmonary circulation. As the postcapillary pressures increase to between 16 and 19 mm Hg, redistribution of blood flow to the upper lobes occurs. As the pressure continues to increase, interstitial pulmonary edema will develop at pressures of 20 to 25 mm Hg, and alveolar edema will develop when the pressure is between 25 and 30 mm Hg. These pressure values occur in patients who have not had long-standing obstruction to flow across the mitral valve orifice. Those patients with long-standing severe mitral stenosis may have little or no abnormality of the pulmonary vascularity, with high postcapillary pulmonary pressures. These patients may also have coexistent pulmonary arterial hypertension secondary to precapillary hypertension.

RADIOGRAPHIC FINDINGS

There are a number of clues in the radiographic diagnoses of mitral stenosis. Depending on the severity and duration of the stenosis, the pulmonary vasculature may reveal redistribution, interstitial edema, or alveolar edema (Fig. 112–14). Left atrial enlargement can be assessed on the frontal radiograph by noting a "double density" to the right of the spine. This represents displacement of the right inferior border of the left atrium due to enlargement of the body of the left atrium (Fig. 112–14). The distance between the midpoint of the double density and the midpoint of the left mainstem bronchus (the "left atrial dimension") should be less than 7.5 cm in an adult male and less than 7.0 cm in an adult female (Fig. 112–14). Left atrial enlargement is present with a discrete convex bulge to the superior posterior cardiac contour below the carina on the lateral chest radiograph (Fig. 112–14). Enlargement of the left atrial appendage should be looked for carefully, since this is a good marker of previous rheumatic heart disease. The left atrial appendage is visible when it enlarges as a discrete convexity along the left heart border between the main pulmonary artery and the "shoulder" of the heart formed by the left ventricle (Figs. 112–14 and 112–15). In isolated mitral stenosis, the aorta is often small as a result of decreased forward cardiac output (Figs. 112–14 and 112–15). Mitral valve calcification may be present and is best assessed on the lateral radiograph or at fluoroscopy (Figs 112–14 and 112–15). In the absence of right ventricular failure and other serious valve lesions of the aortic or tricuspid valve, the cardiothoracic ratio is usually normal or nearly normal (Figs. 112–14 and 112–15). The severity of the mitral lesion can be assessed by the density of calcification of the valve and the degree of pulmonary venous hypertension. In patients with long-standing mitral stenosis, the wall of the left atrium may calcify in response to the large pressure gradient across the mitral valve and the fibrotic changes related to the rheumatic process (Fig. 112–16). There is an increased incidence of atrial fibrillation and left atrial thrombus in these patients. Pulmonary arterial hypertension secondary to precapillary hypertension is suggested on the plain radiograph when there is enlargement of the central pulmonary arteries (Fig. 112–14) and right ventricular enlargement (Fig. 112–16). The degree of mitral stenosis is usually severe in these patients. Clues to the presence of concomitant tricuspid valve disease or aortic valve disease in patients with mitral stenosis reside in finding right heart or ascending aortic enlargement, respectively (Figs. 112–16 and 112–17).

ECHOCARDIOGRAPHIC FINDINGS

M-mode, two-dimensional, and Doppler echocardiographic techniques are all useful in the evaluation of mitral stenosis. In approximately 90 per cent of patients with mitral stenosis, the M-mode study will demonstrate flattening of the E-F slope, decreased diastolic excursions of the mitral leaflets, thickening of the leaflets, and concordant anterior movement of the anterior and posterior leaflets during systole (Fig. 112–18). The size of the left atrium can be accurately measured and serves as an index of severity of the mitral stenosis (Fig. 112–18). A left atrial myxoma can be excluded from the M-mode studies by noting the absence of multiple dense echoes posterior to the anterior leaflet of the mitral valve during diastole.

The size of the left atrium and a direct assessment of mitral valve anatomy can be accomplished using two-dimensional echocardiog-

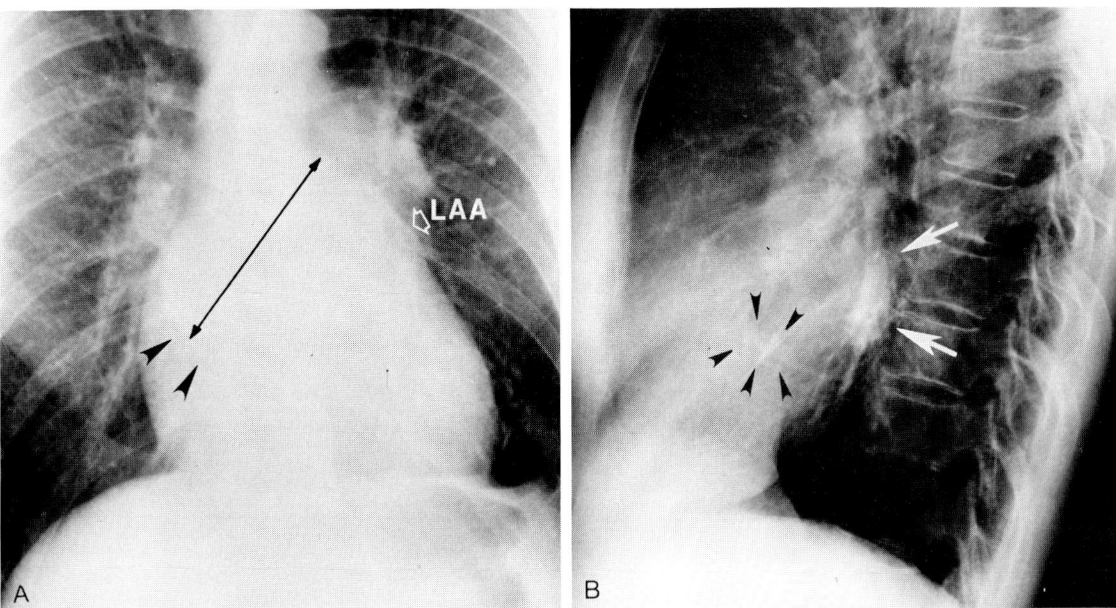

Figure 112–14. Mitral stenosis. PA *(A)* and lateral *(B)* chest radiographs. PA view shows upper lobe vascular redistribution and some increase in interstitial markings in the lungs consistent with moderate pulmonary venous hypertension. Left atrial enlargement is noted as a "double density" along the right heart border *(arrowheads)*. The method of measuring the left atrial dimension is indicated by the double-headed arrow. In this patient the measurement was 9 cm. Note the enlargement of the left atrial appendage (LAA—*arrow*). On the lateral view, there is a discrete posterior bulge along the superior posterior cardiac border *(arrows)* indicating left atrial enlargement. Note also the faint calcification in the mitral valve *(arrowheads)*.

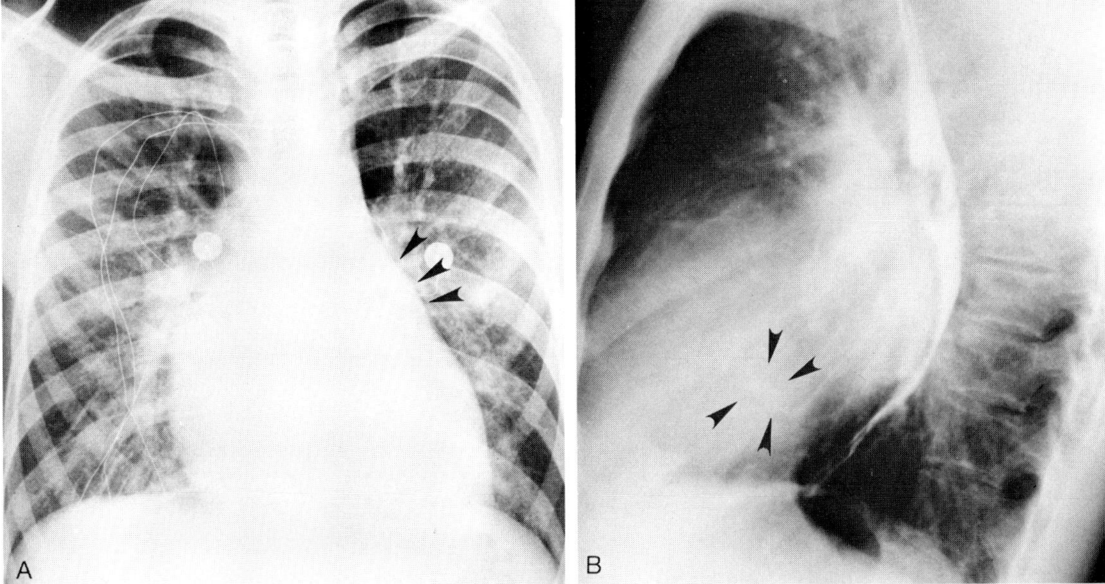

Figure 112–15. Mitral stenosis. PA *(A)* and lateral *(B)* chest radiographs. The PA view shows moderate to severe pulmonary venous hypertension, normal heart size, and enlargement of the left atrial appendage *(arrowheads)*. On the lateral view, the left atrial enlargement is well-defined by the barium in the esophagus. Note also the presence of calcification in the mitral valve *(arrowheads)*. Note that in both this patient and the one illustrated in Figure 112–14, the thoracic aorta is normal in size. Both of these patients had isolated mitral stenosis.

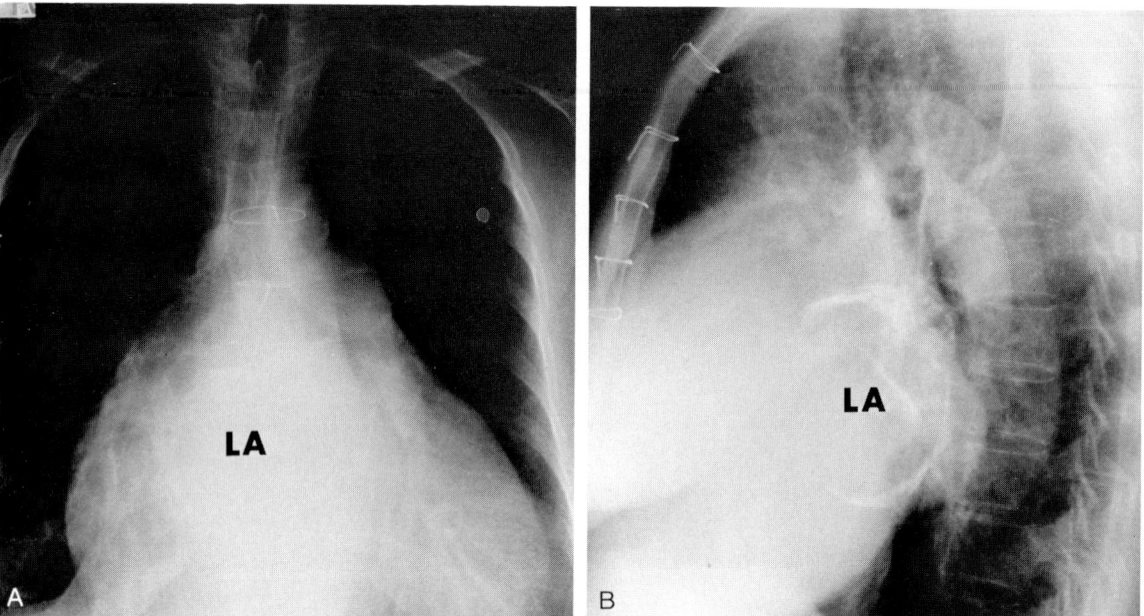

Figure 112–16. Mitral stenosis and tricuspid regurgitation. PA *(A)* and lateral *(B)* chest radiographs. The patient had previous mitral commissurotomy through a median sternotomy and was subsequently lost to follow-up. On re-evaluation, recurrent mitral stenosis and severe tricuspid regurgitation were present. Note the significant cardiac enlargement (especially the right heart) on both views. Note also the curvilinear calcification in the left atrium (LA) on both PA and lateral projections.

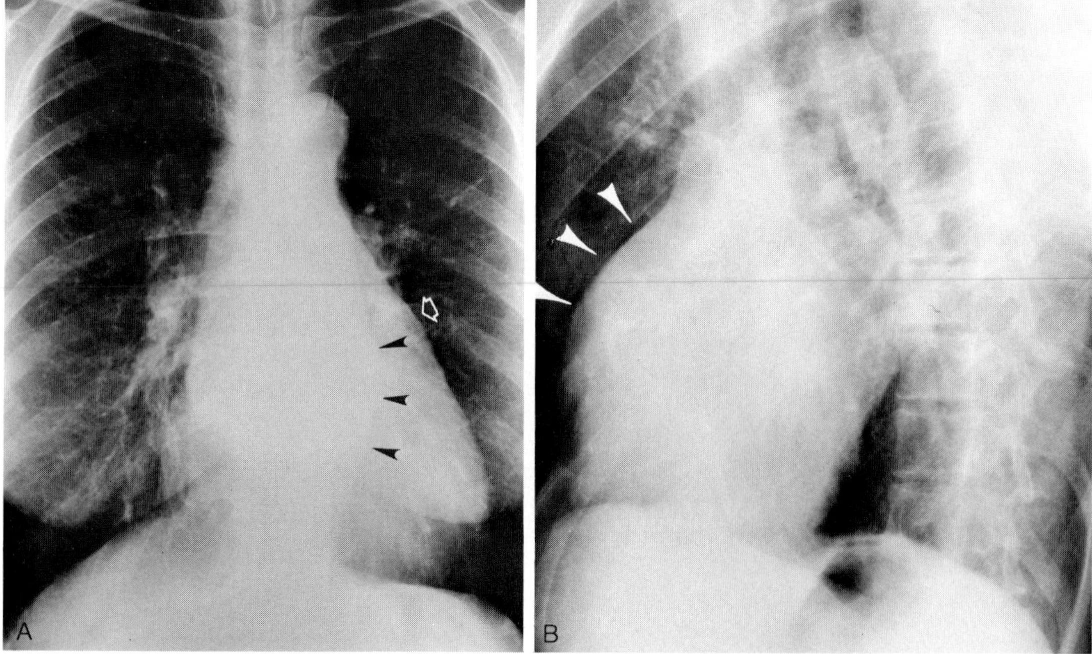

Figure 112–17. Mitral stenosis, tricuspid regurgitation, and aortic regurgitation. PA *(A)* and LAO *(B)* chest radiographs. Features of rheumatic mitral valvular disease are present with enlargement of the left atrium and left atrial appendage *(arrow)*. Note the significant tortuosity of the descending aorta on the PA view *(arrowheads)* and significant right heart enlargement *(arrowheads)* on the LAO projection. These findings suggest additional regurgitant lesions of the tricuspid and aortic valves.

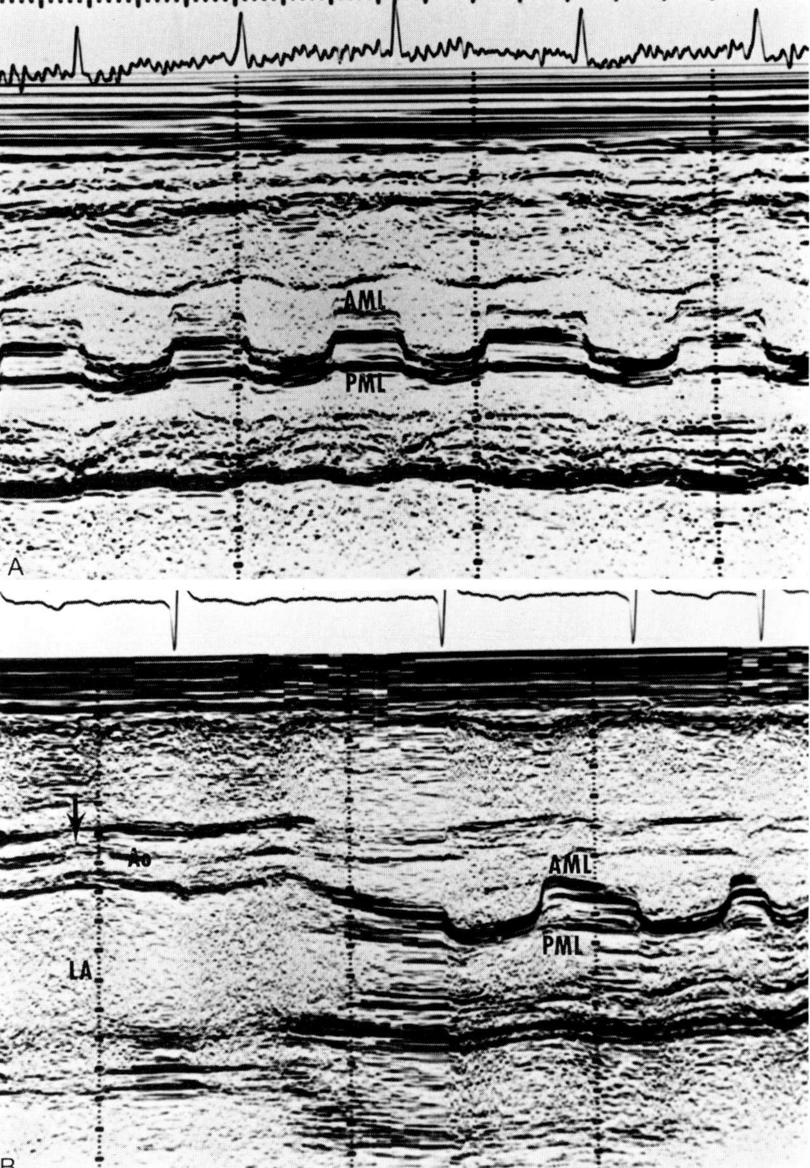

Figure 112–18. Mitral stenosis. *A,* M-mode echocardiographic cut at the tips of the mitral valve leaflets, demonstrating the thickened anterior mitral leaflet (AML) and posterior mitral leaflet (PML) with parallel leaflet motion and reduced leaflet excursion. *B,* M-mode echocardiographic sweep demonstrating the aorta (Ao) and enlarged left atrium (6 cm) (LA) in this patient with mitral stenosis and aortic stenosis. The aortic valve excursion is severely restricted *(arrow).* Note the thickened anterior mitral leaflet (AML) and posterior mitral leaflet (PML) with parallel leaflet motion and severely restricted leaflet excursion.

raphy (Fig. 112–19). The valve area can be computed directly from cross-sectional images of the mitral valve orifice during diastole (Fig. 112–19). The excursion of the leaflets can be assessed along with any evidence of fibrosis and calcification of the leaflets. If the AP diameter of the left atrium exceeds 5.0 cm by either M-mode or two-dimensional echocardiographic examination, the incidence of atrial fibrillation, left atrial thrombus, and systemic embolization is increased.

Doppler echocardiographic techniques can be used to assess the severity of stenosis present in mitral valve disease similar to the application of Doppler techniques to aortic stenosis (Fig. 112–20). Equation (2) can be used to derive the pressure gradient across the mitral valve. It is also possible to directly derive the area of the mitral valve orifice by using the so-called mitral pressure half-time. The half-time is defined as the time required for the transvalvular gradient to fall to half its initial value (Fig. 112–20):

$$t_{1/2} = V_1/(2)^{1/2} \quad (5)$$

The $t_{1/2}$ is the mitral pressure half-time, and V_1 is the initial diastolic velocity across the mitral valve orifice. The mitral valve area (MVA) can then be determined by the following expression:

$$MVA = 220/t_{1/2} \quad (6)$$

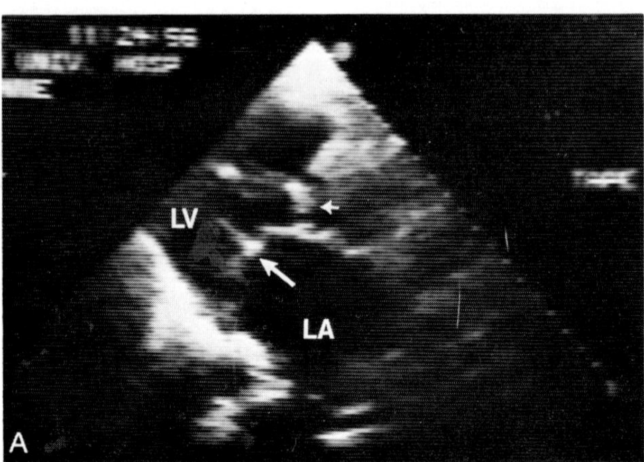

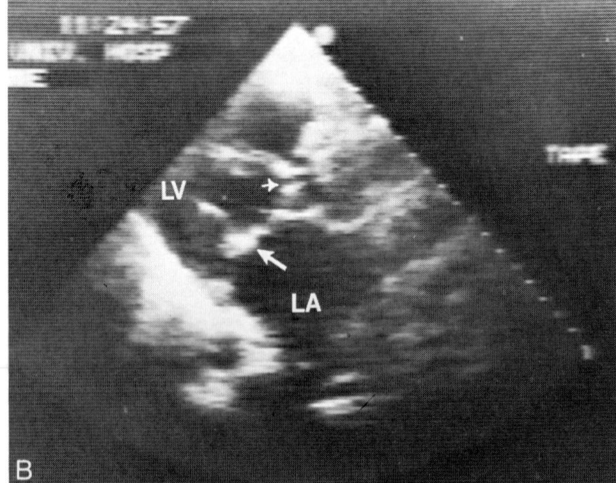

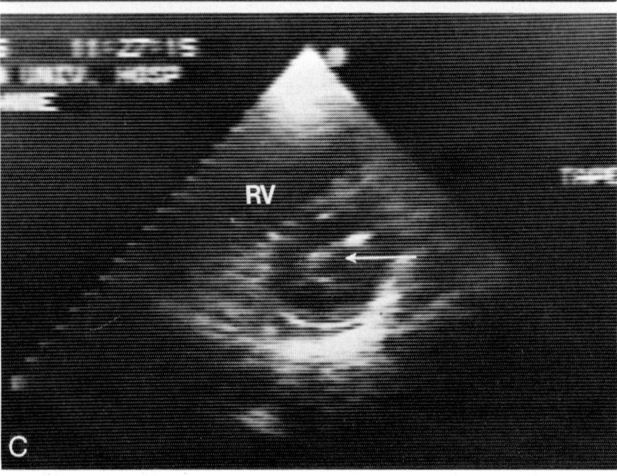

Figure 112–19. Mitral stenosis and aortic stenosis. Long-axis echocardiographic view of the heart in diastole demonstrating a small left ventricle (LV) and a significantly enlarged left atrium (LA). The aortic valve is thickened and calcified *(small arrow)*. The mitral valve is thickened and calcified, and diastolic mitral leaflet excursion is severely limited *(large arrow)*. *B*, Echocardiographic long-axis view in the same patient as *A*, demonstrating the large left atrium (LA) and the left ventricle (LV) in **systole**. The aortic valve leaflet excursion is severely limited *(small arrow)*. Thickened and calcified mitral valve leaflets are present *(large arrow)*. *C*, Short-axis echocardiographic view in **diastole**. Note the severely limited mitral leaflet excursion producing a very small mitral orifice size *(arrow)*.

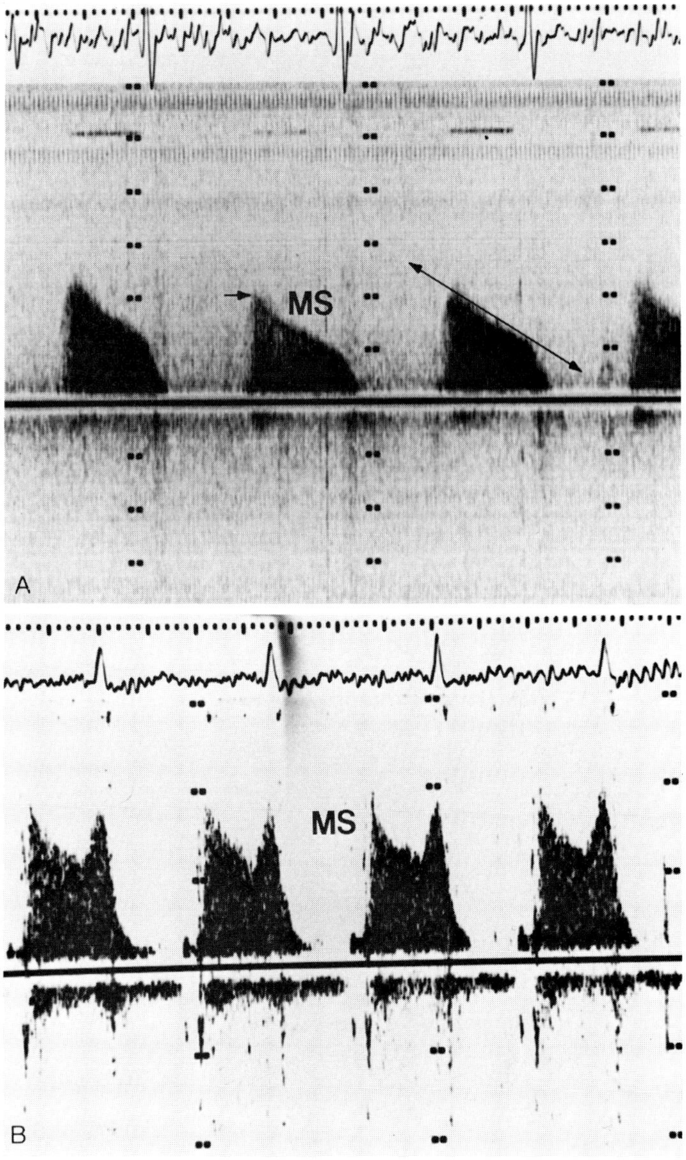

Figure 112–20. Mitral stenosis. *A,* Continuous-wave Doppler recording of the left ventricular inflow velocity from the left ventricular apex in a patient with severe mitral stenosis. Note the high-peak LV inflow velocity *(small arrow).* The slow drop in velocity *(long arrow)* indicates a gradual decrease in the pressure gradient between the left atrium and left ventricle. This is indicative of severe mitral stenosis. The pressure half-time can be used to calculate the mitral valve area from this velocity profile. *B,* Continuous-wave Doppler of mitral stenosis in a patient with sinus rhythm. There are two peaks of left ventricular inflow, the first during passive ventricular filling and the second during atrial systole.

Studies using Doppler techniques have achieved good correlation of MVA determinations with the results of cardiac catheterization, with regression coefficient equal to 0.87. Determination of MVA using Doppler techniques may be more accurate than with two-dimensional echocardiographic techniques in those patients who have undergone mitral valve commissurotomy. The Doppler-derived MVA may be more accurate than the cardiac catheterization-derived MVA value in patients who have significant mitral regurgitation.

ANGIOCARDIOGRAPHIC FINDINGS

The technique usually used to evaluate the mitral valve is ventriculography in the 30 to 40 degree RAO projection. "Forward" pulmonary angiography may be required in rare cases to define the level of obstruction in patients suspected of having mitral stenosis, left atrial myxoma, left atrial thrombus, or cor triatriatum (Fig. 112–21). It is, however, unreliable in assessing the severity of the obstruction. The severity of the lesion is determined hemodynamically by obtaining simultaneous pulmonary capillary wedge pressures and left ventricular inflow tract pressures as well as cardiac output. These data can be used in the formula of Gorlin and Gorlin to calculate the MVA. The angiographic findings at left ventriculography in patients with rheumatic mitral stenosis include calcified, hypokinetic, and domed mitral valve leaflets (Figs. 112–21 and 112–22). The left atrium will appear enlarged, and the left ventricle may be small with a slightly reduced ejection fraction (Fig. 112–22). The mitral valve leaflets will appear thickened and nodular and may appear to attach directly to the papillary muscle. There is usually associated scarring and retraction of the chordae tendineae, which may appear to pull the posteromedial papillary muscle toward the base of the heart. Subvalvular scarring may mimic vegetations on the tips of the mitral valve leaflets, and the subvalvular portion of the left ventricle (the posterobasilar segment in the RAO projection) is frequently hypokinetic owing to this scarring (Fig. 112–22*A*).

Mitral Regurgitation

Mitral regurgitation can develop as a result of previous rheumatic heart disease; mitral valve prolapse ("floppy mitral valve"); or damage or degeneration of any portion of the mitral apparatus: the annulus, the chordae tendineae, or the papillary muscles. Etiologies

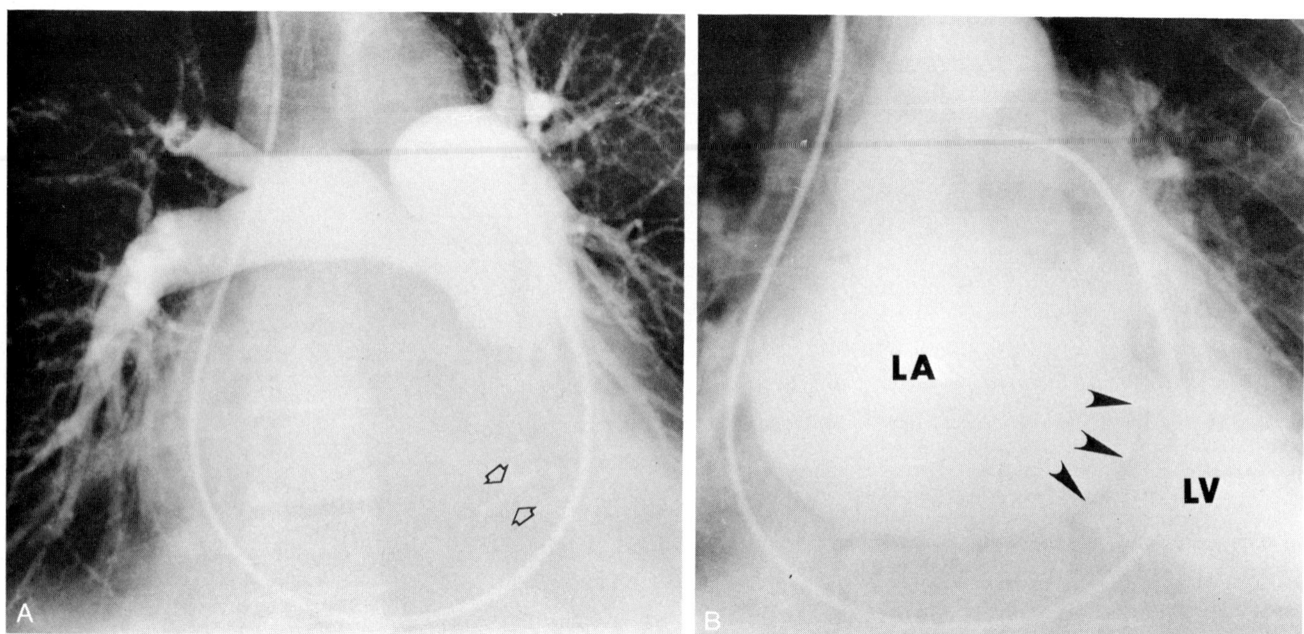

Figure 112–21. Mitral stenosis. *A,* Pulmonary angiogram, AP view, and *(B)* levo phase of pulmonary angiogram, AP view. Note the dilated central pulmonary arteries in the pulmonary arterial phase of the study. Calcification is noted in the mitral valve *(arrows)*. On the levo phase portion of the angiogram, note the dilated left atrium (LA) and the thickened and domed mitral valve *(arrowheads)*. Note also the relatively small left ventricle (LV).

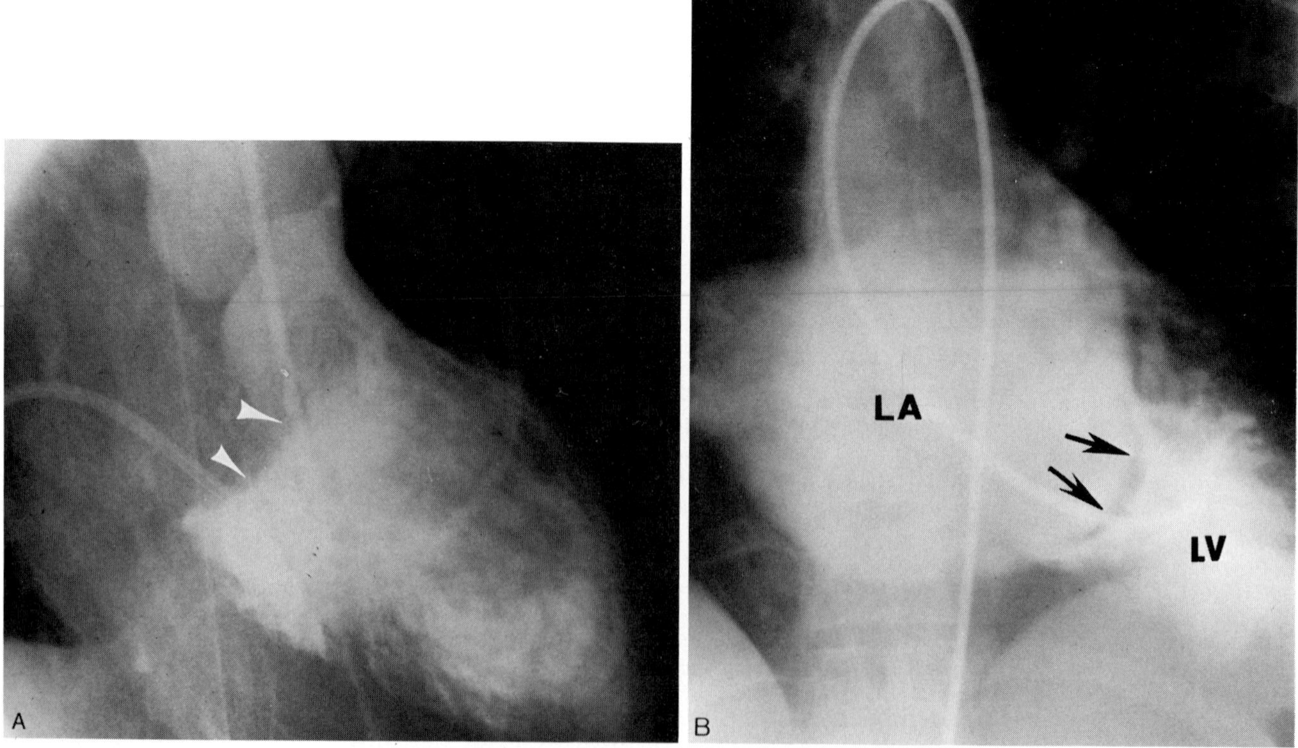

Figure 112–22. Mitral stenosis. *A,* RAO cine left ventriculogram and *(B)* PA cine left ventriculogram in a second patient. In the RAO projection filmed in systole, note the domed mitral valve *(arrowheads)*. The ventricle is normal in size, and there is no evidence of mitral regurgitation. In the PA projection, note the thickened domed mitral valve *(arrows)* and the large left atrium (LA) and small left ventricle (LV). There is significant (3+/4+) mitral regurgitation.

in the latter category include infection, ischemia, and trauma. The pathophysiologic changes that occur with mitral regurgitation are initiated by the backward flow of blood from the left ventricle into the left atrium during left ventricular systole. The increased volume of blood that is under elevated pressure causes the left atrium to dilate to a greater extent in mitral regurgitation than it does in mitral stenosis. The dilatation of the left atrium is a compensatory mechanism that protects the pulmonary capillary bed from postcapillary hypertension. Patients with mitral regurgitation typically will have more left atrial dilatation and less pulmonary venous hypertension than patients with mitral stenosis. In mitral regurgitation, the left ventricular diastolic volume increases markedly with little increase in left ventricular diastolic pressure until myocardial failure develops.

In acute mitral regurgitation from rupture of a papillary muscle or chordae tendineae, the volume of the regurgitation may be so large that the left atrium and left ventricle essentially become one chamber. As a result, left ventricular pressures are reflected directly back into the pulmonary vascular bed. The acute pulmonary venous hypertension that develops may produce intractable pulmonary edema and create an emergent surgical situation.

RADIOGRAPHIC FINDINGS

The chest radiograph in patients with long-standing mitral regurgitation typically shows mild pulmonary venous hypertension and left atrial and left ventricular enlargement (Fig. 112–23). The left ventricular enlargement is generally significant enough to produce moderate to marked cardiomegaly (cardiothoracic ratio $>$ 0.55). In acute mitral regurgitation due to injury to the chordae tendineae or papillary muscles, the left atrium and left ventricle may appear

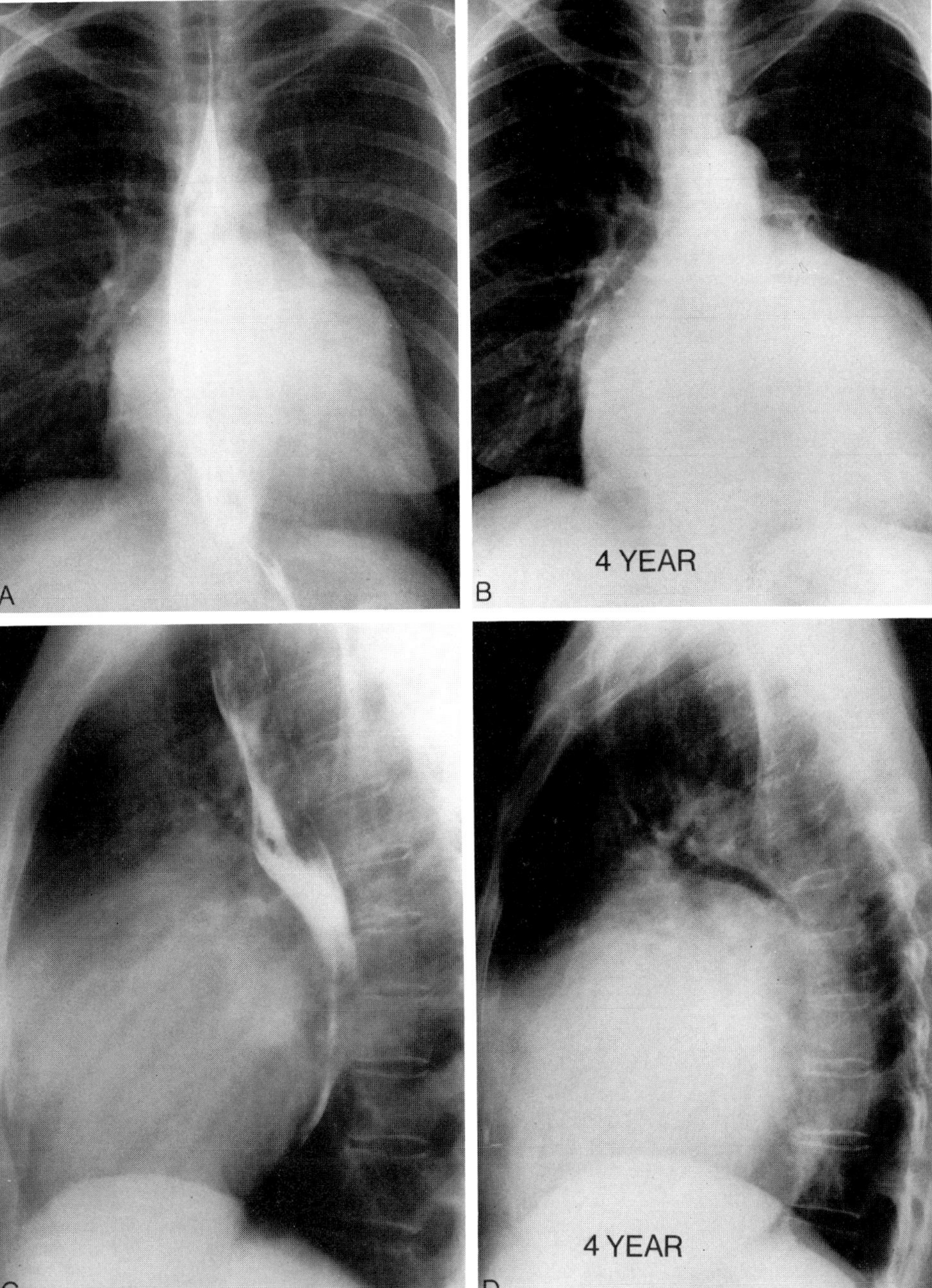

Figure 112–23. Mitral regurgitation. *A* and *B*, PA and *(C* and *D)* lateral chest radiographs in a patient with rheumatic mitral regurgitation. Initial PA and lateral films show normal pulmonary vascularity and cardiomegaly with significant left atrial enlargement. This progresses to massive left atrial enlargement on the four-year follow-up films. Note that the pulmonary vascularity remains normal during this interim.

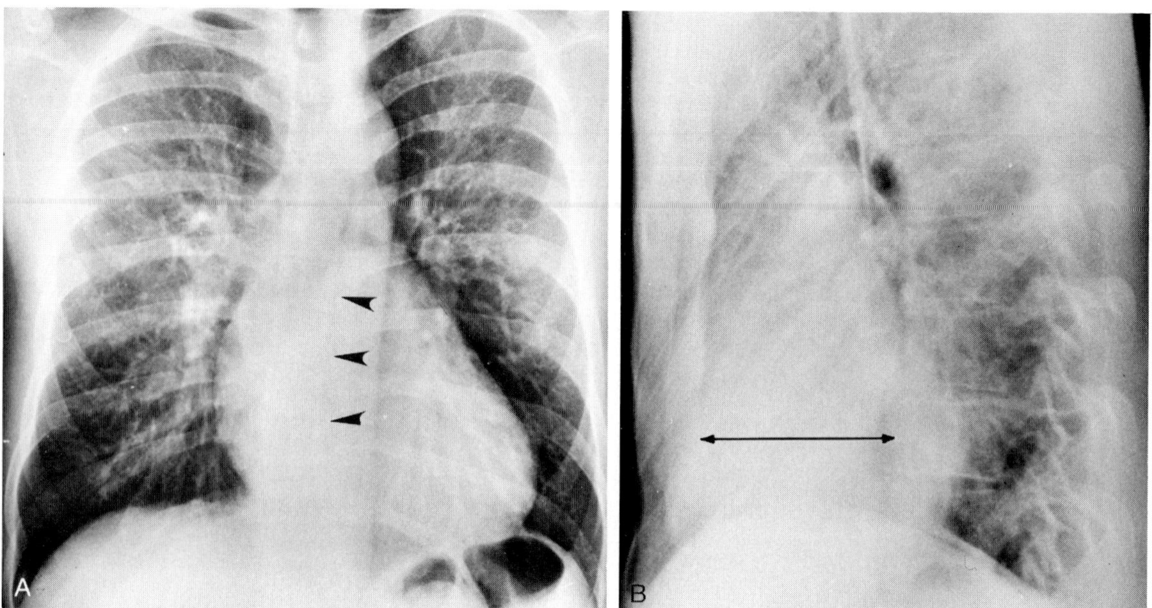

Figure 112–24. Mitral valve prolapse. PA *(A)* and lateral *(B)* chest radiographs demonstrating essentially normal PA film with the exception of mild dextroscoliosis of the thoracic spine *(arrowheads).* On the lateral view, note the marked narrowing of the AP dimension *(double arrow)* and the relatively straight thoracic spine. These skeletal abnormalities are very common in patients with mitral valve prolapse.

normal in size while the lung fields show signs of pulmonary edema. The left atrial appendage will usually be enlarged in patients with a history of previous rheumatic heart disease (Fig. 112–23). In a patient with mitral valve prolapse, the left atrium will not be enlarged, but a large percentage of these patients will have associated skeletal abnormalities such as scoliosis or straightening of the thoracic spine, narrow anteroposterior chest dimension, or pectus excavatum deformity of the sternum (Fig. 112–24). Marfan's syndrome may be associated with mitral regurgitation from mitral valve prolapse. The skeletal features of Marfan's syndrome, including thoracic cage deformities, may also be present on the chest radiograph. Elderly patients with calcification of the mitral annulus may have associated mild mitral regurgitation. The typical C-shaped annular calcification may be appreciated on the lateral chest film (Fig. 112–25).

In patients with an enlarged atrial appendage and suspected history of rheumatic heart disease, mitral regurgitation is most likely the dominant mitral valve lesion when there are marked left atrial and left ventricular enlargement and only mild changes of postcapillary pulmonary hypertension. Patients with congestive (dilated) and hypertrophic obstructive cardiomyopathies often have associated mild mitral regurgitation (see Chapter 114).

ECHOCARDIOGRAPHIC FINDINGS

M-mode, two-dimensional, and Doppler echocardiographic techniques can be used to evaluate mitral regurgitation. The nonspecific findings include left atrial enlargement and left ventricular enlargement. In nonrheumatic mitral regurgitation, the excursion and closing velocity (E-F slope) of the mitral valve are frequently increased.

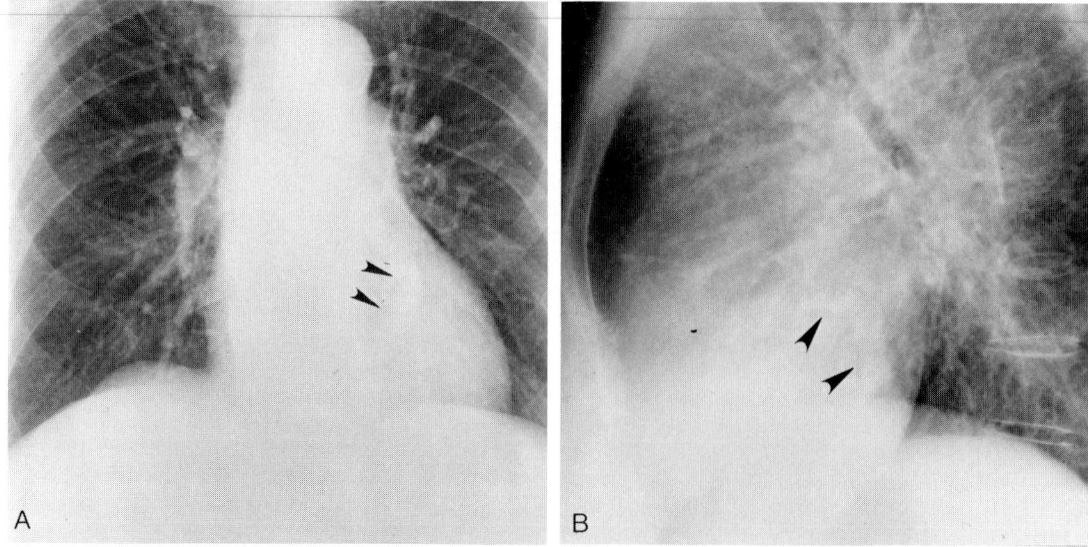

Figure 112–25. Mitral annular calcification. PA *(A)* and lateral *(B)* chest radiographs in an elderly patient demonstrating curvilinear calcification in the typical location of the mitral annulus *(arrowheads).*

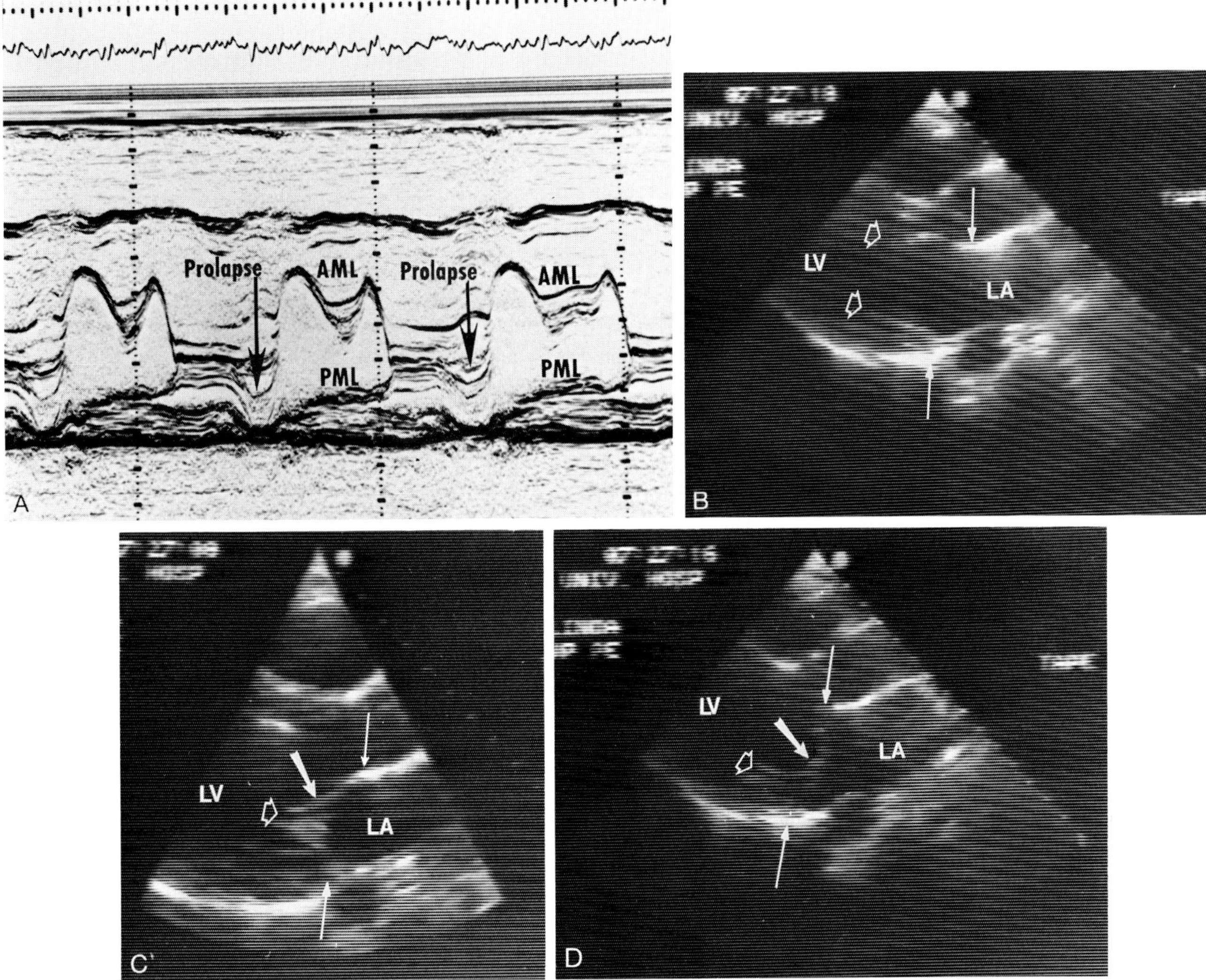

Figure 112–26. Mitral valve prolapse. *A,* M-mode echocardiographic cut through the tips of the mitral valve leaflets in a patient with mitral valve prolapse. There are multiple linear echoes on the anterior mitral leaflet (AML) and posterior mitral leaflet (PML). Note the posterior systolic motion of the mitral valve leaflets *(arrows)*, which is diagnostic of mitral valve prolapse. *B,* Echocardiographic long-axis view in **diastole** of a patient with mitral valve prolapse demonstrating the left ventricle (LV) and the left atrium (LA). The anterior and posterior mitral valve leaflets are marked by *small arrows. C,* Echocardiographic long-axis view in **early systole**. The *small arrows* again point out the base of the anterior and posterior mitral valve leaflets. The *open arrow* demonstrates the tips of the anterior and posterior mitral valve leaflets. The *larger solid arrow* demonstrates the mid-portion of the anterior mitral valve leaflet. *D,* Echocardiographic long-axis view in **late systole**. The *small arrows* again depict the base of the anterior and posterior mitral valve leaflets. The *open arrow* is located at the tips of the anterior and posterior mitral valve leaflets. The *larger solid arrow* demonstrates the significant late systole caudal motion of the anterior mitral valve leaflet in this patient with mitral valve prolapse.

Certain specific causes of mitral regurgitation such as mitral valve prolapse, flail leaflet, or bacterial endocarditis with valve vegetations may be delineated on M-mode and two-dimensional echocardiographic examinations (Fig. 112–26). The degree of compensation of the left ventricle can also be assessed by noting the velocity of shortening of the posterior wall, extent of shortening, and ejection fraction.

Doppler echocardiographic techniques are being used to quantitate the amount of regurgitant flow and to evaluate the regurgitant fraction present in patients with mitral regurgitation as well as in those with aortic regurgitation (Fig. 112–27). The use of Doppler techniques should increase the ability of physicians to quantitate and follow these patients in the future.

ANGIOCARDIOGRAPHIC FINDINGS

The examination of the mitral valve for regurgitation is usually accomplished by obtaining a left ventriculogram in the 30 to 40 degree RAO position. The purpose of the left ventriculography in this case is to grade the severity of the disease and to make a specific diagnosis if possible (Figs. 112–28 and 112–29). The filming of the patient should include both the left atrium and the left ventricle. The following scheme is often used to subjectively grade the degree of mitral regurgitation:

Grade 1: A small amount of contrast passes into the left ventricle, but the posterior wall of the left atrium is not opacified.

Grade 2: There is faint opacification of the entire left atrium, and the contrast clears from the atrium in one or two beats.

Grade 3: There is complete opacification of the left atrium, but the degree of opacification is less than the contrast passing into the aorta. The left atrium and the left ventricle are enlarged. The contrast that fills the left atrium clears in two or three beats after the injection.

Grade 4: There is opacification of the pulmonary veins, with the left atrium as densely opacified as the left ventricle. There is enlargement of the left atrium and left ventricle. The blood that is

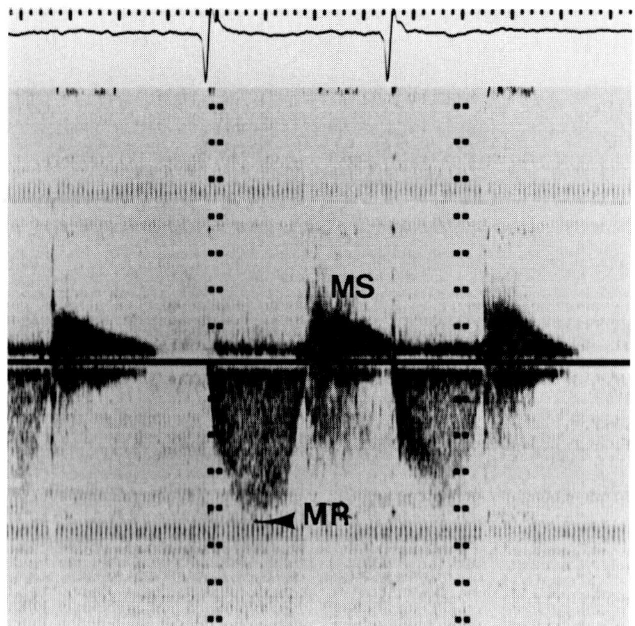

Figure 112–27. Mitral stenosis and regurgitation. Continuous-wave Doppler imaging of the mitral valve in this patient with mitral stenosis (MS) demonstrates a high-velocity mitral regurgitation jet (MR—*arrowhead*).

ejected from the left ventricle appears to go as much into the left atrium as into the aorta.

As with any such visual analysis, there are problems with this subjective assessment of mitral regurgitation. In acute mitral regurgitation, there may not be any enlargement of the left atrium or left ventricle. The smaller volume of these chambers in this situation requires less contrast to densely opacify the left atrium. In long-standing disease, the left atrium and left ventricle may be markedly enlarged, and the amount of contrast material injected must be increased to compensate for the larger chambers involved (Fig. 112–28). The amount of contrast needed is often not known exactly prior to the examination. The amount of mitral regurgitation seen at the time of left ventriculography is also affected by left ventricular afterload, arrhythmias, and the length of diastole. The amount of mitral regurgitation may be underestimated in the presence of an atrial septal defect, because of the washout into the right atrium. The regurgitant lesion is best evaluated by calculating the regurgitant fraction from the angiographic and hemodynamic cardiac outputs. The last technique is not valid if aortic regurgitation or depressed left ventricular wall motion is present.

In most cases of mitral regurgitation the regurgitant stream is quite wide unless there is eccentric fusing of the mitral commissures, in which case the regurgitant stream may be eccentric and narrow. The amount of left atrial and left ventricular dilatation present will depend on the duration and severity of the mitral valve disease. In rheumatic valvulitis, there is scarring, calcification, thickening, and contracture of the valve elements. The valve may appear similar to the stenotic mitral valve. Bacterial endocarditis that involves a nonrheumatic valve and produces mitral regurgitation may be indistinguishable from endocarditis that involves a rheumatic mitral valve unless vegetations can be seen arising from the valve leaflets themselves.

In mitral prolapse, the underlying derangement of the valve that allows regurgitation to occur is elongation of the cusps and chordae that leads to redundant and exuberant valve tissue. The resultant "floppy" valve shows multiple scallops on the posterior leaflet with elongation of the chordae and expansion of the area of the leaflets to allow parts of the mitral valve to enter the left atrium (Fig. 112–29). This will produce mitral regurgitation if the abnormality is severe enough. When pathologic and angiographic studies are compared, the incidence of mitral valve prolapse in the general population is about 5 per cent. The diagnosis of mitral valve prolapse can be made when the amount of the mitral valve leaflets passing posterior to the plane of the mitral annulus exceeds 2 mm. Mild mitral regurgitation is often associated with mitral annular calcification (Fig. 112–30). Mitral valve prolapse may coexist with annular calcification (Fig. 112–30).

Mitral regurgitation can result from rupture of the chordae in patients with rheumatic heart disease, ischemic heart disease, or bacterial endocarditis. The chordae arising from the posteromedial papillary muscle are most often involved, and more than half of the ventriculograms show prolapse of the leaflets ("flail" mitral valve), more commonly the posterior leaflet (Fig. 112–31). Rupture of the head of a papillary muscle may occur from acute myocardial infarction, chest trauma, or endocarditis. The posteromedial papillary muscle is most often involved because it receives poorer collateral circulation than does the anterolateral muscle. The left ventriculogram may show segmental wall motion abnormalities adjacent to

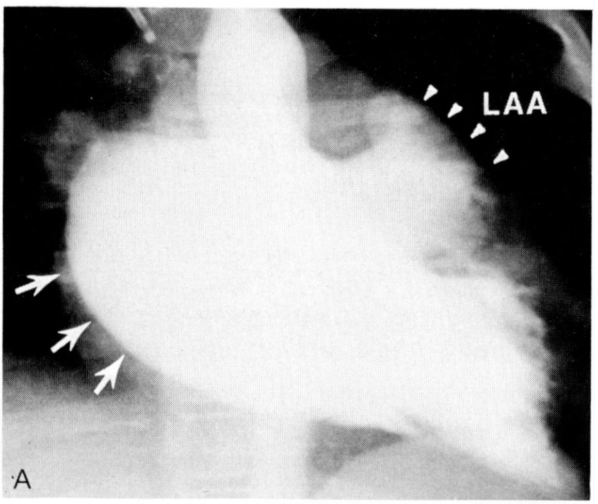

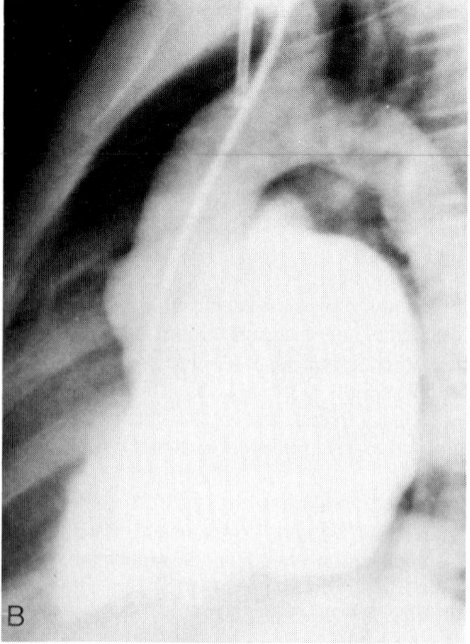

Figure 112–28. Mitral regurgitation. *A,* PA and *(B)* lateral left ventriculograms in a patient with rheumatic mitral regurgitation. In *A,* there is 4+/4+ regurgitation into an enlarged left atrium *(arrows).* Note the regurgitation into the left atrial appendage (LAA—*arrowheads),* which is also dilated.

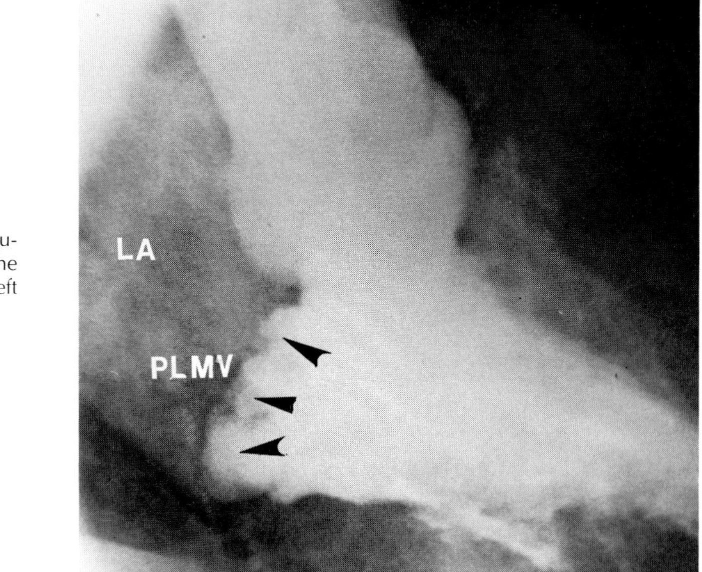

Figure 112–29. Mitral valve prolapse. Forty-degree RAO left ventriculogram demonstrates marked redundancy of the posterior leaflet of the mitral valve (PLMV—*arrowheads),* which is protruding into the left atrium (LA). There is a small amount of mitral regurgitation present.

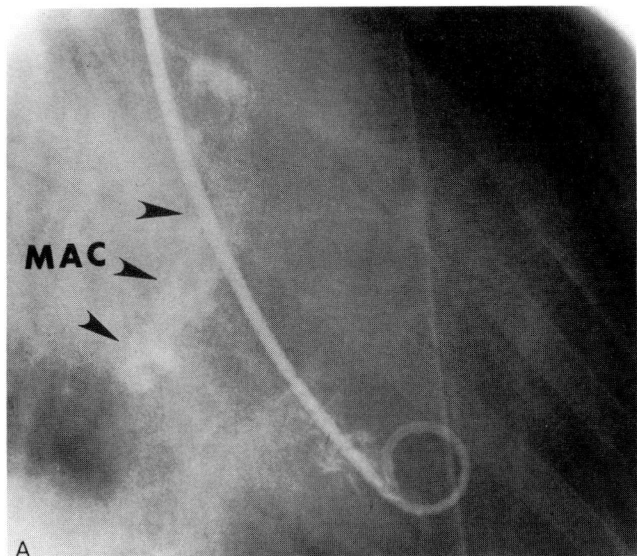

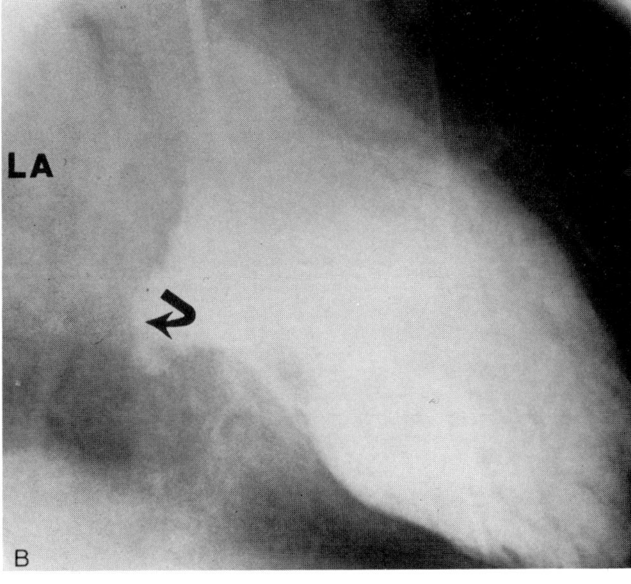

Figure 112–30. Mitral annular calcification. *A,* Cine fluorographic imaging of a 40-degree RAO projection and *(B)* left ventriculogram in 40-degree RAO projection. Prior to appearance of contrast material, note the heavy calcification in the mitral anulus (MAC—*arrowheads).* After contrast administration, note mild prolapse of the posterior leaflet of the mitral valve *(arrow)* and a small amount of mitral regurgitation into the left atrium (LA).

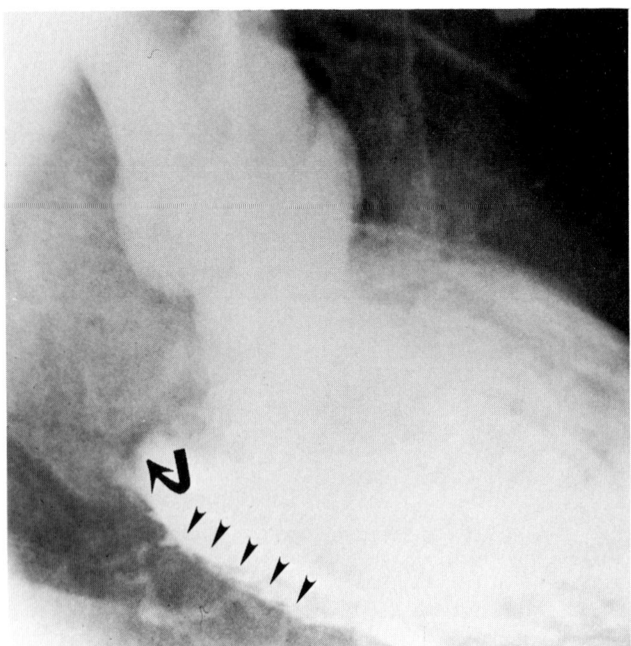

Figure 112–31. Papillary muscle dysfunction. Forty-degree RAO left ventriculogram in systole demonstrates mild prolapse of the posterior leaflet of the mitral valve *(curved arrow).* Segmental wall motion abnormality was noted with posterior basilar wall akinesis *(arrowheads).* There is a small amount of mitral regurgitation into the left atrium. This patient had a previous occlusion of the right coronary artery and an inferior wall myocardial infarction.

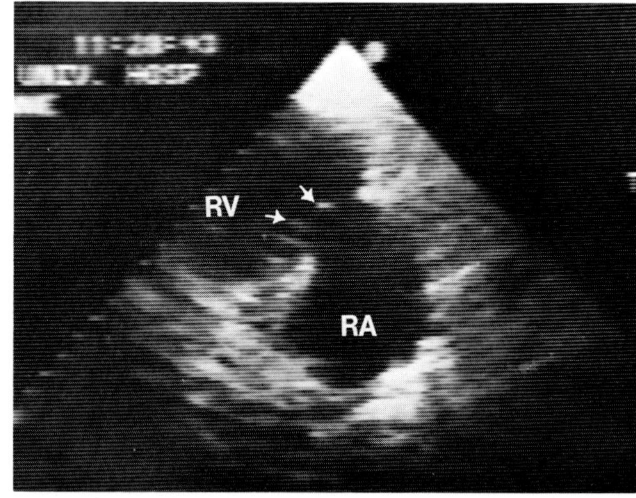

Figure 112–32. Tricuspid valve stenosis. Echocardiographic right ventricular inflow view demonstrating the right atrium (RA) and the right ventricle (RV) in diastole in a patient with severe rheumatic heart disease and rheumatic tricuspid stenosis. Note the severe limitation of tricuspid leaflet excursion *(arrows).*

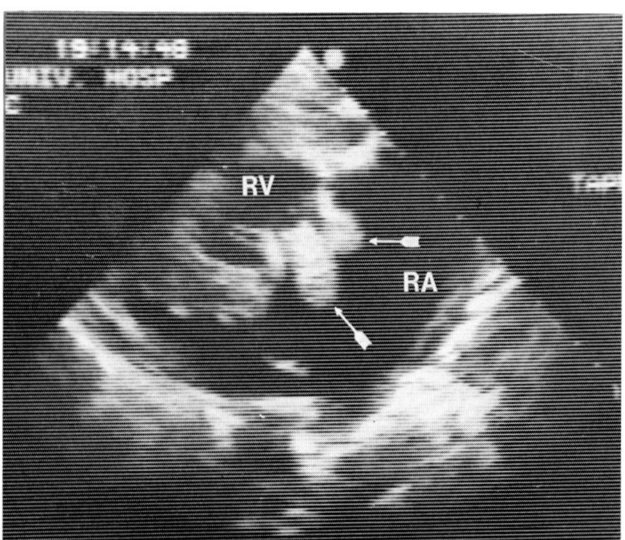

Figure 112–33. Tricuspid valve endocarditis. Echocardiographic RV inflow view in a young drug abuser with infective endocarditis and severe tricuspid regurgitation. Note the right atrium (RA) and right ventricle (RV) and two large tricuspid valve vegetations prolapsing into the right atrium in systole.

the injured papillary muscle, prolapse of valve leaflets, or flail leaflets (Fig. 112–31). Both valve leaflets are affected in rupture of a papillary muscle, since there are chordae that attach both anterior and posterior leaflets to each papillary muscle.

TRICUSPID VALVE

Rheumatic heart disease, bacterial endocarditis, and prolapse can affect the tricuspid valve much as they do the mitral valve. Acquired tricuspid valve disease is usually secondary to rheumatic heart disease, although carcinoid syndrome and external masses have also been implicated. The hallmarks of tricuspid stenosis are enlargement of the right atrium and thickening of the tricuspid valve leaflets (Fig. 112–32). Doming of the leaflets may be seen on echocardiograms and angiocardiograms if the lesion is severe. If tricuspid regurgitation is present, the right ventricle will be enlarged as well (see Fig. 112–16*A*). About 50 per cent of patients with mitral valve prolapse will also have tricuspid valve prolapse. Echocardiography and Doppler echocardiography can identify the etiology and assess the severity of tricuspid regurgitation (Fig. 112–33).

The valve is best evaluated on angiocardiograms in the 30-degree RAO projection. The angiocardiographic scheme for assessing the degree of tricuspid regurgitation is as follows:

Grade 1: Small regurgitant jet projecting back into the right atrium during systole

Grade 2: Persistent opacification of the right atrium by the regurgitant jet

Grade 3: Dense opacification of the entire right atrium by the regurgitant jet from the right ventricle

Grade 4: Dense opacification of the right atrium and both the superior and inferior venae cavae

Bibliography

Ascah KJ, Stewart WJ, Levine RA, Weyman AE: Doppler-echocardiographic assessment of cardiac output. Radiol Clin North Am 23:659–670, 1985.

Green CE, Kelley MJ, Higgins CB: Etiologic significance of enlargement of the left atrial appendage in adults. Radiology 142:21–27, 1982.

Higgins CB, Reinke RT, Jones NE, et al: Left atrial dimensions on the frontal thoracic radiograph: A method of assessing left atrial enlargement. AJR 130:251, 1978.

Kelley MJ, Elliott LP, Shulman ST, et al: The significance of the left atrial appendage in rheumatic heart disease. Circulation 54:146, 1976.

Lachman AS, Roberts WC: Calcific deposits in stenotic mitral valves: Extent and relation to age, sex, degree of stenosis, cardiac rhythm, previous commissurotomy and left atrial body thrombus from study of 164 operatively excised valves. Circulation 57:808, 1978.

Miller SW: Cardiac Angiography. Boston, Little, Brown, 1984.

Newell JD, Higgins CB, Kelley MJ: Radiographic-echocardiographic approach to acquired heart disease: Diagnosis and assessment of severity. Radiol Clin North Am 18:387–409, 1980.

Schwartz A, Vienola PA, Walker HJ, et al: Echocardiographic estimation of aortic-valve gradient in aortic stenosis. Ann Intern Med 89:329, 1978.

Sherrid MV, Clark RD, Cohn K: Echocardiographic analysis of left atrial size before and after operation in mitral valve disease. Am J Cardiol 43:171, 1979.

Stamm RB, Martin RP: Quantification of pressure gradients across stenotic valves by Doppler ultrasound. J Am Coll Cardiol 2:707–718, 1983.

Warth DC, Stewart WJ, Block PC, Weyman AE: A new method to calculate aortic valve area without left heart catheterization. Circulation 70:978–983, 1984.

113 Coronary Artery Disease

RADIOGRAPHIC EVALUATION

CURTIS E. GREEN and LOWELL F. SATLER

EVALUATION OF THE PATIENT WITHOUT TYPICAL ANGINA

Identification of the asymptomatic patient with significant coronary artery disease (CAD) and evaluation of the patient with atypical chest pain remain difficult tasks. None of the simple, noninvasive tests for CAD is sufficiently accurate to reliably exclude its presence, and the more sophisticated tests are either too expensive or impractical for routine screening. Furthermore, the predictive value of the noninvasive tests is a function of the prevalence of the disease in the population being investigated, which in these instances is fairly low. One must therefore carefully select patients for screening procedures based on the likelihood of their having disease as predicted by risk factor analysis.

Chest Radiography

Although not a sensitive test for CAD, chest radiography can be quite useful when certain findings are present. No other test except right heart catheterization is capable of evaluating the pulmonary vasculature for the presence of pulmonary venous hypertension (PVH) that can result from left ventricular failure (LVF). In some patients, this may be the very first clue as to the presence of ischemic heart disease. Occasionally calcium can be identified in the coronary arteries (Fig. 113–1*A*) and if present suggests significant CAD, as will be discussed later. Absence of calcium on a chest radiograph has no significance, since chest radiography is very insensitive to its presence. Calcium in the myocardium is almost pathognomonic for previous myocardial infarction. This may be either amorphous or curvilinear and does not necessarily indicate the presence of either an aneurysm or a thrombus (Fig. 113–1*B*). Left ventricular aneurysms are most frequently caused by myocardial infarction and can be diagnosed when there is an abnormal bulge along the cardiac border; however, they may present without any radiographic findings. The combination of curvilinear calcium and a bulge along the heart border is unlikely to be caused by anything but an aneurysm.

Cardiac Fluoroscopy

Fluoroscopic examination of the heart is an infrequently used but potentially valuable tool for the detection of occult CAD. Part of

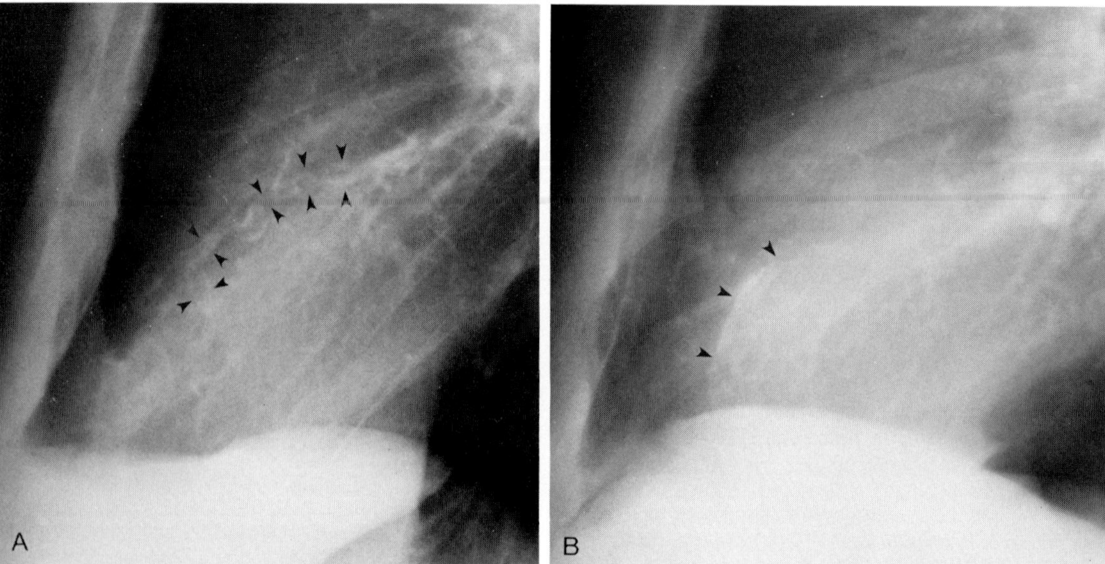

Figure 113–1. Cardiac calcification. *A,* Coronary artery calcification *(arrowheads). B,* Calcified myocardium in a left ventricular aneurysm *(arrowheads).*

the reason that it has fallen into disuse is the misconception that it is helpful for evaluation of cardiac pulsations, something for which it is poorly suited. Fluoroscopy is an excellent way to look for coronary and other cardiac calcium deposits. Coronary artery calcium is strongly correlated with the presence of CAD, especially in patients younger than 55 years of age. Studies have shown this to be true in both hyperlipidemic and normolipemic subjects. The combination of fluoroscopically detectable coronary calcium and a positive exercise test indicates a greater than 80 per cent likelihood of significant CAD.

Coronary Angiography

The point at which one should proceed to coronary angiography in the evaluation of the patient with atypical chest pain depends on the personal philosophy of the attending physician and the necessity for absolute certainty in knowing whether or not CAD is present. In most patients, one or more noninvasive tests that are completely normal eliminate the need for angiography. In some patients, however, the need to know outweighs the risk of the procedure and the cost. An example would be a military pilot who cannot fly until completely cleared medically. Unfortunately, in a large number of patients the noninvasive tests are equivocal and the patient proceeds from one to the next without anyone being willing to say that nothing further need be done. At this point, one is left with two options: a trial of medical therapy or coronary angiography.

EVALUATION OF THE PATIENT WITH TYPICAL ANGINA PECTORIS

There remains a great deal of controversy concerning the relative roles of coronary angiography and the noninvasive tests in patients with typical angina. Part of this is due to a failure to appreciate that coronary angiography and the noninvasive studies do not evaluate the same thing. Angiography looks at coronary artery morphology; radionuclide studies and exercise echocardiography evaluate function and/or physiology. As will be discussed further in this chapter, functional or physiologic tests serve two very important purposes: assessment of the likelihood of CAD and assessment of the functional significance of known CAD. In the patient with typical angina pectoris who is not a candidate for medical therapy or in whom such therapy has already failed, one can make a strong argument for performing coronary angiography before any functional tests. On the other hand, when one is not certain whether chest pain is really angina or when medical therapy is the first choice for treatment, noninvasive evaluation of function is entirely appropriate and can guide therapy as well as indicate the need for angiography.

Chest Radiography

The chest radiograph serves much the same purpose in patients with typical angina as in those in whom the diagnosis is less clear. Again, the most important function is evaluation of the pulmonary vasculature to detect mild degrees of LVF that may be clinically inapparent. Assessment of heart size is both less reliable and less important in this regard than is detection of PVH. It is crucial to look for calcium in the myocardium or aortic valve, as these suggest a specific etiology for chest pain.

Cardiac Fluoroscopy

Although more sensitive and specific than the chest radiograph for the identification of cardiac calcification, fluoroscopic examination of the heart is of limited usefulness in the patient with typical angina pectoris since the identification of calcium in the coronary arteries does not substantially increase the probability of significant CAD over that suggested by symptoms. If there is any suspicion of calcific aortic stenosis, however, fluoroscopy should be performed unless an echocardiogram is already ordered or cannot be performed.

Coronary Angiography

Selective coronary cineangiography remains the standard for the definition of coronary anatomy and is unlikely to be replaced in the foreseeable future. There are significant limitations to angiography that must be appreciated if diagnostic accuracy is to be maximized. All efforts should be made to eliminate as many sources of error as possible. These include strict quality control of processing and x-ray equipment, use of angled views, and tailoring of radiographic technique to match the anatomy and view. If any part of the system breaks down, the results of the study may be misleading.

At this point, it should be mentioned that *selective* views must be obtained. Intravenous digital subtraction angiography has been thoroughly discredited. Selective digital subtraction angiography has also not proved to be very useful with the coronary arteries because of masking problems due to cardiac motion. Unresolved is the question of whether selective digital coronary angiography without subtraction will be as good as cine. At the present time, there remain significant problems with permanent image storage and television resolution. However, digital replay is extremely valuable in the laboratory as a tool for instant replay, and digital processing can be useful for on-line quantitation of coronary stenoses when evaluating for possible angioplasty.

FACTORS AFFECTING THE ACCURACY OF CORONARY ANGIOGRAMS

Like all angiographic techniques, coronary angiography produces a "luminogram"—that is, it does not visualize the wall of the vessel, only its lumen. Because of this, even good-quality angiograms may underestimate the amount of narrowing since coronary atherosclerosis is a diffuse process with localized exacerbations. As a result, what appear to be discrete stenoses may in fact represent more narrowing than is evident (Fig. 113–2). If the vessel is underfilled because of inadequate injection of contrast material or poor flow across a high-grade stenosis, this problem can be accentuated resulting in underestimation of narrowing and distal vessel size.

A second major problem is the relative tortuosity of the coronary arteries and the propensity for vessels to overlap. Because of the eccentricity of many coronary stenoses, one would ideally like to visualize each major segment from at least two directions, but vessels are frequently obscured, foreshortened, or both, making this goal unattainable. As a result, almost every angiogram is a compromise between taking too many views and risking missing a stenosis.

MEASUREMENT OF CORONARY ARTERY STENOSES

Grading of the severity of coronary arterial narrowing is about as much art as science. The process is made substantially easier and more accurate by quality angiography, but all of the problems discussed above become quite apparent when it comes time to interpret the pictures.

The time-honored method for assessing the severity of a stenosis in a coronary artery is to measure the percentage luminal diameter narrowing (Fig. 113–2). This is subject to several significant limitations but is clearly the most time-efficient method and in many cases suffices for clinical work. When one uses this technique, two assumptions are made: the edge of the vessel can be accurately determined and the normal luminal size is known. As it turns out, the human eye is a pretty good discriminator of vessel edges on good-quality angiograms but is not so good at transposing the diameter of the narrowed segment onto that of the "normal" segment. This leads to the common phenomenon of overestimation of coronary stenoses by the visual technique. This particular problem can for the most part be avoided by using some type of caliper, either EKG or electronic, to compare the two segments. For clinical use, where it does not matter whether a stenosis is 60 per cent or 70 per cent, the former works quite nicely. Determining the diameter of the reference (normal) segment is a bit more difficult and fraught with the potential for error. For starters, there is almost never a segment that is completely free of atherosclerotic narrowing, so we almost always end up comparing the stenosis to an area that is itself narrow. This results in underestimation of the true degree of stenosis. Secondly, the reference segment may be ectatic, resulting in overestimation of narrowing. In addition, changes in coronary tone will cause greater constriction of normal segments than of diseased ones, also resulting in underestimation.

Another decision that the interpreter must make is whether to measure a stenosis in the view where it looks the worst or to average two views. The first assumes that the lesion is relatively symmetrical (rarely true) and the second that it is seen equally well in both views. Some observers have taken to calculating luminal cross-sectional area in an attempt to overcome the asymmetry issue, but this requires assumption of some geometric model for the stenosis in addition to its being seen in both views. Few angiographers have found percentage area narrowing to be a useful concept, but pathologists routinely use it since they can directly measure area by sectioning the vessel.

In clinical work, it is rarely important to determine the exact degree of narrowing and for the most part it suffices to give a range of narrowing for each stenosis, for example, 25 to 50 per cent or 75 to 90 per cent, or to use the nearest 10 per cent. This uncertainty is not usually due to inability to determine where the vessel edge is located, but because we cannot be confident of the size of the normal vessel. When coronary narrowing is so obviously diffuse as to preclude the possibility of any normal reference segment, one can only describe the vessel as severely or mildly diffusely diseased using the overall size of the vessel to estimate which of these is the case (Fig. 113–3).

In recent years, evaluation of coronary interventions has given rise to a need for more accurate determination of lumen size and for the ability to detect small changes in vessel size over time. Quantitative coronary angiography (QCA) seeks to provide a means of doing so. QCA uses computed analysis of digitized coronary angiograms to compare the size of the lumen in the region of a stenosis with both a reference segment and a standard, usually a coronary catheter. Under optimal circumstances, lumen size can be determined to a fraction of a millimeter with good reproducibility. One must keep in mind, however, that the computer does not know normal vessel caliber in more than the human observer. Furthermore, poor cine quality, failure to maximally dilate the coronary arteries, poor calibration of catheters, and poor choice of cine frame for analysis can make the data highly suspect. Nevertheless, QCA is an important tool for the analysis of the results of the new techniques in angioplasty and thrombolysis and is far superior to the anecdotal reports that fill the literature.

ANGIOGRAPHIC MANIFESTATIONS OF CORONARY ARTERY DISEASE

Discrete Stenosis. The most commonly seen pattern of coronary artery narrowing is that of one or more discrete stenoses

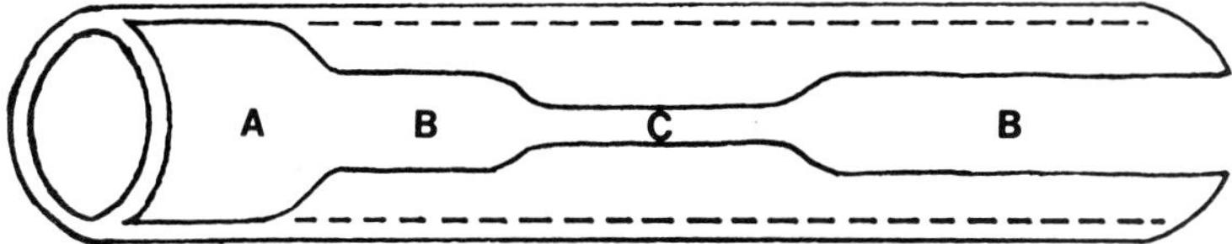

Figure 113–2. Schematic representation of a segment of coronary artery with luminal narrowing of two degrees of severity. If the section labeled A represents the normal vessel caliber, then B has a 50 per cent reduction in luminal diameter, and C is narrowed 75 per cent. If, however, one assumes B to be normal, then C is narrowed only 50 per cent.

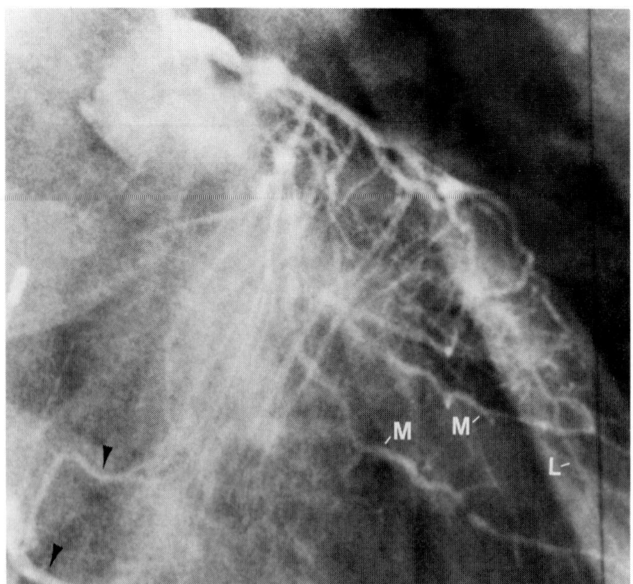

Figure 113–3. Severe, diffuse coronary artery narrowing is present in virtually every branch of the coronary artery. There is also collateral filling of the distal right coronary artery (RCA) branches *(arrowheads).*

(Fig. 113–4). As mentioned above, these are discrete only in a relative sense, since there is usually generalized coronary narrowing. Patients with discrete narrowing of the coronary arteries can be divided into groups based on the number of major vessels with significant narrowing—that is, single-vessel, double-vessel, or triple-vessel disease. Left main coronary artery stenosis is put in a separate category because of its prognostic significance. This division into one-, two-, and three-vessel disease is somewhat arbitrary, since it does not take into account the variability in the amount of myocardium distal to a stenosis. Also, there is not universal agreement as to what constitutes a significant stenosis. Some angiographers consider any stenosis of 50 per cent or greater to be significant, whereas others require 70 per cent narrowing. Animal studies support the notion that a 50 per cent stenosis can be significant under conditions of increased coronary flow.

Discrete stenoses may be either isolated or sequential. The former is more likely when the angina is recent in onset. Patients with a long history of angina are far more likely to have either multiple focal stenoses or diffuse narrowing. Stenoses are most frequently found in the proximal portions of vessels or near bifurcations.

Complete occlusion of one or more coronary arteries can be present in the absence of myocardial infarction owing to the presence of collaterals (Fig. 113–5). Although in some patients collaterals are available virtually immediately, they are more likely to be present when there has been chronic, high-grade stenosis of the artery. Collateral flow and antegrade flow frequently coexist, in which case the distal vessel may not fill completely because of "competitive flow" (Fig. 113–6). One must be very circumspect about calling stenoses in vessels filled from more than one source. In rare instances, even the left main coronary artery can completely occlude without causing infarction, although this is usually accompanied by the patient's demise.

DIFFUSE NARROWING. Diffuse narrowing of a coronary artery is more difficult to recognize and evaluate than is discrete narrowing. Unless the degree of luminal narrowing is quite pronounced, it is likely to be overlooked (see Fig. 113–3). When evaluating diffuse narrowing, one tends to judge a vessel by the size of nearby vessels, which should be similar in size. This is a matter of judgment and is fraught with the potential for error. It is important to note the size of a vessel distal to a discrete stenosis and whether it appears to be diffusely diseased. This may affect the advisability of surgical revascularization, since the surgeon may have a very difficult time anastomosing a vein graft to a small and/or badly diseased coronary artery. One clue to diffuse narrowing is the presence of calcium in the wall of the artery outside the visualized lumen. Unless it is obvious that the calcified segment is markedly ectatic, it is reasonable to use the calcium as the true vessel diameter, since coronary artery calcium is located in the vessel's intima.

Coronary ectasia is a manifestation of CAD that may be clinically important in some patients. It is not uncommon to see mild degrees of coronary artery dilatation in patients with coronary stenoses, but some patients will have marked ectasia involving all the coronary arteries (Fig. 113–7). These patients have a prognosis similar to those with triple-vessel disease but are in general not helped by coronary artery bypass. Coronary ectasia complicates the interpretation of the coronary angiogram because it effectively eliminates any normal area to which stenoses can be compared.

Coronary spasm can occur as an isolated entity or in addition to atherosclerotic narrowing (Fig. 113–8). Spasm can also be induced at the tip of the coronary catheter, especially in the right coronary artery. Because spasm can mimic atherosclerotic narrowing, it is a good idea to give intracoronary nitroglycerin to patients with coronary stenoses to eliminate the possibility of spasm.

CORONARY COLLATERALS. Collateral blood supply to completely or partially obstructed coronary arteries is a major determinant of the physiologic result of the obstruction and one of the reasons why the clinical presentation of coronary artery disease is so variable. Collaterals can be either inter- or intracoronary and can develop on the epicardial surface, in the myocardium, or through the ventricular or atrial septa. Collateral blood supply can also, on rare occasions, come from the bronchial or pericardial arteries.

Intracoronary collaterals connect the proximal portion of an occluded vessel to a distal segment in close proximity to it. These can be recognized by their tortuous appearance and course outside that expected for the native vessel (Fig. 113–9). It may be difficult to distinguish between complete occlusion with intracoronary collaterals and high-grade (>90 per cent) stenosis of a vessel.

Intercoronary collaterals (Figs. 113–5 and 113–10 through 113–13) can exist between separate coronary arteries or between

Text continued on page 1811

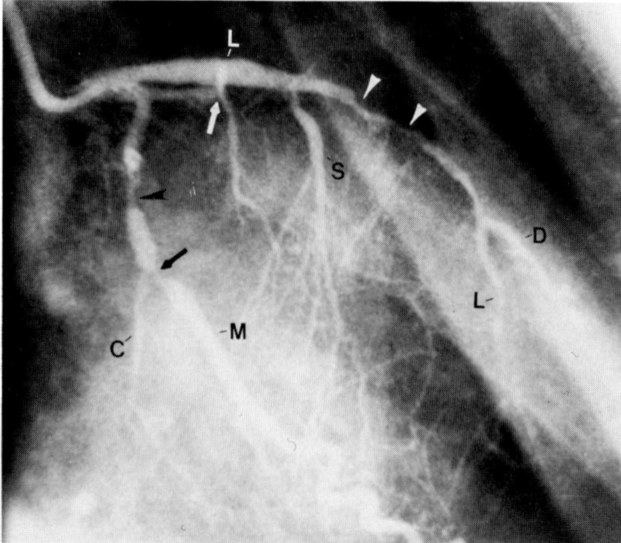

Figure 113–4. RAO view of the left coronary artery (LCA) showing **sequential stenoses** in the circumflex *(black arrowhead)* and second obtuse marginal *(black arrow).* There is also a long stenosis in the LAD *(white arrowheads)* as well as complete occlusion of the first obtuse marginal *(white arrow).* (C = distal circumflex; D = diagonal; L = distal LAD; M = second obtuse marginal; S = septal.)

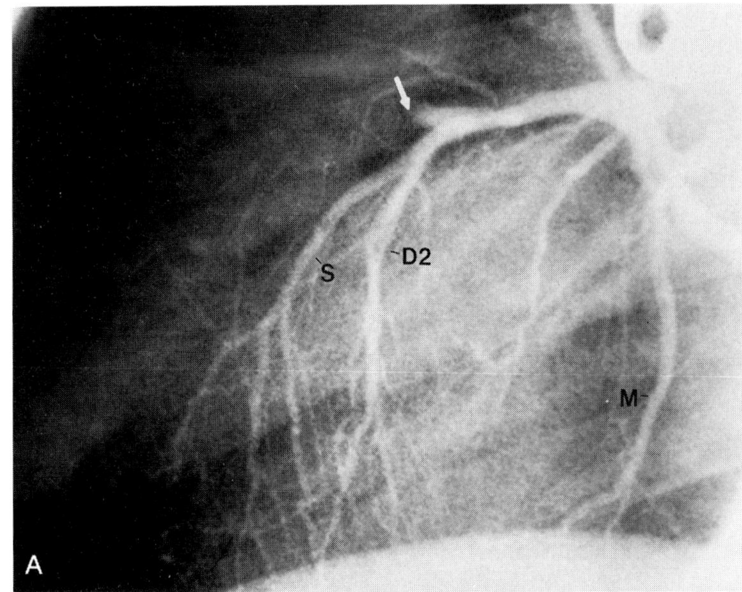

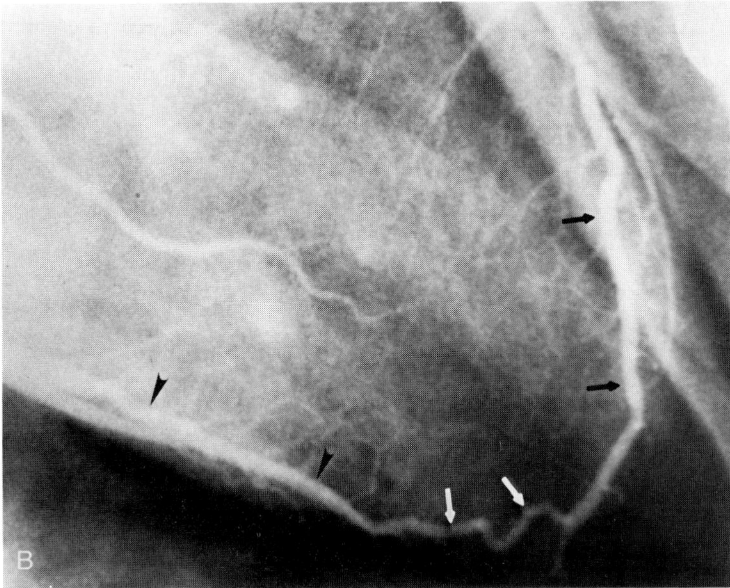

Figure 113–5. *A,* Lateral view of the LCA demonstrates **complete occlusion of the mid-LAD** *(arrow).* (D2 = second diagonal; M = first obtuse marginal; S = septal.) *B,* RAO view after injection of the RCA shows **good collateral filling of the distal LAD** *(black arrows)* from the PDA *(arrowheads)* through a collateral *(white arrows)* coursing around the apex. Note that the collateral is as large as the native vessels.

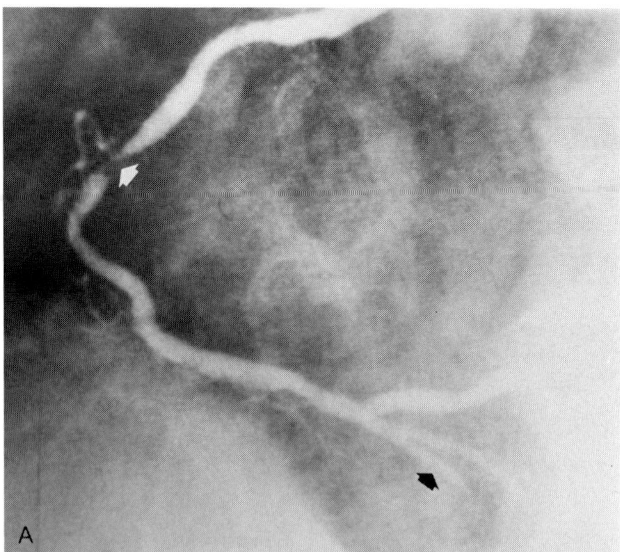

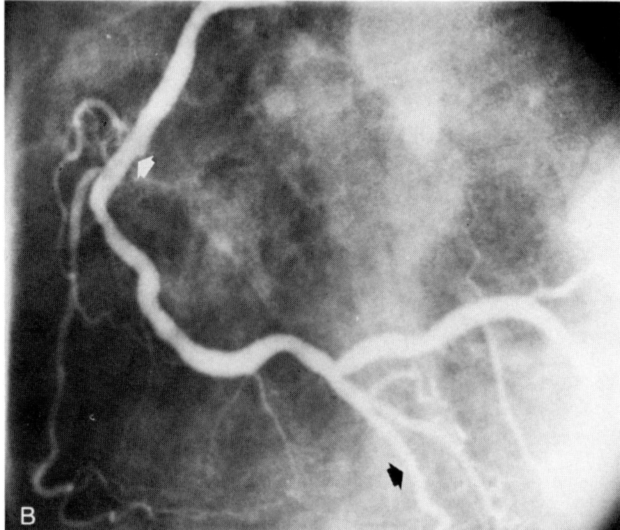

Figure 113–6. *A,* LAO views of the RCA demonstrating **reciprocating flow in the PDA.** Before angioplasty there is a high-grade stenosis of the mid-RCA *(white arrow),* and the PDA *(black arrow)* is incompletely filled because of significant collateral flow from the LCA. *B,* Following angioplasty, there is minimal residual narrowing *(white arrow),* and the PDA *(black arrow)* fills completely.

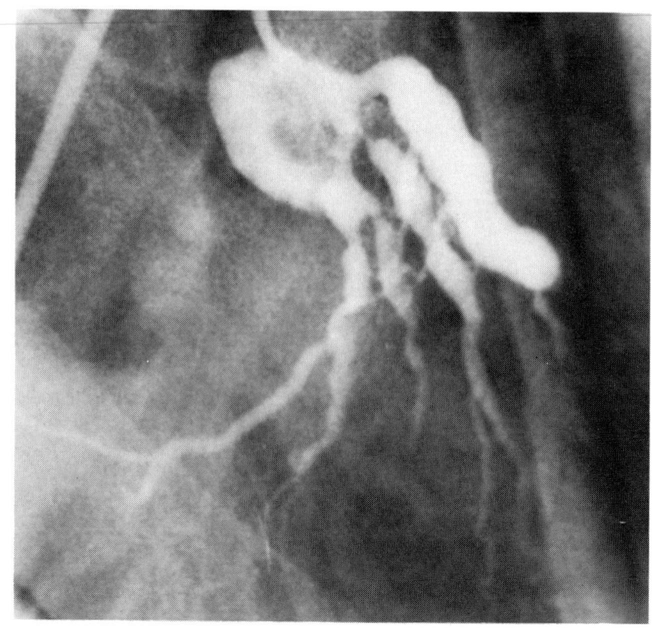

Figure 113–7. Severe coronary artery ectasia involving the LAD and circumflex arteries.

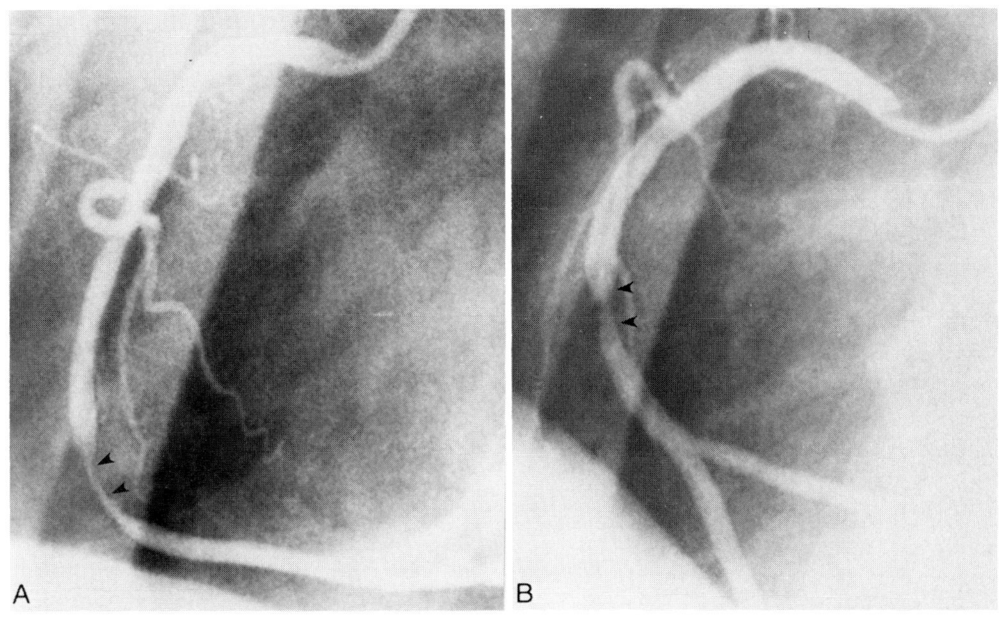

Figure 113–8. *A,* **Spontaneous spasm of the distal RCA.** Initially there is a long 80 per cent stenosis of the distal RCA *(arrowheads). B,* Following intracoronary administration of nitroglycerin, the degree of narrowing is markedly reduced *(arrowheads).*

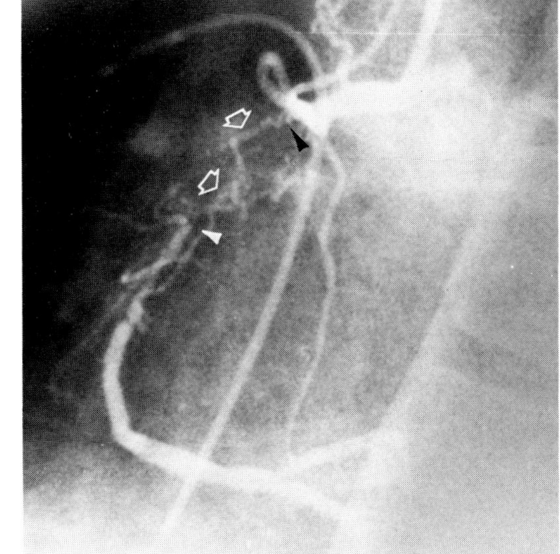

Figure 113–9. LAO view of the RCA showing **complete occlusion of the proximal RCA** *(black arrowhead)* with antegrade (''jump'') collaterals *(arrows)* reconstituting the distal vessel *(white arrowheads).*

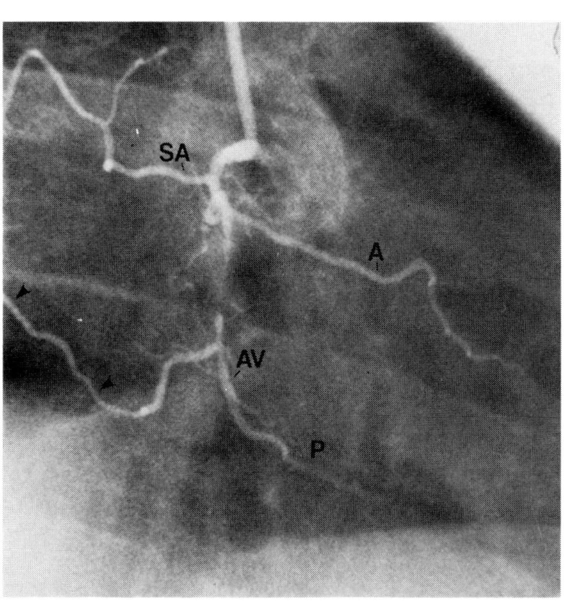

Figure 113–10. RAO view of the RCA showing a **Kugel's collateral** *(arrowheads)* from the proximal RCA via the sinoatrial node artery (SA) to the atrioventricular node artery (AV). (A = acute marginal; P = posterior descending artery.)

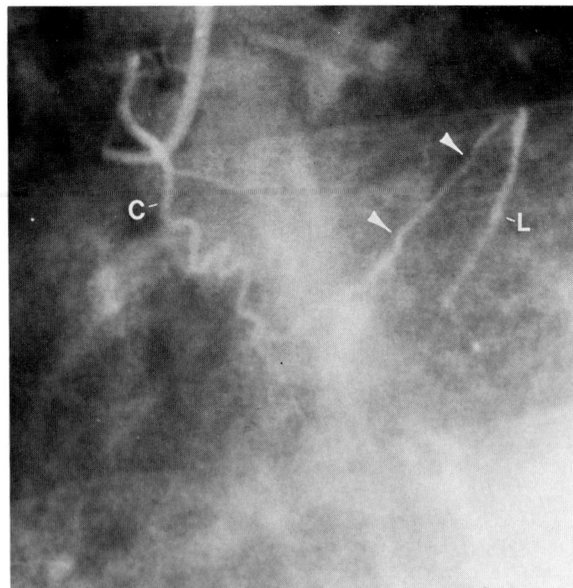

Figure 113–11. LAO view of the RCA demonstrating a collateral *(arrowheads)* from the conus artery (C) to the LAD (L). In this case, the conus artery was inadvertently selectively injected.

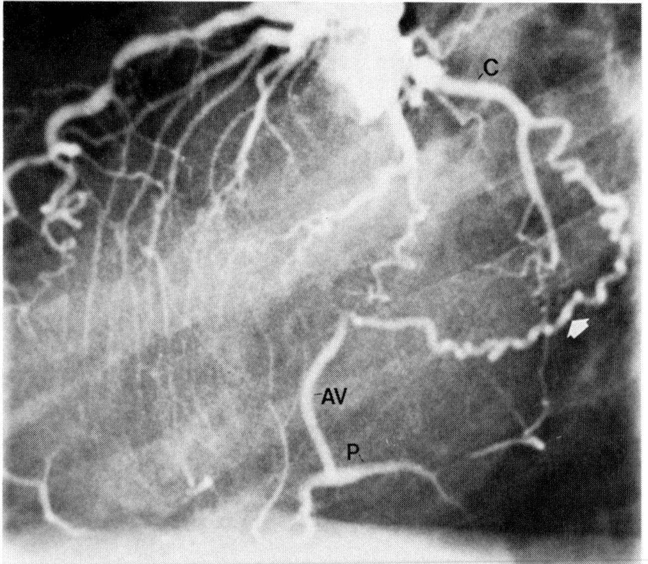

Figure 113–12. Lateral view of the LCA showing a large collateral *(arrow)* from the circumflex (C) to the atrioventricular node artery (AV) via the atrioventricular groove. (P = posterolateral segment artery.)

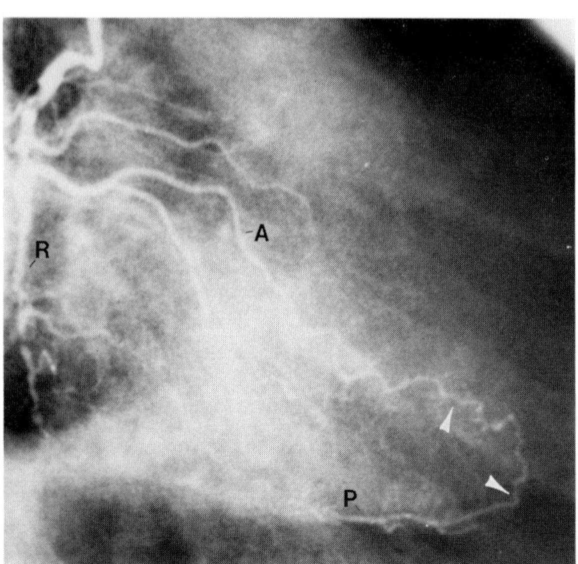

Figure 113–13. Acute marginal (A) to PDA (P) collateral *(arrowheads)*. The mid RCA (R) is severely diseased.

TABLE 113–1. CORONARY COLLATERALS

1. Proximal RCA and distal RCA	a. SANA to AVNA through the atrial septum (Kugel's artery (Fig. 113–10)
	b. Conus artery or early acute marginal to the PDA or late acute marginal (Fig. 113–13)
2. RCA and Cx	a. PLSA to distal circumflex via the atrioventricular groove (Fig. 113–12)
	b. PLB to OM
3. RCA and LAD	a. Conus artery to proximal LAD (Fig. 113–11)
	b. Acute marginal to LAD
	c. PDA to LAD around apex (Fig. 113–5)
	d. PDA to LAD through septum
4. Proximal LAD and distal LAD	a. Proximal diagonal to distal diagonal
6. Proximal Cx and distal Cx	a. Proximal OM and distal OM
	b. Atrial circumflex to distal Cx

AVNA = atrioventricular node artery; Cx = circumflex; LAD = left anterior descending; PDA = posterior descending; PLB = posterolateral branch; PLSA = posterolateral segment artery; OM = obtuse marginal; RCA = right coronary artery; SANA = sinoatrial node artery.

branches of the same artery. They usually have a tortuous appearance and are small, although occasionally they may become so large as to be confused with the native vessels (see Fig. 113–5). The major coronary collateral pathways are described in Table 113–1. When describing coronary arteriograms, it is important to make note of important collaterals and also to determine whether they are jeopardized by stenoses in their vessels of origin.

EVALUATION OF THE PATIENT WITH ACUTE MYOCARDIAL INFARCTION

Chest Radiography

The plain chest radiograph plays an important role in the evaluation of the patient with acute myocardial infarction from a prognostic viewpoint based on the appearance of the pulmonary vasculature and lung fields on the initial film. The degree of PVH correlates well with the severity of myocardial damage and thus the prognosis of the patient. This should be based solely on the appearance of the pulmonary vasculature, since heart size may remain normal in the face of acute LV decompensation. For this reason, it is important that an upright film be obtained if at all possible, since early PVH will be manifested as redistribution of the pulmonary vasculature without signs of interstitial edema, and on a supine film redistribution is not a valid sign of increased pulmonary venous pressure. The chest radiograph also plays an important role in helping to determine the results of therapeutic and diagnostic interventions in the patient with acute myocardial infarction. In this setting, there may be a lack of direct clinical and radiographic correlation as reflected in the pulmonary vasculature. This appears to relate to the 6 to 24 hour time lag necessary for fluid shifts in the lungs.

Coronary Angiography

Over the past ten years, numerous trials of thrombolytic therapy for acute myocardial infarction have demonstrated the short- and long-term benefits of intervention. Similarly, several trials have also shown immediate coronary angioplasty to benefit certain groups of patients. Because of this, patients are frequently taken for coronary angiography during or shortly after acute myocardial infarction. Intravenous administration of thrombolytic agents such as t-PA and streptokinase has been shown to be as effective as intra-arterial administration, obviating the need for immediate catheterization, but a substantial number of patients will have ongoing ischemia and can benefit from emergency angioplasty or coronary bypass surgery. There is, however, debate among cardiologists about the necessity for post-thrombolytic intervention and the necessity for routine post–myocardial infarction catheterization that is unlikely to be resolved. Most cardiologists will send a patient to the laboratory for post-infarction angina and many also consider a non–Q wave myocardial infarction an equally valid indication for study since these patients have a poorer prognosis than do those with Q-wave infarctions.

EVALUATION OF THE PATIENT WITH PREVIOUS INFARCTION

Chest Radiography

As with the patient with acute infarction, the most important role for plain chest radiography in patients with previous infarction is in the evaluation of left ventricular failure. This is particularly important in patients who do not manifest myocardial ischemia as angina but rather have left ventricular failure as an anginal equivalent. Of course, one should also look for signs of a left ventricular aneurysm (Fig. 113–14), but the absence of such signs does not mean that one

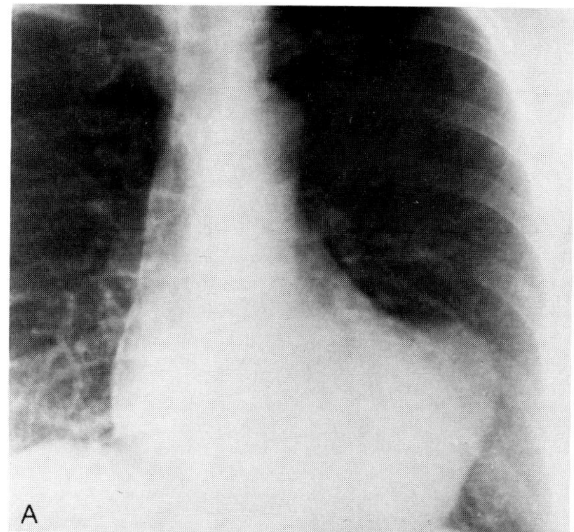

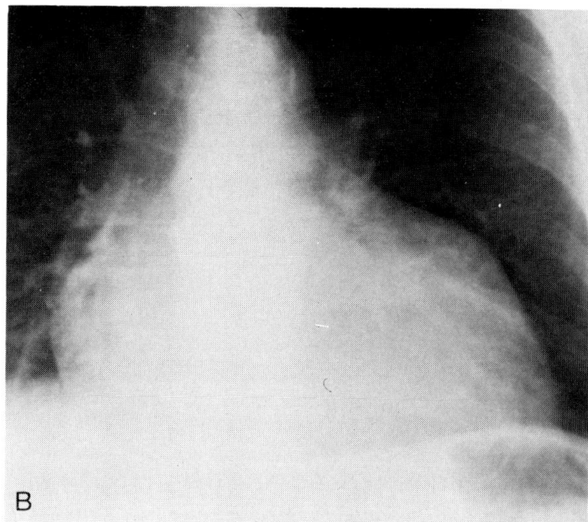

Figure 113–14. *A* and *B,* PA chest radiographs in two patients with left ventricular aneurysms. In *A,* the bulge along the left heart border is more pronounced.

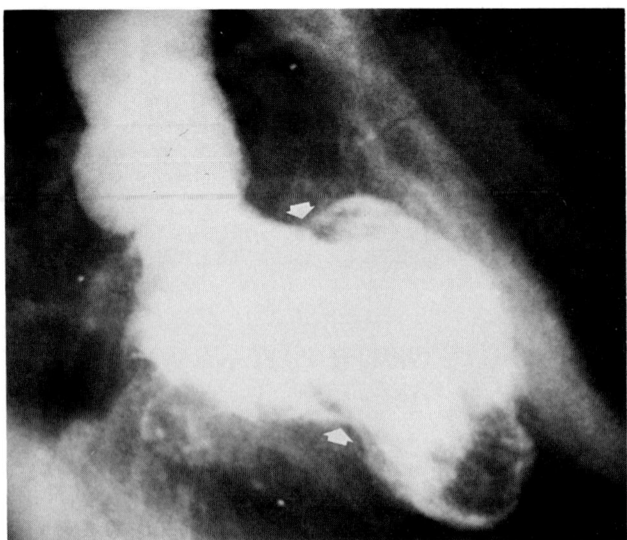

Figure 113–15. Left ventriculogram in the RAO view. There is an aneurysm of the anterolateral and apical segments with its neck *(arrows)* clearly demarcated on this systolic frame. The large filling defect in the apex represents a mural thrombus.

is not present. If the patient has had multiple previous infarcts, the chest radiograph may resemble that of a patient with dilated cardiomyopathy—that is, normal pulmonary vasculature or mild pulmonary venous hypertension and cardiomegaly. Left atrial enlargement in these patients may occur secondary to either poor LV compliance or mitral regurgitation from papillary muscle dysfunction and/or ventricular dilatation.

Cardiac Catheterization

Coronary angiography and left ventriculography can be helpful in the management of some patients with previous myocardial infarction. The patient most likely to benefit is the one with postinfarction angina. This is a potentially disastrous situation, since the patient may have already lost a significant amount of myocardium, and the loss of further muscle may result in cardiogenic shock or chronic LV failure. Because of this, there is ample reason to study these patients on an urgent or even emergent basis. One may find that the only vessel in jeopardy is the infarct-related vessel, in which case one can choose to try medical therapy or to perform angioplasty. On the other hand, there may be myocardium jeopardized by lesions in other vessels that may have become ischemic because it is supplied by collaterals from the infarct-related vessel or because myocardial work has increased to compensate for the infarcted myocardium. In these cases, the patient may require angioplasty or coronary bypass surgery.

Concomitant left ventriculography is important in these patients. Not only does it give important information about wall motion and the amount of mitral regurgitation present, but also LV end-diastolic pressure can be measured. If possible, it is wise to obtain biplane ventriculograms or two single-plane ventriculograms in the right anterior oblique (preferably 45-degree) and cranial left anterior oblique views, since wall motion abnormalities may be present in one and absent in the other. LV mural thrombi and aneurysms may also be identified (Fig. 113–15).

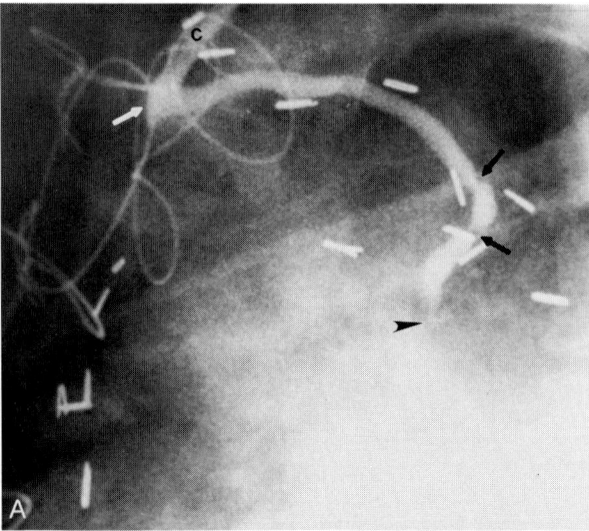

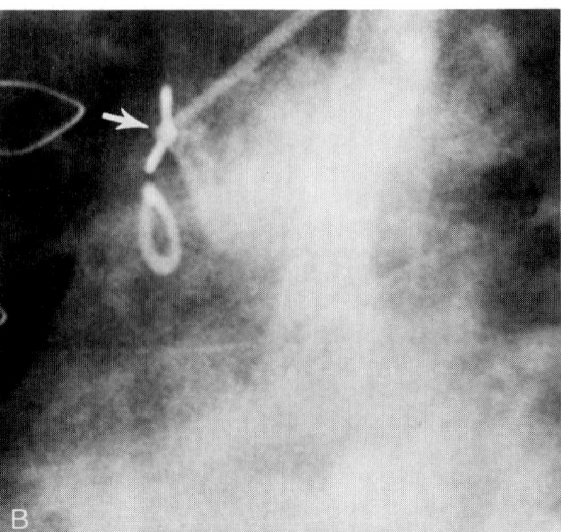

Figure 113–16. Coronary artery bypass graft stenoses. *A,* There are two high-grade stenoses *(arrows)* of the distal portion of the graft as well as at the distal anastomosis *(arrowhead).* Filling of the native vessel was extremely low. (C = catheter tip). *B,* Graft occlusion at its origin from the ascending aorta.

EVALUATION OF PATIENTS FOLLOWING CORONARY BYPASS SURGERY

Chest Radiography

The plain chest radiograph serves the same purpose in this group as in patients with previous myocardial infarction. Serial films are the most helpful, since what could be considered normal on a single examination may have changed significantly and thus reflect an abnormality.

Cardiac Catheterization

Although both computed tomography and intravenous digital subtraction angiography have been used to evaluate graft patency, neither has met with universal success, and selective angiography remains the only means of definitively evaluating the status of coronary artery bypass grafts.

Post-bypass angina or LV failure can result from any of the following: (1) graft stenosis, (2) graft occlusion, (3) progression of disease in ungrafted vessels, (4) grafts placed proximal to significant stenoses, (5) perioperative infarction, and (6) graft spasm. Angina in the early postoperative period is most likely due to graft occlusion or a misplaced graft, whereas late angina is usually due to graft occlusion or stenosis or to progression of disease. Venous grafts seem to be particularly susceptible to atherosclerosis and are usually diseased after several years. Internal mammary grafts have better long-term patency.

When one is evaluating saphenous vein coronary artery bypass grafts, it is important to visualize the proximal and distal anastomoses. This may require angled views. It is more difficult to ascertain the significance of a stenosis in a venous graft than in a native coronary artery, since there is obviously no relationship between the size of the vein and myocardial blood flow requirements, as one presumes is true in the native circulation; however, high-grade stenoses are more than likely significant (Fig. 113–16*A*). Occlusion of a vein graft (Fig. 113–16*B*) can occur either distally, in which case the proximal portion of the graft usually thromboses, or proximally. In the latter case, it may be difficult to cannulate the stump of the graft, and aortography may be useful in identifying the occlusion.

Internal mammary artery-to-coronary artery grafts are usually performed using the left internal mammary artery. It should be selectively cannulated if possible, and particular attention should be paid to the distal anastomosis.

Bibliography

Aldrich RF, Brensike JF, Battaglini JW, et al: Coronary calcifications in the detection of coronary artery disease and comparison with electrocardiographic exercise testing. Circulation 59:113, 1979.

Battler A, Karliner JS, Higgins CB, et al: The initial chest x-ray film in acute myocardial infarction: Relation of initial hemodynamic data and predictive value for early and late mortality. Circulation 61:1004, 1980.

Green CE, Kelley MJ: A renewed role for fluoroscopy in the evaluation of cardiac diseases. Radiol Clin North Am 18:345, 1980.

Green CE, Kelley MJ, Higgins CB, Bookstein JJ: Acquired coronary-to-bronchial artery communication: A possible cause of coronary steal. Cathet Cardiovasc Diagn 7:191, 1981.

Grondin CM, Campeau L, Lesperance J, et al: Comparison of late changes in internal mammary artery and saphenous vein grafts in two consecutive series of patients 10 years after operation. Circulation 70 (Suppl I):1-208, 1984.

Higgins CB, Kelley MJ, Green CE, et al: Physiologic-angiographic correlates of coronary arterial stenoses in resting and intensely vasodilated states. Invest Radiol 17:444, 1982.

Kelley MJ, Huang EK, Langou RA: Correlation of fluoroscopically detected coronary artery calcification with exercise testing in asymptomatic men. Radiology 129:1, 1978.

Kelley MJ, Newell JD: Chest radiography and cardiac fluoroscopy in coronary artery disease. Cardiovasc Clin 1:575, 1983.

Langou RA, Kelley MJ, Huang EK, et al: Predictive accuracy of coronary artery calcification and positive exercise test in asymptomatic non-hyperlipidemic men for coronary artery disease. Am J Cardiol 45:400, 1980.

Markis JE, Joffe CD, Cohn PF, et al: Clinical significance of coronary arterial ectasia. Am J Cardiol 37:217, 1976.

Oliver MG, Morley P, Samuel E, et al: Detection of coronary artery calcification during life. Lancet 1:891, 1964.

Waller BF, Rubin RC, McGrath FC, et al: Coronary calcium—a clue to angiographic underestimation of coronary luminal narrowing. Am Heart J 103:1071, 1982.

RADIONUCLIDE EVALUATION

MICHAEL W. HANSON and R. EDWARD COLEMAN

CLINICAL UTILITY OF RADIONUCLIDE STUDIES

The major utilization of radioisotope techniques in cardiology is in patients with coronary artery disease (CAD). The radioisotope techniques are used for several different purposes, including the detection of significant disease, the location of the disease, the determination of significance of lesions noted at coronary angiography, and the determination of prognosis.

When considering the proper clinical use of a diagnostic test, at least two factors must be taken into account: the probability before the diagnostic test that the patient has CAD (pretest probability) and the properties of the test (sensitivity and specificity). The probability is expressed as the chance that a given condition exists. The statement that a patient has a 90 per cent chance of having significant CAD means that 90 of 100 similar patients will have significant CAD determined at coronary angiography. The sensitivity of a test is the fraction of patients with the disease who have positive results. The specificity of a test is the fraction of patients without the disease who have negative results. The probability of disease after a test (post-test probability) is highly dependent on the pretest probability.

The post-test probability of disease can be determined if the sensitivity and specificity of the test and the patient's pretest probability of disease are known. Thomas Bayes published a treatise in 1763 that included equations for determining the post-test probability of disease. If the test result is positive, the post-test probability is calculated by the following equation:

$$p(D+\,|T+) = \frac{p(T+\,|D+) \times p(D+)}{p(T+\,|D+) \times p(D+) + p(T+\,|D-) \times p(D-)}$$

where $p(D+\,|T+)$ is the post-test probability that the disease is present when the test is positive, $p(T+\,|D+)$ is the sensitivity, $p(D+)$ is the pretest probability of disease, $p(T+\,|D-)$ is the probability that the test is positive if the disease is not present (1-specificity), and $p(D-)$ is the pretest probability that the disease is

TABLE 113–2. APPROACH TO DIAGNOSIS OF CORONARY ARTERY DISEASE*

Pretest probability of disease	10–40%					40–60%				60–90%				
Stress EKG	Neg Follow-up	Pos RS1				Not done				Neg RS1				Pos Cath
Radionuclide Study 1 (RS1)		Neg Follow-up	Equiv RS2		Pos Cath	Neg Follow-up	Equiv RS2		Pos Cath	Neg Follow-up	Equiv RS2		Pos Cath	
Radionuclide Study 2 (RS2)			Neg Follow-up	Pos Cath			Neg Follow-up	Pos Cath			Neg Follow-up	Pos Cath		

*Modified from Rozanski A, Berman DS: The efficacy of cardiovascular nuclear medicine exercise studies. Semin Nucl Med 17:104–120, 1987.

not present. If the test result is negative, the post-test probability is calculated by the following equation:

$$p(D+ \mid T-) = \frac{p(T- \mid D+) \times p(D+)}{p(T- \mid D+) \times p(D+) + p(T- \mid D-) \times p(D-)}$$

where $p(D+ \mid T-)$ is the post-test probability that the disease is present when the test is negative, $p(T- \mid D+)$ is the probability that the test result is negative if the disease is present (l-sensitivity), and $p(T- \mid D-)$ is the specificity.

These equations can be used to demonstrate the effect of the pretest probability on the post-test probability. Using the exercise-redistribution thallium-201 study as an example and the average of results from a large number of thallium studies (sensitivity = 84 per cent; specificity = 94 per cent), abnormal test results are relatively unreliable when the pretest probability of disease is low. If the test is applied to a population with a low prevalence of disease, the false-positive rate is very high, even if the test has a 90 per cent sensitivity and specificity. At a 10 per cent prevalence of CAD, the false-positive rate of patients with an abnormal test is 50 per cent; in a population of 10,000, a total of 900 (10 per cent × 10,000 × 0.90) would have an appropriately abnormal response, and 910 (10 per cent of 9100) patients without disease would have an abnormal response (false-positive rate of 910/1810 × 100 = 50 per cent). Furthermore, negative test results are unreliable when the pretest probability of disease is high. These results are common to all diagnostic tests, and only a perfect test (sensitivity = 100 per cent, specificity = 100 per cent) would not be affected by the pretest probability of disease.

The ability to use Bayes' rule for determining post-test probability of disease depends upon the ability to characterize the probability of disease prior to performing the test. Several studies have documented the ability to estimate the likelihood of CAD based on several clinical factors. The factors that have been found to be important in determining pretest probability are age, sex, presence and quality of angina pectoris (typical, atypical, or nonanginal), presence or absence of historic or EKG evidence of previous myocardial infarction, presence or absence of ST and T-wave changes, history of diabetes mellitus, history of smoking, and history of abnormal blood lipids. Algorithms have been developed using these characteristics to accurately predict the likelihood of significant CAD at coronary angiography.

Several studies have documented the use of the bayesian approach in evaluating patients with suspected CAD. Thallium imaging in patients with a 10 to 90 per cent probability of CAD results in a marked increase in the proportion of patients with a high (90 per cent) or low (10 per cent) probability of CAD. The results of exercise radionuclide ventriculography correctly decreased the probability of disease in 85 per cent of normal patients and correctly increased the probability of disease in 72 per cent of patients with CAD.

When evaluating radionuclide studies as diagnostic tests for detecting CAD, their efficacy has been determined by comparison with results of coronary angiography. A discordancy between the results of radionuclide studies and coronary angiography does not mean that the radionuclide study is wrong, since coronary angiography is not a perfect test for defining anatomic lesions or blood flow. Other methods, such as prognosis, have been used for determining the efficacy of these studies.

The utility of a test is best determined by the additional information it provides compared with the conventional clinical information. Several studies have now documented the additional information available from radionuclide studies. In studies comparing thallium stress-redistribution imaging and exercise electrocardiography, thallium studies were more sensitive (84 per cent compared with 62 per cent) and more specific (94 per cent compared with 83 per cent). Ventricular function and wall motion studies have been demonstrated to provide information additional to the clinical variables for determining likelihood of significant CAD. In patients without a high pretest probability of disease, 32 per cent could be diagnosed with a 90 per cent probability of disease, and 42 per cent could be diagnosed with an 85 per cent probability of disease after radionuclide ventriculography. Thus, most patients with a low or intermediate pretest probability of disease will need additional testing for a definitive diagnosis of CAD.

Rozanski and Berman have outlined their approach to the use of diagnostic testing of patients with suspected CAD (Table 113–2). Owing to the limitations of the diagnostic tests, patients with a pretest probability of less than 10 per cent or greater than 90 per cent are not studied, since too many false-positive and false-negative results occur in these groups. Stress electrocardiography is the first procedure except in patients in whom it is nondiagnostic, such as those with left bundle branch block or those taking digoxin, and in patients with a 40 to 60 per cent pretest probability of disease, since the post-test likelihood of disease will not be changed enough to categorize these patients as having or not having disease. The stress electrocardiogram is cheaper to perform than the radionuclide studies. A negative stress test in patients with a low pretest probability of disease and a positive stress test in patients with a high pretest likelihood of disease are definitive enough for patient management. The 40 to 60 per cent pretest probability group, the 10 to 40 per cent group with a positive stress electrocardiographic response, and the 60 to 90 per cent group with a negative stress electrocardiographic response are best evaluated with a radionuclide study. Depending on the outcome of the first radionuclide study, a second radionuclide study may be needed to determine management.

RADIONUCLIDE STUDIES IN ACUTE MYOCARDIAL INFARCTION

Myocardial infarct imaging with technetium-99m (^{99m}Tc) pyrophosphate is accurate in the detection of acute myocardial infarction. Scans become positive 12 to 24 hours following the onset of infarction, and the maximum positivity is usually observed 48 to 72 hours later. The scans become negative 10 to 14 days following the acute event.

Transmural infarction is associated with abnormal imaging in approximately 95 per cent of patients. The sensitivity for subendocardial myocardial infarction is less than that for transmural infarction. The specificity of infarct imaging is 90 per cent or greater if the causes of diffuse activity from cardiac blood pool and other causes of focal uptake outside the heart are recognized.

The clinical use of myocardial infarct imaging is limited. It is indicated for patients with suspected acute myocardial infarction and pre-existing abnormal electrocardiograms such as left bundle branch block, postoperative patients who have abnormal enzyme levels that are difficult to interpret, recently injured patients, and patients presenting several days after chest pain when the enzyme levels may have returned to normal. The ability of the enzyme MB-CK to accurately detect patients with acute myocardial infarction has greatly reduced the number of myocardial infarct imaging studies performed.

Thallium-201 imaging has been used to select patients in a high-risk category after acute myocardial infarction. The circumferential profiles of the patients were compared with those of normals. Nonsurvivors had significantly larger thallium defects than did survivors.

Gated blood pool imaging can also identify high-risk patients in the coronary care unit (Fig. 113–17). In the same group of patients studied with thallium imaging, an ejection fraction of 35 per cent on the gated blood pool study provided the best discriminator predicting mortality. Forty-seven per cent of nonsurvivors had ejection fractions of 35 per cent or less, whereas 96 per cent of survivors had ejection fractions greater than 35 per cent. These studies demonstrate that radionuclide imaging in patients with acute infarction can stratify patients according to risk. Either the thallium study or the ejection fraction as a single index was better than clinical variables in determining prognosis.

Radionuclide studies are being used for prognostication after myocardial infarction. The results of the studies are used in the formulation of appropriate management of these patients. Predischarge thallium imaging has been used to detect functionally significant multivessel disease and residual myocardial ischemia within the zone of infarction in patients surviving an acute myocardial infarction. The thallium imaging is useful in determining additional disease in arteries other than the vessel associated with the acute event. Patients with acute infarction who are at high risk for subsequent ischemic events include those with defects in more than one vascular distribution, evidence of redistribution, and increased lung uptake of thallium. Most patients who die or have another infarction during the first year after discharge from an uncomplicated infarction have one or more of the imaging findings suggesting a high risk on the predischarge study. Patients with a normal thallium study or a single defect in the area of infarction without redistribution have a 2 per cent mortality rate and a 6 per cent total cardiac event rate, including death, recurrent infarction, and unstable angina during a 15-month period following infarction. More than 50 per cent of the patients who had one of the findings putting them at high risk on the predischarge exercise study had a cardiac event during the 15-month period. The thallium study separated the high- and low-risk groups better than exercise testing alone.

Exercise ventricular function studies have been performed prior to the hospital discharge to stratify patients into high- and low-risk groups after myocardial infarction. Survivors of acute myocardial infarction were studied with rest and exercise ventricular function studies to determine the value of these studies in predicting specific events, including death, recurrent acute infarction, coronary care unit readmission for unstable chest pain, and medically refractory angina after acute myocardial infarction. Ejection fractions at rest and exercise were significantly associated with time to death. Both

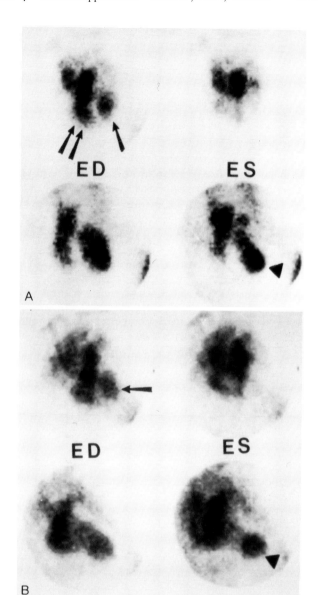

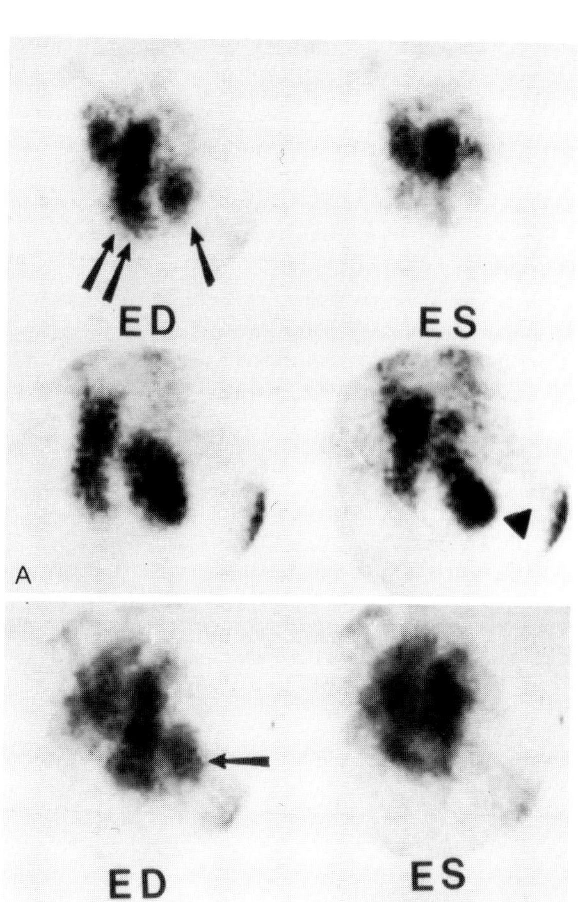

Figure 113–17. End-diastolic (ED) and end-systolic (ES) images from a patient with an ejection fraction of 75 per cent *(upper images)* and a patient with an ejection fraction of 30 per cent *(lower images)* in the best septal *(A)* and anterior *(B)* views. The two arrows identify the right ventricle, and the single arrow identifies the left ventricle. Both ventricles on the upper images have almost no activity remaining at end-systole. The lower images demonstrate dyskinesis of the left ventricular apex *(arrowhead)*. Good contraction is noted at the base of the left ventricle, and the anterior view demonstrates a "neck" to the anteroapical dyskinetic segment. The good basilar contraction, diastolic deformity, focal dyskinetic segment, and "neck" are characteristic of an aneurysm.

the rest and exercise ejection fractions added significant prognostic information to the clinical assessment. The change in the ejection fraction from rest to exercise predicted the time to coronary artery bypass graft surgery for medically refractory angina before and after adjustment for the clinical descriptors. The change in ejection fraction did not predict death or other nonfatal events. Significant correlations were found between the rest and exercise ventricular function study and a variety of clinical descriptors previously reported to have prognostic significance. With an exercise ejection fraction less than 45 per cent, fatality increased dramatically. Mortality at two years was 11 per cent with an exercise ejection fraction of 30 per cent, and 56 per cent with an exercise ejection fraction of 15 per cent.

THALLIUM-201 IMAGING IN THE DETECTION OF CORONARY ARTERY DISEASE

The physiologic principle by which thallium detects CAD relates to the relationship of thallium distribution to myocardial blood flow. Variations in coronary blood flow in different coronary vessels result in different thallium concentrations in the myocardium supplied by those vessels. Since myocardial blood flow is generally normal, even with significant CAD, some method is used to increase blood flow for diagnostic imaging studies. This increase in blood flow can be induced physiologically from increased demand, such as by exercise, or pharmacologically with intravenous dipyridamole or adenosine. Both physiologic and pharmacologic methods can increase myocardial blood flow severalfold, usually to three or four times normal. If a coronary artery is significantly stenosed, blood flow to the myocardium supplied by that vessel cannot increase to the same degree as to the myocardium supplied by a normal artery. Damaged myocardium (areas of previous infarction) cannot accumulate thallium.

Since the thallium does not remain fixed in the myocardium after the initial accumulation, a continuous exchange occurs between the myocardial and blood pool thallium. Redistribution occurs as thallium continues to exchange between the myocardium and blood pool. Redistribution occurs by the wash-out of thallium from the normal myocardium and the wash-in of thallium to defects present on the stress image but no longer ischemic during the redistribution period. Areas of damaged myocardium will not accumulate thallium during the exercise or redistribution imaging studies (Table 113–3). Redistribution images are obtained three to four hours after the exercise injection (Figs. 113–18 to 113–20).

The low sensitivity and predictive value of a negative stress electrocardiogram have limited its use except in certain clinical situations. The sensitivity of the stress electrocardiogram, using the criterion of 1.0 mm or greater of horizontal or downsloping ST-segment depression, varies from 47 to 81 per cent among symptomatic patients referred for possible CAD. A summary of studies from the literature demonstrates a sensitivity of 83 per cent and a specificity of 90 per cent for thallium studies. In these same patients, the stress electrocardiogram has a 58 per cent sensitivity and an 82 per cent specificity.

Several factors relate to the sensitivity and specificity of thallium studies (Tables 113–4 and 113–5). To obtain the best results, the patient should undergo exercise to the predicted heart rate to increase myocardial blood flow. However, if the patient is unable to reach the target heart rate, the thallium study is more frequently abnormal than is the exercise electrocardiogram. The reported sensitivity for detecting one-, two-, and three-vessel disease is 80, 83, and 96 per cent, respectively. Circumflex CAD is more difficult to detect than right or left anterior descending CAD. Distal stenoses or stenoses of branch arteries are also more difficult to detect than are proximal lesions in the three major vessels. The effect of collaterals on thallium imaging is controversial. Some studies have shown more abnormalities on the thallium image in the distribution of occluded arteries not supplied by collateral vessels, but other studies have shown comparable abnormalities, even in the presence of collateral vessels. As with most imaging studies, considerable interobserver variability exists in the interpretation of thallium studies. Interpretation of the study by multiple observers can improve the sensitivity and specificity. The sensitivity of the thallium study may be lower in women than in men, but this discrepancy has not been well-documented.

It has become increasingly important in the clinical setting to be able to distinguish viable from nonviable myocardium. So-called hibernating, viable myocardium that can demonstrate wall motion abnormalities, an absence of wall thickening during ventricular systole, and reduced perfusion at rest can be difficult to identify and distinguish from nonviable myocardium. Standard stress-redistribution thallium imaging protocols may overestimate these segments as demonstrating a complete zone of infarction when the three to four hour redistribution image fails to show significant improvement in perfusion, compared with the defect identified on the immediate stress image. Alternative techniques have, therefore, been described in thallium-201 imaging to assist in the identification of these areas of profoundly ischemic, yet viable, myocardial tissue. One such technique involves the acquisition of a redistribution image at 24 hours after the injection of thallium-201. Using this technique, Kiat et al reported that 57 per cent of persistent defects on standard four-hour redistribution images were reclassified as viable, based on the repeated 24-hour image. Although this technique improves the ability to define regions of profound ischemia, the two-day requirement is often not practical and the image quality at 24 hours may be less than optimal. A second technique that has been described for assessment of myocardial viability with thallium-201 involves the reinjection of a second dose of radionuclide approximately 5 to 10 minutes prior to standard redistribution imaging. Using single photon emission computed tomography (SPECT) imaging, Dilsizian et al studied 140 patients with this technique. The immediate stress image was followed by a standard 3 to 4 hour redistribution image. The patients were then reinjected with 1 mCi

TABLE 113–3. INTERPRETATION OF THALLIUM STUDY

Exercise Image	Redistribution Image	Interpretation
Normal	Normal	Normal
Defect	Normal	Coronary artery disease Ischemia without previous infarction
Defect	Partial normalization	Coronary artery disease Previous infarction and ischemia
Defect	Defect	Coronary artery disease Previous infarction

TABLE 113–4. CAUSES OF FALSE-POSITIVE THALLIUM-201 STUDIES

1. Underestimation of coronary artery disease on coronary angiography
2. Misinterpretation of images such as normal apical thinning
3. Exercise-induced spasm
4. Complete left bundle branch block in absence of coronary artery disease
5. Other cardiac pathology such as sarcoidosis
6. Defect in inferoposterior wall on 70-degree LAO view due to diaphragmatic attenuation
7. Attenuation by breast or enlarged right ventricular blood pool

TABLE 113–5. CAUSES OF FALSE-NEGATIVE THALLIUM-201 STUDIES

1. Inadequate exercise
2. Single vessel disease
3. Circumflex, diagonal, and distal vessel stenosis
4. Collaterals
5. Overestimation of coronary artery disease on coronary angiography
6. Triple-vessel disease with diffuse ischemia
7. Delay between time of injection and imaging

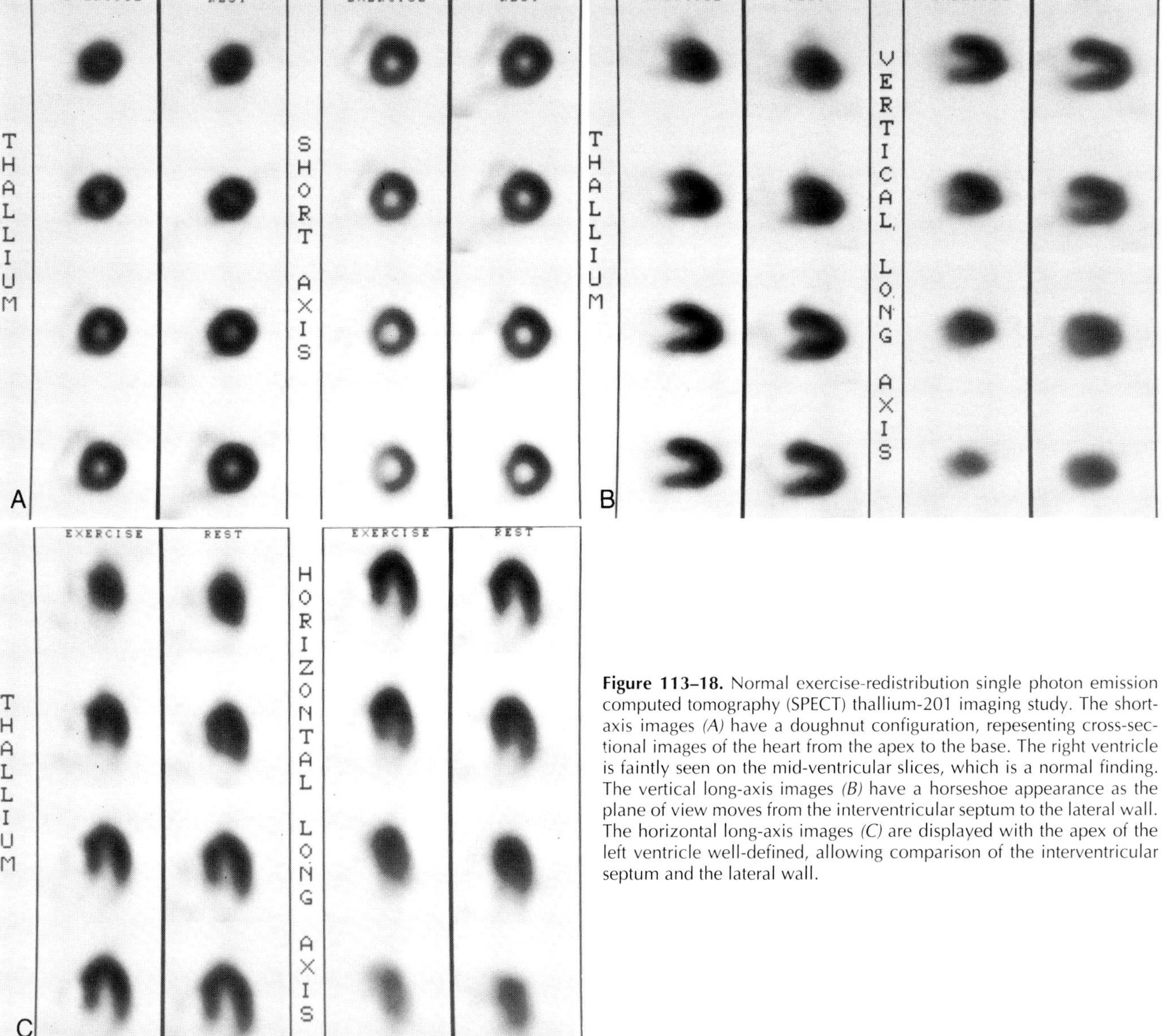

Figure 113–18. Normal exercise-redistribution single photon emission computed tomography (SPECT) thallium-201 imaging study. The short-axis images *(A)* have a doughnut configuration, repesenting cross-sectional images of the heart from the apex to the base. The right ventricle is faintly seen on the mid-ventricular slices, which is a normal finding. The vertical long-axis images *(B)* have a horseshoe appearance as the plane of view moves from the interventricular septum to the lateral wall. The horizontal long-axis images *(C)* are displayed with the apex of the left ventricle well-defined, allowing comparison of the interventricular septum and the lateral wall.

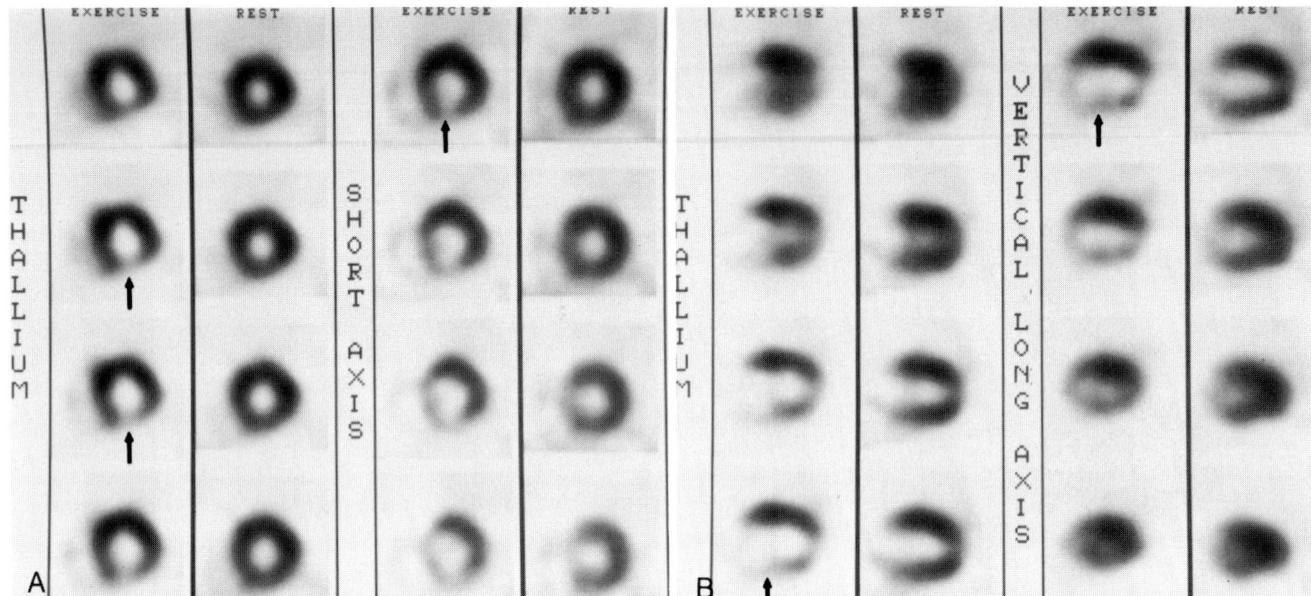

Figure 113–19. Abnormal exercise-redistribution SPECT thallium-201 imaging study in a 46-year-old man with coronary artery disease and a prior myocardial infarction. The exercise short-axis images *(A)* and the vertical long-axis images *(B)* demonstrate a perfusion defect in the inferior wall of the left ventricle *(arrows).* The redistribution images in these same planes demonstrate a complete normalization of tracer in these locations. These findings demonstrate reversible exercise-induced ischemia in the inferior wall of the left ventricle, implicating significant coronary artery disease in the vascular distribution of the right coronary artery.

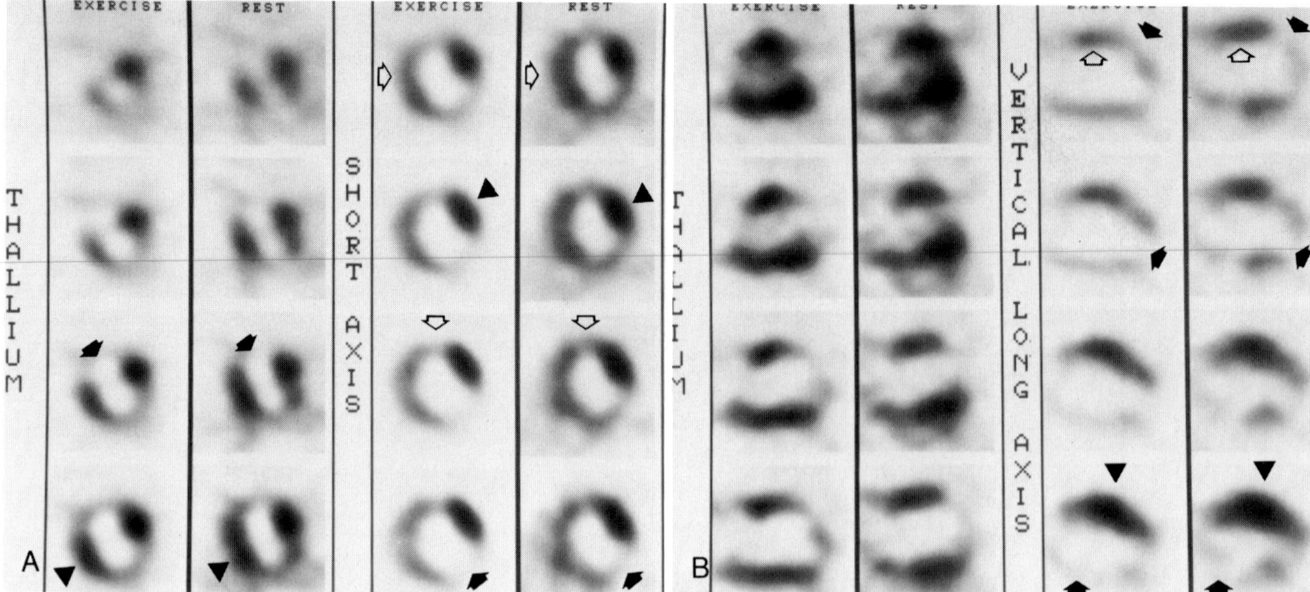

Figure 113–20. Abnormal exercise-redistribution SPECT thallium-201 imaging study in a 64-year-old man who has had multiple myocardial infarctions and two cardiac arrests. The short-axis images *(A)* and the vertical long-axis images *(B)* demonstrate a dilated left ventricle with complex, markedly abnormal myocardial perfusion patterns. At stress, the most normal myocardium is the anterolateral wall and the inferior aspect of the interventricular septum *(triangles).* Perfusion defects are seen in the remaining myocardium. The defects in the apex, low anterior wall, and posterolateral wall are not significantly different between the stress and redistribution images *(closed arrows).* These findings are consistent with completed infarction in these locations. The perfusion defects in the high anterior wall and the mid to upper interventricular septum show minimal improvement at redistribution *(open arrows).* Although these areas are also mostly infarcted myocardium, the findings suggest some degree of superimposed residual ischemia in these locations.

(37 MBq) of thallium-201 and myocardial perfusion imaging was repeated. Of 43 patients with fixed defects, 27 (63 per cent) had additional filling-in of the defect on the reinjection image. Therefore, the reinjection technique provides improved accuracy in thallium-201 evaluation of myocardial viability that is more practical than the 24-hour redistribution imaging technique.

Abnormal thallium images without significant CAD on the coronary arteriogram can be related to several causes (see Table 113–4). Abnormal septal activity on the exercise image that normalizes on the redistribution image has been described in patients with left bundle branch block without significant CAD. Attenuation by the diaphragm, breast, or enlarged right ventricle should be considered in the interpretation of the studies. Myocardial diseases other than CAD, such as sarcoidosis, can cause abnormalities on thallium imaging.

TECHNETIUM-99M–LABELED PERFUSION AGENTS IN THE DETECTION OF CORONARY ARTERY DISEASE

Two ^{99m}Tc-labeled myocardial perfusion agents have been approved for clinical use by the FDA. These agents differ considerably from thallium-201 in their pharmacokinetic properties and imaging characteristics (see Chap. 105). One of these agents is ^{99m}Tc sestamibi (Cardiolite), an isonitrile compound with favorable biologic properties for myocardial imaging. The other agent in this group is ^{99m}Tc teboroxime (Cardiotec), a neutral lipophilic complex of boronic acid that is extracted into the myocardium in relation to coronary artery blood flow but has rapid myocardial clearance.

Several comparative studies have been performed to evaluate the usefulness of these radiopharmaceuticals. In the detection of CAD, studies with both planar and SPECT methods have shown the diagnostic accuracy of ^{99m}Tc sestamibi, ^{99m}Tc teboroxime, and thallium-201 to be equivalent.

One of the major advantages of the ^{99m}Tc-labeled agents is the ability to assess left ventricular function with a first-pass RNA study at the time of the injection of tracer at rest and with exercise, thus providing functional and perfusion data for analysis in patients with known or suspected CAD (Fig. 113–21). Studies reported by Jones et al and Larock et al suggest that combining the assessment of myocardial perfusion with that of left ventricular function can improve diagnostic and prognostic information obtained from these studies.

^{99m}Tc sestamibi has been successful in determining the location and size of acute myocardial infarctions and has been used to evaluate patients during acute ischemic syndromes. Gregoire and Theroux studied 26 patients during spontaneous chest pain suggestive of unstable angina pectoris. Due to the pharmacokinetic characteristics of sestamibi, imaging could be performed later when the patients were more stable, yet still reflect the status of coronary artery blood flow at the time of the injection of tracer. In this setting, compared with coronary angiography, ^{99m}Tc sestamibi SPECT imaging had a sensitivity of 96 per cent and a specificity of 76 per cent for the detection of CAD. Sestamibi has been used to assess the efficacy of thrombolytic therapy by comparing the perfusion image reflecting blood flow before thrombolytic therapy was given with repeat studies performed at 18 to 48 hours and 6 to 14 days after therapy. In the cardiac catheterization laboratory, sestamibi has been used to evaluate the area of myocardium at risk during brief episodes of ischemia induced by balloon occlusion during percutaneous transluminal coronary angioplasty. Due to its rapid clearance from the myocardium and the logistics for imaging, ^{99m}Tc teboroxime has not been used for the evaluation of patients in the acute setting.

PHARMACOLOGIC STRESS TESTING

The inability of a patient to exercise to an adequate predetermined heart rate may result in a false-negative radionuclide functional or perfusion scan. Several alternatives to treadmill or bicycle exercise have been proposed, including hand-grip exercise, arm ergometer exercise, isometric exercise, rapid atrial pacing, and cardiac stress using pharmacologic agents. Currently, the most accepted alternative to standard exercise is the use of pharmacologic stress agents. These pharmacologic alternatives offer the opportunity to study patients who are unable to exercise well or who cannot exercise at all due to a variety of circumstances, including othropedic problems; poor physical conditioning; or medications, such as beta blockers, which limit the heart rate response to exercise.

Two pharmacologic agents that have been used with thallium myocardial perfusion imaging are intravenous dipyridamole (Persantine) and intravenous adenosine. Both of these agents have been demonstrated to be as accurate as exercise-redistribution studies in identifying patients with significant CAD. Some patients who receive intravenous dipyridamole or adenosine for the thallium study will have clinical ischemia (angina and/or electrocardiographic changes). In a review of five reports in the literature with a total of 215 patients who had both exercise and dipyridamole thallium-201 imaging, the overall sensitivity for both studies was 79 per cent, while the specificity for the dipyridamole study was 95 per cent and specificity for the exercise study was 92 per cent in the detection of CAD. Dipyridamole-thallium imaging has also been shown to have prognostic information in patients with recent myocardial infarction and has been used for risk stratification and prognosis. In postinfarction patients, evidence of a reversible defect outside of the zone of infarct has a sensitivity of 63 per cent and a specificity of 75 per cent for subsequent cardiac events. Leppo et al reported that in patients with uncomplicated myocardial infarction, a reversible perfusion defect on dipyridamole-thallium imaging was the best predictor of future cardiac events. Younis et al reported on 107 asymptomatic patients with coronary disease. A reversible thallium-201 defect was the only significant predictor of a subsequent cardiac event (myocardial infarction or death). Of 13 patients who died or had a nonfatal myocardial infarction, 12 had a reversible defect, while all 36 patients with a normal scan had no cardiac events during 14 months of follow-up. Dipyridamole-thallium studies are also useful in stratifying the risk of patients referred for vascular surgery. Ischemic events occurred in patients demonstrating reversible defects on preoperative imaging, whereas no ischemic events occurred in patients with no thallium redistribution.

Verani et al have reported thallium-201 imaging with intravenous adenosine to have a sensitivity of 83 per cent and a specificity of 94 per cent in the diagnosis of CAD, with most of the false-negative studies occurring in patients who had single-vessel disease. Gupta et al reported similar findings with adenosine thallium-201 SPECT imaging and reported a sensitivity of 83 per cent, a somewhat lower specificity of 87 per cent, and a predictive accuracy for the adenosine study of 84 per cent. These values were all equivalent to the exercise thallium-201 studies in the same group of patients.

VENTRICULAR FUNCTION STUDIES IN THE DETECTION OF CORONARY ARTERY DISEASE

Ventricular function is closely related to myocardial blood flow. An immediate result of myocardial ischemia is loss of function. Early studies, using contrast and radionuclide ventriculography, demonstrated that functional abnormalities occurring with exercise could be used to detect significant CAD in patients with chest pain. Borer et al and Jones et al used radionuclide angiocardiographic

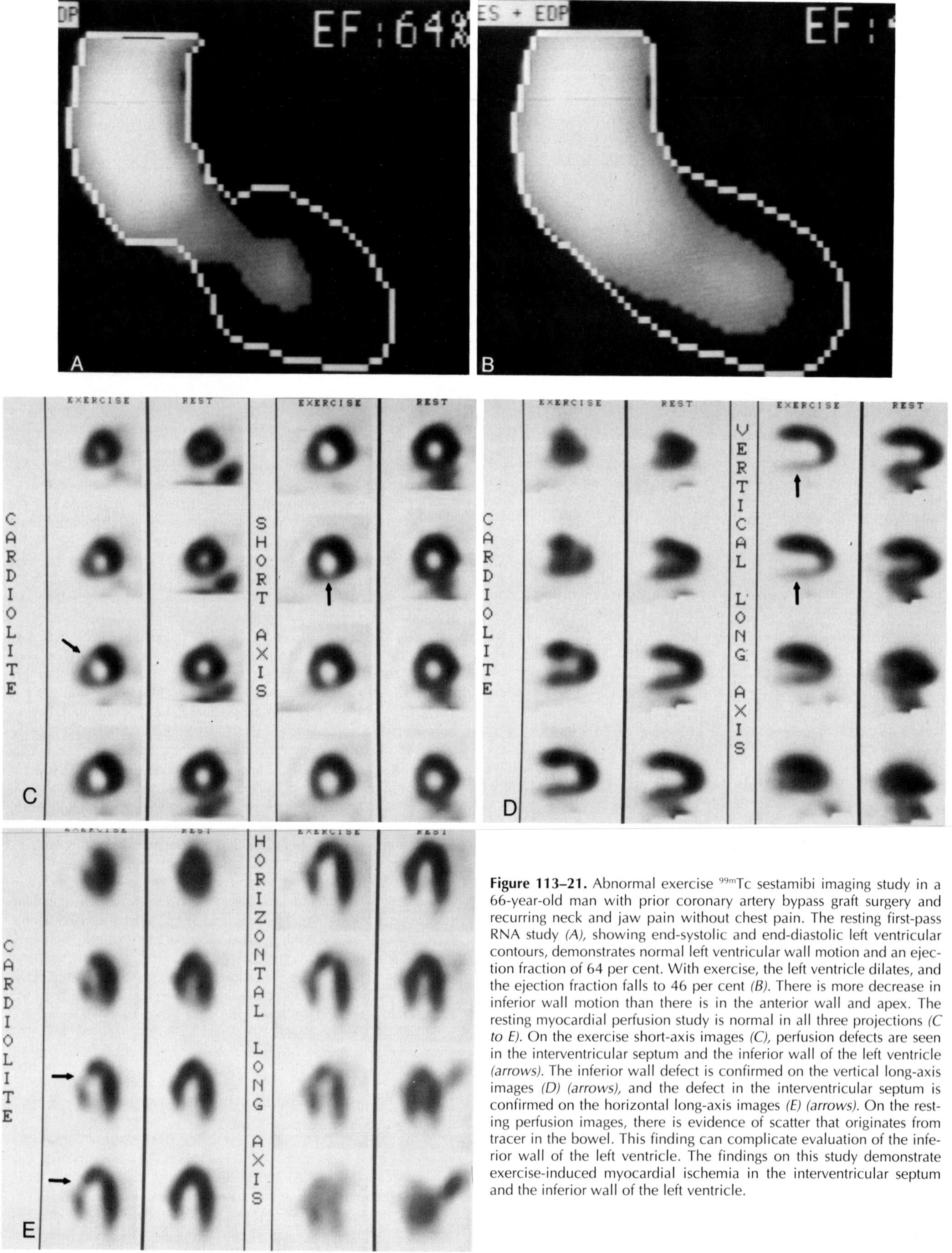

Figure 113–21. Abnormal exercise ^{99m}Tc sestamibi imaging study in a 66-year-old man with prior coronary artery bypass graft surgery and recurring neck and jaw pain without chest pain. The resting first-pass RNA study *(A)*, showing end-systolic and end-diastolic left ventricular contours, demonstrates normal left ventricular wall motion and an ejection fraction of 64 per cent. With exercise, the left ventricle dilates, and the ejection fraction falls to 46 per cent *(B)*. There is more decrease in inferior wall motion than there is in the anterior wall and apex. The resting myocardial perfusion study is normal in all three projections *(C to E)*. On the exercise short-axis images *(C)*, perfusion defects are seen in the interventricular septum and the inferior wall of the left ventricle *(arrows)*. The inferior wall defect is confirmed on the vertical long-axis images *(D) (arrows)*, and the defect in the interventricular septum is confirmed on the horizontal long-axis images *(E) (arrows)*. On the resting perfusion images, there is evidence of scatter that originates from tracer in the bowel. This finding can complicate evaluation of the inferior wall of the left ventricle. The findings on this study demonstrate exercise-induced myocardial ischemia in the interventricular septum and the inferior wall of the left ventricle.

TABLE 113–6. DETERMINATION OF OPTIMAL CRITERIA OF EXERCISE RESPONSE FOR DIAGNOSIS OF CORONARY ARTERY DISEASE IN PATIENTS WITH NORMAL RESTING EJECTION FRACTION

	173 Men		56 Women		229 Patients	
Criteria	Sensitivity	Specificity	Sensitivity	Specificity	Sensitivity	Specificity
1. Rest-to-exercise increase in EF less than 5%	82%	73%	78%	46%	81%	60%
2. Rest-to-exercise change in EF 6% less than predicted	85%	81%	50%	71%	79%	76%
3. Exercise-induced wall motion abnormality	56%	96%	38%	88%	53%	92%
4. Exercise end-systolic volume increased more than 20 ml	48%	96%	34%	79%	46%	88%
5. Criteria 2, 3, or 4	89%	79%	56%	54%	84%	66%

techniques to demonstrate that most persons without significant CAD increase their ejection fraction during exercise, and most patients with documented CAD decrease their ejection fraction with exercise. These studies suggest that deterioration of left ventricular function during exercise is highly sensitive and specific for diagnosing CAD. However, these studies did not include a large group of patients presenting for diagnosis of chest pain.

Jones et al evaluated rest and exercise radionuclide angiocardiographic measurements of left ventricular function in 496 patients who underwent cardiac catheterization for chest pain. First-pass radionuclide angiocardiography was performed using upright bicycle exercise. An exercise treadmill test was performed within three months of catheterization and the radionuclide study in 248 of the 496 patients. The optimal diagnostic criteria for a normal response were determined, excluding patients with insignificant CAD, patients taking propranolol within 24 hours of the study, and patients not achieving an adequate exercise (Table 113–6).

This study found that a resting ejection fraction of less than 50 per cent suggested CAD. Previous studies had suggested that a 5 per cent or greater increase in ejection fraction from rest to exercise was the normal left ventricular response to stress. This study determined that the predicted change in ejection fraction (EF) during exercise for men was as follows:

$$EF = 0.45 - 0.5\ (\text{EF at rest}) - 0.002\ (\Delta\ \text{EDVI})$$

where Δ EDVI is the rest-to-exercise change in end-diastolic volume index. The equation predicting EF for women was:

$$EF = 0.385 - 0.5\ (\text{EF at rest}) - 0.002\ (\Delta\ \text{EDVI})$$

Any patient whose exercise EF was 6 per cent or more below that predicted was considered to have CAD. The sensitivity and specificity of the various criteria are included in Table 113–6. When the optimal criteria were applied to the entire population, the sensitivity was 87 per cent and the specificity 58 per cent. When these criteria were applied prospectively to 221 consecutive patients having radionuclide angiocardiography and cardiac catheterization, the sensitivity was 87 per cent and the specificity 54 per cent. The specificity of the test in the 56 women in the study was 45 per cent.

Some of the problems with using ventricular function studies in evaluating patients with chest pain have been identified (Tables 113–7 to 113–9). Several technical factors are important to consider when evaluating radionuclide ventricular function studies (Table 113–7). The study must be technically adequate before an interpretation of the study can be made. A study of healthy normal volunteers has demonstrated the inability to increase the exercise ejection fraction by 0.05 in persons over age 60. The prevalence of an inability to increase the exercise ejection fraction by at least 0.05 was 95 per cent of the normal subjects by the eighth through tenth decades. Patients with left bundle branch block and normal coronary arteries or insignificant CAD decrease their exercise ejection fraction as a group. The individual responses are quite variable, with some increasing and others decreasing their ejection fraction. Focal wall motion abnormalities may occur with exercise in these patients. Patients with rate-dependent left bundle branch block and no evidence of cardiac disease can also decrease their ejection fraction and develop wall motion abnormalities with exercise.

The low specificity of a failure to increase ejection fraction in women appears to be related to a fundamental difference in the cardiac responses of men and women to upright exercise. A group of normal female volunteers had no change in their ejection fraction from rest to exercise, whereas a group of normal male volunteers increased their ejection fraction by more than 0.05 in 14 of 15 subjects. Only 7 of 16 women increased their ejection fraction by that amount. These normal women increased their cardiac output by increasing their end-diastolic volume.

The diagnostic sensitivity of the exercise radionuclide angiogram is significantly reduced if the exercise acquisition is not obtained at peak exercise. This decreased sensitivity was demonstrated when two groups of patients with exercise-induced ischemia were studied using first-pass radionuclide angiography so that a second exercise acquisition could be obtained within one minute of a first exercise acquisition. In one group, the second study was obtained with a reduction in workload to 50 per cent of the maximum. In the second group, the second exercise study was obtained after a 200 kpm per minute reduction in workload. In the group with the 50 per cent

TABLE 113–7. CONDITIONS ASSOCIATED WITH TECHNICALLY INADEQUATE VENTRICULAR FUNCTION STUDIES

1. Inadequate bolus (first-pass studies)
2. Poor red blood cell label (gated studies)
3. Very irregular atrial fibrillation (may do better with exercise, since rhythm will be more regular)
4. Multiple atrial or ventricular premature contractions
5. Gating problem

TABLE 113–8. PATIENT GROUPS THAT MAY HAVE A REST-TO-EXERCISE DECREASE IN EJECTION FRACTION IN THE ABSENCE OF SIGNIFICANT CORONARY ARTERY DISEASE

1. Age >65 years
2. Women
3. Left bundle branch block
4. Rate-dependent left bundle branch block
5. Valvular heart disease
6. Cardiomyopathy

TABLE 113–9. CAUSES OF A REST-TO-EXERCISE INCREASE IN EJECTION FRACTION IN PATIENTS WITH SIGNIFICANT CORONARY ARTERY DISEASE

1. Failure to reach target heart rate
2. Exercise study acquired after peak exercise (less than maximal workload)
3. Inadequate exercise heart rate due to poor effort, poor physical condition, or beta blocker

reduction in workload, the sensitivity for the detection of CAD would have been reduced from 100 to 52 per cent. In the group with a 200 kpm per minute workload reduction, the sensitivity would have been reduced from 100 to 70 per cent. The increase in ejection fraction with the decreased workload occurred even in patients with ST-segment changes persisting during both acquisitions. Since an exercise blood pool study takes approximately two minutes to acquire, the length of time a patient can maximally exercise must be carefully anticipated so that the entire acquisition is obtained during the peak workload. If part of the acquisition is obtained at a reduced workload, the sensitivity of the study is reduced.

COMPARISON OF THALLIUM-201 AND TECHNETIUM-99m LABELED AGENTS AND VENTRICULAR FUNCTION STUDIES

Myocardial perfusion studies with thallium-201 or with ^{99m}Tc-labeled agents and ventricular function studies are all acceptable methods of evaluating patients with known or suspected CAD. None of these methods is clearly superior to the others. All of these methods have similar sensitivities when performed appropriately, using good techniques. The specificity of the perfusion studies may be better than the ventricular function studies, especially in women. However, there has not been a carefully controlled study to demonstrate the superiority of perfusion imaging in evaluating women with chest pain. Most institutions have developed one of these techniques for use in their institution, and the other techniques have assumed a lesser role. Perfusion imaging with either thallium-201 or ^{99m}Tc-labeled agents (with first-pass RNA) is more commonly used in most institutions for the detection of ischemic CAD than is the multigated acquisition technique. One study demonstrated that SPECT perfusion imaging provided more information than the exercise treadmill test or first-pass ventricular function analysis, but that the ventricular function study did provide independent information. The ability to combine analysis of function and perfusion with the ^{99m}Tc-labeled agents provides information that is not available from either study alone.

CONCLUSIONS

Radionuclide studies have an important role in the evaluation of patients with suspected or documented coronary artery disease. The clinical applications of these techniques have expanded during the last several years. The technical limitations need to be realized when ordering the studies. These tests need to be used with the understanding of Bayes' theorem. Both perfusion and ventricular function studies provide additional information to the stress electrocardiogram in the diagnosis of coronary artery disease. These radionuclide studies also provide prognostic information beyond that of the clinical descriptors. More quantitative techniques may make these studies even more useful in the future.

Bibliography

Becker LC, Silverman KJ, Bulkley BH, et al: Value of early thallium-201 scintigraphy and gated blood pool imaging for predicting mortality in patients with acute myocardial infarction. Ann NY Acad Sci 77:450–469, 1982.

Beller GA, Gibson RS: Sensitivity, specificity and prognostic significance of noninvasive testing for occult or known coronary disease. Prog Cardiovasc Dis 29:241–270, 1987.

Berman DS, Kiat H, Maddahi J: The new Tc-99m myocardial perfusion imaging agents: Tc-99m sestamibi and Tc-99m teboroxime. Circulation 84(3); (Suppl I): I-7–I-21, 1991.

Borer JS, Miller D, Schreiber T, et al: Radionuclide cineangiography in acute myocardial infarction: Role in prognostication. Semin Nucl Med 17:89–94, 1987.

Borges-Neto S, Coleman RE, Potts JM, Jones RH: Combined exercise radionuclide angiography and single photon emission computed tomography perfusion studies for assessment of coronary artery disease. Semin Nucl Med 21:223–229, 1991.

Boucher CA, Brewster DC, Darling RC, et al: Determination of cardiac risk by dipyridamole-thallium imaging before peripheral vascular surgery. N Engl J Med 312:389–394, 1985.

Gibbons RJ, Lee KL, Pryor D, et al: The use of radionuclide angiography in the diagnosis of coronary artery disease—a logistic regression analysis. Circulation 68:740–746, 1983.

Gupta NC, Esterbrooks DJ, Hilleman DE, Mohiuddin SM: Comparison of adenosine and exercise thallium-201 single-photon emission computed tomography (SPECT) myocardial perfusion imaging. Jour Am Coll Cardiol 19(2):248–257, 1992.

Jones RH, McEwan P, Newman GE, et al: Accuracy of diagnosis of coronary artery disease by radionuclide measurement of left ventricular function during rest and exercise. Circulation 64:586–601, 1981.

Kotler TS, Diamond GA: Exercise thallium-201 scintigraphy in the diagnosis and prognosis of coronary artery disease. Ann Intern Med 113(9):684–702, 1990.

Leppo JA: Dipyridamole-thallium imaging: The lazy man's stress test. J Nucl Med 30:281–287, 1989.

Melvin JA, Piret LJ, Vanbutsele RJM, et al: Diagnostic value of exercise electrocardiography and thallium myocardial scintigraphy in patients without previous myocardial infarction: A Bayesian approach. Circulation 63:1019–1024, 1981.

Morris KG, Palmeri ST, Califf RM, et al: Value of radionuclide angiography for predicting specific cardiac events after acute myocardial infarction. Am J Cardiol 55:318–324, 1985.

Rozanski A, Berman DS: The efficacy of cardiovascular nuclear medicine exercise studies. Semin Nucl Med 17:104–120, 1987.

114 Diseases of the Myocardium

Michael J. Kelley

Heart disease affecting the heart muscle has been termed *cardiomyopathy*. The cardiomyopathies in adults can be classified into two main groups—the primary and the secondary forms. In primary cardiomyopathies, the pathologic process involves the myocardium rather than the valves and the cause is unknown and not part of a disorder affecting other organs. Secondary cardiomyopathies are conditions in which the cause is known or in which the heart disease is a manifestation of a systemic disease process. The term *ischemic cardiomyopathy* has been used to refer to myocardial disease in which the etiology is severe, chronic coronary artery disease.

Three functional subgroups of primary cardiomyopathy are identified by certain pathophysiologic abnormalities. In order of frequency they are (1) dilated or "congestive" cardiomyopathy, (2) hypertrophic cardiomyopathy, and (3) restrictive cardiomyopathy. The secondary cardiomyopathies include entities in which the heart is one of the targets for a systemic disease such as amyloidosis (the most common), hemochromatosis, glycogen storage disease, Friedreich's ataxia, sarcoid, Fabry's disease, or scleroderma.

DILATED CARDIOMYOPATHY

The two key characteristics of dilated cardiomyopathy are increased left ventricular chamber size and reduced left ventricular systolic performance. Left ventricular filling pressure is usually elevated owing to the poorly contracting left ventricle. The right ventricle and both atria are frequently dilated. The cardiac enlargement is often accompanied by congestive heart failure.

In most cases of dilated cardiomyopathy, the etiology is unknown, but many cases probably represent the end result of myocardial damage produced by a variety of metabolic, infectious, or toxic agents, including alcohol. The clinical course is characterized by progressive deterioration, with most patients succumbing within four years after the onset of symptoms.

Postmortem examination of the heart reveals enlargement and dilatation of all four chambers and intrinsically normal cardiac valves. The left ventricle frequently contains thrombi, and the coronary arteries are usually normal. Microscopic examination discloses interstitial and perivascular fibrosis and myocardial cell degeneration.

Radiographic Findings

Most symptomatic patients with dilated cardiomyopathy present with cardiomegaly and left ventricular and left atrial enlargement (Figs. 114–1 and 114–2). The left atrial appendage is usually not enlarged, and the aorta is normal. Pulmonary venous hypertension is often present but appears less severe than the degree of cardiomegaly (Figs. 114–1 and 114–2). The right heart is frequently enlarged (Fig. 114–3). When right heart failure supervenes, the azygos vein and superior vena cava may be dilated (Fig. 114–3). The aorta is invariably normal (Figs. 114–1 to 114–3). The heart size may occasionally assume gigantic proportions and simulate the appearance of a large pericardial effusion (Fig. 114–4).

Patients with ischemic cardiomyopathy secondary to severe coronary artery disease can present with clinical, electrocardiographic, and radiographic features similar to those with a dilated cardiomyopathy. Since the prognosis and therapy of these two types of patients may vary considerably, it is advantageous to separate them into their appropriate diagnostic categories. Chest fluoroscopy has proved helpful in identifying coronary artery calcification in those patients with an ischemic basis for the cardiomyopathy. Occasionally, the chest radiograph will provide this information (Fig. 114–5). In the secondary forms of cardiomyopathy, features of the underlying systemic disease may be manifested on the chest radiograph (Fig. 114–6).

Echocardiographic Findings

Both M-mode and two-dimensional echocardiography aid in the assessment of left ventricular dysfunction in dilated cardiomyopathy. Besides excluding concomitant valvular or pericardial disease, they are useful in evaluating the size of the ventricles and the thickness of their walls. There is left ventricular enlargement in both end-diastole and end-systole (Fig. 114–7), and the ejection fraction and fractional fiber shortening are reduced. Approximately 30 per cent of patients will have echo-detected ventricular thrombus. Valve motion may reflect a low cardiac output state and reduced myocardial performance. This is manifested by premature closure of the semilunar valves and delayed end-diastolic closure and reduced opening velocity of the atrioventricular valves. Some patients have regional wall motion abnormalities that may be indistinguishable from ischemic cardiomyopathy and therefore, in these patients, an absolute distinction cannot be made by echocardiography alone.

Radionuclide Studies

Thallium-201 imaging at rest and following exercise is of only limited value in distinguishing left ventricular enlargement due to

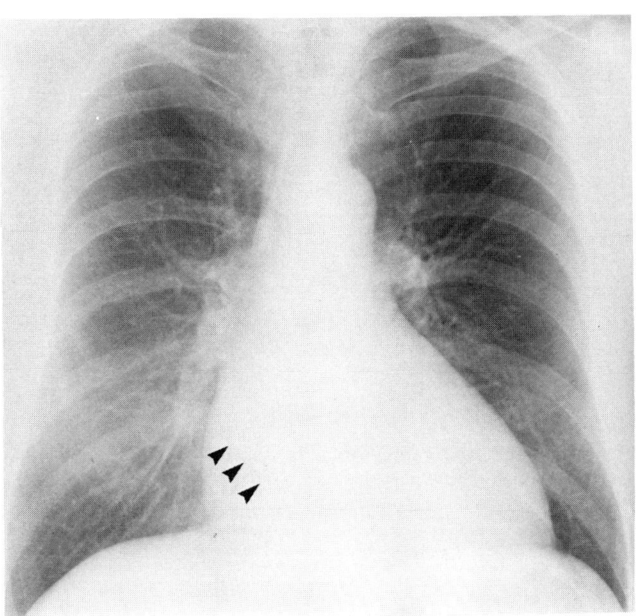

Figure 114–1. Dilated cardiomyopathy. Posterolateral chest radiograph demonstrates upper lobe vascular redistribution (mild pulmonary venous hypertension) and cardiomegaly with left ventricular and left atrial *(arrowheads)* enlargement. The thoracic aorta appears normal.

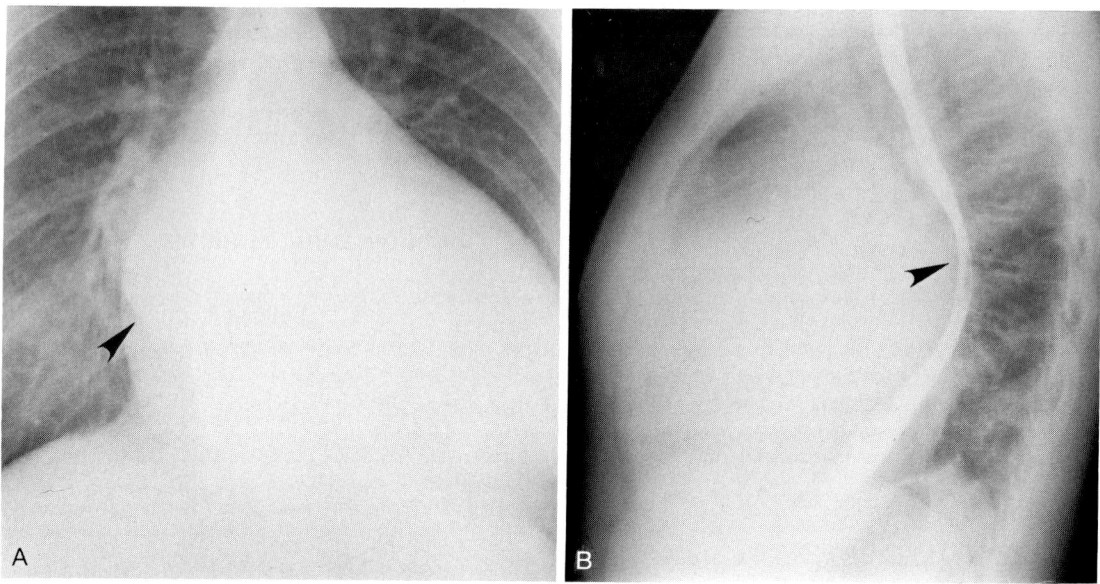

Figure 114–2. Dilated cardiomyopathy. *A,* Posteroanterior (PA) chest radiograph. *B,* Lateral view. The degree of pulmonary venous hypertension is greater than in Figure 114–1. There is marked cardiomegaly with left ventricular and left atrial enlargement *(arrowhead)*. The aorta appears normal.

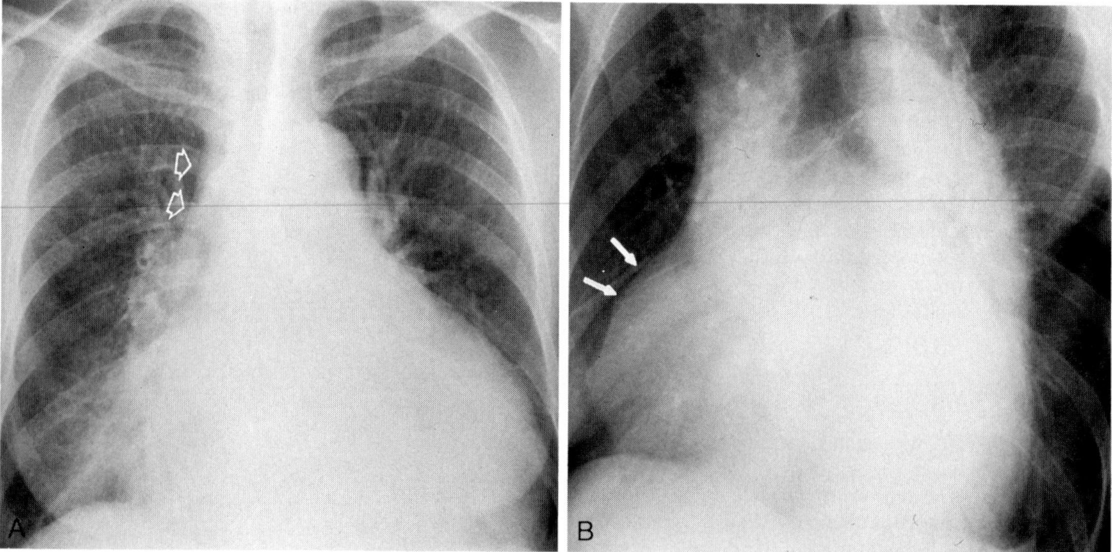

Figure 114–3. Dilated cardiomyopathy. *A,* PA chest radiograph. *B,* Left anterior oblique (LAO) view. Moderate pulmonary venous hypertension and cardiomegaly are present. In this patient with biventricular heart failure, note the prominent azygos vein and superior vena cava *(arrows)* in the PA view and right heart enlargement *(arrows)* in the LAO view.

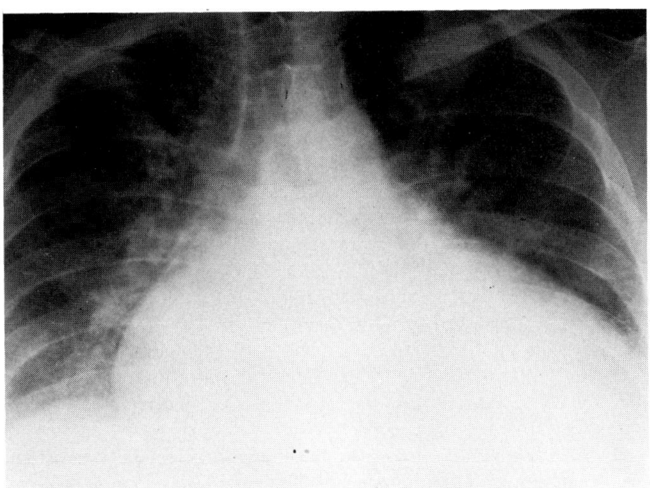

Figure 114–4. Dilated cardiomyopathy. PA chest radiograph shows massive cardiomegaly simulating a pericardial effusion.

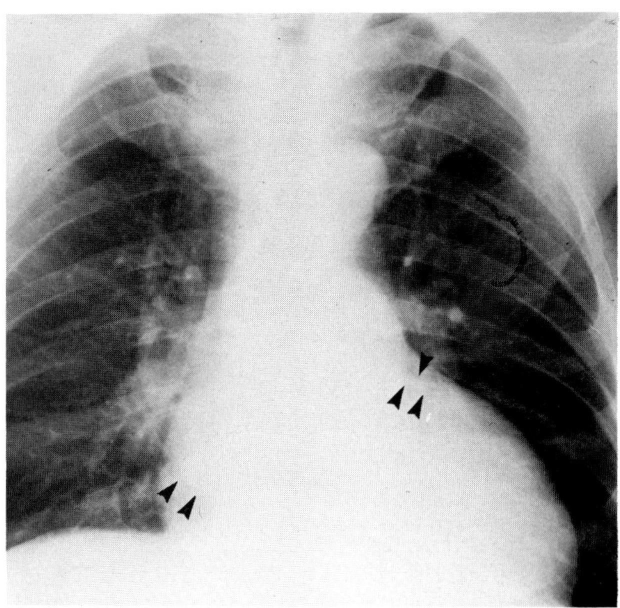

Figure 114–5. Ischemic cardiomyopathy. PA chest radiograph reveals mild pulmonary venous hypertension (redistribution) and left ventricular and left atrial *(double arrowheads)* enlargement. Left coronary artery calcification is evident just medial to the concavity of the mid–left heart border *(three arrowheads)*.

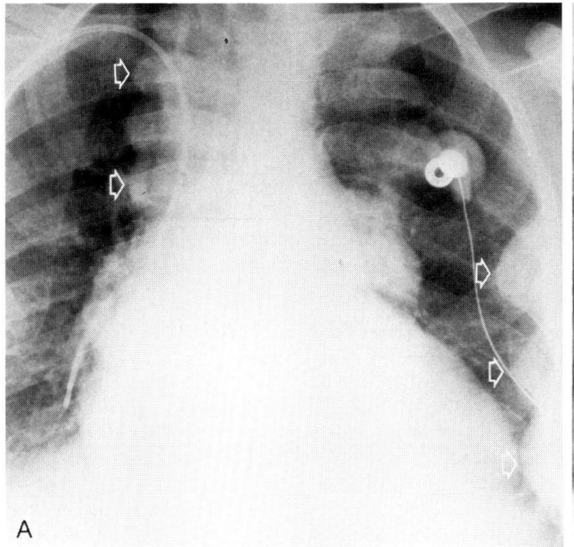

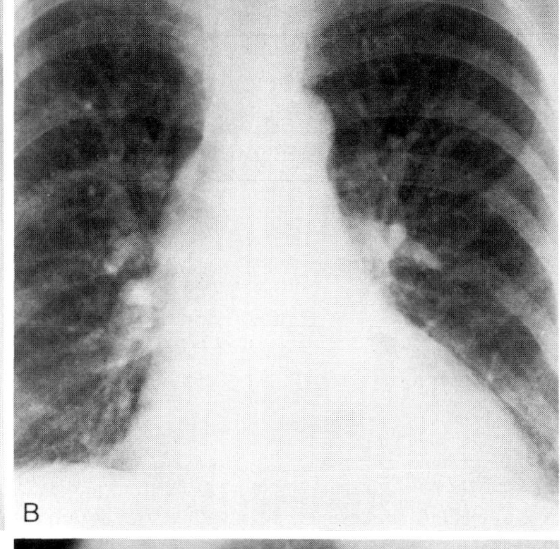

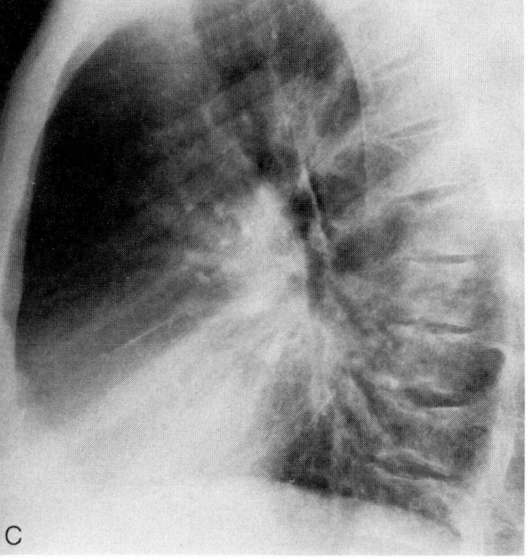

Figure 114–6. *A,* **Secondary cardiomyopathies.** Two patients with severe anemia. PA chest radiograph in a patient with thalassemia. Cardiomegaly is evident, and there are numerous extrapleural densities along the left chest wall and right paraspinous region *(arrows)*, indicating sites of extramedullary hematopoiesis. PA *(B)* and lateral *(C)* chest radiographs in a patient with sickle cell anemia. Pulmonary venous hypertension and cardiomegaly are present. Note the typical features of sickle cell anemia in the thoracic spine (biconcave centra, osteoporosis, and sparse, sclerotic trabeculae).

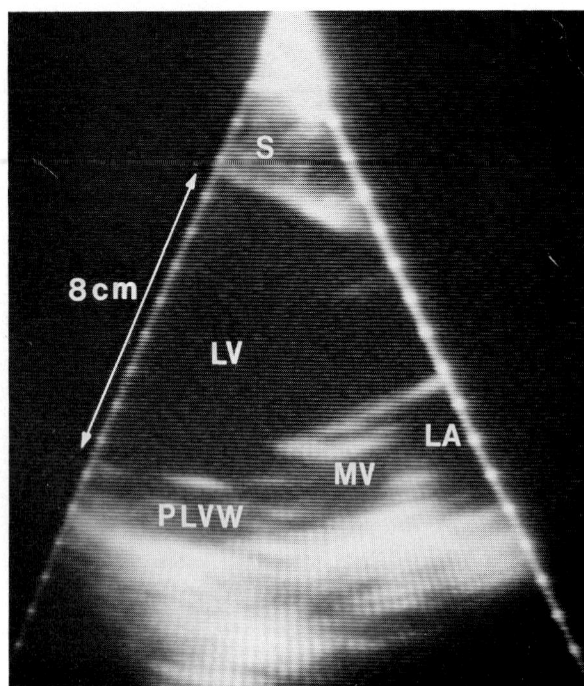

Figure 114–7. Dilated cardiomyopathy. Two-dimensional long-axis view echocardiogram taken in systole demonstrates dilated (8 cm) left ventricular cavity (LV) with thinning of the posterior left ventricular wall (PLVW) and septum (S). (LA = left atrium; MV = mitral valve.)

dilated cardiomyopathy from that due to coronary artery disease, since both conditions may be associated with resting and postexercise perfusion defects. Since the coronary patients may have had multiple infarctions and usually have three-vessel coronary disease, the thallium scan may be difficult to interpret.

Radionuclide studies of the left ventricle in patients with dilated cardiomyopathy reveal elevated end-diastolic and end-systolic volumes, regional wall motion abnormalities, and reduced ejection fractions. This technique may be helpful in following the patient's response to therapy. Serial radionuclide assessment of left ventricular performance is also of value in the initial assessment and subsequent follow-up of patients who are receiving certain medications for treatment of malignancy. Medications such as doxorubicin (Adriamycin) may lead to the development of a cardiomyopathic state, and the radionuclide studies have been shown to be helpful in identifying patients at risk for this complication.

Angiocardiographic Findings

The left ventricle in patients with dilated cardiomyopathy is significantly enlarged, with marked reduction in wall motion (Fig. 114–8). Filling defects in the apex of the left ventricle may occasionally be observed. Mild mitral regurgitation is often present. Coronary arteriography usually reveals normal vessels (Fig. 114–8).

HYPERTROPHIC CARDIOMYOPATHY

There are two subgroups of hypertrophic cardiomyopathy—the obstructive and the nonobstructive types. Both forms are characterized by asymmetrical septal hypertrophy (septal thickness 1.3 or more times the posterior wall thickness), a small left ventricular cavity, reduced left ventricular diastolic compliance, and normal to increased left ventricular systolic function. The myopathic process is associated with myocardial cell disarray and increased connective tissue content.

In hypertrophic obstructive cardiomyopathy (HOCM), a dynamic pressure gradient in the subaortic area divides the left ventricle into a high-pressure apical region and a lower-pressure subaortic region. Thus, the term *idiopathic hypertrophic subaortic stenosis* (IHSS) was initially used to describe this disorder. The hypertrophy typically affects the septum, resulting in *asymmetrical septal hypertrophy* (ASH). The level of obstruction is frequently at the point where the papillary muscles abut the septum, obliterating the mid–left ventricular cavity. The anterior leaflet, the chordae, and the anterior papillary muscle of the mitral apparatus move anteriorly in systole (instead of posteriorly). This abnormal *systolic anterior motion* (SAM) is thought to be due to a Venturi effect created by increased left ventricular outflow turbulence, resulting in a lower pressure in the left ventricular outflow tract that pulls the anterior mitral apparatus forward.

Hypertrophic cardiomyopathy is apparently genetically transmitted as an autosomal dominant trait. The majority of patients experience no symptoms.

Radiographic Findings

The findings are variable. Pulmonary vascularity is usually normal in the asymptomatic patient and may be redistributed in patients with dyspnea. The heart size may vary from normal to markedly enlarged. There does not appear to be any correlation between the heart size and the severity of the left ventricular outflow gradient. Straightening or convexity of the mid–left heart border may be seen (Fig. 114–9) and is thought to be related to septal hypertrophy. Since mitral regurgitation invariably exists when obstruction is present in hypertrophic cardiomyopathy, left atrial enlargement is frequently observed (Fig. 114–9). Calcification of the mitral annulus has been reported in hypertrophic obstructive cardiomyopathy. The thoracic aorta is usually normal.

Echocardiographic Findings

The classic echocardiographic feature of hypertrophic cardiomyopathy is left ventricular hypertrophy. The finding of a thickened septum that is 1.3 or more times the thickness of the posterior wall (measured in diastole) leads to the diagnosis of asymmetric septal hypertrophy (ASH) (Fig. 114–10). The septum is at least 15 mm in thickness (normal < 11 mm). The left ventricular outflow tract is narrowed by the thickened interventricular septum anteriorly and the anterior leaflet of the mitral valve posteriorly. When a pressure gradient exists, there is abnormal systolic anterior motion (SAM) of the anterior leaflet of the mitral valve. Other echocardiographic findings in HOCM include (1) reduced septal motion, (2) reduced rate of closure of the mitral valve in mid-diastole, and (3) partial systolic closure or systolic fluttering of the aortic valve.

Radionuclide Studies

Thallium-201 myocardial imaging can be used to determine the relative thickness of the septum and free wall when echocardiographic evaluation is technically difficult. Gated radionuclide ventriculography permits evaluation of the size and motion of the septum and left ventricle. This is best appreciated in the steep left anterior oblique projection.

Magnetic Resonance Imaging

Qualitative and quantitative evaluation of ventricular dysfunction in hypertrophic cardiomyopathy with magnetic resonance imaging

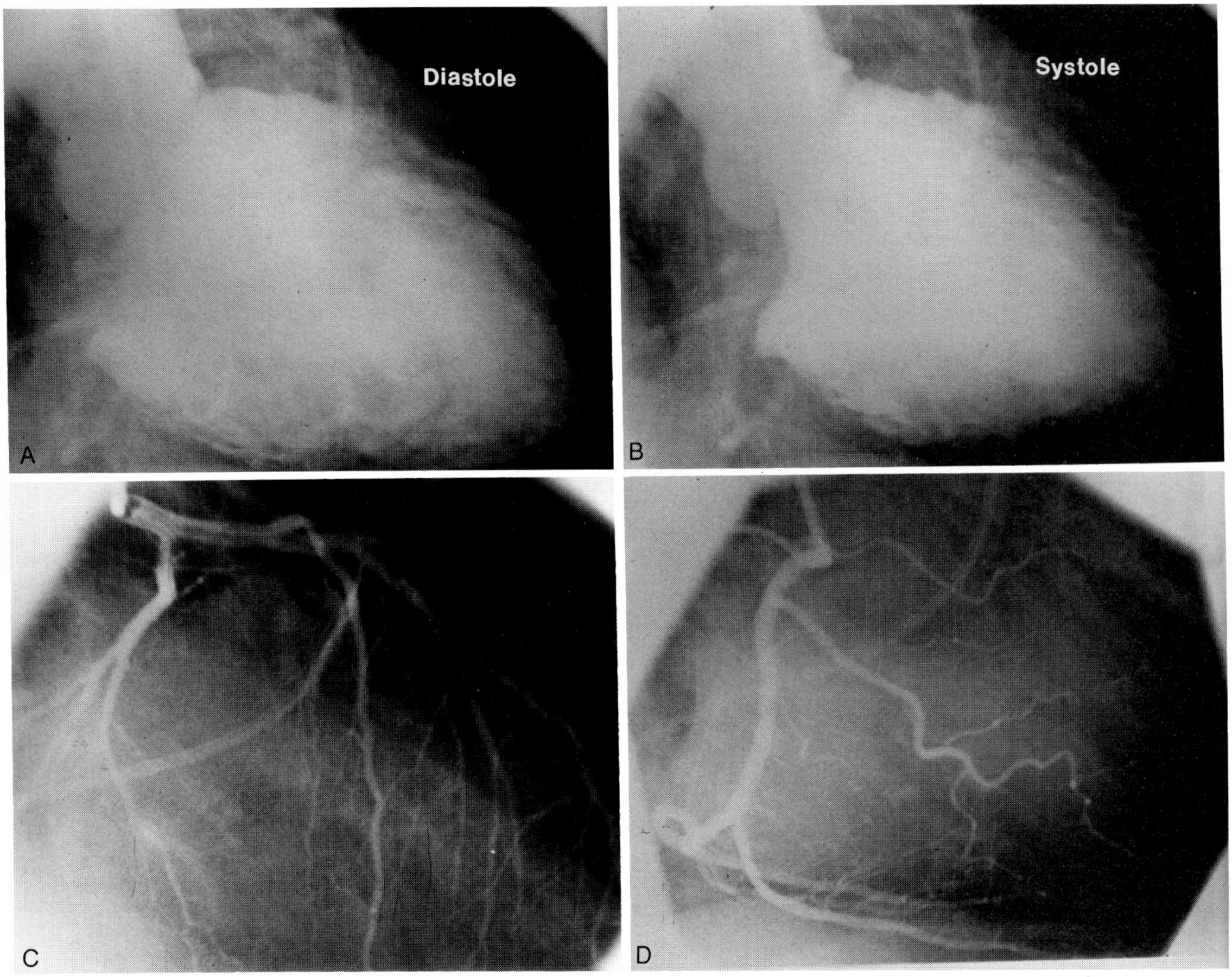

Figure 114–8. Dilated cardiomyopathy. Left ventriculogram in right anterior oblique projection in *(A)* diastole and *(B)* systole. Diffuse severe hypokinesis is noted involving all wall segments. The ejection fraction was calculated at 20 per cent. Left *(C)* and right *(D)* coronary angiograms in the same patient are normal.

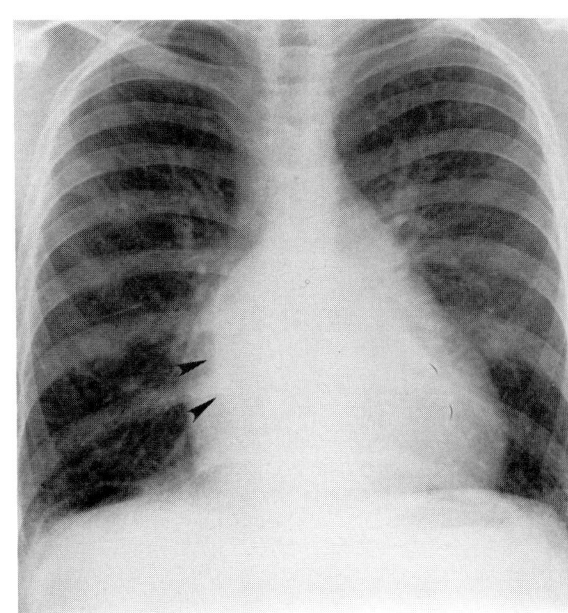

Figure 114–9. Hypertrophic cardiomyopathy. PA chest radiograph demonstrates pulmonary vascular redistribution, normal heart size, straightened left heart border, and left atrial enlargement *(arrowheads)*.

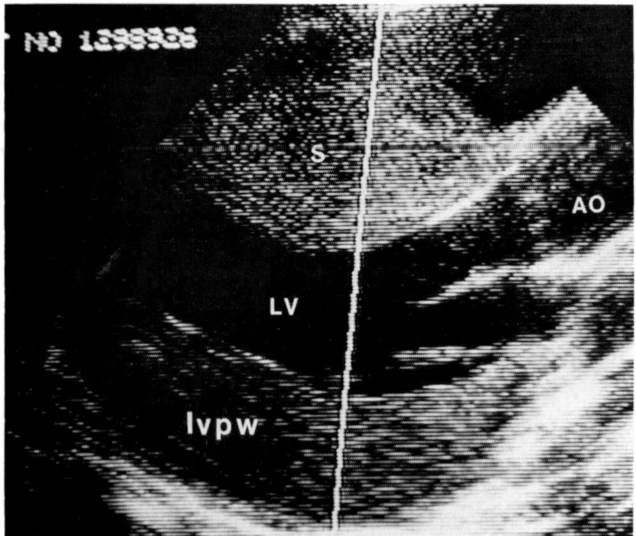

Figure 114–10. Hypertrophic obstructive cardiomyopathy. Two-dimensional echocardiogram shown in precordial long-axis view. There is asymmetrical hypertrophy of the septum (s) and the posterior left ventricular wall (lvpw). (AO = aorta; LV = left ventricular cavity.) (Courtesy of Patricia Burrows, M.D., and Jeffrey Smallhorn, M.D., Toronto, Canada.)

(MRI) is one of the more common indications for this modality. Gated static, mutilevel spin-echo as well as gated dynamic, gradient-echo (''cine'') techniques have been employed.

Angiocardiographic Findings

The right anterior oblique left ventricular angiocardiogram in hypertrophic obstructive cardiomyopathy frequently demonstrates hypertrophied papillary muscles that cause obliteration of the left ventricular cavity in systole. Mitral regurgitation, usually of a mild degree, is best assessed in this projection (Fig. 114–11). The diagnostic angiographic features, however, require a cranial left anterior oblique left ventriculogram. In this view, in systole, the hypertrophied septum impinges on the left ventricular outflow tract. The anterior leaflet of the mitral valve, instead of moving posteriorly, moves anteriorly into the outflow tract and contacts the hypertrophied septum (Fig. 114–11). At the point of this contact a V- or W-shaped radiolucent line may be visualized. This represents the abnormally moving mitral apparatus as it contacts the septum. In patients with symmetric or nonobstructive hypertrophic cardiomyopathy, the left ventriculogram will demonstrate signs of hypertrophy but a normal systolic relationship between the mitral valve and the septum.

RESTRICTIVE CARDIOMYOPATHY

Of the three major subgroups of the cardiomyopathies, the restrictive variety is the least common in western countries. The functional hallmark of the restrictive cardiomyopathies is abnormal disastolic function due to rigid ventricular walls that impede ventricular filling. These ventricles are characterized primarily by abnormal stiffness. Systolic emptying of the ventricles is usually unimpaired. The restrictive cardiomyopathies share with constrictive pericarditis normal or nearly normal systolic function and abnormal ventricular filling. The characteristic hemodynamic feature in both conditions is the ventricular pressure tracing, which shows a deep and rapid early decline at the onset of diastole and a rapid plateau in early diastole.

The most common primary restrictive cardiomyopathy in the United States is a nondilated myopathy associated with reduced ventricular compliance and normal systolic ventricular function. Ventricular dimensions are normal, and the atria are dilated. Other less common primary forms are associated with Löffler's endocarditis (eosinophilia, fever, ventricular thrombus) or endomyocardial fibrosis.

Amyloid heart disease is the most common secondary restrictive cardiomyopathy. The disease usually appears in elderly patients who present with predominant right heart failure. The myocardium is usually uniformly thickened, and pericardial effusion is not uncommon. Other causes of secondary restrictive cardiomyopathy include hemochromatosis, glycogen storage disease, endomyocardial fibrosis, and neoplastic infiltration.

Radiographic Findings

In the most common clinical presentation of cardiac amyloidosis, there is congestive heart failure due to systolic dysfunction. Moderate cardiomegaly is often demonstrated on the chest radiograph. This form of the disease cannot be distinguished clinically from congestive cardiomyopathy. A second presentation of cardiac amyloidosis is that of a restrictive cardiomyopathy, with right-sided congestive failure dominating the clinical picture. The heart size in these patients is usually normal, but the superior vena cava and azygos vein may be enlarged (Fig. 114–12).

Echocardiographic Findings

In cardiac amyloid, increased thickness of the walls of the ventricles and a normal to small-sized left ventricular cavity are noted. Wall excursions may be reduced. The ventricular walls may demonstrate a ''granular'' appearance, presumably due to amyloid deposition.

Hemodynamic/Angiographic Findings

The hemodynamic features of restrictive cardiomyopathy simulate those of chronic constrictive pericarditis. In both conditions the ventricular pressure tracing shows a dip and rapid early decline at the onset of diastole, with a rapid rise to a plateau in early diastole. This dip and plateau have been called the ''square root sign'' and are manifested in the atrial pressure tracing as a prominent Y descent followed by a rapid rise and plateau.

Although the presence of pericardial calcification (best detected by fluoroscopy or computed tomography) is neither absolutely sensitive nor specific for constrictive pericarditis, its presence in a patient in whom the diagnosis rests between constrictive cardiomyopathy and constrictive pericarditis lends strong support to the latter diagnosis.

In contrast to the early accelerated diastolic filling found in constrictive pericarditis, the left ventricle in cardiac amyloid is marked by an impaired rate of early diastolic filling due to the stiff ventricle. This finding requires a frame-by-frame analysis of the left ventriculogram.

The movement of the coronary arteries in systole and diastole has been noted to be impaired in constrictive pericarditis. This may serve as another differentiating point in difficult cases. In some patients, the final diagnosis can be made only after endomyocardial biopsy or exploratory thoracotomy.

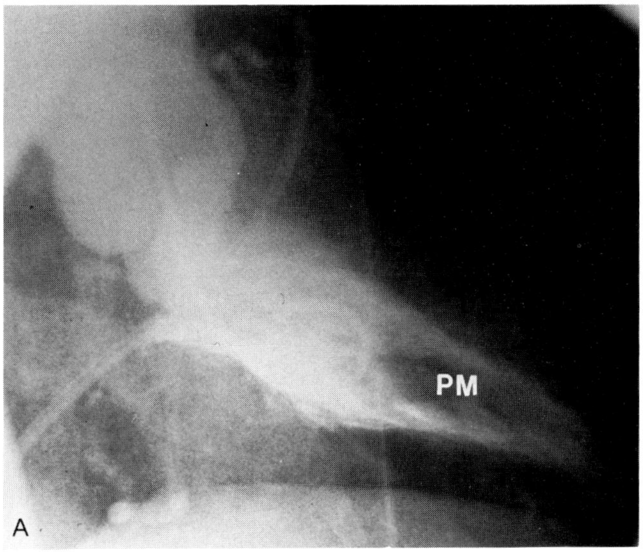

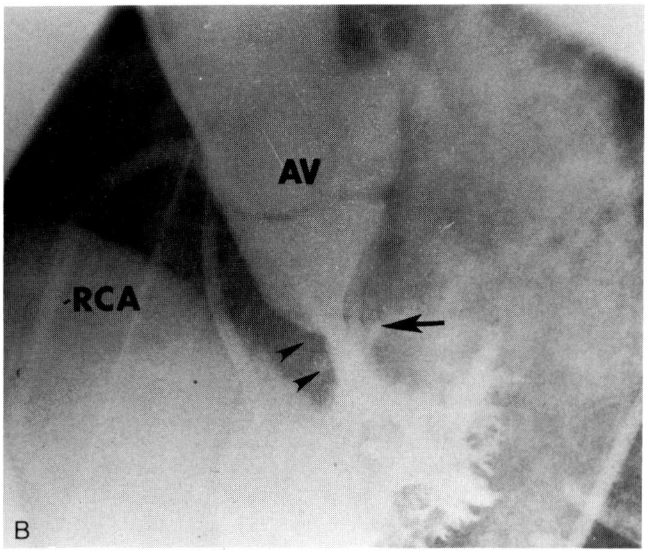

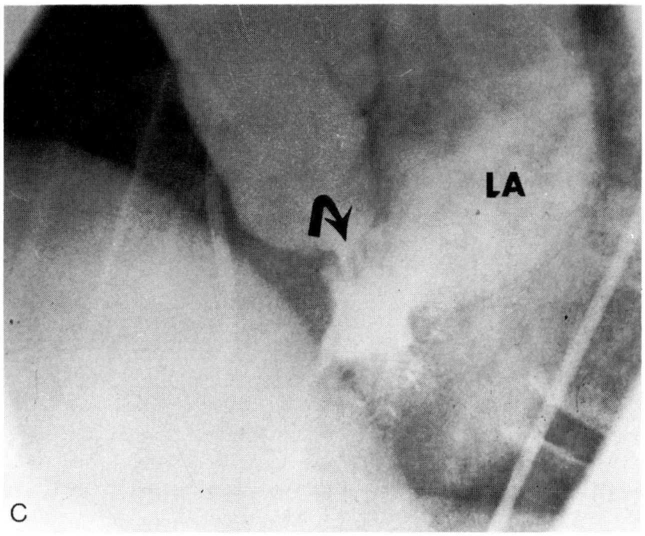

Figure 114–11. Hypertrophic obstructive cardiomyopathy. *A,* RAO cine left ventriculogram and cranial LAO cine left ventriculogram in mid *(B)* and late *(C)* systole. In the RAO view, a hypertrophied posteromedial papillary muscle (PM) is present. In the LAO view *(B),* in mid-systole, the hypertrophied septum *(arrowheads)* together with the anterior leaflet of the mitral valve *(arrow)* impinges on the left ventricular outflow tract. This corresponds to the systolic anterior motion (SAM) seen on the echocardiogram (see Fig. 114–10). In the LAO view *(C),* in late systole, the anterior leaflet of the mitral valve contacts the septum, creating a W-shaped radiolucent line *(curved arrow).* Note the significant amount of mitral regurgitation into the slightly enlarged left atrium (LA). (AV = aortic valve; RCA = right coronary artery.)

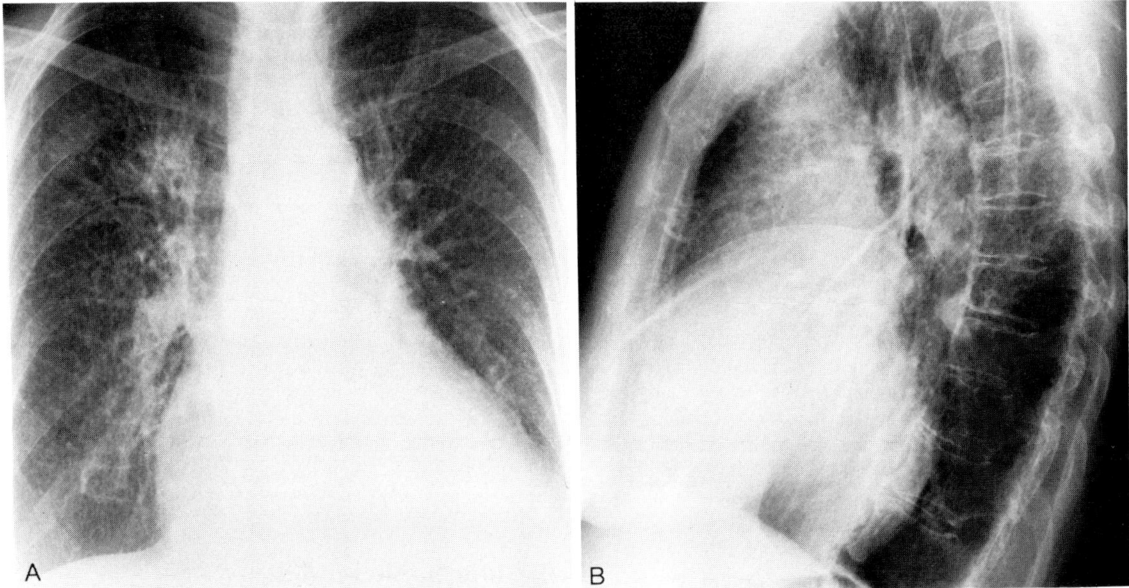

Figure 114–12. Restrictive cardiomyopathy. *A,* PA view. *B,* Lateral view. Moderate pulmonary venous hypertension and cardiomegaly are present. Myocardial biopsy revealed amyloid infiltration.

Bibliography

Alexander J, Dainak N, Berger HJ, et al: Serial assessment of doxorubicin cardiotoxicity with quantitative radionuclide angiocardiography. N Engl J Med 301:1143, 1979.

Alexander J, Kelley MJ, Cohen LS, Langou RA: The angiographic appearance of the coronary arteries in constrictive pericarditis. Radiology 131:609, 1979.

Benotti JR, Grossman W, Cohn PF: The clinical profile of restrictive cardiomyopathy. Circulation 61:1206, 1980.

Clark CE, Henry WL, Epstein SE: Familial prevalence and genetic transmission of idiopathic hypertrophic subaortic stenosis. N Engl J Med 289:709, 1973.

Goodwin JF: Congestive and hypertrophic cardiomyopathies. A decade of study. Lancet 1:731, 1970.

Green CE, Kelley MJ, Higgins CB: Etiologic significance of enlargement of the left atrial appendage in adults. Radiology 142:21, 1982.

Greenberg J, Boucher CA, Okada RD, et al: Incidence of regional wall motion abnormalities in primary congestive cardiomyopathy. J Am Coll Cardiol 1:723, 1983.

Hansen AT, Eskildsen P, Gotzsche H: Pressure curves from the right auricle and right ventricle in chronic constrictive pericarditis. Circulation 3:881, 1951.

Henry WL, Clark CE, Griffith JM, et al: Mechanism of left ventricular outflow obstruction in patients with obstructive asymmetrical septal hypertrophy (idiopathic hypertrophic subaortic stenosis). Am J Cardiol 35:337, 1975.

Hirschmann JV: Pericardial constriction. Am Heart J 96:110, 1978.

Johnson AD, Laiken SL, Shabetai R: Non diagnosis of ischemic cardiomyopathy by detection of coronary artery calcification. Am Heart J 96:521, 1978.

Kelley MJ, Jaffe CC, Kleinman CS: Cardiac Imaging in Infants and Children. Philadelphia, WB Saunders Company, 1982, pp 233, 242.

Kelley MJ, Newell JD: Chest radiography and cardiac fluoroscopy in coronary artery disease. Cardiol Clin 1983, Vol 1, No 4.

Krozon I, Glassman E: Mitral ring calcification in idiopathic hypertrophic subaortic stenosis. Am J Cardiol 42:60, 1978.

Prohost GM, Vignola PA, McKusick KE, et al: Hypertrophic cardiomyopathy. Evaluation by gated cardiac blood pool scanning. Circulation 55:92, 1977.

Reeder GS, Tajik AJ, Seward JB: Left ventricular mural thombosis—echocardiographic diagnosis. Mayo Clin Proc 56:82–86, 1981.

Seward JB, Tajik AJ: Primary cardiomyopathies: Classification, pathophysiology, clinical recognition and management. Cardiovasc Clin 10:199, 1980.

Siqueira-Filho AG, Cunha CL, Tajik AJ, et al: M-mode and two-dimensional echocardiographic features in cardiac amyloidosis. Circulation 63:188, 1981.

Tyberg TI, Goodyer AV, Hurst VW III, et al: Left ventricular filling in differentiating restrictive amyloid cardiomyopathy and constrictive pericarditis. Am J Cardiol 47:791, 1981.

White RD, Paschal CB, Tkach JA, Carvlin MJ: Functional cardiovascular evaluation by magnetic resonance imaging. Top Magn Reson Imaging 2:31–48, 1990.

White RD, Ehman RL, Weinreb JC: Cardiovascular MR imaging: Current level of clinical activity. JMRI 2:365–370, 1992.

115 Diseases of the Pericardium

Michael J. Kelley

The clinical signs and symptoms of pericardial disease are usually diagnostic. The differential diagnosis, however, includes a variety of other conditions such as acute myocardial infarction, pleurisy, spontaneous pneumothorax, and mediastinal emphysema. As part of the diagnostic work-up of these diseases and those directly affecting the pericardium, the chest radiograph, the echocardiogram, and certain angiographic techniques play an important role. The following discussion will describe the various imaging features of a variety of diseases involving the pericardium.

Anatomy of the Pericardium

The pericardium consists of two components: a serous membrane (the visceral pericardium) that covers the outside of the heart and extends beyond the atria and ventricles onto the great vessels for 2 or 3 cm and a serous lined fibrous sac (the parietal pericardium). These two layers are closely apposed to each other in the healthy state, separated only by enough serous fluid (up to 50 ml) to make their surfaces slippery. Since the two surfaces are not attached, there is a potential space between them (the pericardial cavity). The reflection of the visceral pericardium around the vena cava and the pulmonary veins creates a U-shaped cul-de-sac in the dorsal wall of the pericardial cavity (the oblique pericardial sinus). Dorsally, between the arterial and venous attachments of the visceral pericardium there is a pericardium-lined passage, the transverse pericardial sinus. Caudal to the transverse sinus, the pericardium incompletely surrounds the pulmonary veins. The parietal pericardium is attached in varying degrees to all the structures surrounding it. Fibrous ligaments attach it ventrally to the manubrium and xiphoid process and dorsally to the vertebral column. The sac is attached to the central tendon and left side of the diaphragm.

The normal pericardium cannot be distinguished from the heart on the chest radiograph unless it is calcified or (rarely) if air occupies the pericardial sac. In the latter case, one can appreciate this thin membrane and its relationship to the heart and great vessels (Fig. 115–1). On the posteroanterior (PA) chest film, the cranial attachments of the pericardium are (from right to left) the lower third of the superior vena cava, the mid-portion of the ascending aorta, and the upper third of the pulmonary trunk. In some patients a pleuropericardial accumulation of fat may be observed as a density separate from the cardiopericardial silhouette. This "fat pad" appears as a triangular, semilucent density in the anterior cardiophrenic angle (Fig. 115–2). It is more frequently seen in obese patients and more common in the left cardiophrenic angle.

PERICARDIAL EFFUSION

Pericardial effusions may result from noninflammatory conditions such as heart failure, uremia, trauma (hemopericardium), connective tissue disease, or malignancy. Pericardial effusions typically accompany inflammation of the pericardium. Patients with acute pericarditis usually have typical chest pain. It is retrosternal or precordial and radiates to the trapezius and neck. It is aggravated by lying supine or breathing deeply and relieved by sitting up and leaning forward. Occasionally the pain may mimic that of acute myocardial infarction. The characteristic and pathognomonic finding is a pericardial friction rub. Etiologies of acute pericarditis include rheumatic heart disease; tuberculous, fungal, or viral infections; uremia; radiation; and drug hypersensitivity.

Radiographic Findings

The chest radiograph in patients with pericardial effusion may provide clues to the underlying etiology in cases of pericarditis

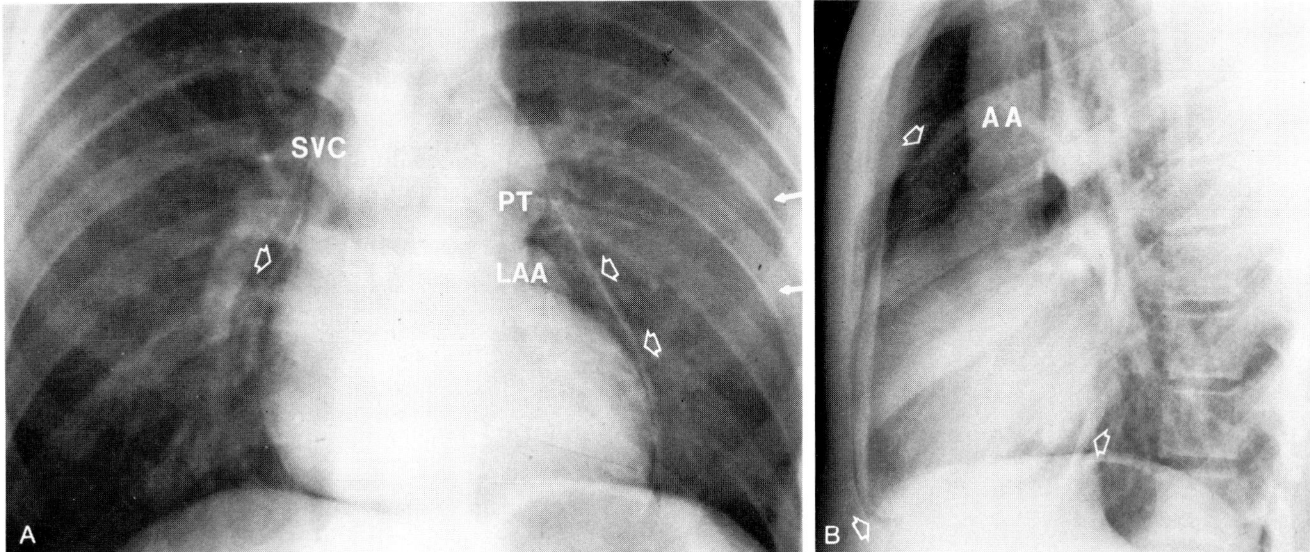

Figure 115–1. Pneumopericardium. *A,* Posteroanterior (PA) chest radiograph. *B,* Lateral view. Radiographs obtained of patient following stab wound to chest. Air within the pericardial sac delineates its relationship *(open arrows)* to the cardiac chambers and great vessels. Moderate left pneumothorax is also present *(arrows).* (AA = ascending aorta; LAA = left atrial appendage; PT = pulmonary trunk; SVC = superior vena cava.) (Courtesy of George Curry, M.D., Dallas, TX.)

secondary to tuberculosis, bacterial pneumonia, or malignancy. Radiographic and fluoroscopic findings of effusion may not be positive if the pericardial cavity contains less than 200 ml of fluid. When fluid collects in the pericardial cavity, the parietal pericardium is displaced outward and the cardiopericardial silhouette increases in size. As the normal pericardial attachments are displaced outward, the recesses between the various chambers and great vessels become obliterated. The increased fluid also has a damping effect on normal cardiac pulsations.

Findings of pericardial effusion at fluoroscopy include a uniform decrease in pulsations of the heart and a decreased ratio of pulsations from the heart as compared with the descending thoracic aorta. One may observe an increase in mediastinal width up to the level of the cranial pericardial attachments when the patient is moved from the erect into the Trendelenburg position as fluid shifts cranially. In the setting of the cardiac catheterization laboratory, when the question of possible cardiac perforation by a catheter arises, the absence of any change in the size and shape of the cardiopericardial silhouette during deep inspiration or following the Valsalva maneuver suggests the accumulation of blood within the pericardium.

In patients with large pericardial effusions (at least 250 ml), the chest radiograph usually demonstrates a symmetrically enlarged cardiopericardial silhouette. This appearance has been characterized as the "flask" or "water bottle" configuration (Fig. 115–3). The

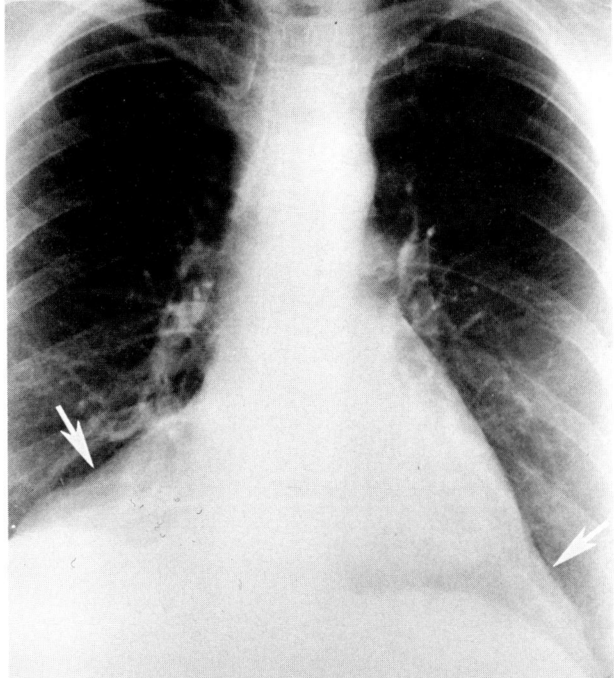

Figure 115–2. Pericardial fat pads. PA chest radiograph reveals triangular fat densities in the anterior cardiophrenic angles *(arrows).*

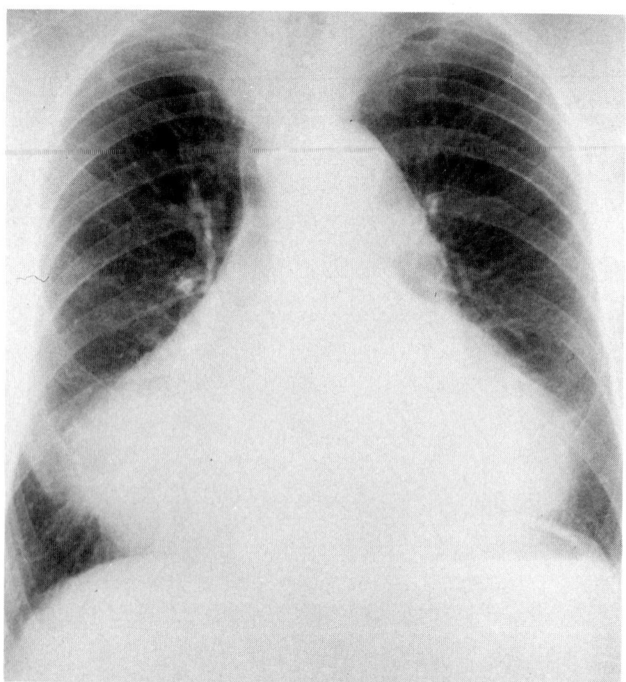

Figure 115–3. Pericardial effusion. PA chest radiograph shows symmetrical enlargement of the cardiopericardial silhouette, resulting in a "flask" or "water bottle" configuration. Note that the cardiac contours are smoothed out, the hilar vessels are obscured, and the cardiophrenic angles are acute. Note also that these findings exist against a background of normal pulmonary vascularity.

normal great vessel contours are smoothed out and the hilar vessels are obliterated. The cardiophrenic angles show acute rather than obtuse angles (Fig. 115–3). On the lateral view, there may be loss of the retrosternal "clear" space. Another radiographic clue to the presence of pericardial effusion is a rapid change in heart size (Fig. 115–4) or the presence of cardiomegaly without the usual radiographic findings of congestive heart failure (Figs. 115–3 and 115–4).

A more reliable radiographic sign of pericardial effusion is visualization of a water density separating the epicardial from the substernal fat "stripes" on the lateral chest film—the "epicardial fat pad sign." Normally, the layer of fat that accumulates over the anterior surface of the heart with increasing age is projected on end as a radiolucent band on the lateral chest radiograph. If the retrosternal soft tissues contain a moderate amount of fat, a second (often indistinguishable) radiolucent band exits anterior to the pericardium (Fig. 115–5). When fluid accumulates in the pericardial cavity, it creates a curvilinear water density between these two radiolucent fat "stripes" (Fig. 115–5). This water density should not exceed 2 mm in width and can be more accurately evaluated at fluoroscopy. In patients who have suspected pericardial effusion, the fat pad sign can be used to explain an increase in the cardiopericardial silhouette (Fig. 115–6). Absence of the fat line(s) has no significance. This sign is found in 15 to 25 per cent of patients with pericardial effusions. Another reliable sign, the "differential density" sign, has been described in patients with echocardiographically proven pericardial effusions. The findings consist of an increase in radiolucency at the margin of the heart (Fig. 115–7). It is observed most fre-

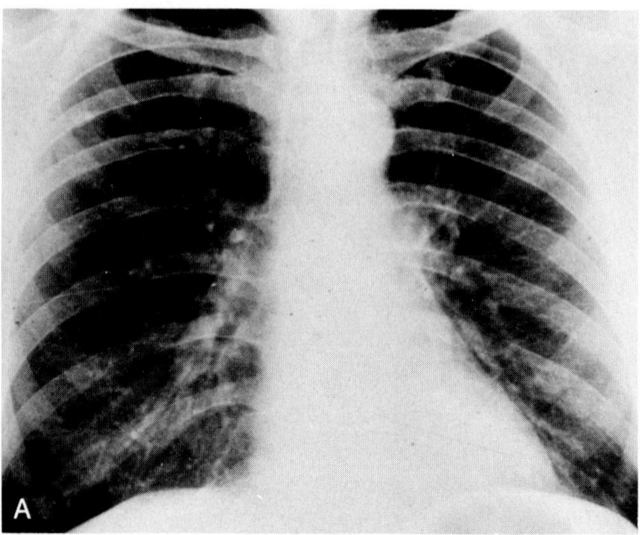

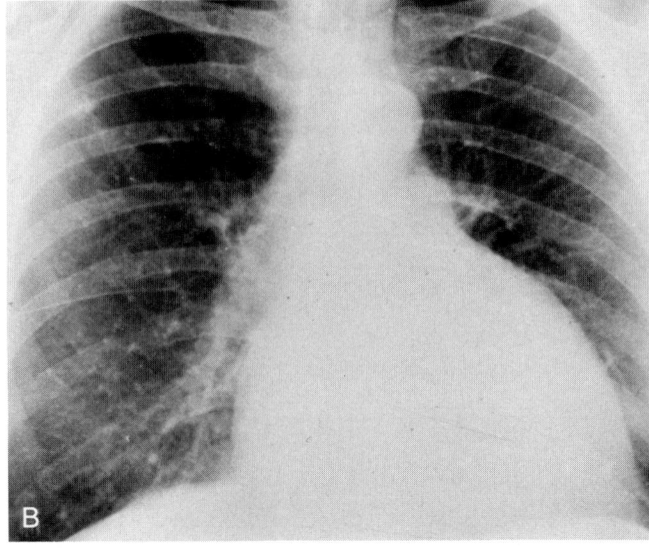

Figure 115–4. Pericardial effusion. *A* and *B*, PA chest radiographs obtained at a three-month interval. The patient had a pericardial friction rub and a moderate pericardial effusion by echo at the time of the second radiograph. This rapid change in the size of the cardiopericardial silhouette with no change in the normal pulmonary vascular pattern should suggest the diagnosis of pericardial effusion.

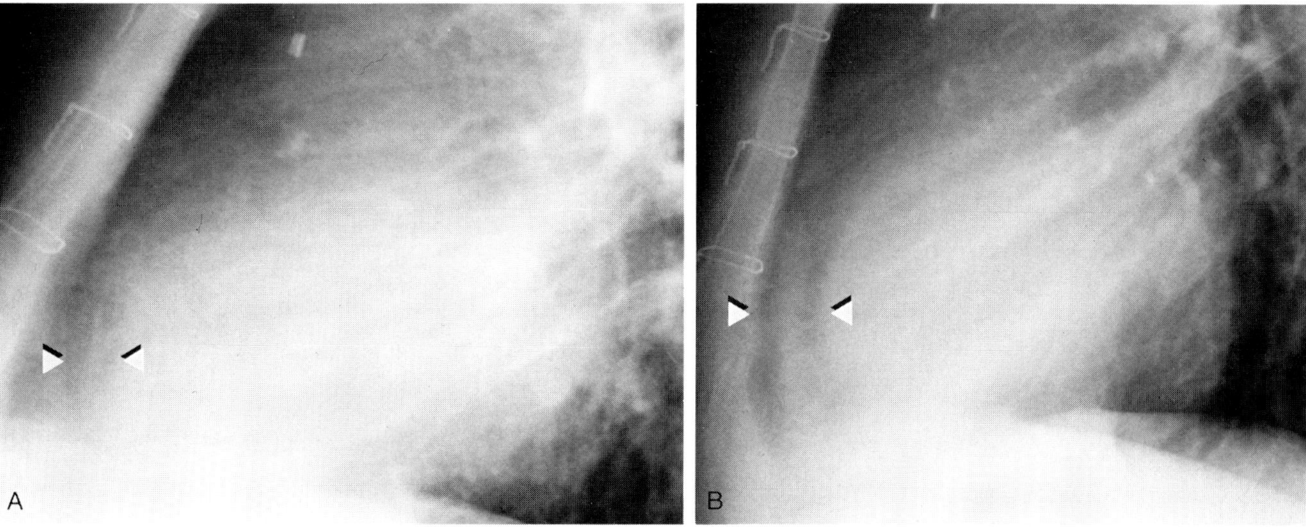

Figure 115–5. Pericardial effusion. Lateral chest radiographs in a patient who had previous coronary artery bypass graft surgery. *A,* The retrosternal tissue contains a moderate amount of fat, and this allows the thin (2 mm) pericardial water density to be distinguished from the deeper fat overlying the surface of the heart *(arrowheads)*. *B,* The patient has developed a moderate pericardial effusion and the water density has increased to 1.5 cm, reflecting fluid in the pericardial sac *(arrowheads)*. (Courtesy of J. T. T. Chen, M.D., Durham, NC.)

quently on the PA chest radiograph near the cardiac apex but may also be seen within the posterior aspect of the cardiopericardial silhouette on the lateral view or along the right atrial border. The basis for this sign is thought to relate to the slight difference in contrast that exists between pericardial fluid and the blood and muscle of the heart.

Echocardiographic Findings

Echocardiography is the most accurate and rapid method for detecting and quantifying pericardial effusion. Accumulation of pericardial fluid creates an anechoic space between the posterior left ventricular wall and the posterior parietal pericardium. In larger effusions, a similar echo-free space exists between the anterior right ventricular wall and the anterior parietal pericardium and chest wall.

The technique is semiquantitative: very small effusions (50 to 100 ml) are imaged only posteriorly, with separation of pericardial and epicardial echoes only in systole; small to moderate effusions (100 to 300 ml) are imaged only posteriorly throughout the cardiac cycle; and large effusions (300 ml) are imaged both anteriorly and posteriorly (Fig. 115–8). Because of the oblique pericardial sinus, the echo-free space disappears behind the left atrium unless massive pericardial effusion is present (Fig. 115–8*A*).

Echocardiography is usually accurate in the diagnosis of pericardial effusion. Occasionally the diagnosis may be confused with a left pleural effusion, an unusually large left atrium, a pulmonary infiltrate, or a large hiatus hernia. Two-dimensional echocardiography is particularly useful in separating pleural effusions from pericardial effusions (Fig. 115–8). Moderate to large pericardial effusions are associated with an excessive swinging of the heart, which may create the false-positive appearance of mitral prolapse or paradoxical septal motion.

Other Imaging Modalities

Computed tomography has been used to image pericardial effusions (Fig. 115–9). This technique may be particularly useful for distinguishing coexisting pleural effusion, for evaluating pericardial thickening and tumor invasion, and for identifying pericardial calcification.

At cardiac catheterization, when contrast is injected into the right atrium, the distance between the outer border of the right atrium and the right atrial chamber should not exceed 5 mm. A separation greater than this suggests a pericardial effusion. Large pericardial effusions may flatten or give a concave appearance to the lateral right atrial border. Manipulation of the catheter tip against the lateral right atrial wall can also define this distance.

The water density representing the myocardium that surrounds the left ventricular cavity during left ventriculography should not exceed 2 cm. In the absence of left or right ventricular hypertrophy (which can increase this value), a thickness greater than 2 cm suggests the presence of a significant pericardial effusion.

Since the coronary arteries lie within the epicardium, when they are opacified during coronary arteriography, they serve as a marker for the epicardium. An abnormally wide separation (> 5 mm) between the coronary arteries and the surrounding cardiac surface suggests a pericardial effusion. This is best seen in the left anterior oblique view of angiograms of the circumflex obtuse marginal branches or the right coronary acute marginal branches.

Other methods that have been utilized to detect pericardial effusion include (1) radionuclide blood pool scanning, (2) intravenous carbon dioxide infusion into the right atrium, and (3) pericardiocentesis with instillation of air. The latter technique may uncover masses within the pericardial space (Fig. 115–10). These methods, however, are rarely used today because of the accurate assessment of the pericardial space by echocardiography.

CARDIAC TAMPONADE

An increase in pressure within the pericardial sac due to fluid accumulation results in cardiac tamponade. This is characterized by an elevation of intracardiac pressures, a limitation of ventricular diastolic filling, and a reduction in stroke volume. The classic triad of cardiac tamponade is a rise in venous pressure, a fall in arterial pressure, and a small quiet heart. These findings, however, apply primarily to tamponade that is of rapid onset, such as that occurring following direct or indirect cardiac trauma. Clinical features include an abnormal inspiratory decline in systolic blood pressure greater than 10 mm Hg (pulsus paradoxus) and dyspnea. The most frequent etiologies of cardiac tamponade are malignancy and idiopathic peri-

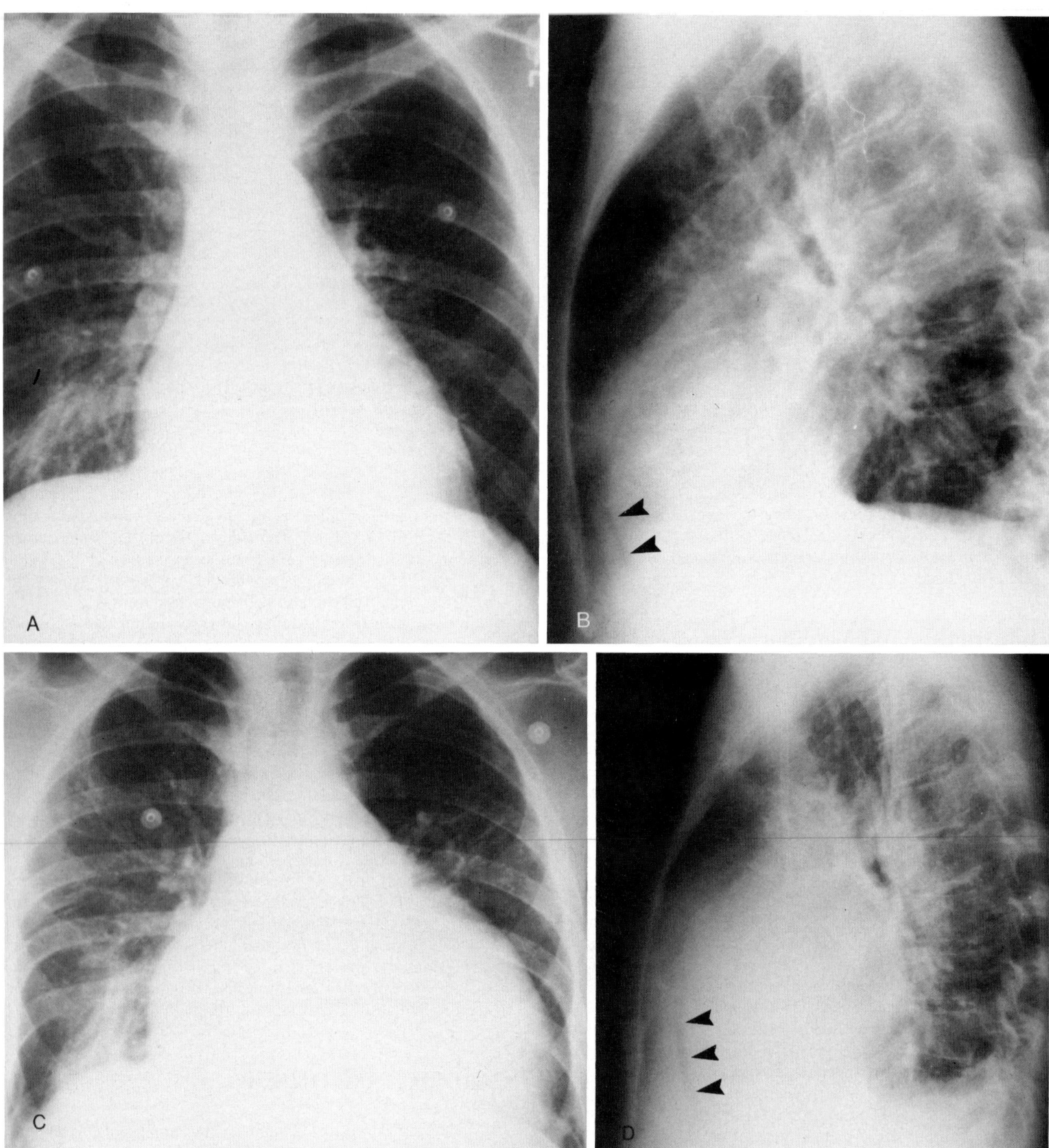

Figure 115–6. "Fat pad sign." *A,* PA chest radiograph shows a normal-sized cardiopericardial silhouette, but lateral view *(B)* demonstrates a positive fat pad sign *(arrowheads).* As the cardiopericardial silhouette increases in *C,* the fat pad sign increases as well, *D (arrowheads)* indicating an increase in the pericardial fluid volume.

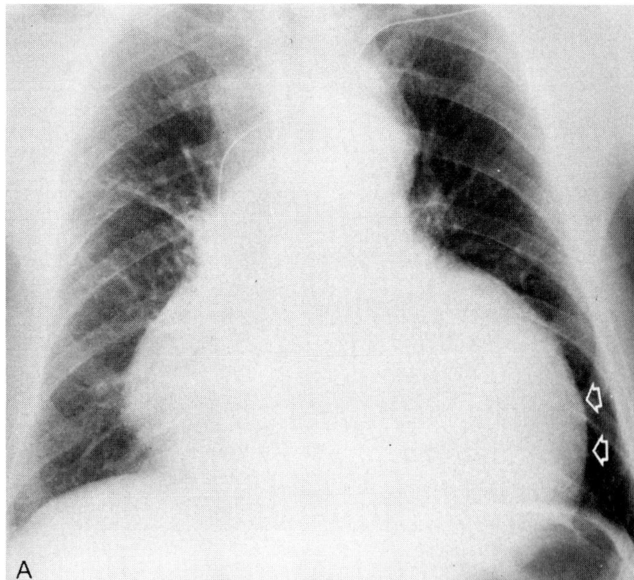

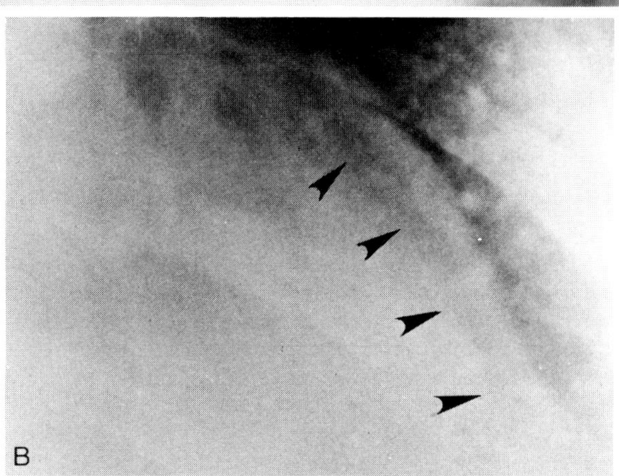

Figure 115–7. Pericardial effusion. PA chest radiographs. *A,* Symmetrical enlargement of the cardiopericardial silhouette. Note the radiolucency along the left lateral margin of the heart *(arrows).* This is an example of the differential density sign of pericardial effusion. *B,* A close-up view of the left heart border of another patient with echocardiogram showing moderate pericardial effusion. Note the curvilinear radiolucency along the left cardiac border *(arrowheads).*

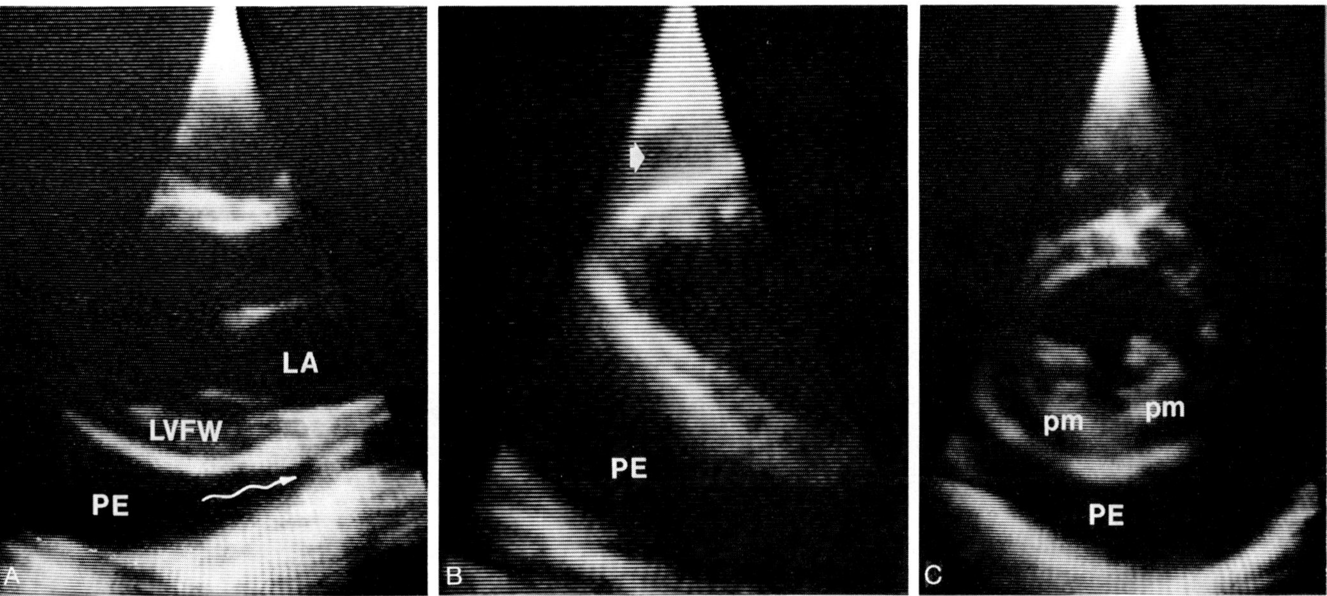

Figure 115–8. Large pericardial effusion. *A* and *B,* Two-dimensional echocardiograms in long-axis view. *C,* Two-dimensional echocardiogram in short-axis view. The echo-free space posterior to the left ventricular free wall (LVFW) represents pericardial effusion (PE). Note that in *A,* the fluid projects behind the left atrium (LA—*arrow*), and in *B,* the fluid projects anteriorly *(arrow)* as well as posteriorly. (pm = papillary muscles.)

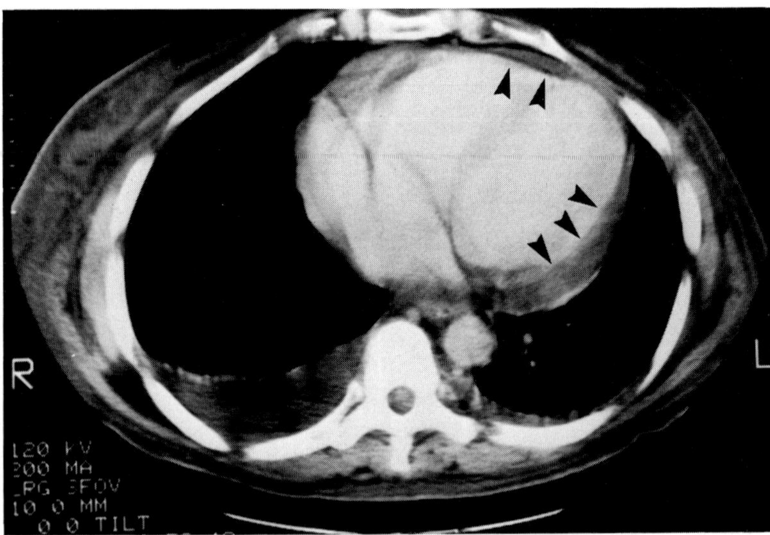

Figure 115–9. Pericardial effusion. Computed tomographic image following intravenous contrast administration. Fluid density representing moderate pericardial effusion is easily distinguished from epicardial fat *(arrowheads)* and contrast-containing left ventricle and right ventricle. Note the right pleural effusion.

carditis. Other causes include pericarditis associated with uremia and myocardial infarction and diagnostic procedures complicated by cardiac perforation.

Radiographic Findings

There are no radiographic features diagnostic of cardiac tamponade. In fact, the chest film in acute hemopericardium due to cardiac rupture or laceration may be entirely normal. If more than 250 ml accumulates slowly, radiographic features previously described for large pericardial effusions may be present. A rapid change in heart size when correlated with the above clinical features is highly suggestive of tamponade (Fig. 115–11). In acute tamponade, fluoroscopically visualized cardiac pulsations are either markedly diminished or absent.

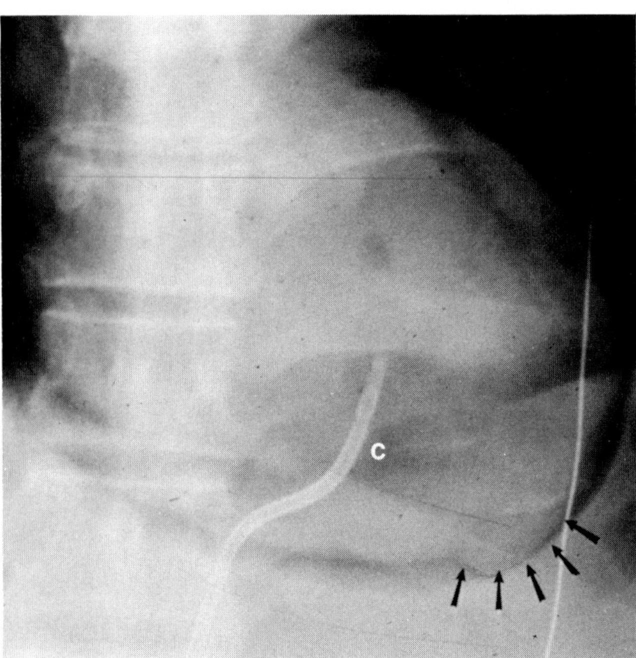

Figure 115–10. Intentional pneumopericardium. Air was instilled through a catheter (c) following pericardiocentesis to define the pericardial space. A mass is seen extending from the epicardial surface of the heart into the pericardial space *(arrows)*. This patient had recurrent pericardial effusions secondary to metastatic carcinoma. The mass proved to be a metastatic implant at autopsy.

Echocardiographic Findings

In the patient with jugular venous distention in whom cardiac tamponade is a possibility, echocardiography (if readily available) should be performed prior to pericardiocentesis. The echocardiogram helps to document the presence and magnitude of the pericardial effusion. The absence of effusion essentially eliminates the diagnosis of tamponade. The other entities that cause elevated systemic venous pressure can be differentiated. These include cardiac muscle dysfunction, constrictive pericarditis, and right ventricular infarction. When cardiac tamponade is excluded by the echocardiogram, the potentially risky pericardiocentesis procedure can be avoided.

Clues to the diagnosis of cardiac tamponade provided by the echocardiogram include early systolic movement of the anterior right ventricular wall, a sudden posterior motion of the interventricular septum during inspiration, and an exaggerated inspiratory increase and expiratory decrease in right ventricular size. These changes, however, are not specific, and a single echocardiogram cannot predict the presence or severity of cardiac tamponade.

CONSTRICTIVE PERICARDITIS

Constrictive pericarditis exists when a thickened, fibrotic, and adherent pericardium restricts diastolic filling of the heart. The disease usually relates to an initial episode of acute pericarditis with effusion, then slowly progresses through a subacute stage to a chronic stage with symmetrical thickening and fibrous scarring of the pericardium and obliteration of the pericardial space. In developed countries, tuberculosis can be found by histologic methods in less than 20 per cent of patients with constrictive pericarditis. The largest number of cases are of undetermined etiology. Other nontubercular etiologies include viral pericarditis, chronic renal failure, connective tissue disorders, neoplastic pericardial infiltration or metastasis, mediastinal irradiation, and cardiac trauma.

In classic constrictive pericarditis, the heavily fibrosed pericardium restricts diastolic filling of all chambers and determines the diastolic volume of the heart. An important and almost invariable

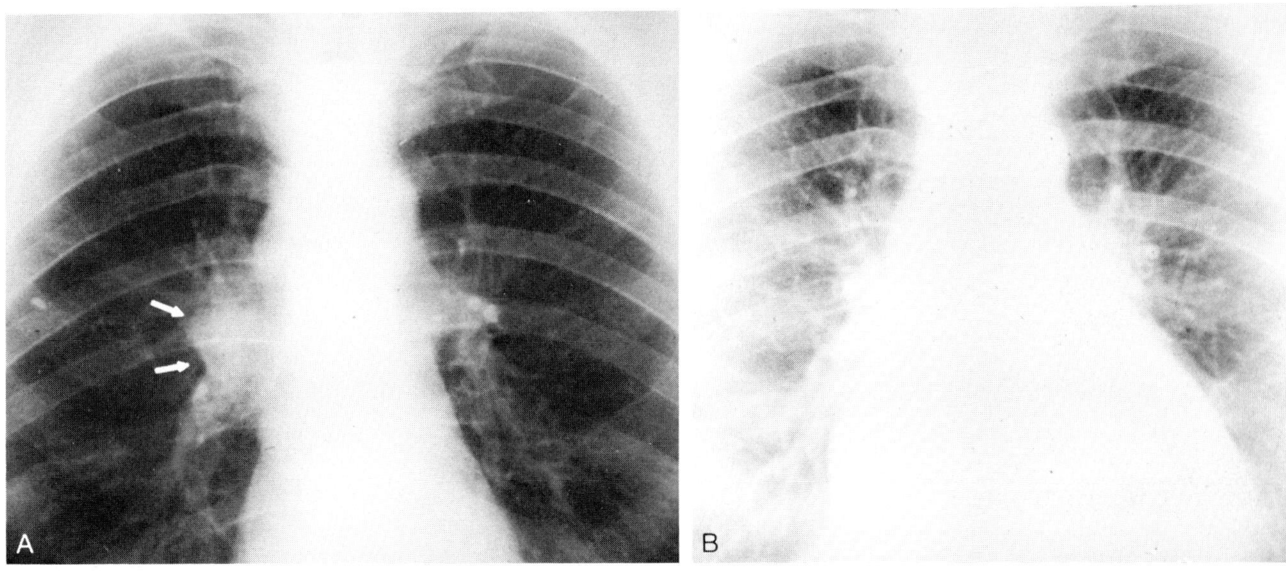

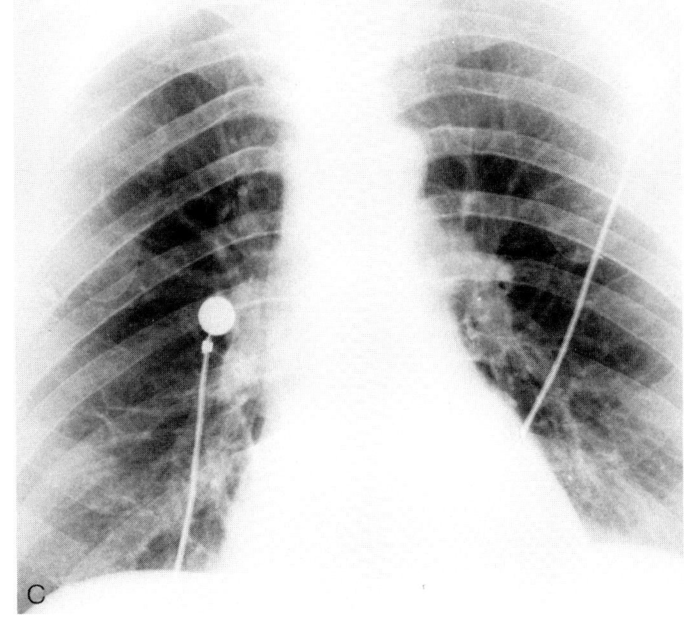

Figure 115–11. Cardiac tamponade. PA chest radiographs. This patient with small cell carcinoma involving the right hilum (note mass in A—*arrows*) was undergoing radiation therapy. *B* was obtained one week after *A* while the patient was experiencing symptoms and signs of cardiac tamponade. It shows a significant increase in the size of the cardiopericardial silhouette. *C* was obtained after pericardiocentesis and radiation therapy. Bloody fluid containing tumor cells was removed at the time of pericardiocentesis, suggesting that the lung tumor had invaded the pericardium.

physiologic consequence of constrictive pericarditis is elevation and equilibration of diastolic pressures in all four cardiac chambers as well as elevation of venous pressure. This results in hepatomegaly and ascites. Increase in neck vein size with inspiration (Kussmaul's sign) may also be present.

Radiographic Findings

Radiographic findings in constrictive pericarditis depend on the severity and chronicity of the condition. Since left atrial pressure is commonly elevated between 15 and 30 mm Hg, there is evidence of redistribution of pulmonary flow and occasionally interstitial edema (Fig. 115–12). The heart is enlarged in two thirds of patients. The left atrium is frequently enlarged. The right superior mediastinum may be prominent owing to dilatation of the superior vena cava and azygos vein (Fig. 115–12), a reflection of elevated systemic venous pressure. The above changes give a "straightened" appearance to the right and left cardiac borders (Fig. 115–12). Pericardial calcification is seen on the chest radiograph or at fluoroscopy in 40 to 50 per cent of patients. The appearance is that of linear or plaque-like calcific densities overlying the right ventricle, in the atrioventricular grooves, and extending to the left posterior cardiac surface (Fig. 115–13). This is best appreciated in the lateral view (Figs. 115–12 and 115–13). Pericardial calcification, however, is not pathognomonic for constrictive pericarditis, as it may be present in the absence of the altered hemodynamics that characterize this disease; i.e., a calcified pericardium is not necessarily a constricted one. Although usually unnecessary, fluoroscopy may be helpful in distinguishing pericardial calcification from calcification within the myocardium (left ventricular aneurysm), left ventricular cavity (mural thrombosis), or mitral annulus.

Echocardiographic Findings

In the absence of a pericardial effusion, it may be difficult to differentiate the thickened pericardium of constrictive pericarditis

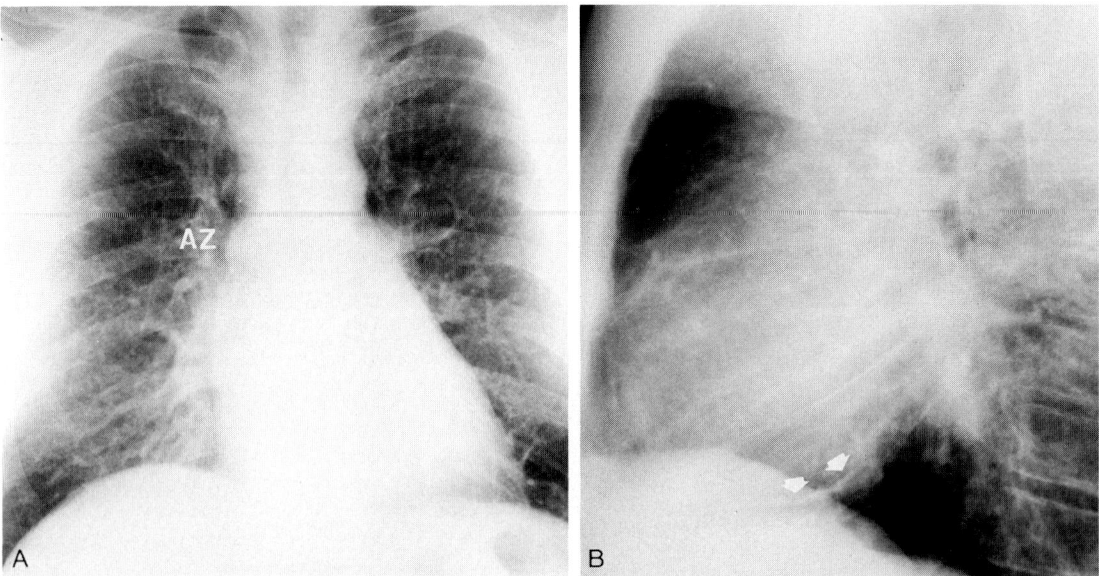

Figure 115–12. Constrictive pericarditis. *A,* PA chest radiograph. *B,* Lateral view. There are redistribution of pulmonary blood flow and interstitial edema. The right and left heart borders are straightened, and the azygos vein (AZ) is enlarged. The lateral view shows a small amount of calcification in the posterior pericardium *(arrows).*

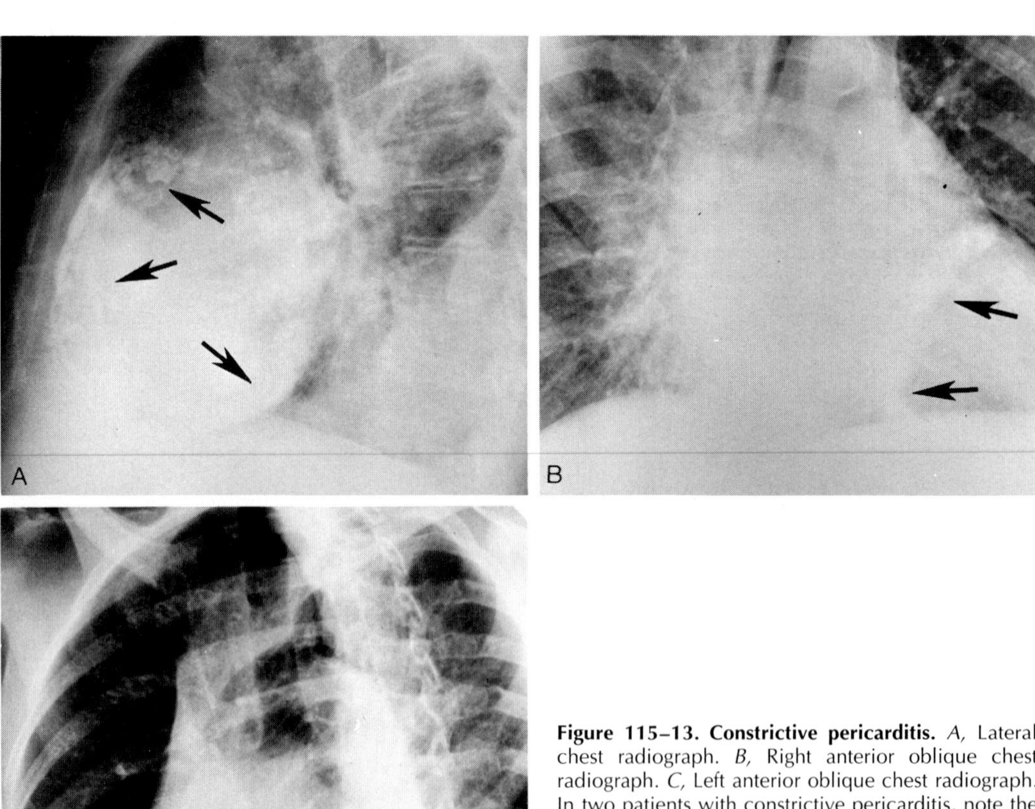

Figure 115–13. Constrictive pericarditis. *A,* Lateral chest radiograph. *B,* Right anterior oblique chest radiograph. *C,* Left anterior oblique chest radiograph. In two patients with constrictive pericarditis, note the plaque-like and linear pericardial calcification in *A (arrows)* and the concentration of calcification in the atrioventricular groove in *B* and *C (arrows).*

from a thickened left ventricular posterior wall. Two patterns have been described on echocardiography. One consists of two echodense parallel lines (representing visceral and parietal pericardium) separated by a small anechoic space of at least 1 mm; another consists of multiple dense echoes in the pericardium. Like pericardial calcification on the chest film, the presence of pericardial thickening alone is not diagnostic of constrictive pericarditis. Other features that are seen in the majority of patients with constrictive pericarditis include premature pulmonic valve opening (due to high right ventricular early diastolic pressure), reduced motion of the left ventricular posterior wall, and systolic flattening and abrupt posterior motion of the interventricular septum. Two-dimensional echocardiography may show an immobile and dense pericardium, bulging of the interventricular septum into the left ventricle during inspiration, and dilatation of the inferior vena cava and hepatic veins.

Angiographic Findings

Most patients in whom constrictive pericarditis is suspected undergo cardiac catheterization and angiocardiography. The goals in this evaluation are (1) to document the elevated and virtually equal (within 5 mm Hg) diastolic filling pressures, (2) to determine the effect of constriction on both stroke volume and cardiac output, (3) to assess myocardial systolic function, and (4) to help distinguish between constrictive pericarditis and restrictive cardiomyopathy. The latter condition, owing to a variety of infiltrative myocardial processes, may mimic constrictive pericarditis hemodynamically in terms of pressure determinations, depression of stroke volume and cardiac output, and impaired diastolic filling. Angiographically, the right atrial border may be straightened in both conditions. The cardiac walls may be thickened because of the presence of a thickened pericardium (in constrictive pericarditis) or myocardium (in restrictive cardiomyopathy).

Certain angiographic findings may be helpful in distinguishing constrictive pericarditis from restrictive cardiomyopathy. The crista supraventricularis (the muscle wall of the right ventricular outflow tract) moves normally during lateral right ventriculography in constrictive pericarditis but does not move in patients with restrictive cardiomyopathy. When coronary cineangiography is performed in the normal patient or in those with restrictive cardiomyopathy, the coronary arteries show a coiling and uncoiling motion during systole and diastole (Fig. 115–14). A lack of this normal mobility is frequently seen when coronary angiography is performed in patients with constrictive pericarditis (Fig. 115–14). The pathologic basis for this angiographic finding appears to be that constrictive pericarditis frequently involves the epicardium. The coronary arteries are therefore "struck down" by the scarring process and have limited mobility. Normal movement of the coronary arteries in patients with known constrictive pericarditis suggests that there is no epicardial involvement by the thickened pericardium. This finding may suggest the diagnosis of constrictive pericarditis in unsuspected cases, in cases in which right heart pressures are not obtained, or in those in which hemodynamic values are atypical or confusing. It may also help to distinguish constrictive pericarditis from restrictive cardiomyopathy, with their similar hemodynamic findings but entirely different prognosis and therapeutic approaches.

POSTMYOCARDIAL INFARCTION/ POSTPERICARDIOTOMY SYNDROME

The postmyocardial infarction syndrome as described by Dressler is an acute illness characterized by fever, pericarditis, pleuritis, and arthralgias that occurs in approximately 4 per cent of patients weeks to months after an acute myocardial infarction. This syndrome is distinguished from the pericarditis that commonly occurs during the first few days after myocardial infarction. The etiology of Dressler's syndrome is unknown, but an autoimmune mechanism in which the antigen is necrotic heart muscle is postulated. The chest radiograph frequently reveals an enlarged cardiopericardial silhouette secondary to pericardial effusion and pleural effusions. Transient pulmonary infiltrates and pleural effusion may be present.

The postpericardiotomy syndrome is identified by the appearance of fever, pericarditis, and pleuritis two to four weeks after cardiac surgery involving manipulation of the pericardium. An average incidence of 30 per cent following cardiac surgery has been reported. A similar clinical syndrome has been reported following cardiac perforation by a catheter or pacemaker, blunt chest trauma, and epicardial pacemaker implantation. Like the etiology of Dressler's syndrome, that of postpericardiotomy syndrome is hypothesized to be an autoimmune reaction directed toward the epicardium by antimyocardial antibodies. A viral infection may be a triggering or accompanying factor.

The chest radiograph demonstrates bilateral pleural effusions in two thirds of patients. Transient enlargement of the cardiopericardial silhouette is present in half the patients, whereas pulmonary infiltrates are noted in about one tenth.

CONGENITAL ANOMALIES OF THE PERICARDIUM

Absence of the Pericardium

Absence of the pericardium most frequently involves the left pericardium. The defect may be either partial or complete. In the partial variety, there is no pericardium covering the region of the left atrial appendage and the pulmonary trunk. Although patients are usually asymptomatic, sudden death secondary to herniation of cardiac structures with resultant cardiac strangulation has been described. About 30 per cent of cases of partial pericardial defect are associated with other congenital anomalies, such as patent ductus arteriosus, atrial septal defect, tetralogy of Fallot, bronchogenic cyst, and pulmonary sequestration.

In the partial form of absence of the pericardium, there is a discrete bulge in the region of the pulmonary trunk and left atrial appendage, and the pulmonary trunk may show an unusually distinct appearance (Fig. 115–15). In the complete form, the chest radiograph shows a marked leftward placement of the cardiac silhouette and a prominent main pulmonary artery. There is interposition of lung tissue between the aorta and pulmonary trunk and between the left hemidiaphragm and the inferior left cardiac border (Fig. 115–16).

Echocardiograms in complete absence of the left pericardium are similar to those seen in conditions associated with right heart volume overload, with paradoxical anterior motion of the septum in systole. Two-dimensional echocardiography helps to exclude other congenital anomalies.

Pericardial Cysts

True cysts of the pericardium are rare and represent persistence of the ventral and parietal pericardial recesses. Radiographically, these appear as smooth, well-circumscribed densities that blend with the cardiac silhouette, causing an unusual prominence along its border. When they occur superiorly, they may be mistaken for mediastinal or pulmonary masses.

Pleuropericardial cysts are more common and are situated in the cardiophrenic angles—60 per cent on the right and 40 per cent on

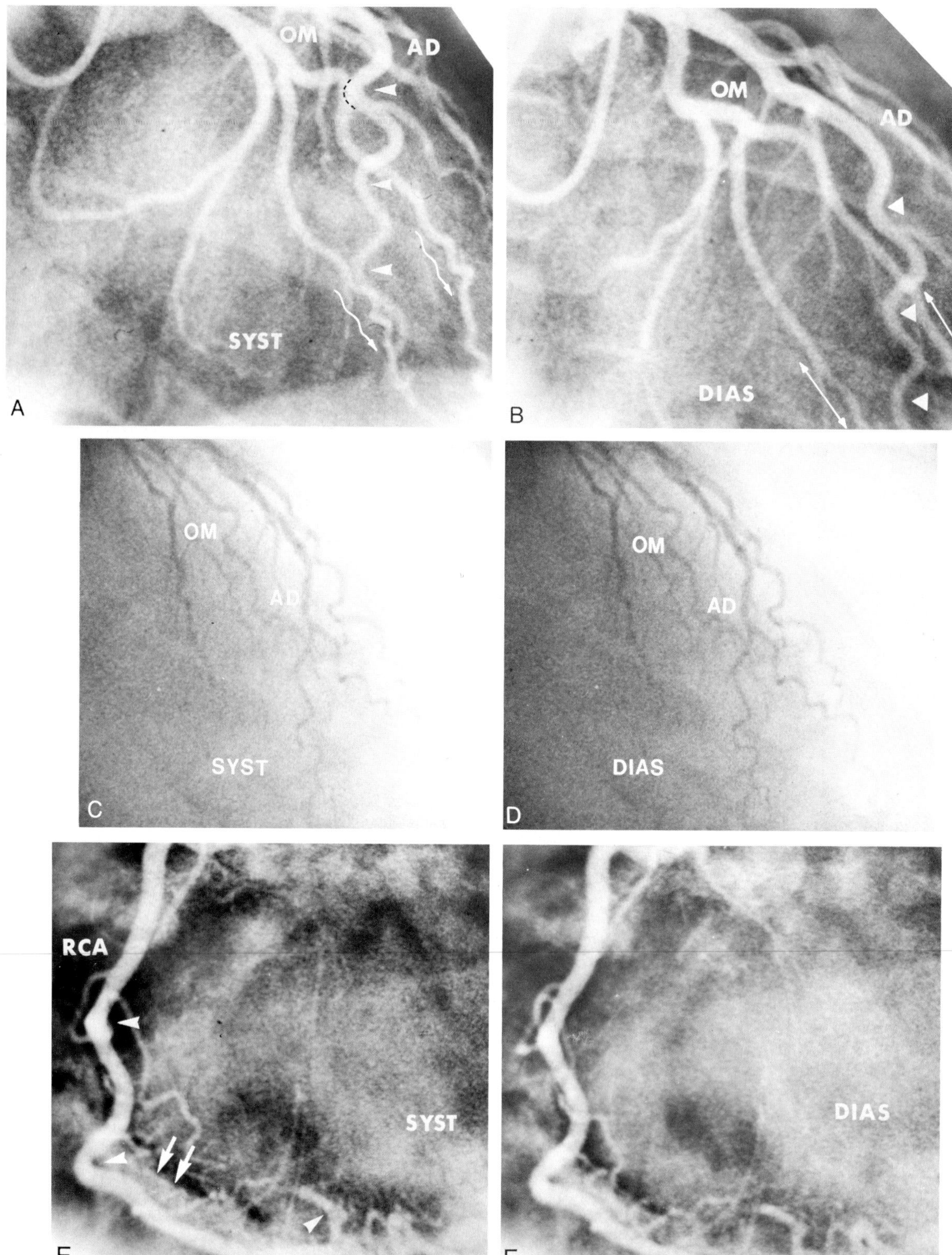

Figure 115–14. Cine frames from left coronary arteriograms performed in right anterior oblique projection **in a patient with restrictive cardiomyopathy.** Note the normal "coiling" and "uncoiling" *(arrowheads and long arrows)* of the anterior descending (AD) and obtuse marginal (OM) branches in *(A)* systole (SYST) and *(B)* diastole (DIAS). *C* and *D,* Left coronary arteriograms performed in right anterior oblique projection in a patient with constrictive pericarditis. Branches of the anterior descending (AD) and obtuse marginal (OM) appear essentially identical in both *(C)* systole (SYST) and *(D)* diastole (DIAS). *E* and *F,* Right coronary arteriograms performed in left anterior oblique projections in a patient with calcific constrictive pericarditis. Both the main right coronary artery (RCA) and small marginal branches *(arrowheads)* show lack of coiling in *(E)* systole (SYST) and *(F)* diastole (DIAS). Note the presence of calcium *(two arrows)* along the base of the heart.

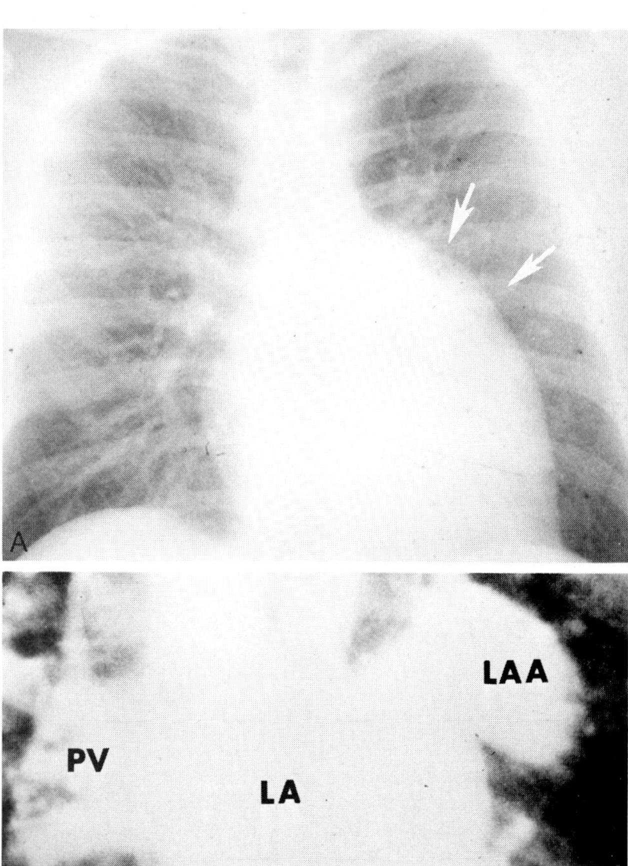

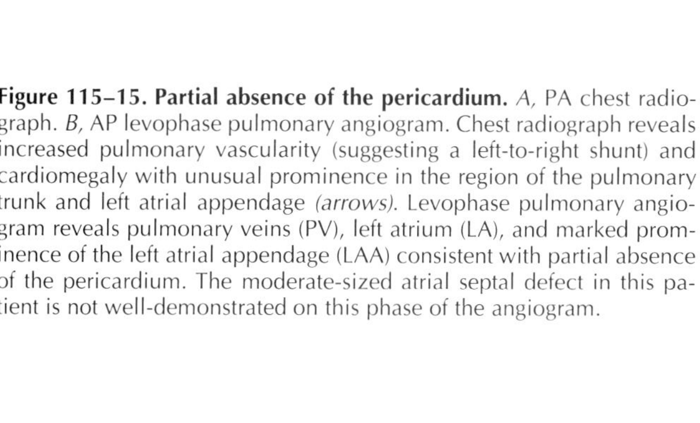
Figure 115–15. Partial absence of the pericardium. *A,* PA chest radiograph. *B,* AP levophase pulmonary angiogram. Chest radiograph reveals increased pulmonary vascularity (suggesting a left-to-right shunt) and cardiomegaly with unusual prominence in the region of the pulmonary trunk and left atrial appendage *(arrows).* Levophase pulmonary angiogram reveals pulmonary veins (PV), left atrium (LA), and marked prominence of the left atrial appendage (LAA) consistent with partial absence of the pericardium. The moderate-sized atrial septal defect in this patient is not well-demonstrated on this phase of the angiogram.

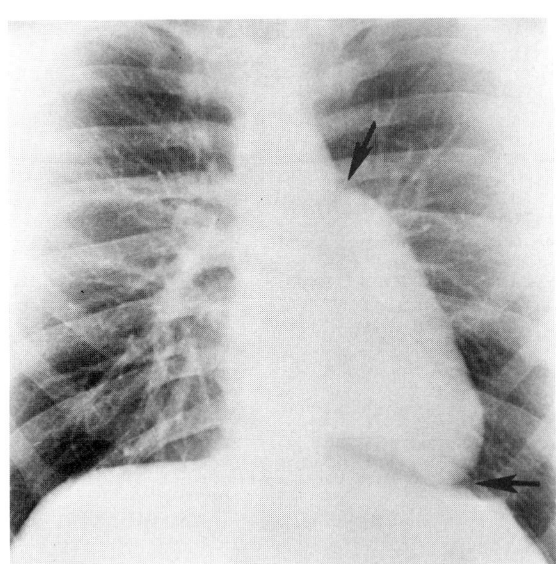

Figure 115–16. Complete absence of the pericardium. PA chest radiograph shows leftward placement of the cardiac silhouette, a prominent pulmonary trunk, and interposition of lung tissue between the aorta and pulmonary trunk and between the left hemidiaphragm and inferior cardiac border *(arrows).*

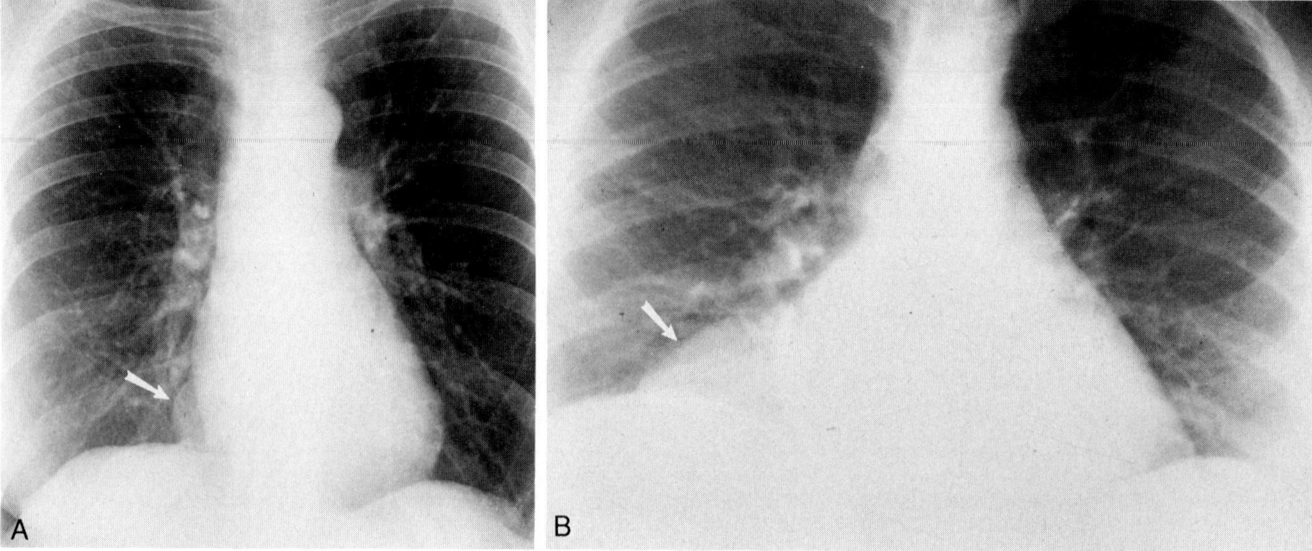

Figure 115–17. Pleuropericardial cysts. PA chest radiographs demonstrate well-circumscribed, lucent curvilinear densities abutting the right heart border and adjacent hemidiaphragm *(arrows).*

the left. These are well-circumscribed, relatively lucent densities that usually touch the anterior wall and adjacent hemidiaphragm (Fig. 115–17). When enlarged they may have a pointed upper border. Their larger size and rounded appearance help to distinguish these cysts from pericardial fat pads.

Pericardial cysts typically come to medical attention after discovery on a chest radiograph. They must be distinguished from solid tumors, true or false cardiac aneurysms, or congenital diaphragmatic herniations. A cyst can be distinguished from solid tumor by echocardiography, contrast-enhanced computed tomography, or magnetic resonance imaging. Angiography may occasionally be required to differentiate a cyst from an aneurysm, particularly if the former is in an unusual location such as the hilum or superior mediastinum.

Bibliography

Alexander J, Kelley MJ, Cohen LS, Langou RA: The angiographic appearance of the coronary arteries in constrictive pericarditis. Radiology 131:609, 1979.

Carsky EW, Mauceri RA, Azimi F: The epicardial fat pad sign: Analysis of frontal and lateral chest radiographs in patients with pericardial effusion. Radiology 137:303, 1980.

Chandraratna PAN, Aronow WS, Imaizumi T: Role of echocardiography in detecting the anatomic and physiologic abnormalities of constrictive pericarditis. Am J Med Sci 283:141, 1982.

Chang LW, Grollman JH Jr: Angiographic differentiation of constrictive pericarditis and restrictive cardiomyopathy due to amyloidosis. AJR 130:451, 1978.

Dressler W: The post-myocardial infarction syndrome. A report of forty-four cases. Arch Intern Med 103:28, 1959.

Engle MA, Klein AA, Hepner S, Enlers KH: The postpericardiotomy and similar syndromes. Cardiovasc Clin 7:211, 1976.

Fowler NO: Physiology of cardiac tamponade and pulsus paradoxus. Physiological, circulatory and pharmacologic responses in cardiac tamponade. Mod Concepts Cardiovasc Dis 47:115, 1978.

Guberman BA, Fowler NO, Engel PJ, et al: Cardiac tamponade in medical patients. Circulation 64:633, 1981.

Higgins CB: MR of the heart: Anatomy, physiology and metabolism. AJR 151:239–248, 1988.

Higgins CB, Byrd BF, McNamara MT, et al: Magnetic resonance imaging of the heart: A review of the experience in 172 subjects. Radiology 155:671–679, 1985.

Kiminsky ME, Rodan BA, Osborne DR, et al: Postpericardiotomy syndrome. Am J Radiol 138:503, 1982.

Lane EJ Jr, Carsky EW: Epicardial fat: Lateral plain film analysis in normals and in pericardial effusion. Radiology 91:1, 1968.

Lewis BS: Real time two-dimensional echocardiography in constrictive pericarditis. Am J Cardiol 49:1789, 1982.

Martins JB, Kerber RE: Can cardiac tamponade be diagnosed by echocardiography? Circulation 60:737, 1979.

Nasser WK, Helmen C, Tavel ME, et al: Congenital absence of the left pericardium: Clinical, electrocardiographic, radiographic, hemodynamic and radiographic findings in six cases. Circulation 41:469, 1970.

Parameswaran R, Goldberg H: Echocardiographic quantitation of pericardial effusion. Chest 83:767, 1983.

Peters RW, Scheinman MM, Raskin S, Thomas AN: Unusual complications of epicardial pacemakers. Am J Cardiol 45:1088, 1980.

Pulvaneswary M: Constrictive pericarditis: Clinical, hemodynamic and radiologic correlation. Australas Radiol 26:53, 1982.

Rogers CI, Seymour EQ, Brock JG: Atypical pericardial cyst location: The value of computed tomography. J Comput Assist Tomogr 4:683, 1980.

Schnittger F, Bowden RE, Abrams J, Popp RL: Echocardiography: Pericardial thickening and constrictive pericarditis. Am J Cardiol 42:388, 1978.

Tehranzadeh J, Kelley MJ: Differential density sign of pericardial effusion. Radiology 133:23, 1979.

Wolverson MK, Grides RD, Sundaram M, et al: Demonstration of unsuspected malignant disease of the pericardium by computed tomography. CT 4:330, 1980.

Wong BY, Lee KR, MacArthur RI: Diagnosis of pericardial effusion by computed tomography. Chest 81:177, 1982.

116 Diseases of the Thoracic Aorta

Ina L. D. Tonkin

This chapter describes a variety of imaging modalities used to detect conditions that affect the thoracic aorta. In many of the lesions presented, the diagnosis can readily be made by using digital subtraction angiography, computed tomography, echocardiography, and magnetic resonance imaging. The definitive diagnosis is often made by vascular imaging with angled projections. The use of these other imaging modalities in conjunction with the chest radiographic findings will be emphasized.

AORTIC ANEURYSM

In a true thoracic aortic aneurysm, all three layers of the aortic wall protrude outward from the lumen. A pseudoaneurysm is usually produced by trauma and is essentially a perforation of the aorta, with the outer wall being composed of the adventitia and the outer one third of media.

Atherosclerotic Aneurysms

The cardinal features of atherosclerosis are (1) dilatation, (2) elongation, and (3) calcification. Pathologic exaggeration of the first feature results in an aneurysm. Aneurysms of the thoracic aorta may be classified according to (1) their location (sinus of Valsalva, ascending aorta, aortic arch, or descending aorta); (2) their cause (congenital, atherosclerotic, luetic, mycotic); and (3) their anatomy (saccular, fusiform, or dissecting). In the past, aneurysms in the ascending aorta were most frequently due to syphilis. However, in the last 35 years, atherosclerosis has become the most common etiologic agent of aneurysms of the ascending aorta.

RADIOGRAPHIC FINDINGS. A posteroanterior chest radiograph may show dilatation or prominence of the ascending aorta with calcification within the aneurysmal segment. There may be fusiform or saccular dilatation of the aorta (Fig. 116–1). Generally, in the posteroanterior projection, there is widening of the aorta to the right, and the aortic knob is grossly dilated. In the left anterior oblique or lateral projection, the diameter of the aorta is increased. Atherosclerotic aneurysms may involve the aortic arch or descending thoracic aorta. Isolated aneurysms of the descending thoracic aorta may present as a left hilar mass on chest radiograph (Fig. 116–2).

ANGIOGRAPHIC FINDINGS. A negative thoracic aortogram does not absolutely exclude an aneurysm from the diagnosis, since nonfilling due to organized clot and thrombus may occur. These aneurysms may be saccular or fusiform (Fig. 116–2*B* to *D*) and may extend to the abdominal aorta with extensive calcification. Retrograde aortography with injection of contrast material into the root of the aorta will demonstrate the aneurysm; rarely, the extent of the aneurysm may not be shown because of contained thrombus. It is important to image the entire thoracic aorta and abdominal aorta to exclude multiple aneurysms.

Syphilitic Aneurysms and Aortitis

Syphilis typically involves the aortic root, the adjacent portions of the ascending aorta, and, rarely, other portions of the thoracic aorta. It is rare in the abdominal aorta. The syphilitic process often involves the aortic valve ring and produces dilatation with calcification, shortening, and thinning of the aortic cusps. Generally, there is aortic valvar regurgitation. Another complication is weakening of the smooth muscle and elastic tissue in the aortic wall with replacement by fibrous tissue. This frequently leads to aneurysm formation. A thin, rim-like calcification of the aneurysm is often seen, but this is not pathognomonic for syphilitic aortitis. Calcium is most frequently found with atherosclerotic aneurysms and can also be found in association with calcific aortic stenosis and rheumatic aortic regurgitation. The serology of the patient as well as the clinical history should be evaluated for possible syphilitic aortitis.

RADIOGRAPHIC FINDINGS. The plain chest radiograph will generally show prominence and dilatation of the ascending aorta with a thin rim of calcification (Fig. 116–3*A* and *B*). Frequently, the calcification extends to the aortic valve with dilatation of the sinuses.

ANGIOGRAPHIC FINDINGS. Retrograde aortography or digital subtraction angiography (DSA) is the most reliable radiographic procedure for diagnosing syphilitic aortitis. The ascending aorta is excessively dilated with involvement of the sinuses of Valsalva. Aortic valve regurgitation may be present (Fig. 116–3*C*). Longstanding syphilitic aortic aneurysms may erode anteriorly through the chest wall or sternum. This can be diagnosed by computed tomography or magnetic resonance imaging (Fig. 116–4).

Mycotic Aneurysms

Only about 2.5 per cent of all aneurysms are of mycotic origin, but these aneurysms deserve special consideration because of their

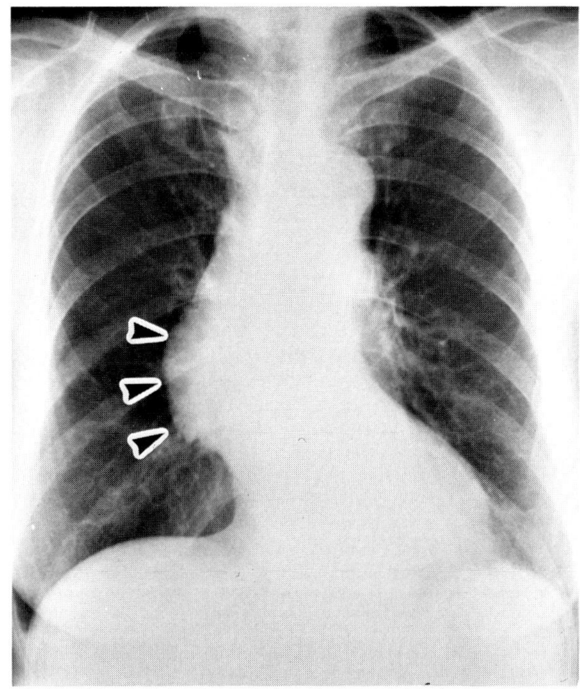

Figure 116–1. Posteroanterior (PA) chest radiograph in a 50-year-old woman with **atherosclerotic aneurysm of the ascending aorta**. Note the irregular contour and density of the ascending aorta *(arrowheads)*.

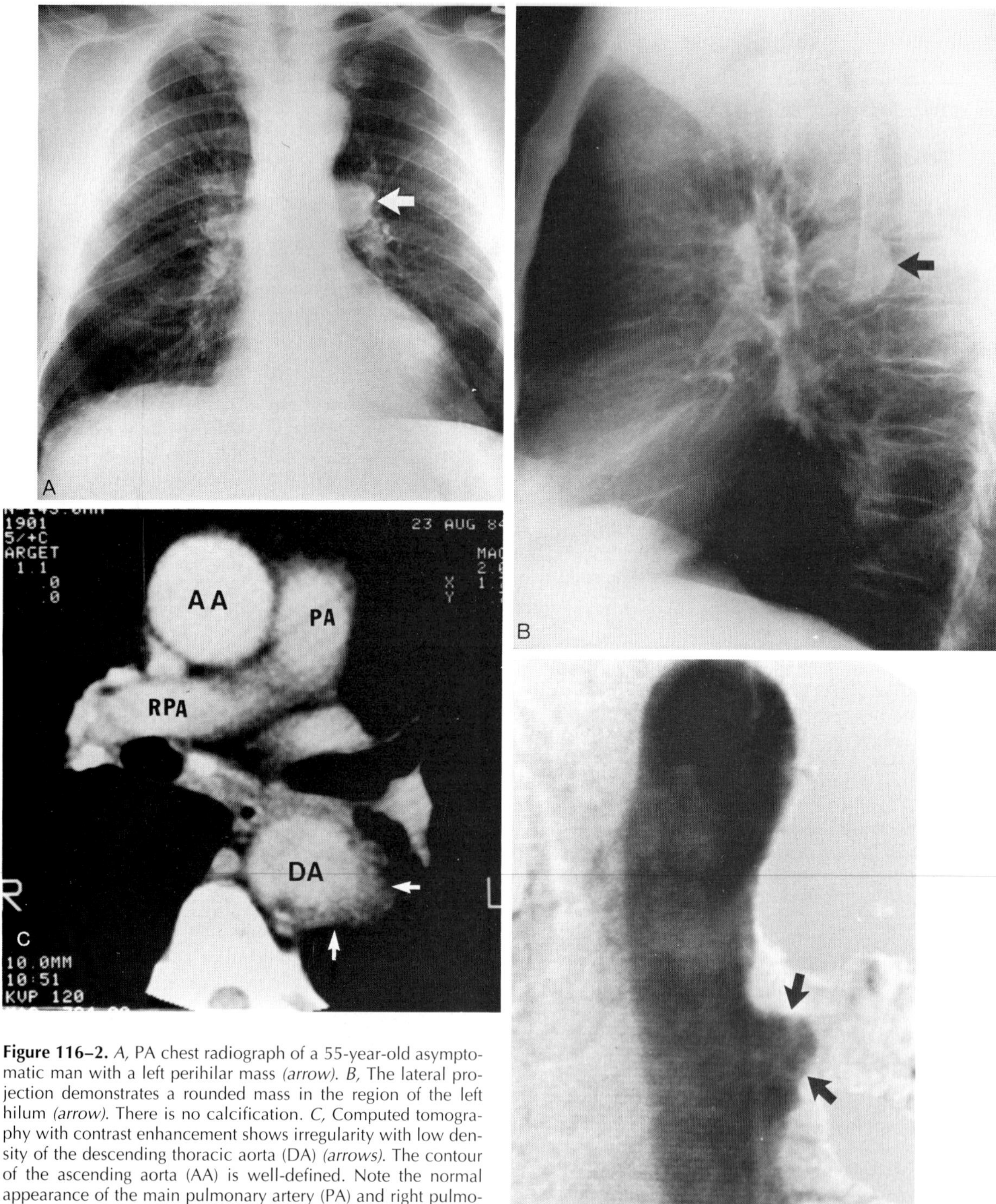

Figure 116–2. *A,* PA chest radiograph of a 55-year-old asymptomatic man with a left perihilar mass *(arrow). B,* The lateral projection demonstrates a rounded mass in the region of the left hilum *(arrow).* There is no calcification. *C,* Computed tomography with contrast enhancement shows irregularity with low density of the descending thoracic aorta (DA) *(arrows).* The contour of the ascending aorta (AA) is well-defined. Note the normal appearance of the main pulmonary artery (PA) and right pulmonary artery (RPA). *D,* Intra-arterial digital subtraction angiography performed in the anteroposterior (AP) projection imaging the descending thoracic aorta. This study confirms a **saccular aneurysm of the descending thoracic aorta** that was partially filled with thrombus *(arrows).* (Courtesy of Morris J. Gavant, M.D., University of Tennessee, Memphis, The Health Science Center.)

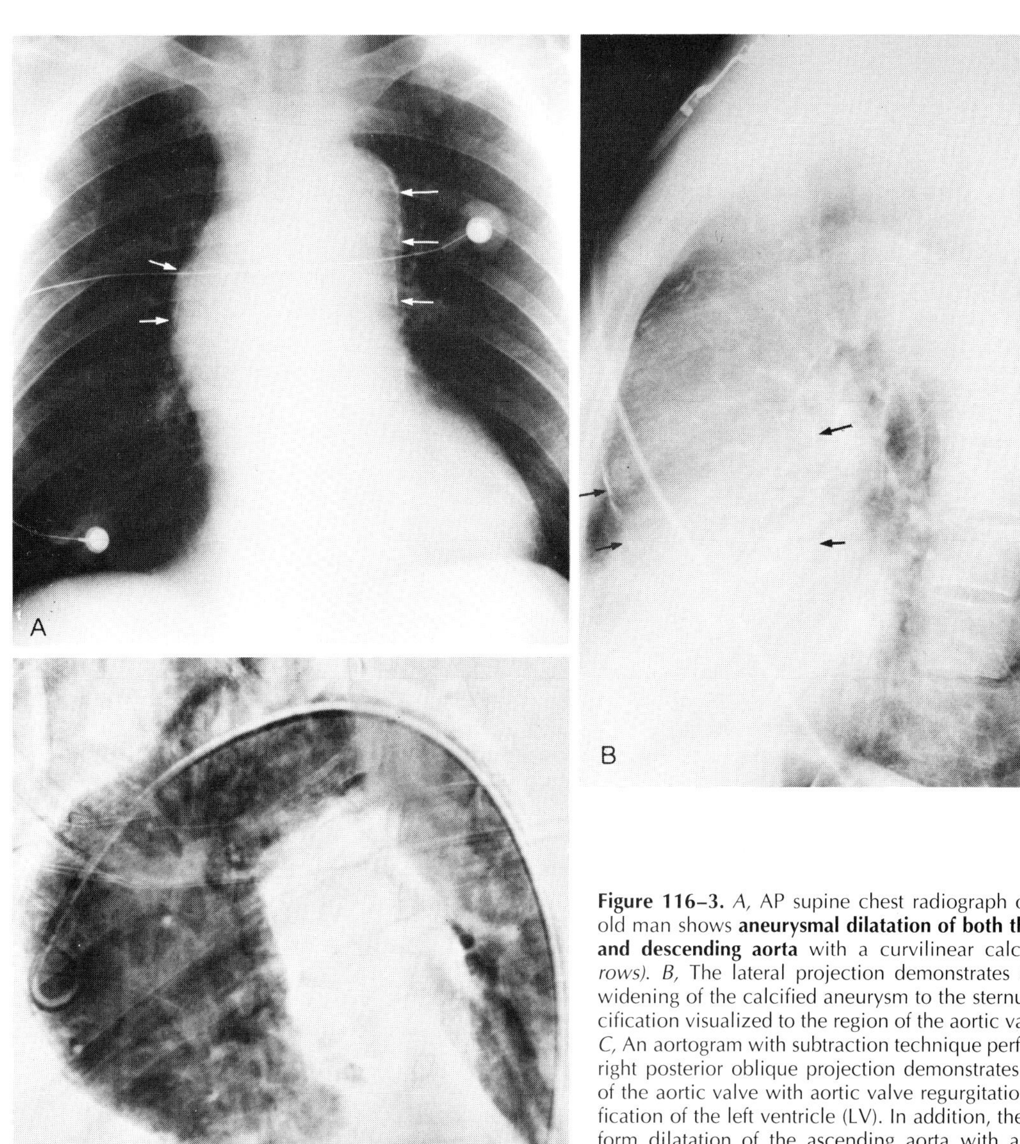

Figure 116–3. *A,* AP supine chest radiograph of a 60-year-old man shows **aneurysmal dilatation of both the ascending and descending aorta** with a curvilinear calcification *(arrows). B,* The lateral projection demonstrates an extensive widening of the calcified aneurysm to the sternum, with calcification visualized to the region of the aortic valve *(arrows). C,* An aortogram with subtraction technique performed in the right posterior oblique projection demonstrates abnormality of the aortic valve with aortic valve regurgitation and opacification of the left ventricle (LV). In addition, the diffuse fusiform dilatation of the ascending aorta with a thin rim of calcification is suggestive of a **syphilitic aneurysm**. The serology was positive in this patient.

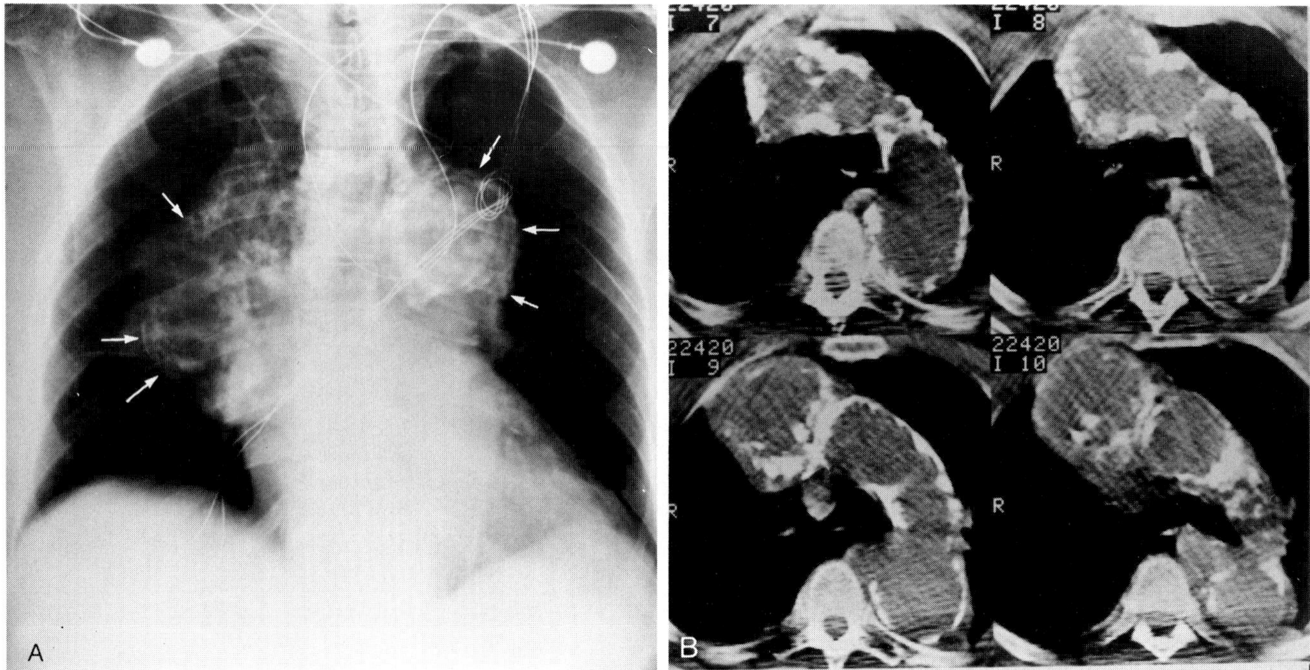

Figure 116–4. *A,* AP portable chest radiograph of an 84-year-old man demonstrates a markedly enlarged ascending and descending aorta with extensive curvilinear calcifications *(arrows). B,* Consecutive computed tomographic slices through the chest show the extent of the **aneurysm of the thoracic aorta,** which has eroded partially into the chest wall. The serology was positive for syphilis in this patient. (Case contributed by Allen K. Tonkin, M.D., Baptist Memorial Hospital, Memphis, TN.)

rapid progression and poor outcome if not recognized early. Mycotic aneurysms are produced by bacterial, fungal, or other infectious agents. Aortic mycotic aneurysms are more often secondary to septicemia and are most commonly seen in the ascending aorta.

ANGIOGRAPHIC FINDINGS. The diagnosis is usually established by retrograde aortography or DSA. Because septic emboli can be dislodged, care should be exercised in examining affected patients. In most circumstances, it is desirable to see the entire aorta (Fig. 116–5), and contrast material should be injected in the ascending portion of the aorta with filming in two projections, preferably

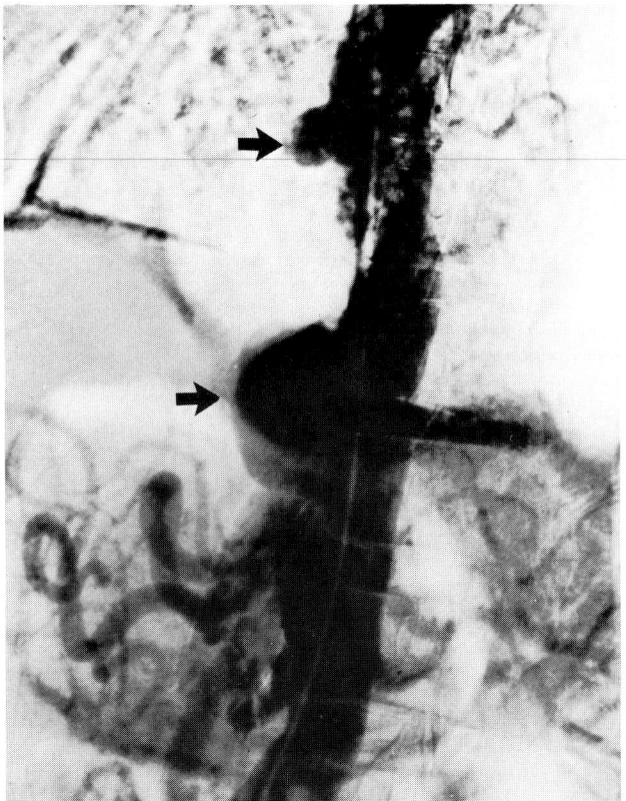

Figure 116–5. A right posterior oblique projection of the lower thoracic and abdominal aorta (subtraction technique) of a drug abuser shows two **mycotic aneurysms of the descending thoracic aorta** *(arrows).*

the right posterior oblique and posteroanterior positions. An accurate diagnosis is essential before surgical correction is undertaken.

Aneurysms of the Sinus of Valsalva

Congenital aneurysms of the sinus of Valsalva are now being diagnosed more frequently. The underlying defect is failure of the medial wall of the aorta to meet or be anchored in the aortic ring, thus leaving a weakened area in the aortic wall. Systemic blood pressure over a period of years causes the weakened area to bulge and eventually rupture. Generally, these aneurysms are congenital; however, they may be secondary to trauma, cystic medial necrosis, bacterial infection, or syphilitic aortitis. They present in the first to fifth decade, most commonly in the teenager and young adult. When an aneurysm of the sinus of Valsalva ruptures, the right sinus of Valsalva most frequently ruptures into the right ventricle, and the noncoronary sinus of Valsalva most frequently ruptures into the right atrium. Patients may have chest pain and acute congestive heart failure with a continuous murmur. These lesions have a frequent association with ventricular septal defect, coarctation of the aorta, and subvalvular aortic stenosis.

Radiographic Findings. Since the sinuses of Valsalva lie deep within the heart, aneurysms of these structures produce no change in the cardiac contour until rupture occurs, or unless there is an additional associated lesion. After rupture, depending on the size of the shunt, cardiomegaly and increased pulmonary flow may be seen. Initially, the right side of the heart enlarges, and later the left ventricle may be overloaded and enlarged (Fig. 116–6*A*). Catheterization of the right side of the heart demonstrates a step-up in oxygen saturation between the vena cava and right atrium or right ventricle, depending on the site of the rupture.

Angiographic Findings. Left ventriculography and aortography are essential for defining the cardiac anatomy, especially if there is a suspected ventricular septal defect. Multiple projections of the aorta are essential for defining the exact sinus defect and the location of rupture (Fig. 116–6*B* and *C*). The diagnosis can also be suspected by history, by the chest radiographic appearance, and by two-dimensional echocardiography (Fig. 116–7). It is important to demonstrate the exact anatomic sinus involved and to locate the site of rupture so that surgical repair with ligation of the aneurysm and plication of the aortic valve can be performed through the chamber into which the aneurysm has ruptured.

Dissecting Aortic Aneurysms

An aortic dissection is a separation of the intima and adventitia that usually occurs at the junction between the middle and outer third of the media. The dissection may involve a localized area of the aortic circumference or the entire circumference. A three-barrel or three-channeled aortic dissection may rarely occur, with one true lumen and two false lumens.

The standard classifications for dissecting thoracic aneurysms commonly used are DeBakey's and Daily's (Fig. 116–8). Type I is the most common. The dissection begins in the ascending aorta and extends across the aortic arch and distally, often to the iliac arteries. In Type II, the most common lesion in Marfan's syndrome, the dissection is limited to the ascending aorta. Types I and II correspond to Group A of Daily et al. In Type III (Group B of Daily), the dissection begins in the thoracic aorta just distal to the left subclavian artery and extends a variable distance. Type III is often due to trauma. Acute Type A dissections make up approximately 66 per cent, Type B about 33 per cent.

Radiographic Findings. The radiographic findings described in aortic dissection include (1) widening of the superior mediastinum, (2) an enlarged aortic arch or irregular aortic contour (see Fig. 116–12*A* and *B*), (3) displacement of the trachea to the right, (4) displacement of the nasogastric tube in the esophagus to the right, (5) irregularity of the descending thoracic aorta (see Fig. 116–14), (6) a left apical pleural effusion, and (7) a para-aortic mass. The chest radiograph may also be normal (Fig. 116–9). Although an increase in aortic wall thickness of more than 4 mm may be a diagnostic criterion for dissecting aneurysm of the thoracic aorta (Fig. 116–10), other explanations exist. The differential diagnosis of an increase in aortic wall thickness also includes normal fat, atherosclerotic disease with intraluminal clot formation, sclerosing aortitis, and neoplasms surrounding the wall of the thoracic aorta.

Acute cardiomegaly may be caused by one of the complications of aortic dissection. This usually is associated with Type I and II dissections, when they involve the aortic valve with resultant acute aortic regurgitation or when the dissection extends into the pericardium with resultant cardiac tamponade.

Angiographic and Computed Tomographic Findings. The angiographic findings of aortic dissection include *direct signs* of a linear radiolucency or intimal flap, a double channel showing the false and true channel, and visualization of the entry and re-entry site (see Fig. 116–9*B* and *C*). The *indirect signs* include a narrowed true lumen, thickening of the aortic wall, and an abnormal catheter position that does not extend to the posterior aspect of the thoracic aorta. In addition, aortic regurgitation or aortic branch involvement may be seen with aortography of the ascending and descending aorta (see Fig. 116–9*B* and *C*). The ascending aortogram may be performed with biplane large-film angiography or with 35-mm biplane cineangiography. The latter may improve diagnostic capabilities by allowing easier visualization of intimal flaps, intimal tears, or retrograde dissection. It also allows for better evaluation of the aortic valve and assessment of aortic regurgitation. An abdominal aortogram should be performed in order to evaluate possible renal artery or other branch involvement (see Fig. 116–9*D*).

Patients who have had chronic dissections of the aorta are prone to redissection, extension of the dissection, aortic aneurysm, and aortic rupture. Computed tomography with contrast medium enhancement provides a convenient noninvasive method for follow-up of these patients. Computed tomography can demonstrate redissection, aneurysmal dilatation of the aorta, and delayed filling of the false lumen (Fig. 116–10*C*). This is also an excellent noninvasive modality for observing these critically ill patients postoperatively. Computed tomography can also be used to detect acute dissections (Fig. 116–11).

In Type II aortic dissections, involvement is limited to the ascending aorta. This is frequently associated with cystic medial necrosis with or without Marfan's syndrome (Fig. 116–12*A* and *B*). The Type II dissection with aortic valve involvement will frequently require a prosthetic aortic valve with graft replacement. The most important late complication of composite aortic grafts and reimplantation of coronary arteries is hemorrhage at the anastomotic site. This can be evaluated with aortography, cineangiography, DSA, computed tomography, and magnetic resonance imaging (Figs. 116–13 and 116–14).

The Type III dissection that occurs distal to the left subclavian artery may be post-traumatic in origin or may be caused by hypertension and long-standing atherosclerosis or other conditions predisposing the patient to weakness of the aortic wall (Fig. 116–15).

TRAUMA TO THE THORACIC AORTA AND GREAT VESSELS

Trauma to the chest generally involves blunt or crushing trauma as opposed to perforating trauma (laceration, rupture, or penetrating wounds). Eighty to 90 per cent of patients with aortic injuries after blunt chest trauma die immediately; the remainder live long enough

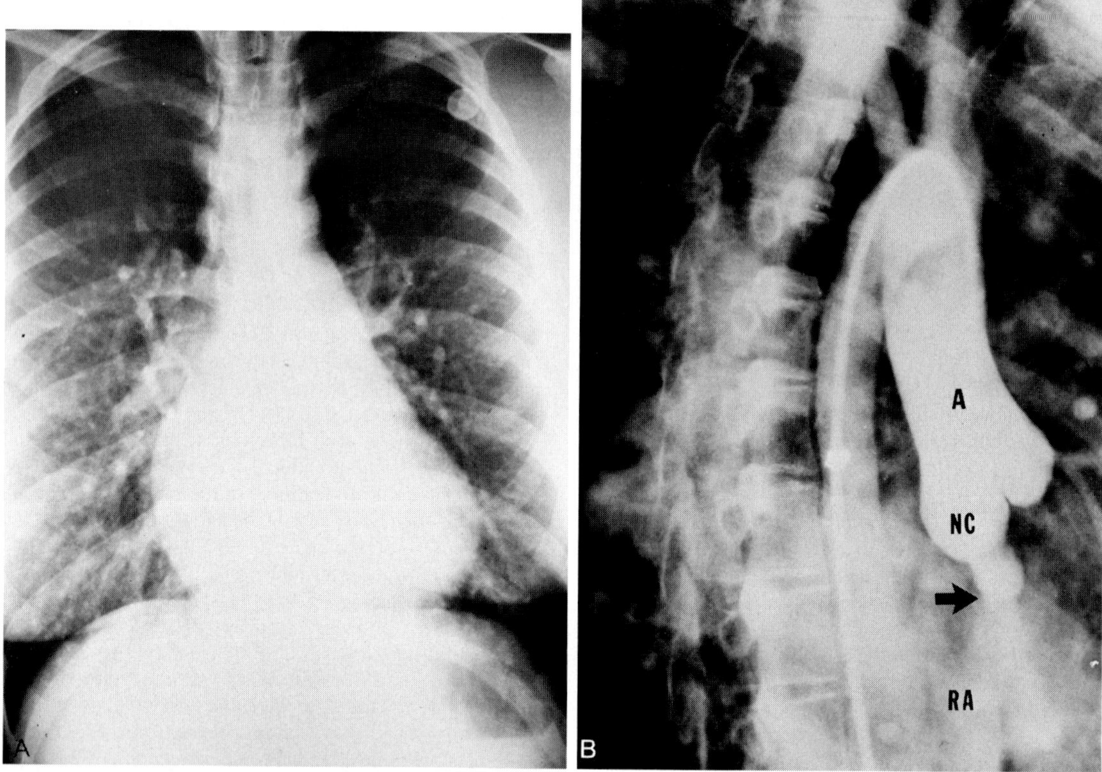

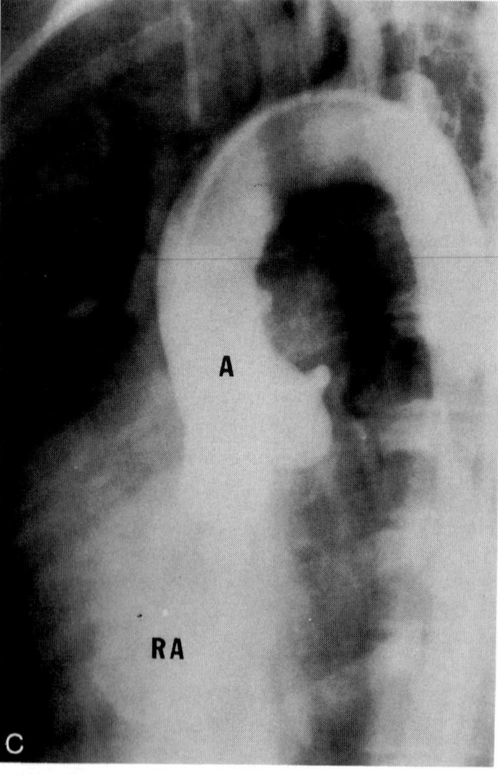

Figure 116–6. *A,* The PA chest radiograph of a 27-year-old woman shows increased vascularity and enlargement of the right side of the heart. *B,* The thoracic aortogram (A) in the right anterior oblique projection shows a **ruptured sinus of Valsalva aneurysm** *(arrow)* involving the noncoronary (NC) sinus, with rupture into the right atrium (RA). *C,* The simultaneous biplane left anterior oblique aortogram also demonstrates the ruptured sinus of Valsalva aneurysm with contrast material entering the right atrium (RA).

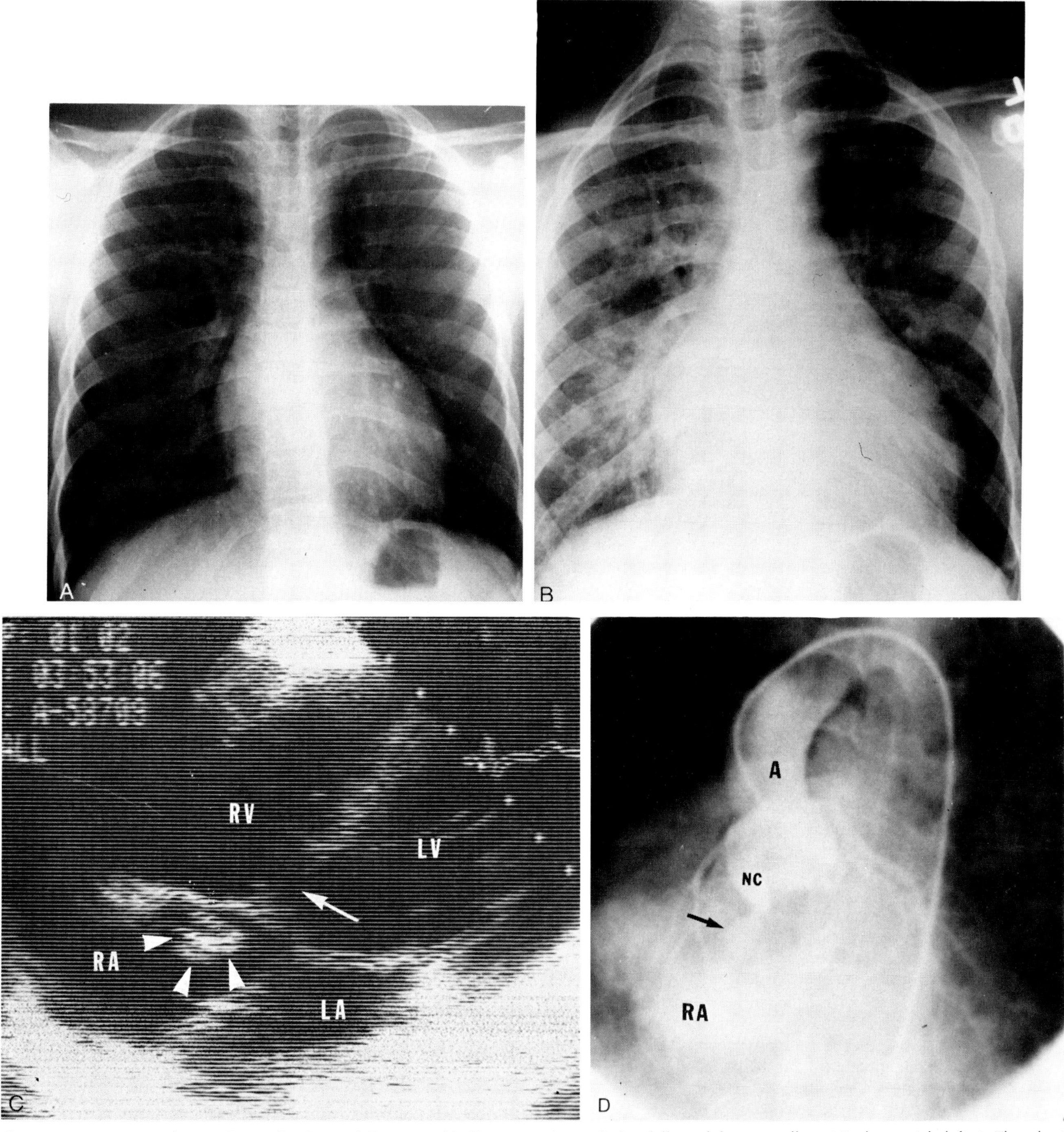

Figure 116–7. *A,* PA chest radiograph of an adolescent with Down syndrome being followed for a small ventricular septal defect. The chest radiograph is essentially normal. *B,* Approximately three years later, the patient had developed a new continuous murmur and signs of congestive heart failure. Note the increase in pulmonary vascularity and cardiac size. *C,* The four-chamber echocardiogram demonstrates an echodense structure *(arrowheads)* in the right atrium (RA). This was identified as a **sinus of Valsalva aneurysm** after cardiac catheterization. In addition, there is a small ventricular septal defect *(large arrow).* (LA = left atrium; LV = left ventricle; RV = right ventricle.) *D,* The cineaortogram (A) in a left anterior oblique projection demonstrates a ruptured sinus of Valsalva aneurysm with a fistula *(arrow)* from the noncoronary (NC) sinus of Valsalva to the right atrium (RA).

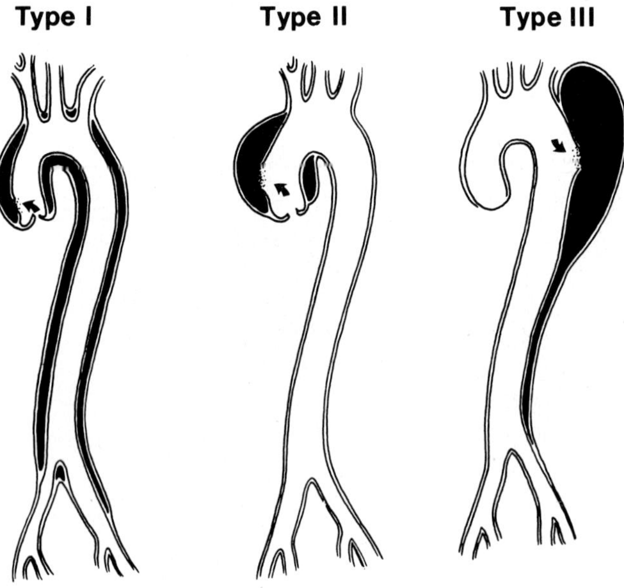

Figure 116–8. Modification of DeBakey's classification of dissecting thoracic aneurysms. The three types of aneurysms are illustrated. Types I and II correspond to Group A of Daily et al. In Type III (Group B of Daily), the dissection originates distal to the left subclavian artery, and the ascending aorta is not involved.

for the injury to be diagnosed. Of these, 80 per cent survive if surgery is performed. Only 2 to 5 per cent will survive blunt chest trauma and subsequently develop chronic traumatic aortic aneurysms if untreated.

Injury to the aorta is usually caused by rapid deceleration and vertically oriented chest trauma during a motor vehicle accident, with resultant shearing and torsion at the supravalvular ascending aorta (5 to 10 per cent) and at the isthmus of the aorta (approximately 90 per cent). Increase in intraluminal pressure applied along the entire length of the thoracic aorta makes it susceptible to injury from blunt chest trauma. However, these forces have to be extremely high in order to cause aortic rupture. The innominate artery appears to be the most susceptible of the brachiocephalic vessels to avulsion, at a site just beyond its point of origin.

Radiographic Findings. The chest radiograph will give the first clue to the diagnosis in the majority of cases of aortic trauma. Whenever possible, a chest radiograph should be obtained in the upright posteroanterior projection. The radiographic findings include widening of the mediastinum (most frequent abnormality), loss of definition of the aortic arch, inferior displacement of the trachea and esophagus to the right, left (and occasionally right) hemothorax, left apical pleural cap, and filling of the clear space between the aortic arch and main pulmonary artery (Fig. 116–16).

An additional sign of chest trauma includes extensive pleural effusion in the left side of the chest. This may be related either to hemorrhage or hemothorax after trauma or to rupture of the thoracic duct and chylothorax. A chylothorax may either result from blunt chest trauma or be secondary to iatrogenic trauma such as surgical repair of a coarctation of the aorta, repair of complete transposition of the great arteries, or palliative Blalock-Taussig shunt.

Angiographic Findings. Aortography will most readily allow aortic rupture and tear to be diagnosed (Fig. 116–16). It will also define the number of tears present, since approximately 15 to 20 per cent of cases have multiple aortic injuries. The most frequent location of the traumatic rupture of the thoracic aorta is below the aortic isthmus. The aortogram may be normal in trauma patients with a widened anterior mediastinum. In these cases, the mediastinal widening on the chest radiograph is often due to tearing of the veins or small arteries. The innominate artery is injured three times more often than the other branches of the aortic arch. Clinically, this presents as decreased pulses in the right arm. Occasionally, aortic dissection may involve the left subclavian artery. Selective aortography of the major branch vessels may be necessary for accurate diagnosis.

Pseudoaneurysms secondary to rupture into the adventitia occur in 2 to 5 per cent of patients who survive aortic trauma and rupture. These traumatic aneurysms may be heavily calcified but are considered unstable and may rapidly enlarge and rupture. When a calcified aneurysm is suspected on the plain radiograph (see Fig. 116–15), aortography should be performed with subsequent surgical correction and replacement of the aneurysm with a graft. Traumatic pseudoaneurysms of the thoracic aorta usually occur distal to the left subclavian artery at the aortic isthmus. Some aneurysms may be seen in unusual locations, including the aortic arch and descending thoracic aorta (Fig. 116–17).

TAKAYASU'S ARTERITIS

Takayasu's arteritis is a primary arteritis of undetermined etiology that affects the aorta, proximal portions of its major branches, and the pulmonary arteries. It can produce stenosis, occlusion, dilatation, or aneurysm. It most commonly affects young women but also occurs in men.

The diagnosis may be suggested from the plain radiograph when there is segmental or generalized dilatation of the thoracic aorta with some irregularity. There may be prominence of the main and intrapulmonary arteries. In addition, rib notching may result from intercostal collateral circulation to occluded subclavian arteries.

The definitive diagnosis is made by angiography or DSA. Occlusive changes may be visualized with areas of post-stenotic dilatation (Fig. 116–18). Additional angiographic features include aneurysms, dissecting aneurysms, aortic insufficiency, and a subclavian steal syndrome. In addition, stenoses of the pulmonary arteries, celiac and mesenteric arteries, and renal arteries have been reported. Patients with renal artery stenoses may present with severe hypertension (Fig. 116–18). Renal artery lesions occur in Takayasu's arteritis in 25 to 75 per cent of the reported cases.

Acknowledgment

The secretarial assistance of Ms. Debbie Johnson is gratefully acknowledged.

Text continued on page 1860

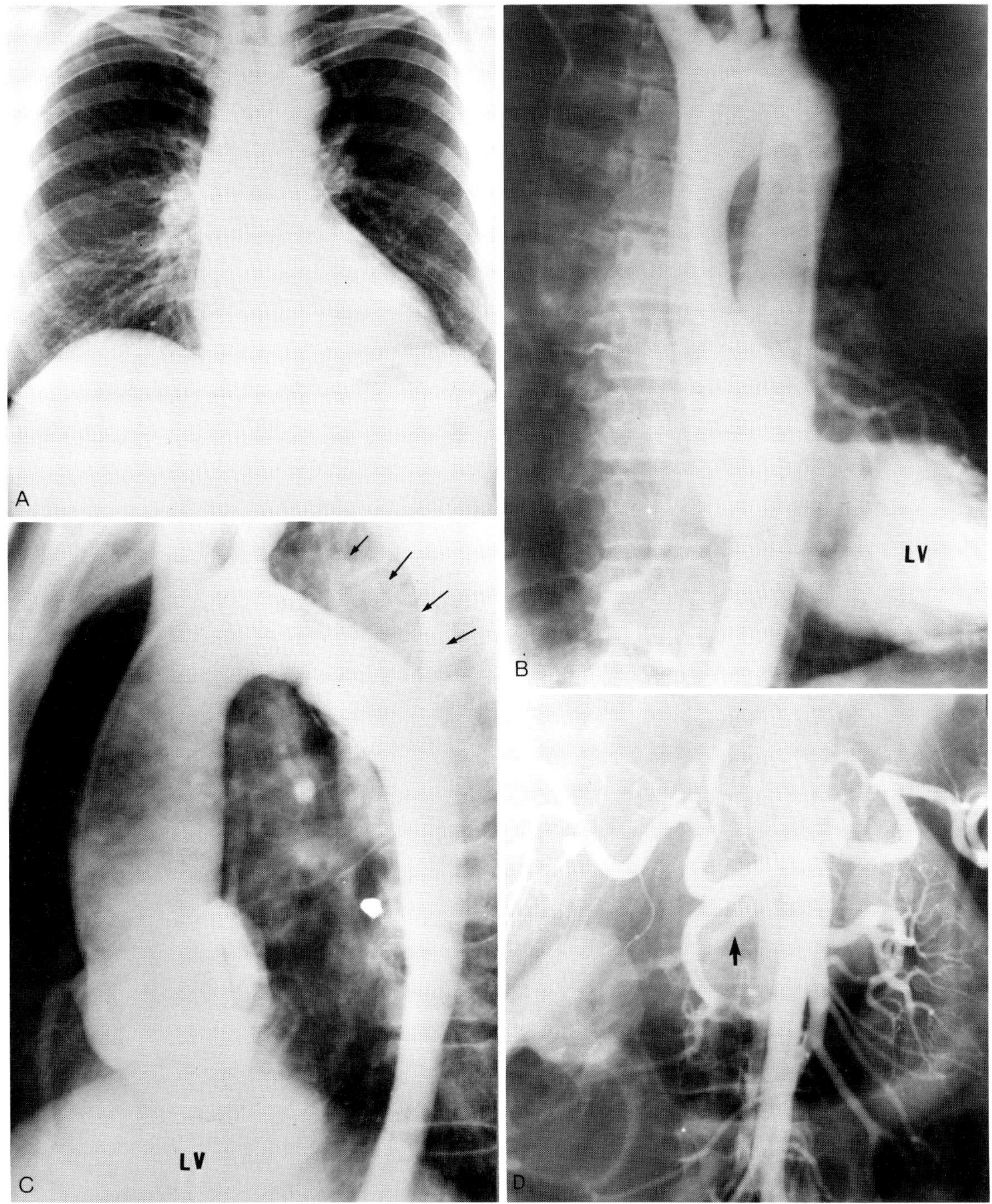

Figure 116–9. *A,* This 56-year-old woman had sharp midline back pain and a new diastolic murmur of aortic regurgitation. The chest radiograph is essentially normal. *B,* The AP thoracic aortogram shows evidence of a **Type I aortic dissection** beginning at the aortic valve. The catheter is in the densely opacified true channel, and there is filling of the left ventricle (LV). *C,* The lateral projection shows opacification of the true channel, with severe aortic valvar regurgitation and opacification of the left ventricle (LV). There is late filling of the false channel *(arrows)*. *D,* In Type I dissections, it is important to evaluate the abdominal aorta. The aortogram demonstrates that the right renal artery is filling from the false channel *(arrow)*.

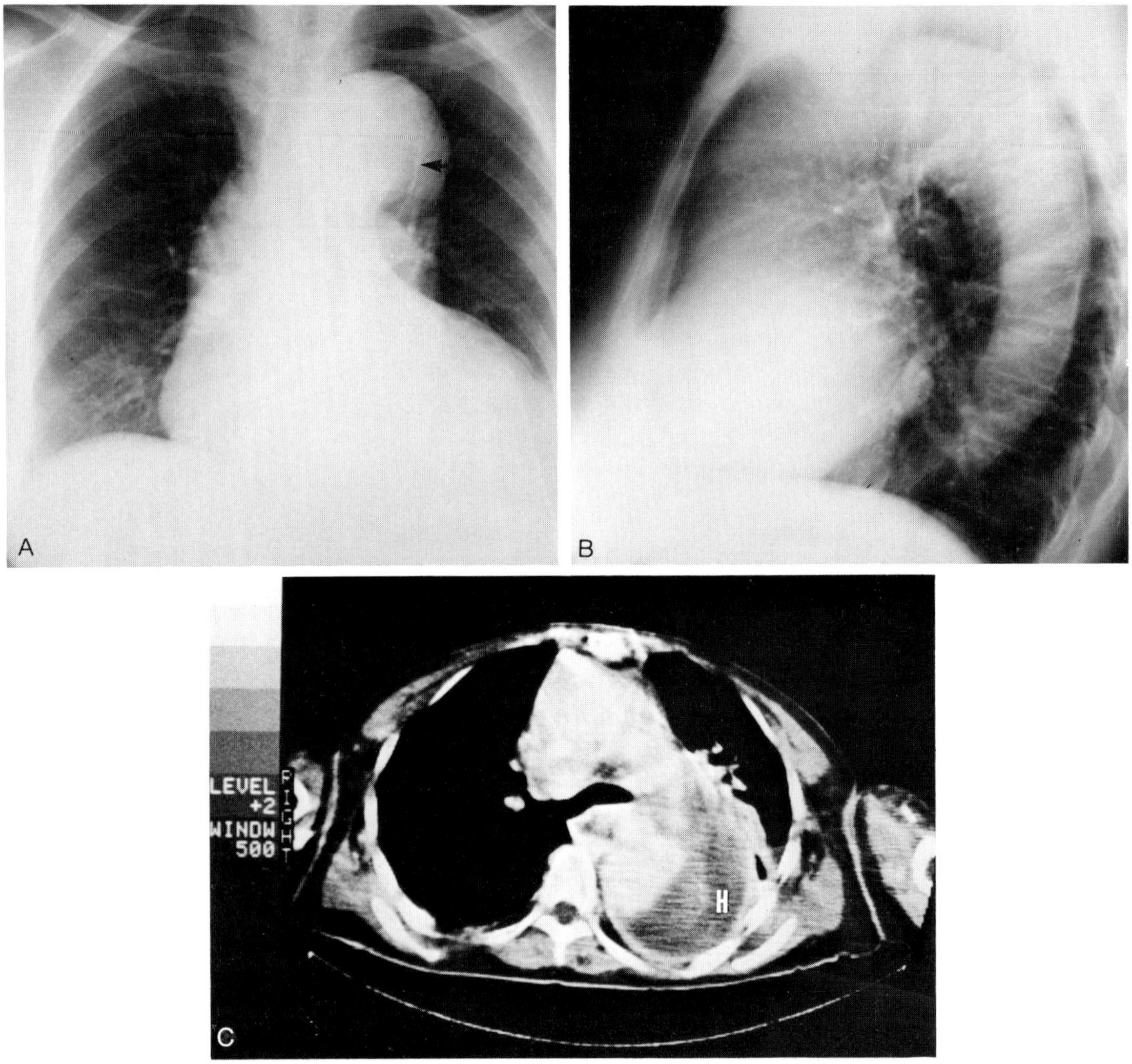

Figure 116–10. Aortic aneurysm. *A,* PA chest radiograph of a 50-year-old woman with a long-standing history of hypertension shows a widened ascending aorta and aortic arch and an enlarged left ventricle. Note the calcification along the intima of the aortic arch *(arrow),* with extension of the adventitia. *B,* The lateral projection shows widening of the ascending aorta compatible with an aortic aneurysm. *C,* A CT scan of the thoracic aorta shows a low-density area compatible with hematoma (H) involving the descending aorta in this patient with aortic aneurysm.

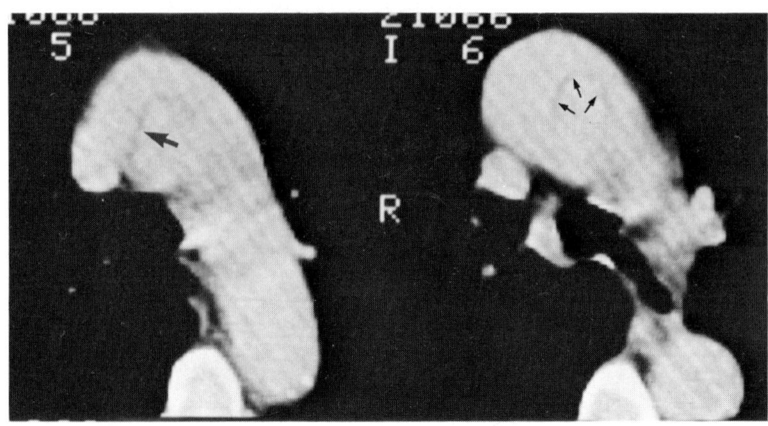

Figure 116–11. Acute aortic dissection can be diagnosed by computed tomography, as in this 50-year-old woman with acute thoracic pain and visualization of the intimal flap on CT *(arrows).* (Case contributed by Allen K. Tonkin, M.D., Baptist Memorial Hospital, Memphis, TN.)

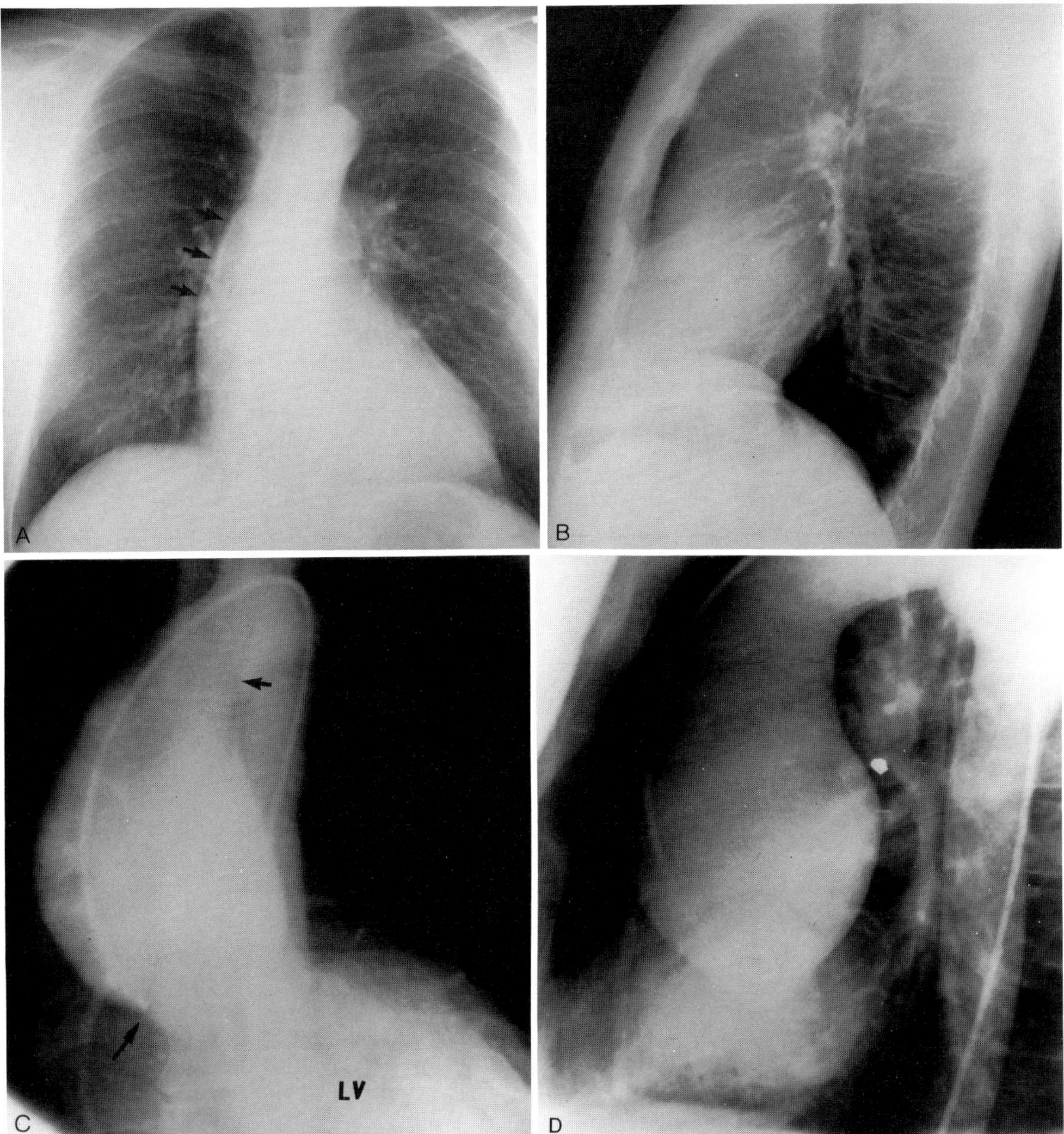

Figure 116–12. *A,* PA chest radiograph in a 42-year-old man with **cystic medial necrosis** shows a classic configuration of a dilated ascending aorta *(arrows)* and an enlarged left ventricle. This patient had a known history of hypertension and a new diastolic murmur. *B,* The lateral projection also shows filling of the retrosternal space by a dilated ascending aorta. *C,* The AP thoracic aortogram shows evidence of a **Type II aortic dissection** extending from the ascending aorta to the arch *(arrows)*. There is a saccular symmetrical dilatation of the ascending aorta and sinuses of Valsalva, with severe aortic valvar regurgitation and opacification of the left ventricle (LV). *D,* The lateral projection also demonstrates symmetrical fusiform dilatation of the entire ascending aorta diagnostic of cystic medial necrosis.

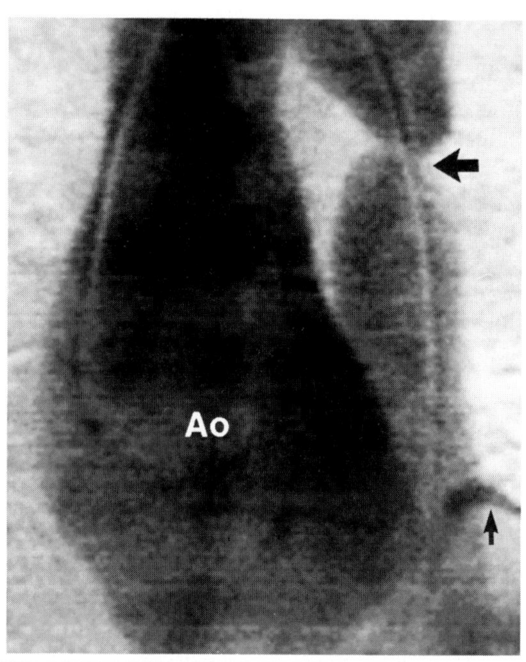

Figure 116–13. Intra-arterial digital subtraction angiography was performed in the AP projection on a 17-year-old male with symmetrical dilatation of the ascending aorta (Ao) and is compatible with **cystic medial necrosis**. Note the coarctation of the aorta *(large arrow)*. The take-off of the left coronary artery *(small arrow)* is also visible. This study was performed with 50 per cent dilute contrast material.

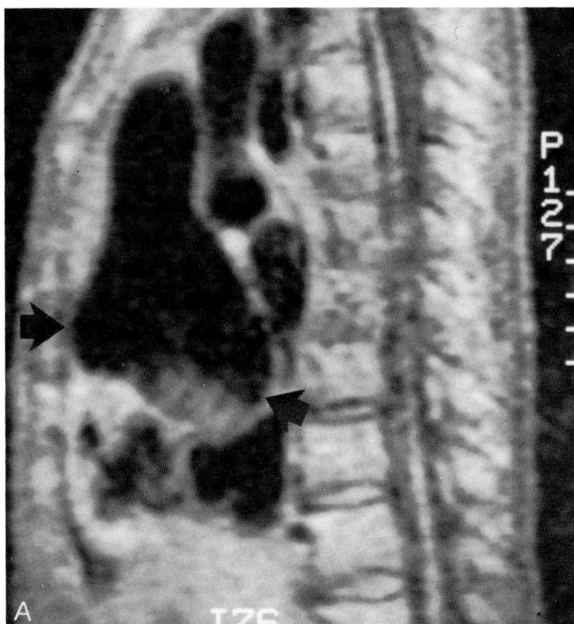

Figure 116–14. *A,* The sagittal view of the MRI of a 17-year-old male with cystic medial necrosis and Marfan's syndrome demonstrates annuloaortic ectasia *(arrows)* and a dilated ascending aorta. *B,* The patient underwent a median sternotomy with placement of a St. Jude valve and graft into the ascending aorta. He returned with chest pain. The chest radiograph shows a normal-sized heart. *C,* The lateral projection demonstrates the St. Jude prosthetic valve in the aortic projection *(arrow).*

Illustration continued on following page

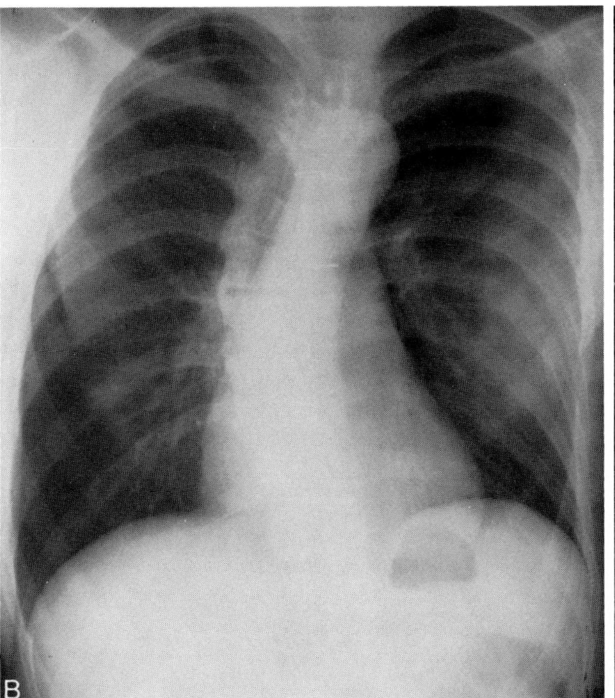

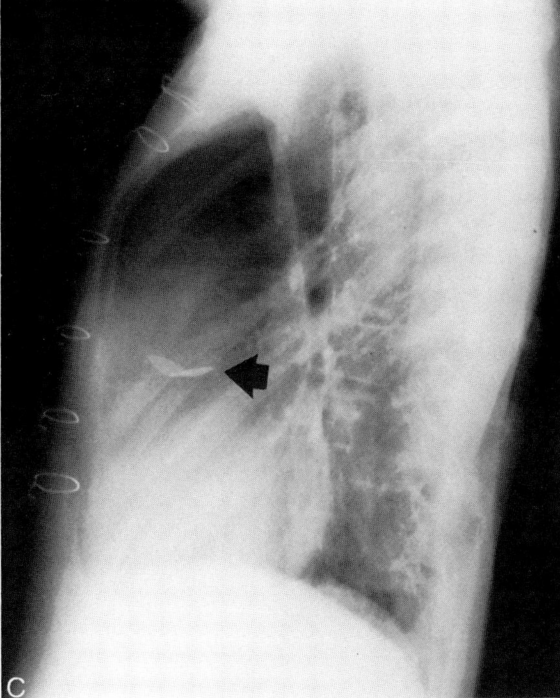

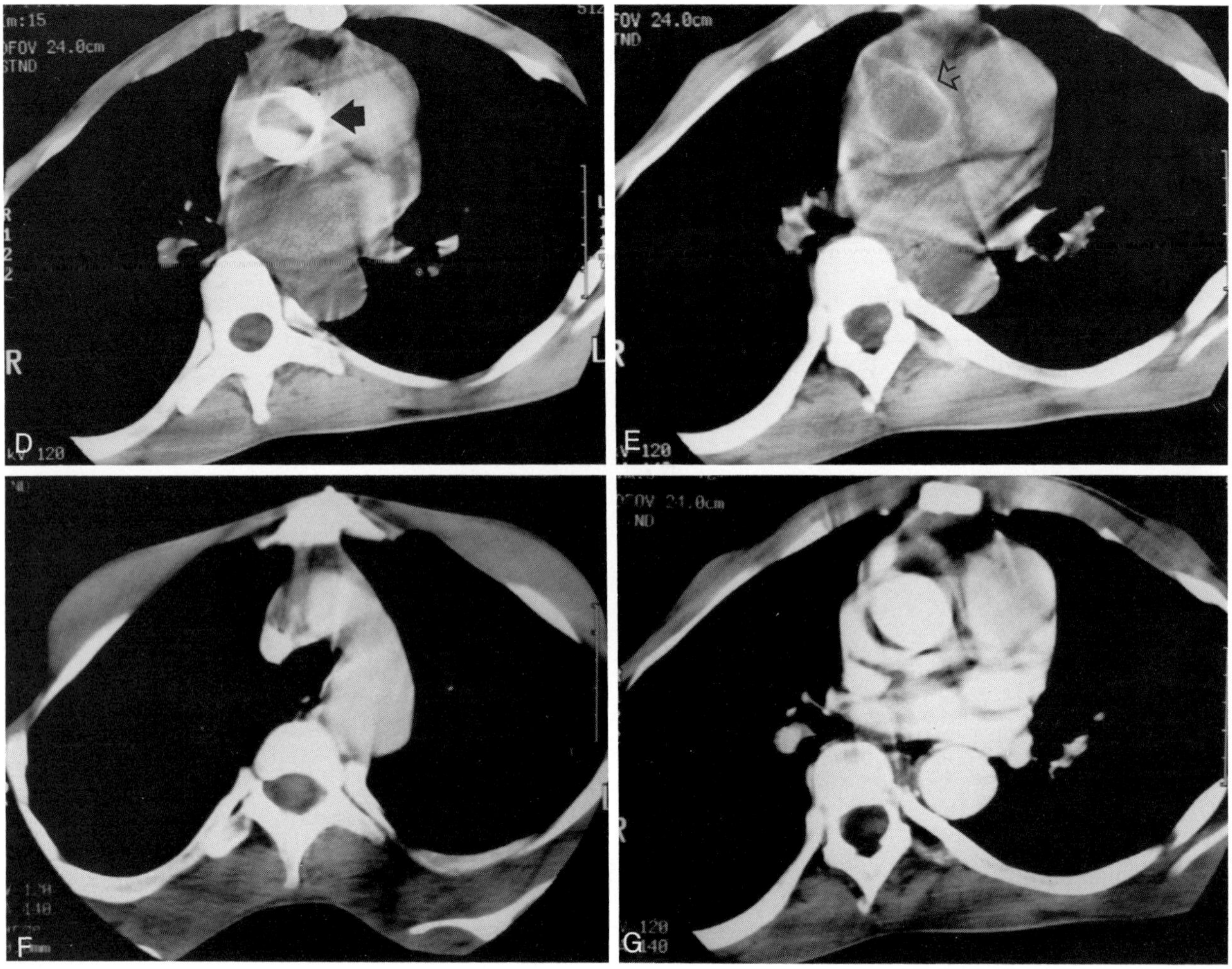

Figure 116–14 *Continued. D,* A CT scan demonstrates the prosthetic St. Jude valve *(arrow). E,* A higher slice of the CT scan shows the graft of the ascending aorta *(open arrow). F,* The upper descending thoracic aorta is somewhat dilated in this hypertensive patient. *G,* With contrast enhancement at a lower level, one notices the outer diameter of the adventitia, which is left in place with the contrast media in the central dense portion of the ascending aorta.

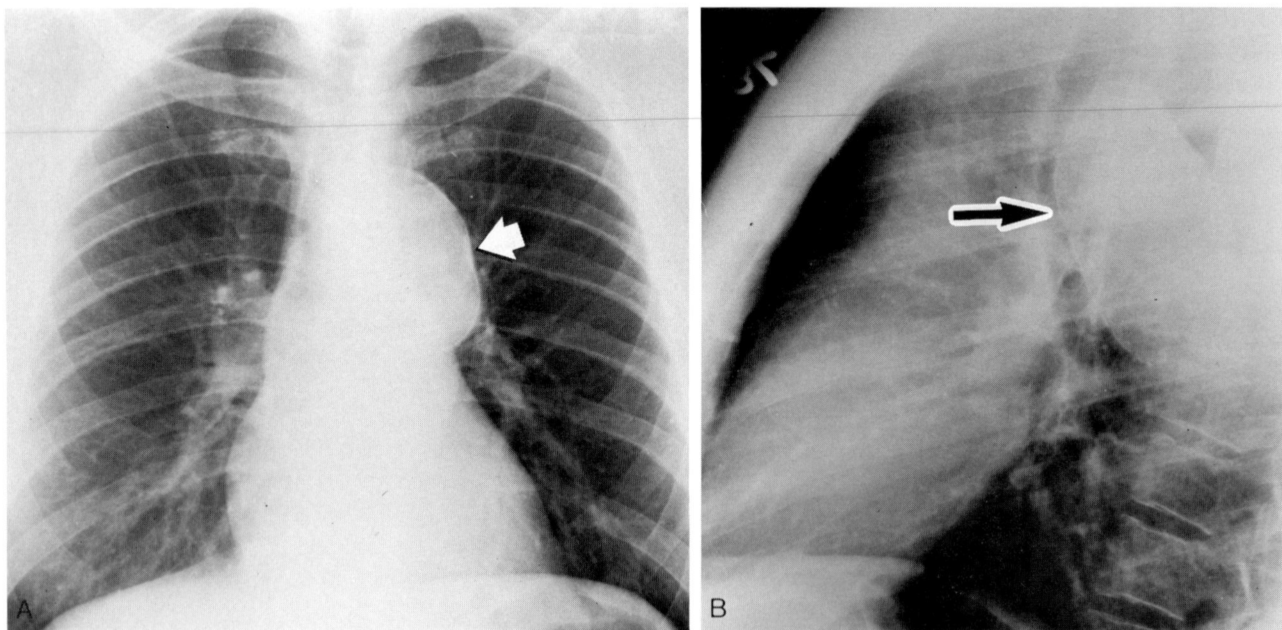

Figure 116–15. *A,* PA view of the chest of a 41-year-old man shows a calcified **Type III aortic dissection**. The calcification extends from the upper descending aorta distal to the take-off of the left subclavian artery *(arrow). B,* The lateral projection demonstrates the fusiform and calcified aneurysm *(arrow)* involving the descending aorta in this patient with a history of long-standing hypertension.

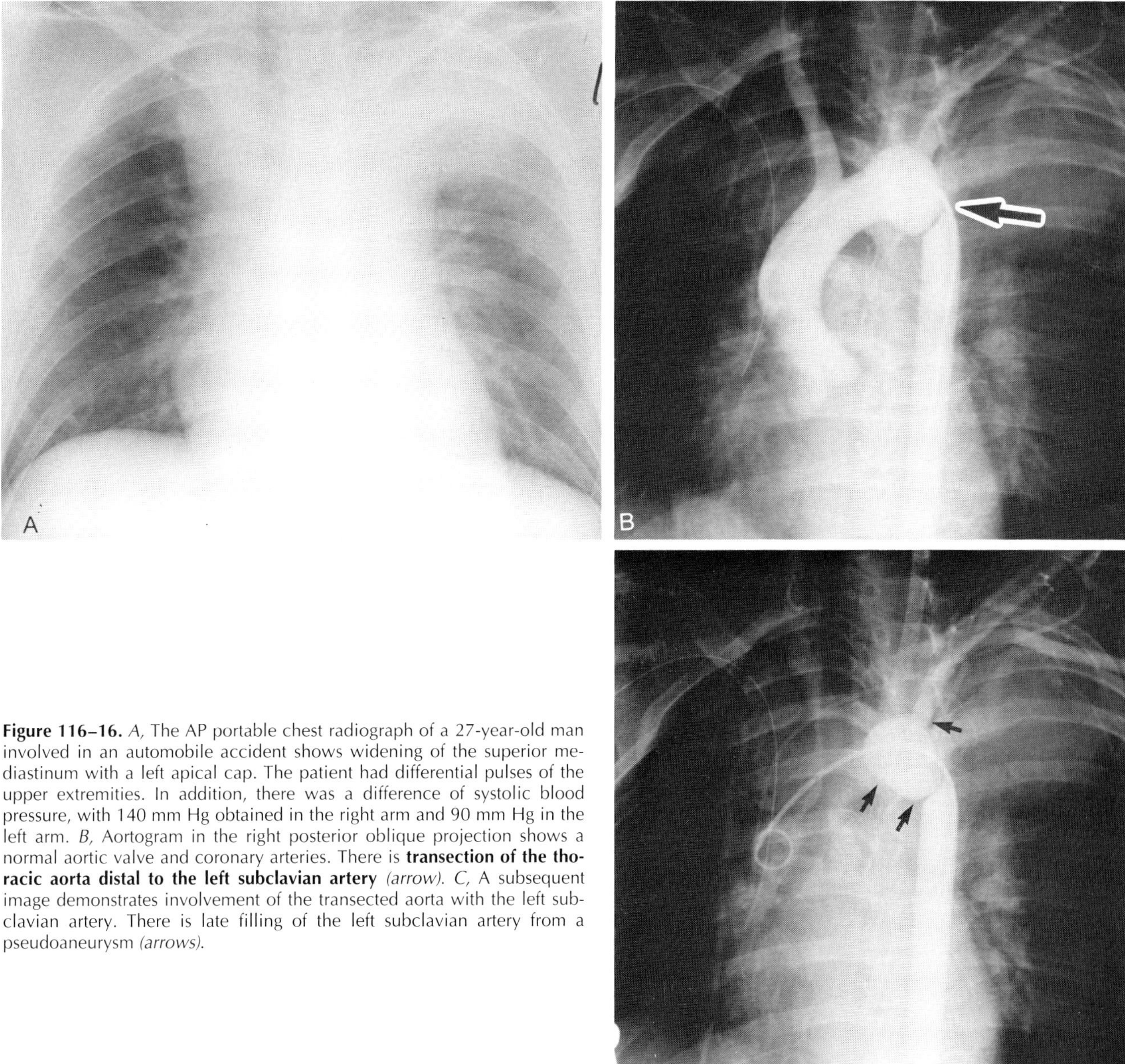

Figure 116–16. *A,* The AP portable chest radiograph of a 27-year-old man involved in an automobile accident shows widening of the superior mediastinum with a left apical cap. The patient had differential pulses of the upper extremities. In addition, there was a difference of systolic blood pressure, with 140 mm Hg obtained in the right arm and 90 mm Hg in the left arm. *B,* Aortogram in the right posterior oblique projection shows a normal aortic valve and coronary arteries. There is **transection of the thoracic aorta distal to the left subclavian artery** *(arrow). C,* A subsequent image demonstrates involvement of the transected aorta with the left subclavian artery. There is late filling of the left subclavian artery from a pseudoaneurysm *(arrows).*

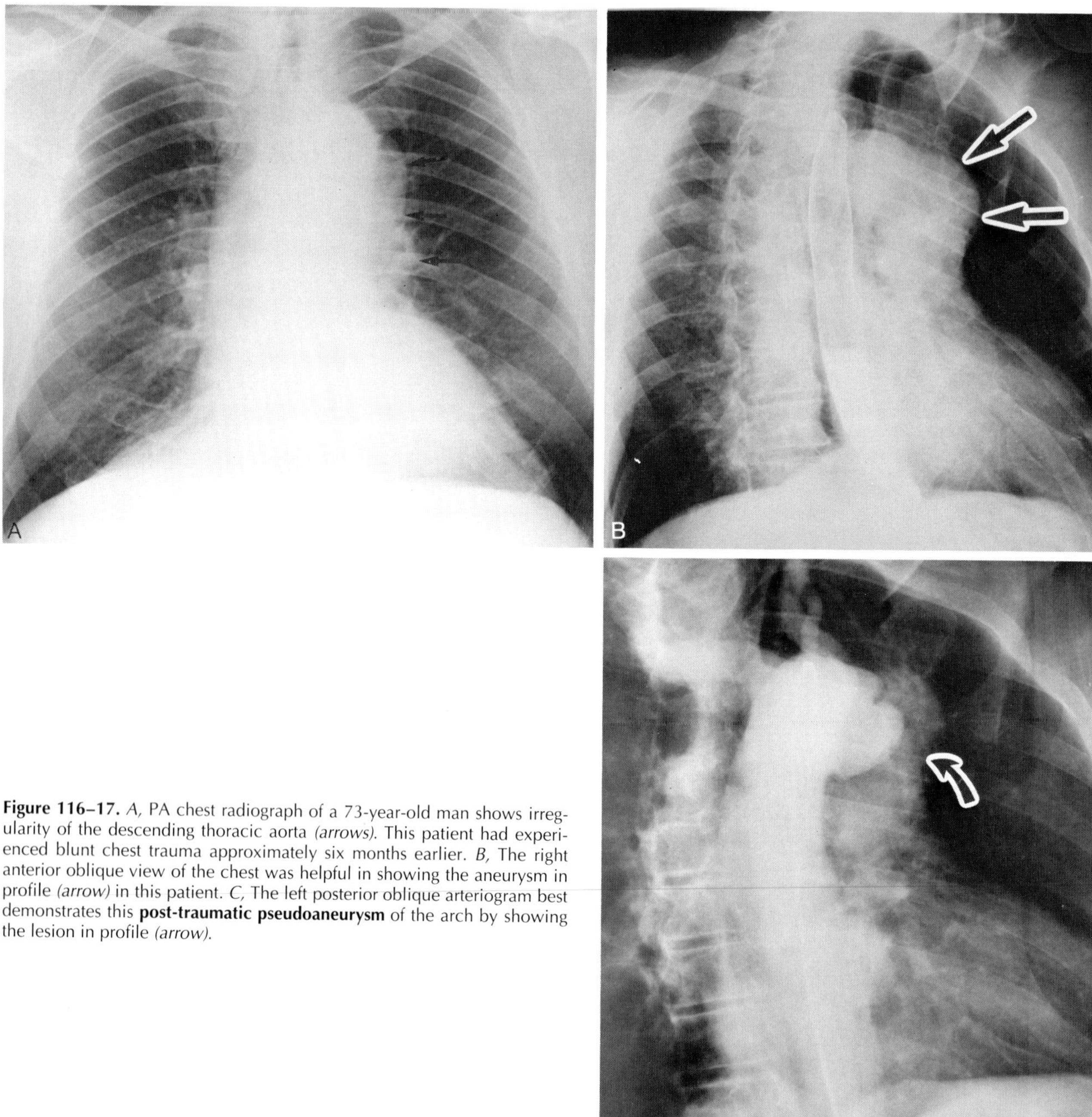

Figure 116–17. *A,* PA chest radiograph of a 73-year-old man shows irregularity of the descending thoracic aorta *(arrows).* This patient had experienced blunt chest trauma approximately six months earlier. *B,* The right anterior oblique view of the chest was helpful in showing the aneurysm in profile *(arrow)* in this patient. *C,* The left posterior oblique arteriogram best demonstrates this **post-traumatic pseudoaneurysm** of the arch by showing the lesion in profile *(arrow).*

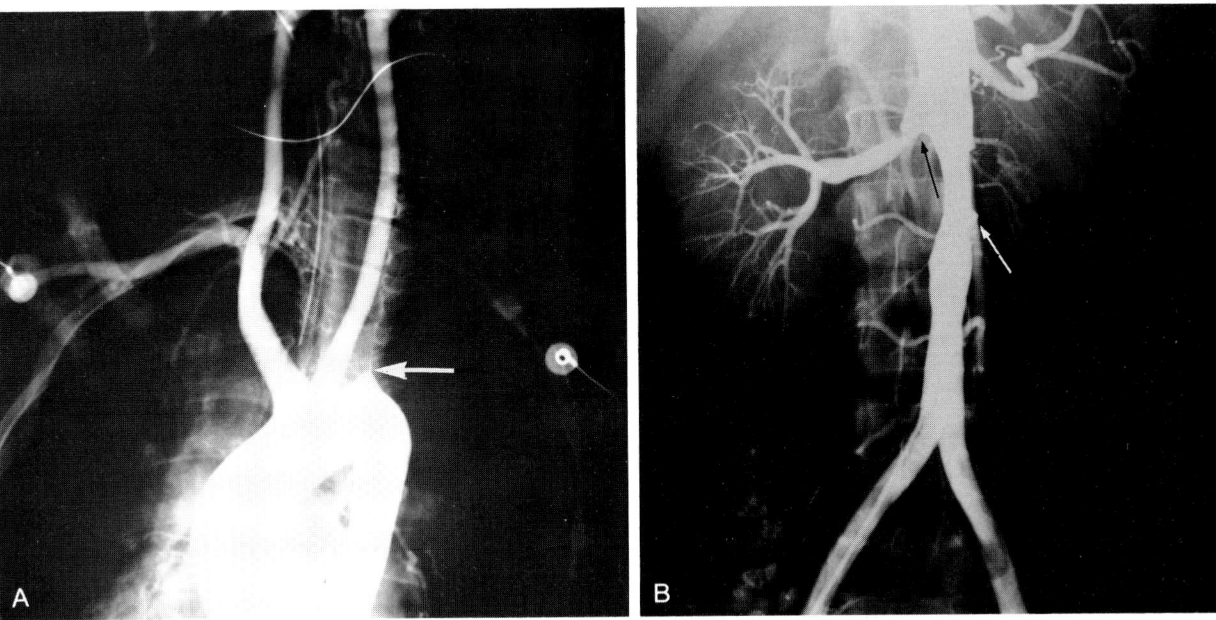

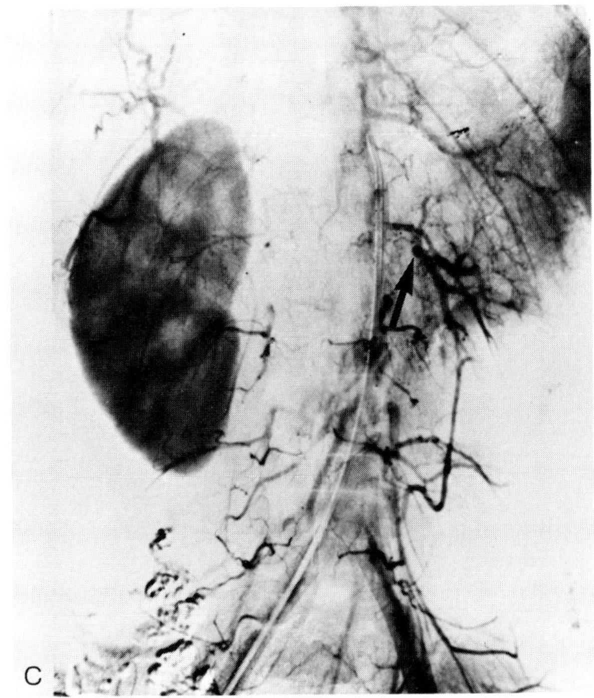

Figure 116–18. *A,* This 14-year-old female presented with severe hypertension and a nonpalpable pulse in the left arm. The thoracic aortogram demonstrates complete occlusion of the left subclavian artery *(arrow).* A left subclavian steal was visualized on subsequent films. *B,* The abdominal aortogram demonstrates a severe stenosis of the right renal artery *(black arrow)* with complete occlusion of the origin of the left renal artery *(white arrow).* In addition, there is some irregularity of the lower abdominal aorta secondary to **Takayasu's arteritis**. *C,* The later phase of the aortogram was subtracted to demonstrate the left intrarenal branches *(arrow)* that have developed from collateral flow.

Bibliography

Amparo EG, Higgins CB, Hricak H, Sollitto R: Aortic dissection: Magnetic resonance imaging. Radiology 155:399–406, 1985.

Cooley RN, Schrieber MH: Congenital anomalies of the heart and great vessels. In Radiology of the Heart and Great Vessels, 3rd ed. Baltimore, Williams and Wilkins, 1980.

Daily PO, Trueblood HW, Stinson FB, et al: Management of acute aortic dissections. Ann Thorac Surg 10:237, 1970.

Daniels DL, Maddison FE: Ascending aortic injury: An angiographic diagnosis. AJR 136:812, 1981.

Dinsmore RE, Willerson JT, Buckley MJ: Dissecting aneurysm of the aorta. Aortographic features affecting prognosis. Radiology 105:567, 1972.

Earnest F IV, Muhm JR, Sheedy PF II: Roentgenographic findings in thoracic aortic dissection. Mayo Clin Proc 54:43, 1979.

Eisen S, Elliott LP: The roentgenology of cystic medial necrosis of the ascending aorta. Radiol Clin North Am 6:437, 1968.

Godwin JD, Turley K, Herfkens RJ, et al: Computed tomography for follow-up of chronic aortic dissections. Radiology 139:655, 1981.

Gomes AS: MRI of congenital heart disease. Cardiovascular Imaging in Categorical Course Syllabus of ARRS. 90th Annual Meeting American Roentgen Ray Society, Washington, DC, 22–38, 1990.

Gutierrez FR, Gowda S, Ludbrook PA, et al: Cineangiography in the diagnosis and evaluation of aortic dissection. Radiology 135:759–761, 1980.

Higgins CB, Reinke RT: Nonsyphilitic etiology of linear calcification of the ascending aorta. Radiology 113:609, 1974.

Higgins CB, Silverman NR, Harris RD, et al: Localized aneurysms of the descending thoracic aorta. Clin Radiol 26:475, 1975.

Hirsch JH, Carter SJ, Chikos PM, et al: Traumatic pseudoaneurysms of the thoracic aorta: Two unusual cases. AJR 130:157, 1978.

Kersting-Sommerhoff BA, Sechtem UP, Schiller NB, et al: MR imaging of the thoracic aorta in Marfan patients. J Comput Assist Tomogr 11(4):633–639, 1987.

McGoon DC: Cardiac Surgery. Philadelphia, FA Davis, 1982.

Price JE Jr, Gray RK, Grollman JH Jr: Aortic wall thickness as an unreliable sign in the diagnosis of dissecting aneurysm of the thoracic aorta. AJR 113:710, 1971.

Simeone JF, Minagi H, Putman CE: Traumatic disruption of the thoracic aorta: Significance of the left apical extrapleural cap. Radiology 117:265, 1975.

Soto B, Harman MA, Ceballos R, et al: Angiographic diagnosis of dissecting aneurysm of the aorta. AJR 116:146, 1972.

Tonkin IL, Marin-Garcia J, Paul RN, et al: Ruptured sinus of Valsalva aneurysm in children: A report of two cases and literature review. Cardiovasc Intervent Radiol 7:78–83, 1984.

Tonkin ILD: Radiography of diseases involving the aortic valve and thoracic aorta. Symposium on Chest Radiography for the Cardiologist. Cardiovasc Clin 1:625–683, 1983.

Tonkin ILD: Pediatric Cardiovascular Imaging. Philadelphia, WB Saunders Company, 1992.

Winkler ML, Higgins CB: MRI of perivalvular infectious pseudoaneurysms. AJR 147:253–256, 1986.

Wojtowycz M: Thoracic Aortography and Bronchial Angiography in Interventional Radiology and Angiography. Handbooks in Radiology, 1990, pp 117–145.

117 Diseases of the Peripheral Vascular System

Julius H. Grollman, Jr., Robert J. Cassling, and Antoinette S. Gomes

OCCLUSIVE PERIPHERAL VASCULAR DISEASE

Atherosclerosis

Atherosclerotic peripheral vascular disease, the most common vascular affliction, can begin at an early age but generally manifests clinically after age 40. Atherosclerotic plaques tend to be eccentrically located within the vessel lumen, have irregular contours, and may be focal or diffuse in nature. The involved vessels are often tortuous and can exhibit focal or diffuse dilatations (aneurysms). Vascular wall calcification is frequent. Small outpouchings filled by contrast material may indicate ulceration within the plaque. In order to accurately assess the degree of vessel luminal narrowing, two orthogonal projections should be obtained.

Experimentally appreciable changes in pressure and flow do not occur until the cross-sectional area of a vessel has been reduced by more than 75 per cent, which corresponds to at least a 50 per cent reduction in diameter. Owing to the many and varied collateral pathways, however, different arteries will tolerate varying degrees of luminal narrowing before symptoms are produced.

Atherosclerotic occlusion of the arterial tree is a chronic indolent process manifested by progressive luminal narrowing prior to the actual occlusion. Consequently, the onset of ischemic symptoms is often gradual. The extent and severity of symptoms are related to the location of the occlusion and whether there has been time for the development of collateral vessels. At first, symptoms tend to be exertional in nature and resolve with rest. Claudication of the buttocks, hips, thighs, and calf is common. Rest pain is an ominous sign of hypoxemia secondary to severe vascular insufficiency. Acute ischemic symptoms may develop rapidly after ulceration of a nonobstructing plaque with secondary thrombosis occluding the vessel. Leriche's syndrome manifests as an inability to maintain an erection, lower extremity weakness, muscular atrophy, and absent distal pulses and is a result of severe stenosis or obliteration of the aortic bifurcation.

Aortic occlusion occurs most commonly in the distal abdominal aorta, often with retrograde propagation of thrombus up to the level of the renal arteries (Fig. 117–1). Since the development of occlusion is gradual, symptoms may be surprisingly minimal and may remain stable for years. Obstructions in the pelvis may occur anywhere throughout the common and external iliac arteries. The most common site of major atherosclerotic involvement below the inguinal ligament is in the distal superficial femoral artery at the adductor hiatus. The popliteal and infrapopliteal arteries are also commonly involved.

It is important for the angiographer to be aware of potential collateral pathways in order to place the catheter properly for accurate assessment of the patency or degree of involvement of the vessels distal to the occlusion. Without contrast entering the major collateral vessels, the downstream runoff vessels will not be accurately assessed.

Many potential anastomotic arcades exist between the aorta and pelvic vessels. In infrarenal aortic occlusions, the inferior mesenteric artery (IMA) is also frequently occluded. In this situation, the

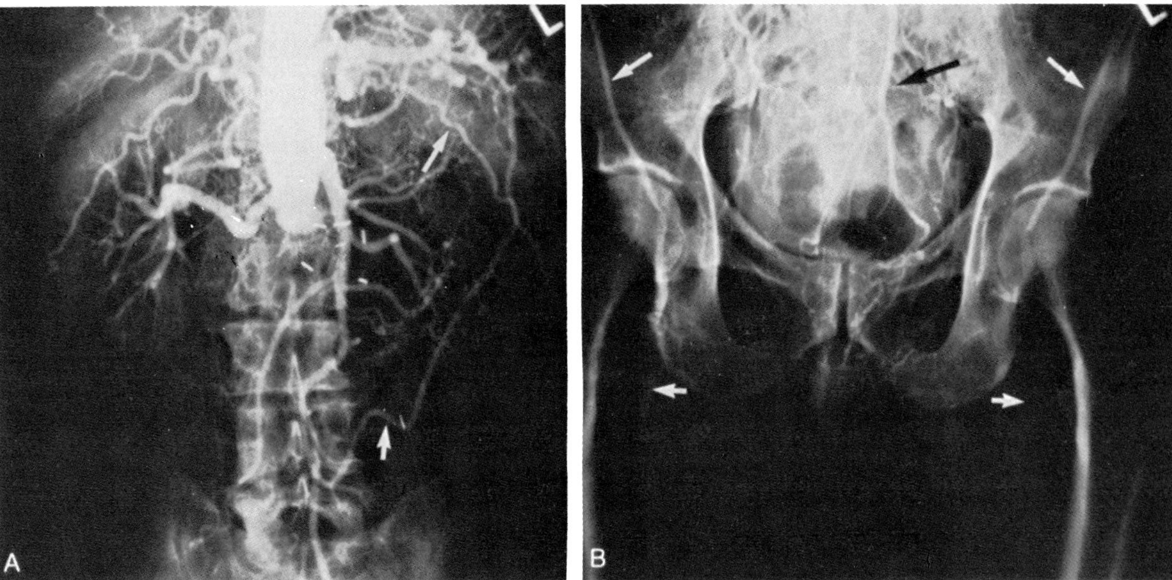

Figure 117–1. *A,* Typical **total aortic occlusion below the renal arteries causing Leriche's syndrome** (a left nephrectomy had previously been performed). Note the large intercostal arteries bilaterally. The marginal artery of Drummond *(long arrow)* provides communication between the left branch of the middle colic artery of the superior mesenteric artery and the left colic branch of the inferior mesenteric artery *(short arrow). B,* Delayed filming of the pelvis shows filling of the inferior mesenteric artery and superior hemorrhoidal artery *(black arrow).* The right and left deep circumflex iliac arteries *(long white arrows)* reconstitute common femoral arteries bilaterally with subsequent filling of the profunda femoral arteries *(short white arrows).* The abrupt decrease in contrast density in the common femoral arteries is due to competitive filling of nonopacified blood from the inferior epigastric arteries, which are a continuation of the internal mammary arteries.

superior mesenteric artery (SMA) may form the first segment of a complicated collateral network supplying the pelvis. The left branch of the middle colic artery arising from the SMA forms an arcade with the left colic branch of the IMA (arc of Riolan). Blood then flows retrogradely down the left colic branch into the superior hemorrhoidal branch of the IMA, which anastomoses with the middle hemorrhoidal branch of the internal iliac artery to feed the external iliac artery (Fig. 117–1). Another collateral network between the superior and inferior mesenteric arteries is through the arcade of Drummond (Fig. 117–1), an anastomotic marginal colonic artery that forms an arcade along the mesenteric surface of the colon giving off vasa recta to the bowel and anastomosing with the middle colic artery. Intercostal arteries will also bring blood to the pelvis via communications with the iliac circumflex and inferior epigastric arteries, branches of the distal external iliac artery. A final but very important collateral pathway is by the internal mammary arteries, which arise from the subclavian arteries and anastomose with the inferior epigastric arteries. This pathway is not demonstrated with aortic injections beyond the origin of the left subclavian artery but is frequently suggested by "wash-out" in the common femoral arteries due to inflow of unopacified blood (Fig. 117–1). With distal infrarenal aortic occlusions, the lumbar arteries may anastomose with the iliolumbar branches of the internal iliac artery, allowing retrograde flow into the external iliac artery and/or to the femoral vessels. If the external iliac artery is also blocked, the branches of the internal iliac vessel can form communications with the femoral system via internal pudendal and superior gluteal artery collaterals to the femoral circumflex arteries. The middle sacral artery may develop communications with internal iliac branches as well.

External iliac or common femoral artery occlusions are collateralized via superior and inferior gluteal artery anastomoses with the lateral femoral circumflex branch of the deep femoral artery (Fig. 117–2). The superficial femoral artery is commonly occluded at its origin and as it leaves the adductor canal just above the knee. Collateral vessels from the distal profunda femoral artery will often typically reconstitute the popliteal artery at varying levels above the knee. Geniculate and sural collaterals will cross the knee joint with popliteal and very proximal tibial artery occlusions. More distal tibial and peroneal artery blockages will collateralize each other through muscular branches that also will reconstitute the dorsal pedal and plantar arteries of the the foot.

Inflammatory Peripheral Vascular Occlusive Disease

Vascular narrowing and occlusions may be secondary to other causes. A vessel that shows smooth segmental or diffuse narrowing

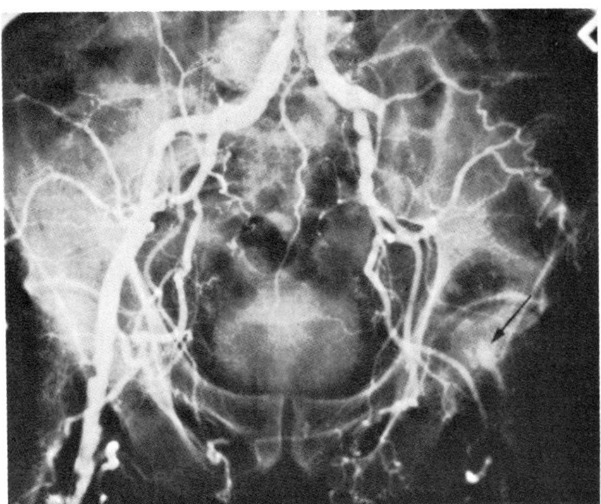

Figure 117–2. Occlusion of the left external iliac and common femoral arteries. Blood flow to the distal common femoral artery *(long arrow)* is via the deep circumflex iliac artery *(short arrow),* which receives collateral vessels from the iliolumbar and superior gluteal artery branches of the internal iliac artery. Other branches of the hypogastric, obturator, internal pudendal, and inferior gluteal arteries also collateralize the common femoral artery.

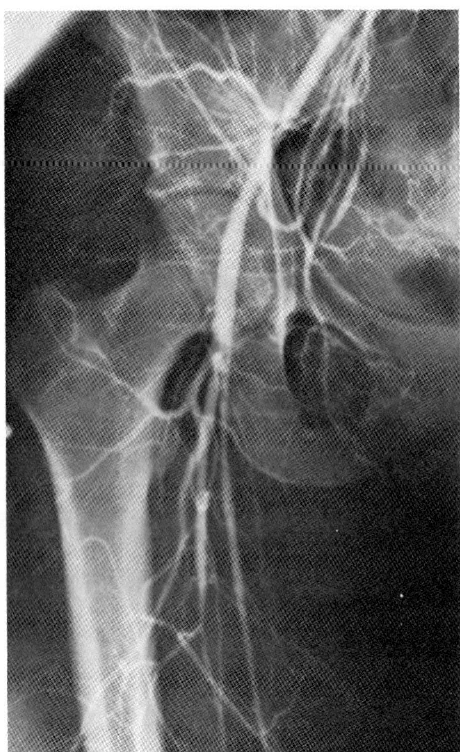

Figure 117–3. Vasculitis in patient with ergotism and peripheral ischemia. Note the long, smooth, segmental narrowings of the common, superficial, and profunda femoral arteries.

rather than the more characteristic irregular stenosis of atherosclerosis should suggest an alternative cause.

VASCULITIS. Various inflammatory processes exist that may involve any of the peripheral and visceral vessels, including the aorta, but that are relatively uncommon causes of vascular obstruction (Fig. 117–3). They can be associated with collagen diseases (discussed later in this chapter), drug reactions, radiation injury, and bacterial infections.

Severe arteriospastic conditions can occur as an idiosyncratic reaction to certain drugs such as ergotamines, lysergic acid, and narcotics. Necrotizing angiitis has been described with methamphetamine abuse.

Late effects of radiation include segmental arterial stenoses and occlusion secondary to endothelial damage and arterial wall ischemia from obliteration of the vasa vasorum. Often, there is superimposed thrombosis and secondary atherosclerosis, making angiographic distinction from primary atherosclerosis difficult. The clinical history and localization of the disease process to the field of radiation will suggest the diagnosis.

Infectious arteritis is uncommon now because of antibiotic availability. Syphilitic aortitis and arteritis, previously the most commonly encountered bacterial disease, is now very rare. Tuberculosis of arteries is usually secondary to extension from tuberculous involvement of the surrounding tissues. Direct arterial involvement begins as a periarteritis and may progress to an obliterative endarteritis or thrombosis. A variety of organisms may involve the arteries primarily, leading either to a panarteritis with occlusion or, more commonly, to a mycotic aneurysm. When endocarditis is the principal etiology, enterococcus and *Streptococcus* are the prevailing organisms. *Staphylococcus* is now the most common pathogen in mycotic aneurysms. *Salmonella* and *Escherichia coli* are also causative organisms.

TAKAYASU'S ARTERITIS. This disease is seen predominantly in young Asian women. In its early active phase, it may present with fever and arthritis; later, symptoms of vascular occlusion may be experienced. It most often involves the aortic arch and brachiocephalic vessels but can also involve the distal aorta and its branches. Pulmonary arterial involvement is common. Smooth, long segmental narrowing of the aorta and its proximal branches is typically seen on angiography. Symptoms are related to the sites of stenosis and can include extremity claudication and stroke, which in the case of the brachiocephalic arteries are referred to as the "aortic arch syndrome."

GIANT CELL ARTERIES. Seen in older patients, this disease involves large, medium, and small arteries with frequent involvement of the aorta and the temporal, ophthalmic, and brachiocephalic arteries (Fig. 117–4). Any vessel, however, may be involved. Sclerotic changes may be seen in the aorta, but dilatation is the primary angiographic finding. Occlusions of the brachiocephalic arteries oc-

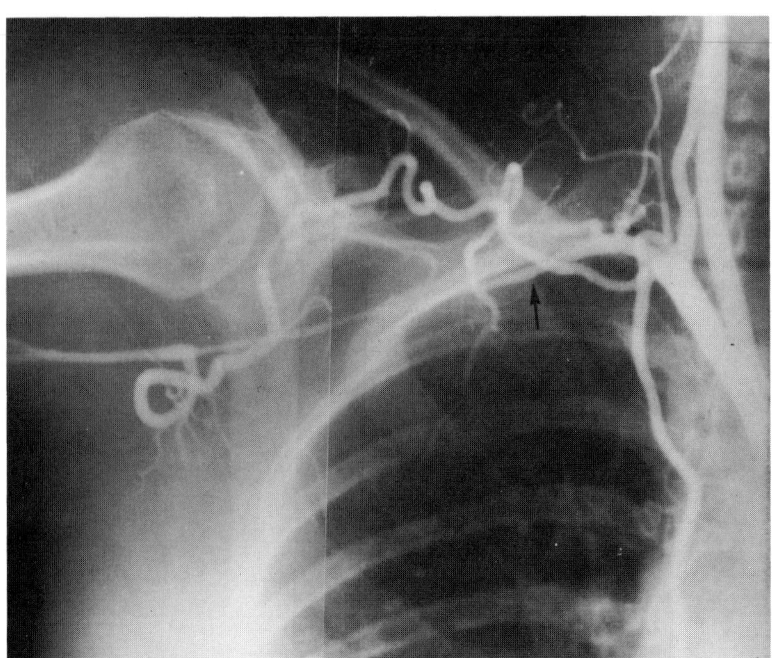

Figure 117–4. Giant cell arteritis resulting in an elongated smooth stenosis beginning in the mid–right subclavian artery *(arrow)* and extending into the axillary artery. This appearance is typical of giant cell arteritis. The process was bilateral in this patient.

cur but are relatively rare. This process may be angiographically indistinguishable from Takayasu's arteritis. Small vessels such as the temporal artery show segmental stenoses and dilations.

Thromboangiitis Obliterans (Buerger's Disease). Thromboangiitis obliterans is a segmental inflammatory process involving medium and small vessels in the hands and feet. It is predominantly seen in young male smokers, particularly those of Asian or Near Eastern ancestry. Angiography shows absence of typical atherosclerosis with abrupt distal occlusions. The collateral vessels have a typical corkscrew appearance due to partial recanalization of the thrombosed vessels as well as development of vasa vasorum.

Thromboembolic Disease

Vascular occlusion may also be caused by thrombosis, either secondary to a primary disease process or due to embolism from a distant source. The acute angiographic appearance of a thromboembolism is generally an abrupt occlusion, sometimes with a meniscus shape. Within a few hours, clot retraction will occur, producing the characteristic appearance of a worm-like filling defect or "railroad tracking" as contrast medium enters the separation between the clot and the vessel wall. With secondary thrombosis, the primary process may be masked, but the appearance of adjacent arterial segments may give a clue. Acute thrombosis superimposed on a chronic atherosclerotic process is a very common presentation.

Embolization from a distant source is usually associated with atrial fibrillation, myocardial infarction with mural thrombus, and bacterial endocarditis. Aortic aneurysms and ulcerated atheromatous plaques may also embolize clot or plaque fragments. Rarely, tumor embolization may occur after arterial invasion by an adjacent neoplasm or from a primary tumor such as a left atrial myxoma.

Primary Diseases of Connective Tissue

There is a broad group of abnormalities of connective tissue that primarily involve arteries. Arteriography is frequently instrumental in their diagnosis.

Fibromuscular Dysplasia. This disease or group of diseases of unknown etiology most frequently affects the main renal arteries. Other arteries may also be involved, including the aorta and the carotid, vertebral, brachial, coronary, celiac, mesenteric, iliac, and femoral arteries (Fig. 117–5). Fibromuscular dysplasia has been histologically classified according to the dominant layer of arterial involvement: intimal, medial, or adventitial. The intimal type is a fibroplasia. The medial type may be one of three kinds: fibroplasia with aneurysms, fibromuscular hyperplasia, or subadventitial fibroplasia. The adventitial type is a periarterial fibroplasia. Angiographically, the involvement may be focal, multifocal, or tubular, with or without aneurysm formation. Dissection can occur if the internal elastic lamina is interrupted.

Collagen Diseases. Distinctive arteriographic abnormalities have been described in rheumatoid arthritis, polyarteritis nodosa, and scleroderma. In *rheumatoid arthritis*, both occlusive and hypervascular changes occur in the small arteries, particularly in the extremities. In *polyarteritis nodosa*, the medium and small muscular arteries of many organs may be involved in a fibrinoid necrosis that may result in small aneurysms. With healing, the intima becomes thickened, progressing to localized stenosis and occlusion. In *scleroderma* (progressive systemic sclerosis), the arterial changes are variable histologically and, unfortunately, may be seen in other disorders. Subintimal fibrosis and stenosis of the mesenteric and pulmonary arteries have been described. Nonspecific intimal thickening may be seen in renal interlobar arteries. Main renal arterial stenosis and dilatation have also been described.

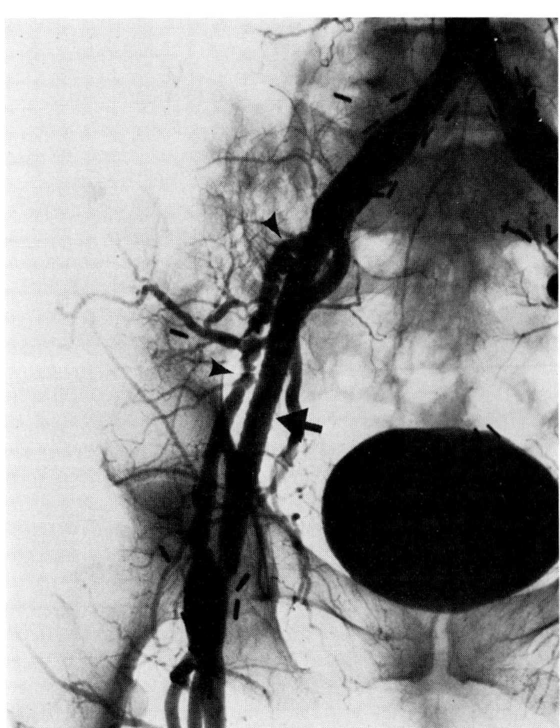

Figure 117–5. Medial fibroplasia *(arrowheads)* with aneurysms involving the external iliac arteries, right only shown. The patient had severe bilateral thigh and calf claudication, for which bilateral common iliac to external iliac bypasses were performed. *Arrow* indicates right graft.

Arteriospastic Disease. Peripheral small vessel arterial spasm occurs in Raynaud's phenomenon. Raynaud's phenomenon may be an isolated finding (Raynaud's disease) or may occur as a symptom of a more severe condition, such as any occlusive disease, collagen diseases, trauma, frostbite, neurogenic disease, drugs, and intravascular coagulation or aggregation. In its milder form, Raynaud's phenomenon is entirely one of spasm. If associated with a more severe process, however, secondary occlusive arterial changes may develop. Thus, if an angiogram demonstrates fixed occlusive change in a patient with clinical findings of arteriospasm, a more severe disease should be considered. Intra-arterial vasodilators and/or warming of the extremity by immersion in warm water is necessary to obtain diagnostic angiographic studies.

Cystic Adventitial Degeneration. This rare disease, occurring in relatively young men, may produce claudication. It has been described primarily in the popliteal artery but also rarely in the external iliac, femoral, radial, and ulnar arteries. There is a gelatinous degeneration of the arterial wall leading to cyst formation localized to the adventitia with subsequent extrinsic occlusion. Characteristically, the artery above and below the diseased segment is normal. The diagnosis can only be suggested arteriographically, but it can be confirmed by ultrasound and computed tomography. Surgical or percutaneous aspiration of the cystic lesion with relief of the extrinsic occlusion can be curative.

Hereditary Disorders of Connective Tissue. A fairly sizable group of syndromes have as their basis a genetically determined abnormal production or metabolism of collagen tissue. Some of these disorders have primary arterial manifestations.

Pseudoxanthoma elasticum is a rare hereditary disease, the basic defect being an abnormal production of elastica that leads to involvement of multiple organ systems. Clinically, redundant skin folds with pseudoxanthomatous yellowish papules are noted. Of interest is the primary involvement of the arteries, especially in the extremities. Pathologically, the medium-sized and small arteries are involved by replacement of the elastic tissue of the media with calcium deposits. Premature atherosclerotic changes may be superimposed on the primary process. The pathologic process is more prominent in the upper extremities, but because of the excellent collateral circulation there are usually few if any symptoms. Intermittent claudication may occur in the lower extremities, even in childhood. The arteries may become calcified, and angiographic studies demonstrate irregular narrowing progressing to occlusion of the smaller arteries, including the cerebral, coronary, visceral, and peripheral arteries. Gastrointestinal hemorrhage secondary to angiomatous malformations in the visceral branches is relatively frequent in this disorder.

Idiopathic *cystic medial necrosis* typically involves the ascending aorta, but can also involve the peripheral arteries, including the coronary, carotid, subclavian, and renal arteries. Complications consist of aneurysm formation and dissecting hematoma.

Ehlers-Danlos syndrome is due to a defect in the organization of collagen tissue causing extreme tissue fragility. As a result, patients with this syndrome are prone to spontaneous rupture of major arteries, aneurysm formation, and acute aortic dissection. Arteriography carries a significant risk of arterial laceration and hemorrhage.

Homocystinuria is due to an inborn error of metabolism in which primary involvement of the medium-sized and larger arteries is common. Transverse intimal striations occur secondary to fibrous intimal proliferation with fragmentation of the adjacent elastic tissue. This abnormality predisposes to thrombosis, which can be fatal. Any vessel can be involved, including veins. Because even minor trauma such as a venipuncture may be complicated by thrombosis, it is believed that angiography is contraindicated in these patients.

Extrinsic Arterial Compression Syndromes

Thoracic Outlet Syndrome. Neurovascular symptoms in the upper extremities may result from compression of the brachial plexus and subclavian artery and vein by the scalenus anticus or subclavius muscle and a cervical or first thoracic rib. The angiographic diagnosis is best accomplished by selective subclavian injection with the patient placing his or her arm in a position that reproduces symptoms or with the arm abducted and externally rotated. Adson's maneuver, which consists of holding the shoulders back and down, turning the head sharply to the affected side and having the patient hold a breath in deep inspiration, is the most commonly known test for this syndrome. However it is an unreliable test positive in only approximately 2% of patients with thoracic outlet syndrome and in a small percentage of normal patients.

Correlation of the angiographic findings with the clinical symptoms is extremely important as, unfortunately, typical defects in the region of the costoclavicular tunnel during hyperabduction may occur in essentially asymptomatic patients. The diagnosis is best made clinically. Angiography is indicated in patients with a reduced upper extremity pulse or blood pressure or when a complication such as aneurysm or thrombus formation with occlusion or peripheral embolism is suspected.

Extracranial Cephalic Arterial Compression. Severe extrinsic abnormalities resulting in reduction of cerebral blood flow and ischemic symptoms have been described. Basilar artery insufficiency can be caused by impingement of a cervical osteoarthritic spur on the vertebral artery.

Transient occlusion of the vertebral artery at its entrance into the sixth cervical transverse foramen may occur secondary to compression by adjacent cervical muscles when the head turns to the contralateral side. This maneuver should be performed during angiography if the symptoms of cerebral ischemia are considered related to head position.

Kinking of vessels, particularly the carotid artery, resulting in mechanical stenosis has also been described. One must be careful about making this diagnosis because this finding is occasionally seen in asymptomatic patients.

Celiac Axis Compression Syndrome. Compression of the celiac axis by the median arcuate ligament of the diaphragm may be associated with postprandial epigastric pain. The etiology of the pain is uncertain. Initially vascular insufficiency with intestinal angina was suggested, but this has been challenged because the syndrome may occur even though the SMA and IMA are patent. Generally, complicating flow factors must appear before true vascular insufficiency occurs—for example, obstruction of the mesenteric arteries or decreased cardiac output. Compression of the adjacent celiac ganglion has therefore been proposed as the cause of the syndrome.

The angiographic diagnosis is best made on a lateral or steep (70-degree) left posterior oblique abdominal aortogram. There is dorsocaudal displacement of the celiac trunk with smooth eccentric impression on its anterior wall, maximized in deep expiration with decrease in inspiration. Rarely, compression of the superior mesenteric and renal artery by extrinsic fibrotic bands from the diapragm has been described.

Popliteal Artery Entrapment Syndrome. This rare syndrome, occurring primarily in relatively young adult men, consists of intermittent claudication typically due to entrapment of the abnormally coursing popliteal artery by the medial head of the gastrocnemius muscle and, less commonly, by other variant abnormal courses of the popliteal artery. Entrapment by fascial slips encompassing a normally positioned popliteal artery has also occurred. Angiographically, the diagnosis may be made either by recognizing the defect of an extrinsic band crossing the popliteal artery or by an unusual medial deviation of the popliteal artery. Compression occasionally may be documented only when there is vigorous plantar or dorsiflexion of the foot; thus the angiographer must consider this diagnosis in young patients with typical claudication and relatively normal arteries.

ANEURYSMS

Abdominal Aortic Aneurysms

Atherosclerotic Aneurysms. The majority of abdominal aneurysms are atherosclerotic in origin and almost always involve the aorta distal to the origin of the renal arteries. They are characteristically saccular or fusiform in configuration. Occasionally these aneurysms are more extensive with involvement of the suprarenal aorta and even the thoracic aorta (referred to as an thoracoabdominal aortic aneurysm). Also commonly seen are atherosclerotic aneurysms of the renal and splenic arteries, which are typically fusiform in shape. Atherosclerotic aneurysms of the other visceral branches are much less common. Rarely, inflammatory atherosclerotic abdominal aneurysms occur, their etiology being uncertain. Their angiographic appearance is similar to that of noninflammatory atherosclerotic aneurysms. Ultrasound (US), computed tomography (CT), and magnetic resonance imaging (MRI) are helpful in establishing their diagnosis by showing thickening of the aortic wall. The increased periaortic soft-tissue density of inflammatory aneurysms may enhance on contrast CT studies.

False Aneurysms (Pseudoaneurysms). False aneurysms are not surrounded by the usual three layers of the vessel wall but only by the adventitia and surrounding tissues. They are most commonly seen at the site of anastomosis of a vascular graft to native artery but also may occur following trauma, including catheterization procedures. Characteristically, they have a narrow neck and are saccular in nature. Pancreatitis with pseudocyst formation may erode the splenic artery, resulting in a false aneurysm.

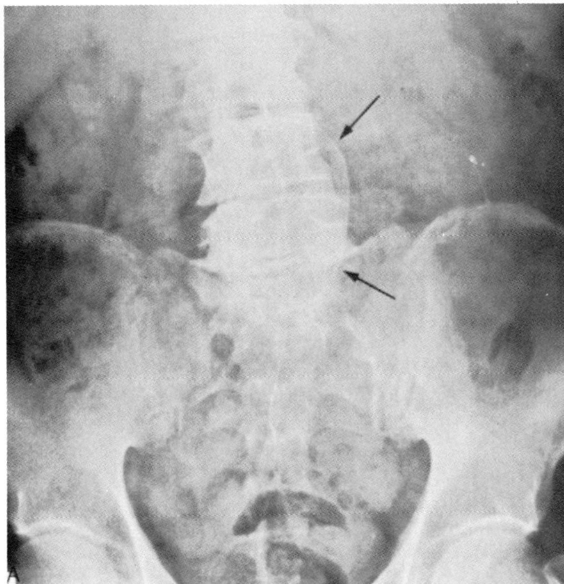
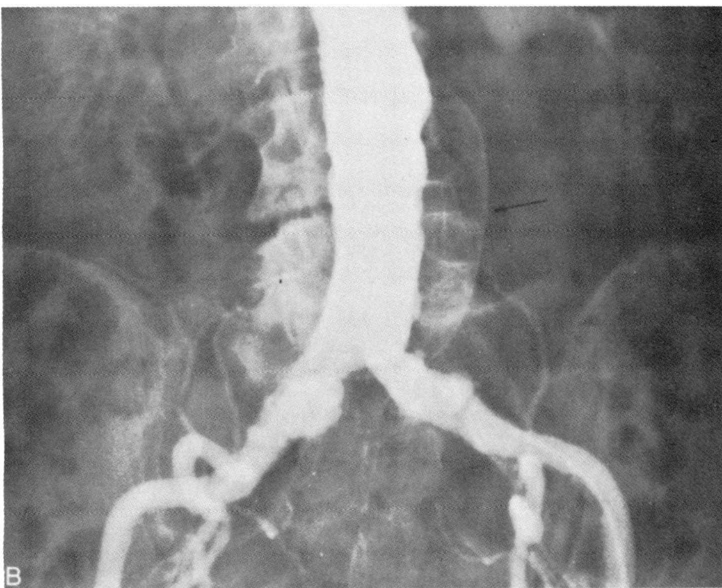

Figure 117–6. Aortic abdominal aneurysm. *A,* Anteroposterior abdominal radiograph demonstrates a heavily calcified lower abdominal aortic aneurysm *(arrows). B,* Angiogram shows the patent lumen of the aneurysm. Thrombus is present between the opacified lumen and the calcified wall *(arrows)* of the aneurysm.

MYCOTIC ANEURYSMS. These aneurysms are typically false and are secondary to an infectious process that weakens the arterial wall. Therefore, they are usually focal and saccular in nature and often appear relatively suddenly with rapid enlargement. They have a tendency to rupture. Aneurysms of the mesenteric arteries are usually due to blood-borne nonhemolytic *Streptococcus, Staphylococcus,* or *Salmonella.*

DISSECTING HEMATOMA. Abdominal aortic aneurysms due to dissecting hematoma are almost invariably extensions of thoracic dissection. Clinical diagnosis is usually suggested by the presence of a previously existing dissecting hematoma of the thoracic aorta. Aortographic diagnosis may be difficult unless a contrast injection is made into the thoracic aorta. This is particularly true if the false channel is thrombosed. Contrast-enhanced CT and MRI may more easily demonstrate the pathologic process.

IMAGING OF ABDOMINAL ANEURYSMS. Although abdominal aortic aneurysms are typically discovered clinically by the presence of a pulsatile abdominal mass, the diagnosis is frequently incidently suggested by mural calcification seen on routine anteroposterior and lateral abdominal radiographs (Fig. 117–6*A*), or demonstration during abdominal US, CT, and MRI. Angiography is currently the most effective way to view the internal dimensions of the aneurysm and to demonstrate the status of the renal artery origins and the other visceral branches (Fig. 117–6*B*). Involvement of the IMA by the aneurysm and extension of the aneurysm into the iliac arteries can be easily visualized. On the other hand, angiography may grossly underestimate the true size of the aneurysm because mural thrombus partially obscures the true lumen. Rarely, the aneurysmal nature of the aorta is obscured by the mural thrombus, giving the appearance of a nearly normal aorta. In these cases, the aneurysm is suggested by the absence of the lumbar and inferior mesenteric arteries. Selective arteriography may be necessary to define the location and extent of aneurysms of the branches of the abdominal aorta.

Conventional cross-sectional imaging techniques are superior in determining the actual size of aneurysms and the presence of mural thrombus but are less effective in identifying visceral or iliac artery involvement as compared to angiography. Ultrasound with color flow and CT give detailed cross-sectional information and are reliable imaging screening tests. With US, two planes are generally scanned. Supine transverse scans from the xiphoid process to the aortic bifurcation are performed first to give a general idea of the longitudinal course of the aorta and to mark the width of the aneurysm. Longitudinal scans characterize the length and depth of the aneurysm as well as possible iliac extension (Fig. 117–7). The presence of gas or barium in the gastrointestinal tract interferes with penetration of the US beam and can result in a nondiagnostic study. Accuracy by US in identifying abdominal aneurysms is approximately 95 per cent. An aortic measurement of 3 cm or greater in either the anteroposterior or transverse diameter should be considered suspicious for an aneurysm.

Computed tomography (Fig. 117–8*A*) can be used to measure directly the actual diameter of the aneurysm and to identify the relationship between the aneurysm and other major vascular structures. Mural thrombus is easily seen, as are the retroperitoneal structures. In a leaking aneurysm, retroperitoneal blood can be detected (Fig. 117–8*B*). With CT, postsurgical anatomy can be accurately displayed and complications such as hemorrhage, infection, thrombosis, or pseudoaneurysm formation diagnosed accurately.

Magnetic resonance imaging is useful for the diagnosis of aneurysms. Without contrast media, it can image the entire aneurysm and mural thrombus and show its relation to the origins of adjacent branches such as the renal arteries. It provides better visualization of the iliac arteries than is afforded by CT, since multiple planes are available. T_1-weighted spin-echo and 2D and 3D MR angiographic techniques appear to offer information comparable with that of angiographic techniques. Spiral CT angiography also promises to be useful in the diagnosis of abdominal aneurysms.

PERIPHERAL ARTERIAL ANEURYSMS. Aneurysms of the lower extremities are generally secondary to atherosclerosis. Peripheral aneurysms may also be caused by trauma and infection (mycotic). Pseudoaneurysms may occur at any surgical anastomosis. Isolated iliac aneurysms are uncommon and are usually an extension of an aortic aneurysm. Aneurysms may involve the femoral and the popliteal artery and may present as a palpable mass. In addition, femoral aneurysms frequently present with distal embolization whereas popliteal aneurysms frequently present with acute thrombosis or distal embolization causing lower leg ischemia. Acute

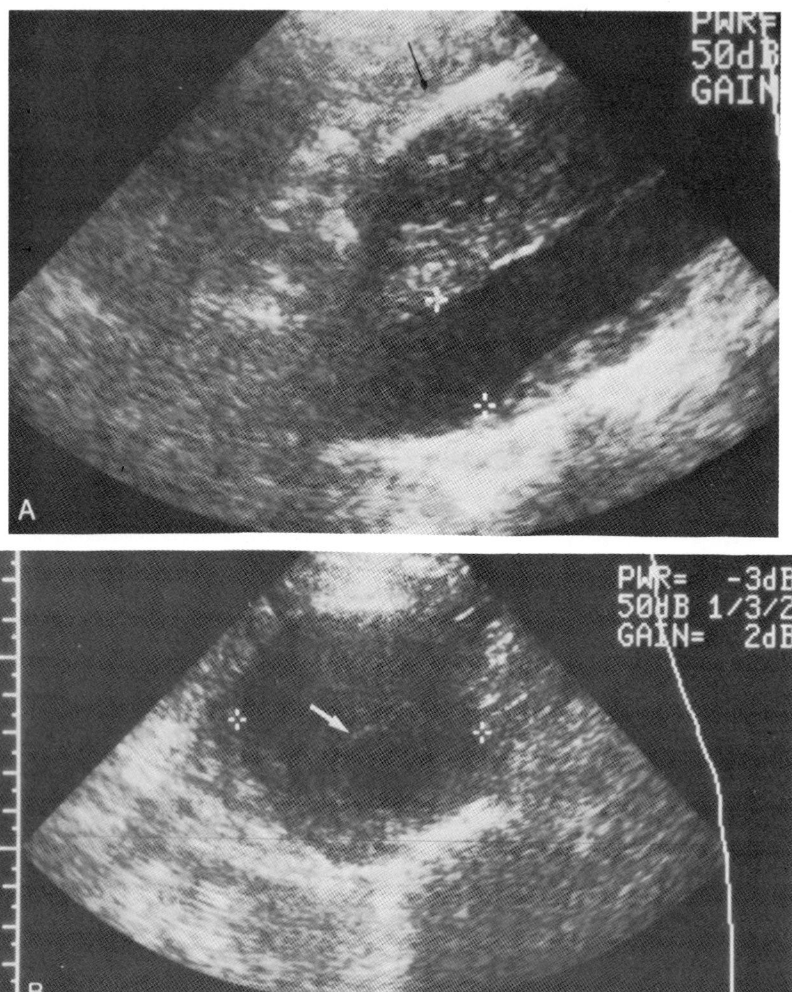

Figure 117–7. Ultrasound of an abdominal aneurysm. *A*, Longitudinal ultrasound of an abdominal aortic aneurysm with calipers measuring the true lumen of the aneurysm. The outer wall of the aneurysm is well-demonstrated *(arrow)*, as is the mural thrombus. *B*, Transverse ultrasound of the abdominal aorta in the same patient clearly demonstrates the actual aneurysm diameter, which is marked by the calipers. The centimeter markers on the left of the image indicate a 6-cm transverse diameter. The true lumen is well seen *(arrow)*.

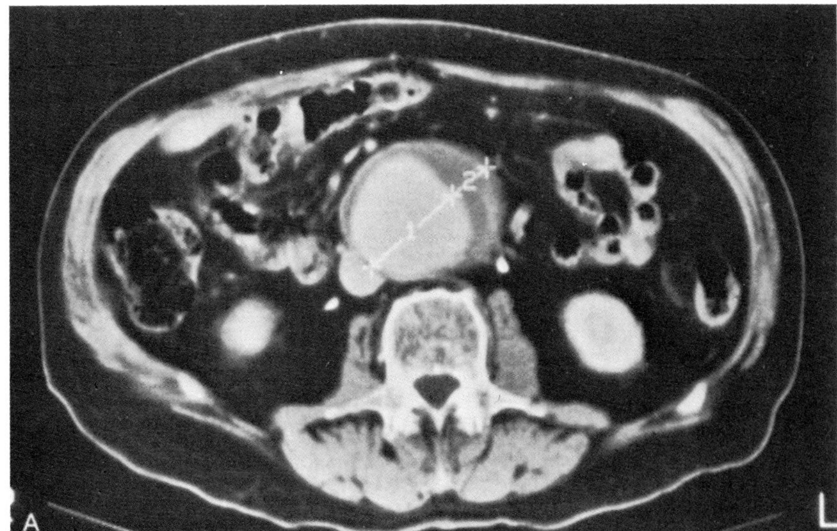

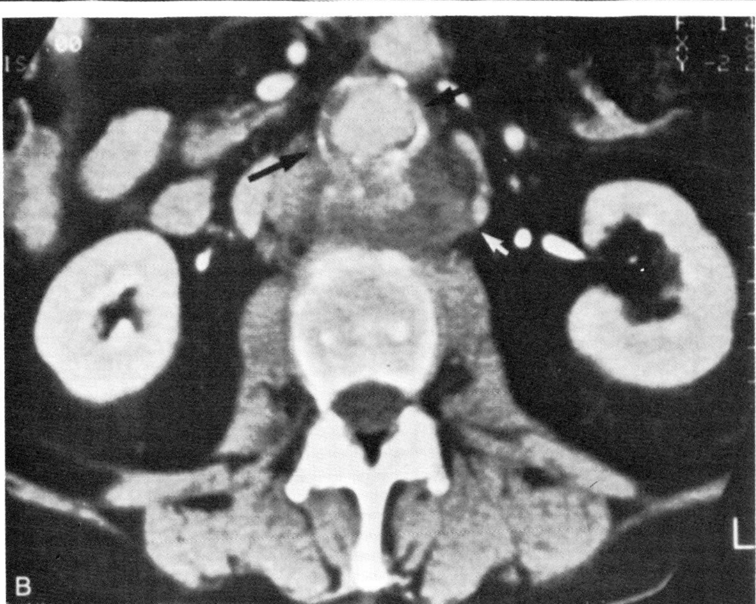

Figure 117–8. Computed tomographic images of an aortic aneurysm. *A,* The true lumen (1) and outer wall (2) are well seen. *B,* Leaking aortic aneurysm. Calcifications line the aortic wall *(black arrows).* Note the amorphous density of extravasated blood in the retroperitoneum, which is displacing the aorta anteriorly *(white arrow).*

pain may also be related to rapid expansion or dissection of the aneurysm. Ultrasound is very useful in defining the etiology of a thigh or popliteal mass.

The *arteria magna syndrome* is a condition characterized by widespread arterial dilatation, elongation, and tortuosity. It is associated with larger localized aneurysms at multiple sites, including the abdominal aorta and the iliac, femoral, and popliteal arteries. Typically, these patients have bounding pulses and very slow arterial flow.

PERIPHERAL ARTERIAL TRAUMA

The angiographic findings in arterial trauma can vary greatly. Direct injury to the vascular tree occurs most commonly as a result of penetrating or blunt trauma or as a result of adjacent fracture. In pelvic trauma, angiography can serve as both a diagnostic and a therapeutic modality. In the presence of massive pelvic hemorrhage, detection of the actual bleeding site at surgery is quite difficult. Often the proximal internal iliac artery is ligated blindly, leaving potential distal collateral communications to supply the bleeding vessel. Arteriography can readily demonstrate a bleeding artery by revealing the site of contrast extravasation (Fig. 117–9). Selective catheterization of the bleeding artery can then be performed, followed by transcatheter embolization.

The distal superficial femoral artery is often injured because of its proximity to bone and its position in the relatively fixed abductor canal. The popliteal artery is also fixed behind the knee and is prone to injury by knee dislocations and fractures, although penetrating trauma is more common.

The most common finding at arteriography following trauma is spasm evidenced by segmental, elongated contractions of the vessel with slowed flow through the affected region. Stretching and displacement of vessels are often seen and are secondary to soft-tissue edema or hematoma. The mechanism of secondary injury is overstretching of the affected artery. The intimal layer ruptures prior to the medial or adventitial layers. Localized subintimal dissection may cause partial or complete occlusion with thrombosis. Transection of the vessel occurs when all three layers are torn.

Edema in the muscle compartments of the extremities may be caused by trauma resulting in major soft-tissue injury with hemorrhage or, less commonly, by acute obstruction of a major artery supplying a compartment. There is acute swelling, resulting in a

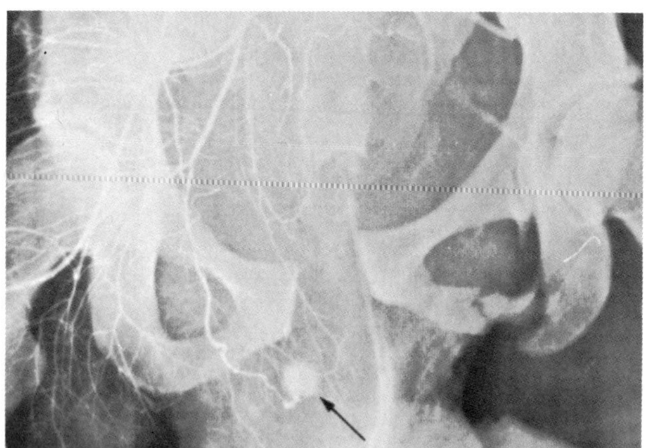

Figure 117–9. Multiple pelvic fractures and extravasation of contrast from an active bleeding site from the internal pudendal artery *(arrow)*. Bleeding was also demonstrated from the left internal iliac artery (not shown). Both vessels were successfully embolized.

vicious cycle of increasing ischemia with extrinsic compression by the surrounding edematous muscles resulting in a further reduction in perfusion. The condition is referred to as a compartment syndrome, the anterior tibial compartment syndrome being the most common. Emergency fasciotomy may be required to relieve the process and prevent serious nerve and muscle necrosis.

Pseudoaneurysm and arteriovenous (AV) fistula may occur. An AV fistula develops when penetrating trauma pierces both an artery and its adjacent vein simultaneously and a communication develops between the two. An AV fistula may be associated with a false aneurysm, or there may be a clean endothelial channel formed in a chronic AV communication. Clinically, most patients have a bruit over the fistula, and there may be signs of venous hypertension with varicosities in the area. Branham's sign (bradycardia on manual compression of the fistula) may be elicited.

The clinical state of the peripheral pulses distal to the site of trauma is often an unreliable indicator of the extent of proximal vascular injury. Pulses may be reduced when only vascular spasm is present and conversely may be present with more severe injury. Because of the disparity between the physical and angiographic findings, some surgeons recommend routine performance of angiography when major vessels pass through the region of trauma in spite of the low yield of positive findings.

CONGENITAL ARTERIOVENOUS MALFORMATIONS

Congenital arteriovenous malformations (AVMs) comprise a spectrum of vascular abnormalities that occur as a result of an arrest or maldevelopment during embryogenesis of the vascular system. The defect in embryogenesis may occur at any phase, and congenital AVMs may therefore have a wide spectrum of appearances. They may appear as cavernous hemangiomas that show structural similarity to the capillary network stage, involve mature channels with large arteriovenous communications, occur as pure venous angiodysplasias, or contain a mixture of elements.

The hemodynamic consequences depend upon the size of the fistulous communications and the degree of arteriovenous shunting. Large shunts result in increased stroke volume and circulating blood volume and can lead to cardiomegaly and congestive heart failure. Cutaneous manifestations are common.

Angiographically, those AVMs with large arteriovenous shunts typically show an increased number of feeding vessels, with early arteriovenous shunting into enlarged veins. If capillary vessels predominate, such as in a capillary hemangioma, the feeding arteries tend to be normal in size, but a dense capillary blush is usually present with puddling of contrast (Fig. 117–10). The large draining veins may be normal or mildly abnormal. Arteriography is the modality that best determines the nature and full extent of these lesions and should be performed prior to surgical treatment, as these lesions are often larger and more extensive than appreciated on physical examination. MRI is also a frequently used method for assessing their location and extent.

PERIPHERAL ARTERY SURGERY

Surgical or endovascular intervention is indicated when claudication becomes disabling or rest ischemia is present as manifested by rest pain in the foot or ischemic ulceration. Preoperative noninvasive vascular testing, especially with duplex color flow US, may be helpful in determining the relative location and severity of the occluded segments. Angiography is, however, an essential part of the preoperative evaluation, providing precise information about the diseased segment and delineating the status of the runoff vessels to the foot.

Common surgical procedures consist of bypass grafts and thromboendarectomy. The three most common graft materials are woven Dacron, autologous vein, and tubular expanded polytetrafluoroethylene (PTFE, or Gore-Tex). Dacron is used primarily in the aortoiliac region, whereas autologous vein and PTFE are used in the extremities. Two types of anastomoses are used: end-to-end and end-to-side. The former is employed primarily in the aorta and requires aortic transection suitable only when there is adequate retrograde flow to the internal iliac vessels by way of the distal anastomoses. Otherwise, end-to-side anastomoses are used.

Axillofemoral grafts, which avoid entering the abdominal cavity, are reserved for high-risk patients with rest ischemia due to combined aortoiliac and infrainguinal disease. Femoropopliteal bypass grafts require both adequate inflow of blood from the proximal aortoiliac vessels and continuity of the distal popliteal segment with any of its three terminal branches to the foot. Autologous saphenous

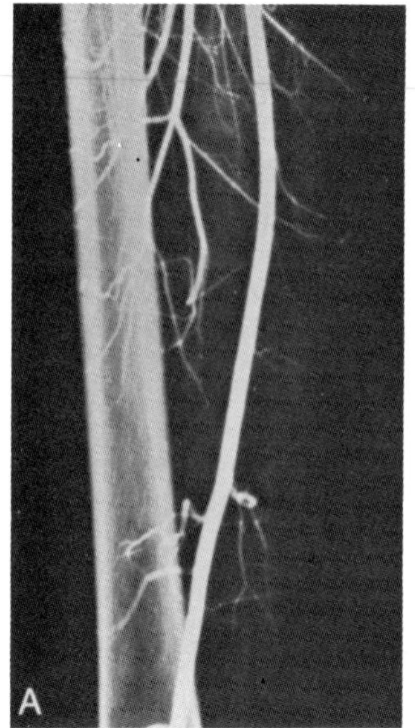

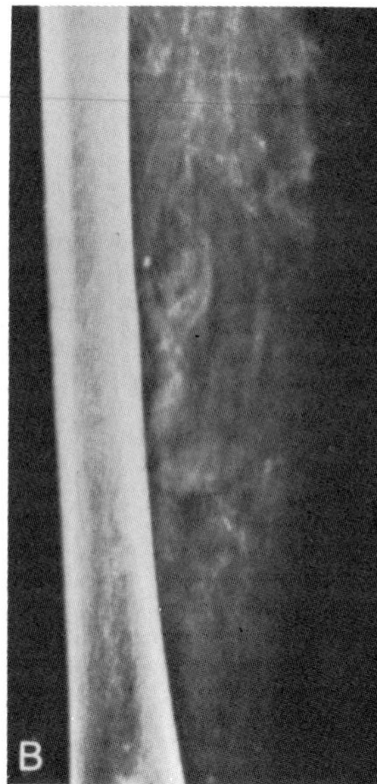

Figure 117–10. Arteriovenous malformation. *A*, Patient with cavernous hemangioma of the thigh. Typically the arterial phase is normal. *B*, Delayed films show characteristic abnormal parenchymal stain.

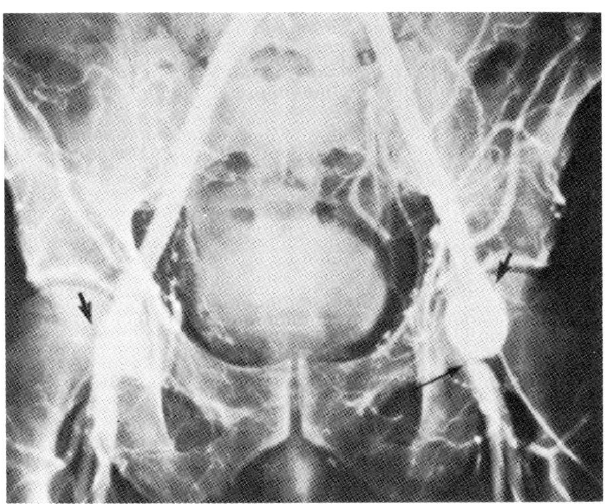

Figure 117–11. Aorto-bifemoral grafts from bilateral pseudoaneurysms at the distal anastomoses *(short arrows)*. Note the stenosis distally on the left *(long arrow)*.

vein is considered to be the graft material of choice, with PTFE the best synthetic alternative. Bypasses to the proximal popliteal artery above the knee joint have a high success rate, whereas bypasses below the knee, although successful, have a higher failure rate, felt to be due to the trauma of knee bending. Infrapopliteal bypasses (to the tibial and peroneal branches) are performed only when femoropopliteal bypass is not possible and usually only for limb salvage in severe ischemic states.

Thromboendarterectomy is reserved for short accessible stenoses or occlusions such as the common femoral and carotid bifurcations or combined with bypass procedures to ensure a patent anastomosis. Thrombectomy is employed for thromboembolic disorders, usually with assistance of the Fogarty balloon catheter.

Graft occlusion or thrombosis may be secondary to an unsatisfactory anastomosis or inadequate inflow or runoff. In the angiographic evaluation of aortoiliac grafts, it is essential to view the proximal and distal graft anastomoses for stenosis or anastomotic pseudoaneurysm formation. Anastomotic pseudoaneurysm formation is an occasional postoperative complication and occurs as a result of partial separation at a suture line. Perianastomotic fibrotic tissue prevents immediate hemorrhage and forms a capsule around the hematoma, which gradually enlarges owing to intra-arterial pressure. The fibrous capsule may rupture, causing enlargement of the mass or erosion to the exterior. Static flow within the false aneurysm results in partial filling of the lumen with thrombus (Fig. 117–11). Infection may also cause a pseudoaneurysm.

Any patient with fever and a paraprosthetic mass must be presumed to have an infected graft. Gallium or indium-labeled white blood cell scanning may be helpful. Vascular prosthesis replacing or bypassing the aorta are prone to erosion into adjacent hollow structures, resulting in an aortoenteric fistula with gastrointestinal bleeding and sepsis. The third and fourth portions of the duodenum and the proximal jejunum that lie directly over an aortic suture line and the proximal portion of the graft are the most common sites for development of this complication. The fistula results from pressure necrosis of the bowel caused by pulsation of the prosthetic graft. Damage to the bowel wall may lead to local perforation and contamination of the graft anastomosis by enteric bacteria. Disruption of the suture line is then inevitable. Arteriography may demonstrate a pseudoaneurysm, but detection of actual bleeding is unusual. Computed tomographic scanning and barium studies are usually more helpful.

Although many surgeons are uncomfortable with the catheterization of a prosthetic graft, it is relatively safe in experienced hands and has a lower morbidity than the transaxillary or transbrachial approach. Strict sterile technique is mandatory. Technically, the puncture in the groin is more difficult because of postsurgical scarring and occasionally the native artery is entered rather than the graft itself. Repuncture at a different level and angle may be necessary. Once passage of the wire into the graft is ensured, a vascular sheath should be placed through which the procedure is performed. Use of a catheter alone, particularly if it is made of polyethylene, may result in entrapment in the prosthetic fiber mesh. Prophylactic antibiotics are recommended if the sheath is left in place for interventional studies.

PERIPHERAL VENOUS DISEASE

Thoracic, abdominal, and upper and lower extremity venography is most commonly performed to evaluate venous patency. Obstruction is most commonly due to thrombus, but tumor invasion or extrinsic compression by ligaments, retroperitoneal and mediastinal fibrosis, neoplasms, and rarely lipomatosis are other causes.

Acute venous thrombosis will appear as an intraluminal filling defect outlined by a rim of contrast material. Vessel recanalization may occur with time, resulting in stringy-appearing vessels with loss of valves.

The superior vena cava and inferior vena cava, (IVC) are also generally studied to evaluate obstruction. Thrombus, extrinsic compression, and primary or secondary tumor invasion all may cause obstruction (Fig. 117–12). Prior to placing an IVC filter, the IVC should be visualized to determine its size and to localize any thrombus. In addition, the level of entrance of the renal veins should be determined as well as the presence of significant venous anomalies such as a double IVC.

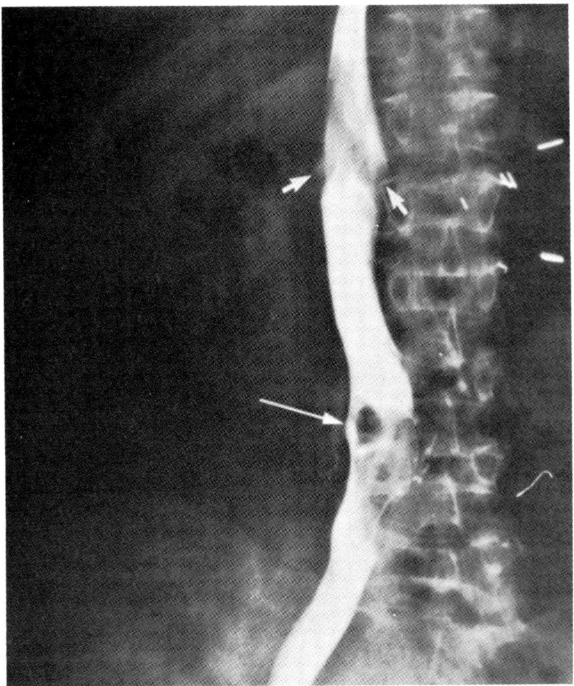

Figure 117–12. Inferior vena cavogram. Clot is present in the proximal inferior vena cava *(long arrow)*. Note the flow defects at L2, from wash-in of unopacified blood from the renal veins *(short arrows)*. These defects were variable from film to film and should not be misinterpreted as clots, which are constant from film to film.

Bibliography

Brewster DC: Direct reconstruction for aortoiliac occlusive disease. In Rutherford RB (ed): Vascular Surgery, 3rd ed. Philadelphia, WB Saunders, 1989, pp 667–691.

Bron KM: Femoral arteriography. In Abrams HL (ed): Angiography, 3rd ed. Boston, Little, Brown, 1983, pp 1835–1877.

Cliff MM, Soulen RL, Finestone AJ: Mycotic aneurysms—a challenge and a clue. Review of ten-year experience. Arch Intern Med 126:977–982, 1970.

Crawford ES, Bomberger RA, Glaeser DH, et al: Aortoiliac occlusive disease: Factors influencing survival and function following reconstructive operations over a twenty-five year period. Surgery 90:1055–1067, 1981.

Gaines VD, Ramchandani P, Soulen RL: Popliteal entrapment syndrome. Cardiov Intervent Radiol 8:156–159, 1985.

Grollman JH Jr, Barker WF: Extrinsic arterial compression syndromes. In Barker WF (ed): Peripheral Arterial Disease, 2nd ed. Philadelphia, WB Saunders Company, 1975.

Lande A, Rossi P: The value of total aortography in the diagnosis of Takayasu's arteritis. Radiology 114:287–297, 1975.

Malone JM, Moore WS, Goldstone J: The natural history of bilateral aortofemoral bypass grafts for ischemia of the lower extremities. Arch Surg 110:1300–1306, 1975.

Mannick JA, Whittemore AD: Aortoiliac occlusive disease. In Moore WS (ed): Vascular Surgery: A Comprehensive Review, 3rd ed. New York, Grune and Stratton, 1991, p 350.

May AG, Van de Berg L, DeWeese JA, Rob CG: Critical arterial stenosis. Surgery 54:250–258, 1963.

Ravitch MM: Hypogastic artery ligation in acute pelvic trauma. Surgery 56:601–602, 1964.

Wade GL, Smith DC, Mohr LL: Follow up of 50 consecutive angiograms obtained utilizing puncture of prosthetic vascular grafts. Radiology 146:663–667, 1983.

Weaver FA, Yellin AE, Bauer M, et al: Is arterial proximity a valid indication for arteriography in penetrating extremity trauma? A prospective analysis. Arch Surg 125:1256–1260, 1990.

118 Cardiac Pacemakers and Prosthetic Valves

James T. T. Chen

In the treatment of heart disease, the use of cardiac pacemakers and prosthetic valves is now commonplace. To ensure the proper placement and function of these devices, radiology plays an important role.

CARDIAC PACEMAKERS

The clinical application of artificial cardiac pacing began when a patient in ventricular asystole was successfully resuscitated by external electric stimulation. Considerable advances in pacemaker systems have been made in the last three decades. Currently in the United States, about 500,000 patients have implanted pacemakers. The indications for pacing are (1) to treat patients with bradycardias and tachycardias and (2) to pace-map various atrial and ventricular sites in the differential diagnosis of arrhythmias.

A pacemaker consists of three parts: (1) the power source or pulse generator, (2) the conducting wires, and (3) the electrodes by which the electric stimuli are delivered to the endocardium or the myocardium. The wires and the electrodes are collectively called the pacing lead. Cardiac pacemakers may be used temporarily or permanently. When the stimuli are directed to the endocardium, the electrodes are introduced transvenously into the right atrium or ventricle or both. To deliver the stimuli to the myocardium, the electrodes are implanted transmediastinally on the ventricles.

Modern pacemakers are capable of performing two basic functions. They stimulate (pace) the heart and recognize (sense) the intrinsic cardiac impulses. The information obtained by the latter function is used to modulate the timing of the succeeding pacemaker stimulus. Consequently, the pacer responds and coordinates with the spontaneous cardiac electric events.

There are two kinds of pacing electrodes: unipolar and bipolar. In unipolar systems, only the cathode is placed in the heart; the anode, which is the metallic housing of the pulse generator, is located away from the heart. Bipolar systems place both the anode and the cathode electrodes inside the heart.

To ensure proper placement of the pacemaker and to maintain its normal functions after implantation, radiologic examinations, in addition to clinical and electrocardiographic assessments, play an important role.

Demand Ventricular Pacemaker

Today the most frequently implanted pacemaker is the demand ventricular pacemaker. It senses the ventricular activity and paces the ventricle only when the need arises. The proper position of transvenous ventricular pacemaker electrodes is depicted by line "b" in Figure 118–1 and by pacing lead "b" in Figure 118–2.

In a well-positioned posteroanterior view of a patient without right ventricular enlargement, the tip of the pacing lead should be at, but medial to, the right ventricular apex, which is situated about midway between the midline of the chest and the cardiac apex. In this position, the tip is usually entrapped by the trabeculae and moves synchronously with and at the same amplitude as the ventricular wall. Any excessive play within the cardiac chamber indicates dislodgement of the electrodes. When the tip is more lateral to the midpoint, the question of perforation of the right ventricular wall should be raised. When the pacing lead is more than 60 per cent laterad from the midline to the left ventricular apex, myocardial perforation should be seriously considered. The electrodes may actually lie in the pericardium (dotted line "c" in Figs. 118–1 and 118–3). This can cause excessive or erratic movements of the electrodes asynchronous with the ventricle. The electric stimuli may be delivered to the left hemidiaphragm instead of the ventricle, or the pacemaker may continue to work, work intermittently, or fail altogether.

The pulmonary arterial position of the electrodes may be in the main trunk or one of its branches (Fig. 118–1, line "a"). Again,

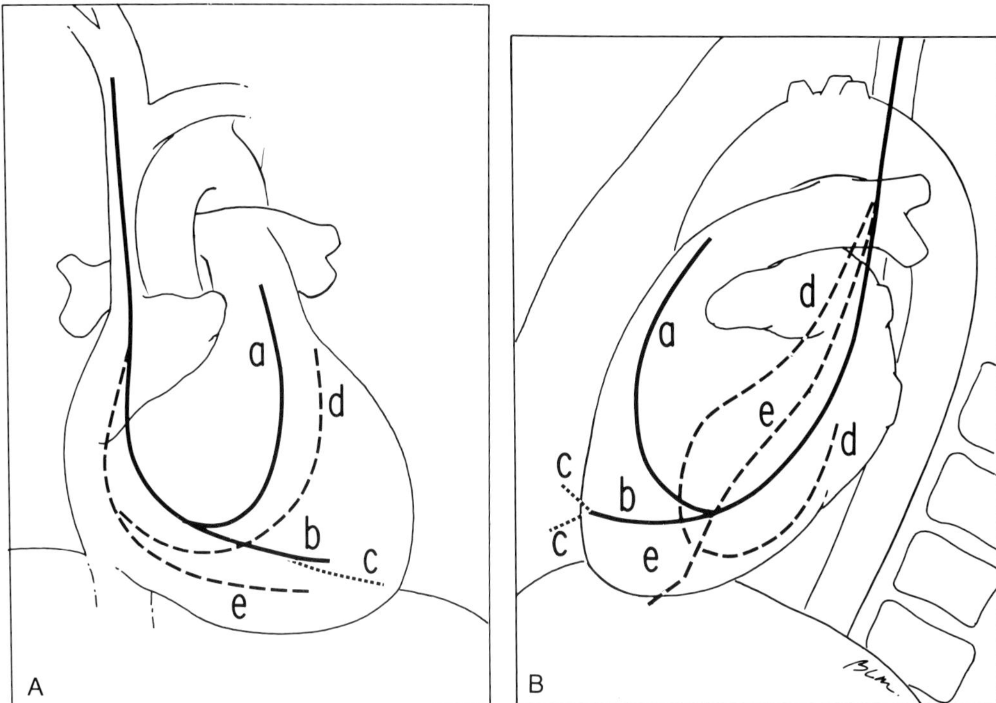

Figure 118–1. *A*, Posteroanterior (PA) presentation of **catheter positions in ventricular pacing**. (*A* from Hewitt MJ, Chen JTT, Ravin CE, Gallagher JJ: Coronary sinus atrial pacing: Radiographic considerations. AJR 136:323, 1981. © 1981, American Roentgen Ray Society.) *B*, Lateral presentation. (a = pulmonary artery position; b = right ventricular apex position; c = pericardial position following myocardial perforation; d = great cardiac vein position; e = middle cardiac vein position.)

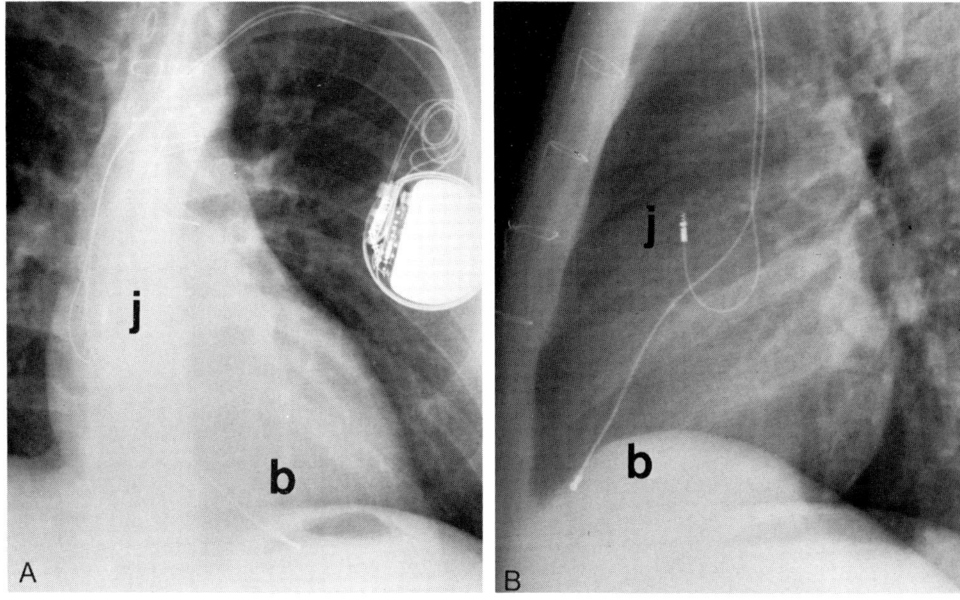

Figure 118–2. *A*, PA view of **normal transvenous atrioventricular sequential pacing catheters**. "j" and "b" denote atrial and ventricular catheters, respectively. *B*, Lateral view.

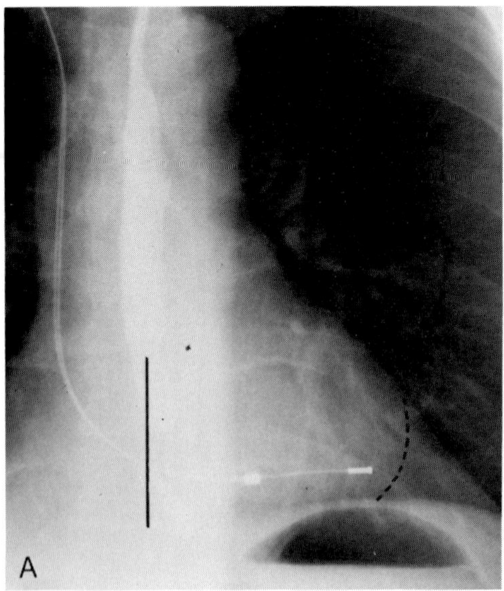

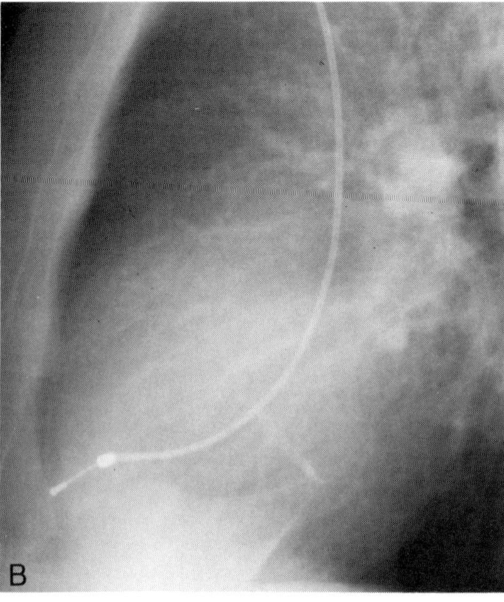

Figure 118–3. *A,* PA view of a patient with **pacemaker failure**. The pacing catheter is situated beyond the confines of the right ventricle. The tip of the pacing lead is too far left of the midline *(solid line),* approaching the left ventricular apex *(broken line). B,* The tip of the electrode is obviously outside the myocardium, through the subepicardial fat stripe into the pericardium.

such malpositions are frequently accompanied by impaired pacemaker function.

In the lateral view, the tip of the pacing lead should be pointing to the anterior costophrenic sulcus behind the sternum (Fig. 118–1*B*, line "b"; and Fig. 118–2*B*, lead "b"). It should be interior and posterior to the subepicardial fat stripe, which is the divider between the myocardium and the pericardium. Once the tip is beyond the fat stripe, it has perforated the ventricle and intruded into the pericardium (Fig. 118–3*B*). Further protrusion out of the chamber may cause an upward or downward deflection of the lead (Fig. 118–1*B*, dotted line "c"; and Fig. 118–3*B*). The pulmonary arterial position of the electrodes in the lateral view is depicted by line "a" in Figure 118–1*B*.

In rare instances, perforation of the right ventricle may cause cardiac tamponade. Most such perforations, however, are not accompanied by significant bleeding, and no specific treatment is indicated other than withdrawal and reposition of the lead.

Coronary Sinus Atrial Pacing

Transvenous atrial pacing via an electrode placed in the coronary sinus has become commonplace for both diagnosis and therapy of cardiac arrhythmias. Atrial and atrioventricular sequential pacing has the advantage of restoring natural cardiac function and output by preserving atrioventricular synchrony.

The coronary sinus represents the persistent left horn of the sinus venosus. It runs in the posterior part of the left atrioventricular groove and is approximately 23 mm long and 10 mm in diameter. There are five major tributaries of the coronary sinus: (1) great cardiac vein, (2) middle cardiac vein, (3) posterior left ventricular vein, (4) oblique vein of Marshall, and (5) small cardiac vein. The electrodes in coronary sinus pacing are most commonly seen in either the great cardiac vein (Fig. 118–4) or the middle cardiac vein (Fig. 118–5). Since all cardiac veins, including the coronary sinus, are embedded in the subepicardial fat stripes, the electrodes within the veins are actually outside the myocardium when viewed tangentially on the radiograph (Fig. 118–4*B*). This appearance should not be interpreted as cardiac perforation.

When the pacing lead extends from the right atrium via the coronary sinus into the great cardiac vein, it follows the left atrioventricular groove, forming a gentle smooth curve leftward, posteriorly, and superiorly (Fig. 118–4). Such a typical radiographic appearance helps prevent echocardiographic misinterpretation of a coronary sinus lead as a left atrial mass.

When the lead extends from the right atrium via the coronary

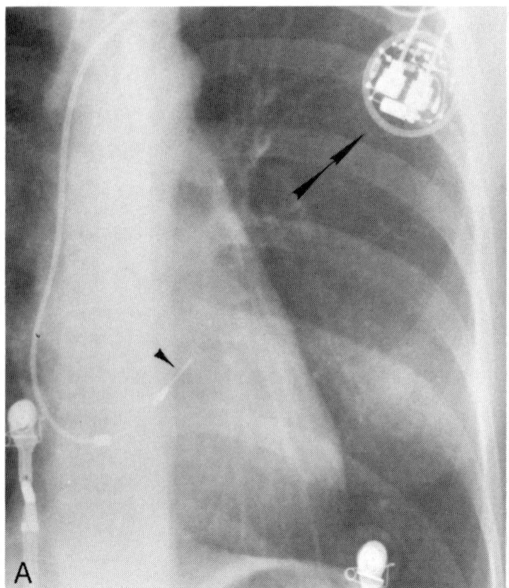

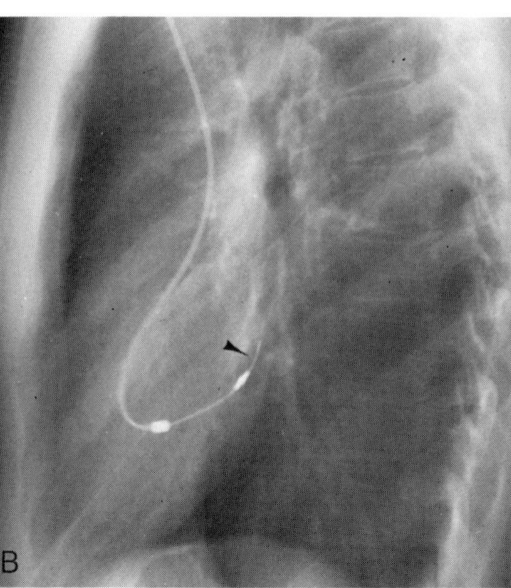

Figure 118–4. *A,* PA view. **Normal position of coronary sinus catheter with its tip in the great cardiac vein**. The flexible tip *(arrowhead)* extends beyond the electrode to prevent dislodgement and to avoid ventricular pacing. Attached to the chest wall is the radiofrequency pacemaker control *(long arrowheads). B,* In the lateral view, the wire appears quite peripheral *(arrowhead)* in position, lying in the subepicardial fat along the left atrioventricular groove.

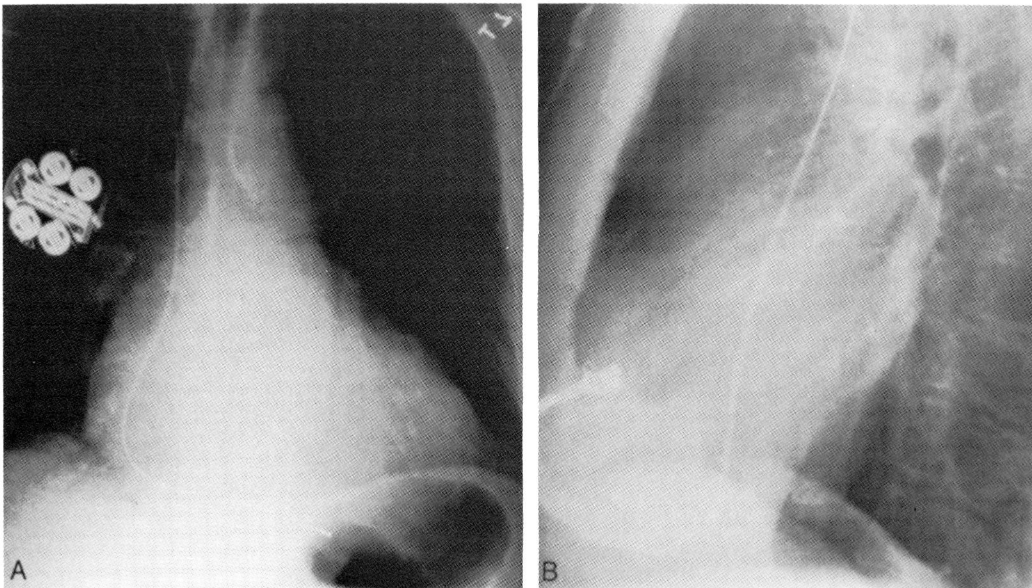

Figure 118–5. *A*, PA view of **pacing catheter in middle cardiac vein**. Note the position of the pacing lead below the tricuspid valve with its tip in the subepicardial fat outside the myocardium. *B*, Lateral view. Note the straight course of the pacing lead and anterior turn at the termination. (*A* and *B* from Hewitt MJ, Chen JTT, Ravin CE, Gallagher JJ: Coronary sinus atrial pacing: Radiographic considerations. AJR 136:323, 1981. © 1981, American Roentgen Ray Society.)

sinus into the middle cardiac vein, it pursues a route lower than the tricuspid valve, bending leftward and inferiorly in the posteroanterior view and inferiorly and forward in the lateral view. In either view, the pacing lead lies between the myocardium and epicardium in the posterior interventricular groove (Fig. 118–5). Without the lateral radiograph, the coronary sinus position of the pacing lead is difficult to distinguish from the right ventricular position (compare Fig. 118–2*A* with Fig. 118–5*A*).

Right Atrial Pacing

Another site for atrial pacing is in the right atrial appendage. The atrial J lead can be easily and expeditiously implanted in the appendage using lateral view fluoroscopy and rechecking in the posteroanterior view. The normally positioned lead should be pointing anteriorly and medially (see Fig. 118–2, lead "j").

Atrioventricular Sequential Pacing

The modern atrioventricular sequential pacemakers sense and pace both the atria and the ventricles, thereby preserving the normal atrioventricular synchrony and the cardiac output. The normal position of each pacing lead is depicted in Figure 118–2.

Persistent Left Superior Vena Cava

The incidence of persistent left superior vena cava is from 0.3 to 0.5 per cent in the general population but 4.5 per cent in patients with congenital atrioventricular conduction defects. The left superior vena cava represents the persistent left cardinal venous system. It drains primarily into the coronary sinus and secondarily via the left brachiocephalic vein into the right-sided superior vena cava. The normal position of a pacing catheter in the left superior vena cava is depicted in Figure 118–6.

Transmediastinal Pacing

In addition to the aforementioned transvenous pacing procedure, the heart can also be paced transmediastinally by implanting the electrodes directly into the left ventricular myocardium (Figs. 118–7 to 118–9). Two techniques are used in this regard—open thoracotomy and percutaneous implantation through the chest wall.

Twiddler's Syndrome

Whether in the chest or abdominal wall, the pulse generator may change position spontaneously within a capacious packet. More commonly, however, rotation of the generator is caused by the patient's habitually twiddling the pacemaker. A change in the position of the generator may twist the pacing lead and ultimately displace or break the electrode (Fig. 118–7).

Fracture of the Lead

With the newer models, breakage of a wire or electrode is infrequent. It usually occurs at a fixation point: near the generator, across the intercostal space, or at the point of insertion (Fig. 118–8). Subtle breakage of a wire within an intact cover of insulating material may be difficult to detect. Fluoroscopy and multiple spot films in various projections may help clarify the confusion. On the other hand, some bipolar leads may show radiopaque discontinuity that is of no clinical significance. This is known as pacemaker lead pseudofracture (Fig. 118–9).

PROSTHETIC VALVES

Two types of artificial cardiac valves are currently in use for both the semilunar and the atrioventricular positions. They are (1) mechanical and (2) tissue valves. The former are more durable than

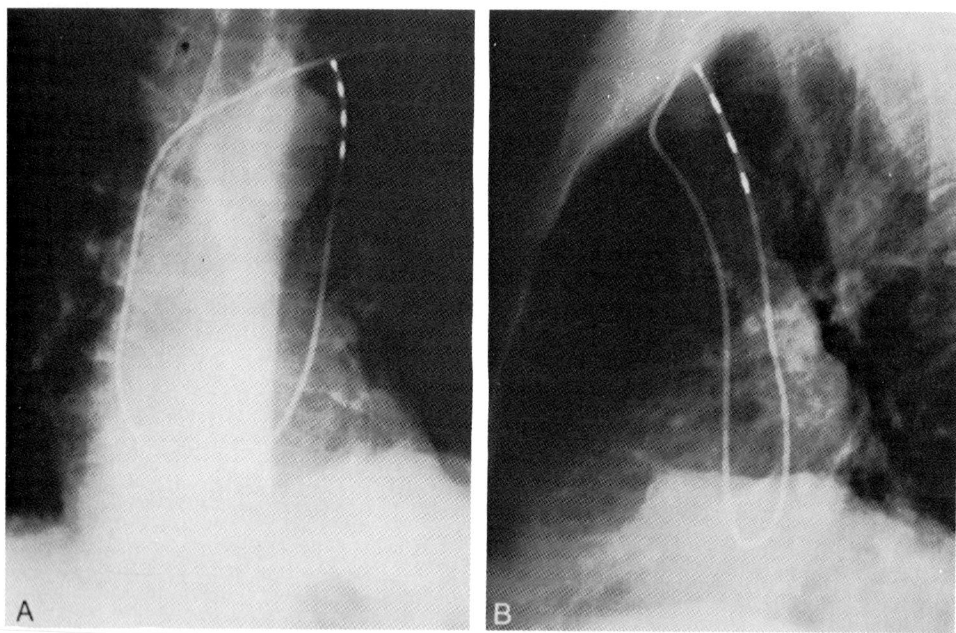

Figure 118–6. *A*, PA view of the pacing catheter in persistent left superior vena cava. *B*, Lateral view. (*A* and *B* from Hewitt MJ, Chen JTT, Ravin CE, Gallagher JJ: Coronary sinus atrial pacing: Radiographic considerations. AJR 136:323, 1981. © 1981, American Roentgen Ray Society.)

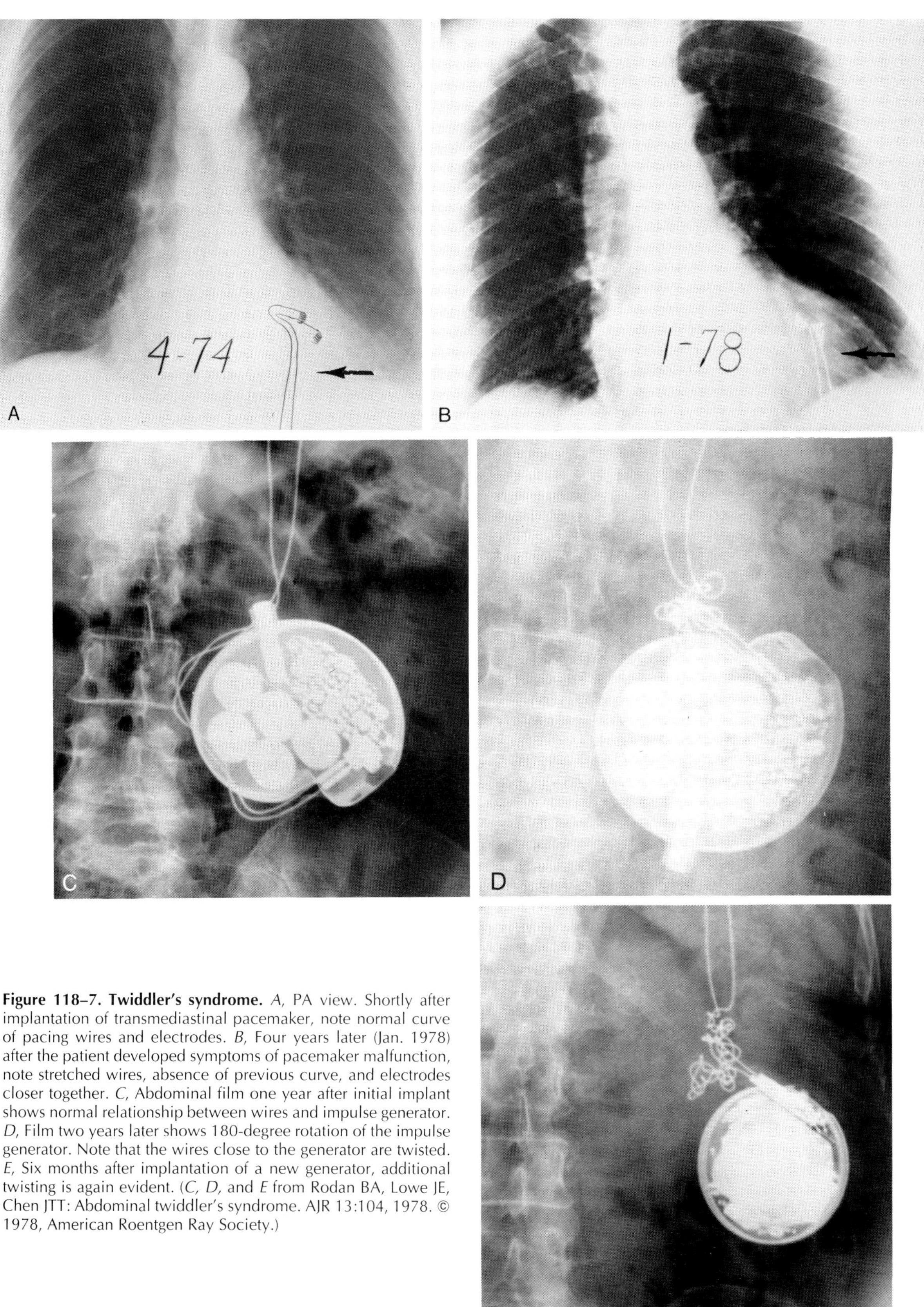

Figure 118–7. Twiddler's syndrome. *A*, PA view. Shortly after implantation of transmediastinal pacemaker, note normal curve of pacing wires and electrodes. *B*, Four years later (Jan. 1978) after the patient developed symptoms of pacemaker malfunction, note stretched wires, absence of previous curve, and electrodes closer together. *C*, Abdominal film one year after initial implant shows normal relationship between wires and impulse generator. *D*, Film two years later shows 180-degree rotation of the impulse generator. Note that the wires close to the generator are twisted. *E*, Six months after implantation of a new generator, additional twisting is again evident. (*C, D,* and *E* from Rodan BA, Lowe JE, Chen JTT: Abdominal twiddler's syndrome. AJR 13:104, 1978. © 1978, American Roentgen Ray Society.)

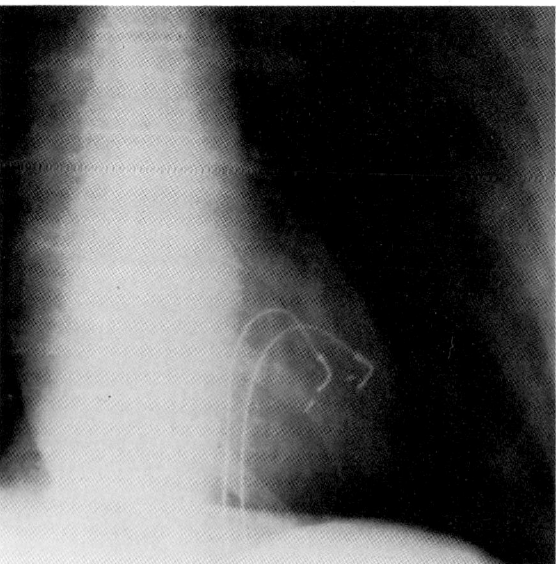

Figure 118–8. PA view of the **transmediastinal pacemaker**. Note the fractured electrodes.

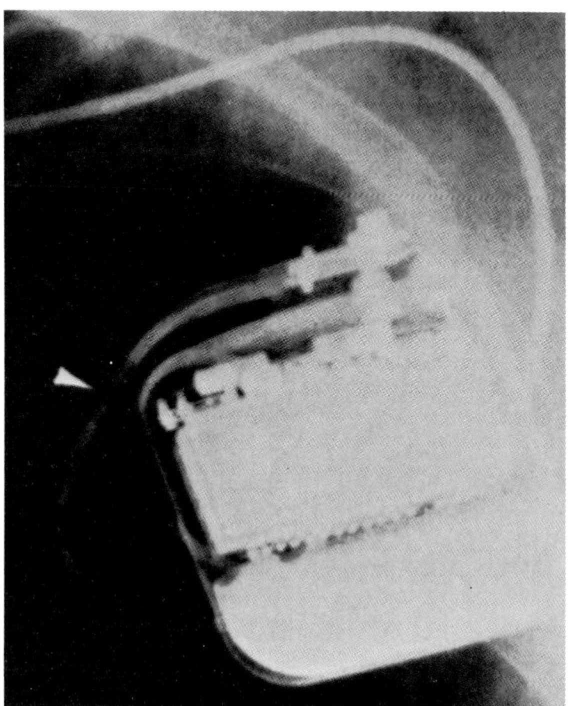

Figure 118–9. Anteroposterior view of a **Pacesetter model 820**. The radiolucent area noted in the proximal portion of the lead is the point where the support coil terminates just prior to the bifurcation of the leads. The small wires seen within the radiolucent area represent the inner distal winding of the coil conductor (*arrowhead*). (From Steiner RM, Morse DP, Tegtmeyer CJ: Pacemaker lead pseudofracture. Radiology 143:793, 1982. Reproduced with permission.)

the latter, but have the disadvantage of dependence on long-term anticoagulants. Tissue valves, on the other hand, have a much lower thrombogenicity, eliminating the need for long-term anticoagulation. The major drawback of tissue valves is their tendency to early deterioration, necessitating reoperation in a few years. This problem is particularly serious in the pediatric population. The main pathologic feature in the young is a rapidly developing calcific stenosis of the tissue valve.

The radiologist plays an important role in identifying an artificial valve and in detecting its malfunctions.

Identification of Prosthetic Valves

The mechanical prostheses can be classified into three major types. They are (1) the caged-ball, (2) the caged-disc, and (3) the tilting-disc types.

The caged-ball type is exemplified by the Starr-Edwards valves (Fig. 118–10). The caged-disc type is represented by the Beall valve (Fig. 118–11). The tilting-disc type includes the Björk-Shiley (Fig. 118–12) and the St. Jude (Fig. 118–13) valves.

The tissue valves can be classified into two types: the porcine valves and the bovine pericardial valve. Porcine valves include the Hancock (Fig. 118–12) and the Carpentier-Edwards (Fig. 118–14)

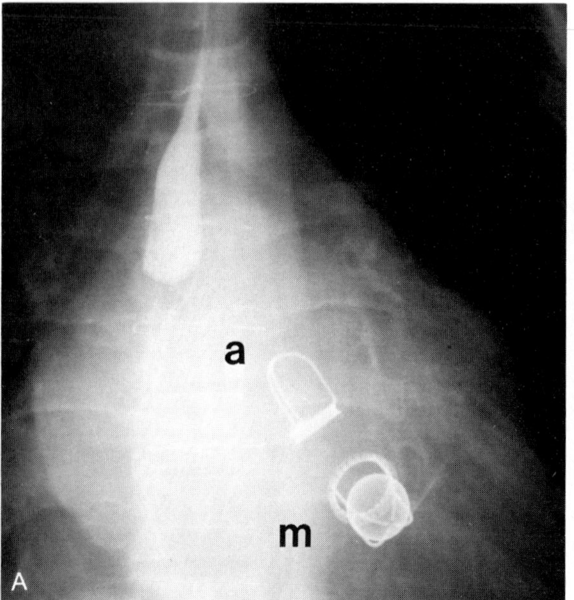

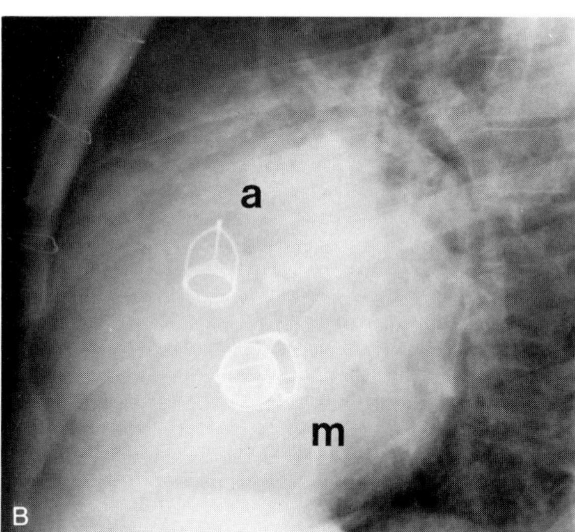

Figure 118–10. Two **Starr-Edwards prostheses**, one in the mitral (m) and the other in the aortic (a) position. *A*, PA view. *B*, Lateral view.

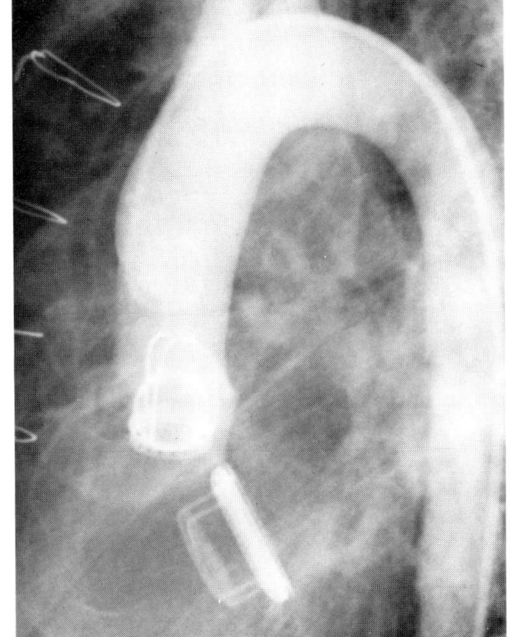

Figure 118–11. A **Beall caged-disc prosthesis** in the mitral position and a **Starr-Edwards caged-ball prosthesis** in the aortic position are well-imaged on the lateral view. The aortogram is normal.

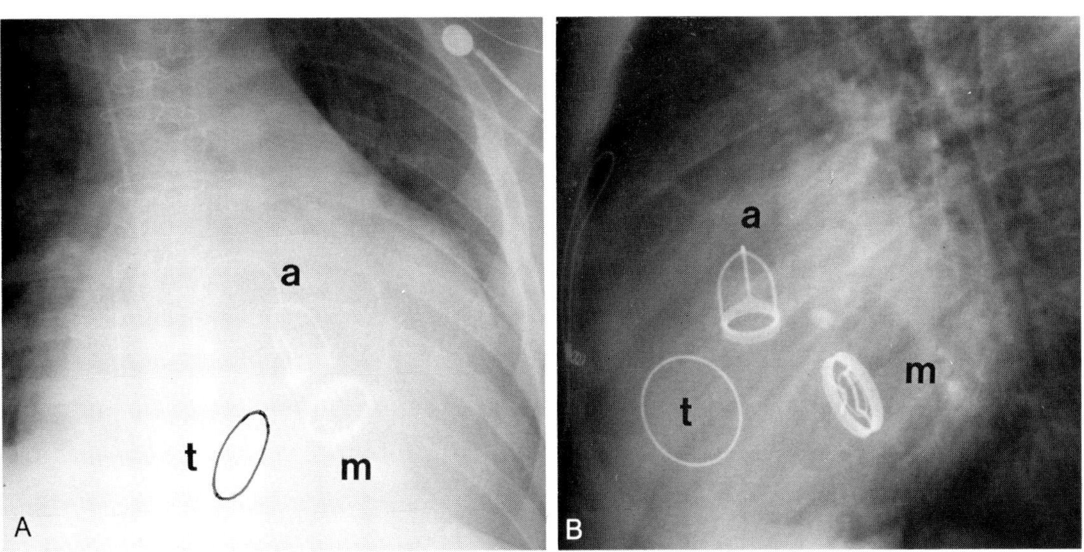

Figure 118–12. A patient with long-standing rheumatic heart disease. A **Starr-Edwards valve** is in the aortic (a) position, a **Björk-Shiley valve** is in the mitral (m) position, and a **Hancock porcine valve** is in the tricuspid (t) position. *A*, PA view. *B*, Lateral view.

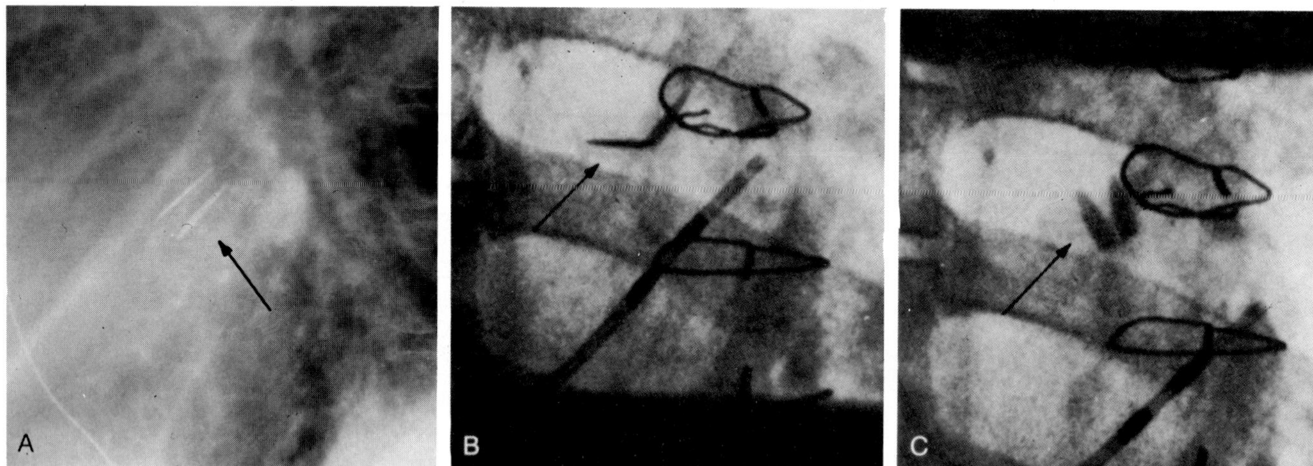

Figure 118–13. *A,* A **St. Jude mitral valve** is seen in the open position—the two leaflets of the valve are caught in profile as two parallel lines of increased density *(arrow).* When the valve is in the closed position or when the leaflets are viewed en face, they become invisible. *B,* A side view of a St. Jude valve with its two leaflets caught in the closed position *(arrow). C,* A side view of the same leaflets caught in the open position *(arrow).* (*B* and *C* reproduced with permission from Kotler MN, et al: The role of noninvasive technique in the evaluation of the St. Jude cardiac prosthesis. In DeBakey M (ed): Advances in Cardiac Valves. New York, Yorke Medical Books, 1983.)

valves. The bovine pericardial valve is called the Ionescu-Shiley valve (Fig. 118–15).

For annuloplasty of both the mitral and tricuspid valves, the Carpentier ring, a flexible incomplete ring, is used (Fig. 118–16). This technique is most suited to the treatment of patients with isolated regurgitation, with dilatation of the annulus, and without calcium in the leaflets.

Detection of Prosthetic Malfunctions

Malfunctions of the cardiac prostheses can be diagnosed or suggested either by radiographic techniques alone or by correlating them with clinical and echocardiographic findings.

PROSTHETIC INSTABILITY

A well-seated and well-functioning prosthesis moves to and fro in the direction of the blood flow with only a negligible tilt between the two phases of the cardiac cycle. A phasic prosthetic tilt greater than 12 degrees or a rocking movement of the valve is indicative of prosthetic instability with loosening of the surgical sutures. An unstable prosthesis is almost always associated with regurgitation of that valve. The causes of prosthetic instability include faulty surgical technique, infective endocarditis, and tissue deterioration in the bed of the prosthesis as frequently encountered in patients with mitral valve prolapse or Marfan's syndrome.

PARAVALVULAR LEAK

Leaking around a prosthetic valve may or may not be associated with prosthetic instability, depending on the site and the extent of tissue damage and in turn on the number of sutures pulling loose from the annulus. In the absence of an unstable prosthesis, a paravalvular leak is manifested only by signs of valvular regurgitation.

VALVULAR REGURGITATION

Valvular regurgitation without prosthetic instability usually results from cuspal tears and perforations of the tissue valves and

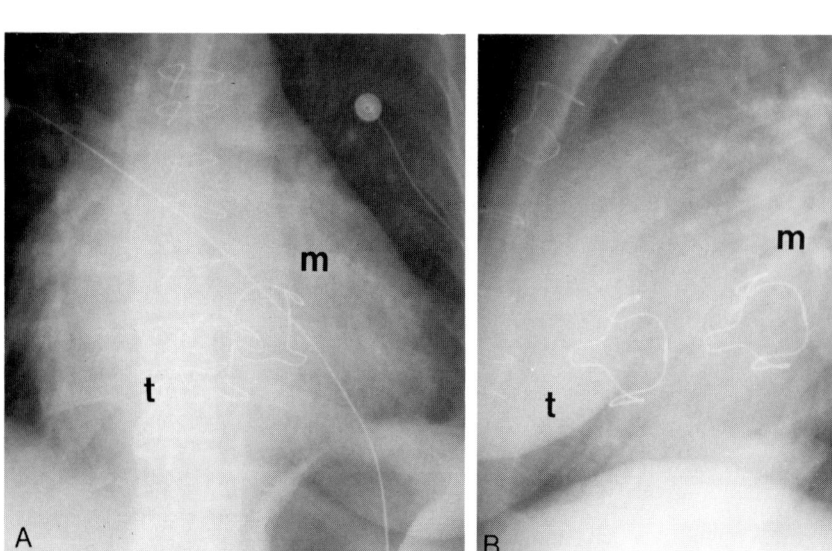

Figure 118–14. Patient with rheumatic mitral stenosis and tricuspid regurgitation. Both valves were replaced. A **Carpentier-Edwards porcine valve** is seen in the mitral (m) and tricuspid (t) position. *A,* PA view. *B,* Lateral view.

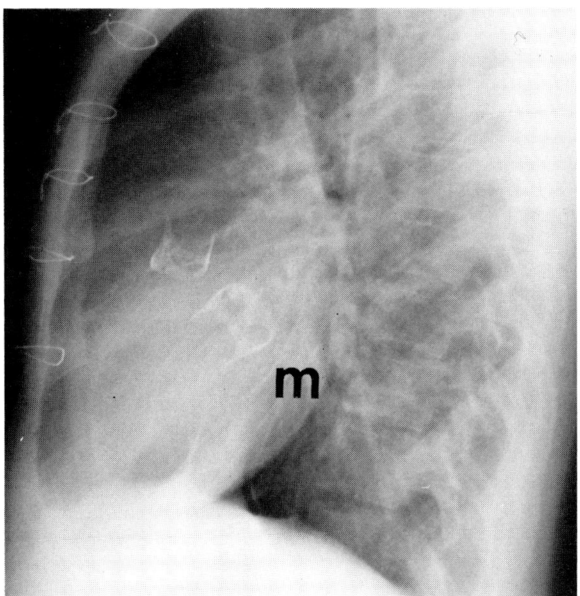

Figure 118–15. Two **Ionescu-Shiley valves** are seen in the lateral view, one in the mitral (m) and the other in the aortic position.

from thrombosis, degeneration, or wear of the mechanical valves. Caged-disc valves are known to leak as a result of grooving or erosion of the disc poppets. A more serious condition results when a deformed disc cocks into a fixed position, causing massive valvular regurgitation. In the older models of caged-ball prostheses, excessive wear of the poppet may allow it to dislodge from the cage. Swelling of such a poppet from lipid infiltration may cause its impaction in the cage. Thrombus in a mechanical valve may cause valvular stenosis or regurgitation or both. In the case of double valve replacement, the stent or ring of the mitral prosthesis may prevent the aortic poppet from seating in diastole, thereby causing aortic regurgitation.

Cases with outlet strut fracture involving the Björk-Shiley valve have been reported. These patients usually experience a sudden onset of profound heart failure. The auscultatory clicks of the prosthetic valve are lost. Instead of using time-consuming cardiac catheterization, the diagnosis should promptly be made by identifying the defective strut and the disc embolus on well-penetrated radiographs of the chest and abdomen. Emergency surgery should be performed immediately under such circumstances.

With the increasing popularity of the bileaflet St. Jude prosthesis for cardiac valve replacement, some rare but serious complications relating to such implantations have been documented. Owing to mechanical failure of the prosthesis, a 12-year-old boy suddenly lost one of the two leaflets, causing severe mitral regurgitation. Two patients developed obstruction to one of the two leaflets in the aortic position and died. These complications can be promptly diagnosed by a simple fluoroscopic observation and videotape recording.

The radiographic signs of aortic regurgitation are dilatation and hyperkinesis of both the left ventricle and the aorta prior to cardiac decompensation. Following congestive heart failure, the left ventricle loses its contractility and dilates further. By then, pulmonary edema is usually present.

The hallmark of mitral regurgitation is a combination of dilatation and hyperkinesis of the left-sided cardiac chambers prior to cardiac decompensation. Following left-sided heart failure, increased cardiomegaly, pulmonary edema, and loss of left ventricular contractility will become evident.

Radiographic signs of tricuspid regurgitation include dilatation of right-sided cardiac chambers with increased right atrial expansion during ventricular contraction and evidence of systemic venous hypertension.

VALVULAR STENOSIS

Obstruction of a prosthetic valve may result from calcification of a tissue valve and thrombotic stenosis of a mechanical valve. In either case, the decreased or absent excursion of a ball or disc poppet can be observed on fluoroscopy and recorded on videotape. A calcified prosthetic valve is identified more easily by fluoroscopy than by radiography. Another mechanical problem causing stenosis of a prosthetic valve has to do with the prosthetic size disproportion. When a mitral prosthesis is too big for the left ventricle, for instance, the movement of the poppet may be limited, causing obstruction to left atrial emptying and, less commonly, also obstructing the outflow tract of the left ventricle. When an excessively large valve prosthesis is implanted in the aortic position, emptying of the left ventricle may be impaired.

Aortic stenosis secondary to prosthesis dysfunction manifests itself radiographically as left ventricular dilatation associated with pulmonary venous congestion. Mitral stenosis secondary to an obstructed prosthetic valve manifests itself as left atrial and right ventricular enlargement associated with pulmonary venous hypertension. Prosthetic tricuspid valve stenosis results in systemic venous hypertension with dilatation of the right atrium and the systemic veins, which pulsate excessively during ventricular diastole.

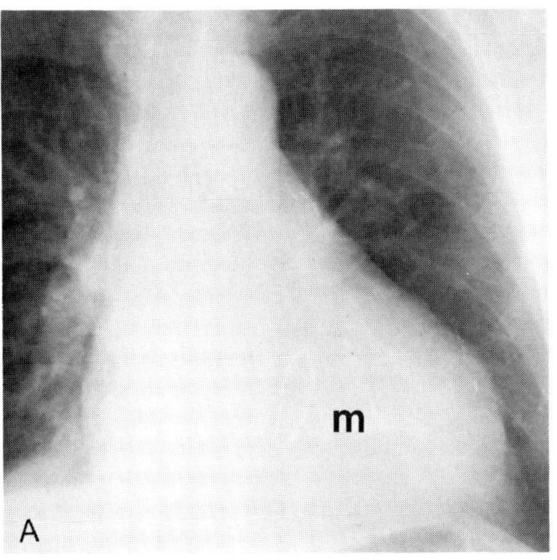

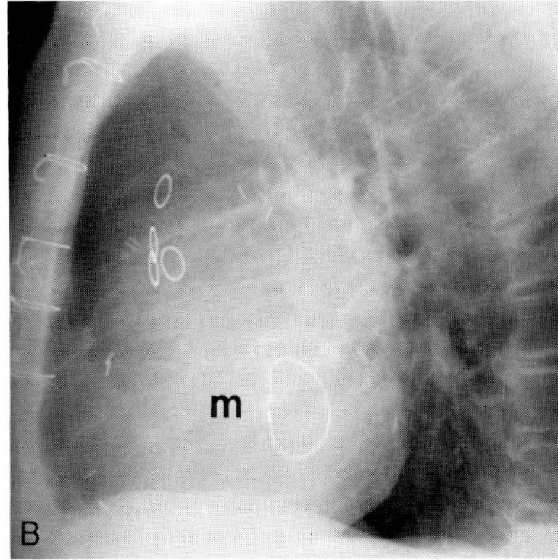

Figure 118–16. A patient with **post–myocardial infarction mitral regurgitation.** A Carpentier annuloplasty ring was implanted in the mitral position (m) at the time of coronary bypass graft surgery. *A*, PA view. *B*, Lateral view.

Bibliography

Bognolo DA, Vijayanagar RR, Eckstein PF: Atrial and atrioventricular sequential pacing, rationale and clinical experience. J Fla Med Assoc 66:1028, 1979.

Bognolo DA, Vijayanagar R, Eckstein PF, et al: Implantation of permanent transvenous atrial J lead using lateral view fluoroscopy. Ann Thorac Surg 31:574, 1981.

Cohn LH, Gallucci V: Cardiac bioprostheses. Proceedings of the Second International Symposium. New York, Yorke Med Books, 1982.

DeBakey M: Advances in Cardiac Valves, Clinical Perspectives. New York, Yorke Med Books, 1983.

Guit GL, vanVoorthuisen AE, Steiner RM: Outlet strut fracture of the Björk-Shiley mitral valve prosthesis. Radiology 154:298, 1985.

Hanabergh E, Rahim A, Agatston A, et al: Coronary sinus pacer lead simulating left atrial mass. J Ultrasound Med 1:83,1982.

Hewitt MJ, Chen JTT, Ravin CE, Gallagher JJ: Coronary sinus atrial pacing: Radiographic considerations. AJR 136:323, 1981.

McAlpine WA: The Heart and Coronary Arteries: An Anatomic Atlas for Clinical Diagnosis, Radiologic Investigation and Surgical Treatment. New York, Springer, 1976.

Morse D, Steiner RM: The Pacemaker and Valve Identification Guide. Garden City, NY, Medical Examination Publishing Co., 1978.

Ormond RS, Rubenfire M, Anbe DT, et al: Radiographic demonstration of myocardial penetration by permanent endocardial pacemakers. Radiology 98:35, 1971.

Rodan BA, Lowe JE, Chen JTT: Abdominal twiddler's syndrome. AJR 131:1084, 1978.

Ross EM, Roberts WD: A precaution when using the St. Jude medical prosthesis in the aortic valve position. Am J Cardiol 54:231, 1984.

Sabiston DC Jr, Spencer FC (eds): Surgery of the Chest, 5th ed. Philadelphia, WB Saunders Company, 1990, pp 1597–1634.

Sorkin RP, Schaurmann BJ, Simon AB: Radiographic aspects of permanent cardiac pacemakers. Radiology 119:281, 1976.

Steiner RM, Morse DP, Tegtmeyer CJ: Pacemaker lead pseudofracture. Radiology 143:793, 1982.

Willis J (ed): Complications of convexo-concave heart valves. FDA Drug Bull 14:22, 1984.

Zipes DP, Barold SS: Cardiac pacemakers. In Braunwald EW (ed): Heart Disease: A Textbook of Cardiovascular Medicine, 4th ed. Philadelphia, WB Saunders Company, 1992.

Zoll P: Resuscitation of the heart in ventricular standstill by external electric stimulation. N Engl J Med 247:768, 1952.

IMAGING THE FEMALE PATIENT

The following section deals with imaging problems that are unique to the female patient. The fact that we have such a section in a textbook of this nature represents in part the profound and continuing impact of the development of the newer imaging modalities on our way of thinking about long-standing medical problems. However, one must not attribute the new ways of dealing with these problems entirely to the development of these new modalities. There has been a basic change in the level of intensity with which we view medical problems, and this new self-criticism, coupled with an increased public awareness of some diseases and interest in a higher standard of medical care, has led us to reexamine critically certain traditional diseases. Mammography is one of the best examples for which an emphasis on another facet of the disease—early detection—has been brought about by both changes in technology and an understanding of the disease itself. The same is true of the approach to prenatal diagnosis, which has been greatly influenced both by the development of sonography and by our ways of thinking about prenatal problems.

The following chapters present much of the current information regarding imaging problems of the female patient. Available information is constantly being refined as schemes are re-evaluated and our technology improves. Just as the difference between the information in this section and that presented in standard textbooks of 10 or 15 years ago is enormous, we can also anticipate significant changes over the next several years which will revise much of what is presented in this section. However, the major new trends are now apparent, and future changes undoubtedly will be along the lines set forth in the following chapters.

JAMES D. BOWIE

The Pregnant Patient

119 Ultrasonic Imaging in Obstetrics

Rudy E. Sabbagha

The last 15 years have witnessed marked enhancement in the resolution of ultrasonic images. The use of dynamic (real-time) equipment in the form of linear array and sector transducers has also simplified sonography, particularly in the fields of obstetrics and gynecology. The reasons are related to two factors. First, scanning of a moving target, such as the fetus, is easier with dynamic transducers. Second, sector transducers (a) can be angled to the adnexal areas to image the ovaries and (b) can help the sonographer distinguish a pelvic mass from bowel, the latter frequently exhibiting peristalsis.

The rapid progress in ultrasonic imaging has resulted in an exponential increase in the data that can be recovered from the examination of the pregnant uterus. Although acquisition of a large body of information can, on specific occasions, be beneficial in patient management, controversy has erupted about how much information should be gathered by one ultrasound study. With the rise in medicolegal litigation, professional liability will undoubtedly increase when either too few or too many data are reported, especially since the predictive values of normal and abnormal ultrasonic findings are not fully defined.

The need for sonographers to spend additional time in ruling out the presence of all anomalies on every fetus is being questioned by many physicians. There is concern about the following points:

1. Execution of ultrasonic studies for anomalies by nonphysician professionals and by physicians inexperienced in the diagnosis of anomalies because their practice deals mainly with normal pregnancies.
2. Unnecessarily subjecting low-risk pregnant women to a more prolonged examination and additional ultrasonic intensity for the detection of anomalies, when the incidence of birth defects in that group is quite low.
3. Cost-effectiveness of testing every pregnancy for anomalies when the overall yield is small.
4. Remuneration for these tests by third-party payers.
5. Lack of manifestation of a variety of anomalies at 16 to 18 weeks' gestation, an interval commonly used for initial scans. For example, duodenal atresia, intestinal obstruction, polycystic renal disease, heterozygous achondroplasia, late-onset hydrocephalus, and microcephalus are conditions that frequently become ultrasonically apparent only past 20 and sometimes 30 weeks of pregnancy.

THE ULTRASOUND EXAMINATION

To formulate some guidelines about the ultrasound examination, the Section of Obstetrical and Gynecological Ultrasonographers (SOGU) of the American Institute of Ultrasound in Medicine defined the following two categories the standard and second-opinion ultrasonic studies.

In the standard study, data are collected regarding (1) gestational age and fetal growth; (2) number of fetuses; (3) presence of fetal heart motion; (4) qualitative estimate of amniotic fluid volume; (5)

placental position and, where applicable, placental grade; (6) survey of fetal anatomy for gross anomalies; and (7) pelvic mass, if present.

A second-opinion study by an expert ultrasonographer is encouraged when an abnormal finding is suspected in either the mother or the fetus.

Second-opinion studies imply that some abnormality is already suspected. However, in situations in which the examiner fails to detect a fetal anomaly, a second-opinion study is not requested and the benefit of an expert consultation is lost. A scenario like this one can lead to endless complications, especially if the woman in question is at high risk for fetal anomalies.

Women who are more likely to have fetal anomalies should have targeted imaging for fetal anomaly (TIFFA) examinations by physician ultrasonographers with wide experience in the diagnosis of birth defects. In this group of women, TIFFA studies are not only indicated but are also cost-effective. The indications for TIFFA studies include (1) history of a defect, (2) elevated α-fetoprotein (AFP) in maternal serum or in amniotic fluid, (3) intrauterine growth retardation (IUGR), (4) insulin-dependent maternal diabetes mellitus, (5) breech presentation at term, (6) polyhydramnios or oligohydramnios, and (7) suspicion of an anomaly in the course of a standard ultrasound study.

Of interest are our findings regarding the outcome of TIFFA examinations in women referred for the evaluation of an anomaly diagnosed elsewhere. First, 60 per cent of referrals with a diagnosis of hydrocephaly were in fact normal. Second, 28 per cent of fetuses with a diagnosis of urethral obstruction had another abnormality—a mesoderm defect of the abdominal wall and urinary system, a condition for which diversion shunts are contraindicated. Third, 17 per cent of referrals because of anencephalus were normal.

AFP and Ultrasound

As analysis of maternal serum for AFP concentration becomes a routine antenatal screening test by 16 weeks, the ultrasonographer will be called on more frequently to offer an explanation for abnormal values. When serum AFP is elevated, a standard ultrasound study should be performed. If AFP level remains high after correcting for dates, TIFFA examination should be performed to determine whether the test is falsely elevated. This is necessary because, in a recent report by Hobbins et al., the offspring in 14 of 28, or 50 per cent, of pregnancies with abnormal AFP in amniotic fluid (a condensation of thousands of pregnant women with elevated serum AFP) were devoid of overt anomalies. In another report by Milunsky and Sapirstein, 9 of 16, or 50.6 per cent, of pregnancies with high amniotic fluid AFP and positive acetylcholinesterase delivered normal babies. A low maternal serum AFP ($\leq$0.4 multiples of the median) is also associated with an increased incidence of Down syndrome.

Ultrasound Examinations Placed in Perspective

The ultrasonographer should continually place the ultrasonic findings in their proper perspective. In this regard, a number of areas should be critically looked at:

1. Necessity of calculating the cephalic index or the femur length/biparietal diameter (FL/BPD) ratio in all pregnancies.
2. Prediction of fetal weight on every fetus regardless of its size.
3. Routine averaging of multiple parameters to define pregnancy dates.
4. Whether to measure actual circumferences of the head and body or to calculate an approximate circumference measurement from two or more diameters.
5. When to use the biophysical profile.
6. Existing controversy over the definition of and meaning of oligohydramnios.
7. Controversy over the accuracy of the femur in predicting dates.

Cephalic Index, Head Circumference, and FL/BPD Ratio

Dolichocephaly rarely occurs under 26 weeks' gestation, when dating the pregnancy by ultrasound is considered reliable. Even if it did occur then, the variation in dates produced by side-to-side flattening of the fetal head will be incorporated within the two standard deviation limits defining the range in the accuracy of cephalometry.

Dolichocephaly is more likely to occur in the presence of factors that increase intrauterine pressure, such as multiple pregnancy and oligohydramnios. Logically, determination of the cephalic index or head circumference should be limited to those conditions, and after 26 weeks' gestation.

The FL/BPD ratio can be low or high in many normal fetuses when the BPD and femur values are in opposite directions from their respective means; i.e., one parameter is one standard deviation above the mean, and the other is one standard deviation below the mean. Thus, to avoid confusion and false alarm it makes sense to relate FL and BPD measurements, obtained at specific intervals in gestation, to their normal growth curves.

Fetal Weight Predictions

Depending on the formula used, the accuracy of fetal weight prediction falls between 15 and 20 per cent of actual weight per kilogram. For example, in a 1000-g fetus the error will be 150 g. On the other hand, predicting fetal weight in the range of 4000 g carries an error of 600 g. Formulas targeted to estimate the weight of large fetuses may reduce the error to $\pm$12 per cent.

Averaging Multiple Parameters to Date Pregnancies

Routinely averaging different parameters to define the length of pregnancy is not only redundant but can also lead to errors when there is altered fetal growth.

1. When two or more parameters predict dates closely, averaging is unnecessary, since any predictor can be used. However, the fact that the estimates are in agreement indicates that the probability of that end point is more certain (Bayes' theorem).
2. In asymmetric IUGR, it is imperative that a head measurement be used, since the abdominal circumference by definition is small and the femur can also be shortened. Averaging parameters in this condition of altered growth will dilute the effect of the best predictor, namely, head size.
3. In symmetric IUGR, averaging any number of parameters is useless because all measurements are small and falsely predict a less mature fetus. A detailed menstrual history in such women is often found to be helpful.

How to Measure Circumferences

Actual circumference measurements of the head and body remain the most sensitive methods in differentiating normal from abnormal growth.

The Biophysical Profile

At the present time the test for biophysical profile should not be routinely requested, particularly if (1) a standard ultrasound examination was previously performed and (2) the nonstress test was normal. Additionally, the biophysical profile score will be more reliable if the test is to be performed only on women not receiving medication known to suppress the central nervous system and performed approximately 1.5 to 2 hours after meals because fetal breathing is commonly observed then. If breathing is absent during this interval, the likelihood that the fetus is compromised versus simply in a sleep cycle is increased.

Controversy in the Definition and Meaning of Oligohydramnios

Although the initial findings by Manning et al. suggested that estimates of amniotic fluid equal to or less than 1 cm indicated oligohydramnios, Chamberlain et al. as well as other investigators recently changed this definition to 2 or even 3 cm.

The finding of oligohydramnios is more significant in selected pregnancies at high risk for IUGR, the risk determined either clinically or by abnormal ultrasonic biometry or both. Under such circumstances, Manning et al. found that oligohydramnios (amniotic fluid 1.0 cm or less) is predictive of IUGR in approximately 90 per cent of cases.

In contrast, in a retrospective study of women who delivered undergrown neonates, Hoddick et al. reported that the "1 cm sign" was a poor predictor of IUGR, since it was only found in 4 of 52, or 7.7 per cent, of such pregnancies.

In another well-controlled study conducted by Philipson et al., the predictive value of oligohydramnios in unselected pregnancies was reported to be 40 per cent, and the sensitivity, projected to the whole pregnant population, was poor, namely, 16 per cent. These authors defined oligohydramnios as paucity of amniotic fluid in all areas with evidence of fetal crowding.

Recently, the amniotic fluid index (sum of largest packet in four quadrants) has been more frequently utilized; a level ≤ 5.0 is associated with adverse perinatal outcome.

Controversy Relative to the Accuracy of the Femur Length in Dating Pregnancy

Initial reports by O'Brien and Queenan suggested that the femur is an accurate predictor of dates within a margin of approximately seven days, until 23 weeks of pregnancy. After this interval the accuracy is lost. Hadlock et al. more or less confirmed these findings, although they reported the accuracy to fall within 10 days until approximately 26 weeks' gestation.

Subsequently, Jeanty et al. published the results of a very extensive study and showed that the accuracy of the femur was the same throughout pregnancy but the range of accuracy was wide, two standard deviations encompassing 2.8 weeks.

The History

Finally, the sonographer should rely heavily on the history and try to elicit the reason for the referral directly from the patient. The following examples illustrate the importance of the history in conducting or interpreting the ultrasound examination:

1. A woman is referred in the third trimester of pregnancy to rule out twins. The physician's concern is rapid growth of the fundal height. Twins are ruled out. However, the BPD is found to correlate with 37 weeks rather than 33 menstrual weeks. The patient states that she always gives birth to very large babies. In the interpretation of the report the sonographer should take into account the fact that in this specific case fetal age can be as little as 33 weeks, the reason for the discrepancy between the ultrasound and menstrual dates being related to the presence of a large fetus, one less mature than mean BPD charts indicate.

2. The diagnosis of symmetric IUGR should be seriously considered in a woman when menstrual dates point to 36 weeks but all fetal parameters indicate a gestational age of 32 weeks.

3. In a woman who previously had tubal ligation and now presents with a positive pregnancy test, ectopic gestation should be meticulously sought.

4. In a woman with a history of menstrual irregularities, a thick endometrial cavity should not be assumed to represent an intrauterine device (IUD); she should be asked whether an IUD had been previously inserted.

Bibliography

Chamberlain PF, Manning FA, Morrison I, et al: Ultrasound evaluation of amniotic fluid volume. I. The relationship of marginal and decreased amniotic fluid volumes to perinatal outcome. Am J Obstet Gynecol 150:245–249, 1984.

Griffiths DM, Gough MH: Dilemmas after ultrasonic diagnosis of fetal abnormality. Lancet 1:623, 1985.

Haddow JE, Wald NJ (eds): Alpha-fetoprotein screening: The current issues, a report of the Third Scarborough Conference. Scarborough, ME, Foundation for Blood Research, 1981.

Hadlock FP, Harrist RB, et al: Ultrasonically measured fetal femur length as a predictor of menstrual age. AJR 138:875, 1982.

Hadlock FP, Harrist RB, Sharman RS, et al: Estimation of fetal weight with the use of head, body, and femur measurements—A prospective study. Am J Obstet Gynecol 151:333–337, 1985.

Hobbins JC, Venus I, Tortora M, et al: Stage II ultrasound examination for the diagnosis of fetal abnormalities with an elevated amniotic fluid alpha-fetoprotein concentration. Am J Obstet Gynecol 142:1026–1029, 1982.

Hoddick WH, Callen PW, Filly RA, Creasy RK: Ultrasonographic determination of qualitative fluid volume in intrauterine growth retardation: Reassessment of the 1 cm rule. Am J Obstet Gynecol 149:758, 1984.

Hutson JM, McNay M, MacKenzie JR, et al: Antenatal diagnosis of surgical disorders by ultrasonography. Lancet 1:621, 1985.

Jeanty P, Rodesch F, Delbeke D, Dumont JE: Estimation of gestational age from measurements of fetal long bones. J Ultrasound Med 3:75–79, 1984.

Manning FA, Hill LM, Platt LD: Qualitative amniotic fluid volume determination—antepartum detection of intrauterine growth retardation. Am J Obstet Gynecol 139:254, 1981.

Milunsky A, Sapirstein VS: Prenatal diagnosis of open neural tube defects using the amniotic fluid acetylcholinesterase assay. Obstet Gynecol 59:1, 1982.

O'Brien GD, Queenan JT: Growth of the ultrasound fetal femur length during normal pregnancy. Am J Obstet Gynecol 141:833, 1981.

Phelan JP, Ahn MO, Smith CV, et al: Amniotic fluid index measurements during pregnancy. J Reprod Med 32:601, 1987.

Philipson EH, Sokol RJ, Williams T: Oligohydramnios: Clinical associations and predictive value for intrauterine growth retardation. Am J Obstet Gynecol 146:271, 1983.

Rutherford SE, Phelan JP, Smith CV, et al: The four quadrant assessment of amniotic fluid volume. An adjunct to antepartum fetal heart rate testing. Obstet Gynecol 70:353, 1987.

Sabbagha RE: Intrauterine growth retardation avenues of future research in diagnosis and management by ultrasound. Semin Perinatol 8:1, 1984.

Sabbagha RE, Minogue J, Tamura RK, Hungerford SA: Estimation of BW by the use of ultrasound formulas targeted to large, appropriate, and SGA fetuses. Am J Obstet Gynecol 160:255, 1989.

Sabbagha RE, Sheikh Z, Tamura RK, et al: Predictive value, sensitivity, and specificity of targeted imaging for fetal anomalies in gravid women at high risk for birth defects. Am J Obstet Gynecol 152:822, 1985.

120 The Use of Diagnostic Ultrasound Imaging in Pregnancy*

From crude initial studies in the 1950s, ultrasonography in pregnancy has become a highly developed technology capable of detecting many fetal structural and functional abnormalities. It has found application in detecting ectopic pregnancy and multiple pregnancy, assessing fetal life and function, diagnosing physical anomalies, and guiding physicians as they make efforts to treat the fetal patient. The advent of ultrasound has overcome many of the diagnostic limitations of radiography and has virtually eliminated the need for fetal exposure to ionizing radiation.

With these advantages and marked improvements in the technology and equipment, the use of ultrasound in obstetric practice has grown rapidly. The procedure is available in nearly all hospitals, and many physicians have acquired equipment for use in their offices. Furthermore, because of the absence of clinically perceived risk of ultrasound and its usefulness in assessing structural anomalies, multiple pregnancy, and fetal size and gestational age, many practitioners have begun to advocate its routine use as a screening device in all pregnancies.

Lack of risk has been assumed because no adverse effects have been demonstrated clearly in humans. However, other evidence dictates that a hypothetical risk must be presumed with ultrasound. Likewise, the efficacy of many uses of ultrasound in improving the management and outcome of pregnancy also has been assumed rather than demonstrated, especially its value as a routine screening procedure.

On the basis of the collective experience of members of the panel, the material presented, and the literature review that was conducted, we conclude that in obstetric practice in the United States, use of diagnostic ultrasound imaging has an expanding role, and its use is becoming widespread. Information on the extent of use of diagnostic ultrasound in pregnancy was available from single institutions and states agencies, marketing studies, the office survey conducted by the American College of Obstetricians and Gynecologists, and the 1980 National Natality Survey. These data lead to estimates of the percentage of pregnant women exposed to at least one ultrasound examination, ranging from a low of 15 per cent to a high of 40 per cent. There is reason to believe that all of these sources seriously underestimate the true extent of exposure to ultrasound, since they do not necessarily include exposure via Doppler devices, including those used to listen to fetal heart tones and in antepartum and intrapartum fetal heart rate monitoring.

Exposure to imaging devices in the recent past has been to static scanners, real-time equipment of the linear array type, and mechanical sector scanners. The quantity used most often to report instrumentation output is intensity. Typical time average value ranges of intensity are 0.1 to 60 mW/sq cm (spatial average, temporal average intensity) and 1 to 200 mW/sq cm (spatial peak, temporal average intensity). The spatial peak, pulse average intensity typically ranges from 1 to 200 mW/sq cm for such pulsed ultrasound equipment.

The time average intensities of the typical obstetric Doppler devices used to listen to the fetal heart and for fetal heart rate monitoring in the antepartum and intrapartum period are within the same range as for pulsed equipment. These systems operate in the continuous wave mode, viz, 0.2 to 20 mW/sq cm (spatial average, temporal average intensity) and 0.6 to 80 mW/sq cm (spatial peak, temporal average intensity). As new technologies and applications evolve, for example, measurement of blood flow using pulsed Doppler, exposure levels may be substantially higher.

Manufacturers of ultrasound equipment introduced into United States commerce are required to report outputs to the FDA. We recommend that these quantities be measured and reported to the user in a form consistent with the requirements of the AIUM/NEMA Safety Standard for Diagnostic Ultrasound Equipment.

Dose is a quantitative measure of an agent that is given or imparted and combines quantities such as intensity and exposure time. No dose quantity has been identified for ultrasound. Variation in tissue properties between individuals as well as scanning conditions influence dose in an unpredictable way. For all practical purposes, fetal dose cannot be quantitated precisely. For this reason, there are no data on the dose to either the mother or the fetus in the clinical setting. Documentation of dwell time and type of machine and transducer used would begin to address this problem. It is recommended that at least this specific exposure information be recorded for each examination. Thus, it is important that each exposure to ultrasound by all Doppler and imaging devices be recorded.

Ultrasound has been used in a wide variety of clinical situations to aid in managing pregnancy. For each of these applications, there is literature recording the clinical experience from various centers, with evidence of the benefits ultrasound has had in each respective application, although these applications have not been subjected to the rigorous evaluation provided by a randomized, controlled clinical trial. The following should not be considered circumstances in which use of diagnostic ultrasound imaging is mandatory. Rather, where significant clinical questions exist, the resolution of which would alter the remainder of prenatal care, ultrasound can be of benefit for the following:

1. *Estimation of gestational age for patients with uncertain clinical dates, or verification of dates for patients who are to undergo scheduled elective repeat cesarean delivery, indicated induction of labor, or other elective termination of pregnancy.* Ultrasonographic confirmation of dating permits proper timing of cesarean delivery or labor induction to avoid premature delivery.
2. *Evaluation of fetal growth* (e.g., when the patient has an identified etiology for uteroplacental insufficiency, such as severe preeclampsia, chronic hypertension, chronic renal disease, severe diabetes mellitus, or for other medical complications of pregnancy where fetal malnutrition, i.e., intrauterine growth retardation [IUGR] or macrosomia, is suspected). Following fetal growth permits assessment of the impact of a complicating condition on the fetus and guides pregnancy management.
3. *Vaginal bleeding of undetermined etiology in pregnancy.* Ultrasound often allows determination of the source of bleeding and status of the fetus.
4. *Determination of fetal presentation* when the presenting part cannot be adequately determined in labor or the fetal presentation is variable in late pregnancy. Accurate knowledge of presentation guides management of delivery.
5. *Suspected multiple gestation* based on detection of more than

*Taken from the National Institutes of Health, Food and Drug Administration Consensus Development Conference Consensus Statement, February 6–8, 1984. Excerpts contributed by Stephen W. Smith.

one fetal heart beat pattern, fundal height larger than expected for dates, and/or prior use of fertility drugs. Pregnancy management may be altered in multiple gestation.

6. *Adjunct to amniocentesis.* Ultrasound permits guidance of the needle to avoid the placenta and fetus, to increase the chance of obtaining amniotic fluid, and to decrease the chance of fetal loss.

7. *Significant uterine size/clinical dates discrepancy.* Ultrasound permits accurate dating and detection of such conditions as oligohydramnios and polyhydramnios, as well as multiple gestation, IUGR, and anomalies.

8. *Pelvic mass* detected clinically. Ultrasound can detect the location and nature of the mass and aid in diagnosis.

9. *Suspected hydatidiform mole* on the basis of clinical signs of hypertension, proteinuria, and/or the presence of ovarian cysts felt on pelvic examination or failure to detect fetal heart tones with a Doppler ultrasound device after 12 weeks. Ultrasound permits accurate diagnosis and differentiation of this neoplasm from fetal death.

10. *Adjunct to cervical cerclage placement.* Ultrasound aids in timing and proper placement of the cerclage for patients with incompetent cervix.

11. *Suspected ectopic pregnancy* or when pregnancy occurs after tuboplasty or prior ectopic gestation. Ultrasound is a valuable diagnostic aid for this complication.

12. *Adjunct to special procedures* such as fetoscopy, intrauterine transfusion, shunt placement, in vitro fertilization, embryo transfer, or chorionic villi sampling. Ultrasound aids instrument guidance, which increases safety of these procedures.

13. *Suspected fetal death.* Rapid diagnosis enhances optimal management.

14. *Suspected uterine abnormality* (e.g., clinically significant leiomyomata or congenital structural abnormalities, such as bicornuate uterus or uterus didelphys, etc.). Serial surveillance of fetal growth and state enhances fetal outcome.

15. *Intrauterine device (IUD) localization.* Ultrasound guidance facilitates removal, reducing chances of IUD-related complications.

16. *Ovarian follicle development surveillance.* This facilitates treatment of infertility.

17. *Biophysical evaluation for fetal well-being* after 28 weeks of gestation. Assessment of amniotic fluid, fetal tone, body movements, breathing movements, and heart rate patterns assists in the management of high-risk pregnancies.

18. *Observation of intrapartum events* (e.g., version/extraction of second twin, manual removal of placenta, etc.). These procedures may be done more safely with the visualization provided by ultrasound.

19. *Suspected polyhydramnios or oligohydramnios.* Confirmation of the diagnosis is permitted, as well as identification of the cause of the condition in certain pregnancies.

20. *Suspected abruptio placentae.* Confirmation of diagnosis and extent assists in clinical management.

21. *Adjunct to external version from breech to vertex presentation.* The visualization provided by ultrasound facilitates performance of this procedure.

22. *Estimation of fetal weight and/or presentation in premature rupture of membranes and/or premature labor.* Information provided by ultrasound guides management decisions on timing and method of delivery.

23. *Abnormal serum alpha-fetoprotein (AFP) value* for clinical gestational age when drawn. Ultrasound provides an accurate assessment of gestational age for the AFP comparison standard and indicates several conditions (e.g., twins, anencephaly) that may cause elevated AFP values.

24. *Follow-up observation of identified fetal anomaly.* Ultrasound assessment of progression or lack of change assists in clinical decision making.

25. *Follow-up evaluation for suspected placenta previa.*

26. *History of previous congenital anomaly.* Detection of recurrence may be permitted, or psychologic benefit to patients may result from reassurance of no recurrence.

27. *Serial evaluation of fetal growth in multiple gestation.* Ultrasound permits recognition of discordant growth, guiding patient management and timing of delivery.

28. *Evaluation of fetal condition in late registrants for prenatal care.*

Accurate knowledge of gestational age assists in pregnancy management decisions for this group.

The information presented in the material reviewed by the panel, including the studies of Bennett, Eik-Nes, Bakketeig, Grennert, and others, allowed no consensus that routine ultrasound examinations for all pregnancies improved perinatal outcome or decreased morbidity or mortality. There was, however, evidence that there was a higher rate of detection of twins and congenital malformations, as well as more accurate dating of pregnancy, but without significant evidence of improved outcome. The evidence with respect to the number of antepartum days of hospitalization and induction rates was contradictory among the various trials. The data on perinatal outcome were inconclusive. The panel recognized the inadequacy of the clinical trials on which these conclusions are drawn. Furthermore, it is acutely aware of the difficulty associated with conducting ideally controlled clinical trials and the large numbers of patients that must be included to uncover differences between control and experimental groups for a morbid event that occurs infrequently and spontaneously in the control population.

The panel concludes that diagnostic ultrasound for pregnant women improves patient management and pregnancy outcome when there is an accepted medical indication. Randomized, controlled clinical trials would be the best way in the United States to determine the efficacy of routine screening of all pregnancies.

The panel conducted an extensive review of the primary literature on this subject and of reports by the Bureau of Radiological Health (1976), Food and Drug Administration (1982), World Health Organization (1982), and the National Council on Radiation Protection and Measurements (1984). A number of epidemiologic studies tend to support the safety of diagnostic ultrasound exposure to humans. In particular, in the three randomized clinical trials in which half of the women were exposed routinely to ultrasound, there was no association of routine ultrasound exposure to birth weight. In the two studies that addressed the subject, no association of ultrasound exposure with hearing loss was observed. On the other hand, many of the studies reporting on the safety of diagnostic ultrasound in humans were considered inadequate to address many other important issues because of technical problems in conducting such research.

Some of the more than 35 published animal studies suggest that in utero ultrasound exposure can affect prenatal growth. When teratologic effects have been found, energies capable of causing significant hyperthermia have usually existed.

A number of biologic effects have been observed following ultrasound exposure in various experimental systems. These include reduction in immune response, change in sister chromatid exchange frequencies, cell death, change in cell membrane functions, degradation of macromolecules, free radical formation, and reduced cell reproductive potential. It should be noted that (1) some of the studies employed energy levels greater than would be expected to exist in clinical use; (2) in vitro exposure conditions to ultrasound used in many of the experiments are hard to place in perspective for risk assessment; (3) some of the observations, for example, changes in sister chromatid exchange frequency and induction of chromosomal abnormalities, have not been reproducible, tending to refute the original findings. Nevertheless, some of the reported effects cannot be ignored or overlooked and deserve further study as outlined below. The existence of these studies is one of the factors that contributed to our decision that routine ultrasound screening cannot be recommended at this time.

From the body of information reviewed, taking into account the available literature on bioeffects, data on clinical efficacy, and with concern for psychosocial, economic, and legal/ethical issues, it is the consensus of the panel that ultrasound examination in pregnancy should be performed for a specific medical indication. The data on clinical efficacy and safety do not allow a recommendation for routine screening at this time.

Ultrasound examinations performed solely to satisfy the family's desire to know the fetal sex, to view the fetus, or to obtain a picture of the fetus should be discouraged. In addition, visualization of the fetus solely for educational or commercial demonstrations without medical benefit to the patient should not be performed.

Prior to an ultrasound examination, patients should be informed of the clinical indication for ultrasound, specific benefit, potential risk, and alternatives, if any. In addition, the patient should be supplied with information about the exposure time and intensity, if requested. A written form may expedite this process in some cases. Patient access to educational materials regarding ultrasound is strongly encouraged. All settings in which these examinations are conducted should assure patients' dignity and privacy.

Given that the full potential of diagnostic ultrasound imaging is critically dependent on examiner training and experience, the panel recommends minimum training requirements and uniform credentialing for all physicians and sonographers performing ultrasound examinations. All health care providers who use this modality should demonstrate adequate knowledge of the basic physical principles of ultrasound, equipment, record keeping requirements, indications, and safety.

It is critical, in view of the existing data and the special considerations affecting fetal and embryonic development, to encourage and support a sustained research effort aimed specifically at test systems that can help provide a better data base for developing reasonable estimates of bioeffects and of risk. In particular, we recommend the following:

1. The study of fundamental mechanisms leading to bioeffects.
2. Laboratory experiments that focus especially on those cellular processes that are most likely to be affected during embryonic and fetal development.
3. Postnatal studies in animals after in utero exposure to ultrasound.
4. Exploration of interactions between administered ultrasound and such developmentally significant agents as drugs, nutrition, ionizing radiation, hyperthermia, and hypoxia.
5. Development of improved dosimetry.

A long-term follow-up of infants involved in a randomized clinical trial would help clarify questions about the effect of ultrasound on development in humans, and other epidemiologic studies using a wide variety of methods should be considered. Studies of the psychosocial, ethical, and legal aspects of ultrasound use are also needed.

Further nonexperimental studies that seek to establish the clinical efficacy of ultrasound should address the question of its contribution to reducing morbidity and mortality. Randomized, controlled clinical trials of routine ultrasound screening in pregnancy should be conducted in the United States.

Bibliography

Bakketeig LS, Brodtkorb C, Eik-Nes SH, et al: Screening by ultrasound during pregnancy—a randomized control trial. Presentation to Diagnostic Ultrasound Panel, NIH, June 1983.

Bennett MJ, Little G, Dewhurst J, Chamberlain G: Predictive value of ultrasound measurement in early pregnancy: A randomized controlled trial. Br J Obstet Gynecol 89:338–341, 1982.

Eik-Nes SH, Okland O: Ultrasound screening of pregnant women—a prospective randomized study. Presentation to Diagnostic Ultrasound Panel, NIH, June 1983.

Grennert L, Persson PH, Gennser G: Benefits of ultrasonic screening of a pregnant population. Acta Obstet Gynecol Scand (Suppl) 78:5–14, 1978.

121 Normal First Trimester

Alan V. Cadkin

Optimal examination of an intrauterine pregnancy (IUP) requires the use of a high-resolution real-time scanner, a vaginal probe, and meticulous scan technique.

TWO TO SEVEN WEEKS OF GESTATION

Conception occurs at two weeks' gestation (menstrual age). A tiny blastocyst forms and usually implants within the endometrium of the upper portion of the uterus between days 21 and 24, at which time the serum beta-subunit human chorionic gonadotropin (hCG) value becomes positive and a decidual reaction occurs throughout the endometrium. The decidua basalis underlies the conceptus, while the decidua capsularis covers its luminal surface. The remainder of the endometrium lining the uterine cavity is the decidua parietalis, which is usually 4 to 10 mm thick. It usually consists of an outer hyperechoic zone and an inner hypoechoic zone (Fig. 121–1), although it may be almost entirely hyperechoic. Vascular flow may be noted in the decidua. A thin hyperechoic line may be seen in the expected location of the uterine cavity where the inner layer of the decidua is in apposition to itself (Fig. 121–1).

The first *specific* diagnostic sonographic finding indicating the presence of an IUP (whether viable or nonviable) is the visualization of the decidua–chorionic sac (i.e., an intrauterine gestational [chorionic] sac that is surrounded in part by the decidua parietalis) between days 32 and 35. The mean serum beta-subunit hCG is approximately 500 to 1500 mIU/ml, depending on the reference standard used, the equipment, and the skill of the sonographer. The gestational sac consists of a uniformly hyperechoic sphere composed of the chorion and chorionic villi, which completely surround the anechoic gestational sac fluid (Fig. 121–1). The chorionic sac is more echogenic than the decidua parietalis, and its hyperechoic wall ranges from 1.5 to 6 mm in thickness between five and seven weeks' gestation.

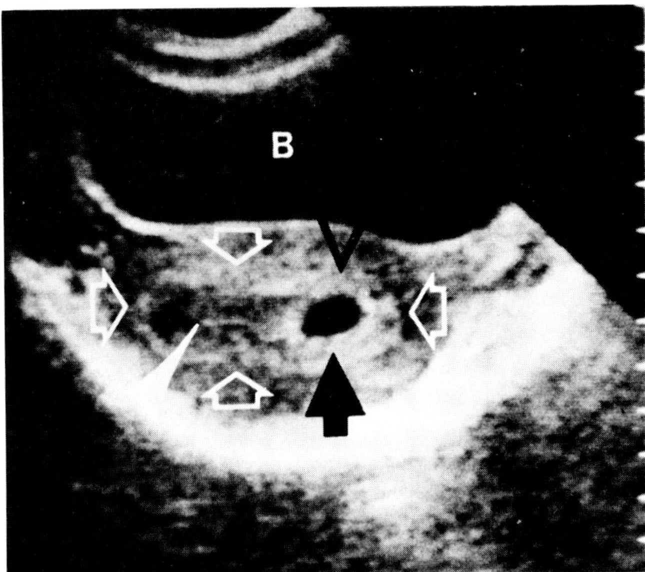

Figure 121–1. Six weeks' gestation with decidua–chorionic ring sign. The decidua *(open white arrows)* surrounds the chorionic ring *(solid black arrow)*. The decidua consists of an outer hyperechoic zone and an inner hypoechoic zone. The uterine cavity line is seen just to the reader's right of the *solid white arrowhead,* while fluid in the uterine cavity (pseudosac) is just to the reader's left of the *solid white arrowhead.* Implantation appears to be at the site of the *open black arrowhead.* (B = urinary bladder.)

By day 38, the decidua–chorionic sac should be easily seen, with a mean sac diameter of 6 to 9 mm. The mean gestational sac fluid diameter (mean sac diameter) is the average of the length, width, and depth on perpendicular sonograms through the largest portion of the gestational sac. The diameters are measured from sac-fluid to fluid-sac interfaces. The secondary yolk sac may be detected as a 2 to 4 mm spherical fluid-filled structure that appears as two parallel linear or curvilinear thin echoes (or a completely circular echo) within the periphery of the gestational sac between days 33 and 38.

At six weeks (day 42), the yolk sac is seen as a 3 to 4 mm circular cystic structure surrounded by a thick hyperechoic wall (Fig. 121–2). Early embryonic cardiac activity may be noted contiguous to the yolk sac, with a mean embryonic heart rate (EHR) of 110 beats per minute, and the mean sac diameter is slightly less than 12 mm (fluid volume of 0.9 ml).

By day 46, the crown-rump length (CRL) is 6 mm, and embryonic cardiac activity should be easily detected. By seven weeks, the CRL is 9 to 10 mm, the mean EHR is 130 beats per minute, and the mean sac diameter is 21 mm. The amnion, if seen, is initially closely applied to the embryo and is thinner and less echogenic than the yolk sac (Fig. 121–2).

EIGHT TO TEN WEEKS

The chorionic villi at the implantation site proliferate and will form the future placenta. This chorion frondosum produces a crescentic, uniformly hyperechoic area along a portion of the gestational sac wall that measures between 7 and 12 mm in thickness (Fig. 121–3). The chorionic villi under the decidua capsularis degenerate and cause this portion of the gestational sac wall to become thin (chorion laeve) (see Fig. 121–3).

By eight weeks, the amnion may be seen as a thin-walled structure surrounding the embryo and amniotic fluid. At normal sensitivity (gain) settings, the amnion may be seen only where it is perpendicular to the sound beam (see Fig. 121–3). By increasing the gain, the entire amnion may be demonstrated (see Fig. 121–2). The chorionic fluid (which may contain some scattered linear low-level echoes) contains the yolk sac and surrounds the amnion. The embryo may show early limb development, and sections through the cranium may demonstrate one or more midline cystic areas due to normal development of the ventricular system (Fig. 121–4).

At nine weeks, the CRL is slightly less than 25 mm, and the mean EHR is 175 beats per minute. By nine weeks, primary ossification of the clavicle, mandible, and maxilla occurs and produces strong echoes within the embryo.

Between nine and 10 weeks, the following should be observed:

1. The embryo is usually C-shaped or slightly flexed (see Fig. 121–3), and the CRL should be measured when the embryo is in this resting position. The embryo has a bipolar appearance, with the head comprising approximately half the CRL. Embryonic movement should be detected.
2. The chorion frondosum is almost always distinguishable from the thinner chorion laeve and surrounding decidua (see Fig. 121–3).
3. The umbilical cord, which is a few millimeters thick and somewhat similar in length to the embryo, should be easily demon-

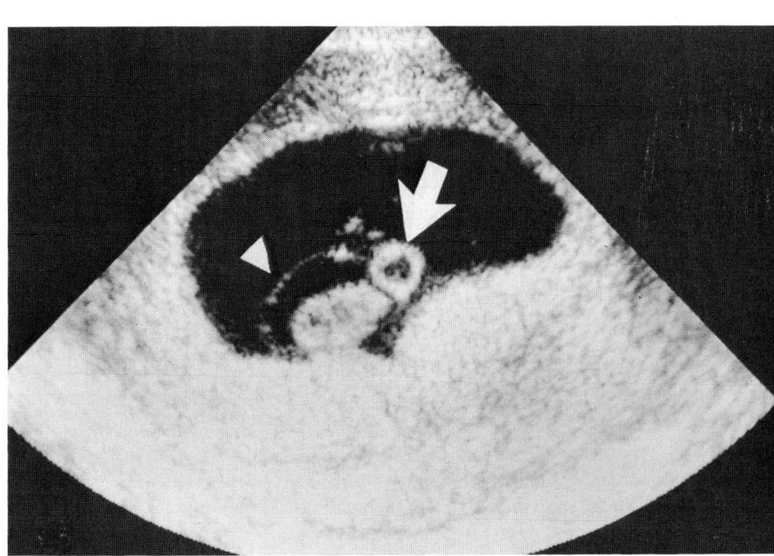

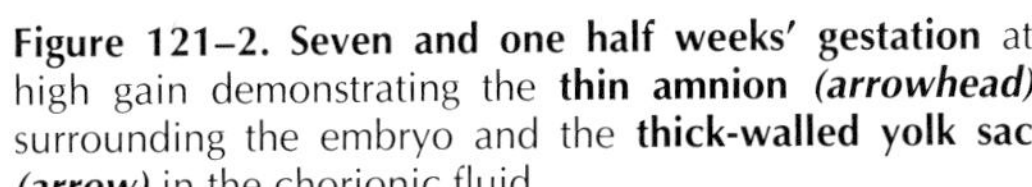
Figure 121–2. Seven and one half weeks' gestation at high gain demonstrating the **thin amnion *(arrowhead)*** surrounding the embryo and the **thick-walled yolk sac *(arrow)*** in the chorionic fluid.

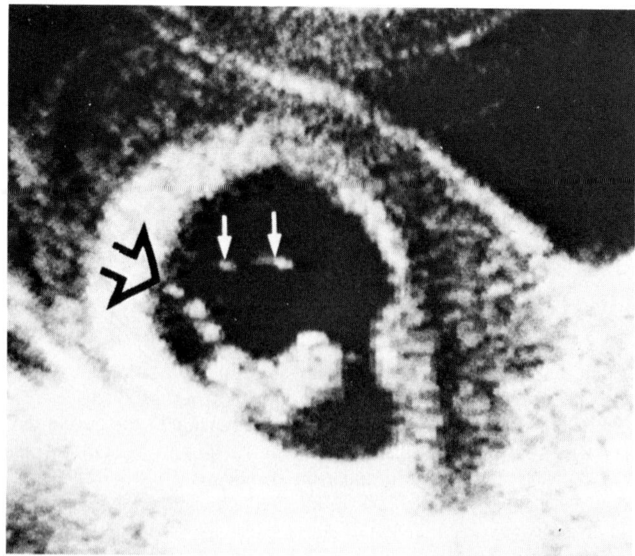

Figure 121–3. Nine weeks' gestation demonstrating the umbilical cord *(open black arrow)* connecting the chorion frondosum (which is surrounding and enclosing the *open black arrow)* to the embryo (note "C" shape). Portions of the amnion *(white arrows)* demarcate the ventral chorionic cavity from the posterior amniotic cavity. The thin chorion laeve is opposite the placental site.

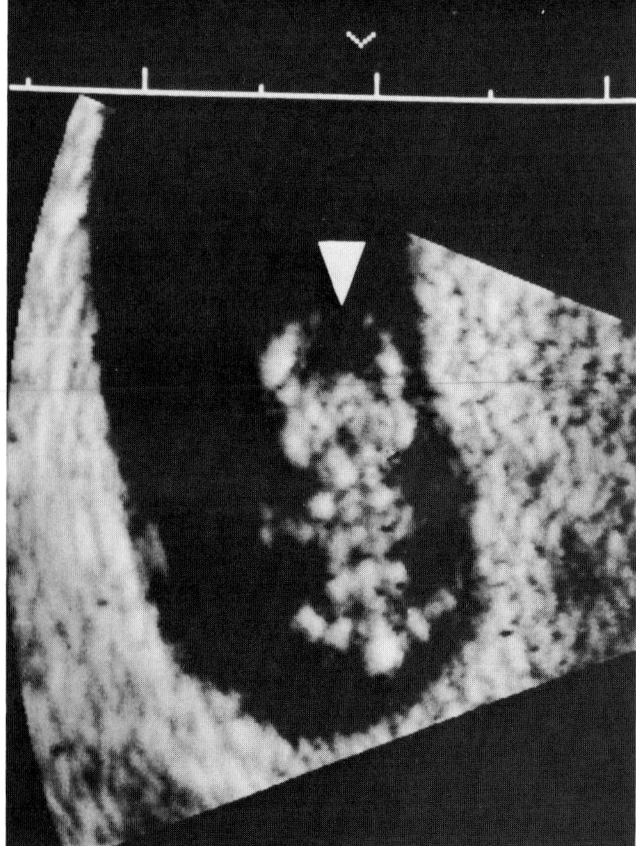

Figure 121–4. Eight weeks' gestation demonstrating a coronal section of the embryo with a **normal intracranial cystic ventricular structure *(arrowhead)*** and **small limb buds** adjacent to the body.

strated when searched for (see Fig. 121–3). There is mild hyperechoic thickening of the cord just before its abdominal insertion due to the normal physiologic hernia of bowel, which disappears by 12 weeks.

4. The falx and echogenic choroid plexus appear, and the yolk sac measures about 5 mm.

At 10 weeks, the gestational sac fills the uterine cavity and the embryonic period is ending, since major organogenesis is complete except for external genitalia. A sonolucent nuchal fold of 3 mm or less is normal.

A small anechoic or complex, predominantly hypoechoic collection of fluid or blood may be seen in the residual endometrial cavity in some IUPs, possibly because of implantation bleeding or the residuum of degenerated chorion laeve (see Fig. 121–1). This pseudosac or crescent, which is contiguous to the gestational sac, can be used to indicate the presence of an IUP (when an embryo is not apparent) and should not be labeled a blighted twin.

ELEVEN TO FOURTEEN WEEKS

There is loss of the gestational sac appearance; however, the placenta is clearly defined and consists of moderately strong homogeneous echoes (Fig. 121–5). The placenta increases in thickness and circumference and covers one third to one half the internal surface of the uterus. Placenta previa can be excluded in some patients when the placental-cervical relationship is clearly defined.

The amnion and chorion become contiguous; however, small pockets of chorionic fluid are usually demonstrable and most commonly persist into the early second trimester.

The fetus demonstrates rapid growth (doubles in length) and there is further differentiation of the organs and tissues. The fetal limbs are easily seen, the spine becomes visible, and the fetal face becomes humanoid in appearance (Fig. 121–6). The appendicular long bones, scapula, ilium, phalanges, and skull bones begin to ossify. The biparietal diameter can be easily measured, and the midline echo should be seen (at 12 weeks the biparietal diameter [BPD] =

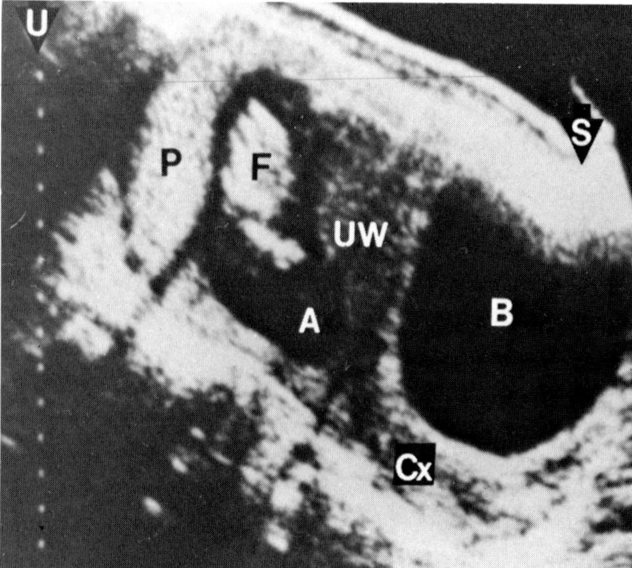

Figure 121–5. Twelve weeks' gestation with fundal placenta (P) and thickened uterine wall (UW) inferiorly. (F = fetus; A = amniotic fluid; Cx = cervix; B = bladder; U = umbilicus; S = symphysis pubis.)

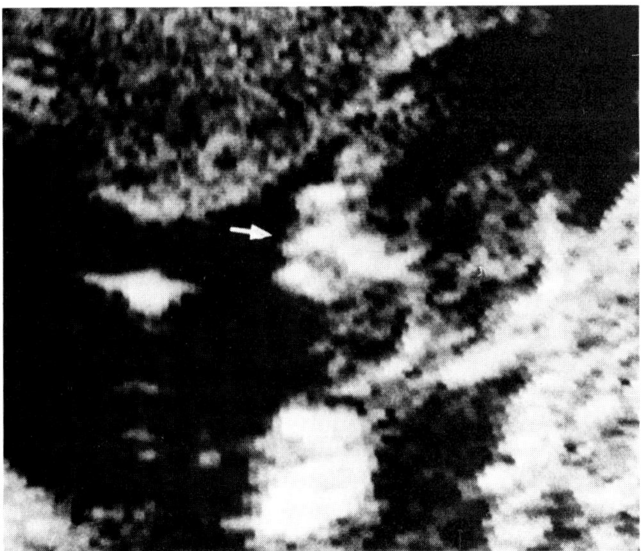

Figure 121–6. Thirteen weeks' gestation demonstrating fetal profile with exquisite detail of face. *Arrow* points to the lips.

19 mm). The external genitalia are fully differentiated between 13 and 14 weeks, at which time the BPD is 28 mm and the mean EHR is 150 beats per minute.

Of interest, the normal gestational sac increases in volume from a mean of 1 ml at six weeks' gestation to 30 ml at 10 weeks' gestation to 100 ml at 13 weeks' gestation.

UTERUS

The myometrium, which consists of uniform medium-strength internal echoes, must entirely surround the pregnancy before a diagnosis of an IUP can be rendered. Myometrial (Braxton-Hicks) contractions may be seen throughout the first trimester as a localized thickening of (see Fig. 121–5), or a rounded mass within, the uterine wall (Fig. 121–7). Their echogenicity is very similar or identical to that of normal myometrium (allowing for relative echo enhancement), and they may persist for as long as 30 minutes. They are usually spontaneous, imperceptible to the patient, and can occur anywhere within the myometrium. The external contour of the uterus remains smooth without distortion; however, the gestational sac or placenta may bulge inward (sometimes markedly) (see Fig. 121–7).

Contractions should not be confused with fibroids that in general are less echogenic, less homogeneous, may have poor sound transmission, may distort the external uterine contour, and are persistent. A bicornuate uterus can be distinguished from a contraction by recognizing a central decidual reaction in the nonpregnant horn.

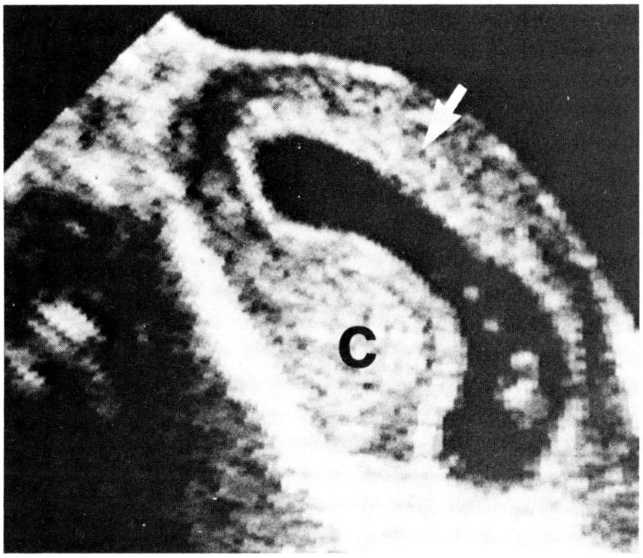

Figure 121–7. Nine weeks' gestation with a posterior contraction (C) indenting the gestational sac. The placenta *(arrow)* is anterior.

MULTIPLE GESTATION

Late division of a fertilized ovum may produce a monochorionic sac that can be diamniotic or monoamniotic. One should search carefully for more than one embryo (in a six- to eight-week size gestational sac) in order not to miss an early multiple pregnancy.

If there appears to be more than one sac, each sac should exhibit the decidua–chorionic sac criteria before a diagnosis of multiple gestation is made, so that a collection of fluid or blood in the endometrial cavity surrounded by decidua (pseudosac) is not labeled a blighted twin.

Obviously, multiple gestation can be correctly diagnosed whenever more than one live fetus is demonstrated.

GESTATIONAL AGE

Gestational age can be estimated in normal IUPs with an accuracy better than ±4 days as follows:

1. Prior to visualization of embryonic cardiac activity with a mean sac diameter (MSD) of less than 15 mm: Gestational age (days) = 30 + MSD (mm) but not to exceed 42 days.
2. From six to nine weeks' gestation: Gestational age (days) = 40 + CRL (mm) when there is normal embryonic cardiac activity.
3. After nine weeks, use the CRL chart by Robinson and Fleming (Table 121–1).

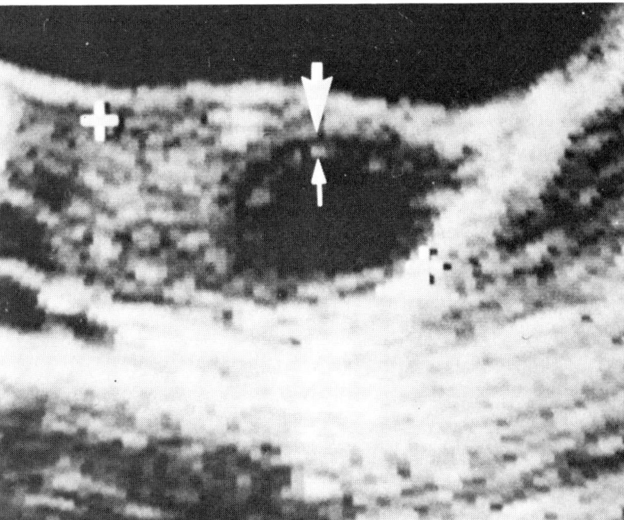

Figure 121–8. Corpus luteum cyst is located in the lateral half of the ovary *(plus sign)*. Note the "halo" between the *arrows* at the outer margin of the cyst and the contiguous normal ovarian parenchyma.

TABLE 121–1. MEAN CROWN-RUMP LENGTH (CRL) AND THE CORRESPONDING GESTATIONAL AGE

Menstrual Maturity (weeks + days)	Mean CRL (mm)*	Menstrual Maturity (weeks + days)	Mean CRL (mm)*
9 + 0	23.5	10 + 4	38.4
9 + 1	25.0	10 + 5	39.9
9 + 2	26.2	10 + 6	41.4
9 + 3	27.4	11 + 0	43.0
9 + 4	28.7	11 + 1	44.6
9 + 5	30.0	11 + 2	46.2
9 + 6	31.3	11 + 3	47.8
10 + 0	32.7	11 + 4	49.5
10 + 1	34.0	11 + 5	51.2
10 + 2	35.5	11 + 6	52.9
10 + 3	36.9	12 + 0	54.7

*CRL values are devised from regression analysis.
From Robinson HP, Fleming JEE: A critical evaluation of sonar crown-rump length measurements. Br J Obstet Gynaecol 82:702, 1975.

The CRL or embryonic length is the longest axis of the embryo or fetus when it is in a normal resting state (i.e., not hyperflexed or hyperextended). Do *not* include the yolk sac, umbilical cord, extremities, or amnion in the CRL measurement. Between 12 and 14 weeks, the biparietal diameter can be used to date pregnancy with an accuracy of ±1 week.

CORPUS LUTEUM CYST

A corpus luteum cyst, which is normal, is commonly identified in the first trimester, and usually regresses by 16 weeks. It is commonly 1 to 3 cm in diameter, but, rarely, may be as large as 8 to 10 cm. The cyst wall is usually thin but can be thick and hyperechoic. The presence of an intraovarian hypoechoic "halo" surrounding the corpus luteum cyst may be noted in many patients (Fig. 121–8). The interior of the cyst may be anechoic, contain low-level echoes due to blood, or it may contain short, scattered, linear echoes, interlacing thin or thick strands, or a nonshadowing soft-tissue mass due to blood clot. Multiple cysts may occur in one or both ovaries in patients who received infertility drugs, and, rarely, with normal intrauterine pregnancies.

Bibliography

Cadkin AV, McAlpin J: The decidua–chorionic sac: A reliable sonographic indicator of intrauterine pregnancy prior to detection of a fetal pole. J Ultrasound Med 3:539–548, 1984.
Moore KL: The Developing Human. Philadelphia, WB Saunders Company, 1982.
Timor-Tritsch IE, Blumenfeld Z, Rottem S: Sonoembryology. In Timor-Tritsch IE, Rottem S (eds): Transvaginal Sonography. New York, Elsevier Science, 1991, pp 225–298.

122 Complications of Early Pregnancy

David A. Nyberg and Faye C. Laing

The growth and development of an intrauterine pregnancy are frequently affected by a variety of disorders, particularly during the first trimester. Complications of early pregnancy include spontaneous or threatened abortion, ectopic pregnancy, hydatidiform degeneration, and concurrent uterine or adnexal masses. Because patients may present with similar signs and symptoms, most commonly pelvic pain, vaginal bleeding, or a palpable mass, pelvic sonography is a valuable adjunct to the clinical examination.

CLINICAL PRESENTATION

Spontaneous abortion is defined as the natural termination of an intrauterine pregnancy prior to 20 gestational weeks. It occurs commonly, affecting about 10 to 20 per cent of observed pregnancies. Many more pregnancies (estimated at 50 per cent) result in subclinical abortion prior to or at the time of implantation. Ultrasound plays no role in the evaluation of these occult abortions. Clinically apparent spontaneous abortions occur most often in the first trimester, particularly before 12 weeks. More than 60 per cent of these early abortuses have chromosomal anomalies. Although the etiology of chromosomally normal abortions is usually unknown, maternal factors that have been implicated include smoking, toxins and drugs, pelvic irradiation, febrile illnesses, and some medical diseases, including diabetes mellitus. Coexisting intrauterine contraceptive devices greatly increase the risk of abortion, intrauterine infections, and premature rupture of membranes. Causative factors of recurrent abortion include hormonal deficiency, immunologic factors, and uterine abnormalities.

The term *threatened abortion* is a clinically descriptive phrase applied to patients during the first 20 weeks of pregnancy who have vaginal bleeding and a closed cervix. Approximately 20 per cent of all pregnant women experience these symptoms in early pregnancy. By definition, the term *threatened abortion* assumes viability of the embryo, although the eventual outcome is uncertain. If all patients with threatened abortion are analyzed, approximately one half have their pregnancies terminate in spontaneous abortion, while the other half have a normal outcome. There is no known effective treatment to ensure a normal outcome.

SONOGRAPHIC FINDINGS

When presented with the clinical problem of threatened abortion, the sonologist must attempt to answer two questions: (1) Is an intrauterine pregnancy (IUP) present? (2) If an IUP is present, is it normal? Much of the information required to answer the first question may be found in Chapters 121 and 123. In this chapter, we address the second question.

TABLE 122–1. DIFFERENTIAL DIAGNOSIS OF SPECIFIC SONOGRAPHIC FINDINGS IN WOMEN WITH A POSITIVE PREGNANCY TEST

Sonographic Finding	Differential Diagnosis
Empty uterus	Normal intrauterine pregnancy (3 to 5 weeks) Recent spontaneous abortion Ectopic pregnancy
Intrauterine debris	Incomplete spontaneous abortion Intrauterine blood Molar pregnancy
Sac, no embryo	Viable intrauterine pregnancy (5 to 6.5 weeks) Nonviable intrauterine pregnancy Pseudogestational sac of ectopic pregnancy
Embryo, no cardiac motion	Nonliving intrauterine pregnancy*
Embryo, cardiac motion	Living intrauterine pregnancy

*Cardiac motion may occasionally be absent for an embryo measuring 4 mm or less. For larger embryos, a potential pitfall is blood clot.

Complete/Incomplete Abortion

Both the terminology and the sonographic findings of nonviable pregnancies vary with the time of the ultrasound relative to the abortion process (Table 122–1). If the abortion is complete, the uterus appears empty and has a relatively thin endometrium. The differential diagnosis for this appearance (assuming a positive pregnancy test) includes an early normal IUP (3 to 5 menstrual weeks) or an ectopic pregnancy. Correlation with the menstrual history and serial human chorionic gonadotropin (hCG) levels will usually reveal the correct diagnosis.

An abortion-in-progress is usually visible as a distorted gestational sac in the lower uterus or cervix. Rescanning a short time later may show continued egress or even complete expulsion of the gestational sac. The typical ultrasound features as well as clinical evaluation usually permit an abortion-in-progress to be distinguished from a cervical ectopic pregnancy.

If the abortion is incomplete, a variable amount of tissue is identified within or adjacent to the endometrium. The gestational sac, if present, appears collapsed and angular. Variable amounts of disorganized echogenic debris and/or fluid are usually present. A thickened endometrium (>5 mm) may be the only clue to retained products. Color flow imaging may be helpful by showing prominent flow in areas of retained trophoblastic tissue. Uterine curettage is indicated when retained gestational tissue is identified or when vaginal bleeding persists.

Living Embryo

Although the individual prognosis varies with embryonic age, maternal age, and the clinical presentation, most women with symptoms of a threatened abortion who show a living embryo on sonography can be counseled that the risk of subsequent abortion is less than 10 to 20 per cent. Mortality rates as high as 20 to 30 per cent have been reported in studies using transvaginal sonography (TVS) among women with vaginal bleeding and a living embryo at six weeks. These differences reflect the facts that most pregnancy losses occur during early pregnancy and TVS can detect cardiac motion at an earlier stage of pregnancy.

TABLE 122–2. SONOGRAPHIC FINDINGS ASSOCIATED WITH A POOR PROGNOSIS IN ASSOCIATION WITH A LIVING EMBRYO (POSITIVE CARDIAC ACTIVITY)

Bradycardia (<90 beats per minute)
Growth retardation
Discrepancy in size of embryo and gestational sac, or first trimester "oligohydramnios"
?Perigestational hemorrhage (a large amount)

Several sonographic factors have been found to be associated with a poor prognosis, even in the presence of a living embryo (Table 122–2). These include embryonic bradycardia (<90 beats per minute), growth delay, and first trimester oligohydramnios. First trimester growth delay, or "growth retardation," may be demonstrated by an unexpectedly small embryo compared with the menstrual history or subnormal growth of the embryo or gestational sac with serial sonograms. First trimester oligohydramnios, seen as a small gestational sac compared with the size of the embryo (Fig. 122–1), frequently accompanies growth delay. The clinical significance of subchorionic hemorrhage, which may be seen in up to 25 per cent of women with symptoms of threatened abortion, is more controversial. Some studies have reported a higher risk of spontaneous abortion when such hemorrhages are identified, whereas other studies have found a greater risk only if the hemorrhage is large. Most small hemorrhages resolve without clinical sequelae unless clinical symptoms persist, in which case the risk of preterm labor may be increased.

Embryonic (Fetal) Demise

*Embryonic demise** (Fig. 122–2) refers to a discrete embryo in which the absence of cardiac activity is clearly documented.

**Embryonic demise* refers to demise occurring at less than 10 weeks; *fetal demise* refers to the absence of cardiac activity in a fetus that is developmentally 10 or more menstrual weeks (eight weeks post-conception).

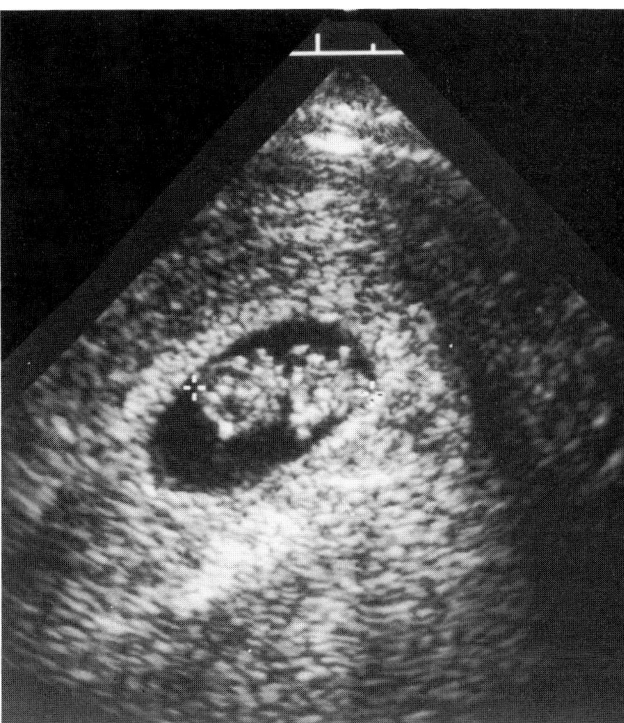

Figure 122–1. First trimester oligohydramnios. Scan at 9 weeks by menstrual history shows a crown-crump length of 1.7 cm, corresponding to 8.1 weeks. The gestational sac (mean diameter, 1.8 cm) is small relative to the size of the embryo. Fetal demise occurred one week later.

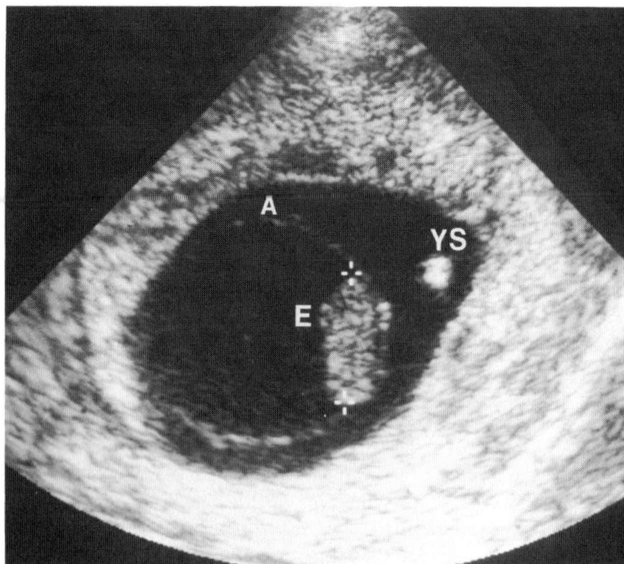

Figure 122–2. Embryonic demise. Transvaginal scan at 11 weeks by menstrual history in a woman with vaginal spotting shows a non-living embryo (E). Note calcified yoke sac (YS). (A = amnion.)

Blighted ovum, or *anembryonic pregnancy* (discussed next), refers to a gestational sac in which the embryo either failed to develop or died at a stage too early to visualize. These terms are preferred over the clinical term *missed abortion*, which does not adequately describe development of the conceptus. Because overlap between the various terms may occur, however, any abnormal condition may also be described as a nonviable, unsuccessful or failed IUP.

Cardiac activity is reliably identified with transabdominal ultrasound after seven weeks' gestation and with TVS after 46 menstrual days (6.5 weeks). When TVS is used, cardiac activity is usually detected as soon as the embryo is large enough to measure. Occasionally, however, cardiac activity cannot be appreciated in very small embryos that measure less than 5 mm in crown-rump length (CRL). For this reason, caution should be exercised when the embryo is small and the gestational sac otherwise appears normal. If cardiac activity is absent and the CRL is 5 mm or longer, embryonic demise can be reliably diagnosed.

Blighted Ovum

A blighted ovum (anembryonic pregnancy) is a gestational sac in which the embryo either failed to develop or died at a very early stage (Figs. 122–3 and 122–4). When the embryo is very small, however, the distinction between blighted ovum and early embryonic demise is often difficult. TVS can clearly detect a nonliving embryo (embryonic demise) in some patients who would be classified as having a blighted ovum on transabdominal sonography alone.

A blighted ovum should be distinguished from a potentially viable gestational sac before 6.5 menstrual weeks, when the embryo is simply too small to resolve. In patients with threatened abortion who subsequently are diagnosed as having a nonviable pregnancy, the menstrual history usually exceeds embryologic development by several weeks. Because the menstrual history is often unreliable or uncertain, however, it is preferable to use other independent criteria for distinguishing normal from abnormal gestations. Sonographic criteria that are useful for diagnosing blighted ova include a large "empty" sac with the absence of a living embryo, the absence of a normal yolk sac, a thickened and expanded amnion, an enlarged yolk sac, and an abnormal choriodecidual reaction (Table 122–3). It may be difficult to distinguish an expanded amnion from an enlarged yolk sac when only one membrane is identified. However, in the absence of a living embryo, either finding indicates a nonviable gestation.

Treatment

Uterine curettage is usually recommended when sonography demonstrates embryonic demise, blighted ovum, or incomplete spontaneous abortion. Although most women eventually abort, delay in treatment can cause prolonged bleeding, infection, unnecessary psychologic stress, and medical expense. The presence of retained gestational products also represents an obstacle to successful implantation of subsequent pregnancies. In women with clinical symptoms and ultrasound findings consistent with a recent complete spontaneous abortion, the need for uterine curettage may be obviated. However, uterine curettage is indicated if vaginal bleeding is persistent despite the negative ultrasound findings.

If there is any doubt regarding the potential viability of a particular pregnancy, it can be resolved with serial sonography and/or hCG levels. A normal gestational sac grows approximately 1 mm per day (range, 0.71 to 1.75 mm per day). Embryonic growth is also approximately 1 mm in length per day. HCG levels should double every two to three days during early pregnancy.

PELVIC MASSES

Pelvic masses discovered during pregnancy are a unique diagnostic and therapeutic challenge. Because clinical evaluation may be difficult, sonographic examination is often invaluable in order to confirm the presence of a mass and to determine its size and echo texture. In general, as the uterus enlarges and distorts normal anatomic relationships, pelvic masses become more difficult to detect both clinically and sonographically. Similar to evaluation in a nongravid patient, sonographic assessment of a pelvic mass should attempt to characterize it as cystic, solid, or complex and to determine whether its origin is uterine or adnexal. Serial sonography can be useful for determining growth or regression of a mass. If possi-

TABLE 122–3. SONOGRAPHIC FINDINGS ASSOCIATED WITH FAILED INTRAUTERINE PREGNANCIES

Embryo
Absence of cardiac motion in embryos 5 mm or larger
Absence of cardiac motion after 6.5 menstrual weeks
Yolk sac
Large yolk sac (or amnion) without a visible embryo
Calcified yolk sac
Large gestational sac
> 18 mm lacking a living embryo
> 10 mm lacking a visible yolk sac
Shape
Irregular or bizarre
Position
Low
Trophoblastic reaction
Irregular
Absent double decidual sac finding
Thin trophoblastic reaction (≤2 mm)
Intratrophoblastic venous flow
Growth
Gestational sac growth of ≤0.6 mm/day
Absent embryonic growth
Human chorionic gonadotropin (hCG) correlation
Discrepancy between sac size and hCG level

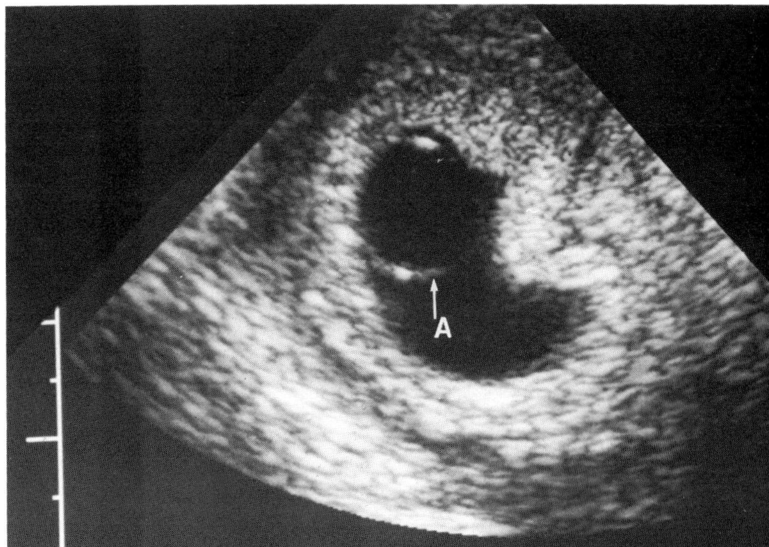

Figure 122–3. Blighted ovum. Transvaginal scan at 10 weeks by menstrual history shows an abnormal shape of the gestational sac. An expanded amnion (A) is identified within the gestational sac. No embryo was present. Note that it may be difficult to distinguish an enlarged yolk sac from an expanded amnion.

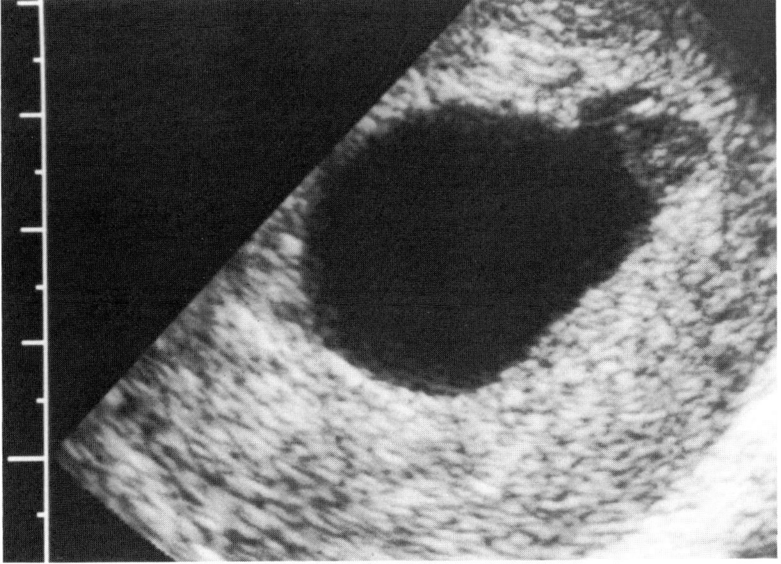

Figure 122–4. Blighted ovum. Transvaginal scan at 11 weeks by menstrual history shows an abnormal gestational sac. Note enlarged gestational sac (mean diameter, 2.5 cm); poor choriodecidual reaction; abnormal sac shape; and absence of embryo, yolk sac, or amnion.

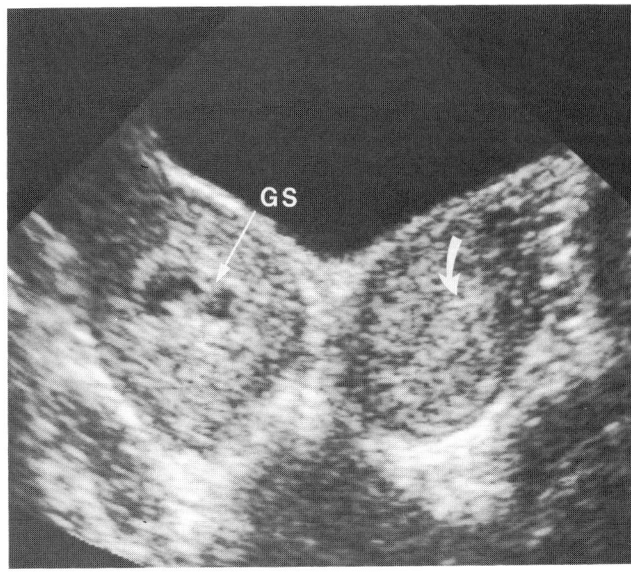

Figure 122–5. A transverse scan of a **bicornuate uterus** demonstrates a gestational sac (GS) in the right uterine horn and a decidual reaction in the left horn (*curved arrow*).

ble, pelvic masses should be managed conservatively during pregnancy, especially during the first and third trimesters, when, respectively, the threat of a spontaneous abortion and premature labor is the greatest. Masses less than 5 cm in diameter that are not enlarging are usually observed.

Functional corpus luteum cysts are by far the most common adnexal "masses" associated with pregnancy during the first and second trimesters. The symptomatic corpus luteum cyst is also a common cause of pelvic pain in women with a living embryo/fetus during the first and second trimester. Although corpus luteum cysts are generally less than 4 cm in diameter, they can become much larger. They usually resolve by 16 weeks but can occasionally persist to the third trimester. The sonographic appearance of a corpus luteum cyst is variable. The outer wall is typically smooth and thin. Internal echoes and linear strands may be seen within the cyst from hemorrhage.

Persistence or enlargement of a cystic mass after 20 weeks should suggest other possibilities, including a cystic neoplasm; paraovarian cyst; endometrioma; or degenerated, pedunculated fibroid. Ovarian cystadenoma and benign cystic teratoma (dermoid) are the most common tumors found among these patients.

Uterine leiomyomata (fibroids) are the most common solid pelvic mass associated with pregnancy. These benign tumors may enlarge dramatically during pregnancy as the result of estrogen stimulation. The most rapid growth of fibroids usually occurs during the first half of pregnancy. Although fibroids are usually asymptomatic, they may be associated with an increased risk of spontaneous abortion and placental abruption and may cause clinical symptoms on the basis of size, degeneration, and/or hemorrhage. Fibroids occupying the lower pelvis may also obstruct vaginal delivery.

Uterine fibroids typically appear as heterogeneous, hypoechoic masses that produce acoustic attenuation. Calcification, hemorrhage, or infarction may alter this appearance. Fibroids should be distinguished from focal uterine contractions, which are typically less discrete, do not produce acoustic attenuation, and are associated with thickening of the myometrium. However, distinguishing fibroids from focal uterine contractions occasionally may be difficult. A follow-up or delayed scan will resolve this dilemma, since focal contractions typically resolve within 30 to 60 minutes.

Occasionally, a congenital uterine anomaly can be taken for a pelvic mass. The most common anomaly to present in this manner is a bicornuate or didelphys uterus, which is due to failure of fusion of the müllerian ducts. During the first trimester, ultrasound can suggest the presence of a uterine duplication (Fig. 122–5). Typically, the gestational sac is seen in one horn and decidual reaction in the second horn. As the gravid uterine horn enlarges with advancing gestational age, the nongravid horn may be difficult if not impossible to visualize.

CONCLUSION

Ultrasound has an essential role in the evaluation of patients during the first trimester to determine whether the pregnancy is progressing normally. Visualization of a living embryo carries a good prognosis that usually results in the birth of a normal infant. On the other hand, demonstration of an abnormal or nonviable pregnancy can initiate appropriate management.

Bibliography

Bromley B, Harlow BL, Laboda LA, Benacerraf BR: Small sac size in the first trimester: A predictor of poor fetal outcome. Radiology 178:375–377, 1991.

Horrow MM: Enlarged amniotic cavity: A new sonographic sign of early embryonic death. AJR 158:359–362, 1992.

Levi CS, Lyons EA, Lindsay DJ: Early diagnosis of nonviable pregnancy with endovaginal US. Radiology 167:383–385, 1988.

Levi CS, Lyons EA, Zheng XH, et al: Endovaginal US: Demonstration of cardiac activity in embryos of less than 5.0 mm in crown-rump length. Radiology 176:71–74, 1990.

Lindsay DJ, Lovett IS, Lyons EA, et al: Yolk sac diameter and shape at endovaginal US: Predictors of pregnancy outcome in the first trimester. Radiology 183:115–118, 1992.

Nyberg DA, Laing FC: Threatened abortion and abnormal intrauterine pregnancy. In Nyberg DA, Hill LM, Bohm-Velez M, Mendelsohn E (eds): Transvaginal Sonography. Chicago, Year Book Publishers, 1992, pp 85–103.

123 The Diagnosis of Ectopic Pregnancy

Faye C. Laing

In the past 20 years, improvements in medicine have helped to conquer or ameliorate the ravages of many morbid physical conditions. Unfortunately for many, ectopic pregnancy is not one of those conditions. Instead, its incidence appears to be increasing, the diagnosis is more often missed than made by the initial examining physician, and it is responsible for 3 to 7 per cent of maternal deaths. Early detection of ectopic pregnancy is hampered because clinical findings are nonspecific and because, until recently, no specific tests or imaging techniques for suggesting the correct diagnosis have been available.

The past decade has witnessed the introduction, development, and dissemination of two diagnostic aids that can lead to earlier detection of ectopic pregnancy. These include highly sensitive and specific pregnancy tests, and high-resolution, real-time ultrasonography. The recent addition of vaginal probes as well as spectral and color Doppler has greatly improved ultrasound's ability to detect ectopic pregnancy.

In this chapter the role of ultrasonography in making the diagnosis of ectopic pregnancy is discussed and its relationship to the newer pregnancy tests is considered. The appropriate use of laboratory tests and ultrasonography may allow earlier detection of ectopic pregnancy, which in turn may lead to a diminution in the role of maternal morbidity and mortality.

CLINICAL CONSIDERATIONS

A rather dramatic global variation exists regarding the incidence of ectopic pregnancy. At one extreme are the statistics in Kingston, Jamaica, where one ectopic pregnancy occurs for every 28 deliveries; at the other end of the spectrum are the figures from the midwestern United States, where one ectopic pregnancy occurs for every 280 deliveries. Most often its frequency is reported to be between 0.5 and 1 per cent of all pregnancies.

The occurrence of ectopic implantation is closely related to the prevalence of salpingitis. Indeed, up to 50 per cent of patients with ectopic pregnancy have either a history of or pathologic evidence for pelvic inflammatory disease. Although tubal damage most often results from primary infection, it can also occur after nongynecologic pelvic inflammation, such as appendicitis, and it can result from tubal surgery for reconstructive purposes or for an antecedent ectopic gestation.

In patients with an ectopic pregnancy, the migration of the fertilized ovum into the uterus is delayed or prevented. Instead, as occurs in 95 per cent of patients with ectopic pregnancy, the implantation is within a fallopian tube, particularly the ampullary (most common) or isthmic (second most common) portion. Interstitial implantations are unusual (3 to 4 per cent of ectopic pregnancies) but are the most serious owing to delayed rupture with associated massive hemorrhage. In up to one third of cases, transmigration of the ovum occurs, with implantation in the contralateral tube. This can cause a confusing clinical picture, with a corpus luteum cyst palpated on the side opposite the acute symptoms.

The classic clinical triad for ectopic pregnancy typically develops three to five weeks after a missed menstrual period and consists of pain, irregular vaginal bleeding, and an adnexal mass. Because the pain is so varied in intensity, duration, and location, it is frequently attributed to other organ systems. Tubal rupture, which occurs in 80 to 90 per cent of patients, is heralded by a sudden dramatic exacerbation of pain. Amenorrhea and irregular vaginal bleeding are present approximately 70 per cent of the time and are usually attributed to hormonal fluctuations. An adnexal mass is palpated approximately 40 per cent of the time.

A major problem is that the classic triad is totally nonspecific. In fact, only 10 to 15 per cent of patients with the triad have an ectopic pregnancy. Most patients with these clinical findings are not even pregnant and have pelvic inflammatory disease, a ruptured ovarian cyst, or pain of unknown etiology. Furthermore, of patients with ectopic pregnancy, fewer than 50 per cent have the classic triad. It is obvious, therefore, that clinical evaluation of these patients plays a very limited role.

DIAGNOSTIC CONSIDERATIONS

Traditional diagnostic evaluation consists of a urine pregnancy test and/or culdocentesis. Recently, more accurate pregnancy tests, ultrasonography, and laparoscopy have been added to the diagnostic armamentarium.

Pregnancy Tests

All pregnancy tests are based on detecting human chorionic gonadotropin (hCG) in either urine or serum. Analysis of the molecular configuration of this glycoprotein has revealed it to consist of an alpha and a beta chain. Although the beta chain is unique to this molecule, the alpha chain is very similar in configuration to that of other hormones, including luteinizing hormone, follicle-stimulating hormone, and thyroid-stimulating hormone. HCG is normally elaborated by trophoblastic tissue beginning eight days after conception. Its concentration roughly doubles every two days, and it peaks at a level of 100,000 mIU/ml during the sixth week after conception.

Since the introduction of an antiserum specific for the beta chain in 1972, there has been progressive development of highly sensitive and specific serum radioimmunoassay (RIA) pregnancy tests, which can detect HCG concentrations as low as 1 mIU/ml serum. The advantages of RIA tests over previously used immunologic pregnancy tests include the fact that (1) they are specific for HCG, (2) they can detect the low levels of hCG present in patients with ectopic pregnancy, (3) a negative test excludes a gestational event, and (4) quantitative levels have specific clinical implications.

Ultrasonography

Because of ultrasound's ability to image the uterus and adnexa noninvasively, it has assumed a leading role in the evaluation of patients who are suspected of ectopic pregnancy. A wide spectrum of ultrasonographic findings can be observed in these patients. Visualization of a living ectopic pregnancy, ectopic fetal head, or ectopic gestational sac is relatively unusual, occurring in perhaps 10 per cent of cases when an abdominal approach is used. Because of improved resolution, vaginal transducers can detect a living ectopic pregnancy 21 to 28 per cent of the time (Fig. 123–1). A completely normal examination in which the uterus contains a normal central cavity echo, the adnexa lack masses, and free intra-abdominal fluid is absent occurs in approximately 20 per cent of cases when an abdominal approach is used and in approximately 0 to 8 per cent of cases when a vaginal approach is used.

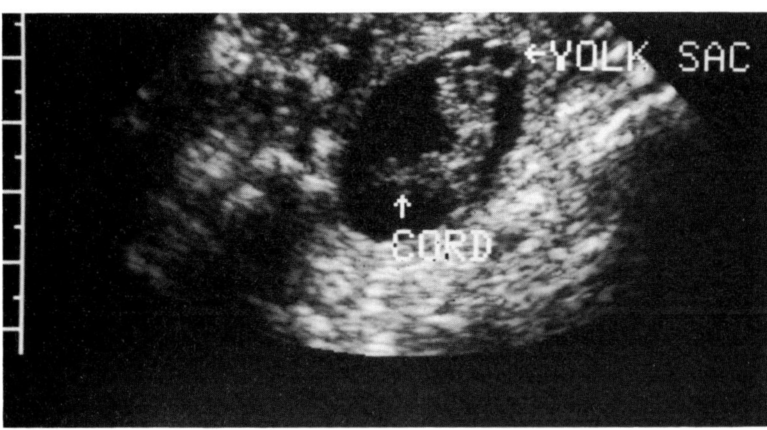

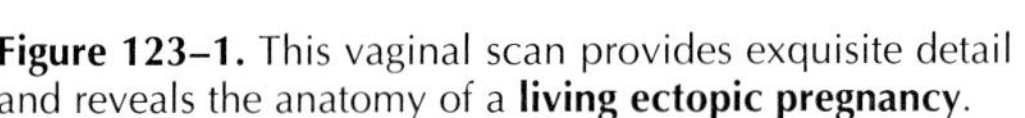
Figure 123–1. This vaginal scan provides exquisite detail and reveals the anatomy of a **living ectopic pregnancy**.

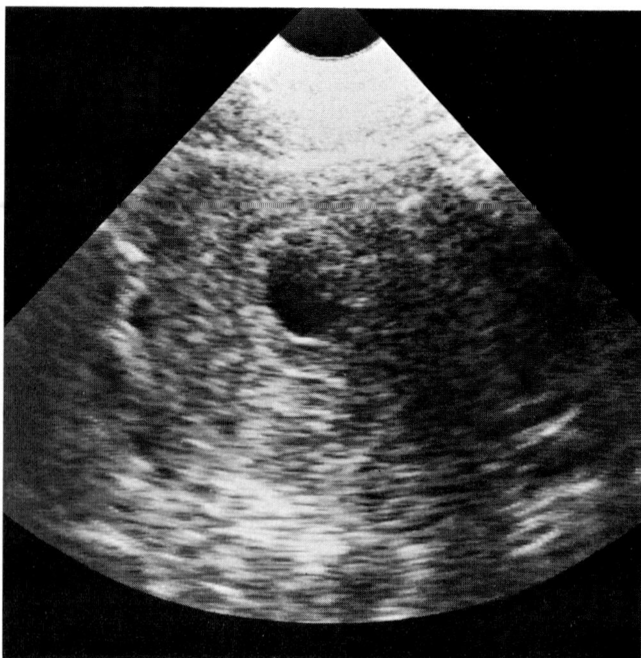

Figure 123–2. An **intrauterine fluid collection** is seen with surrounding decidual changes. This was due to a blighted ovum.

In ideal circumstances, a serum RIA test is obtained before ordering untrasonography. If the test result is negative, a gestational event, either intrauterine or extrauterine, is excluded. If the test is positive, ultrasonography should be performed in an effort to determine the location of the pregnancy. The most common observation is a normal intrauterine pregnancy, which statistically excludes an ectopic pregnancy. Because ultrasonography effectively excludes an ectopic pregnancy by identifying an intrauterine gestation, its major purpose should be evaluation of the uterine contents.

Uterine Changes

If fetal movements are visible within an intrauterine gestational sac, the probability of a concomitant extrauterine pregnancy is one in 15,000 to 30,000 pregnancies. If an intrauterine fluid collection is detected but no fetal pole is seen, three diagnostic possibilities exist. First, an abnormal intrauterine pregnancy may be present, in which case the fluid is due to a blighted ovum (Fig. 123–2). Second, an ectopic pregnancy may be present with an associated decidual cast (Fig. 123–3). Although decidual changes are visible in 50 per cent of patients with ectopic pregnancy, pseudogestational sacs occur in only 20 per cent of patients with ectopic pregnancy. Third, the intrauterine fluid collection may be due to a normal early intrauterine pregnancy, before visualization of the fetus.

Endovaginal imaging is very useful for differentiating a pseudogestational sac of an ectopic pregnancy from an early normal intrauterine pregnancy (when the fetal pole is not yet visible). A normal gestational sac that is only 3 to 4 mm in diameter can be differentiated from a pseudogestational sac by noting that the products of conception are normally within the decidualized endometrium, whereas a pseudosac is located within the uterine cavity (Fig. 123–4). Slightly later in pregnancy two closely spaced concentric lines become visible around a portion of the normal gestational sac (but are not present around a pseudogestational sac, Fig. 123–5). This "double decidual sac" finding can be observed when the mean gestational sac diameter is 1 cm or more. Gestational morphology indicates that the double lines detected by ultrasonography represent the decidua parietalis (decidua vera) and adjacent decidua capsularis (see Chapter 121). In comparison, the pseudogestational sac of ectopic pregnancy is composed of a single decidual layer and appears as a single echogenic ring.

The final uterine appearance that can be seen in patients at risk for ectopic pregnancy is a normal to slightly enlarged uterus with a

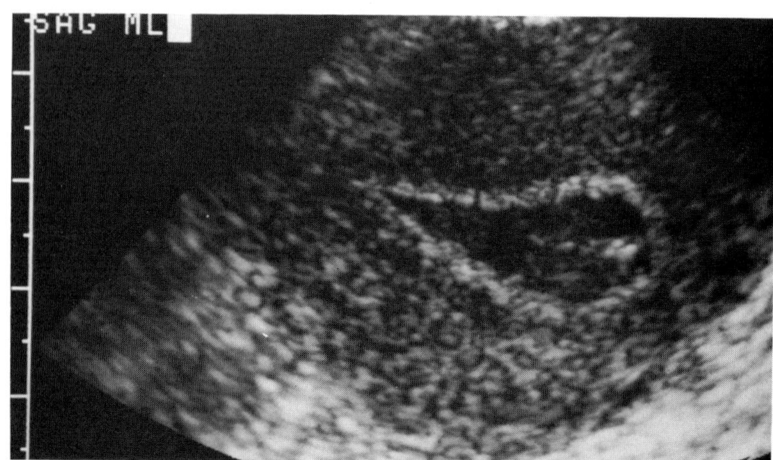

Figure 123–3. This **intrauterine fluid collection** is due to a decidual cast associated with an ectopic pregnancy.

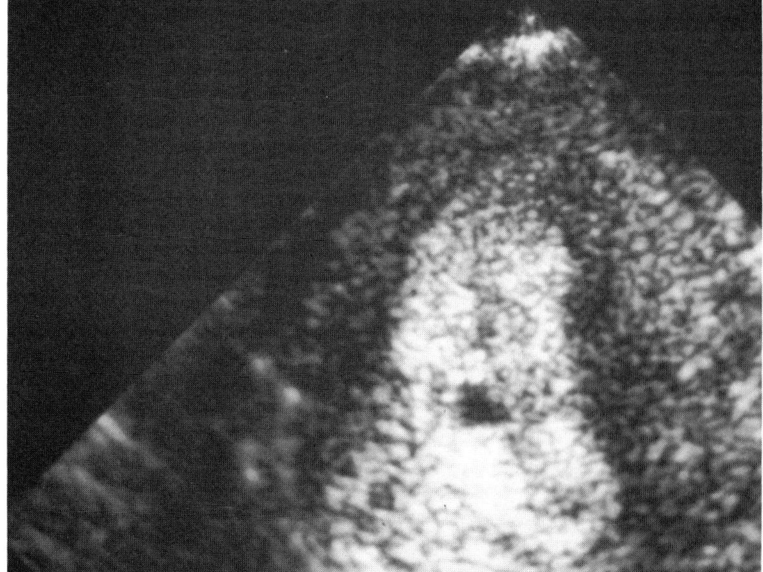

Figure 123–4. This vaginal scan demonstrates the **intradecidual location of an early normal intrauterine pregnancy**. Note that it is located next to the uterine cavity. (From Laing FC: Abnormal first-trimester pregnancy. In Rifkin MD, Charboneau JW, Laing FC (eds): Syllabus special course: Ultrasound 1991. Oak Brook, IL, RSNA Publications, 1991, pp 93–102.)

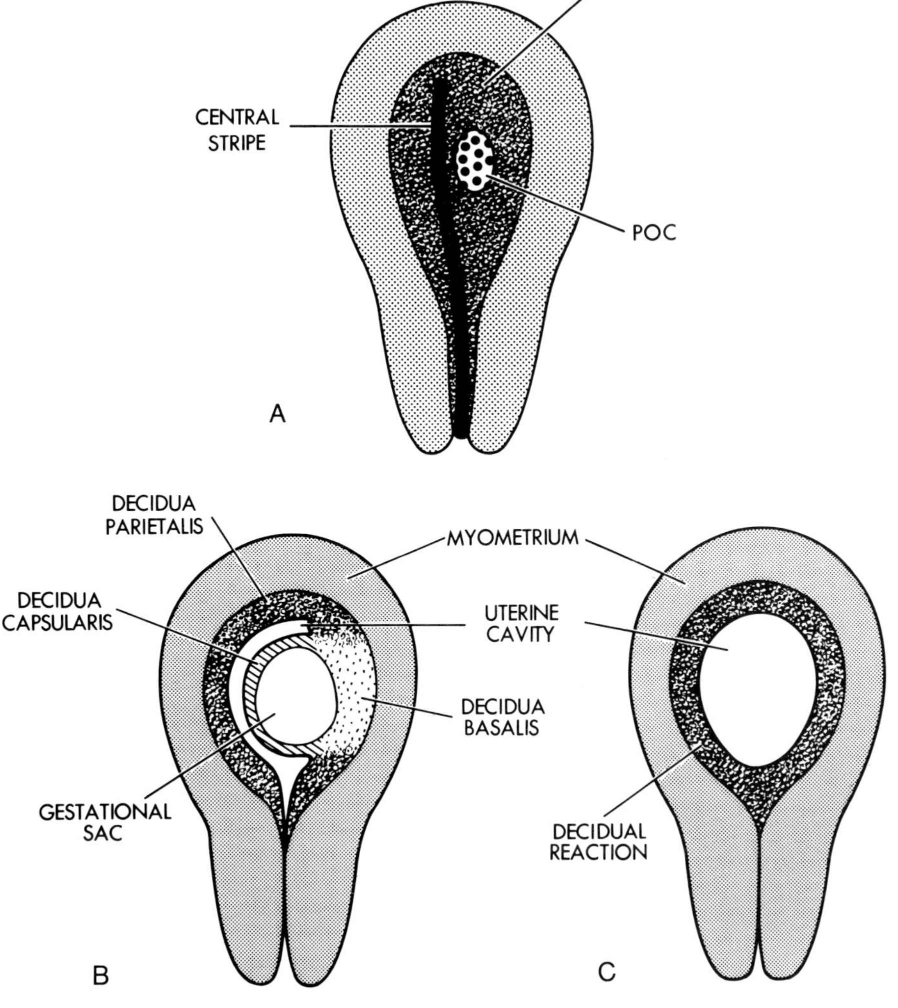

Figure 123–5. *A*, **Uterine appearance of a very early intrauterine pregnancy**, as seen on a vaginal scan. Note that the sac is located within the decidual reaction and is not in the uterine cavity. (*A* from Laing FC: Abnormal first-trimester pregnancy. In Rifkin MD, Charboneau JW, Laing FC (eds): Syllabus special course: Ultrasound 1991. Oak Brook, IL, RSNA Publications, 1991, pp 93–102.) *B*, Early intrauterine pregnancy, as seen on a transabdominal scan. It demonstrates the closely apposed decidua capsularis and the decidua parietalis, which account for the double decidual sac sign and allow the diagnosis of an intrauterine pregnancy to be made. *C*, Depiction of a pseudogestational sac of ectopic pregnancy. High-amplitude echoes may be seen surrounding an intrauterine fluid collection due to a decidual reaction. (*B* and *C* from Nyberg DA, Laing FC, Filly RA, et al: Ultrasonographic differentiation of the gestational sac of early intrauterine pregnancy from the pseudogestational sac of ectopic pregnancy. Radiology 146:755–759, 1983, with permission.)

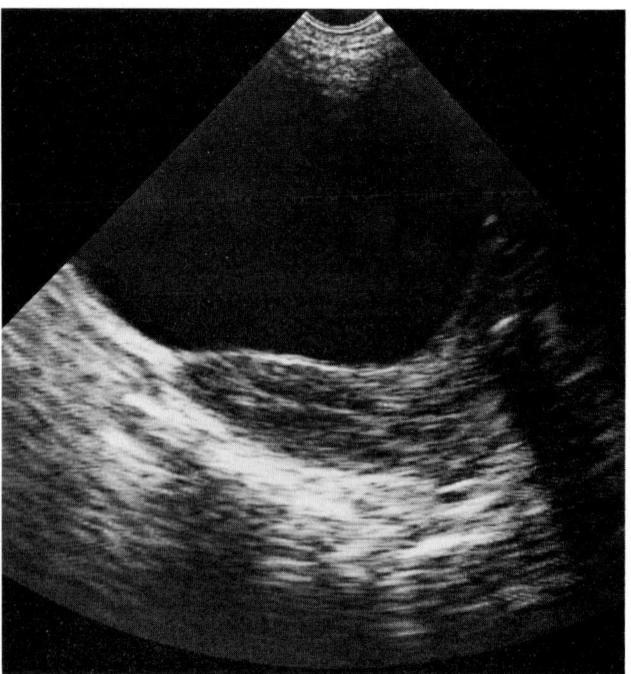

Figure 123–6. A **normal central cavity echo** is seen in the uterus of this patient who was found to have an ectopic pregnancy.

normal central cavity echo (Fig. 123–6). In patients whose pregnancy test is positive, the diagnostic possibilities include (1) a very early intrauterine pregnancy, (2) a recent abortion, and (3) an ectopic pregnancy. A normal central cavity echo occurs in approximately 50 per cent of patients with ectopic pregnancy.

If the RIA pregnancy test is positive and the uterus lacks an intradecidual implantation site or a "double decidual sac" finding, the patient should be considered at risk for ectopic pregnancy. If the patient does not desire her pregnancy, uterine evacuation should be performed and the presence or absence of chorionic villi should be noted. If chorionic villi are present, an intrauterine pregnancy has occurred. If chorionic villi are absent, serial hCG determinations may help to distinguish an ectopic pregnancy from a recent abortion. In patients who desire their pregnancy, the clinical status should determine whether serial tests (pregnancy test and/or ultrasound) should be performed or urgent laparoscopy is required.

Adnexal Changes

Because nonpregnant patients, those with intrauterine gestations, and those with ectopic pregnancies frequently have adnexal masses, it is often difficult to assess the clinical significance of these masses. Although visualizing an extrauterine living fetus is specific for ectopic pregnancy, this finding is unusual (see Fig. 123–1). It is important to correlate the presence of an adnexal mass with the uterine appearance, the clinical examination, and the result of the RIA pregnancy test. Vaginal transducers and Doppler ultrasound are greatly improving the ability to evaluate the adnexa. In an effort to detect an ectopic pregnancy, it is important to look for a dilated fallopian tube, complex mass, and/or gestational sac that is separate from the ovary (Fig. 123–7). Vaginal transducers can visualize an adnexal ring in approximately 65 to 76 per cent of cases and an extrauterine embryo or yolk sac in up to one third of cases. Color and pulsed Doppler evaluation are also proving useful by localizing ectopic trophoblastic tissue, with its characteristic low-resistance, high-velocity arterial flow pattern (Fig. 123–8).

Cul-de-Sac Changes

Although small quantities of cul-de-sac fluid can be seen with vaginal probes in up to 31 per cent of patients with intrauterine pregnancies, the presence of cul-de-sac fluid in a patient who is clinically and sonographically in the at-risk category suggests that an ectopic pregnancy is present and it is either leaking or rupturing. Like adnexal masses, however, cul-de-sac fluid in and of itself is nonspecific and must be interpreted in light of the clinical findings, the result of an RIA pregnancy test, and the appearance of the uterus. Occasionally, a patient with an intrauterine pregnancy may have cul-de-sac fluid as a result of a ruptured or hemorrhagic corpus luteum cyst, or it may be due to a concurrent inflammatory process. If cul-de-sac fluid is visualized shortly after a culdocentesis has been performed, it may have been iatrogenically introduced.

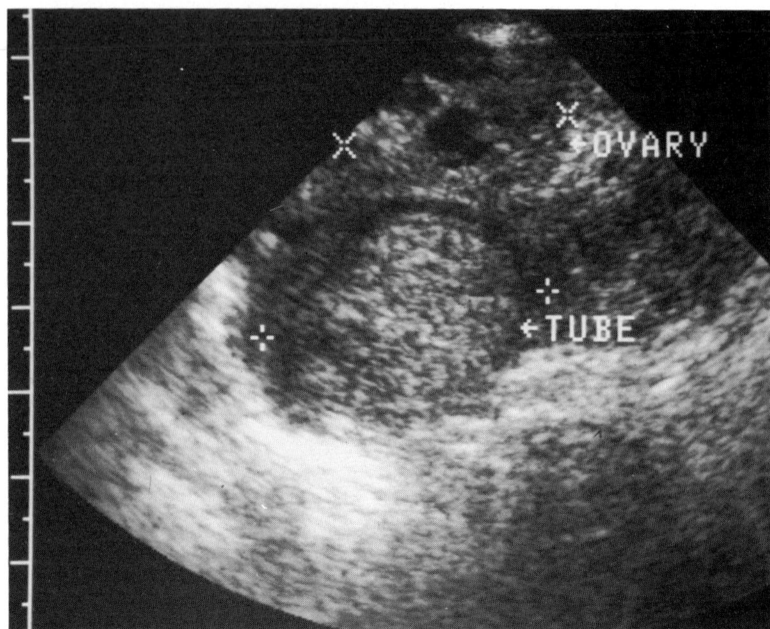

Figure 123–7. This patient has an **ectopic pregnancy**. The vaginal scan reveals a rounded echogenic mass that is due to a dilated fallopian tube (cut in cross-section) that contains echogenic blood. Note that the mass is located adjacent to a normal-appearing ovary.

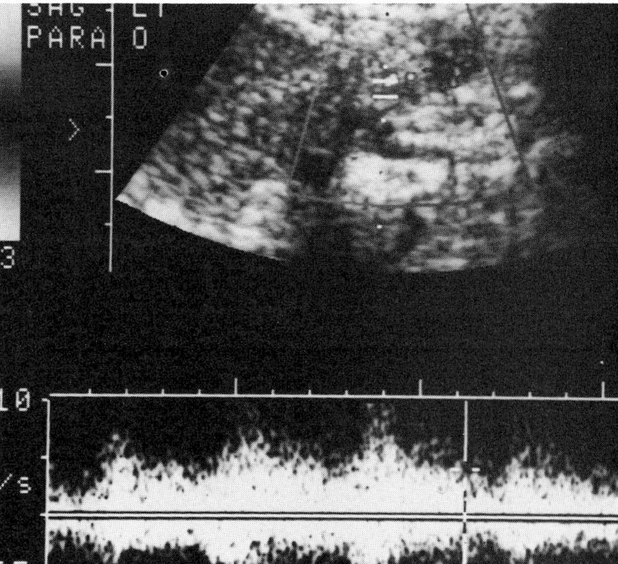

Figure 123–8. This vaginal ultrasound examination revealed a para-ovarian echogenic mass. The pulsed Doppler signal revealed a characteristic low-resistance, high-velocity arterial flow pattern, indicative of ectopic trophoblastic tissue.

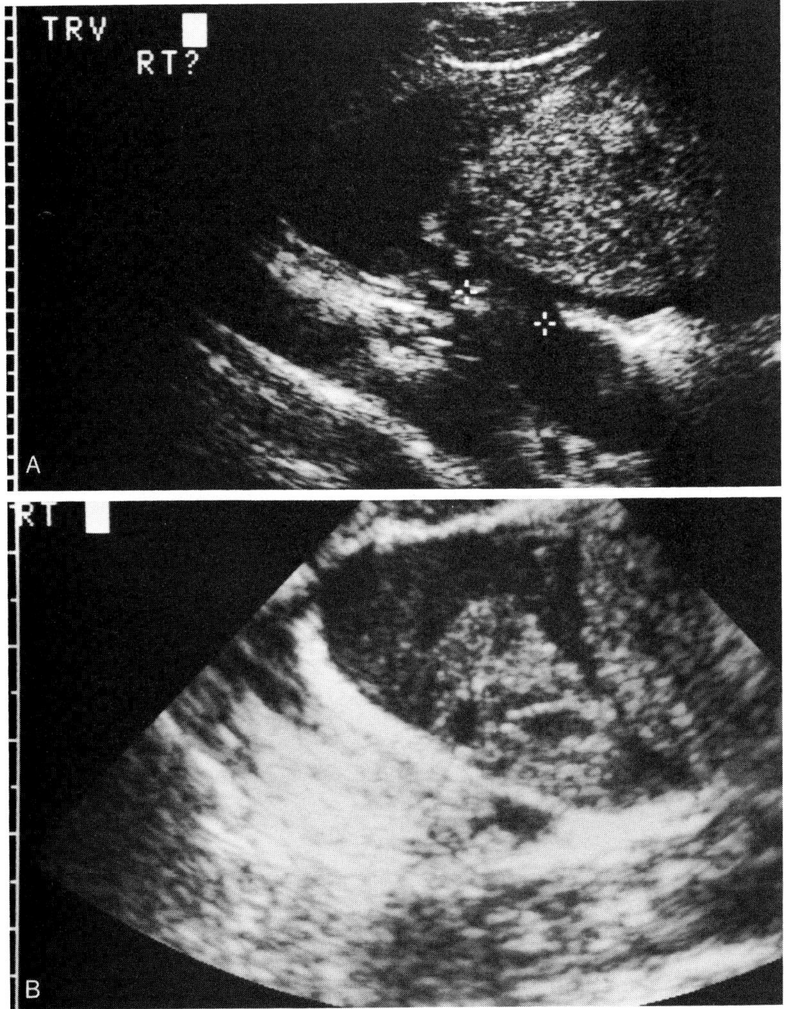

Figure 123–9. *A*, This transverse scan of the right adnexal region was obtained using a transabdominal approach. **Echo-free fluid** is visible adjacent to the right ovary (between gradicule markers). *B*, A vaginal scan of the same patient reveals that the **fluid is echogenic**. In a patient with a positive pregnancy test and no evidence for an intrauterine pregnancy, this appearance is highly suggestive of a hemoperitoneum.

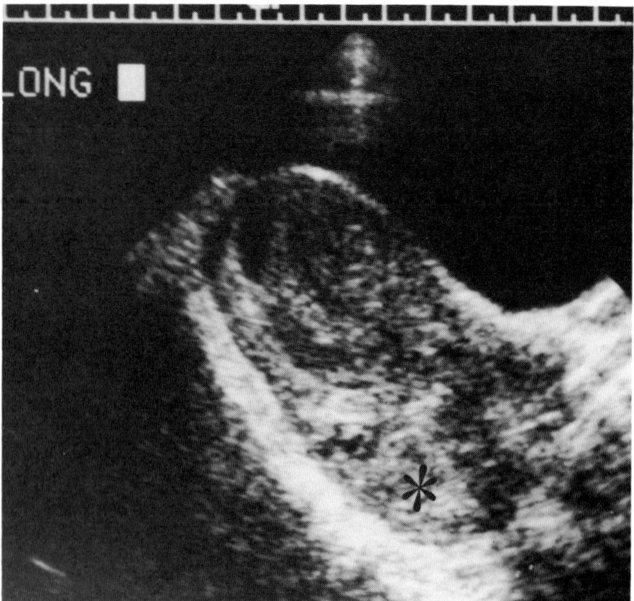

Figure 123–10. A sagittally oriented transabdominal scan reveals **intensely echogenic clot in the cul-de-sac** (*asterisk*).

Technical factors are important for detecting small collections of cul-de-sac fluid. If the urinary bladder is overdistended, the fluid can be displaced out of the cul-de-sac and be totally invisible, or it may appear as a characteristic triangular fluid configuration adjacent to the uterine fundus. In a patient suspected of ectopic pregnancy, it is best to rescan the pelvis after the patient voids and to use a vaginal transducer. In addition to examining the cul-de-sac, one should also use an abdominal approach and scan the paracolic gutters and right subhepatic space (Morison's pouch) in an effort to uncover free intra-abdominal fluid.

The typical ultrasound appearance for hemoperitoneum is fluid that contains varying amounts of particulate echogenic material. Although this finding may be subtle, endovaginal scanning makes it easier to detect (Fig. 123–9). Echogenic fluid occurs in about 56 per cent of patients with ectopic pregnancy and has a positive predictive value for diagnosing hemoperitoneum of 93 per cent. Clot is frequently intensely echogenic and has been shown to have the same or greater echo intensity as uterine myometrial echoes in 60 per cent of cases (Fig. 123–10). This appearance can be mistaken for a solid, echogenic mass.

ULTRASONOGRAPHY VIS-A-VIS BETA–HUMAN CHORIONIC GONADOTROPIN PREGNANCY TESTS

The necessity of obtaining both the pregnancy test and ultrasound examination is frequently questioned. Whether both studies are required depends to some degree on individual philosophy, but more on the clinical condition of the patient. For example, if a patient arrives in the emergency department in a state of hypovolemic shock, the most expeditious route is to perform a culdocentesis, which, if positive, necessitates urgent laparotomy. Neither a pregnancy test nor ultrasonography is warranted.

If the patient's clinical condition is semiacute and she has a suspicious history and physical examination, a pregnancy test should be obtained in addition to ultrasonography. In patients with a positive test, the result of ultrasonography is frequently crucial because it can determine whether the pregnancy is intrauterine or extrauterine.

If the patient's condition is not acute and she is clinically stable, one could argue that a quantitative serum pregnancy test should be obtained initially. The logic to this approach is that failure to identify an intrauterine gestation when the hCG value exceeds the discriminatory level places the patient at risk for an ectopic pregnancy. (The discriminatory level is the level of hCG at which a normal intrauterine gestational sac should always be visible.) Although the discriminatory level of hCG varies somewhat from one ultrasound department to another, and also depends on the standard against which hCG is measured, there is no question that comparing the ultrasound findings with the quantitative hCG level can be very helpful in diagnosing ectopic pregnancy. Typical discriminatory hCG levels for identifying a normal intrauterine gestational sac when an abdominal approach is used are 1800 mIU/ml (2nd International Standard [IS]) or 3240 mIU/ml (International Reference Preparation [IRP]). Because of improved ability to detect smaller gestational sacs, vaginal scanning has lowered the discriminatory hCG levels to 1000 mIU/ml (2nd IS) or 1800 mIU/ml (IRP). If an intrauterine gestational sac is not seen but the level of hCG is beneath the discriminatory level, the differential diagnosis includes an early normal intrauterine pregnancy, a recent abortion, or an ectoptic pregnancy. Depending on the patient's clinical status, she could be observed for several days (and have serial hCG determinations), or laparoscopy should be considered. If serial hCG values are increasing but fail to show a normal doubling pattern, either an abnormal intrauterine pregnancy or an ectopic pregnancy is present. Under these circumstances, a uterine dilation and curettage should be performed to determine the presence or absence of chorionic villi. Although ultrasonography could be omitted in these cases, most gynecologists elect to scan these patients to assess more com-

CONCLUSION

The combined use of a serum RIA pregnancy test and high-resolution ultrasound allows a more direct diagnosis of ectopic pregnancy. Clinical suspicion is mandatory if the early diagnosis of ectopic pregnancy is to be made. The combination of a positive pregnancy test and lack of evidence for an intrauterine pregnancy is suggestive of an ectopic pregnancy (although an abnormal or a very early intrauterine pregnancy could also have these findings). It is impossible to recommend a specific systematic approach for any given patient. The pattern of management depends on available equipment, the presence or absence of adnexal or cul-de-sac findings, and, of course, the clinical status of the patient.

Bibliography

Cacciatore B, Stenman UH, Ylostalo P: Comparison of abdominal and vaginal sonography in suspected ectopic pregnancy. Obstet Gynecol 73:770–774, 1989.

Dashefsky SM, Lyons EA, Levi CS, et al: Suspected ectopic pregnancy: Endovaginal and transvesical US. Radiology 169:181–184, 1988.

Dillon EH, Feyock AL, Taylor KJW: Pseudogestational sacs: Doppler US differentiation from normal or abnormal intrauterine pregnancies. Radiology 176:359–364, 1990.

Emerson DS, Cartier MS, Altieri LA, et al: Diagnostic efficacy of endovaginal color Doppler flow imaging in an ectopic pregnancy screening program. Radiology 183:413–420, 1992.

Filly RA: Ectopic pregnancy: The role of sonography. Radiology 162:661–668, 1987.

Fleischer AC, Pennell RG, McKedd MS, et al: Ectopic pregnancy: Features at transvaginal sonography. Radiology 174:375–378, 1990.

Kurjak A, Zalud I, Schulman H: Ectopic pregnancy: Transvaginal color Doppler of trophoblastic flow in questionable adnexa. J Ultrasound Med 10:685–689, 1991.

Kadar N, DeVore G, Romero R: Discriminatory hCG zone: Its use in the sonographic evaluation for ectopic pregnancy. Obstet Gynecol 58:156–161, 1981.

Laing FC: Abnormal first-trimester pregnancy. In Rifkin MD, Charboneau JW, Laing

FC (eds): Syllabus Special Course: Ultrasound 1991. Oak Brook, IL, RSNA Publications, 1991, pp 93–102.
Mahony BS, Filly RA, Nyberg DA, Callen PW: Sonographic evaluation of ectopic pregnancy. J Ultrasound Med 4:221, 1985.
Nyberg DA, Filly RA, Mahony BS, et al: Early gestation: Correlation of hCG levels and sonographic identification. AJR 144:951–954, 1985.
Nyberg DA, Hughes MP, Mack LA, et al: Extrauterine findings of ectopic pregnancy at transvaginal US: Importance of echogenic fluid. Radiology 178:823–826, 1991.
Nyberg DA, Laing FC, Filly RA, et al: Ectopic pregnancy: Diagnosis by sonography correlated with hCG levels. J Ultrasound Med 6:145–150, 1987.
Nyberg DA, Laing FC, Filly RA, et al: Ultrasonographic differentiation of the gestational sac of early intrauterine pregnancy from the pseudogestational sac of ectopic pregnancy. Radiology 146:755–759, 1983.
Nyberg DA, Mack LA, Jeffrey RB, et al: Endovaginal sonographic evaluation of ectopic pregnancy: A prospective study. AJR 149:1181–1186, 1987.
Nyberg DA, Mack LA, Laing FC, Jeffrey RB: Early pregnancy complications: Endovaginal sonographic findings correlated with human chorionic gonadotropin levels. Radiology 167:619–622, 1988.
Pellerito JS, Taylor KJW, Quedens-Case C, et al: Ectopic pregnancy: Evaluation with endovaginal color flow imaging. Radiology 183:407–411, 1992.
Rempen A: Vaginal sonography in ectopic pregnancy. J Ultrasound Med 7:381–387, 1988.
Taylor KJW, Ramos IM, Feyock AL, et al: Ectopic pregnancy: Duplex Doppler evaluation. Radiology 173:93–97, 1989.
Thorsen MK, Lawson TL, Aiman EJ, et al: Diagnosis of ectopic pregnancy: Endovaginal vs transabdominal sonography. AJR 155:307–310, 1990.

124 Ultrasound Imaging of Normal Fetal Anatomy

Richard A. Bowerman

Fetal scanning can be divided into three components. First, measurement of specific fetal anatomic structures is necessary to determine fetal gestational age, assess fetal growth, and define the dimensions of certain structures (Table 124–1). Second, documentation of specific structures encompassing portions of all anatomic regions or organ systems is performed to exclude the majority of detectable major anomalies (Table 124–2). Finally, there is an implicit requirement to survey the portions of the fetus not covered by the preceding examinations for textural abnormalities, mass lesions either within the normal confines of the body or protruding from or deforming a body surface, structural deficiencies, etc.

Initial scanning should determine head and spine position to identify left-right-sidedness in the fetus and to simplify subsequent delineation of specific anatomic structures. Optimal fetal imaging can be limited by adverse fetal position, maternal obesity, early or advanced gestational age, oligohydramnios, and marked polyhydramnios.

HEAD AND NECK

Measurements derived in this region include the biparietal diameter (BPD), head circumference (HC), cisterna magna, and ventricular atrium. The structures documented include the cavum septum pellucidum (CSP). The remaining brain, including the cerebral hemispheres and cerebellum, should be evaluated in addition to the bony orbits and soft tissues of the face and neck.

The osseous structures of the skull base and calvarium can be well delineated from the late first trimester. The BPD and HC are key measurements for the assignment of gestational age and evaluation of growth and weight. Both parameters are derived from an axial image of the head through the brain at the level of the thalami and CSP (Fig. 124–1). If the cranial configuration is either dolichocephalic (narrow and long) or brachycephalic (wide and short), the BPD measurement may be erroneous. This can be predicted by the use of the Cephalic Index, defined as the ratio of the BPD to the occipitofrontal diameter. When this value lies outside a range of .74 to .83, the HC is a better predictor of gestational age than the BPD.

The posterior fossa is visualized by angling the probe down posteriorly from the axial plane used for BPD/HC measurement. The cerebellar hemispheres and midline vermis are readily identified anterior to the cisterna magna (Fig. 124–2). Measurements of both the depth of the cisterna magna (normal range is 3 to 10 mm) and the transverse width of the cerebellum are useful in detecting pathology.

The cerebral hemispheres are sonographically echopenic, in marked contrast to the echogenic choroid plexus, which is seen within the developing ventricles (Figs. 124–3 and 124–4). The ventricle/choroid plexus complex appears quite prominent relative to the brain until approximately 19 to 20 weeks, when rapid brain growth leads to increasing cerebral cortical thickness. With the exception of the frontal horn, and later the developing occipital horn, the choroid plexus normally fills the lateral ventricle from medial to lateral wall. Ventricular walls may be difficult to see unless outlined by fluid or oriented perpendicular to the scan plane,

TABLE 124–1. STANDARD FETAL MEASUREMENTS

Biparietal diameter
Head circumference
Abdominal circumference
Femur length
Ventricular atrium
Cisterna magna

TABLE 124–2. FETAL ANATOMY TO DOCUMENT

Heart (four-chamber view)
Stomach
Bladder
Kidneys/renal area
Anterior abdominal wall
Spine
Cavum septum pellucidum

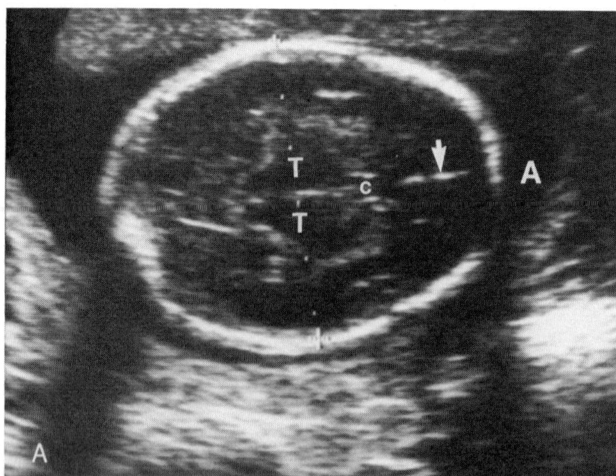

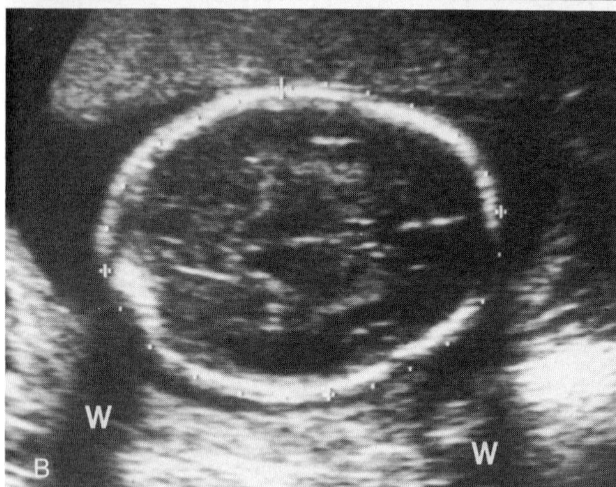

Figure 124–1. *A*, Axial image shows hypoechoic thalami (T), midline cavum septum pellucidum (c), and anterior echo from the falx cerebri and/or interhemispheric fissure (*arrow*). (A = anterior.) For biparietal diameter (BPD) measurement, the calipers (+) are placed on the outer margin of the near calvarial echo and the inner margin of the far calvarium. *B*, On the same image, the head circumference (HC) is determined at the outer margin of the calvarium, circumferentially. (W = distal shadowing arising from the margins of the calvarium.)

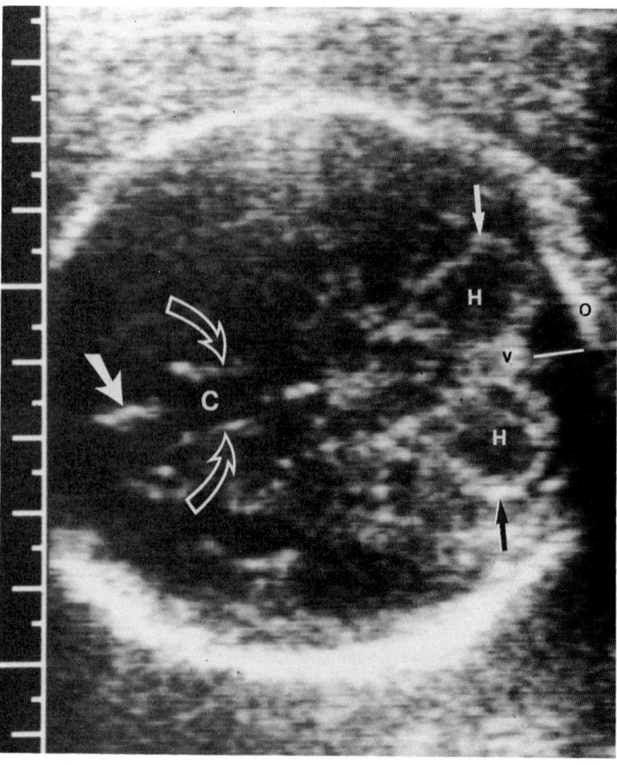

Figure 124–2. Angled axial scan shows the hypoechoic cerebellar hemispheres (H) and midline echogenic vermis (v). *Straight arrows* demarcate transverse cerebellar diameter. The cisterna magna is measured (*white bar*) from the vermis to the occipital bone (o). The cavum septum pellucidum (C) is delineated by echogenic walls (*curved arrows*). The *slanted arrow* indicates the falx/interhemispheric fissure.

Figure 124–3. Axial mid (*A*) and (*B*) high scans of the brain at 15.5 weeks show the large echogenic choroid plexus (p) filling the lateral ventricles from medial to lateral walls, except in the frontal horns (*arrows* indicate walls). The echo-poor cerebral hemispheres (b) surround the ventricular system and should not be mistaken for fluid-containing spaces.

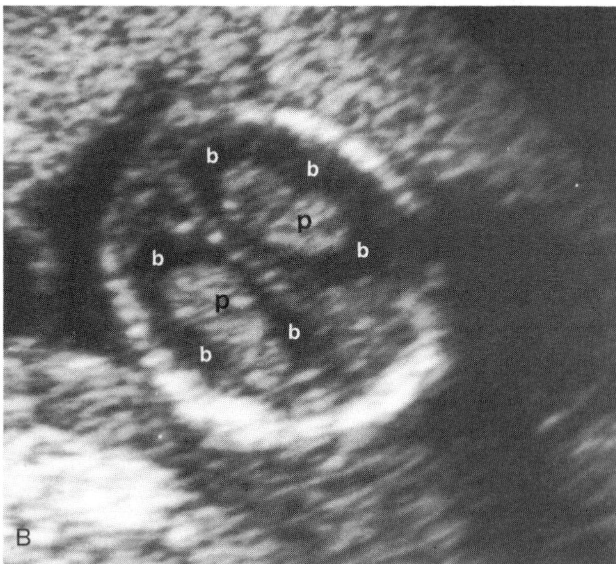

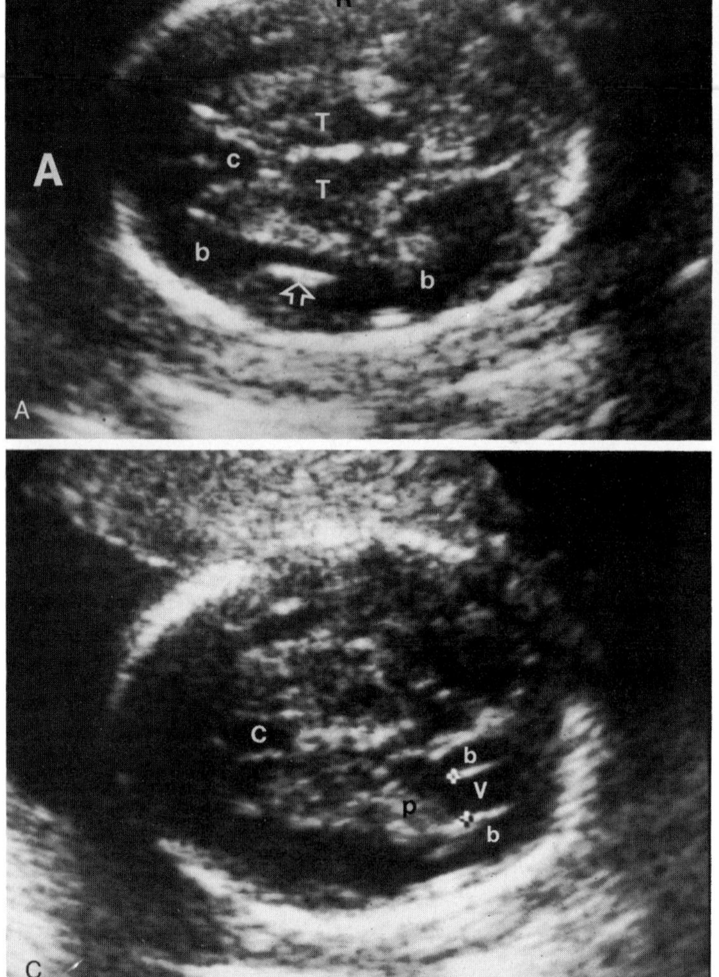

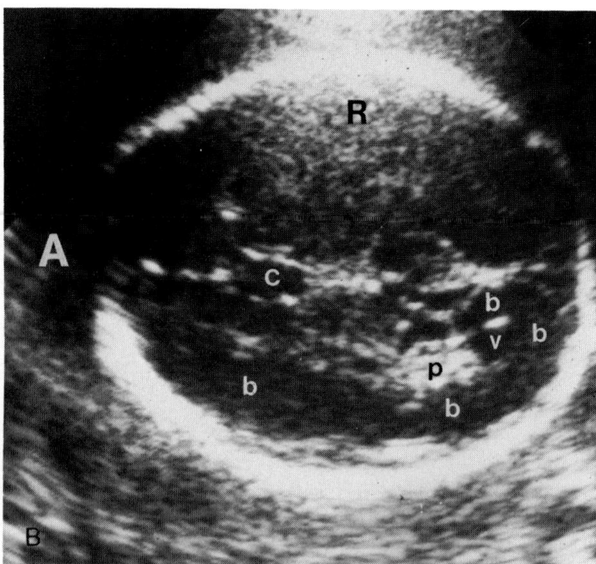

Figure 124–4. Axial images, 22 weeks. *A,* Intracranial anatomy is evaluated primarily in the dependent hemisphere since reverberations (R) from bone obscure the non-dependent side. The cerebral hemisphere is echopenic (b). A bright echo (*arrow*) marks the interface between insular cortex and the lateral sulcus, a patulous subarachnoid space that becomes the sylvian fissure. (T = thalami; c = cavum septum pellucidum; A = anterior.) *B,* Higher section delineates the choroid plexus (p) anterior to the occipital horn (v), both surrounded by echopenic brain (b). *C,* The atrium of the lateral ventricle is measured (+) from medial to lateral ventricular walls (v).

where they are recognized by their linear echogenic nature. Several measurements have been proposed to detect ventriculomegaly. The current preference is to determine the width of the atrium of the lateral ventricle on an axial image above that obtained for a BPD/HC (Fig. 124–4). Normal values are 7.6 mm (=/− 6 mm), with measurements of greater than 10 mm considered abnormal. Because reverberation artifact obscures the near side of the brain, the described intracranial anatomy is primarily noted only in the dependent hemisphere.

The CSP is a fluid-filled midline structure located between the lateral ventricles, best seen anterior to the thalami (see Fig. 124–2). A normal appearance of the CSP implies that the cerebral midline structures are intact, excluding certain midline central nervous system anomalies.

Within the face, structures that can be routinely imaged include the bony orbits, nose, lips, chin, tongue, toothbuds, maxilla, and mandible (Fig. 124–5). Sagittal, coronal, and/or axial scan planes may be necessary to image the target area. An axial or coronal image of the orbits allows for measurement of the outer orbital diameter, which correlates with gestational age and may be used to detect hypo-/hypertelorism (Fig. 124–6). Imaging of the nasolabial region is important to exclude anterior facial clefts (Fig. 124–7).

The fluid-filled hypopharynx, trachea, and major vessels can often be identified within the neck. Most important, however, is the confirmation of smooth, echogenic cutaneous surfaces, which will exclude a protruding neck mass.

SPINE

The spine as seen sonographically comprises three echogenic ossification centers within each vertebral segment. The anterior center is the developing vertebral body, while the paired posterior ossifications lie at the junction of the lamina and pedicle. Seen in longitudinal section, the spine appears as two rows of roughly parallel echogenic ossification centers (Figs. 124–8, 124–10, and 124–11). The classic appearance of the spine on transverse sonograms is three punctate echogenic ossification centers in a triangular configuration (Figs. 124–9 and 124–12). There is variability, however, in the appearance of these centers. They appear more linear in the cervical and thoracic spine than in the lumbosacral region. With advancing gestational age and associated skeletal ossification, the vertebral configuration becomes ring-like at all levels.

Transverse imaging of all segments from cervical to sacral is generally believed to be the most sensitive means to examine the

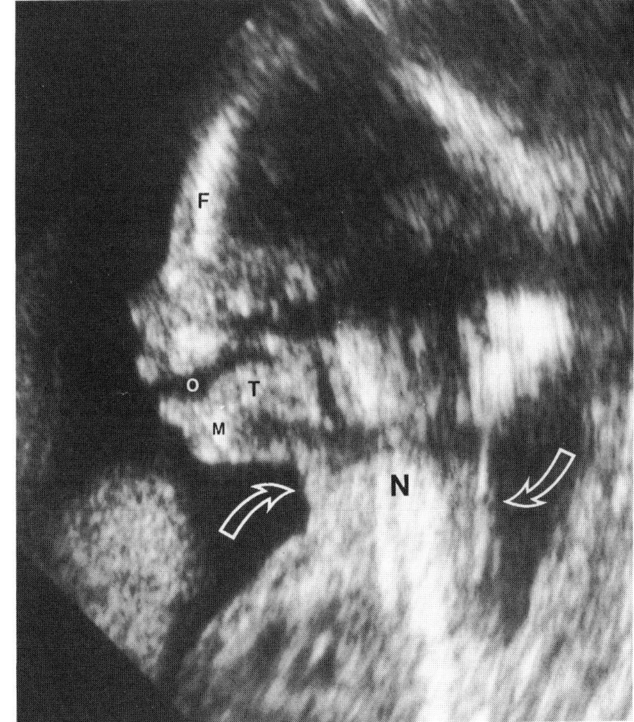

Figure 124–5. Face profile shows the frontal bone (F), nose, lips, and chin. The tongue (T) is outlined by amniotic fluid (o). (M = mandible.) Note echogenic cervical spine (N) and soft tissues of neck (*arrows*).

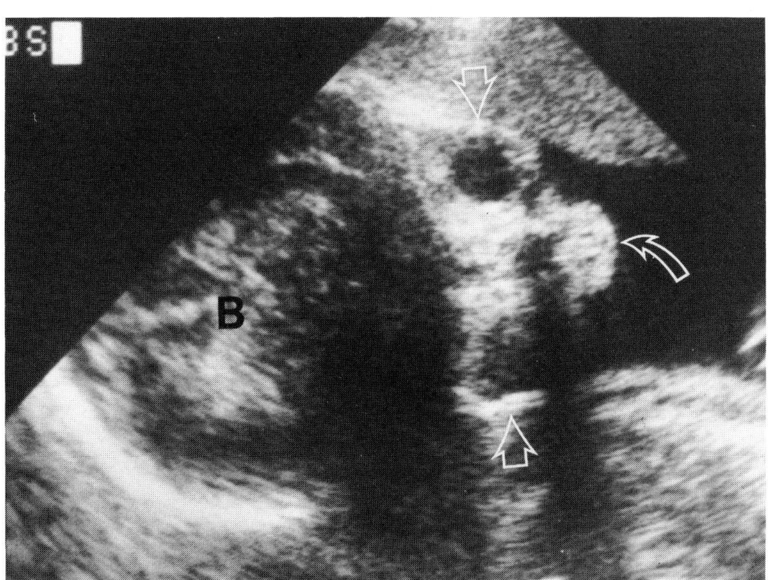

Figure 124–6. *Arrows* indicate lateral margins of bony orbits on angled axial section of face, which includes nose (*curved arrow*) and brain (B).

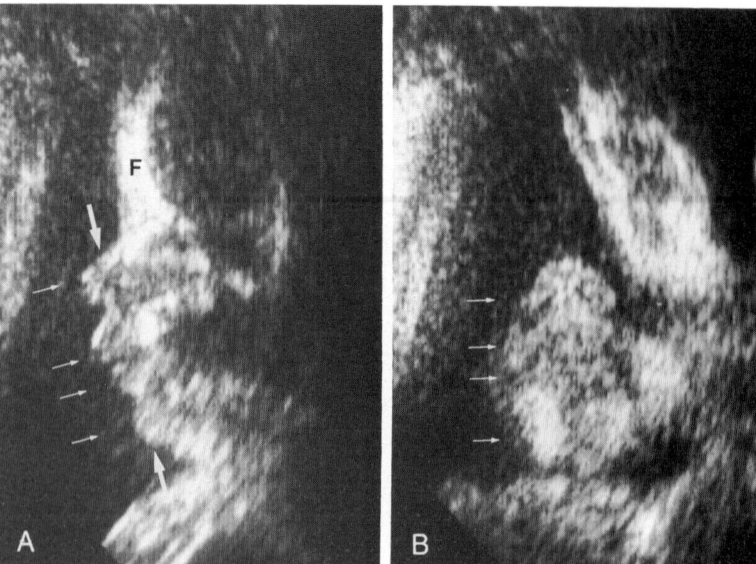

Figure 124–7. Sagittal (*A*) and coronal (*B*) images show the nose, upper/lower lips, and chin (*small arrows*). *Large arrows* in *A* delineate scan plane for *B*. (F = forehead.)

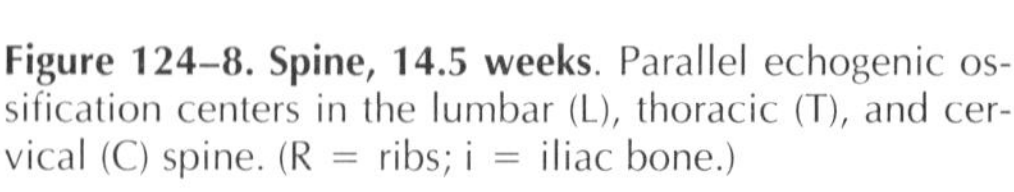

Figure 124–8. Spine, 14.5 weeks. Parallel echogenic ossification centers in the lumbar (L), thoracic (T), and cervical (C) spine. (R = ribs; i = iliac bone.)

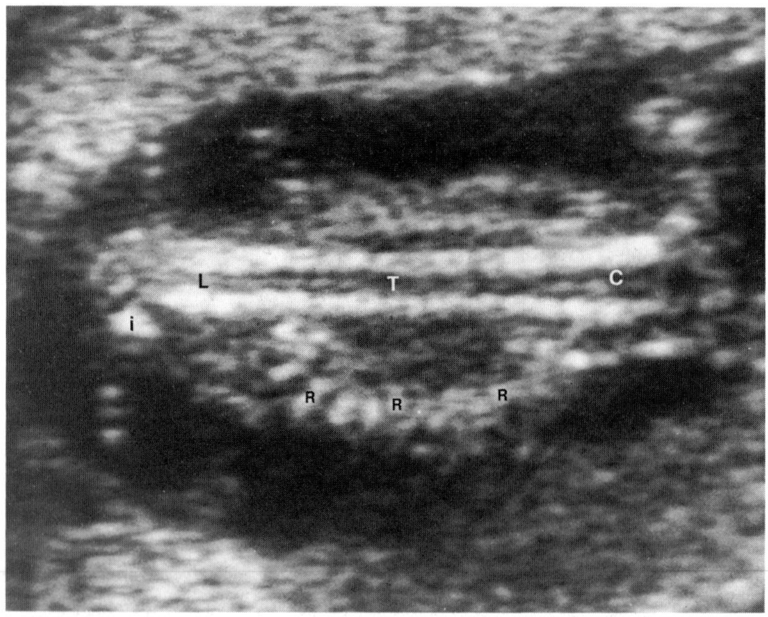

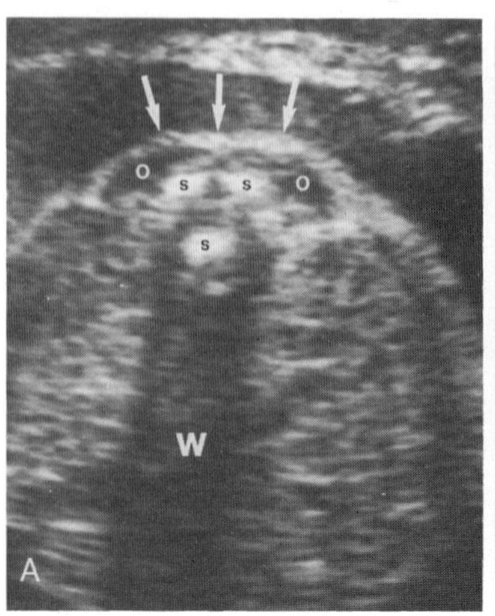

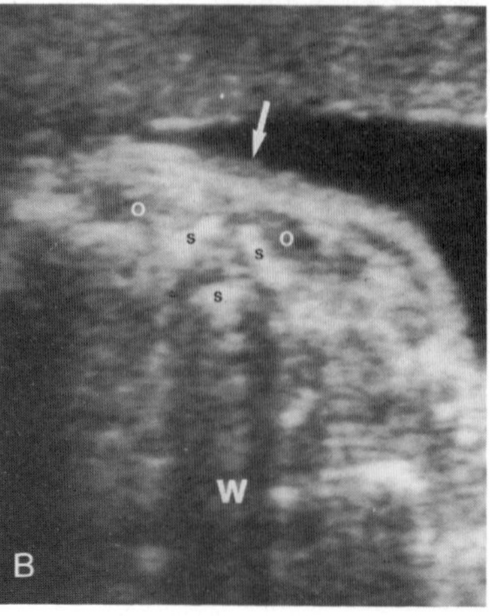

Figure 124–9. Axial spine images show (*A*) classic three punctate echogenic ossification centers (s), casting a distal shadow (W), and (*B*) linear appearance (s) of the posterior elements. Note posterior hypoechoic paraspinal musculature (o) and echogenic skin/subcutaneous tissues (*arrows*).

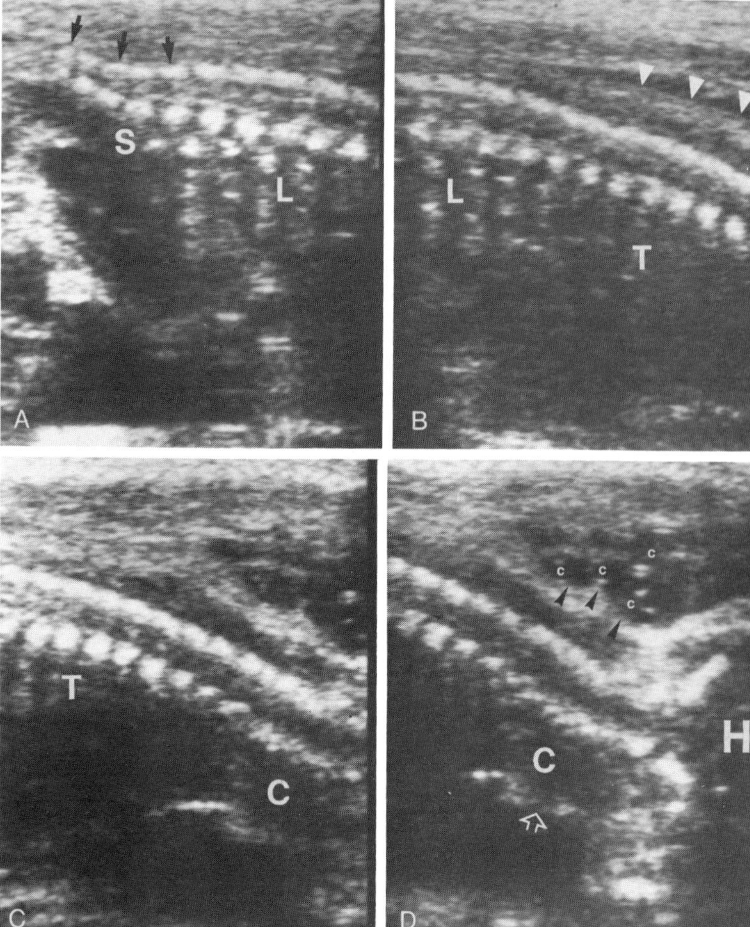

Figure 124–10. *A* to *D,* Sequential parasagittal scans of ossification centers within the sacral (S), lumbar (L), thoracic (T), and cervical (C) spine. In *A,* the tapered, posteriorly curving configuration of the sacrum is apparent (*arrows*). In *B,* the posterior skin surface is readily delineated when outlined by amniotic fluid (*white arrowheads*). In *D,* note anterior neck (*open arrow*) and posteriorly, the soft tissues of the neck (*black arrowheads*) distorted by multiple loops of the umbilical cord (c). This should not be mistaken for a cervical mass such as a hygroma. (H = head.)

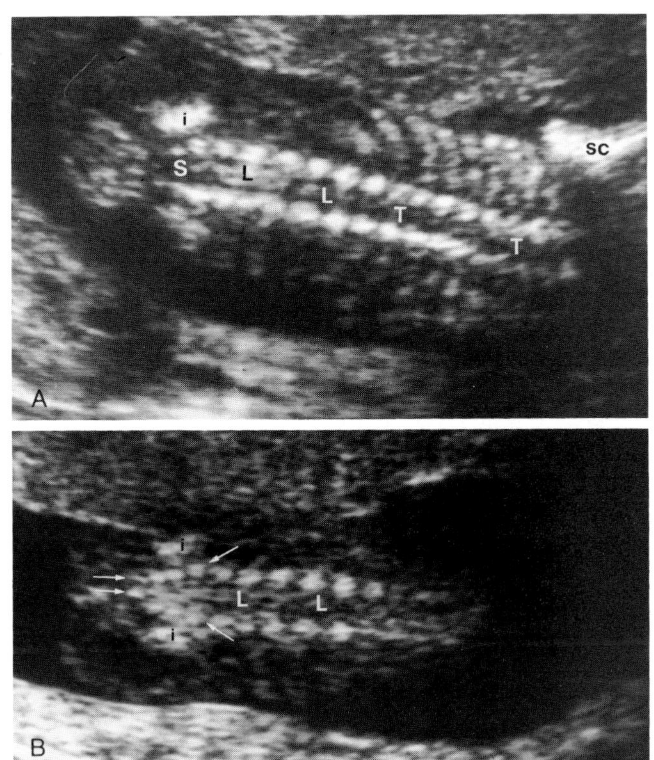

Figure 124–11. *A,* Coronal images through the posterior ossification centers of the upper sacral (S), lumbar (L), and lower/mid-thoracic (T) spine show mild widening in the lumbar region. *B,* The tapering sacral elements (*arrows*) can be difficult to image simultaneously due to the overlying iliac bones (i).

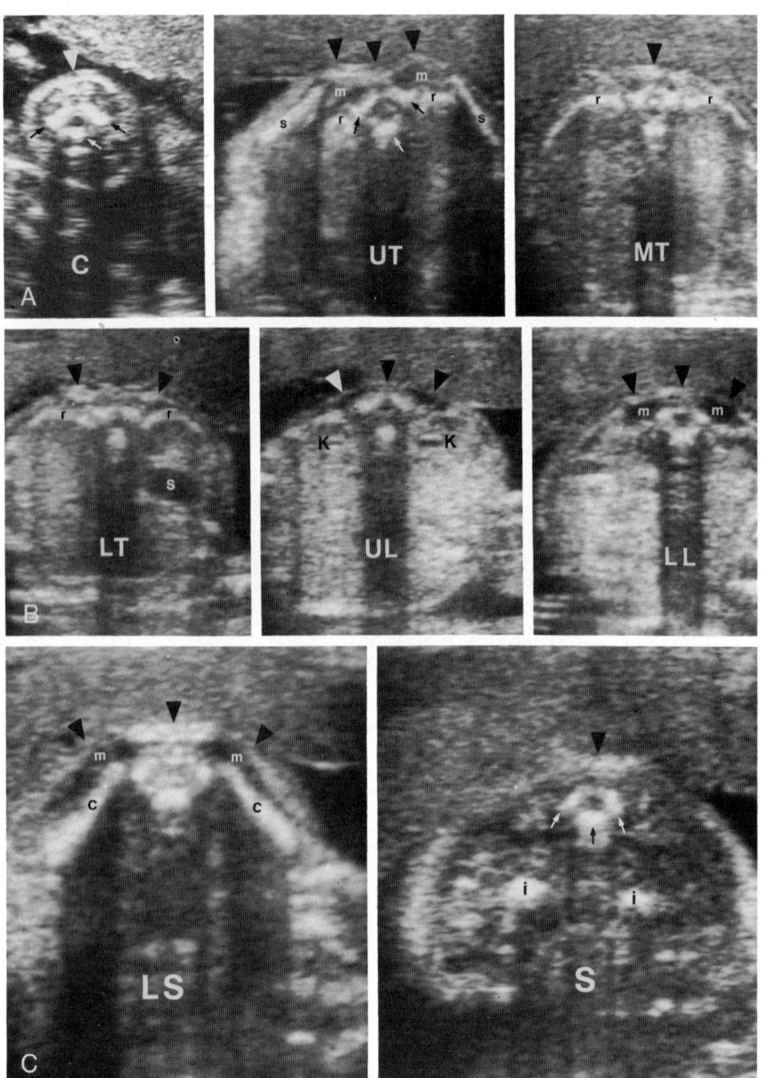

Figure 124–12. *A* to *C,* Sequential axial scans document the appearance of the three ossification centers and adjacent soft tissues in the cervical (C), upper thoracic (UT), mid-thoracic (MT), lower thoracic (LT), upper lumbar (UL), lower lumbar (LL), lumbosacral (LS), and sacral (S) spine. (*Arrows* delineate centers on several scans.) Paraspinal musculature (m) is thicker by the scapulae (s), iliac crests (c), and in the cervical and lower lumbar regions. (r = ribs.)

spine. Any widening between the posterior ossification centers or defect in the hypoechoic paraspinal muscles or echogenic posterior soft tissues suggests a neural tube defect. Longitudinal scans provide a useful overall perspective and may confirm findings noted in the transverse plane.

THORAX

The bony thorax is composed of the thoracic spine, ribs, scapulas, and clavicles, all readily identified because of their inherent subject contrast with adjacent structures. However, because these bones become more mineralized with advancing gestational age, imaging of the underlying intrathoracic structures becomes progressively more difficult. Cardiac anatomy is best delineated when the fetal chest is directed anteriorly. A sonographic window is created that avoids the calcified and shadowing posterior aspects of the ribs. Cartilage, which forms the anterior rib cage, is hypoechoic and allows good sound transmission (Figs. 124–13 and 124–14).

Evaluation of the heart should begin with confirmation of cardiac activity and assessment of rate and rhythm. The normal fetal heart rate is 120 to 160 beats per minute.

The four-chamber view of the heart is the basic image used to detect cardiac and other intrathoracic abnormalities. This axial scan through the lower thorax shows the heart, lungs, and adjacent bony thorax (Fig. 124–15). Cardiac displacement can be detected secondary to noncardiac intrathoracic masses or primary cardiac malposition. The thoracic circumference is also measured at this level. Although this measurement is difficult to obtain with consistency, a low value may indicate pulmonary hypoplasia. The primary value of the four-chamber view is in the evaluation of cardiac anatomy, however. When the four-chamber view is normal, approximately 70 per cent of major cardiac anomalies are excluded.

The heart occupies about one third of the cross-sectional area of the thorax, lying roughly in the mid-anterior chest. The cardiac apex should be directed to the left, which is easily detected by determining the position of the ventricles. The ventricles have thicker walls than the atria and are the chambers into which the AV valves are seen to open. The right ventricle is the most anterior chamber and is approximately equal to the left ventricle in size. The interventricular septum is seen separating these chambers. Intraventricular echoes are the papillary muscles and, on the right, the moderator band at the apex. The left atrium is the most posterior cardiac chamber, separated from the equal-sized right atrium by the interatrial septum. The foramen ovale, which allows right-to-left flow of fetal blood, is readily identified within the atrial septum. The adjacent membranous septum primum, which balloons into the lumen of the left atrium, prevents retrograde left-to-right flow (Fig. 124–16). Sensitivity for the detection of cardiac defects is increased

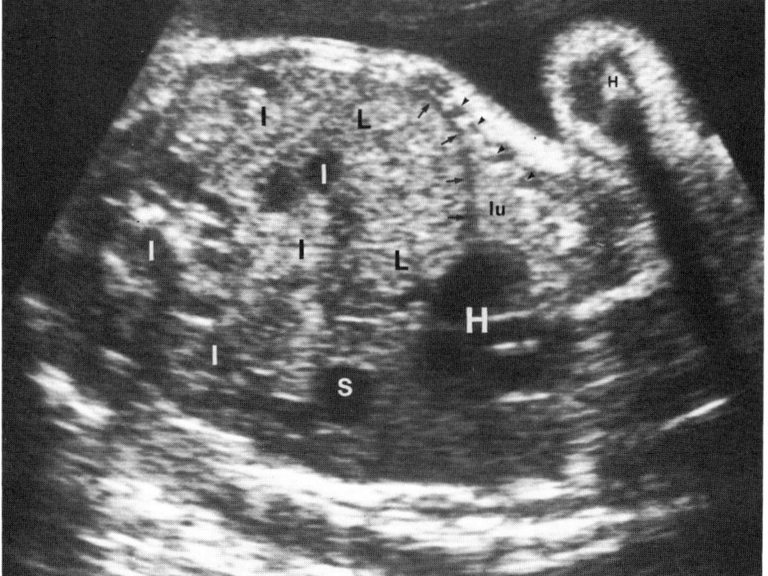

Figure 124–13. Heart (H), lung (lu), and cartilaginous ribs (*arrowheads*) lie in the thorax superior to the diaphragm (*arrows*). Within the abdomen, the stomach (S) is in the left upper quadrant while much of the abdominal cavity is filled with liver (L) and bowel (I) of varying sonographic character. (H = humerus.)

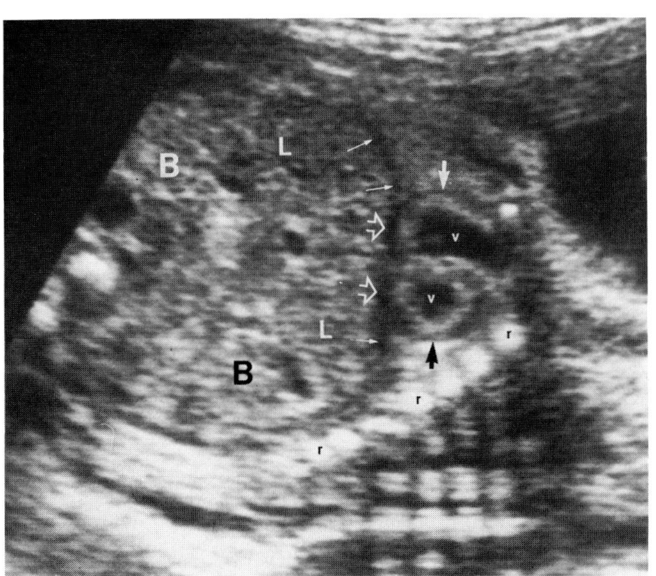

Figure 124–14. The heart (*large solid arrows*) in short-axis view demonstrates ventricular cavities (v), intraventricular septum, and ventricular free walls. The thin hypoechoic rim is a normal component of the myocardium, not an effusion. The diaphragm (*thin arrows*) appears thicker when contiguous with such hypoechoic myocardium (*open arrows*). Note echogenic, calcified ribs (r), casting distal shadows that obscure underlying structures. (L = liver; B = bowel.)

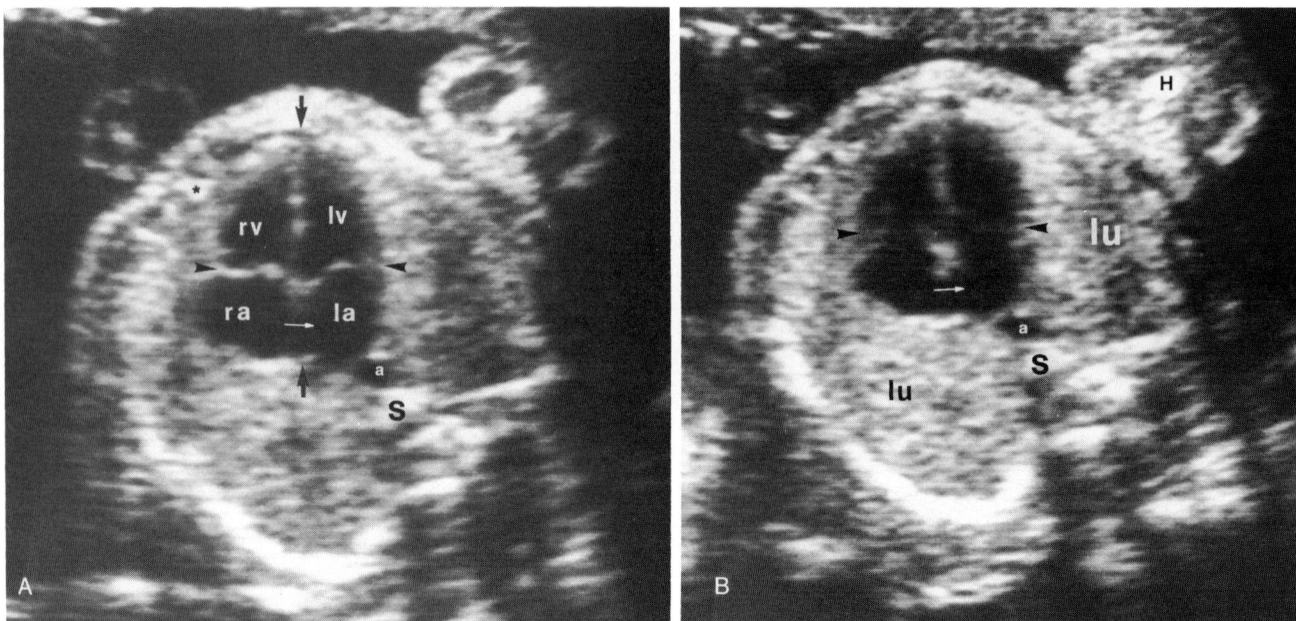

Figure 124–15. Heart, four chamber view. *A,* The AV valves (*arrowheads*) are closed, separating the right and left ventricles (rv, lv) from their respective atria (ra, la). The foramen ovale (*white arrow*) and intracardiac septa (*black arrows*) are noted. (S = spine; *asterisk* = sternal ossification center.) *B,* The AV valves (*arrowheads*) are open, being less apparent during their intraventricular excursions. (lu = lungs; H = humerus.)

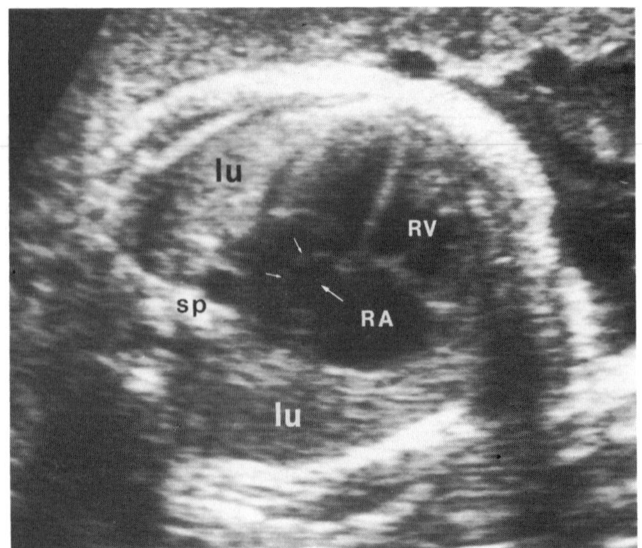

Figure 124–16. Four-chamber view shows foramen ovale (*large arrow* indicates direction of blood flow) within the atrial septum. The septum primum (*small arrows*) protrudes into the left atrium; (RV = right ventricle; RA = right atrium; lu = lung; sp = spine.)

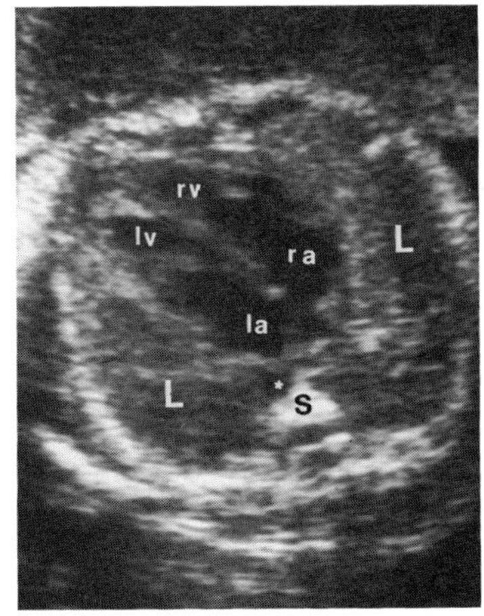

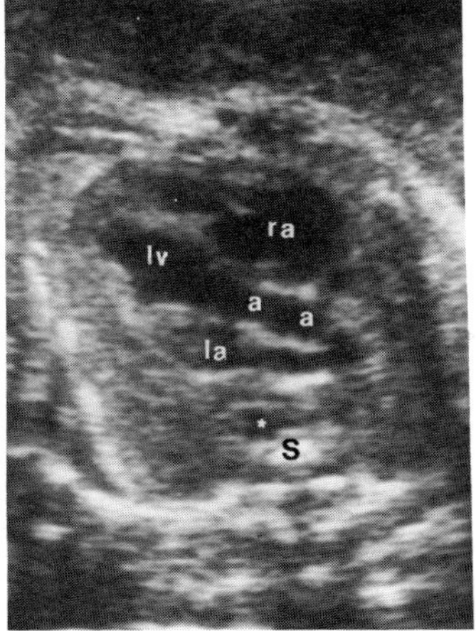

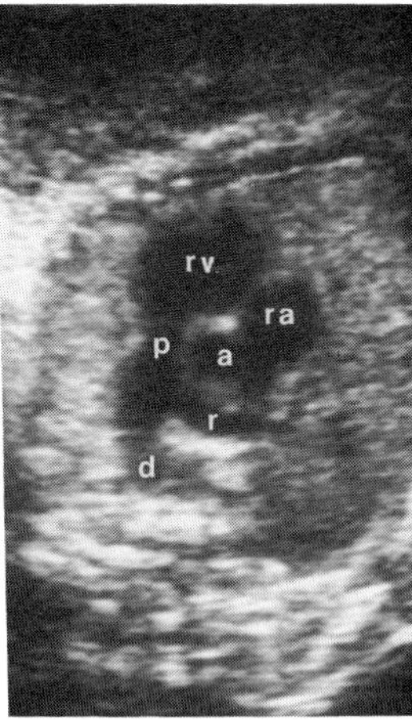

Figure 124–17. *A*, Four-chamber view for orientation. (rv = right ventricle; lv = left ventricle; ra = right atrium; la = left atrium; L = lung; s = spine; *asterisk* = descending aorta.) Angling superiorly. *B*, The aorta (a) is seen arising from the left ventricle. *C*, The main pulmonary artery (p) arises from the right ventricle, then divides into a right pulmonary artery (r) that passes posterior to the aorta (a) and a left pulmonary artery that connects with the ductus venosus (d) that leads to the descending aorta.

when additional views of the ventricular outflow tracts/great vessels are obtained (Fig. 124–17).

The remainder of the thorax is filled by the lungs, which appear as homogeneous, midlevel echogenic structures. They are separated from the intra-abdominal structures by the diaphragm (see Figs. 124–13, 124–14, and 124–16). The diaphragm is hypoechoic, as are the other muscles in the body.

ABDOMEN AND PELVIS

The basic abdominal/pelvic survey includes documentation of the stomach, bladder, kidneys/renal area, and cord insertion site, as well as an abdominal circumference measurement.

The abdominal circumference measurement is key to fetal growth evaluation. It is derived from an axial scan through the fetal liver at the level where the midline umbilical vein enters the portal venous system (Fig. 124–18). Only a short segment of the umbilical vein deep within the liver should be included in the image, because a longer segment indicates an oblique section through the vein as it courses inferiorly toward the umbilicus. Measurement is taken at the skin surface circumferentially.

The stomach is recognized as a fluid-filled viscus in the left upper quadrant (Fig. 124–19). Failure to see a stomach beyond 14 weeks is highly suggestive of a fetal anomaly. The bladder is identifiable in the low pelvis as an anterior midline cystic structure (Fig. 124–20). Recent emptying may necessitate scanning over as long as a 45 to 90 minute interval to document the bladder's presence. Other fluid-filled structures that may be delineated within the abdomen include the gallbladder, umbilical vein, other large blood vessels, the renal collecting systems, and bowel in the late second and third trimesters. The detection of other fluid collections within the abdomen is suspicious for fetal pathology.

The gallbladder should not be mistaken for the umbilical vein, because this could lead to mismeasurement of the abdominal circumference. It is typically somewhat teardrop shaped, in contrast to the uniform caliber of the umbilical vein, and lies at the inferior edge of the liver, extending from the porta hepatis to a position to the right of midline (Fig. 124–21). Contrary to the midline-positioned umbilical vein, the gallbladder will not be seen to penetrate the abdominal wall.

The kidneys, difficult to identify before 17 to 18 weeks, are identified as bilateral, hypoechoic, paraspinal structures with a central, somewhat more echogenic sinus complex. In the late second and third trimesters, the collecting system often contains small quantities of fetal urine. Normally the renal pelvis measures less than 1 cm in the anteroposterior dimension (Fig. 124–22).

The anterior abdominal wall at the level of the cord insertion should be imaged to confirm a normal-sized umbilical cord of uniform width entering the abdomen, with no adjacent masses (Fig. 124–23). Two small umbilical arteries and the one umbilical vein are noted in the cord either near the insertion or in a free-floating loop (Fig. 124–24).

The liver occupies a large portion of the upper abdomen, with the left lobe quite prominent in the fetus (see Fig. 124–19*A*). Most of the rest of the abdomen/pelvis is filled with bowel. In the early second trimester, the bowel is of midlevel to increased echogenicity. In the late second and third trimesters, hypoechoic meconium-filled colon and, occasionally, fluid-containing loops of small bowel are noted (see Figs. 124–13 and 124–19 *B*).

Adrenal glands are often imaged as thin sonolucent structures with a central linear echo, in a paraspinal/suprarenal location. The right gland is posterior to the IVC, while the left gland is more variable in position and more difficult to discern (Fig. 124–25).

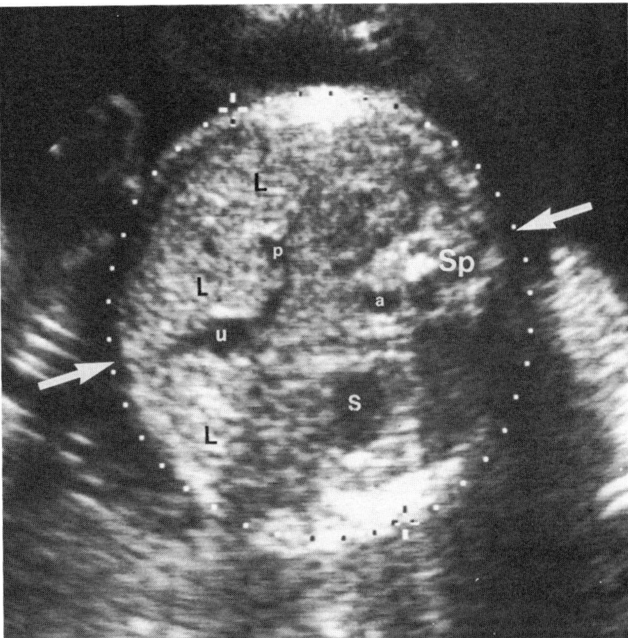

Figure 124–18. Abdominal circumference measurement derived from an axial image through liver (L) at junction of umbilical vein (u) and portal venous system (p). The circumference can also be calculated by averaging the transverse (+) and anteroposterior (*arrows*) diameters of the abdomen and multiplying this value by 3.14.

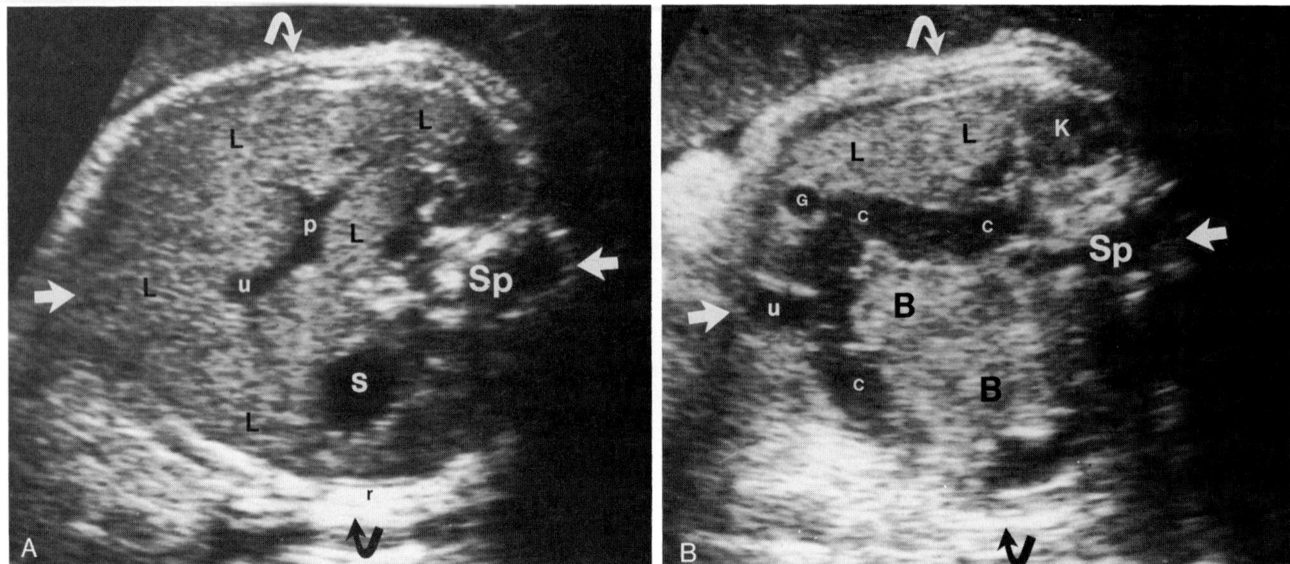

Figure 124–19. *A,* Axial image of upper abdomen shows stomach (S) and the liver (L) (u = umbilical vein; p = portal vein; r = rib, Sp = spine.) *Arrows* delineate cutaneous margins, poorly seen anteriorly and posteriorly due to refractive shadowing. *B,* Axial image of the mid-abdomen shows the inferior liver (L) with the anteriorly positioned umbilical vein (u) and gallbladder (G). Prominent, hypoechoic loops of colon (c) and heterogeneous small bowel (B) fill the central abdomen. (K = right kidney.)

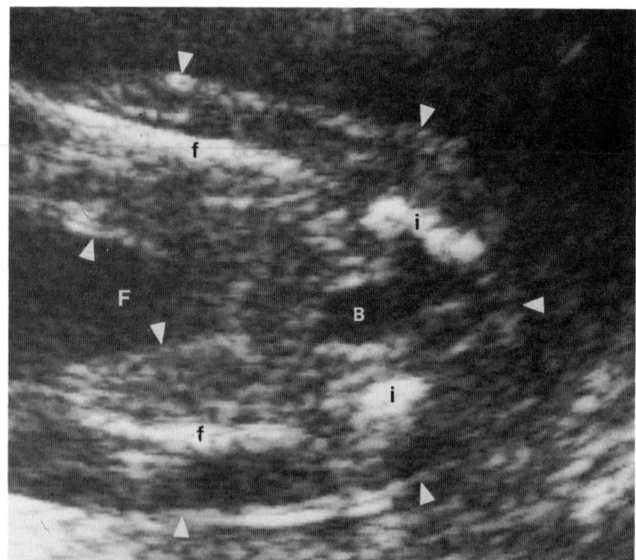

Figure 124–20. Axial image of pelvis through iliac crests (i) shows the anterior, midline fluid-filled bladder (B). The femora (f) are noted within the soft tissues of the thighs. *Arrowheads* delineate skin surfaces. (F = amniotic fluid.)

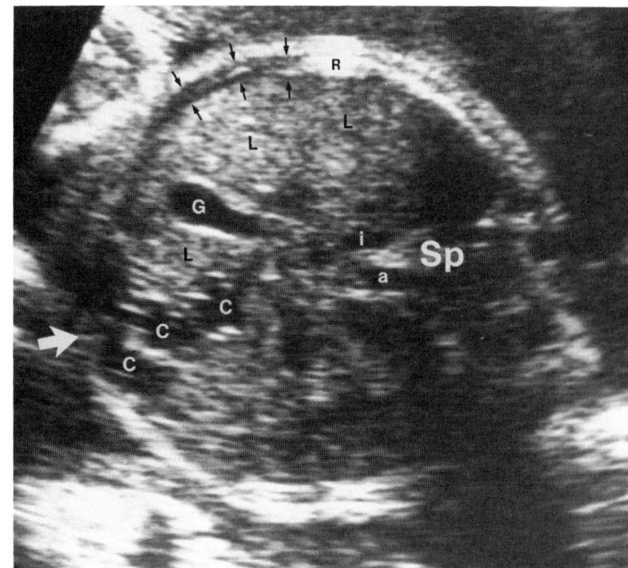

Figure 124–21. Axial section of the mid-abdomen shows the gallbladder (G) in the right upper quadrant. The aorta (a) and inferior vena cava (i) are anterior to the spine (Sp). The abdominal wall musculature (*small arrows*) is hypoechoic, seen external to the liver (L) and deep to the echogenic subcutaneous tissues. It is contiguous with muscles surrounding ribs (R) superiorly. (c = colon; *large arrow* indicates anterior midline.)

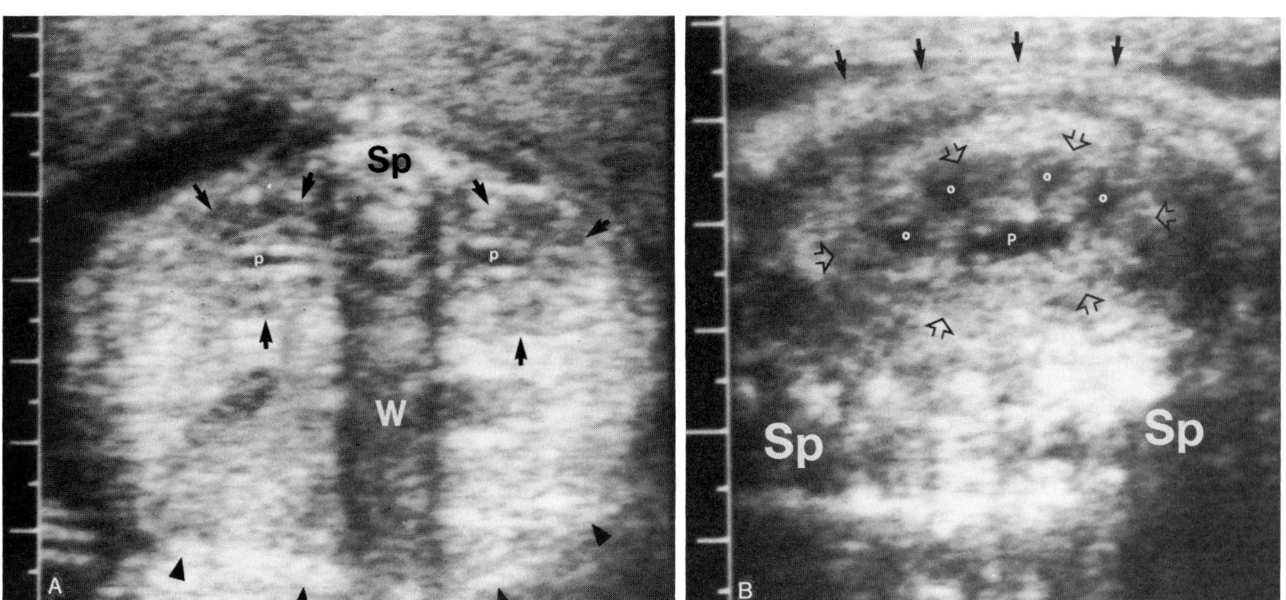

Figure 124–22. *A*, Axial image shows the spine (Sp) with shadowing (W) and the hypoechoic paraspinal kidneys (*arrows*). The renal pelvis (p) contains urine. *B*, Coronal image of the kidney (*open arrows*) shows hypoechoic pyramids (o) surrounded by mid-level echogenic cortex, and the central pelvis (p). *Closed arrows* indicate lateral abdominal wall. (Sp = spine.)

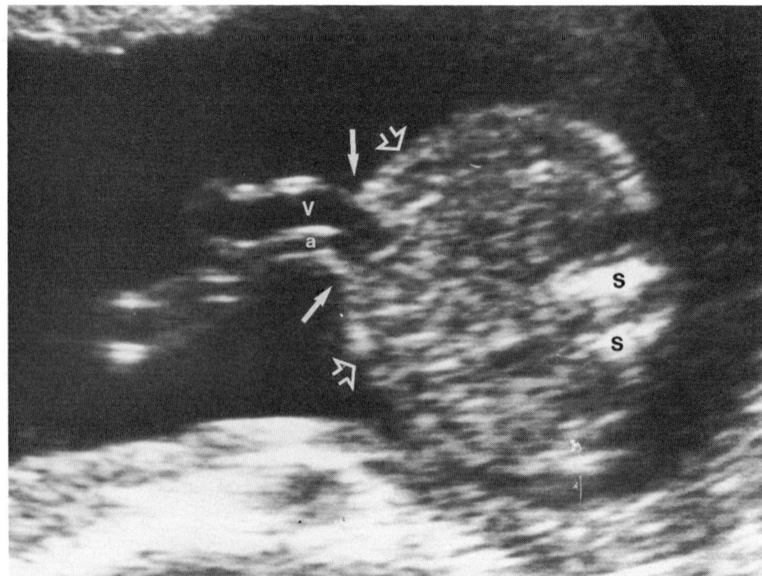

Figure 124–23. Axial image shows the umbilical cord (V = vein; a = artery) entering the abdomen (*long arrows*). The adjacent abdominal wall (*open arrows*) is intact. (s = spine.)

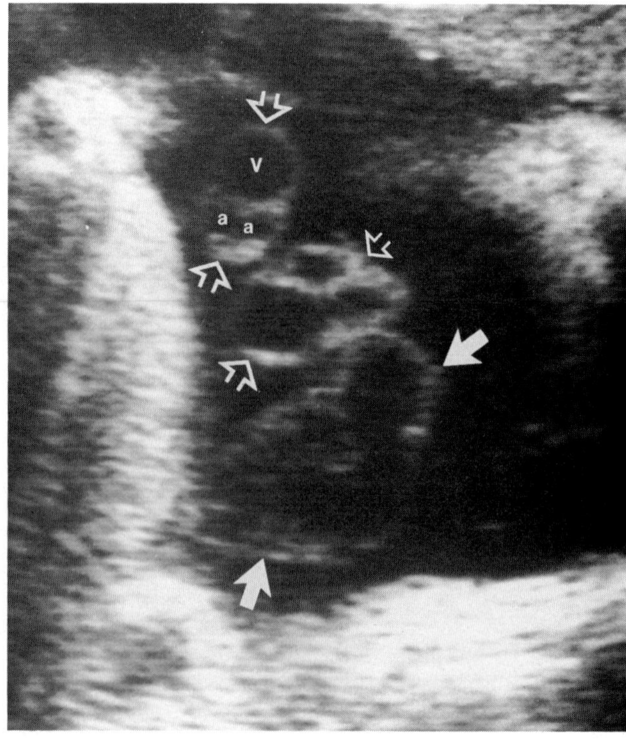

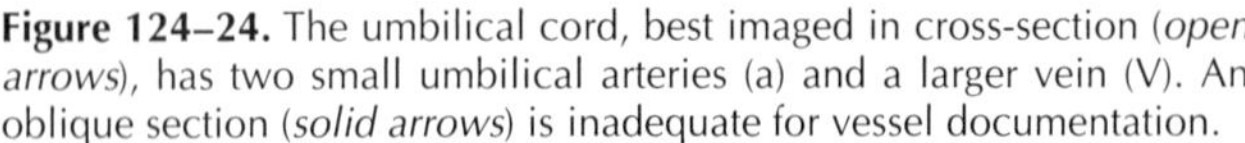

Figure 124–24. The umbilical cord, best imaged in cross-section (*open arrows*), has two small umbilical arteries (a) and a larger vein (V). An oblique section (*solid arrows*) is inadequate for vessel documentation.

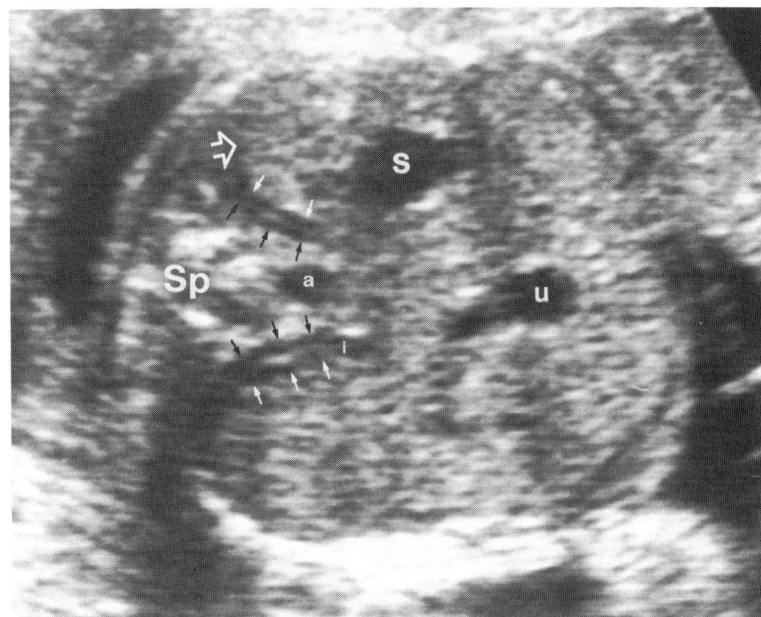

Figure 124–25. The adrenal glands (*small arrows*) are seen posterior to the inferior vena cava (i) and medial to the spleen (*open arrow*). (s = stomach; u = intrahepatic umbilical vein; Sp = spine; a = aorta.)

When the adjacent kidney is absent, the normally prominent fetal adrenal gland may resemble a kidney.

GENITALIA

Male and female genitalia are similar embryologically until about 12 to 13 weeks' gestational age, and even beyond that time there is often marked similarity. Beyond 18 to 19 weeks, assuming adequate visualization of the perineum, fetal gender can usually be assigned with a high degree of certainty. Although specific gender assignment can be made earlier, many indeterminate scans will occur in this age range.

Axial or coronal scans with varying degrees of angulation to avoid adjacent structures are necessary to see the perineum. The earliest finding in the male is identification of a penis, seen as a solid tubular structure projecting between the thighs (Fig. 124–26*A*). Occasionally the umbilical cord is found between the thighs, but its fluid-filled nature differentiates it from the penis. Through the second trimester, the scrotum becomes increasingly apparent as a bulbous soft tissue structure at the base of the penis. Testicles, which are echogenic, descend into the scrotum during the seventh month. Small isolated hydroceles are usually of no concern clinically (Fig. 124–26*B*).

Imaging the early female genitalia reveals a pattern of parallel linear echos that represent the interfaces at the margins of the labia (Fig. 124–27*A*). In the third trimester, the labia majora are more pronounced as fuller soft-tissue structures between which the thinner echos of the labia minora may occasionally be seen (Fig. 124–27*B*).

EXTREMITIES

Ossification of the long bones commences in the first trimester, making these echogenic structures readily identifiable due to their subject contrast with adjacent soft tissues. Before ossification, the cartilaginous components of the skeleton are sonographically hypoechoic, a feature readily appreciated in the epiphyses of the long bones. Similarly, the carpus is nonossified prenatally, while, within the foot, the calcaneus and talus begin ossification in the late second trimester.

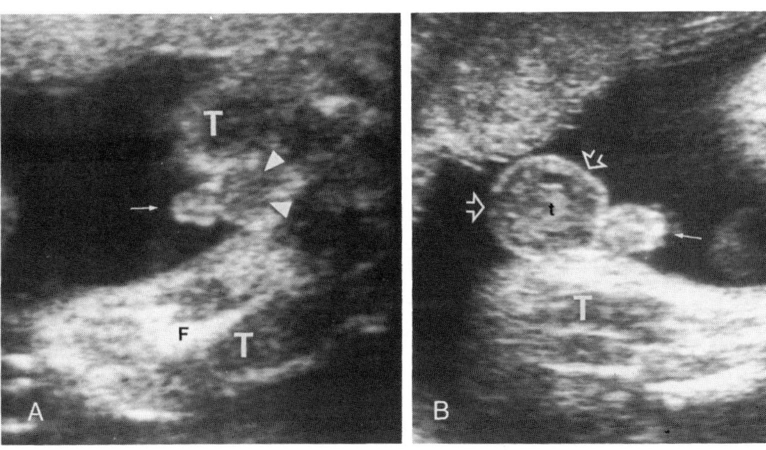

Figure 124–26. *A*, Penis (*arrow*) and scrotum (*arrowheads*) between the thighs (T), 26 weeks. (F = femur.) *B*, Penis (*arrow*) and scrotum (*open arrows*) with a slightly echogenic testicle (t) and a small hydrocele at 32 weeks.

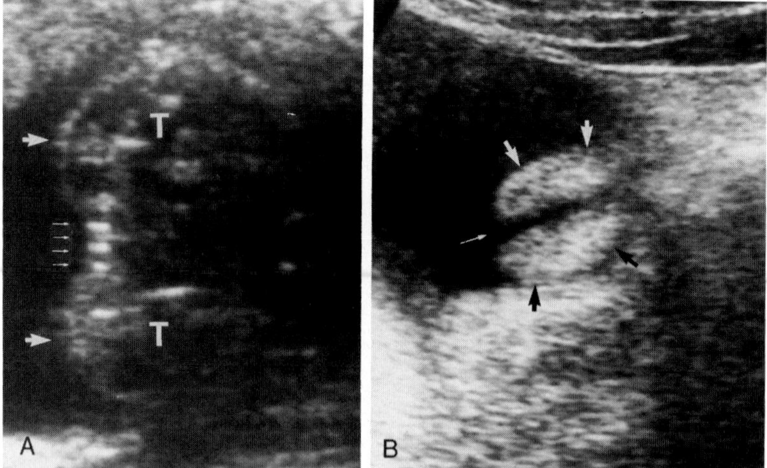

Figure 124–27. *A*, Parallel linear echos (*small arrows*) between the thighs (T, *large arrows*) represent the edges of the labia majora, 20 weeks. *B*, Off-axial image at 36 weeks shows the prominent soft tissues of the labia majora (*large arrows*) with a midline separation (*thin arrow*).

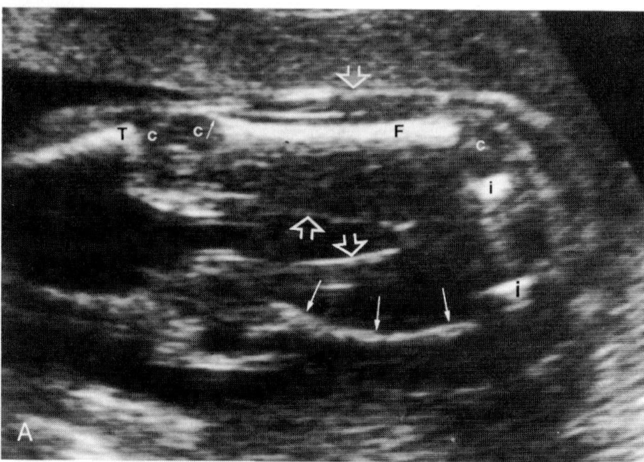

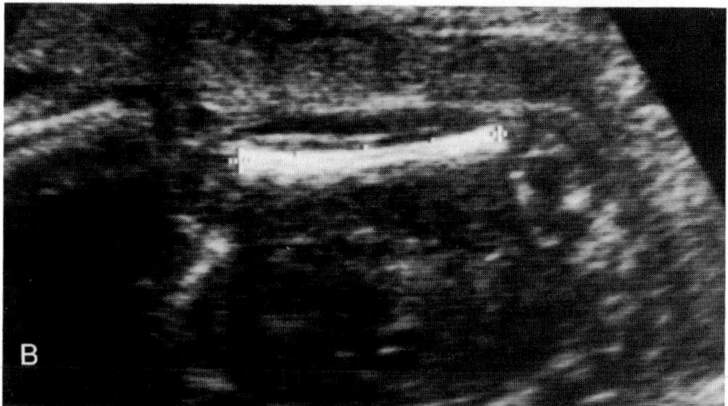

Figure 124–28. *A*, Femur (F) is identified adjacent to pelvic structures (i = ischial bones). The cartilaginous epiphyses (c) of the femur and proximal tibia (T) are sonographically hypoechoic. An echogenic "spike" (*short arrow*) distally is a cartilage–soft tissue interface and should not be included in femur meassurement. The medial aspect of the femur is curved relative to the lateral surface, illustrated on the poorly seen dependent femur (*thin arrows*). Skin margins of the thighs are noted (*open arrows*). *B*, Ossified portion of femur is measured (+) on an image where bone and distal shadowing are relatively uniform in echotexture.

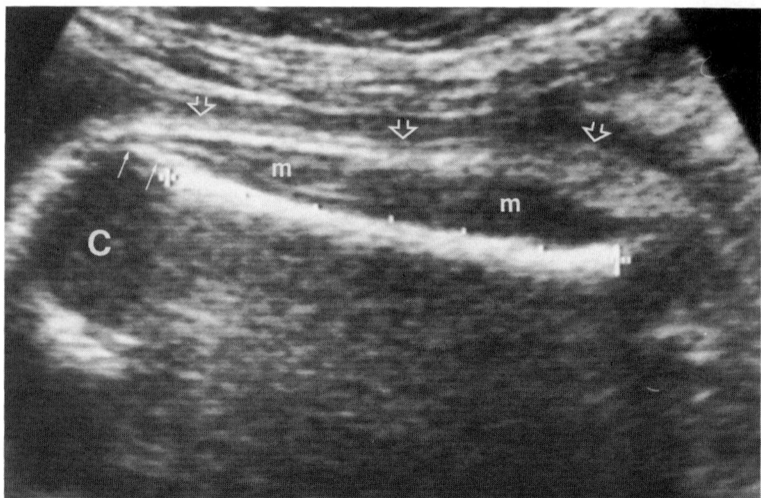

Figure 124–29. Ossified femoral shaft is marked for measurement (+), excluding the distal femur "spike" (*thin arrows*). Hypoechoic thigh muscles (m) lie deep to the subcutaneous and cutaneous tissues (*open arrows*).

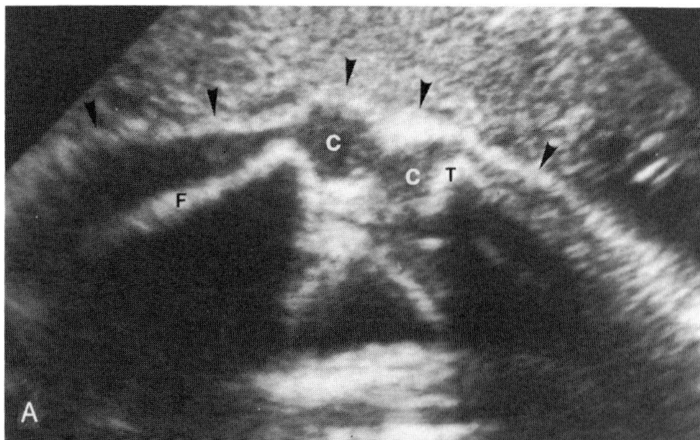

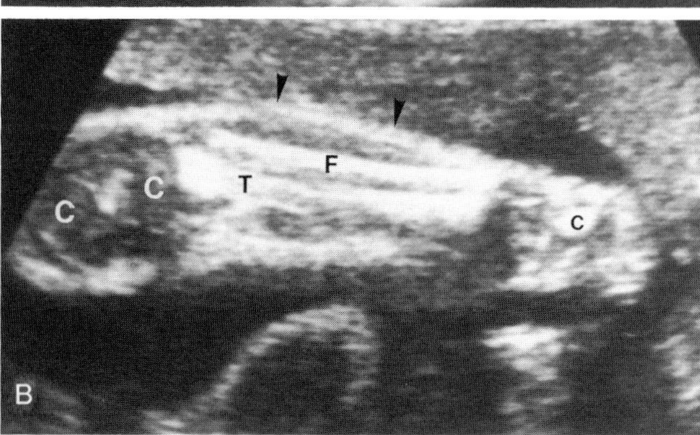

Figure 124–30. *A*, Longitudinal image of knee shows distal femur (F) and proximal tibia (T) with their articular cartilages (c). *Arrowheads* indicate skin surfaces anteriorly. *B*, Scanning distally reveals the tibia (T) and fibula (F). Specific individual bone measurements are possible. (c = calcaneus.)

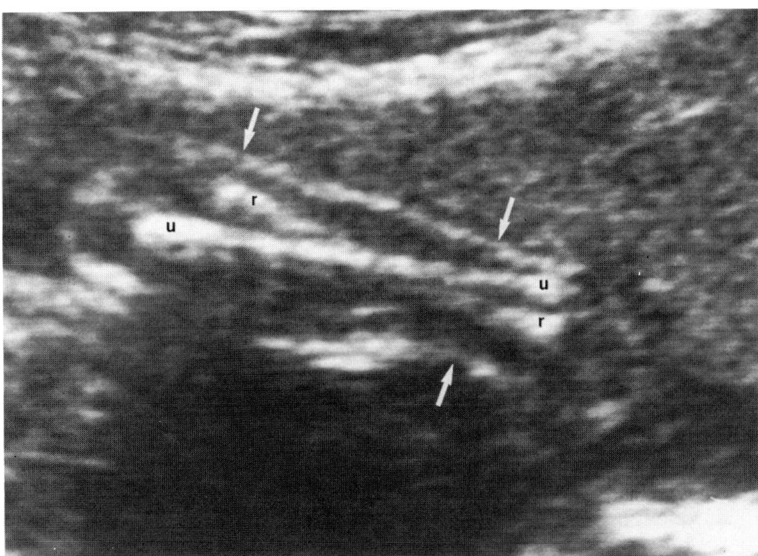

Figure 124–31. The radius (r) and ulna (u) are in a pronated position. While the ulna extends further into the elbow, both terminate at about the same level in the wrist. *Arrows* mark skin margins.

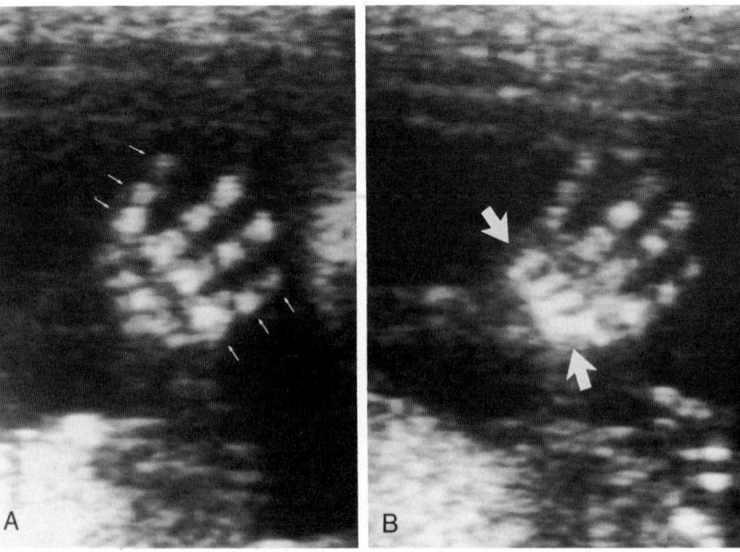

Figure 124–32. Hand. *A*, Individual phalanges (*arrows*) can usually be identified. *B*, Slight probe movement optimizes images of the metacarpals (*arrows*).

The femur length is the only routinely documented long-bone measurement. It is used in the assessment of fetal age and growth as well as a screen for generalized skeletal dysplasias. Only the ossified portion of the femur is measured, from its proximal end near the greater trochanter to its far end at the distal metaphysis. It should appear uniformly echogenic and cast a distal shadow to ensure the correct plane (Figs. 124–28 and 124–29).

Although documentation of all four extremities is not necessary, the presence of grossly normal bones and soft tissues to the levels of the hands and feet should be confirmed during real-time scanning. Imaging of specific bones is possible by careful progression from one segment to the next (e.g., scanning from the pelvis to the femur), then rotation of the probe as necessary through the cartilages of the knee to image the tibia/fibula and further distally the foot (Fig. 124–30). Long-bone length and configuration, joint alignment, and soft tissues can all be evaluated (Fig. 124–31). With optimal fetal positioning, individual digits can be imaged (Fig. 124–32).

Bibliography

Bowerman RA: Atlas of Normal Fetal Ultrasonographic Anatomy. St. Louis, Mosby-Year Book, 1992.

Cardoza JD, Goldstein RB, Filly RA: Exclusion of fetal ventriculomegaly with a single measurement: The width of the lateral ventricular atrium. Radiology 169:711–714, 1988.

Filly RA, Simpson GF, Linkowski G: Fetal spine morphology and maturation during the second trimester: Sonographic evaluation. J Ultrasound Med 6:631–636, 1987.

Kurtz, AB, Goldberg BB: Obstetrical Measurements in Ultrasound, A Reference Manual. Chicago, Year Book, 1988.

Mahoney BS, Callen PW, Filly RA, et al: The fetal cisterna magna. Radiology 153:773–776, 1984.

Mahoney BS, Filly RA: High resolution sonographic assessment of the fetal extremities. J Ultrasound Med 3:489–498, 1984.

McGahan JP: Sonography of the fetal heart: Findings on the four-chamber view. AJR 156:547–553, 1991.

Pretorius DH, Gosink BB, Clautice-Engle T, et al: Sonographic evaluation of the fetal stomach: Significance of nonvisualization. AJR 151:987–989, 1988.

Standards and Guidelines for Performance of the Antepartum Obstetrical Examination. Bethesda, MD, American Institute of Ultrasound in Medicine, 1990.

125 Miscellaneous Fetal Abnormalities

James D. Bowie

Any sonographic examination of the pregnant patient entails three separate tasks. The first is a general survey of the pregnancy. This includes evaluation of the number of fetuses present; their position; the placenta, cord, and membranes; the amount of amniotic fluid; and the uterus and adnexas. The second requires measurement of various fetal structures in an attempt to establish gestational age; determine or monitor fetal growth; and, in some cases, estimate fetal size or proportion. The third task is to evaluate the fetus by examination of either its structure, i.e., imaging of gross anatomy, or its activity, which may indicate functional capabilities.

As suggested in the first two chapters in this section, which of these tasks receives top priority depends on the clinical problems being evaluated. The precision with which an individual problem can be defined often also establishes the capacity to answer it. Unfortunately, many nonobstetricians, including radiologists, feel very uncomfortable with the clinical problems posed by the pregnant patient. The following chapters deal with some of these problems but certainly not every clinical question that an imager may encounter.

Patients are referred to sonographers for evaluation of a variety of potential morphologic malformations. The most common reason is evaluation regarding a positive family history of a significant fetal abnormality, usually affecting a previous sibling. Other reasons include a positive screening test, such as abnormal maternal serum alpha-fetoprotein; suspicion of a defect on prior ultrasound; and known risk factors. This latter category includes maternal age, exposure to drugs or toxins, and certain maternal disease conditions.

In these patients the abnormalities most frequently detected sonographically involve (1) the neural axis, (2) the urinary tract, (3) the gastrointestinal tract, (4) various fetal masses, (5) the limbs, and (6) the heart and great vessels. Most of these abnormalities are discussed in separate chapters in this section. This chapter deals with the syndromes that affect multiple organ systems, chromosomal abnormalities, and various but relatively frequent fetal masses not described elsewhere. This is by no means an exhaustive treatment of these disorders, and the reader is directed to the suggested reading at the end of the chapter for more detailed information.

FETAL MASSES

Most fetal masses are covered in other sections. Those involving the surface of the fetus include cystic hygromas, lymphangiomas, hemangiomas, and some teratomas. Intrathoracic masses that have been described include cystic adenomatoid malformation of the lung and pulmonary cysts. Teratomas have been described in intracranial, cervical, intrathoracic, abdominal, and sacrococcygeal locations (Fig. 125–1). Organ extrophies and neural tube defects belong in this group, and the reader should remember that when these two abnormalities occur in association with amniotic bands, their location and appearance can be very atypical.

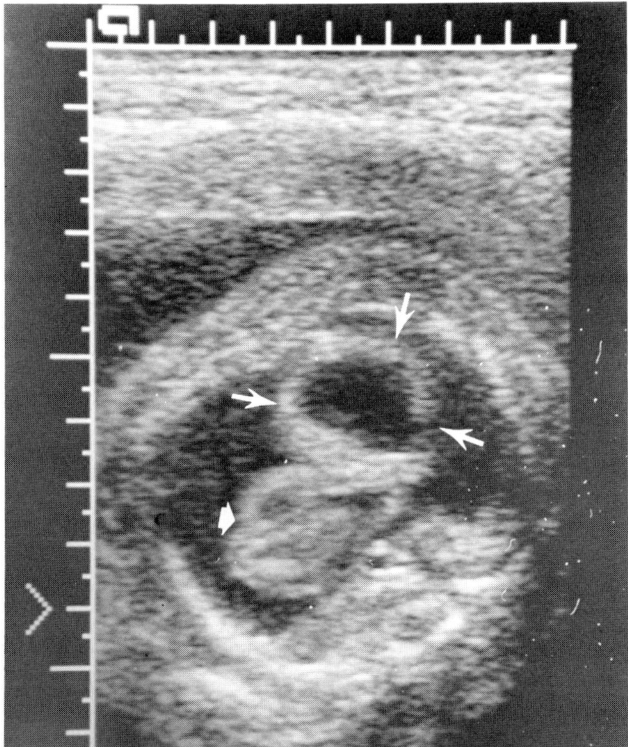

Figure 125–1. A mediastinal teratoma *(arrows)* displaces the heart posteriorly *(arrowhead)*. The hypoechoic region around these two structures is pleural fluid, and the skin thickening is a result of hydrops.

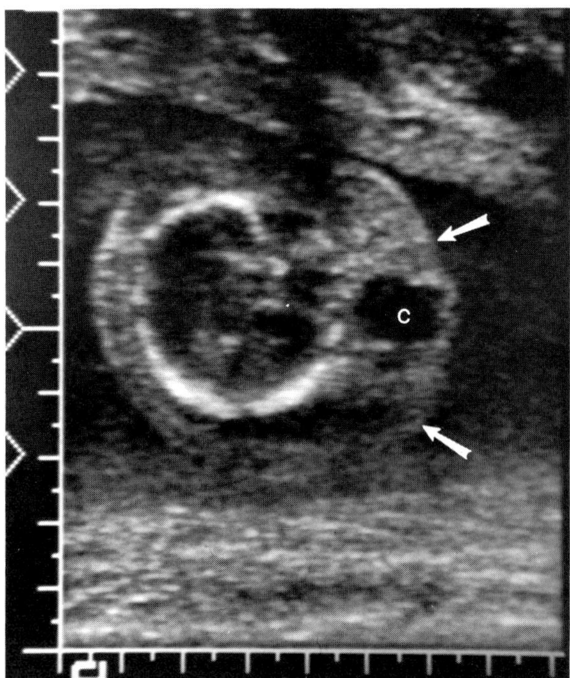

Figure 125–2. Small cystic hygroma (C) and marked subcutaneous edema *(arrows)* in a fetus with Turner's syndrome.

Cystic Hygromas

Cystic hygromas are among the more frequently encountered fetal masses. They have been diagnosed as early as the first trimester. In approximately 70 to 75 per cent of cases of intrauterine cystic hygromas, the chromosomal pattern is 45XO (Turner's syndrome); about 20 per cent are 46XX; and 1 to 6 per cent are 46XY. Cystic hygromas are also associated with fetal alcohol syndrome, trisomies 18 and 21, deletion of the short arm of 18 (18 p-syndrome), and Noonan's syndrome. Noonan's syndrome resembles Turner's syndrome in its expression, i.e., short stature, broad forehead, micrognathia, web neck, and right-sided congenital heart disease, but mental deficiency occurs more frequently in Noonan's syndrome than in Turner's syndrome. It may be familial but has no identified chromosomal abnormality, and the inheritance pattern is not determined. Cystic hygromas are typically found posterior and lateral in the neck (Fig. 125–2). Sonographic visualization of a midline septum in a posterolateral cystic neck mass in the absence of a bony defect distinguishes a cystic hygroma from an encephalocele. In larger cystic hygromas multiple septa are often seen, and in smaller ones the characteristic septum may be difficult to identify. Sometimes these masses are so large that they are mistaken for the amniotic cavity itself by inexperienced examiners.

Intradermal lymphangiectasia, or fetal edema, may occur in association with cystic hygroma, and is associated with a poor prognosis. Cystic hygromas occur in the lateral neck, axilla, groin, and mediastinum, but, to my knowledge, their in utero appearance has not been described. In theory, hemangiomas of the skin could be mistaken for cystic hygroma, but all published cases of facial hemangiomas have been echogenic masses that do not resemble the fluid collection of cystic hygroma. Cutaneous hemangiomas in other areas, however, may be echolucent and, when seen in association with asymmetric limb hypertrophy, are part of the Klippel-Trenaunay-Weber syndrome. Asymmetric limb hypertrophy is also seen with some congenital tumors and the neurocutaneous syndromes.

LUNG MASSES

Fetal lung masses are usually either cystic adenomatoid malformations (CAMs) of the lung (Fig. 125–3) or various lung cysts. Intrathoracic bowel segments secondary to a diaphragmatic hernia or a diaphragmatic or mediastinal teratoma may be mistaken for a fetal lung mass. A dilated bronchus has been described as an echo-free pulmonary mass and an extralobar pulmonary sequestration as an echogenic pulmonary mass. The latter two conditions appear to be rare.

CAMs may be divided into three types, each of which has different sonographic appearances. Type I is largely hypoechoic and consists of single or multiple large cysts. Type II contains multiple small cysts that are usually recognized sonographically. It is useful to distinguish this type, since it is frequently associated with additional renal and gastrointestinal abnormalities of the fetus. In type III, the lesion is noncystic sonographically, but the microscopic cysts create innumerable interfaces with the sonographic beam. The lesion therefore appears as an echogenic lung mass. In most cases of CAM there are associated fetal hydrops and polyhydramnios, which are associated with a poor prognosis; however, type I in the absence of hydrops has a generally better prognosis.

DIAPHRAGMATIC HERNIA

In about three fourths of cases, diaphragmatic hernia occurs on the left side. More than 90 per cent of left diaphragmatic hernias occur through the foramen of Bochdalek. About half of these infants have associated malformations, usually involving the central nervous system (CNS). Sonographically, the major features are polyhydramnios, mediastinal displacement, and inability to show normal upper abdominal anatomy. While sonographers are encouraged to look for normal fetal diaphragms, most antenatal diagnoses of diaphragmatic hernia are made either on the basis of the above indirect signs or by seeing fetal stomach, bowel, or gallbladder displaced to the level of the heart. Since slight obliquity in the scan plane can give the appearance of displaced abdominal organs, this condition can be very difficult to diagnose.

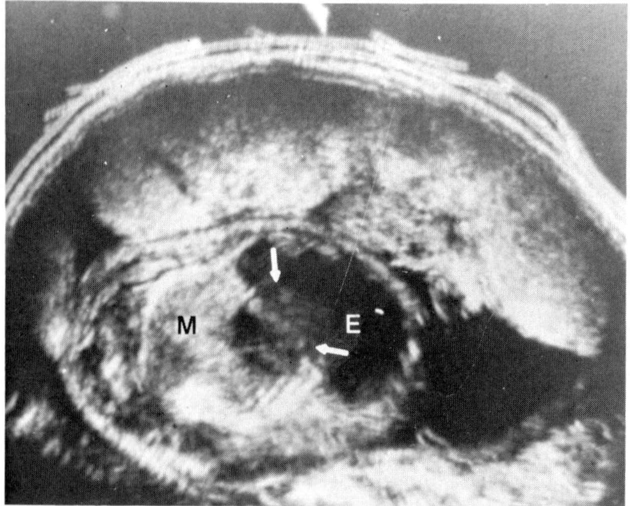

Figure 125–3. A solid-appearing mass (M) is seen to the side of the fetal heart *(arrows)*. A pleural effusion (E) is present as well. This fetus had a **cystic adenomatoid malformation of the lung.**

PLEURAL EFFUSION

The presence of fluid in the fetal pleural space is usually the result of a more generalized process such as fetal hydrops. It has been described in conjunction with diaphragmatic hernia and occasionally occurs as an isolated phenomenon. An isolated pleural effusion usually results from abnormal development of the thoracic duct, which leads to chylothorax in the newborn. There may be associated polyhydramnios, and the effusion can be small or large, unilateral or bilateral. The overall mortality associated with a fetal pleural effusion is about 15 per cent but is worse when the effusions are large or bilateral or develop early in pregnancy.

CHROMOSOMAL ABNORMALITIES

The major role of sonography in these disorders is to provide guidance for amniocentesis or chorionic villi sampling. It has been mentioned that cystic hygromas may suggest Turner's syndrome and, recently, that thickening of the skin over the posterior neck may suggest Down's syndrome. About half of the babies with Down's syndrome have congenital heart disease, the most common of which are atrioventricular canal, ventriculoseptal defect, and atrial septal defect. Careful antenatal echocardiography may detect these lesions.

Triploidy (69XXX or 69XXY) may affect as many as 1 per cent of conceptuses. The great majority spontaneously abort early in pregnancy, and survival beyond 22 weeks is rare, with no reported survival beyond the neonatal period. The chapter on gestational trophoblastic disease (Chap. 142) should be reviewed for this condition. The most salient sonographic feature is early intrauterine growth retardation (IUGR) with body asymmetry; i.e., the head is larger than the abdomen. There is usually oligohydramnios, and the placenta may be thick or hydropic. CNS abnormalities are common, including hydrocephaly, holoprosencephaly, micro-ophthalmia, and hypertelorism. Other abnormalities may include low-set posterior ears, micrognathia, syndactyly, ambiguous genitalia, congenital heart defects, pulmonary hypoplasia, and renal dysplasia.

MULTIPLE ORGAN SYSTEMS

Drugs

One major group of fetuses with multiple organ system involvement is those affected by mutagens (drugs, chemicals, infections, and maternal disease). Only a brief survey of these problems can be offered here. The most frequently used drugs today are alcohol and tobacco. Both have been shown to produce adverse effects on the fetus. It is not clear how much alcohol is required to affect the fetus, but there does seem to be a relationship between heavier doses and worse outcomes. The major features of the fetal alcohol syndrome are IUGR, facial dysmorphogenesis, and CNS abnormalities (usually mental retardation). Cardiac defects (atrial septal defect, ventricular septal defect, and tetralogy of Fallot) may also be seen. The facial dysmorphogenesis should be of interest to sonographers, since at least some of the features may be apparent, including microcephaly, maxillary hypoplasia, micrognathia, and cleft palate. Although there has been some suggestion that tobacco use in pregnancy is associated with an increased incidence of abruptio placentae, placenta previa, or cleft lip and palate in the fetus, the major effect of this drug is IUGR. Other drugs that may produce effects on the fetus are too numerous to cover in this chapter. Warfarin, phenytoin, diazepam, and the polychlorinated biphenyls are among the drugs that have especially severe fetal effects.

Infectious Agents

Infectious agents that produce adverse fetal effects include rubella, varicella, toxoplasmosis, cytomegalovirus, and syphilis. The role of sonography in detecting whether a fetus is affected by these conditions is unknown. Both cytomegalovirus and toxoplasmosis have been associated with fetal hydrops as well as fetal periventricular calcifications and occasional hydrocephalus. Toxoplasmosis and rubella have been associated with microcephaly and with micro-ophthalmia in some affected infants. Early rubella infection is associated with congenital cardiac defects. All intrauterine infections have been associated with early IUGR.

Diabetes Mellitus

It is well-recognized that the infant of a diabetic mother is at much greater risk for a variety of complications, including macrosomia, small left colon, and respiratory distress syndrome. It is less well-recognized but equally important to remember that these fetuses are at increased risk for a wide variety of congenital anomalies. The mechanism for these abnormalities is unknown, but the renal and cardiac systems are often affected and the caudal regression syndrome seems to be the one most unique to children of diabetic mothers. Perhaps as many as one sixth of babies born to diabetic mothers have some evidence of the caudal regression syndrome. Most of these are very mild and consist of minor coccygeal or sacral defects. Sacral agenesis, however, is relatively common, and the more severe forms include agenesis of lower vertebral segments and sireniform (mermaid) malformations. This last condition is characterized by rotation and fusion of the lower extremities and absence or fusion of the fibulas. It is associated with bilateral renal agenesis, blind-ending colon, and absence of the external genitalia and anus. The caudal regression syndrome is also associated with meningocele, hypoplastic femur, arthrogryposis, and urinary tract abnormalities (Fig. 125–4). It may also be related to the VATER association of abnormalities (vertebral anomalies, ventricular septal defects, anal atresia, tracheoesophageal fistula with esophageal atresia, dysplasia of the radius, renal anomalies, and several other anomalies including single umbilical artery).

Other Syndromes That Affect Multiple Organ Systems

Although the VATER association appears to be more than a random one, there is no known mechanism or etiology for it and the pattern of occurrence appears to be sporadic.

Most of the important conditions that affect multiple organ systems in utero have been mentioned above or are described in other chapters. Several of the remaining conditions are autosomal recessive and appear to be closely related to each other. For example, Jeune's syndrome is either related to or part of a spectrum of Ellis–van Creveld syndrome. Both have asphyxiating thoracic dysplasia as a feature that is seen sonographically as a flat anteroposterior dimension of the chest. Both may also have renal abnormalities and both are short-limbed dwarf syndromes but, unlike Jeune's syndrome, Ellis–van Creveld syndrome has polydactyly and about half of patients with Ellis–van Creveld syndrome have congenital heart disease. Robert's syndrome is closely related to Meckel-Gruber syndrome and has a spectrum of presentations, but usually there are an occipital encephalocele and dysplastic kidneys. In both of these conditions, the kidneys are large and echogenic sonographically. Meckel's syndrome may also be associated with microcephaly, hydrocephaly, hypotelorism, cleft lip, and cleft palate. Campomelic dysplasia is another autosomal recessive condition associated with cleft palate but primarily characterized by abnormally short limbs that are bowed anteriorly. Absent scapula, macrocephaly, and hydronephrosis are also seen in campomelic dysplasia.

Amniotic Disruption Complex

One condition that affects multiple organs deserves special mention. This has been given a number of names, including amniotic band syndrome, limb/body wall deficiency syndrome, and amniotic band sequence (Fig. 125–5). The importance of recognizing this condition is that its occurrence is sporadic, yet its protean manifestations cause it to be mistaken for other conditions with increased recurrence risks. Often the sonographer is more instrumental in suggesting the correct diagnosis than is the pathologist. The syndrome is seen in association with fibrous mesodermic bands from the chorionic side of the amnion. This is the reason disruption of the amnion has been hypothesized to be a cause of the disease. Some of the associated defects are easy to understand, since entanglement of the fetal extremities by the bands appears to cause amputations or distal edema of the extremity. Other defects are seen that are harder to explain, and a band may not always be seen as an obvious cause.

Some findings that suggest this syndrome are asymmetric amputations of extremities or extremity edema, syndactyly originating distally; gastroschisis in an unusual location or with exteriorization of liver; asymmetric anencephaly or lateral encephaloceles; unusual clefting of the face, lips, or palate; and scoliosis or postural deformities. If sought sonographically, the bands can usually be seen. These may not correspond to the identified defects but are attached to the fetus and either move with it or restrict its movement. These bands must be distinguished from other intrauterine membranes that are independent of the fetus. Oligohydramnios is often present in these cases, making identification of the bands difficult. However, polyhydramnios may also occur, and amniotic fluid volume is not a distinguishing feature.

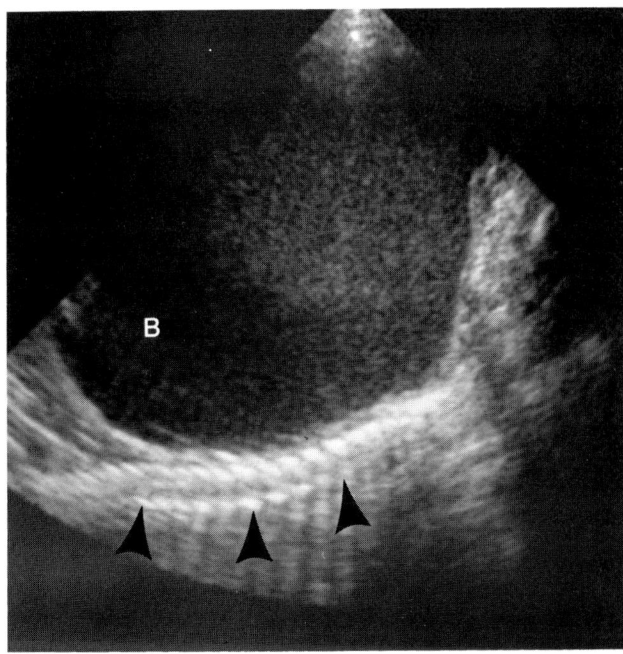

Figure 125–4. The fetal spine can be seen posteriorly *(arrowheads)*. The entire fetal abdomen contained a large fluid structure with swirling echogenic contents (B). This proved to be a massively distended fetal bladder in a fetus with anal atresia, urethral atresia, and sacral agenesis as part of the caudal regression syndrome.

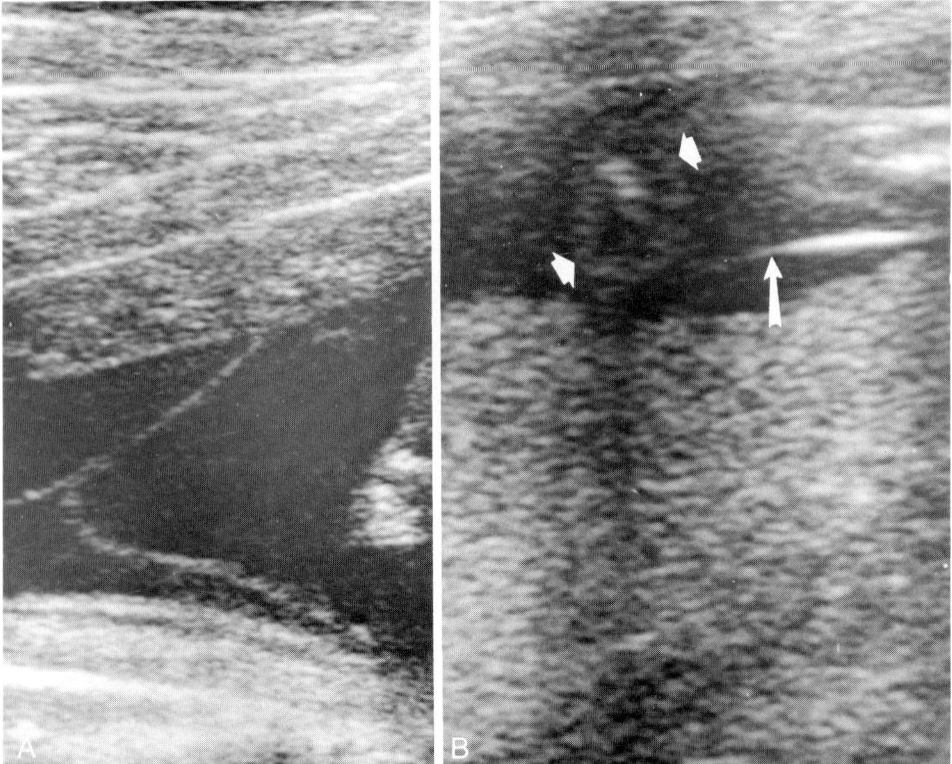

Figure 125–5. *A,* **Multiple bands** are seen within the amniotic cavity. *B,* **One band** *(arrow)* was seen to be adherent to a fetal limb *(arrowheads*). The fetus was born with amputation of several digits of the affected hand.

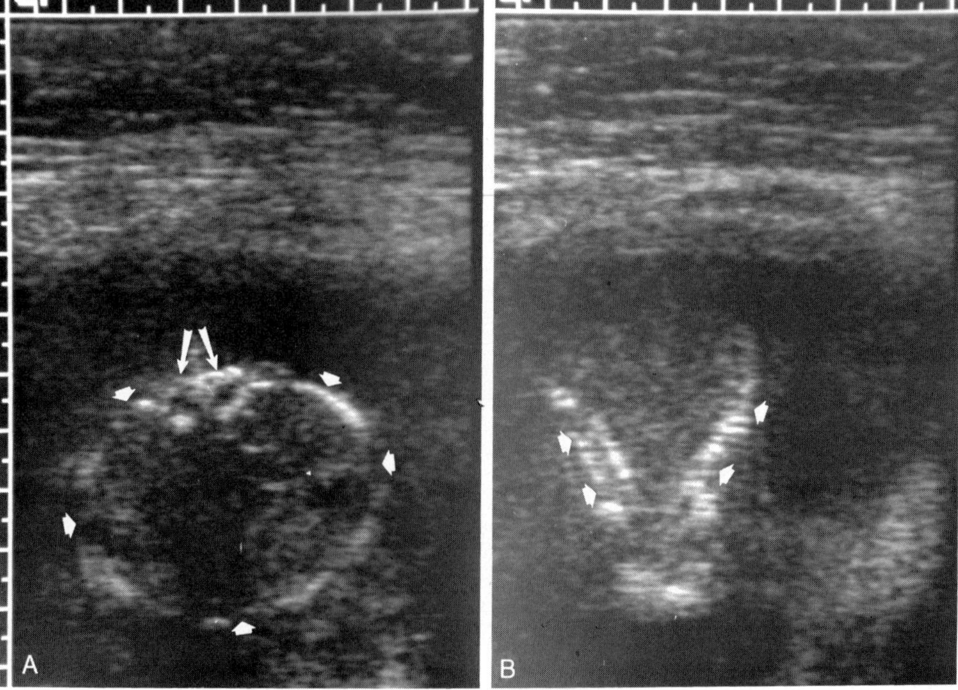

Figure 125–6. *A,* The outlined oval (*short arrows*) is **two conjoined fetal heads** with a small rudimentary face marked by the closely placed orbits *(arrows). B,* **Two separate spines** *(arrowheads)* are seen to connect at the base of the conjoined head. Four lower extremities were also observed.

CONJOINED TWINS

Conjoined twins is a rare event that results from late twinning of a single zygote. The estimated incidence of this phenomenon is between 1 in 50,000 and 1 in 100,000 births. In the two most common forms of conjoining, the twins are face to face and joined at the anterior chest (thoracopagus) or abdomen (omphalopagus). The next most common forms of conjoined twins are side-by-side attachment or facing away and joined at the ischia (ischiopagus) or buttocks (pygopagus). Combinations that involve joining at the head are less common and may include joining of other portions of the body (Fig. 125–6). Sonographically, signs have been described such as observing a fixed relative position of twins, but the real distinguishing feature is demonstration of continuity of skin between the two fetuses. The goal of the sonographer is to identify the organs that are conjoined and to predict the extent of involvement. This cannot always be done accurately, but the sonographer can be extremely useful in giving information that is necessary for the perinatal decisions involved in this rare condition.

FETAL HYDROPS AND ASCITES

It is not always possible for the ultrasound examiner to distinguish between fetal hydrops, which is a generalized edema state in the fetus (Fig. 125–7), and fluid collections limited to a single space, such as pleural effusions or ascites. This distinction should be made whenever possible, however. In addition, the sonographer must be careful not to mistake conditions that result in thickening of the subcutaneous tissue for fetal hydrops. This can happen with thanatophoric dwarfs, lymphangiectasia, and macrosomatic fetuses.

Hydrops fetalis has a rather poor overall survival, estimated to be from one fourth to one third of those affected. It has traditionally been divided into immune causes and nonimmune causes. Most cases of immune hydrops are the result of Rh sensitization. With increasing use of RhoGAM, non-Rh immune hydrops becomes a higher percentage of these cases. The two most common causes of non-Rh immune hydrops are anti-B and anti-Kell antibodies.

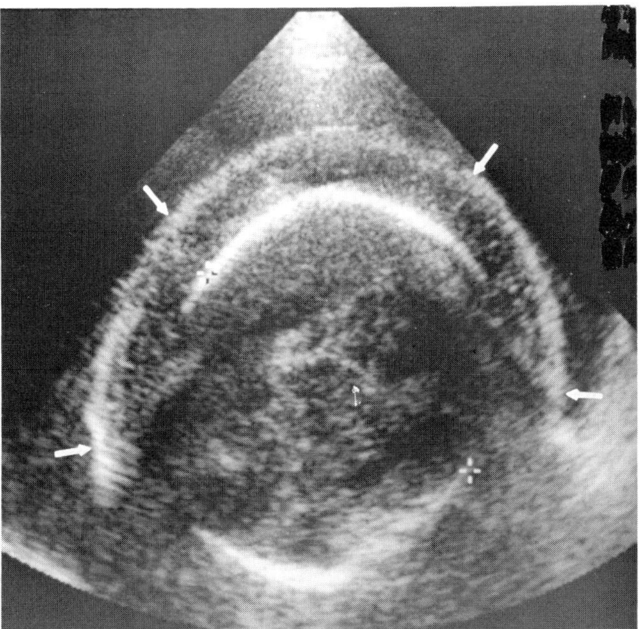

Figure 125–7. Marked edema of the fetal scalp *(arrows)* is noted in this hydropic fetus. *Asterisks* are on the fetal skull.

TABLE 125–1. CAUSES OF FETAL HYDROPS

I. Cardiac
  A. Arrhythmias
  B. Structural abnormalities
    1. Tetralogy of Fallot
    2. Hypoplastic left heart
    3. Ebstein's anomaly
    4. Subaortic stenosis
    5. ASD, VSD
    6. Cardiac and mediastinal tumors
II. Pulmonary
  A. Cystic adenomatoid malformation of the lung
  B. Pulmonary lymphangiectasia
  C. Pulmonary hypoplasia
III. Renal
  A. Congenital nephrosis
  B. Renal dysplasia
  C. Renal vein thrombosis
IV. Hematologic
  A. Alpha-thalassemia (homozygous)
  B. Hemophilia A
V. Vascular
  A. Twin-twin transfusions
  B. Fetal-maternal bleed
  C. Fetal arteriovenous malformations (sacral teratomas)
VI. Congenital Anomalies
  A. Chromosomal
    1. Trisomy 13
    2. Trisomy 18
    3. Trisomy 21
    4. Turner's syndrome
    5. XX/XY mosaicism
  B. Other
    1. Achondroplasia
    2. Lymphangiectasia
    3. Pterygium syndrome
    4. Cystic hygroma
VII. Intrauterine Infections
  A. TORCH
  B. Leptospirosis
  C. Congenital hepatitis
  D. Chagas' disease
VIII. Miscellaneous
  A. Myotonic dystrophy
  B. Fetal neuroblastomatosis
  C. Storage diseases
IX. Maternal
  A. Diabetes
  B. Toxemia
X. Placental/Umbilical Cord
  A. Umbilical vein thrombosis
  B. Chorionic vein thrombosis
  C. Placental chorioangioma
XI. Idiopathic and Other

Causes of nonimmune hydrops are so numerous as to defy classification, although many attempts have been made. Table 125–1 is a composite of two classifications. Virtually the entire fetus, umbilical cord, and placenta must be studied carefully by the sonographer in these cases. The most important observation the sonographer can make is the presence of a cardiac arrhythmia, since this may be a reversible cause of fetal hydrops. The tachyrhythmias (supraventricular tachycardia and atrial flutter) and bradyrhythmias (heart blocks) have both been associated with fetal hydrops. Other diagnoses that can be made sonographically to explain fetal hydrops include structural heart defects, cardiac masses, cystic adenomatoid malformation of the lung, pulmonary hypoplasia, lymphangiectasia, multiple pterygium syndrome, mediastinal teratomas, sacral teratomas, and achondroplasia. In addition, umbilical vein thrombosis and chorioangioma of the placenta are detectable by ultrasound. Thus it bears repeating that the entire fetus, cord, and placenta need to be examined in these cases.

The clinical evaluation of patients with fetal hydrops begins with a thorough ultrasound, maternal blood grouping, antibody screen, Kleihauer-Betke test, and serology. Depending on these results, TORCH titers (toxoplasmosis, rubella, cytomegalovirus, and herpes simplex), a G-6-PD test, hemoglobin electrophoresis, antinuclear antibody titers, a glucose tolerance test, and even fetal amniotic fluid for karyotype and delta O.D.-450 need to be considered.

Fetal ascites in the absence of hydrops usually results from abnormalities of the gastrointestinal or genitourinary system of the fetus. Common gastrointestinal causes of fetal ascites include small bowel atresias, perforations, and volvulus. The genitourinary causes are usually related to obstruction, often at the bladder outlet. Other causes include familial cirrhosis, systemic infections (especially toxoplasmosis and cytomegalovirus), chylous ascites, and torsion of ovarian cysts. Unfortunately, in many cases the cause is never determined. Fetal ascites has been described as disappearing spontaneously with no known cause in rare instances.

Bibliography

Campbell S, Pearce JM: The prenatal diagnosis of fetal structural anomalies by ultrasound. Clin Obstet Gynecol 10:475–506, 1983.

Chervenak FA, Isaacson G, Tortora M: A sonographic study of fetal cystic hygromas. J Clin Ultrasound 13:311–315, 1985.

Hill LM: Effects of drugs and chemicals on the fetus and newborn (2 parts). Mayo Clin Proc 59:707–716, 755–765, 1984.

Jones KL: Smith's Recognizable Patterns of Human Malformation, 4th ed. Philadelphia, WB Saunders Company, 1988.

Mahony BS, Filly RA, Callen PW, Golbus MS: The amniotic band syndrome: Antenatal sonographic diagnosis and potential pitfalls. Am J Obstet Gynecol 152:638, 1985.

McKusick's Mendelian Inheritance in Man, 6th ed. Baltimore, Johns Hopkins University Press, 1983.

126 Prenatal Diagnosis of Anomalies of the Central Nervous System

Gianluigi Pilu, Roberto Romero, Antonella Perolo, and Giampaolo Grisolia

Due to both the frequency and severity of congenital anomalies arising from or involving the central nervous system, the interrogation of this area of fetal anatomy has always been a source of major concern for obstetrics sonographers.

In the early 1970s, prenatal diagnosis was possible for only a small group of catastrophic lesions. In more recent years, rapid advances in ultrasound technology have resulted in the introduction of gray-scale imaging and high-resolution, real-time ultrasound, allowing the identification of very subtle details of fetal anatomy. Nevertheless, the prominent developmental changes that occur in the cerebrum well beyond the end of embryogenesis and throughout the entire gestation have proved to be a significant source of confusion for sonographers, and it took years before the different fetal intracranial structures could be accurately mapped.

At present, the different appearance of the fetal brain in the different gestational ages is well-understood. Nomograms of the normal size of the head, ventricular system, and selected parts of the cerebrum, including the frontal lobe and cerebellum, have been developed to assist the early recognition of intracranial anomalies. The recent introduction of transvaginal high-resolution sonography has extended diagnosis into the first trimester. A rational approach to the evaluation of the fetal brain in the second and third trimester has also been standardized, allowing routine screening for the vast majority of cerebral abnormalities.

In this chapter, we review the principles of embryogenesis and gestational development of the brain and provide guidelines for sonographic identification and management of fetal abnormalities.

EMBRYOGENESIS AND DEVELOPMENTAL ANATOMY OF THE CENTRAL NERVOUS SYSTEM

The differentiation and development of the neural axis have been extensively reviewed. In this section, we do not try to give a comprehensive overview of this exceedingly complex topic. Rather, we focus on those aspects of embryogenesis that are relevant for the understanding of congenital abnormalities amenable to prenatal diagnosis. We also consider the morphologic modifications that normally occur during the first half of pregnancy that can be recognized with ultrasound.

The nervous system originally derives from the neural plate, a dorsal thickening of the ectoderm that can be recognized as early as the 14th day of development. The essential steps leading to the formation and early differentiation of the cerebrum are summarized in Figure 126–1. The faster growth rate of the lateral portions of the plate results in the formation of two longitudinal folds demarcating an internal groove. The folds fuse with each other in the midline, starting the transformation of the groove into a tube at about the midportion of the embryonic disk. Closure proceeds then cephalad and caudally. From 20 to 24 days the neural tube is almost entirely closed, the only exception being two openings at the extremities—the anterior and posterior neuropores. The anterior neuropore undergoes obliteration first, followed by the posterior neuropore at about

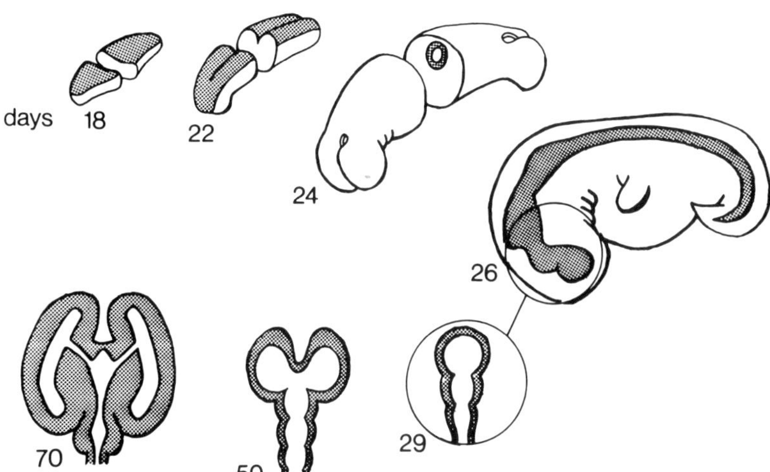

Figure 126–1. Schematic representation of human central nervous system development. Two main stages can be recognized. The first one, commonly referred to as dorsal induction, leads to the closure of the neural tube. The second stage, ventral induction, leads to the sagittal sedimentation and differentiation of the nervous axis.

24 to 26 days. This first stage of nervous development is often referred to as *dorsal induction.*

At 26 days, the rostral portion of the neural tube is cleaved along the horizontal planes, giving rise to the three primary vesicles of the brain: the prosencephalon, mesencephalon, and rhombencephalon. Two further cleavages occur in the following weeks, leading to the subdivision of the prosencephalon into the telencephalon and diencephalon and subdivision of the rhombencephalon into the metencephalon and myelencephalon.

The cerebral hemispheres originate from two paired diverticula ballooning out of the telencephalon. At the same time, the diencephalon—the primordium of the optic thalami—gives rise to two anterior paired diverticula; the optic bulbs; and two unpaired buds on the median plane, the anterior neurohypophysis and the posterior pineal body. The mesencephalon will form the cerebral peduncles and quadrigeminal plate. The metencephalon will develop into the pons, cerebellum, and rostrad portion of the fourth ventricle, while the myelencephalon will give origin to the medulla oblongata and caudad portion of the fourth ventricle.

Cleavage of the primitive cerebrum along four horizontal planes, leading to the formation of the five primary cerebral vesicles, results in constriction and in secondary enlargements of the cavity of the neural tube that will originate in time the ventricular system. The cavity contained within the telencephalon (the telocele) undergoes paired symmetrical division and diverticulation along the sagittal plane, with the formation of two distinct cavities that will give rise to the lateral ventricles. This process of paired diverticulation is commonly referred to as *ventral induction*, and it is closely related to the development of the median facial structures.

Cavities are now formed within the cerebrum. The cavities contained within the diencephalon (the diocele), mesencephalon (the mesocele), and metencephalon-myelencephalon (the metacele and myocele) form the third ventricle, aqueduct of Sylvius, and fourth ventricle, respectively. The remaining portion of the neural tube cavity develops into the ependymal canal, which runs within the spinal cord. At this time in gestation, transvaginal sonography with a high-frequency probe can consistently reveal significant details of the developing brain vesicles (Fig. 126–2).

The inward rotation of the rapidly growing hemispheres enfolds the thin membranous roof of the telocele (the thela choroidea) deep into the brain. The hemispheres are now separated by a thin mesenchymal layer that is the primordium of the falx cerebri. The cerebral cortex is quite thin at this point in gestation, most of the hemispheres being occupied by the primitive ventricular cavities. At about the sixth week of gestation, the medial wall of the lateral ventricles is seen bulging within the cavity, forming a fold that is rapidly covered by pseudostratified epithelium and molded by the proliferation of the underlying blood vessels into a villous structure—the choroid plexus. Both anatomic studies on animal models and sonographic investigation of the human fetus in utero have outlined the generous size of the choroid plexus, which fills the lateral ventricles almost entirely from about eight to 16 weeks. The peculiar echogenicity of this structure in vivo (Fig. 126–3) has been attributed to its high glycogen content, which is thought to represent a major energetic supply for the rapidly growing cerebrum.

While the choroid plexuses decrease in size relative to both brain mass and ventricular volume, the lateral ventricles are stretched and molded by the many developing processes occurring within the forebrain (growth of cerebral lobes, basal ganglia and thalami, and formation and deepening of the cerebral sulci). Assessment of the developmental anatomy of the ventricular system in the fetus has depended mainly on complex dissection procedures and barium casting techniques. More recently, real-time ultrasound has allowed documentation of the observations previously made on abortion specimens in a large number of living fetuses (Fig. 126–4). By the fourth month of gestation, the lateral ventricles are large in size compared with the cortex and intracranial cavity. At this time, the bodies and the frontal horns are short, the atrium being by far the most prominent portion. Both ontogenetically and phylogenetically, the last modification in the shape of the lateral ventricle to occur is the formation of the occipital horns, because only higher mammals and mature fetuses have an occipital lobe large enough to allow a well-defined internal cavity. The lateral ventricles are fully developed at about the 30th week of gestation. Because the fetus usually lies on one side inside the amniotic cavity, ultrasound examination of the intracranial contents mainly relies on axial scans. The obstetric sonographer should be familiar with the tomographic anatomy of the brain. Two axial planes that can be easily obtained in the vast majority of fetuses enable a proper assessment of the relevant cerebral anatomy. The first section plane is especially useful for assessing the integrity of the lateral ventricles (Fig. 126–5). By using this scanning plane, nomograms of frontal horns and atria have been established. The internal width of the atrium is constant between 15 weeks and term and has a mean value of 6 to 7 mm, with a standard deviation of less than 1 mm. Clinical studies suggest that a measurement of less than 10 mm is indicative of normalcy.

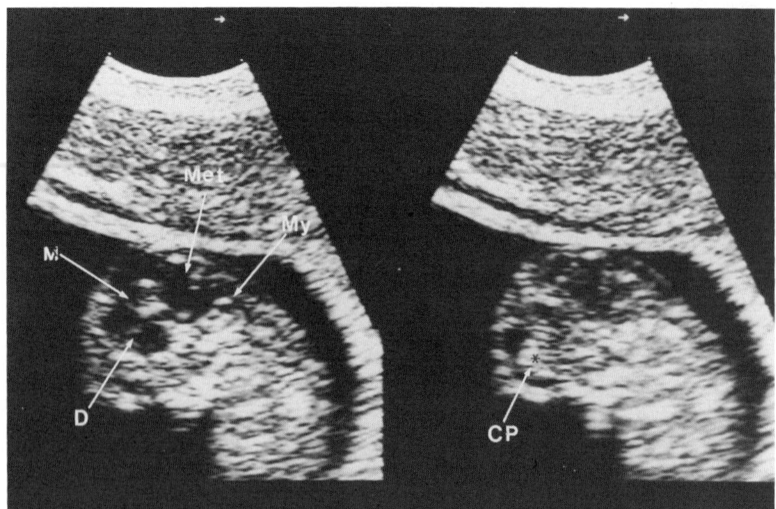

Figure 126–2. Sagittal views of the brain of an embryo at 9 weeks' menstrual age obtained with a 6.5-mHz vaginal transducer. In the midsagittal view *(left)*, the convolutions of the primary cerebral vesicles are easily recognized. From rostrad to caudad, the diencephalon (D), mesencephalon (M), metencephalon (Met), and myelencephalon (My) are seen. In the right panel, the scanning plane was moved slightly lateral to demonstrate the bright glomus of the choroid plexus (CP) within the developing hemisphere.

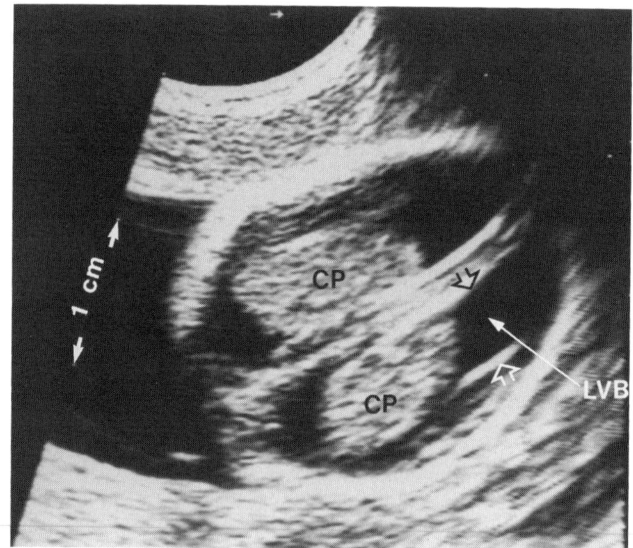

Figure 126–3. Axial scan of the brain of a fetus at 14 weeks' gestational age obtained with a 6.5-mHz vaginal transducer. The large, bright choroid plexus (CP) dominates the cerebral appearance. Notice the wide body of lateral ventricles (LVB) and the thin unlabeled cortex.

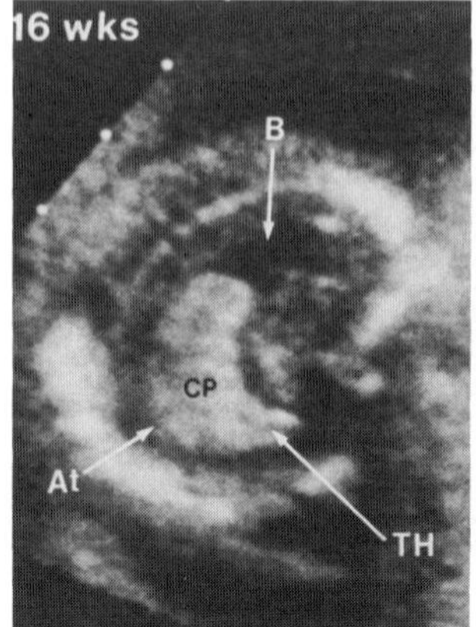

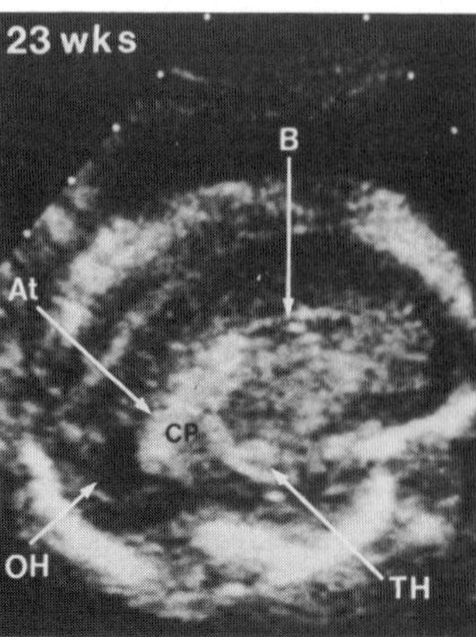

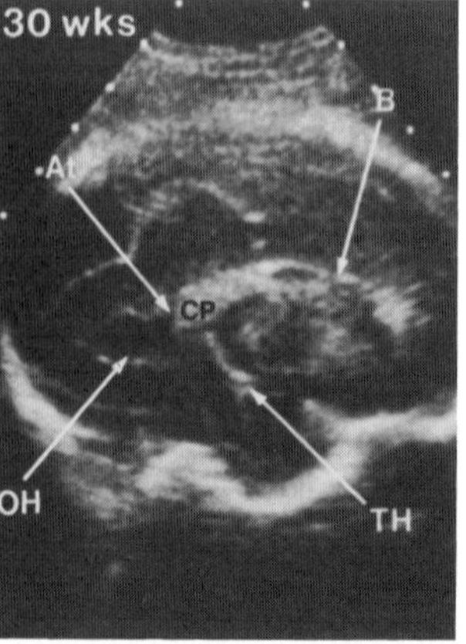

Figure 126–4. Parasagittal scans of the fetal head at 16, 23, and 30 weeks obtained with standard transabdominal sonography with either 5- or 3.5-mHz transducers. Note the modifications in the size and shape of the body (B), atrium (At), and temporal horns (TH) of lateral ventricles. At 16 weeks, the atrium is prominent and it ends blindly posteriorly, the occipital horn (OH) appearing only at about mid-gestation. At any gestational interval, the choroid plexus (CP) is seen filling the atrium entirely.

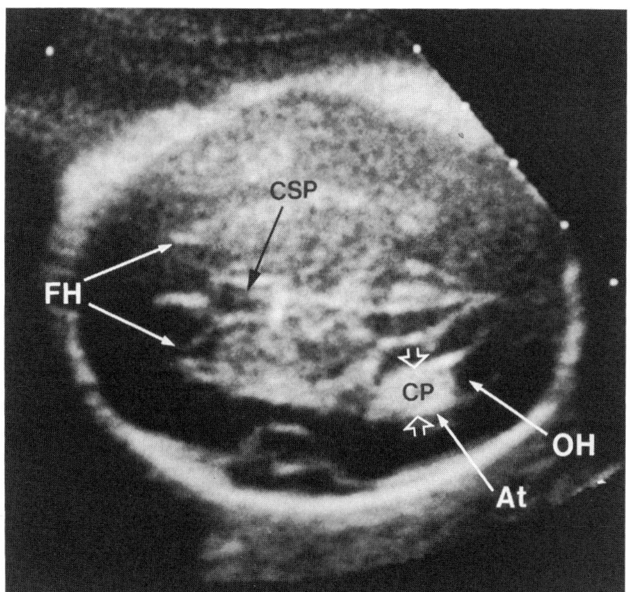

Figure 126–5. Axial scan of the fetal head at the level of frontal horns (FH), atria (At) and occipital horns (OH) of lateral ventricles. The choroid plexus (CP) fills the atrium entirely, being closely apposed to both the medial and lateral wall *(open arrows)*. (CSP = cavum septi pellucidum.) The vein of Galen cistern is seen as a triangular sonolucent space demarcated on both sides by the medial surface of the occipital lobes. Within this cistern, the great cerebral vein of Galen is clearly seen. Incomplete opercularization of the insula results in a wide fluid-filled fossa extending centrally on both sides of the brain.

Moving the transducer slightly caudad it is possible to image the plane that is commonly used for measuring the biparietal diameter and head circumference (Table 126–1). Eventually, a posterior angulation of the transducer allows demonstration of the posterior fossa structures (Fig. 126–6). A nomogram of the transverse cerebellar diameter is displayed in Table 126–1.

A few other anatomic structures will be considered in this section. The cavum septi pellucidi is a fluid-filled cavity between the leaves of the septum pellucidum. The cavum is largely patent in the fetus (see Figs. 126–5 and 126–6), and it decreases progressively in size during gestation, being sonographically recognizable in 40 to 60 per cent of normal newborn infants.

The distinctive feature of the human brain prior to the 22nd week of gestation is a peculiar smoothness. Only the calcarine and parieto-occipital fissures are discernible. In the following eight weeks, the rapid growth of the cerebral cortex leads to the formation of the rolandic fissure and of the cingulate, frontal, and parietal sulci. The formation of cortical convolutions proceeds steadily up to the 40th week, when tertiary sulci can be finally seen. Evaluation of the convolutional pattern is a well-established method to assess maturity in both pathologic and neonatal ultrasound studies. Cerebral sulci can be appreciated sonographically in utero as well (Fig. 126–7). However, adequate visualization requires the use of transfontanellar coronal and sagittal scans. Because these views can be obtained only in a minority of cases, this otherwise promising approach to the intrauterine estimation of fetal maturity has important limitations.

Development of the brain results in a conspicuous modification of the subarachnoid cisterns. Knowledge of the normal sonographic anatomy of the subarachnoid space is useful in both avoiding misinterpretation of normal sonograms and differentially diagnosing

TABLE 126–1. NOMOGRAM OF THE BIPARIETAL DIAMETER (BPD), HEAD CIRCUMFERENCE (HC), AND TRANSVERSE CEREBELLAR DIAMETER (TCD) THROUGHOUT GESTATION

	BPD			HC			TCD		
Week	.05th p	.50th p	.95th p	.05th p	.50th p	.95th p	.05th p	.50th p	.95th p
14	23	28	32	79	103	128	13	16	19
15	27	31	36	92	117	141	14	16	19
16	30	35	39	105	130	154	15	17	20
17	34	38	43	118	143	168	15	18	21
18	37	42	46	131	156	180	16	19	22
19	40	45	49	144	168	193	17	19	22
20	44	48	53	156	181	205	17	20	23
21	47	51	56	168	193	217	18	21	24
22	50	55	59	180	204	229	19	22	25
23	53	58	62	191	215	240	20	23	26
24	56	61	65	201	226	251	21	24	26
25	59	64	68	212	236	261	22	24	27
26	62	67	71	222	246	271	22	25	28
27	65	70	74	231	256	280	23	26	29
28	68	72	77	240	265	289	24	27	30
29	70	75	79	248	272	298	25	28	30
30	73	77	82	257	281	306	25	28	31
31	75	79	84	264	289	314	26	29	32
32	77	82	86	271	296	321	27	30	33
33	79	84	88	279	303	328	28	31	33
34	81	86	90	285	310	335	28	31	34
35	83	87	92	292	316	341	29	32	35
36	84	89	93	298	322	347	30	33	36
37	86	90	95	303	328	353	30	33	36
38	87	91	96	309	333	358	31	34	37
39	88	93	97	314	339	363	32	35	37
40	89	93	98	319	344	368	32	35	38

congenital anomalies. The extracortical space overlying the cerebral convexities is very prominent early in gestation and decreases steadily starting from about the fifth month until it becomes of minimal dimensions in the adult. Before the sixth month of gestation, the frontal and temporal lobes adjacent to the insula—the opercula—are separated by an ample space, the base of which is the insula (see Fig. 126–5). The opercula progressively get closer until they meet to form the Sylvian fissure. The beginning of Sylvian fissure demarcation is already visible at 22 weeks of gestation. However, it is not until 32 to 34 weeks of gestation that the opercularization is complete. The cistern of the vein of Galen (or the quadrigeminal cistern), which lies in the angle between the superior surfaces of the cerebellum and mesencephalon, can be seen on sonographic scans as early as the 15th week (see Fig. 126–6). The cisterna magna, which is situated between the inferior surface of the cerebellum and the posterior aspect of the medulla oblongata, can be consistently visualized with ultrasound. The width of the cisterna magna depends on gestational age between 15 and 40 weeks and is normally less than 10 mm.

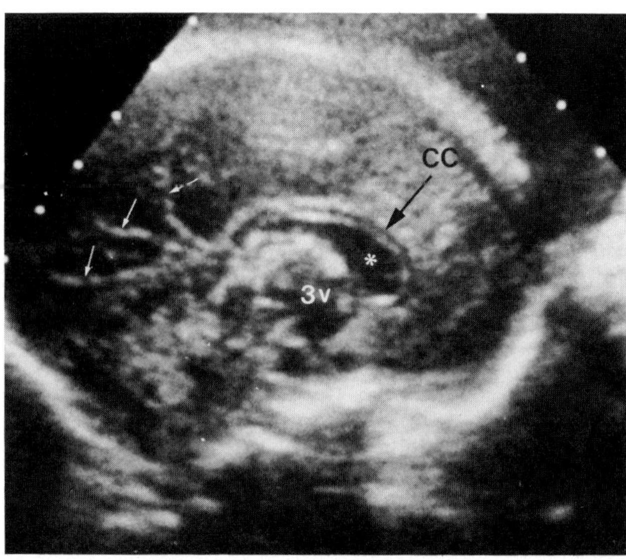

Figure 126–7. Midsagittal scan of the fetal head at 29 weeks. The corpus callosum (CC) is seen as a thin sonolucent crescent interposed between the echogenic pericallosal cistern and the patent cavum septi pellucidum *(asterisk)*. Anteriorly to the third ventricle (3v), the chiasmatic cistern is seen. Well-developed cerebral sulci (parieto-occipital, calcarine, and collateral) are seen on the medial surface of the hemisphere *(white arrows)*.

HYDROCEPHALUS

Congenital hydrocephalus arises in most cases from an obstruction in the normal pathway of the cerebrospinal fluid. The incidence ranges between 0.3 and 1.5 in 1000 births in different series. Hydrocephalus can result from pathologic entities that differ both in etiology and in clinical course. In a series of 205 infants with congenital isolated hydrocephalus, aqueductal stenosis was found in 43 per cent, communicating hydrocephalus in 38 per cent, and Dandy-Walker malformation in 13 per cent. However, pediatric data may not apply to cases recognized before birth. Fetal ventriculomegaly usually enters one of three main entities: simple hydrocephalus (which may result from aqueductal stenosis or communicating hydrocephalus); Dandy-Walker malformation; and hydrocephalus associated with other cerebral anomalies, most frequently disorders of dorsal induction, disorders of ventral induction, and disruptive lesions.

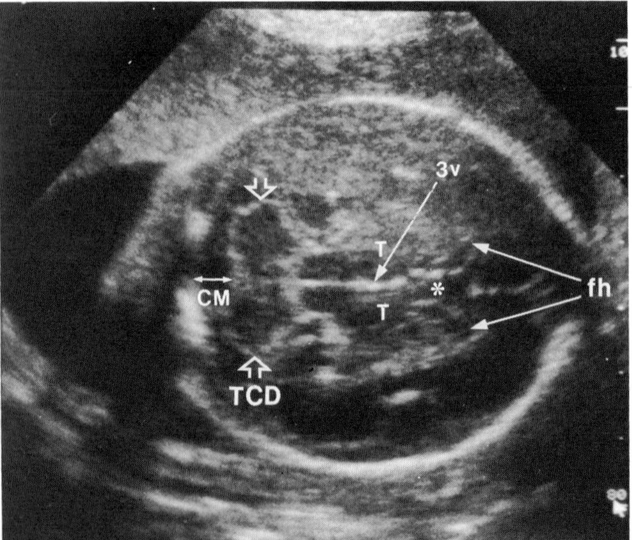

Figure 126–6. Axial scans of the fetal head demonstrating the posterior fossa. The normally generous cisterna magna (CM) outlines the cerebellum. Measurement of transverse cerebellar diameter (TCD) is demonstrated. (T = thalami; 3v = third ventricle; fh = frontal horns; *asterisk* = cavum septi pellucidum.)

Both congenital infections and genetic factors are involved in the pathogenesis of aqueductal stenosis. Infectious agents include toxoplasmosis, syphilis, cytomegalovirus, mumps, and influenza virus. Many familial cases indicate an X-linked pattern of transmission that is thought to account for 25 per cent of lesions occurring in males. A multifactorial etiology has also been suggested. Infections result in gliotic stenosis of the aqueduct. True malformations include narrowing and forking (multicanalization) and, less frequently, a transverse septum obstructing the lumen. In an autopsic series, 50 per cent of cases of aqueductal stenosis were due to gliosis, 46 per cent to forking, and 4 per cent to simple narrowing. Congenital tumors such as gliomas, pinealomas, and meningiomas cause aqueductal stenosis by external compression. Outlet obstruction of the third ventricle results in enlargement of the third and lateral ventricles. The degree of ventriculomegaly, even if variable, is severe in the vast majority of cases. Neurosurgical series of treated infants indicate a mortality rate between 10 and 30 per cent. In one study, only 50 per cent of infants developed a normal intelligence following surgical correction. In a more recent series, the mean IQ of treated infants was 71.

Communicating hydrocephalus usually results from failure of reabsorption of cerebrospinal fluid. It has been found in cases of agenesis or blockage of arachnoid granulation due to subarachnoid hemorrhage; venous occlusion of the superior sagittal sinus, torcular Herophili, or lateral sinuses; and overproduction of cerebrospinal fluid by a choroid plexus papilloma. A multifactorial etiology with a recurrence risk of 1 to 2 per cent has been suggested. Communicating hydrocephalus in its most typical manifestation is characterized by a variable degree of enlargement of the entire ventricular system associated with dilatation of the subarachnoid spaces. However, a radiologic study outlining the natural history of this lesion has demonstrated that, in the earliest stage, enlargement is confined to the subarachnoid channels overlying the cerebral hemispheres. In a further stage, a simultaneous dilatation of both the subarachnoid spaces and the ventricular system is seen. Eventually, only ventriculomegaly can be demonstrated.

According to recent experience, isolated communicating hydrocephalus carries a good prognosis. In a series of 13 treated infants, no deaths occurred and the intelligence was normal in all cases.

It should be stressed that the traditional view that considers stenosis of the aqueduct and communicating hydrocephalus as two separate entities has been challenged, and it has been postulated that ventriculomegaly may be the cause instead of the consequence of aqueductal stenosis.

The etiology of Dandy-Walker malformation is still unclear. Genetic factors probably play a major role. Familial cases have been reported by many authors. They seem to indicate that an autosomal recessive transmission is implicated in at least some instances. More recently, this view has been challenged, and a multifactorial etiology with an empiric recurrence risk of 1 to 5 per cent has been advocated. Dandy-Walker malformation is frequently associated with other nervous system abnormalities, such as agenesis of corpus callosum, heterotopia, polymicrogyria, agyria and macrogyria, systemic anomalies such as congenital heart disease (mainly ventricular septal defects), polydactyly-syndactyly, cleft palate, and polycystic kidneys, and it may be a part of a number of genetic and nongenetic syndromes that have been extensively reviewed.

Dandy-Walker malformation is featured by the association of three distinct anomalies: hydrocephalus, a retrocerebellar cyst, and a defect in the cerebellar vermis through which the posterior fossa cyst communicates with the fourth ventricle. The embryology of this lesion is still unclear. In the original view of Dandy and Taggart and Walker, the condition was secondary to primary atresia of the exit foramina of the fourth ventricle, which progressively lead to disruption of the cerebellar vermis. Other authors have suggested that the primary disorder is a defective formation of the cerebellar vermis resulting in secondary maldevelopment and atresia of the foramina of the fourth ventricle. Eventually, it was postulated that Dandy-Walker malformation results from embryonic ventriculomegaly, which would lead to an abnormal expansion of the primordia of the roof of the fourth ventricle.

In spite of the classical definition of Dandy-Walker malformation, it has been demonstrated that in 80 per cent of cases hydrocephalus is absent at birth and develops only after several months or years. This observation is relevant for the obstetric sonographer because it indicates that the Dandy-Walker malformation cannot be excluded on the basis of the absence of ventriculomegaly alone. Recent pediatric series indicate that treated infants have an overall mortality rate ranging between 10 and 30 per cent and an IQ above 80 in 30 to 40 per cent of cases.

The issue of prenatal diagnosis of hydrocephalus by sonography has been addressed by many investigators. As macrocrania usually does not develop until late in gestation, head measurements are unreliable and the identification of hydrocephalus should depend on the direct demonstration of the enlargement of the ventricular system. Nomograms of the normal size of the frontal horns, atria, and occipital horns of the lateral ventricles throughout gestation are now available. There is evidence indicating that probably the most effective approach relies on visualization of the atria of lateral ventricles. Under normal conditions, the glomus of the choroid plexus is closely apposed to both the medial and lateral wall of lateral ventricle, and this relationship is itself indicative of normalcy (see Fig. 126–5). In a minority of cases, a slight disproportion is found between the medial wall and the choroid plexus. Under this condition, measurement of the internal width of the atrium is suggested. This measurement is normally less than 10 mm between 15 weeks and term. It has also been suggested that fetal ventriculomegaly should be divided into two different categories: mild ventriculomegaly (atrial width between 10 and 15 mm) and overt hydrocephalus (atrial width > 15 mm). The clinical significance of mild ventriculomegaly (Fig. 126–8) per se is uncertain. However, there is plenty of evidence indicating that this condition is associated with an excess of both nervous and nonnervous anomalies and chromosomal aberrations as well. Interestingly enough, most of the anomalies found in these cases are subtle and would probably otherwise escape detection. The list includes spina bifida, agenesis of corpus callosum, and minor holoprosencephaly. Overt hydrocephalus is usually associated with obstruction to cerebrospinal fluid turnover (Fig. 126–9). Under these circumstances, the site of the obstruction may be inferred by identifying the enlarged portion of the ventricular system. Marked dilatation of the lateral and third ventricles suggests aqueductal stenosis. Tetraventricular enlargement in the presence of a normal cerebellar vermis associated with distention of the subarachnoid cisterns suggests communicating hydrocephalus. A defect in the cerebellar vermis through which the fourth ventricle communicates with a posterior fossa cyst indicates Dandy-Walker malformation (Fig. 126–10). Differentiation of the anatomic type of hydrocephalus should always be attempted, because each form carries a different prognosis. In most cases, however, distinction between aqueductal stenosis and communicating hydrocephalus is not possible.

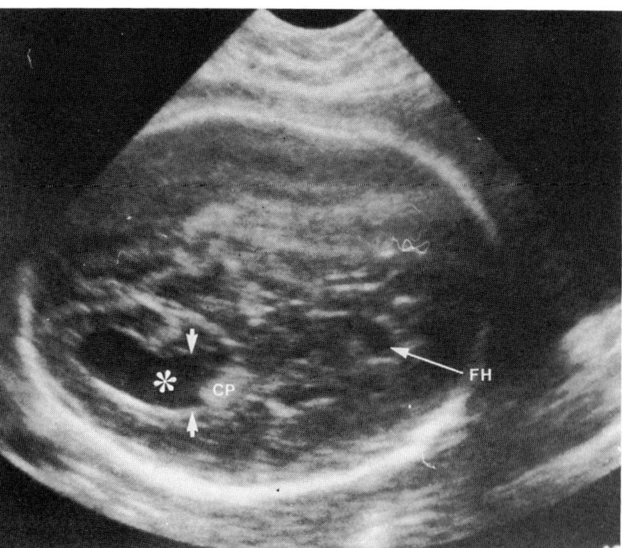

Figure 126–8. Mild idiopathic ventriculomegaly in a third trimester fetus. The atrial width (arrowheads) is 12 mm, and the choroid plexus (CP) is clearly detached from the medial wall of the ventricle. Mild ventriculomegaly was confirmed at birth by transfontanellar sonography. The neurologic examination was otherwise normal. (FH = frontal horns.)

Many researchers have tried to correlate the outcome of ventriculomegalic infants with the extent of ventricular enlargement. Measurements such as the frontal cerebral mantle thickness and the brain mass (calculated on the basis of the frontal cerebral mantle thickness and the occipitofrontal diameter) were used. All these studies uniformly indicated that the prognosis cannot be predicted on the basis of a quantitative evaluation of the spared cerebral cortex. Many reports indicate that even infants with a cerebral mantle thickness of a few millimeters sometimes develop a normal or superior intelligence following treatment. At present, the outcome of affected infants seems to depend more on the nature of the underlying lesion than on the degree of ventriculomegaly.

Difficulties in establishing a reliable prognosis in utero are reflected in uncertainties in electing the proper obstetrical management. When the diagnosis of hydrocephalus is made before viability, many parents are likely to request termination of pregnancy. In continuing pregnancies, many authors believe that delivery at fetal maturation and prompt neurologic treatment will maximize the chances of survival and normal development for the affected infants. A cesarean section is recommended in those cases with associated macrocrania. Because the chance of a normal intellectual development does not appear too remote, cephalocentesis to allow vaginal delivery in cases of fetopelvic disproportion is strongly contraindicated, in view of the significant risk associated with such a procedure.

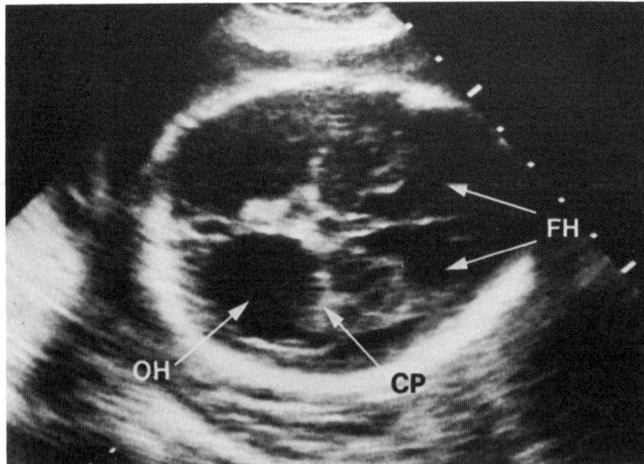

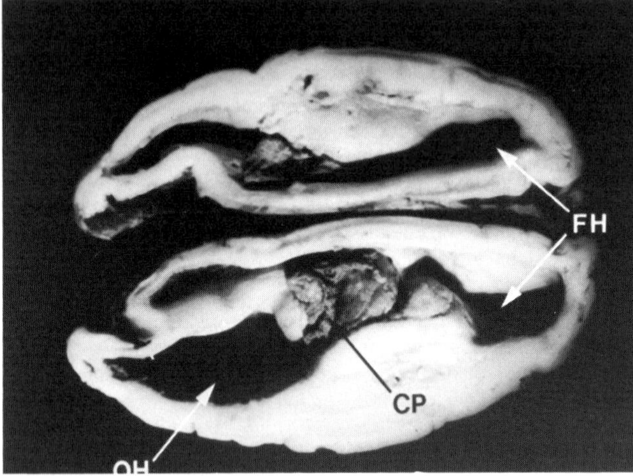

Figure 126–9. Overt hydrocephalus in a midtrimester fetus. The atrial width was 20 mm. Pathology was compatible with aqueductal stenosis. (FH = frontal horns; CP = choroid plexus; OH = occipital horns.)

It should be stressed that one of the factors that influence the outcome of hydrocephalic fetuses is the possible association with other important life-threatening anomalies. In our experience, the incidence of severe associated anomalies, including chromosomal aberrations and extranervous malformations, is almost 30 per cent. In view of these figures, an effort to identify associated anomalies should always be made before aggressive obstetrical management is considered. Detailed examination of the entire fetal anatomy by high-resolution ultrasound, echocardiography, and karyotyping is strongly recommended. If severe anomalies are found, suggesting that postnatal survival is unlikely, a conservative management can be offered to the parents.

Intrauterine treatment of congenital obstructive hydrocephalus by ventriculoamniotic shunting was suggested in the 1980s. However, the experience on human fetuses was not encouraging. The Registry of the International Society of Fetal Medicine and Surgery indicates that of a total of 44 fetuses who underwent shunting between 1982 and 1985, the procedure-related death rate was 10 per cent. Fifty-three per cent of survivors had severe handicap, 12 per cent had mild handicap, and only 35 per cent were developing normally at follow-up.

DISORDERS OF DORSAL INDUCTION

The incidence of neural tube defects varies considerably according to geographic and ethnic factors. A figure of 1 in 1000 to 2000 births is commonly quoted for the general population. In South Wales, the frequency rises to about 7 in 1000 births. The etiology is multifactorial, with a recurrence risk of 1 to 5 per cent after the birth of one affected child.

Two pathogenetic hypotheses have been suggested. Failure of closure of the anterior (anencephaly) or the posterior neuropore (spina bifida) has been postulated by the vast majority of authors. Others have postulated a secondary opening of the already-formed neural tube after embryonic hydrocephalus.

In anencephaly, the cranial vault as well as the telencephalic and diencephalic structures are absent. Necrotic remnants of the brain stem and rhombencephalic structures are covered by a vascular membrane. Associated malformations are common and include spina bifida, cleft lip, cleft palate, clubfoot, and omphalocele. Polyhydramnios is frequently found.

Spina bifida is divided into types: occulta and aperta. Spina bifida occulta is characterized by vertebral schisis covered by normal soft tissues. Large defects are usually associated with pigmented and dimpled lesions overlying skin and subcutaneous lipomas. Spina bifida aperta is characterized by a defect of the skin, underlying soft tissues, and vertebral arches exposing the neural canal. The defect may be covered by a thin meningeal membrane (meningocele). In the presence of neural tissue inside the sac, the lesion is referred to as a *myelomeningocele*, a term often used to indicate all cases of spina bifida aperta. The defect may vary considerably in size. The lumbar, thoracolumbar, or sacrolumbar areas are most frequently affected. Spina bifida aperta is almost always associated with a typical intracranial malformation (Arnold-Chiari or Chiari type II malformation) consisting of displacement of the cerebellar vermis, fourth ventricle, and medulla oblongata through the foramen magnum inside the upper cervical canal. Hydrocephalus of variable degree is present in virtually all cases of spina bifida aperta. Hydrocephalus is thought to arise from the low position of the exit foramina of the fourth ventricle, which can be either obstructed by the surrounding bony structures or open inside the spinal canal. In the latter case, the cerebellum impacted within the posterior fossa would prevent the return of cerebrospinal fluid to the intracranial subarachnoid spaces and reabsorption sites. Deformities and obstruction of the aqueduct are found in almost all cases and are

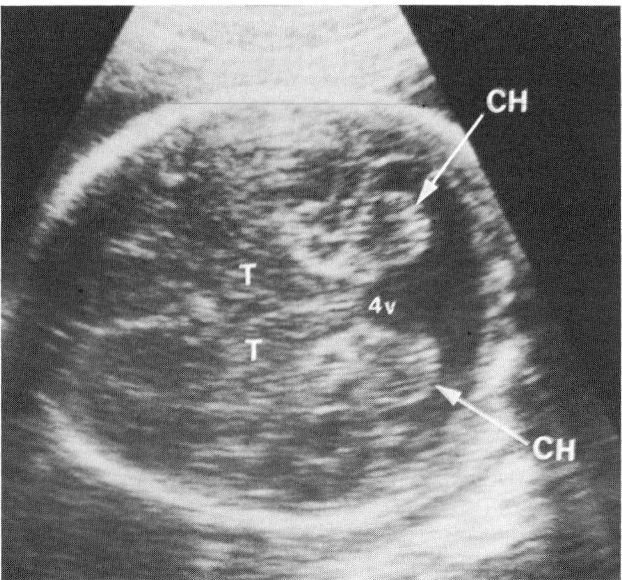

Figure 126–10. Fetal Dandy-Walker malformation. A wide defect is seen at the level of the cerebellar vermis. Through this defect, the cystic cisterna magna amply communicates with the area of the fourth ventricle (4v). The cerebellar hemispheres (CH) are widely separated. (T = thalami.)

thought to derive from the external compression operated by the enlargement of the lateral ventricles. Infants with spina bifida aperta often have associated anomalies, such as kyphoscoliosis and clubfoot.

Anencephaly is invariably fatal. The outcome for infants with spina bifida is dictated by the site and extension of the lesion. The mortality is high, the seven-year survival rate being only 40 per cent despite early treatment. Many survivors suffer from significant disabilities, such as lower limb paralysis or dysfunction and incontinence. The association of spina bifida and severe hydrocephalus was traditionally considered a poor prognostic factor for intellectual development. More recent studies indicate that in many cases, control of intracranial hypertension by shunting results in a normal or even superior intelligence.

The association between fetal neural tube defects and elevated amniotic and maternal serum alpha-fetoprotein and amniotic acetylcholinesterase is well-established. The combined use of alpha-fetoprotein determination and ultrasound as a screening tool for the prenatal diagnosis of these lesions has been advocated and is presently routinely used in several countries, including Great Britain and United States.

Anencephaly was the first congenital anomaly recognized in utero by ultrasound. The diagnosis is easy and relies on the demonstration of the absence of the cranial vault. Because the fetal head can be positively identified by modern ultrasound equipment as early as the first trimester, particularly when transvaginal high-resolution sonography is used, anencephaly is recognizable in this period (Fig. 126–11).

We are not aware of cases of spina bifida occulta diagnosed in utero by ultrasound. It seems unlikely that such lesions can be detected even by the most experienced operators. Open defects can be recognized by demonstrating the defect of the neural arches and overlying soft tissues (Figs. 126–12 and 126–13). The accuracy of ultrasound in predicting fetal spinal lesions is a critical issue. It is clear that the predictive value of the technique largely depends on the quality of the equipment, the experience of the operator, and the amount of time dedicated to any single patient. No data are available with regard to level 1, not-targeted examinations. However, there is little doubt that the sensitivity of these examinations is quite low. Level 2 examinations on patients at risk for either familial history or elevated alpha-fetoprotein yield a much greater accuracy. The use of sonography for antenatal detection of spina bifida was first suggested in the early 1970s. In the original study, ultrasound was successful in identifying one affected fetus and ruling out lesions in one normal fetus, and it failed to recognize a lumbosacral defect in a third fetus. Ten years later, most referral centers reported a sensitivity and specificity of level 2 ultrasound of close to 100 per cent. Both the increased experience of the operators and the introduction of high-resolution, real-time ultrasound equipment were probably responsible for this dramatic diagnostic improvement.

Sonologists have recently focused on the evaluation of intracranial anatomy in fetuses with spina bifida. Several reports indicate that typical cranial signs are consistently found. These findings include frontal bossing (the "lemon sign"; Fig. 126–14); hypoplasia of the posterior fossa structures, attested by an abnormal configuration of the cerebellum (the "banana sign"); an abnormally reduced transverse cerebellar diameter; failure to recognize the cerebellum; and obliteration of the cisterna magna (Fig. 126–15). These signs are easily demonstrated by even less experienced so-

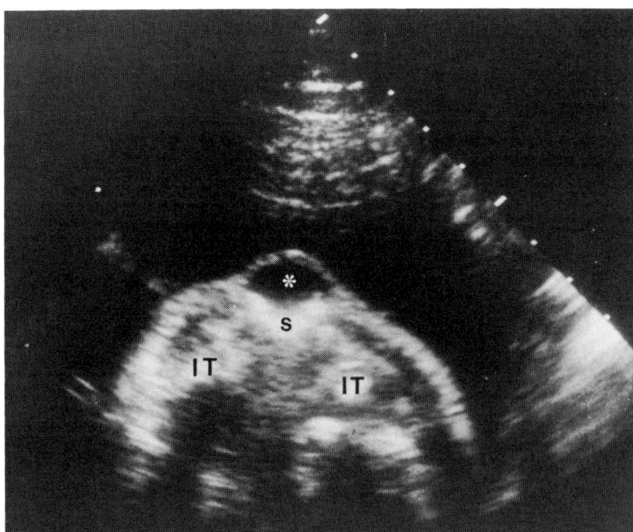

Figure 126–12. Transverse view of the sacrum (S) in a midtrimester fetus with **myelomeningocele** *(asterisk)*. (IT = ischial tuberosities.)

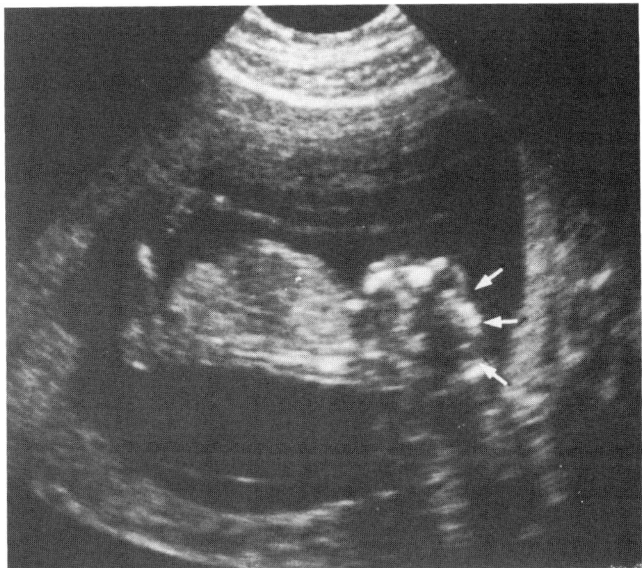

Figure 126–11. Anencephaly demonstrated by transvaginal sonography in a fetus at 12 weeks' gestational age.

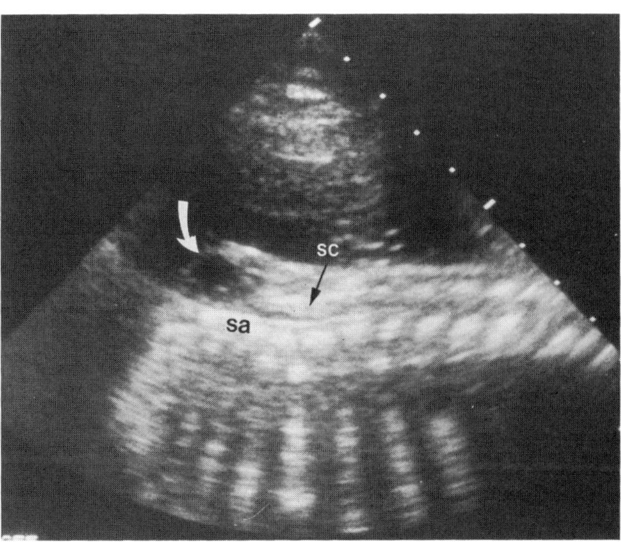

Figure 126–13. Sagittal view in the same case as seen in Figure 126–12, demonstrating that the spinal cord (sc) is involved in the lesion. (sa = sacrum; *arrow* = the cystic myelomeningocele.)

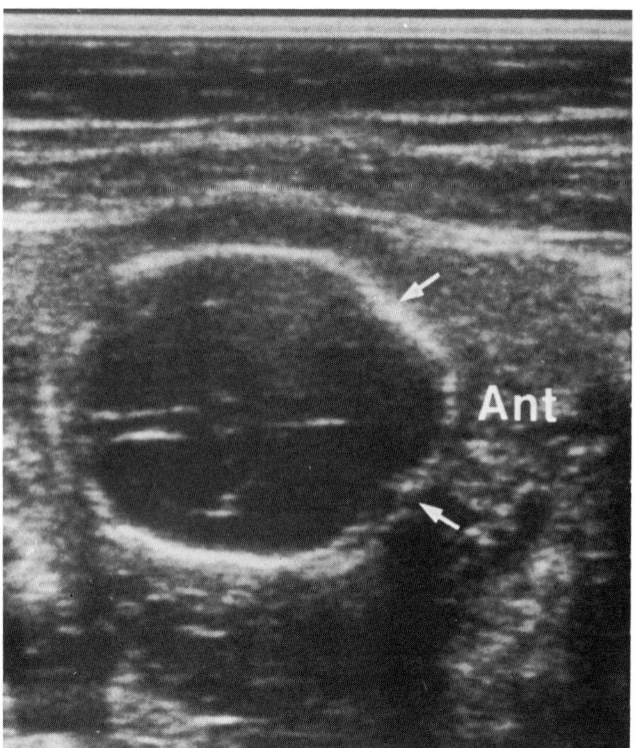

Figure 126–14. Frontal bossing *(arrows)* in a midtrimester fetus with spina bifida: **the "lemon sign."**

nographers and are therefore potentially useful for sonographic mass screening of spina bifida.

Because anencephaly is an invariably fatal lesion, termination of pregnancy can be offered at any time in pregnancy. When the diagnosis of spina bifida is made prior to viability, termination of pregnancy can be offered to the parents. When this is refused or in cases recognized later or in gestation, an attempt to identify the site and the extent of the lesion should be made to assess a tentative prognosis. Options should be discussed with the couple. Several reports have indicated that birth injury is frequent in fetuses with spina bifida and represents a major prognostic shortcoming. Cesarean delivery is recommended by several authorities, although clear-cut benefit is still unproven.

The term *cephalocele* indicates a protrusion of intracranial contents through a bony defect of the skull. The etiology is unknown. The observation that cephaloceles may occur in families with a history of neural tube defects suggests that the anomalies are somewhat related. Cephaloceles may occur either as isolated defects or as a part of genetic and nongenetic syndromes. Classical examples include Meckel's syndrome (autosomal recessive transmission, also featured in microcephaly, polydactyly, polycystic kidneys, and multiple visceral anomalies) and the amniotic band syndrome (sporadic, featured in asymmetrical and/or multiple cephaloceles, gastroschisis, facial clefts, amputation, and ring constrictions of the limbs). In most cases, the lesion arises from the midline, in the occipital area; less frequently it arises from the parietal or frontal bones. Encephaloceles are characterized by the presence of brain tissue inside the lesion. When only meninges protrude, the term *cranial meningocele* should be used. Cephaloceles often cause impaired cerebrospinal fluid circulation and hydrocephalus. Massive encephaloceles may be associated with microcephaly. The outcome is mainly related to the presence or absence of brain tissue inside the lesion. Encephaloceles carry a neonatal mortality rate of about 40 per cent and an incidence of intellectual impairment and neurologic sequelae of 80 per cent. Infants with cranial meningoceles are reported to develop a normal intelligence in 60 per cent of cases.

Fetal cephaloceles should be suspected when a paracranial mass is seen on sonography. The diagnosis of encephaloceles is easy, because the presence of brain tissue inside the sac is striking on ultrasound. Differentiation of a cranial meningocele from soft-tissue edema or a cystic hygroma of the neck may be difficult. Demonstration of the bony defect in the skull would allow a proper diagnosis, but cranial meningoceles are often associated with extremely small (a few millimeters) defects that are not amenable to antenatal sonographic recognition. There are certain clues that can be sought to assist a correct diagnosis. Cranial cephaloceles are very often associated with ventriculomegaly. Cystic hygromas arise from the region of the neck, have multiple internal septations and a thick wall, and are often associated with generalized soft-tissue edema and hydrops. Some cephaloceles protrude through the base of skull inside the pharynx. These lesions are obviously inaccessible to prenatal ultrasound identification unless derangement of intracranial morphology is present. Because cephaloceles are often associated

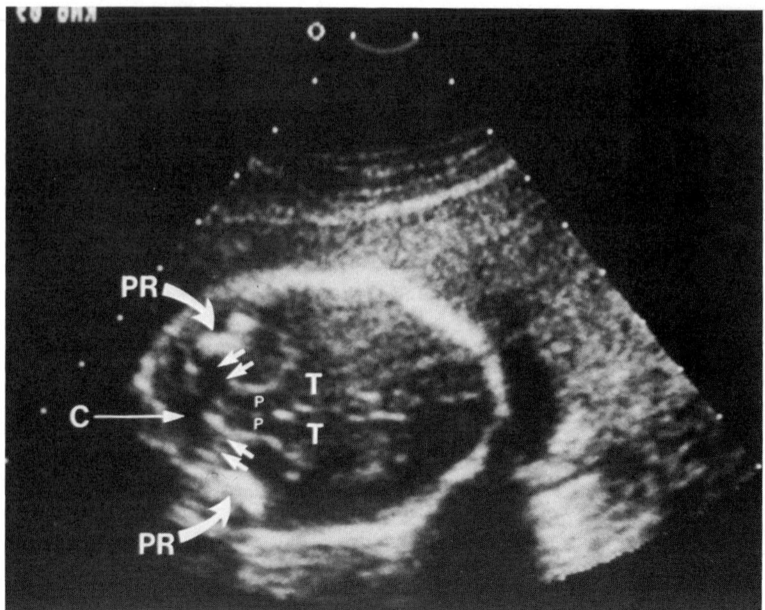

Figure 126–15. Posterior fossa in a midtrimester fetus with spina bifida. As a consequence of Arnold-Chiari malformation, the small cerebellum (C) is displaced downward and appears obscured by the petrous ridges of the temporal bone (PR). (T = thalami; P = cerebral peduncles.)

with other anomalies, a careful investigation of the entire fetal anatomy is recommended.

Termination of pregnancy can be offered prior to viability. In continuing pregnancies, a cesarean section should be considered to avoid birth trauma. However, because infants with massive encephaloceles and microcephaly have a dismal prognosis, conservative management can be offered in these cases.

DISORDERS OF VENTRAL INDUCTION

The term *ventral induction* refers to the interrelated developmental events that occur in the embryonic forebrain starting from the fifth week of gestation and lead to the separation of the cerebral hemispheres and the formation of the midline structures. The differentiation of these nervous structures is closely related to the development of the mid-face. Disorders of ventral induction include a group of midline cerebral defects that encompass a wide spectrum of severity and are typically associated with craniofacial malformations.

Holoprosencephaly

Holoprosencephaly is a complex developmental anomaly of the telencephalic and diencephalic structures. Its incidence is unknown, because milder forms are probably unrecognized. Two subtypes of this anomaly, cyclopia and cebocephaly, have been reported to occur in 1 in 40,000 and 1 in 16,000 births, respectively. An incidence of 4 in 1000 abortions has also been reported, suggesting a high intrauterine fatality rate for this defect. The etiology is heterogeneous. In most cases, the anomaly is isolated and sporadic. In other cases, chromosomal abnormalities have been found, as well as other congenital anatomic deformities such as anencephaly, encephalocele, Di George's syndrome, and Meckel's syndrome. Several familial cases suggest genetic inheritance with autosomal dominant transmission. The overall recurrence risk is 6 per cent.

Holoprosencephaly is the consequence of a failed diverticulation of the embryonic prosencephalon into its components, the cerebral hemispheres and the diencephalic structures. The primary disorder seems to reside in the prechordal mesenchyma, which is thought to induce both cleavage of the primitive forebrain and development of the median facial structures (orbits, nose, median upper lip, and palate). This concept provides an explanation of the typical association between brain anomalies and facial dysmorphism seen in this malformation sequence. Failure of the forebrain to undergo paired symmetrical division along the sagittal plane and diverticulation results in varying degrees of fusion of the cerebral structures. In alobar holoprosencephaly, the most severe type, the interhemispheric fissure and the falx cerebri are totally absent; there is a single primitive ventricle (holoventricle); the thalami are fused on the midline; and the third ventricle, neurohypophysis, olfactory bulbs, and tracts are absent. In semilobar holoprosencephaly, the two cerebral hemispheres are partially separated posteriorly, but there is still a single ventricular cavity. In both the alobar and semi-lobar forms, the roof of the ventricular cavity (the thela choroidea), normally enfolded within the brain, may balloon out between the cerebral convexity and the skull to form a cyst of variable size—the dorsal sac. Alobar and semi-lobar holoprosencephaly are often associated with microcephaly and less frequently with macrocephaly, which is invariably due to internal obstructive hydrocephalus. In the lobar variety, the interhemispheric fissure is well-developed posteriorly and anteriorly, but there is still a variable degree of fusion of the cingulate gyrus and of the lateral ventricles and the septum pellucidum is absent. The facial anomalies are pleomorphic. According to the most popular classification, five categories can be recognized: cyclopia, which is featured by a single eye or partially divided eyes in a single orbit; arhinia; median cleft palate and/or lip; median philtrum-premaxilla anlage; and flat nose. Cyclopia and ethmocephaly are invariably associated with alobar holoprosencephaly. Cebocephaly and median cleft lip may be found in either the alobar or semi-lobar variety. Median philtrum-premaxilla anlage is indicative of either semi-lobar or lobar varieties. It should be stressed that infants with any kind of holoprosencephaly may have a normal face.

The invariably poor prognosis for infants affected by alobar and semi-lobar holoprosencephaly is well-established. Infants with the lobar variety may have both a normal life span and a normal intelligence even if precise prognostic figures are not available.

Several cases of sonographic antenatal diagnosis of holoprosencephaly have been reported in the literature. The most valuable finding was the single primitive ventricle (Fig. 126–16). Demonstration of facial anomalies strengthens the diagnosis of holoprosencephaly based on central nervous system findings. Conversely, should any of the aforementioned facial features be serendipitously encountered, a careful examination of the intracranial contents is recommended.

The ultrasonic findings of semi-lobar holoprosencephaly are very similar to those of the alobar variety. In newborns, semi-lobar holoprosencephaly can be identified surely by visualizing well-developed occipital horns. The lobar variety of holoprosencephaly can be identified by demonstrating fusion and squaring of the roof of the frontal horns (Fig. 126–17).

When either alobar or semi-lobar holoprosencephaly is identified in utero, termination of pregnancy could be offered prior to viability. A conservative management is strongly recommended in continuing pregnancies. The prognosis of lobar holoprosencephaly is unclear, and this is reflected in the uncertainty as to the obstetric management.

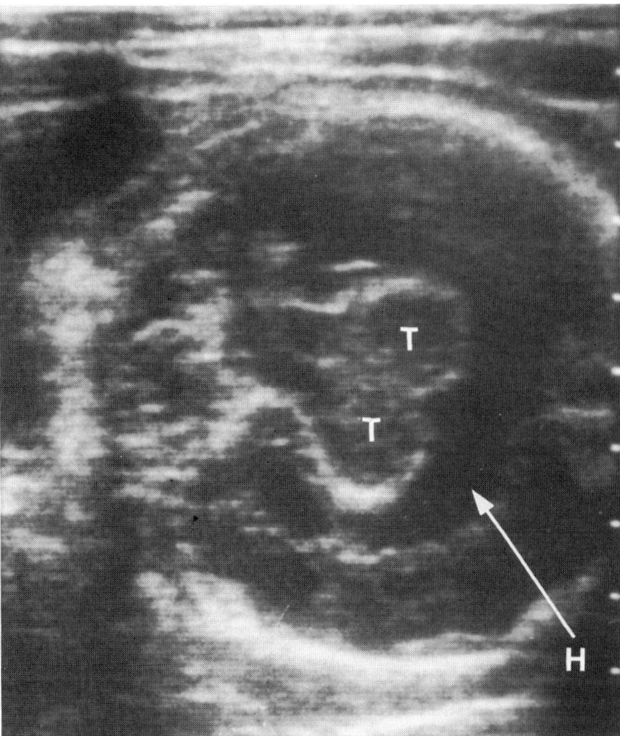

Figure 126–16. Fetal alobar holoprosencephaly. There is a single rudimentary crescent-shaped ventricular cavity (H) delineating typically bulb-shaped thalami (T).

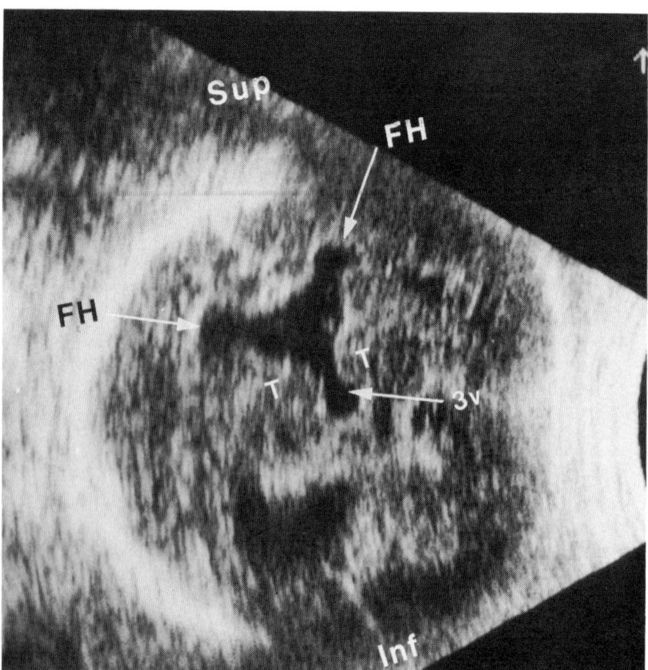

Figure 126–17. In this fetus, **lobar holoprosencephaly** is inferred by the mid-coronal view of the brain demonstrating a wide central fusion of the frontal horns (FH) with the inferior third ventricle (3v). The flattened roof of the frontal horns and bulb-like thalami (T) can also be noted.

Agenesis of the Corpus Callosum

The corpus callosum is a white matter structure connecting the two cerebral hemispheres. Embryologically it derives from the massa commissuralis, which is formed by fusion of the lateral margins of the groove that separates the two primitive telencephalic ventricles. The anterior portion of the corpus callosum is the first one to be formed. Growth proceeds caudally, the definitive configuration of the corpus callosum being assumed only by the 20th week. Agenesis may be complete or partial. In the latter case, aplasia affects the posterior portion, which is ontogenetically the last one to be formed. The incidence of agenesis of the corpus callosum is highly controversial. Figures ranging from 1 in 100 to 1 in 19,000 have been reported. The etiology is unknown. Agenesis of the corpus callosum can be found in association with chromosomal aberrations (trisomy 13 and 18), mostly as a part of the holoprosencephalic malformative sequence. Various teratogens can produce agenesis of the corpus callosum in animal models. The familial cases reported in the literature suggest a marked genetic heterogeneity, with evidence supporting autosomal dominant, autosomal recessive, and X-linked inheritance as well. Agenesis of the corpus callosum may be a part of genetic syndromes, such as Aicardi's syndrome (seizures, chorioretinal lacunas, mental retardation, microcephaly, and vertebral anomalies; sex-linked dominant inheritance), Andermann's syndrome (mental retardation and progressive motor neuropathy; autosomal recessive transmission), acrocallosal syndrome (mental retardation, macrocephaly, and polydactyly; autosomal recessive transmission), and F.G. syndrome (mental retardation, macrocephaly, and hypotonia). The high frequency of associated malformations suggests that agenesis of the corpus callosum may be a part of a widespread developmental disturbance. Associated central nervous system anomalies, including microcephaly, abnormal convolutional patterns, neural tube defects, Dandy-Walker malformation, and aplasia or hypoplasia of the pyramidal tracts are found in 80 per cent of the cases. Systemic anomalies including a variety of musculoskeletal, cardiovascular, genitourinary, and gastrointestinal malformations were found in 60 per cent of cases.

The criteria for the postnatal diagnosis of agenesis of the corpus callosum by diagnostic imaging techniques such as ventriculography, computed tomography, transfontanellar ultrasound, and magnetic resonance imaging are well-established. They mainly depend on the demonstration of the alterations of the cerebral architecture that are typically found in this condition. The bodies of the lateral ventricles are invariably widely separated, and the atria and occipital horns are enlarged (colpocephaly). The third ventricle is frequently enlarged and dorsally extended, being found at the same level as or higher than the bodies of lateral ventricles.

Antenatal diagnosis of agenesis of the corpus callosum is difficult. In our experience, the most valuable sonographic finding is the demonstration of an abnormal configuration of the lateral ventricles. The wide separation of the bodies of lateral ventricles and the enlargement of the atria result in a very typical image (Fig. 126–18). Dorsal extension of the third ventricle allows a specific diagnosis, but it is an inconsistent finding, as it was present in only 50 per cent of our cases (Fig. 126–19). A very valuable, although inconstant, finding is widening of the interhemispheric fissure, which results in triplication of the midline echo (see Figs. 126–17 and 126–18). Meticulous scanning may also allow at times direct demonstration of the absence of the corpus callosum.

Establishing a reliable prognosis for agenesis of the corpus callosum is extremely difficult. Many patients suffer from mental retardation and neurologic abnormalities including increased muscle tone and seizures and are psychologically abnormal. However, in some cases the condition is totally asymptomatic. It is likely that disabilities depend more on the amount and extent of associated anomalies than on agenesis of the corpus callosum. No specific figures are available at present. Difficulties in assessing the prognosis are reflected in the uncertainty as to parental counseling and obstetrical management. A careful search for associated anomalies, including echocardiography and karyotyping, is mandatory. However, it should be stressed that the ability of prenatal ultrasound to identify several of the anomalies classically associated with agenesis of the corpus callosum, such as abnormal convolutional patterns, has not been tested yet. Abnormalities of the pyramidal tracts, which may cause significant disability, are obviously unpredictable. Termination of pregnancy can be offered before viability, but the parents should be informed that there is a chance of an entirely normal intellectual and neurologic development. In continuing pregnancies, no specific obstetric management is required. Agenesis of the corpus callosum may be associated with macrocephaly. In these cases, a cesarean delivery is indicated without doubt.

DESTRUCTIVE CEREBRAL LESIONS

Porencephaly

The term *porencephaly* refers to a condition in which cystic cavities form within the brain matter. They may form as the result of either a morphogenetic disorder (true porencephaly or schizencephaly) or an intrauterine or postnatal destructive process (pseudoporencephaly or encephaloclastic porencephaly). The cavities usually communicate with the ventricular system, the subarachnoid space, or both. The developmental form is often bilateral and symmetrical. A unilateral lesion is usually found in pseudoporencephaly. In both pseudoporencephaly and encephaloclastic porencephaly, there is a wide variability in the size of the lesion. Hydrocephalus is frequently associated.

True porencephaly and congenital pseudoporencephaly are severe anomalies with dismal prognoses. The vast majority of patients are affected by severe mental retardation and important neurologic sequelae, such as blindness and tetraplegia.

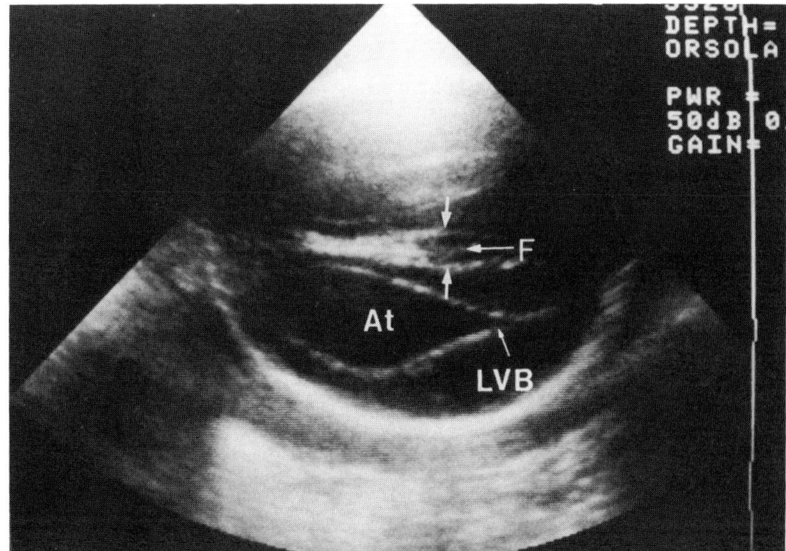

Figure 126–18. Typical configuration of lateral ventricles in a fetus with agenesis of the corpus callosum. The atria of lateral ventricles (At) are considerably enlarged; the bodies of lateral ventricles (LVB) are normal in size but widely separated. Enlargement of the interhemispheric fissure results in triplication of the midline echo. (F = falx cerebri.)

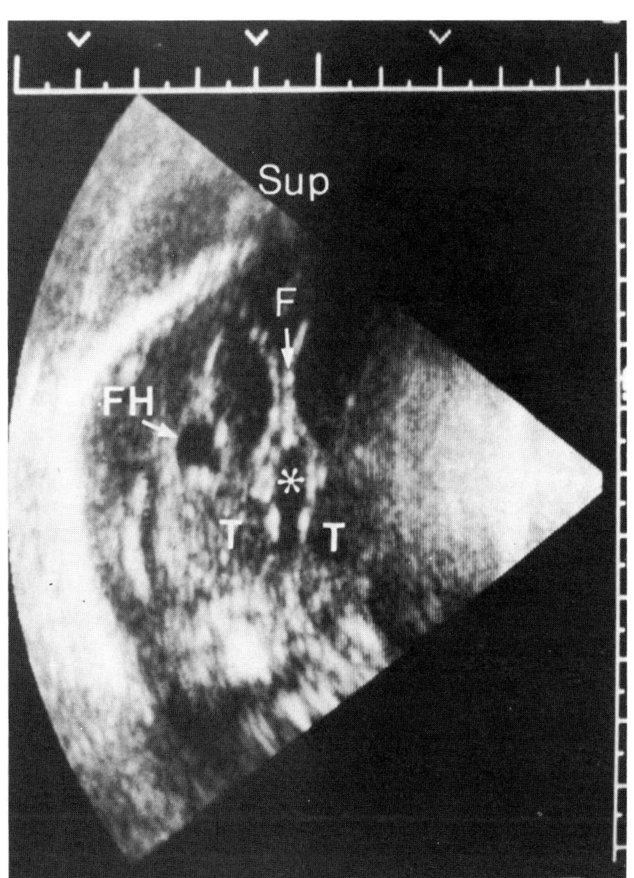

Figure 126–19. Coronal scan in the same case as seen in Figure 126–18. Upward displacement of the third ventricle *(asterisk)* that can be seen at the same level of frontal horns (FH) is demonstrated. The close proximity between the third ventricle and the superior falx cerebri (F) excludes the presence of the corpus callosum. The interhemispheric fissure is typically enlarged.

Prenatal sonographic identification of intracerebral cystic cavities is easy, but the differential diagnosis with intracranial cysts of different nature, such as arachnoid cysts and congenital tumors, may be impossible. When a confident diagnosis of porencephaly is made before viability, termination of pregnancy should be offered to the parents. In continuing pregnancies, a conservative obstetric management is recommended.

Hydranencephaly

Hydranencephaly is thought to result from an intrauterine destructive process and may be considered an extreme form of pseudoporencephaly. Most of each cerebral hemisphere is absent, and the intracranial cavity is filled with fluid. Remnants of the temporal and occipital lobes can be found. The brain stem and rhombencephalic structures are usually spared. The head may be small, of normal size, or extremely enlarged. The etiology is heterogeneous. Congenital infections including toxoplasmosis and cytomegalovirus and intrauterine strangulation or atresia of the internal carotid arteries have been reported. Prognosis is severe. Long survival has been reported. Obviously, however, these infants are incapable of any intellectual achievement.

Even if replacement of intracranial structures with fluid is easily detected by antenatal sonography, a certain identification of hydranencephaly may be difficult. The differential diagnosis includes severe hydrocephalus and holoprosencephaly. However, even in the most devastating forms of ventriculomegaly, it is possible to demonstrate the falx cerebrii and some spared cortex. In alobar holoprosencephaly, the falx is absent, but a crescent-shaped frontal cortex can usually be seen. In hydranencephaly, the falx is, in the vast majority of cases, absent or incomplete. In our experience, the most valuable finding for a specific diagnosis is the demonstration of the bulb-like brain stem, which, in the absence of the surrounding cortex, bulges inside the fluid-filled intracranial cavity (Fig. 126–20). The sonographic appearance is somewhat similar to that of the hypoplastic thalami that can be seen in cases of alobar or semilobar holoprosencephaly. Obviously, confusion between holoprosencephaly and hydranencephaly is uneventful, because both conditions have a dismal prognosis, and the obstetrical management does not differ.

MICROCEPHALY

The definition of microcephaly is highly controversial. Some authors suggest using as a diagnostic criterion a head circumference 2 standard deviations below the mean, but others believe that a threshold of −3 standard deviations should be used. Differences in diagnostic modalities probably account for the wide variability of the incidence of this condition. Figures ranging from 1.6 in 1000 births to 1 in 25,000 to 50,000 can be found in the literature. The etiology is extremely heterogeneous. Microcephaly should be considered not a separate entity but rather a symptom of many etiologic disturbances. Genetic and environmental causative factors are both well-accepted, and the reader is referred to the extensive reviews on the subject. A widely accepted classification distinguishes two main categories: (a) microcephaly resulting from nongenetic insults such as infections, anoxia, radiations, etc., and (b) genetic microcephaly, which includes all those cases in which microcephaly is a part of an inherited syndrome.

Microcephalic individuals share in common a typical disproportion in size between the splanchnocranium and neurocranium. The forehead is sloping. The correlation between a small head circumference and reduced brain mass and total cell number is well-established. The cerebral hemispheres are affected to a larger extent than the diencephalic and rhombencephalic structures. Abnormal convolutional patterns (macrogyria, microgyria, and agyria) are frequently found. The ventricles may be enlarged. Microcephaly is frequently found in cases of porencephaly, lissencephaly, and holoprosencephaly.

Establishing a reliable prognosis for infants affected by microcephaly is difficult. Associated anomalies obviously have a major influence on the outcome. Controversial clinical data exist with regard to isolated microcephaly. Infants with a head circumference below −2 standard deviations are found to have a normal or borderline intellect in 50 per cent of cases. A normal intelligence was found in 80 per cent and 30 per cent of infants with a head circumference below −2 and −3 standard deviations below the mean, respectively. Even if it is hard to derive precise prognostic figures from these studies, there is evidence indicating that a small head size does not necessarily imply mental retardation.

Many difficulties arise in attempting to identify fetal microcephaly. The utility of head measurement alone is limited, because head

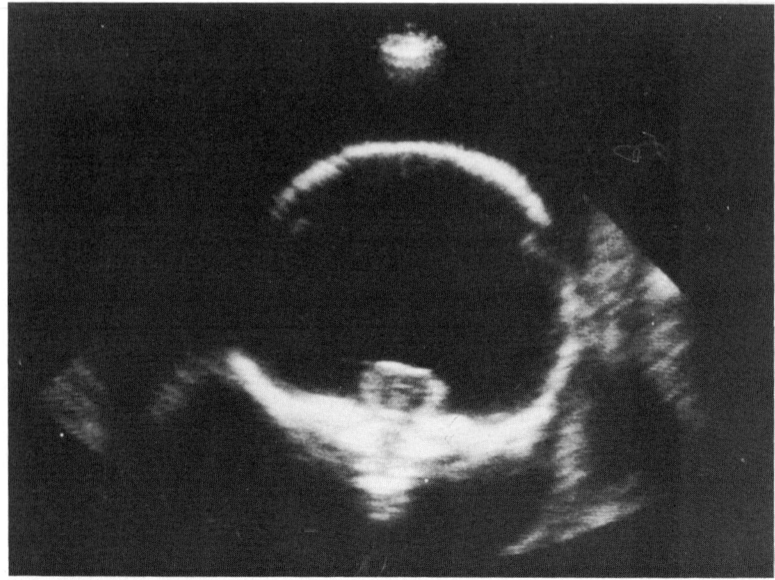

Figure 126–20. Hydranencephaly. The cerebral hemispheres are entirely replaced by fluid. The brain stem appears relatively spared.

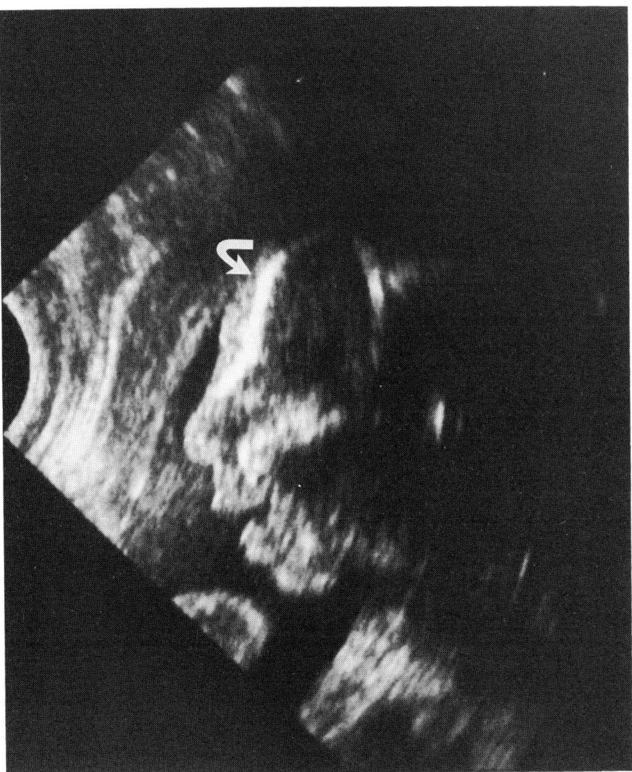

Figure 126–21. Severe sloping of the forehead *(arrow)* is demonstrated in this fetus with **microcephaly**.

measurement can be markedly biased by factors such as incorrect dating or intrauterine growth retardation. Furthermore, the natural history of fetal microcephaly is largely unknown. A progressive intrauterine development of the lesion has been seen in some cases with normal cranial size in the midtrimester. This observation is in agreement with our own experience. Nevertheless, recognition before viability is of paramount importance because microcephaly has genetic implications and many couples with a positive familial history demand prenatal diagnosis. A comparison of biometric parameters such as the head circumference:abdominal circumference ratio and the femur length:biparietal diameter ratio has been suggested. Nevertheless, both false-positive and false-negative diagnoses have been reported. It is clear that the predictive value of ultrasound biometry has several limitations at present. A qualitative evaluation of the intracranial structures is a very useful adjunct to biometry, because cerebral malformations are found in a significant proportion of infants with microcephaly. The impression of a sloping forehead may increase the index of suspicion in dubious cases (Fig. 126–21).

CHOROID PLEXUS CYSTS

Prenatal sonographic identification of choroid plexus cysts has been reported with increasing frequency over the last few years (Fig. 126–22). The incidence of this finding is probably between 1 and 3 per cent of midtrimester fetuses. Although the pediatric literature indicates that small choroid plexus cysts have no clinical significance, it would seem that their detection in utero may increase the risk of chromosomal aberrations, particularly trisomy 18. A survey of the presently available prospective series suggests that the risk is in the range of 1 to 5 per cent.

There does not seem to be a clear-cut association between the size of the cyst and the risk of chromosomal aberrations, which are found even with very small cysts. Disappearance of the cyst documented at serial scans is not reassuring, because this occurs in cases with aneuploidy. Most fetuses with trisomy 18 have associated malformations that are easily detected with ultrasound, congenital heart disease and skeletal abnormalities being the most frequent findings.

Identification of a choroid plexus cyst is without doubt an indication for a careful survey of fetal anatomy. There is controversy at present over whether karyotype determination should be offered to the parents in cases in which no associated anomalies can be detected. There is, however, no doubt that in the presence of a normal karyotype the prognosis is excellent. Because a handful of cases in which a disproportionate increase of cyst size with symptoms of intracranial pressure have been described in the neurosonological literature, a follow-up scan at the onset of the third trimester may be indicated to demonstrate regression or disappearance of the cyst.

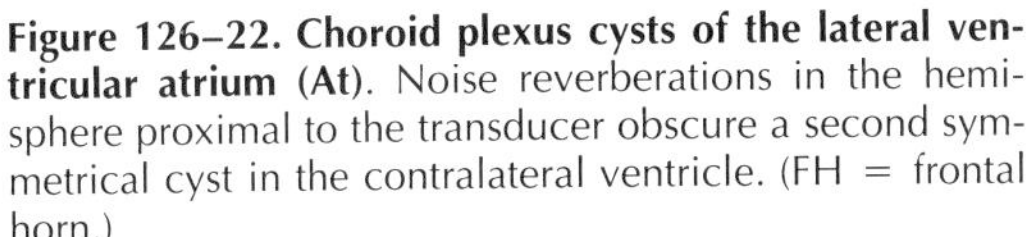

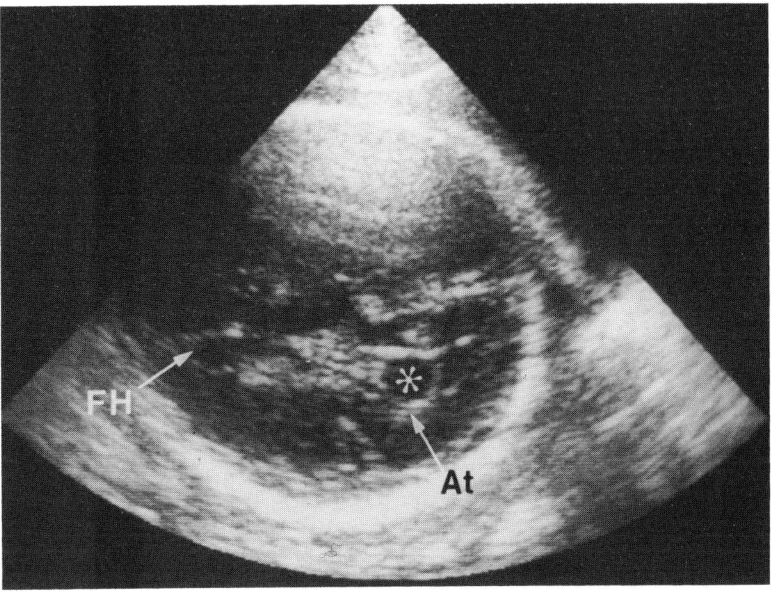

Figure 126–22. Choroid plexus cysts of the lateral ventricular atrium (At). Noise reverberations in the hemisphere proximal to the transducer obscure a second symmetrical cyst in the contralateral ventricle. (FH = frontal horn.)

CONCLUSION

Modern ultrasound technique has unique value in the evaluation of the normal and abnormal fetal central nervous system very early in pregnancy. A large number of congenital anomalies can be consistently recognized. The criteria for identification of nervous malformations are well-established. However, it should be stressed that many uncertainties exist as to parental counseling and obstetrical management. At present, the prognostic figures derived by pediatric studies are used in most instances. It is important to realize that these figures may not apply to the fetus. The natural histories of many congenital anomalies are still unknown. The establishment of reliable prognostic figures to be applied to affected fetuses and the development of precise guidelines for obstetrical management appear to be a priority for the next decade.

Bibliography

Benacerraf BR, Harlow B, Frigoletto JD: Are choroid plexus cysts an indication for second trimester amniocentesis? Am J Obstet Gynecol 160:1207, 1989.

Campbell S, Johnstone FD, Holt EM, et al: Anencephaly: Early ultrasonic diagnosis and active management. Lancet 2:1226, 1972.

Chervenak FA, Rosenberg J, Brightman RC, et al: A prospective study of the accuracy of ultrasound in predicting fetal microcephaly. Obstet Gynecol 69:908, 1987.

Chudleigh P, Pearce MJ, Campbell S: The prenatal diagnosis of transient cysts of the fetal choroid plexus. Prenat Diagn 4:135, 1984.

Cuomo Perpignano M, Cohen HL, Klein VR, et al: Fetal choroid plexus cysts: Beware the smaller cyst. Radiology 182:715, 1992.

Filly RA, Chinn DH, Callen PW: Alobar holoprosencephaly. Ultrasonographic prenatal diagnosis. Radiology 151:455, 1984.

Filly RA, Cardoza JD, Goldstein RB, et al: Detection of central nervous system anomalies: A practical level of effort for a routine sonogram. Radiology 172:403, 1989.

Filly RA, Goldstein RB, Callen PW: Fetal ventricle: Importance in routine obstetric sonography. Radiology 181:1, 1991.

Fiske CE, Filly RA: Ultrasound evaluation of the normal and abnormal fetal neural axis. Radiol Clin North Am 20:285, 1982.

Gabrielli S, Reece EA, Pilu G, et al: The clinical significance of prenatally diagnosed choroid plexus cysts. Am J Obstet Gynecol 160:1207, 1989.

Goldstein I, Reece EA, Pilu G, et al: Cerebellar measurement using sonography in the evaluation of fetal growth and development. Am J Obstet Gynecol 156:1065, 1987.

Goldstein RB, LaPidus AS, Filly RA, et al: Mild lateral cerebral ventricular dilatation in utero: Clinical significance and prognosis. Radiology 176:237, 1990.

Mahony BS, Callen PW, Filly RA, et al: The fetal cisterna magna. Radiology 153:773, 1984.

Manning FA, Harrison MR, Rodeck E, et al: Catheter shunts for fetal hydronephrosis and hydrocephalus. Reports of the International Fetal Surgery Registry. N Engl J Med 315:336, 1986.

Myrianthopoulos NC: Epidemiology of central nervous system malformations. In Vinken PJ, Bruyn GW (eds): Handbook of Clinical Neurology. Amsterdam, Elsevier, 1977, pp 139–171.

Nicolaides KH, Campbell S, Gabbe SG, et al: Ultrasound screening for spina bifida: Cranial and cerebellar signs. Lancet 2:72, 1988.

Pilu G, DePalma L, Romero R, et al: The fetal subarachnoid cisterns: An ultrasound study with report of a case of congenital communicating hydrocephalus. J Ultrasound Med 5:365, 1986.

Pilu G, Reece EA, Romero R, et al: Prenatal diagnosis of cranio-facial malformations by sonography. Am J Obstet Gynecol 155:45, 1986.

Pilu G, Romero R, Reece EA, et al: Subnormal cerebellum in fetuses with spina bifida. Am J Obstet Gynecol 158:1052, 1988.

Pilu G, Reece EA, Goldstein I, et al: Sonographic evaluation of the normal developmental anatomy of the fetal cerebral ventricles: II. The atria. Obstet Gynecol 73:250, 1989.

Pilu G, Sandri F, Perolo A, et al: Prenatal diagnosis of lobar holoprosencephaly. Ultrasound Obstet Gynecol 2:88, 1992.

Pilu G, Goldstein I, Reece EA, et al: Sonography of fetal Dandy-Walker malformation: A reappraisal. Ultrasound Obstet Gynecol 2:151, 1992.

Sandri F, Pilu G, Cerisoli M, et al: Sonographic diagnosis of agenesis of the corpus callosum in the fetus and newborn infant. Am J Perinatol 5:226, 1988.

Siedler DE, Filly RA: Relative growth of the higher fetal brain structures. J Ultrasound Med 6:573, 1987.

127 Ultrasound Studies of Fetal Cardiac Anatomy

Kathryn L. Reed

With advances in ultrasound technology, the human fetal heart has become accessible to noninvasive investigation. Methods currently in use include two-dimensional linear array and sector scanning, M-mode echocardiography, and Doppler echocardiography. Sahn et al. and Allan et al. conducted studies to establish normal dimensions of the fetal heart using two-dimensional and M-mode examinations. Normal cardiac anatomy has been the subject of other investigations, and fetal cardiac function has been studied with M-mode and Doppler technique. Finally, the abnormal human heart has been investigated in an effort to improve both management and understanding of the high-risk fetus and newborn. This chapter focuses on the study of the normal human fetal heart.

Fetal cardiac anatomy and physiology differ from that found in the adult in several significant aspects. Anatomically, the foramen ovale and ductus arteriosus are patent in the fetus. The right ventricle has larger dimensions and a more spherical shape in cross-section than in the adult. Physiologically, blood flows in parallel through both ventricles simultaneously in the fetus, rather than in a serial pattern, as it does in the adult. The right ventricle pumps a larger amount of blood than does the left and ejects it primarily across the ductus arteriosus into the systemic circulation, rather than into the pulmonary artery branches. The left ventricle receives blood from the pulmonary veins, but the major source of blood is the left atrium via the foramen ovale. Blood is then pumped into the ascending aorta and carotid arteries. Other physiologic differences in the fetus include increases in heart rate and volume flow and decreases in the partial pressure of oxygen, oxygen saturation, blood pressure, and peripheral resistance.

FETAL CARDIAC ANATOMY

The fetal heart should always be approached in the context of the surrounding fetus and mother. At our institution we begin each cardiac examination with a brief history of the pregnancy, to determine the primary reason for the investigation and potential special areas of investigation. A complete ultrasound examination is then performed, obtaining information about the number and lie of the fetus(es), the position of the fetus, the location of the placenta , and the amount of amniotic fluid. Measurements of the fetus include biparietal diameter, head circumference, abdominal diameters and circumference, and femur length. A general anatomic investigation includes the fetal head, neck, spine, chest, bladder, kidneys, stomach, and limbs.

The examination of the fetal heart includes a four-chamber view, a long-axis/great-vessel view, a short-axis/great-vessel view, and a view of the great-vessel arches.

Four-Chamber View

The four-chamber view is usually obtained by turning the transducer to a transverse position across the fetal body at the level of the heart (Figs. 127–1 and 127–2). The anatomy that can be examined in this view includes the right and left ventricles, the tricuspid and mitral valves, and the ventricular and atrial septa. The foramen ovale or "left atrial" flap can be used to identify the left atrium. The tricuspid valve usually inserts lower on the ventricular septum than does the mitral valve. The left ventricle is closest to the spine. A slight angling of the view reveals the left ventricular outflow tract and the ascending aorta (Fig. 127–3). Further angling of the transducer reveals the main pulmonary artery as it exits the right ventricle (Fig. 127–4).

Long-Axis/Great-Vessel View

This view is obtained in the sagittal direction and is most easily arrived at by finding the vena cava, which is parallel to the spine. When the vena cava is identified, the tricuspid valve can usually be seen, along with the right atrium and right ventricle (Fig. 127–5). The pulmonary outflow tract is often visible exiting from the anterior portion of the right ventricle. Between the pulmonary artery and the vena cava, the ascending aorta can be identified, although it arises from a different plane.

Short-Axis/Great-Vessel View

The short-axis/great-vessel view is found at a 45-degree angle to the two previous views. In this view, the pulmonary artery is seen encircling the aorta (Fig. 127–6).

Great-Vessel Arches

The aortic arch can be seen in a sagittal plane. It is distinguished from the pulmonary artery "arch" (the ductus arteriosus) in two ways. First, the carotid arteries can be seen as they branch from the

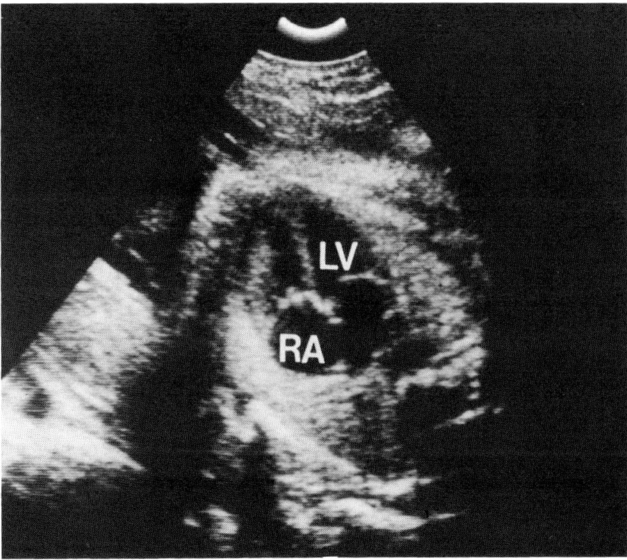

Figure 127–1. Four-chamber view of the human fetal heart. The spine is at 4 o'clock. (RA = right atrium; LV = left ventricle.)

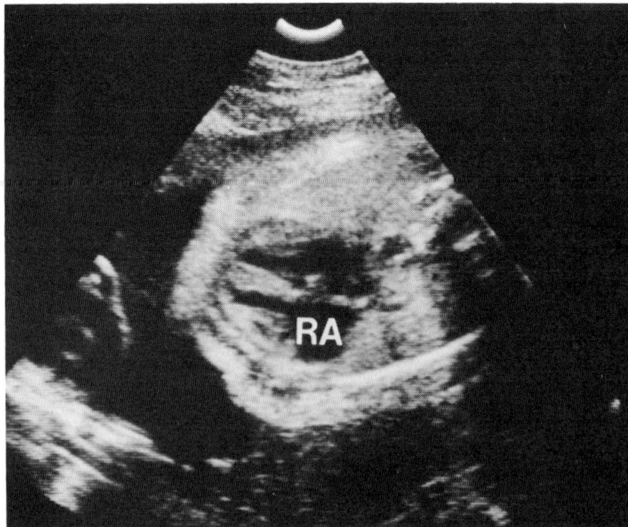

Figure 127–2. Four-chamber view of the human fetal heart from the same fetus as in Figure 127–1. The spine is now at 2 o'clock. Note the more thickened appearance of the myocardium, and ventricular septum. (RA = right atrium.)

transverse aortic arch. Second, the aortic arch has a tighter curve to it, whereas the pulmonary arch arises more anterior and lower than the aortic arch (Fig. 127–7).

Other Views

The fetus is often quite active during an examination and provides an excellent opportunity to view the three dimensions of the heart in ways difficult to reproduce in the neonate.

These views of cardiac anatomy are useful in several ways. The presence of normal structures is generally assured. In addition, comparisons of right and left ventricles, tricuspid and mitral valves, and pulmonary artery and aortic diameters can be made. The presence of abnormal ratios between the structures compared can be an indication of the presence of an anomaly.

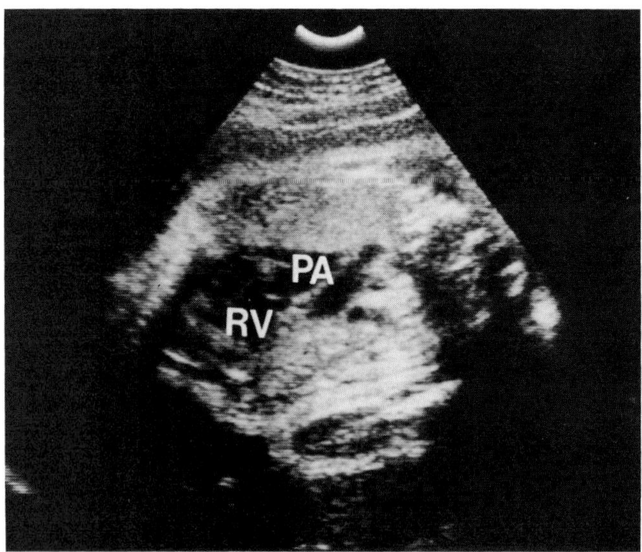

Figure 127–4. Right ventricle (RV) and main pulmonary artery (PA) from the same fetus as in Figures 127–1 to 127–3.

ABNORMALITIES

Fetal echocardiography is used in a variety of clinical settings to establish the presence of normal cardiac anatomy or to identify abnormalities of cardiac structure or function.

Abnormalities that challenge the echocardiographer of the neonate can be even more difficult to identify or exclude in the fetus. Small ventricular septal defects, minor valvular abnormalities, and anomalous pulmonary venous return are examples of lesions that are difficult or impossible to discover.

Congenital Abnormalities

Nearly every congenital abnormality identifiable by ultrasound after birth can be seen in the fetus, with the exceptions of a patent

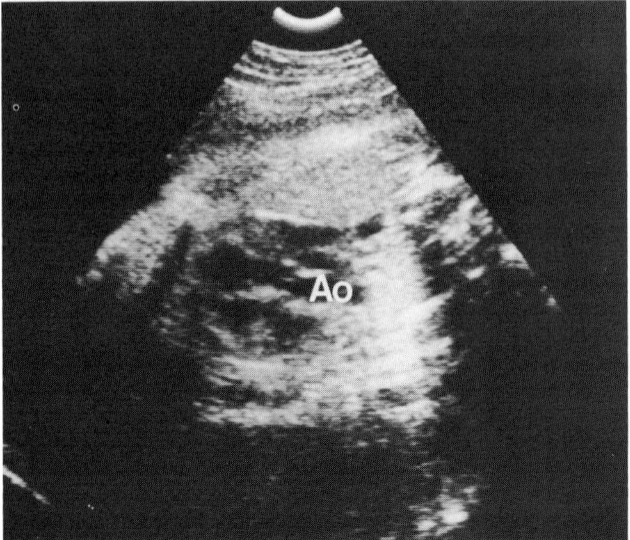

Figure 127–3. Left ventricle and ascending aorta (Ao) from the same fetus as in Figures 127–1 and 127–2.

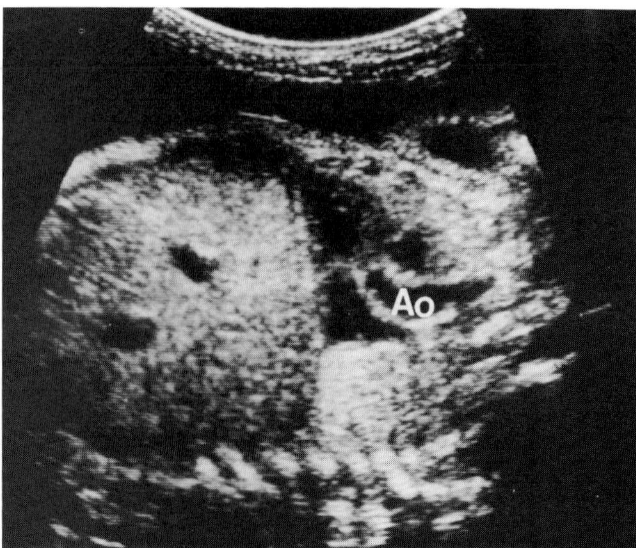

Figure 127–5. Long-axis/great-vessel view from the same fetus as in prior figures. The transducer is now more sagittal than transverse. The aorta (Ao) may be seen as two bright walls; anterior to this, the pulmonary valve may be seen. The right atrium and superior vena cava are seen posteriorly.

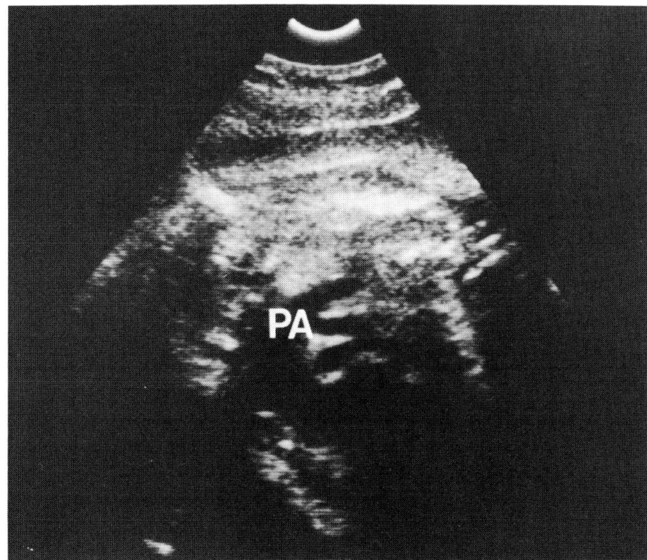

Figure 127–6. Short-axis/great-vessel view from the same fetus as in prior figures. The aorta is now seen as a circular shape around which the pulmonary artery (PA) curves.

foramen ovale and a patent ductus arteriosus, which are normal in the fetus. Identification of cardiac abnormalities prior to delivery enables parents and medical personnel to prepare for an outcome different from normal, to monitor the fetus carefully prior to birth, and to select delivery times and places for optimal newborn evaluation and management. If a cardiac abnormality is identified in the fetus, a careful search for other anatomical abnormalities should be made and a karyotype of the fetus considered, since there is an association of cardiac with other anatomical defects and chromosomal abnormalities, all of which might affect fetal prognosis and pregnancy management. An abnormal four-chamber view may be the first evidence of an abnormality in a fetus (Fig. 127–8).

Growth Failure

Fetuses with suboptimal intrauterine environments may develop abnormalities of vascular and cardiac function. Changes in the velocity of blood through the umbilical artery may be measured using Doppler ultrasound, and cardiac changes (e.g., ventricular dilatation, hypertrophy, and pericardial effusions) may be seen. Velocities of blood through the heart may also change as the condition progresses.

Arrhythmias

Fetuses are less accessible to the usual techniques for identifying arrhythmias (i.e., electrocardiography), and therefore two-dimensional, M-mode, and Doppler ultrasound techniques are used to identify fetal cardiac arrhythmias and to assess the cardiovascular responses. M-mode ultrasound, in which a cursor is placed across an atrial structure and a ventricular structure simultaneously, is used to identify timing of wall motion and thus the type of arrhythmia present (Fig. 127–9).

The majority of fetal arrhythmias consist of irregular heart rates due to premature atrial and ventricular contractions, which are usually benign. In a small percentage of fetuses with premature contractions, fetal cardiac anomalies are found; in some fetuses, a sustained tachyarrhythmia develops, which requires further attention.

Sustained tachyarrhythmias may be observed, or they may be treated either indirectly, by treating the mother with antiarrhythmic agents, or directly, by administering medication into the fetal umbilical vein.

Sustained bradycardias are accompanied by cardiac anomalies in 30 per cent of fetuses. Mothers of fetuses with complete heart block should be tested for lupus and anti-Ro and anti-La antibodies. Many fetuses tolerate heart block well; treatment for fetuses that develop heart failure (effusions or hydrops) has been disappointing.

Other Indications

Fetal echocardiography is also performed in fetuses with hydrops, since many cases of nonimmune hydrops are cardiac in origin. Twin fetuses may develop twin-transfusion syndrome with cardiac failure from either hypervolemia or hypovolemia. Fetuses of mothers treated for preterm labor with prostaglandin synthetase inhibition should be examined for evidence of ductal constriction, since the ductus arteriosus is known to be sensitive to prostaglandins.

Mothers whose fetuses are recommended for study include those with a history of a congenital heart lesion in themselves or a child

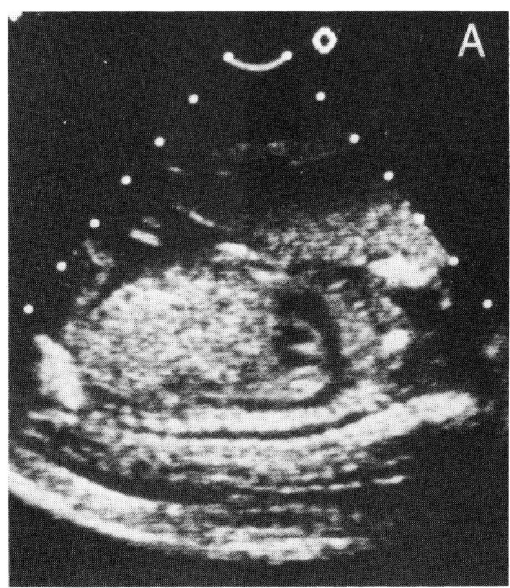

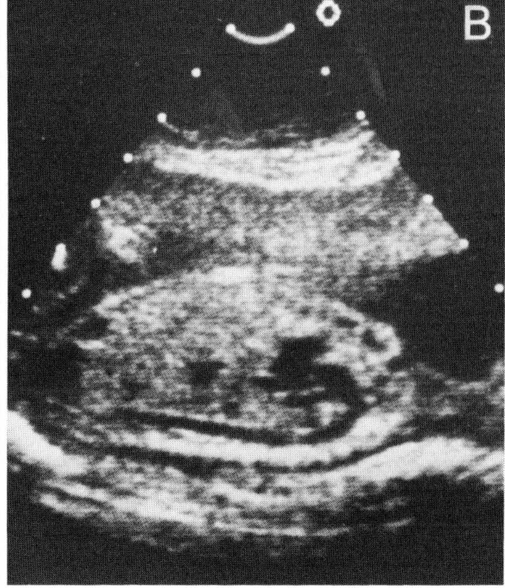

Figure 127–7. The great vessel arches view. The ductal arch *(A)* begins more anteriorly and forms a more flattened arch lower in the fetal chest than does the aortic arch *(B)*; cerebral vessels are seen exiting the transverse aortic arch. (From Reed KL, Anderson CF, Shenker L: Fetal Echocardiography: An Atlas. Reprinted by permission of Wiley-Liss, a division of John Wiley and Sons, Inc., © 1988.)

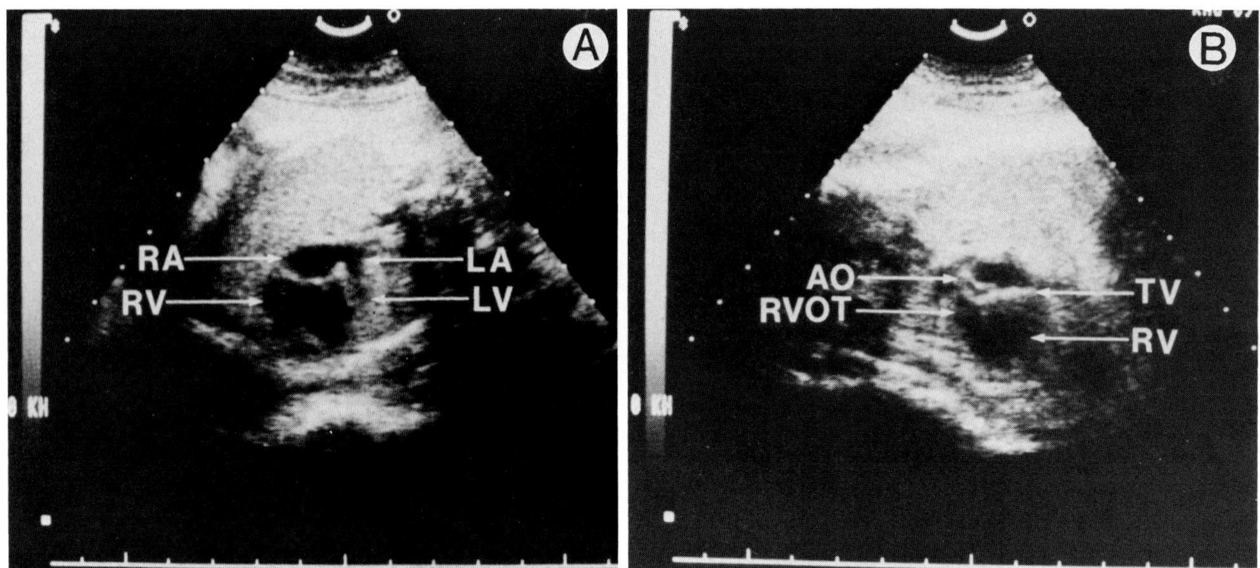

Figure 127–8. Four-chamber *(A)* and long-axis *(B)* views from a fetus with a **hypoplastic left ventricle**. (RA = right atrium; LA = left atrium; RV = right ventricle; LV = left ventricle; AO = aorta; RVOT = right ventricular outflow tract; TV = tricuspid valve.) (From Reed KL, Anderson CF, Shenker L: Fetal Echocardiography: An Atlas. Reprinted by permission of Wiley-Liss, a division of John Wiley and Sons, Inc., © 1988.)

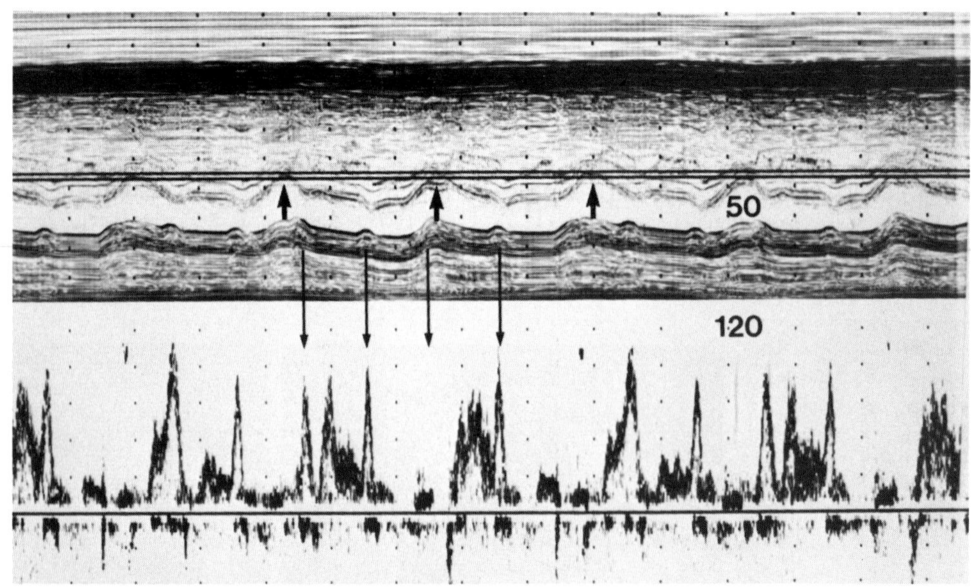

Figure 127–9. M-mode *(upper frame)* and two-dimensional Doppler ultrasound tracing *(lower frame)* from a fetus with **complete heart block**. The ventricular rate *(large arrows)* is 50 bpm; the atrial rate *(narrow arrows)* is 120 bpm. (From Reed KL, Anderson CF, Shenker L: Fetal Echocardiography: An Atlas. Reprinted by permission of Wiley-Liss, a division of John Wiley and Sons, Inc., © 1988.)

or relative, women with predisposing diseases such as diabetes, women exposed to teratogens known to cause cardiac pathology, and those with fetuses with abnormalities discovered during pregnancy.

Fetuses should be studied as early as 14 to 16 weeks' gestation (a four-chamber view is possible at this age) and again at 26 to 27 weeks. As the fetus grows, the examination can become more difficult, since the fetus often lies left side down and the heart is shadowed by spine and ribs.

In summary, the fetal heart is now available for noninvasive examination. Differences in fetal and adult anatomy and physiology should be considered when performing these studies. Anatomy can be determined by using both standard and unorthodox views, as available on the basis of fetal position. Certain abnormalities cannot be excluded on the basis of current scanning capabilities. The study of the human fetal heart not only provides ongoing care for the high-risk fetus, but also is an area of continuing research about normal cardiac anatomy and physiology.

Bibliography

Allan LD: Manual of Fetal Echocardiography. Boston, MTP Press, 1986.

Allan LD, Joseph MC, Boyd EGCA, et al: M-mode echocardiography in the developing human fetus. Br Heart J 47:573, 1982.

Allan LD, Tynan MJ, Campbell S, et al: Echocardiographic and anatomical correlates in the fetus. Br Heart J 44:444, 1980.

DeVore GR, Donnerstein RL, Kleinman CS, et al: Fetal echocardiography I: Normal anatomy as determined by real-time-directed M-mode ultrasound. Am J Obstet Gynecol 144:249, 1982.

Kleinman CS, Donnerstein RL, DeVore GR, et al: Fetal echocardiography for evaluation of in utero congestive heart failure. N Engl J Med 306:568, 1982.

Reed KL: Fetal arrhythmias: Etiology, diagnosis, pathophysiology, and treatment. Semin Perinatol 13:294–304, 1989.

Reed KL, Anderson CF, Shenker L: Fetal Echocardiography: An Atlas. New York, Wiley/Liss, 1988.

Reed KL, Meijboom EJ, Sahn DJ, et al: Cardiac Doppler flow velocities in human fetuses. Circulation 68:278, 1983.

Romero R, Pilu G, Jeanty P, et al: Prenatal Diagnosis of Congenital Anomalies. Norwalk, CT, Appleton & Lange, 1988.

Sahn DJ, Lange LW, Allen HD, et al: Quantitative real-time cross-sectional echocardiography in the developing normal human fetus and newborn. Circulation 62:588, 1980.

128 Fetal Anomalies of the Abdomen and Abdominal Wall

Lewis H. Nelson

Many congenital structural anomalies, syndromes, and genetic anomalies are associated with abnormalities of the fetal abdominal wall or intra-abdominal structures. This chapter discusses common ultrasonographic findings associated with these abdominal defects. Table 128–1 may serve as a guide to the differential diagnosis until the sonographer develops an individualized approach.

Table 128–2 compares the features of the more common anterior abdominal wall defects of omphalocele (Figs. 128–1 to 128–3) and gastroschisis (Fig. 128–4). Extrophy of the bladder also produces an abdominal wall defect but does not result in an exophytic mass or group of echoes exterior to the wall. In omphalocele, eventration of abdominal contents occurs through the umbilical ring into a sac covered by peritoneum. In gastroschisis, on the other hand, extrusion of bowel occurs through a paramedian defect, generally to the right of the fetal umbilicus. Identification of the normal umbilical cord insertion (Fig. 128–4*A* and *C*), therefore, is important in distinguishing gastroschisis from a ruptured omphalocele. If the umbilical cord does not appear to end in the abdominal wall but in a mass of floating loops of bowel, then the fetus may have a ruptured omphalocele. Contents of the mass anterior to the abdominal wall other than bowel, such as liver, nearly always imply an omphalocele. Rarely, a large umbilical hernia may contain liver and be confused with an omphalocele.

Occasionally an omphalocele may be part of Beckwith-Wiedemann syndrome, which consists of omphalocele, macroglossia, and macrosomia with some degree of polyhydramnios, renal hyperplasia, renal medullary dysplasia, adrenal cytomegaly, pancreatic islet-cell hyperplasia, facial nevus flammeus, and severe neonatal hypoglycemia. These infants can do well with proper prenatal preparations for delivery to protect the abdominal wall defect and to avoid severe neonatal hypoglycemia. If an omphalocele is diagnosed, genetic amniocentesis may provide additional information that can be helpful in patient management, since many large omphaloceles occur in chromosomally abnormal fetuses. If the omphalocele is associated with limb deficiencies or kyphoscoliosis, the anterior mass may be displaced posteriorly to such a degree that it resembles a sacrococcygeal teratoma (Fig. 128–5).

Deficient abnormal abdominal musculature associated with urinary tract anomalies and cryptorchidism has been called the prune-

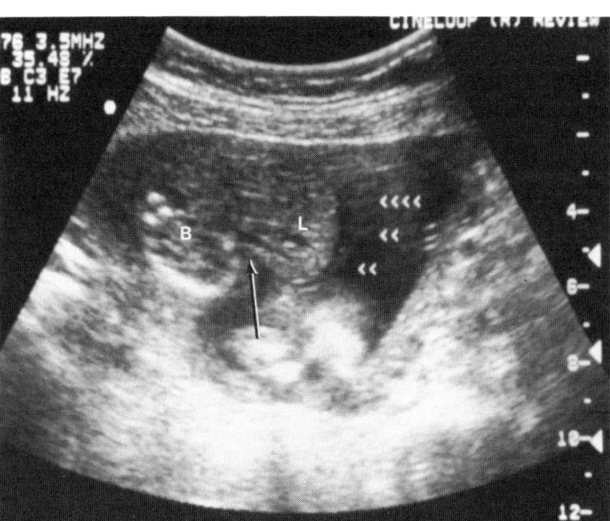

Figure 128–1. Omphalocele. The fetal liver (L) is in the sac (<) protruding through the abdominal wall defect (*arrow*) in the fetal body (B).

TABLE 128–1. GROUPING OF ANOMALIES ACCORDING TO LOCATION AND MULTIPLICITY OF ANECHOIC AREAS

GROUP	ULTRASOUND FINDINGS	ANATOMIC AREAS	ASSOCIATED FINDINGS
1	Single pelvic sonolucency	A. Normal bladder, usually consistently visible after 16 to 18 weeks	A. Absence implies renal dysfunction (scan hour to observe function): oligohydramnios
		B. Peritoneal cyst	
		C. Mesodermal/ovarian cysts	
		D. Enlarged bladder	D. Outlet obstruction: posterior urethral valves (males), bladder neck obstruction, hypotonic atony, MMIPS*: Prune-belly syndrome: elongated abdominal cross-section
2	Single abdominal sonolucency	A. Normal stomach	
		B. Omental cyst	
		C. Gastric outlet obstruction (usually multiple)	C. Peristalsis: helpful in identifying as gastrointestinal; polyhydramnios
3	Multiple abdominal sonolucencies	A. Normal bowel	A. Normal amniotic fluid volume
		B. "Double bubble"	B. Duodenal atresia; polyhydramnios
		C. Other multiple areas	C. Imperforate anus, meconium ileus, Hirschsprung's disease, meconium pseudocyst
		D. Bowel floats in fluid	D. Ascites
		E. Any of group 1	E. Oligohydramnios usually present in A or D of Group 1
4	Posterior abdominal sonolucencies	A. Generally renal, multicystic	A. Hydroureter, hydronephrosis, paranephric pseudocyst: IPKD†, multicystic kidney, oligohydramnios if bilateral
		B. Any of group 2	B. Polyhydramnios
5	Intrathoracic sonolucencies	A. Single or multiple	A. Pleural fluid, teratoma, chylothorax, intrathoracic cyst, cystic adenomatoid malformation
		B. Defect in diaphragm	B. Diaphragmatic hernia—adjacent to heart
6	Extraperitoneal or extrathoracic sonolucencies and sonodensities (multiple or single)	A. Dorsal	A. Neural tube defects: elevated alpha-fetoprotein; hydrocephaly and polyhydramnios frequently present
		B. Ventral	B. Omphalocele, gastroschisis, extrophy of fetal organs (usually elevated alpha-fetoprotein), lymphatic anomalies
		C. Posterolateral	C. Cystic hygroma
		D. Neck	D. Teratoma, goiter

*Megacystis-microcolon-hypoperistalsis syndrome.
†Infant polycystic kidney disease.

TABLE 128–2. COMPARISON OF OMPHALOCELE AND GASTROSCHISIS

	OMPHALOCELE	GASTROSCHISIS
Location	Anterior to fetus	Anterior to fetus
Covering	Membrane or membrane remnant	No membrane
Echoes	More solid appearance	Multiple floating anechoic areas
Contents	Portion of bowel, usually other abdominal contents	Bowel only
Umbilical cord	Involved	Not involved
Associated abnormalities	Gastrointestinal, cardiac	Few (Meckel's malrotations)
Chromosomal abnormalities	Frequent	Rare
Miscellaneous	If ruptures, resembles gastroschisis	Thickened bowel wall because of reaction to amniotic fluid
	Beckwith-Wiedemann syndrome	
	Limb/body wall deficiency syndrome	
	Pentalogy of Cantrell	

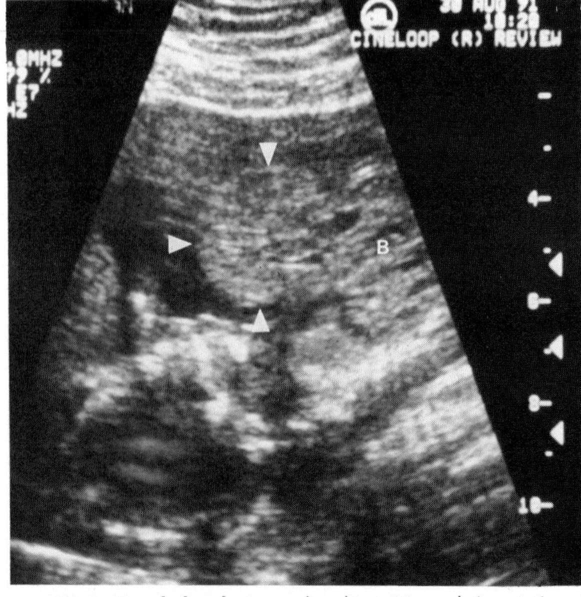

Figure 128–2. Omphalocele (*arrowheads*) at 16 weeks' gestation. The sac is as large as the fetal body (B).

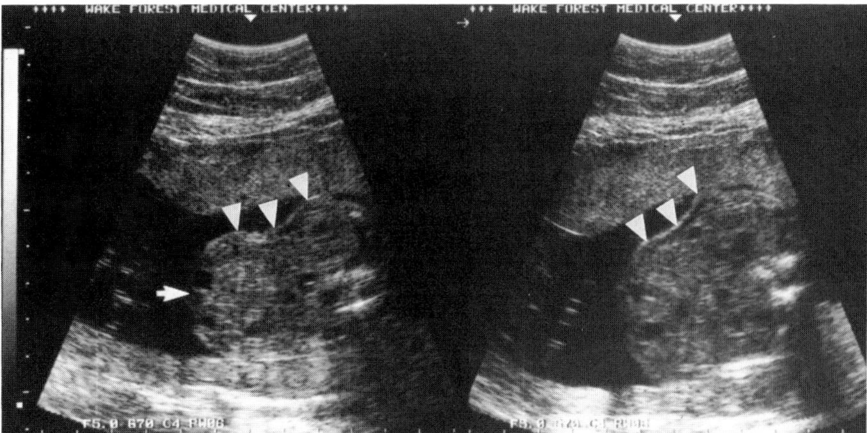

Figure 128–3. Pseudo-omphalocele. *A,* The false omphalocele (*arrow in A*) disappeared within 10 minutes. *B,* The abdomen returning to a normal contour. Note that the skin (*arrowheads in A and B*) is intact and contiguous.

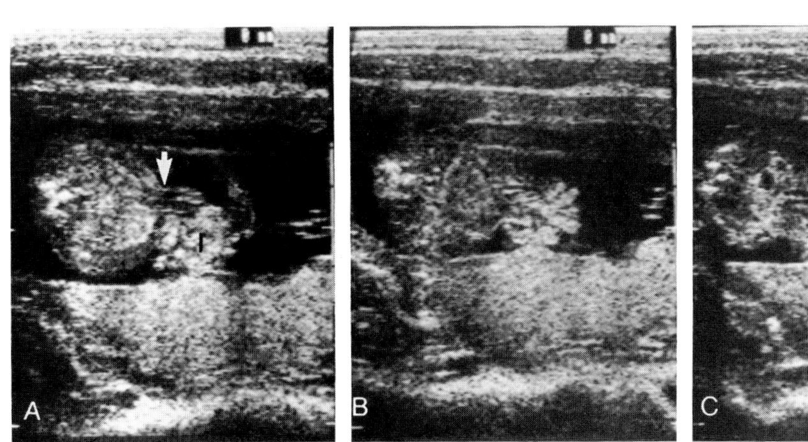

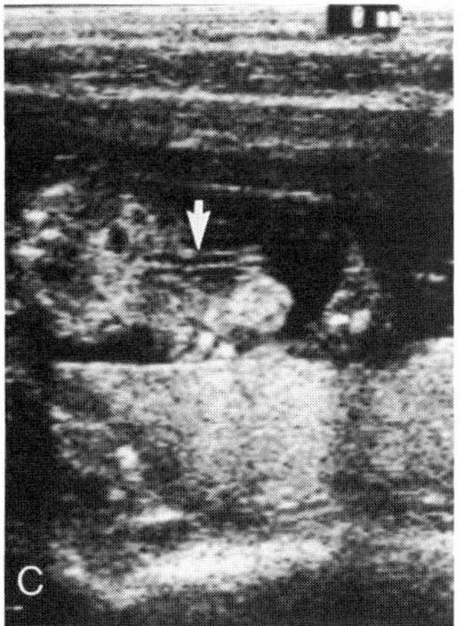

Figure 128–4. *A* to *C,* **Gastroschisis.** Matted loops of fetal intestines (I) are outside the fetal body (B). Visualization of the umbilical cord insertion site (*arrows in A and C*) confirms the diagnosis.

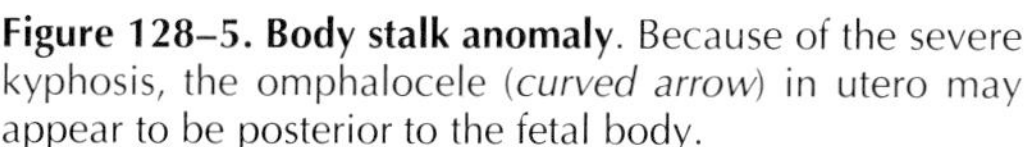

Figure 128–5. Body stalk anomaly. Because of the severe kyphosis, the omphalocele (*curved arrow*) in utero may appear to be posterior to the fetal body.

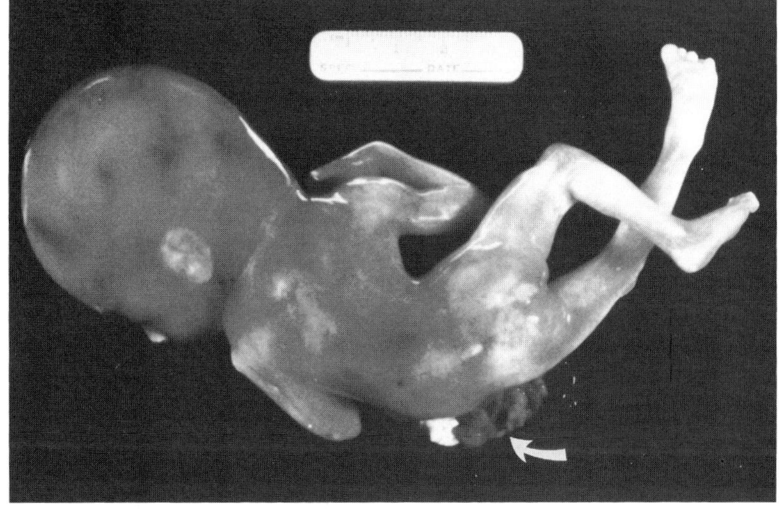

belly syndrome because the thinned anterior abdominal wall of the neonate gives the wrinkled appearance of a prune. In utero, the absence of muscle tone allows the usual roundness of the fetal abdomen to distort to a markedly elliptical shape. The presence of multiple intra-abdominal cystic echoes and oligohydramnios suggestive of a urinary tract anomaly in association with a lax fetal abdominal wall should suggest prune-belly syndrome. Since the majority of these infants are males with undescended testes, one should look for fetal sex and an empty scrotal sac, recognizing that in normal babies there is variability of the time of testicular descent.

Normally the fetal stomach and bladder are readily seen as the largest anechoic areas in the abdomen because of their liquid contents. The fetal gallbladder and fluid-filled segments of bowel are smaller and should not be confused with stomach and bladder. Clues to gastrointestinal tract abnormalities may be the absence of fluid in the stomach and the appearance of additional anechoic areas such as the second fluid collection (analogous to the "double bubble" sign on a postnatal radiograph) of duodenal atresia.

The absence of fluid in the stomach may mean esophageal atresia, especially when associated with polyhydramnios and absence of fluid in other portions of the fetal gut (Fig. 128–6). The converse is not true, however, since esophageal atresia is frequently associated with degrees of respiratory tract—to—gastrointestinal tract fistulas that enable amniotic fluid to reach the gastrointestinal tract via the fetal trachea.

In duodenal atresia, associated with the "double bubble" sign (Fig. 128–7), one can visualize the increased peristalsis associated with duodenal atresia and trace the duodenal bulb to the stomach with real-time ultrasound (Fig. 128–8). Duodenal atresia can be fatal to the neonate because of aspiration and electrolyte imbalance. Of particular significance is the fact that trisomy 21 occurs in approximately 30 per cent of infants with duodenal atresia. Other associated anomalies include malrotation of the gut, congenital heart disease, tracheo-esophageal fistulas, and renal malformations. Unfortunately, a single ultrasound study prior to 28 to 29 weeks' gestation may not eliminate the diagnosis of duodenal atresia in a normal-appearing fetus. Serial scans should be performed if a subsequent fetus is at risk for recurrence. Of serious consequence unless recognized is the combination of duodenal and esophageal atresia. In this instance, the stomach may be massively dilated beyond that found in duodenal atresia above.

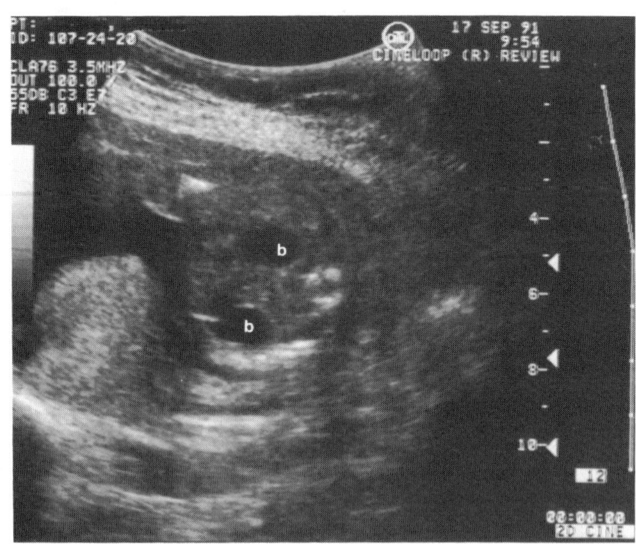

Figure 128–7. The large anechoic areas of the "**double bubble**" **sign (b)** are seen in the fetal abdomen.

As the number of dilated loops of bowel seen on ultrasound increases, the probability that the obstruction is more distal in the gastrointestinal tract also increases. Such entities include distal small bowel and anal atresia or obstruction of the distal colon from functional etiologies (Figs. 128–9 and 128–10). The differential diagnosis of a multicystic appearing mass in the fetal abdomen should include hydronephrosis with dilated ureters. As previously mentioned, amniotic fluid volume assists in this distinction; genitourinary obstruction, depending on the degree of severity, tends to be associated with diminished amniotic fluid volume, whereas gastrointestinal obstruction frequently leads to increased amounts of amniotic fluid. Bowel obstruction typically does not affect the normal-appearing bladder and kidneys.

In addition to the increased number of dilated segments of bowel, the presence of calcified particles within the bowel should suggest lower bowel obstruction and possible rupture. After rupture, intracavitary or intraluminal calcifications can occur (Figs. 128–11 and

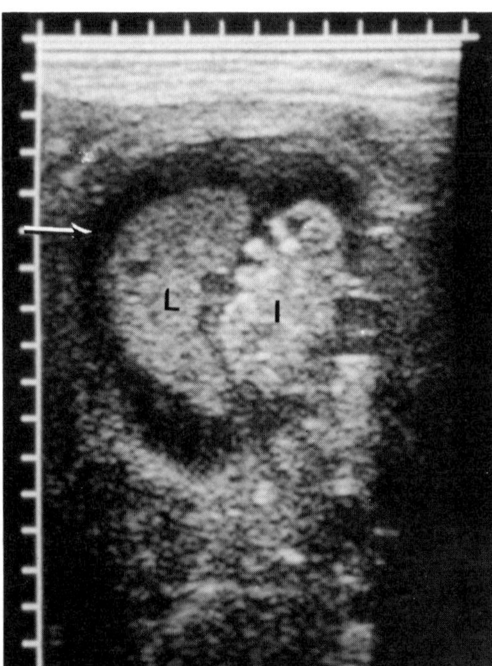

Figure 128–6. No fluid is seen in the fetal intestines (I), which, with the liver (L), are floating free in ascitic fluid (*arrow*) in a 32-week fetus with **esophageal atresia and ascites**.

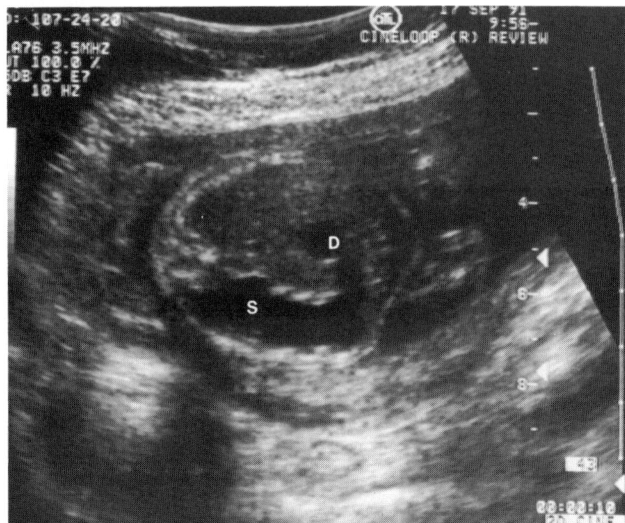

Figure 128–8. By rotating the scanner, **the dilated stomach (S) and a portion of the duodenum (D)** can be imaged.

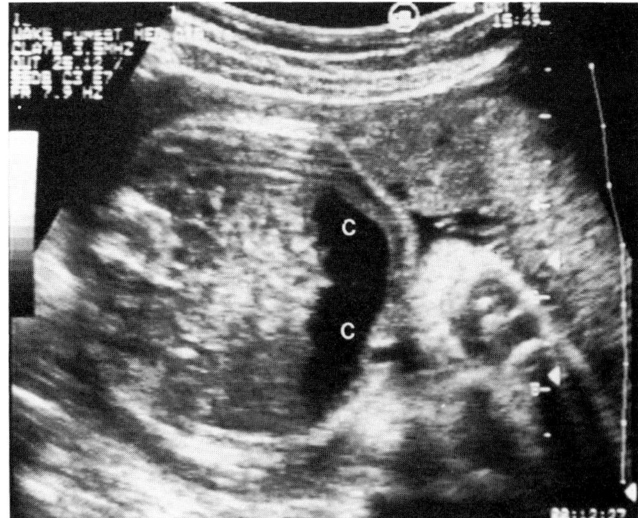

Figure 128–9. Portions of a **dilated transverse colon (C)** are seen at approximately 25 weeks' gestation.

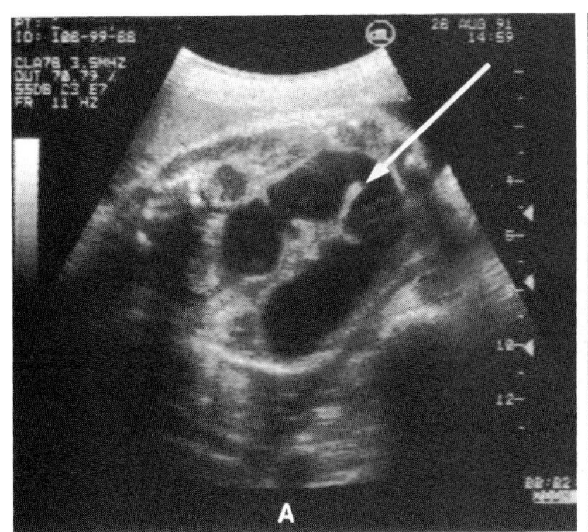

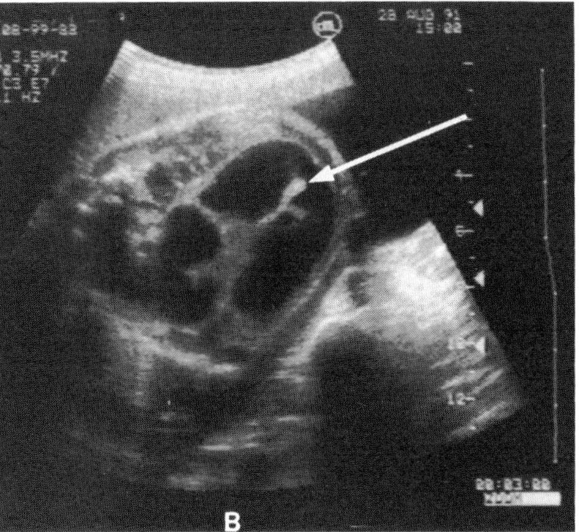

Figure 128–10. *A* and *B*, **Large dilated segment of fetal bowel**. During the approximately 23 seconds that elapsed between the two images, a peristaltic wave (*arrow*) could be observed.

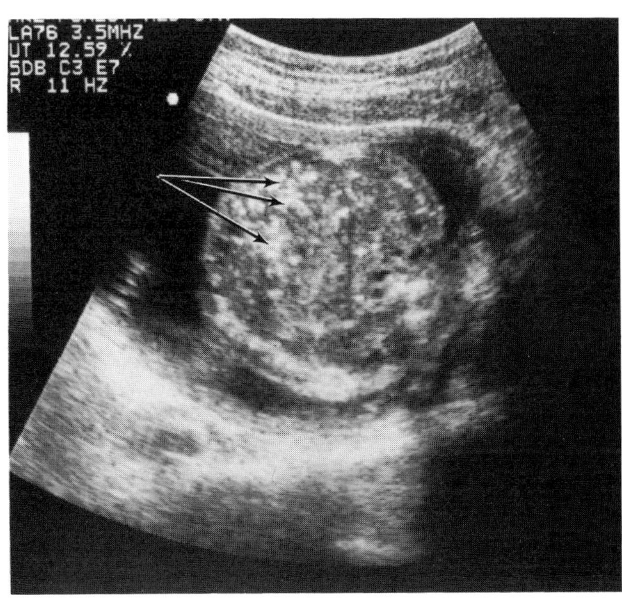

Figure 128–11. Intra-abdominal calcifications (*arrows*) generally associated with fetal bowel rupture secondary to mechanical (atresia) or functional (Hirschsprung's disease) obstruction. (Courtesy of Dr. Mac Ernest.)

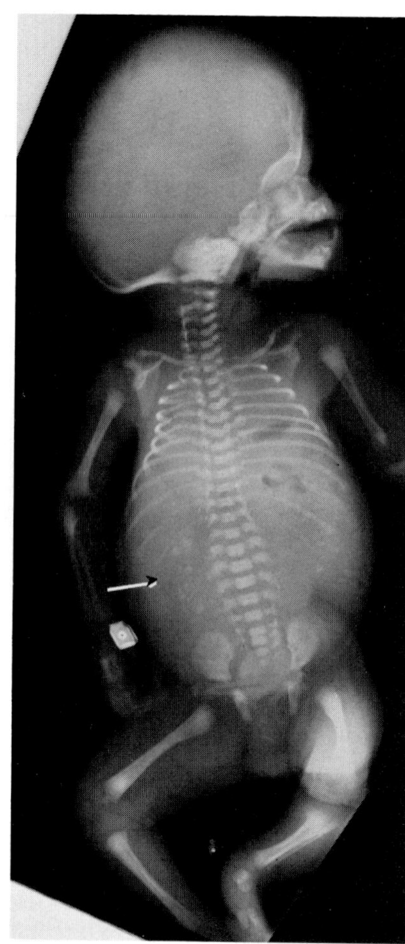

Figure 128–12. A roentgenogram showing **small flecks of calcium (*arrow*).** There is also hydrocephaly and dysraphism of the lumbosacral spine.

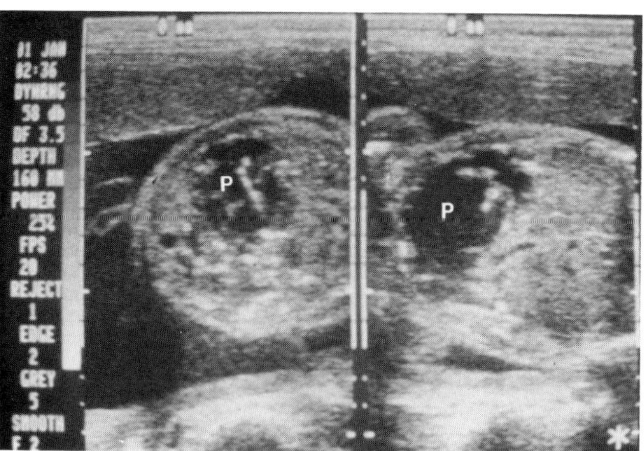

Figure 128–13. Two different views of a **meconium pseudocyst (P).**

128–12). One may see a swirling motion of these calcifications, which is caused by bowel peristalsis. Unfortunately, since these intraluminal calcifications occur only rarely and the fetal colon may be quite prominent in the absence of obstruction, the antenatal sonographic diagnosis of colonic, rectal, or anal obstruction frequently remains elusive.

If the fetal gastrointestinal tract ruptures in utero, meconium may escape and cause an intense peritoneal reaction that will seal off the sterile meconium. The resultant structure, a meconium pseudocyst (Fig. 128–13), will appear as a large anechoic area with dense borders and some degree of acoustic shadowing from calcifications of the meconium. This increased echogenicity and shadowing separate a normal stomach from a pseudocyst.

Other anechoic masses have been described in the fetal abdomen and pelvis. These may represent ovarian cysts in the female fetus, paranephric pseudocysts, or teratomas. Ovarian cysts may be of little consequence (Fig. 128–14), but the paranephric pseudocyst

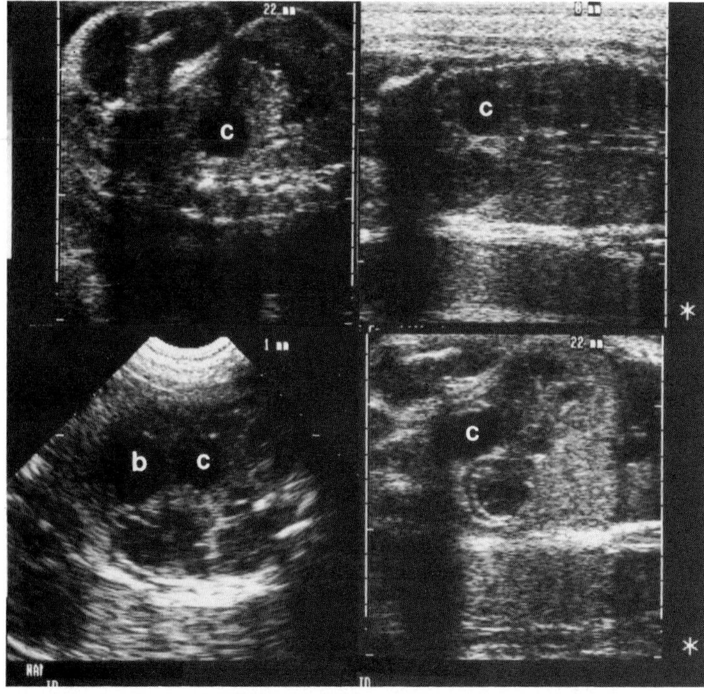

Figure 128–14. Multiple views of an **ovarian cyst (c).** Over time, the fetal bladder (b) volume changes, which assists in identification of the bladder.

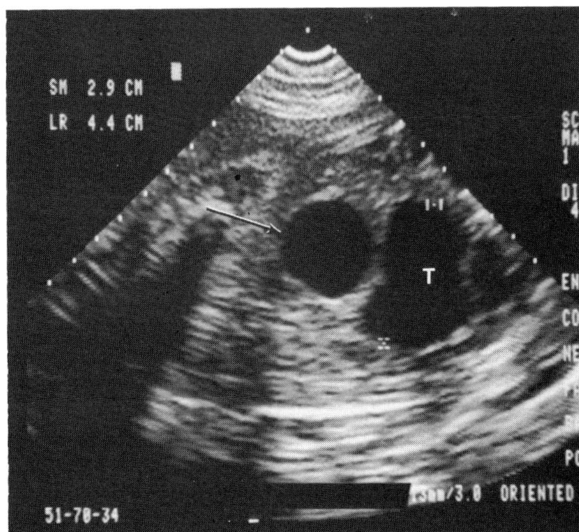

Figure 128–15. A large anechoic mass proven to be a **cystic teratoma (T)** noted separate from the fetal bladder (*arrow*). The mass gradually increased in size. The fetal bladder was identified by a variable volume over one hour of scanning.

(urinoma) can be confused with hydronephrosis and portends severe obstructive uropathy. Callen et al. found a nonfunctioning ipsilateral kidney in four of five cases of paranephric pseudocyst. Teratomas frequently contain cystic areas. Not all of these teratomas will be extrinsic to the fetus but can be pelvic-abdominal (Fig. 128–15) and must be differentiated from fetal bladder and ovarian cysts. The fetal bladder will have a variable volume during an hour of scanning.

Anomalies of the fetal abdominal wall and abdomen frequently do not exist in isolation and require diligence in identifying all normal anatomy present and monitoring physiologic functions such as peristalsis or voiding. Despite the differential diagnostic characteristics described herein, it may still not be possible to assign a specific label to a group of findings until the infant is delivered and further diagnostic techniques are feasible (Table 128–3).

TABLE 128–3. COMPLEMENTARY DIAGNOSTIC TESTS IN EVALUATING FETAL ABDOMINAL WALL AND ABDOMINAL ANOMALIES

Amniocentesis	Chromosomes, viral cultures, alpha-fetoprotein Amniogram
Percutaneous umbilical blood sampling	Chromosomes, fetal blood studies
Real-time ultrasound	Fetal movement and concomitant movement of mass Fetal swallowing Peristalsis Voiding
Aspiration of fluid-filled structures	Chemical analysis of contents Reaccumulation time Occasionally therapeutic
Maternal abdominal roentgenogram (rarely indicated)	Calcifications

Bibliography

Bean WJ, Calonje MA, Aprill CN, Geshner J: Anal atresia: A prenatal ultrasound diagnosis. J Clin Ultrasound 6:111, 1978.
Berdon WE, Baker DH, Wigger HJ, Blanc WA: The radiologic and pathologic spectrum of the prune belly syndrome. Radiol Clin North Am 15:83, 1977.
Callen PW, Bolding D, Filly RA, Harrison MR: Ultrasonographic evaluation of fetal paranephric pseudocysts. J Ultrasound Med 2:209, 1983.
Garris J, Kangarloo H, Sarti D, et al: The ultrasound spectrum of prune-belly syndrome. J Clin Ultrasound 8:117, 1980.
McCook TA, Felman AH: Esophageal atresia, duodenal atresia, and gastric distention: Report of two cases. AJR 131:167, 1978.
McGahan JP, Hanson F: Meconium peritonitis with accompanying pseudocyst: Prenatal sonographic diagnosis. Radiology 148:125, 1983.
Nelson LH, Clark CE, Fishburne JI, et al: Value of serial sonography in the in utero detection of duodenal atresia. Obstet Gynecol 59:657, 1982.
Pretorius DH, Meier PR, Johnson ML: Diagnosis of esophageal atresia in utero. J Ultrasound Med 2:475, 1983.
Schaffer RM, Barone C, Friedman AP: The ultrasonographic spectrum of fetal omphalocele. J Ultrasound Med 2:219, 1983.
Shalev E, Weiner E, Zuckerman H: Prenatal ultrasound diagnosis of intestinal calcifications with imperforate anus. Acta Obstet Gynecol Scand 62:95, 1983.
Stephenson SR, Weaver DD: Prenatal diagnosis—A compilation of diagnosed conditions. Am J Obstet Gynecol 141:319, 1981.
Wrobleski D, Wesselhoeft C: Ultrasonic diagnosis of prenatal intestinal obstruction. J Pediatr Surg 14:598, 1979.

129 Fetal Urinary Tract Abnormalities

Barry S. Mahony

Genitourinary lesions constitute the majority of causes for neonatal abdominal masses. Careful antenatal sonographic evaluation of the fetal abdomen and pelvis will detect many fetal genitourinary abnormalities. Renal anomalies are often incidental findings, however, and many are not detected unless a complete sonographic examination is performed routinely. For this reason, the American Institute of Ultrasound in Medicine, the American College of Radiology, and the American College of Obstetricians and Gynecologists recommend evaluation of the fetal bladder and renal regions as components of a basic obstetric ultrasound during the second and third trimesters of pregnancy.

After detection of a fetal genitourinary anomaly, each of the components of the genitourinary system should be evaluated. Knowing the normal sonographic appearance of the fetal genitourinary system and the expected ultrasound features of the different anomalies assists in this task.

THE NORMAL FETAL URINARY TRACT

In the second and third trimesters, amniotic fluid volume is largely dependent on fetal urination. Therefore, an assessment of the quantity of amniotic fluid constitutes the initial evaluation of

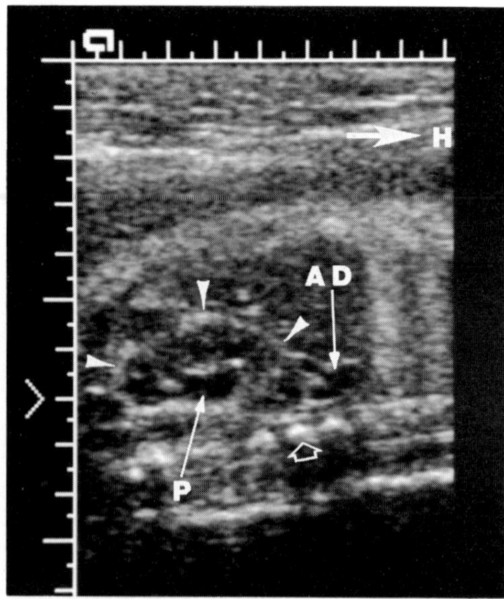

Figure 129–1. Coronal real-time sonogram of the fetal abdomen demonstrates the fetal kidney *(arrowheads)* in its paraspinous location (*open arrow* = fetal spine). The kidney is outlined by the echogenic retroperitoneal fat. Note the small amount of fluid in the renal pelvis (P); this amount of minimal fetal pyelectasis is frequently present. Also note the fetal adrenal gland (AD), which is normally relatively prominent in the fetus. (H = toward the fetal head.)

the fetal genitourinary system. A normal amniotic fluid volume implies the presence of at least one functioning kidney.

Normal fetal kidneys may be identified in their paraspinous location as early as 12 to 14 menstrual weeks. In longitudinal section the fetal kidneys are elliptical in shape, and in transverse section they are circular structures adjacent to the lumbar spinal ossification centers (Fig. 129–1). As pregnancy advances, the echogenic retroperitoneal fat that surrounds the kidneys assists in their sonographic visualization. The hypoechoic fetal renal pyramids are arranged in anterior and posterior rows surrounding the central renal sinus. The echo intensity of the normal fetal renal cortex usually approximates or may even be slightly greater than that of the surrounding tissues, permitting visualization of the relatively echopenic pyramids. Identification of the characteristic arrangement of the hypoechoic pyramids in anterior and posterior rows avoids any confusion between them and parenchymal cysts. Within the central pelvocalyceal system, a small amount of fluid is commonly seen in the absence of obstruction.

Normal measurements for renal length, width, thickness, volume, and circumference as a function of menstrual age have been reported and correspond to renal size obtained on stillborn fetuses. As general guidelines of renal size, the normal fetal kidney is approximately twice as long as it is wide and the renal length (in mm) is approximately equal to the gestational age (in weeks). For example, at 30 weeks the normal fetal kidney measures approximately 30 mm long and 15 mm in anteroposterior width. Diminution in renal size is more difficult to establish than is renal enlargement because the renal border may be partially obscured and difficult to distinguish from the adjacent adrenal.

Nondilated fetal ureters have not been routinely identified. However, the normal fetal urinary bladder has been shown as early as 10 to 12 weeks. Since the fetus normally fills and empties the urinary bladder every 30 to 45 minutes, the bladder is frequently seen to increase in size and to empty during the course of a sonographic examination. At 32 weeks the maximum fetal bladder volume should not exceed 10 ml, but it increases rapidly so that it is approximately 40 ml at term. Similarly, fetal urine volume production, calculated by measuring change in bladder volume with time, increases from 9.6 ml/hour at 30 weeks to 27.3 ml/hour at 40 weeks. Observation of filling and emptying of the fetal-urinary bladder confirms that urine is being produced. The normal fetal urinary bladder has a very thin or virtually invisible wall and occupies an anterior midline position within the fetal pelvis. The urinary bladder is usually spherical or elliptical in configuration. Observing a change in volume of the urinary bladder permits differentiation between it and other cystic pelvic structures. The urethra may be identified extending the length of an erect fetal penis, but in females or males with a flaccid penis, the normal urethra is difficult to identify.

GENITOURINARY ANOMALIES

Hydronephrosis

Hydronephrosis is the most common cause of an abdominal mass in the newborn. Antenatal sonography detects fetal hydronephrosis of varying extent from minimal pyelectasis to severe hydronephrosis with virtually complete loss of renal parenchyma. With careful assessment, the level of urinary tract obstruction can be localized by sonography.

Measurements of the anteroposterior diameter of the renal pelvis and kidney, as well as assessment of caliectasis after 19 weeks, provide useful prognostic information regarding the degree of dilatation. A pelvic diameter of less than 10 mm and a ratio between the pelvic diameter and kidney diameter of less than 50 per cent in the absence of rounded calyces is probably physiologic and rarely progresses. On the other hand, a diameter of the renal pelvis of more than 10 to 15 mm and a ratio between the pelvic diameter and kidney diameter of more than 50 per cent with rounded calyces indicate significant pyelocaliectasis that frequently requires surgical management.

As the severity of pyelocaliectasis progresses, the calyces dilate further and the parenchyma thins (Fig. 129–2). In severe cases, only a large paraspinous cystic structure is seen, and distinction between other abdominal masses may be difficult. As a general rule, however, if the mass touches the fetal spine it likely originates from the genitourinary system. In some cases of severe hydronephrosis, rupture of the urinary tract may produce a perinephric urinoma or lead to fetal urinary ascites, both of which may decompress the urinary tract. A perinephric urinoma is a large unilocular cystic flank mass touching the fetal spine (Fig. 129–3).

Site of Obstruction

If urinary tract obstruction is present, certain sonographic features allow one to determine the site of obstruction. This information is necessary if antenatal or prompt postnatal surgical management is contemplated. Even if early surgical intervention is not deemed necessary, antenatal diagnosis of urinary tract obstruction permits increased surveillance so that the patient does not return as an infant or child with loss of renal function from progression of an obstructive lesion that had been clinically silent.

Ureteropelvic junction obstruction is the most common cause of neonatal hydronephrosis. In ureteropelvic junction obstruction the renal pelvis, infundibula, and calyces are dilated. Only a single fluid-filled structure with a thin rim of surrounding parenchyma is present in severe cases. The ureters are nondilated and, therefore, not seen sonographically. If the contralateral kidney is normal, the amniotic fluid volume is normal and the urinary bladder fills and empties normally, even if the degree of obstruction is severe enough to cause renal damage on the ipsilateral side.

In some cases, unequivocal fetal pyelocaliectasis without hydroureter (compatible with ureteropelvic junction obstruction) has been detected antenatally, but a sonogram obtained on the first day fol-

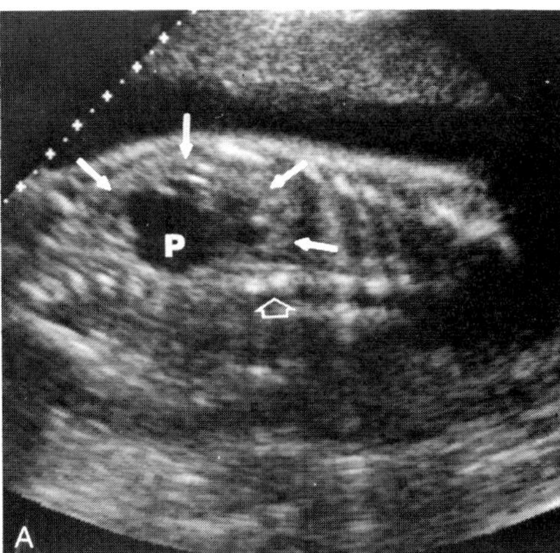

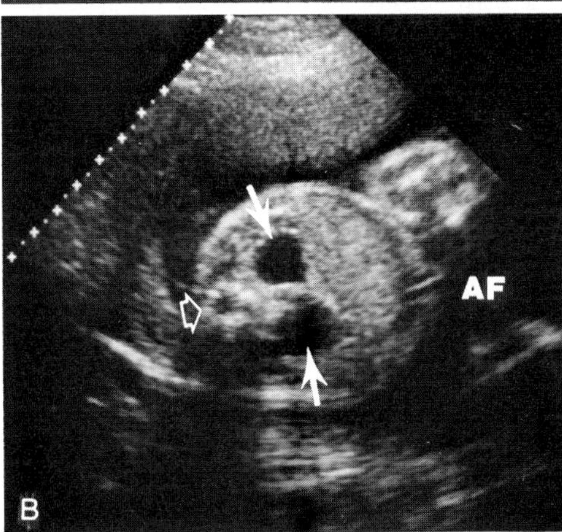

Figure 129–2. *A*, Coronal scan of the fetal abdomen with **unilateral ureteropelvic junction obstruction** displays moderate pyelocaliectasis *(small arrows)*. (P = Renal pelvis; *open arrow* = fetal spine.) *B*, Axial scan of another fetus shows bilateral dilatation of the renal pelvis and infundibula *(arrows)* in this fetus with **bilateral ureteropelvic junction obstruction**. Since a normal amount of amniotic fluid (AF) is present, one may infer that the obstruction is not complete. (*Open arrow* = fetal spine.)

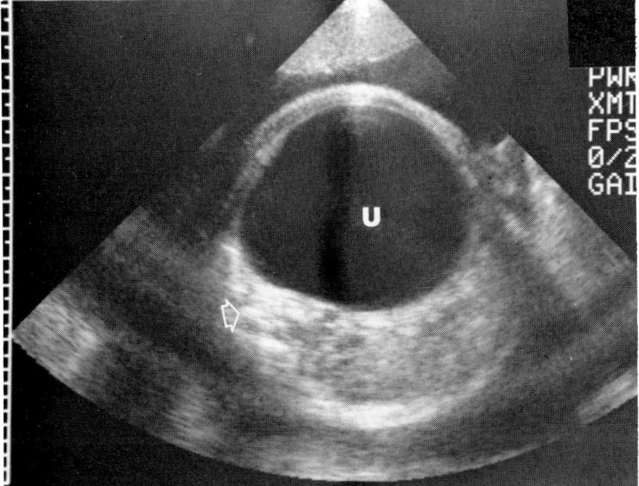

Figure 129–3. This fetus had a **left ureteropelvic junction obstruction** and a large, unilocular fluid-filled left paraspinous mass representing a **perinephric urinoma** (U) caused by urinary tract rupture. *(Open arrow* = fetal spine.)

lowing birth showed no evidence of hydronephrosis. This is assumed to be secondary to relative neonatal dehydration, because studies obtained several days later again confirm the presence of unilateral hydronephrosis. A normal renal sonogram in a newborn who had unequivocal hydronephrosis in utero, therefore, should be repeated late in the first week postpartum to confirm the diagnosis of urinary tract obstruction.

Ureteropelvic junction obstruction, when present, occurs bilaterally in approximately 30 per cent of cases (Fig. 129–2*B*). Asymmetric involvement is most common, and fortunately, only rarely does severe bilateral ureteropelvic junction obstruction occur. If there is severe bilateral ureteropelvic junction obstruction, oligohydramnios will be present and the urinary bladder may be empty. Unilateral ureteropelvic junction obstruction may be associated with contralateral multicystic dysplastic kidney or renal agenesis. Both of these will produce profound oligohydramnios if the ureteropelvic junction is severe.

Obstruction at the ureterovesical junction in the fetus is rare. Usually this results from an ectopic ureterocele associated with ureteric duplication and obstruction of an upper pole renal moiety. Sonography visualizes dilatation of the obstructed ureter leading to a hydronephrotic upper pole. A serpentine fluid-filled structure touching the fetal spine and originating from the renal pelvis distinguishes hydroureter from fluid-filled bowel. When ureterovesical junction obstruction is secondary to ectopic ureterocele, the hydronephrotic upper pole moiety may displace the unobstructed lower pole inferiorly. The urinary bladder volume is normal. Ectopic ureterocele is bilateral in approximately 15 per cent of cases. Unless the obstruction is both severe and bilateral, the amount of amniotic fluid is normal. Ureteroceles may be seen as cystic structures within or adjacent to the collapsed urinary bladder in rare cases. Rarely cystic structures in the fetal pelvis, such as an ovarian cyst, hydrocolpos, or an anterior meningocele, may be mistaken for the urinary bladder. If the midline pelvic fluid collection fills and empties over a 30 to 45 minute period, however, it is the urinary bladder rather than another cystic pelvic mass.

A common cause of obstruction of the urinary bladder and obstructive uropathy in the male fetus is posterior urethral valves. Although severely affected male fetuses demonstrate a broad spectrum of findings, a dilated posterior urethra and dilated, thick-walled urinary bladder represent strong evidence of posterior urethral valvar obstruction (Fig. 129–4*A*). In this condition hydroureter is usually more pronounced than is pyelocaliectasis but either of these findings occurs in only approximately 40 per cent of cases (Fig. 129–4*B*). Urine ascites or uriniferous perirenal pseudocysts (urinomas) from spontaneous decompression of the urinary tract may occur in association with bladder outlet obstruction as early as the beginning of the second trimester of pregnancy.

When one considers the diagnosis of posterior urethral valvar obstruction, the fetal perineum should be examined to determine the sex. When male genitalia cannot be documented in cases with massive distention of the fetal urinary bladder, either caudal regression anomaly or megacystic intestinal hypoperistalsis syndrome should be considered. Both occur in either gender, but the latter is more common in females.

Severe urethra-level obstruction may dilate the bladder to the point that it distends the fetal abdomen and elevates the hemidiaphragms. Urine ascites may also distend the abdominal wall, resulting in lax abdominal musculature characteristic of the prune-belly syndrome. Oligohydramnios probably represents the overriding feature indicative of a poor prognosis because of its association with pulmonary hypoplasia, a common cause of death in neonates with severe obstructive uropathy. Among fetuses with urethra-level obstruction and oligohydramnios, approximately 95 per cent subsequently die. If oligohydramnios occurs in urinary tract obstruction it is usually secondary to severe and persistent obstruction that does not permit egress of fluid from the fetal urinary tract. It may also result from diminished renal function in the absence of persistent

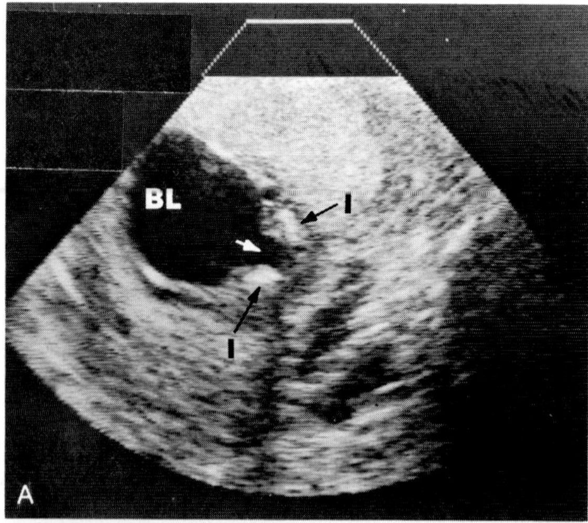

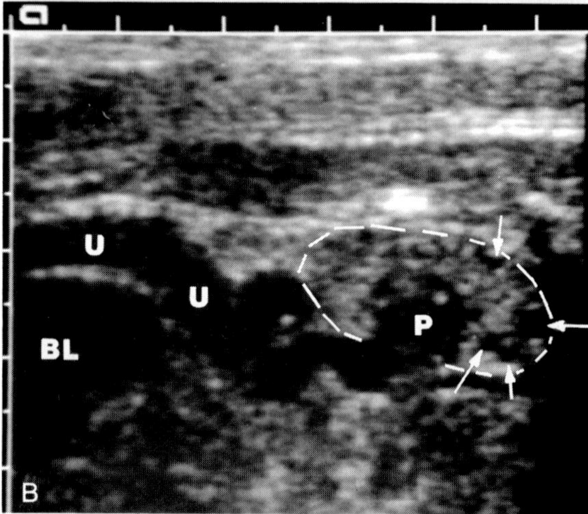

Figure 129–4. *A,* Scan of the fetal pelvis with **posterior urethral valvar obstruction** shows a dilated urinary bladder (BL) and dilated posterior urethra *(small arrow)* pointing toward the fetal perineum. Oligohydramnios is present, an indicator of a poor prognosis. (I = fetal iliac alae.) *B,* This magnified parasagittal scan of another fetus with **posterior urethral valvar obstruction** demonstrates a tortuous, dilated ureter (U) leading to a minimally dilated renal pelvis (P). Note the small renal parenchymal cysts *(arrows),* which, in the setting of obstructive uropathy, indicate the presence of renal dysplasia. The dashed line outlines the approximate border of the dysplastic kidney. (BL = a portion of the dilated urinary bladder.)

obstruction. Aspiration of fetal urine and catheter measurement of fetal urine production can indicate whether the predominant problem is lack of egress of fluid from the urinary tract or from diminished renal function. However, increased fetal risk accompanies these procedures.

Renal Dysplasia

Accurate prediction of irreversible renal damage is important, since any beneficial effect of fetal urinary tract decompression presupposes that the kidney has not already suffered extensive irreversible damage. Renal dysplasia, defined as abnormal parenchymal development from anomalous differentiation of metanephric tissue, suggests irreversible renal damage. Functional capacity of an affected kidney depends on the extent and severity of the dysplasia. Renal dysplasia is characterized pathologically by disorganized epithelial structures surrounded by abundant fibrous tissue. Although cortical cysts are often present, this is not a necessary finding.

In fetal kidneys with obstructive uropathy, sonographic demonstration of renal cysts correlates with the presence of dysplasia (Figs. 129–4*B* and 129–5). If renal cysts are not seen by ultrasound, however, renal dysplasia cannot be excluded. The intensity of fetal renal echogenicity provides a less accurate prediction of renal dysplasia than does visualization of renal cortical cysts. Increased renal echogenicity yields a specificity of only 80 per cent and an accuracy of a positive prediction of 89 per cent for dysplasia. Importantly, not all fetal kidneys that are of greatly increased echogenicity are dysplastic.

Multicystic Dysplastic Kidney

In a multicystic dysplastic kidney, the renal pelvis and ureter are usually atretic and little if any renal function exists. One may consider this entity to represent urinary tract obstruction at its most extreme. The distal ureter may occasionally be dilated in proximal ureteral atresia, and the renal pelvis may be dilated in distal ureteral atresia. In multicystic dysplasia (1) the reniform contour is lost; (2) numerous cysts of variable sizes without identifiable communication or anatomic arrangement exist; and (3) tissue resembling possible renal parenchyma, if present, is interspersed between the cysts (Fig. 129–6). The gross pathologic appearance of a multicystic dysplastic kidney correlates with this sonographic appearance.

In 30 to 40 per cent of patients with multicystic dysplastic kidneys the contralateral kidney is diseased. Even when one cannot adequately visualize the contralateral kidney, a normal amount of amniotic fluid and normal emptying and filling of the fetal urinary bladder imply normal contralateral renal function. Approximately 10 per cent of patients with a multicystic dysplastic kidney have hydronephrosis of the other kidney, usually from ureteropelvic junction obstruction (Fig. 129–6*B*). The degree of obstruction in these cases determines the amount of amniotic fluid, since the obstructed kidney is the only potentially functional one. Profound oligohydramnios and absence of fetal urinary bladder filling in the setting

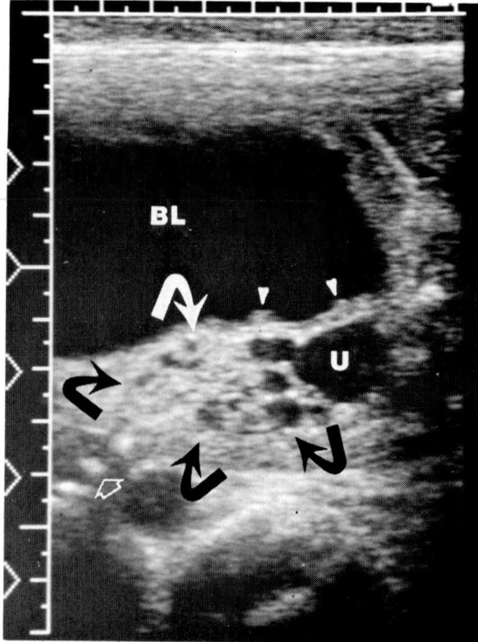

Figure 129–5. Oblique scan of the fetal pelvis with **posterior urethral valvar obstruction** displays the markedly dilated, thick-walled urinary bladder (BL) with trabeculations *(arrowheads).* The dilated ureter (U) leads to an echogenic kidney *(curved arrows)* that contains numerous small cortical cysts indicative of renal dysplasia. No amniotic fluid is present. (*Open arrow* = a portion of the fetal spine.)

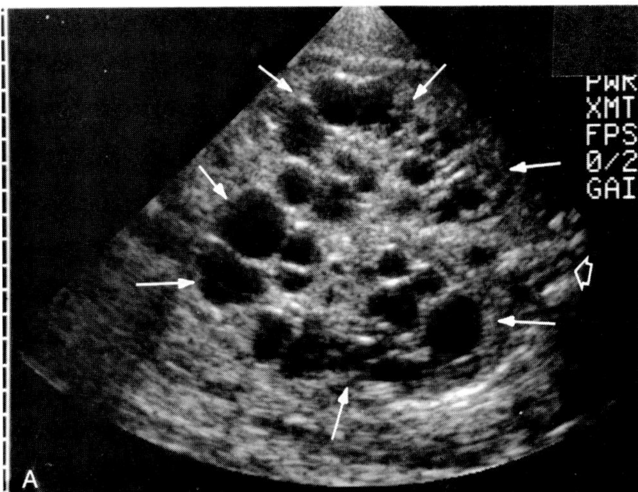

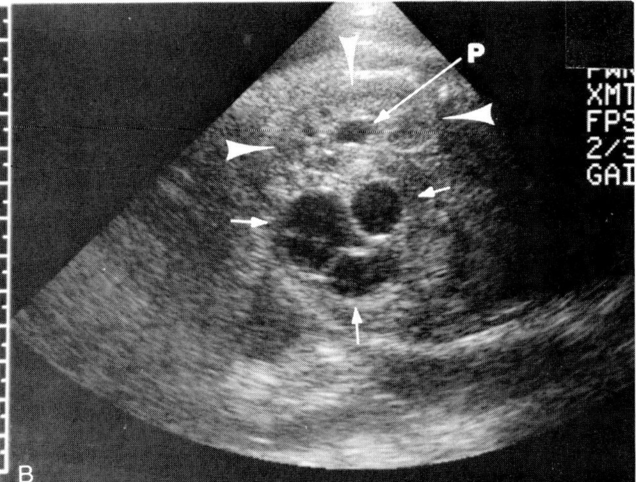

Figure 129–6. *A,* These bilateral masses *(small arrows),* which almost fill the fetal abdomen but touch the spine *(open arrow),* represent **bilateral multicystic dysplastic kidneys** on this axial sonogram of the fetal abdomen. The masses contain numerous, variably sized cysts without anatomic arrangement or identifiable communication. Since these are nonfunctional kidneys, the absence of amniotic fluid helps to distinguish multicystic dysplastic kidney from other causes of intra-abdominal fluid collections, such as proximal small bowel obstruction, in which polyhydramnios would be evident. *B,* Axial scan of the fetal abdomen demonstrates a portion of a **unilateral multicystic dysplastic kidney** *(small arrows)* as well as the contralateral kidney *(arrowheads),* which exhibits minimal pyelectasis (P). Once the diagnosis of unilateral multicystic dysplastic kidney has been made, attention must be directed to the contralateral kidney, since this is the only potentially functional kidney.

of multicystic dysplasia suggest either bilateral multicystic dysplasia, which occurs in approximately 20 per cent of cases, or, rarely, concomitant contralateral renal agenesis. The absence of functioning renal tissue in either circumstance renders these combinations lethal. If only a unilateral multicystic dysplastic kidney is seen but no contralateral kidney is identified, then the diagnosis of contralateral renal agenesis or severe hypoplasia can be made if the conditions of oligohydramnios and absent fetal bladder are present.

Infantile Polycystic Kidney Disease

Infantile polycystic kidney disease (IPKD), which is inherited in an autosomal recessive manner, exhibits a variable degree of renal involvement. The antenatal sonographic diagnosis of IPKD has been made as early as 17 menstrual weeks. This disorder is characterized by medullary ectasia resulting in numerous 1 to 2 mm cysts of nonobstructed renal collecting tubules and leading to bilaterally enlarged kidneys. The sonographic appearance of IPKD in the fetus and neonate is one of bilaterally enlarged kidneys that are of increased echogenicity relative to the adjacent structures but maintain their reniform shape (Fig. 129–7). The cortex may be echogenic early in pregnancy, but later the medullae are echogenic and are surrounded by a peripheral rim of hypoechoic renal cortex. The numerous tiny cysts are usually too small to be seen sonographically but produce multiple interfaces that result in the characteristic diffusely increased renal echogenicity. Visualization of distinct fetal renal cysts suggests cystic dysplasia rather than IPKD, although late in pregnancy macroscopic cysts may be seen in IPKD. Because of diminished renal function the renal pelves, ureters, and bladder are not distended.

If bilaterally enlarged kidneys are seen in a fetus at risk for IPKD, the diagnosis of the syndrome should be made. However, a normal sonogram early in gestation of a fetus at risk for IPKD does not assure absence of this genetic disease. The fetal urinary tract may appear sonographically normal before 19 to 20 menstrual weeks, but at 24 to 25 menstrual weeks the ultrasound shows unequivocally enlarged echogenic kidneys. It is not entirely clear why this happens but it is possible that, at least in some cases, the pathologic abnormality in IPKD expresses itself only following completion of nephron induction.

If the maternal history indicates no genetic risk for IPKD, visualization of enlarged fetal kidneys raises the possibility of bilateral mesoblastic nephromas or congenital metabolic diseases, such as glycogen storage disease or tyrosinosis. These conditions might be difficult to distinguish from IPKD. However, oligohydramnios and absence of urine within the bladder would favor IPKD over the other entities and would signify a poor prognosis.

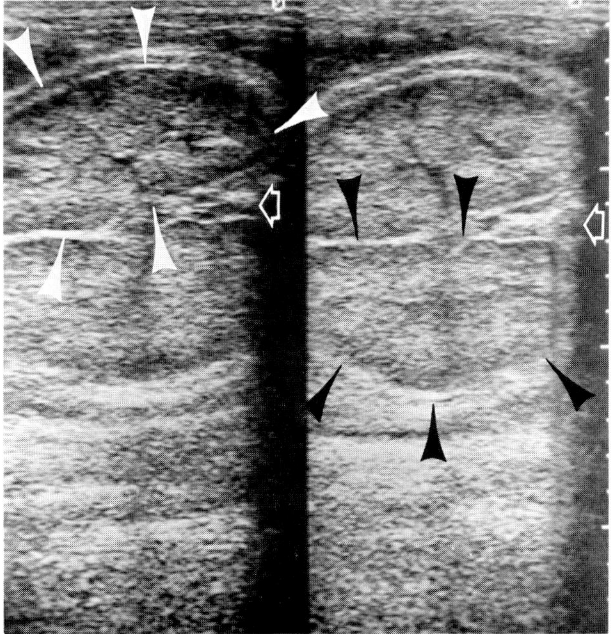

Figure 129–7. Dual image axial scans of a fetus at 33 menstrual weeks with **infantile polycystic kidney disease** displays bilaterally enlarged kidneys *(arrowheads)* that fill almost the entire fetal abdomen but maintain their reniform contour. A thin rim of echopenic cortex surrounds the echogenic medullae. Oligohydramnios is present. (*Open arrows* = fetal spine.)

Renal Agenesis or Severe Hypoplasia

Bilateral renal agenesis or severe bilateral renal hypoplasia, resulting in absence of renal function, represents a severe and lethal form of renal disease. Sufficiently early identification of this lethal condition allows elective termination. The incidence of bilateral renal agenesis is about one in 4000 births; it is more common in males than in females. The etiology is thought to be a disturbance of the mesonephric duct, causing failure of the metanephric blastema to differentiate and resulting in a failure of the kidney and ureter to form. Absence of urine production results in severe oligohydramnios and leads to pulmonary hypoplasia, which is the major cause of immediate death in these infants.

The important sonographic observations for diagnosis of absence of renal function prior to 20 menstrual weeks include (1) severe oligohydramnios and (2) absence of urine within the fetal urinary bladder. Unfortunately, the oligohydramnios increases the difficulty of imaging these fetuses. Because of this, nonvisualization of the urinary bladder is more significant than apparent visualization of the kidneys, since fetal adrenal glands or bowel may be mistaken for kidneys and may produce the erroneous impression that fetal kidneys are present. Identification of medullary pyramids is the most reliable way to distinguish a kidney from either the bowel or the adrenal glands, since neither the bowel nor the adrenals simulate this appearance. Hypoplastic kidneys may be identified when present, but the sonographic and clinical appearance is otherwise identical to that of bilateral renal agenesis. Absence of urine in the fetal urinary bladder over a 60 to 90 minute observation period provides evidence of fetal anuria or severe oliguria.

CONCLUSION

Careful evaluation of the fetal abdominal contents and amount of amniotic fluid often enables an accurate antenatal diagnosis when a genitourinary abnormality is detected. In obstructive uropathy, the site of obstruction may be delineated. In the setting of fetal urinary tract pathology, sonographic demonstration of oligohydramnios predicts a poor prognosis, and, if obstructive uropathy is present, cortical renal cysts predict the presence of severe dysplasia.

Bibliography

Arger PH, Coleman BG, Mintz MC, et al: Routine fetal genitourinary tract screening. Radiology 156:485, 1985.

Avni EF, Thoua Y, Van Gansbeke, et al: Development of the hypodysplastic kidney: Contribution of antenatal US diagnosis. Radiology 164:123, 1987.

Grannum PW: The genitourinary tract. In Nyberg DA, Mahony BS, Pretorius DH (eds): Diagnostic Ultrasound of Fetal Anomalies: Text and Atlas. Chicago, Year Book Medical Publishers, 1990, pp 433–491.

Grignon A, Filiatrault D, Homsy Y, et al: Ureteropelvic junction stenosis: Antenatal ultrasonographic diagnosis, postnatal investigation, and follow-up. Radiology 160:649, 1986.

Hashimoto BE, Filly RA, Callen PW: Multicystic dysplastic kidney in utero: Changing appearance on US. Radiology 159:107, 1986.

Hill LM: Abnormalities of amniotic fluid. In Nyberg DA, Mahony BS, Pretorius DH (eds): Diagnostic Ultrasound of Fetal Anomalies: Text and Atlas. Chicago, Year Book Medical Publishers, 1990, pp 38–66.

Hoddick WK, Filly RA, Mahony BS, et al: Minimal fetal renal pyelectasis. J Ultrasound Med 4:85, 1985.

Jeanty P, Dramanix-Wilmet M, Elkhazen N, et al: Measurement of fetal kidney growth on ultrasound. Radiology 144:159, 1982.

Kleiner B, Callen PW, Filly RA: Sonographic analysis of the fetus with ureteropelvic junction obstruction. AJR 148:359, 1987.

Kleiner B, Filly RA, Mack L, et al. Multicystic dysplastic kidney: Observations of contralateral disease in the fetal population. Radiology 161:27, 1986.

Lawson TL, Foley WD, Berland LL, et al: Ultrasonographic evaluation of the kidneys. Analysis of normal size and frequency of visualization as related to stage of pregnancy. Radiology 138:153, 1981.

Lebowitz RL, Griscom NT: Neonatal hydronephrosis: 147 cases. Radiol Clin North Am 15:49, 1977.

Mahony BS, Callen PW, Filly RA: Fetal urethral obstruction: US evaluation. Radiology 157:221, 1985.

Mahony BS, Callen PW, Filly RA, et al: Progression of infantile polycystic kidney disease in early pregnancy: J Ultrasound Med 3:277, 1984.

Mahony BS, Filly RA, Callen PW, et al: Fetal renal dysplasia: Sonographic evaluation. Radiology 152:143, 1984.

Zerres K: Genetics of cystic kidney disease: Criteria for classification and genetic counseling. Pediatr Nephrol 1:397, 1987.

130 Fetal Skeletal Abnormalities

Barry S. Mahony and Peter W. Callen

High-resolution antenatal sonography clearly depicts the fetal skeleton. In the later stages of the embryonic period (eight postconception weeks, 10 menstrual weeks), osteogenesis of the appendicular skeleton commences when the mid-shaft of the long bones converts from a cartilaginous model into bone. It is this primary ossification center that sonography images first, often before the end of the first trimester when adequate size and intrinsic subject contrast enable delineation of numerous limb structures.

Primary ossification of the clavicle and mandible begins at eight menstrual weeks; by 11 menstrual weeks, all of the appendicular long bones, the scapula, ilium, and phalanges have begun to ossify and may be seen sonographically. During the fourth month of gestation (approximately 13 to 16 menstrual weeks), the ischium, metacarpals, and metatarsals ossify. The pubis, tarsal calcaneus, and talus ossify during the fifth and sixth months. Ossification of the remaining tarsals and of all the carpal bones does not occur until after birth.

At later stages of development (in most instances not until postnatal life), a similar process converts the most central and oldest cells of the cartilaginous epiphyses into the secondary ossification centers, which in turn are visible sonographically. Only the secondary ossification centers of the distal femur and proximal tibia and, less often, the proximal humerus appear prenatally; the remaining secondary ossification centers do not appear until after birth.

The amount of amniotic fluid, fetal position, and fetal motion dictate which portions of the fetal appendicular skeleton may be imaged sonographically. Extremities can be well seen as early as the beginning of the second trimester of pregnancy when they are bathed in adequate amounts of amniotic fluid in the focal zone of the transducer and are not shadowed by other fetal parts. Whereas observation of each fetal bone is neither practical nor necessary in the vast majority of obstetric sonograms, when a specific indication exists, persistence and patience usually permit adequate visualization to predict the presence or absence of many extremity abnormalities.

THE NORMAL FETAL SKELETON

The primary ossification centers of the shoulder and pelvis provide excellent anatomic landmarks. Imaging of the scapula in the long axis coronally produces a Y configuration, whereas the scapula manifests a triangular configuration when imaged posteriorly. The distal clavicle, although among the first bones to ossify, is usually not well seen in projections other than a posterior view of the shoulder because of shadowing from the flexed fetal head and from the mandible. Visualization of the ilium, ischium, and pubis assists in localization of pelvic structures such as the urinary bladder and the caudal end of the spine.

During the course of a real-time examination the fetus may flex, extend, abduct, and adduct the extremities. Since the humerus is often adducted against the fetal thorax and the femur is frequently flexed at approximately 90 degrees to the long axis of the spine, the length of these long bones may be readily measured. The ends of the primary femoral and humeral ossification centers flare slightly to join the larger echopenic epiphyses, giving the long bones a slightly bowed appearance.

Several scans obtained in the long axis of the bone should be obtained to ensure optimal long bone measurement. Either electronic or mechanical calipers, placed at the ends of the highly echogenic primary ossification center, assist in measurement. Correlation of the long bone measurement with published measurements and with other indicators of gestational age (i.e., last menstrual period, biparietal diameter, previous sonographic evaluation) optimizes gestational age assessment. Furthermore, a fetus whose bones measure greater than two standard deviations below the mean for a known menstrual age may be suspected of dwarfism (Table 130–1).

Prior to 22 menstrual weeks, the humeral length corresponds closely to the femoral length, but as gestation progresses the femur becomes longer relative to the humerus. It should be understood, however, that published measurements of the fetal long bones correspond to measurements only of the ossified diaphyses. Epiphyseal cartilage, although visible sonographically at the ends of the long bones, has not been included in fetal long bone measurements. Furthermore, skeletal measurements obtained from an initial sonogram during the third trimester of pregnancy are of limited value in the assessment of menstrual age because of significant biologic variability in fetal size.

The more proximal extent of the ulna at the elbow distinguishes the ulna from the radius. At the wrist, however, the two bones end at the same level. Demonstration of this relationship effectively excludes limb reduction anomalies that characteristically foreshorten the distal radius. Unlike the radius and ulna, the tibia and fibula end at the same level proximally as well as distally.

The carpals and tarsals, except the calcaneus and talus, do not ossify until after birth. The ossified metacarpals, metatarsals, and phalanges, as well as their cartilaginous ends, however, can be readily imaged and enumerated by the middle of the second trimester of pregnancy. Their cartilaginous ends produce echopenic gaps between the ossified diaphyses.

The foot length nearly equals the femur length, so the femur length/foot length ratio remains near unity during the second and

TABLE 130–1. BIPARIETAL DIAMETERS AND BONE LENGTHS AT DIFFERENT MENSTRUAL AGES*

Menstrual Age (Weeks)	Biparietal Diameter	Femur	Tibia	Fibula	Humerus	Radius	Ulna
13	2.3 (0.3)	1.1 (0.2)	0.9 (0.2)	0.8 (0.2)	1.0 (0.2)	0.6 (0.2)	0.8 (0.3)
14	2.7 (0.3)	1.3 (0.2)	1.0 (0.2)	0.9 (0.3)	1.2 (0.2)	0.8 (0.2)	1.0 (0.2)
15	3.0 (0.1)	1.5 (0.2)	1.3 (0.2)	1.2 (0.2)	1.4 (0.2)	1.1 (0.1)	1.2 (0.1)
16	3.3 (0.2)	1.9 (0.3)	1.6 (0.3)	1.5 (0.3)	1.7 (0.2)	1.4 (0.3)	1.6 (0.3)
17	3.7 (0.3)	2.2 (0.3)	1.8 (0.3)	1.7 (0.2)	2.0 (0.4)	1.5 (0.3)	1.7 (0.3)
18	4.2 (0.5)	2.5 (0.3)	2.2 (0.3)	2.1 (0.3)	2.3 (0.3)	1.9 (0.2)	2.2 (0.3)
19	4.4 (0.4)	2.8 (0.3)	2.5 (0.3)	2.3 (0.3)	2.6 (0.3)	2.1 (0.3)	2.4 (0.3)
20	4.7 (0.4)	3.1 (0.3)	2.7 (0.2)	2.6 (0.2)	2.9 (0.3)	2.4 (0.2)	2.7 (0.3)
21	5.0 (0.5)	3.5 (0.4)	3.0 (0.4)	2.9 (0.4)	3.2 (0.4)	2.7 (0.4)	3.0 (0.4)
22	5.5 (0.5)	3.6 (0.3)	3.2 (0.3)	3.1 (0.3)	3.3 (0.3)	2.8 (0.5)	3.1 (0.4)
23	5.8 (0.5)	4.0 (0.4)	3.6 (0.2)	3.4 (0.2)	3.7 (0.3)	3.1 (0.4)	3.5 (0.2)
24	6.1 (0.5)	4.2 (0.3)	3.7 (0.3)	3.6 (0.3)	3.8 (0.4)	3.3 (0.4)	3.6 (0.4)
25	6.4 (0.5)	4.6 (0.3)	4.0 (0.3)	3.9 (0.4)	4.2 (0.4)	3.5 (0.3)	3.9 (0.4)
26	6.8 (0.5)	4.8 (0.4)	4.2 (0.3)	4.0 (0.3)	4.3 (0.3)	3.6 (0.4)	4.0 (0.3)
27	7.0 (0.3)	4.9 (0.3)	4.4 (0.3)	4.2 (0.3)	4.5 (0.2)	3.7 (0.3)	4.1 (0.2)
28	7.3 (0.5)	5.3 (0.5)	4.5 (0.4)	4.4 (0.3)	4.7 (0.4)	3.9 (0.4)	4.4 (0.5)
29	7.6 (0.5)	5.3 (0.5)	4.6 (0.3)	4.5 (0.3)	4.8 (0.4)	4.0 (0.5)	4.5 (0.4)
30	7.7 (0.6)	5.6 (0.3)	4.8 (0.5)	4.7 (0.3)	5.0 (0.5)	4.1 (0.6)	4.7 (0.3)
31	8.2 (0.7)	6.0 (0.6)	5.1 (0.3)	4.9 (0.5)	5.3 (0.4)	4.2 (0.3)	4.9 (0.4)
32	8.5 (0.6)	6.1 (0.6)	5.2 (0.4)	5.1 (0.4)	5.4 (0.4)	4.4 (0.6)	5.0 (0.6)
33	8.6 (0.4)	6.4 (0.5)	5.4 (0.5)	5.3 (0.3)	5.6 (0.5)	4.5 (0.5)	5.2 (0.3)
34	8.9 (0.5)	6.6 (0.6)	5.7 (0.5)	5.5 (0.4)	5.8 (0.5)	4.7 (0.5)	5.4 (0.5)
35	8.9 (0.7)	6.7 (0.6)	5.8 (0.4)	5.6 (0.4)	5.9 (0.6)	4.8 (0.6)	5.4 (0.4)
36	9.1 (0.7)	7.0 (0.7)	6.0 (0.6)	5.6 (0.5)	6.0 (0.6)	4.9 (0.5)	5.5 (0.3)
37	9.3 (0.9)	7.2 (0.4)	6.1 (0.4)	6.0 (0.4)	6.1 (0.4)	5.1 (0.3)	5.6 (0.4)
38	9.5 (0.6)	7.4 (0.6)	6.2 (0.3)	6.0 (0.4)	6.4 (0.3)	5.1 (0.5)	5.8 (0.6)
39	9.5 (0.6)	7.6 (0.8)	6.4 (0.7)	6.1 (0.6)	6.5 (0.6)	5.3 (0.5)	6.0 (0.6)
40	9.9 (0.8)	7.7 (0.4)	6.5 (0.3)	6.2 (0.1)	6.6 (0.4)	5.3 (0.3)	6.0 (0.5)
41	9.7 (0.6)	7.7 (0.4)	6.6 (0.4)	6.3 (0.5)	6.6 (0.4)	5.6 (0.4)	6.3 (0.5)
42	10.0 (0.5)	7.8 (0.7)	6.8 (0.5)	6.7 (0.7)	6.8 (0.7)	5.7 (0.5)	6.5 (0.5)

*Mean values (cm); value of 2 standard deviations in parentheses.

From Merz E, Kim-Kern M-S, Pehl S: Mensuration of fetal limb bones in the second and third trimesters. J Clin Ultrasound 15:175, 1987. Reprinted by permission of John Wiley and Sons, Inc., copyright © 1987.

third trimesters. This femur/foot length ratio remains near unity for normal small fetuses or for growth-retarded fetuses, but it is abnormally low for fetuses affected by skeletal dysplasia.

At approximately 29 to 35 menstrual weeks, ossification of the distal femoral epiphysis begins in the center of the epiphyseal cartilage. The ossification enlarges centrifugally as gestation progresses. Ossification of the central portion of the proximal tibial epiphysis begins approximately two to three weeks after the appearance of the ossification center in the distal femoral epiphysis. The proximal tibial secondary ossification center enlarges more rapidly than does its distal femoral counterpart during the last few weeks of gestation and for several weeks following birth.

SHORT-LIMBED DYSPLASIAS, HYPOMINERALIZATION SYNDROMES, AND LIMB REDUCTION ABNORMALITIES

Antenatal sonography provides an ideal means of measuring the length of fetal extremity bones. The high subject contrast of the fetal ossification center enables sonography to image the bone. When contained within the focal zone of the transducer, sonography images the bone free of distortion and magnification. The absence of ionizing radiation enables the sonographer to obtain numerous images in varying planes of section. Standard values for length of the fetal long bones, especially the femur, assist in prediction of menstrual age (Table 130–1).

Discordance of fetal femoral length with gestational age, as determined by calvareal size, menstrual dates, and/or previous examinations, assists in detection of many short-limbed bone dysplasias prior to 22 menstrual weeks. Although some bone dysplasias do not show definitively shortened bone length early in gestation, a shortened femoral length confirms the presence of dwarfism but is nonspecific for the type of dwarfism. Similar degrees of limb foreshortening may be seen, for example, in such dissimilar conditions as achondrogenesis, homozygous achondroplasia, camptomelic dysplasia, homozygous recessive osteogenesis imperfecta, and congenital hypophosphatasia.

Pedigree analysis, in conjunction with sonography, often assists in prenatal distinction among the various short-limbed dwarf syndromes. If the sonogram is performed because of a specific genetic risk (i.e., diastrophic dwarfism or chondroectodermal dysplasia), detection of shortened limb bones suggests recurrence. In the absence of a familial short-limbed dysplasia, however, serendipitous discovery of shortened limbs on a sonogram performed for obstetric indications requires a careful search for other characteristic features which, when present, permit confident antenatal diagnosis of the specific form of dwarfism. Radiographs often do not clarify these situations, since they suffer from limitations caused by overlapping structures, fetal motion, and variable magnification. In the absence of characteristic sonographic features, a definitive diagnosis of a specific dwarf syndrome usually requires postpartum examination with radiographs.

Among the congenital short-limbed dysplasias that occur either sporadically or in an autosomal recessive pattern, thanatophoric dwarfism, heterozygous achondroplasia, achondrogenesis, and osteogenesis imperfecta are most common, but many others can be detected with prenatal ultrasound. Characteristic features of syndromes occasionally exist and permit potential antenatal sonographic distinction of the specific syndrome and assessment of prognosis. For example, achondrogenesis and camptomelic dysplasia are uniformly lethal in the neonatal period. Individuals affected with homozygous recessive osteogenesis imperfecta, thanatophoric dwarfism, or congenital hypophosphatasia rarely survive. In the absence of complications, on the other hand, the prognosis for both function and survival of a person with heterozygous achondroplasia is normal.

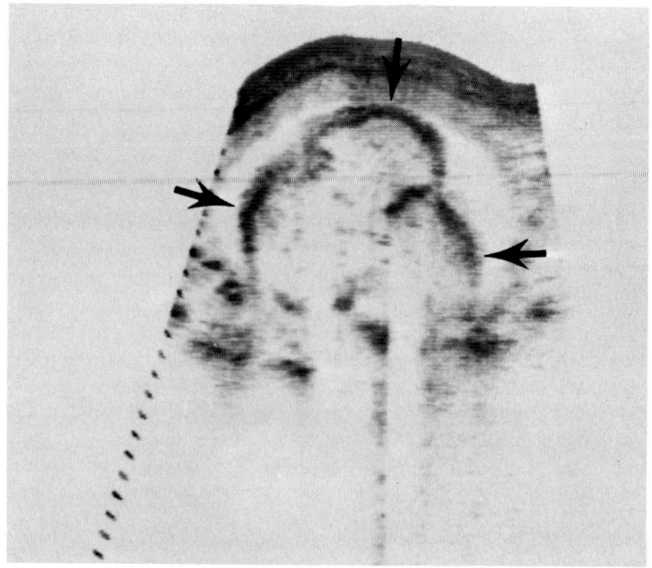

Figure 130–1. Axial sonogram of the fetal head demonstrates the trilobed appearance characteristic of the **cloverleaf skull deformity** *(arrows)*. Other scans confirmed marked femoral shortening in this fetus with thanatophoric dwarfism. (Reproduced from Mahony BS, Filly RA, Callen PW, Golbus MS: Thanatophoric dwarfism with the cloverleaf skull: A specific antenatal sonographic diagnosis. J Ultrasound Med 4:151–154, 1985, with permission.)

Approximately 14 per cent of thanatophoric dwarfs have the cloverleaf skull deformity, a severely enlarged trilobed head presumably caused by intrauterine closure of the coronal, lambdoid, and squamous sutures. The cloverleaf skull deformity is readily apparent on the antenatal sonogram (Fig. 130–1). Although the cloverleaf skull deformity may occur in a variety of syndromes, it occurs only in short-limbed dwarfs who have either homozygous achondroplasia or thanatophoric dwarfism. No confusion should exist between homozygous achondroplasia and thanatophoric dwarfism, since the parents of thanatophoric dwarfs are of normal stature, whereas the parents of a fetus with homozygous achondroplasia are readily recognizable as achondroplastic dwarfs. Detection of a short-limbed dwarf with the cloverleaf skull deformity whose parents are of normal stature, therefore, enables a confident antenatal diagnosis of thanatophoric dwarfism.

In heterozygous achondroplasia, unlike other short-limbed dysplasias, the length of the fetal femora shows a characteristic growth curve (Fig. 130–2). Until approximately 20 menstrual weeks the femora are normal in length but then fall away from the normal curve and pass below the 99 per cent prediction interval at approximately 24 to 25 menstrual weeks. Fetuses at genetic risk for recurrent heterozygous achondroplasia that demonstrate this typical growth curve can be suspected to be heterozygous achondroplastic dwarfs, although other skeletal dysplasias may produce femoral shortening late in gestation. Unfortunately, antenatal sonographic diagnosis of heterozygous achondroplasia on this basis requires sequential scans over an extended period commencing early in gestation.

The bowing of the extremity long bones, characteristic of camptomelic dysplasia, can be detected sonographically. Detection of this feature, in conjunction with other findings of camptomelic dysplasia such as an elongated skull and hypoplasia of the scapulae and cervical spine, may permit antenatal diagnosis of this syndrome in the absence of a familial risk.

Certain features occasionally permit distinction among the short-limbed dysplasias characterized by hypomineralization of bone, i.e.,

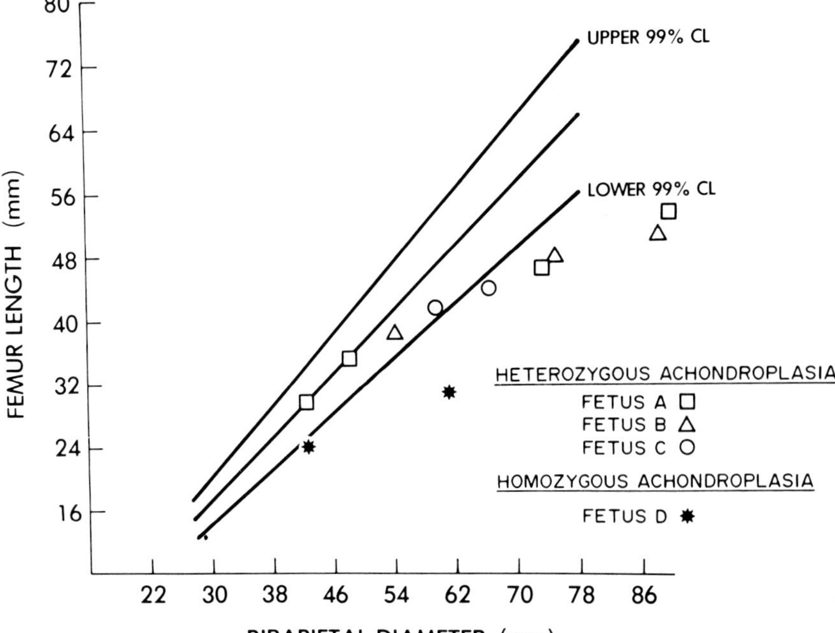

Figure 130–2. Graph demonstrating the **growth patterns of three heterozygous achondroplastic dwarfs and one homozygous achondroplastic dwarf.** The solid lines indicate the mean and prediction intervals at a 99 per cent confidence limit in normal fetuses. (Reproduced from Filly RA, Golbus MS: Ultrasonography of the normal and pathologic fetal skeleton. In Callen PW (ed): Ultrasonography in Obstetrics and Gynecology. Philadelphia, WB Saunders Company, 1983, p 89.)

achondrogenesis, homozygous recessive osteogenesis imperfecta, and congenital hypophosphatasia. Since the extent of calcification necessary to produce a sonographically normal-appearing bone is undetermined, caution must be exercised in the exclusion of each of these syndromes that result in hypomineralization of bone.

A fetus with achondrogenesis may exhibit absent vertebral body ossification but normal calvareal ossification (Fig. 130–3). The absent or severe delay in calvareal ossification characteristic of severe hypophosphatasia and homozygous recessive osteogenesis imperfecta has been described in achondrogenesis, but a well-ossified

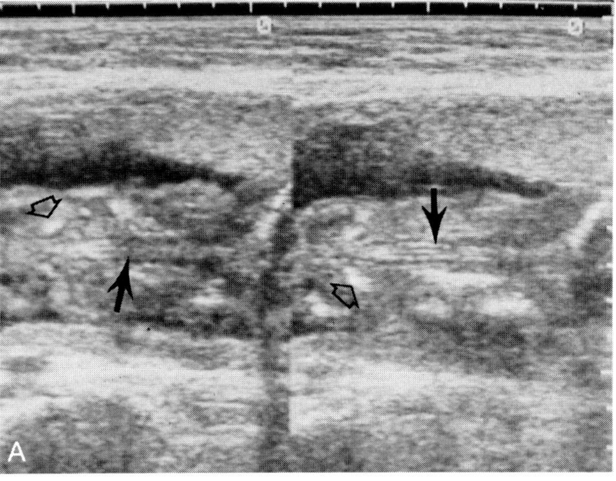

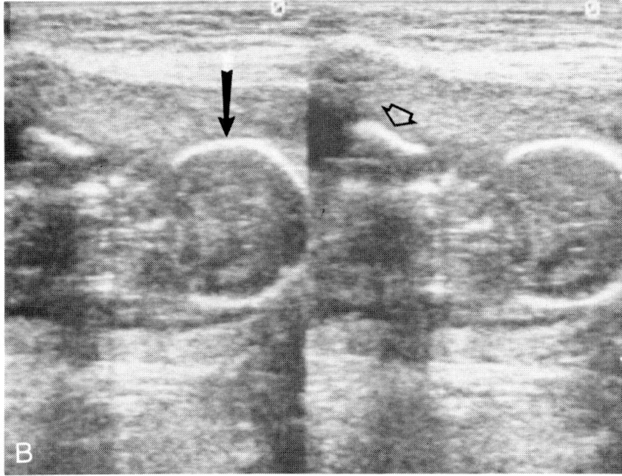

Figure 130–3. *A,* Sonograms obtained at approximately 19 menstrual weeks that demonstrate characteristic features of **achondrogenesis.** Coronal sonograms display the lucent spinal canal *(closed arrows),* visible because of the absence of spinal ossification. Iliac ossification appears normal *(open arrows). B,* Sonographs obtained along the long axis of the humerus demonstrate shortening of the humerus *(open arrow)* and normal calvareal ossification *(closed arrow).* Other scans showed marked femoral shortening. (Reproduced from Mahony BS, Filly RA, Cooperberg PL: Antenatal sonographic diagnosis of achondrogenesis. J Ultrasound Med 3:333–335, 1984, with permission.)

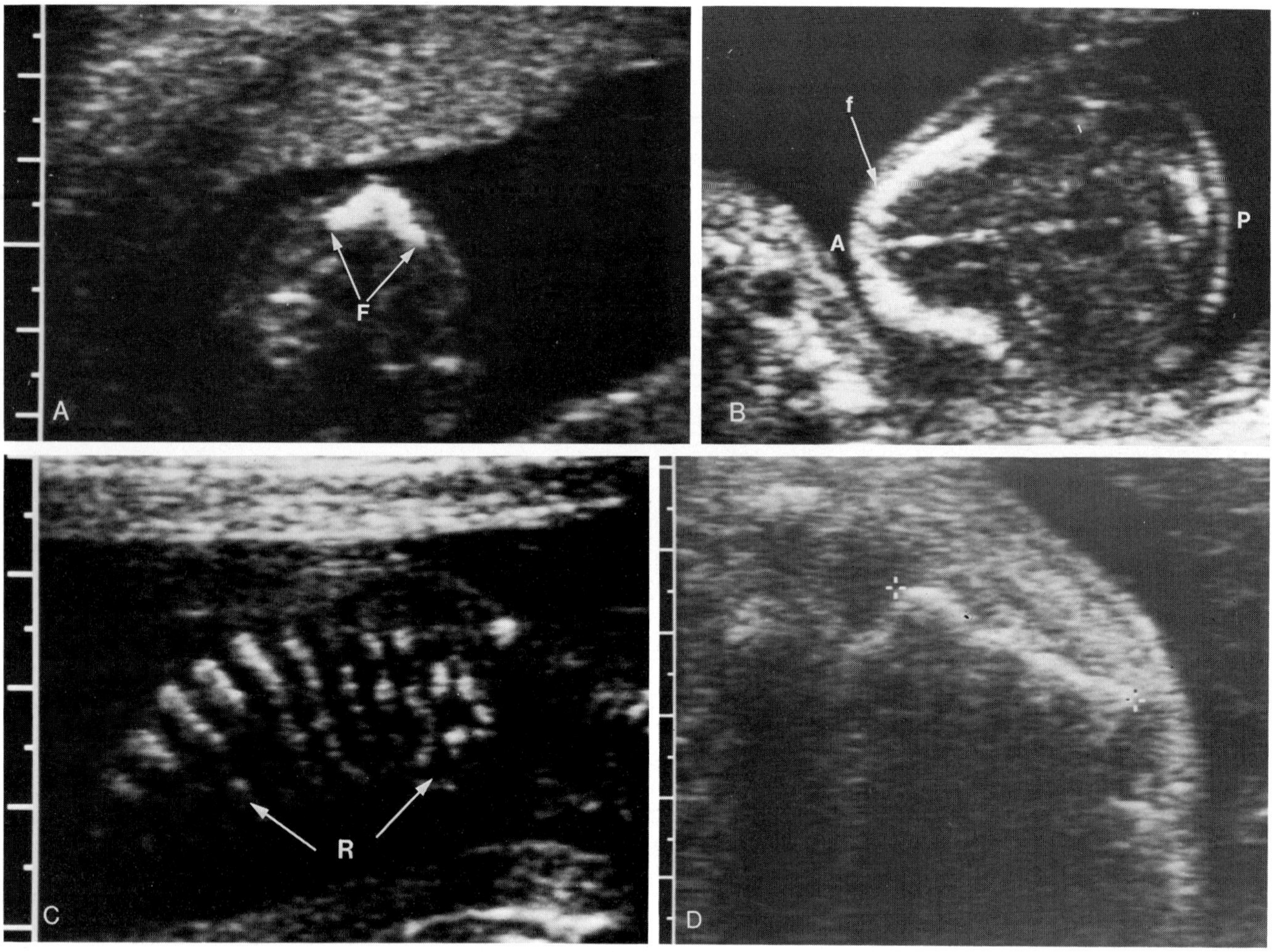

Figure 130–4. Antenatal sonogram showing characteristic features of **homozygous recessive osteogenesis imperfecta.** *A,* Femur at 18 weeks is shortened and sharply angulated secondary to a mid-shaft fracture. (F = femur.) *B,* Axial scan of the head shows ossification only of the frontal bone. Degrees and distribution of hypomineralization vary in homozygous recessive osteogenesis imperfecta. (A = anterior; P = posterior; f = frontal bone.) *C,* Parasagittal scan of the chest demonstrates multiple rib fractures and decreased rib echogenicity. (R = ribs.) *D,* The femur (graticules) in a different fetus at 36 weeks is shortened (3.3 cm = mean for 20.5 weeks) and apparently thickened with a wavy appearance, probably secondary to the "accordion" effect of numerous fractures with callus formation.

calvarium sonographically differentiates achondrogenesis from the other two entities. Numerous cases of homozygous recessive osteogenesis imperfecta have been reported. The characteristic features include (1) severely shortened limb bones with sharp angulation or with apparent thickening secondary to numerous fractures and subsequent callus formation; (2) hypomineralization of bone, either diffuse or focal; and (3) multiple rib fractures (Fig. 130–4). Unlike the thickened bones of homozygous recessive osteogenesis imperfecta, the limb bones in congenital hypophosphatasia tend to be delicate or may even be absent.

For a fetus with a genetic risk for a limb reduction anomaly, detailed sonographic evaluation of the fetal limbs may detect a focal absence of bone. Aplasia or hypoplasia of the radius should be readily apparent, since the radius will not end at the same level distally as the ulna. If specifically sought, antenatal sonography should detect other major limb reduction abnormalities (i.e., amelia, hemimelia, or phocomelia) or postural changes (clubfoot or clubhand [Fig. 130–5]). Furthermore, a detailed examination may occasionally detect polydactyly (Fig. 130–6). Subtle hypoplasias or syndactyly may be extremely difficult to discern. One may exclude the presence of syndactyly of the hand if the fetus splays open the fingers in question or clasps the hand together and interdigitates the fingers, but in the absence of these occurrences one may only infer the possibility of syndactyly.

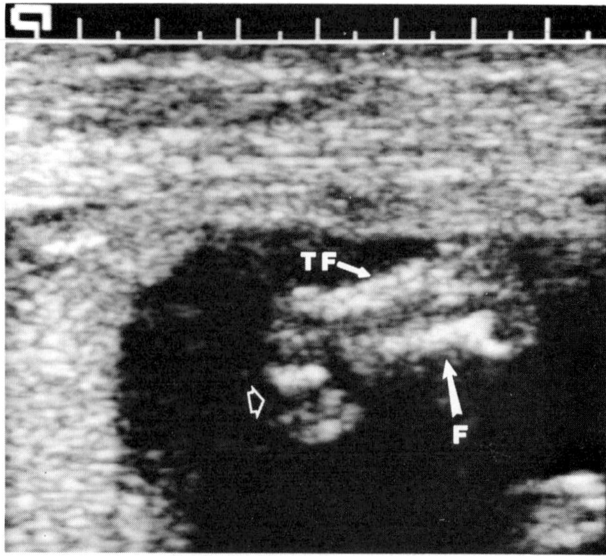

Figure 130–5. Sonogram performed at 16 menstrual weeks in a fetus with **multiple pterygium syndrome** shows talipes equinovarus (club foot: *open arrow*). (TF = tibia and fibula; F = femur.)

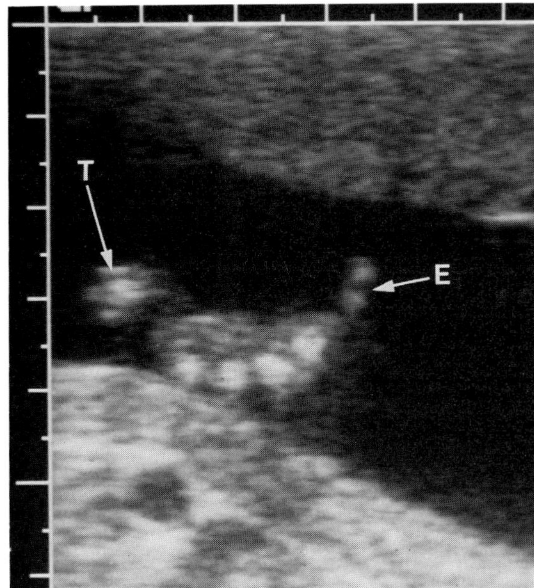

Figure 130–6. Sonogram through the base of the fetal hand demonstrates **postaxial polydactyly.** (E = extra digit; T = thumb.)

Even in the absence of a genetic risk, the detection of a limb reduction deformity may assist in the antenatal diagnosis of a specific entity. Amniotic band syndrome, for example, is a nonheritable cause of various fetal malformations including the limbs, craniofacial region, and trunk. Rupture of the amnion leads to entrapment of fetal parts by fibrous mesodermic bands that emanate from the chorionic side of the amnion. Entrapment of fetal parts by the bands may cause amputation or slash defects in nonembryologic distributions. Even when the aberrant bands of tissue are not visualized, characteristic fetal deformities in nonembryologic distributions provide evidence strongly suggestive of the amniotic band syndrome.

In summary, antenatal sonography accurately depicts the fetal skeleton. Even in the absence of a genetic risk, measurement of fetal long bones enables detection of short-limbed dysplasias, and observation of characteristic features occasionally permits distinction among several of the dwarf and hypomineralization syndromes. Detailed sonographic examination may reveal focal skeletal abnormalities when a familial risk exists or when findings suspicious for amniotic band syndrome are present.

Bibliography

Brons JTJ, Van der Harten HJ, Wladimiroff JW, et al: Prenatal ultrasonographic diagnosis of osteogenesis imperfecta. Am J Obstet Gynecol 159:176, 1988.
Campbell J, Henderson A, Campbell S: Fetal femur/foot length ratio: A new parameter to assess dysplastic limb reduction. Obstet Gynecol 72:181, 1988.
Hegge FN, Prescott GH, Watson PT: Utility of a screening examination of the fetal extremities during obstetrical sonography. J Ultrasound Med 5:639, 1986.
International nomenclature of constitutional diseases of bone. AJR 131:352, 1978.
Jeanty P, Romero R, d'Alton M, et al: In utero sonographic detection of hand and foot deformities. J Ultrasound Med 4:595, 1985.
Kurtz AB, Filly RA, Wapner RJ, et al: In utero analysis or heterozygous achondroplasia: Variable time of onset as detected by femur length measurements. J Ultrasound Med 5:137, 1986.
Mahony BS, Filly RA: High resolution sonographic assessment of the fetal extremities. J Ultrasound Med 3:489, 1984.
Mahony BS, Filly RA, Callen PW, et al: Thanatophoric dwarfism with the cloverleaf skull: A specific antenatal sonographic diagnosis. J Ultrasound Med 4:151, 1985.
Mahony BS, Filly RA, Cooperberg PL: Antenatal sonographic diagnosis of achondrogenesis. J Ultrasound Med 3:333, 1984.
Mahony BS: The extremities. In Nyberg DA, Mahony BS, Pretorius DH (eds): Diagnostic Ultrasound of Fetal Anomalies: Text and Atlas. Chicago, Year Book, 1990, pp 492–562.
Merz E, Kim-Kern M-S, Pehl S: Ultrasonic mensuration of fetal limb bones in the second and third trimester. J Clin Ultrasound 15:175, 1987.
Oriole IM, Castilla EE, Barbosa JG: Birth prevalence rates of skeletal dysplasias. J Med Genet 23:328, 1986.
Pretorius DH, Rumack CM, Manco-Johnson ML, et al: Specific skeletal dysplasias in utero: Sonographic diagnosis. Radiology 159:237, 1986.
Sirtori M, Ghidini A, Romero R, et al: Prenatal diagnosis of sirenomelia. J Ultrasound Med 8:83, 1989.
Spranger JW, Langer LO, Weidemann H-R: Bone dysplasias: An atlas of constitutional disorders of skeletal development. Philadelphia, WB Saunders Company, 1981.

131 Amniotic Fluid Volume Abnormalities: Ultrasonic Evaluation

John W. Seeds and Charles M. McCurdy, Jr.

Amniotic fluid normally surrounds the fetus, highlighting fetal soft-tissue anatomy. Both excesses and deficiencies of amniotic fluid should alert the clinician to possible structural or metabolic abnormalities of the fetus or mother. Diagnostic ultrasound can be an important tool, both in the detection of abnormalities of amniotic fluid volume and in the diagnosis of certain fetal malformations that may be related to these amniotic fluid volume complications of pregnancy. This chapter will first review normal amniotic fluid dynamics, then explore the clinical and ultrasonic basis for the diagnosis of an abnormality of amniotic fluid volume, and finally examine those fetal organ systems commonly related to volume derangements, including illustrative examples of specific anomalies.

AMNIOTIC FLUID DYNAMICS

Human pregnancy demonstrates continuous growth and development. Both the water and dissolved constituents of amniotic fluid are constantly exchanging across fetal surfaces, maintaining a net equilibrium of volume that itself is slowly changing as pregnancy progresses. Early in pregnancy, the maintenance of amniotic fluid volume does not require fetal renal function because both transudation and bulk flow of water occur across virtually all fetal and membrane surfaces and are responsible for volume homeostasis. It is uncertain exactly when during human pregnancy fetal renal function becomes necessary for continued amniotic fluid volume support. Early theories that with fetal skin keratinization at about 24 weeks, fetal renal function assumes a primary role in amniotic fluid production are inconsistent with recent reports of severe oligohydramnios detected at 18 to 20 weeks in cases of fetal renal agenesis, urinary obstruction, or renal dysplasia. Such findings strongly suggest that fetal renal function is necessary for amniotic fluid volume maintenance from about 18 weeks.

The accurate measurement of amniotic fluid volume is not a simple task. Perhaps the best attempt to measure amniotic fluid volume in normal pregnancy was reported by Queenan in 1972 using a para-aminohippuric acid dilution technique in Rh-isoimmunized women undergoing amniocentesis for diagnostic purposes who later proved to have been carrying unaffected Rh-negative infants. His data (Fig. 131–1) demonstrate a consistent increase in amniotic fluid volume to about 32 weeks and then a subtle drop in volume after that until delivery. The variability of the data is significant, and Table 131–1 summarizes the reported upper and lower limits of normal for various gestational ages. The sonographic assessment of amniotic fluid volume is largely subjective. A subjective visual appreciation in amniotic fluid volume hinges on the relative relationship of amniotic fluid to the fetal mass. Figure 131–2 correlates the average amniotic fluid volume for a given gestational age with the average fetal mass at the same gestational age. It may be seen that there is normally more amniotic fluid mass than fetus up to about 24 weeks, and that although the average amniotic fluid volume continues to increase to a peak of about a liter at 32 weeks, fetal mass exceeds fluid volume after 26 or 27 weeks.

The amniotic fluid index (AFI), a semi-quantitative sonographic assessment of amniotic fluid volume, was introduced in 1987. This method of estimating amniotic fluid volume utilizes measurement of vertical pockets of amniotic fluid in each of four quadrants divided by maternal surface landmarks (e.g., umbilicus and linea nigra) and addition of the four values. The normal range for advanced gestations is between 5 and 20 cm. Subsequently, normal values have been established for pregnancies beyond 15 weeks' gestation with values above the 95th percentile (polyhydramnios) and below the 5th percentile (oligohydramnios) defined as abnormal.

After about 18 weeks, fetal urine production becomes vital and primary to the maintenance of amniotic fluid volume. Ultrasonic volumetric studies of fetal bladder filling rates performed in the third trimester of normal pregnancy suggest that the fetus produces about 5 cc of urine per kilogram per hour, or about 450 cc of urine per day near term. It is not known if these data may be precisely extrapolated to the younger fetus during the second trimester, but it is accepted that fetal urine production and swallowing probably maintain a similar balance in the smaller infant as well. Another possible source of fluid is lung effluent, as some observers have shown significant fetal tracheal fluid production and a consistent outward flow from fetal lungs near term. It is likely that fluid production by the lungs occurs predominantly late in gestation.

TABLE 131–1. AMNIOTIC FLUID VOLUME

Lower limit	125 cc at 15 wks − 2SD 250 cc at 20 wks 400 cc at 28–38 wks
Upper limit	300 cc at 16 wks 800 cc at 20 wks 1200 cc at 28 wks 2000 cc at 32–36 wks 1500 cc at 40 wks

CLINICAL INDICATIONS FOR SONOGRAPHY

The most common indication for referral of a pregnancy patient for sonography, second to a request for gestational age assignment, is a clinical impression of a uterine size/date discrepancy. The clinical basis for diagnosing such a discrepancy is the observation that in a normal pregnancy the uterine height, measured in centimeters above the pubic symphysis (Fig. 131–3), is approximately equal to the gestational age in weeks, between 20 and 35 weeks. In studying the growth of fundal height in normal pregnancies, the lower limit of normal is about 4 cm less than gestational age in weeks, and the upper limit about 2 cm more than gestational age. Deviation from these norms is adequate clinical justification for referral for sonographic evaluation.

This uterine measurement reflects the aggregate mass of fetus, fluid, placenta, and uterus and may, therefore, indicate an abnormality of any of these when it exceeds or falls short of expected dimensions. In a large number of cases, a discrepancy will be the result of inaccurate dates. In some, however, a fetal malformation and/or an amniotic fluid volume excess or deficiency will be found.

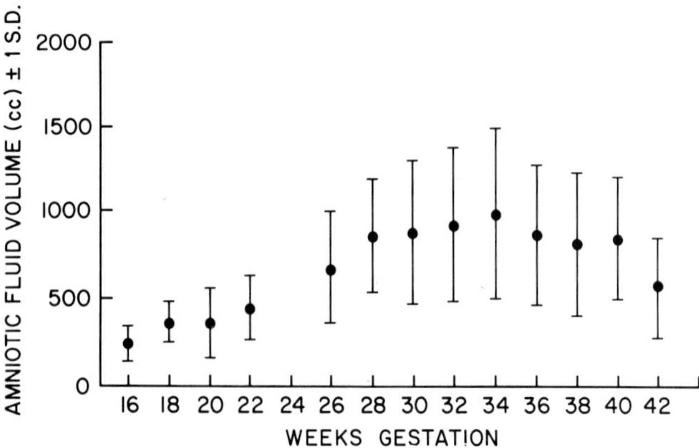

Figure 131–1. Average amniotic fluid volume (± 1 standard deviation) determined by dilution techniques in normal pregnancies.

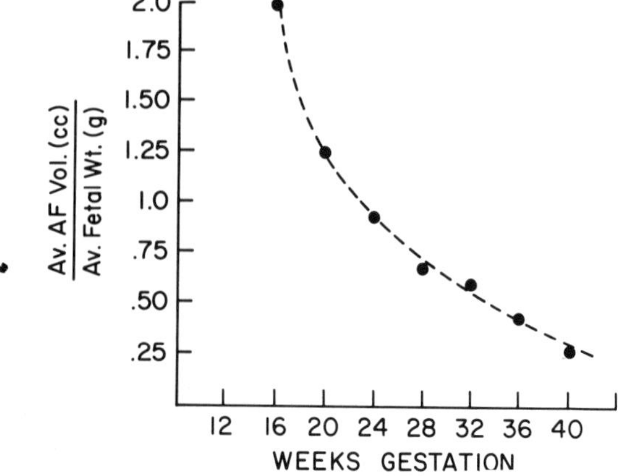

Figure 131–2. Relative relationship between average amniotic fluid volume and average fetal weight at various gestational ages.

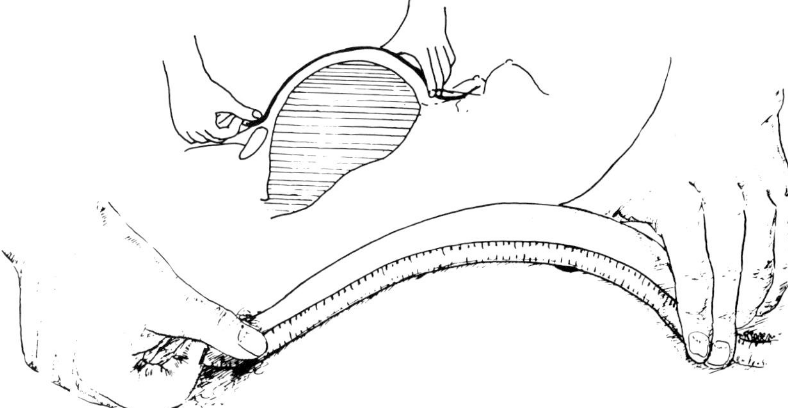

Figure 131–3. Clinician measuring the fundal height of a pregnant uterus.

HYDRAMNIOS

Hydramnios (polyhydramnios) indicates an excess of amniotic fluid and complicates from 1 in 200 to 1 in 100 pregnancies. The traditional definition of hydramnios requires a volume of 2000 cc, but accurate volume determination is clinically invasive and cumbersome and usually unnecessary. Whenever uterine size exceeds normal limits for gestational age and sonographic fetal dimensions (biparietal diameter and femur length) are appropriate for gestational age, with the excess uterine size seen on sonography (Fig. 131–4) due to amniotic fluid, a clinical diagnosis of hydramnios is made. Such a diagnosis carries major prognostic significance, because serious clinical consequences of hydramnios include premature labor, maternal respiratory or renal embarrassment, and even uterine rupture. Close clinical surveillance is indicated in cases of hydramnios to detect evidence of maternal or fetal compromise that might require delivery; however, clinical intervention is limited. Both therapeutic amniocentesis to remove excess fluid and relieve pressure, and pharmacologic inhibition of labor contractions often seen with the overdistention of hydramnios, are seldom indicated and offer only short-term benefit. Therapeutic amniocentesis may lead to labor, abruptio placentae, or spontaneous rupture of membranes, and rapid reaccumulation is the rule. Inhibition of labor secondary to uterine overdistention may also result in abruptio placentae or even uterine rupture. Therefore, clinical management involves mainly close maternal and fetal observation and careful sonographic examination of fetal morphology, with consideration of delivery if either mother or fetus is seen to deteriorate.

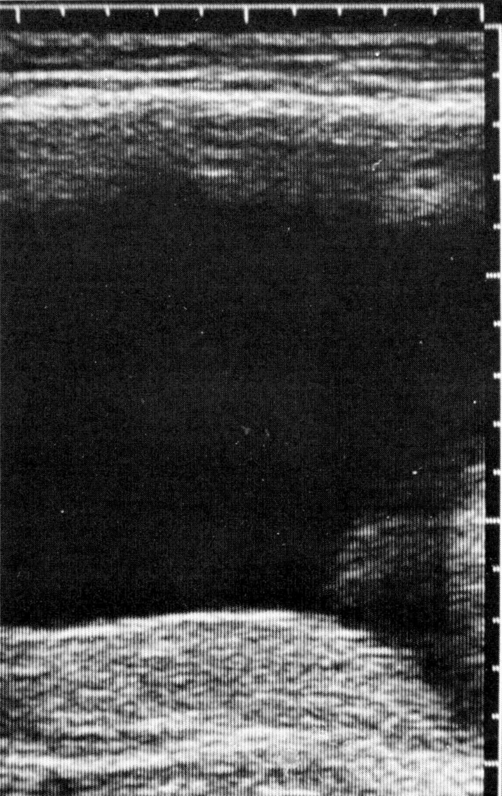

Figure 131–4. Typical ultrasonic appearance of **severe hydramnios.** Large anechoic areas of amniotic fluid in a large-for-dates uterus with appropriate fetal dimensions.

Hydramnios may result from a variety of circumstances. About 10 per cent of cases involve multiple gestation. Another 38 per cent are associated with diabetes mellitus or Rh isoimmunization, and about a third are idiopathic. Although only about 22 per cent of cases overall are associated with fetal malformation, once diabetes, Rh isoimmunization, and multiple pregnancy are excluded, fetal anomalies are found in almost half of the remaining cases. Because many of the associated malformations are potentially detectable with sonography, a careful fetal morphologic examination is necessary whenever hydramnios is diagnosed.

An imbalance in the equilibrium of amniotic fluid volume may be the result of overproduction or diminished removal. Fetal organ systems that may manifest malformations associated with hydramnios, therefore, are those that might alter effective uptake of amniotic fluid or central nervous system defects that might result in overproduction of urine owing to diminished antidiuretic hormone secretion (see Table 131–1). Accurate prenatal diagnosis of many of these malformations might be important to fetal survival by providing warning and thereby allowing time for maternal referral and/or planned, controlled delivery at a center where immediate neonatal therapy is available. Therefore, the sonographic study of the pregnancy complicated by hydramnios becomes a careful search for associated fetal malformations.

Hydramnios-Associated Malformations

Central Nervous System

Both anencephaly (Fig. 131–5) and hydrocephalus (Figs. 131–6 and 131–7) may be seen with excess amniotic fluid. Although at one time the relationship was thought to be due to damaged or absent muscular control, resulting in decreased fetal swallowing, more recent information suggests that often the volume of fluid

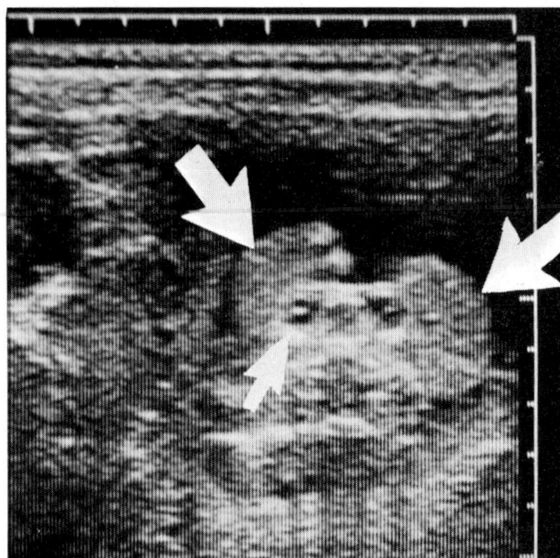

Figure 131–5. A frontal view of an **anencephalic fetus.** The *large arrows* indicate masses of neural tissue originating from the base of the skull of this anencephalic infant, and the *small arrow* indicates one of the two orbits that are seen in this view.

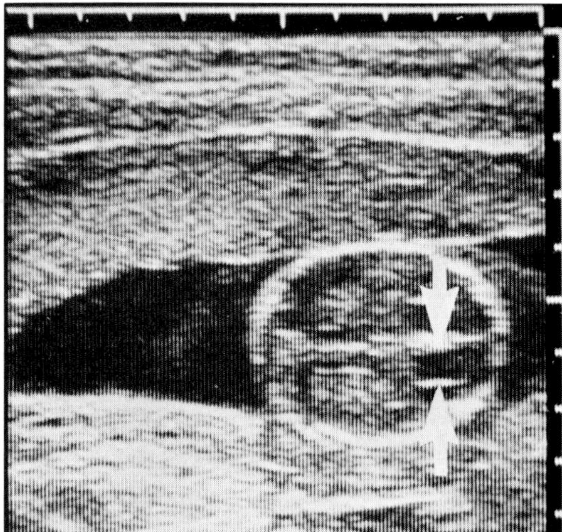

Figure 131–7. This biparietal view of a 17-week fetus demonstrates the anterior horns of the lateral ventricles. The *arrows* indicate one anterior horn appropriate for measurement. A specific image should be rejected unless both lateral horns can be seen simultaneously and appear symmetrical.

swallowed by such a fetus is not only normal, but increased. Therefore, it has been suggested that the mechanism involves a central defect in antidiuretic hormone production and an actual increase in fetal urine production. Ultrasonic findings of increased fetal bladder filling rates in such cases appear to support such a mechanism.

Abnormalities of the Fetal Chest

Proximal bowel obstruction is well known to be associated with hydramnios. The most proximal part of the bowel is the esophagus. Hydramnios may be seen with absolute, partial, or functional obstruction of the esophagus or duodenum. The fetal stomach normally occupies the left upper fetal abdomen (Fig. 131–8). Esophageal atresia in the absence of a tracheoesophageal fistula would prevent visualization of the fetal stomach on repeated or prolonged observations (Fig. 131–9).

Intrathoracic pressure may be increased with some abnormalities, and the increased pressure is often used to explain the associated hydramnios because of at least partial functional esophageal obstruction. Hydramnios is, therefore, seen with congenital fetal pleural effusions (Fig. 131–10) and global cardiomegaly (Fig. 131–11). Specific enlargement of the left atrium has also been seen with hydramnios, presumably on the basis of esophageal compression

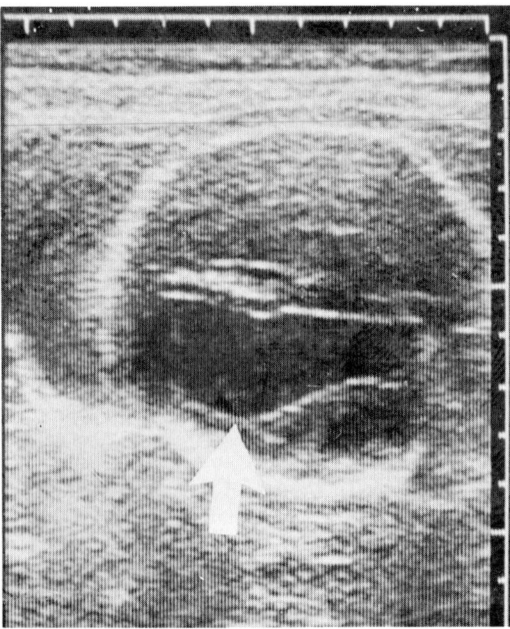

Figure 131–6. Hydrocephalus. Frequently, the posterior or occipital regions of the lateral ventricles are more severely dilated than the frontal horns, as indicated here.

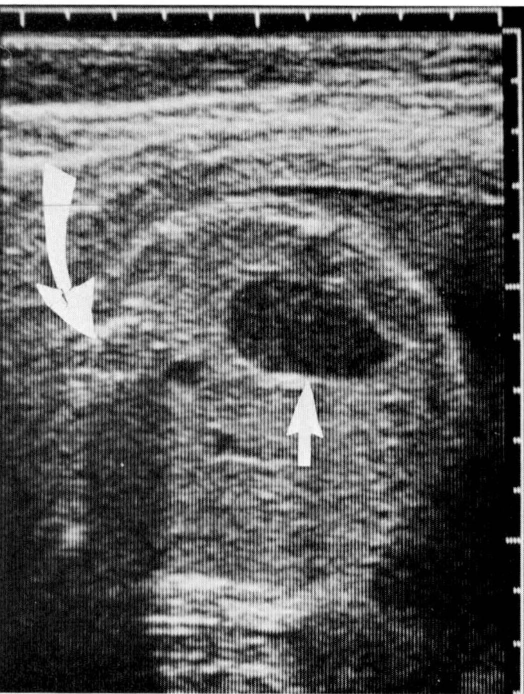

Figure 131–8. Transverse scan of **the upper abdomen of a normal fetus.** The *curved arrow* indicates the spine, with a typical acoustic shadow. The *small arrow* indicates a normal stomach on the left side of the upper abdomen.

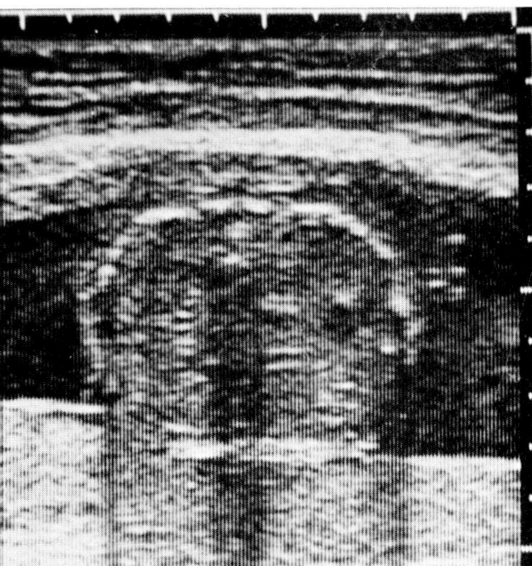

Figure 131–9. A transverse view of the upper abdomen of a fetus with **esophageal atresia.** Polyhydramnios is not well demonstrated in this view, but no stomach is seen on this and repeated examinations.

(Fig. 131–12). Hydramnios is also seen with cystic adenomatous malformation of the lung. The association of diaphragmatic hernia with hydramnios may be due to increased intrathoracic pressure or to mechanical distortion of the gastroesophageal junction within the chest. Anytime an anechoic cystic area is seen above the fetal diaphragm to the left side of the fetal heart with a shift of the fetal mediastinum, diaphragmatic hernia is the most likely diagnosis. Myotonic dystrophy, an autosomal dominant inheritable muscular disease, is consistently associated with hydramnios, probably because of chronic esophageal muscular weakness.

Finally, cardiac arrhythmias may lead to hydramnios, perhaps secondarily through pump failure and hydrops fetalis (Fig. 131–13). Such rhythm disturbances may be assessed with M-mode fetal echocardiography and can result from either structural abnormalities or conduction blockage. An intermittent complete heart block would result in irregular nonconduction of atrial beats (Fig. 131–14). Certain supraventricular tachyarrhythmias resulting in failure on a rate basis may be successfully treated in utero with maternally administered cardiac drugs; therefore, the accurate diagnosis of the lesion can have significant clinical implications.

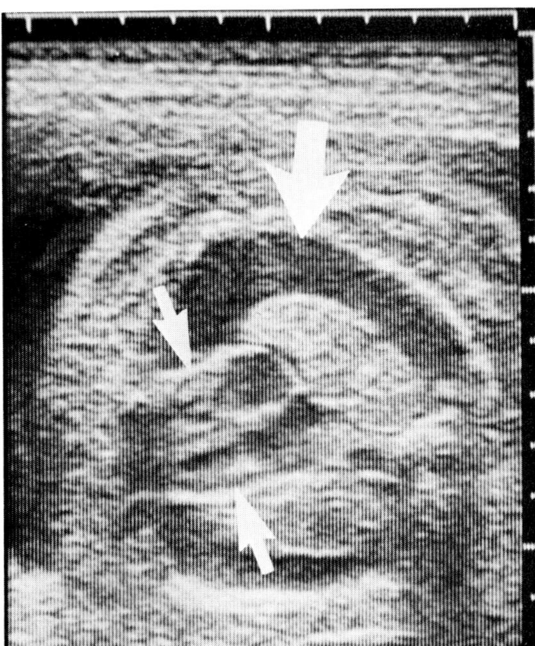

Figure 131–10. A transverse view of the chest of a fetus with **bilateral pleural effusions.** The *large arrow* indicates the effusion on the right side of the fetal chest, and the *smaller arrows* indicate the lateral margins of the cardiac ventricles. This patient presented with acute hydramnios.

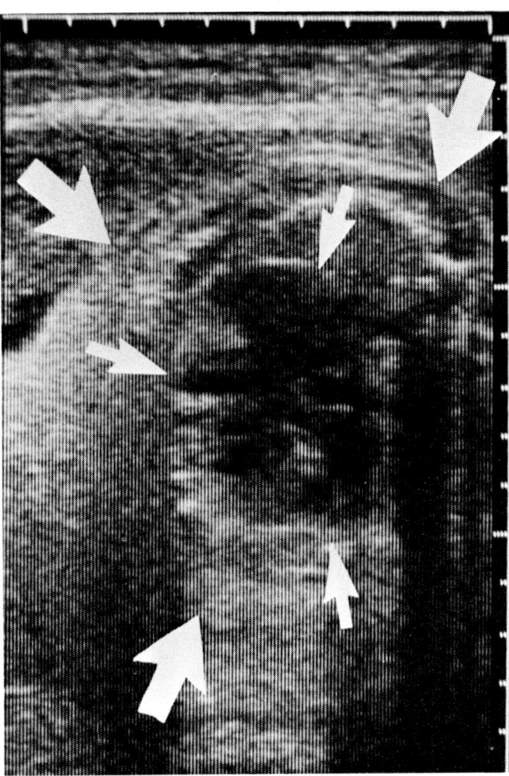

Figure 131–11. This transverse scan of the chest of this fetus demonstrates **cardiomegaly.** The *large arrows* indicate the margins of the chest and the *small arrows* indicate the margins of the heart. The average cardiac diameter divided by the average chest diameter should not exceed 0.55. This patient presented with hydramnios.

Abdominal Lesions

Stomach outflow obstruction is usually associated with hydramnios. The coincident appearance of a pregnancy complicated by hydramnios, and a large, sometimes irregular double cystic mass of the upper fetal abdomen strongly suggests obstruction of the duodenum (Fig. 131–15). The etiology may be duodenal atresia, an annular pancreas, or even intraluminal duodenal webs, but the prenatal ultrasonic image will be similar.

Ventral wall defects such as gastroschisis or omphalocele (Fig. 131–16) are also sometimes associated with hydramnios, although for different reasons. Partial mechanical obstruction at or near the site of herniation presumably leads to impaired function and secondary hydramnios in the case of omphalocele. Certainly a similar mechanism may be at work in many instances of gastroschisis, but because no membrane protects the herniated viscera from amniotic fluid in gastroschisis, an intense serosal inflammatory reaction is seen in the bowel wall, probably contributing to decreased effective function. This bowel wall inflammatory reaction in cases of gastroschisis produces an echogenic thickening of the bowel wall visible on scan. A diagnosis of a ventral wall defect carries important implications for the fetus because 30 to 50 per cent of infants

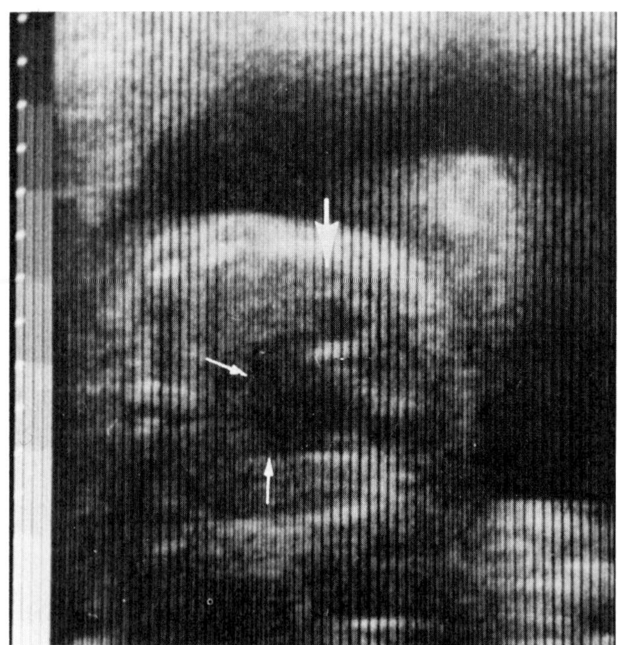

Figure 131–12. In this transverse scan of the chest of a fetus of a patient who presented with hydramnios, **the left ventricle was enlarged and hypoactive and the left atrium was severely dilated.** The *larger arrow* indicates the thickened wall of the left ventricle, and the *smaller arrows* indicate the extent of the left atrium.

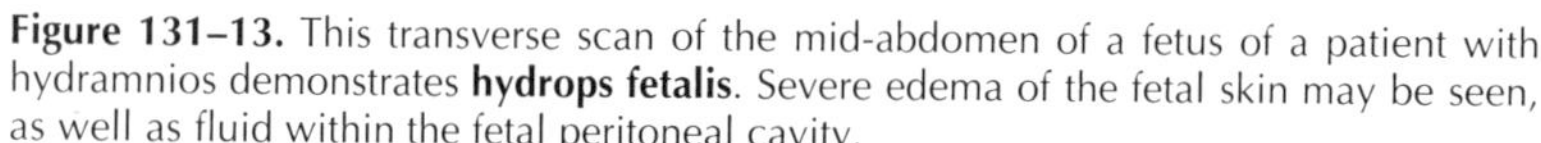

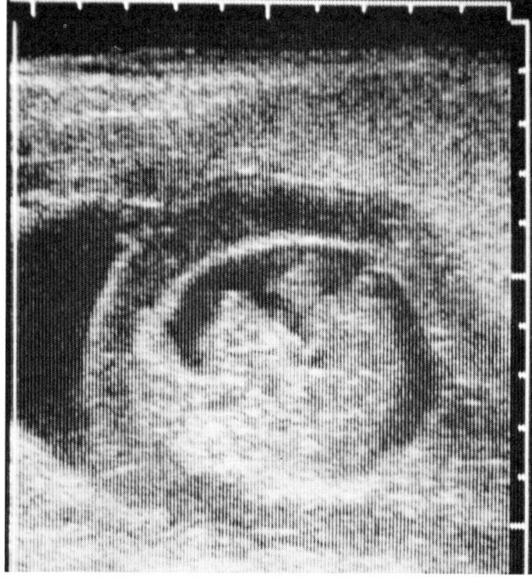

Figure 131–13. This transverse scan of the mid-abdomen of a fetus of a patient with hydramnios demonstrates **hydrops fetalis**. Severe edema of the fetal skin may be seen, as well as fluid within the fetal peritoneal cavity.

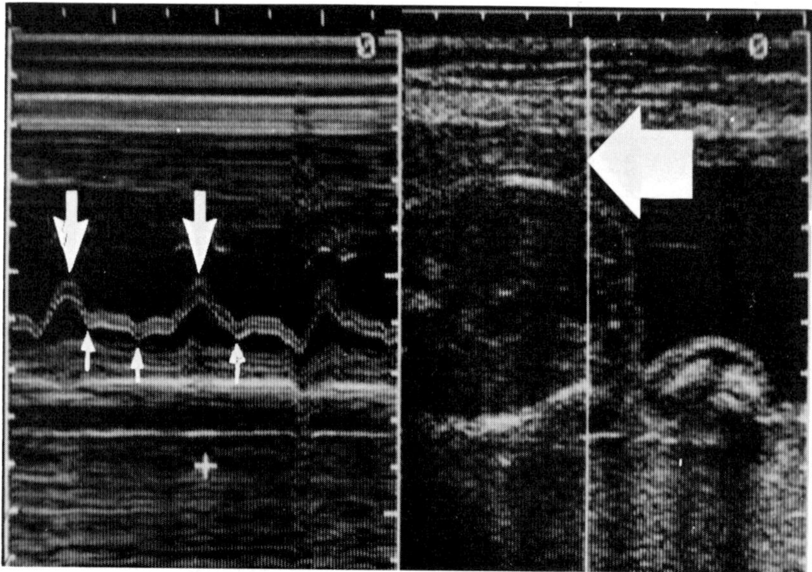

Figure 131–14. This fetal echocardiogram was performed on a patient with a large-for-dates uterus. The *large arrow* indicates the location of the M-mode beam. On the left side of the echocardiogram, the *small arrows* indicate atrial activity occurring at a rate of approximately 120 atrial beats per minute. The *larger arrows,* however, indicate an irregular ventricular activity of less than 60 beats per minute. This disassociation, which is visible on M-mode echocardiography, is indicative of a complete heart block.

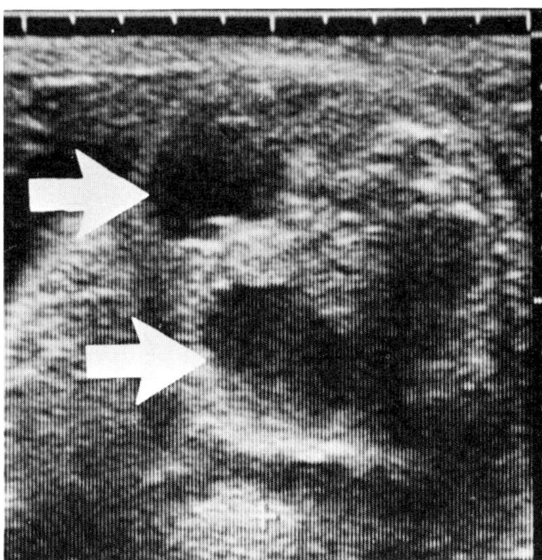

Figure 131–15. Transverse scan of the upper abdomen of a fetus of a patient with hydramnios. The typical double anechoic masses of **duodenal obstruction** may be seen. This patient underwent corrective surgery following delivery and was found to have intraluminal duodenal webs.

with omphalocele have serious associated anomalies, whereas only 11 per cent of fetuses with gastroschisis are otherwise malformed.

Finally, nonspecific fetal intra-abdominal mass lesions extrinsic to the bowel may be associated with hydramnios. Large renal cysts may result from ureteropelvic junction obstruction and can be associated with displacement and dysfunction of the proximal bowel (Fig. 131–17). Hydramnios may result in a similar fashion from congenital fetal megacolon (Fig. 131–18) or even fetal ovarian cysts or omental masses. Spontaneous fetal bowel perforation with resulting meconium peritonitis is also associated with hydramnios (Fig. 131–19).

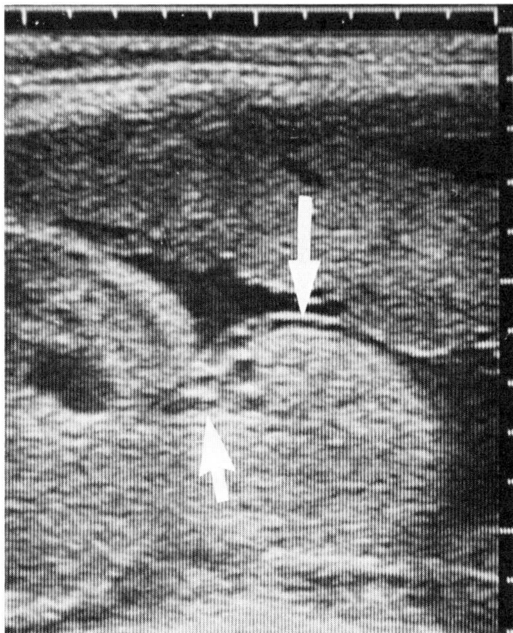

Figure 131–16. Transverse scan at the level of the umbilicus at approximately 32 weeks of a fetus with an **omphalocele.** The *longer arrow* indicates the membrane surrounding the soft tissue of the omphalocele, which is typical of this lesion. The *shorter arrow* indicates one of the umbilical vessels actually entering the fetal abdomen from the omphalocele.

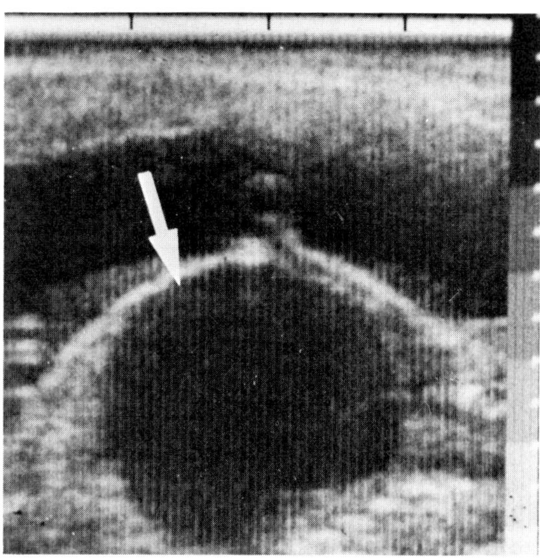

Figure 131–17. This is a longitudinal scan of the abdomen of a fetus at 32 weeks with a very large cystic abdominal mass. This mass proved to be a **perirenal cyst associated with ureteropelvic junction obstruction.**

Twin-Twin Transfusion Syndrome

An unusual complication of monochorionic twinning is twin-twin transfusion syndrome. This situation results as a consequence of abnormal placental vessel anastomoses leading to abnormal perfusion of one twin at the expense of the donor twin. At birth these twins are significantly disparate with regard to weight and central hematocrit. Approximately 1 per cent of monochorionic twin gestations will be complicated by acute twin-twin transfusion syndrome. This severe variant is manifest by acute onset of polyhydramnios in the recipient twin and severe oligohydramnios in the

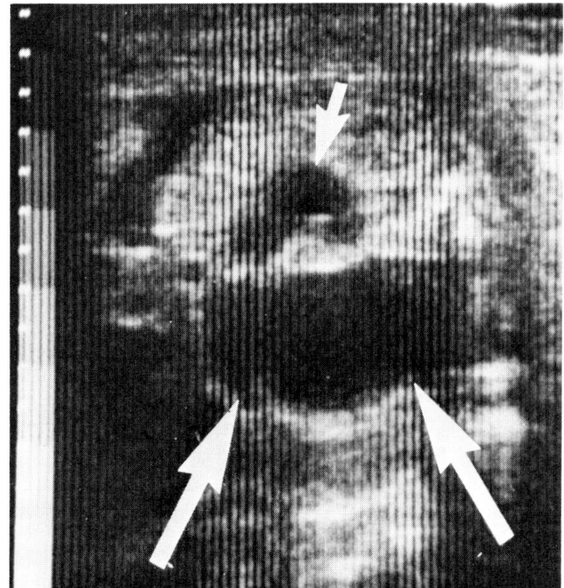

Figure 131–18. This transverse scan of the mid-abdomen of a fetus of a patient with hydramnios demonstrates an irregular large cystic mass of the fetal abdomen, which proved to be a **congenital fetal megacolon**.

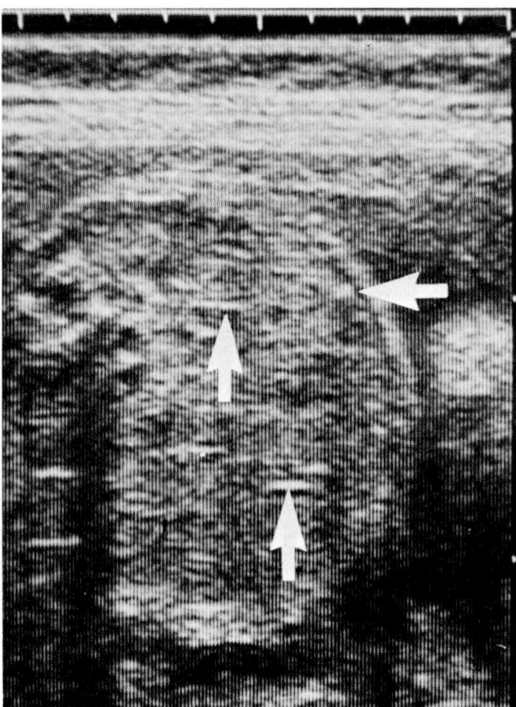

Figure 131–19. A transverse scan of the mid-abdomen of the fetus of a patient with hydramnios who proved to have **meconium peritonitis** at birth. The *arrows* indicate increased echogenicity within the fetal abdomen. Fetal intraperitoneal calcifications are typical indications of fetal meconium peritonitis.

donor, or "stuck," twin. Acute twin-twin transfusion syndrome usually occurs between 16 and 28 weeks, and sonographic evidence of recipient twin cardiac failure (e.g., mitral valve regurgitation, effusions, ascites, and hydrops) is common. In contrast to the chronic form of twin-twin transfusion, perinatal mortality with acute twin-twin transfusion without intervention approaches 100 per cent.

Therapeutic amniocentesis is the primary mode of treatment for twin-twin transfusion remote from term. Correction of the amniotic fluid volume surrounding the recipient twin in theory relieves the increased intrauterine pressure that accentuates the abnormal perfusion dynamics present in twin-twin transfusion syndrome. Elliot and coworkers have reported a perinatal survival greater than 75 per cent in cases of acute twin-twin transfusion treated with aggressive, repeated amniocenteses.

Indications for Further Ultrasonography

In summary, a clinical diagnosis of hydramnios based on large-for-dates uterus, ultrasonic fetal dimensions consistent with dates, and a subjectively increased amniotic fluid volume, or AFI greater than 20 cm, should lead to a careful sonographic examination of the fetal cranial, thoracic, and abdominal anatomy.

OLIGOHYDRAMNIOS

Whenever the uterine size is more than 4 cm smaller than expected for gestational age, and sonography demonstrates that there is little or no amniotic fluid present (Fig. 131–20), oligohydramnios is the likely diagnosis. Although some authors have defined severe oligohydramnios as absence of a pocket of fluid of at least 1 cm in greatest dimension, this is a very restrictive definition. Most observers accept a definition of oligohydramnios that includes crowding of fetal small parts and fetal/uterine contact throughout most of the uterus, or AFI less than 5 cm. Depending on the clinical circumstances and gestational age, oligohydramnios suggests a very poor prognosis for the pregnancy. Severe oligohydramnios may result from fetal malformation, chronic distress as seen in severe growth retardation, or chronic rupture of membranes.

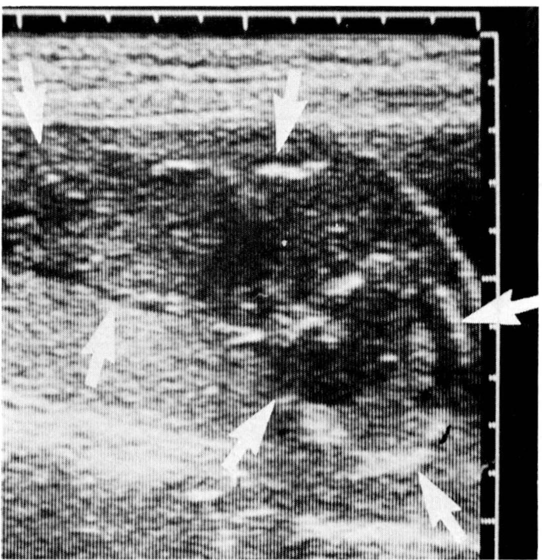

Figure 131–20. A longitudinal scan of a 20-week pregnant uterus demonstrating **almost complete absence of amniotic fluid.** The *arrows* indicate the outline of the fetus, and no pockets of amniotic fluid are seen.

Because fetal urine is the prime constituent of amniotic fluid after about 18 weeks, fetal renal abnormalities should be suspected when severe oligohydramnios is seen in early pregnancy, and in fact, serious renal impairment has been reported in half of such cases. Renal agenesis is a common finding, as well as obstruction (Fig. 131–21), various forms of renal dysplasia (Fig. 131–22), or more

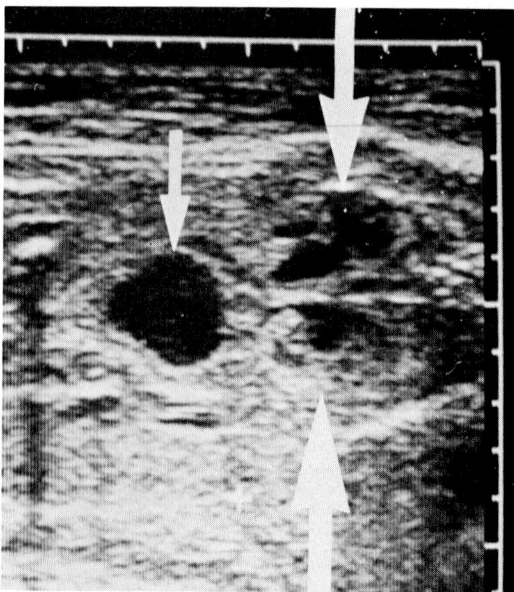

Figure 131–21. Longitudinal scan of the trunk of the fetus of a patient with severe oligohydramnios. The *smaller arrow* indicates a dilated fetal bladder, and the *large arrows* indicate longitudinal images of both hydronephrotic kidneys. This fetus was later found to have **posterior urethral valves in a bladder outlet obstruction syndrome.**

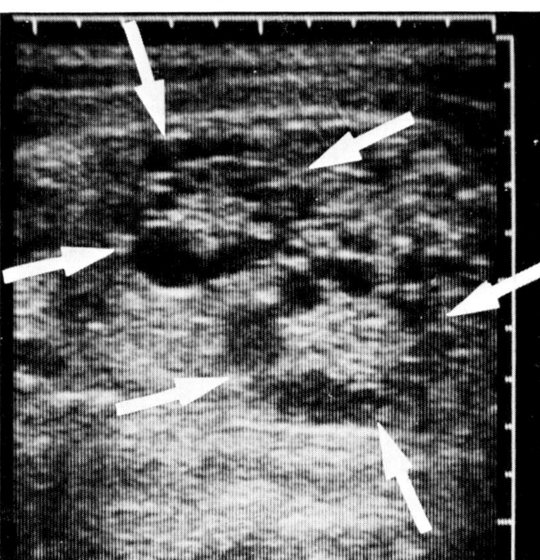

Figure 131–22. A transverse scan of the mid-abdomen of the fetus of a patient with severe oligohydramnios in the third trimester. The arrows indicate the outlines of both kidneys, which proved to have **multicystic renal dysplasia.**

complex malformations (Fig. 131–23). Table 131–2 summarizes the malformations associated with severe oligohydramnios found early in the second trimester.

Fetal prognosis in early severe oligohydramnios is guarded, not only because of the implications of the primary lesion but also because of the secondary effects of sustained severe oligohydramnios on fetal limb and lung development. Pulmonary hypoplasia is a lethal abnormality often seen in pregnancies complicated by chronic severe oligohydramnios. In fact, the majority of neonatal deaths result from pulmonary failure related to hypoplasia. There is now no reliable method of assessing prenatally the risk of pulmonary hypoplasia, but a strong suspicion of the condition may be drawn from the finding of a disproportionately large cardiac/thoracic ratio, suggesting underdeveloped lungs.

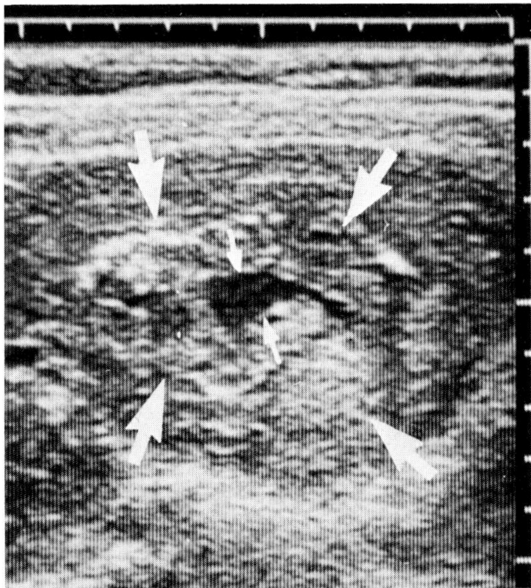

Figure 131–23. This transverse scan of a 17-week pregnant uterus with severe oligohydramnios demonstrates an irregular cystic mass of the fetal mid-abdomen. The *large arrows* indicate the outline of the fetal trunk, and the *small arrows* indicate the extent of the irregular fetal abdominal mass. The mass proved to represent confluence between **an obstructed bladder and an obstructed large colon.**

TABLE 131–2. FETAL ABNORMALITIES NOTED WITH EARLY SEVERE OLIGOHYDRAMNIOS

URINARY TRACT
Renal agenesis
Multicystic dysplasia
Urethral obstruction
Polycystic dysplasia
OTHERS
Cytogenetic abnormalities
Triploidy
Isochromosome X
Severe intrauterine growth retardation
Prune-belly syndrome
Impending fetal death
Ruptured membranes

Although renal agenesis is an important prenatal diagnosis, it is often difficult to make with confidence owing to poor image quality secondary to absence of amniotic fluid. Furthermore, because adrenal hyperplasia is a common associated finding in these infants, there is the danger that the sonographer may believe there are kidneys where there are none. Identification of a bladder is not necessarily irrefutable proof of the presence of functional renal tissue either, inasmuch as the bladder is usually physically present with renal agenesis and may often contain enough tissue transudate to be seen sonographically without renal tissue.

It is, therefore, often difficult or impossible to precisely identify prenatally the etiology of a severe mid-trimester oligohydramnios, but experience has shown that the prognosis for such a pregnancy is poor. Severe oligohydramnios later in pregnancy might relate to a variety of nonanomalous circumstances, such as ruptured membranes or growth retardation. Either of these situations can also benefit from sonographic surveillance of fetal growth or well-being. Furthermore, fetal limb and trunk movements and breathing movements are dynamic data concerning fetal well-being in the case of growth retardation and severe oligohydramnios that can be important to the clinican caring for the patient. Severe oligohydramnios, therefore, whether early or late, is ominous and may signify either fetal malformation or serious distress.

Bibliography

Alexander ES, Spitz HB, Clark RA: Sonography of polyhydramnios. AJR 138:343, 1982.

Elliot JP, Urig MA, Clewell WH: Aggressive therapeutic amniocentesis for treatment of twin-twin transfusion syndrome. Obstet Gynecol 77:537, 1991.

Moore TR, Cayle JE: The amniotic fluid index in normal human pregnancy. Am J Obstet Gynecol 162:1168, 1990.

Phelan JP, Smith CV, Broussard P, et al: Amniotic fluid volume assessment with the four-quadrant technique at 36–42 weeks' gestation. J Reprod Med 32:540, 1987.

Queenan JT, Thompson W, Whitfield CR, et al: Amniotic fluid volumes in normal pregnancies. Am J Obstet Gynecol 114:34, 1972.

Ray D, Berger N, Ensor R: Hydramnios in association with unilateral fetal hydronephrosis. J Clin Ultrasound 10:82, 1982.

Seeds AE: Current concepts of amniotic fluid dynamics. Am J Obstet Gynecol 138:575, 1980.

Skovbo P, Smith-Jensen S: Ultrasonic scanning and fetography of polyhydramnios. Acta Obstet Gynecol Scand 60:51, 1981.

Zamah NM, Gillieson MS, Walters JH, et al: Sonographic detection of polyhydramnios: A five-year experience. Am J Obstet Gynecol 143:523, 1982.

132 The Role of Fetal Biometry in Obstetric Sonography

Frank P. Hadlock

The use of ultrasound as a diagnostic tool in obstetrics has expanded rapidly in recent years, primarily because of the tremendous amount of information it can provide. In general, the information gained from an ultrasound examination is based on critical observations and/or measurements. Examples of key *observations* are fetal number, fetal presentation, presence or absence of cardiac activity, presence or absence of certain fetal anomalies, placental location and maturation, amniotic fluid volume assessment, and abnormalities of the uterine wall (e.g., fibroids) or adnexa (e.g., ovarian cyst). The observation process also plays a key role in mensuration, in that it is used to identify the images from which measurements will be made.

Mensuration has been applied in obstetric sonography to the fetus, the amniotic fluid volume, the placenta volume, and the total intrauterine volume. At present, the most important of these measurements are those of the fetus, because they can provide accurate information on fetal age and size. Knowledge of fetal age allows the obstetrician to plan elective deliveries within the time frame of a term pregnancy (38 to 42 weeks), and it allows him or her to institute measures that will optimize fetal outcome in cases in which labor ensues before 38 weeks or after 42 weeks. Evaluation of fetal size in utero is important in recognition and proper measurement of accelerated or retarded fetal growth; knowledge of fetal age is also important in identifying these entities because the normal range of fetal size changes with advancing menstrual age.

ESTABLISHING NORMAL REFERENCE DATA

At present the most effective method of assessing fetal size and age using ultrasound is through fetal biometry, in which fetal sonographic measurements are evaluated using statistical methods. The measurements made from ultrasound images can be one dimensional (i.e., linear), two dimensional (i.e., area), or three dimensional (i.e., volume). Because of their simplicity and their proven clinical usefulness, linear measurements are used most commonly in obstetric sonography. Although there are a number of fetal images that could be chosen for purposes of measurement, those most commonly used today for estimation of fetal size and age are a longitudinal axis through the fetal head and trunk (crown-rump length), axial images of the fetal head and abdomen, and a longitudinal image of the fetal femur (Figs. 132–1 and 132–2).

In order to assess fetal age or size using biometry, one must establish the normal range of measurements for a given fetal parameter for each week in gestation. This is accomplished by studying a population of fetuses in women who know precisely their menstrual history and/or conceptual dates, and in whom there are no complications of pregnancy that may alter fetal growth (e.g., hypertension, diabetes). The study population can be examined in longitudinal fashion, in which each fetus is measured multiple times throughout pregnancy, or by cross-sectional analysis, in which each fetus is examined only once in pregnancy. Theoretically, the longitudinal studies should provide better data on the true shape of the growth curve expected for subsequent fetuses, whereas the cross-sectional studies may have an advantage in defining the normal range for a given parameter at any point in pregnancy.

The data are evaluated by regression analysis, with size as the dependent variable, and the predicted mean value and the variation around the mean are defined for each week in gestation. Such data provide normal values for evaluating fetal growth in subsequent sonographic examinations. The data are then re-evaluated, with age as the dependent variable and the measurements as an independent variable, and prediction of age based on a given fetal measurement can be obtained. Estimates of the overall variability (range of error) in predicting age from a given measurement can be made by evaluation of the standard deviation of the regression equation, if it is uniform throughout the time frame studied, or by calculation of the observed variability of the population studied at each week in gestation. When using data from fetal studies generated in the manner described, one must be certain that the population characteristics, the equipment specifications, and the imaging and measurement methodology are appropriate for one's own laboratory.

ESTIMATION OF FETAL AGE

Fetal age should theoretically begin at conception, and conceptual age and gestational age are synonymous terms that can be used to define age calculated from the point of conception. In clinical practice, it is unusual for patients to know the exact date of conception, whereas it is quite common to know the beginning of the first day of the last menstrual period. It is for this reason that obstetricians typically date pregnancies by menstrual age, which is based on counting from the first day of the last menstrual period. The major limitation of this system is that it assumes that all patients ovulate and conceive in mid-cycle, which clearly is not always the case. In patients who are known to ovulate early in their cycle, use of menstrual age will underestimate fetal age, whereas for patients who ovulate late in the cycle, data based on menstrual age may overestimate fetal age. In any case, the term *menstrual age* will be used exclusively in this chapter in reference to establishing the duration of pregnancy by ultrasound.

Estimates of fetal age using ultrasound are most accurate in the first half of pregnancy and are less accurate as one approaches term. This is thought to be due to the fact that there is very little biologic variability in actual size in the first half of pregnancy whereas as term approaches, individual variations in fetal size become more pronounced. Pregnancies are most accurately dated using ultrasound by measurement of the fetal crown-rump length (CRL) between 8 and 12 menstrual weeks. The first step in the procedure is taking the average crown-rump measurement from three independent images; one can then refer to published tables (Table 132–1) for an estimation of fetal age or one can simply solve a regression equation such as the one from Nelson: menstrual age (days) = 51.008 + 0.6 CRL (mm). Estimates of menstrual age obtained in this way should be accurate to within ± 5 days in 95 per cent of cases, and in our experience the accuracy should be within ± 7 days in virtually all normal pregnancies. MacGregor has demonstrated that the accuracy (± 2 SD) can be expressed as ± 9 per cent of the

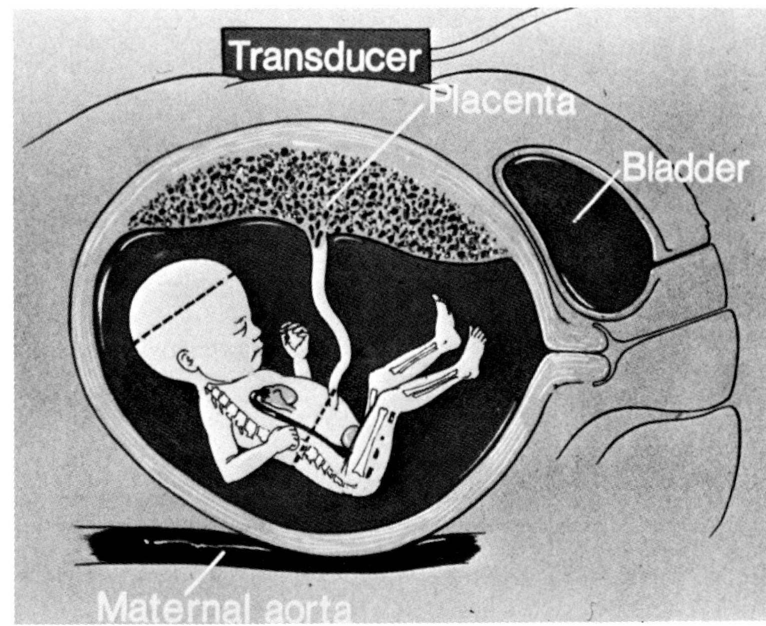

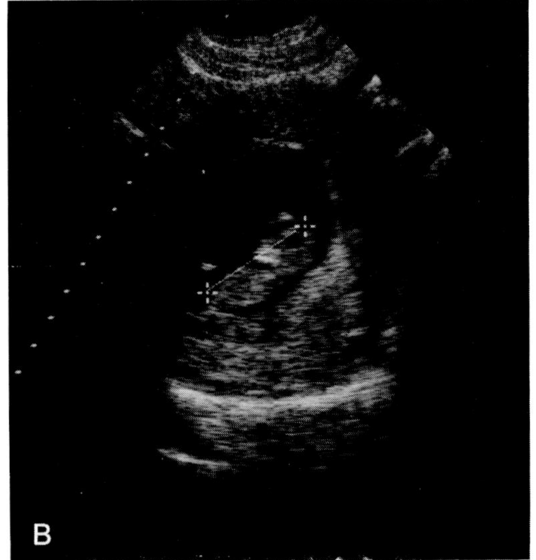

Figure 132–1. *A,* **The crown-rump length (CRL)** is measured along the longitudinal axis of the fetus from the top of the head to the bottom of the rump. The proper image planes for measurements of the fetal head, abdomen, and femur are indicated by *dashed lines. B,* Demonstrates a CRL measurement of 38 mm in a fetus at 10.5 menstrual weeks. In this case, the head is to the right and the rump to the left.

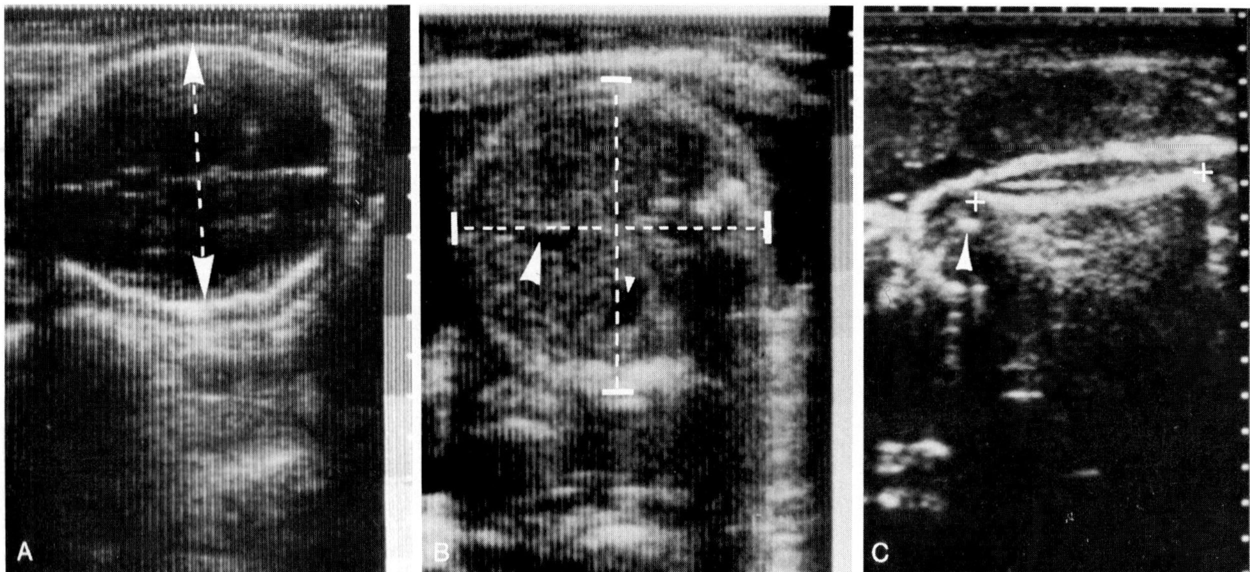

Figure 132–2. *A,* An axial section through the fetal head at the level indicated in Figure 132–1. The biparietal diameter is measured from leading edge to leading edge (outer to inner), as indicated by the *connected arrowheads.* The head circumference can be measured directly along the outer margin of the calvarium, or it can be estimated from the short and long axes (measured outer to outer) using the formula for calculating the circumference of an ellipse: $\text{CIRC} = 4.443\sqrt{\left(\frac{D1}{2}\right)^2 + \left(\frac{D2}{2}\right)^2}$. *B,* The section of the fetal abdomen in Figure 132–1. Important landmarks are the umbilical portion of the left portal vein *(large arrowhead)* and the fetal stomach *(small arrowhead).* The circumference can be measured directly along the outer margin, or it can be calculated using the ellipse approximation formula from the short and long axes measured outer to outer *(dotted lines). C,* The femur length image in Figure 132–1. The caliper markers (+) indicate proper measurement technique. Note that the ossification center of the distal femoral epiphyses *(arrowhead)* is not included in this measurement.

TABLE 132–1. PREDICTED MENSTRUAL AGE (WKS) FROM CROWN-RUMP LENGTH (CRL)

CRL (cm)	MA (wks)	CRL (cm)	MA (wks)	CRL (cm)	MA (wks)	CRL (cm)	MA (wks)	CRL (cm)	MA (wks)	CRL (cm)	MA (wks)
0.2	5.7	2.2	8.9	4.2	11.1	6.2	12.6	8.2	14.2	10.2	16.1
0.3	5.9	2.3	9.0	4.3	11.2	6.3	12.7	8.3	14.2	10.3	16.2
0.4	6.1	2.4	9.1	4.4	11.2	6.4	12.8	8.4	14.3	10.4	16.3
0.5	6.2	2.5	9.2	4.5	11.3	6.5	12.8	8.5	14.4	10.5	16.4
0.6	6.4	2.6	9.4	4.6	11.4	6.6	12.9	8.6	14.5	10.6	16.5
0.7	6.6	2.7	9.5	4.7	11.5	6.7	13.0	8.7	14.6	10.7	16.6
0.8	6.7	2.8	9.6	4.8	11.6	6.8	13.1	8.8	14.7	10.8	16.7
0.9	6.9	2.9	9.7	4.9	11.7	6.9	13.1	8.9	14.8	10.9	16.8
1.0	7.1	3.0	9.9	5.0	11.7	7.0	13.2	9.0	14.9	11.0	16.9
1.1	7.2	3.1	10.0	5.1	11.8	7.1	13.3	9.1	15.0	11.1	17.0
1.2	7.4	3.2	10.1	5.2	11.9	7.2	13.4	9.2	15.1	11.2	17.1
1.3	7.5	3.3	10.2	5.3	12.0	7.3	13.4	9.3	15.2	11.3	17.2
1.4	7.7	3.4	10.3	5.4	12.0	7.4	13.5	9.4	15.3	11.4	17.3
1.5	7.9	3.5	10.4	5.5	12.1	7.5	13.6	9.5	15.3	11.5	17.4
1.6	8.0	3.6	10.5	5.6	12.2	7.6	13.7	9.6	15.4	11.6	17.5
1.7	8.1	3.7	10.6	5.7	12.3	7.7	13.8	9.7	15.5	11.7	17.6
1.8	8.3	3.8	10.7	5.8	12.3	7.8	13.8	9.8	15.6	11.8	17.7
1.9	8.4	3.9	10.8	5.9	12.4	7.9	13.9	9.9	15.7	11.9	17.8
2.0	8.6	4.0	10.9	6.0	12.5	8.0	14.0	10.0	15.9	12.0	17.9
2.1	8.7	4.1	11.0	6.1	12.6	8.1	14.1	10.1	16.0	12.1	18.0

MA = menstrual age. The 95% confidence interval is ± 8% of the predicted age.

From Hadlock FP, Shah YP, Kanon DJ, Lindsey JV: Fetal crown-rump length: Reevaluation of relation to menstrual age (5–18 weeks) with high-resolution real-time US. Radiology 182:501–505, 1992.

predicted value throughout the first trimester of pregnancy. The only serious limitation of this method is that it does not allow one to study the fetal anatomy in detail, so that anomalies in fetal development will typically be missed at this stage in pregnancy. However, a 1990 study (Timor-Tritsch et al, 1990) suggests that the use of the vaginal probe may allow detection of some anomalies in the first trimester of pregnancy.

In the second and third trimesters, the fetal crown-rump length is extremely difficult to measure, and its accuracy in predicting age is also compromised because of individual variations in fetal size. The primary measurements that have been used to estimate age in the second and third trimesters are the biparietal diameter (BPD), head circumference (HC), abdominal circumference (AC), and femur length (FL). As with the crown-rump length, measurements of these fetal parameters can be translated into fetal age estimations using any of several published tables, or one can solve the regression equation upon which a table is based. Provided in Table 132–2 are regression equations for predicting menstrual age from any of these four fetal parameters used alone or in combination. The biparietal diameter and femur length in combination should provide excellent estimates of fetal age between 12 and 20 weeks, whereas after 20 weeks the head circumference and femur length combination should provide the best estimates of fetal age. The head circumference is substituted for the BPD after 20 weeks because it is more shape-independent than the BPD, thus less subject to errors due to molding of the fetal head. If the BPD is used for dating after 20 weeks, we recommend the shape correction method of Doubilet be used routinely. In our laboratory we use all four measurements throughout the second and third trimesters. One can arrive at an estimate of fetal age based on multiple parameters by simply averaging the individual estimates of age, but this is more easily accomplished by solving the regression equations by use of programmed microcomputers. The variability in predicting menstrual age using any of the four parameters individually or in combination is provided in Table 132–3. In general, the 95 per cent confidence interval for predicting age between 12 and 18 weeks is ± 8 days, between 18 and 30 weeks approximately ± 11 days, and between 30 and 42 weeks approximately ± 18 days. The variability can also be expressed as ± 9 per cent of the predicted value for the individual parameters, and ± 7 per cent for the multiple-parameter models throughout gestation. One must remember, however, that in 5 per cent of cases, the errors in age estimate will fall outside of the confidence bounds listed in Table 132–3.

A number of other measurements of the fetus have been introduced as potential estimators of menstrual age. These include measurements of the fetal orbits, cerebellum, spine, foot, and other long bones. For most of these measurements, good studies of the variability in predicting age have not been reported to date, and for those in which variability estimates are available, there is no apparent increase in the accuracy of age estimates using these methods. Because the limiting factor in menstrual age estimates from fetal biometry is the genetic variation in actual fetal size as pregnancy advances, we feel it is unlikely that additional biometric parameters will add to the accuracy of age estimation using ultrasound. It is possible, however, that certain nonbiometric observations such as amniotic fluid volume, degree of placental maturation, appearance of the fetal external ear, and presence or absence of certain epiphyseal ossification centers may play a role in increasing the accuracy of age estimates based on fetal biometry.

EVALUATION OF FETAL GROWTH

As indicated in the introduction, the expected value and its variability have been established for a number of fetal growth parameters (Table 132–4). In evaluating fetal growth one must know menstrual age precisely because the normal measurement values and their variability change with advancing menstrual age. The primary purpose for evaluating fetal size is to determine if there is evidence of retarded (IUGR) or accelerated (macrosomia) fetal growth. At term, absolute fetal size is also important in that it may affect management decisions such as mode of delivery.

In order to assess the normalcy of fetal size at a given point in gestation, one must be aware of established definitions for retarded and accelerated fetal growth. In clinical practice, fetal growth retardation is defined as a fetal weight below the tenth percentile for age, whereas fetal macrosomia is defined as a weight above the ninetieth percentile for age in the peer population. Fetal weight can be estimated from fetal measurements using ultrasound, but the limited accuracy (± 2 standard deviations = ± 16 to 25 per cent) could lead to a high number of false-positive and false-negative diagnoses. The studies on estimation of fetal weight using ultrasound have been enlightening, however, in that they have demonstrated consistently that the fetal abdominal circumference is the single fetal parameter most closely related to fetal weight. For this reason, we feel that estimates of the normalcy of fetal nutrition should focus primarily on the abdominal circumference. Measurements more than two standard deviations below the mean for age are highly suspicious for growth retardation, and serial scanning at two-week intervals is recommended as follow-up in such cases. Abdominal circumference measurements more than three standard deviations below the mean are considered unequivocal sonographic evidence of IUGR, and appropriate clinical measures, including early delivery (if fetal lung maturity can be demonstrated), are recommended.

Abdominal circumference measurements more than two standard deviations above the mean are considered very suspicious for evidence of macrosomia, and measurements more than three standard deviations above the mean are considered unequivocal evidence of fetal macrosomia. In such cases, repeat scans near term are done to confirm continuation of the abnormal growth pattern, and fetal weight estimates (which also take into account head size and femur length) are used to give the clinician an estimate of fetal size in clinically defined units, namely grams. Even with the limitations in accuracy of fetal weight estimation using this method in our laboratory (± 2 standard deviations = ± 16 per cent), fetal weight estimates above 4500 g are considered extremely strong evidence of macrosomia at term (Table 132–5). As with growth-retarded fetuses, macrosomic fetuses experience a high degree of perinatal morbidity and mortality in comparison with the peer population, and for this reason some clinicians now feel that fetuses that demonstrate a macrosomic pattern early in the third trimester should have delivery before they exceed 4000 g in weight (provided fetal lung maturity can be demonstrated), to avoid the potential trauma associated with delivery.

Evaluation of fetal measurements other than the abdominal circumference can also be quite useful in that they can define abnormal growth (unrelated to nutritional status) that may be limited to a particular part of the fetal body. For example, the fetal head circumference is known to be a good index of fetal head size, and measurements more than three standard deviations below the mean are highly suggestive of fetal microcephaly. Similarly, measurements more than three standard deviations above the mean should be viewed with suspicion for fetal hydrocephalus, which can be better detected by direct evaluation of the fetal ventricular system. Evaluation of fetal long bone length, particularly femur length, has been useful in detecting abnormal growth of the fetal skeleton. Measurements of femur length more than three standard deviations below the mean for age, particularly in parents of normal stature, should be viewed with extreme suspicion as evidence of retarded skeletal growth.

When evaluating the normalcy of fetal growth in patients with uncertain dates, the sonographer is extremely limited because he or she has no objective criteria against which to assess fetal size on a single examination. In cases of this type, it is very important to

TABLE 132–2. REGRESSION EQUATIONS FOR PREDICTING MENSTRUAL AGE (MA) FROM FETAL MEASUREMENTS (14–42 WKS)

Fetal Measurements (cm)	Regression Equation	Standard Deviation (wks)	Maximum Error (wks)	R^2 (%)
BPD	MA = 9.54 + 1.482 (BPD) + 0.1676 $(BPD)^2$	1.36	5.1	96.7
HC	MA = 8.96 + 0.540 (HC) + 0.0003 $(HC)^3$	1.23	4.1	97.3
AC	MA = 8.14 + 0.753 (AC) + 0.0036 $(AC)^2$	1.31	4.6	96.9
FL	MA = 10.35 + 2.460 (FL) + 0.170 $(FL)^2$	1.28	4.9	97.1
BPD, AC	MA = 9.57 + 0.524 (AC) + 0.1220 $(BPD)^2$	1.18	3.8	97.5
BPD, HC	MA = 10.32 + 0.009 $(HC)^2$ + 1.3200 (BPD) + 0.00012 $(HC)^3$	1.21	3.5	97.4
BPD, FL	MA = 10.50 + 0.197 (BPD) (FL) + 0.9500 (FL) + 0.7300 (BPD)	1.10	3.6	97.8
HC, AC	MA = 10.31 + 0.012 $(HC)^2$ + 0.3850 (AC)	1.15	4.3	97.6
HC, FL	MA = 11.19 + 0.070 (HC) (FL) + 0.2630 (HC)	1.04	3.3	98.0
AC, FL	MA = 10.47 + 0.442 (AC) + 0.3140 $(FL)^2$ − 0.0121 $(FL)^3$	1.11	3.8	97.8
BPD, AC, FL	MA = 10.61 + 0.175 (BPD) (FL) + 0.2970 (AC) + 0.7100 (FL)	1.06	3.4	98.0
HC, BPD, FL	MA = 11.38 + 0.070 (HC) (FL) + 0.9800 (BPD)	1.04	3.2	98.1
HC, AC, FL	MA = 10.33 + 0.031 (HC) (FL) + 0.3610 (HC) + 0.0298 (AC) (FL)	1.03	3.4	98.1
HC, AC, BPD	MA = 10.58 + 0.005 $(HC)^2$ + 0.3635 (AC) + 0.02864 (BPD) (AC)	1.14	4.0	97.7
BPD, HC, AC, FL	MA = 10.85 + 0.060 (HC) (FL) + 0.6700 (BPD) + 0.1680 (AC)	1.02	3.2	98.1

BPD = biparietal diameter; MA = menstrual age; HC = head circumference; AC = abdominal circumference; FL = femur length.
Reprinted from Hadlock FP, Deter RL, Harrist RB, Park SK: Estimating fetal age: Computer-assisted analysis of multiple fetal growth parameters. Radiology 152:497–501, 1984, with permission.

TABLE 132–3. SUBGROUP VARIABILITY IN PREDICTING MENSTRUAL AGE USING THE REGRESSION EQUATIONS IN TABLE 132–2

	Subgroup Variability (±2 SD) in Weeks				
Fetal Parameters	12–18 Weeks (N = 43)	18–24 Weeks (N = 69)	24–30 Weeks (N = 76)	30–36 Weeks (N = 95)	36–42 Weeks (N = 78)
BPD	±1.19	±1.73	±2.18	±3.08	±3.20
HC	±1.19	±1.48	±2.06	±2.98	±2.70
AC	±1.66	±2.06	±2.18	±2.96	±3.04
FL	±1.38	±1.80	±2.08	±2.96	±3.12
BPD, AC	±1.26	±1.68	±1.92	±2.60	±2.88
BPD, HC	±1.08	±1.49	±1.99	±2.86	±2.64
BPD, FL	±1.12	±1.46	±1.84	±2.60	±2.62
HC, AC	±1.20	±1.52	±1.98	±2.68	±2.52
HC, FL	±1.08	±1.34	±1.86	±2.52	±2.28
AC, FL	±1.32	±1.64	±1.88	±2.66	±2.60
BPD, AC, FL	±1.20	±1.52	±1.82	±2.50	±2.52
BPD, HC, FL	±1.04	±1.35	±1.81	±2.52	±2.34
HC, AC, FL	±1.14	±1.46	±1.86	±2.52	±2.34
HC, AC, BPD	±1.21	±1.58	±1.94	±2.60	±2.52
BPD, HC, AC, FL	±1.08	±1.40	±1.80	±2.44	±2.30

BPD = biparietal diameter; HC = head circumference; AC = abdominal circumference; FL = femur length.
Reprinted from Hadlock FP, Deter RL, Harrist RB, Park SK: Estimating fetal age: Computer-assisted analysis of multiple fetal growth parameters. Radiology 152:497–501, 1984, with permission.

TABLE 132–4. PREDICTED FETAL MEASUREMENTS AT SPECIFIC MENSTRUAL AGES

Menstrual Age (wks)	Biparietal Diameter (cm)*	Head Circumference (cm)†	Abdominal Circumference (cm)‡	Femur Length (cm)§
12.0	1.7	6.8	4.6	0.7
12.5	1.9	7.5	5.3	0.9
13.0	2.1	8.2	6.0	1.1
13.5	2.3	8.9	6.7	1.2
14.0	2.5	9.7	7.3	1.4
14.5	2.7	10.4	8.0	1.6
15.0	2.9	11.0	8.6	1.7
15.5	3.1	11.7	9.3	1.9
16.0	3.2	12.4	9.9	2.0
16.5	3.4	13.1	10.6	2.2
17.0	3.6	13.8	11.2	2.4
17.5	3.8	14.4	11.9	2.5
18.0	3.9	15.1	12.5	2.7
18.5	4.1	15.8	13.1	2.8
19.0	4.3	16.4	13.7	3.0
19.5	4.5	17.0	14.4	3.1
20.0	4.6	17.7	15.0	3.3
20.5	4.8	18.3	15.6	3.4
21.0	5.0	18.9	16.2	3.5
21.5	5.1	19.5	16.8	3.7
22.0	5.3	20.1	17.4	3.8
22.5	5.5	20.7	17.9	4.0
23.0	5.6	21.3	18.5	4.1
23.5	5.8	21.9	19.1	4.2
24.0	5.9	22.4	19.7	4.4
24.5	6.1	23.0	20.2	4.5
25.0	6.2	23.5	20.8	4.6
25.5	6.4	24.1	21.3	4.7
26.0	6.5	24.6	21.9	4.9
26.5	6.7	25.1	22.4	5.0
27.0	6.8	25.6	23.0	5.1
27.5	6.9	26.1	23.5	5.2
28.0	7.1	26.6	24.0	5.4
28.5	7.2	27.1	24.6	5.5
29.0	7.3	27.5	25.1	5.6
29.5	7.5	28.0	25.6	5.7
30.0	7.6	28.4	26.1	5.8
30.5	7.7	28.8	26.6	5.9
31.0	7.8	29.3	27.1	6.0
31.5	7.9	29.7	27.6	6.1
32.0	8.1	30.1	28.1	6.2
32.5	8.2	30.4	28.6	6.3
33.0	8.3	30.8	29.1	6.4
33.5	8.4	31.2	29.5	6.5
34.0	8.5	31.5	30.0	6.6
34.5	8.6	31.8	30.5	6.7
35.0	8.7	32.2	30.9	6.8
35.5	8.8	32.5	31.4	6.9
36.0	8.9	32.8	31.8	7.0
36.5	8.9	33.0	32.3	7.1
37.0	9.0	33.3	32.7	7.2
37.5	9.1	33.5	33.2	7.3
38.0	9.2	33.8	33.6	7.4
38.5	9.2	34.0	34.0	7.4
39.0	9.3	34.2	34.4	7.5
39.5	9.4	34.4	34.8	7.6
40.0	9.4	34.6	35.3	7.7

*BPD = $-3.08 + 0.41\ (MA) - 0.000061\ MA^3$; $r^2 = 97.6\%$; 1 SD = 3 mm.
†HC = $-11.48 + 1.56\ (MA) - 0.0002548\ MA^3$; $r^2 = 98.1\%$; 1 SD = 1 cm.
‡AC = $-13.3 + 1.61\ (MA) - 0.00998\ MA^2$; $r^2 = 97.2\%$; 1 SD = 1.34 cm.
§FL = $-3.91 + 0.427\ (MA) - 0.0034\ MA^2$; $r^2 = 97.5\%$; 1 SD = 3 mm.
BPD = biparietal diameter; HC = head circumference; AC = abdominal circumference; FL = femur length; MA = menstrual age.
Reprinted from Hadlock FP, Deter RL, Harrist RB, Park SK: Estimating fetal age: Computer-assisted analysis of multiple fetal growth parameters. Radiology 152:497–501, 1984, with permission.

TABLE 132–5. IN UTERO FETAL WEIGHT STANDARDS AT ULTRASOUND

Menstrual Week	Percentiles (g)				
	3rd	10th	50th	90th	97th
10	26	29	35	41	44
11	34	37	45	53	56
12	43	48	58	68	73
13	55	61	73	85	91
14	70	77	93	109	116
15	88	97	117	137	146
16	110	121	146	171	183
17	136	150	181	212	226
18	167	185	223	261	279
19	205	227	273	319	341
20	248	275	331	387	414
21	299	331	399	467	499
22	359	398	478	559	598
23	426	471	568	665	710
24	503	556	670	784	838
25	589	652	785	918	981
26	685	758	913	1068	1141
27	791	876	1055	1234	1319
28	908	1004	1210	1416	1513
29	1034	1145	1379	1613	1724
30	1169	1294	1559	1824	1949
31	1313	1453	1751	2049	2189
32	1465	1621	1953	2285	2441
33	1622	1794	2162	2530	2703
34	1783	1973	2377	2781	2971
35	1946	2154	2595	3036	3244
36	2110	2335	2813	3291	3516
37	2271	2513	3028	3543	3785
38	2427	2686	3236	3786	4045
39	2576	2851	3435	4019	4294
40	2714	3004	3619	4234	4524

From Hadlock FP, Harrist RB, Martinez-Poyer J: In utero analysis of fetal growth: A sonographic weight standard. Radiology 181:129–133, 1991.

evaluate body proportionality using body ratios, which have been demonstrated to be essentially age-independent between 21 and 42 weeks. The first step in this process is evaluation of fetal head shape by use of the cephalic index (short axis/long axis × 100; normal = 78 ± 8). If this ratio is normal, one should measure the femur length/BPD ratio (FL/BPD × 100 = 79 ± 8). If this measurement is abnormally low one should view the femur measurement with suspicion for possible dwarfism, which can be evaluated in serial growth studies; if this ratio is abnormally high, one should view the head measurement with suspicion for possible microcephaly, and again this should be documented on serial growth studies. If the femur length/BPD ratio is normal, one can measure the femur length/abdominal circumference ratio (FL/AC × 100 = 22 ± 2). If the other body ratios have been normal and this ratio is low, one should be suspicious that the abdominal measurement indicates possible macrosomia, and serial growth studies at three-week intervals should be instituted. If this measurement is high, the possibility of compromise of abdominal growth secondary to growth retardation should be considered, and this should be confirmed again with serial growth studies at three-week intervals.

CONCLUSIONS

It should be obvious from the foregoing discussion that mensuration of fetal size, particularly the three major fetal body components (i.e., head size, abdominal size, femur length) can provide an enormous amount of information about both the size and age of the fetus. In determining fetal age using ultrasound after the first trimester, emphasis should be placed on head size and femur length, whereas in evaluating the normalcy of fetal size at a specific menstrual age, emphasis should be placed primarily on the abdominal circumference. Inherent in the use of these measurements is the understanding that stringent observation criteria have been used to ensure that the anatomy of the structures measured is normal. For example, one would obviously not use head size as an index of fetal age if hydrocephalus is demonstrated.

It is extremely important to understand that it is difficult, if not impossible, to establish both age and size by a single ultrasound examination. For example, if one attempted to do this in a symmetrically growth-retarded or accelerated fetus, the abdominal circumference would be very likely to be at the fiftieth percentile for the age established by head circumference and femur length. In fetuses whose growth is asymmetrically retarded or accelerated, it may be possible to suspect abnormal fetal growth if the abdominal circumference value is abnormally high or low for the age established by head circumference and femur length, particularly if the femur length/abdominal circumference ratio is abnormal. In such cases, the index of suspicion for growth retardation would be even higher if one observed oligohydramnios or decreased fetal movement, whereas early fetal macrosomia might be suspected (if the AC were high for the age established by head circumference and femur length, and the FL/AC ratio is low) if observations of polyhydramnios or excessive subcutaneous fat were observed. In either case, however, serial sonographic studies with attention to growth of the abdominal circumference would be required to confirm the diagnosis.

In recent years, the use of microcomputers for evaluation of data from obstetric sonograms has been outlined in several reports. It is our belief that in the future the regression equations for age and growth determination will be stored in such computers, and that the sonographer will make six linear measurements using electronic calipers (BPD, short and long axes of the head and abdomen measured outer to outer, and femur length), and will also indicate certain key observations such as oligohydramnios or polyhydramnios, placental maturation, and presence or absence of the distal femoral epiphyses or proximal tibial epiphyses; the computer will then analyze body proportionality based on cephalic index, FL/BPD ratio, and FL/AC ratio and will calculate age, weight, and weight percentile based on the appropriate measurements. The efficacy of such a system will depend on the ability of the clinician to make accurate measurements from appropriate images and to put the computer-generated evaluation into an appropriate clinical context.

Bibliography

Doubilet PM, Greenes RA: Improved prediction of gestational age from fetal head measurements. AJR 142:797, 1984.

Drumm JE, Clinch J, MacKenzie G: The ultrasonic measurement of fetal crown-rump length as a method of assessing gestational age. Br J Obstet Gynaecol 83:417–421, 1976.

Hadlock FP: Sonographic estimation of fetal age and weight. Radiol Clin North Am 28(1):39–50, 1990.

Hadlock FP, Deter RL, Harrist RB: Sonographic detection of abnormal fetal growth patterns. In Platt LD (ed): Clinical Obstetrics and Gynecology. Philadelphia, Harper and Row, 1984, pp 342–351.

Hadlock FP, Deter RL, Harrist RB, Park SK: The use of ultrasound to determine fetal age—a review. Med Ultrasound 7:95–103, 1983.

Hadlock FP, Deter RL, Harrist RB, Park SK: Estimating fetal age: Computer-assisted analysis of multiple fetal growth parameters. Radiology 152:497–501, 1984.

Hadlock FP, Harrist RB, Carpenter RJ, et al: Sonographic estimation of fetal weight. Radiology 150:535–540, 1984.

Hadlock FP, Harrist RB, Martinez-Poyer J: In utero analysis of fetal growth: A sonographic weight standard. Radiology 181:129–133, 1991.

Hadlock FP, Shah YP, Kanon DJ, Lindsey JV: Fetal crown-rump length: Reevaluation of relation to menstrual age (5–18 weeks) with high-resolution real time US. Radiology 182:501–505, 1992.

Mac Gregor SN, Tamura RK, Sabbagha RE, et al: Underestimation of gestational age by conventional crown-rump length dating curves. Obstet Gynecol 70:344–348, 1987.

Nelson LH: Comparison of methods for determining crown-rump measurement by real-time ultrasound. J Clin Ultrasound 9:67, 1981.

Timor-Tritsch IE, Peisner DB, Raju S: Sonoembryology: An organ-oriented approach using a high-frequency vaginal probe. J Clin Ultrasound 18:286–298, 1990.

133 Ultrasound Evaluation for Intrauterine Growth Retardation

Barbara S. Hertzberg

Evaluation for intrauterine growth retardation (IUGR) presents one of the most challenging diagnostic dilemmas in obstetric ultrasound. Perinatal morbidity and mortality are dramatically increased in fetuses affected by IUGR, yet diagnosis is complicated by inconsistencies in definition, the ever-growing list of biometric parameters used to assign gestational age and monitor fetal growth, as well as lack of consensus among experts regarding the optimal approach to diagnosis. This chapter will examine the definition of IUGR, present a pragmatic approach for identifying the "at risk" fetus using ultrasound measurements, and describe the use of Doppler ultrasound in the evaluation of IUGR.

GENERAL CONCEPTS

Small for Gestational Age

The conventional definition of IUGR is fetal weight below the tenth percentile for gestational age. This definition, however, has a number of inherent difficulties when an attempt is made to apply it to the clinical setting. Critical examination of the definition indicates that the affected fetus is more precisely termed *small for gestational age* (SGA) than *growth retarded.* The SGA group represents a heterogeneous population that is not limited to fetuses with pathologic restrictions on growth. Furthermore, fetuses with pathologic restrictions on growth who weigh above the tenth percentile for gestational age but never achieve their full potential are, by definition, excluded from the SGA group. Thus, although the concept of small for gestational age is central to the definition of IUGR, SGA and pathologic growth retardation are not synonymous.

With this in mind, let us examine the small for gestational age population in more detail. This population can be divided into three subgroups based on the underlying process that causes the fetus to be SGA (Fig. 133–1). The three subgroups are (1) normal fetuses with low, but normal genetic growth potential; (2) fetuses with pathologic restrictions on *intrinsic* growth potential; and (3) fetuses in whom growth has been adversely affected by factors *extrinsic* to the fetus. This subdivision is important because the increased risks of perinatal morbidity and mortality associated with IUGR do not apply to the subgroup of normal fetuses who are SGA owing to low inherent growth potential. The purpose of the SGA definition is to identify a group of pregnancies at risk for increased complications who may benefit by increased antenatal surveillance and timed early delivery. This classification, however, neither is all-inclusive of the targeted population, nor does it detect only fetuses who have the potential to benefit from intervention. Detection of an SGA fetus by ultrasound measurements identifies the pregnancy *at risk* for IUGR, but does not necessarily indicate that pathologic restrictions to growth are operative.

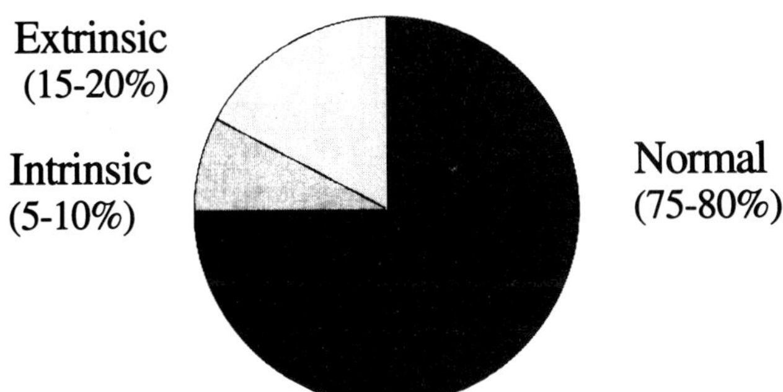

Figure 133–1. Subgroups of **small for gestational age (SGA)** fetuses based on etiology.

The subgroup of normal fetuses who are SGA because of low, but normal genetic growth potential accounts for approximately 75 to 80 per cent of fetuses who are SGA by ultrasound measurements. Thus, the majority of SGA fetuses are not at increased risk for perinatal morbidity and mortality.

On the other hand, fetuses who exhibit lower than expected growth as a result of pathologic restrictions on *intrinsic* growth potential comprise only approximately 5 to 10 per cent of the SGA population. This group of intrinsically abnormal fetuses can be further subdivided based on the etiology of intrinsic growth restriction, as follows: (1) chromosomal abnormality (e.g., trisomy 13, 18, 21, triploidy); (2) major congenital abnormality (e.g., renal agenesis, short-limbed dysplasia); (3) severe early extrinsic insult resulting in permanent intrinsic abnormality—i.e., in utero infection, drug or teratogen exposure. This intrinsically abnormal group tends to present earlier in gestation than do other forms of growth retardation, and owing to the severe, irreversible nature of the underlying processes involved, the prognosis is usually fixed at the time of detection. Thus, affected fetuses typically do not benefit from timed early delivery, and the value of ultrasound in these cases lies in defining the etiology, and distinguishing this group from the subgroup that derives potential benefit from increased antenatal surveillance and timed early delivery, that is, the SGA pregnancy in which fetal growth has been adversely affected by factors *extrinsic* to the fetus.

A multitude of factors extrinsic to the fetus, such as maternal hypertension, smoking, diabetes, inadequate maternal nutrition, placental infarction, and placental abruption can impair fetal growth. These entities have been collectively referred to as *uteroplacental dysfunction,* and typically present relatively late in pregnancy (third trimester or late second trimester). This group is thought to account for approximately 15 to 20 per cent of SGA fetuses, and owing to the increased perinatal risks posed by remaining in an unfavorable intrauterine environment, has the potential to benefit from increased antenatal surveillance and timed early delivery. Thus, from a practical standpoint, this is the group that the obstetrician is targeting when ultrasound is requested to "rule out IUGR."

Low Birth Weight

The term *low birth weight* (LBW) should not be interchanged with the concepts of SGA or IUGR. LBW babies subdivide into two main groups: (1) premature infants whose low birth weight occurs solely because they were born early, but who are above the 10th percentile for gestational age; and (2) infants who are truly SGA, i.e., weight below the 10th percentile for gestational age. Additionally, there is an overlap group of LBW infants who exhibit characteristics of both groups because they are both premature and

SGA. The division of LBW infants into two main groups is important because the "premie" subgroup would have benefited by remaining in the intrauterine environment as long as possible, whereas only fetuses in the SGA subset have the potential to benefit from timed early delivery.

Symmetrical vs Asymmetrical Growth Retardation

SGA fetuses have been divided into two other subgroups based on whether the entire fetus is proportionately small for gestational age—i.e., *symmetrical* growth retardation, or whether selected body parts (particularly the abdomen) are preferentially more affected than others—termed *asymmetrical* growth retardation. Although there are exceptions, the fetus whose growth is intrinsically limited tends to exhibit a symmetrical form of IUGR, with a proportionate reduction in size of all body parts. Conversely, asymmetrical growth restriction tends to be associated with growth impairment that occurs later in pregnancy, secondary to extrinsic limitations ("uteroplacental dysfunction"). In the asymmetrical form the abdomen is particularly severely diminished, in part from reduced subcutaneous fat but largely owing to reduced glycogen stores in the fetal liver, which constitutes the bulk of the fetal abdomen. On the other hand the brain, and consequently the head, are said to be "spared." This sparing is presumed due to reflex redistribution of blood flow to the head of the compromised fetus.

The concepts of symmetrical and asymmetrical IUGR have been challenged. There are many exceptions to the tendency for early or intrinsic insults to result in early-onset "symmetrical" growth reduction and uteroplacental dysfunction to cause late-onset "asymmetrical" growth restriction. In fact it is probably unusual for asymmetrical growth retardation to occur in a pure form. Although the abdomen is predominantly affected in asymmetric IUGR, head size is also frequently compromised, albeit to a lesser extent. Furthermore, although severe IUGR due to uteroplacental dysfunction may start out with an asymmetrical biometric profile, if allowed to progress, the process restricting growth can become so severe it eventually affects head size and fetal length to a sufficient extent that the profile converts to a symmetrical one. Even the concept that severe early insults or intrinsic defects such as chromosomal abnormalities cause symmetrical IUGR is not an infallible one. As an example, triploid fetuses are characterized by early-onset growth retardation that exhibits a distinct head to body disproportion (Figs. 133–2*A* and *B*). Thus, although groups of IUGR fetuses exhibit biometric profiles that tend to be either "symmetrical" or "asymmetrical," these are not absolute concepts, but rather, growth restriction results in a wide spectrum of body proportions.

APPROACH TO IDENTIFY THE SGA FETUS

Sonographic identification of the SGA fetus poses a complex, challenging problem, and as a result, there is lack of consensus on the optimal approach to diagnosis. The approach that will be presented here is an attempt to optimize detection of the SGA fetus without adding undue complexity to the measurement and calculation process. This approach is not the only acceptable one, but rather, numerous other schemes are available for evaluating this question. As our understanding of this complex topic evolves, new

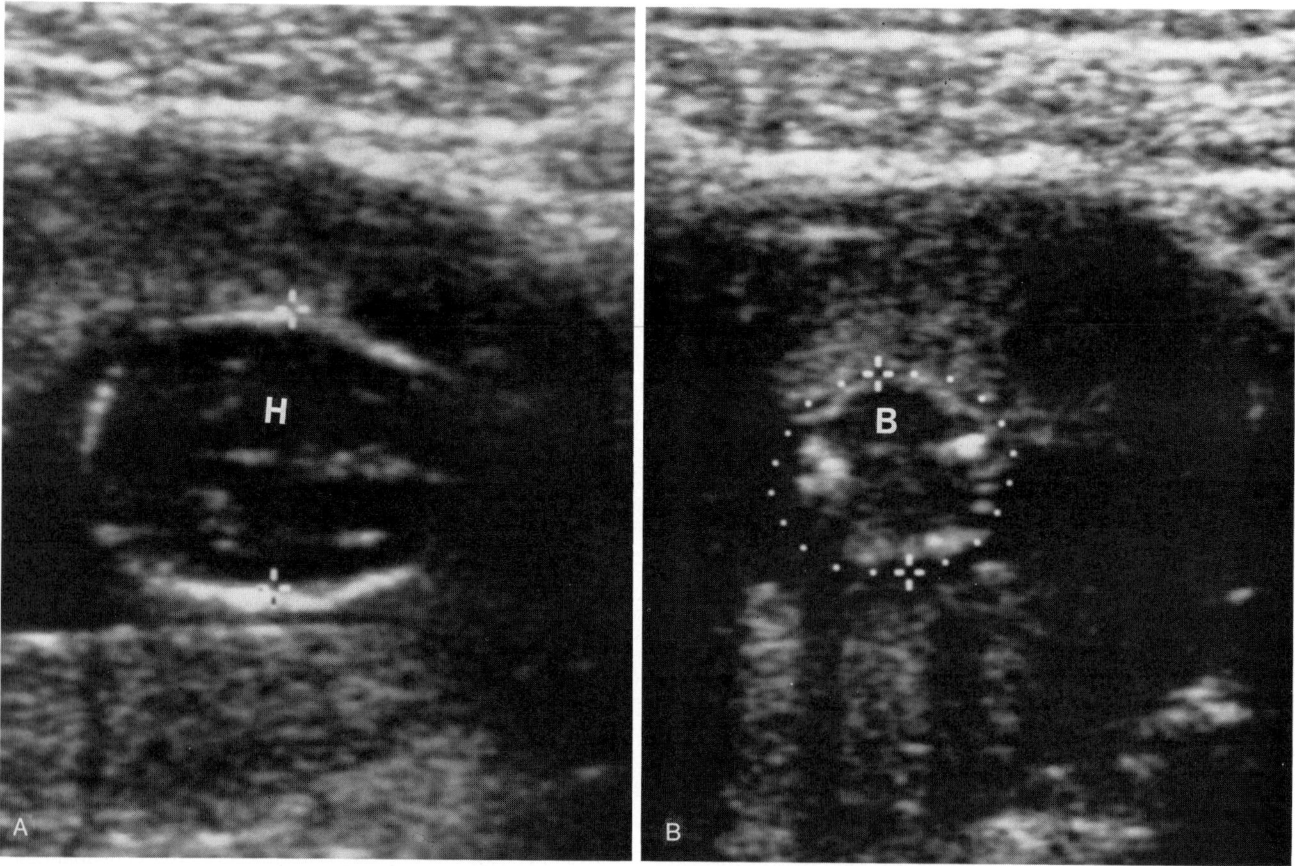

Figure 133–2. *A* and *B*, Pronounced head (H)–body (B) size discrepancy in a fetus with early-onset **intrauterine growth retardation (IUGR)** due to triploidy.

schemes will undoubtedly replace existing ones. The reader is reminded that ultrasound measurements are not actually intended to diagnose IUGR, but rather to identify a subgroup of fetuses who are likely to be SGA, and as a result, are "at risk for IUGR." Sonographic identification of the SGA population is not perfect, and even if it were, many SGA fetuses do not have pathologic restrictions on growth.

Estimation of Gestational Age

Inasmuch as the focus of ultrasound in evaluating for IUGR is to detect the SGA fetus, the first step in any scheme to address the question of IUGR is to estimate gestational age. The accuracy of all determinations made beyond this point, by definition, depends on how accurate the initial estimation of gestational age was. This represents a major stumbling block in many cases. Use of the first day of the last menstrual period (LMP) can be notoriously misleading. In the absence of convincing historical information (in vitro fertilization, artificial insemination, ovulation induction, etc.) or an early ultrasound examination estimating gestational age, it may not be possible to estimate gestational age with any degree of certainty. Without an estimated gestational age to use as a standard to evaluate fetal size, one cannot determine if a particular fetus is small for gestational age, and analysis for potential IUGR is limited to evaluation of indirect measures such as ratios of body proportions or interval growth (discussed below).

The approach we use to estimate gestational age and evaluate fetal size requires measurement of four fetal biometric parameters: the biparietal diameter (BPD), head circumference (HC), femur length (FL), and abdominal circumference (AC). Combinations of these parameters are used to estimate gestational age and evaluate fetal size. The crown-rump length is utilized for sonographic estimates of gestational age during the first trimester. During the second trimester, prior to 20 weeks, the estimated gestational ages (EGAs) corresponding to the BPD and FL are averaged to give a best EGA. After 20 weeks, we average together the EGAs that correspond to the HC and FL (see Table 132–4). Perhaps even more important than the selection of parameters used to estimate gestational age is the concept that *once an estimated gestational age is established, it should almost always be used as the standard in subsequent studies of the fetus.* Unless an error is discovered in the original measurement or calculation process, redefining the EGA using subsequent sonograms introduces more error in setting the age, and dilutes the real value of subsequent studies, which is to see if growth deviates from the expected.

Evaluation of Fetal Size

Once an estimated gestational age has been assigned, the next step is to determine if fetal size is appropriate for age. Multiple individual parameters or combinations of parameters can be analyzed to determine if fetal size is appropriate. Our preference is to evaluate the estimated fetal weight and the abdominal circumference (AC). The AC is thought to be the most sensitive single parameter available to estimate fetal size. To maximize its accuracy, one must perform this measurement in a consistent reproducible manner, using a cross-section of the fetal abdomen at the level of the liver. The AC image should demonstrate a rounded configuration to the fetal abdomen, containing a crescentic tubular structure corresponding to the confluence of the right and left portal veins (Fig. 133–3*A*). Scans that reveal an ovoid contour to the abdomen or demonstrate a long straight segment of portal vein extending into the abdomen from the anterior abdominal wall are likely to represent oblique sections that overestimate abdominal size (Fig. 133–3*B*). The exceptions are when oligohydramnios or other conditions that distort abdominal shape are present.

The measured abdominal circumference is compared with the expected AC for a given gestational age in order to determine the percentile level or number of standard deviations from the mean. This gives an indication of how the measured AC deviates from the AC expected for the gestational age assigned to the fetus. Conversion to a standard deviation or percentile can be done by referring to a table or via computer program (Table 133–1). In doing so, it is important to recognize that some published reference tables are expressed in terms of standard deviations from the mean and others give percentiles, but the two are not equivalent (Table 133–2).

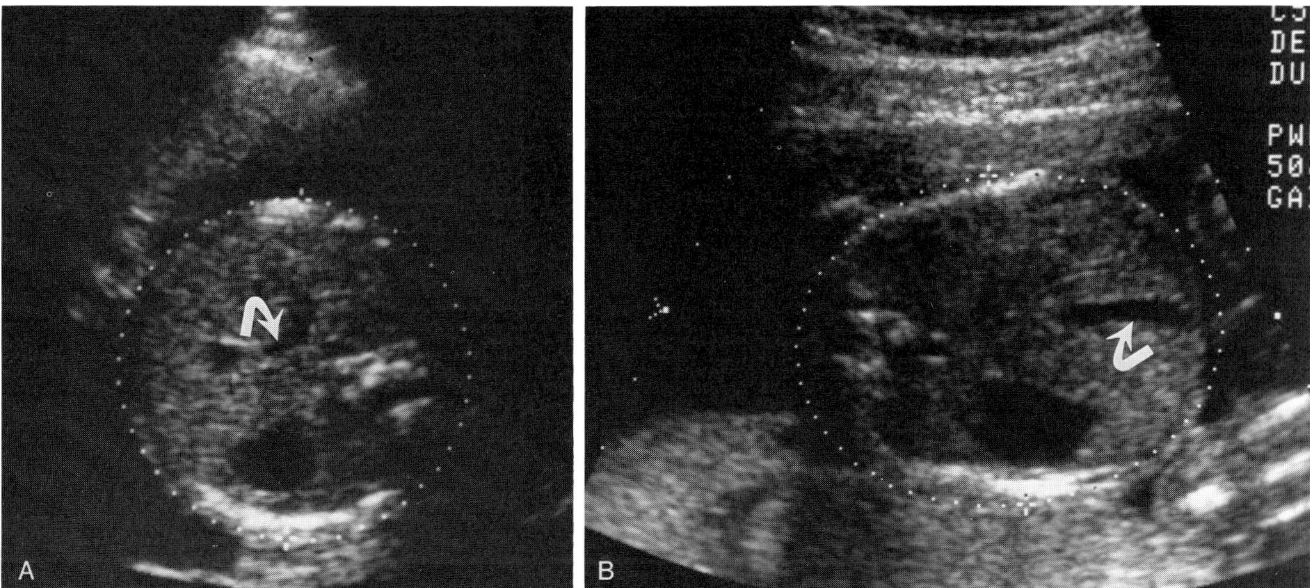

Figure 133–3. *A,* **Correct scan plane for abdominal circumference measurements.** The confluence of the right and left portal veins *(arrow)* is seen as a crescentic tubular structure. Also note round shape of abdomen. *B,* **Incorrect scan plane for abdominal circumference measurement.** In this image of the fetal abdomen, the shape of the abdomen is ovoid (compare with round configuration in *A*), and a long, straight segment of portal vein *(arrow)* is seen extending into the abdomen from the anterior abdominal wall. This is an oblique scan plane that tends to overestimate the abdominal circumference.

TABLE 133–1. ABDOMINAL CIRCUMFERENCE (AC) COMPARED WITH GESTATIONAL AGE—NUMBER OF STANDARD DEVIATIONS FROM THE MEAN

Abdominal Circumference (mm)	Estimated Gestational Age (Weeks)																			
	22	**23**	**24**	**25**	**26**	**27**	**28**	**29**	**30**	**31**	**32**	**33**	**34**	**35**	**36**	**37**	**38**	**39**	**40**	**41**
175	0.00	−0.89	−1.64	−2.33	−2.97	−3.52	−4.06	−4.57	−5.14	−5.67	−6.53	−7.12	−7.54	−7.89	−8.05	−8.53	−9.19	−9.42	−10.28	−11.24
178	0.24	−0.67	−1.43	−2.13	−2.77	−3.33	−3.88	−4.40	−4.97	−5.50	−6.35	−6.94	−7.37	−7.72	−7.89	−8.37	−9.03	−9.26	−10.11	−11.06
180	0.40	−0.52	−1.29	−2.00	−2.65	−3.21	−3.76	−4.29	−4.86	−5.39	−6.24	−6.82	−7.26	−7.61	−7.79	−8.26	−8.92	−9.16	−10.00	−10.94
182	0.56	−0.37	−1.14	−1.87	−2.52	−3.09	−3.65	−4.17	−4.74	−5.28	−6.12	−6.71	−7.14	−7.50	−7.68	−8.16	−8.81	−9.05	−9.89	−10.82
184	0.72	−0.22	−1.00	−1.73	−2.39	−2.97	−3.53	−4.06	−4.63	−5.17	−6.00	−6.59	−7.03	−7.39	−7.58	−8.05	−8.70	−8.95	−9.78	−10.71
186	0.88	−0.07	−0.86	−1.60	−2.26	−2.85	−3.41	−3.94	−4.51	−5.06	−5.88	−6.47	−6.91	−7.28	−7.47	−7.95	−8.59	−8.84	−9.67	−10.59
188	1.04	0.07	−0.71	−1.47	−2.13	−2.73	−3.29	−3.83	−4.40	−4.94	−5.76	−6.35	−6.80	−7.17	−7.37	−7.84	−8.49	−8.74	−9.56	−10.47
190	1.20	0.22	−0.57	−1.33	−2.00	−2.61	−3.18	−3.71	−4.29	−4.83	−5.65	−6.24	−6.69	−7.06	−7.26	−7.74	−8.38	−8.63	−9.44	−10.35
192	1.36	0.37	−0.43	−1.20	−1.87	−2.48	−3.06	−3.60	−4.17	−4.72	−5.53	−6.12	−6.57	−6.94	−7.16	−7.63	−8.27	−8.53	−9.33	−10.24
194	1.52	0.52	−0.29	−1.07	−1.74	−2.36	−2.94	−3.49	−4.06	−4.61	−5.41	−6.00	−6.46	−6.83	−7.05	−7.53	−8.16	−8.42	−9.22	−10.12
196	1.68	0.67	−0.14	−0.93	−1.61	−2.24	−2.82	−3.37	−3.94	−4.50	−5.29	−5.88	−6.34	−6.72	−6.95	−7.42	−8.05	−8.32	−9.11	−10.00
198	1.84	0.81	0.00	−0.80	−1.48	−2.12	−2.71	−3.26	−3.83	−4.39	−5.18	−5.76	−6.23	−6.61	−6.84	−7.32	−7.95	−8.21	−9.00	−9.88
200	2.00	0.96	0.15	−0.67	−1.35	−2.00	−2.59	−3.14	−3.71	−4.28	−5.06	−5.65	−6.11	−6.50	−6.74	−7.21	−7.84	−8.11	−8.89	−9.76
202	2.16	1.11	0.30	−0.53	−1.23	−1.88	−2.47	−3.03	−3.60	−4.17	−4.94	−5.53	−6.00	−6.39	−6.63	−7.11	−7.73	−8.00	−8.78	−9.65
204	2.32	1.26	0.44	−0.40	−1.10	−1.76	−2.35	−2.91	−3.49	−4.06	−4.82	−5.41	−5.89	−6.28	−6.53	−7.00	−7.62	−7.89	−8.67	−9.53
206	2.48	1.41	0.59	−0.27	−0.97	−1.64	−2.24	−2.80	−3.37	−3.94	−4.71	−5.29	−5.77	−6.17	−6.42	−6.89	−7.51	−7.79	−8.56	−9.41
208	2.64	1.56	0.74	−0.13	−0.84	−1.52	−2.12	−2.69	−3.26	−3.83	−4.59	−5.18	−5.66	−6.06	−6.32	−6.79	−7.41	−7.68	−8.44	−9.29
210	2.80	1.70	0.89	0.00	−0.71	−1.39	−2.00	−2.57	−3.14	−3.72	−4.47	−5.06	−5.54	−5.94	−6.21	−6.68	−7.30	−7.58	−8.33	−9.18
212	2.96	1.85	1.04	0.13	−0.58	−1.27	−1.88	−2.46	−3.03	−3.61	−4.35	−4.94	−5.43	−5.83	−6.11	−6.58	−7.19	−7.47	−8.22	−9.06
214	3.12	2.00	1.19	0.27	−0.45	−1.15	−1.76	−2.34	−2.91	−3.50	−4.24	−4.82	−5.31	−5.72	−6.00	−6.47	−7.08	−7.37	−8.11	−8.94
216	3.28	2.15	1.33	0.40	−0.32	−1.03	−1.65	−2.23	−2.80	−3.39	−4.12	−4.71	−5.20	−5.61	−5.89	−6.37	−6.97	−7.26	−8.00	−8.82
218	3.44	2.30	1.48	0.53	−0.19	−0.91	−1.53	−2.11	−2.69	−3.28	−4.00	−4.59	−5.09	−5.50	−5.79	−6.26	−6.86	−7.16	−7.89	−8.71
220	3.60	2.44	1.63	0.67	−0.06	−0.79	−1.41	−2.00	−2.57	−3.17	−3.88	−4.47	−4.97	−5.39	−5.68	−6.16	−6.76	−7.05	−7.78	−8.59
222	3.76	2.59	1.78	0.80	0.07	−0.67	−1.29	−1.89	−2.46	−3.06	−3.76	−4.35	−4.86	−5.28	−5.58	−6.05	−6.65	−6.95	−7.67	−8.47
224	3.92	2.74	1.93	0.93	0.20	−0.55	−1.18	−1.77	−2.34	−2.94	−3.65	−4.24	−4.74	−5.17	−5.47	−5.95	−6.54	−6.84	−7.56	−8.35
226	4.08	2.89	2.07	1.07	0.33	−0.42	−1.06	−1.66	−2.23	−2.83	−3.53	−4.12	−4.63	−5.06	−5.37	−5.84	−6.43	−6.74	−7.44	−8.24
228	4.24	3.01	2.22	1.20	0.47	−0.30	−0.94	−1.54	−2.11	−2.72	−3.41	−4.00	−4.51	−4.94	−5.26	−5.74	−6.32	−6.63	−7.33	−8.12
230	4.40	3.19	2.37	1.33	0.60	−0.18	−0.82	−1.43	−2.00	−2.61	−3.29	−3.88	−4.40	−4.83	−5.16	−5.63	−6.22	−6.53	−7.22	−8.00
232	4.56	3.33	2.52	1.47	0.73	−0.06	−0.71	−1.31	−1.89	−2.50	−3.18	−3.76	−4.29	−4.72	−5.05	−5.53	−6.11	−6.42	−7.11	−7.88
234	4.72	3.48	2.67	1.60	0.87	0.07	−0.59	−1.20	−1.77	−2.39	−3.06	−3.65	−4.17	−4.61	−4.95	−5.42	−6.00	−6.32	−7.00	−7.76
236	4.88	3.63	2.81	1.73	1.00	0.20	−0.47	−1.09	−1.66	−2.28	−2.94	−3.53	−4.06	−4.50	−4.84	−5.32	−5.89	−6.21	−6.89	−7.65
238	5.04	3.78	2.96	1.87	1.13	0.33	−0.35	−0.97	−1.54	−2.17	−2.82	−3.41	−3.94	−4.39	−4.74	−5.21	−5.78	−6.11	−6.78	−7.53
240	5.20	3.93	3.11	2.00	1.27	0.47	−0.24	−0.86	−1.43	−2.06	−2.71	−3.29	−3.83	−4.28	−4.63	−5.11	−5.68	−6.00	−6.67	−7.41
242	5.36	4.07	3.26	2.13	1.40	0.60	−0.12	−0.74	−1.31	−1.94	−2.59	−3.18	−3.71	−4.17	−4.53	−5.00	−5.57	−5.89	−6.56	−7.29
244	5.52	4.22	3.41	2.27	1.53	0.73	0.00	−0.63	−1.20	−1.83	−2.47	−3.06	−3.60	−4.06	−4.42	−4.89	−5.46	−5.79	−6.44	−7.18
246	5.68	4.37	3.56	2.40	1.67	0.87	0.13	−0.51	−1.09	−1.72	−2.35	−2.94	−3.49	−3.94	−4.32	−4.79	−5.35	−5.68	−6.33	−7.06
248	5.84	4.52	3.70	2.53	1.80	1.00	0.25	−0.40	−0.97	−1.61	−2.24	−2.82	−3.37	−3.83	−4.21	−4.68	−5.24	−5.58	−6.22	−6.94
250	6.00	4.67	3.85	2.67	1.93	1.13	0.38	−0.29	−0.86	−1.50	−2.12	−2.71	−3.26	−3.72	−4.11	−4.58	−5.14	−5.47	−6.11	−6.82
252	6.16	4.81	4.00	2.80	2.07	1.27	0.50	−0.17	−0.74	−1.39	−2.00	−2.59	−3.14	−3.61	−4.00	−4.47	−5.03	−5.37	−6.00	−6.71
254	6.32	4.96	4.15	2.93	2.20	1.40	0.63	−0.06	−0.63	−1.28	−1.88	−2.47	−3.03	−3.50	−3.89	−4.37	−4.92	−5.26	−5.89	−6.59
256	6.48	5.11	4.30	3.07	2.33	1.53	0.75	0.06	−0.51	−1.17	−1.76	−2.35	−2.91	−3.39	−3.79	−4.26	−4.81	−5.16	−5.78	−6.47
258	6.64	5.26	4.44	3.20	2.47	1.67	0.88	0.18	−0.40	−1.06	−1.65	−2.24	−2.80	−3.28	−3.68	−4.16	−4.70	−5.05	−5.67	−6.35
260	6.80	5.41	4.59	3.33	2.60	1.80	1.00	0.30	−0.29	−0.94	−1.53	−2.12	−2.69	−3.17	−3.58	−4.05	−4.59	−4.95	−5.56	−6.24
262	6.96	5.56	4.74	3.47	2.73	1.93	1.13	0.42	−0.17	−0.83	−1.41	−2.00	−2.57	−3.06	−3.47	−3.95	−4.49	−4.84	−5.44	−6.12
264	7.12	5.70	4.89	3.60	2.87	2.07	1.25	0.55	−0.06	−0.72	−1.29	−1.88	−2.46	−2.94	−3.37	−3.84	−4.38	−4.74	−5.33	−6.00
266	7.28	5.85	5.04	3.73	3.00	2.20	1.38	0.67	0.06	−0.61	−1.18	−1.76	−2.34	−2.83	−3.26	−3.74	−4.27	−4.63	−5.22	−5.88
268	7.44	6.00	5.19	3.87	3.13	2.33	1.50	0.79	0.17	−0.50	−1.06	−1.65	−2.23	−2.72	−3.16	−3.63	−4.16	−4.53	−5.11	−5.76
270	7.60	6.15	5.33	4.00	3.27	2.47	1.63	0.91	0.29	−0.39	−0.94	−1.53	−2.11	−2.61	−3.05	−3.53	−4.05	−4.42	−5.00	−5.65
272	7.76	6.30	5.48	4.13	3.40	2.60	1.75	1.03	0.40	−0.28	−0.82	−1.41	−2.00	−2.50	−2.95	−3.42	−3.95	−4.32	−4.89	−5.53
274	7.92	6.44	5.63	4.27	3.53	2.73	1.88	1.15	0.51	−0.17	−0.71	−1.29	−1.89	−2.39	−2.84	−3.32	−3.84	−4.21	−4.78	−5.41
276	8.08	6.59	5.78	4.40	3.67	2.87	2.00	1.27	0.63	−0.06	−0.59	−1.18	−1.77	−2.38	−2.74	−3.21	−3.73	−4.11	−4.67	−5.29
278	8.24	6.74	5.93	4.53	3.80	3.00	2.13	1.39	0.74	0.04	−0.47	−1.06	−1.66	−2.17	−2.63	−3.11	−3.62	−4.00	−4.56	−5.18
280	8.40	6.89	6.07	4.67	3.93	3.13	2.25	1.52	0.86	0.13	−0.35	−0.91	−1.54	−2.06	−2.53	−3.00	−3.51	−3.89	−4.44	−5.06
282	8.56	7.04	6.22	4.80	4.07	3.27	2.38	1.64	0.97	0.22	−0.24	−0.82	−1.43	−1.94	−2.42	−2.89	−3.41	−3.79	−4.33	−4.94
284	8.72	7.19	6.37	4.93	4.20	3.40	2.50	1.76	1.09	0.31	−0.12	−0.71	−1.31	−1.83	−2.32	−2.79	−3.30	−3.68	−4.22	−4.82
286	8.88	7.33	6.52	5.07	4.33	3.53	2.63	1.88	1.20	0.40	0.00	−0.59	−1.20	−1.72	−2.21	−2.68	−3.19	−3.58	−4.11	−4.71
288	9.04	7.48	6.67	5.20	4.47	3.67	2.75	2.00	1.31	0.49	0.11	−0.47	−1.09	−1.61	−2.11	−2.58	−3.08	−3.47	−4.00	−4.59
290	9.20	7.63	6.81	5.33	4.60	3.80	2.88	2.12	1.43	0.58	0.21	−0.35	−0.97	−1.50	−2.00	−2.47	−2.97	−3.37	−3.89	−4.47
292	9.36	7.78	6.96	5.47	4.73	3.93	3.00	2.24	1.54	0.67	0.32	−0.24	−0.86	−1.39	−1.89	−2.37	−2.86	−3.26	−3.78	−4.35
294	9.52	7.93	7.11	5.60	4.87	4.07	3.13	2.36	1.66	0.76	0.42	−0.12	−0.74	−1.28	−1.79	−2.26	−2.76	−3.16	−3.67	−4.24
296	9.68	8.07	7.26	5.73	5.00	4.20	3.25	2.48	1.77	0.84	0.53	0.00	−0.63	−1.17	−1.68	−2.16	−2.65	−3.05	−3.56	−4.12
298	9.84	8.22	7.41	5.87	5.13	4.33	3.38	2.61	1.89	0.91	0.63	0.10	−0.51	−1.06	−1.58	−2.05	−2.54	−2.95	−3.44	−4.00
300	10.00	8.37	7.56	6.00	5.27	4.47	3.50	2.73	2.00	1.02	0.74	0.21	−0.40	−0.94	−1.47	−1.95	−2.43	−2.84	−3.33	−3.88
302	10.16	8.52	7.70	6.13	5.40	4.60	3.63	2.85	2.11	1.11	0.84	0.31	−0.29	−0.83	−1.37	−1.84	−2.32	−2.74	−3.22	−3.76
304	10.32	8.67	7.85	6.27	5.53	4.73	3.75	2.97	2.23	1.20	0.95	0.41	−0.17	−0.72	−1.26	−1.74	−2.22	−2.63	−3.11	−3.65
306	10.48	8.81	8.00	6.40	5.67	4.87	3.88	3.09	2.34	1.29	1.05	0.51	−0.06	−0.61	−1.16	−1.63	−2.11	−2.53	−3.00	−3.53
308	10.64	8.96	8.15	6.53	5.80	5.00	4.00	3.21	2.46	1.38	1.16	0.62	0.05	−0.50	−1.05	−1.53	−2.00	−2.42	−2.89	−3.41
310	10.80	9.11	8.30	6.67	5.93	5.13	4.13	3.33	2.57	1.47	1.26	0.72	0.15	−0.39	−0.95	−1.42	−1.89	−2.32	−2.78	−3.29
312	10.96	9.26	8.44	6.80	6.07	5.27	4.25	3.45	2.69	1.56	1.37	0.82	0.26	−0.28	−0.84	−1.32	−1.78	−2.21	−2.67	−3.18
314	11.12	9.41	8.59	6.93	6.20	5.40	4.38	3.58	2.80	1.64	1.47	0.92	0.36	−0.17	−0.74	−1.21	−1.68	−2.11	−2.56	−3.06
316	11.28	9.56	8.74	7.07	6.33	5.53	4.50	3.70	2.91	1.73	1.58	1.03	0.46	−0.06	−0.63	−1.11	−1.57	−2.00	−2.44	−2.94
318	11.44	9.70	8.89	7.20	6.47	5.67	4.63	3.82	3.03	1.82	1.68	1.13	0.56	0.05	−0.53	−1.00	−1.46	−1.89	−2.33	−2.82
320	11.60	9.85	9.04	7.33	6.60	5.80	4.75	3.94	3.14	1.91	1.79	1.23	0.67	0.15	−0.42	−0.89	−1.35	−1.79	−2.22	−2.71
322	11.76	10.00	9.19	7.47	6.73	5.93	4.88	4.06	3.26	2.00	1.89	1.33	0.77	0.26	−0.32	−0.79	−1.24	−1.68	−2.11	−2.59
324	11.92	10.15	9.33	7.60	6.87	6.07	5.00	4.18	3.37	2.09	2.00	1.44	0.87	0.36	−0.21	−0.68	−1.14	−1.58	−2.00	−2.47
326	12.08	10.30	9.48	7.73	7.00	6.20	5.13	4.30	3.49	2.18	2.11	1.54	0.97	0.46	−0.11	−0.58	−1.03	−1.47	−1.89	−2.35

TABLE 133–1. ABDOMINAL CIRCUMFERENCE (AC) COMPARED WITH GESTATIONAL AGE—NUMBER OF STANDARD DEVIATIONS FROM THE MEAN *Continued*

Abdominal Circumference (mm)	Estimated Gestational Age (Weeks)																			
	22	**23**	**24**	**25**	**26**	**27**	**28**	**29**	**30**	**31**	**32**	**33**	**34**	**35**	**36**	**37**	**38**	**39**	**40**	**41**
328	12.24	10.44	9.63	7.87	7.13	6.33	5.25	4.42	3.60	2.27	2.21	1.64	1.08	0.56	0.00	−0.47	−0.92	−1.37	−1.78	−2.24
330	12.40	10.59	9.78	8.00	7.27	6.47	5.38	4.55	3.71	2.36	2.32	1.74	1.18	0.67	0.11	−0.37	−0.81	−1.26	−1.67	−2.12
332	12.56	10.74	9.93	8.13	7.40	6.60	5.50	4.67	3.83	2.44	2.42	1.85	1.28	0.77	0.22	−0.26	−0.70	−1.16	−1.56	−2.00
334	12.72	10.89	10.07	8.27	7.53	6.73	5.63	4.79	3.94	2.53	2.53	1.95	1.38	0.87	0.32	−0.16	−0.59	−1.05	−1.44	−1.88
336	12.88	11.04	10.22	8.40	7.67	6.87	5.75	4.91	4.06	2.62	2.63	2.05	1.49	0.97	0.43	−0.05	−0.49	−0.95	−1.33	−1.76
338	13.04	11.19	10.37	8.53	7.80	7.00	5.88	5.03	4.17	2.71	2.74	2.15	1.59	1.08	0.54	0.06	−0.38	−0.84	−1.22	−1.65
340	13.20	11.33	10.52	8.67	7.93	7.13	6.00	5.15	4.29	2.80	2.84	2.26	1.69	1.18	0.65	0.17	−0.27	−0.74	−1.11	−1.53
342	13.36	11.48	10.67	8.80	8.07	7.27	6.13	5.27	4.40	2.89	2.95	2.36	1.79	1.28	0.76	0.28	−0.16	−0.63	−1.00	−1.41
344	13.52	11.63	10.81	8.93	8.20	7.40	6.25	5.39	4.51	2.98	3.05	2.46	1.90	1.38	0.86	0.39	−0.05	−0.53	−0.89	−1.29
346	13.68	11.78	10.96	9.07	8.33	7.53	6.38	5.52	4.63	3.07	3.16	2.56	2.00	1.49	0.97	0.50	0.06	−0.42	−0.78	−1.18
348	13.84	11.93	11.11	9.20	8.47	7.67	6.50	5.64	4.74	3.16	3.26	2.67	2.10	1.59	1.08	0.61	0.18	−0.32	−0.67	−1.06
350	14.00	12.07	11.26	9.33	8.60	7.80	6.63	5.76	4.86	3.24	3.37	2.77	2.21	1.69	1.19	0.72	0.29	−0.21	−0.56	−0.94
352	14.16	12.22	11.41	9.47	8.73	7.93	6.75	5.88	4.97	3.33	3.47	2.87	2.31	1.79	1.30	0.83	0.41	−0.11	−0.44	−0.82
354	14.32	12.37	11.56	9.60	8.87	8.07	6.88	6.00	5.09	3.42	3.58	2.97	2.41	1.90	1.41	0.94	0.53	0.00	−0.33	−0.71
356	14.48	12.52	11.70	9.73	9.00	8.20	7.00	6.12	5.20	3.51	3.68	3.08	2.51	2.00	1.51	1.06	0.65	0.13	−0.22	−0.59
358	14.64	12.67	11.85	9.87	9.13	8.33	7.13	6.24	5.31	3.60	3.79	3.18	2.62	2.10	1.62	1.17	0.76	0.27	−0.11	−0.47
360	14.80	12.81	12.00	10.00	9.27	8.47	7.25	6.36	5.43	3.69	3.89	3.28	2.72	2.21	1.73	1.28	0.88	0.40	0.00	−0.35
362	14.96	12.96	12.15	10.13	9.40	8.60	7.38	6.48	5.54	3.78	4.00	3.38	2.82	2.31	1.84	1.39	1.00	0.53	0.14	−0.24
364	15.12	13.11	12.30	10.27	9.53	8.73	7.50	6.61	5.66	3.87	4.11	3.49	2.92	2.41	1.95	1.50	1.12	0.67	0.29	−0.12
366	15.28	13.26	12.44	10.40	9.67	8.87	7.63	6.73	5.77	3.96	4.21	3.59	3.03	2.51	2.05	1.61	1.24	0.80	0.43	0.00
368	15.44	13.41	12.59	10.53	9.80	9.00	7.75	6.85	5.89	4.01	4.32	3.69	3.13	2.62	2.16	1.72	1.35	0.93	0.57	0.13
370	15.60	13.56	12.74	10.67	9.93	9.13	7.88	6.97	6.00	4.13	4.42	3.79	3.23	2.72	2.27	1.83	1.47	1.07	0.71	0.31
372	15.76	13.70	12.89	10.80	10.07	9.27	8.00	7.09	6.11	4.22	4.53	3.90	3.33	2.82	2.38	1.94	1.59	1.20	0.86	0.46
374	15.92	13.85	13.04	10.93	10.20	9.40	8.13	7.21	6.23	4.31	4.63	4.00	3.44	2.92	2.49	2.06	1.71	1.33	1.00	0.62
376	16.08	14.00	13.19	11.07	10.33	9.53	8.25	7.33	6.34	4.40	4.74	4.10	3.54	3.03	2.59	2.17	1.82	1.47	1.14	0.77
378	16.24	14.15	13.33	11.20	10.47	9.67	8.38	7.45	6.46	4.49	4.84	4.21	3.64	3.13	2.70	2.28	1.94	1.60	1.29	0.92
380	16.40	14.30	13.48	11.33	10.60	9.80	8.50	7.58	6.57	4.58	4.95	4.31	3.74	3.23	2.81	2.39	2.06	1.73	1.43	1.08
382	16.56	14.44	13.63	11.47	10.73	9.93	8.63	7.70	6.69	4.67	5.05	4.41	3.85	3.33	2.92	2.50	2.18	1.87	1.57	1.23
384	16.72	14.59	13.78	11.60	10.87	10.07	8.75	7.82	6.80	4.76	5.16	4.51	3.95	3.44	3.03	2.61	2.29	2.00	1.71	1.38
386	16.88	14.74	13.93	11.73	11.00	10.20	8.88	7.94	6.91	4.84	5.26	4.62	4.05	3.54	3.14	2.72	2.41	2.13	1.86	1.54
388	17.04	14.89	14.07	11.87	11.13	10.33	9.00	8.06	7.03	4.93	5.37	4.72	4.15	3.64	3.24	2.83	2.53	2.27	2.00	1.69
390	17.20	15.04	14.22	12.00	11.27	10.47	9.13	8.18	7.14	5.02	5.47	4.82	4.26	3.74	3.35	2.94	2.65	2.40	2.14	1.85

This table was generated with a computer program. To use the table, choose the column containing the measured AC (in mm) from the shaded area on the left, and the column containing the estimated gestational age (in menstrual weeks) from the top shaded area. The value at the intersection of these two columns is the number of standard deviations the measured AC is above or below (−) the mean AC for gestational age.

Table courtesy of Louis Humphrey and James D. Bowie, MD, Duke University Medical Center. Reprinted with permission from 1991 Special Course Syllabus in Ultrasound, Intrauterine Growth Retardation, RSNA Publications.

A multitude of different thresholds have been used to identify the SGA fetus. This variation exists because as the cut-off level is increased, the sensitivity for detecting IUGR increases, but the specificity and predictive value of a positive test decrease. Our approach is to use the 10th percentile (−1.28 SD) as the threshold level for interpreting the AC. If the AC falls below this cut-off, the fetus is considered SGA and is said to be at risk for IUGR.

A second way to identify the SGA fetus is to compute an estimated fetal weight and compare it with the expected weight for the assigned gestational age. The concept of using fetal weight to evaluate fetal size is intuitively appealing because the definition of the SGA fetus is based on weight; thus it follows that estimated weight is the parameter most closely related to the definition. Unfortunately, the in utero estimation of fetal weight is far from perfect.

TABLE 133–2. CONVERTING BETWEEEN PERCENTILES AND STANDARD DEVIATIONS

Percentiles	Standard Deviations
25th	(−) 0.68
20th	(−) 0.84
15th	(−) 1.04
10th	(−) 1.28
5th	(−) 1.64
2.28th	(−) 2.00

Courtesy of James D. Bowie, MD, Duke University Medical Center. Reprinted with permission from 1991 Special Course Syllabus in Ultrasound, Intrauterine Growth Retardation, RSNA Publications.

There is no consensus on the ideal formula for estimating weight, and the accuracy of currently available formulas is marred by inaccuracies in obtaining fetal body measurements, variability in fetal densities and relative body proportions from fetus to fetus, as well as by the possibility of weight alterations occurring during the transition from intrauterine to extrauterine life. The Shepard formula is commonly used to calculate an estimated fetal weight (EFW). This formula utilizes a combination of two parameters, the BPD and AC, and has been summarized in a convenient to use tabular form (Table 133–3). Using the Shepard formula, if the estimated fetal weight is below the 5th percentile for gestational age (Table 133–4), it is abnormal and the fetus is considered to be at greater risk for IUGR than the at-risk fetus with an abnormal AC but an EFW above the 5th percentile.

The Shepard formula considers only head and abdomen size in calculating fetal weight. Although there is evidence to suggest that inclusion of the femur length, a predictor of fetal height, in weight formulas may improve the accuracy of weight determinations, this has not been consistently confirmed. Weight formulas that utilize three or more parameters tend to be complex, and do not lend themselves to the tabular format shown in Table 133–3. They can, however, be incorporated into clinical practice through use of a computer program.

To summarize this approach to evaluating the question of IUGR in the fetus with sufficient data to assign a gestational age, the first step is to estimate gestational age. Having done that, the measured AC is compared with the expected AC for the assigned estimated gestational age. If it is below a predetermined threshold level (the 10th percentile), the fetus is considered to be "at risk for IUGR." If, in addition, the estimated fetal weight is below the 5th percentile

TABLE 133–3. ESTIMATED FETAL WEIGHTS IN "ESTIMATED GRAMS," DERIVED FROM THE SHEPARD FORMULA

Biparietal Diameter (mm)	Abdominal Perimeter (mm)																							
	40	**45**	**50**	**55**	**60**	**65**	**70**	**75**	**80**	**85**	**90**	**95**	**100**	**105**	**110**	**115**	**120**	**125**	**130**	**135**	**140**	**145**	**150**		
30	80	83	87	91	95	99	104	108	113	118	123	129	135	141	147	154	161								
31	83	86	90	94	98	103	107	112	117	122	128	133	139	145	152	159	166	173	181						
32			93	97	102	105	111	116	121	128	132	138	144	150	157	164	171	178	186						
33			97	101	105	110	115	120	125	130	136	142	148	155	162	169	176	184	192						
34			100	104	109	114	119	124	129	135	141	147	153	160	167	174	182	190	198	206	215				
35					113	118	123	128	134	139	145	152	158	165	172	180	187	195	204	213	222				
36					117	122	127	132	138	144	150	157	163	170	178	185	193	202	210	219	229				
37					121	126	131	137	143	149	155	162	169	176	183	191	199	208	217	226	235	245	256		
38							136	142	148	154	160	167	174	182	189	197	206	214	223	233	243	253	263		
39							141	146	153	159	166	173	180	187	195	203	212	221	230	240	250	260	271		
	70	**75**	**80**	**85**	**90**	**95**	**100**	**105**	**110**	**115**	**120**	**125**	**130**	**135**	**140**	**145**	**150**	**155**	**160**	**165**	**170**	**175**	**180**		
40	145	152	158	164	171	178	186	193	202	210	219	228	237	247	257	268	279								
41			163	170	177	184	192	200	208	217	226	235	245	255	265	276	288	299	312						
42			169	176	183	190	198	205	215	223	233	242	252	262	273	264	296	308	321						
43			174	182	189	197	205	213	222	231	240	250	260	270	281	293	305	317	330						
44			180	188	195	203	211	220	229	238	247	257	268	279	290	302	314	326	340	353	368				
45					202	210	218	227	236	245	255	265	276	287	299	311	323	336	349	363	378				
46					208	217	225	234	244	253	263	274	285	296	308	320	333	346	359	374	389				
47					215	224	233	242	251	261	271	282	293	305	317	329	342	356	370	384	400	415	432		
48							240	250	259	269	280	291	302	314	326	339	352	366	381	395	411	427	444		
49							248	258	268	278	289	300	312	324	336	349	363	377	392	407	422	439	456		
	100	**105**	**110**	**115**	**120**	**125**	**130**	**135**	**140**	**145**	**150**	**155**	**160**	**165**	**170**	**175**	**180**	**185**	**190**	**195**	**200**	**205**	**210**	**215**	**220**
50	256	256	276	287	298	309	321	334	346	360	374	388	403	418	434	451	468	486	505						
51			285	296	307	319	331	344	357	370	385	399	414	430	447	464	481	500	519						
52			294	305	317	329	341	354	368	381	396	411	426	443	459	477	495	513	533						
53			304	315	327	339	352	365	379	393	408	423	439	455	472	490	508	527	547	568	589				
54					337	350	363	376	390	405	420	435	451	468	486	504	522	542	562	583	605				
55					348	360	374	388	402	417	432	448	464	482	499	518	537	557	577	598	620				
56					359	372	385	399	414	429	445	461	478	495	513	532	552	572	593	614	637	660	684		
57							397	412	426	442	458	474	492	509	528	547	567	587	609	631	654	677	702		
58							409	424	439	455	471	488	506	524	543	562	583	604	625	648	671	695	720		
59									453	469	485	503	520	539	558	578	599	620	642	665	689	713	739	765	792

	140	145	150	155	160	165	170	175	180	185	190	195	200	205	210	215	220	225	230	235	240	245	250		
60	466	483	500	517	536	554	574	594	615	637	659	683	707	732	758	784	812								
61	480	497	514	532	551	570	590	611	632	654	677	701	725	751	777	804	832								
62			530	548	567	587	607	628	650	672	696	720	745	770	797	825	853	883	913						
63			545	564	583	603	624	645	668	691	714	739	764	790	818	846	875	905	936						
64			561	580	600	621	642	664	686	709	734	759	784	811	839	867	897	927	959						
65					617	638	660	682	705	729	753	779	805	832	860	889	919	950	982	1,015	1,050				
66					635	657	678	701	725	749	774	800	826	854	882	912	942	974	1,006	1,040	1,075				
67					654	675	698	721	745	769	795	821	848	876	905	935	966	998	1,031	1,065	1,100	1,137	1,174		
68							717	741	765	790	816	843	870	899	928	959	990	1,023	1,056	1,091	1,127	1,164	1,202		
69							738	762	786	812	838	865	893	922	952	983	1,015	1,048	1,082	1,117	1,154	1,191	1,230		
	170	**175**	**180**	**185**	**190**	**195**	**200**	**205**	**210**	**215**	**220**	**225**	**230**	**235**	**240**	**245**	**250**	**255**	**260**	**265**	**270**	**275**	**280**	**285**	**290**
70	758	783	806	834	861	888	917	946	977	1,008	1,041	1,074	1,109	1,144	1,181	1,219	1,258	1,299	1,340						
71			830	857	884	912	941	971	1,002	1,034	1,067	1,101	1,136	1,172	1,209	1,248	1,287	1,328	1,371						
72			853	880	908	936	966	996	1,028	1,060	1,094	1,128	1,164	1,200	1,238	1,277	1,317	1,359	1,402						
73					932	961	991	1,022	1,054	1,087	1,121	1,156	1,192	1,229	1,268	1,307	1,348	1,390	1,433	1,478	1,524				
74					958	987	1,018	1,049	1,081	1,115	1,149	1,185	1,221	1,259	1,298	1,338	1,379	1,422	1,456	1,511	1,558				
75					983	1,013	1,044	1,076	1,109	1,143	1,178	1,214	1,251	1,290	1,329	1,370	1,411	1,455	1,499	1,545	1,592	1,641	1,691		
76							1,072	1,104	1,138	1,172	1,208	1,244	1,282	1,321	1,361	1,402	1,444	1,488	1,533	1,579	1,627	1,676	1,727		
77							1,100	1,133	1,167	1,202	1,238	1,275	1,313	1,353	1,393	1,435	1,478	1,522	1,568	1,615	1,663	1,713	1,764		
78							1,129	1,163	1,197	1,233	1,269	1,307	1,346	1,385	1,426	1,469	1,512	1,557	1,603	1,651	1,700	1,750	1,802	1,855	1,910
79									1,228	1,264	1,301	1,339	1,379	1,419	1,461	1,503	1,547	1,593	1,639	1,688	1,737	1,788	1,840	1,894	1,950
	210	**215**	**220**	**225**	**230**	**235**	**240**	**245**	**250**	**255**	**260**	**265**	**270**	**275**	**280**	**285**	**290**	**295**	**300**	**305**	**310**	**315**	**320**	**325**	**330**
80	1,260	1,296	1,334	1,373	1,412	1,453	1,495	1,539	1,583	1,629	1,677	1,725	1,775	1,827	1,880	1,934	1,990								
81			1,367	1,407	1,447	1,488	1,531	1,575	1,620	1,667	1,715	1,764	1,814	1,866	1,920	1.975	2,032	2,090	2,150						
82			1,402	1,441	1,482	1,524	1,568	1,612	1,658	1,705	1,753	1,803	1,854	1,907	1.961	2,017	2,074	2,133	2,193						
83			1,437	1,477	1,519	1,561	1,605	1,650	1,697	1,744	1,793	1,843	1,895	1,948	2,003	2,059	2,117	2,175	2,237	2,300	2,365				
84					1,556	1,599	1,643	1,689	1,736	1,784	1,834	1,885	1,937	1,991	2,046	2,103	2,161	2,221	2,282	2,346	2,411				
85					1,594	1,638	1,683	1,729	1,776	1,825	1,875	1,927	1,979	2,034	2,090	2,147	2,206	2,265	2,328	2,392	2,458				
86							1,723	1,770	1,818	1,867	1,918	1,970	2,203	2,078	2,134	2,192	2,252	2,313	2,375	2,440	2,506	2,574	2,644		
87							1,764	1,811	1,860	1,910	1,961	2,014	2,068	2,123	2,180	2,238	2,298	2,360	2,423	2,488	2,555	2,623	2,694		
88							1,806	1,854	1,903	1,954	2,005	2,059	2,113	2,169	2,227	2,286	2,346	2,406	2,472	2,538	2,605	2,674	2,745	2,817	2,892
89									1,947	1,998	2,051	2,104	2,160	2,216	2,274	2,334	2,395	2,457	2,522	2,588	2,656	2,725	2,797	2,870	2,945
	250	**255**	**260**	**265**	**270**	**275**	**280**	**285**	**290**	**295**	**300**	**305**	**310**	**315**	**320**	**325**	**330**	**335**	**340**	**345**	**350**	**355**	**360**	**365**	**370**
90	1,993	2,044	2,067	2,151	2,207	2,264	2,323	2,383	2,445	2,508	2,573	2,639	2,707	2,778	2,849	2,923	2,999								
91			2,145	2,199	2,256	2,313	2,372	2,433	2,495	2,559	2,624	2,692	2,760	2,831	2,903	2,977	3,054	3,132	3,212						
92			2,193	2,249	2,305	2,364	2,423	2,484	2,647	2,611	2,677	2,745	2,814	2,885	2,958	3,033	3,109	3,188	3,268						
93			2,243	2,299	2,356	2,415	2,475	2,537	2,600	2,665	2,731	2,799	2,869	2,941	3,014	3,089	3,166	3,245	3,326	3,409	3,494				
94					2,406	2,467	2,526	2,590	2,654	2,719	2,786	2,855	2,925	2,997	3,071	3,147	3,224	3,304	3,385	3,468	3,554				
95					2,461	2,521	2,582	2,645	2,709	2,775	2,842	2,912	2,982	3.055	3,129	3,205	3,283	3,363	3,445	3,526	3,614				
96							2,637	2,701	2,765	2,832	2,900	2,969	3,041	3,114	3,188	3,265	3,343	3,423	3,505	3,590	3,676	3,764	3,854		
97							2,694	2,757	2,823	2,890	2,958	3,028	3,100	3,173	3,248	3,325	3,404	3,485	3,567	3,652	3,738	3,827	3,918		
98									2,881	2,949	3,018	3,088	3,160	3,234	3,310	3,387	3,466	3,547	3,630	3,715	3,802	3,891	3,982	4,075	4,170
99									2,941	3,009	3,078	3,149	3,222	3,296	3,372	3,450	3,530	3,611	3,695	3,780	3,867	3,956	4,047	4,141	4,236
100									3,002	3,071	3,141	3,212	3,285	3,360	3,436	3,514	3,594	3,676	3,760	3,845	3,933	4,022	4,114	4,207	4,303

Reprinted with permission from Jeanty P, Cantraine F, Romero R, et al: A longitudinal study of fetal weight growth. J Ultrasound Med 3:321–328, 1984.

TABLE 133–4. SHEPARD FORMULA—WEIGHT AGAINST GESTATIONAL AGE

Weeks	Percentile		
	5th	50th	95th
9	44	45	46
10	46	48	51
11	50	54	59
12	57	63	71
13	67	77	90
14	81	96	116
15	100	122	151
16	125	155	196
17	155	197	253
18	192	247	322
19	237	307	404
20	288	377	499
21	346	456	607
22	411	545	728
23	484	644	862
24	563	753	1010
25	650	871	1172
26	745	1000	1347
27	847	1139	1536
28	957	1288	1740
29	1074	1448	1958
30	1199	1618	2189
31	1331	1798	2434
32	1468	1984	2688
33	1608	2176	2950
34	1750	2369	3213
35	1888	2557	3469
36	2017	2734	3711
37	2131	2890	3925
38	2221	3016	4100
39	2276	3099	4225
40	2287	3131	4290

Reprinted with permission from Jeanty P, Cantraine F, Romero R, et al: A longitudinal study of fetal weight growth. J Ultrasound Med 3:321–328, 1984.

for gestational age, the likelihood of IUGR is further increased. These steps assume gestational age can be estimated with a reasonable degree of certainty but do not work when gestational age is in doubt.

The Pregnancy with a Poor Estimate of Gestational Age

In pregnancies with poor estimates of gestational age, sonographic evaluation for growth retardation is severely hampered. Evaluation of ratios of body proportions or serial scans measuring interval growth may permit diagnosis of growth aberrations, but the accuracy of ultrasound is limited in these situations. Body proportion ratios were developed in an attempt to establish an age-independent measure of fetal size that could be used in the large number of fetuses in whom it is not possible to reliably estimate gestational age.

The most commonly used age-independent ratio is the FL/AC, although other alternatives include the FL/TC (thigh circumference) and the tibia length/calf circumference ratios. We prefer the FL/AC ratio because the levels for obtaining the abdominal circumference and femur length images are more precisely defined and readily reproducible than the levels for thigh and calf circumference measurements. Another commonly employed ratio is the HC/AC, but this ratio varies with gestational age, and as such requires knowledge of the gestational age for interpretation. Thus, although the HC/AC ratio provides an index of whether growth retardation is symmetrical or asymmetrical, it cannot be used to identify the SGA fetus when gestational age is unknown.

The value for a normal FL/AC remains relatively constant after 21 menstrual weeks, with a mean of 22 ± 2 (2 SD). The 90th percentile of 23.5 is usually used as the upper limits of normal for the FL/AC. An elevated FL/AC indicates that the abdomen is relatively small compared with the femur, a combination that is commonly present in fetuses with asymmetrical IUGR. The most obvious pitfall of this ratio is it cannot detect the symmetrically growth retarded fetus. Additionally, there is much overlap in the FL/AC ratios obtained on growth-retarded and normal fetuses, so there is no cut-off that yields both high sensitivity and high specificity.

Once a fetus with an abnormal FL/AC has been detected, follow-up studies need to focus on specific body parameters rather than on serial FL/AC ratios. Conversion of an abnormal FL/AC to normal is not necessarily a good sign. Although it could potentially indicate improvement in the growth retardation process, another possibility is that growth suppression has become so severe that growth of bone length has been as severely compromised as abdominal growth, i.e., the pattern has converted from one of asymmetrical to symmetrical growth retardation.

Despite the problems inherent in using the FL/AC ratio, there is little else available to assess the appropriateness of fetal size on the basis of a single third-trimester sonogram when a good estimate of gestational age is not available. Another approach is to perform serial ultrasonography at two- to three-week intervals. To allow for technical differences in measurements from one study to another, one should not perform serial measurements more frequently than every two weeks. A progressive fall in the standard deviation or percentile level for the AC, or lack of expected increase in EFW, can be used as indications of an aberration in growth. Unfortunately, the optimal cut-off levels for diagnosing inadequate interval growth of the AC and EFW are not well defined.

ROLE OF DOPPLER ULTRASOUND

Sonographic detection of an SGA fetus signals the need for increased antenatal surveillance. Such surveillance generally consists of serial sonography to evaluate interval growth, and tests of fetal well-being. Tests of well-being are used in an attempt to detect fetal compromise and optimize the timing of delivery. These tests include biophysical profiles, non-stress tests, contraction stress tests, and Doppler interrogation of the maternal-fetal circulation. The remainder of this discussion concentrates on the use of Doppler ultrasound.

Compared with measurements of fetal size, Doppler ultrasound is a more rapidly changing parameter that lends itself to repeated sampling at shorter time intervals. By providing an indication of fetal well-being that is independent of fetal size, a normal result on a Doppler examination can be reassuring in the normal fetus who is SGA owing to low genetic growth potential but is not compromised.

Doppler techniques have been used to interrogate a variety of blood vessels in the maternal-fetal circulation, including the umbilical artery, uterine arteries and their branches, umbilical vein, fetal descending aorta, renal arteries, internal carotid arteries, and middle cerebral arteries. Of these, the umbilical arteries are the vessels that have been the most intensely studied to date and receive the widest clinical use.

The umbilical arteries transport blood from the fetal descending aorta to the placenta. In the placenta they form a rich capillary network that allows for slow, low-resistance flow, with a long time for exchange of nutrients and oxygen. This is reflected in a waveform that exhibits continuous positive flow during diastole (Fig. 133–4). In normal pregnancies the umbilical artery circulation

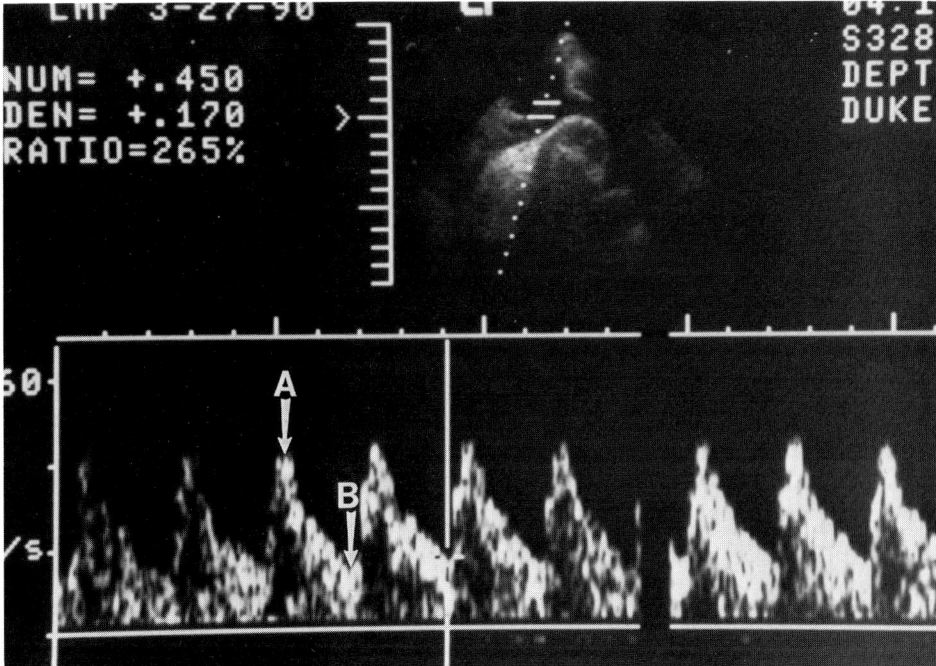

Figure 133–4. Normal Doppler tracing of umbilical artery demonstrates continuous positive blood flow during diastole. The A/B ratio is calculated by dividing peak systole (A) by end-diastole (B).

evolves as gestational age advances, developing progressively lower resistance to flow, manifested by increased diastolic velocities relative to systole.

On the other hand, in some pregnancies affected by such disorders as IUGR or chromosomal abnormalities, resistance to blood flow is abnormally elevated so the diastolic component of the umbilical artery waveform is lower than expected relative to systole (Fig. 133–5). It has been hypothesized that the decrease in placental blood flow which accompanies this circulatory change results in inadequate opportunity for exchange of nutrients and oxygen, limitations on fetal growth, and hypoxia. The waveform alterations seen in such pregnancies correlate with a histologic lesion in the placenta consisting of obliteration of small muscular arteries in the villi. Similarly the progressive decline in resistance that occurs as normal pregnancies proceed is associated with an increasing number of small arterial channels in placental villi.

The main efficacy of Doppler has been in evaluating for fetal compromise and aiding in timing delivery of fetuses who are at risk for IUGR based on biometric parameters. Although it was also hoped that Doppler techniques would be useful in screening for IUGR, such screening has been shown to have a very low yield when applied to the general population.

A variety of indices have been used to quantitate the relationship between systolic and diastolic blood flow, but because the various ratios have similar accuracies in evaluating for growth retardation or fetal compromise, the A/B ratio (peak systolic divided by end-diastolic velocity, or S/D ratio), which is the simplest to obtain, is the one most extensively used (see Fig. 133–4). A compilation of

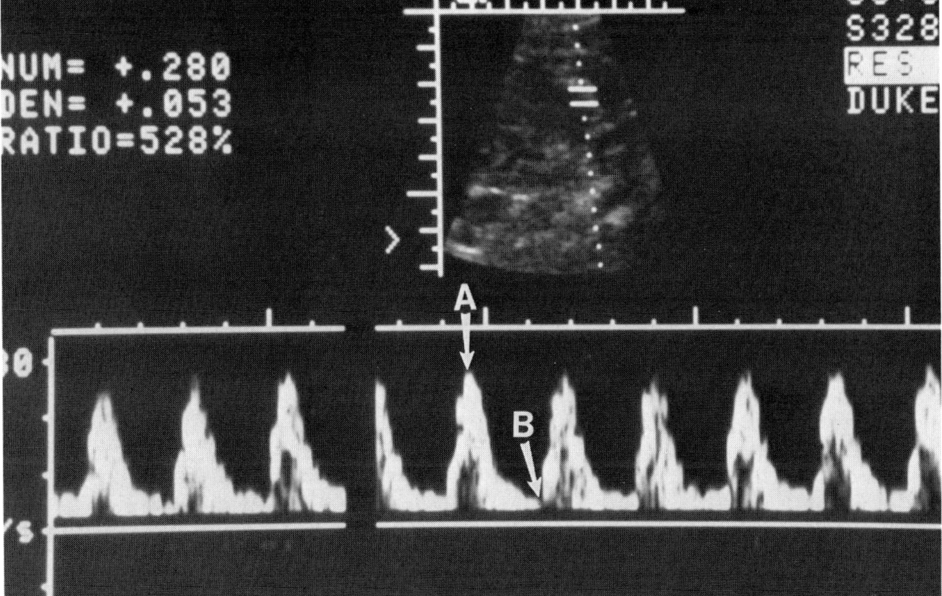

Figure 133–5. Abnormal umbilical artery Doppler tracing in a fetus with an elevated A/B ratio demonstrates diminished end-diastolic flow (B) relative to peak systolic flow (A).

TABLE 133–5. UMBILICAL ARTERY FLOW A/B RATIO

WEEKS	MEAN	UPPER LIMIT
24	3.5	4.25
25	3.4	4.1
26	3.3	3.9
27	3.2	3.75
28	3.1	3.7
29	3.0	3.6
30	2.9	3.5
31	2.85	3.45
32	2.8	3.4
33	2.7	3.3
34	2.6	3.15
35	2.55	3.1
36	2.45	3.0
37	2.4	2.9
38	2.35	2.8
39	2.3	2.65
40	2.2	2.5

Courtesy of Dr. James D. Bowie, Duke University Medical Center. This table represents a composite of graphs found in the references by Trudinger et al, Stuart et al, and Erskine and Ritchie.

Reprinted with permission from 1991 Special Course Syllabus in Ultrasound, Intrauterine Growth Retardation, RSNA Publications.

normal A/B ratios and upper limits based on several studies is listed in Table 133–5. As gestational age increases, both the mean and upper limits of normal for the A/B ratio progressively decrease. As a general rule of thumb, at 26 weeks' gestation and beyond, any value above 4 is elevated, and any value below 2.5 is within the normal range. Additionally, a multitude of variables including fetal heart rate, fetal activity state, fetal breathing motions, fetal movements, uterine contractions, and sampling site affect the shape of the waveforms obtained from the umbilical arteries. Whenever possible, measurements should be obtained in the midportion of the umbilical cord, during periods of fetal inactivity, in the absence of fetal breathing motion.

Detection of absent or reversed end-diastolic flow in the umbilical artery is a particularly worrisome finding, associated with perinatal death rates as high as 50 to 90 per cent. Although some authors recommend that absent or reversed diastolic flow indicates the need for immediate delivery, if the fetus is very premature, decisions regarding delivery must be balanced with gestational age and other clinical factors.

Like the umbilical artery circulation, the fetal cerebral circulation is altered in compromised fetuses. Although the umbilical arteries and the fetal descending aorta exhibit an increase in vascular resistance, the internal carotid and middle cerebral arteries show decreased resistance with abnormally low indices. These changes are thought to be due to a compensatory mechanism whereby increased resistance in the fetal body and placenta and decreased resistance in the brain shunt blood to the brain in order to spare the cerebrum.

In closing, it should be stressed that just as the biometric parameters used to evaluate for IUGR are not interpreted in a vacuum, abnormal Doppler values must be considered in the context of gestational age, clinical data, and other tests of fetal well-being. An abnormal Doppler value indicates only that there is abnormal resistance to blood flow in the maternal-fetal circulation. The potential consequences of abnormal flow (restricted growth, fetal hypoxia, etc.) may not be operative at the time of sampling. Fetal compromise depends on a multitude of factors, including the severity of circulatory compromise, its duration, the underlying etiology, as well as the compensatory response by the fetus. An abnormal Doppler study indicates that the fetus is at risk to develop compromise, but not every pregnancy with an abnormal Doppler study has an adverse outcome, nor does every growth-retarded fetus display abnormal waveforms. Despite these limitations, there is a clear-cut association between abnormal umbilical artery Doppler values and adverse pregnancy outcomes. It is hoped that the incorporation of Doppler evaluation of the umbilical artery circulation into surveillance of pregnancies at risk for IUGR will help to decrease perinatal morbidity and mortality.

Bibliography

Abramowicz JS, Warsof SL, Sherer DM, et al: Value of a random single Doppler study of the umbilical artery for predicting perinatal outcome. J Ultrasound Med 10:337–339, 1991.

Beattie RB, Dornan JC: Antenatal screening for intrauterine growth retardation with umbilical artery Doppler ultrasonography. Br Med J 298:631, 1989.

Benson CB, Belville JS, Lentini JF, et al: Intrauterine growth retardation: Diagnosis based on multiple parameters—a prospective study. Radiology 177:499–502, 1990.

Benson CB, Boswell SB, Brown DL, et al: Improved prediction of intrauterine growth retardation with use of multiple parameters. Radiology 168:7–12, 1988.

Benson CB, Doubilet PM: Doppler criteria for intrauterine growth retardation: Predictive values. J Ultrasound Med 7:655–659, 1988.

Benson CB, Doubilet PM: "Head sparing" in fetuses with intrauterine growth retardation: Does it really occur? Radiology 161(P):75, 1986.

Benson CB, Doubilet PM, Saltzman DH, Jones TB: FL/AC ratio: Poor predictor of intrauterine growth retardation. Invest Radiol 20:727–730, 1985.

Bowie JD: Fetal growth. In Callen PW (ed): Ultrasonography in Obstetrics and Gynecology. Philadelphia, WB Saunders Company, 1988, pp 65–82.

Brown HL, Miller JM Jr, Gabert HA, Kissling G: Ultrasonic recognition of the small-for-gestational-age fetus. Obstet Gynecol 69:631–635, 1987.

Bruinse HW, Sijmons EA, Reuwer PJHM: Clinical value of screening for fetal growth retardation by Doppler ultrasound. J Ultrasound Med 8:207–209, 1989.

Campbell S, Thomas A: Ultrasound measurement of the fetal head to abdomen circumference ratio in the assessment of growth retardation. Br J Obstet Gynaecol 84:165, 1977.

Carroll BA: Duplex Doppler systems in obstetric ultrasound. Radiol Clin North Am 28:189–203, 1990.

Chambers SE, Hoskins PR, Haddad NG, et al: A comparison of fetal abdominal circumference measurements and Doppler ultrasound in the prediction of small-for-dates babies and fetal compromise. Br J Obstet Gynaecol 96:803–808, 1989.

Crane JP, Beaver HA, Cheung SW: Antenatal ultrasound findings in fetal triploidy syndrome. J Ultrasound Med 4:519–524, 1985.

Dobson PC, Abell DA, Beischer NA: Mortality and morbidity of fetal growth retardation. Aust N Z J Obstet Gynaecol 21:69, 1981.

Erskine RLA, Ritchie JWK: Umbilical artery blood flow characteristics in normal and growth-retarded fetuses. Br J Obstet Gynaecol 92:605–610, 1985.

Eyck JV, Wladimiroff JW, Noordam MJ, et al: The blood flow velocity waveform in the fetal internal carotid and umbilical artery; its relation to fetal behavioural states in the growth retarded fetus at 37–38 weeks gestation. Br J Obstet Gynaecol 95:473–477, 1988.

Ferrazzi E, Vegni C, Bellotti M, et al: Role of umbilical Doppler velocimetry in the biophysical assessment of the growth retarded fetus—answers from neonatal morbidity and mortality. J Ultrasound Med 10:09–315, 1991.

Giles WB, Trudinger BJ, Baird PJ: Fetal umbilical artery flow velocity waveforms and placental resistance: Pathological correlation. Br J Obstet Gynaecol 92:31–38, 1985.

Guzman ER, Schulman H, Karmel B, Higgins P: Umbilical artery Doppler velocimetry in pregnancies of less than 21 weeks' duration. J Ultrasound Med 9:655–659, 1990.

Hadlock FP: Sonographic estimation of fetal age and weight. Radiol Clin North Am 28(1):39–50, 1990.

Hadlock FP, Deter RL, Harrist RB, et al: A date-independent predictor of intrauterine growth retardation: Femur length/abdominal circumference ratio. AJR 141:979–984, 1983.

Hadlock FP, Deter RL, Rossavik IK: Detection of abnormal fetal growth patterns: Intrauterine growth retardation and macrosomia. In Athey PA, Hadlock FP (eds): Ultrasound in Obstetrics and Gynecology, 2nd ed. St. Louis, CV Mosby, 1985, pp 38–59.

Hadlock FP, Harrist RB, Carpenter RJ, et al: Sonographic estimation of fetal weight—the value of femur length in addition to head and abdomen measurements. Radiology 150:535–540, 1984.

Hendricks SK, Sorensen TK, Wang KY, Bushnell JM: Doppler umbilical artery waveform indices—normal values from fourteen to forty-two weeks. Am J Obstet Gynecol 161:761–765, 1989.

Hohler CW: Ultrasound diagnosis of intrauterine growth retardation. In Sanders RC, James AE (eds): The Principles and Practice of Ultrasonography in Obstetrics and Gynecology, 3rd ed. Norwalk, CT, Appleton-Century-Crofts, 1985, pp 157–173.

Jeanty P, Cantraine F, Romero R, et al: A longitudinal study of fetal weight growth. J Ultrasound Med 3:321–328, 1984.

Kay HH, Carroll BA, Bowie JD, et al: "Non-uniformity" of fetal umbilical systolic/diastolic ratios as determined with duplex Doppler sonography. J Ultrasound Med 8:417–420, 1989.

Lugo G, Cassady G: Intrauterine growth retardation—clinicopathologic findings in 233 consecutive infants. Am J Obstet Gynecol 109:615, 1970.

Manning FA, Hohler C: Intrauterine growth retardation: Diagnosis, prognostication, and management based on ultrasound methods. In Fleischer AC, Romero R, Man-

ning FA, et al (eds): The Principles and Practice of Ultrasonography in Obstetrics and Gynecology, 4th ed. Norwalk, CT, Appleton and Lange, 1991, pp 331–347.
Mehalek KE, Rosenberg J, Berkowitz GS, et al: Umbilical and uterine artery flow velocity waveforms—effect of the sampling site on Doppler ratios. J Ultrasound Med 8:171–176, 1989.
Mires G, Dempster J, Patel NB, Crawford JW: The effect of fetal heart rate on umbilical artery flow velocity waveforms. Br J Obstet Gynaecol 94:665–669, 1987.
Mulders LG, Wijn PF, Jongsind HW, Hein PR: A comparative study of three indexes of umbilical blood flow in relation to prediction of growth retardation. J Perinat Med 15:3–12, 1987.
Newnham J, Patterson L, James I, Reid S: The effect of heart rate on Doppler flow velocity systolic-diastolic ratios in umbilical and uteroplacental arterial waveforms. Early Hum Dev 21:21–29, 1990.
Newnham JP, Patterson LL, James IR, et al: An evaluation of the efficacy of Doppler flow velocity waveform analysis as a screening test in pregnancy. Am J Obstet Gynecol 162:403–410, 1990.
Rochelson B, Schulman H, Farmakides G, et al: The significance of absent end-diastolic velocity in umbilical artery velocity waveforms. Am J Obstet Gynecol 156:1213–1218, 1987.
Satoh S, Lauanagi T, Fukuhara J, et al: Changes in vascular resistance in the umbilical and middle cerebral arteries in the human intrauterine growth retarded fetus, measured with pulsed Doppler ultrasound. Early Hum Dev 20:213–220, 1989.
Shepard MJ, Richards VA, Berkowitz RL, et al: An evaluation of two equations for predicting fetal weight by ultrasound. Am J Obstet Gynecol 142:47–54, 1982.
Selbing A, Wichman K, Ryden G: Screening for detection of intra-uterine growth retardation by means of ultrasound. Acta Obstet Gynecol Scand 63:543–548, 1984.
Spencer JAD, Price J, Lee A: Influence of fetal breathing and movements on variability of umbilical Doppler indices using different numbers of waveforms. J Ultrasound Med 10:37–41, 1991.
Stuart B, Drumm J, Fitzgerald DE, Duignan NM: Fetal blood velocity waveforms in normal pregnancy. Br J Obstet Gynaecol 87:780–785, 1980.
Thompson RS, Trudinger BJ, Cook CM: Doppler ultrasound waveform indexes: A/B ratio, pulsatility index and Pourcelot ratio. Br J Obstet Gynaecol 95:581–588, 1988.
Trudinger BJ, Cook CM, Collins L: Fetal umbilical artery flow velocity waveforms and placental resistance: Clinical significance. Br J Obstet Gynaecol 92:23–30, 1985.
Villar J, Belizan JM: The timing factor in the pathophysiology of the intrauterine growth retardation syndrome. Obstet Gynecol Survey 37:499–506, 1982.
Vintzileos AM, Neckles S, Campbell WA, et al: Ultrasound fetal thigh-calf circumferences and gestational age-independent fetal ratios in normal pregnancy. J Ultrasound Med 4:287–292, 1985.
Warsof SL, Cooper DJ, Little D, Campbell S: Routine ultrasound screening for antenatal detection of intrauterine growth retardation. Obstet Gynecol 67:33–39, 1986.
Wilcox AJ: Intrauterine growth retardation: Beyond birthweight criteria. Early Hum Dev 8:189–193, 1983.
Wladimiroff JW, Tonge HM, Stewart PA: Doppler ultrasound assessment of cerebral blood flow in the human fetus. Br J Obstet Gynaecol 93:471–475, 1986.
Woo JSK, Liang ST, Lo RLS: Significance of an absent or reversed end diastolic flow in Doppler umbilical artery waveforms. J Ultrasound Med 6:291–297, 1987.
Yarkoni S, Reece A, Wan M, et al: Intrapartum fetal weight estimation: a comparison of three formulas. J Ultrasound Med 5:707–710, 1986.
Yarlagadda P, Willoughby L, Maulik D: Effect of fetal heart rate on umbilical arterial Doppler indices. J Ultrasound Med 8:215–218, 1989.

134 Ultrasound of the Placenta

Beverly A. Spirt and Lawrence P. Gordon

The early gestational sac is characterized sonographically by a hyperechoic rim representing the chorionic villi, surrounded by the lacunar space containing maternal blood (Fig. 134–1). Absence or disruption of the hyperechoic rim is indicative of an abnormal pregnancy (Fig. 134–2). Beginning at about 5 weeks menstrual age, the villi opposite the implantation site normally regress; the remaining villi (chorion frondosum) along with the decidua basalis form the early placenta. At sonography, the placenta has a diffuse granular texture produced by echoes emanating from the villous tree, which is bathed in maternal blood. The fetal surface of the placenta, or "chorionic plate," is visible as a distinct line of echoes. The echo pattern of the placenta is distinct from that of the retroplacental myometrium, which appears relatively hypoechoic when compared with the placenta (Fig. 134–3).

Maternal blood enters the intervillous space via spiral arterioles, which are too small to be seen sonographically. Venous drainage occurs along the base of the placenta as well as in the septa (Fig. 134–3).

Placental septa, composed of decidua and trophoblast, extend from the basal plate toward the fetal surface during the third month of gestation. These divide the maternal surface into 15 to 20 lobes, which have no known physiologic significance. At term, up to 19 per cent of placentas contain septal cysts, thought to result from obstructed venous drainage. These are of no clinical significance.

PLACENTAL CALCIFICATION

The echo pattern of the placenta does not change significantly from the end of the first to the beginning of the third trimester. At this time, physiologic calcification can be detected as echogenic foci primarily in the basal plate and septa and, to a lesser degree, in the perivillous and subchorionic spaces (Fig. 134–4). The incidence of placental calcification increases exponentially with advancing

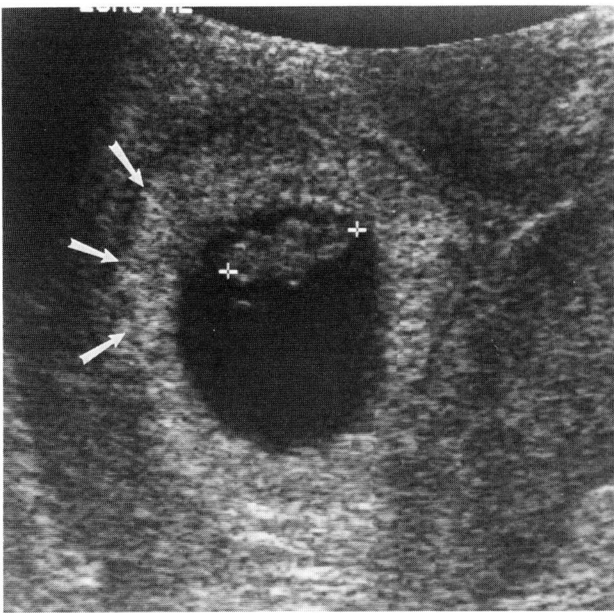

Figure 134–1. Early pregnancy. Sagittal scan at 7.5 weeks shows gestational sac with hyperechoic rim *(arrows)*. (Cursors = fetus.)

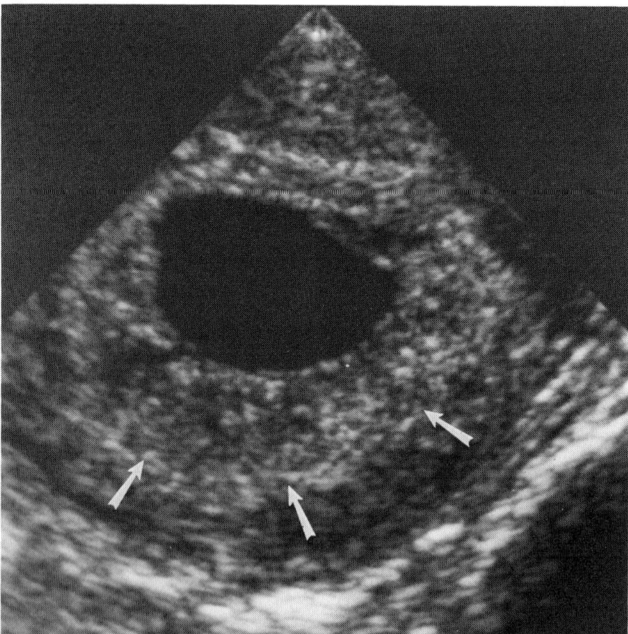

Figure 134–2. Blighted ovum. Endovaginal scan at 6.5 weeks' amenorrhea shows abnormal gestational sac with inhomogeneous rim *(arrows)* containing hypoechoic spaces in which flow was demonstrated. No fetus was present.

gestational age, beginning at about 29 weeks. Placental calcification is also more common in women of lower parity, and in deliveries occurring in summer or early fall. Postmature placentas do not show increased calcification. The presence or degree of placental calcification has no proven pathologic or clinical significance.

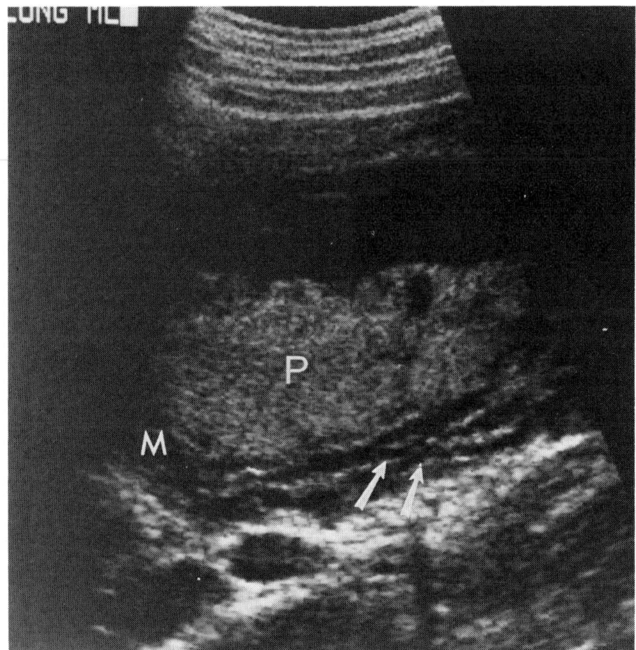

Figure 134–3. Normal placenta. Sagittal scan at 19.6 weeks shows typical echotexture of the posterior placenta (P). Note relatively hypoechoic retroplacental myometrium (M). Retroplacental tubular structures represent draining veins *(arrows).*

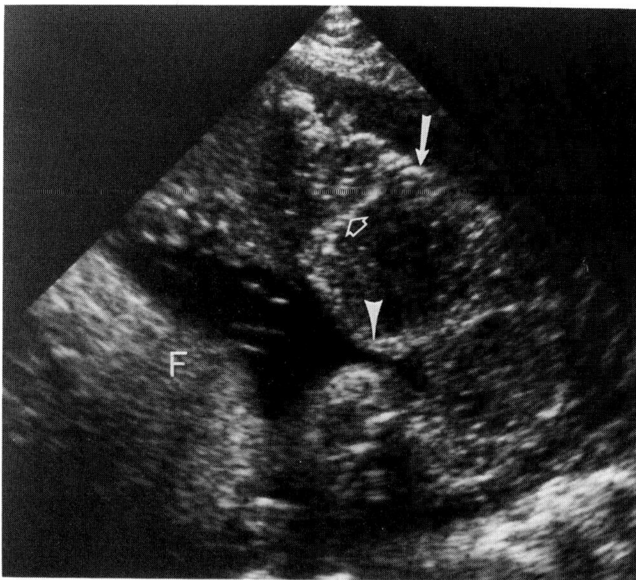

Figure 134–4. Calcification. At 38 weeks, anterior placenta shows prominent calcification in the basal plate *(arrow),* septa *(open arrow),* and subchorionic space *(arrowhead).* (F = fetus.)

CONTRACTIONS AND BLADDER EFFECT

Temporary variations in the shape of the placenta and myometrium occur with different degrees of bladder filling, and with myometrial contractions. A moderately full bladder is useful for optimal transabdominal imaging prior to 16 weeks. However, overdistention of the bladder often compresses the anterior wall of the uterus against the posterior wall, artificially elongating the cervix and mimicking placenta previa (Fig. 134–5). Braxton-Hicks contractions, which are imperceptible to the mother, cause transient thickening of the placenta and myometrium (Fig. 134–6) and commonly mimic placenta previa as well (Fig. 134–7). It is important to rescan the patient after an interval of 20 minutes to one hour in order to distinguish a contraction from a leiomyoma or retroplacental hematoma, and/or to exclude the diagnosis of placenta previa. Leiomyomas, which may vary in echotexture from hypoechoic to echogenic and complex, usually do not change in size over a short period of time. Retroplacental hematomas also vary in echotexture, and can occur in the absence of external bleeding. They may lead to diffuse intravascular coagulopathy.

SUCCENTURIATE LOBE

Permanent variations in shape that may be diagnosed sonographically include succenturiate lobes (Fig. 134–8). These occur in up to 8 per cent of placentas, and are important because of the association with retained placenta and vasa previa (Fig. 134–9).

PLACENTA PREVIA

A placenta that covers part or all of the internal cervical os is called placenta previa (Fig. 134–10). This condition is a cause of third trimester bleeding, and necessitates a cesarean section. True placenta previa occurs in approximately 0.3 to 1 per cent of births.

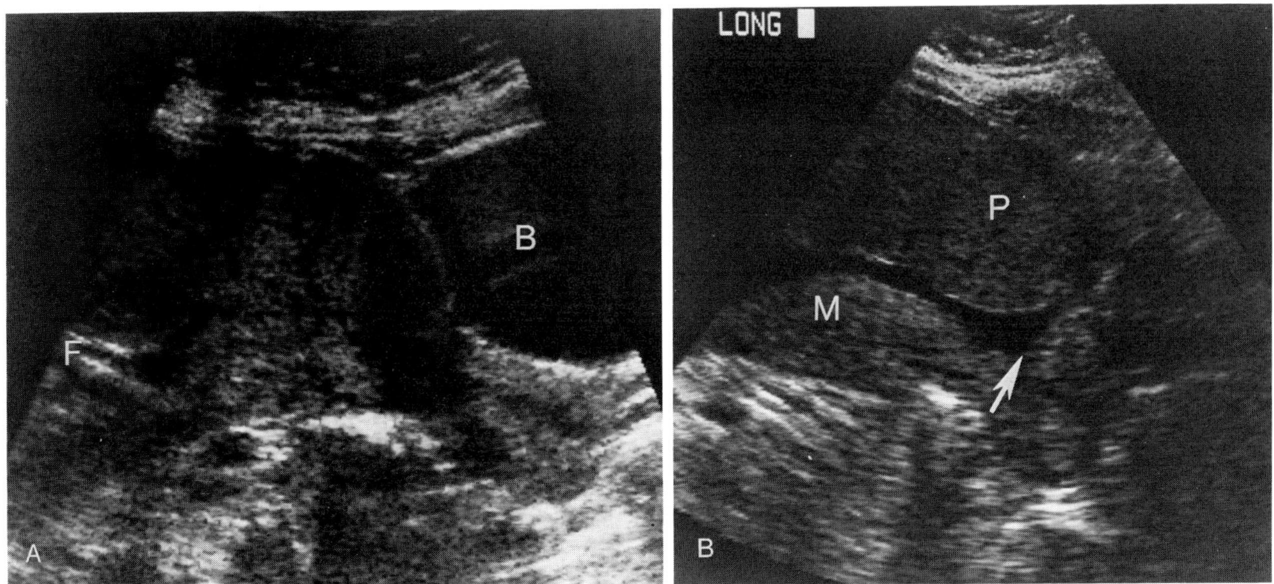

Figure 134–5. Bladder effect. *A,* Sagittal scan at 22.5 weeks shows apparent placenta previa. (B = maternal bladder; F = fetus.) *B,* Following voiding, the anterior placenta (P) is seen to be well away from the internal os of the cervix *(arrow).* (M = myometrium.) (*A* and *B* from Spirt BA, Gordon LP: Imaging of the placenta. In Taveras JM, Ferrucci JT (eds): Radiology. Philadelphia, JB Lippincott, 1992.)

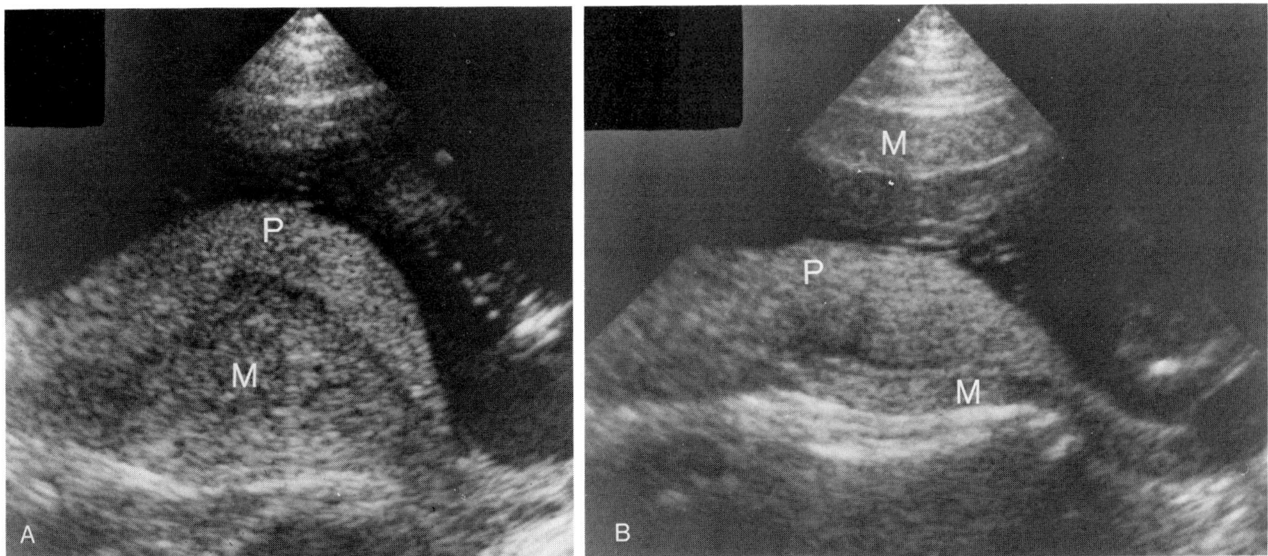

Figure 134–6. Contraction. *A,* Sagittal scan at 15 weeks shows posterior placenta (P) and retroplacental myometrium (M) distorted by contraction. *B,* Twenty minutes later, the contraction is gone.

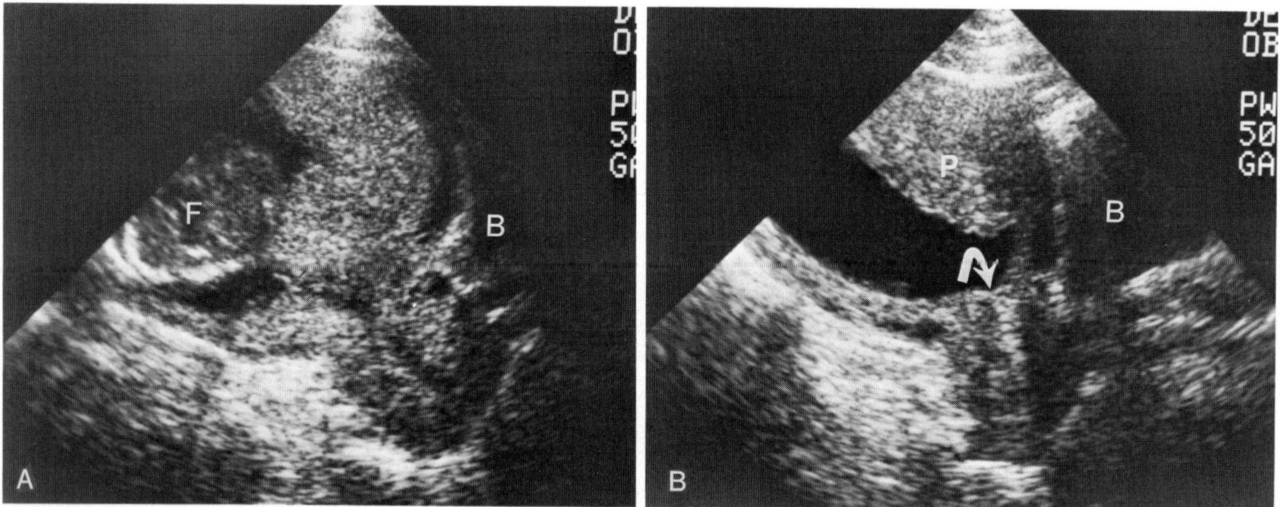

Figure 134–7. Contraction mimicking placenta previa. *A,* Sagittal midline scan at 18.5 weeks shows apparent placenta previa. (F = fetus; B = maternal bladder.) *B,* Repeat scan 28 minutes later shows that the anterior placenta (P) is well away from the internal os *(curved arrow)* of the cervix. (*A* and *B* from Spirt BA, Gordon LP: Sonography of the placenta. In Fleischer AC, Romero R, Manning FA et al (eds): The Principles and Practice of Ultrasonography in Obstetrics and Gynecology, 4th ed. East Norwalk, CT, Appleton and Lange, 1991, pp. 133–157.)

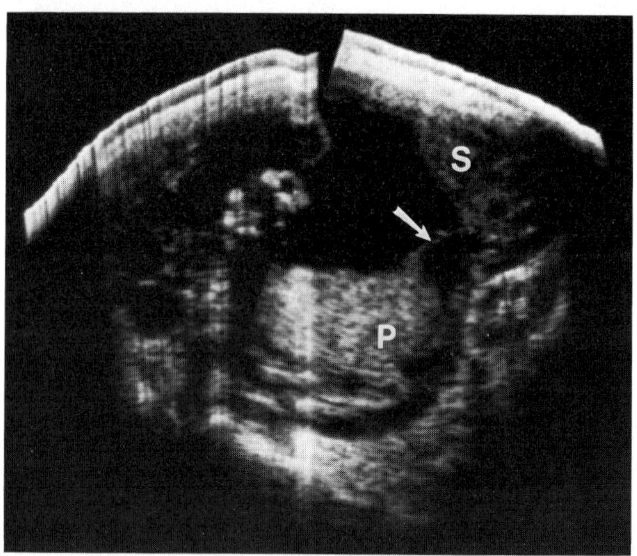

Figure 134–8. Succenturiate lobe. Transverse static scan at 28 weeks shows posterior placenta (P) with left anterior succenturiate lobe (S). (*Arrow* = membranes elevated over anechoic space representing subchorionic hematoma, confirmed at delivery.) (From Spirt BA, Kagan EH, Gordon LP, et al: Antepartum diagnosis of a succenturiate lobe. Sonographic and pathologic correlation. J Clin Ultrasound 9:139–140, 1981. Reprinted by permission of John Wiley & Sons, Inc. Copyright © 1981.)

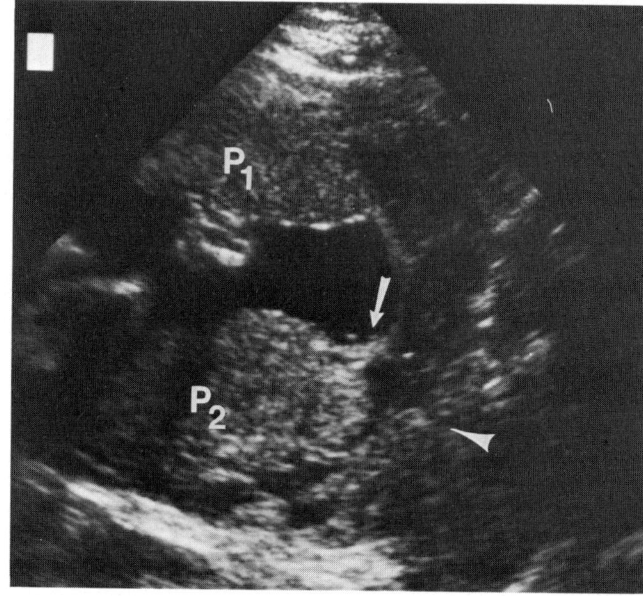

Figure 134–9. Vasa previa. Midline sagittal scan at 25 weeks shows vessel *(arrow)* overlying internal cervical os *(arrowhead).* Placenta was on the left, with anterior (P_1) and posterior (P_2) extensions. Vasa previa was confirmed at cesarean section.

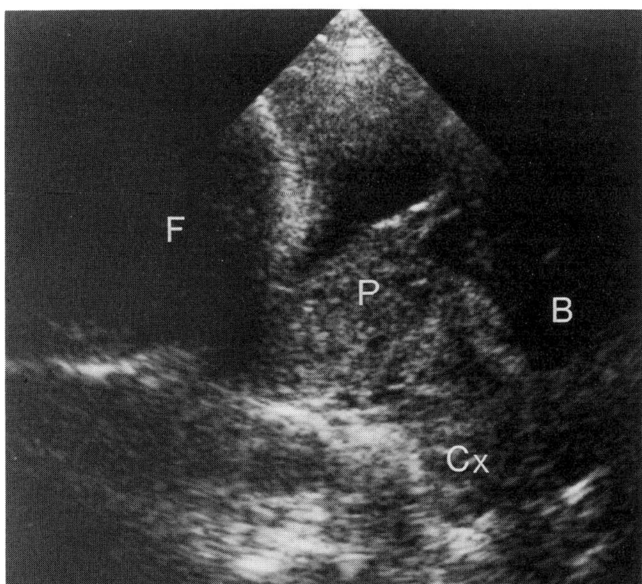

Figure 134–10. Placenta previa. Midline sagittal scan at 34 weeks shows placenta previa. (F = fetal head; P = placenta; Cx = cervix; B = maternal bladder.)

False-positive sonographic diagnoses of placenta previa are common, due to either an overdistended bladder or contractions in the lower segment of the uterus in the late first and early second trimesters. Thus in the case of suspected placenta previa, it is important to rescan the patient after voiding, and/or after at least 20 minutes to one hour.

It is useful to determine the relationship of the placenta to the internal os of the cervix prior to 20 weeks. After that time, the cervix may be obscured by the fetal head. The transvaginal probe or, if bleeding has occurred, transperineal scanning may be used to establish the diagnosis of placenta previa in the late second or third trimester.

There is an increased incidence of placenta previa in women who smoke, and in patients with a prior history of abortion, placenta previa, or cesarean section. Placenta previa is found in approximately 30 per cent of cases of placenta creta, a condition in which deficiency of the decidua results in adherence to (placenta accreta), invasion of (placenta increta), or penetration through (placenta percreta) the myometrium. Placenta creta occurs more frequently in patients with a history of prior cesarean section, uterine scars of other etiology, increasing parity, and prior manual removal of the placenta. It results in severe hemorrhage, with a 14 per cent incidence of uterine rupture; hysterectomy is usually indicated. At sonography, the usual retroplacental myometrial "stripe" may be absent. Multiple anechoic/hypoechoic spaces with visible flow are seen within the placenta, without a corresponding pathologic lesion (Fig. 134–11). This may be a function of the aberrant blood flow caused by absence of the normal decidual circulation.

SIZE

Circumferential enlargement continues into the third trimester. Variation in size of the placenta occurs in maternal and fetal disorders. Large placentas are found with hemolytic disease of the newborn, maternal anemia, and maternal diabetes (Fig. 134–12). Placentas from pre-eclamptic mothers tend to be small. Small placentas are also associated with small-for-dates infants; this does not imply a cause-and-effect relationship. The placenta is a fetal organ, and its size therefore corresponds to the size of the baby.

NORMAL MACROSCOPIC LESIONS

Subchorionic hypoechoic/anechoic spaces that sometimes contain flow can be seen from the second trimester on in up to 15 per cent of obstetric sonograms (Figs. 134–13 and 134–14). These correlate with the presence of subchorionic fibrin at delivery and are of no clinical significance. Intraplacental hypoechoic/anechoic lesions that are single or few in number usually represent either intervillous thromboses (Fig. 134–15) or perivillous fibrin (Fig. 134–16). Intervillous thromboses contain both fetal and maternal red cells. They are thought to be due to leakage of fetal cells through a villous tear, which presumably stimulates the maternal coagulation process. Intervillous thrombi are of no apparent clinical significance except in cases of Rh incompatibility, in which they may lead to maternal sensitization. Perivillous fibrin deposits have no known clinical significance. Hypoechoic/anechoic intraplacental lesions seen at sonography sometimes correspond to blood-filled spaces at delivery (Fig. 134–17). These represent areas of pooling or stasis of blood, probably an early stage in the formation of either intervillous thrombosis or perivillous fibrin.

Placental infarcts, which result from coagulation necrosis of villi and occur most commonly at the base of the placenta, cannot be detected at sonography unless they are complicated by hemorrhage.

HYDATIDIFORM MOLE

Multiple diffuse intraplacental anechoic lesions are abnormal. These usually represent hydatidiform change, which may be separated into two groups: the classic hydatidiform mole, and the partial mole with alternate areas of hydatidiform change and normal villi. Hydatidiform mole is believed to result from abnormal fertilization of an empty ovum by a single sperm, with duplication of the haploid paternal chromosomes, or dispermy. The placenta is completely replaced with dilated, hydropic villi. At sonography, the uterus is filled with solid material containing multiple anechoic spaces (Fig. 134–18), which enlarge with advancing gestational age.

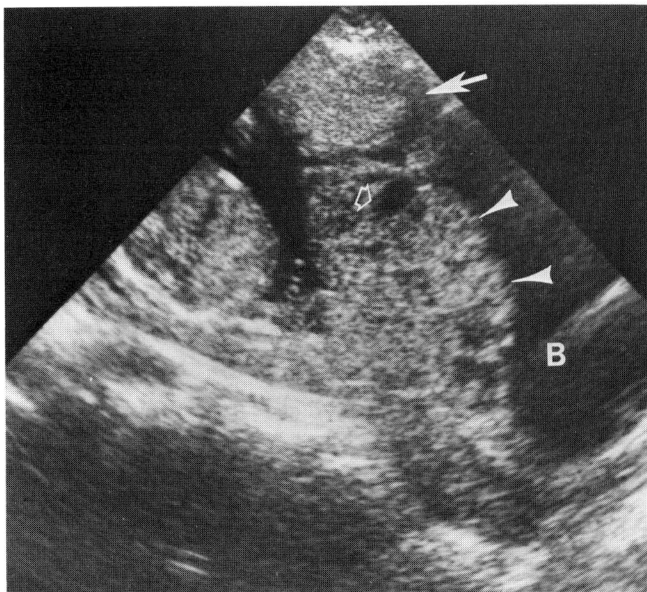

Figure 134–11. Placenta percreta. Midline sagittal scan at 20.5 weeks shows anterior placenta previa. Note retroplacental myometrium *(arrow),* which disappears inferiorly *(arrowheads)* where placenta invades myometrium. Multiple prominent hypoechoic areas were seen within the placenta *(open arrow).* (B = maternal bladder.) (Courtesy of Medical Imaging Department, Crouse Irving Memorial Hospital, Syracuse, NY.)

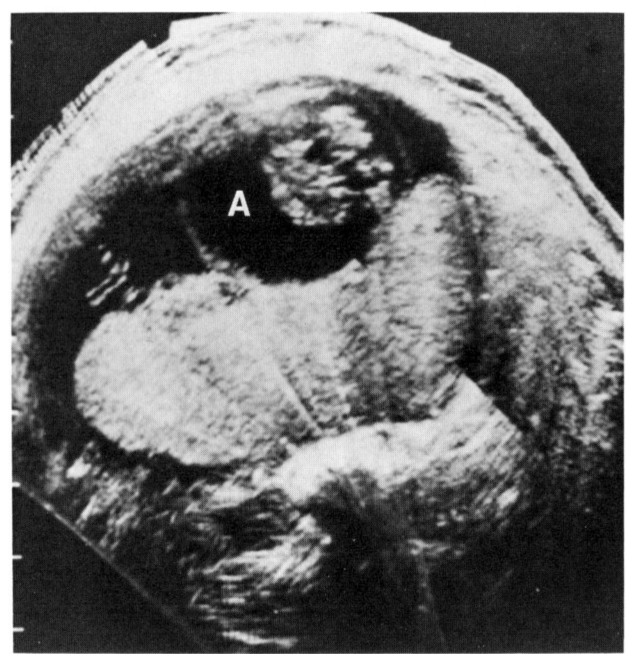

Figure 134–12. Maternal-fetal Rh incompatibility. Transverse scan at 28 weeks shows markedly enlarged placenta. Note fetal ascites (A). (Courtesy of Dr. Edward Bell, Syracuse, NY. From Spirt BA, Gordon LP: Sonography of the placenta. In Fleischer AC, Romero R, Manning FA, et al (eds): The Principles and Practice of Ultrasonography in Obstetrics and Gynecology, 4th ed. East Norwalk, CT, Appleton and Lange, 1991, pp. 133–157.)

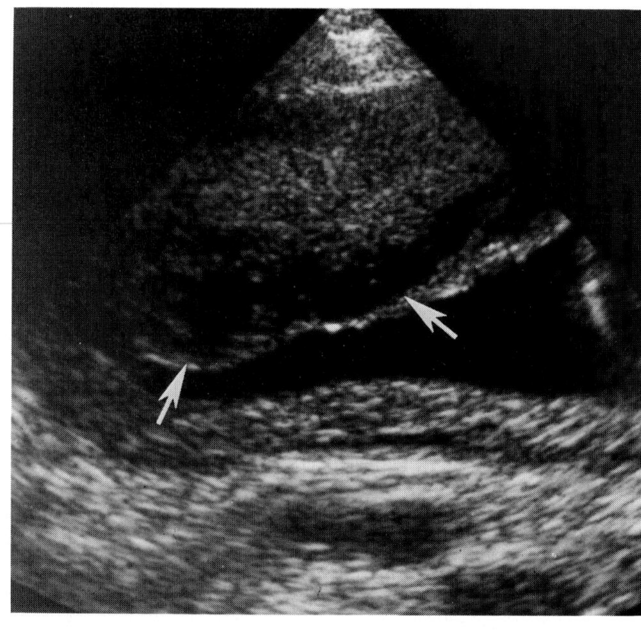

Figure 134–13. Subchorionic fibrin deposition. Sector scan at 17 weeks shows anechoic/hypoechoic subchorionic lesion *(arrows),* with flow demonstrated at real-time sonography. This correlated with a laminated fibrin deposit at delivery.

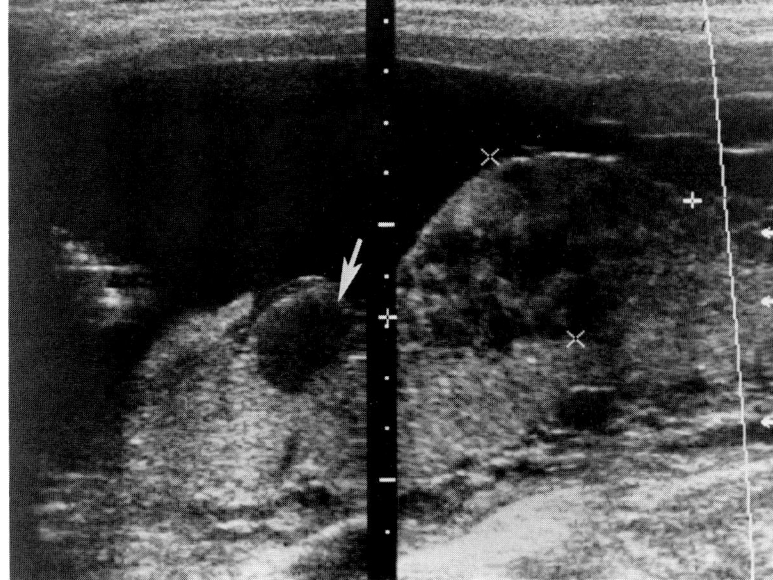

Figure 134–14. Subchorionic fibrin deposition. Sagittal scan at 26.4 weeks shows large complex subchorionic lesion *(cursors)* with adjacent smaller lesion *(arrow)*; both correlated with subchorionic fibrin deposition at delivery.

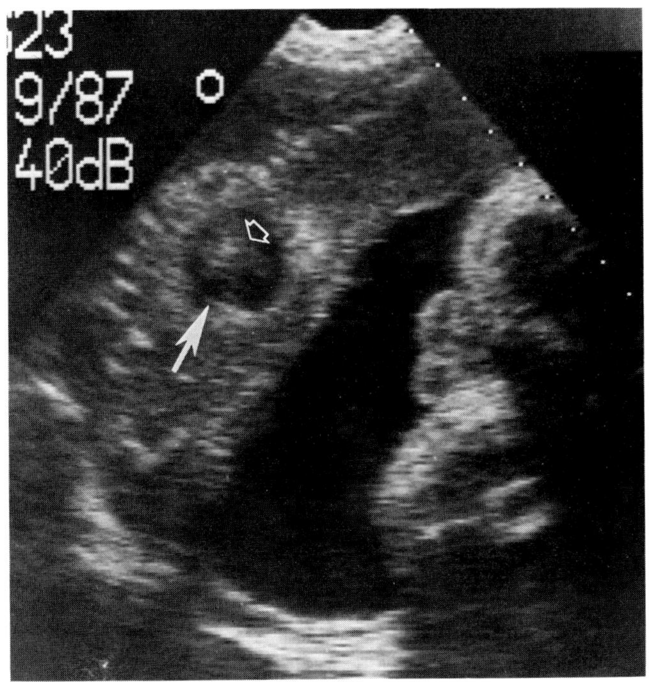

Figure 134–15. Intervillous thrombosis. Sagittal scan at 37 weeks shows hypoechoic intraplacental lesion *(arrow)* with flow *(open arrow)* visible at real-time examination. At delivery, a combination of semi-liquid blood and laminated fibrin was found, consistent with intervillous thrombosis. (Courtesy of Dr. John McKennan, Mohawk Valley General Hospital, Ilion, NY. From Spirt BA, Gordon LP: Sonography of the placenta. In Fleischer AC, Romero R, Manning FA, et al (eds): The Principles and Practice of Ultrasonography in Obstetrics and Gynecology, 4th ed. East Norwalk, CT, Appleton and Lange, 1991, pp. 133–157.)

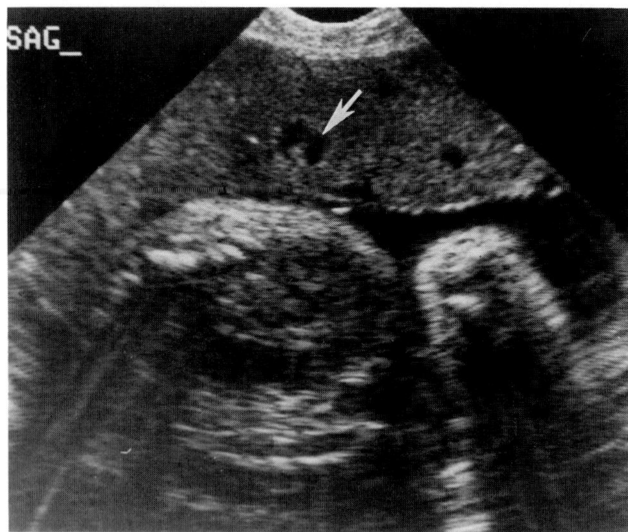

Figure 134–16. Perivillous fibrin deposition. Sagittal scan at 35 weeks shows hypoechoic intraplacental lesion *(arrow)* with echogenic area within, corresponding to perivillous fibrin deposition at delivery. (From Spirt BA, Gordon LP: Sonography of the placenta. In Fleischer AC, Romero R, Manning FA et al (eds): The Principles and Practice of Ultrasonography in Obstetrics and Gynecology, 4th ed. East Norwalk, CT, Appleton and Lange, 1991, pp. 133–157.)

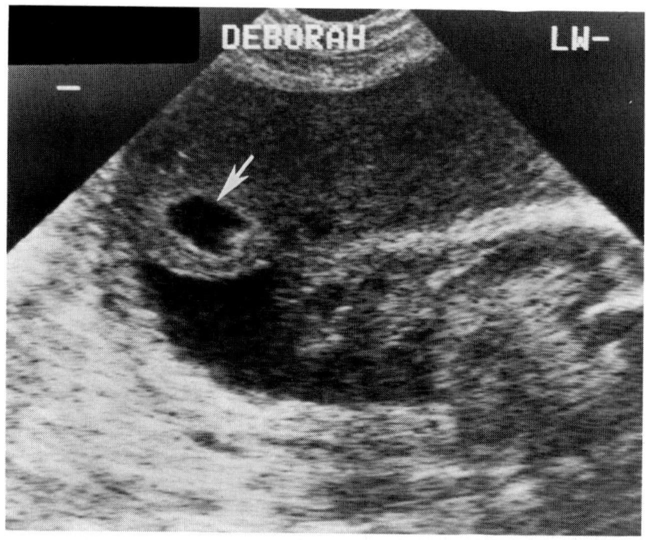

Figure 134–17. "Maternal lake." Sector scan at 35 weeks, same patient as in Figure 134–16. Anechoic intraplacental lesion *(arrow)* corresponded to blood-filled space at delivery; the blood fell out upon sectioning the placenta. (From Spirt BA, Gordon LP: The placenta. In Rumack CM, Wilson SR, Charbonneau JW (eds): Diagnostic Ultrasound. St. Louis, CV Mosby, 1991, pp. 935–953.)

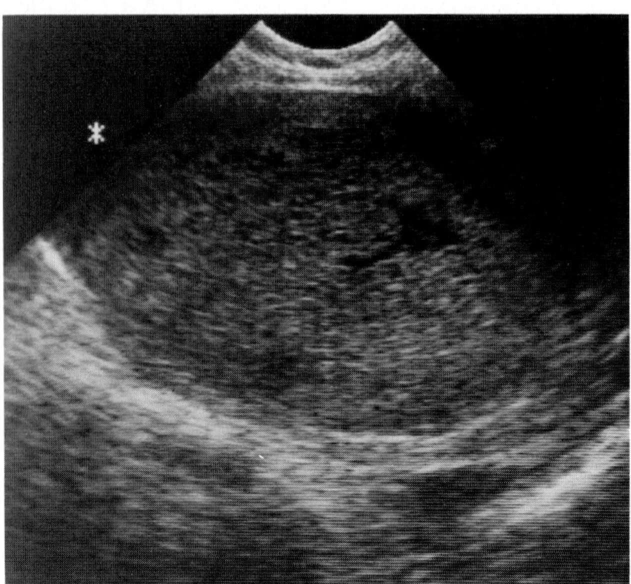

Figure 134–18. Hydatidiform mole. Sagittal scan shows the uterus filled with material containing multiple tiny anechoic spaces, typical of hydatidiform mole. (From Spirt BA, Gordon LP: Practical aspects of placental evaluation. Semin Roentgenol 26:32–49, 1991.)

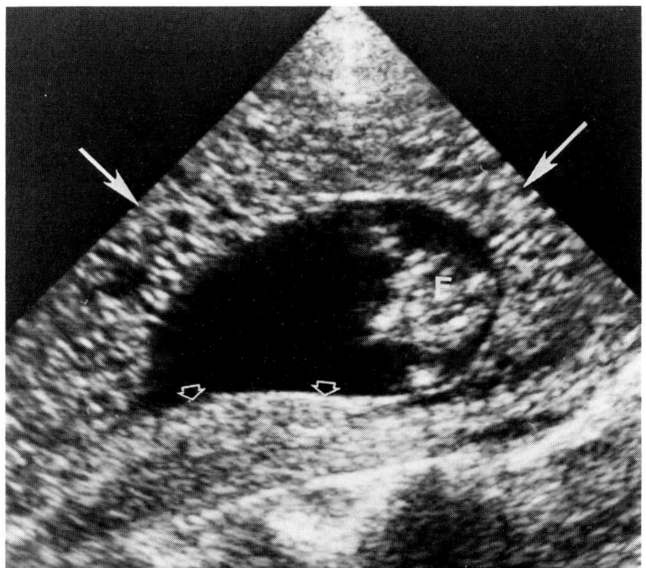

Figure 134–19. Hydatidiform mole and coexistent fetus. Transverse scan at 13 weeks shows large anterior mass *(arrows)* containing multiple tiny anechoic spaces, and separate posterior placenta *(open arrow)*. (F = fetus.) (Courtesy of Medical Imaging Department, Crouse Irving Memorial Hospital, Syracuse, NY. From Spirt BA, Gordon LP: Practical aspects of placental evaluation. Semin Roentgenol 26:32–49, 1991.)

Transvaginal sonography is useful to confirm the presence of early hydatidiform mole, when the vesicles may be too small to distinguish transabdominally. Bilateral ovarian enlargement with multiple theca lutein cysts sometimes occurs in the presence of a hydatidiform mole, in reaction to the high circulating levels of human chorionic gonadotropin (hCG). A fetus coexistent with a hydatidiform mole may occur in the case of multiple fertilization with one ovum empty. In this situation, a normal placenta is found along with the fetus and mole (Fig. 134–19). Rarely, an embryo may be found with a complete mole, without evidence of a twin gestation.

PARTIAL MOLE

With partial mole, a fetus may be present that is usually triploid (69 chromosomes). The placenta is large, with multiple anechoic lesions (Fig. 134–20). Partial moles often present clinically with early onset of pre-eclampsia in the second trimester. Both cytogenetic analysis and monitoring of chorionic gonadotropin levels are warranted because cases of partial mole have been reported that progressed to persistent trophoblastic disease requiring chemotherapy.

CHORIOANGIOMA

There are two nontrophoblastic primary tumors of the placenta: the chorioangioma, which is relatively common, and the rare teratoma. The chorioangioma is a vascular malformation that is usually small and not readily detectable without careful sectioning of the placenta. At sonography, a large tumor appears well-circumscribed, with a complex echo pattern (Fig. 134–21). It may be associated with fetal hydrops, cardiomegaly, and congestive heart failure.

ANTEPARTUM HEMORRHAGE

Bleeding from placenta previa and acute abruption occurs close to term, while chronic retroplacental hemorrhage can occur as early as the first trimester. Retroplacental hemorrhage may result in (1) external bleeding without a significant intrauterine hematoma, (2) a retroplacental hematoma with or without external bleeding, or (3) formation of a submembranous hematoma that may be at a distance from the placenta, with or without external bleeding. Sonographic examination in cases of antepartum bleeding may be negative if most of the bleeding is external. A retroplacental hemorrhage may appear as a hypoechoic or complex mass at sonography. Blood that accumulates beneath the membranes at a distance from the placenta will appear as a hypoechoic or anechoic collection under the elevated membranes (Fig. 134–22). The clinical significance of retro-

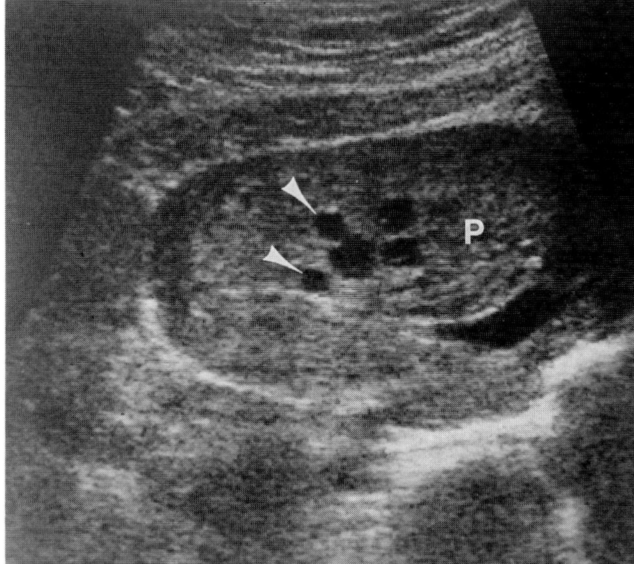

Figure 134–20. Triploidy. Sagittal scan at 15 weeks' amenorrhea shows enlarged anterior placenta (P) with multiple anechoic lesions of varying size *(arrowheads)*. There was fetal demise; chromosomal analysis confirmed triploidy.

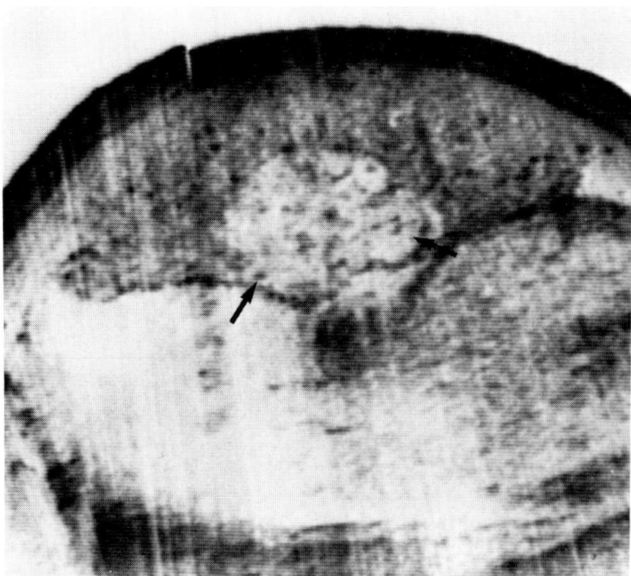

Figure 134–21. Chorioangioma. Transverse static image at 34 weeks shows complex subchorionic mass *(arrows)*, confirmed as chorioangioma at delivery.

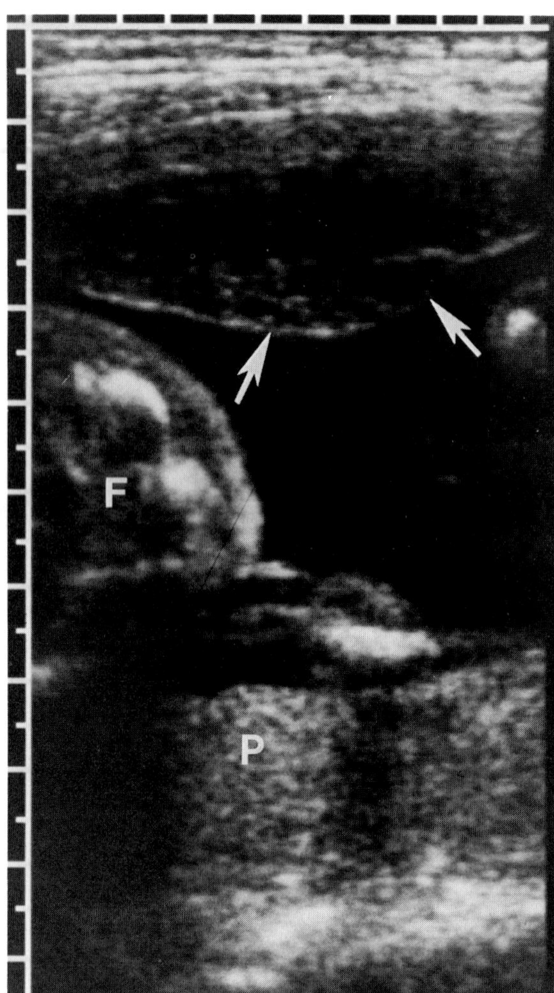

Figure 134–22. Submembranous hematoma. Sagittal scan at 19 weeks shows anterior hypoechoic submembranous collection *(arrows)*. The placenta (P) is posterior. (F = fetus.) The patient had been bleeding. The collection decreased in size on subsequent examinations. At delivery, a corresponding submembranous collection of fibrin was found.

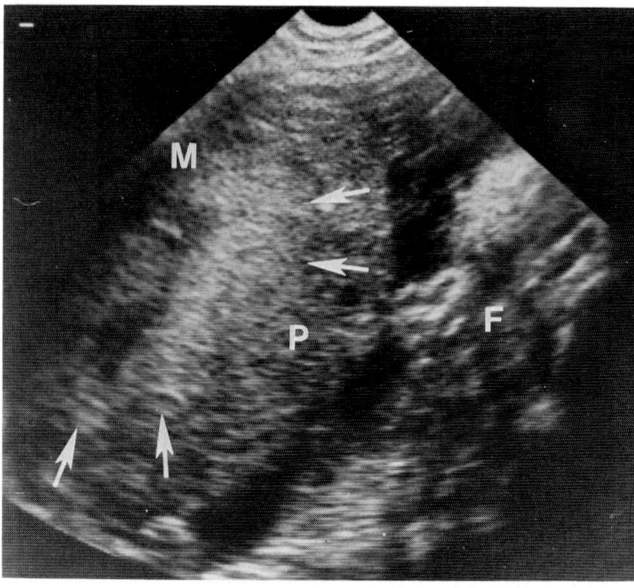

Figure 134–23. Abruptio placentae. Sagittal sector scan at 35 weeks in a hypotensive patient who was bleeding shows inhomogeneous collection *(arrows)* between placenta (P) and myometrium (M). (F = fetus.) At cesarean section, 75 per cent abruption was found. (Courtesy of Medical Imaging Department, Crouse Irving Memorial Hospital, Syracuse, NY. From Spirt BA, Gordon LP: The placenta. In Rumack CM, Wilson SR, Charbonneau JW (eds): Diagnostic Ultrasound. St. Louis, CV Mosby, 1991, pp. 935–953.)

placental hemorrhage depends upon the size and extent of the lesion. Disseminated intravascular coagulopathy may occur in some cases as a result of tissue injury.

ABRUPTIO PLACENTAE

Abruptio placentae refers to acute separation of part or all of the placenta from the myometrium, resulting in serious hemorrhage and shock. If the patient is sufficiently stable to undergo sonography prior to delivery, an echogenic retroplacental collection may be found that causes the placenta to appear artifactually thickened (Fig. 134–23).

Bibliography

Artis AA, Bowie JD, Rosenberg ER, Rauch RF: The fallacy of placental migration: Effect of sonographic techniques. AJR 144:79–81, 1985.

Fox H: Pathology of the Placenta. In Bennington JL (ed): Major Problems in Pathology, vol VII. London, WB Saunders Company Ltd, 1978.

Fox H: General pathology of the placenta. In Fox H (ed): Haines and Taylor Obstetrical and Gynaecological Pathology, 3rd ed. Edinburgh, Churchill-Livingstone, 1987, pp 972–1000.

Harris RD, Simpson WA, Pet LR, et al: Placental hypoechoic/anechoic areas and infarction: Sonographic-pathologic correlation. Radiology 176:75–80, 1990.

Mazur MT, Kurman RJ: Gestational trophoblastic disease. In Kurman RJ (ed): Blaustein's Pathology of the Female Genital Tract, 3rd ed. New York, Springer-Verlag, 1987, pp 835–875.

Nyberg DA, Mack LA, Benedetti TJ: Placental abruption and placental hemorrhage: Correlation of sonographic findings with fetal outcome. Radiology 164:357–361, 1987.

Spirt BA, Gordon LP: The placenta as an indicator of fetal maturity: Fact and fancy. Semin Ultrasound 5:290–297, 1984.

Spirt BA, Gordon LP: The placenta. In Rumack CM, Wilson SR, Charbonneau JW (eds): Diagnostic Ultrasound. St. Louis, Mosby–Year Book, 1991, pp 935–953.

Spirt BA, Gordon LP, Kagan EH: Intervillous thrombosis: Sonographic and pathologic correlation. Radiology 147:197–200, 1983.

Spirt BA, Kagan EH, Rozanski RM: Sonolucent areas in the placenta: Sonographic and pathologic correlation. AJR 131:961–965, 1978.

135 General Obstetric Sonography

James D. Bowie

Each ultrasound study of a pregnant patient can be looked upon as three separate tasks. The first is a general survey of the pelvic contents and related structures, second is a detailed examination of the fetus, and third is obstetric measurements. Much of this information is conveyed in other chapters, especially those dealing with measurements and detailed examination of the fetus. Despite the attention these two problems deserve, there remains much valuable clinical information to be produced by a general survey at the beginning of each obstetric examination. Chapters on amniotic fluid volume and the placenta cover some of this material and should be reviewed in conjunction with this chapter.

The general survey is today most often done with real-time equipment. Although this provides for greater speed and ease of examination than did older static B-scan equipment, it is extremely important for the examiner to use a systematic approach to assure that all of the appropriate areas are imaged. A random placement of the transducer with the goal of seeing the fluid, placenta, and fetus is to be discouraged. One of many systematic approaches is to begin in the midline with a sagittal scan plane, with the transducer just cephalad to the symphysis pubis, and examine all adjacent areas by rocking the transducer to either side. The transducer can then be moved to a more cephalic position and the rocking motion repeated. Repositioning the transducer along this sagittal line should be done until all uterine and pelvic contents are examined. Then a right and a left parasagittal scan series can be performed in a similar manner. After the sagittal series, transverse views can be taken essentially by turning the transducer 90 degrees and slowly sliding it along each of the sagittal scan planes. In addition to determining placental location and fluid volume and counting the number of fetuses, it is important to be sure that certain areas have either been seen or a strong attempt made to visualize them. These areas include the uterine cervix, the umbilical cord (especially the insertions of the cord into both the placenta and the fetus), the retroplacental area and margins of the placenta, the uterine wall, and the adnexal regions. In some cases it is useful to examine the maternal kidneys, although this is not recommended as part of the obstetric routine. The following discussion deals with some of the important findings that can be discovered in this survey.

TWINS

Because suspected twins and a uterus that is large for dates are both indications for obstetric sonograms, the finding of multiple gestation is not unusual. Because of selective referral this is seen by the sonographer with somewhat more frequency than the usual 1 in 90 reported incidence. The actual incidence of twins varies in different locations from as often as 1 in 30 to as rare as 1 in 200 pregnancies. This variation is due to the different frequencies of dizygotic twins, which vary with race, increasing age, increasing parity, and use of certain drugs. The frequency of monozygotic twins is relatively uniform at about 1 in 250 pregnancies.

Most twins are separated by a membrane, which the sonographer should make every attempt to visualize (Fig. 135–1). In all dizygotic twins and in monozygotic twins with early division of the zygote, the membrane consists of two layers of chorion and two layers of amnion. If the twinning occurs after implantation for monozygotic twins, the membrane consists of only two layers of amnion. Rarely with very late twinning there is no amniotic membrane between the embryos. This monoamniotic condition probably occurs in less than 1 per cent of all twins.

Thus in the first trimester most twins are identified as being present in two separate gestational sacs. If they appear to be contained in one sac, the very thin amnion that will form a separating membrane should be looked for. Positive diagnosis of monoamniotic twins can be made only when no separating membrane is seen and crossing or interlocking of fetal parts is seen that would not be possible if a separating membrane were present.

Because a membrane occurs in all dizygotic twins and most monozygotic twins, presence of a membrane does not distinguish between these two conditions. The presence of two placentas sepa-

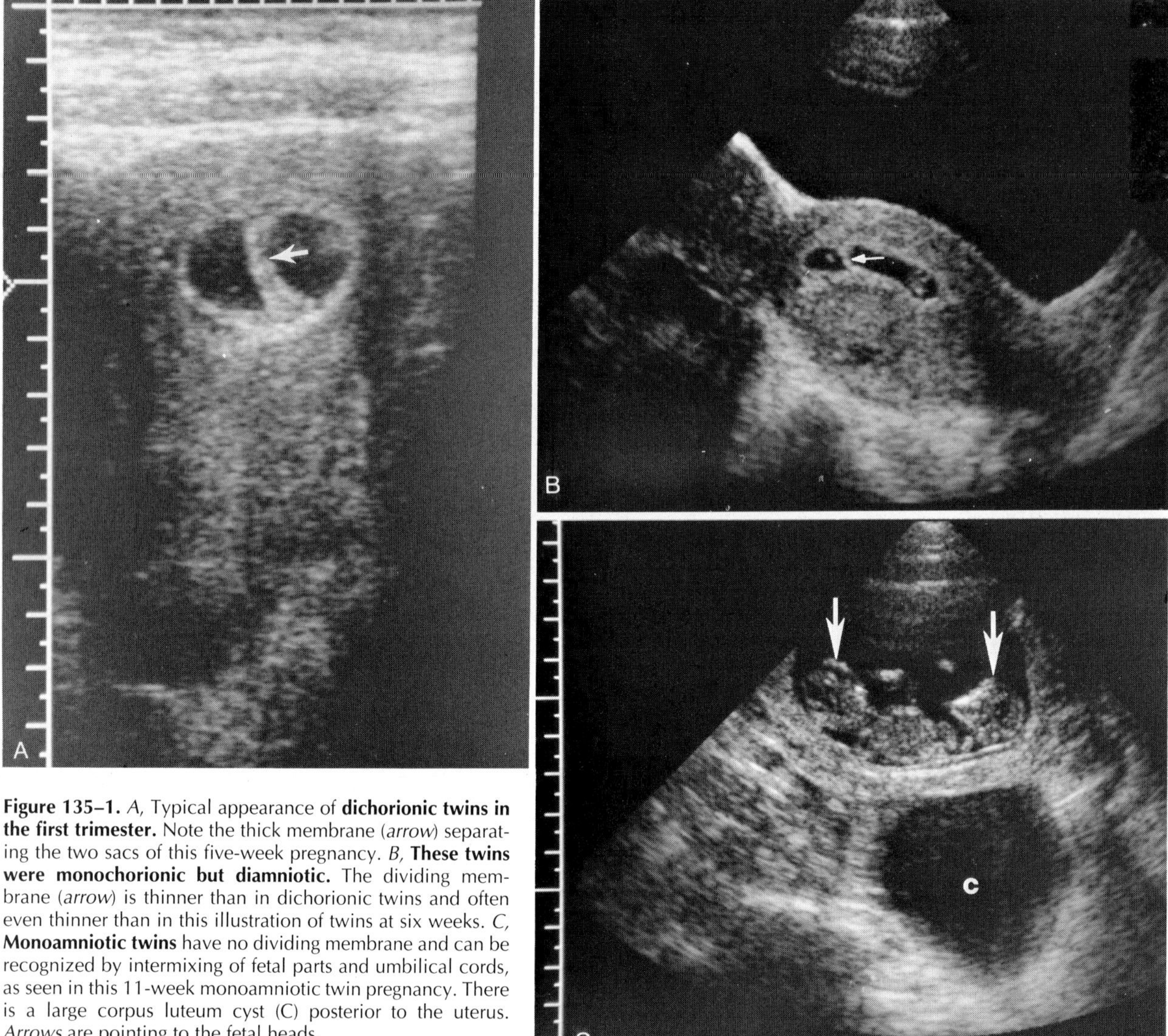

Figure 135–1. *A,* Typical appearance of **dichorionic twins in the first trimester.** Note the thick membrane (*arrow*) separating the two sacs of this five-week pregnancy. *B,* **These twins were monochorionic but diamniotic.** The dividing membrane (*arrow*) is thinner than in dichorionic twins and often even thinner than in this illustration of twins at six weeks. *C,* **Monoamniotic twins** have no dividing membrane and can be recognized by intermixing of fetal parts and umbilical cords, as seen in this 11-week monoamniotic twin pregnancy. There is a large corpus luteum cyst (C) posterior to the uterus. *Arrows* are pointing to the fetal heads.

rate from each other suggests diamniotic dichorionic twins but does not distinguish between monozygotic and dizygotic twins. The only way we know to positively make this distinction by sonography prenatally is to identify one twin to be of a different sex than the other, which indicates dizygotic twins.

However, the presence of a membrane is important to note because of the much greater risk of monoamniotic twins for cord accidents, twin-to-twin transfusions, and difficult deliveries because of locking of one twin to the other. More importantly, the failure to identify a membrane may be a result of marked oligohydramnios in one amniotic space. When this occurs the membrane is collapsed around one twin and difficult to identify (Fig. 135–2). In the absence of a clearly seen membrane this condition should be suspected and both fetuses watched to see if they are clearly moving freely in the amniotic fluid. If one seems to stay in a relatively fixed position, it should be watched while the maternal position is changed. If this does not stimulate a significant repositioning of the fetus, it should be studied in detail for the presence of membrane closely applied to it. This is a highly significant finding that is virtually diagnostic of fetal distress of the affected twin. Often, if followed serially, the other twin will develop polyhydramnios and fetal hydrops. When this happens it is likely that the underlying mechanism is a twin-to-twin transfusion.

Growth patterns of twins and of multiple gestations in general are poorly understood. Because most twins are dizygotic, it is usual to find some discrepancy in growth between the two fetuses as the pregnancy progresses. Even when this occurs in monozygotic twins it is not clear that it represents an abnormal growth pattern. Various sonographic standards have been suggested to diagnose twin "discordance," but our policy has been to look at each fetus individually for evidence of growth retardation. If one has sonographic criteria for growth retardation but the other does not, this represents significant discordance in growth patterns.

Several investigators have suggested that different growth standards be used for twins than for singleton pregnancies. This is because as a group, twins tend to have less growth in the third trimester and are associated with a much greater incidence of growth retardation as well as prematurity. The danger of using such special charts for twins is that it may reduce our sensitivity to growth retardation and fetal distress.

Singleton growth standards should be applied to twins whenever gestational age is well established, and every effort should be made to establish this when twins are a clinical possibility. There is some possible advantage in using growth parameters developed specially for twins when the question is one of gestational age and the first ultrasound examination takes place in the third trimester. Because

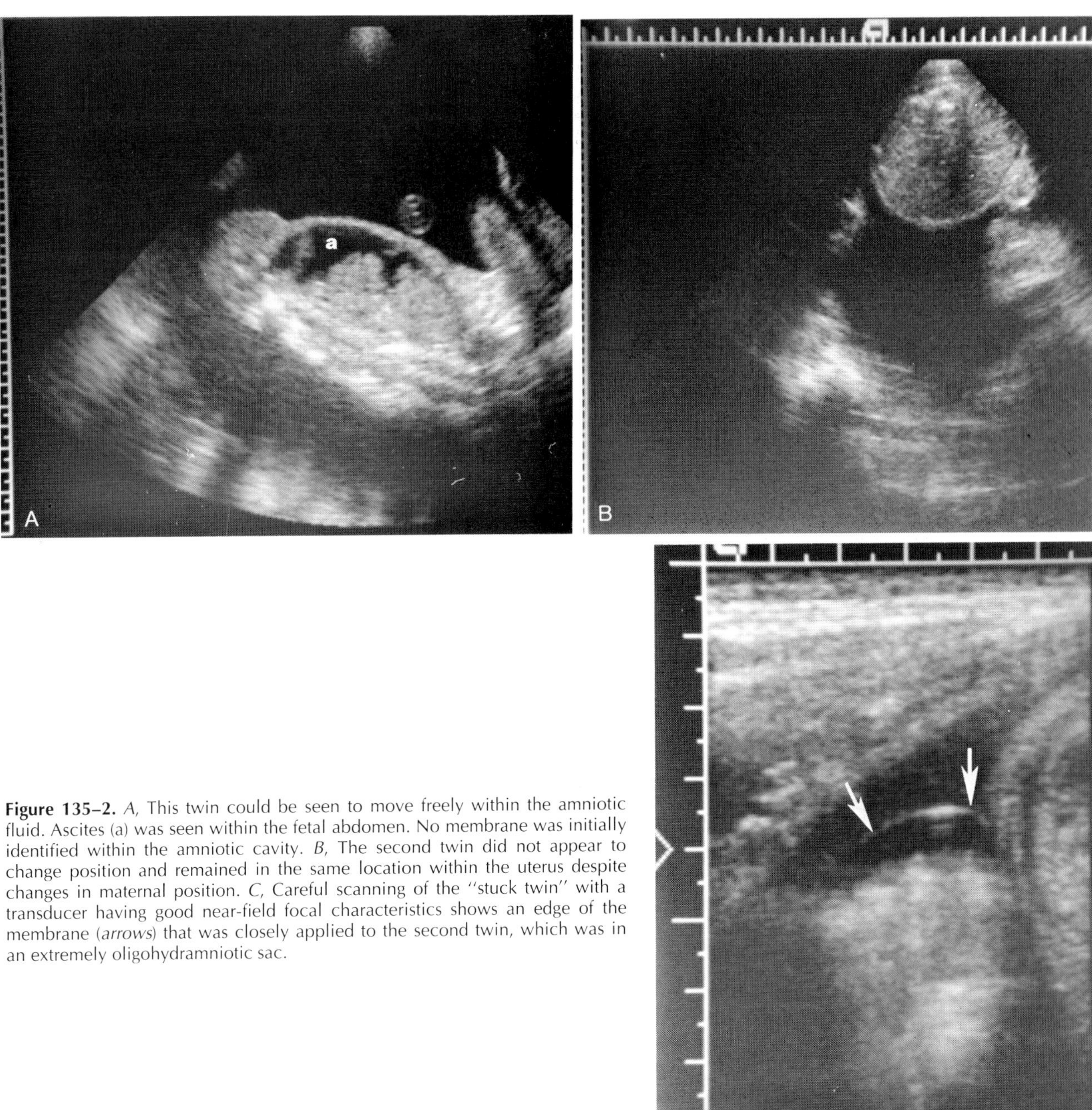

Figure 135–2. *A,* This twin could be seen to move freely within the amniotic fluid. Ascites (a) was seen within the fetal abdomen. No membrane was initially identified within the amniotic cavity. *B,* The second twin did not appear to change position and remained in the same location within the uterus despite changes in maternal position. *C,* Careful scanning of the "stuck twin" with a transducer having good near-field focal characteristics shows an edge of the membrane (*arrows*) that was closely applied to the second twin, which was in an extremely oligohydramniotic sac.

estimating gestational age is so difficult in these circumstances and other parameters are more important, it is unlikely the special charts for twins will improve the range of the estimated gestational age.

Much of what has been said about twins applies to cases of more than two fetuses. In these situations the majority of the fetuses are from different zygotes, although it is possible for the group to include a monozygotic pair. Different growth patterns are frequent and management of these pregnancies can be very difficult; severe prematurity is usually the end result.

FETAL POSITION

Determining fetal position is not difficult with current equipment. The sonographer generally needs only to describe the basic orientation of the fetus. The essential possibilities are head down, breech down, or transverse. The head down position is not synonymous with a vertex position and, in fact, the subtype of presentation can only be predicted when the patient is in labor and confirmed by physical examination. From a cephalic position, chin, brow, occiput, and vertex presentations are all possible, just as from a breech position, single or double footing as well as complete and frank breech presentations are all possible. Most of these presentations are self-explanatory, but the reader should be reminded that the frank breech occurs when both legs are extended. The single breech occurs when one leg is extended and one knee is flexed (this is also called an incomplete breech). The complete breech occurs when both knees are flexed (this is sometimes called a double breech). Because the actual presenting part cannot be predicted until labor begins, the sonographer should be satisfied to describe fetal position as cephalic, breech, or transverse.

The breech position is more often associated with a dolichocephalic head but has little significance until late in pregnancy. Transverse positions have been associated with a number of disorders, and the sonographer is obligated to look for them when this condition is observed. Among the possible disorders are fetal anomalies, uterine fibroids, and placenta previa.

UTERINE CERVIX

Study of the uterus properly should begin by seeing the uterine cervix. This structure appears as a solid mass of soft tissue projecting posteriorly from the uterus into the pelvis (Fig. 135–3). It can be visualized either through the urine-filled bladder or by using the amniotic fluid as an acoustic pathway. In the former case the cervix is invariably distorted by false elongation and reduction in anterior-posterior extent. Additionally, the full bladder can compress an abnormal internal os and prevent dilatation of the internal os from being visible sonographically. On the other hand, visualization of the cervix with an empty bladder using amniotic fluid as a window is difficult technically, becomes increasingly difficult as the pregnancy progresses, and is almost impossible in cases of severe oligohydramnios. Every effort should be made to visualize the cervix through the amniotic fluid with an empty bladder prior to 26 weeks of gestation and after that time, either with a partially filled bladder or empty bladder as is necessary.

The undistorted cervix, with an empty maternal bladder, is roughly square in shape. The endocervical canal measured from the internal os to a line projected along the posterior vagina is from 2.2 to 4 cm in length. If it is greater than 4 cm some degree of distortion, due to either bladder filling or myometrial contraction, can be assumed to be occurring, and if it is under 2.2 cm it is abnormally short. This latter condition we have seen most often in women exposed to DES as a fetus or in women with pregnancies consistent with ''incompetent'' cervix. Large tubular structures are frequently seen to either side of the cervix. These represent the enlarged tortuous pelvic veins returning blood from the uterus and placenta. A normal variant is the protruding cervix, which represents a myometrial contraction occurring at the internal os. ''Funneling'' of the internal os results in shortening of the endocervical canal and can be seen with an incompetent cervix and early labor (Fig. 135–4). Rarely nabothian cysts are seen in the cervix. Often these appear to be in the proximal vagina and should not be mistaken for vaginal fluid. These are benign inclusion cysts that can be seen in both pregnant and nonpregnant women.

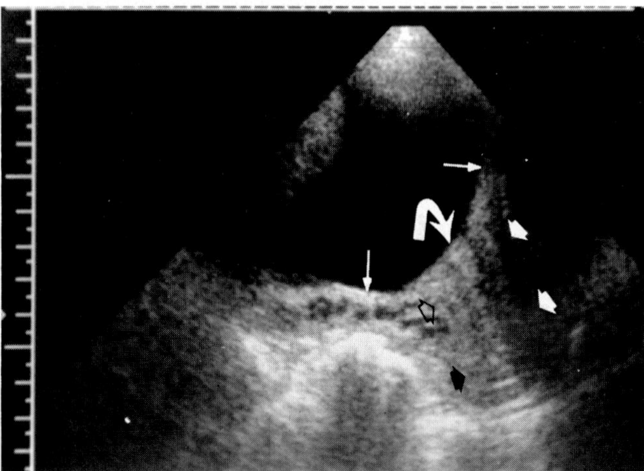

Figure 135–3. Longitudinal section through the lower uterus in a 28-week pregnancy. The cervix is the muscular portion of myometrium projecting posteriorly (*short arrows*). The internal os is marked by echogenic material (probably mucous/glandular interfaces) within the endocervical canal (*curved arrow*). The thin myometrium is seen extending away from the cervix (*arrows*). Behind the posterior myometrium are multiple uterine wall vessels, which are frequently seen near the cervix.

PLACENTA PREVIA

A primary reason to identify the cervix and especially the internal os is to determine the presence or absence of placenta previa. This condition exists when a portion of the placenta overlies the cervix and results in late second and third trimester vaginal bleeding. This usually occurs as a result of abruption of the placental portion overlying the cervix and can be life-threatening, especially during active labor. Prior to the use of sonography there was no really accurate technique to determine the presence of placenta previa other than by digital examination when the cervix was dilated enough. This necessitated rather carefully controlled circumstances that permitted the prompt administration of intravascular volume expanders and emergency cesarean section.

Sonography has changed a great deal of this. Careful demonstration of the internal os and surrounding cervix with no placenta covering this area virtually completely excludes the possibility of a placenta previa. This is what sonographic examination does best. False-negative studies do occur but are almost always a result of failure to visualize this area completely. There are two common ways this happens. First, the placenta can be located along one side of the uterus but only the lower anterior or posterior border is seen owing to inadequate sonographic examination technique. Because the visualized placental margin is away from the region of the cervix, the absence of a placenta previa is assumed. Because the cervix itself is not visualized, the more central laterally placed position of the placenta that crosses it is not identified. In the second circumstance, the cervix is also not seen and the lower margin of the placenta is identified some distance away from it. In this case there will be an accessory lobe (succenturiate) of the placenta which crosses a portion of the cervix. The key steps to diagnosing placenta previa are, in both of these situations, to find the lowest margin of the placenta and to visualize the internal os of the cervix. When both cannot be shown clearly, then some element of doubt must remain.

Because of the importance of seeing the cervix with suspected placenta previa, it is often necessary to use Trendelenburg's position, or, with the obstetrician's help, to elevate the lower fetal body part. If it is not possible to safely do this, demonstration that the body part is closely applied to the cervix is presumptive evidence against placenta previa. If the placenta is posterior, another useful landmark is the sacral prominence. If the fetal parts are less than 1.5 cm from this, it can be assumed that no placenta is interposed. The converse assumptions are somewhat more tenuous because fetal parts may not be immediately adjacent to the cervix or may be more than 1.5 cm from the sacral promontory in the absence of any intervening tissue or that tissue may not be placenta (e.g., a fetal limb or uterine leiomyomata). The definitive diagnosis can be made only when the cervix, its internal os, and the lower margin of placenta are seen.

Much confusion seems to exist concerning false-positive diagnosis of placenta previa with ultrasound. This is due in part to the high frequency of false-positive diagnoses of placenta previa. It has been shown recently that the great majority of these false-positive diagnoses are a result of compression of the lower uterus by a distended maternal urinary bladder. The remainder of the false-positive diagnoses are almost all a result of distortion of the lower uterus by myometrial contractions. These are often difficult to recognize and their distorting influence is apparent only when patients are studied for a long time (one to two hours) during one visit or serially over several days. Because some degree of elongation and

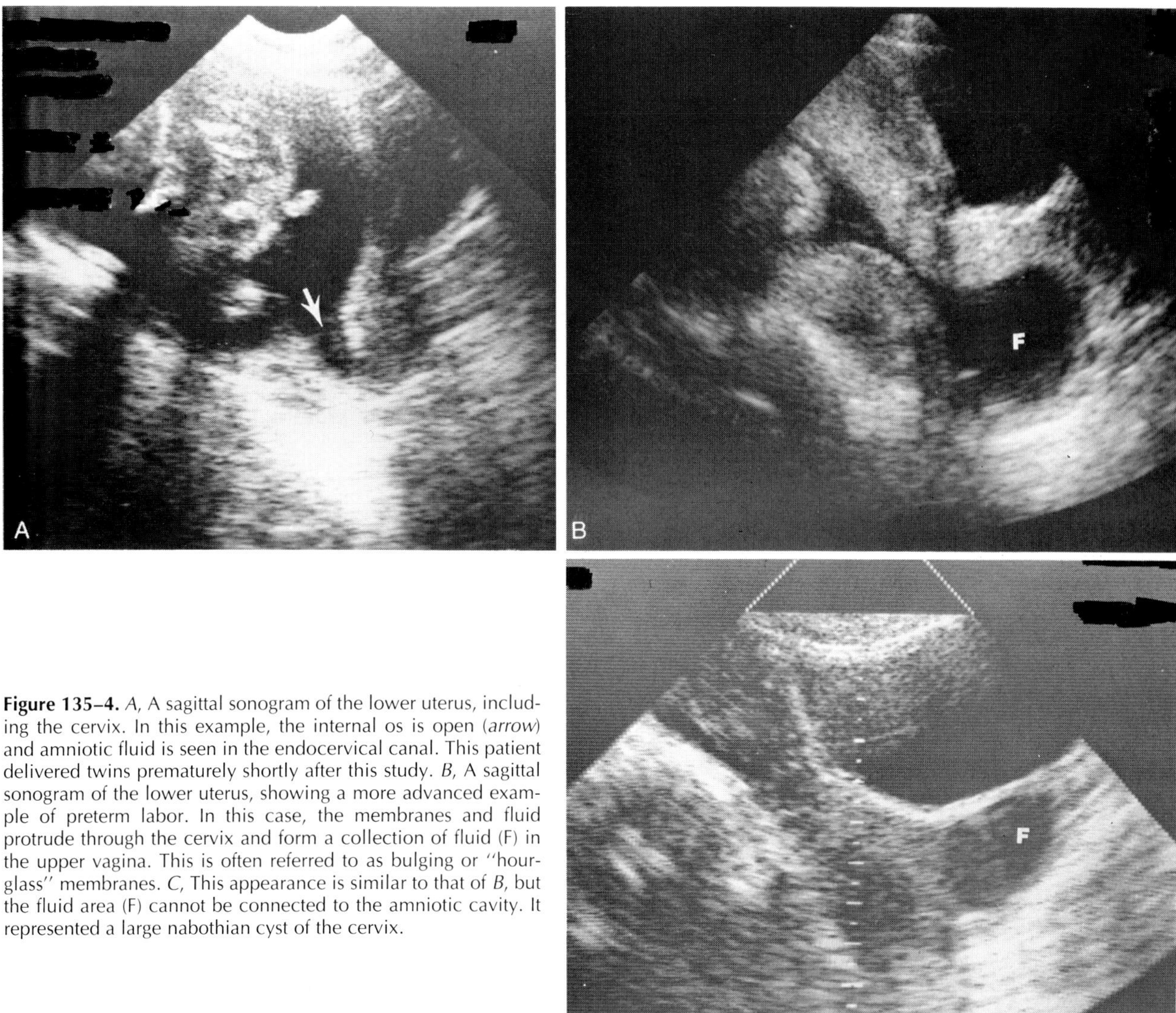

Figure 135–4. *A*, A sagittal sonogram of the lower uterus, including the cervix. In this example, the internal os is open (*arrow*) and amniotic fluid is seen in the endocervical canal. This patient delivered twins prematurely shortly after this study. *B*, A sagittal sonogram of the lower uterus, showing a more advanced example of preterm labor. In this case, the membranes and fluid protrude through the cervix and form a collection of fluid (F) in the upper vagina. This is often referred to as bulging or "hourglass" membranes. *C*, This appearance is similar to that of *B*, but the fluid area (F) cannot be connected to the amniotic cavity. It represented a large nabothian cyst of the cervix.

thinning of the lower uterus undoubtedly occurs as pregnancy advances, a placenta that is only a few millimeters away from the cervix in the early second trimester can be several centimeters away at term. This should not be referred to as "placental migration" or "dynamic placentation." Because the uterus is relatively smaller and myometrial thinning has not occurred, the distorting influences of bladder filling and myometrial contractions are greater early in pregnancy than later. Thus, a false-positive ultrasound is more likely when the distances involved approach the resolution of the equipment and, in fact, are mostly a phenomenon of early pregnancy.

Taking care to examine the cervix with an empty bladder and in the absence of myometrial contractions almost eliminates false-positive diagnosis of placenta previa in early pregnancy. The remainder are usually recognized with subsequent scans, which are recommended after any diagnosis of placenta previa. Myometrial contractions away from the cervix are recognized by their failure to bulge the external contour of the uterus, by the fact that they are more echogenic than typical leiomyomata, and by their transient nature. When they involve the region of the cervix they appear to elongate the cervix and should be suspected whenever the endocervical canal measures more than 4 cm with an empty bladder. They can also be recognized when the myometrium appears focally thicker where it joins the cervix than in another area such as the fundus. Care should be taken to identify leiomyomata as a focal cause of myometrial thickening (Fig. 135–5).

Classifications of placenta previa have traditionally been based on physical examination. We have proposed a classification based on the sonographic findings (Fig. 135–6). By defining the margin of the cervix internally as the projection of a line parallel to its exterior side and identifying the edge of the internal os as a projection of the border of the endocervical canal, these landmarks can be used. If the placental edge touches but does not cross the margin of the cervix, this is a low-lying placenta. If the placenta crosses this margin but not the border of the internal os, this is a marginal placenta previa. If one border of the internal os but not the other is crossed, this is a partial placenta previa. If both sides of the internal os are crossed, this is a complete placenta previa. These can be further subdivided into posterior, anterior, etc., and central complete previa. Because low-lying placentas and some marginal placenta previas may deliver vaginally, this is a useful distinction, but even marginal placenta previa can be associated with significant hemorrhage.

After evaluation of the cervix, the entire uterine wall should be examined to the extent possible. Some of the useful information in distinguishing focal myometrial contractions from uterine leiomyo-

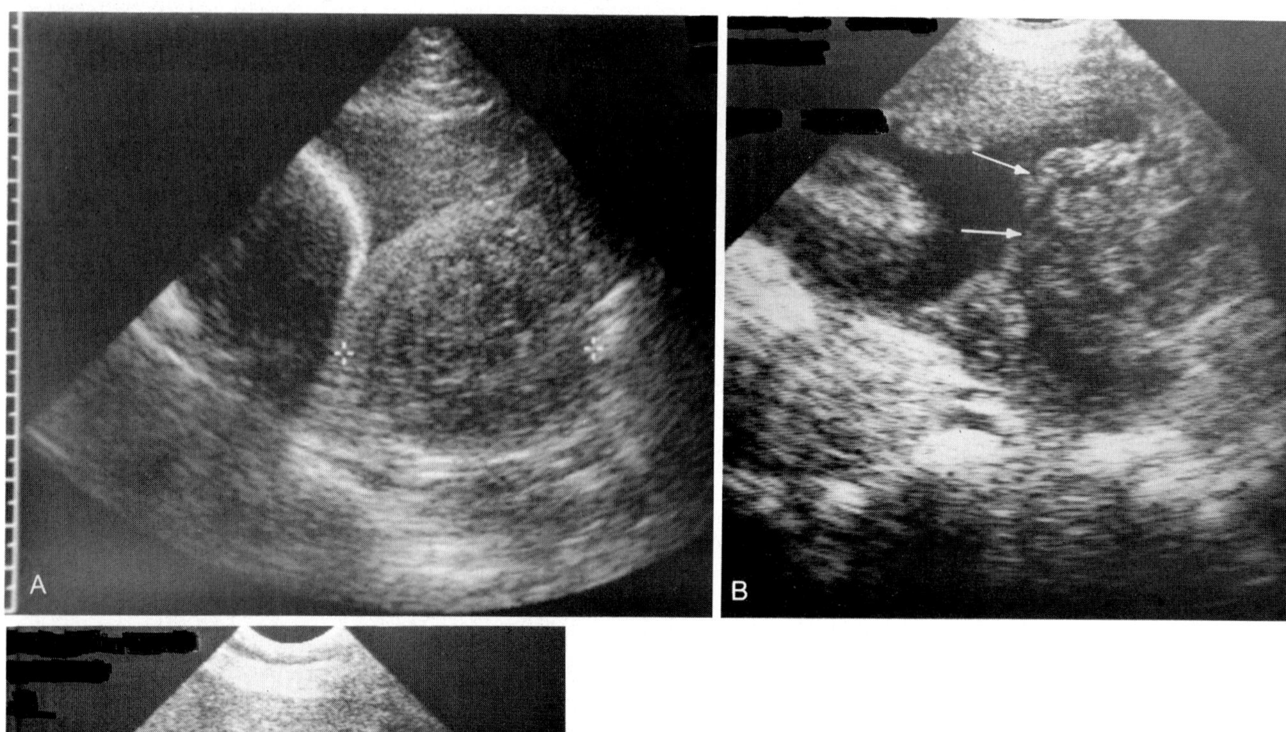

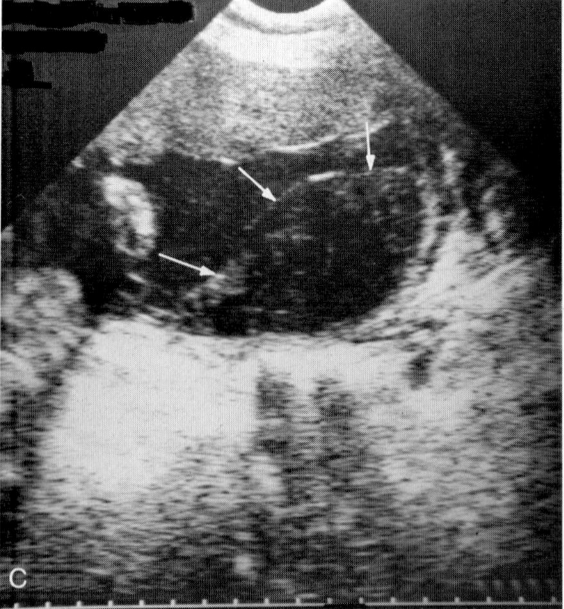

Figure 135–5. *A,* A **large leiomyoma** *(between asterisks)* is seen in the lower uterus. Without careful inspection, this could be mistaken for a portion of placenta and the false-positive diagnosis of placenta previa given. *B,* Echogenic material (*arrows*) extending into the lower uterus could be mistaken for placenta. During real-time study, this had a "gelatinous" movement when struck by the fetus. *C,* The same echogenic area (*arrows*) as in *B* one week later. This clot from a placental abruption is now hypoechoic, and the margin of the anterior placenta is easier to identify.

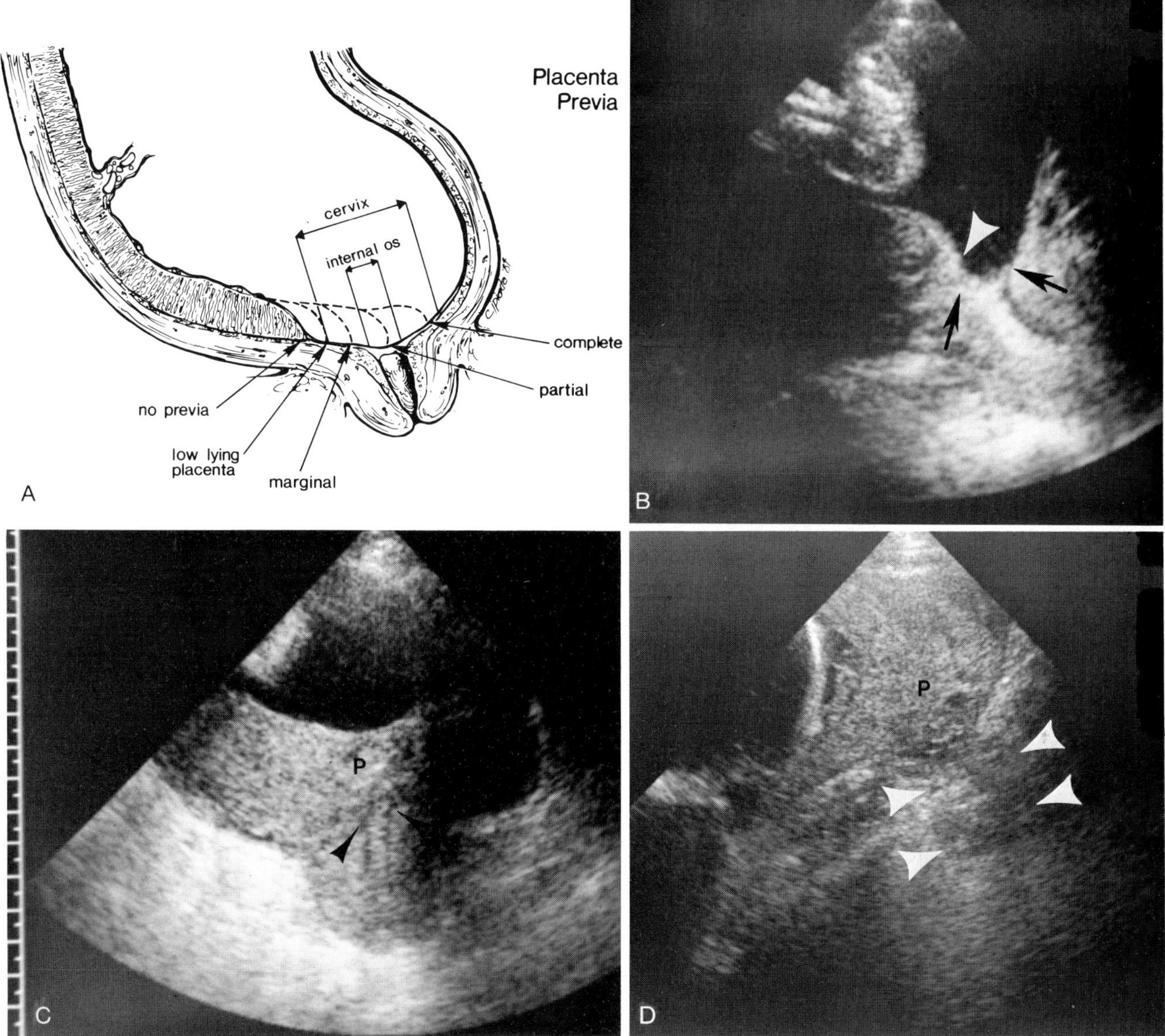

Figure 135–6. *A,* Diagram for our system of evaluating extent of placenta previa with an empty bladder. The outer lines establish the outer margins of the cervix and the inner lines the margins of the internal os. *B,* Example of a partial placenta previa. The edge of the placenta (*arrowhead*) just crosses the edge of the internal os (*arrows*). *C,* Example of a posterior complete placenta previa. The placenta (P) completely crosses both edges of the internal os (*arrows*). *D,* Example of a central complete placenta previa. The placenta (P) completely fills the lower uterus. Only part of the cervix (*arrowheads*) can be seen, and the endocervical canal is not well shown.

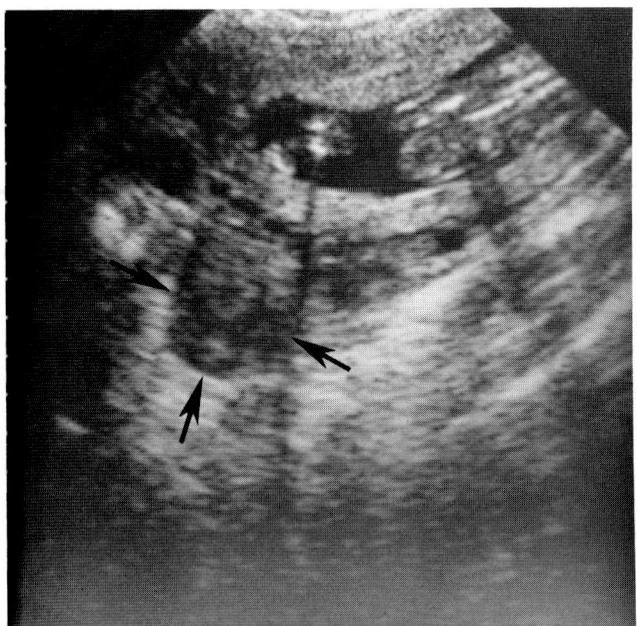

Figure 135–7. Note the large mass seen posterior to the uterus (*arrows*). This proved to be a **uterine leiomyoma.**

mata has already been given. This distinction is of prognostic significance because the presence of focal contractions is a normal phenomenon and that of leiomyomata is a significant risk to the outcome of the pregnancy. Leiomyomata are frequently more hypoechoic than usual in the pregnant uterus, but the echogenicity is highly variable (Fig. 135–7). Nevertheless, they account for virtually all solid masses of the pregnant uterine wall. The size, number, and location of these masses should be noted. Even though some of these will grow with advancing pregnancy, most do not change significantly. There is an increased incidence of both placental abruption and premature labor in patients with leiomyomata in pregnancy. The risks for both phenomena are greater when a leiomyoma is present with a diameter over 3 cm or when leiomyomata are present in a subplacental position.

PELVIC MASSES

The other common mass to be seen during an initial survey is a cystic pelvic mass. These are usually the result of a corpus luteum cyst of pregnancy and are recognized in up to 40 per cent of normal pregnancies by sonography in the first trimester. These are usually simple cysts, less than 5 cm in diameter, but they may have thick walls, occasional septations, or internal echoes, and rarely are up to 10 to 12 cm in diameter. Because cystic tumors can be discovered in pregnant women as well as nonpregnant women, differentiation of normal corpus luteum cysts from a possible tumor is difficult. Certainly a larger size and presence of internal structure make any pelvic mass more likely to be neoplastic. The recommendation in the majority of cases in which a pelvic mass is seen is to monitor the mass by a study at 14 weeks. If the mass persists or has enlarged, it is very suspicious and after one more month, surgical exploration is suggested to determine the nature of the mass.

Bibliography

Artis AA, Bowie JD, Rosenberg ER, Rauch RF: The fallacy of placental migration: Effect of sonographic techniques. AJR 144:79–81, 1985.

Barss VA, Benacerraf BR, Frigoletto FD: Ultrasonographic determination of chorion type in twin gestation. Obstet Gynecol 66:779–783, 1985.

Leopold GE: Antepartum obstetrical ultrasound examination guidelines. J Ultrasound Med 5:241–242, 1986.

Persson PH, Kullander S: Long-term experience of general ultrasound screening in pregnancy. Am J Obstet Gynecol 8:942–947, 1983.

136 Postpartum Sonography

Beatrice L. Madrazo and Mark E. Baker

NORMAL SONOGRAPHIC ANATOMY

During the early stages of our clinical research on the value of sonography in the postpartum period, we evaluated 25 asymptomatic patients who had undergone spontaneous vaginal deliveries. Evaluation of this group of patients allowed us to establish the normal sonographic parameters for the postpartum uterus. Table 136–1 lists these values.

Sonographic evaluation of the postpartum uterus is easily accomplished owing to the large uterine size and its anterior and cephalad position outside of the pelvis proper. The postpartum uterus exhibits homogeneous, medium-intensity echoes throughout its walls. Oc-

TABLE 136–1. NORMAL SONOGRAPHIC PARAMETERS OF THE POSTPARTUM UTERUS

Parity	No. of Patients	Normal Values	Uterine Size (cm) L	AP	W	End. Cavity (cm) AP Thickness	Uterine Wall (cm)
Primipara	20	Range	16.5–25	7–10	8.5–14	0.5–1.2	3–5
Multipara	14	Range	19–22	7–11	9–13.5	0.5–1.3	4.1–6.5

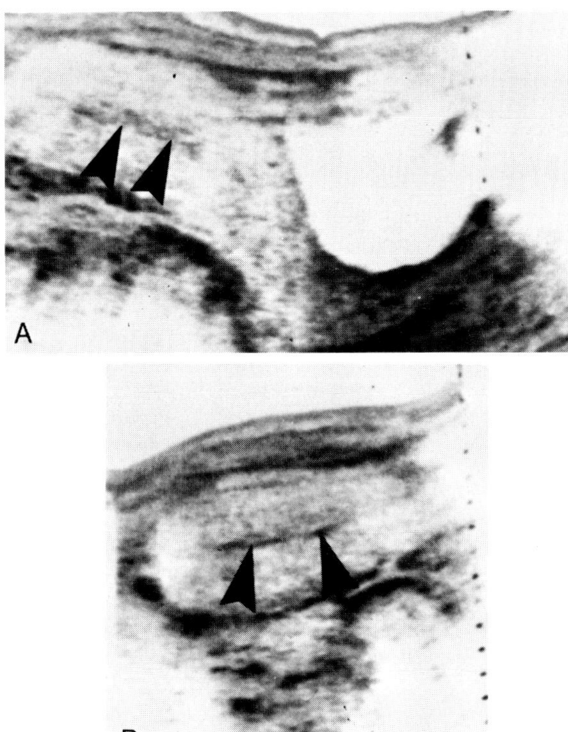

Figure 136–1. Normal postpartum uterus. Longitudinal (*A*) and transverse (*B*) pelvic sonograms show the collapsed uterine cavity as a thick echogenic stripe *(arrowheads)*.

casionally tubular, round, or ovoid areas of sonolucency are present in the myometrium representing the enlarged myometrial vessels. The endometrial cavity is seen by sonography as a central linear group of echoes of higher intensity than the myometrium (Fig. 136–1). Early in the post-delivery period, a small amount of echo-free (fluid) or echogenic material (blood clots) may be present within the uterine cavity. This results in a small degree of separation of the cavity walls, but in our experience with normal post-delivery patients, the separation of the cavity walls never exceeded 13 mm. No focal areas of enlargement of the cavity should exist. The previous site of placental implantation cannot be discriminated from other surface areas of the endometrial cavity. Only small amounts of endometrial cavity air should be seen one to two days postpartum, unless instrumentation has occurred.

Over 200 postpartum patients have been evaluated with sonography at our institution. We have visualized the broad ligaments on an occasional patient but have failed to visualize the ovaries in all these patients. We postulate that this lack of display of the ovaries is due to their extrapelvic position and obscuration by gas-filled bowel loops. In our series of normal post-delivery patients, only one patient had visible fluid in the posterior cul-de-sac, of a small amount.

Sonographic evaluation of the post–cesarean section uterus requires knowledge of the surgical technique. Currently, the lower uterine segment transverse incision is the most common form of cesarean section. In most institutions, the abdominal incision is a low transverse approach. The abdominal wall layers (i.e., subcutaneous tissue, anterior rectus fascia, and peritoneum) are rapidly opened. The lower uterine segment is visualized, and the peritoneal fold between the uterine serosa and bladder serosa is identified. This is elevated and incised. Using blunt dissection, one elevates the posterior wall of the bladder away from the uterus, exposing the lower uterine segment where a transverse incision is made. After delivery, the uterine wound is closed using a continuous lock stitch in both the deep and superficial layers (a first and second layer closure). Then the peritoneum is closed, with the rectus fascia and subcutaneous tissues following.

Normally, the abdominal wound should show no mass in the subcutaneous space. It is important to assess this space with a high-frequency transducer with a short focal zone or, if unavailable, using a water bath technique. The uterine wound interposed between the posterior aspect of the bladder and the anterior portion of the lower uterine segment can, with practice, be easily identified as an oval, relatively homogeneous region of different echogenicity (i.e., increased or decreased) when compared with the uterine myometrium (Fig. 136–2). This region is symmetrical and oval and measures approximately 3 to 5 cm in lateral dimension, 1 to 2 cm in AP dimension, and 3 to 5 cm in longitudinal length. Within this area, focal, quite small areas of high-amplitude echoes with distal shadowing may be seen; these represent sutures. It has been our experience that findings compatible with gas are not normally present within the endometrial scar. As for the uterus itself, endometrial cavity gas is not normal, two days following cesarean section, unless the patient has been recently instrumented (postpartum dilatation and curettage [D&C], endometrial biopsy/culture). Cul-de-sac fluid is not routinely visualized following cesarean section.

POSTPARTUM HEMORRHAGE

During delivery and the first two hours thereafter, the average blood loss is approximately 500 ml. A blood loss in excess of 500

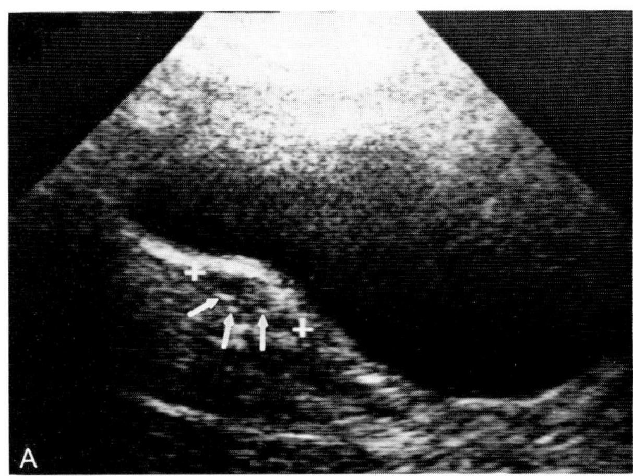

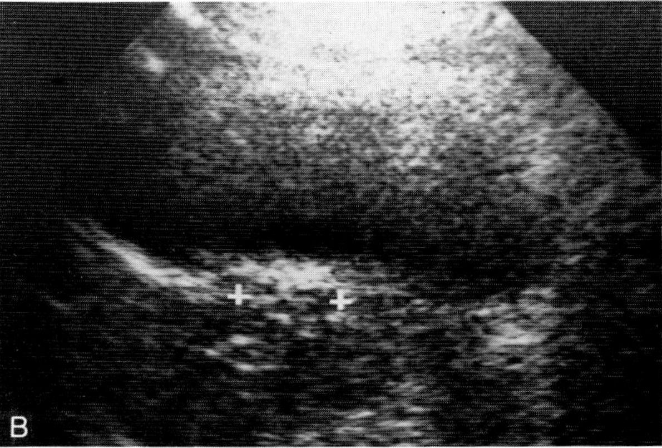

Figure 136–2. Normal, post–low-transverse incision, cesarean section. Longitudinal (*A*) and transverse (*B*) pelvic sonograms show the uterine incision site (between +'s) as an oval symmetrical area of different echogenicity when compared with adjacent uterus. Bright echoes (*arrows*) within the incision represent sutures.

TABLE 136–2. POSTPARTUM HEMORRHAGE—PREDISPOSING FACTORS

1. Malnutrition
2. Toxemia of pregnancy
3. Multiparity
4. Uterine overdistention (large fetus, multiple pregnancy, hydramnios)
5. Prolonged labor
6. General anesthesia
7. Intrauterine manipulations
8. Rapid delivery
9. Blood coagulopathy
10. Use of estrogens to suppress lactation

ml is by definition postpartum hemorrhage. The reported incidence of this complication is variable, ranging from 1 to 4 per cent.

Table 136–2 lists predisposing factors to postpartum hemorrhage. Excessive uterine enlargement such as might occur with multiple gestation, large fetus, or pregnancy associated with hydramnios may result in uterine overdistention and failure of uterine contraction following delivery. Other factors such as toxemia, prolonged labor, rapid delivery, and uterine manipulations are also implicated as causative factors in postpartum hemorrhage. Occasionally, a blood coagulopathy may result in hemorrhage owing to copious bleeding from the placental implantation site.

Following separation of the placenta from the endometrium, the natural uterine involution following delivery serves to control the bleeding from the implantation site. Local factors at the level of the bleeding myometrial vessels lead to the development of thrombi with resulting occlusion of their lumen and involution of these vessels. These hemostatic events will occur and control the bleeding provided that all events take place in their normal sequence: uterine contraction, thrombosis of myometrial vessels, and healing of the implantation site. Any factor or factors that interfere with this normal series of events (such as retained products of conception, infection, and failure of the uterus to contract) result in postpartum hemorrhage.

By far the two most common causes of postpartum hemorrhage are uterine atony and retained products of conception. A third and less severe cause of postpartum hemorrhage is undetected laceration of the cervix, vagina, or perineum.

Uterine atony refers to failure of the uterus to contract following delivery of the fetus, placenta, and membranes. Immediately following delivery, the uterine fundus descends from its subxiphoid position to attain a position just cephalad to the umbilicus. During the first week postpartum, uterine weight decreases from 1000 to 500 g, and the uterus descends further toward the pelvis, lying midway between the umbilicus and the symphysis pubis. Sonographically, an atonic uterus is indistinguishable from the normal involuting, postpartum uterus.

The presence of an enlarged, soft uterus following delivery in a patient with hemorrhage is managed by external uterine massage and compression of the uterus in an attempt to expel from the cavity any retained products of conception or blood clots. If these maneuvers fail to control the hemorrhage, intravenous infusion of oxytocic drugs is used to induce uterine contraction. True uterine atony is a self-limiting process that usually responds to external uterine massage and administration of oxytocic drugs.

Persistence of uterine hemorrhage following these standard forms of management for post-delivery bleeding suggests that an associated problem exists. In most cases, the hemorrhage is secondary to retained products of conception within the uterine cavity. Retention of placental fragments, blood clots, or secundines (membranes) will lead to postpartum hemorrhage.

Sonography is a noninvasive imaging method that can rapidly assess the uterine cavity for retained products of conception. Table 136–3 lists the sonographic findings seen in patients with postpartum hemorrhage secondary to retained products of conception.

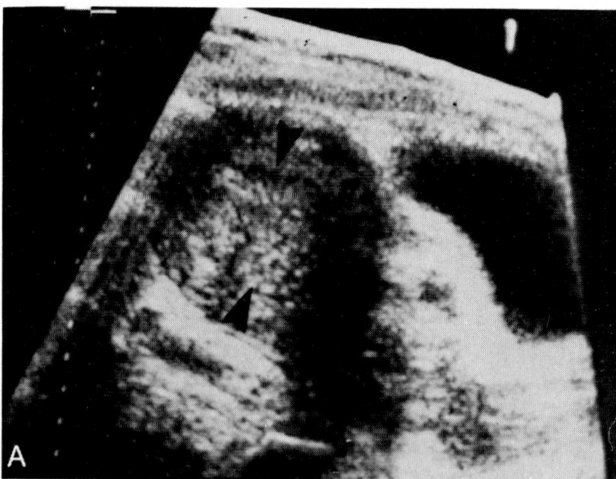

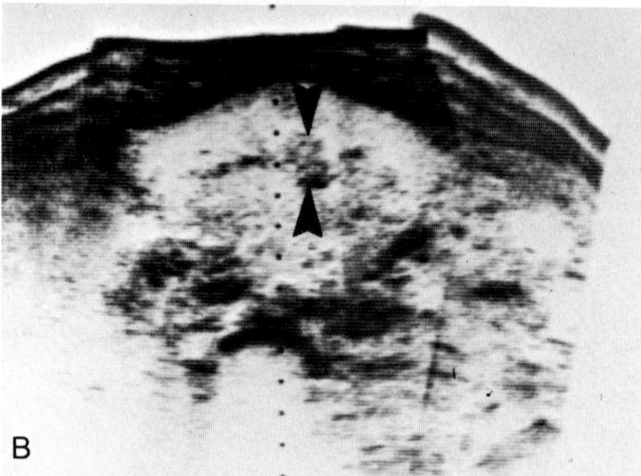

Figure 136–3. Retained products of conception. Longitudinal (*A*) and transverse (*B*) pelvic sonograms of different patients show expansion of the uterine cavity by an echogenic mass (*arrowheads*). In *A*, note the stippled echo pattern of fragment.

Discrete retained placental fragments present as echogenic round or oval intracavitary areas with a stippled echo pattern (Fig. 136–3). A less echogenic rim may be seen peripheral to the placental fragment. Associated findings include acoustic shadowing (lack of sound transmission) due to calcifications within the retained placental piece, fluid, and gas pockets. Lysis of the placental piece may occur, and a mixture of echogenic and echo-free areas may coexist.

It becomes almost impossible to differentiate a retained placental fragment from blood clots, and vice versa. However, the useful clinical information obtained by sonography is that the cause of hemorrhage is the presence of retained material in the uterine cavity, be it placental fragments, blood clots, and/or secundines.

In addition to infection, a relatively common complication from cesarean section occurs secondary to inadequate hemostasis. If the lower uterine segment incision is extended too far laterally into abundant vessels, bleeding may not stop. In addition, any bleeding in the uterine wound will be contained in the extraperitoneal space

TABLE 136–3. SONOGRAPHIC APPEARANCE OF RETAINED PLACENTAL FRAGMENTS

1. Echogenic intracavitary tissues, round or oval
2. Stippled echo pattern
3. Associated acoustic shadowing
4. Fluid within the uterine cavity

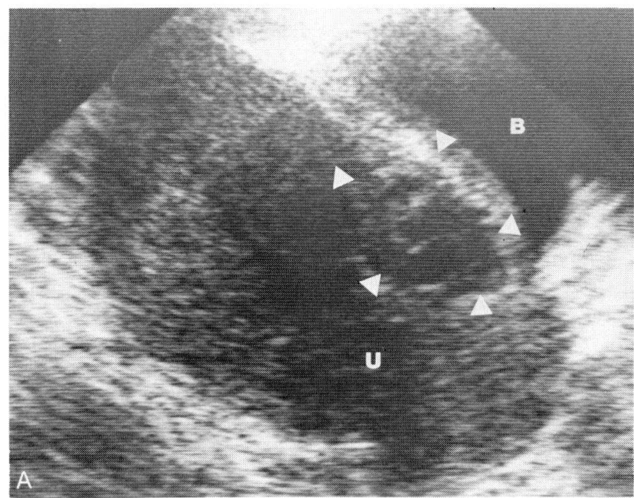

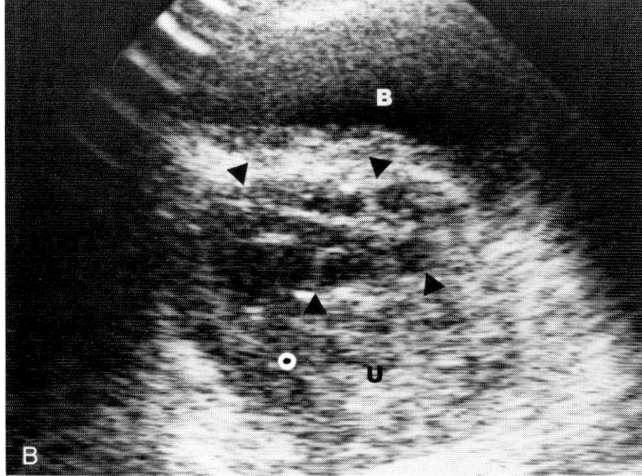

Figure 136–4. Bladder-flap hematoma. Longitudinal (*A*) and transverse (*B*) pelvic sonograms showing an oval/round complex mass (*arrowheads*) interposed between the lower uterine segment (U) and urinary bladder (B).

because the parietal peritoneum has been closed over the uterine wound. Small hematomas collect between the posterior wall of the bladder and the anterior portion of the lower uterine segment—the so-called bladder-flap hematoma. As they enlarge, they can extend laterally along the broad ligaments into the extraperitoneal pelvic fat or subperitoneally around the uterus itself. The most dreaded outcome is an infected hematoma that may require hysterectomy. Another relatively common site of a hematoma is the space between the parietal peritoneum and the rectus fascia in the abdominal wall wound—the so-called subfascial hematoma.

Sonographically, a bladder-flap hematoma presents as a rounded, complex, primarily hypoechoic mass asymmetrically interposed between the posterior wall of the bladder and the lower uterine segment (Fig. 136–4). It is quite well defined, often located at the edge of the incision site, and can be easily distinguished from the normal changes of the uterine wound. When large, it may extend laterally to involve the broad ligament, creating a large mass lateral to the uterus. Further extension into the extraperitoneal pelvis is difficult to assess using sonography, and in our experience CT better defines this. If gas is present within the mass, infection is strongly suggested and a percutaneous aspiration is recommended for confirmation. A subfascial hematoma presents sonographically as a complex mass posterior to the abdominal wall fascia/muscles but anterior to the uterus and bladder (Fig. 136–5). Because the peritoneal lining cannot be visualized, its posterior extent may not be well defined. The most important aspect of this is that it is not intraperitoneal. If infection is suspected, these hematomas are quite easily aspirated using sonographic guidance.

POSTPARTUM INFECTION

Postpartum infection is the most common complication following delivery. It has a reported incidence of 3 to 4 per cent in those patients who undergo spontaneous vaginal deliveries, and a 13 to 27 per cent incidence in the patient who has undergone cesarean section.

Several factors predispose to postpartum infections (Table 136–4). A malnourished, anemic patient is susceptible to infections owing to lack of adequate immune response. Pre-existing infections in the birth canal will be exacerbated following vaginal deliveries. Premature rupture of membranes, prolonged labor, intrapartum vaginal examination, and fetal monitoring are also predisposing factors for postpartum infections. The greater incidence of infections in the post-surgical patient is to be expected because surgical patients are prone to have infections as a postoperative complication.

A very important contributing factor for post-delivery infection is the lochial elimination during the puerperium. The vaginal milieu

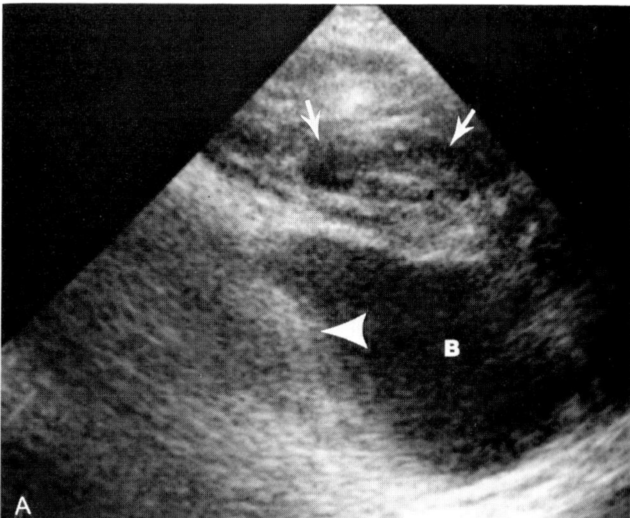

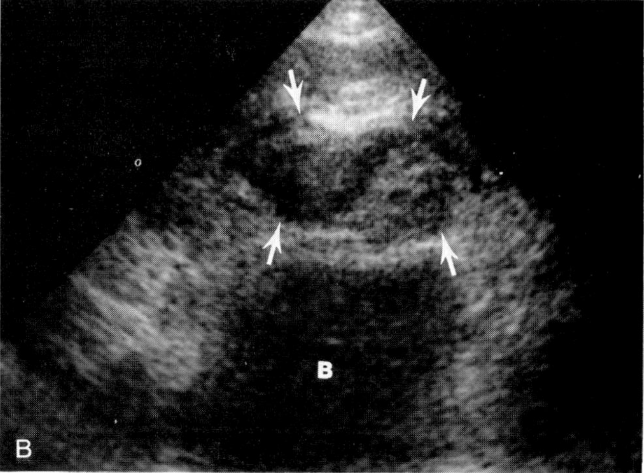

Figure 136–5. Subfascial hematoma. Longitudinal (*A*) and transverse (*B*) pelvic sonograms showing a complex mass (*arrows*) anterior to the urinary bladder (B). Note that the region of the bladder flap (*arrowhead*) is normal.

TABLE 136–4. PUERPERAL INFECTIONS—PREDISPOSING FACTORS

1. Anemia
2. Vaginitis-cervicitis
3. Poor nutrition and hygiene
4. Toxemia
5. Coitus late in pregnancy
6. Premature or early rupture of membranes
7. Prolonged labor and frequent vaginal examinations during labor
8. Intrapartum maternal and fetal monitoring
9. Manual removal of placenta
10. Retention of secundines
11. Lacerations (spontaneous or operative vaginal delivery)
12. Cesarean section

is normally acid, owing to the saprophytic presence of the *Lactobacillus acidophilus* (Doderlein bacilli). The elimination of lochia following delivery results in alkalinization of the vagina, leading to bacterial overgrowth. Ascent of these bacteria from the vagina into the uterine cavity results in infection. The thrombosed vessels at the former placental site of implantation serve as an excellent culture media for bacterial growth.

The most common bacterial groups seen in postpartum endometritis are anaerobic and aerobic streptococci, *Escherichia coli, Bacteroides,* and pyogenic streptococci. A mixed bacterial flora is usually found in cases of endometritis, and this is the rationale behind the use of broad-spectrum antibiotics in cases of postpartum infections.

The post-delivery febrile patient is clinically difficult to manage. Distinguishing between urinary tract infection and endometritis is not usually possible, and in cases of endometritis, blood cultures are seldom positive.

Over the past ten years, we have used sonography to evaluate febrile post-delivery patients. Patients were treated for 48 hours with broad-spectrum antibiotics, and those who showed no response to treatment or were readmitted to the hospital during the puerperium with suspected endometritis and/or wound infection were referred to our services for sonographic evaluation. Table 136–5 lists the sonographic findings in patients with endometritis.

Of the 98 patients evaluated, 77 had intracavitary uterine infections. In 31 patients, sonograms were normal. The clinical diagnosis and management of these patients were for endometritis. Their response to therapy is presumptive evidence that the source of infection was indeed the uterine cavity. We feel that this group of false-negative sonograms in these cases of endometritis represents

TABLE 136–5. SONOGRAPHIC FINDINGS IN PATIENTS WITH ENDOMETRITIS

CONDITION	NO. OF PATIENTS
Dilated uterine cavity with echogenic tissues	10
Dilated uterine cavity with echogenic tissues and gas	2
Dilated uterine cavity with fluid	22
Dilated uterine cavity with fluid and gas	2
Gas within uterine cavity	5
Normal uterine cavity with fluid in the cul-de-sac	3
Fluid collection around uterine incision	5
Gas within or around uterine incision	4
Hematoma in broad ligament	2
Hematoma or abscess formation in abdominal incision	11
Possible ovarian vein thrombophlebitis	1
Normal sonograms (false-negatives)	31
TOTAL	98

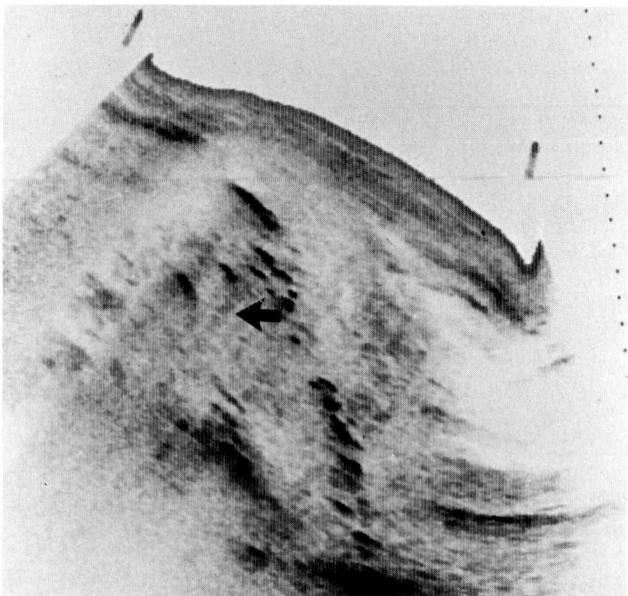

Figure 136–6. Endometritis. Transverse pelvic sonogram showing high-intensity intracavitary echoes with associated "ring down" (*arrow*) due to endometrial gas.

those cases of mild to moderate endometritis in which exudation was small, not resulting in either separation of the uterine cavity walls or retention of secretions within the cavity. Therefore, there was a lack of sonographic findings in this group of patients.

The other 46 patients had sonographic findings consistent with endometritis, such as dilated uterine cavity, intracavitary echogenic collections, fluid, and gas. Gas pockets are readily demonstrated on sonograms owing to their characteristic attenuating effects on sound transmission. Common gas-producing bacteria in cases of endometritis are *E. coli* and *Clostridium perfringens (welchii).* We always assess patients suspected of having endometritis by sonography prior to any surgical manipulations such as D&C. Figures 136–6 and 136–7 illustrate the sonographic findings in cases of endometritis.

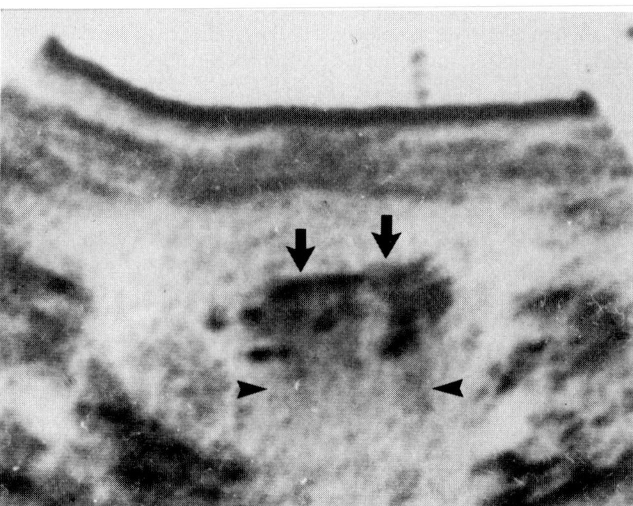

Figure 136–7. Endometritis with retained products of conception. Transverse pelvic sonogram showing high-intensity intracavitary echoes (*arrows*) with associated "ring down" (*arrowheads*). D&C revealed infected, retained products of conception.

In post-cesarean patients, endometrial infection is suspected when fluid and/or gas is present in the endometrial cavity. Infection of a bladder-flap or subfascial hematoma can be confirmed only by percutaneous aspiration, but the presence of gas within a hematoma is very suspicious.

As we have mentioned at the beginning of this chapter, in our experience with 25 uncomplicated postpartum patients we saw fluid in the cul-de-sac in one patient. In 3 of 98 patients with postpartum infection, fluid in the cul-de-sac was the only abnormality noted by sonography. We feel that these three patients with endometritis clinically had spillage of exudates from the uterine cavity via the fallopian tube into the peritoneal cavity. Another possible explanation would be production of a peritoneal exudate due to the presence of an infectious pelvic process.

CONCLUSION

The most significant contribution sonography makes to the care of the postpartum woman is in its ability to assess, in a noninvasive fashion, the uterine cavity for retained products of conception, endometritis, and infectious processes of the abdominal and uterine incisions of post-cesarean section patients.

Bibliography

Baker ME, Bowie JD, Killam AP: Sonography of post-cesarean section bladder-flap hematoma. AJR 144:757–759, 1985.

Baker ME, Kay HH, Mahony BS, et al: Sonography of the low transverse incision cesarean section: A prospective study. Submitted for publication.

Dewhurst CJ: Secondary post-partum hemorrhage. Br J Obstet Gynaecol 73:53, 1966.

Fausten D, Minkoff H, Schaffer R, et al: Relationship of ultrasound findings after cesarean section to operable morbidity. Obstet Gynecol 66:195–198, 1985.

Lee CY, Madrazo BL, Drukker BH: Ultrasonic evaluation of the post-partum uterus in the management of post-partum bleeding. Obstet Gynecol 58:227, 1981.

Rome RM: Secondary post-partum hemorrhage. Br J Obstet Gynaecol 82:289, 1975.

Vorherr H: Puerperal genitourinary infection. In Sciarra JJ (ed): Gynecology and Obstetrics. Philadelphia, Harper and Row, 1982, pp 7–29.

Wiener MD, Bowie JD, Baker ME, Kay HH: Sonography of post-cesarean section subfascial hematoma. AJR 148:907–910, 1987.

Gynecology

137 Clinical Considerations in Imaging the Nonpregnant Female Patient

James F. Holman

The most important diagnostic aid in the approach to a patient with a suspected gynecologic disorder is a well-taken history. This point is emphasized at the outset because medicine is now practiced in an environment so technology-oriented that attention to such a basic principle is easily overlooked. Given that the history is the foundation upon which the diagnostic approach is based, the pelvic examination is the gold standard of physical diagnosis in gynecology. The pelvic examination may be considered our least invasive test, whereas exploratory laparotomy would probably be acknowledged as our most invasive diagnostic test. In the past two decades, the laparoscope has become an essential diagnostic tool, much less invasive than an exploratory laparotomy. Nevertheless, it usually requires a general anesthetic and certainly is considerably more invasive than a pelvic examination. Bridging the gap between simple palpation and direct visualization, ultrasonography and computed tomography of the pelvis have emerged as important, noninvasive adjuncts in our diagnostic armamentarium. The utility of ultrasound in obstetrics has far outstripped its use in gynecology, and there remain significant deficiencies in our knowledge about its application to gynecology. However, the limitations of a pelvic examination point to an obvious need to expand and refine the contemporary role of imaging procedures in the diagnosis of gynecologic disorders.

PELVIC ANATOMY

Prerequisite to any diagnostic approach to gynecologic disorders is some understanding of reproductive anatomy and physiology. Basic information regarding both of these subjects will be reviewed.

VAGINA. The vagina is a fibromuscular structure extending from the vulva to the uterus. Its axis is usually directed toward the sacrum, and it is normally easily visible sonographically as a characteristic echogenic stripe. It is normally a closed, potential space, but under certain situations it will easily accommodate several hundred milliliters of blood or fluid. It is located between the colon and bladder. The posterior vaginal wall is longer than the anterior wall and under ultrasound it can be seen to extend behind and above the uterine cervix.

UTERUS. The uterus is a solid muscular organ that in the adult measures approximately $6 \times 4 \times 3$ cm in the longitudinal, transverse, and anteroposterior dimensions, respectively. Size is influenced by parity, being larger in a multiparous than in a nulliparous female. In most parous women the corpus is twice the length of the cervix, but in both premenarchal girls and postmenopausal women this relationship is usually reversed. With an empty bladder the uterus is most commonly in an anterior position, but as it is viewed sonographically, the full bladder usually results in a horizontal (to the table) position. A markedly retroverted uterus frequently obscures sonographic visualization of the endometrium.

The fallopian tubes originate from the cornual portions of the uterus and are normally about 12 cm in length. The isthmic (proximal) portion is considerably narrower than the ampullary (distal) tube. In most women normal fallopian tubes are not reliably demonstrated by ultrasound, but under pathologic conditions they may be obvious.

OVARIES. The ovaries are attached to the uterus by the utero-ovarian ligament, which attaches below and posterior to the uterotubal junction. The opposite pole or hilum contains the ovarian vessels, which enter from a superolateral position. These vessels, as well as the uterine vessels, are usually visible on ultrasound. Ovarian position in relation to the uterine fundus may vary, being either above, beside, or below the level of the fundus. They may also be side by side in the posterior cul-de-sac (the space between the uterus and colon and the most dependent portion of the pelvic cavity). In most women both ovaries are easily visible on ultrasound. The degree of bladder fullness influences ovarian position and visibility. Occasionally, overfilling of the bladder elevates the ovaries out of the pelvis and makes visualization difficult. They may be further obscured by pelvic adhesions as well as their position in relation to the uterus.

REPRODUCTIVE PHYSIOLOGY

The menstrual cycle in women of reproductive age is a dramatic, dynamic system of complex interactions among the hypothalamic, pituitary, and ovarian axes. The endocrinology of this system is characterized by rising gonadotropin levels early in the follicular phase of the cycle that produce, initially, increasing estrogen levels. Estrogen production of sufficient magnitude triggers the luteinizing hormone (LH) surge at mid-cycle, resulting in ovulation about 24 hours later. Progesterone production increases significantly at ovulation, heralding the luteal phase. The follicle releasing the ovulated ovum (now designated the corpus luteum) then becomes the steroid hormone factory for the second half of the menstrual cycle. It produces chiefly progesterone and estrogen, normally for two weeks, then undergoes involution resulting in rapidly declining steroid hormone levels that culminate in the menstrual period. These events recur at monthly intervals about 400 times during the reproductive life span of most women.

In the female pelvis the ovaries and uterus undergo predictable anatomic changes in response to these endocrinologic events. By about cycle day 5 or 6 in a normally ovulating woman, the chosen ovulatory follicle has begun to establish dominance over several other follicles among a developing cohort. This follicle measures about 10 mm by cycle day 7 or 8, and it increases in size approximately 3 mm per day, developing to a peak preovulatory size of 20 ± 4 to 5 mm. Given that the mean diameter of the normal ovary is 3 cm, the development of a 2-cm preovulatory follicle affords a dramatic change in ovarian morphology that is easily visualized sonographically.

The appearance of the newly formed corpus luteum is not nearly as characteristic as the preovulatory follicle. The corpus luteum appearance on ultrasound may vary from soft-tissue density to a very cystic structure, sometimes not readily distinguishable from a preovulatory follicle. Despite this definite variability in appearance of the ovulated follicle, sonographic monitoring of ovulation is an invaluable tool, particularly during ovulation induction. It provides evidence, other than hormonal, that follicle collapse and presumably oocyte release have occurred. And, during ovulation induction, ultrasonography provides important information regarding the number and size of stimulated follicles.

Cervical mucus also changes during the menstrual cycle. It is very scanty in amount following ovulation but during the preovulatory period it increases in amount and becomes clear and watery immediately prior to ovulation. A very echogenic line can usually be seen in the endocervix until the immediate preovulatory period when a lucent canal appears in most women. Another mid-cycle development is fluid in the cul-de-sac (estimated to be 5 to 10 ml), which can be seen in many women following ovulation.

SELECTED GYNECOLOGIC DISORDERS

There are probabaly two main reasons the gynecologist considers ordering a pelvic ultrasonogram. The first is to evaluate a palpable pelvic abnormality; the second is to exclude a pelvic abnormality in a woman who is either difficult to examine or whose clinical picture suggests pathology that cannot be appreciated on examination. Some of the more common specific clinical entities that may be evaluated by ultrasound will be reviewed with attention to pathogenesis, anatomic findings, the clinical picture, and useful information that may be derived from ultrasound.

Pelvic Inflammatory Disease

Depending on population characteristics, pelvic inflammatory disease (PID) certainly is one of the more common gynecologic problems for which sonography may be performed. The incidence of PID has changed dramatically in recent years, as has its microbiology. An ascending gonococcal infection was formerly thought to be the most common route of infection, but in the past decade the roles of *Chlamydia* and mixed anaerobic infections have become recognized. It is thought that a transient endometritis precedes the salpingitis and oophoritis that usually follow. An exudative process involving the tubal epithelium may produce permanent damage and subsequent infertility. Occasionally pyosalpinges (pus-filled fallopian tubes) occur but a more common residual is hydrosalpinges, both of which can certainly be visualized sonographically.

In a more advanced stage, a tubo-ovarian abscess may occur that probably results from leakage of pus from the distal tube with a significant collection. The tube and ovary form most of the abscess wall, although bowel and omentum are also frequently involved in the inflammatory complex.

It is frequently difficult for the clinician on pelvic examination to distinguish between a pus-containing abscess and an inflammatory complex that does not contain a frank abscess. Prognosis and management are different in the two entities in that a large abscess is less likely to respond to antibiotics and more likely to require surgery.

Although in our experience there is not a distinct, typical sonographic picture characteristic of PID, clinically useful information can be obtained in certain cases. The distinction regarding abscess versus no abscess may be made. Furthermore, abscess size may be followed as an indication of response to antibiotics. And hydrosalpinges, which are more of a chronic than an acute sequela, can be seen.

Uterine Leiomyomas

Another common clinical entity encountered by the gynecologist is the uterine leiomyoma, frequently incorrectly termed a *fibroid.* These benign tumors are composed primarily of muscle, but they contain varying amounts of fibrous connective tissue. They seem to be somehow steroid hormone (principally estrogen)–related in that they are essentially never found prior to menarche, and they almost never enlarge and usually diminish in size following the menopause. It has been estimated that by the fifth decade of life, 40 per cent of women may have leiomyomas, but there are population differences, with a three- to nine-fold higher occurrence rate in blacks.

Their pathogenesis is not well understood. However, their apparent responsiveness to estrogen is an interesting and oft described phenomenon. It has been generally held that leiomyomas frequently enlarge following exogenous estrogen administration or during pregnancy in response to rising estrogen levels. However, the assessment of size changes has been largely determined by pelvic examination, not a highly discriminating method of measurement. With ultrasonography these tumors can be accurately measured, and a study using sonographic monitoring of tumor size during pregnancy has challenged our existing dogma. It is likely that with an accurate, noninvasive way of monitoring their size, some of our ideas about these tumors may change.

Myomas are frequently described in terms of location within the uterine wall—submucous, intramural, or subserosal. They may also be described as pedunculated (with a stalk), intraligamentary (extending into the broad ligament), or ''parasitic'' (a detached tumor deriving its blood supply from omentum or adjacent organs).

Their gross appearance and consistency are highly variable. They are usually firm and fairly dense, but they may undergo various types of degeneration and contain liquefied material, or undergo hemorrhage into the tumor. Calcification of leiomyomas is commonly seen, usually in postmenopausal women. Malignant change is rare. These tumors may vary in size from several millimeters to as large as 30 pounds, and they are commonly multiple in number.

Women with myomas usually present clinically with a pelvic mass (or enlarged uterus), with abnormal bleeding, or with pain or pressure symptoms. Large myomas are usually palpable, but it may be difficult for the clinician to distinguish between a myoma extending into the adnexal area and an adnexal mass, an important clinical distinction. Small myomas, on the other hand, may not be palpable but may be the unrecognized source of abnormal uterine bleeding, particularly if submucous in location. Surgery, either a myomectomy or hysterectomy, is the usual treatment of choice, but asymptomatic myomas that are not large may merely be observed.

Given the clinical problems cited, the benefit of ultrasound assessment of women with myomas is obvious. Sonography may be used to document their presence or location as well as to monitor change in size.

Endometriosis

Endometriosis is a common gynecologic disorder that is defined as the presence of endometrial tissue in locations other than the uterine lining. It is an interesting but enigmatic disease about which there are several theories of pathogenesis. One, which does not explain all cases but which is most universally accepted, is that it occurs in response to retrograde menstruation. Although retrograde menstruation is probably more common than has been previously appreciated, it is likely that not all women who experience retrograde menstruation develop endometriosis. Why some do and others do not is still an unanswered question.

Consistent with the idea of retrograde menstruation is the finding that endometriosis occurs in dependent areas of the pelvis. Common sites of involvement are the uterosacral ligaments, serosal surfaces of the posterior and anterior cul-de-sacs, and ovaries. Serosal implants may range from tiny, superficial lesions that are barely visible to larger coalesced areas 2 to 3 cm in size that induce adhesions in adjacent peritoneum or other pelvic organs. Ovarian endometriosis may also vary from small superficial implants to large, multiloculated "chocolate cysts" that usually contain a tarry, syrupy fluid resembling old motor oil.

It is generally thought, although not unequivocally established, that endometriosis is hormonally responsive, just as is the endometrium from which it derives. It is definitely hormonally responsive to the extent that it does not occur prior to menarche and disappears following either menopause or bilateral oophorectomy. Uncommonly it may be supported by exogenous estrogens in the absence of ovaries.

Affected women usually come to the gynecologist's attention because of pain, a pelvic mass, or infertility. The amount of pain cannot necessarily be correlated with the severity of the disease. Infertility in cases of moderate or severe endometriosis is usually related to anatomic distortions that interfere with ovum pick-up or tubal transport. The etiology of infertility in women with mild endometriosis is a matter of current debate, and some investigators question that there is a correlation.

Similar to the findings in PID, it has been our experience that there is not a typical sonographic picture diagnostic of pelvic endometriosis. Given the variability of extent and pathologic changes seen in the disease, it is not surprising that ultrasound findings are not pathognomonic. Pelvic inflammatory disease is the most commonly associated differential diagnostic entity, but an ectopic pregnancy, particularly a chronic ectopic, may also present with similar sonographic findings. A β-hCG assay can almost always rule in or out ectopic pregnancy. Ultrasound may be of significant benefit in following the progress of the disease or response to treatment in a female with known endometriosis. Treatment is usually either hormonal suppression or surgery.

Adnexal Masses

Although it is not a specific entity, the adnexal mass is a common physical finding in gynecology. Imaging of ovarian tumors will be discussed in detail in Chapters 144 and 145; however, some general comments from the viewpoint of a gynecologist will be made. Literally, *adnexa* refers to the ovaries; however the concept of an adnexal mass to the gynecologist is more generic and refers to any mass (structure larger than ovary) in the region of the ovary.

The most common adnexal mass in women during their reproductive years is the "functional" cyst. Such a cyst results from ovarian follicle development and is termed either a *follicular* (arising from a preovulatory follicle) or a *luteal* (arising from a postovulatory follicle) cyst. These cysts are more often single structures that usually range in size from 5 mm to 10 cm. It is also important to keep in mind that the normal preovulatory follicle is about 20 mm in diameter. The luteal cyst is likely to contain blood that may demonstrate echogenic properties on sonography. Both of these cysts are common and are almost always managed expectantly, rarely requiring surgery.

Other adnexal masses may include any of the previously discussed entities. It is also not uncommon that bowel or bowel contents are perceived by the gynecologist as adnexal masses. Tubal pathology ranging from a hydrosalpinx or hematosalpinx to a tubal pregnancy also falls into this diagnostic category. Para-ovarian cysts are not uncommon, as are hydatid cysts (attached to the tubal fimbria).

Ultrasound may be an important diagnostic study for a number of reasons. One of the more common indications is to establish whether, in fact, such a mass exists. Furthermore, additional information may be obtained regarding their characteristics, such as size, shape, cystic versus solid or complex, relationship to either uterus or bowel, and other associated pelvic findings (e.g., cul-de-sac fluid or uterine enlargement).

THERAPEUTIC PROCEDURES

Because, typically, the radiologist performs the diagnostic pelvic ultrasound and the gynecologist performs therapeutic procedures, the two modalities have traditionally been separated. Sonographically directed amniocentesis and removal of intrauterine devices have been described for some time. However, we have begun to appreciate the potential for ultrasound as a visual guide for various gynecologic procedures.

Passing an instrument into the uterus is a blind procedure that presents a risk of uterine perforation, particularly in certain clinical situations. We have found ultrasound to be of benefit with difficult dilatations and curettages (D&C); in evacuation of uterine contents in conditions associated with an enlarged uterus, which carries a higher risk of uterine perforation (e.g., retained products of conception during the postpartum period, evacuation of a hydatidiform mole); during embryo transfer in the in vitro fertilization (IVF) procedure; and for transvesical follicle aspiration in women with pelvic adhesions who are in the IVF program. There are most certainly many other potential applications for ultrasound-directed gynecologic procedures.

With time and additional experience, the role of ultrasound in the approach to the woman with a gynecologic problem will probably be expanded and become better defined. At present, our patients will be better served by close communication and direct interaction between radiologists and gynecologists, and the possibilities for acquiring new knowledge will definitely be enhanced.

Bibliography

DeCherney AH, Romero R, Polan ML: Ultrasound in reproductive endocrinology. Fertil Steril 37:323, 1982.

Hall DA, Hann LE, Ferucci JT, et al: Sonographic morphology of the normal menstrual cycle. Radiology 133:185, 1979.

Kistner RW: Gynecology: Principles and Practice. Chicago, Year Book Medical Publishers, 1979.

Reeves RD, Drake TS, O'Brien WF: Ultrasonographic versus clinical evaluation of a pelvic mass. Obstet Gynecol 55:551, 1980.

138 Normal Computed Tomographic Anatomy of the Pelvis with Ultrasound and MRI Correlations

Elias Kazam, Yong Ho Auh, Elizabeth Ramirez de Arellano, William A. Rubenstein, Kenneth Zirinsky, and John A. Markisz

With the widespread availability of ultrasound (US), computed tomography (CT), and magnetic resonance imaging (MRI), sectional anatomy—already a valuable tool for the interpretation of conventional radiographs—has acquired added significance. In this chapter we review briefly the normal CT anatomy of the pelvis, with US-MRI correlations. For the purpose of this discussion, the pelvis is divided arbitrarily into two major components: the greater pelvis, which extends from the first sacral vertebra to the level of the upper acetabula, where the iliac, pubic, and ischial bones unite; and below it, the lesser pelvis, which extends inferiorly to the level of the ischial tuberosities, with its floor being formed by the urogenital diaphragm.

The CT images displayed here were obtained with GE 9800 equipment using 10-mm collimation and scan times of 2 to 3 seconds. Intravenous and oral contrast media were administered routinely, unless contraindicated. The US images were obtained with Accuson or ATL real-time scanners, using the highest frequency transducers, usually 3.5 mHz, which provided adequate penetration. Endovaginal and endorectal scans, performed with 5 mHz and 7 mHz transducers, provided improved spatial and textural detail. Color and spectral Doppler were valuable for assessing the vascularity of the pelvic organs, and for studying the pelvic side walls. The MRI scans were obtained with a 1.5-Tesla (T) magnet (GE Signa), or a .5-T scanner (Technicare Teslacon), using spin-echo (SE) techniques. Multiple-slice, multiple-echo images were obtained routinely—usually in the transverse plane, with echo times (TE) of 30 and 70 msec, and intersequence intervals (TR) of 1500 to 2500 msec. Additional images were usually obtained in the sagittal and/or coronal planes, using a single-echo, multiple-slice technique (TR = 500 msec/TE = 30 msec). Multi-echo T_2-weighted sagittal and/or coronal images were occasionally added to this protocol. For all the spin-echo (SE) images in this chapter, TR and TE are indicated as follows: (SE TR [msec]/TE [msec]). Slice thickness was 7.5 mm for all studies. The interslice gap was 2.5 mm for single-echo images, and 5.0 mm for the multiple-echo images. The sagittal images illustrated here are displayed with the subject's head oriented to the reader's left, whereas the transverse and coronal images are displayed with the subject's right side oriented to the reader's left side. A brief description of the major structures and the organs appears below.

THE BLOOD VESSELS

Just above the inlet to the greater pelvis, the abdominal aorta divides into two common iliac arteries that diverge as they extend inferiorly. At the L4 (fourth lumbar) and upper L5 vertebrae, the common iliac arteries lie in front of the vena cava, medial to the psoas muscles (Fig. 138–1*A*). Below this level they lie anterior to the common iliac veins. Between the L5 and S1 (first sacral) vertebrae, the common iliac arteries divide further into external and internal iliac branches (Fig. 138–1*B*).

The external iliac arteries course forward and laterally, anterolateral to the external iliac veins, to the inguinal ligaments, where they become the femoral arteries (Fig. 138–1*B* to *D*; see Figs. 138–6, 138–7, 138–11*A*, 138–14, 138–15, and 138–16*A* and *B*). Thus, the external iliac vessels diverge progressively from their internal iliac counterparts as they course inferiorly within the pelvis, medial to the psoas muscles. Two important external iliac branches are identifiable on CT and MRI demarcating the internal inguinal ring and the proximal inguinal canal:

1. The inferior epigastric artery and vein arise from, or drain into, their parent external iliac vessels just above the inguinal ligament. They extend anterosuperiorly along the medial margin of the internal inguinal ring to the anterior abdominal wall, where they course behind the rectus abdominis muscles (see Figs. 138–6, 138–11*A*, and 138–14*A* and *B*). Indirect inguinal hernias enter the internal inguinal ring lateral to the proximal inferior epigastric vessels, whereas direct inguinal hernias lie medial to these vessels.
2. The deep circumflex iliac vessels ascend anterolaterally from the external iliac vessels, behind the inguinal ligament and the internal inguinal ring, to the anterosuperior iliac spines (see Figs. 138–6, 138–11*A*, and 138–14*A*, and 138–17*A*). The spermatic cord may be visualized within the proximal inguinal canal anterior to these vessels (see Figs. 138–15*A* and 138–17*A*).

The internal iliac arteries course posteroinferiorly, in front of the internal iliac veins (see Fig. 138–1*B* to *D*), to the inferior margins of the sacroiliac joints, where they divide into anterior and posterior trunks as follows:

1. The anterior trunk gives rise to vesical, uterine, prostatic, and rectal branches (see Figs. 138–4, 138–5*C*, 138–11*A*, and 138–14*C* and *D*). These course with their corresponding venous plexuses, lateral to the organs they supply, within the visceral layer of the pelvic fascia. The terminal branches of the anterior trunk are the internal pudendal and inferior gluteal arteries (see Figs. 138–7, 138–8*A*, 138–11*A*, 138–12, 138–14, 138–15*A* and *D*, and 138–16*B*). Both exit the greater sciatic foramen below the piriformis muscle, accompanied by the internal pudendal and inferior gluteal veins, the pudendal nerve, and the sciatic nerve. The inferior gluteal vessels then continue downward, along with the sciatic nerve (see Fig. 138–15*D*), into the back of the thigh, whereas the internal pudendal vessels and pudendal nerve curve inward through the lesser sciatic foramen, to run in the pudendal canal at the medial borders of the obturator internus muscles.
2. The posterior trunk gives rise to iliolumbar, lateral sacral, and superior gluteal branches. The iliolumbar vessels course anterior to the sacrum, behind the obturator nerve, to supply the iliacus and psoas muscles (see Fig. 138–1*B* and *D*). The lateral sacral vessels enter the sacral foramina, whereas the superior gluteal vessels exit the greater sciatic foramen above the piriformis, to supply the gluteal muscles.

In general, the iliac vessels appear denser than muscle (see Figs. 138–1 and 138–7) or isodense with muscle (see Figs. 138–6 and

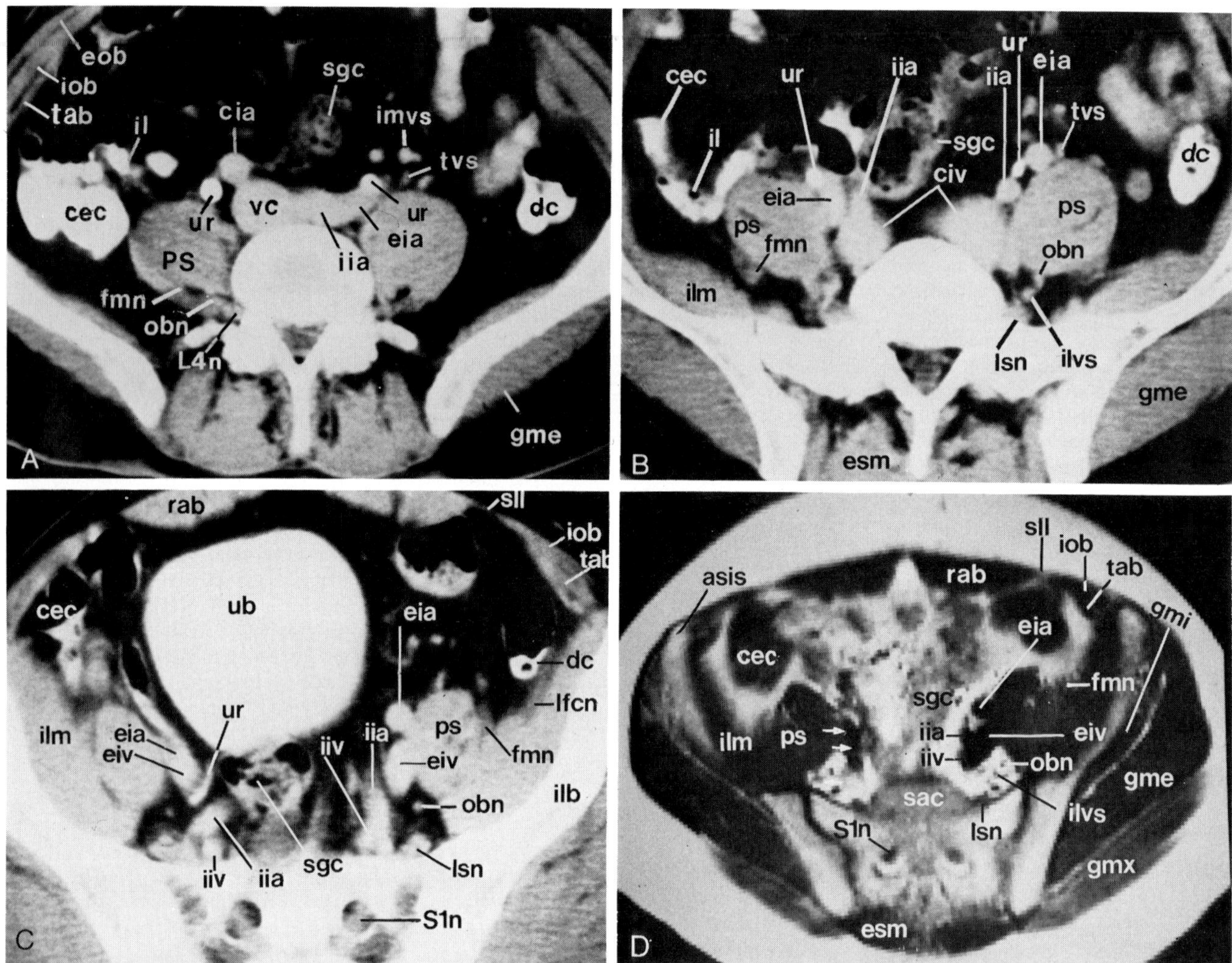

Figure 138–1. The pelvic inlet. *A,* **CT through L5 vertebra.** The right common iliac artery (cia) lies anterior to the inferior vena cava (vc) and right ureter (ur). The left common iliac artery is beginning to divide into external (eia) and internal (iia) branches. (tvs = testicular vessels; imvs = inferior mesenteric vessels; cec = cecum; il = ileum; sgc = sigmoid colon; dc = descending colon.) The femoral (fmn) and obturator (obn) nerves have just emerged from the posteroinferior margin of the psoas muscles (PS). (L4n = fourth lumbar nerve.) The nerves are relatively prominent in this patient with neurofibromatosis, but with no obvious pelvic neural tumors. (eob = external oblique muscle; iob = internal oblique muscle; tab = transversus abdominis muscle; gme = gluteus medius muscle.)

B, **CT through S1 vertebra, 30 mm below *A*.** The left external iliac artery (eia) has moved anterolaterally and is now separated from the left internal iliac artery (iia) by the left ureter (ur). The right common iliac artery has just divided into external (eia) and internal (iia) iliac artery branches. (civ = common iliac veins) The obturator nerves (obn) lie at the posteromedial aspects of the psoas muscles (ps), anterior to the iliolumbar vessels (ilvs). (lsn = lumbosacral trunk.) The femoral nerves (fmn) course between the psoas and iliacus muscles (ilm). (tvs = testicular vessels; esm = erector spinae muscle.)

C, **CT 30 mm below *B*.** The left external iliac artery (eia) now lies just anterior to its corresponding vein (eiv), medial to the psoas muscle (ps). The left internal iliac artery (iia) is contiguous with and just anterior to its corresponding vein (iiv). The right external iliac artery and vein (eia, eiv) are separated from the right internal iliac vessels (iia, iiv) by the right ureter (ur). The lateral femoral cutaneous nerve (lfcn) is visible just behind the descending colon (dc). (ub = urinary bladder; rab = rectus abdominis muscle; sll = semilunar line; ilb = iliac bone.)

D, **MRI of another patient at approximately the level of *C*.** The left external iliac artery (eia) and vein (eiv) have nearly the same configuration as in *C*. (sac = sacrum.) The right external and internal iliac vessels *(arrows)* are not as clearly delineated from each other. Compare with *C* for visualization of nerves, muscles, and bones.

138–14*A* and *C*) on contrast-enhanced CT. They become markedly hyperdense on dynamic CT scans. They lack signal and therefore appear black on MRI (see Figs. 138–1*D*, 138–11*A*, and 138–14*B* and *D*). On sonography, most of the internal iliac vessels are obscured by overlying bowel gas and fat. The external iliac vessels can be demonstrated as echo-poor structures, if the beam is angled laterally through the bladder (see Figs. 138–5*B* and 138–16*B*).

An understanding of sectional vascular anatomy has several clinical applications. First, abnormalities of the iliac vessels, such as aneurysms or venous thrombi, which are detected with sectional imaging, can be localized correctly without resorting to angiography. Second, the inferior epigastric and deep circumflex iliac vessels serve as important markers for the internal inguinal ring and as important collateral pathways in case of venous or arterial obstruction. Finally, since nodes may appear isodense with vessels even on contrast-enhanced CT, a diagnosis of pelvic lymph node enlargement should be made only after the iliac vessels are identified. At times, dynamic contrast-enhanced CT scans are required to differentiate dilated iliac vessels from lymph nodes.

THE PELVIC LYMPH NODES

The pelvic nodes are grouped mainly around the common iliac, external iliac, and internal iliac vessels, with smaller groups along the inferior epigastric, deep circumflex iliac, sacral, and obturator vessels. They may be invisible on normal CT scans, or they may appear as small structures, measuring up to 1 cm in diameter, which are either hypodense or isodense relative to muscles (see Figs. 138–6 and 138–14*A* and *C*). On MRI, lymph nodes appear slightly brighter, or occasionally as bright as muscle (see Fig. 138–14*B* and *D*). In general, lymph nodes may not be visualized with US, unless they are enlarged. However, it is possible to visualize the anterolateral pelvic wall on decubitus views, with the external iliac vessels and adjacent node groups (see Fig. 138–16*B*). The more posterolaterally positioned internal iliac vessels and nodes are difficult to delineate with US.

Normal-sized nodes may be difficult to differentiate from adjacent vessels or nerves, even with the best CT scanners. This is usually of no clinical significance. Of much greater importance is the ability to reliably differentiate enlarged pelvic nodes from adjacent blood vessels and bowel loops. This is especially true at the pelvic inlet, where the common iliac vessels are grouped together (see Fig. 138–1), and the external iliac region, where the psoas muscle and external iliac vessels, or adjacent bowel loops, may be confused with adenopathy on CT. For these reasons, intravenous and oral contrast media are administered routinely in our institution to opacify the blood vessels and hollow viscera on CT. With MRI, the distinction between lymph nodes and vessels is possible because of the characteristically poor signal from blood vessels.

THE PELVIC NERVES

The major pelvic nerve trunks can be seen well with modern CT equipment, and to a lesser degree with MRI. For illustrative purposes, CT scans from a patient with neurofibromatosis and diffusely prominent nerves are included in Figure 138–1*A* to *C*. The same nerves, however, can be clearly visualized by CT and MRI in other patients without neurofibromatosis (see Figs. 138–1*D*, 138–6, 138–14*A* to *D*). These include the following:

The *femoral nerve* can be seen at the L5 level, just as it emerges from the posterior margin of the psoas muscle. At this point it lies lateral to the obturator nerve (see Fig. 138–1*A*). The femoral nerve then courses laterally and anteriorly between the psoas and iliacus muscles, where it can be seen on CT or MRI when surrounded by sufficient fat (see Fig. 138–1*C* and *D*). Just lateral to it at this level, the lateral femoral cutaneous nerve may be visible anterior to the iliacus muscle and behind the distal descending colon or cecum (see Fig. 138–1*C*). More inferiorly, the femoral nerve continues its anterior course, either within or just in front of the fatty groove between the psoas and iliacus muscles. In this latter location it is usually not well seen by CT and is difficult to differentiate from radio-dense iliac fascia in the iliopsoas groove (see Fig. 138–7).

The *obturator nerve* is first visible behind the psoas muscle at the L5 level, where it lies medial to the femoral nerve, lateral to the L4 nerve, and anterior to the iliolumbar vessels (see Fig. 138–1*A*, *B*, and *D*). It then courses anteroinferiorly, in front of the internal iliac vessels and their obturator branches (see Fig. 138–1*C*) and behind the external iliac lymph nodes (see Fig. 138–14*A*). Within the obturator foramen, the obturator nerve courses laterally, adjacent to the bone, and is difficult to differentiate from the obturator vessels or nodes on CT (see Fig. 138–15*B*).

The *L4 nerve* lies posteromedial to the psoas muscle at the L5 level (see Fig. 138–1*A*). A portion of it then joins the L5 nerve below it, to form the lumbosacral trunk (see Fig. 138–1*C* and *D*), which continues posteroinferiorly, in front of the gluteal vessels, to the greater sciatic foramen, where it joins the S1 to S3 nerves to form the sciatic nerve (see Fig. 138–6).

The *sacral nerves* course inferiorly from the sacral foramina (see Fig. 138–1*C* and *D*) into the posterior pelvis. The S1 and S2 nerves are the largest of these. They are accompanied by the inferior gluteal vessels to the greater sciatic foramen, where they join the lumbosacral trunk and the S3 nerve to form the sciatic nerve (see Fig. 138–6).

The *sciatic nerve* is the largest in the body and the most consistently visible with CT or MRI (see Figs. 138–6 and 138–14*A* and *B*). It exits the pelvis through the greater sciatic foramen below the piriformis muscle, and descends into the posterior thigh lateral to the ischial tuberosity, with the inferior gluteal vessels and the posterior femoral cutaneous nerve at its medial aspect (see Fig. 138–12).

The *pudendal nerve* may be seen occasionally with CT or MRI, medial to the inferior gluteal vessels and piriformis muscle (see Fig. 138–14*A* and *B*). It exits the pelvis through the inferior portion of the greater sciatic foramen and then curves inward with the internal pudendal vessels, through the lesser sciatic foramen, to run in the pudendal canal lateral to the ischiorectal fat. Within the canal, the pudendal nerve is usually indistinguishable by CT from its accompanying vessels and the hyperdense fascia that surrounds them (see Fig. 138–12).

In general, nerves appear either hypodense (see Figs. 138–1*C*, 138–6, 138–12, and 138–14*A* and *C*) or isodense (see Figs. 138–1*A* and *B*) relative to muscle on contrast-enhanced CT. On MRI they tend to be brighter than muscle (see Figs. 138–14*B* and *D*) but are sometimes isointense with small vessels (see Fig. 138–1*D*). As mentioned above, small nerves may not be differentiated reliably from contiguous small vessels and lymph nodes with either technique. Nevertheless, an understanding of the sectional anatomy of the pelvic nerves is useful. First, neural tumors, rather than enlarged lymph nodes or unspecified masses, may be diagnosed by CT and correctly localized to their nerves of origin. Secondly, large nerve trunks are less likely to be confused with enlarged lymph nodes, particularly in the retropsoas region at the L5-S1 level (see Fig. 138–1). Finally, nerve compression can be predicted from the CT scan when masses or fluid collections occupy the expected locations of pelvic nerves. Examples of this include compression of the retropsoas nerves by pelvic tumor, of the femoral nerve by hematoma or by an iliopsoas bursa, and of the sciatic nerve by hematoma or bone after posterior fracture-dislocation of the hip.

THE URETERS

The ureters lie anterior or lateral to the common iliac arteries at the inlet to the greater pelvis (see Fig. 138–1*A*). As the common iliac vessels divide, the ureters may course briefly in front of the external iliac artery or vein (see Fig. 138–1*B*) and then between the external and internal iliac vessels (see Fig. 138–1*C*). They descend along the lateral aspect of the pelvis, parallel to the anterior margin of the greater sciatic foramen (see Figs. 138–7 and 138–14*A* and *C*). They then turn anteromedially at the level of the ischial spines and course anterior to the vaginal fornices or seminal vesicles (see Fig. 138–15*A*) to join the urinary bladder. These anatomic markers are helpful for localizing the pelvic ureter on MRI (see Fig. 138–14*D*), ultrasound (see Fig. 138–16*A*), or non-enhanced CT scans, where it is not positively identified by intraluminal contrast media.

THE URINARY BLADDER

The urinary bladder lies within the extraperitoneal fat anterior to the peritoneum. Except for the bladder neck, which is fixed in position behind the pubic symphysis and in front of the upper vagina or prostate (see Fig. 138–13), the bladder is free to glide within the fat around it. Its shape and position are therefore easily variable, depending on the volume of urine within it (see Figs. 138–1*C* and 138–14*C* and *D*). A distended bladder is valuable for both ultrasonic and MRI imaging of the pelvis because it displaces potentially troublesome bowel loops superiorly (see Figs. 138–16*E* and 138–17*C* and *D*). Diagnostic confusion may arise in elderly individuals with bladder diverticula, which may mimic adnexal cysts on sonography if their narrow necks are not demonstrated.

The bladder wall can be delineated with intravesical ultrasound, CT, or MRI. Limitations to these methods include the invasiveness of transvesical ultrasound, the impairment of bladder wall delineation by intraluminal contrast media on CT, and the loss of spatial resolution on T_2-weighted MRI images. The chemical shift artifact can also distort the bladder wall on MRI (see Fig. 138–17). This artifact is attributable to the chemical shift difference between the resonant frequencies of water protons and fat protons. The resonant frequency of fat is shifted to the downfield side of the read-out gradient by about 4 ppm, which is approximately equal to the width of one pixel. Because localization of the signal in the read-out gradient field is dependent on the proton resonant frequencies, the downshifted proton signal from fat is interpreted as having arisen from one pixel further downfield. This leaves the pixel representing the fat that is immediately contiguous to the bladder with a significantly decreased observed intensity. The locus of all such pixels forms a dark line that may be mistaken for thickening of the bladder wall (see Fig. 138–17).

THE PARAVESICAL SPACES

The bladder, ureters, urachus, and obliterated umbilical arteries are surrounded by umbilicovesical fascia, which is analogous to the renal fascia. The umbilicovesical fascia divides the preperitoneal fat into an inner perivesical compartment, analogous to the perirenal space, and a peripheral anterolateral prevesical compartment, analogous to the anterior pararenal space. The prevesical space extends inferiorly behind the pubic symphysis, anterior to the upper prostate or vagina, where it is commonly referred to as the space of Retzius (see Fig. 138–15*B* and *C*). On CT or MRI the umbilicovesical fascia and contiguous peritoneum can be visualized as linear densities along the urachus (median umbilical ligament) and old umbilical arteries (medial umbilical ligaments) (see Figs. 138–6 and 138–14*A* to *C*). These thin folds mark the interface between two potentially large spaces on either side of the peritoneum:

1. Extraperitoneal prevesical collections lie anterior and lateral to the umbilical folds or ligaments, displacing the bladder posteriorly and compressing it from the sides.
2. Intraperitoneal fluid collects behind the umbilical folds, either centrally within the supravesical space posteromedial to the medial umbilical folds, or posterolateral to these folds within the inguinal fossae. In the absence of ascites, the supravesical space is usually occupied by small bowel, whereas the right and left inguinal fossae are occupied by cecum (or terminal ileum) and sigmoid, respectively (see Fig. 138–1*C*). The peritoneal space also extends behind the bladder into the cul-de-sac. In the female, the cul-de-sac is invaginated by the uterus, which divides it into a shallow anterior vesicouterine recess and a deeper posterior rectouterine pouch.

THE FEMALE REPRODUCTIVE SYSTEM

The *uterus* is divisible into a *cervix, body,* and *fundus* (Figs. 138–2 to 138–10). The *cervix* is relatively elongated, extending between the external and internal os, and accounting for one third to nearly one half of the length of the uterus. The external cervical os is best delineated on T_2-weighted MRI, which highlights its relatively bright endocervical portion and surrounding hypointense fibrous stroma (see Figs. 138–9 and 138–11*B*). This same fibrous component appears bright on contrast-enhanced CT, allowing for delineation of the cervix from surrounding upper vagina. On US, the lower cervix is usually indistinguishable from surrounding vagina, unless the vaginal lumen is delineated with air or fluid (see Figs. 138–2 and 138–3). The internal cervical os lies at the junction of uterine cervix and body, and cannot be precisely localized with US, CT, or MRI. The *uterine body* extends between the internal os and the fallopian tubes, accounting for nearly half of the remaining length of the uterus. The *uterine fundus* is the convex upper portion that extends above the entrance of the fallopian tubes (see Figs. 138–2, 138–3, 138–9*A*, and 138–10).

The uterus is usually *anteverted,* with the cervical canal oriented backwards, away from the pubic symphysis (see Figs. 138–2, 138–3, 138–6, and 138–9*A*). A *retroverted* uterus is posteriorly inclined, with the cervix oriented anteriorly towards the pubis (see Fig. 138–7). *Retroflexion,* which often accompanies retroversion, refers to a posterior curvature of the uterus at the junction of its cervix and body. A *bicornuate* uterus is divided into two horns with separate endometrial canals within its body, but a single endocervical canal. An *arcuate* uterus is a variant of uterus bicornis, with only a short vertical depression in the midportion of the fundus. In uterus *bicornis didelphys* there is complete failure of fusion of the embryologic mesonephric ducts, with two separate uterine canals, two cervices, and a septate vagina (Fig. 138–11). There may be associated absence of a kidney.

The anatomic landmarks that are most useful for delineating the uterus on sectional imaging are the uterine ligaments, the endometrium, and the uterine vessels (see Figs. 138–2 to 138–11):

1. The *uterine ligaments* attach the uterus to adjacent pelvic structures. The *broad ligaments* are peritoneal folds that suspend the uterus from the lateral pelvic walls. The lateral tapering of the uterine contours at their broad ligamentous attachments (see Figs. 138–4, 138–5*A* and 5*B*, 138–6 to 138–8, and 138–11) is helpful for distinguishing the uterus from adnexal or other pelvic masses on transverse sections. The *round ligaments* are attached to the anterior uterus just below the fallopian tubes (see Figs. 138–4, 138–5*B*, 138–6 to 138–8, and 138–11*A*). They then course anterolaterally to enter the internal inguinal ring, just lateral to the inferior epigastric vessels (see Figs. 138–6 and 138–11*A*). They are more difficult to detect with ultrasound because of their anteroposterior course parallel to the sound beam. Partial emptying of the bladder and decubitus views are helpful for sonographic demonstration of the round

Text continued on page 2020

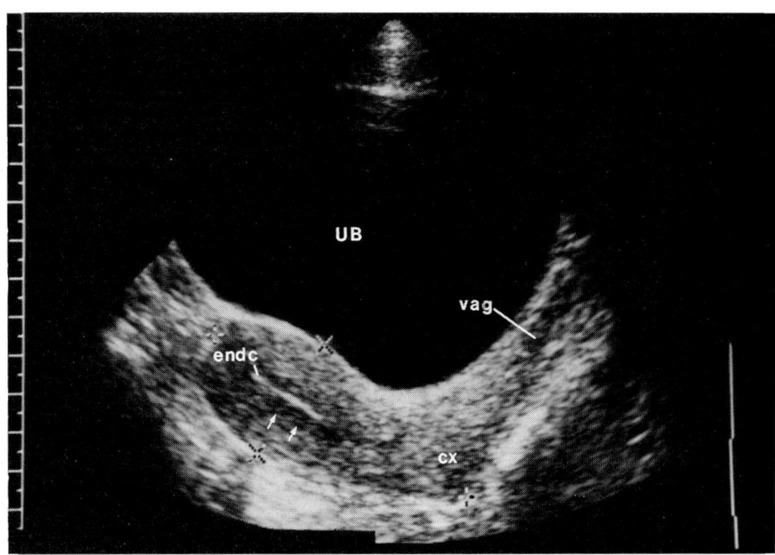

Figure 138–2. Midsagittal sonogram of the uterus two days after the last menstrual period (LMP). Cursors have been placed along the longest and greatest anteroposterior dimensions of the uterus. The endometrial canal (endc) is surrounded by an echo-poor zone *(arrows)*, which, without knowledge of the menstrual history, is consistent with proliferative endometrium and/or inner myometrium (junctional zone). In this case, the echo-poor zone is attributable mainly to inner myometrium. (cx = uterine cervix; vag = vagina; UB = urinary bladder.) (From Kazam E, Ramirez de Arellano E, Rubenstein WA, et al: Sonography of the pelvis and the lower urinary tract: Normal anatomy with CT and MRI correlations. In Shirkhoda A, Madrazo BL (eds): Pelvic Ultrasound. Baltimore, Williams and Wilkins, 1993, pp 1–18.)

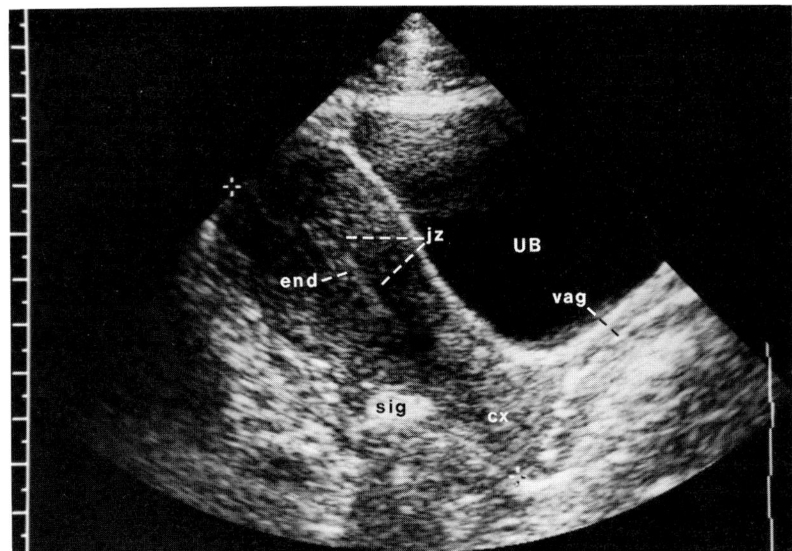

Figure 138–3. Midsagittal uterine sonogram 18 days post-LMP. The endometrium (end) is thicker and more echogenic than in Figure 138–2, but considerably less prominent than in another patient 18 days post-LMP (see Fig. 138–4). (jz = junctional zone.) The vaginal lumen (vag) is clearly demarcated by air, up to its superior aspect, outlining the inferior margin of the uterine cervix (cx). (UB = urinary bladder; sig = sigmoid colonic air.) (From Kazam E, Ramirez de Arellano E, Rubenstein WA, et al: Sonography of the pelvis and the lower urinary tract: Normal anatomy with CT and MRI correlations. In Shirkhoda A, Madrazo BL (eds): Pelvic Ultrasound. Baltimore, Williams and Wilkins, 1993, pp 1–18.)

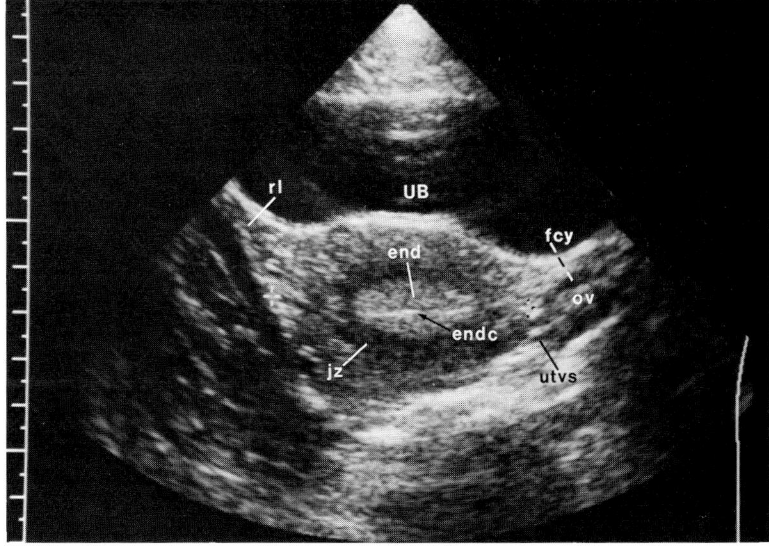

Figure 138–4. Transverse sonogram through the uterine body 18 days post-LMP. The endometrium (end) is significantly thicker and more echogenic than in Figures 138–2 and 138–3. A distinct inner myometrial junctional zone (jz) is visible. Note lateral tapering of uterine contours at attachment of round ligament (rl). (utvs = uterine vessels; ov = left ovary; fcy = ovarian follicle; UB = urinary bladder; endc = endometrial canal.) (From Kazam E, Ramirez de Arellano E, Rubenstein WA, et al: Sonography of the pelvis and the lower urinary tract: Normal anatomy with CT and MRI correlations. In Shirkhoda A, Madrazo BL (eds): Pelvic Ultrasound. Baltimore, Williams and Wilkins, 1993, pp 1–18.)

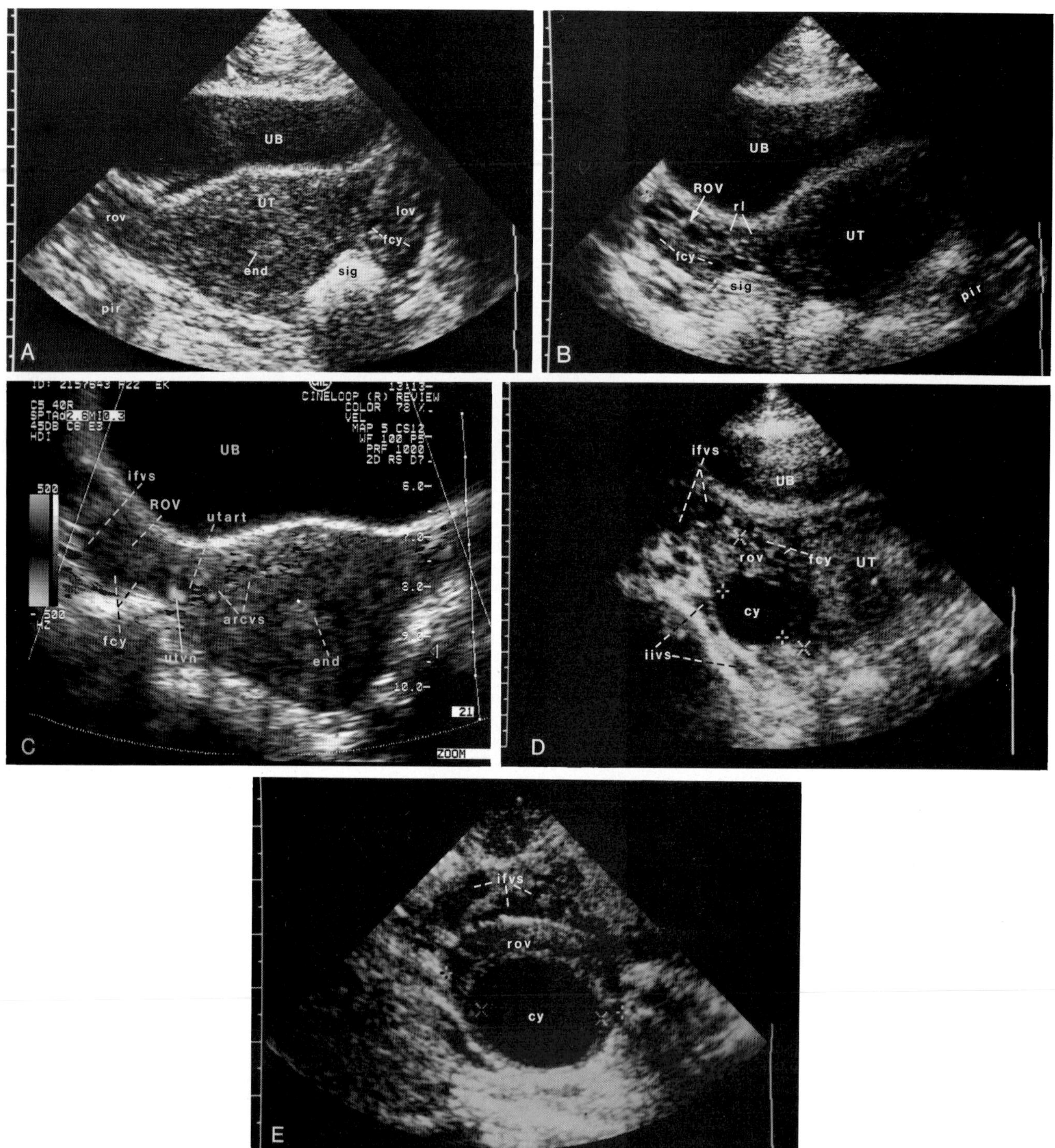

Figure 138–5. Ovarian sonography. *A,* **Transverse supine sonogram** shows the left ovary (lov) partially separated from the uterus by sigmoid colon (sig). Note the echo-poor follicles (fcy) at the periphery of the left ovary. (rov = right ovary; UT = uterus; UB = urinary bladder; pir = piriformis muscle.)

B, **Transverse sonogram in right posterior oblique position.** Visualization of the right ovary (ROV) is markedly improved over Figure 138–4*A*, because the sound beam traverses a shorter path through fluid-filled urinary bladder (UB), nearly perpendicular to the ovary. (fcy = ovarian follicles; UT = uterus; rl = round ligament; sig = sigmoid colon; pir = piriformis muscle.)

C, **Ovarian, uterine, and pelvic vessels.** Color Doppler sonogram of the uterus and right ovary (ROV). Small ovarian follicles (fcy) can be distinguished from adjacent infundibulopelvic vessels (ifvs) and uterine vessels (utart, utvn). The arcuate branches (arcvs) of the right uterine artery (utart) can be seen penetrating the myometrium and coursing toward the midline to anastomose with their contralateral counterparts. These are accompanied by their corresponding veins. (end = secretory endometrium; UB = urinary bladder.)

D and *E,* **The infundibulopelvic vessels.** Transabdominal *(D)* and endovaginal *(E)* sonograms of the same ovary. The infundibulopelvic vessels (ifvs) are clearly separated from the right ovary (rov) by an echogenic linear interface in *E,* but are indistinguishable from ovarian follicles (fcy) in *D.* (cy = ovarian cyst, UT = uterus; iivs = internal iliac vessels; UB = urinary bladder.)

(*A* to *E* from Kazam E, Ramirez de Arellano E, Rubenstein WA, et al: Sonography of the pelvis and the lower urinary tract: Normal anatomy with CT and MRI correlations. In Shirkhoda A, Madrazo BL (eds): Pelvic Ultrasound. Baltimore, Williams and Wilkins, 1993, pp 1–18.)

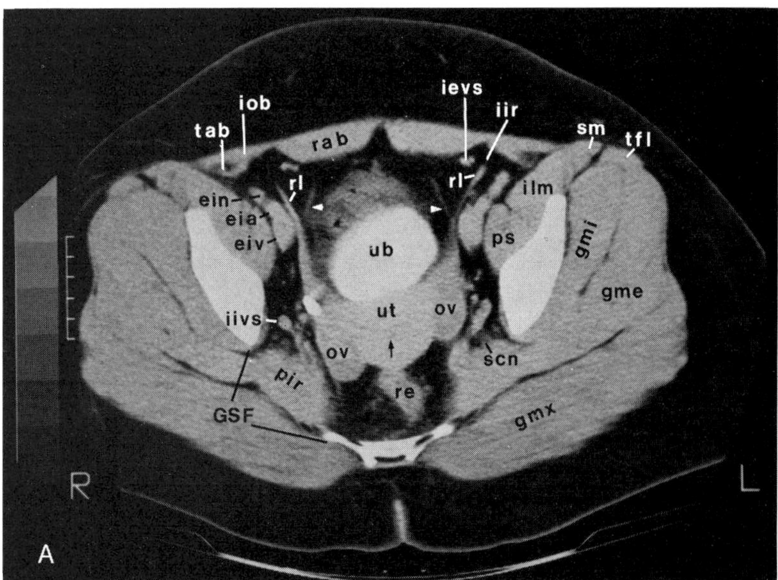

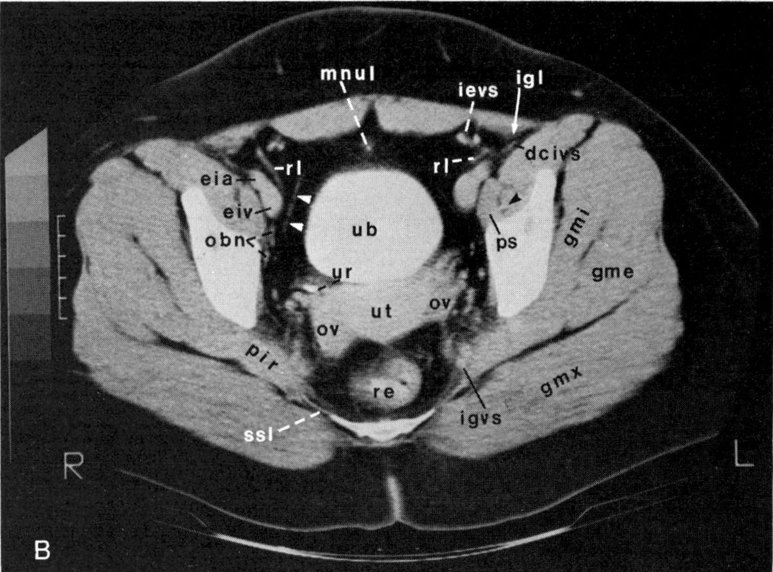

Figure 138–6. CT of the uterus and ovaries. CT scans through the upper *(A)* and lower *(B)* greater sciatic foramen (GSF). The round ligaments (rl) course anterolaterally from their attachments to an anteverted uterus (ut) to enter the internal inguinal ring (iir), lateral to the inferior epigastric vessels (ievs). The deep circumflex iliac vessels (dcivs in *B*) course directly behind the posterior margins of the inguinal canal, contiguous to the inguinal ligament (igl). The ovaries (ov) lie on either side of the uterus, posterolateral to the round ligaments. (*Black arrow* = endometrial lucency; eia = external iliac artery; eiv = external iliac vein; ein = external iliac lymph node; obn = obturator lymph node; iivs = internal iliac vessels; igvs = inferior gluteal vessels; scn = sciatic nerve; ub = urinary bladder; ur = ureter; *white arrowheads* = medial umbilical folds; mnul = median umbilical fold; re = rectum; ilm = iliacus; ps = psoas muscles; *black arrowhead* = radiodense iliac fascia; rab = rectus abdominis; iob = internal oblique; tab = transversus abdominis; pir = piriformis; gmx = gluteus maximus; gme = gluteus medius; gmi = gluteus minimus; tfl = tensor fasciae latae; sm = sartorius muscles; ssl = sacrospinous ligament.) (*A* and *B* from Kazam E, Ramirez de Arellano E, Rubenstein WA, et al: Sonography of the pelvis and the lower urinary tract: Normal anatomy with CT and MRI correlations. In Shirkhoda A, Madrazo BL (eds): Pelvic Ultrasound. Baltimore, Williams and Wilkins, 1993, pp 1–18.)

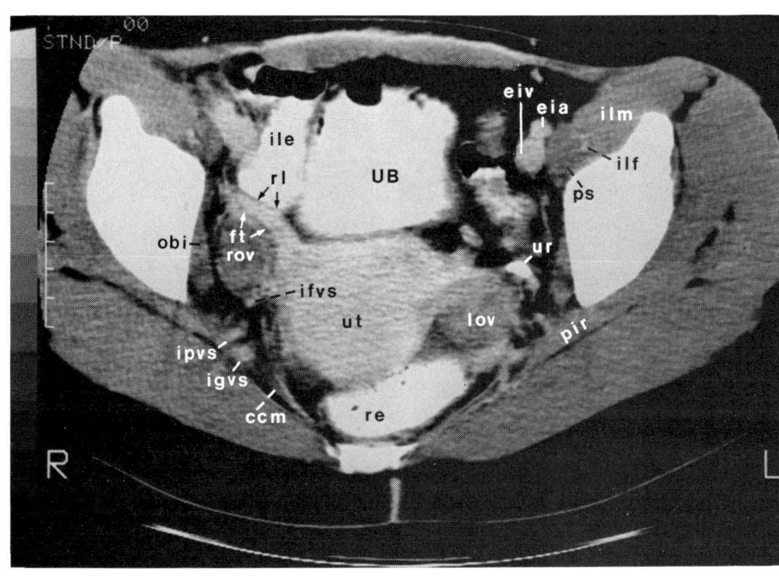

Figure 138–7. Retroverted uterus. CT scan through the lower portion of the greater sciatic foramen. The uterus (ut) is retroverted, with a slightly convex anterior margin. The round ligament (rl) is contiguous to the right fallopian tube (ft). (rov, lov = ovaries; ifvs = ovarian and infundibulopelvic vessels; ur = left ureter; UB = urinary bladder; igvs = inferior gluteal vessels; ipvs = inferior pudendal vessels; re = rectum.) The psoas (ps) and iliacus muscles (ilm) are separated by radiodense iliac fascia (ilf). (eia = external iliac artery; eiv = external iliac vein; obi = obturator internus muscle; pir = piriformis muscle; ile = ileum; ccm = coccygeus muscle.) (From Kazam E, Ramirez de Arellano E, Rubenstein WA, et al: Sonography of the pelvis and the lower urinary tract: Normal anatomy with CT and MRI correlations. In Shirkhoda A, Madrazo BL (eds): Pelvic Ultrasound. Baltimore, Williams and Wilkins, 1993, pp 1–18.)

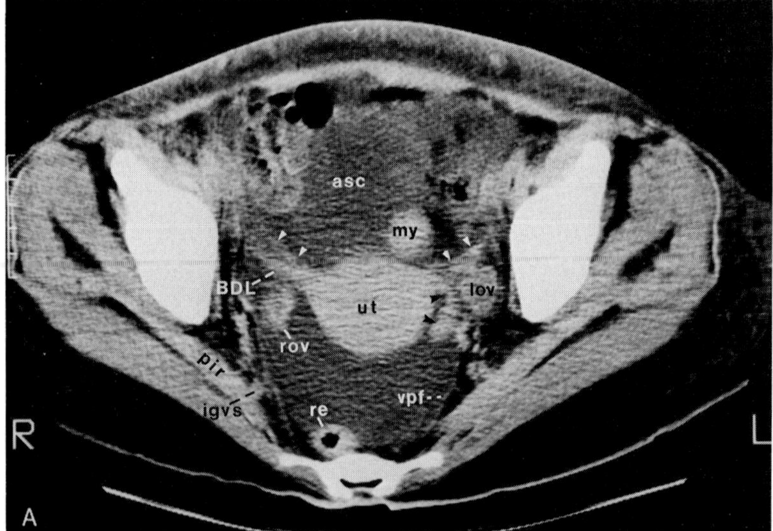

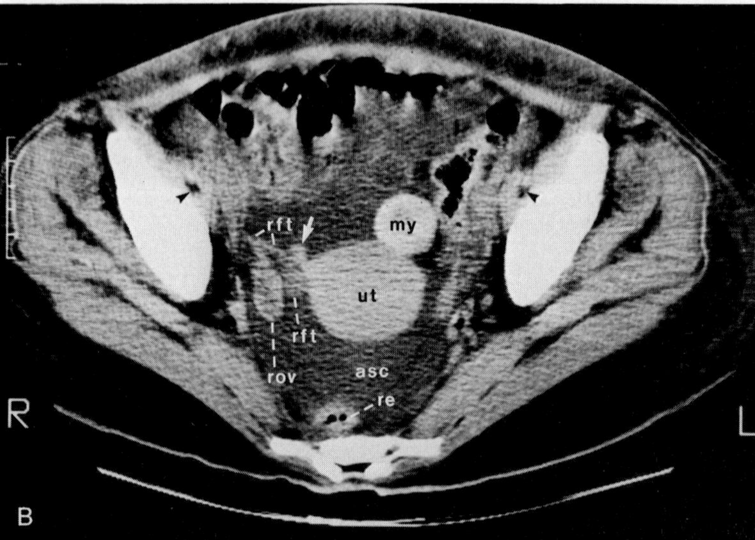

Figure 138–8. Improved CT visualization of fallopian tubes and uterine ligaments in the presence of ascites. *A,* **CT through greater sciatic foramen.** The left fallopian tube *(black arrowheads)* is clearly visible between the uterus (ut) and left ovary (lov). (rov = right ovary; BDL = broad ligament; white arrowheads = round ligament; my = serosal myoma; asc = ascites in supravesical space and cul-de-sac; re = rectum.) The piriformis muscle (pir) exits the greater sciatic foramen as it courses laterally toward the greater trochanter. (igvs = inferior gluteal vessels; vpf = visceral layer of pelvic fascia.)

B, **CT scan 1 cm above** ***A.*** The right fallopian tube (rft) is now visible between the right ovary (rov) and uterus (ut). (my = serosal myoma; *white arrow* = small intraligamentous myoma; *black arrowheads* = fat in groove separating psoas and iliacus muscles.)

(*A* and *B* from Kazam E, Ramirez de Arellano E, Rubenstein WA, et al: Sonography of the pelvis and the lower urinary tract: Normal anatomy with CT and MRI correlations. In Shirkhoda A, Madrazo BL (eds): Pelvic Ultrasound. Baltimore, Williams and Wilkins, 1993, pp 1–18.)

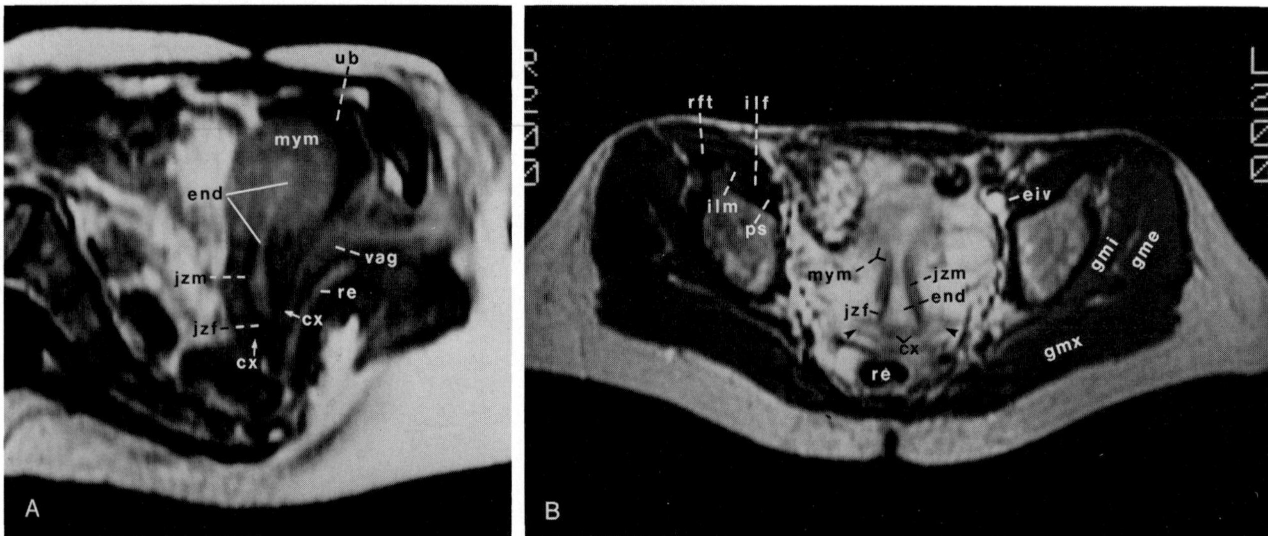

Figure 138–9. Uterine MRI. Sagittal T_1-weighted MRI (1000/25 msec) of an anteverted uterus *(A),* and transverse T_2-weighted MRI (2000/40 msec) *(B).* (mym = fundic myometrium; end = endometrium.) The dark structure peripheral to the endometrium probably represents inner myometrium (jzm) within the uterine body and mainly fibrous tissue (jzf) within the cervix (cx). (vag = vagina; *arrowhead* = vaginal fornix; ub = urinary bladder; re = rectum; ps = psoas muscle; ilm = iliacus muscle.) The iliac fascia (ilf) and rectus femoris tendon (rftn) are hypointense because of their fibrous internal structure *(B).* (gmx = gluteus maximus; gme = gluteus medius; gmi = gluteus minimus; eiv = external iliac vein.) (*A* and *B* from Kazam E, Ramirez de Arellano E, Rubenstein WA, et al: Sonography of the pelvis and the lower urinary tract: Normal anatomy with CT and MRI correlations. In Shirkhoda A, Madrazo BL (eds): Pelvic Ultrasound. Baltimore, Williams and Wilkins, 1993, pp 1–18.)

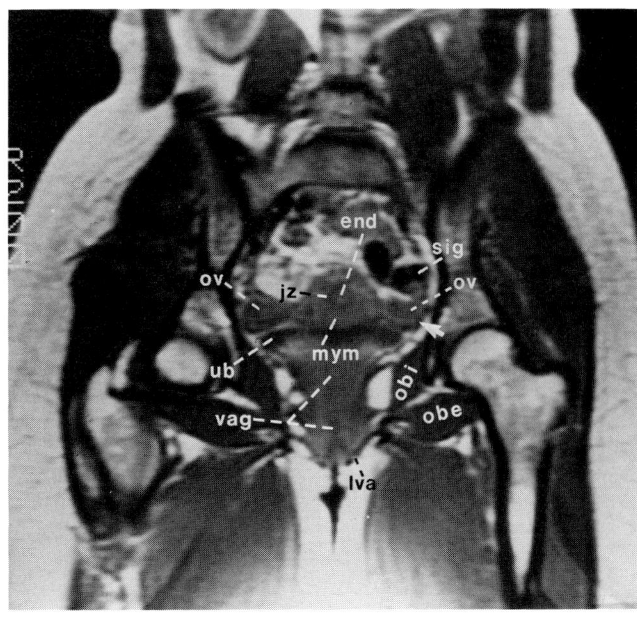

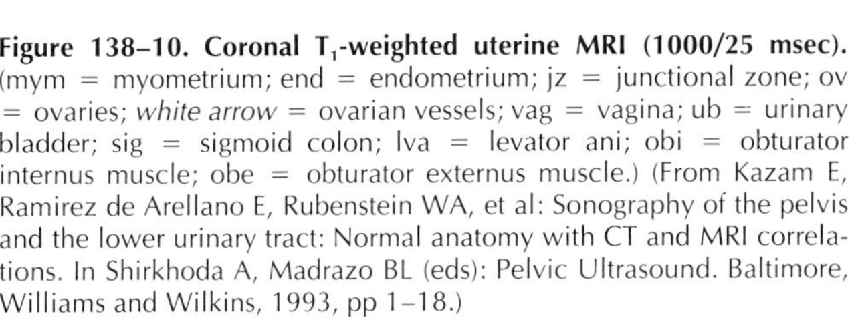

Figure 138–10. Coronal T_1-weighted uterine MRI (1000/25 msec). (mym = myometrium; end = endometrium; jz = junctional zone; ov = ovaries; *white arrow* = ovarian vessels; vag = vagina; ub = urinary bladder; sig = sigmoid colon; lva = levator ani; obi = obturator internus muscle; obe = obturator externus muscle.) (From Kazam E, Ramirez de Arellano E, Rubenstein WA, et al: Sonography of the pelvis and the lower urinary tract: Normal anatomy with CT and MRI correlations. In Shirkhoda A, Madrazo BL (eds): Pelvic Ultrasound. Baltimore, Williams and Wilkins, 1993, pp 1–18.)

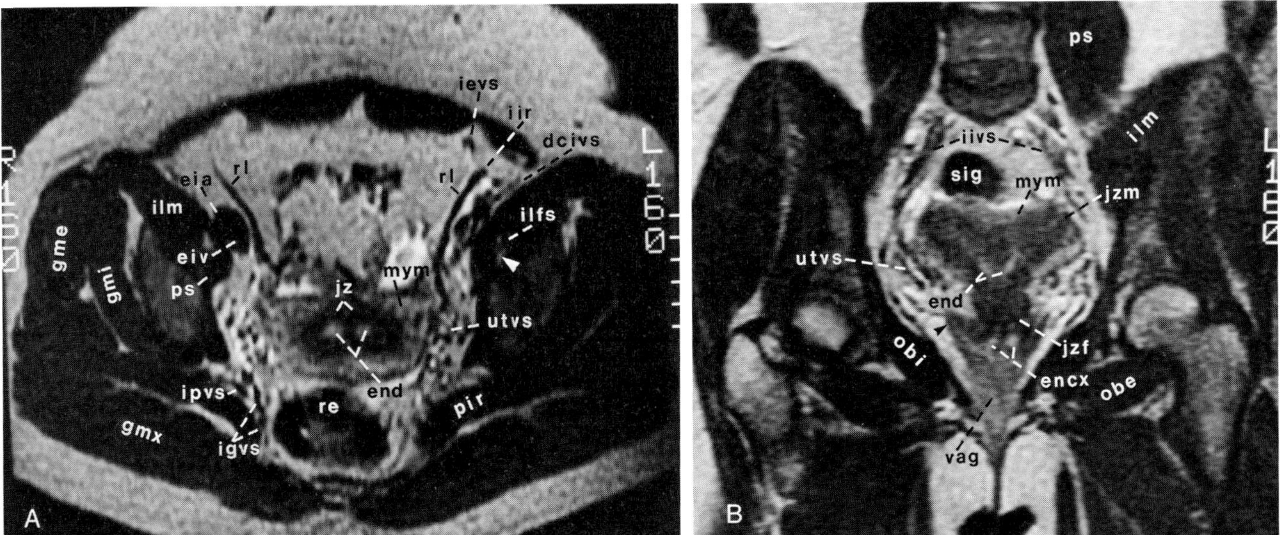

Figure 138–11. MRI of uterus bicornis didelphys. *A,* **Transverse T_2-weighted MRI** (1700/80 msec) of the uterine body shows two clearly demarcated endometrial canals (end), surrounded by a low-intensity junctional zone (jz), and myometrium (mym) of intermediate brightness. The round ligament (rl) courses anterolaterally from the uterus to enter the internal inguinal ring (iir), lateral to the inferior epigastric vessels (ievs). The deep circumflex iliac vessels (dcivs) lie posterior to the proximal inguinal canal. Compare this region with Figure 138–6. (eia = external iliac artery; eiv = external iliac vein.) The psoas (ps) and iliacus (ilm) muscles are separated by a small amount of fat *(arrowhead)* that surrounds the hypointense iliac fascia (ilfs). (utvs = uterine vessels; ipvs = internal pudendal vessels; igvs = inferior gluteal vessels; pir = piriformis; gmx = gluteus maximus; gme = gluteus medius; gmi = gluteus minimus muscle; re = rectum.)

B, **T_2-weighted coronal MRI** (1700/70 msec) of the same uterus shown in *A*. Two endometrial (end) and endocervical (encx) canals are clearly delineated. The junctional zone of inner myometrium (jzm) is continuous with the cervical fibrous tissue (jzf). The vagina (vag) and its superior fornices *(arrowhead)* are clearly shown. (iivs = internal iliac vessels; utvs = uterine vessels; sig = sigmoid colon; obi = obturator internus muscle; obe = obturator externus muscle; ps = psoas muscle; ilm = iliacus muscle.)

(*A* and *B* from Kazam E, Ramirez de Arellano E, Rubenstein WA, et al: Sonography of the pelvis and the lower urinary tract: Normal anatomy with CT and MRI correlations. In Shirkhoda A, Madrazo BL (eds): Pelvic Ultrasound. Baltimore, Williams and Wilkins, 1993, pp 1–18.)

ligaments (see Fig. 138–5*B*). When traced backwards to their uterine attachments, the round ligaments may be helpful for identifying the uterus on transverse sections. Masses that are attached to the posteromedial portion of the round ligament are likely to be uterine in origin, whereas those that lie lateral to the round ligament are usually extrauterine, e.g., adnexal (see Figs. 138–5 to 138–7). Masses lying at the superior or anterior aspect of the uterus, between the two round ligaments, may be either uterine or adnexal (see Fig. 138–8). After abdominoperineal resection of the rectum, the round ligamentous attachments of the posteriorly displaced uterus can help to differentiate it on transverse sections from postoperative fibrosis or recurrent neoplasm.

2. *The endometrium* can be distinguished from the myometrium with US, CT, and MRI. In addition, with T_2-weighted MRI and occasionally US, two myometrial zones can also be differentiated.

The *endometrial canal* is usually visualized as a thin echogenic line on ultrasound (see Figs. 138–2 to 138–4), representing the interface between the apposed layers of the endometrium. The endometrium itself consists of a peripheral *basal* layer and an inner *functional* layer. Although it is not possible to delineate these two layers with current imaging techniques, cyclical changes in the functional layer can be visualized with US.

In the *proliferative phase,* 1 to 2.5 weeks after the onset of menses, the endometrium is usually echo-poor and thickens progressively. Although measurements vary with the observer, and also with the path of the sound beam and the transducer frequency, e.g., transabdominal vs endovaginal imaging, proliferative endometrium may measure up to 8 mm (± 3 mm standard deviation), and is generally echo-poor. Without an accurate menstrual history, it is difficult to differentiate proliferative endometrium from the echo-poor inner myometrium, or junctional zone (see Fig. 138–2). In the secretory phase, 2.5 to 4 weeks after menses, the endometrium continues to thicken, e.g., up to an average total of 11 mm (± 4 mm), and generally becomes more echogenic with posterior acoustic enhancement. The extent of echogenicity and acoustic enhancement vary among patients (see Figs. 138–3 and 138–4). Interestingly, the endometrial lining of the lower two thirds of the cervix does not undergo the same cyclical menstrual changes.

Care must be taken not to mistake the thick secretory endometrium for pathologic change. In general, pathologic states such as endometrial hyperplasia are associated with significantly thicker endometrial measurements than those that appear in the paragraph above. In one report, mean endometrial thickness in patients with endometrial hyperplasia was 19 mm with a range of 8 to 45 mm, vs 5 mm with a range of 2 to 10 mm for the control group (Malpani et al, 1990). Overall, endovaginal US is superior to the transabdominal approach for imaging endometrial abnormalities. On contrast-enhanced CT, the endometrium appears radiolucent, even long after the menopause, and may measure up to 20 mm in thickness (see Fig. 138–6). Correlation with a post-CT sonogram is often helpful if endometrial carcinoma is suspected because of a widened central radiolucency.

The endometrium appears bright on MRI, especally with T_2-weighting, and can be shown to thicken progressively from the proliferative to the secretory phase of the menstrual cycle (see Figs. 138–9 to 138–11). MRI measurements of endometrial thickness tend to be lower than US measurements.

A relatively echo-poor *junctional zone* of inner myometrium may be visualized around the endometrium especially during the secretory phase of the menstrual cycle (see Fig. 138–4). The myometrium within the junctional zone tends to be compact and hypovascular, with slightly less water content than the more peripheral endometrium. This may account for the hypoechoic appearance of the junctional zone on sonography and its relatively low intensity on T_2-weighted MRI. Overall, the junctional zone is better seen with MRI than US because it may not be distinguishable from echo-poor proliferative endometrium sonographically (see Figs. 138–9 to 138–11). The junctional zone is usually thicker and better defined on MRI than on US of the same patient. Because of these factors, MRI is a better imaging tool than US for pathologic processes that involve the junctional zone, such as invasive endometrial carcinoma, adenomyosis, and cervical carcinoma. The junctional zone is usually not visible with CT.

3. The *uterine vessels* are closely applied to the margins of the uterus, and are continuous superolaterally with the infundibulopelvic vessels around the ovaries. They are easiest to see with US or MRI (see Figs. 138–4, 138–5*C,* and 138–11). Each *uterine artery* arises from the corresponding internal iliac artery, and courses medially on the levator ani muscles, anterior to the lower ureter, to reach the lateral border of the cervix. It then ascends within the broad ligament, along the lateral margins of the uterus, giving off *arcuate* branches that penetrate the myometrium and course in its periphery toward the midline to anastomose with their contralateral counterparts (see Fig. 138–5*C*). *Radial arteries* arise from the arcuate arteries and penetrate the myometrium, giving off *spiral arteries* that supply the endometrium. At the superior aspect of the uterus, each uterine artery curves laterally within the broad ligament towards the ovary, where it anastomoses with the ovarian artery to form an *infundibulopelvic plexus.* The uterine veins parallel the arteries.

The uterine vessels enlarge with pregnancy even if it is ectopic. In such cases they are helpful not only for differentiating the uterus from adjacent adnexal masses, but also for suggesting the diagnosis of pregnancy. The uterine vessels may also enlarge during the late secretory phase of the menstrual cycle, and in the presence of pelvic inflammatory disease. High-velocity, turbulent, low-impedance flow, with a relatively large forward diastolic component, has been documented within the peritrophoblastic spiral arteries during pregnancy. This finding has helped to differentiate decidual reaction from intrauterine gestation, and occasionally to localize ectopic pregnancy. Similar flow patterns may be seen with uterine myomas and molar pregnancies.

The *fallopian* or *uterine tubes* extend into the broad ligaments from their point of origin just above and behind the round ligaments. Each tube is approximately 10 cm long, and consists of a 1-cm long *intramural* or *interstitial* segment, a 3-cm long narrow *isthmus,* a 5-cm long tortuous and redundant ampulla, and a 1-cm long trumpet-like *infundibulum* that is fimbriated. Portions of the nondilated tube may be identifiable on transverse CT, especially in the presence of ascites within the para-ovarian fossa (see Figs. 138–7 and 138–8). Coronal MRI may help occasionally to differentiate fallopian tube from ovary.

The *ovaries* lie within the broad ligaments anterior to the ureters and internal iliac vessels (see Figs. 138–5 to 138–8, and 138–10). The portion of the broad ligament that extends from the ovary and infundibulum of the uterine tube to the lateral pelvic wall is known as the *infundibulopelvic ligament* (Fig. 138–5*D* and *E*). If the infundibulopelvic and ovarian ligaments become lax, for example after multiple pregnancies, or if the uterus is retroverted or retroflexed, the ovary may lie posterior to the ureter (see Fig. 138–7). The ovary may also lie above, anterior, or posterior to the uterus. Each ovary has a dual blood supply, derived from the gonadal vessels laterally and the uterine vessels medially. These vessels form a plexus within the infundibulopelvic ligament, which is collectively termed the *infundibulopelvic vessels* (see Fig. 138–5*D* and *E*). The venous components of this network are also named the pampiniform plexus. Low-impedance arterial flow with an increased forward diastolic component has been documented in the ovarian vessels prior to and during ovulation, and also in the presence of the corpus luteum.

The anatomic landmarks that are most valuable for identifying the ovaries on sectional images are the peripheral follicles and/or infundibulopelvic vessels, and the sigmoid colon:

1. The ovaries can be identified positively on sectional images when the multiple cystic follicles at their periphery, or the infundi-

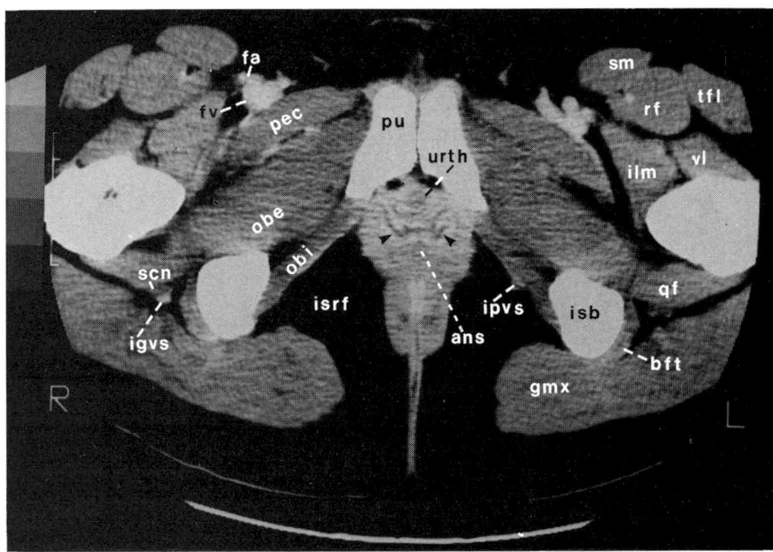

Figure 138–12. CT of urethra and lower vagina. The urethra (urth) has a relatively lucent central portion, due to redundant mucosa within its lumen, and a radiodense rim representing urethral wall musculature. The vagina *(arrowheads)* also has a lucent redundant lumen and bright muscular wall. (ans = anus; isrf = ischiorectal fossa fat; sm = sartorius; rf = rectus femoris; ilm = iliacus; vl = vastus lateralis; qf = quadratus femoris; gmx = gluteus maximus; pec = pectineus; obe = obturator externus; obi = obturator internis muscle.) The common femoral artery (fa) and vein (fv) have already bifurcated into superficial and deep branches on the left. The sciatic nerve (scn) and inferior gluteal vessels (igvs) now course in the posterior thigh. The radiodense biceps tendon (bft) is attached to the ischial tuberosity (isb). The internal pudendal vessels (ipvs) have exited the pelvis and are coursing within the radiodense pudendal canal. (pu = pubic symphysis.) (From Kazam E, Ramirez de Arellano E, Rubenstein WA, et al: Sonography of the pelvis and the lower urinary tract: Normal anatomy with CT and MRI correlations. In Shirkhoda A, Madrazo BL (eds): Pelvic Ultrasound. Baltimore, Williams and Wilkins, 1993, pp 1–18.)

bulopelvic vessels around them are visualized (see Figs. 138–4 to 138–8). The improved spatial resolution of endovaginal sonography, and the availability of relatively sensitive Doppler ultrasound have facilitated the differentiation between follicles and infundibulopelvic vessels (see Fig. 138–5*C* to *E*). US is the method of choice for identifying dominant follicles for in vitro fertilization.

On CT, the infundibulopelvic vessels can be demonstrated with dynamic scanning, and may contain phleboliths in older women. On T_1-weighted MRI, the peripheral follicles and/or infundibulopelvic vessels appear as dark foci (see Fig. 138–10), which may form a black rim at the periphery of the ovary, not to be confused with the chemical shift artifact. The spin-echo technique, with T_2-weighted multiple-slice/multiple-echo images, has the potential for differentiating follicles from infundibulopelvic vessels. As TE increases, follicles become progressively brighter while the vessels may either remain dark or show even echo enhancement. Unfortunately the loss of signal and spatial resolution with longer TE makes it difficult to consistently visualize these small structures on MRI.

Like the uterine vessels, the infundibulopelvic vessels, particularly the pampiniform plexus, enlarge in pregnancy, and should not be mistaken for dilated uterine tubes.

2. The sigmoid colon often indents the grooves between the ovaries and uterus, particularly on the left, and at times, bilaterally. This leads to a characteristic echogenic focus on transverse sonograms (see Fig. 138–5*A* and *B*), which should not be mistaken for calcification.

The *vagina* forms recesses termed *vaginal fornices,* on either side of the uterine cervix, which invaginates its superior portion (see Figs. 138–3, 138–9, 138–10, and 138–11*B*). It is wide in transverse diameter, and extends inferiorly between the bladder neck and urethra in front, and the rectum behind (Figs. 138–12 and 138–13). It is separated from the rectum by the rectovaginal septum, which is formed by fusion of the peritoneal layers around the cul-de-sac. Urine that escapes from the filled bladder in the supine position may gravitate into the vagina, and should not be mistaken for fluid in the cul-de-sac, or for a vesicovaginal fistula.

Given the readily available sagittal and coronal sections, and the ease with which the signal-poor cervix can be differentiated from

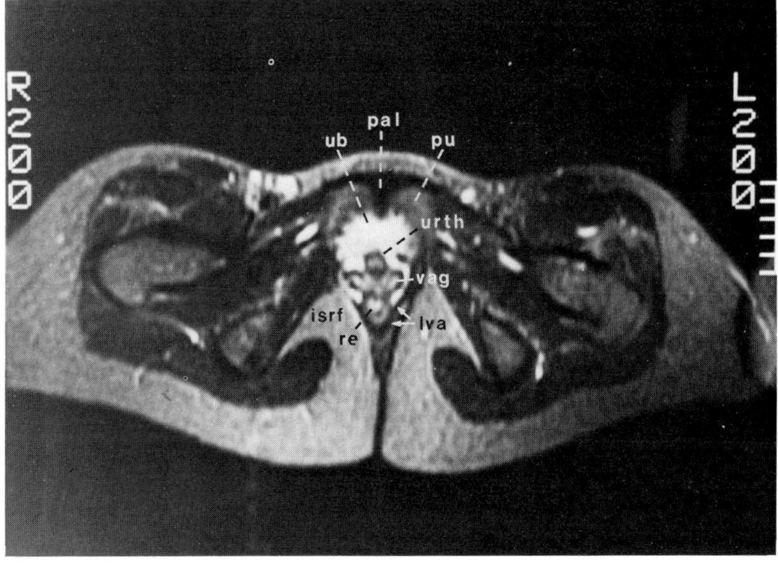

Figure 138–13. MRI of urethra and lower vagina. T_2-weighted transverse scan (1700/80 msec) through the pubic symphysis (pu). The cystic and vascular structures appear bright, while fat—for example, in the ischiorectal fossa (isrf)—has diminished intensity. The urethra (urth) and lower vagina (vag) have dark rims, representing their muscular walls, and relatively bright central lumina due to redundant mucosa. (ub = lower urinary bladder; re = rectum; lva = levator ani muscle; pal = pubic arcuate ligament.) Compare with Figure 138–12. (From Kazam E, Ramirez de Arellano E, Rubenstein WA, et al: Sonography of the pelvis and the lower urinary tract: Normal anatomy with CT and MRI correlations. In Shirkhoda A, Madrazo BL (eds): Pelvic Ultrasound. Baltimore, Williams and Wilkins, 1993, pp 1–18.)

surrounding vagina, MRI is preferable to sonography and CT for demonstrating the extent of vaginal masses and their relationship to the uterine cervix.

The Parametria

Extension of uterine and/or ovarian malignancies into the surrounding peritoneal and extraperitoneal tissues is best detected with CT, in our experience. With its higher spatial resolution, CT is more sensitive to the slight changes in attenuation of the pelvic fat that accompany early tumor extension. The higher sensitivity of CT also applies to the upper abdomen in the detection of omental tumor implants. The presence of infiltrated fat, however, is not necessarily specific for tumor, as it may also be seen with inflammatory disease and after surgery or radiation. With its poorer spatial resolution and the loss of signal at longer TE, MRI has been less reliable for detection of parametrial tumor extension and particularly poor for demonstrating involvement of adjacent bowel. This is because fluid-filled bowel, or bowel with small amounts of intraluminal air, cannot be positively identified on MRI. The increased sensitivity of CT in the parametria also applies to the detection of fluid within the intraperitoneal and extraperitoneal spaces around the bladder and uterus.

THE PELVIC MALE REPRODUCTIVE ORGANS

The *spermatic cord* (see Fig. 138–15*A* and *D*) is formed at the internal inguinal ring by the junction of the vas deferens with the testicular, deferential, and cremasteric vessels, and with the genital, cremasteric, and testicular nerves. Of these structures the vas deferens and testicular vessels are visible on CT and MRI (Fig. 138–14*A* to *C*). The fat within the internal spermatic fascia of the cord is derived in part from the retroperitoneal fat around the testicular vessels and from the prevesical fat around the vas deferens. Occasionally, it may form lipomas within the spermatic cord.

The *vas deferens* lies in the posterior part of the spermatic cord, where it is usually obscured by adjacent structures on CT or MRI. After leaving the cord at the internal inguinal ring, the vas follows a tortuous path, extending first superomedially, and then inferiorly in front of the ureter (see Fig. 138–14*A* to *C*). It then continues its medial course between the bladder and the upper seminal vesicles, where it becomes dilated and tortuous *(ampullary segment)* (Figs. 138–15*A*, 138–16*A*, and 138–17*A*). The terminal portion of the vas is narrowed again. It descends vertically in the midline, medial to the seminal vesicles, and joins the seminal vesicle duct to form the *ejaculatory duct,* which in turn empties into the urethra at the *verumontanum,* or *colliculus seminalis* (see Fig. 138–16*F* and *G*).

The *seminal vesicles* are tubular structures that lie at the superior aspect of the prostate, behind the lower urinary bladder and terminal ureters (see Figs. 138–14*C* and *D*, 138–15*A*, and 138–16*A* and *E*). Each vesicle is approximately 5 cm in maximal dimension, and consists of a coiled, compacted tube, measuring 10 to 15 cm in length, and 3 to 4 mm in diameter. The saccules formed by this tube may contain echo-poor or echogenic fluid on sonography (see Fig. 138–16*A*). These same saccules may appear relatively bright on MRI, and become so bright on T_2-weighted images that the seminal vesicles blend with the surrounding pelvic fat (see Fig. 138–17*A* and *B*). On CT, the saccules may appear isodense with muscle (see Fig. 138–14*C*), or they may be visualized as focal lucencies (see Fig. 138–15*A*), particularly in patients with marked prostatic hypertrophy or ejaculatory duct obstruction. The seminal vesicles lie with the urinary bladder in the perivesical space. They are separated from the rectum by the cul-de-sac superiorly, and by the rectovesical septum (Denonvilliers' fascia) inferiorly. The *seminal vesicle* duct joins with the ipsilateral vas deferens to form the *ejaculatory duct* (see Fig. 138–16*F*).

The *prostate* lies behind the pubic symphysis, posteroinferior to the bladder neck, and anterior to the rectum (see Figs. 138–15*B* and *C*, 138–16*C* to *G*, and 138–17*C* and *D*). It is separated from the rectum by the rectovesical septum, which is formed by fusion of the peritoneal envelopes of the cul-de-sac, analogous to the rectovaginal septum. The prevesical space extends downward, in front of the anterosuperior prostate (see Fig. 138–15*B* and *C*), to the attachments of the puboprostatic ligaments, which form its floor. The prostate is shaped like an inverted cone, with its base directed superiorly toward the bladder neck, and its apex directed inferiorly toward the levator ani and transversus perinei profundi muscles. The urethra courses through the prostate, at first posteroinferiorly *(proximal prostatic urethra),* and then directly inferiorly *(distal prostatic urethra)* at an angle of nearly 35 degrees with the proximal urethra. The verumontanum forms a ridge of tissue in the upper distal urethra, just below its junction with the proximal urethra. The proximal urethra is surrounded by smooth muscle fibers, which form a *preprostatic sphincter,* whereas the distal urethra is surrounded by striated muscle.

The prostate can be divided into a nonglandular *fibromuscular stroma* anterior to the urethra, and a *glandular* portion posterior to the urethra. The glandular portion can be further subdivided into a *central zone* behind the proximal urethra, and a *peripheral zone* behind the distal urethra. In addition, there is a normally diminutive glandular component, termed the *transitional zone,* that lies on either side of the proximal urethra, contiguous to the preprostatic sphincter.

The urethral lumen is visible as an echogenic linear structure on US, especially on midline sagittal views (see Fig. 138–16*F*). Periurethral calcifications often parallel and serve as a guide for the course of the urethra. The lumen and contiguous glandular calcifications have a triangular configuration on transverse sections at the level of the verumontanum (see Fig. 138–16*G*). The *fibromuscular stroma* appears relatively echo-poor on US, radio-dense on contrast-enhanced CT, and hypointense on MRI. The *preprostatic sphincter* around the proximal urethra blends with the fibromuscular portion and has the same appearance on US, CT, and MRI (see Fig. 138–16*D* to *G*). The *transitional zone* on either side of the preprostatic sphincter is normally diminutive and poorly delineated on sectional images, but may be visualized as an echogenic region, particularly if it contains focal calcifications (see Fig. 138–16*C, D,* and *G*). In older males, benign prostatic hyperplasia originates from the transitional zone, with secondary compression and extrinsic narrowing of the peripheral zone.

The *central zone* behind the proximal urethra is relatively echogenic, because it contains larger glands with more calcified corpora amylacea than the peripheral zone—which has intermediate echogenicity (see Fig. 138–16*D* to *G*). It is possible to visualize both the upper central zone and lower peripheral zone on one transverse US section because of cephalocaudad angulation of the sound beam (see Fig. 138–16*C, D,* and *F*). The ejaculatory ducts course through the central zone to empty at the verumontanum (see Fig. 138–16*F*). The ducts of transitional and central zone glands also empty at the verumontanum, whereas peripheral gland ducts empty into the distal urethra. There is a predilection for calcifications to form at the interface between transitional and peripheral zone, in a region called the *surgical capsule* (see Fig. 138–16*G*).

Both the central zone and peripheral zone appear relatively lucent on CT (see Fig. 138–15*B* and *C*) and bright on T_2-weighted MRI. The peripheral zone is the site of origin of nearly 70 to 80 per cent of prostatic carcinomas, compared with 5 to 10 per cent for the central zone, and 10 to 20 per cent for the transitional zone.

Text continued on page 2028

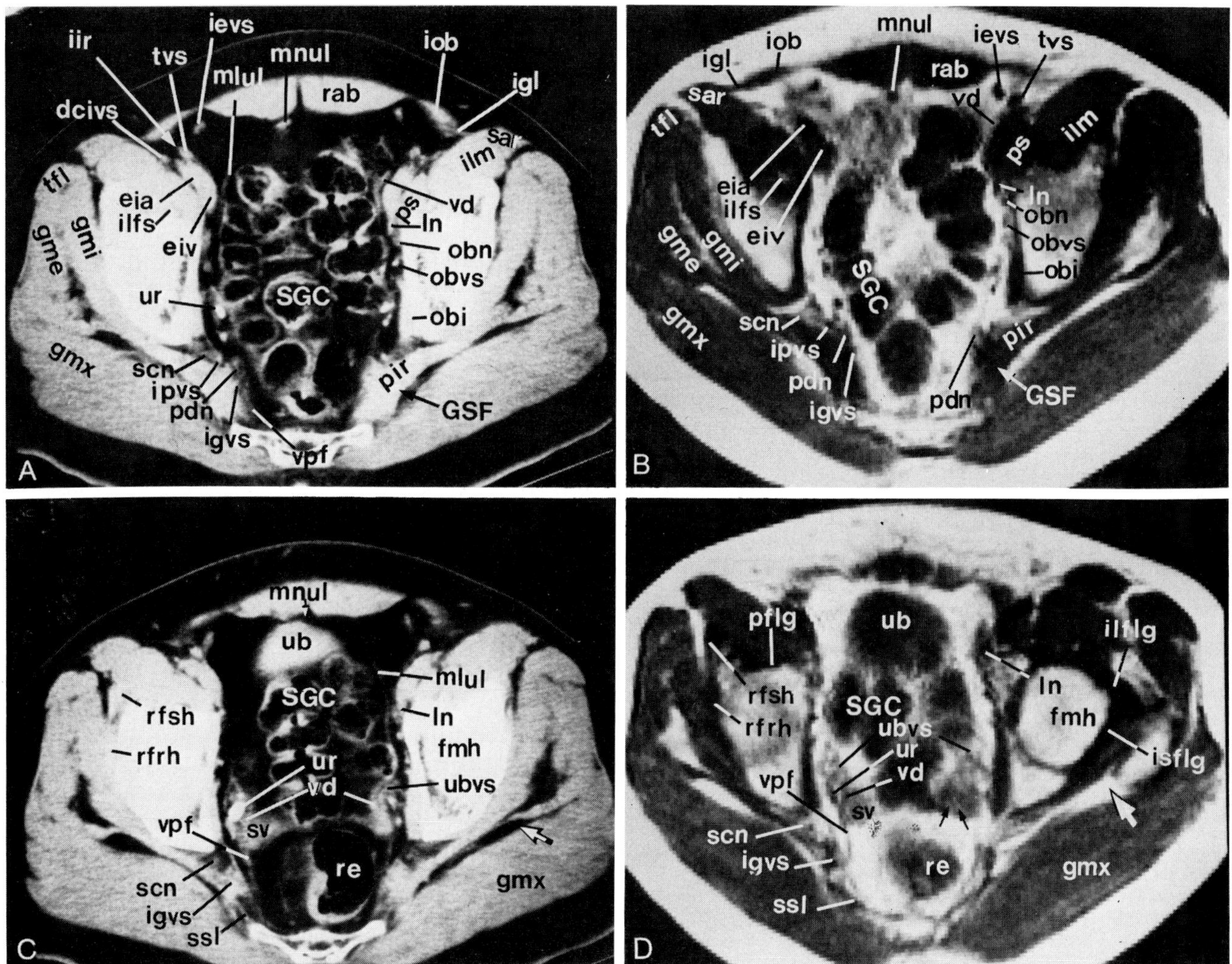

Figure 138–14. The male pelvis. *A* and *B,* **CT *(A)* and MRI *(B)* of same patient through greater sciatic foramen.** The pelvis is occupied mostly by a tortuous sigmoid colon (SGC). (ievs = inferior epigastric vessels; tvs = testicular vessels.) The left vas deferens (vd) courses just medial to the external iliac artery (eia) and vein (eiv) on CT, analogous to the round ligament in Figure 138–6*A*, but is not as clearly delineated on MRI. The external iliac vessels (eia, eiv) blend with the isointense psoas muscle (ps) on MRI but not on CT. The obturator (obn) and sciatic (scn) nerves are well seen with both techniques. (ln = external iliac lymph nodes; obvs = obturator vessels; obi = obturator internus muscle.) The pudendal nerve (pdn) is better seen on MRI *(B)*. The ureter (ur) is indistinguishable from pelvic vessels on MRI.

C and *D,* **CT *(C)* 10 mm below *A* and corresponding MRI *(D)*.** The superior portions of the seminal vesicles (sv) and urinary bladder (ub) are now visible. Fluid-containing saccules within the seminal vesicles appear bright on MRI but are not well visualized on this CT. The vasa deferentia are better seen on CT. The right vas deferens (vd) lies just medial to the ureter (ur). *Small arrows* indicate the left vas deferens. (ubvs = vesical venous plexus.) The femoral head (fmh) appears isointense on MRI, with the fat *(arrow)* anterior to the gluteus maximus muscle (gmx). The tendons of the straight (rfsh) and reflected (rfrh) heads of the rectus femoris muscle, and the pubofemoral (pflg), iliofemoral (ilflg), and ischiofemoral (isflg) ligaments can be differentiated from the brighter adjacent muscles on MRI, unlike the case with CT.

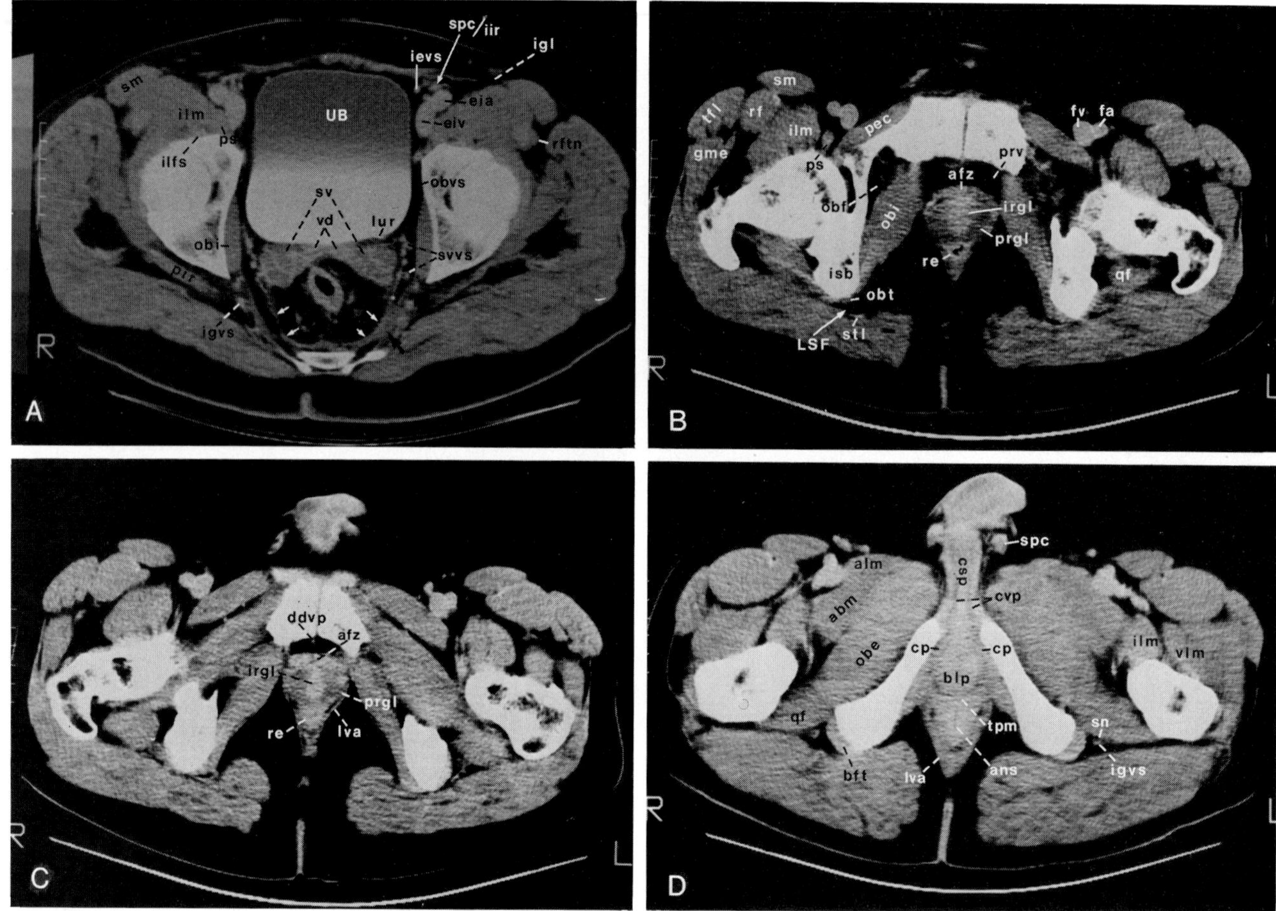

Figure 138–15. CT of male pelvis. *A,* **CT through lower greater sciatic foramen.** The seminal vesicles (sv) have a radiolucent internal structure, representing intraluminal vesicular fluid, with interspersed "septa"—representing the walls of the convoluted tubule and saccules that form each seminal vesicle. (vd = ampullary portions of vas deferens; svvs = seminal vesicle venous plexus; *white arrows* = perirectal fascia; *black arrow* = edema of presacral fat.) The left ureter (lur) is visible at its junction with the urinary bladder (UB). The spermatic cord (spc) lies within the internal inguinal ring (iir), lateral to the inferior epigastric vessels (ievs). (igl = inguinal ligament; eia, eiv = external iliac vessels; obvs = obturator vessels; sm = sartorius muscle; ilm = iliacus muscle; ps = psoas muscle.) The iliac fascia (ilfs) is visible at its attachment to the anterosuperior acetabulum. (obi = obturator internus muscle; pir = piriformis muscle; rftn = rectus femoris tendon; igvs = inferior gluteal vessels.)

B and *C,* **Contrast-enhanced CT scans of upper** ***(B)*** **and lower** ***(C)*** **prostate.** The anterior fibromuscular zone (afz) is deficient in glandular tissue and appears radiodense relative to the peripheral gland (prgl), which represents "central zone" superiorly *(B)* and "peripheral zone" inferiorly *(C).* The inner gland (irgl) is also radiodense, due to enhancing musculature of the preprostatic sphincter around the proximal urethra *(B)* or the striated muscle around the distal urethra *(C).* The urethral lumen is not delineated. The "transitional zone" of proximal periurethral glands is contiguous to, and partially within, the preprostatic sphincter *(B),* but is not separately delineated. (ddvp = deep dorsal vein of penis; prv = prevesical space fat; lva = levator ani muscle; re = rectum; fa = femoral artery; fv = femoral vein; pec = pectineus; ps = psoas; ilm = iliacus; rf = rectus femoris; sm = sartorius; tfl = tensor fasciae latae; gme = gluteus medius; obi = obturator internus; qf = quadratus femoris.) The obturator tendon (obt) exits the pelvis through the lesser sciatic foramen (LSF), between the sacrotuberous ligament (stl) and the ischium (isb).

D, **CT scan below the prostate** shows the bulb of the penis (blp) and the corpora cavernosa (cvp), crura (cp), and corpus spongiosum (csp) of the penis. (spc = spermatic cord; ans = anus; lva = levator ani muscle; tpm = transverse perinei muscle; alm = adductor longus; abm = adductor brevis; obe = obturator externus; ilm = iliacus; qf = quadratus femoris; vlm = vastus lateralis; igvs = inferior gluteal vessels; sn = sciatic nerve; bft = biceps femoris tendon.)

(*A* to *D* from Kazam E, Ramirez de Arellano E, Rubenstein WA, et al: Sonography of the pelvis and the lower urinary tract: Normal anatomy with CT and MRI correlations. In Shirkhoda A, Madrazo BL (eds): Pelvic Ultrasound. Baltimore, Williams and Wilkins, 1993, pp 1–18.)

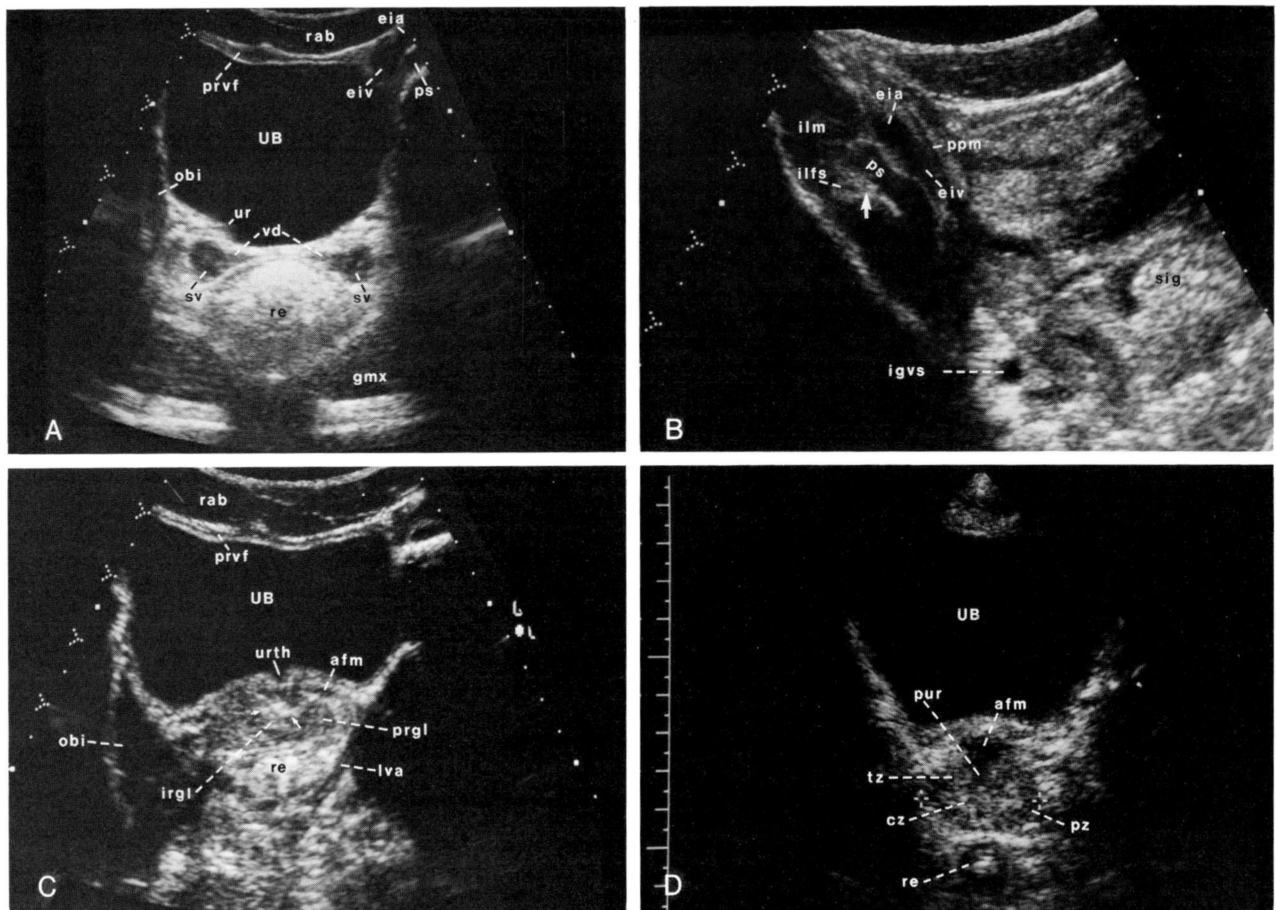

Figure 138–16. Sonography of the male pelvis. *A,* **Transvesical sonogram** shows the seminal vesicles (sv) posterior to the urinary bladder (UB) at the level of the uretero (ur)–vesical junction. The echo-poor texture of the seminal vesicles is attributable to intraluminal fluid, while the short septum-like echogenic interfaces represent the walls of the compacted, saccular tube that forms each seminal vesicle. Compare with Figure 138–15*A*. (vd = ampullary portion of the vas deferens; re = rectum; prvf = prevesical fat; eia = external iliac artery; eiv = external iliac vein; ps = psoas; rab = rectus abdominis; obi = obturator internus; gmx = gluteus maximus.)

B, **Transverse sonogram of lateral pelvic wall.** The psoas (ps) and iliacus (ilm) muscles are separated by echogenic fat *(arrow)* that surrounds the echo-poor iliac fascia (ilfs). Compare with Figures 138–6, 138–7, and 138–11*A*. The external iliac artery (eia) and vein (eiv) lie medial to the psoas muscle and lateral to the interface of parietal peritoneum with extraperitoneal fat (ppm). The posterolateral pelvic wall structures are poorly delineated relative to CT and MRI. (igvs = inferior gluteal vessels; sig = sigmoid colon.)

C, **Transvesical sonogram through the upper prostate with caudad angulation.** The proximal urethra (urth) is visible at the neck of the urinary bladder (UB). The prostatic anterior fibromuscular zone (afm) is relatively echo-poor. The inner gland (irgl) contains echo-poor portions, due to periurethral musculature, and echogenic portions due to calcifications *(arrow)* within the periurethral transitional zone. prgl = peripheral gland; prvf = prevesical fat; (lva = levator ani muscle; re = rectum; obi = obturator internus muscle.)

D, **Transvesical sonogram through midprostate.** The echo-poor anterior fibromuscular zone (afm) is contiguous posteriorly with the echo-poor preprostatic sphincter around the proximal urethra (pur). The transitional zone (tz) and central zone (cz) posteriorly are echogenic relative to the peripheral zone (pz). (re = rectum.)

Illustration continued on following page

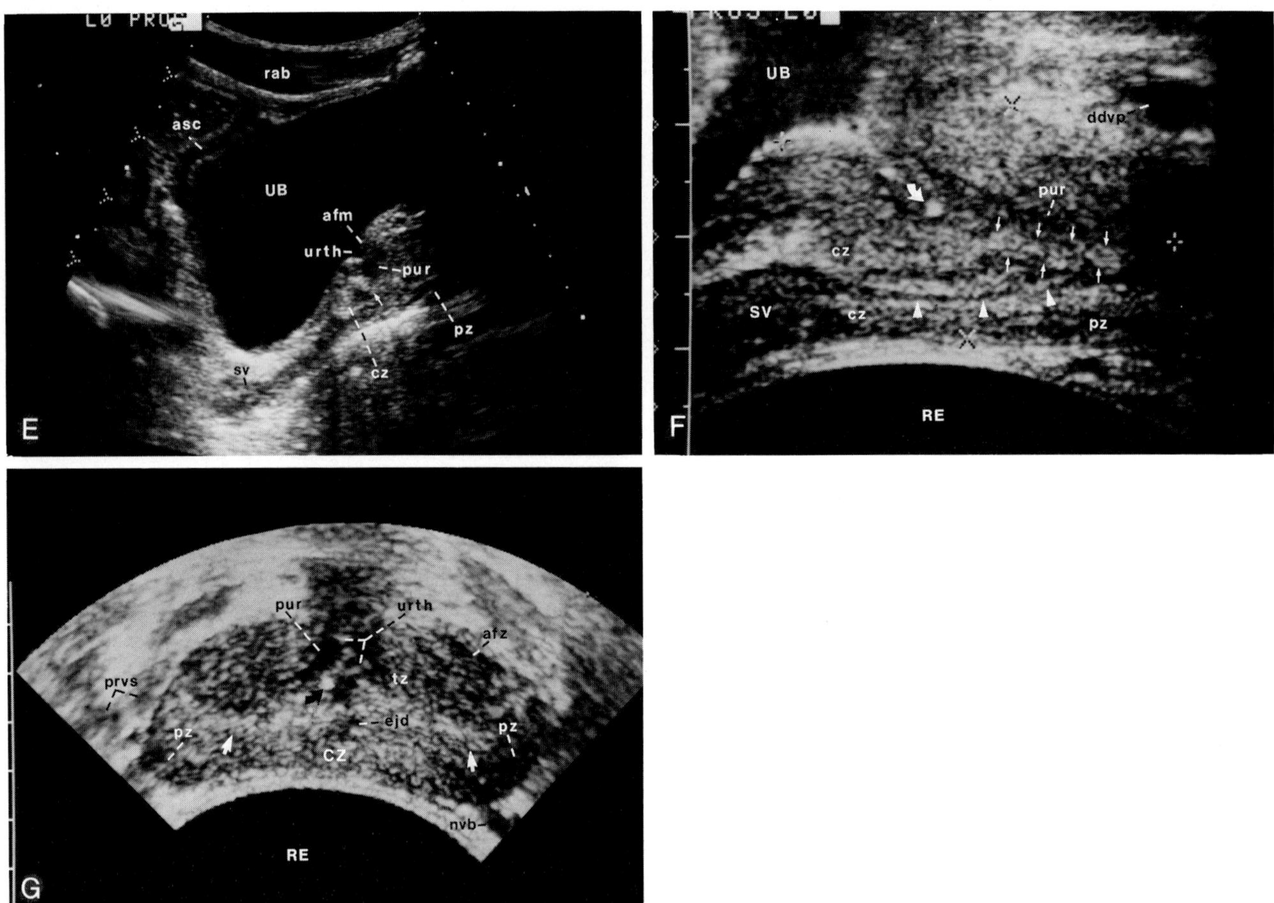

Figure 138–16 *Continued*

E, **Sagittal transvesical sonogram** shows the proximal urethra (urth) at the neck of the urinary bladder (UB). The echo-poor anterior fibromuscular stroma (afm) is continuous with the preprostatic sphincter (pur), which surrounds the proximal prostatic urethra. Calcification in periurethral transitional zone glands is seen *(arrow).* The central zone (cz)—superiorly—is more echogenic than the peripheral zone (pz) inferiorly. (sv = seminal vesicles; asc = small amount of ascites.)

F, **Sagittal transrectal prostatic sonogram.** The lumen of the urethra is echogenic *(arrows),* while the periurethral musculature (pur) is echo-poor. There is focal periurethral calcification *(curved arrow)* within transitional zone glands. The ejaculatory duct *(arrowheads)* can be followed inferiorly, as it courses through the central zone (cz), from the seminal vesicle (SV) to its junction with the urethra. (pz = peripheral zone; UB = urinary bladder; ddvp = deep dorsal vein of the penis; RE = rectal lumen.)

G, **Transverse transrectal upper prostatic sonogram.** The urethral lumen (urth) has a triangular configuration, which is typical at the level of the verumontanum (not delineated). (pur = echo-poor preprostatic sphincter; ejd = left ejaculatory duct.) The transitional zone (tz) and central zone (cz) are relatively echogenic. The peripheral zone (pz) has intermediate echogenicity, and is partially visualized on the same transverse section as the central zone because of cephalocaudad angulation of the beam. Calcifications in periurethral transitional zone glands are seen *(curved arrow).* The echogenic curvilinear interface *(arrows)* between inner prostate and peripheral gland is attributable to calcifications at the surgical capsule. (afz = anterior fibromuscular zone; nvb = neurovascular bundle; prvs = prostatic venous plexus; RE = rectal lumen.)

(*A* to *G* from Kazam E, Ramirez de Arellano E, Rubenstein WA, et al: Sonography of the pelvis and the lower urinary tract: Normal anatomy with CT and MRI correlations. In Shirkhoda A, Madrazo BL (eds): Pelvic Ultrasound. Baltimore, Williams and Wilkins, 1993, pp 1–18.)

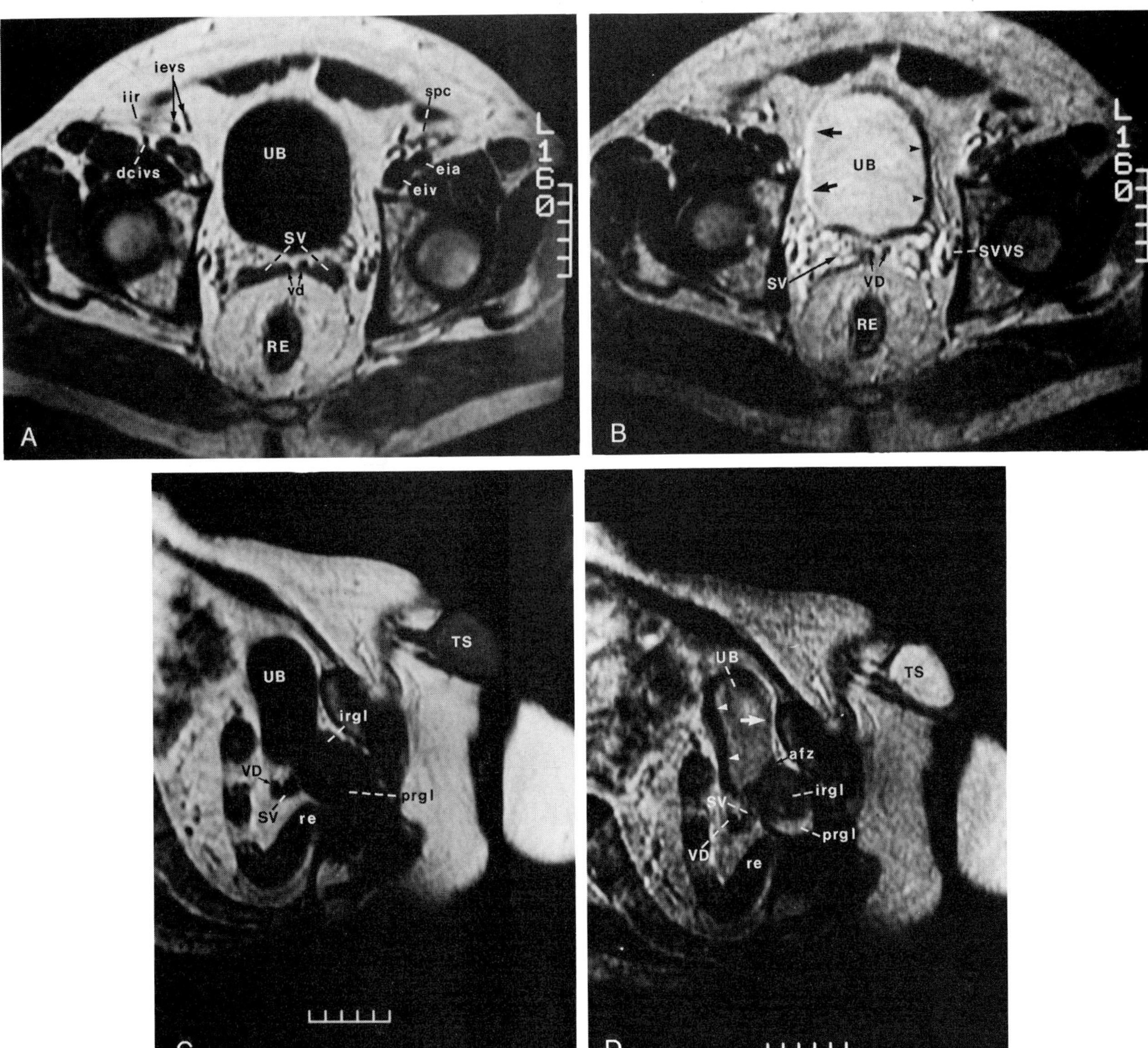

Figure 138–17. MRI of the male pelvis. *A* and *B,* **Transverse MRI through the seminal vesicles.** Intermediate (1700/20 msec, *A*) and T_2-weighted (1700/80 msec, *B*) multiecho images at the same anatomic level. The seminal vesicles (SV) become hyperintense on the T_2-weighted images because of their fluid content. The muscular walls of the ampullary portions of the vas deferens (vd) remain hypointense *(B),* while their small lumens show focal enhancement with T_2-weighting. The seminal vesicle venous plexus (SVVS) and the urinary bladder lumen (UB) also become hyperintense in *B.* Note apparent thickening and hypointensity of the left lateral urinary bladder wall *(arrowheads),* in contradistinction to the bright right lateral wall *(arrows),* due to chemical shift artifact. A similar effect is evident for the lateral walls of the rectum (RE). The vascular and ligamentous structures that demarcate the internal inguinal ring (iir) and proximal inguinal canal are clearly visible *(A):* inferior epigastric (ievs), external iliac (eia, eiv), and deep circumflex iliac (dcivs) vessels. (spc = spermatic cord.)

C and *D,* **Midsagittal MRI of the prostate.** Intermediate (1700/20 msec, *C*) and T_2-weighted (1700/80 msec, *D*) multiecho images through the same anatomic plane. The peripheral glandular portion (prgl) of the prostate becomes hyperintense on the T_2-weighted image. It represents central zone superiorly and peripheral zone inferiorly, although these two zones are otherwise indistinguishable by MRI. The anterior fibromuscular zone (afz) remains hypointense in *D,* while the inner gland (irgl) (representing urethra, periurethral musculature, and transitional zone) shows slightly enhanced intensity on T_2-weighting. (VD = vas deferens; SV = medial seminal vesicle; TS = testicle; re = rectum.) Note pseudothickening *(arrowheads)* of superior wall of urinary bladder (UB) in contradistinction to its inferior wall *(arrow),* due to chemical shift artifact.

(*A* to *D* from Kazam E, Ramirez de Arellano E, Rubenstein WA, et al: Sonography of the pelvis and the lower urinary tract: Normal anatomy with CT and MRI correlations. In Shirkhoda A, Madrazo BL (eds): Pelvic Ultrasound. Baltimore, Williams and Wilkins, 1993, pp 1–18.)

THE INTESTINES

The *cecum* lies in the right lower quadrant anterior to the iliacus muscle (see Fig. 138–1*A* to *D*). Although it is saccular in most patients (see Fig. 138–1*D*), it may occasionally have a conical configuration with a narrow inferior portion (see Fig. 138–1*A* to *C*). The cecum may extend into the pelvis, where it lies in the right inguinal fossa and may herniate through the right inguinal canal. It is intraperitoneal. Fluid, or occasionally ovarian cysts, may be found within the retrocecal recess.

The *appendix,* not illustrated here, may be visualized as a narrow tubular structure posteromedial to the cecum. It may extend into the pelvis, next to the right adnexa. Occasionally, it may be seen posteromedial to the psoas muscle at the L5-S1 level, in close proximity to the retropsoas nerves.

The *distal ileum* is often visualized within the right inguinal fossa (see Fig. 138–7). It may also extend into the cul-de-sac, between the bladder and rectum.

The *distal descending colon* lies in front of the iliacus muscle, just above the acetabular roof (see Fig. 138–1*A* to *D*), where it curves medially to form the sigmoid colon. It may have a complete mesentery, or mesocolon, in 36 per cent of patients. In such cases the left ovary may occasionally be found within its deep lateral or medial paracolic gutters.

The *sigmoid colon* forms a loop that extends anteriorly to the right and then posteriorly on one or both sides of the midline. It may be found within the left inguinal fossa (see Fig. 138–8*B*), at the pelvic inlet above the urinary bladder (see Figs. 138–1*B* and 138–14*A* to *D*), and behind the upper urinary bladder. It frequently indents the grooves between the uterus and the ovaries (see Fig. 138–5*A* to *C*).

The *rectum* begins at approximately the S3 vertebral level (see Figs. 138–8, 138–9, 138–14*C,* and 138–17), and extends inferiorly (see Figs. 138–9*A,* 138–12, 138–13, 138–15, and 138–17) to the anus. The rectal columns, which are prominent longitudinal folds, may be visualized as tiny mucosal ridges on CT of the nondistended distal rectum. Above them, the rectum is typically dilated in its ampullary portion (see Fig. 138–14*C* and *D*). There are prominent transverse folds in the rectal ampulla below the rectosigmoid junction which are best seen with MRI (see Fig. 138–17*C* and *D*). Because of its three small flexures, two to the left and one to the right, the rectum is often found on either side of the midline on CT (see Figs. 138–8 and 138–14*C* and *D*). It is surrounded by perirectal fat and by the visceral layer of the pelvic fascia (see Figs. 138–8*A* and 138–14*C* and *D*), which may become thickened on CT in the presence of perirectal disease.

THE PELVIC MUSCLES

The muscles in and around the pelvis may serve as valuable anatomic landmarks or as pathways for extension of pelvic collections. Occasionally, they may contribute to diagnostic errors on sectional imaging.

The *iliacus* and *psoas muscles* course anterolaterally through the pelvis and exit behind the inguinal ligament to insert via a common tendon onto the lesser trochanter (see Figs. 138–1*A* to *D,* 138–6, 138–7, 138–14*A* to *D,* and 138–15). They are separated from each other by a small fatty groove (see Figs. 138–6 to 138–8, 138–9*B,* 138–11*A,* and 138–14*A*) that contains iliac fascia and the femoral nerve. This fat appears lucent on CT (see Figs. 138–6 to 138–8 and 138–15*A*), bright on MRI (see Fig. 138–11*A*), and echogenic on US (see Fig. 138–16*B*). Radio-dense iliac fascia is often visible within this fat (see Figs. 138–6 to 138–8, 138–14, 138–15*A*). This fascia appears signal-poor on MRI (see Fig. 138–11*A*) and echo-poor on US (see Fig. 138–16*B*). Occasionally, this fatty interface is elongated. In such cases the psoas muscle may mimic enlarged external iliac lymph nodes. Retroperitoneal collections may extend inferiorly along the iliopsoas into the thigh.

The *piriformis muscle* courses from its attachments around the anterior sacral foramina, anterolaterally and inferiorly to exit the greater sciatic foramen (see Figs. 138–6 to 138–8, 138–11*A,* and 138–14*A* to *D*). Above the piriformis, the superior gluteal vessels and nerves also exit the greater sciatic foramen, whereas below it passes the sciatic, pudendal, and posterior femoral cutaneous nerves and the inferior gluteal and internal pudendal vessels. The piriformis inserts on the greater trochanter, in close proximity to the gluteus medius muscle. Although it is occasionally well seen with ultrasound, it is more often obscured, at least partially, by bowel gas or fat (see Fig. 138–5*A*). In such cases the visualized portions of the piriformis should not be mistaken for pathologic lesions. Collections may extend from the pelvis to the buttocks, and vice versa, along the piriformis muscle and through the greater sciatic foramen.

The *coccygeus muscle* courses from the ischial spine to the coccyx in contiguity with the sacrospinous ligament, separating the greater sciatic foramen above from the lesser sciatic foramen below (see Figs. 138–7 and 138–14*C* and *D*). Through the lesser sciatic foramen pass the nerve and tendon of the obturator internus muscle, the pudendal nerve, and the internal pudendal vessels.

The *levator ani muscles* are visible, especially with MRI, in the pelvic floor along the lateral aspects of the prostate and rectum (see Figs. 138–10, 138–13, 138–15*C* and *D,* and 138–16*C*). They are thicker than the visceral pelvic fascia directly above them (see Figs. 138–8*A* and 138–14*C* and *D*).

The *rectus abdominis muscles* are separated from the internal oblique and transversus abdominis muscle by the semilunar line, which contains no muscle fibers (see Figs. 138–1*C* and *D,* 138–6, and 138–14*A* to *D*). Spigelian hernias may occur at this line. The rectus sheath is formed by only a thin layer of transversalis fascia, below a line (arcuate line) that is midway between the pubis and umbilicus. The prevesical space and rectus sheath communicate with each other through this thin layer, along perforating inferior epigastric vessels and nerves.

LIGAMENTS AND TENDONS

The ligaments and tendons appear hyperdense on contrast-enhanced CT because of their highly attenuating and capillary-rich fibrous tissues. As a result, some of these structures may be initially mistaken for blood vessels on CT. These include the sacrospinous ligament between the greater and lesser sciatic foramina (see Figs. 138–6 and 138–14*C*), the sacrotuberous ligament that marks the posterior borders of the greater and lesser sciatic foramina (see Fig. 138–15*B*), and the iliac fascia between the psoas and iliacus muscles (see Fig. 138–7). These same fibrous tissues are devoid of signal on MRI and appear black, like blood vessels (see Fig. 138–14*D*). Fibrous structures that appear so bright on CT that they blend with adjacent bone can be delineated with MRI. These include the tendons of the rectus femoris and biceps femoris muscles (see Fig. 138–14*C* and *D*), the iliofemoral, ischiofemoral, and pubic arcuate ligaments (see Figs. 138–14*C* and *D,* and 138–13), and the lumbosacral fascia.

Bibliography

Auh YH, Rubenstein WA, Markisz JA, et al: Intraperitoneal paravesical spaces: CT delineation with US correlation. Radiology 159:311–317, 1986.

Auh YH, Rubenstein WA, Schneider M, et al: Extraperitoneal paravesical spaces: CT delineation with US correlation. Radiology 159:319–328, 1986.

Brown HK, Stoll BS, Nicosia SV, et al: Uterine junctional zone: Correlation between histologic findings and MR imaging. Radiology 179:409–413, 1991.

Demas B, Hricak H, Jaffe RB: Uterine MR imaging: Effects of hormonal stimulation. Radiology 159:123–126, 1986.

Dillon EH, Feyock AL, Taylor KNW: Pseudogestational sacs: Doppler US differentiation from normal or abnormal intrauterine pregnancies. Radiology 176:359–364, 1990.

Eycleshymer AC, Shoemaker DM: A Cross Section Anatomy. New York, Appleton-Century-Crofts, 1970, pp 86–101, 104–113.

Fleischer AC, Dudley BS, Entman SS, et al: Myometrial invasion by endometrial carcinoma: Sonographic assessment. Radiology 162:307–310, 1987.

Fleischer AC, Kalemeris GC, Entman SS: Sonographic depiction of the endometrium during normal cycles. Ultrasound Med Biol 12:271–277, 1986.

Fleischer AC, Kalemeris GC, Machin JE, et al: Sonographic depiction of normal and abnormal endometrium with histopathologic correlation. J Ultrasound Med 5:445–452, 1986.

Forrest TS, Elyaderani MK, Muilenburg MI, et al: Cyclic endometrial changes: US assessment with histologic correlation. Radiology 167:233–237, 1988.

Haynor DR, Mack LA, Souldes MR, et al: Changing appearance of the normal uterus during the menstrual cycle: MR studies. Radiology 161:459–462, 1986.

Hricak H, Stern JL, Fisher MR, et al: Endometrial carcinoma staging by MR imaging. Radiology 162:297–305, 1987.

Husband JES, Olliff JFC, Williams MP, et al: Bladder cancer: Staging with CT and MR imaging. Radiology 173:435–440, 1989.

Kazam E, Auh YH, Rubenstein WA, et al: Computed tomography of the lower urinary tract and pelvis. In Pollack HM (ed): Clinical Urography. Philadelphia, WB Saunders Company, 1990, pp 407–432.

Kazam E, Ramirez de Arellano E, Rubenstein WA, et al: Sonography of the pelvis and the lower urinary tract: Normal anatomy with CT and MRI correlations. In Shirkhoda A, Madrazo BL (eds): Pelvic Ultrasound. Baltimore, Williams and Wilkins, 1993, pp 1–18.

Malpani A, Singer J, Wolverson MK, Merenda G: Endometrial hyperplasia: Value of endometrial thickness in ultrasonographic diagnosis and clinical significance. J Clin Ultrasound 18:173–177, 1990.

Mark AD, Hricak H, Heinrichs LW, Henderickson MR, Winkler ML, Bachica JA, Stickler JE. Adenomyosis and leiomyoma: differential diagnosis with MR imaging. Radiology 163:527–529, 1987.

McCarthy S, Scott G, Majumdar S, Shapiro B, Thompson S, Lange R, Gore J. Uterine junctional zone: MR study of water content and relaxation properties. Radiology 171:241–243, 1989.

McCarthy S, Tauber C, Gore J: Female pelvic anatomy: MR assessment of variations during the menstrual cycle and with use of oral contraceptives. Radiology 160:119–123, 1986.

Mendelson EB, Bohm-Velez M, Joseph N, Neiman HL: Endometrial abnormalities: Evaluation with transvaginal sonography. AJR 150:139–142, 1988.

Mendelson EB, Bohm-Velez M, Joseph N, Neiman HL: Gynecologic imaging: Comparison of transabdominal and transvaginal sonography. Radiology 166:321–324, 1988.

Mitchell DG, Schonholz L, Hilpert PL, et al: Zones of the uterus: Discrepancy between US and MR images. Radiology 174:827–831, 1990.

Ritchie WGM: Sonographic evaluation of normal and induced ovulation. State of the art. Radiology 161:1–10, 1986.

Salo JO, Kivissari L, Lehtonen T: Comparison of magnetic resonance imaging with computed tomography and intravesical ultrasound in staging bladder ca. Urol Radiol 10:167, 1988.

Scoutt LM, Flynn SD, Luthringer DJ, et al: Junctional zone of the uterus: Correlation of MR imaging and histologic examination of hysterectomy specimens. Radiology 179:403–407, 1991.

Soila KP, Viamonte M Jr, Starewicz PM: Chemical shift misregistration effect in magnetic resonance imaging. Radiology 153:819–820, 1984.

Taylor KJW, Burns PN, Wells PNT, et al: Ultrasound Doppler flow studies of the ovarian and uterine arteries. Br J Obstet Gynecol 92:240–246, 1985.

Tessler FN, Schiller VL, Perrella RR, et al: Transabdominal versus endovaginal pelvic sonography: Prospective study. Radiology 170:553–556, 1989.

Togashi K, Nishimura K, Itoh K, et al: Uterine cervical cancer: Assessment with high-field MR imaging. Radiology 160:431–435, 1986.

Whalen JP: Radiology of the Abdomen: An Anatomic Approach. Philadelphia, Lea & Febiger, 1976.

Williams PL, Warwick R (eds): Gray's Anatomy, 36th ed. Philadelphia, WB Saunders, 1980.

9 Hysterosalpingography

Charles J. Fagan

Hysterosalpingography is an imaging test that utilizes a contrast medium and radiographic techniques to visualize the uterine cavity and lumina of the fallopian tubes. Historically, its major use has been in evaluating the patency of fallopian tubes and normalcy of the uterine cavity in infertile women. As a result, the frequency with which the study is performed has been influenced little by pelvic sonography. Sonography has, however, virtually replaced hysterosalpingography in defining the anatomy of the internal genitalia in the pediatric intersex patient.

TECHNIQUE

Careful technique in the performance of the study is as essential as intelligent analysis of the findings to avoid mistaken diagnoses. The study is usually done on an outpatient basis and safely performed between the seventh and fourteenth days of the menstrual cycle. There are several ways to perform the examination. A thorough method that requires the gynecologist's participation is described as follows:

Initially, an anteroposterior scout radiograph of the pelvis is made. A radiolucent speculum is placed in the vagina and a pelvic examination performed. The vaginal vault is cleaned with an appropriate antiseptic agent. The anterior lip of the cervix is then grasped with a tenaculum so that the uterus can be pulled into a coronal plane. Various types of cannula are attached to the cervix or inserted into the cervical os. These devices form a seal over the external cervical os and establish an avenue through which 3 to 10 ml of aqueous or oil-based contrast material is injected into the uterine cavity by controlled hydrostatic pressure. The whole event is carefully monitored by image-intensified video fluoroscopy so that appropriate frontal and oblique spot films can be made to record sequential opacification of the cervical canal, the uterine cavity, and the lumina of the fallopian tubes. If peritonealization of contrast material is not observed, a post-injection radiograph of the pelvis is made after the patient has been permitted to ambulate for 5 to 10 minutes. Glucagon (2 mg intravenously) may relieve temporary proximal tube obstruction caused by dysfunctional muscular spasm.

The end point of the study, under normal conditions, is opacification of a normal uterine cavity, uterine tubes, and free spillage of contrast materal into the peritoneal cavity (Fig. 139–1).

INDICATIONS

Evaluation of the patency of the fallopian tubes and normalcy of the uterine cavity of infertile women represents the most frequent indication for hysterosalpingography. The major other indications include the following:

1. Search for acquired and congenital uterine abnormalities as underlying causes for repeated second and third trimester abortions.
2. Delineation of fallopian tube nonpatency or renewed continuity following tubal ligation and reconstructive surgery, respectively.
3. Demonstration of uterine fistula (usually secondary to uterine perforation by an IUD, neoplasm, or tuberculosis).
4. Identification of an empty uterus in a suspected abdominal pregnancy.
5. Demonstration of the precise relationship of a pelvic IUD to the uterus.

The latter two indications are appropriate after ultrasound has been unsuccessful in providing the needed information.

TUBAL PATENCY

Fallopian tubes vary in length from 7 to 14 cm and are divided into intramural (interstitial), isthmic, and ampullary segments. The intramural portion is relatively short (1.5 to 3.0 cm) and obliquely oriented and enters the uterus at the apex of the uterine cornu. The longest segment of the tube, the isthmic portion, appears as a fine, thread-like structure. Laterally, the bulbous ampullary portion of the tube is a tortuous or convoluted structure that opens into the peritoneal cavity via a funnel-like diverticulum, the infundibulum (see Fig. 139–1).

Hysterosalpingography remains the principal method to image the lumen of the fallopian tubes. The presence of periadnexal disease is not reliably demonstrated but is inferred from indirect evidence such as delayed spill, localized paratubal collections of contrast material, or recognition that the tube is draped around an adnexal mass (Fig. 139–2). Normal and altered paratubal anatomy is better demonstrated by laparoscopy. The more common conditions associated with nonpatency of the fallopian tubes and demonstrable by hysterosalpingography include total or partial absence of

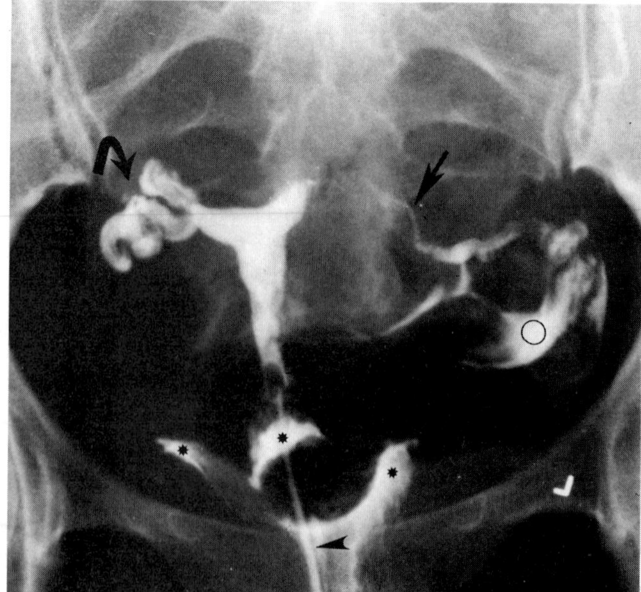

Figure 139–1. Normal hysterosalpingogram. The opacified cavity of the uterine body is triangular in shape. The normal isthmic segments of the fallopian tubes appear as thin, thread-like structures *(arrow)*. The bulbous ampullary portions of the uterine tubes are tortuous and show multiple convolutions *(curved arrow)*. Peritonealization of contrast material has occurred *(circle)*. Opacification of the uterine cavity and fallopian tubes was accomplished, in this case, with a small Foley catheter *(arrowheads)* that inadvertently permitted reflux of contrast material back into the vagina *(asterisks)*.

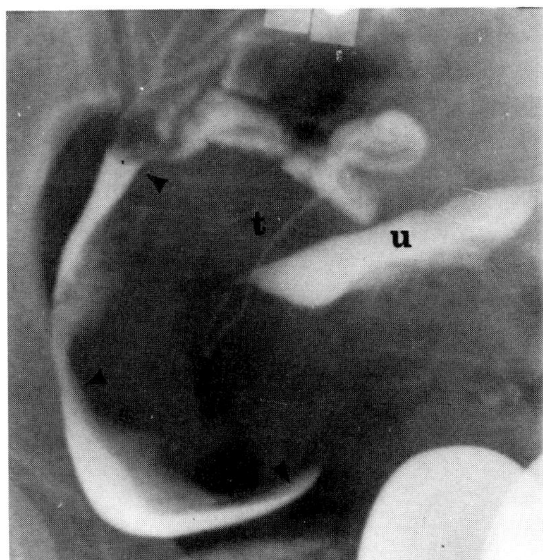

Figure 139–2. Indirect evidence of para-adnexal disease. Contrast material from a patent fallopian tube outlines a large ovarian mass *(arrowheads)*. At laparotomy, the fallopian tube was draped around a 4 × 5 × 5 cm ovarian endometrioma. (U = contrast material in the fundus of the uterine cavity.) (From Fagan CJ: Endometriosis. Radiol Clin North Am 12:109, 1974.)

a tube, nodular isthmic disease, diverticulosis (salpingitis isthmica nodosa), tuberculous salpingitis (Fig. 139–3), tubal polyps, and hydrosalpinx (Fig. 139–4). The latter represents the sequelae of repeated and/or chronic infections that cause obstructing tubal mucosal changes, fibrosis, and adhesions of the fimbriated ends. The status of luminal nonpatency or continuity following tubal ligation and reconstructive surgery, respectively, requires hysterosalpingographic confirmation (Fig. 139–5).

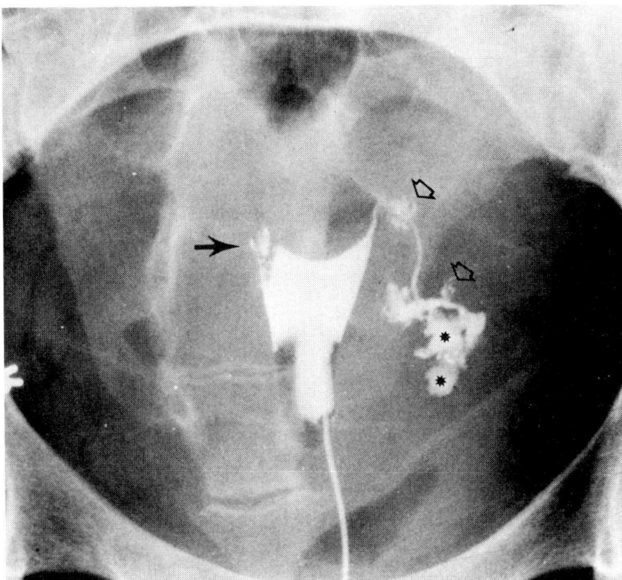

Figure 139–3. Tuberculous salpingitis resembling salpingitis isthmica nodosa. Nodular isthmic disease, from whatever cause, is manifested by interruption of the tubal luminal continuity *(arrow)* and the presence of extraluminal collections of contrast material in diverticula *(open arrows)*. There is no free spill of contrast material into the peritoneal cavity, but rather there is contrast material trapped in peritubal adhesions *(asterisks)*. Salpingitis isthmica nodosa is diverticulosis of the fallopian tubes without luminal obstruction.

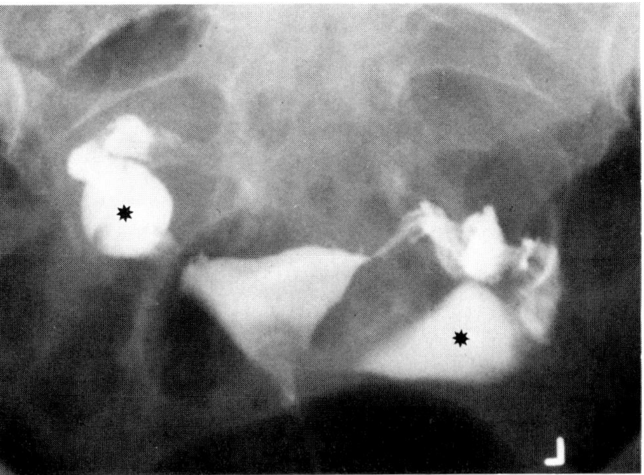

Figure 139–4. Hydrosalpinx. The uterine cavity and immediate proximal segments of the fallopian tubes are normal, but the ampullary ends are grossly dilated, clubbed, and obstructed *(asterisks)*. No peritonealization of contrast material is observed.

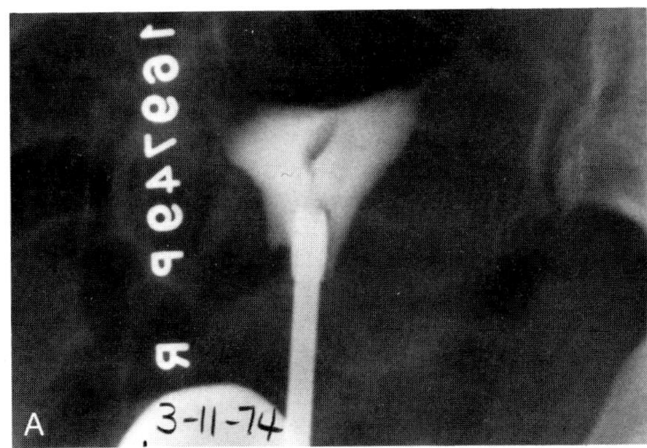

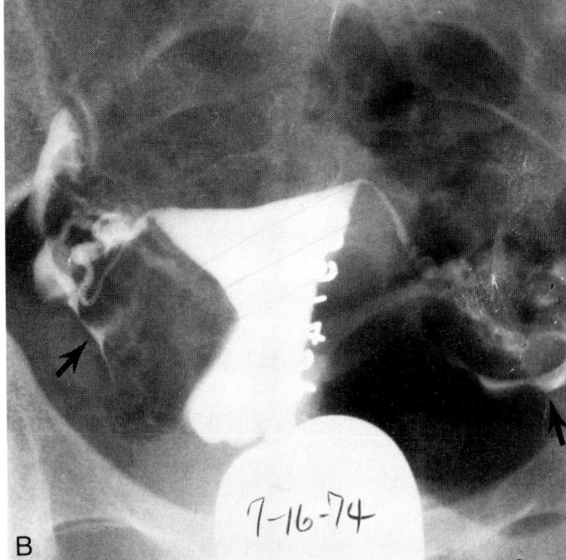

Figure 139–5. Postoperative evaluation of fallopian tube continuity. *A*, The uterine cavity is seen, but neither tube fills, indicating a successful tubal ligation. *B*, This same patient had a repeat hysterosalpingogram four months later after reconstructive tubal surgery. The study now shows normal-appearing, patent tubes. Note peritonealization of contrast material *(arrows)*. (From Schreiber MH, Fagan CJ: Surgical Radiology, Vol 3. Philadelphia, WB Saunders Company, 1974.)

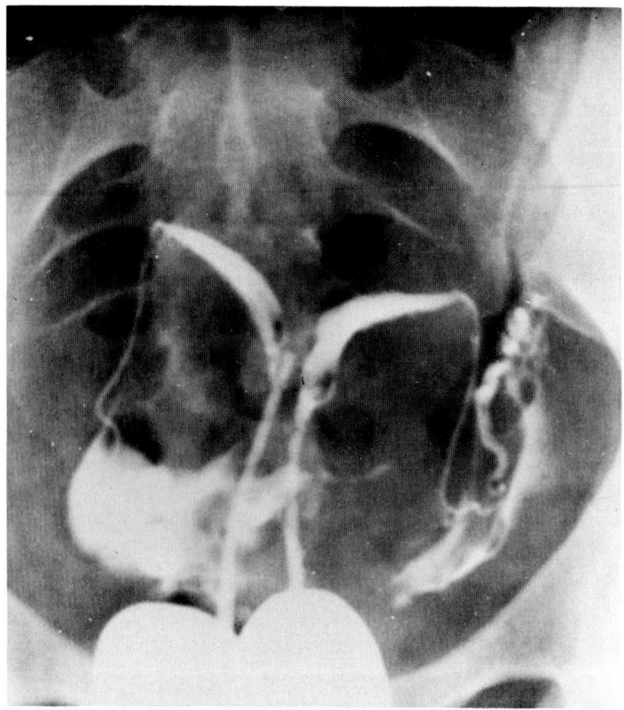

Figure 139–6. Uterine didelphys. The vagina was incompletely septated, but two cannulas are needed to opacify separate uterine horns and normal patent fallopian tubes in this patient.

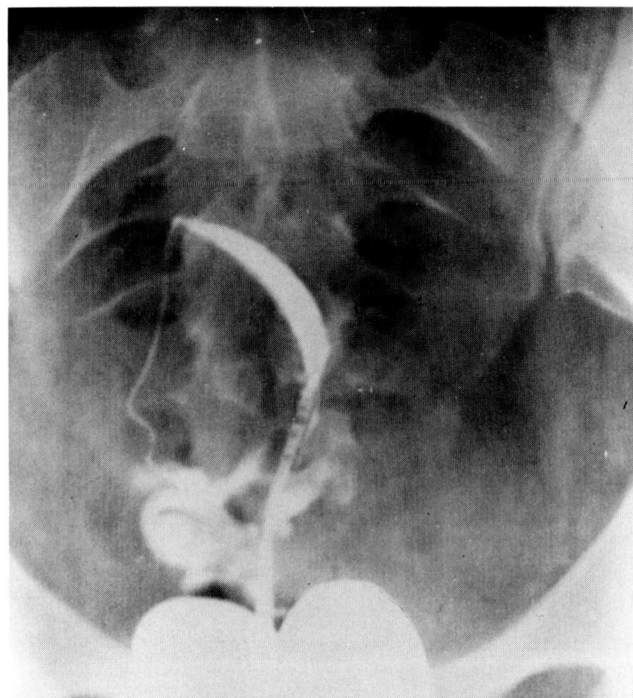

Figure 139–7. Unicornuate uterus. On the right side, a single uterine horn with a normal patent fallopian tube is opacified by a hysterosalpingogram.

UTERINE ANOMALIES AND LESIONS

Hysterographically, the uterine cavity is composed of a spindle-shaped cervical canal, followed by a short, inverted, cone-shaped isthmus and the triangular cavity of the uterine body (see Fig. 139–1).

The uterus, fallopian tubes, and proximal vagina develop from a paired müllerian duct system. Aberrations of early development may give rise to a spectrum of uterine anomalies, the majority of which are referred to as septate anomalies. Most of these uterine defects are nonobstructive and are demonstrable by hysterosalpingography.

Complete failure of fusion of the paired müllerian ducts results in uterine didelphys. Two separate reproductive units are present: an ovary, a fallopian tube, and a partially or completely separated vagina on each side (Fig. 139–6). Complete failure of development of one müllerian duct will result in a true unicornuate or single-horn uterus (Fig. 139–7). Partial arrested development of one müllerian tube may result in a unicornuate uterus with a noncommunicating, rudimentary horn. This condition is not imaged by hysterosalpingography but is identified by carefully conducted pelvic ultrasonography. The most common uterine defect is a bicornuate uterus that results from incomplete müllerian duct fusion. The result is two separate horns partitioned by a uterine septum but joined at a variable distance above the cervix. Various forms of septate and subseptate uteri result from varying degrees of incomplete reabsorption of a common sagittal septum that initially separates the paired müllerian ducts. Externally, the uterus is morphologically normal, but internally, septa of various thicknesses and lengths divide the uterus into two compartments. The septa are seen as negative defects in the uterine cavity that is opacified by a hysterogram. Infantile and arcuate uteri represent the most common nonseptated uterine anomalies. The arcuate uterus has a rounded indentation on its fundal surface that simulates the appearance of a fundal fibroid (Fig. 139–8). A diverticulum-like projection that may or may not communicate with the isthmic portion of the uterine cavity represents still another congenital anomaly, a Gartner's duct cyst (Fig. 139–9). These malformations can reach a large size.

Renal ectopia and agenesis represent common genitourinary anomalies associated with several of these uterine defects. Most

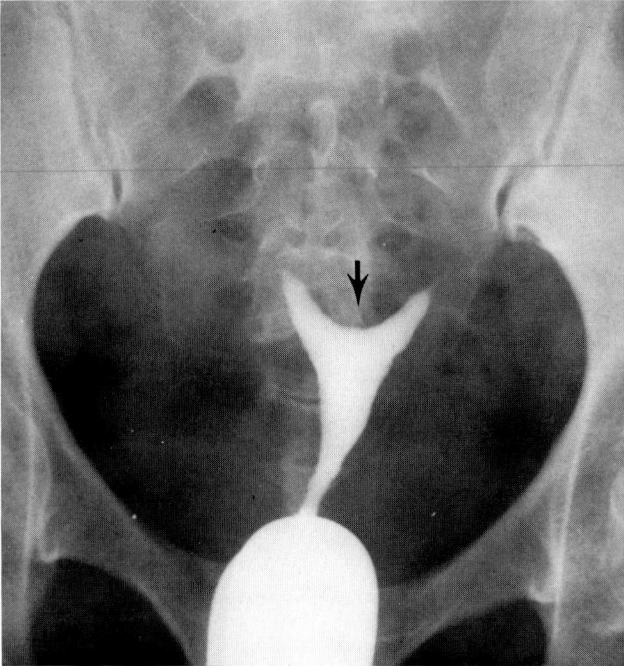

Figure 139–8. Arcuate uterus. Incomplete development of the fundus of the uterus results in a rounded appearance of the fundal portion of the opacified uterine cavity *(arrow)*. A fundal fibroid could simulate this appearance. (Courtesy of MH Schreiber, M.D.)

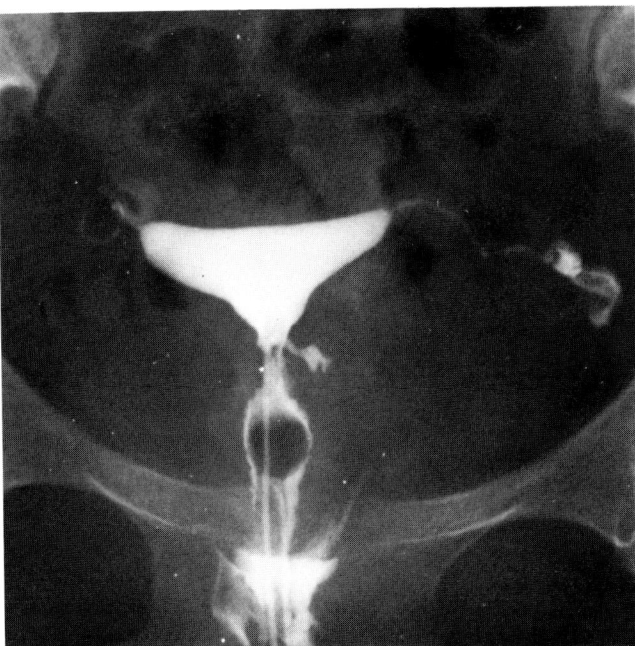

Figure 139–9. Gartner's duct cyst. Opacification of a diverticulum-like projection that communicates with the isthmic portion of the uterine cavity is diagnostic of this congenital anomaly. Not all Gartner's duct cysts communicate with the cervical canal to permit their visualization via hysterosalpingography. (Courtesy of MH Schreiber, M.D.)

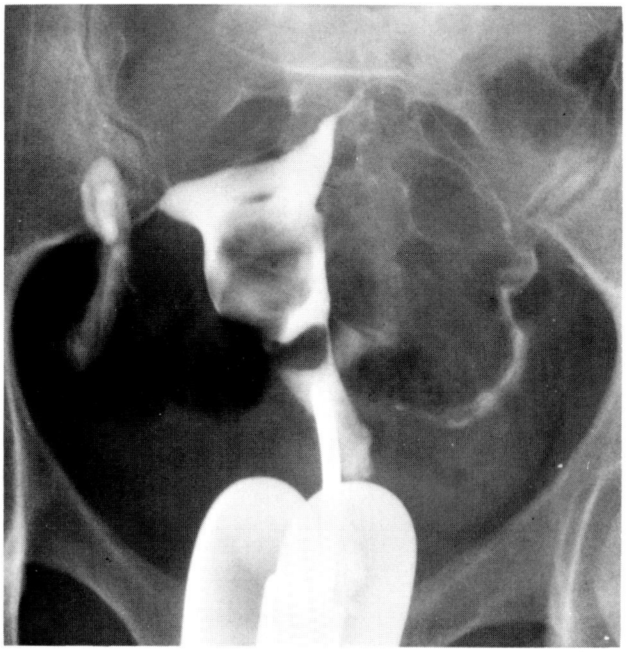

Figure 139–11. Submucosal myomas. Large and small soft-tissue masses, myomas in this case, are manifested by filling defects in the opacified uterine cavity. Intrauterine adhesions could present a similar appearance. (From Schreiber MH, Fagan CJ: Surgical Radiology, Vol 3. Philadelphia, WB Saunders Company, 1974, Chap. 40.)

noncongenital uterine abnormalities demonstrated by hysterosalpingography are manifested by filling defects, distortion, and varying degrees of obstruction of the uterine cavity. Filling defects on hysterography may be caused by myomata, polyps, adhesions, carcinoma, intrauterine pregnancy, and air bubbles. The hysterographic appearance of intrauterine adhesions is variable. The filling defects created by these lesions may be single or multiple, smooth or irregular, and central or peripheral in location (Fig. 139–10). The association of oligomenorrhea or amenorrhea in intrauterine adhesions describes Ascherman's syndrome.

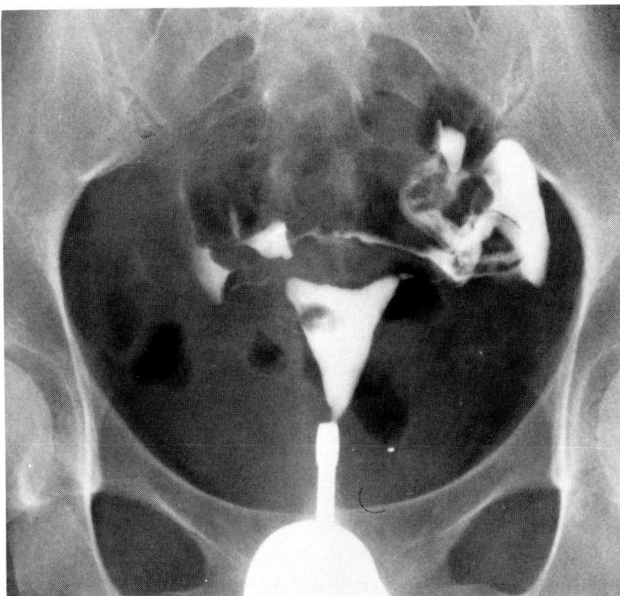

Figure 139–10. Polypoid intrauterine adhesions. This persistent filling defect may be single or multiple, smooth or irregularly contoured, and located anywhere in the uterine cavity. More often, intrauterine adhesions have an irregular contour and are frequently multiple in number, causing considerable deformity of the uterine cavity. (Courtesy of MH Schreiber, M.D.)

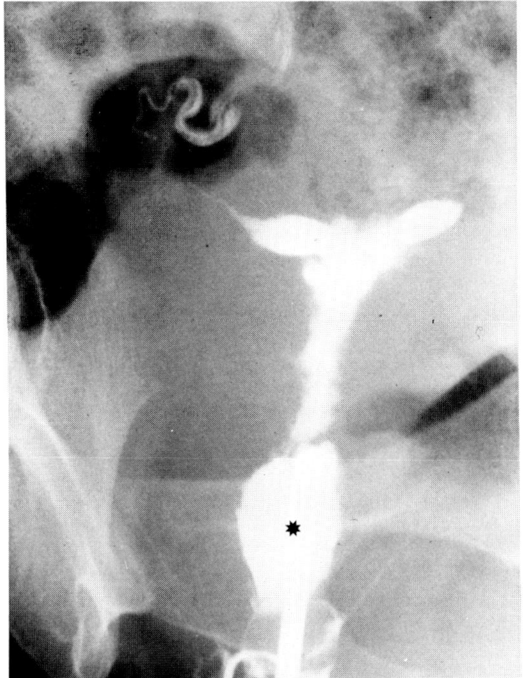

Figure 139–12. Endometritis. The normal, smooth, straight lateral walls of this uterine cavity have been transformed into inflamed, irregular, and serrated surfaces. Note the patulous cervical canal *(asterisk)*.

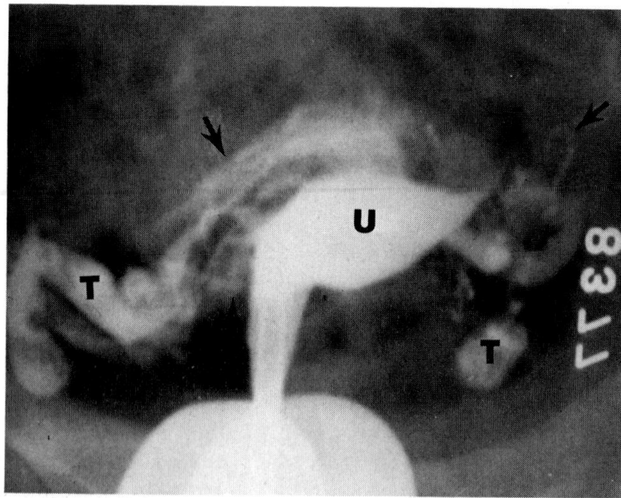

Figure 139–13. Venous intravasation of contrast material. Violation of the endometrium by a cannula or uncontrolled instillation of contrast material can result in opacification of myometrial vessels and lymphatics *(arrows)*. (U = uterine cavity; T = obstructed, dilated fallopian tubes.) (From Schreiber MH, Fagan CJ: Surgical Radiology, Vol 3. Philadelphia, WB Saunders Company, 1974, Chap. 40.)

Myomas may distort the uterine cavity and occlude the cornu, predisposing women to infertility, abnormal bleeding, and spontaneous abortion. More often, a small, submucosal myoma may play the role of an intrauterine device, predisposing women to nonobstructive infertility (Fig. 139–11).

Hysterosalpingography is contraindicated in acute pelvic inflammatory disease (PID), and any uterine changes that might be associated with acute PID are usually overshadowed by adnexal and tubal alterations. However, chronic granulomatous and tuberculous endometritis may result in abnormalities demonstrable on hysterogram, such as contour deformities, stricture formation, and even contrast material intravasation and fistula formation (Fig. 139–12). Inadvertent insertion of the cannula into the myometrium and/or excessive pressure during the instillation of contrast material may result in opacification of myometrial vessels and lymphatics (Fig. 139–13). Although not a desirable result, when water-soluble contrast material is used, venous intravasation is not a serious complication.

Large, complex, and solid pelvic masses may make it impossible to delineate the uterus by pelvic sonography. Hematoceles of chronic ectopic pregnancy and an advanced abdominal pregnancy represent conditions in which there is a need to know if the uterine cavity is empty. The location, size, and morphology of the uterine cavity can be readily identified by a hysterogram (Fig. 139–14).

Hysterosalpingography should remain an important diagnostic procedure for the investigation of several gynecologic conditions.

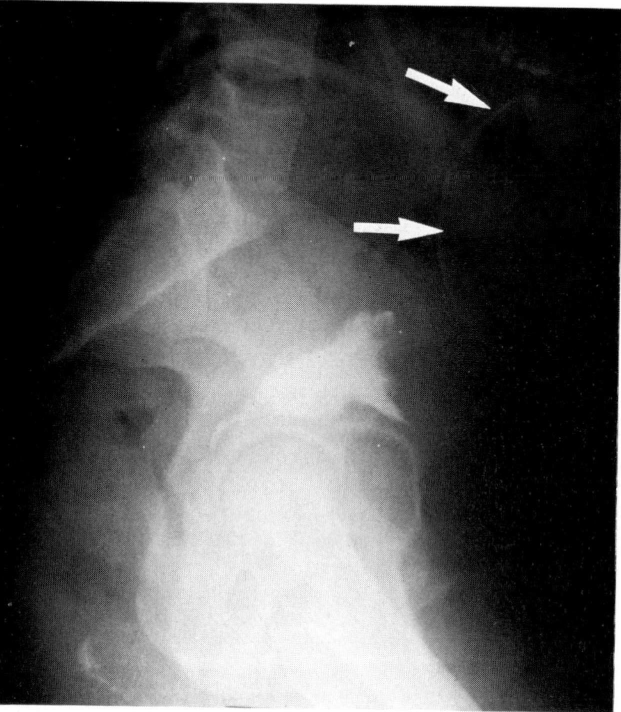

Figure 139–14. Empty uterine cavity and abdominal pregnancy. Large, extrauterine pelvic masses can distort pelvic anatomy sufficiently to preclude visualization of the uterus by ultrasound. The location, size, and morphology of the uterine cavity were readily established by hysterosalpingography in this case. Note the fetal head *(arrows)* of the abdominal pregnancy.

Bibliography

Deutsch AL, Gosink BB: Non-neoplastic gynecologic disorders. Semin Roentgenol 17:269, 1982.

Deutsch AL, Gosink BB: Normal female pelvic anatomy. Semin Roentgenol 17:241, 1982.

Fagan CJ: Endometriosis. Radiol Clin North Am 12:109, 1974.

Horwitz RC, Morton PC, Shaff MI: A radiological approach to infertility—hysterosalpingography. Br J Radiol 52:255, 1979.

Kasby CB: Hysterosalpingography: An appraisal of current indications. Br J Radiol 53:279, 1980.

Krantz KE: Anatomy of the female reproductive system. In Benson RC (ed): Current Obstetric and Gynecologic Diagnosis and Treatment. Los Altos, CA, Lange Medical Publisher, 1980.

Siegler AM: Hysterosalpingography. Fertil Steril 40:139, 1983.

Soules MR, Spadoni LR: Oil versus aqueous media for hysterosalpingography: A continuing debate based on many opinions and few facts. Fertil Steril 38:1, 1982.

Spring DB, Wilson RE, Arsonet GH: Foley catheter hysterosalpingography: A simplified technique for investigating infertility. Radiology 131:543, 1979.

Zanetti E, Ferrari LR, Rossi G: Classification and radiographic features of uterine malformations: Hysterosalpingographic study. Br J Radiol 51:161, 1978.

140 Gynecologic Sonography

Arthur C. Fleischer

There are several applications of sonography in the evaluation of gynecologic disorders. The recent development of transvaginal sonography (TVS) has expanded the role of sonography in a variety of gynecologic disorders. Sonography has an important and established role in the evaluation of pelvic masses, ovarian follicular monitoring, and intrauterine contraceptive device (IUCD) localization. In addition, TVS affords evaluation of the endometrium, myometrium, and ovary, particularly in the postmenopausal woman. It also provides a means of guided aspiration or drainage. The recent addition of color Doppler capabilities and the transabdominal and transvaginal probe extends sonographic evaluation from a purely anatomic to a physiologic basis relative to other pelvic imaging modalities (computed tomography and magnetic resonance imaging). Sonography continues to have an important role in the evaluation of both benign and malignant gynecologic disorders because of its high degree of patient acceptance, its ease of operation, the lack of adverse bioeffects, and the relatively inexpensive cost of the scanners.

INDICATIONS

The most common indications for gynecologic sonography include the following:

1. The evaluation of a palpable or clinically suspected pelvic mass.
   a. Evaluation of origin (i.e., uterine or ovarian).
   b. Determination of internal consistency (i.e., cystic, complex, or solid) and regularity of walls.
   c. Detection of associated abnormalities (i.e., ascites, metastatic lesions).
2. Ovarian follicular monitoring/guided follicular aspiration.
3. IUCD localization and evaluation of associated complications.
4. Evaluation of suspected endometrial or myometrial lesions.

NORMAL ANATOMY AND SCANNING TECHNIQUE

Before the specific indications for sonography as they relate to gynecologic disorders are discussed, the sonographic depiction of the normal pelvic organs and structures, particularly the uterus and ovaries, shall be described.

Optimal transabdominal sonographic (TAS) delineation of the pelvic structures requires that the patient's urinary bladder be fully distended. A distended urinary bladder displaces gas-containing bowel loops from the pelvis and lower abdomen and also places the uterus in a horizontal orientation relative to the incident beam. This allows delineation of the uterus and the adnexa in the most optimal situation, since in this orientation the axial rather than lateral resolution properties of the scanner are used.

Except in specific cases, TVS follows TAS. For TVS, the urinary bladder should be nondistended, and an organ-oriented rather than image plane approach to the pelvic sonographic study should be used.

Because of the close proximity of the probe to the structures to be imaged, TV probes use 5 to 10 mHz. The probe should be properly disinfected before the condom covering is secured to it. The preferred orientation of the image is with the apex of the image at the top of the screen.

The uterus should be used as the point of reference for evaluation of the female pelvis. The size and shape of the uterus vary according to the pubertal, as well as parity, status of the individual (Table 140–1; Fig. 140–1*A* to *E*). Prior to puberty, the uterus is a tubular structure measuring 3 to 4 cm in length and 0.5 to 1 cm in width and anteroposterior dimension, with a relatively thin fundus and a thick and long cervix (Fig. 140–1*A*). In addition, the length of the cervix is two to four times greater than that of the fundus. As puberty is reached, the uterine fundus elongates and thickens and becomes larger than the uterine cervix (Fig. 140–1*B*). At puberty, the cervix-to-fundus ratio is 1:1, compared with the adult configuration, in which the fundus is twice the length and size of the cervix. As a generalization, the normal uterus of a postpubertal nulliparous individual measures approximately 6 to 8 cm in long axis, 4 to 6 cm in transverse, and 3 to 4 cm in anteroposterior dimension. Multiparous individuals have a uterus that is 1 to 2 cm larger in each dimension than that of nulliparous patients (Fig. 140–1*C*). After menopause, the uterus, like the ovary, undergoes a regression in size (Fig. 140–1*D*). The endometrium thins to less than 3 mm in width and becomes atrophic. Retroflexion of the uterus is a normal variant and is most frequently encountered in parous women. In this condition the uterine fundus is directed posteriorly (Fig. 140–1*E*).

A group of linear interfaces which represents the endometrium can be identified within the uterus (Fig. 140–2*B* to *M*). The sonographic appearance of the endometrium varies according to the phase of endometrial development (Fig. 140–2*A*). Although the endometrium can be evaluated with TAS, its texture and thickness is best depicted with TVS (Fig. 140–2*J* to *M*). In the menstrual phase, the endometrium appears as a thin and interrupted central echogenic interface, corresponding to blood and pieces of sloughed endometrium (Figs. 140–2*B* and *J*). As the endometrium begins to form glandular elements in the proliferative phase, it becomes thicker and has relatively hypo- to isoechoic texture (Fig. 140–2*C* and *K*). Immediately after ovulation, an innermost portion of the endometrium becomes hypoechoic, probably secondary to edema within the compactum and spongiosa layers of the functionalis combined with minute amounts of intraluminal secretions. When imaged on a transverse sonogram, the endometrium has a ring configuration, with the hypoechoic area centrally surrounded by an echoic layer (Fig. 140–2*D* and *L*). In the secretory phase, the endometrial glands elongate and secrete mucin and glycogen. In this phase of development, the endometrium has an echogenic appearance and may measure as much as 6 to 7 mm in thickness per layer (up to 14 mm in total width) (Fig. 140–2*E, F, H,* and *M*). Immediately beneath the endometrium is a hypoechoic layer of myometrium. This layer of myometrium is thought to be hypoechoic because of its relatively vascular consistency as well as being more compact than the outer layers of myometrium (Fig. 140–2*G*).

TABLE 140–1. NORMAL UTERINE DIMENSIONS (cm)

	Long	Transverse	Anteroposterior	Relative Length of Cervix: Corpus/Fundus
Prepubertal	3–4	0.5–1	0.5–1	2–4:1
Pubertal (nulliparous)	5.5–8	4.5–6	2.5–3.5	1:1
Adult (parous)	7–9	4.5–6	2.5–3.5	1:2
Postmenopausal	2–4	0.5–1.3	0.5–1.3	1:1

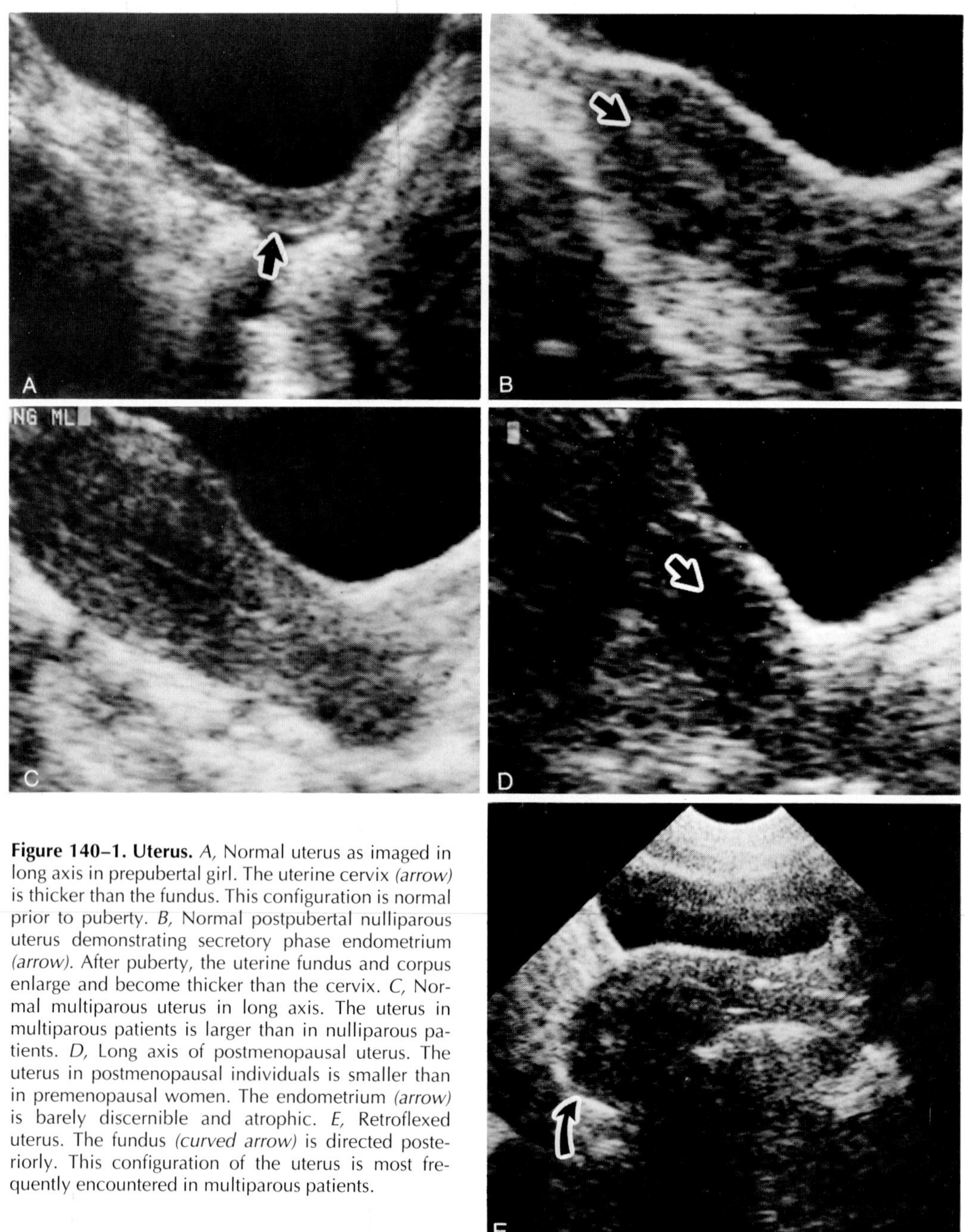

Figure 140–1. Uterus. *A,* Normal uterus as imaged in long axis in prepubertal girl. The uterine cervix *(arrow)* is thicker than the fundus. This configuration is normal prior to puberty. *B,* Normal postpubertal nulliparous uterus demonstrating secretory phase endometrium *(arrow).* After puberty, the uterine fundus and corpus enlarge and become thicker than the cervix. *C,* Normal multiparous uterus in long axis. The uterus in multiparous patients is larger than in nulliparous patients. *D,* Long axis of postmenopausal uterus. The uterus in postmenopausal individuals is smaller than in premenopausal women. The endometrium *(arrow)* is barely discernible and atrophic. *E,* Retroflexed uterus. The fundus *(curved arrow)* is directed posteriorly. This configuration of the uterus is most frequently encountered in multiparous patients.

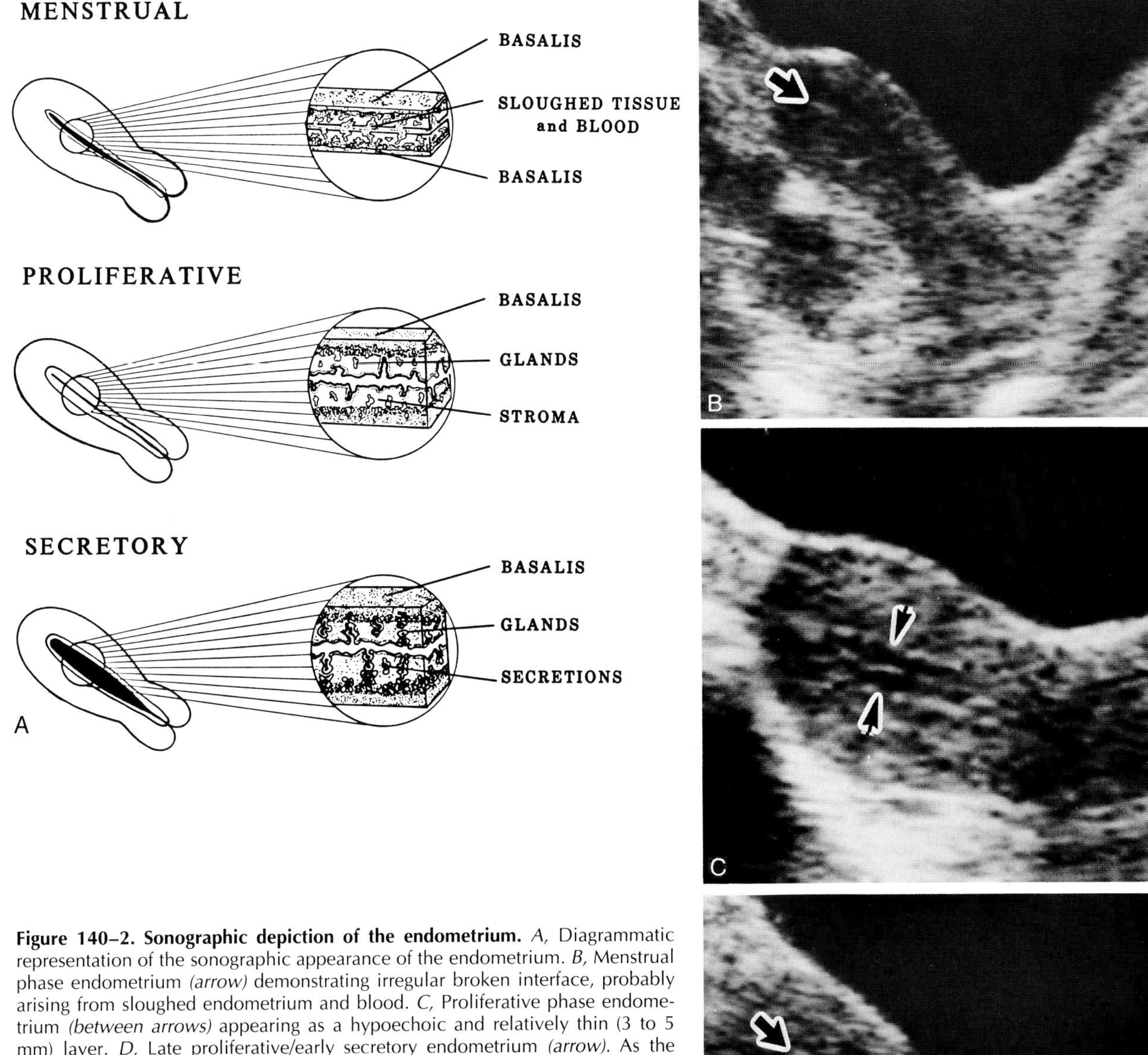

Figure 140–2. Sonographic depiction of the endometrium. *A,* Diagrammatic representation of the sonographic appearance of the endometrium. *B,* Menstrual phase endometrium *(arrow)* demonstrating irregular broken interface, probably arising from sloughed endometrium and blood. *C,* Proliferative phase endometrium *(between arrows)* appearing as a hypoechoic and relatively thin (3 to 5 mm) layer. *D,* Late proliferative/early secretory endometrium *(arrow).* As the secretory or luteal phase approaches, the endometrium becomes more echogenic, probably owing to increased glycogen and mucin within the glands.

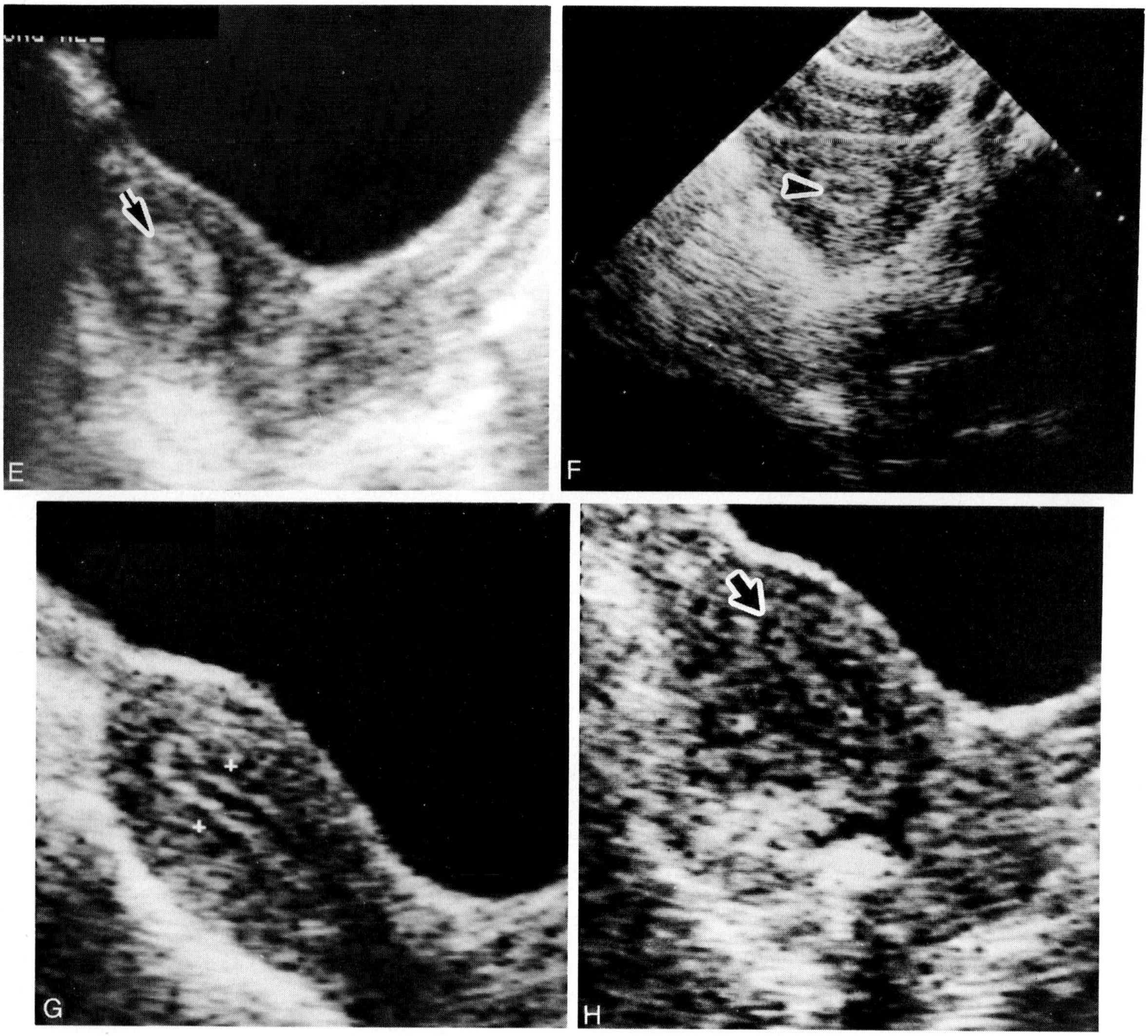

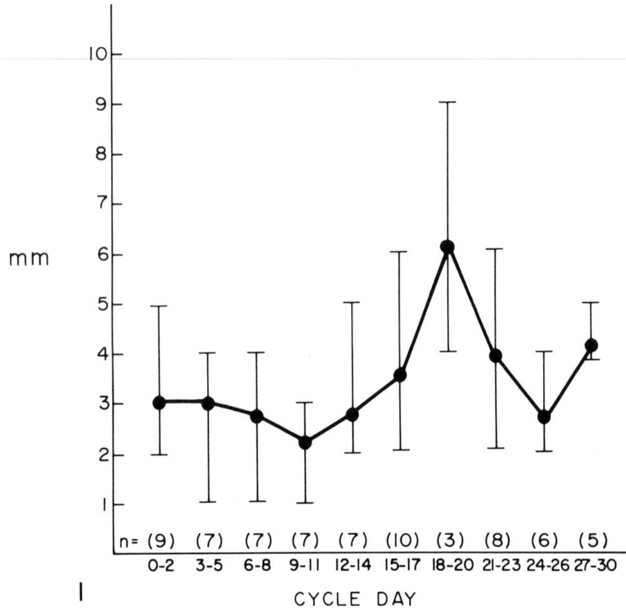

Figure 140–2 *Continued E,* Appearance of the endometrium in the periovulatory period. The endometrium *(arrow)* has a thin hypoechoic internal layer, which probably corresponds to edema in the compactum and spongiosum strata of the functionalis. *F,* Same normal individual as in *E,* scanned in a transverse plane. The endometrium *(arrow)* has a "ring configuration." *G,* Midsecretory phase endometrium *(between cursors)* demonstrating echogenic texture. Echogenicity probably arises from distended glands that contain inspissated secretions. The endometrium is thickest in this phase of development. *H,* Late secretory phase endometrium demonstrating hypoechoic "halo" *(arrow)* surrounding the echogenic layers. This "halo" probably arises from the relatively vascular and compact inner myometrium. *I,* Mean and range of endometrial thickness throughout the cycle in 10 spontaneously ovulating women.

Illustration continued on following page

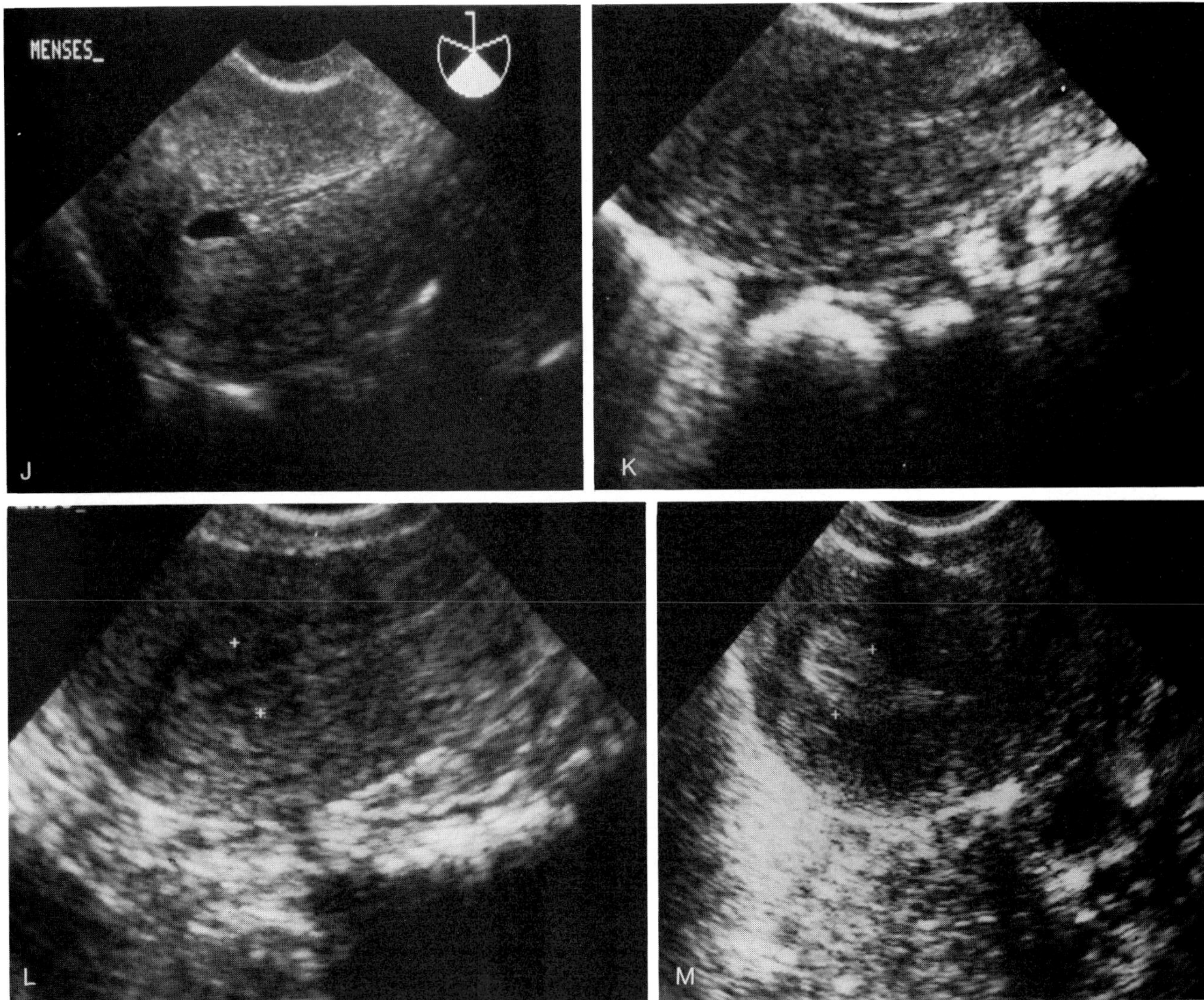

Figure 140–2 *Continued J* to *M,* Transvaginal sonography of cyclic changes in the endometrium. *J,* Menstrual phase. The endometrium is in the process of sloughing. *K,* Early to mid-proliferative phase. The endometrium is isoechoic and the myometrium probably due to the lack of glandular development and homogeneous arrangement. *L,* Midcycle showing a multi-layered appearance *(between cursors).* The functionalis layer is hypoechoic. *M,* Secondary phase showing an echogenic texture probably related to glandular secretion and stromal edema.

As a generalization, the normal-sized ovary is an almond-shaped structure that measures approximately 3 cm in transverse dimension, 2 cm in anteroposterior dimension, and 2 cm in long axis (Fig. 140–3*A* to *C* and *I*). The ovary can measure up to 5 cm in one axis but should maintain its relatively fusiform shape. The volume of the ovary can be calculated using the prolate ellipse approximation by multiplying the long, transverse, and anteroposterior dimensions by 0.523 (Table 140–2). This calculation is useful in the evaluation of clinically suspected polycystic ovary disease.

Sonography can readily detect developing follicles that are greater than 5 to 10 mm in size, owing to the anechoic fluid contained within them (Fig. 140–3*A* and *B*). As with the endometrium, TVS is preferred over TAS for follicular evaluation. A mature follicle typically measures approximately 20 mm in average dimension (Fig. 140–3*D* and *J*). Occasionally, the cumulus oophorus can be detected (see Fig. 140–9*A*). The cumulus appears as a focal bulge from the inner follicular wall and contains the oocyte that is surrounded by a cluster of granulosa cells. After ovulation the wall of the follicle becomes thickened and serrated (Fig. 140–2*M*). Duplex and/or transvaginal color sonography can detect increased arterial flow within the wall of the corpus luteum associated with angiogenesis. Intrafollicular hemorrhage may appear echogenic or hypoechoic depending on the amount of clot organization.

Occasionally, sonography can detect certain uterine and adnexal malformations and/or normal anatomic variants that may clinically mimic pelvic pathology (Fig. 140–4*A* and *B*). For example, a patient with a bicornuate uterus may come to the attention of the sonologist because it is mistaken on pelvic examination for an adnexal mass, or unilateral renal agenesis is detected (Fig. 140–4*B*). In this condi-

Text continued on page 2044

TABLE 140–2. NORMAL OVARIAN DIMENSIONS

	MEAN	RANGE
Greatest Dimension (cm)		
Transverse	3.0	2.5–5.0
Anteroposterior	1.7	1.5–3.0
Longitudinal	1.0	0.1–1.5
Volume (cu cm)		
Prepubertal	0.46	0.1–0.9
Postpubertal	4.0	1.8–5.7

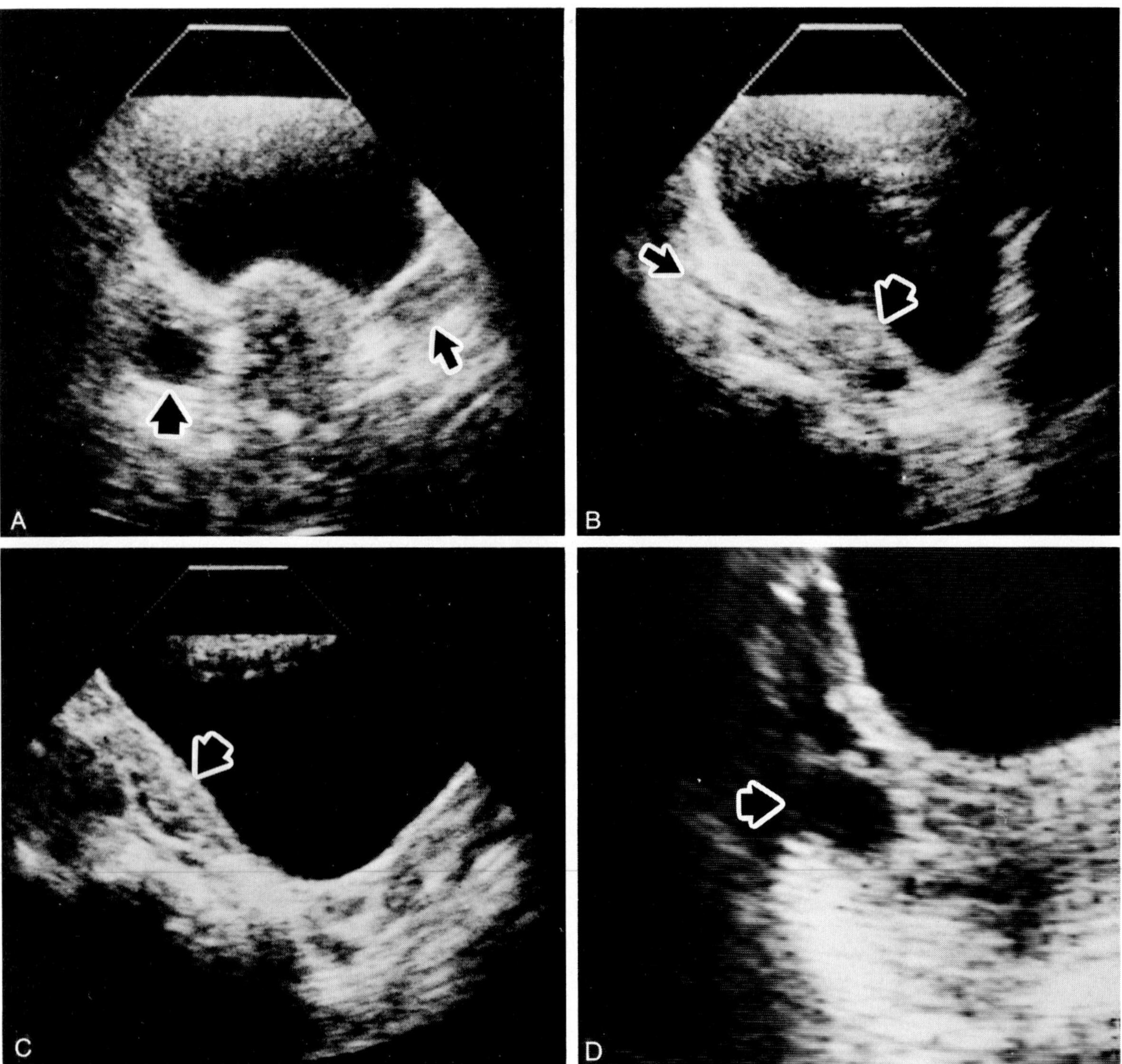

Figure 140–3. Ovaries. *A,* Transverse real-time image demonstrating the uterus and both ovaries. The right ovary contains an immature follicle *(large arrow).* The left *(small arrow)* does not contain any developing follicles. *B,* Long axis of right ovary *(large arrow)* demonstrating an immature follicle. The internal iliac vein *(small arrow)* courses posterior to the ovary. *C,* Long axis of left ovary *(arrow)* of the patient in *B. D,* Magnified sonogram of mature follicle *(arrow)* prior to ovulation.

Illustration continued on following page

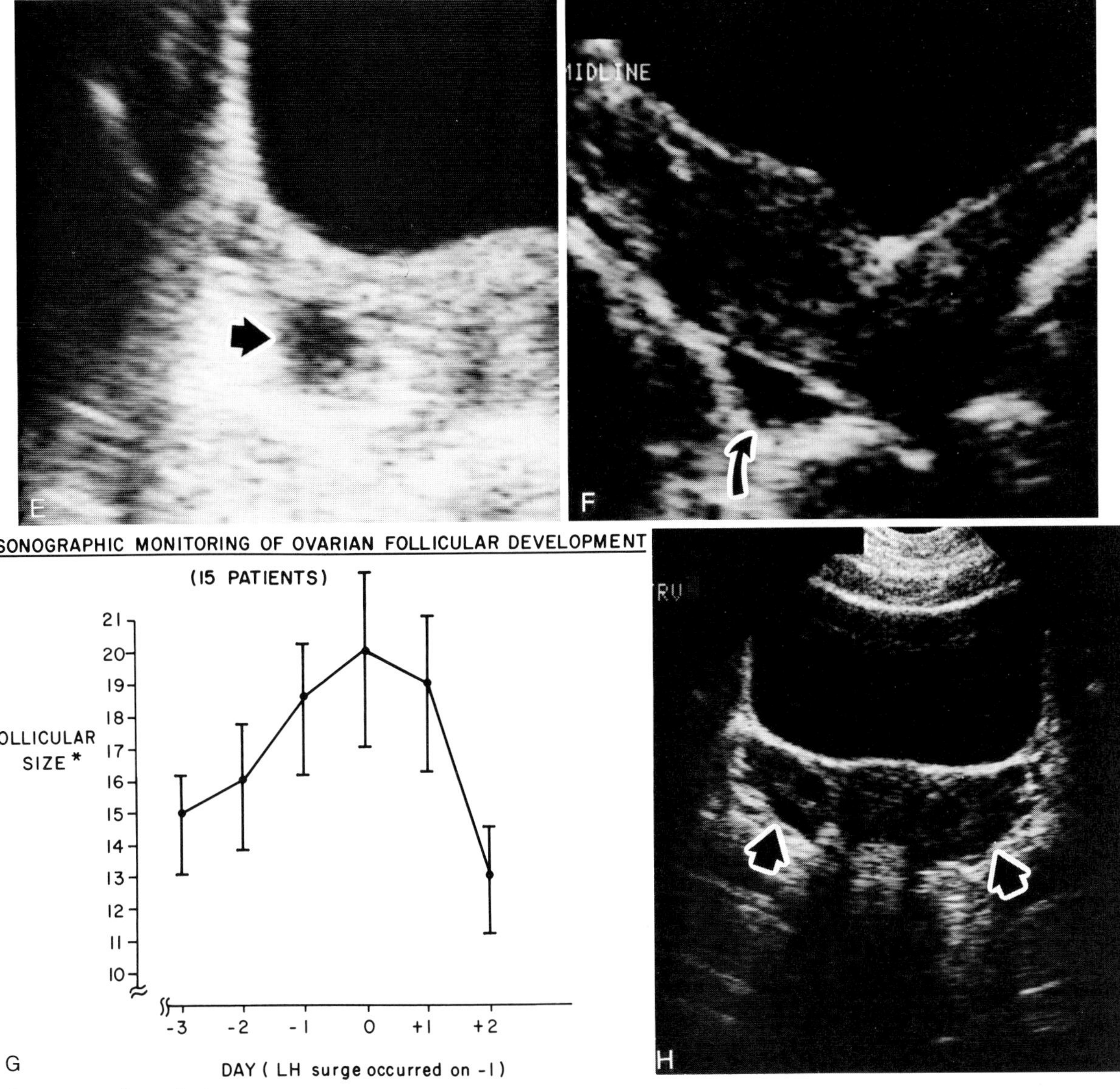

Figure 140–3 *Continued E,* Same patient two days later demonstrating internal echogenicity, probably corresponding to hemorrhage. Also note that the border of the follicle *(arrow)* has become "crenated" or folded upon itself, another sign that ovulation has occurred. *F,* Blood *(arrow)* in cul-de-sac associated with ovulation. *G,* Mean and standard deviation of follicular size in the periovulatory period in 15 spontaneously ovulating women. *H,* Transverse real-time sonogram of patient with bilaterally enlarged ovaries *(arrows)* that contain numerous immature follicles, consistent with sclerotocystic or "polycystic" ovarian disease.

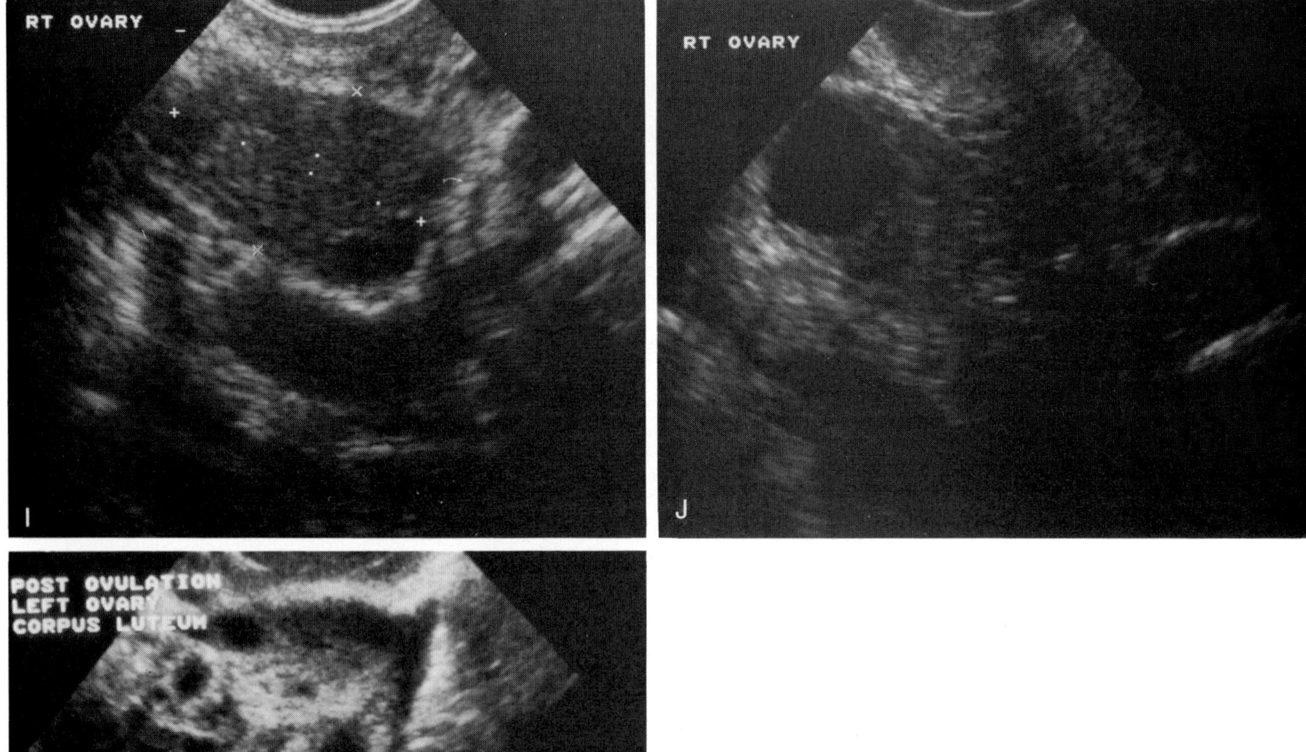

Figure 140–3 *Continued I,* Transvaginal sonogram of normal right ovary *(between cursors)* in early follicular phase. *J,* TVS showing a mature follicle within right ovary. *K,* TVS showing fresh corpus luteum with thickened, serrated wall.

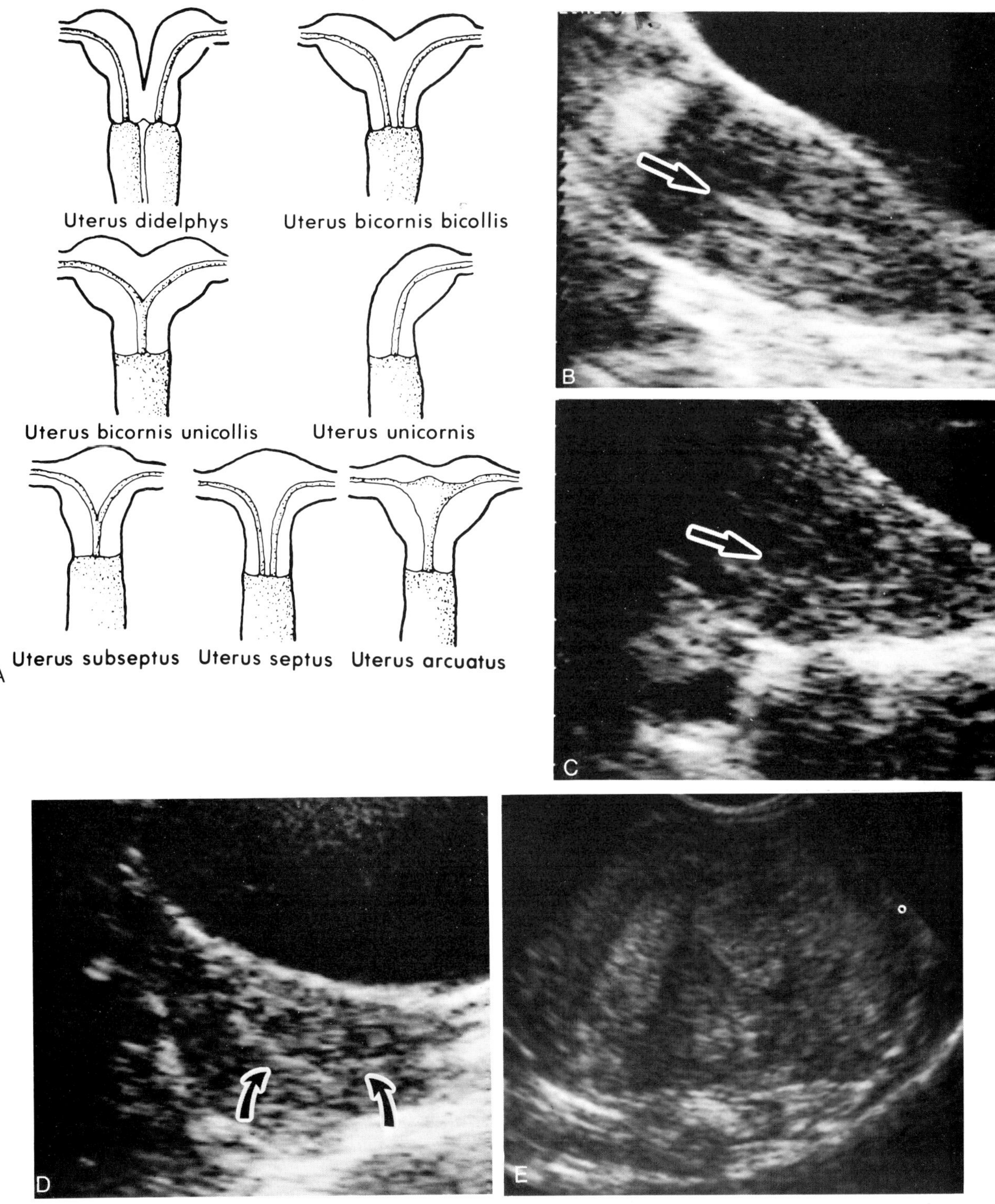

Figure 140–4. Uterine malformations. *A*, Diagram of the variety of uterine malformations. (Courtesy of Peter Callen, M.D.) *B*, Bicornuate uterus. Longitudinal scan taken to the right of midline shows normal uterine outline with centrally located endometrium *(arrow)*. *C*, Same patient as in *B* to the left of the midline shows a structure that has a similar configuration. *D*, On transverse scan, two separate endometrial interfaces can be identified *(arrows)*, confirming that the uterus has two separate lumina. *E*, TVS of bicornuate uterus showing both endometria.

tion, the bilobed outline and double intrauterine lumen can be identified on sonography (Fig. 140–4*B* to *D* and *E*). This condition and other fusion anomalies of the uterus can be associated with unilateral renal agenesis.

Another uterine malformation that can be encountered on sonography is the so-called T-shaped uterus encountered in women whose mothers took diethylstilbestrol during pregnancy. These uteri are wider in the transverse dimension than in the longitudinal plane and have a relatively thin fundus compared with the corpus.

One of the most common anatomic variants of the ovary is the polycystic or sclerocystic ovary. This malformation is usually encountered in girls who experience amenorrhea, hirsutism, and infertility. Although up to a third of these patients have a normal-sized ovary, usually the ovaries are rounded and large and contain several immature (less than 10 mm) follicles along their periphery (Fig. 140–3*F*).

SONOGRAPHIC EVALUATION OF PELVIC MASSES

Although there is some overlap in the sonographic appearance of pelvic masses, the combination of the sonographic data with clinical history can provide relatively specific differential diagnosis. TVS is quite helpful in further identifying the origin and internal consistency of the mass. Several studies have shown increased diagnostic accuracy when TVS was used as an adjunct to conventional TAS. For this discussion, pelvic masses are classified as cystic, complex, and solid (Table 140–3).

TABLE 140–3. SONOGRAPHIC DIFFERENTIAL DIAGNOSES OF PELVIC MASSES*

CYSTIC	COMPLEX	SOLID
Completely cystic	Predominantly cystic	Uterine
Ovarian	Ovarian	Leiomyoma (sarcoma)
Physiologic ovarian cyst	Cystadenoma	Endometrial carcinoma, sarcoma
Cystadenoma	Tubo-ovarian abscess	Extrauterine
Endometrioma	Cystic teratoma	Solid ovarian tumor (1° to 2°) torsed ovary
Tubal	Other	Bowel
Hydrosalpinx	Ectopic pregnancy	Pelvic lymphadenopathy
Other	Predominantly solid	
Paraovarian cyst	Ovarian	
Multiple	Cystadenoma (carcinoma)	
Endometrioma	Germ cell tumor	
Internal echoes	Uterine	
Hemorrhagic ovarian cyst	Degenerated fibroid	
Endometrioma	Other	
Mucinous cystadenoma	Ectopic pregnancy	
Dermoid cyst with sebum		
Septated		
Cystadenoma (carcinoma)		
Mucinous		
Serous		
Papillary		
Endometrioma		
Dermoid cyst		
Hemorrhagic corpus luteum		

*Based on the most common appearance on transabdominal and transvaginal sonography.

Cystic Masses

Several histologic types of masses appear as a cystic adnexal mass (Fig. 140–5*A* to *G*). These include physiologic (follicular and luteal) ovarian cysts, hydrosalpinx, endometrioma, and small ovarian epithelial tumors, to name a few. It is apparent from this list of diagnostic possibilities that the sonographic appearance of a cystic adnexal mass does not always imply the histologic composition of the mass. However, most studies show that a completely smooth walled anechoic cyst has an extremely high chance of being benign.

Follow-up sonograms can detect whether or not a cystic mass has regressed, and this is helpful in confirming the clinical impression of a physiologic ovarian cyst (Fig. 140–5*A* and *B*). Endometriomas may occasionally be differentiated from other types of adnexal cystic masses by their irregular borders and internal echoes corresponding to organized hemorrhage of some of the larger (more than 1 cm) endometriomas (Fig. 140–5*C*).

TVS can be used to ascertain that a cystic mass arises from within the ovary. Identification of papillary excrescence or septa suggests the possibility of malignancy (Fig. 140–6*L*).

Complex Masses

The most common complex adnexal mass encountered on sonography is the dermoid cyst. This type of pelvic mass may have a variety of sonographic appearances, depending on the number and type of predominant tissue contained within the mass (Figs. 140–6*A* to *C* and 140–7*A*). The fat within a dermoid cyst contains elements that appear as echogenic, shadowing material. Calcifications that are present within a dermoid cyst appear as focal areas of echogenicity, usually associated with a distal acoustic shadow. Occasionally, a dermoid cyst can be differentiated from the complex pelvic masses that contain echogenic material on the basis of the fact that the fat within a dermoid cyst layers anteriorly rather than posteriorly as it does in gravity-dependent material such as cellular debris within a papillary cystadenoma (Fig. 140–6*J* and *K*).

An ectopic pregnancy can present as a complex adnexal mass (Fig. 140–6*B*). The sonologist should be aware that this can occur, since ectopic pregnancies, if left undetected, can cause extensive intraperitoneal hemorrhage. Thus, serum pregnancy testing with beta human chorionic gonadotropin (β-hCG) is encouraged in any woman of childbearing age who has a complex adnexal mass. In some cases, even the β-hCG will be negative in chronic ectopic pregnancies. Chronic ectopic pregnancies can appear as solid extrauterine masses owing to the hematoma that results from the gradual erosion of the tube (Fig. 140–7*F*).

Tubo-ovarian abscesses, hematosalpinges, and hemorrhagic corpus luteum cysts can appear as complex adnexal masses (Fig. 140–6*B*). One should be aware that an ectopic pregnancy can coexist with a tubo-ovarian abscess or chronic tubal disease. TVS has an important role in distinguishing a simple hydrosalpinx from a tubo-ovarian abscess. It has also been used as a means of aspirating and treating tubo-ovarian abscesses.

Hemorrhagic corpus luteum cysts have a spectrum of sonographic appearances ranging from anechoic to complex, predominantly solid adnexal masses (Figs. 140–6*F* and 140–7*E*). Patients with this condition usually complain of at least one episode of unusually severe pelvic pain. On TVS, hemorrhagic cysts usually contain internal echoes arising from clotted blood or strands that arise from the clot and course toward the wall.

Another common type of cystic or complex adnexal or pelvoabdominal mass is that created by ovarian epithelial tumors. Ovarian epithelial tumors can range in appearance from totally anechoic to complex masses with solid, irregular, internal components (Figs. 140–5*F* and 140–6*F* and *H*). Completely cystic adnexal masses or pelvoabdominal masses usually represent serous cystadenomas, whereas cystic masses with thin internal septations usually represent

Text continued on page 2052

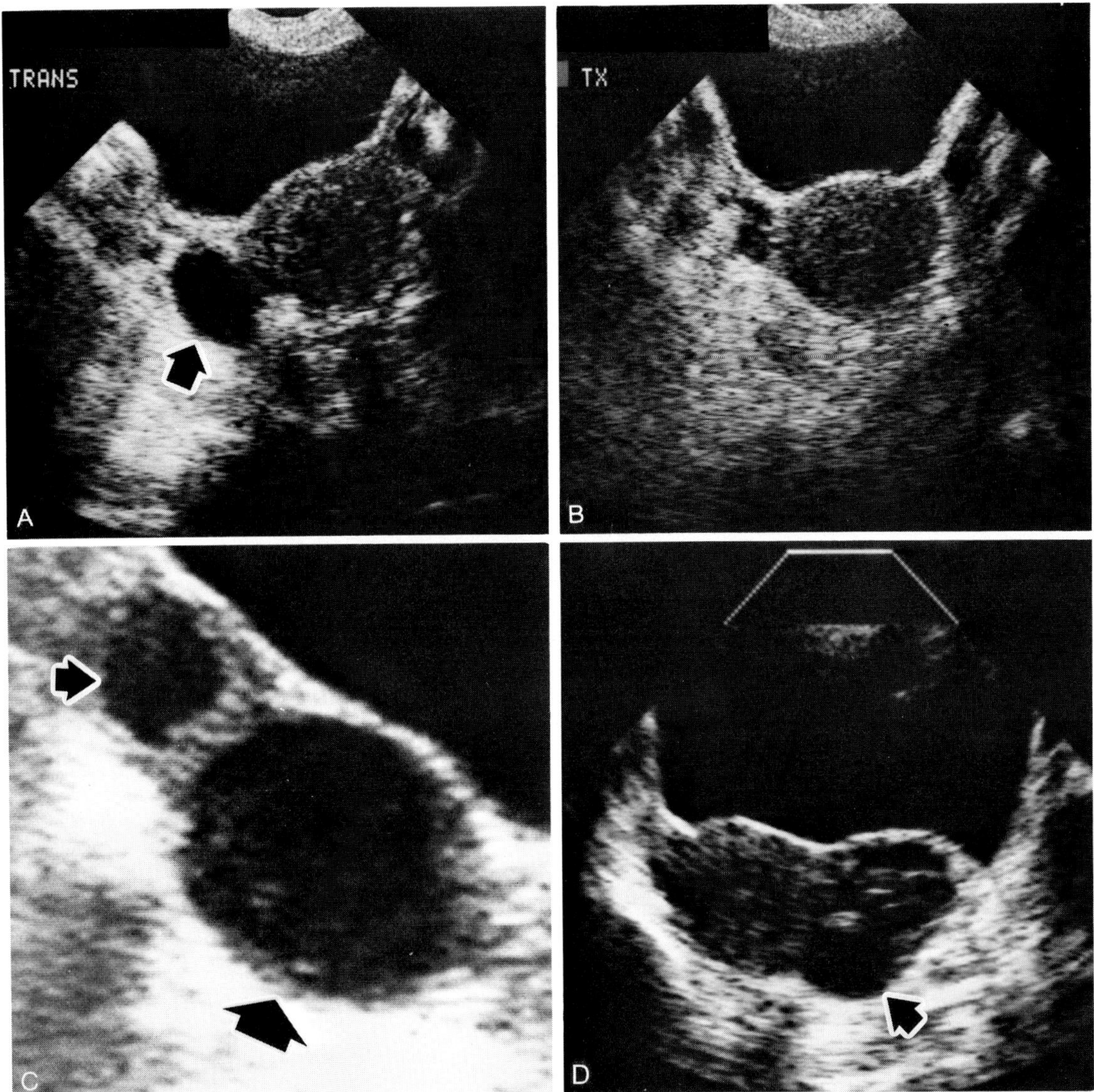

Figure 140–5. Cystic pelvic masses. *A,* Longitudinal real-time sonogram demonstrating completely cystic right adnexal mass *(arrow). B,* This mass (seen in *A*) regressed on follow-up examination two months later and probably represented a follicular cyst. *C,* Magnified longitudinal real-time sonogram demonstrating cystic adnexal mass *(large arrow)* inferior to the left ovary. This mass at laparoscopy was found to represent a paraovarian cyst. The left ovary contained a mature follicle *(small arrow),* which was successfully aspirated for oocyte harvest. *D,* Transverse real-time sonogram of tubo-ovarian abscess appearing as a cystic structure *(arrow)* contiguous with the left ovary.

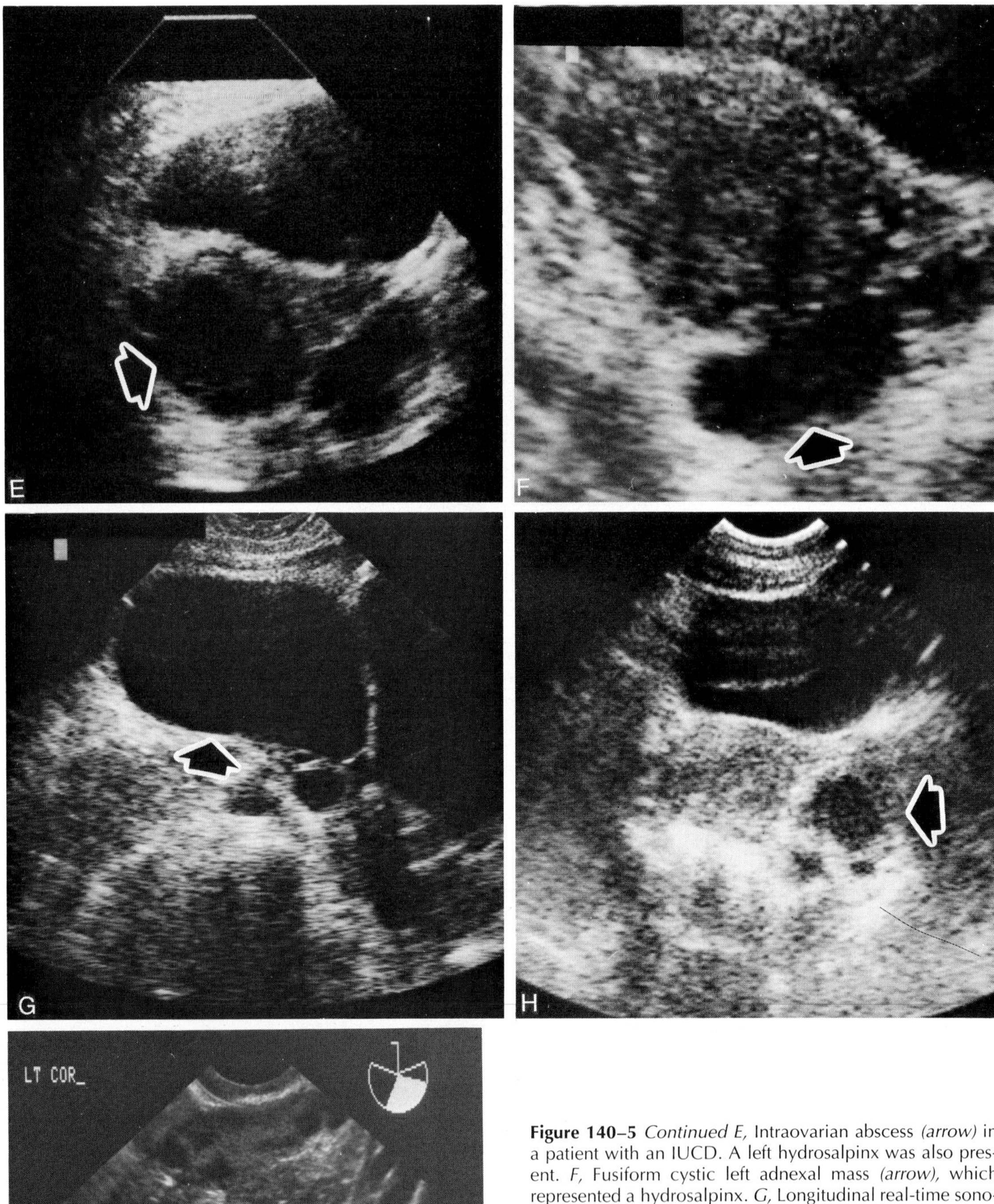

Figure 140–5 *Continued E,* Intraovarian abscess *(arrow)* in a patient with an IUCD. A left hydrosalpinx was also present. *F,* Fusiform cystic left adnexal mass *(arrow),* which represented a hydrosalpinx. *G,* Longitudinal real-time sonogram of a completely cystic pelvoabdominal mass *(arrow)* arising from the left ovary. This represented a serous cystadenoma of the ovary. *H,* Multiple cysts in the left adnexa with internal echoes and irregular borders *(arrow).* These represented multiple endometriomas. These masses may have irregular borders due to surrounding fibrosis. *I,* TVS of paraovarian cyst adjacent to left ovary.

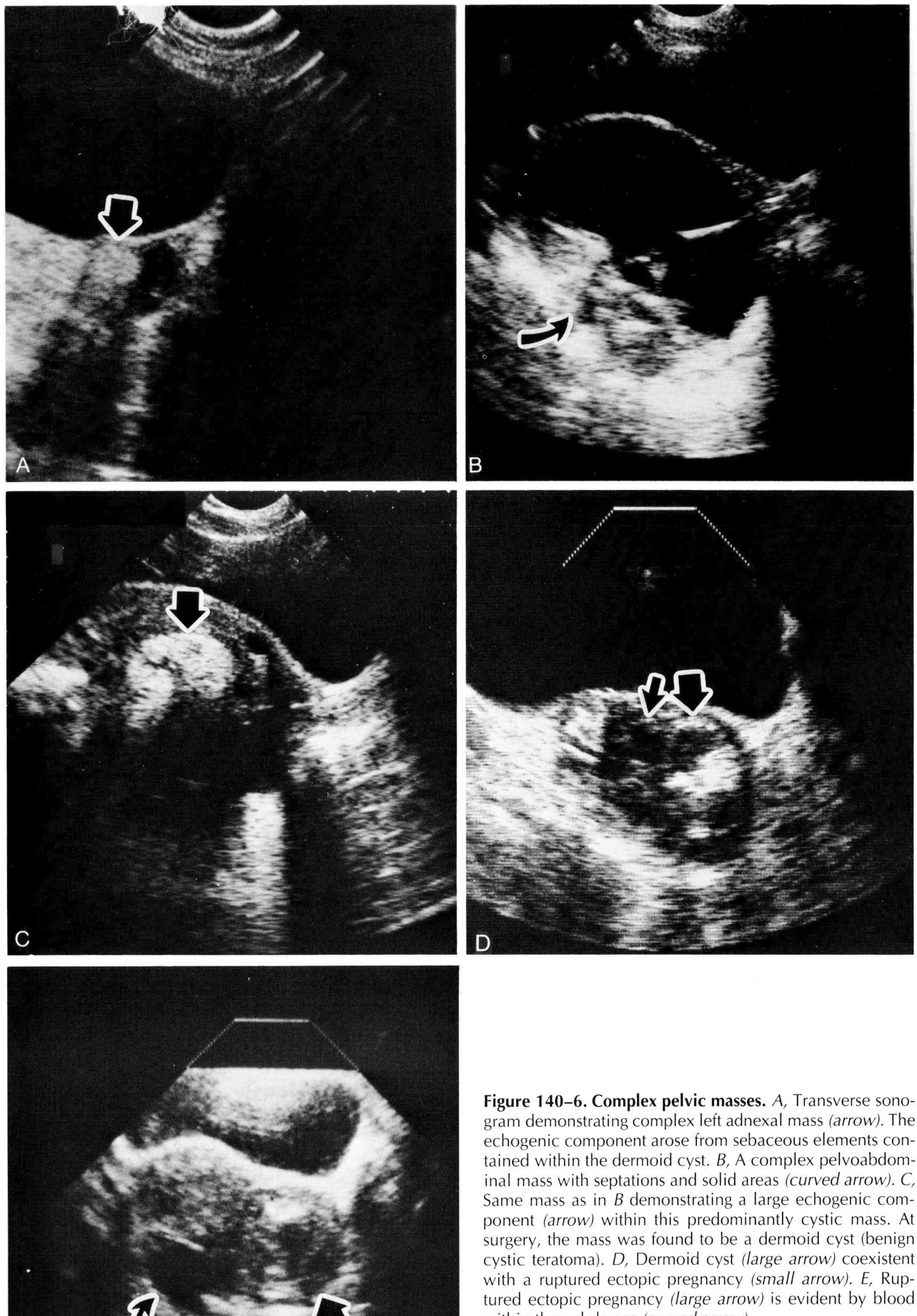

Figure 140–6. Complex pelvic masses. *A,* Transverse sonogram demonstrating complex left adnexal mass *(arrow).* The echogenic component arose from sebaceous elements contained within the dermoid cyst. *B,* A complex pelvoabdominal mass with septations and solid areas *(curved arrow). C,* Same mass as in *B* demonstrating a large echogenic component *(arrow)* within this predominantly cystic mass. At surgery, the mass was found to be a dermoid cyst (benign cystic teratoma). *D,* Dermoid cyst *(large arrow)* coexistent with a ruptured ectopic pregnancy *(small arrow). E,* Ruptured ectopic pregnancy *(large arrow)* is evident by blood within the cul-de-sac *(curved arrow).*

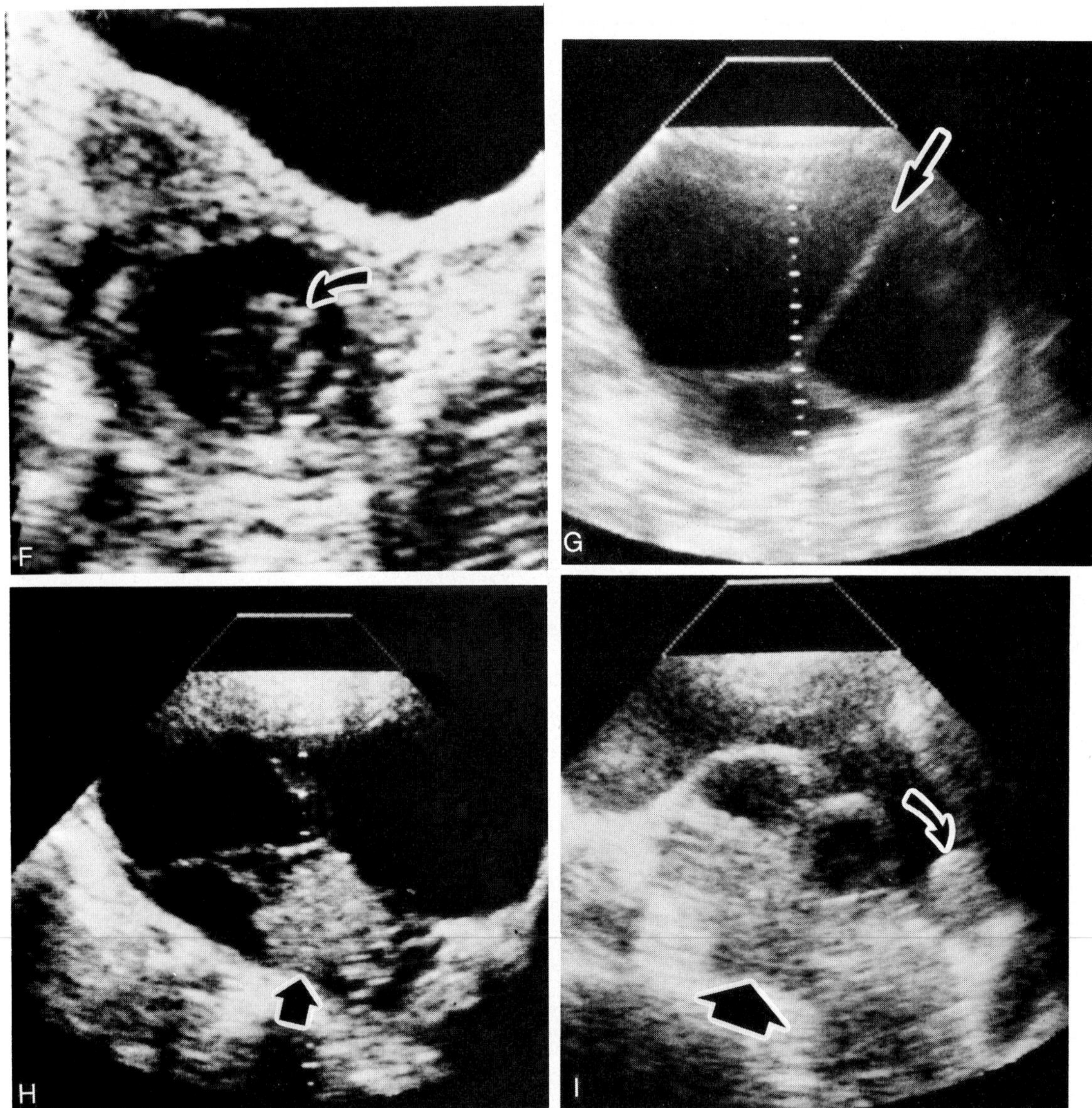

Figure 140–6 *Continued F,* Hemorrhagic corpus luteum cyst with a small amount of organized clot *(arrow).* This organized clot appeared as echogenic material within the cyst. This patient had a false-positive urinary pregnancy test secondary to proteinuria. *G,* Predominantly cystic pelvoabdominal mass within thin internal septa *(arrow).* This is the typical appearance of a mucinous cystadenoma of the ovary. *H,* As compared with *G,* this mass has a large solid component. In general, the more solid and/or irregular the internal components of a mass, the more likely it is to be malignant. This was a papillary cystadenocarcinoma of the ovary. *I,* Complex mass with solid components *(large arrow).* Ascites and serosal metastases *(curved arrow)* were present in this patient with papillary serous cystadenocarcinoma of the ovary.

Illustration continued on following page

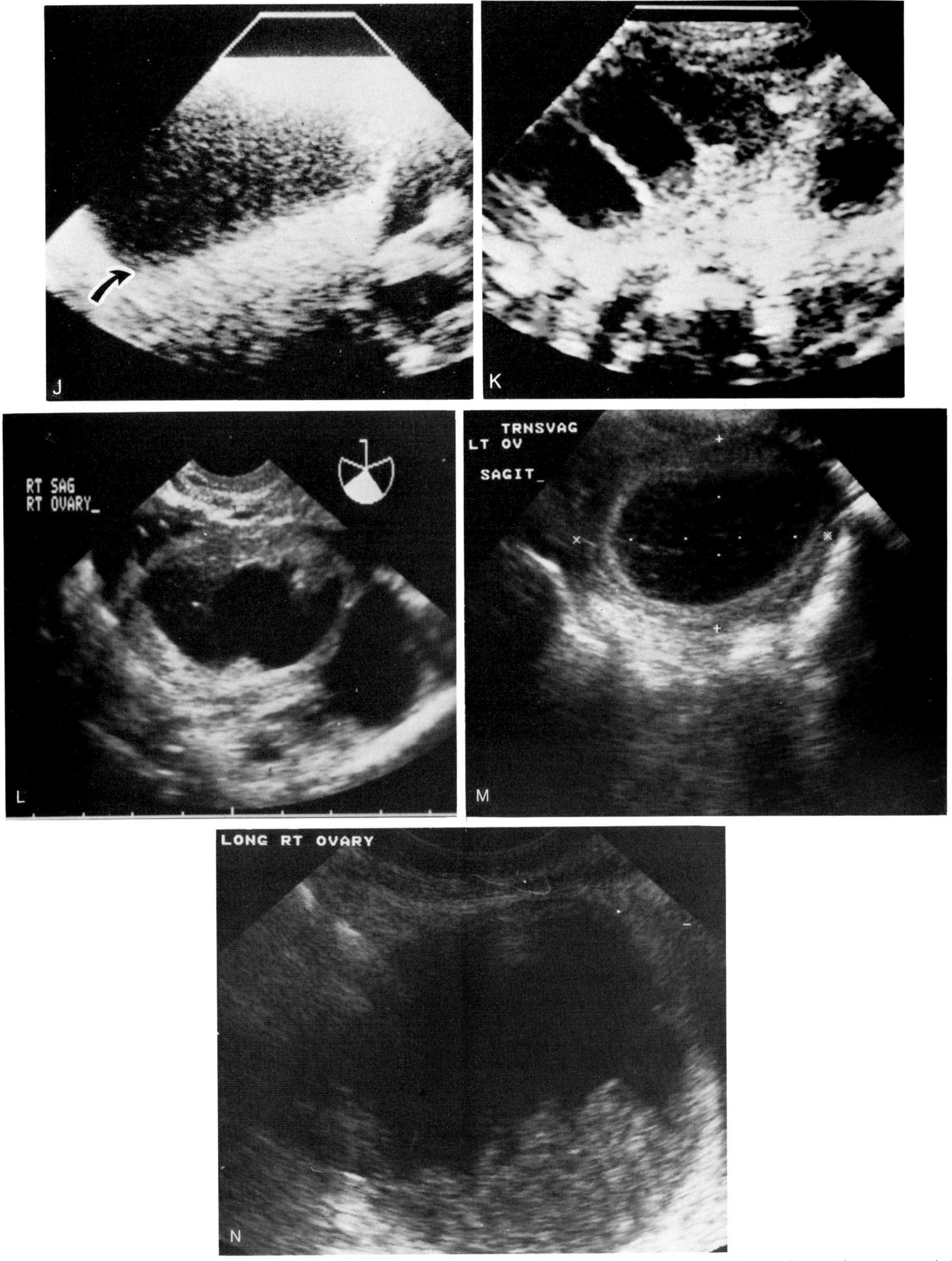

Figure 140–6 *Continued J,* This complex pelvoabdominal mass had a gravity-dependent layer of echogenic material *(curved arrow)* that corresponded to cellular debris within a papillary serous cystadenoma. *K,* Ovarian torsion in an infant girl. The cystic areas were luteinized cysts, probably resulting from in utero exposure to physiologically high levels of maternal estrogen. *L,* TVS of papillary serous cystadenocarcinoma with focally thickened wall and papillary excrescences. *M,* TVS of hemorrhagic ovarian cyst *(between cursors)* with internal echoes arising from clotted blood. *N,* TVS of cystic mass with solid area and papillary excrescences found to represent an ovarian metastasis from a gastrointestinal primary.

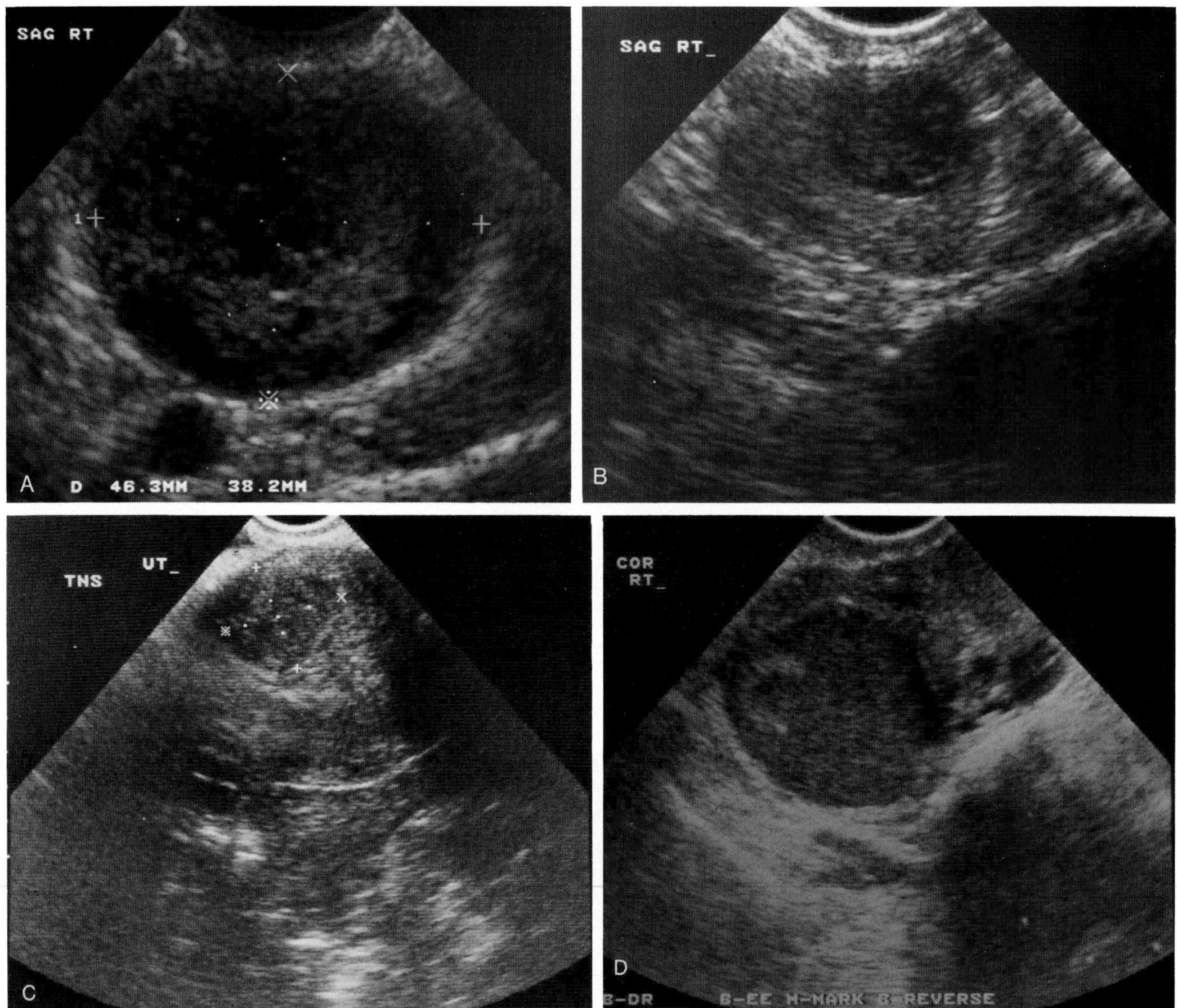

Figure 140–7. Solid pelvic masses. *A,* TVS of solid inhomogeneous mass within right ovary. *B,* Same patient as in *A,* 2 months later showing marked regression of hemorrhagic ovarian cyst. *C,* TVS showing small solid tumor *(between cursors)* within the right ovary found to repress a Sertoli-Leydig cell tumor. *D,* TVS of an endometrioma containing clotted blood. Even though the mass contains internal echoes, there is enhanced through transmission, suggesting its more fluid consistency. *E,* TVS of dermoid cyst containing echogenic sebaceous fluid. *F,* Hemorrhagic ovarian cyst *(arrow)* in a 16-year-old girl with pelvic pain. Organized clot within a cyst appears as echogenic internal material. *G,* Chronic ectopic pregnancy appearing as a solid extrauterine mass *(arrow)*. *H,* Dermoid cyst consisting predominantly of sebaceous liquid. An echogenic focus is also present within the cyst, representing an area of calcification. *I,* Massive stromal edema of the ovary occurring secondary to ovarian torsion. After detorsion of the ovary, it became normal-sized. *I,* Massive stromal edema of the ovary *(between cursors)* occurring secondary to ovarian torsion. After detorsion, the ovary regressed to normal size.

Illustration continued on following page

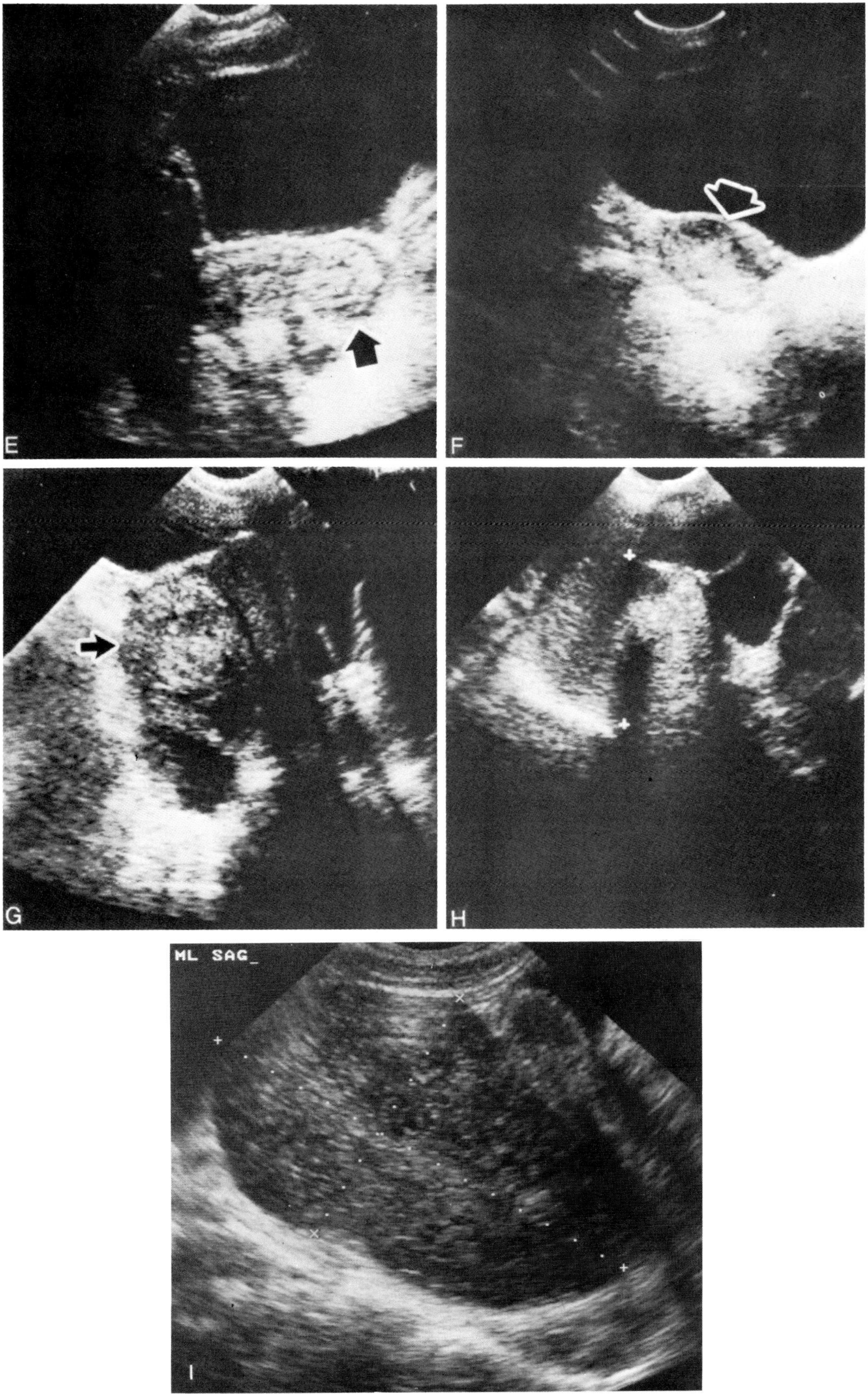

Figure 140–7 *Continued*

mucinous cystadenomas (Figs. 140–5*F* and 140–6*D*). In general, the more irregular the internal septations or the more solid the internal components of a mass, the more likely it is malignant.

TVS has been proposed as a means of detecting ovarian carcinoma. However, since this disease is relatively uncommon, scanning an unselected population of women may not prove worthwhile or cost-effective. Evaluation of patients at risk with conventional or color Doppler TVS seems promising.

Ovarian torsion usually occurs when the ovary contains a mass that potentiates the twisting of the ovarian pedicle. If this torsion is intermittent and does not totally occlude the venous blood flow from the ovary, the ovaries can become massively enlarged and appear as solid masses with internal echogenic areas from internal hemorrhage (Figs. 140–6*K* and 140–7*I*). Long-standing torsion usually results in an enlarged ovary with anechoic areas that represent areas of fibrinolyzed clot. Thus, ovarian torsion has a spectrum of sonographic features ranging from totally anechoic to predominantly solid. The most common appearance is that of a complex, predominantly cystic mass. Color Doppler TVS may offer a means for definitive and early diagnosis of this disorder.

Solid Pelvic Masses

In general, most solid pelvic masses are contiguous with the uterus. Most solid pelvic masses are fibroids. These tumors usually are hypoechoic relative to the normal myometrium and may contain highly echogenic areas arising from calcifications (Fig. 140–7*B*). Occasionally, the whorled configuration of the muscle and connective tissue that compose this tumor can be recognized sonographically. Sonography has an important role in the evaluation of the adnexa in patients with fibroids, since it may be difficult on pelvic examination to detect adnexal disease in a patient with multiple leiomyomas.

Solid masses adjacent to the uterus, such as those arising from intraperitoneal metastasis, may also give the impression of overall enlargement of the uterus similar to that encountered with a fibroid. This finding has been described as an ''indefinite uterus sign'' and has been associated with an increased chance of interpretative error.

As previously stated, most ovarian masses are cystic. A few can be solid, such as those arising from adenocarcinoma or other tumors, such as colon, that are metastatic to the ovary. Occasionally, hemorrhagic ovarian cysts, dermoids, or endometriomas can appear as solid adnexal masses owing to clotted blood contained within them (Fig. 140–7*A* and *C* to *I*).

CONDITIONS ASSOCIATED WITH MALIGNANCY

TVS has enhanced the sonographic detection and evaluation of ovarian and endometrial carcinomas. Although not all postmenopausal ovaries can be visualized with TVS, a negative TVS has excellent predictive value. Conversely, TVS can detect small (<2 cm) lesions and with color Doppler evaluation can assess the relative probability of malignancy. Hopefully, with more extensive use of TVS, diagnosis of ovarian carcinoma can be made earlier.

As opposed to the typically clinically silent presentation of ovarian carcinoma, most patients with endometrial carcinoma present with uterine bleeding. In these patients, TVS can distinguish those patients who will have a negative biopsy (endometrial width <5 mm) from those with hyperplasia or carcinoma. TVS can also be used to assess the relative amount of myometrial invasion in patients with proven endometrial carcinoma.

In patients with a pelvic mass that may be malignant, other areas of the body should be carefully evaluated. These include the paracolic, perihepatic, and cul-de-sac regions for ascites; the peritoneal and omental surfaces for metastasis; the liver for metastasis; and the kidneys for obstructive uropathy (Fig. 140–8*A* to *E*). If no pelvocalyceal distention is documented by sonography, excretory urography may not be necessary, unless the surgeon needs to know the exact course of the ureters.

Since ascites usually occurs as the result of tumor seeding to the peritoneum, malignancy can be inferred when the mass is associated with ascites. However, the absence of ascites does not always indicate that the lesion is benign. Conversely, some benign conditions such as an ovarian fibroma can be associated with ascites and hydrothorax (Meigs' syndrome).

Liver metastases from ovarian carcinoma are most frequently encountered in patients who have been treated and present with recurrent disease. The liver metastases encountered in these patients can range from cystic to solid lesions. Peritoneal seeding of tumor is difficult to detect if the lesions are less than 1 cm or are not surrounded by intraperitoneal fluid. However, when these masses are greater than 2 cm and are associated with ascites, they are readily depicted (Figs. 140–8*C* to *G*). Some metastases from gynecologic tumors can grow within the cul-de-sac. Since they are adjacent to the uterus and have similar echogenicity to the uterus, they may give the impression of overall enlargement of the uterus. As stated previously, this situation can lead to ''the indefinite uterus'' sign and can be encountered whenever a mass of similar echogenicity is situated adjacent to the uterus.

MISCELLANEOUS UTERINE DISORDERS

Sonography has a role in evaluation of some types of uterine disorders. For example, abnormally thick endometrium detected sonographically may be a sign of endometrial pathology (Fig. 140–9*A*). Similarly, abnormally thick and irregular endometrium associated with intraluminal fluid may be an indication of endometrial carcinoma with or without cervical stenosis (Fig. 140–9*B*). Adenomyosis of the uterus, which results from endometriotic myometrial implants, may also appear to result in thickening of the central intrauterine interface. A hypoechoic intraluminal area may be encountered in patients with hematometra within the uterine corpus secondary to cervical or uterine carcinoma (Fig. 140–9*C*). Myometrial invasion of trophoblastic tissue appears as focal echogenic areas within the uterus (Fig. 140–9*D*). Similarly, the relative amount of myometrial invasion for endometrial carcinoma can be detected with TVS (Fig. 140–9*E* and *F*).

OVARIAN FOLLICULAR MONITORING

TVS has an important role in assisting the gynecologic endocrinologist in monitoring the infertile patient during ovulation induction. Specifically, the size, number, and location of developing follicles can be documented using sonography (Fig. 140–10*A* and *B*). In general, most mature follicles range from 18 to 22 mm in average dimension. The success or failure of attempts at ovulation induction can be accurately assessed (Fig. 140–10*C* and *D*). In addition, the presence or absence of ovulation can be implied by the interval development of fluid within the cul-de-sac associated with a follicle that has developed a thickened, crenated border.

GUIDED FOLLICULAR ASPIRATION

TVS is particularly useful for delineation of follicles and for transforniceal follicular aspiration guidance (Fig. 140–10*B*).

Text continued on page 2057

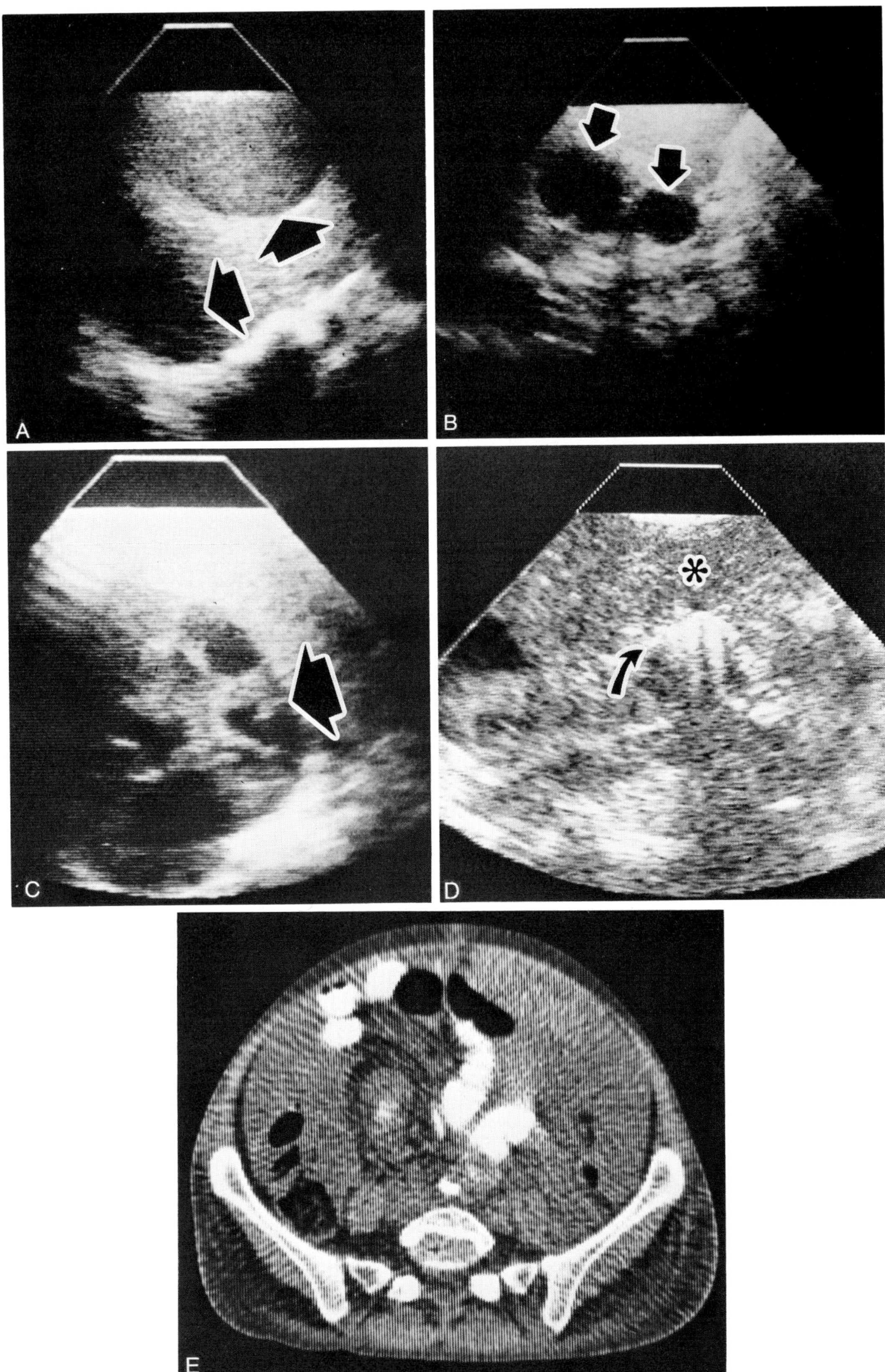

Figure 140–8. Disorders associated with gynecologic malignancy. *A,* Transverse sonogram of the liver demonstrating several large hypoechoic areas *(arrows).* These masses corresponded to metastases from ovarian carcinoma. *B,* Multiple cystic metastases within the liver *(arrows)* in a patient with recurrent disease from a mucinous cystadenocarcinoma of the ovary. As more patients are being successfully treated with chemotherapy, they may present with recurrent disease as evidenced by metastases to the liver. *C,* Complex mass *(arrow)* within the liver arising from metastases associated with mucinous cystadenocarcinoma of the ovary. This metastasis mimics the gross appearance of the primary tumor. *D,* Peritoneal metastases in a patient with uterine carcinoma. The mass *(asterisk)* was outlined inferiorly by gas-filled bowel *(arrow). E,* CT scan of the patient as in *F.* Identification of the peritoneal metastases was difficult owing to surrounding ascites.

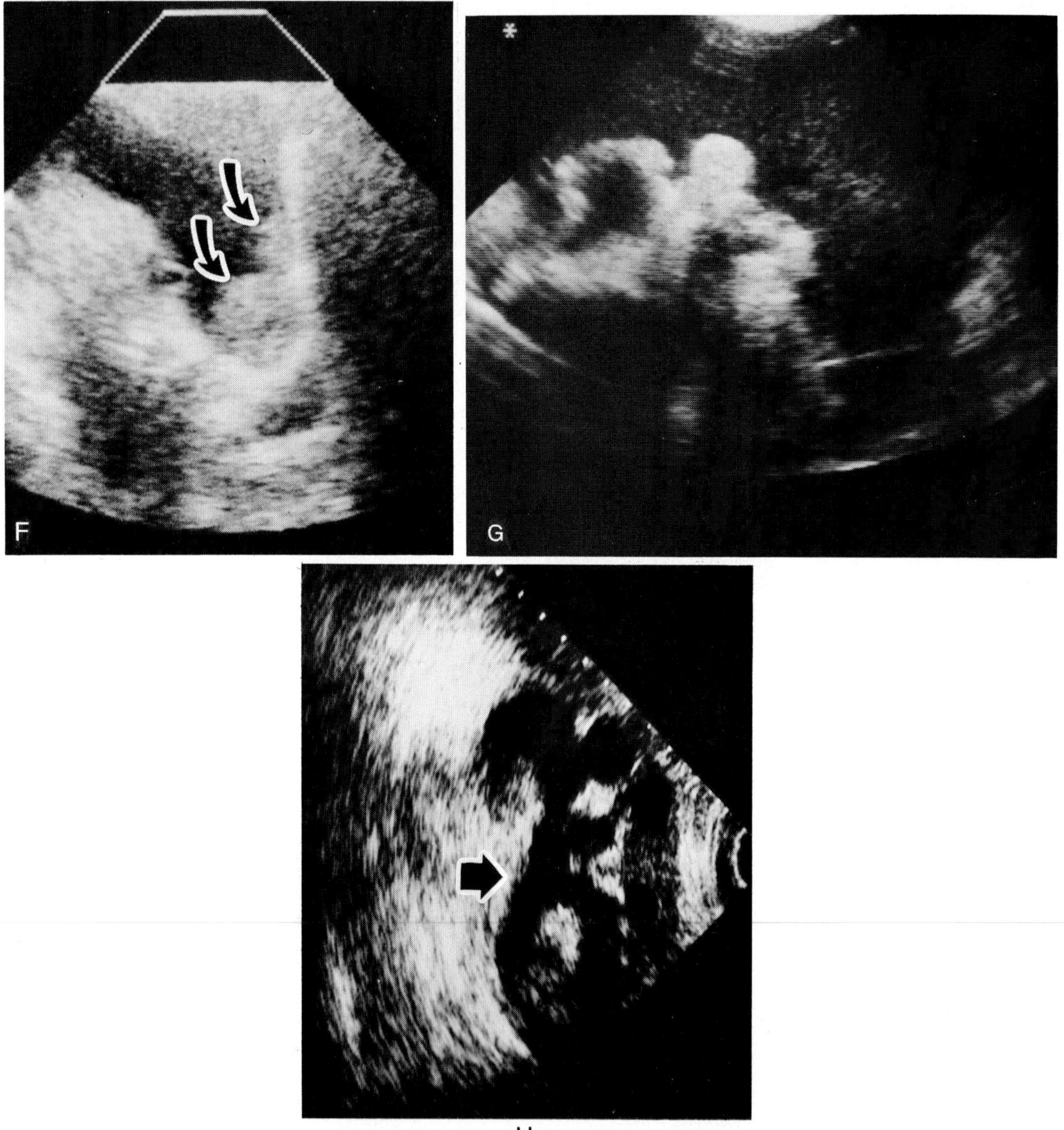

Figure 140–8 *Continued F,* Serosal metastases associated with malignant ovarian carcinoma along the dome of the urinary bladder *(arrows). G,* Pseudomyoma peritonei appearing as echogenic material surrounding loops of matted bowel. *H,* Obstructive uropathy of the left pelvis as imaged in a coronal plane secondary to advanced cervical carcinoma. The presence or absence of abnormal pelvocalyceal distention should be assessed in every patient with a large pelvic mass. Distended pelvis and infundibula are present in this patient *(arrow).*

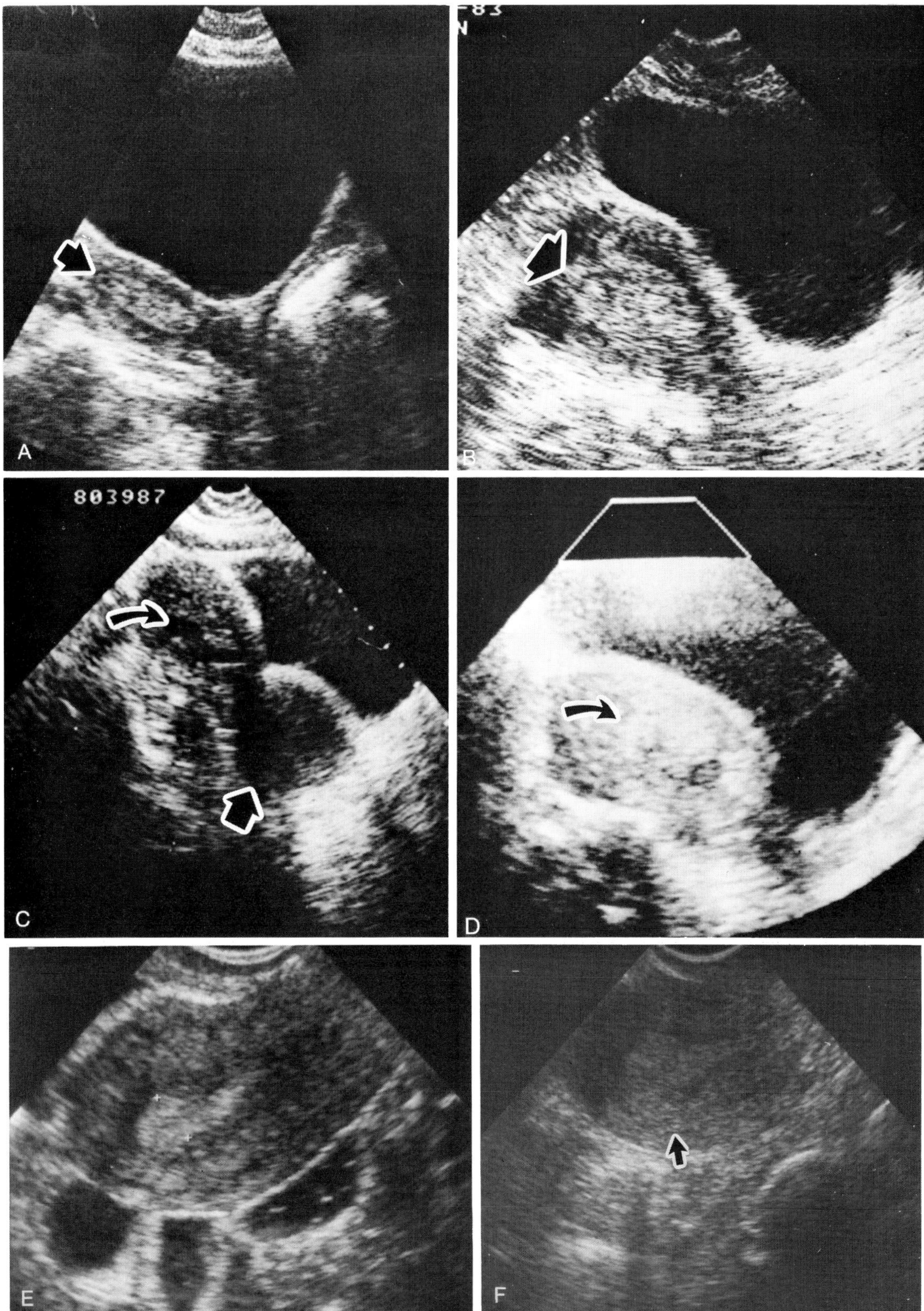

Figure 140–9. Miscellaneous uterine disorders. *A,* Thick and echogenic endometrium *(arrow)* related to retained mucous secretions. Normal endometrial biopsy. *B,* Abnormally thick and irregular endometrium *(arrow)* in a patient with endometrial carcinoma. *C,* Cervical carcinoma *(large arrow)* associated with hematometria *(curved arrow)*. *D,* Choriocarcinoma appearing as multiple echogenic foci *(curved arrow)* within the myometrium. *E,* TVS of echogenic hyperplastic endometrium *(between cursors)*. *F,* TVS of moderately invasive endometrial carcinoma. Note the disruption of the hypoechoic subendometrial halo in area of invasion *(arrow)*.

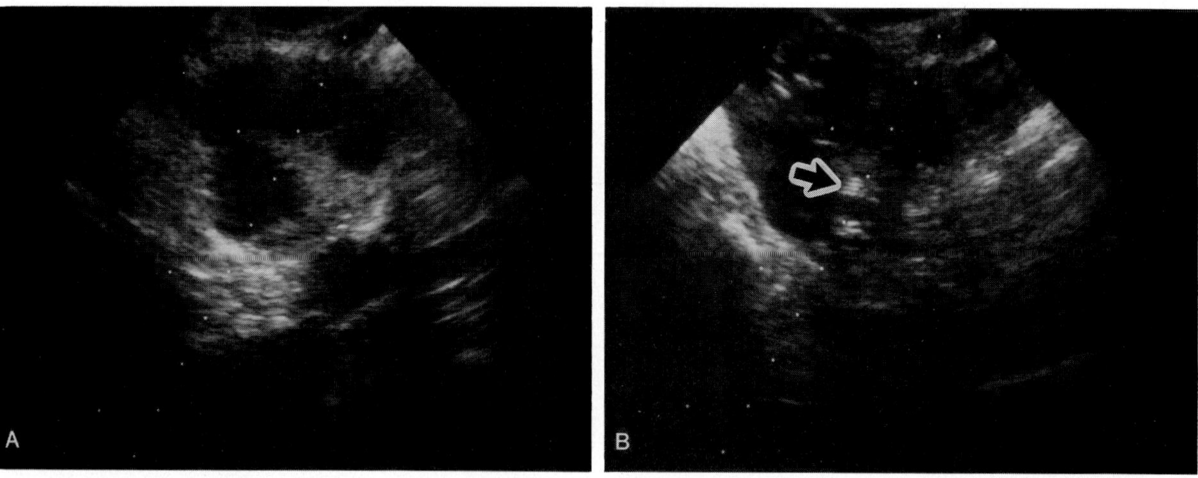

Figure 140–10. Follicular monitoring and aspiration with TVS. *A,* Multiple mature follicles resulting from ovulation induction. *B,* Still frame taken from TVS-guided follicular aspiration shows the echogenic needle tip (*arrow*) within the deflated follicle.

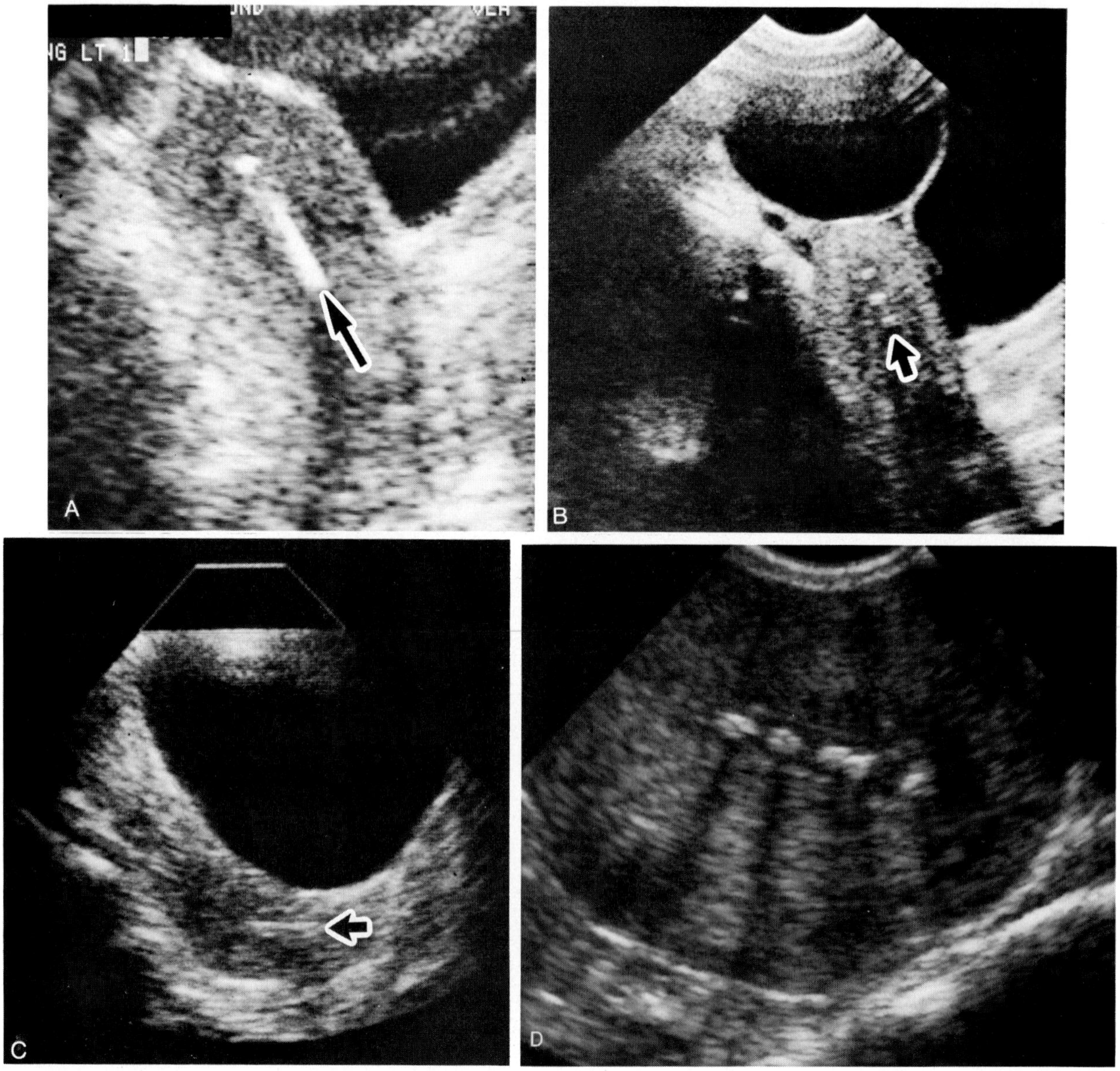

Figure 140–11. Intrauterine contraceptive devices. *A,* Long-axis view demonstrating shaft and horizontal portion of Copper-7 IUCD *(arrow).* The intrauterine contraceptive device should be within the lumen of the fundus and corpus. *B,* Long-axis view of Lippes loop *(arrow)* within the uterus. Multiple echogenic interfaces arise from the strands of the IUCD. This patient also had a completely cystic dermoid cyst superior to the uterine fundus. *C,* Long-axis view of the shaft of a Progestocert IUCD *(arrow).* Since this IUCD does not contain metallic wires, it is not echogenic. *D,* TVS of Lippes loop within the endometrial lumen.

INTRAUTERINE CONTRACEPTIVE DEVICE LOCALIZATION

Sonography is helpful in delineating the location of an IUCD. Normally, the IUCD should be placed within the lumen of the corpus and fundal portions of the uterus (Fig. 140–11*A* to *C*).

Sonography is useful in evaluation of IUCD complications such as concomitant intrauterine pregnancy or uterine perforation. In uterine perforation, the IUCD will be outside of the endometrial lumen and have an abnormal orientation relative to the uterine lumen. Intrauterine pregnancies occurring with an IUCD in place have a reasonable chance of completion. Partial embedding of the IUCD within the myometrium can also be diagnosed in some cases by sonographic depiction of the location of the IUCD relative to the endometrium (Fig. 140–11*A* to *D*).

Bibliography

Bourne T, Campbell S, Steer C, et al: Transvaginal colour flow imaging: A possible new screening technique for ovarian cancer. Br Med J 299:1367–1370, 1989.

Campbell S, Bhan V, Royston P, et al: Transabdominal ultrasound screening for early ovarian cancer. Br Med J 299:1363–1367, 1989.

Fleischer A, Entman S, Gordon A: TV and TA sonography of pelvic masses. J Ultrasound Med Biol 15:529–533, 1989.

Fleischer A, Mendelson E, Bohm-Velez M, Entman S: Transvaginal and transabdominal sonography of the endometrium. Semin US CT MRI 9(2):81, 1988.

Goldstein SR, Nachtigall M, Snyder JR, Nachtigall L: Endometrial assessment by vaginal ultrasonography before endometrial sampling in patients with postmenopausal bleeding. Am J Obstet Gynecol 163:119–123, 1990.

Goldstein SR, Subramanyam B, Snyder JR, et al: The postmenopausal cystic adnexal mass: The potential role of ultrasound in conservative management. Obstet Gynecol 743:8–10, 1989.

Granberg S, Norstrom A, Wikland M: Tumors in the lower pelvis as imaged by vaginal sonography. Gynecol Oncol 37:224–229, 1990.

Osmers R, Volksen M, Schauer A: Vaginosonography for early detection of endometrial carcinoma. Lancet 335:1569–1571, 1990.

Teisala K, Heinonen PK, Punonen R: Transvaginal ultrasound in the diagnosis and treatment of tubo-ovarian abscess. Br J Obstet Gynaecol 97:178–180, 1990.

Van Nagell JR, Higgins RV, Donaldson ES, et al: Transvaginal sonography as a screening method for ovarian cancer—a report of the first 1000 cases screened. Cancer 65:573–577, 1990.

141 Imaging of Uterine Masses and Tumors

James W. Walsh

Diseases of the uterine corpus and cervix are a common cause of lower abdominal distention and pelvic pain, abnormal uterine bleeding, or a pelvic mass in the female patient. Assessment of uterine masses and neoplasms is thus an important aspect of gynecologic imaging. Except for the plain film of the pelvis, noninvasive imaging modalities have virtually replaced the excretory urogram and the barium enema as the best means to evaluate uterine morphology and pathology. Sonography is an important imaging modality for evaluating congenital anomalies of the uterus, endometrial fluid collections, intrauterine contraceptive devices, gestational trophoblastic disease (GTD), leiomyomata, and diseases of the endometrium. When sonography is nondiagnostic, magnetic resonance (MR) is useful for further characterizing congenital anomalies or uterine masses and tumors in pregnant patients. Computed tomography (CT) is currently recommended for evaluating large or complicated leiomyomata, staging advanced cancers of the cervix and endometrium, detecting persistent and metastatic GTD, and evaluating recurrent cervical and endometrial cancers. MR has significant advantages in local staging of clinical Stage I or II cancers of the cervix and endometrium and in differentiating tumor from leiomyomata. MR has also become the procedure of choice in differentiating adenomyosis from leiomyomata and in evaluating the number, size, and location of leiomyomata in pregnant or infertile patients. In this chapter, a multimodality diagnostic approach to the most common uterine masses and tumors is described.

DIAGNOSTIC PITFALLS

Variations in uterine position may be mistaken for a pelvic mass on physical examination or on imaging studies. The normal position of the uterus is forward with a slight angulation of the fundus on the cervix, i.e., anteversion. Retrodisplacements of the uterus may be congenital or acquired owing to adnexal inflammatory disease or to mechanical displacement from a pelvic neoplasm. Retroversion is a retrodisplacement in which the uterus is tilted backward on its transverse axis and is seen in 20 per cent of all females. Retroflexion is a more extreme bending backward of the uterine fundus on the cervix (Fig. 141–1).

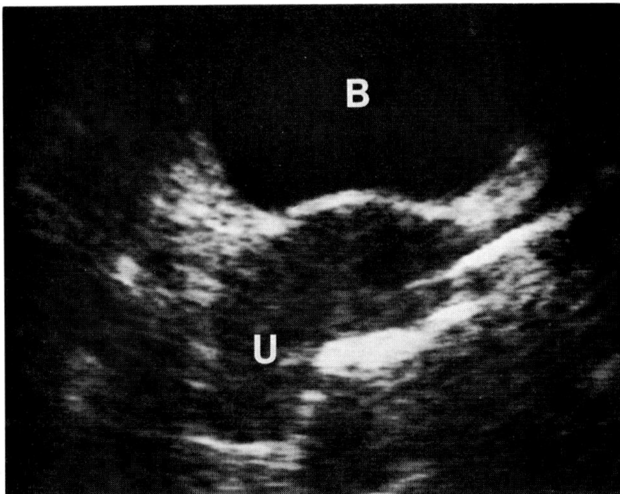

Figure 141–1. Sagittal sonogram through bladder (B) and a retroflexed uterus (U) in a patient with a suspected cul-de-sac mass on pelvic examination.

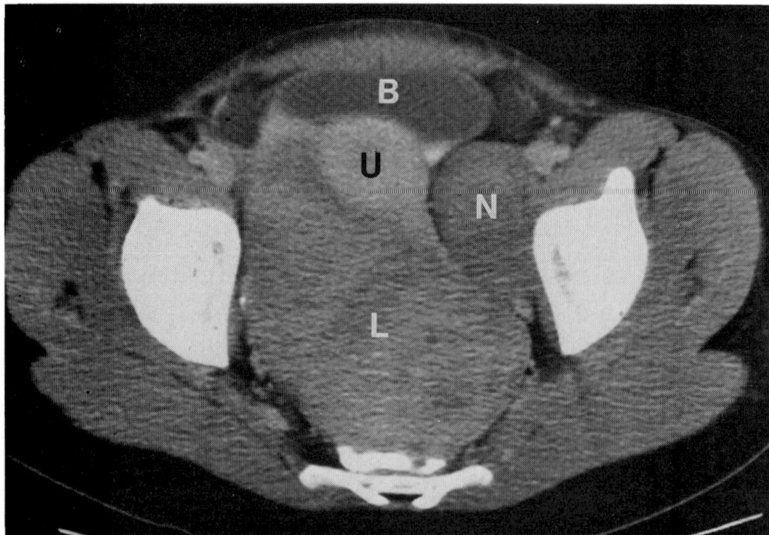

Figure 141–2. CT scan through bladder (B) shows an enlarged left external iliac lymph node (N) and an ovarian lymphoma (L) inseparable from a normal contrast-enhanced uterus (U). (Case courtesy of Jack Scatarige, M.D., Depaul Medical Center, Norfolk, VA.)

Differentiation of uterine from extrauterine masses is a significant problem in pelvic mass diagnosis. On sonography, recognition of the central endometrial echo, a characteristic pear shape, and anatomic relationships to the bladder and vagina are key determinants in distinguishing the uterus from other pelvic structures. On CT, the round, broad, cardinal, or uterosacral ligaments; endometrial cavity; myometrial intravenous contrast enhancement; and midline position between bladder and rectum are key parameters in localizing the uterus. On MR, recognition of the uterine ligaments, uterine zonal anatomy on T_2-weighted images, and midpelvic position on three-dimensional images is usually sufficient to identify the uterus. Inflammatory diseases such as endometriosis or tubo-ovarian abscess commonly obliterate uterine borders and displace the uterus from its midline position. Less commonly, the uterus may be surrounded and invaded by tumors of the ovary (Fig. 141–2). Finally, there may be difficulty in differentiating the uterus from a contiguous solid tumor or from a mass arising in the adjacent broad ligament, e.g., leiomyoma or leiomyosarcoma (Fig. 141–3).

LEIOMYOMATA

Uterine leiomyomata occur in 20 to 40 per cent of women beyond 30 to 35 years of age and are one of the most common causes of an enlarged uterus. They vary considerably in size and number, and multiplicity is common. Leiomyomata are classified by their location into submucous, intramural, or subserous types. Intramural leiomyomata are the most common type and typically distort the uterine outline and cause an irregular, enlarged uterus. Pedunculated subserosal leiomyomata can simulate other solid pelvic masses by protruding into the cul-de-sac or into the paracolic gutters (Figs. 141–4 and 141–5). Occasionally, a giant fibroid uterus may extend up to the umbilicus and cause hydronephrosis by compressing the ureter against the pelvic brim.

A plain abdominal radiograph may be the only study necessary to diagnose a leiomyoma if it shows typical stippled, flocculent, or whorl-like calcifications (Fig. 141–6). In the absence of characteristic plain film findings, sonography is the next imaging procedure

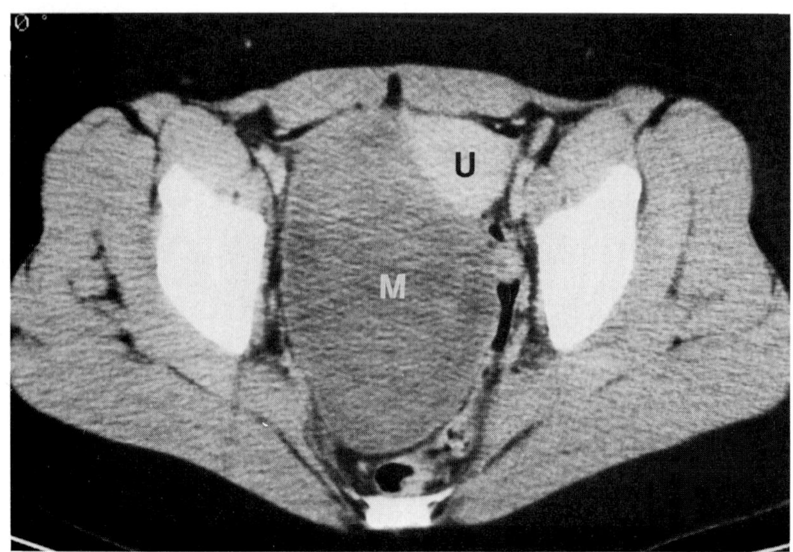

Figure 141–3. Right broad ligament leiomyoma. CT scan through a large heterogeneous solid pelvic mass (M), which is inseparable from the compressed and displaced uterine corpus (U).

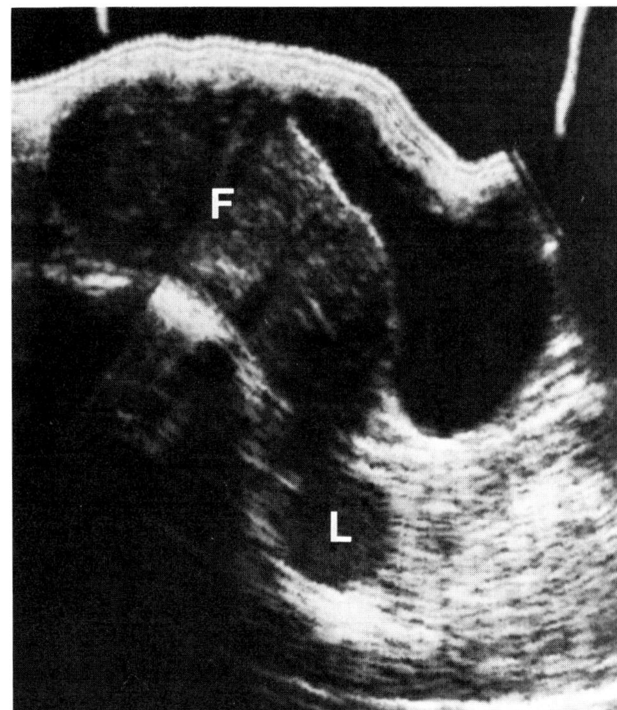

Figure 141–4. Sagittal sonogram of an enlarged fibroid uterus (F) with a pedunculated leiomyoma (L) in the cul-de-sac.

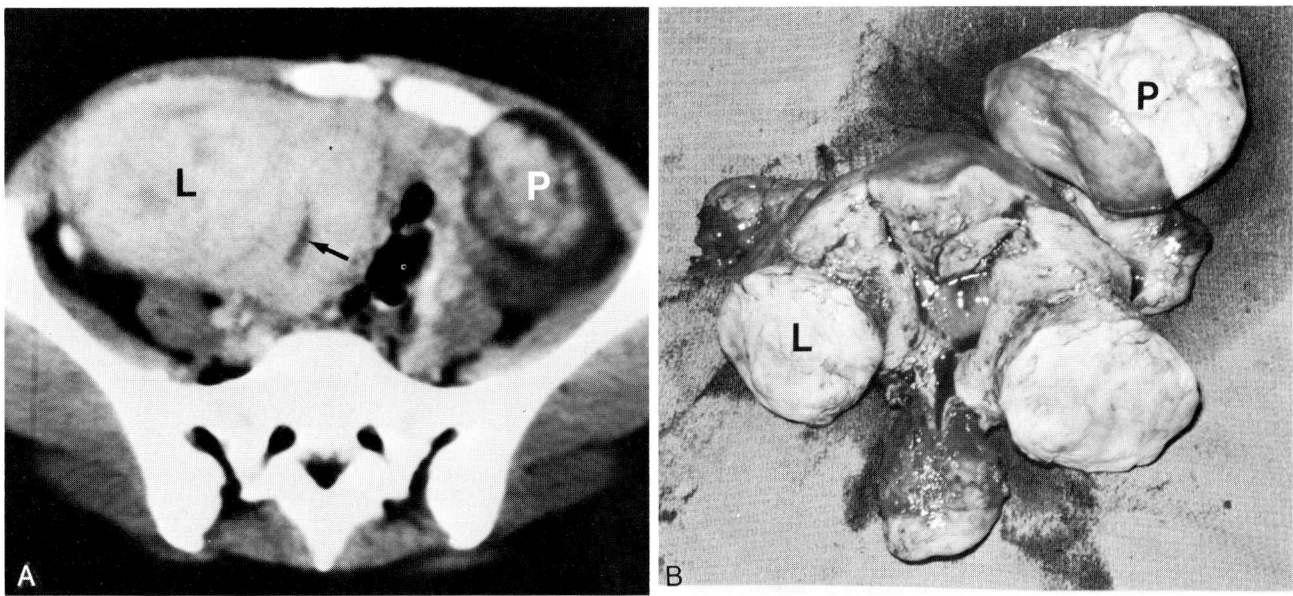

Figure 141–5. *A,* CT scan of an intramural isodense leiomyoma (L) deforming the endometrial cavity *(arrow)* and a pedunculated leiomyoma (P) with a hypodense peripheral rim. *B,* Frontal view of the hysterectomy specimen with the intramural leiomyoma (L) and the pedunculated subserosal leiomyoma (P).

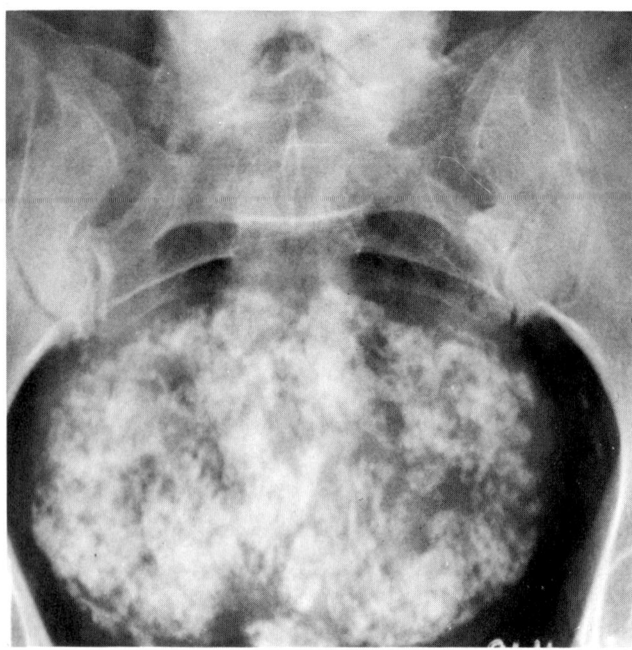

Figure 141–6. Anteroposterior radiograph of a typical densely calcified **leiomyoma.**

of choice. The classic sonographic appearance of a leiomyoma is a focal hypoechoic solid mass associated with irregularity and lobulation of the uterine contour and uterine enlargement (Fig. 141–7). Calcific foci are quite common in leiomyomata and are recognized as bright specular echoes with distal acoustic shadowing. Hyaline, cystic, and fatty degeneration in leiomyomata are uncommon sonographic findings. In some cases of large leiomyomas, sonographic diagnosis may be difficult owing to poor bladder filling from extrinsic mass compression or to overlying gas that obscures the relationship of the leiomyoma to normal portions of the uterus. In such situations, CT may provide a confident diagnosis of a fibroid uterus and exclude an adnexal mass. MR is also useful in distinguishing leiomyomas from other solid pelvic masses when sonography is indeterminate.

With current high-resolution CT scanners and intravenous contrast, it is possible to demonstrate the normal uterine cavity and to differentiate subserosal, intramural, and submucosal leiomyomata. The characteristic CT features of uterine myomata include uterine enlargement with a lobulated and protuberant outer contour, a soft-tissue mass thickening the myometrium and deforming the endometrial cavity, foci of punctate or amorphous coarse calcifications, and a heterogeneous density within the soft-tissue mass (Figs. 141–5 and 141–7). The leiomyomata may be hypodense, isodense, or hyperdense on CT relative to normal contrast-enhanced myometrium (Figs. 141–5, 141–7, and 141–8). Also, subserosal fibroids are commonly surrounded by a hypodense rim attributable to a pseudocapsule of thickened serosa (Fig. 141–5). Pedunculated leiomyomata frequently lie anterior to the aortic bifurcation or laterally

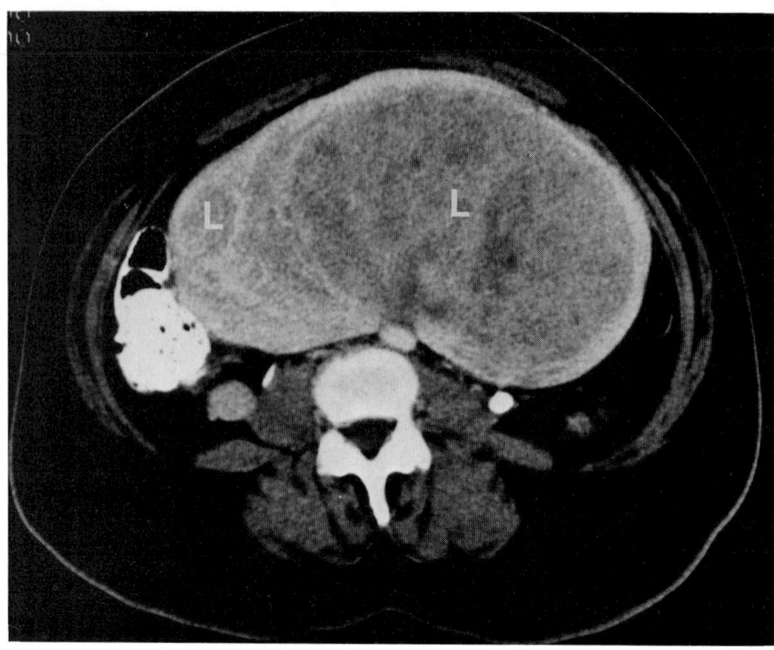

Figure 141–7. CT scan through the lower abdomen shows an enlarged uterus containing several heterogeneous, hypodense leiomyomata (L) surrounded by normal, peripheral, contrast-enhanced myometrium.

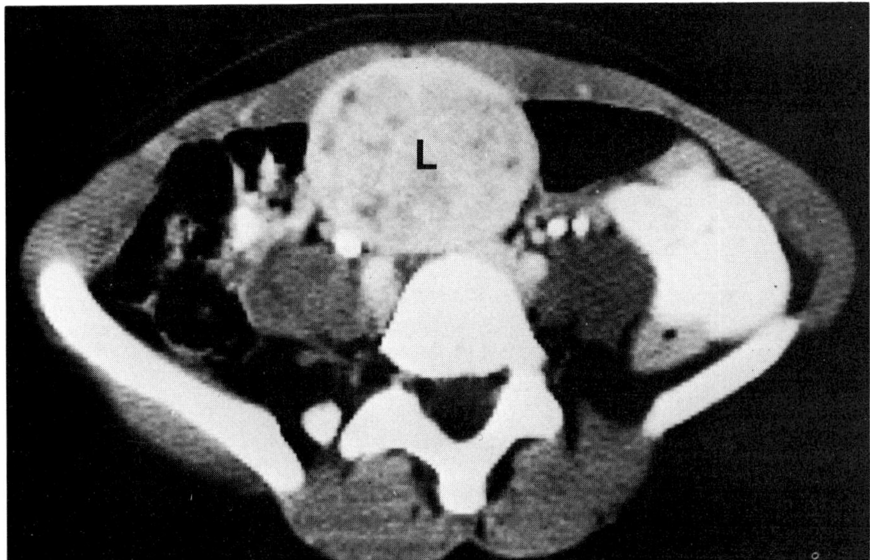

Figure 141–8. CT scan of a hyperdense leiomyoma (L) anterior to contrast-filled common iliac vessels.

in the iliac fossae. The origin of this type of lesion from the uterus may be difficult to determine on the transverse plane of CT.

Unusual manifestations of leiomyomas (e.g., infection; necrosis; infarction; intramural hemorrhage; or cystic, fatty, or sarcomatous degeneration) may simulate a primary cervical or endometrial cancer (Fig. 141–9). Also, a subserosal leiomyoma may herniate from the endometrial cavity, protrude out of the cervical os, and mimic the appearance of cervical cancer.

MR is now commonly used to precisely delineate the number, size, and location of leiomyomas prior to selective myomectomy in pregnant or infertile patients or to monitor therapy with gonadotropin-releasing hormone analogs. Leiomyomas usually have low signal intensity or are isointense compared with myometrium on T_1-weighted images and have low signal intensity on T_2-weighted images (Fig. 141–10). They may be partially or completely hyperintense on T_2-weighted images, depending on the degree of cellularity, hyalinization, and hemorrhage, and hence are indistinguishable from endometrial malignancy.

The differential diagnosis of a uterine corpus mass includes primary and recurrent endometrial malignancy, a leiomyoma, an intrauterine fluid collection, and endometrial extension of a cervical carcinoma. Although the sonographic, CT, and MR appearances of leiomyomata cannot always be differentiated from a uterine cancer, patients with an endometrial malignancy are usually symptomatic because of perimenopausal or postmenopausal bleeding and rarely present with an asymptomatic pelvic mass. In equivocal cases, a fractional dilatation and curettage may be necessary to differentiate a uterine corpus cancer or sarcoma from a leiomyoma.

UTERINE FLUID COLLECTIONS

Small endometrial fluid collections, 1.5 to 5 cm in greatest diameter, may be detected by sonography in nonpregnant patients who have vaginal bleeding or inflammation of the endometrium or

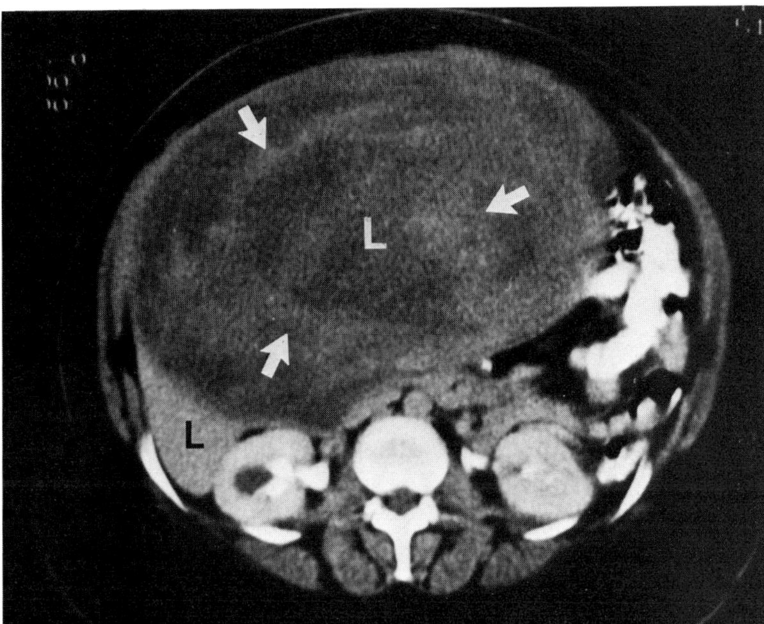

Figure 141–9. CT scan through the inferior liver (L) and kidneys shows a huge, hypodense leiomyoma (L) with whorls of high-density material *(arrows)* due to hemorrhage into a leiomyomatous uterus.

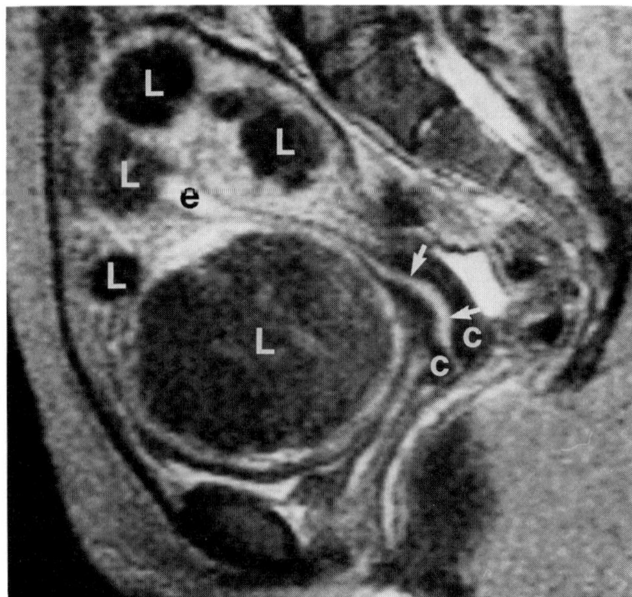

Figure 141–10. Sagittal T_2-weighted spin-echo (2500/90) MR through the normal hypointense anterior and posterior lips of the cervix (c) and hyperintense endocervical canal *(arrows)* and endometrium (e) shows uterine enlargement and myometrial expansion by multiple hypointense intramural leiomyomas (L).

adnexa. The differential diagnosis of these fluid collections includes dysfunctional uterine bleeding, a submucosal leiomyoma, endometritis, endometrial hyperplasia or a polyp, and cancer (Fig. 141–11). Congenital anomalies are the usual cause of vaginal and/or uterine fluid collections in prepubertal and adolescent females. Larger intrauterine fluid collections in adults are usually due to cervical stenosis from senile contraction, primary or recurrent carcinoma of the endometrium or cervix, uterine sarcoma, radiation therapy, or postsurgical scarring. Subsequent accumulation of blood (hematometra), pus (pyometra), or sterile fluid (hydrometra) proximal to the obstruction causes progressive dilatation of the uterus. Sonography, CT, and MR reliably diagnose an obstructed, fluid-filled uterus and differentiate it from other pelvic masses. The size of the uterus and the thickness of the myometrium vary with the amount of endometrial fluid and the degree of uterine distention. In adults, a pyometra or hematometra is usually due to carcinoma of the cervix or endometrium (Figs. 141–12*A* and 141–13*B*).

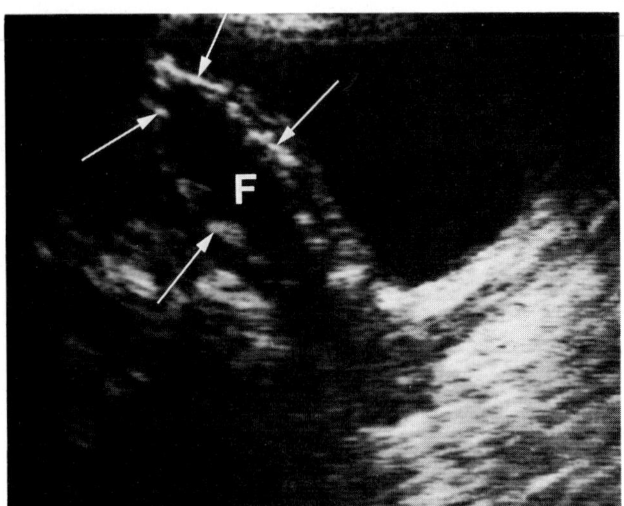

Figure 141–11. Sagittal sonogram of a small endometrial fluid collection (F) surrounded by abnormal hyperechoic endometrium *(arrows)* due to adenosquamous carcinoma of the endometrium in a 64-year-old female with postmenopausal bleeding.

ENDOMETRIAL CARCINOMA AND SARCOMA

Carcinoma of the endometrium is the most common invasive cancer of the female genital tract. Adenocarcinomas comprise 90 to 95 per cent and sarcomas 1 to 3 per cent of endometrial malignancies. Seventy-five per cent of adenocarcinomas occur after age 50, with a peak incidence at age 62. Initial symptoms are intermenstrual or postmenopausal bleeding, and patients usually seek medical attention when the cancer is at an early stage (74 per cent Stage I and 15 per cent Stage II). Diagnosis is established by fractional dilatation and curettage. Clinical staging of uterine corpus malignancy is based on bimanual pelvic examination, sounding the depth of the uterine cavity, cystoscopy, sigmoidoscopy, chest radiography, and excretory urography. MR is the most promising technique for evaluating Stage I and II tumors and differentiating the degree of myometrial invasion.

Indications for CT staging of uterine corpus malignancy are (1) to accurately determine stage in patients with an equivocal pelvic examination or a medical contraindication to surgical staging, (2) to screen for lymphatic or peritoneal metastases in patients with poorly differentiated carcinomas or sarcomas, and (3) to confirm advanced Stage III–IVb cancers. Sonography is not widely used to evaluate these tumors because of its limited ability to detect either parametrial and pelvic sidewall invasion or lymphatic and peritoneal metastases. CT and MR staging criteria are developed from the International Federation of Gynecology and Obstetrics (FIGO) staging classification: Stage I, tumor confined to corpus; Stage II, tumor involving corpus and cervix; Stage III, tumor extension to parametria, adnexae, pelvic sidewall, or pelvic nodes; Stage IVa, bladder or rectal involvement; Stage IVb, metastases to para-aortic lymph nodes, peritoneal cavity, omentum, or liver (Figs. 141–12, 141–14, and 141–15).

CT staging of endometrial malignancy requires intravenous contrast administration to differentiate normal contrast-enhanced myometrium from intrauterine tumor. CT demonstrates endometrial tumor as a hypodense mass in the uterine cavity or myometrium, as a fluid-filled uterus due to tumor obstruction of the endocervical canal, or as a contrast-enhancing lesion in the myometrium. Tumor may be confined to the endometrial cavity and appear as a hypodense polypoid mass surrounded by less dense endometrial fluid, or it may focally invade the myometrium and be highlighted by adja-

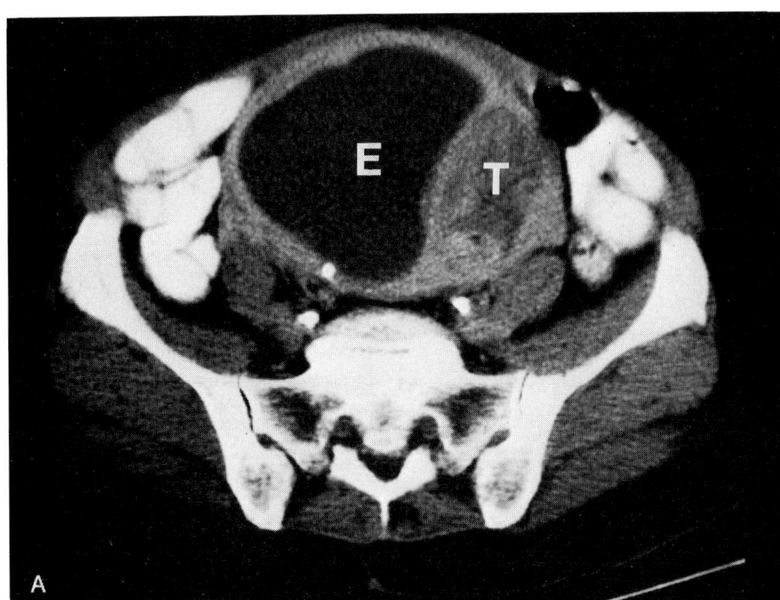

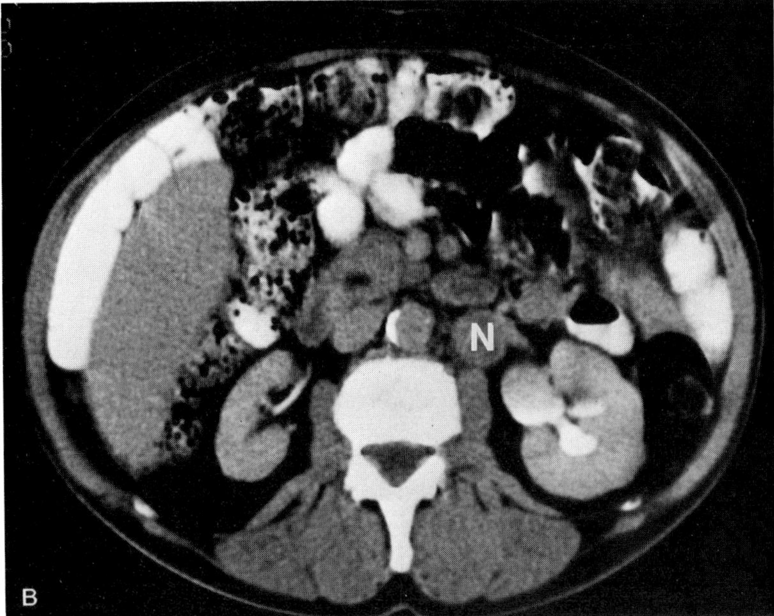

Figure 141–12. Stage IVb endometrial sarcoma. *A,* CT scan at the sacral promontory shows an enlarged uterus with a dilated, fluid-filled endometrial cavity (E) and left myometrial tumor invasion (T). *B,* CT scan through the kidneys shows a left para-aortic lymph node metastasis (N).

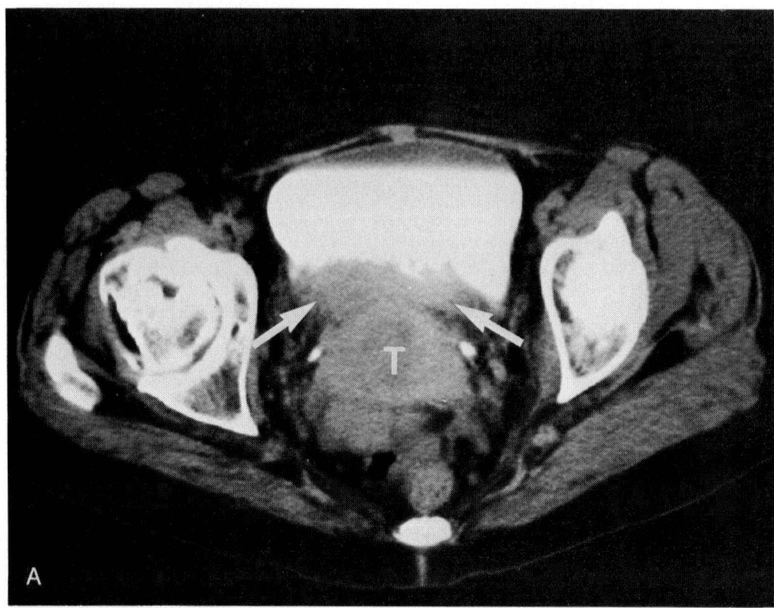

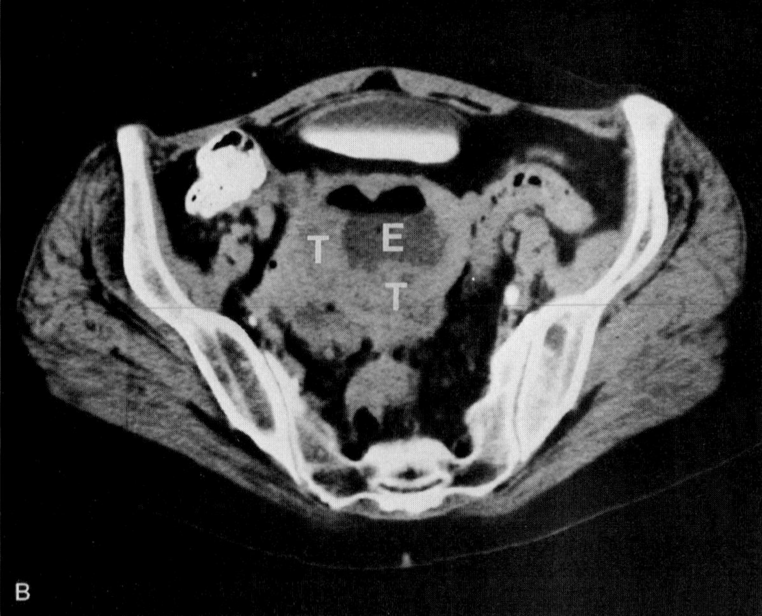

Figure 141–13. Stage IVa cervical cancer. *A,* CT scan through a hypodense cervical tumor (T) shows direct anterior tumor extension *(arrows)* and a nodular posterior bladder wall due to tumor invasion. *B,* CT scan at a higher level shows tumor invasion of the uterine corpus (T) with a dilated endometrial cavity (E) containing an air-fluid level due to an associated pyometra.

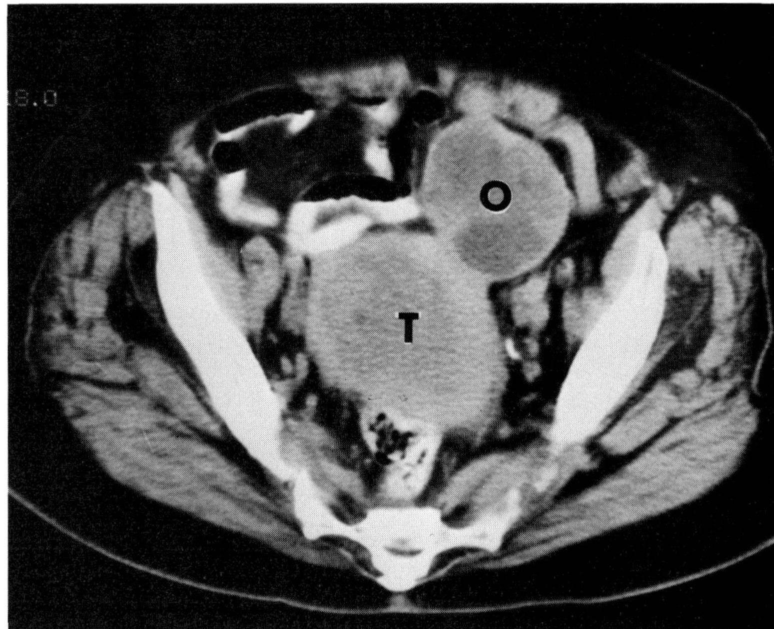

Figure 141–14. Stage III endometrial sarcoma. CT scan through an enlarged uterus with central hypodense tumor (T) and a heterogeneous left ovarian metastasis (O).

cent normal enhanced myometrium (Figs. 141–12*A*, 141–14, and 141–15*B*). Endometrial tumor involvement of the cervix is characterized as cervical enlargement greater than 3.5 cm in diameter and heterogeneous hypodense areas within the fibromuscular cervical stroma (Fig. 141–15*A*). Stage III disease is characterized by parametrial and pelvic sidewall extension or metastatic disease to the ovary and fallopian tube (Fig. 141–14), and Stage IVb disease is indicated by abdominal metastases (Fig. 141–12).

The normal MR appearance of the uterine corpus on T_2-weighted images includes a central high-intensity zone representing the endometrium and a junctional low-intensity zone and a peripheral medium-intensity zone representing the myometrial thickness. Endometrial tumor is best seen on T_2-weighted images as an increased thickness or expansion and lobulation or irregularity of the central high-intensity zone. Superficial myometrial tumor invasion is characterized on T_2-weighted images as an irregular disrupted myometrial-endometrial interface or high–signal intensity tumor in the inner half of the myometrium. An intact junctional zone correlates with tumor confined to the endometrium or superficial invasion of less than 50 per cent of the myometrium. Deep myometrial invasion is indicated by high–signal intensity tumor in the outer half of the myometrium with an intact outer stripe of normal peripheral myometrium. Stage II tumors are characterized by widening and expansion of the cervical canal associated with a heterogeneous cervical stroma signal intensity. Stage III tumors are depicted as trans-serosal tumor extension beyond the outer uterine borders.

CERVICAL CARCINOMA

Carcinoma of the cervix is the sixth most common cancer in females after breast, colorectum, lung, endometrium, and ovary. Although the peak incidence of invasive cancer is at ages 45 to 55, it is not uncommon to see advanced tumors in the 25 to 45 year old age group. Most women are asymptomatic, with leukorrhea or vaginal bleeding and spotting occurring in less than one third. Ninety-five per cent of these cancers are squamous cell carcinomas, and 5 per cent are adenocarcinomas arising from glandular elements in the endocervix. Clinical staging consists of pelvic examination, chest radiography, cystoscopy, excretory urography, sigmoidoscopy, and barium enema. CT and MR have largely replaced the excretory urogram and barium enema for tumor staging because the latter two methods have proven insensitive in evaluating advanced cervical cancer (Stages IIb–IVb). MR is the imaging technique for differentiating Stage Ib from Stage IIb cervical cancer (Fig. 141–16). CT is indicated in evaluating poorly differentiated lesions or large bulky tumors, especially if detection of pelvic and para-aortic lymph node metastases is critical (Fig. 141–17).

Imaging of cervical cancer is considered after the diagnosis is established by cervical biopsy or endocervical curettage. CT is not routinely indicated in clinical Stage Ib–IIa tumors because clinical staging by pelvic examination has a higher accuracy than CT staging. CT has a significant error rate in Stage Ib tumors due to a false-positive diagnosis of parametrial tumor extension. Sonography has not gained widespread acceptance as a staging technique because of its limited ability to detect either local tumor extension into peripelvic fat or lymph node metastases.

CT-MR staging criteria in cervical carcinoma are based on the FIGO staging classification: Stage Ib, tumor confined to cervix; Stage IIb, parametrial tumor extension but not to pelvic sidewall; Stage IIIb, pelvic sidewall extension, pelvic lymph node enlargement greater than 1.5 to 2.0 cm, or hydronephrosis; Stage IVa, bladder or rectal involvement; Stage IVb, para-aortic or inguinal lymph node enlargement or intraperitoneal metastases (Figs. 141–13, 141–17, and 141–18).

The primary goal of CT evaluation is to differentiate a tumor confined to the cervix from a tumor that has infiltrated the adjacent parametrial tissues. CT criteria for a tumor confined to the cervix are (1) smooth, well-defined peripheral cervix margins; (2) absence of prominent parametrial soft-tissue strands or mass; and (3) preservation of the fat plane around the pelvic ureter. The characteristic CT findings of cervical cancer are a solid inhomogeneous mass enlarging the cervix to more than 3 cm in diameter with hypodense areas in the tumor because of necrosis, ulceration, and diminished intravenous contrast enhancement compared with normal cervical stroma (Figs. 141–13*A*, 141–17, and 141–18). Intravenous contrast enhancement is very important to differentiate normal contrast-enhanced peripheral cervical margins from irregular, hypodense borders owing to tumor invasion of paracervical and parauterine fat (Fig. 141–18). Endometrial fluid collections and uterine enlargement may be associated with tumor obstruction of the endocervical canal (Fig. 141–13*B*).

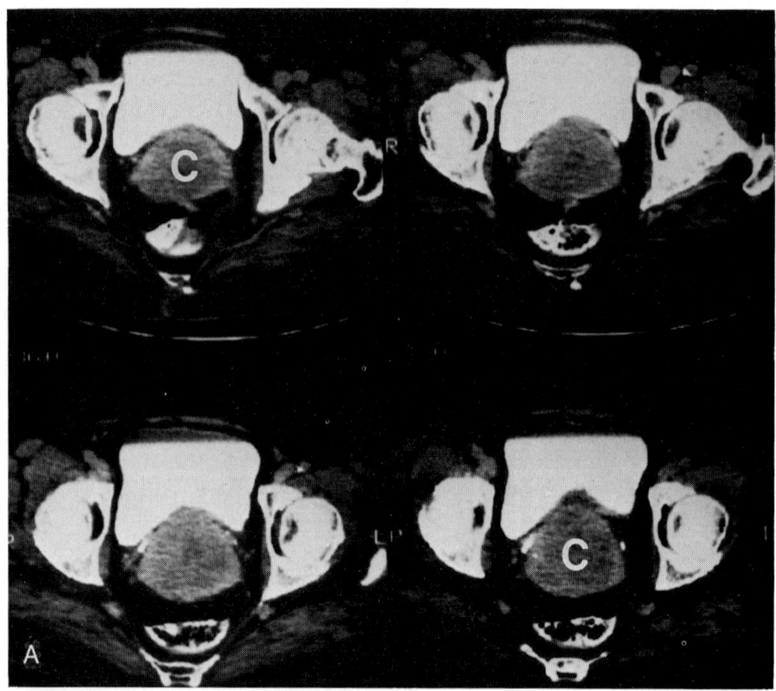

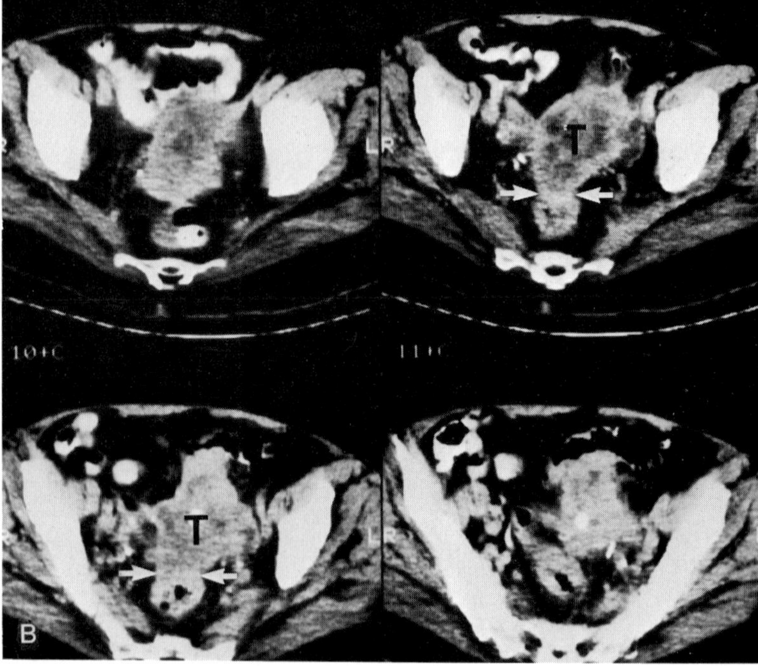

Figure 141–15. Stage IVa endometrial cancer. *A,* Five-mm contiguous CT sections through an enlarged heterogeneous cervix (C) indicating tumor involvement. *B,* Five-mm contiguous CT sections through the heterogeneous hypodense uterine corpus tumor (T) show associated tumor invasion of the sigmoid colon *(arrows),* confirmed by surgery.

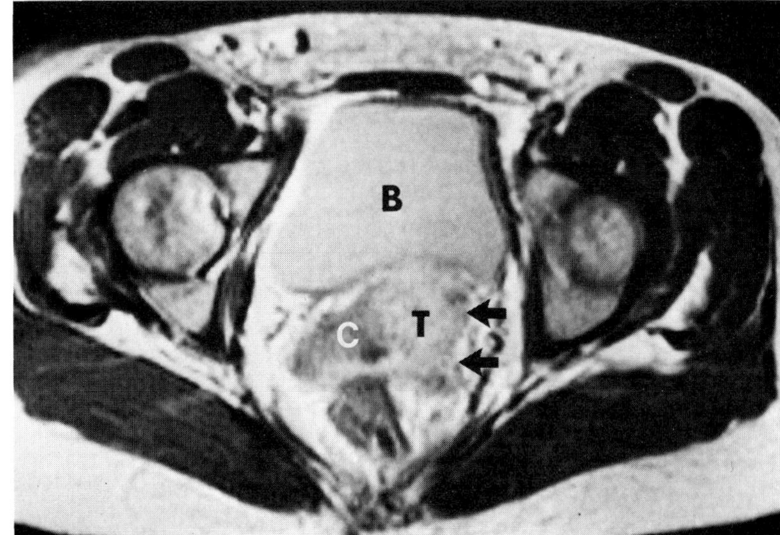

Figure 141–16. Stage IIb cervical cancer. Axial proton density spin-echo (2500/45) MR through the bladder (B) and normal hypointense cervical stroma (c) shows hyperintense tumor (T) replacing the left side of the cervix and extending into the left parametrium *(arrows)*.

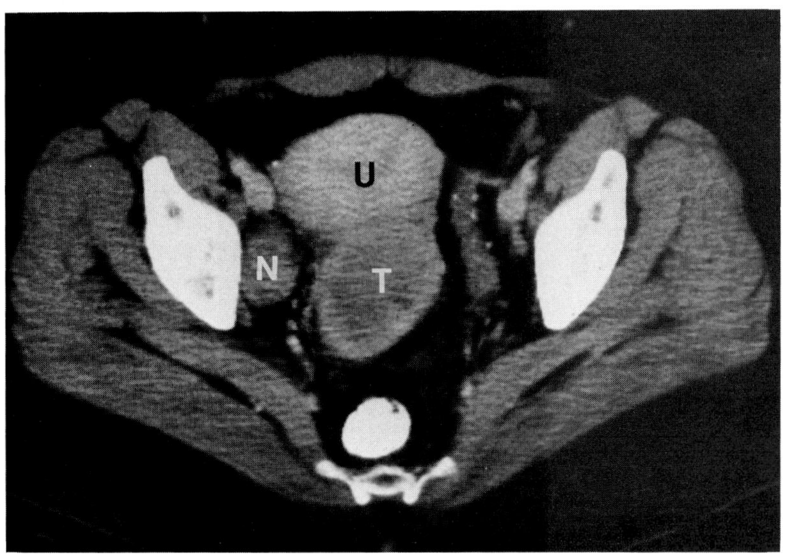

Figure 141–17. Stage IIIb cervical cancer. CT scan through the normal uterine corpus (U) shows a hypodense tumor (T) expanding the endocervix and an associated right obturator lymph node metastasis (N).

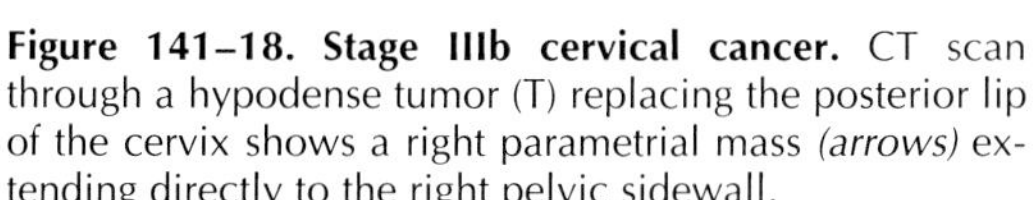

Figure 141–18. Stage IIIb cervical cancer. CT scan through a hypodense tumor (T) replacing the posterior lip of the cervix shows a right parametrial mass *(arrows)* extending directly to the right pelvic sidewall.

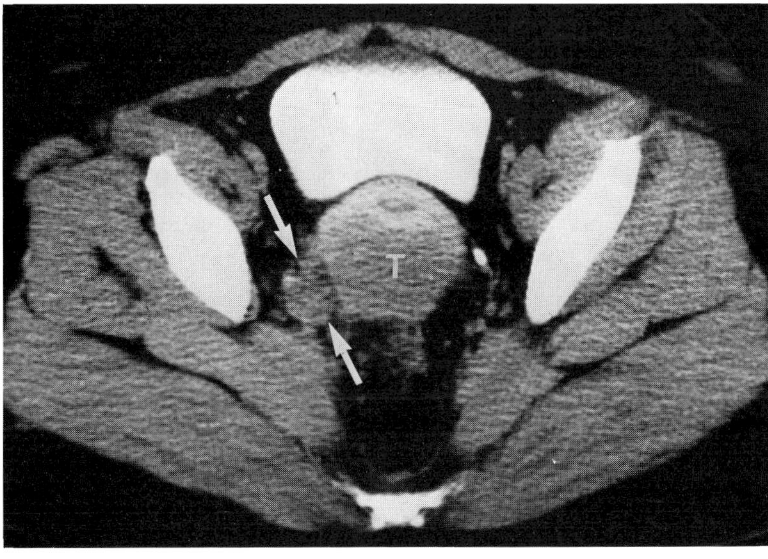

CT criteria for parametrial tumor extension are (1) irregularity and poor definition of the peripheral cervix margins; (2) prominent parametrial soft-tissue strands; (3) an eccentric soft-tissue mass; and (4) obliteration of the periureteral fat plane (Fig. 141–18). The latter two criteria are essential for a definitive CT diagnosis of a stage IIB tumor. Pelvic sidewall tumor extension (Stage IIIb) is characterized by irregular, linear, confluent parametrial soft-tissue mass extending to the obturator internus muscle laterally and/or piriformis muscle posterolaterally (Fig. 141–18). CT detection of hydronephrosis or pelvic adenopathy with or without obvious pelvic sidewall extension also indicates a Stage IIIb tumor (Fig. 141–17). CT criteria for bladder/rectal involvement (Stage IVa) are focal loss of the perivesical/perirectal fat plane accompanied by asymmetrical wall thickening; serrations or nodular indentations along the bladder/rectal wall; an intraluminal tumor mass; or a vesicovaginal fistula (Fig. 141–13*A*).

MR is the preferred imaging technique for evaluating Stage I cancers of the cervix because of the high predictive value of MR determination of tumor confined to the cervix. On T_2-weighted images, the characteristic feature of cervical cancer is a mass with a signal intensity greater than the normal hypointense cervical stroma. An intact area of low–signal intensity stroma around the periphery of the tumor is a reliable indicator that the tumor is restricted to the cervix (Stage Ib). MR criteria for parametrial tumor extension (Stage IIb) include loss of parametrial fat planes on T_1-weighted images and abnormal high–signal intensity tumor extending through a disrupted low–signal intensity ring of the cervix into the parametria or cardinal-uterosacral ligaments on axial T_2-weighted images (Fig. 147–16). MR criteria for pelvic sidewall tumor extension (Stage IIIb) are tumor extending beyond the lateral margins of the cardinal ligaments and loss of the normal low signal intensity of the piriformis or obturator internus muscles on T_2-weighted images. The Stage IVa criterion is segmental loss of the normally low–signal intensity wall of the bladder or rectum on T_2-weighted images. Sagittal MR images are useful in detecting bladder or rectal invasion and vaginal tumor extension.

Bibliography

Casillas J, Joseph RC, Guerra JJ Jr: CT appearance of uterine leiomyomas. RadioGraphics 10:999–1007, 1990.

Dudiak CM, Turner DA, Patel SK, et al: Uterine leiomyomas in the infertile patient: Preoperative localization with MR imaging versus US and hysterosalpingography. Radiology 167:627–630, 1988.

Fleischer AC, Dudley BS, Entman SS, et al: Myometrial invasion by endometrial carcinoma: Sonographic assessment. Radiology 162:307–310, 1987.

Gross BH, Silver TM, Jaffe MH: Sonographic features of uterine leiomyomas: Analysis of 41 proven cases. J Ultrasound Med 2:401–406, 1983.

Hricak H, Rubinstein LV, Gherman GM, Karstaedt N: MR imaging evaluation of endometrial carcinoma: Results of an NCI cooperative study. Radiology 179:829–832, 1991.

Kim SH, Choi BI, Lee HP, et al: Uterine cervical carcinoma: Comparison of CT and MR findings. Radiology 175:45–51, 1990.

Mintz MC, Grumbach K: Imaging of congenital uterine anomalies. Semin Ultrasound CT MR 9:167–174, 1988.

Posniak HV, Olson MC, Dudiak CM, et al: MR imaging of uterine carcinoma: Correlation with clinical and pathologic findings. RadioGraphics 10:15–27, 1990.

Sawyer RW, Walsh JW: CT in gynecologic pelvic diseases. Semin Ultrasound CT MR 9:122–142, 1988.

Togashi K, Ozasa H, Konishi I, et al: Enlarged uterus: Differentiation between adenomyosis and leiomyoma with MR imaging. Radiology 171:531–534, 1989.

Walsh JW: Computed tomography of gynecologic neoplasms. Radiol Clin North Am 30(4):817–830, 1992.

Walsh JW, Jones CM III: Diagnostic imaging techniques in gynecologic oncology. In Hoskins WJ, Perez CA, Young RC (eds): Gynecologic Oncology Principles and Practice. Philadelphia, JB Lippincott, 1992, pp 443–463.

Weinreb JC, Barkoff ND, Megibow A, Demopoulos R: The value of MR imaging in distinguishing leiomyomas from other solid pelvic masses when sonography is indeterminate. AJR 154:295–299, 1990.

Zawin M, McCarthy S, Scoutt L, et al: Monitoring therapy with a gonadotropin-releasing hormone analog: Utility of MR imaging. Radiology 175:503–506, 1990.

142 Imaging of Gestational Trophoblastic Disease

Jeffrey D. Wicks

Imaging examinations play a critical role in the diagnosis, classification, and management of patients with gestational trophoblastic disease (GTD). Diagnostic ultrasound has improved the ability to make an early diagnosis of GTD and in combination with other imaging modalities can accurately determine the presence and extent of metastatic disease.

GTD affects one out of every 1500 to 2000 pregnancies in the United States. The term *gestational trophoblastic disease* denotes the spectrum of disease including classic or complete hydatidiform mole; partial or incomplete hydatidiform mole; mole with co-existent live fetus; invasive or persistent mole; and metastatic GTD, including choriocarcinoma. The biologic behavior and hence the treatment vary with the above categories. Diagnostic imaging is helpful in differentiating between some of these categories and is critical for the staging of metastatic disease. Although diagnostic imaging techniques are crucial in making the diagnosis of GTD, the imaging appearance is at times nonspecific, necessitating histologic and cytogenetic analysis.

The clinical hallmark of GTD is vaginal bleeding in the first trimester or early second trimester. The uterus may be appropriate, large, or small for dates, depending on the category of trophoblastic disease. Levels of the serum beta subunit of human chorionic gonadotropin (β-hCG) are generally elevated. The patient may also have symptoms of hyperemesis gravidarum or pre-eclamptic toxemia. Although thyrotoxicosis has been frequently reported as presenting with a molar pregnancy, clinical manifestations of thyrotoxicosis appear to be infrequent. Prior to the use of diagnostic ultrasound, the diagnosis was often not made until the patient passed vesicular tissue per vagina. Diagnostic ultrasound now permits an earlier diagnosis and in many cases is helpful in distinguishing between some of the above categories of GTD.

In this chapter, I describe the varied sonographic appearances of

GTD at the time of diagnosis and the use of other imaging modalities where appropriate.

COMPLETE OR CLASSIC HYDATIDIFORM MOLE

Complete or classic hydatidiform mole is a distinct subset of GTD. Patients usually present with vaginal bleeding in the late first trimester or early second trimester, and the uterus is large for dates. Hyperemesis gravidarum or symptoms and signs of pre-eclamptic toxemia are other less common presentations. The serum β-hCG is elevated. Because of a wide range of normal values and the association of elevated β-hCG levels with multiple gestations, an elevated β-hCG level itself is not pathognomonic for hydatidiform mole.

Pathologically, the endometrial cavity is filled with vesicular tissue. Histologic analysis shows no fetal tissue or amniotic membranes. There is edematous enlargement of the villi (villous hydrops) and absence of fetal villous blood vessels. There is diffuse trophoblastic proliferation with varying degrees of atypia. Complete or classic hydatidiform mole most commonly has a 46XX genotype.

The typical sonographic appearance of a classic mole is that of an enlarged-for-dates uterus in which the endometrial cavity is filled with relatively echogenic, complex material. Its appearance varies depending on the time of presentation. In the first trimester the clusters of vesicles are small (2 mm or less) and are generally not resolvable. This results in the appearance of a diffusely echogenic, solid-appearing mass occupying the endometrial cavity (Fig. 142–1). With time the vesicles increase in size, reaching 20 mm in the second trimester. This results in a more complex sonographic appearance with hyperechoic solid tissue separated by clusters of anechoic cystic vesicles (Fig. 142–2). Larger fluid-filled, anechoic areas may also be seen, which represent hemorrhagic degeneration of the molar tissue (Fig. 142–3).

Theca lutein cysts have been reported in 20 to 50 per cent of classic hydatidiform moles. They are usually bilateral and multiseptated in appearance (Fig. 142–4). If there is marked uterine enlargement at the time of presentation, the ovaries may be located high in the pelvis or in the lower abdomen and obscured by overlying intestinal gas. In these cases, the theca lutein cysts may not be seen until the first postevacuation follow-up ultrasound examination. Identification of theca lutein cysts at the time of diagnosis will help differentiate GTD from other diseases that may mimic hydatidiform mole, such as degenerating leiomyomata and malignant ovarian tumors or from missed or incomplete abortions. The theca lutein

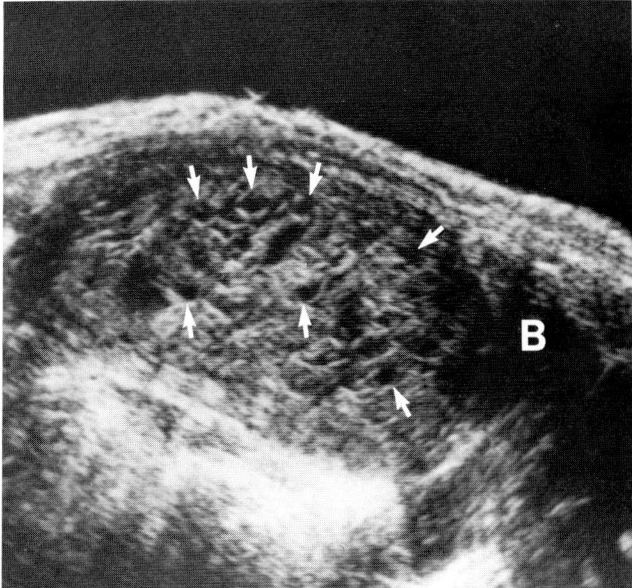

Figure 142–2. Classic hydatidiform mole. Sagittal sonogram of a patient with 15 weeks of amenorrhea, vaginal bleeding, and no audible fetal heart tones. Note the enlarged uterus completely filled with molar tissue. In contrast to Figure 142–1, multiple anechoic, fluid-filled vesicles (*arrows*) are also identified. (B = bladder.)

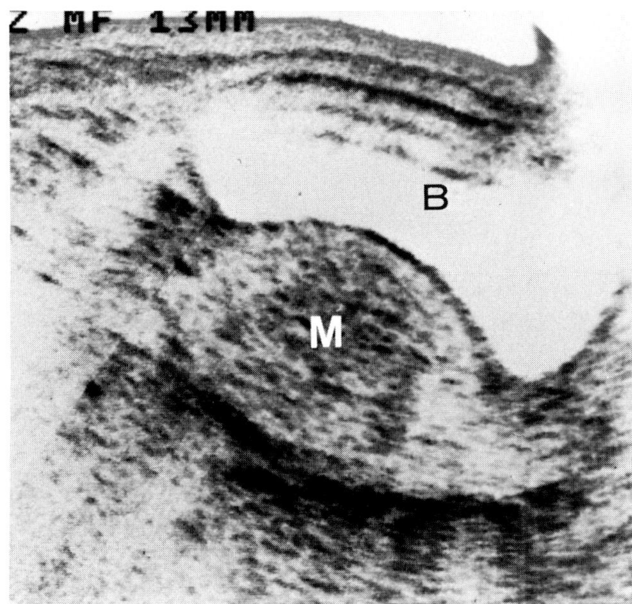

Figure 142–1. Classic hydatidiform mole. Sagittal sonogram of the pelvis in a patient with eight weeks of amenorrhea and vaginal bleeding. The uterus is enlarged, and the endometrial cavity is filled with a diffusely hyperechoic, solid molar tissue (M). (B = bladder.)

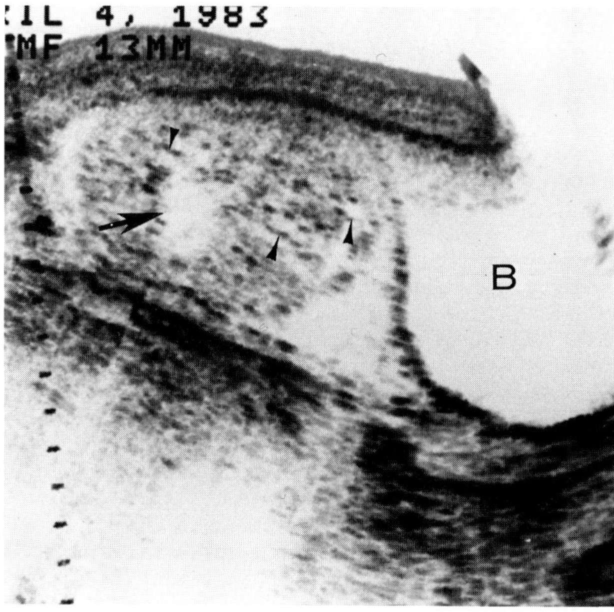

Figure 142–3. Classic hydatidiform mole. Sagittal sonogram of the pelvis of a patient with 10 weeks of amenorrhea and vaginal bleeding. Small vesicles (*arrowheads*) are seen as well as a larger anechoic area secondary to hemorrhage (*arrow*). (B = bladder.)

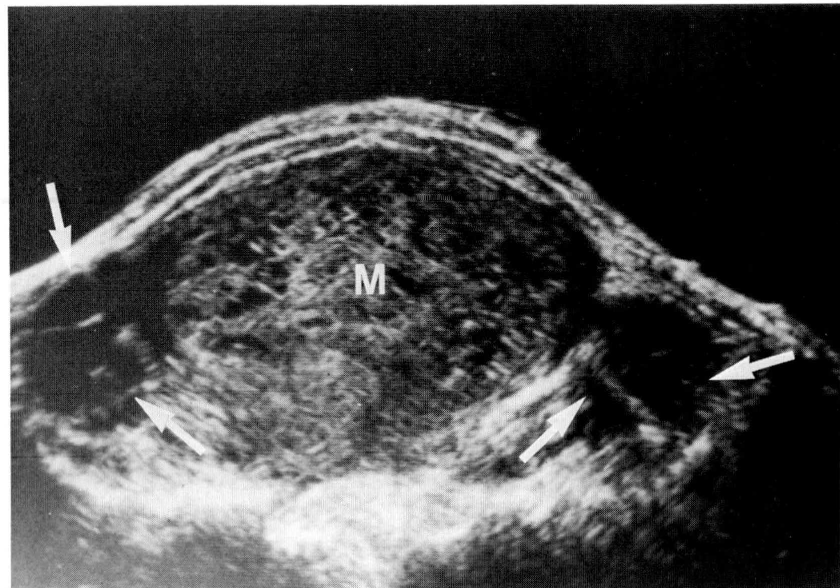

Figure 142–4. Theca lutein cysts. Transverse sonogram shows the enlarged uterus filled with complex, solid molar tissue (M). Bilateral septated theca lutein cysts (*arrows*) are also seen in this second trimester patient.

cysts gradually diminish in size after uterine evacuation but usually lag behind the decline in the serum β-hCG levels.

PARTIAL HYDATIDIFORM MOLE

Partial hydatidiform mole appears to be a separate clinical entity that is characterized pathologically by the presence of fetal tissue and amniotic membranes. There is partial villous hydrops, and fetal villous blood vessels are present. Little or no trophoblastic proliferation is present histologically. There is a very high incidence of gross fetal anomalies and a high incidence of chromosomal abnormalities of the polyploidy type, especially triploidy and trisomy variations. Patients with partial moles tend to present later with a small-for-dates uterus, have relatively lower β-hCG levels that drop to normal quickly following evacuation, and have a lower incidence of persistent disease. The differentiation of partial mole from classic mole is important because partial moles appear to be less often malignant. This may lead some gynecologists to recommend no chemotherapy and not restrict subsequent pregnancy for one year as is the case with a classic mole.

Partial moles have a spectrum of sonographic appearances. The most common is that of a large intact gestational sac surrounded by a thick rim of placenta-like tissue (Fig. 142–5). This tissue may contain multiple well-defined vesicles. The sac itself is empty or contains a small, ill-defined fetal pole. As many as one third of partial moles have an appearance similar to that of a complete or classic mole with solid echogenic tissue separated by multiple fluid-filled vesicles. The least common presentation is that of an irregular heterogeneous group of echoes within the endometrial cavity with or without a deformed gestational sac. The uterus is usually appropriate or small for dates, which somewhat differentiates this condition from classic mole. There has generally been no correlation between the sonographic appearance and the β-hCG level.

As will be discussed, partial mole can be associated with a live fetus. In this situation the fetus is usually growth-retarded. The placenta is only partially involved and appears relatively large compared with the size of the amniotic cavity.

Partial mole is difficult to distinguish sonographically from a missed abortion. The hydropic degeneration that is associated with an early abortion can appear similar to the vesicle formation associated with the partial mole. Careful pathologic analysis of the evacuated tissue is critical to make the distinction.

PERSISTENT HYDATIDIFORM MOLE

The typical treatment for classic hydatidiform mole is complete evacuation of the uterus by suction curettage. Although diagnostic ultrasound can demonstrate a decrease in uterine size and a decrease in the size of the theca lutein cysts following evacuation, a more critical follow-up study is the serum β-hCG level. The β-hCG level should return to normal within 8 to 12 weeks.

Persistent or locally invasive mole typically occurs in a patient

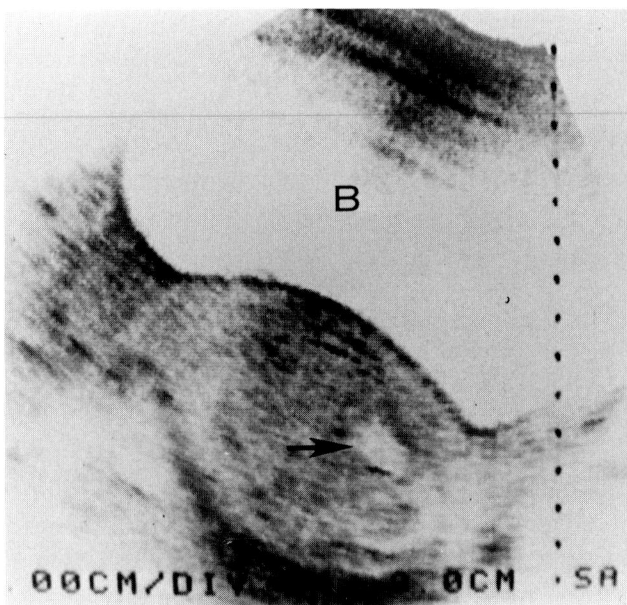

Figure 142–5. Partial hydatidiform mole. Sagittal sonogram of the uterus shows a gestational sac (*arrow*) surrounded by a large amount of solid, molar tissue. (B = bladder.)

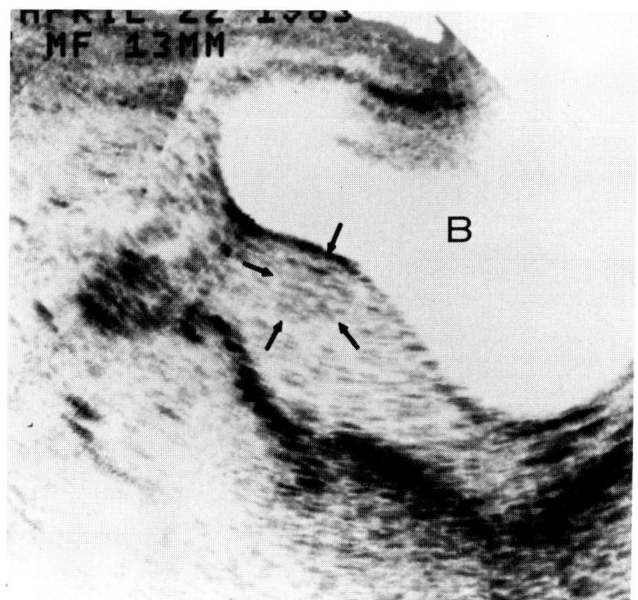

Figure 142–6. Persistent hydatidiform mole. Sagittal sonogram of the pelvis of a patient with persistently elevated β-hCG level six weeks following evacuation. The uterus has returned to normal size. Note the hyperechoic region in the fundus (*arrows*), which proved to be myometrial, invasive mole. (B = bladder.)

who presented with a classic mole and had a suction curettage followed by an initial drop in the serum β-hCG level. One to three months after evacuation, there is a plateauing or even a rise of the β-hCG level. The patient may also have symptoms of vaginal bleeding and persistent uterine enlargement and theca lutein cysts.

Sonographic evaluation in this circumstance may reveal uterine enlargement with hyperechoic areas within the myometrium representing residual or locally invasive molar tissue (Fig. 142–6). Vesicular changes are usually not identifiable, but cystic areas may occasionally be seen secondary to hemorrhage or necrosis (Fig. 142–7). A normal uterine ultrasound is not sufficient to exclude the presence of residual or locally invasive uterine GTD. As many as one third of patients with persistent elevation of the serum β-hCG levels and a normal uterine ultrasound will have microscopic foci of molar tissue at surgery. Transvaginal ultrasound, especially when combined with Doppler or color-flow imaging, will probably offer improved detection capabilities. The role of magnetic resonance imaging has yet to be established, but it may offer improved diagnostic sensitivity as well. The differential diagnosis of rising serum β-hCG level following evacuation includes a normal intrauterine pregnancy. This is readily diagnosed sonographically by five to six menstrual weeks' gestation.

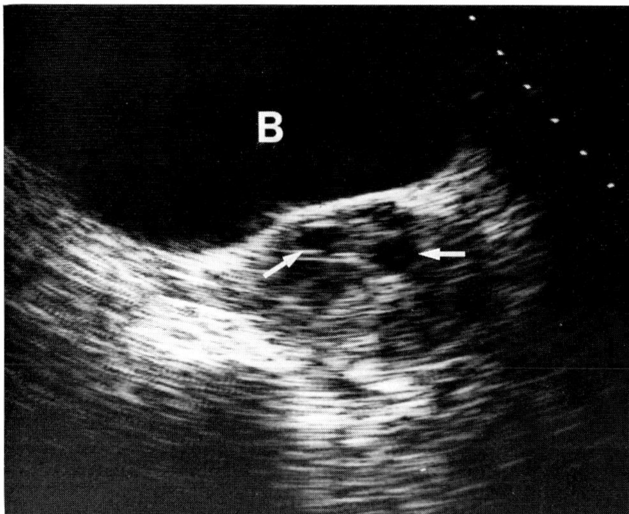

Figure 142–7. Persistent hydatidiform mole. Transverse sonogram of the uterus shows anechoic, cystic areas of hemorrhage or necrosis (*arrows*) in a patient with invasive mole. (B = bladder.)

In addition to repeat dilatation and curettage, these patients require single-agent chemotherapy, usually methotrexate. The response rate is excellent, with cure rates approaching 100 per cent.

COEXISTENT HYDATIDIFORM MOLE WITH LIVE FETUS

Coexistent hydatidiform mole and live fetus is a rare condition with an incidence of between 1 in 10,000 and 1 in 100,000 pregnancies in the United States. This represents less than 5 per cent of all molar pregnancies. The suspected etiology of a classic mole associated with a live pregnancy is that of a biovular twin gestation with one gestation developing normally and the other degenerating into a molar gestation. In this situation, the classic mole develops separate from the normal placenta associated with the fetus. The fetus is usually normal. Patients can present with vaginal bleeding, hyperemesis gravidarum, or pre-eclamptic toxemia. Although live births have been reported with an associated mole, most fetuses die. The potential malignant transformation of molar tissue and commonly associated maternal complications of molar pregnancy account for the usual recommendation for immediate pregnancy intervention.

Sonographically, a normal-appearing placenta and fetus within the amniotic cavity are identified. In addition, molar tissue is seen as a separate structure with varying degrees of vesicular change (Fig. 142–8). Theca lutein cysts may also be present.

A live fetus may also be associated with vesicular changes of a single placenta. The situation is more difficult to evaluate sonographically because it is not possible to distinguish hydropic degeneration from actual molar tissue. Sonographically, one sees partial involvement of the placenta with areas of increased echogenicity

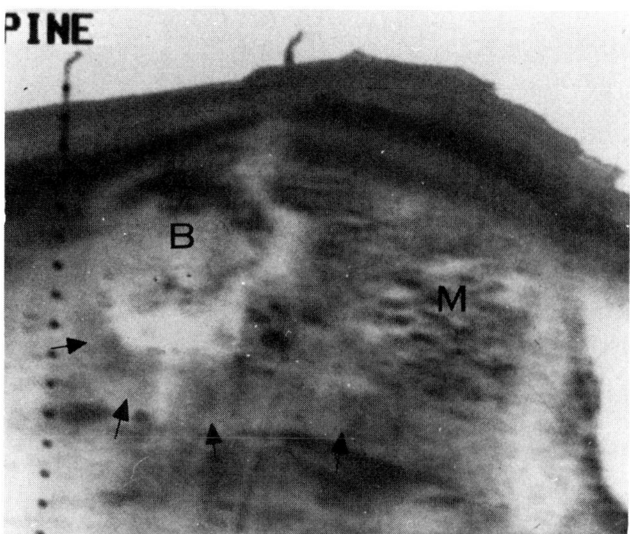

Figure 142–8. Mole with coexistent live fetus. Sagittal sonogram of the uterus shows solid molar tissue (M) in the lower uterus. The fetal body (B) and normal-appearing placenta (*arrows*) are in the fundus. At delivery, the fetus and normal placenta were separate from the hydatidiform mole. (Courtesy of R. Bree, M.D.)

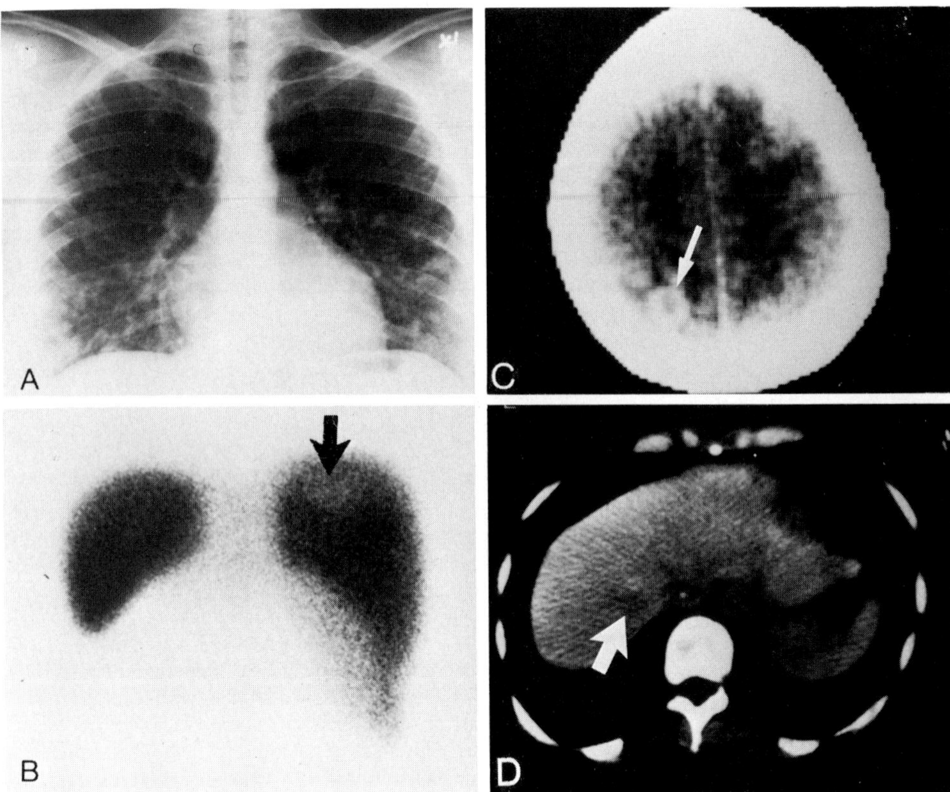

Figure 142–9. Metastatic gestational trophoblastic disease in a patient with choriocarcinoma. *A,* Chest radiograph shows multiple pulmonary nodules. *B,* Liver-spleen scan. *C,* CT scan of the brain shows an enhancing cortical metastatic lesion (*arrow*). *D,* Hepatic CT demonstrates a metastatic lesion (*arrows*).

and small anechoic vesicular spaces. In the case of hydropic degeneration, the cystic areas represent edematous villi as opposed to actual molar tissue. The greater the amount of replacement of normal placenta with vesicular change, the greater the placental insufficiency and risk to the fetus. The single placentas involved with molar tissue rather than hydropic degeneration are most likely of the partial mole variety. β-hCG levels may or may not be elevated. An uncomplicated partial molar pregnancy with a live fetus can be followed closely until fetal viability is assured or until serious maternal complications develop.

METASTATIC GESTATIONAL TROPHOBLASTIC DISEASE

Approximately 3.5 per cent of molar pregnancies are associated with metastases outside the uterus. Ninety-five per cent of these cases are choriocarcinoma on pathologic examination. The most common sites of metastases are the lungs, liver, brain, and extension within the pelvis outside the uterus to the pelvic peritoneum or the vagina. The serum β-hCG level alone at the time of initial diagnosis is not an adequate predictor of which patients will develop metastatic disease. There is no specific sonographic appearance of the tissue within the endometrial cavity to indicate a higher risk for the development of metastatic disease.

Patients with metastatic GTD are divided into low- and high-risk groups. Low-risk patients have metastatic disease limited to the lungs or pelvis and a pretreatment urinary hCG excretion of less than 100,000 mIU/day or serum β-hCG of less than 40,000 mIU/ml. The duration of their disease prior to chemotherapy is less than four months. High-risk patients have metastases to the brain and/or liver or a pretreatment urinary β-hCG titer of greater than 100,000 mIu/day or serum β-hCG or more than 40,000 mIU/ml. Other high-risk factors include a duration of malignancy of more than four months, unsuccessful previous chemotherapy, or antecedent term pregnancy. Low-risk patients can be treated with single-agent chemotherapy. High-risk patients require multiple-agent chemotherapy and may also require adjuvant radiation therapy to specific organs or regions of the body and/or surgery.

Patients with pulmonary metastases alone are considered at a low risk and respond well to single-agent chemotherapy. The embolism of trophoblastic cells is a common occurrence with normal deliveries, and finding trophoblastic cells in the pulmonary vessels of patients with GTD is also considered not uncommon.

All patients with GTD should have a chest x-ray and baseline serum β-hCG level. At the time of initial sonographic examination, evaluation of the liver can also be easily performed. The presence of liver metastases places the patient in a high-risk classification and dictates appropriate treatment. As previously mentioned, the serum β-hCG level should drop to normal by 8 to 12 weeks and is the most sensitive indicator of residual disease or possible metastases. Patients with persistently elevated or rising β-hCG levels following evacuation should have a repeat chest radiograph and pelvic ultrasonography. If the chest radiograph is positive for metastases, computed tomography of the brain, abdomen, and pelvis should also be considered (Fig. 142–9). Computed tomography of the chest may be necessary to clarify suspicious findings on chest radiograph. The serum β-hCG level in the postevacuation state is proportional to the bulk of the residual or metastatic tumor. Even when the β-hCG level has returned to normal, metastases seen on imaging studies may take months to resolve.

Bibliography

Bree RL, Silver TM, Wicks JD, Evans E: Trophoblastic disease with coexistent fetus: A sonographic spectrum. J Clin Ultrasound 6:310–314, 1978.

Munyear TP, Callen PW, Filly RA, et al: Further observations on the sonographic spectrum of gestational trophoblastic disease. J Clin Ultrasound 9:349–358, 1981.

Naumoff P, Szulman AE, Weinstein B, et al: Ultrasonography of partial hydatidiform mole. Radiology 140:467–470, 1981.

Williams AG, Mettler FA, Wicks JD: Utility of diagnostic imaging in the staging of gestational trophoblastic disease. Diag Gynecol Obstet 4:159–163, 1982.

143 Endometriosis and Pelvic Inflammatory Disease

Michael A. Sandler

Endometriosis and pelvic inflammatory disease (PID) are common diseases that occur primarily in women of child-bearing age. They are common causes of infertility and chronic pelvic pain. Sonographic and clinical features are quite variable in each entity, and both are common indications for pelvic sonography. Ultrasound is valuable not only for diagnosis but also to determine the extent of disease and to assess the efficacy of conservative treatment.

ENDOMETRIOSIS

Endometriosis is defined as the presence of actively functioning endometrial tissue outside of the uterus in an aberrant location. The tissue is hormonally dependent and undergoes cyclic changes; bleeding may occur at menstruation. This frequently results in excessive fibrosis that may cause distortion and rarely destruction of adjacent organs.

The ovary and cul-de-sac are the most common sites. Other locations in the pelvis include uterine ligaments, fallopian tubes, rectovaginal septum, bladder, and pelvic peritoneum. Virtually any site within the pelvis may be affected, particularly in widespread endometriosis. Rarely, distal sites such as laparotomy scars, umbilicus, lungs, pleura, extremities, and skin may be involved. A number of theories have been proposed to explain the histogenesis of endometriosis. These include the tubal regurgitation theory, which proposes that at the time of menstruation, endometrial tissue is passed out the tubes in a retrograde manner and is deposited in the pelvis. The coelomic metaplasia theory suggests that the mucosa of the genital tract undergoes metaplasia resulting in endometriosis. Hematogenous spread has been proposed to explain the occurrence in distal sites, such as the extremities or lungs. A combination of these theories is necessary to explain all cases, but the regurgitation theory probably accounts for most lesions of endometriosis.

The symptoms of endometriosis are quite variable, without direct relationship to the findings demonstrated on sonography or laparoscopy. A small amount of disease may produce dramatic symptoms in some patients, whereas others with substantial disease have little discomfort. Pelvic pain is the most common symptom. If there is considerable involvement of the pelvic organs, particularly the uterosacral ligaments, presacral plexus, and the cul-de-sac, dyspareunia and dysmenorrhea may occur. Infertility has been the classic symptom associated with this entity, and as many as 40 to 50 per cent of infertile women have endometriosis. It has been implicated as the only factor causing infertility in 6 to 15 per cent of women. Although endometriosis generally occurs in women between the ages of 20 and 40 years, there are scattered reports in postmenopausal women.

Endometriosis has two different presentations at laparotomy. It may be diffuse with numerous small, typically punctate mulberry nodules scattered throughout the pelvic peritoneum, frequently in the region of the uterosacral ligaments and retrovaginal septum. This appearance generally cannot be recognized on sonograms, although Birnholz has suggested that because of periodic bleeding, a local inflammatory reaction may occur with resultant increase in echogenicity of the peritoneum.

The other form of endometriosis, in which one or more relatively discrete masses are present, is what is commonly identified on sonography. The most common presentation is a spherical mass with shaggy irregular walls having the sonographic properties of a cyst including through transmission (Fig. 143–1). Scattered debris usually can be seen, and occasionally septations are present (Fig. 143–2). It may not be possible to separate a large multiseptated mass from numerous adjacent lesions. Rarely, clumps of echoes are present that probably represent clotted blood. If numerous areas of echogenicity are present, the lesion has the appearance of a mixed mass of solid and cystic elements instead of a cystic one. Through transmission may not be present. Layering of debris may occur with a fluid/fluid level that will maintain the same relationship if the patient is placed in a decubitus position. Birnholz has reported that the swirling of blood elements may be seen if the lesion is palpated while being imaged. Most endometriomas are 4 to 8 cm in diameter, but they may range from 1 or 2 cm to 14 cm or greater. Endovaginal scanning is of some value in the detection of small lesions. Also, this technique may better characterize lesions that are indeterminate on transabdominal scanning and separate them from other structures (Fig. 143–3).

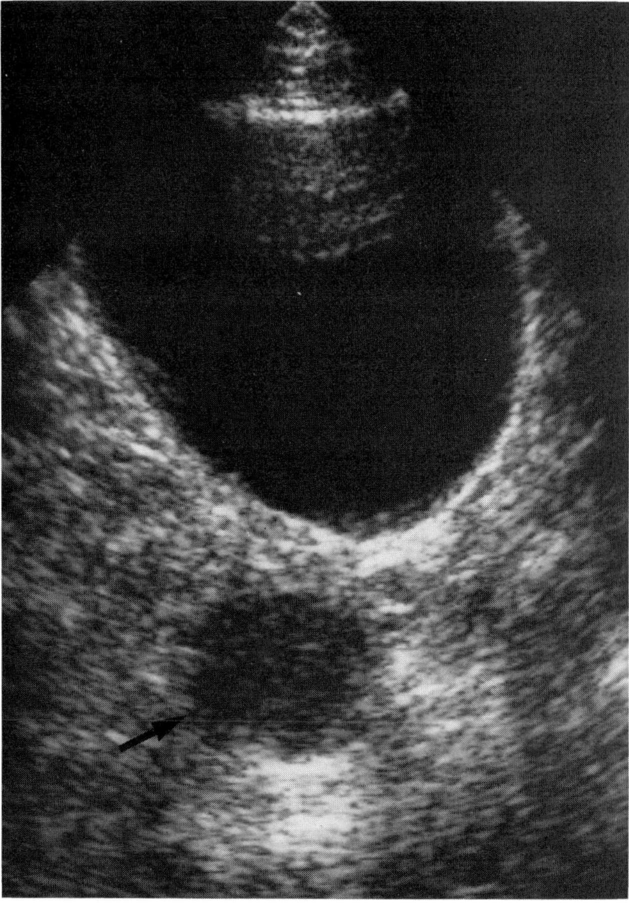

Figure 143–1. Sagittal scan demonstrating **cystic mass** *(arrow)* with irregular walls and debris.

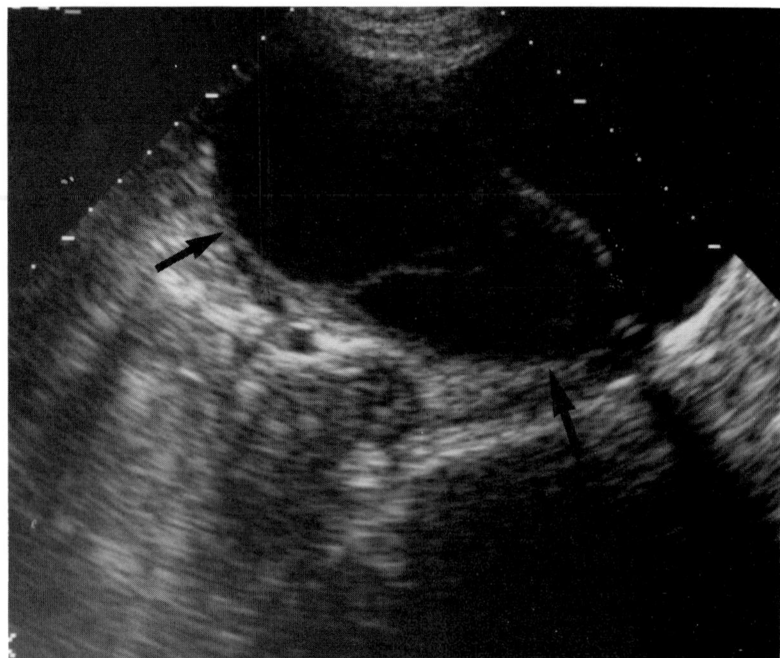

Figure 143–2. Sagittal scan demonstrating **cystic mass** *(arrows)* with septations and debris.

This most typical appearance of an endometrioma, that of a cystic mass containing echoes, is not specific. Any cystic mass containing blood particles, such as hemorrhage within an ovarian cyst or cystadenoma, can have a similar appearance. In addition, typical symptoms may not be present, since an ovarian endometrioma is frequently asymptomatic and may be discovered upon routine pelvic examination. Consequently, without appropriate symptomatology, a specific diagnosis is not possible. However, in patients presenting with infertility, this appearance would be suggestive of endometriosis even if pelvic examination is within normal limits, as has been reported.

Rarely, an endometrioma will have smooth walls and be totally anechoic. In these cases it would be indistinguishable from a simple ovarian cyst. However, unlike endometriomas, simple cysts will usually regress, even if hemorrhage occurs, within several menstrual cycles.

With widespread endometriosis, a great deal of fibrosis may be present in the pelvis, resulting in loss of fascial planes. The uterus may no longer be seen as a distinct entity and will merge with the multiple masses present in the adnexae and cul-de-sac (Fig. 143–4). On the basis of sonography alone it may not be possible to separate this appearance of endometriosis from diffuse PID or extensive ovarian carcinoma, except that fluid in the cul-de-sac is rarely present in endometriosis. These patients may present with a "frozen pelvis" on pelvic examination. However, the clinical setting is substantially different in these entities. With endometriosis there is

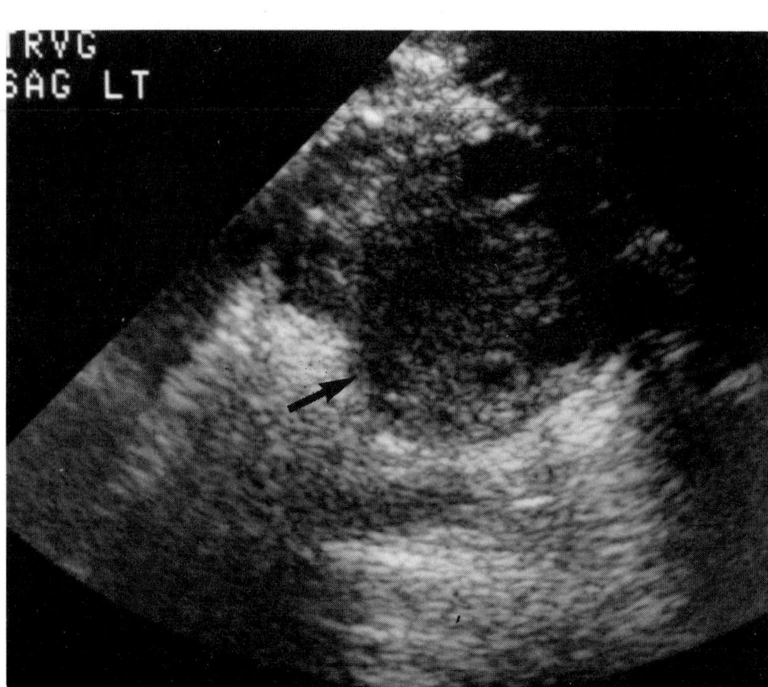

Figure 143–3. Endovaginal scan demonstrating **cystic mass** *(arrow)* containing debris. The findings were unclear on transabdominal scanning.

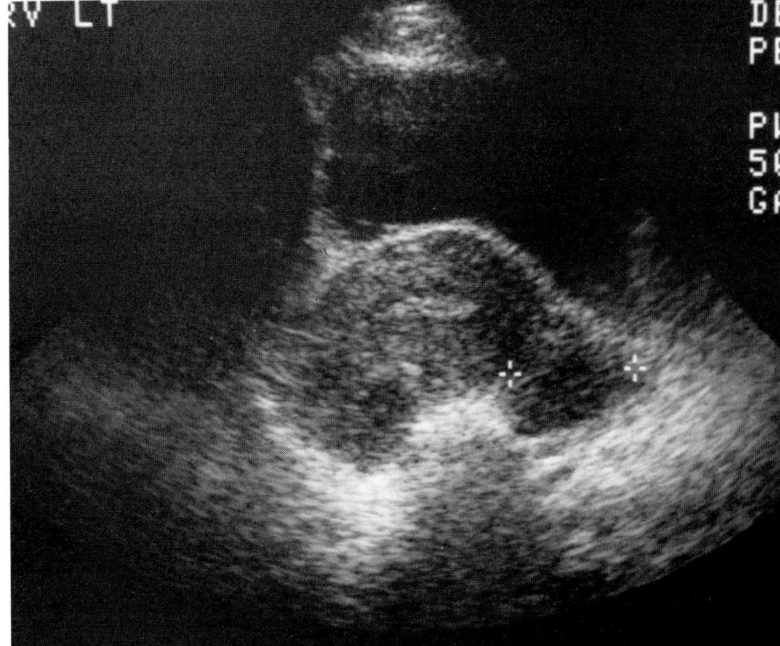

Figure 143–4. Transverse scan demonstrating indistinctness of uterus and adnexa due to extensive **endometriosis.** Electronic calibers indicate left adnexa.

little tenderness on physical examination and no laboratory data to suggest infection or symptoms to indicate widespread ovarian carcinoma.

All endometriomas have various amounts of hemorrhagic debris and fibrin deposition. If this debris is homogeneously distributed, the endometrioma will have a ''solid'' appearance. These ''solid'' endometriomas have a relatively typical appearance of a homogeneous mass with medium-level intensity echoes with or without through transmission, although at surgery they will be identical to lesions appearing cystic on sonography. Solid ovarian carcinomas usually are more inhomogeneous and are sound attenuating, but solid benign ovarian tumors such as thecomas, fibromas, or ovarian cysts with a great deal of hemorrhage may have an identical appearance. There is a small incidence of carcinoma in endometrial deposits, which is termed *endometroid carcinoma.* These lesions are similar in appearance on sonography to ovarian cystadenocarcinomas.

Adenomyosis (internal endometriosis) occurs when the endometrial tissue grows into the myometrium. Endometrial glands and stroma will be present between the muscle bundles. This has been described on sonography as small irregular hypoechoic areas. However, a number of authors have been unable to identify adenomyosis in patients with endometriosis. Therefore, uterine findings are generally not of value in suggesting a diagnosis of endometriosis as opposed to other cystic adnexal masses.

Although in many cases, the sonographic appearance of endometriosis will not be specific, this diagnosis can certainly be suggested in the appropriate clinical circumstance, particularly in the infertile patient. Sonography can also be of value in following patients with known endometriosis who are being treated conservatively with medication.

PELVIC INFLAMMATORY DISEASE

PID is an infection that occurs typically among menstruating, sexually active, nonpregnant women. This entity has assumed even greater importance, since it is increasing in incidence and is recognized as a leading cause of infertility. It is also responsible for a significant rise in the number of ectopic pregnancies.

PID is defined as the clinical entity that occurs as a result of the ascending spread of bacteria from the vagina and cervix to the endometrium, fallopian tubes, and other adjacent pelvic organs. Although there are other causes of pelvic infection, such as uterine manipulation, surgery, and pregnancy, PID generally refers to the sequelae of sexually transmitted disease. PID is caused by sexually transmitted organisms, specifically *Neisseria gonorrhoeae* and *Chlamydia trachomatis,* as well as a polymicrobial spectrum including nongonococcal aerobic and anaerobic organisms. There is a significant difference among these organisms. *N. gonorrhoeae* and *C. trachomatis* are primary pathogens that cause an infection in the normal female genital tract, whereas the others are opportunistic organisms that are not normally pathogens. However, they are able to further injure the genital tract that has already been damaged by a primary pathogen or are passed along by an intrauterine device or nonspecific vaginitis.

The infection begins in the vagina and ascends into the cervix and endometrium. Because of its inherent resistance, the vagina is protected, but a cervicitis or endometritis will result. This will be of a limited duration, since drainage, especially during the menstrual period, will occur. The inflammatory process will then spread to the fallopian tubes, producing an acute suppurative salpingitis that is usually bilateral. If there is spillage out the fimbriated edge of the tube, pelvic peritonitis and abscess formation frequently in the cul-de-sac may occur.

With the initial attack there will be scarring and residual inflammation, but the infection may be eliminated with appropriate antibiotic therapy. However, subsequent superimposed infection, usually with aerobic and anaerobic organisms, in the damaged genital tract may result in well-formed tubo-ovarian abscesses and the formation of hydrosalpinx or pyosalpinx as well as dense adhesions. It has been shown that the possibilities of infertility and ectopic pregnancy increase with each episode of PID.

The most common presenting symptom is pelvic pain, usually exacerbated by movement or sexual intercourse. Vaginal discharge is present in about half the cases, with abnormal vaginal bleeding, dysuria, and gastrointestinal complaints also occurring in a minority

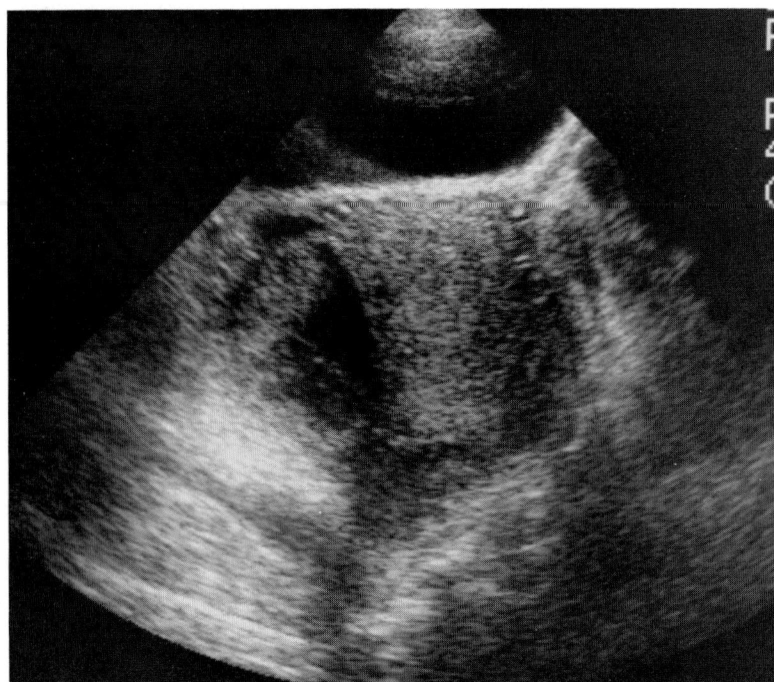

Figure 143–5. Transverse scan demonstrating **right tubo-ovarian abscess and fluid in cul-de-sac and left adnexa with indistinctness of uterus and fullness in left adnexa.**

of patients. Cervical motion tenderness on pelvic examination is present in almost all cases. Unlike other infectious conditions, leukocytosis may be absent in as many as half of the cases of PID, with fever being present in only approximately one third of patients. The lack of fever, leukocytosis, and vaginal discharge in many patients may cause difficulty in distinguishing PID from other causes of acute pelvic pain.

Sonographic findings in PID are quite variable, since there is a wide spectrum of disease. In addition, even with similar pathology, the sonographic features will frequently vary from patient to patient. The initial episode of PID may be associated with minimal if any sonographic findings. Many of these patients are treated with antibiotics and are not referred for sonographic evaluation. A common finding is indistinctness of the uterine outline, which has been referred to as the ''indefinite uterus.'' However, this may be present in other entities, including endometriosis, ovarian carcinoma, and uterine leiomyomas. The endometrial echo may not be present and the uterus may be more hypoechoic than normal and contain a small amount of fluid due to endometritis. If the disease is adequately treated with antibiotics, subsequent sonograms will show a normal uterus. Some cases of acute salpingitis and a number of cases of chronic interstitial salpingitis also may have no sonographic findings, and the ''indefinite uterus'' may be seen in chronic as well as acute disease.

Recurrent infection, particularly with secondary organisms, leads to more significant pathology with widespread sonographic findings. The organisms ascend into the uterus and enter the fallopian tubes, resulting in an acute suppurative salpingitis and pyosalpinx if the tube becomes obstructed. The tubes distend and appear as hypoechoic masses. Inflammation around the fallopian tube and spillage into the peritoneal cavity result in the involvement of the ovary with tubo-ovarian abscess. These have a variable sonographic appearance. At first, the abscess can appear predominantly solid, like inflammatory masses elsewhere in the body, but will become more cystic as necrosis and liquefaction occur (Fig. 143–5). The walls are usually thick, irregular, and shaggy.

In some cases, a significant amount of inflammation may be present without distinct abnormalities. Endovaginal scanning is useful for further evaluation and may detect tubo-ovarian abscesses (Fig. 143–6). For this reason, patients with suspected PID should routinely have endovaginal scanning. In addition, there have been reports of ultrasound-guided transvaginal drainage of tubo-ovarian abscesses.

If the fimbriated end of the tube is obstructed, and after appropriate antibiotic therapy for pyosalpinx, a hydrosalpinx will form with serous fluid instead of purulent material. The tube will distend and the hydrosalpinx will usually appear oval in both transverse and sagittal planes. Occasionally it may be tubular in the sagittal plane, allowing for a specific diagnosis. The walls may be smooth or shaggy (Fig. 143–7). Sonography cannot reliably differentiate pyosalpinx, hydrosalpinx, or tubo-ovarian abscess in some cases unless a distinct fallopian tube or ovary can be identified by endovaginal scanning.

Although PID is a bilateral process, one adnexa may have the predominant findings. The other side may look grossly normal or simply more full and/or hypoechoic than normal particularly on transabdominal scanning. Frequently, the adnexal structures will be poorly defined, but no definite abnormal mass can be identified. In some cases, endovaginal scanning will identify subtle abnormalities that are not apparent on transabdominal scanning. These include an enlarged ovary with indistinct borders and periovarian thickening or fluid collections on that side.

Diffuse PID is also associated with inflammatory fluid in the cul-de-sac resulting from spillage from the fallopian tubes. If the fluid becomes loculated, a peritoneal abscess may form. If it is large and rises out of the pelvis, the peritoneal abscess may be confused with a tubo-ovarian abscess. These abscesses may be poorly defined and simply present as a heterogeneous mass posterior to the uterus, displacing it anteriorly (Fig. 143–8). In some patients, this same appearance will be present in the adnexa, so the entire pelvis will have a disorganized appearance of solid and cystic areas, with none of the normal structures being well-defined or even visualized.

After appropriate antibiotic treatment, the residual of PID may be visualized on sonography. In addition to hydrosalpinx, well-defined fluid collections may form from burned-out tubo-ovarian abscesses. These lesions frequently contain septations and debris and may

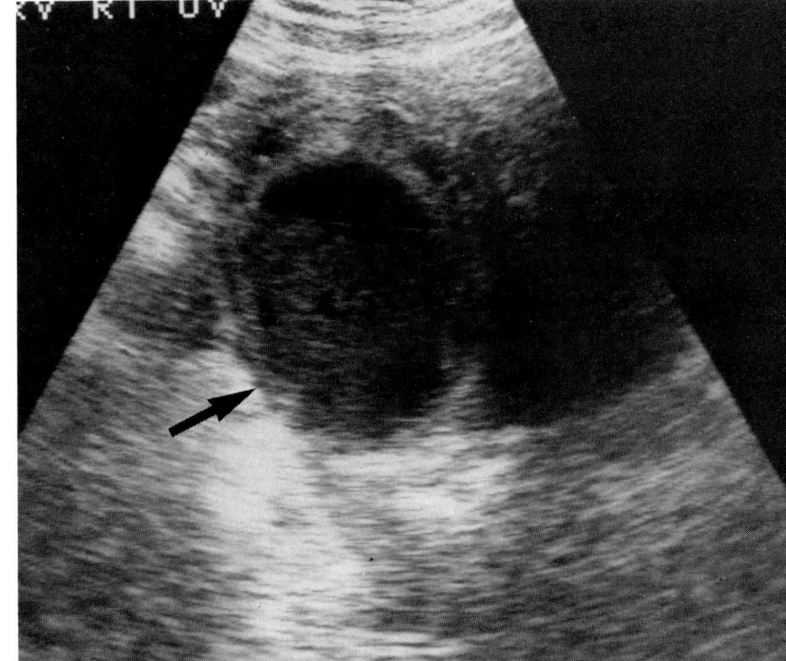

Figure 143–6. Endovaginal scan demonstrating **tubo-ovarian abscess** *(arrow)* with fluid-debris level.

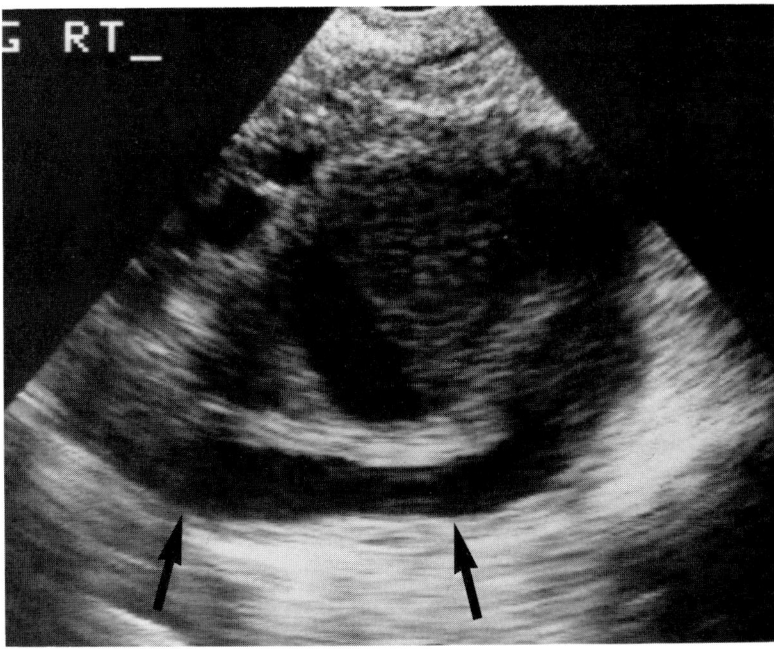

Figure 143–7. Endovaginal scan demonstrating **dilated fallopian tube** *(arrows)*.

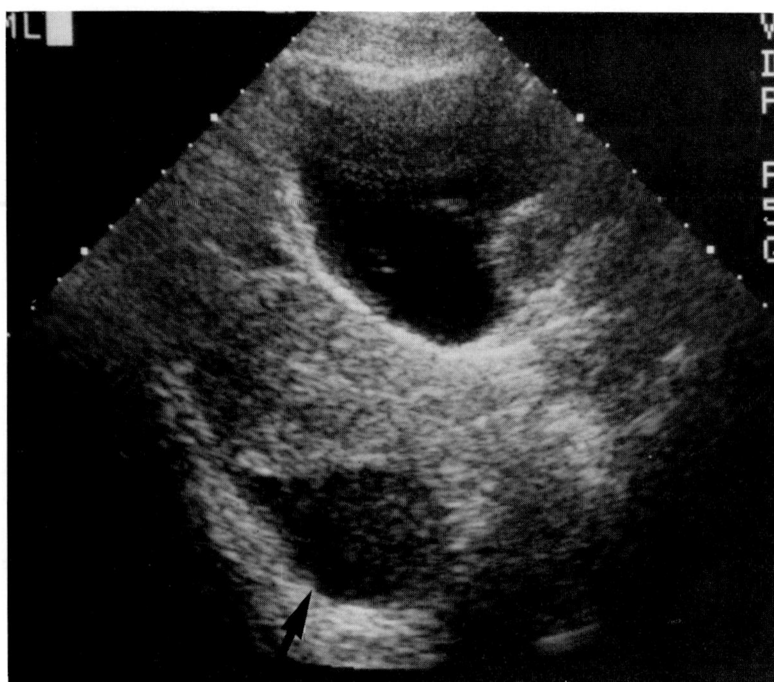

Figure 143–8. Sagittal scan demonstrating **abscess in cul-de-sac** *(arrow).*

appear similar to cystadenomas or occasionally cystadenocarcinomas. Adhesions form within the pelvis, and matted bowel loops may also be present.

The sonographic differential diagnosis for PID includes endometriosis, ruptured ectopic pregnancy, ruptured hemorrhagic ovarian cyst, ovarian torsion, and appendiceal abscess. Although diffuse endometriosis may appear similar to PID, the history and physical examination usually are sufficient to separate these entities. If bleeding from a ruptured ectopic pregnancy fills the cul-de-sac and fluid extends to the other adnexa or a corpus luteum cyst is present, it may appear similar to some cases of PID. Although this appearance is not common for ruptured ectopic pregnancy, culdocentesis may be necessary in some cases to separate these entities. An appendiceal abscess or ruptured hemorrhagic ovarian cyst may cause diffuse changes in the pelvis, similar to PID. The main values of ultrasound in patients with PID are to exclude other diagnoses when the patient presents with pelvic pain without other symptoms and to diagnose abscesses and chronic sequelae.

Bibliography

Endometriosis

Athey PA, Diment DD: The spectrum of sonographic findings in endometriosis. J Ultrasound Med 8:487–491, 1987.

Birnholz JC: Endometriosis and inflammatory disease. Semin Ultrasound 4:184–192, 1983.

Coleman BG, Arger PH, Mulhern CB Jr: Endometriosis and ultrasonic correlation. AJR 132:747–749, 1979.

Goldman SM, Minkin SI: Diagnosing endometriosis with ultrasound, accuracy and specificity. J Reprod Med 25:178–182, 1980.

Sandler MA, Karo JJ: The spectrum of ultrasonic findings in endometriosis. Radiology 127:229–231, 1978.

Walsh JW, Taylor KJW, Rosenfield AT: Gray scale ultrasonography in the diagnosis of endometriosis and adenomyosis. AJR 132:87–90, 1979.

Pelvic Inflammatory Disease

Berland LL, Lawson TL, Foley WD, Albarelli JN: Ultrasound evaluation of pelvic infections. Radiol Clin North Am 20:367–382, 1982.

Birnholz JC: Endometriosis and inflammatory disease. Semin Ultrasound 4:184–192, 1983.

Lipsit ER: Inflammatory disease of the pelvis and postoperative fluid collections. Clin Diagn Ultrasound 15:85–104, 1984.

Patten RM, Vincent LM, Wolner-Hanssen P, Thorpe E Jr: Pelvic inflammatory disease. Endovaginal sonography with laparoscopic correlation. J Ultrasound Med 9:681–689, 1990.

Spiegel RM, Ben-Ora A: Ultrasound of inflammatory disease in the pelvis. Semin Ultrasound 1:41–50, 1980.

Swayne LC, Love MB, Karasick SR: Pelvic inflammatory disease: Sonographic-pathologic correlation. Radiology 151:751–755, 1984.

vanSonnenberg E, D'Agostino HB, Casola G, et al: US-guided transvaginal drainage of pelvic abscesses and fluid collections. Radiology 181:53–56, 1991.

144 Benign Ovarian Disease

Michael R. Clair

The ovary provides the diagnostician a kaleidoscope of pathologies because of the normal physiologic cycle and the expression of nearly 50 different histologic cell types of tumors and tumor-like conditions. Approximately 80 per cent of all ovarian tumors are benign. Table 144–1, a modification of the World Health Organization classification of tumors and tumor-like conditions of the ovary (in conjunction with the International Federation of Gynecology and Obstetrics), serves as an outline to this section.

IMAGING

Imaging of the pelvis is most often performed to confirm the presence of an adnexal abnormality detected during a physical examination. Although ultrasound remains the pre-eminent first choice for imaging the female pelvis, the recent application of a multimodality assessment of pelvic disease including magnetic resonance imaging (MRI) and computed tomography (CT) has proven invaluable in evaluating ovarian pathology. Ultrasound is extremely accurate in determining the size, location, and gross morphology of pelvic or ovarian tumors, although specific histologic characterization is usually not possible. MRI and CT imaging of the pelvis provide additional multiplanar information and a larger field of view than ultrasound, without some of the inherent limitations. Ultrasound, MRI, and CT have demonstrated essentially equal sensitivity and specificity for epithelial tumors, dermoids, and endometriomas. MRI may be helpful in differentiating ovarian from uterine pathology.

The recent emphasis on endovaginal ultrasound reflects the continued modifications in technology that are improving the visualization of the deep pelvic soft tissues. Endovaginal color and spectral Doppler interrogation of an ovarian mass may prove useful in tumor evaluation.

Regardless of the imaging algorithm used to evaluate ovarian pathology, imaging studies should always be interpreted in light of the patient's physical findings and hormonal milieu, and other imaging studies either concurrently or sequentially performed.

TABLE 144–1. BENIGN OVARIAN NEOPLASMS

I. Coelomic (Germinal) Epithelial Neoplasms (and Derivatives)
  A. Serous tumors
  B. Mucinous tumors
  C. Endometrioid
  D. Adenofibroma
  E. Brenner tumors
II. Sex Cord Stromal Neoplasms
  A. Granulosa-thecal-luteal cell tumors
  B. Androblastoma; Sertoli-Leydig cell tumors
  C. Fibroma
III. Germ Cell Neoplasms
  A. Teratoma
IV. Gonadoblastoma
V. Soft-Tissue Tumors Not Specific to Ovary
VI. Unclassified
VII. Tumor-Like Conditions
  A. Pregnancy luteoma
  B. Hyperthecosis
  C. Follicular cyst and corpus luteum cyst
  D. Polycystic ovaries
  E. Endometriosis
  F. Simple cysts
  G. Inflammatory lesions
  H. Paraovarian cysts

Modification of the International Histological Classification of Tumors No. 9. Geneva, World Health Organization, 1973.

OVARIAN NEOPLASMS

The ovary appears remarkably resistant to disease. Ovarian tumors, although less common than functional and true cysts, tend to be of the greatest importance. Benign tumors of the ovary (as well as their malignant and borderline counterparts) may be the nidus of hormonal synthesis, acute surgical emergencies, infertility, and/or obstetric problems.

Benign Ovarian Neoplasms of Coelomic (Germinal) Epithelium and Its Derivatives

As a group, these comprise the greatest majority of ovarian tumors, accounting for approximately 50 to 75 per cent of all adult ovarian tumors. The serous type is slightly more frequent than the mucinous type. Serous and mucinous adenomas are often depicted as cystic pelvic masses of approximately 4 to 20 cm in size at presentation (Fig. 144–1). The sonographic, CT, and MRI features of the cystic component may range from entirely cystic, to very fine uniform internal debris, to large septations and papillations along the inner wall (Fig. 144–2). There does not appear to be any consensus as to whether the presence of internal echogenic material increases the likelihood of malignancy in an individual case. It does appear, however, that the benign serous and mucinous tumors are more likely to be unilocular, with thin septations, few papillations, and little internal debris. Ascites also seems to be less prevalent with benign disease. The size of these tumors also tends to correlate poorly in the individual case with the likelihood of benignity, although larger masses have a greater likelihood of being malignant. The unilocular variety is often histopathologically designated a cystoma and the multilocular variety a cystadenoma.

Serous Cystadenoma

Serous cystadenomas occur most often between the ages of 20 and 50 and account for approximately 30 per cent of all ovarian tumors. Malignant transformation is seen in approximately 30 to 45 per cent of cases. The exact incidence of bilaterality has not been established, but reports have been as high as 50 per cent. The serous cystadenoma is usually a unilocular mass (filled with serous fluid). The borders are usually smooth and well-defined, and sonographically there is usually very good transmission. Fine internal debris, septations, and papillations of the tumor's inner wall may occasionally be seen. The benign tumors may also hemorrhage or be associated with ascites.

Mucinous Cystadenoma

There is considerable overlap in both the clinical and sonographic characteristics of the mucinous and serous tumors. Mucinous tu-

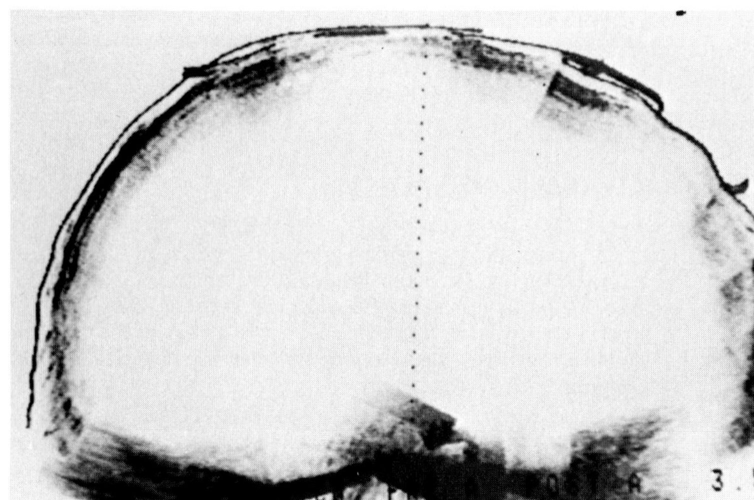

Figure 144–1. Giant serous cystadenoma. The entire mass is cystic, with smooth inner walls and no internal architecture.

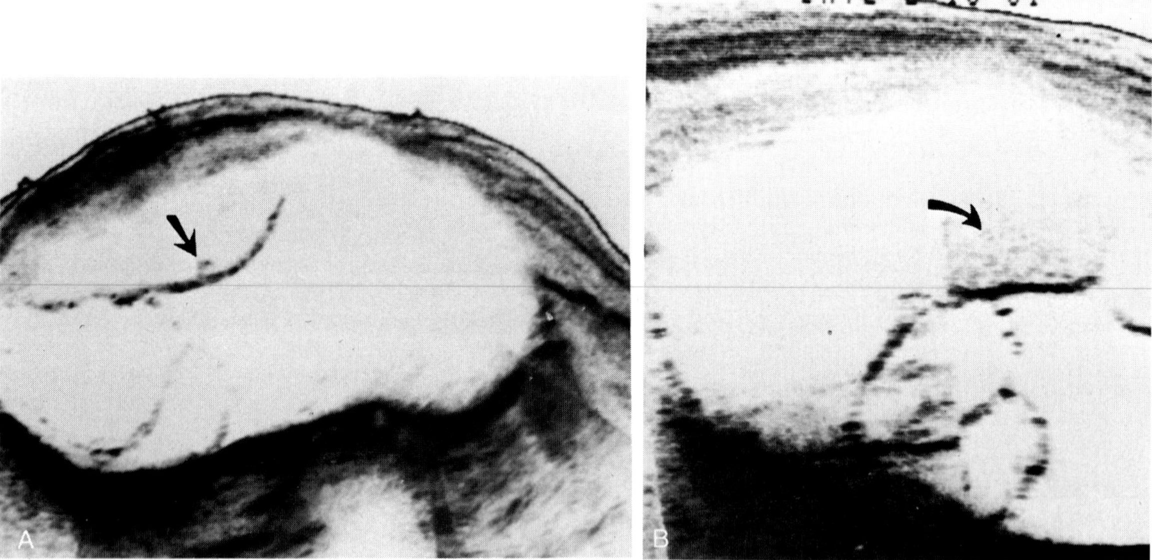

Figure 144–2. Serous cystadenoma. The larger serous tumors tend to multiloculate. Note *(A)* the septal papillations *(straight arrow)* and *(B)* fine echoes *(curved arrow)* demonstrated within several locules.

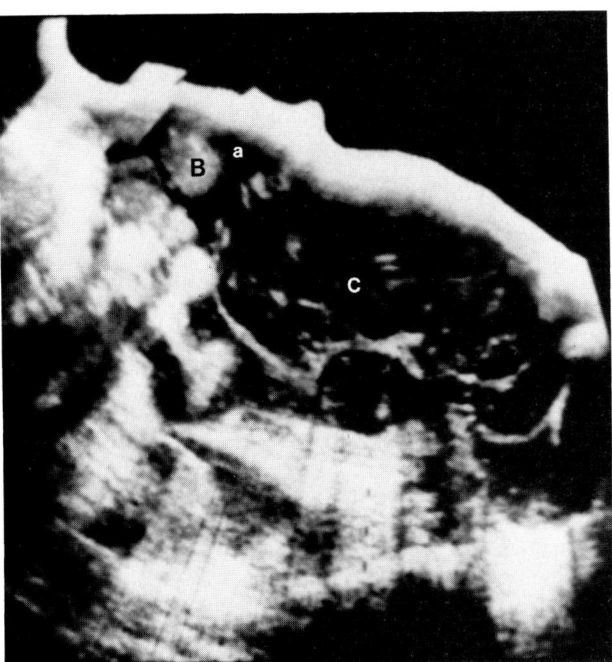

Figure 44–3. Mucinous cystadenoma. A multiloculated cystic mass was surrounded by bowel loops floating within ascites. (B = bowel; a = ascites; C = cystadenoma.)

mors account for approximately 20 per cent of all ovarian tumors and the ratio of benign to malignant type is 7 to 1; they are therefore less commonly malignant than their serous counterparts. Mucinous tumors are often considerably larger than serous tumors and more often are multilocular (Fig. 144–3). Coarse internal debris, thick septa, and papillations are also common (Fig. 144–4). In approximately 5 per cent of cases mucinous tumors may be bilateral. Spontaneous rupture may produce pseudomyxoma peritonei, and intracystic hemorrhage may occur.

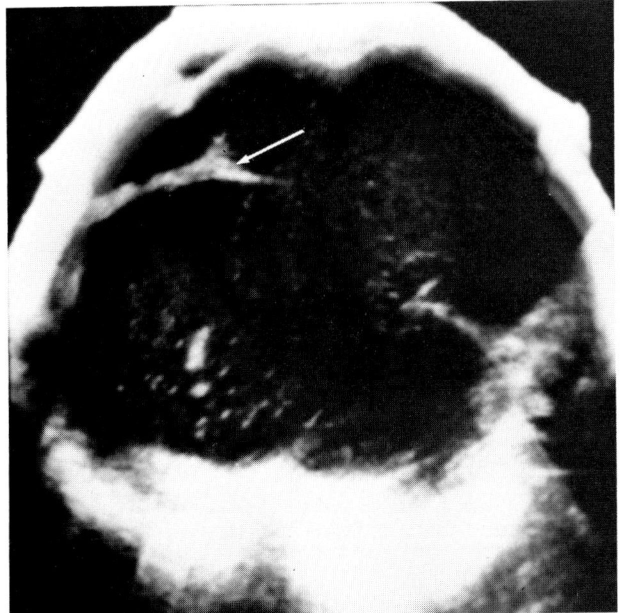

Figure 144–4. Mucinous cystadenoma. Transverse section of a giant tumor with fine particulate matter demonstrated with a high frequency transducer examination. Multiple thick-walled septa are seen *(arrow).*

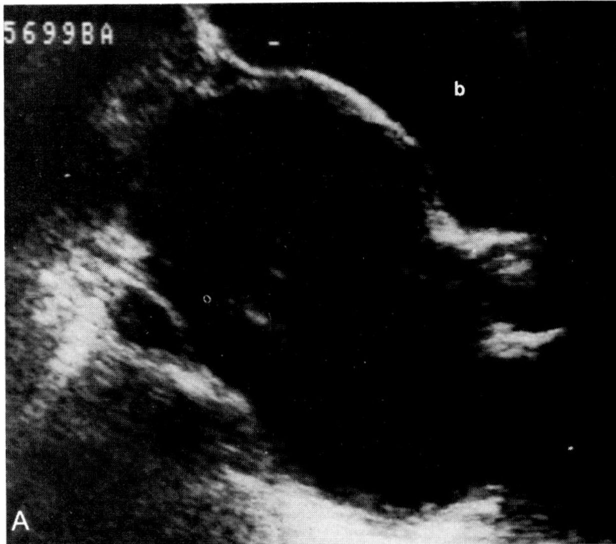

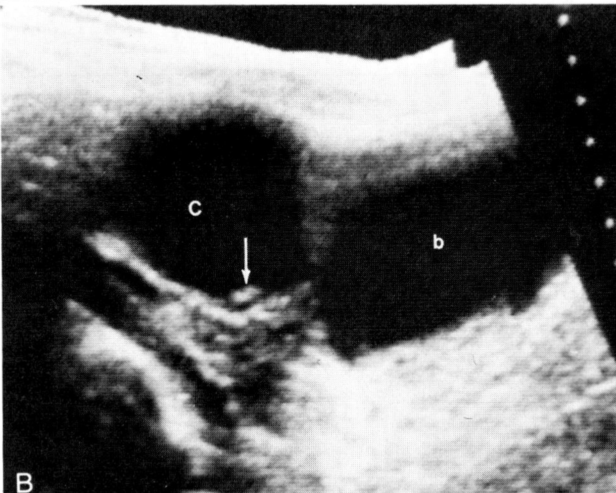

Figure 144–5. *A,* **Cystadenofibroma.** This tumor is mostly cystic with several thin septa. This may be indistinguishable from a serous cystadenoma. (b = bladder.) *B,* **Adenofibroma.** The cystic component (c) was designated serous cystadenoma at pathology with a small papillation *(arrow)* designated an adenofibroma.

Cystadenofibroma and Adenofibroma

Cystadenofibroma and adenofibroma are essentially variants of serous cystadenomas. These tumors are usually small and may be multilocular (Fig. 144–5).

Brenner Tumors

Brenner tumors are very unusual, predominantly solid tumors that account for approximately 2 per cent of all ovarian tumors. They are usually seen in patients older than 50 years of age. They are usually small but may present as large masses with cystic spaces. These tumors are often associated with other epithelial cystomas in the same ovary and with benign teratomas.

Benign Sex Cord and Mesenchymal Tumors

These are tumors of the specialized ovarian gonadal stroma and include all neoplasia originating from either the sex cords of the

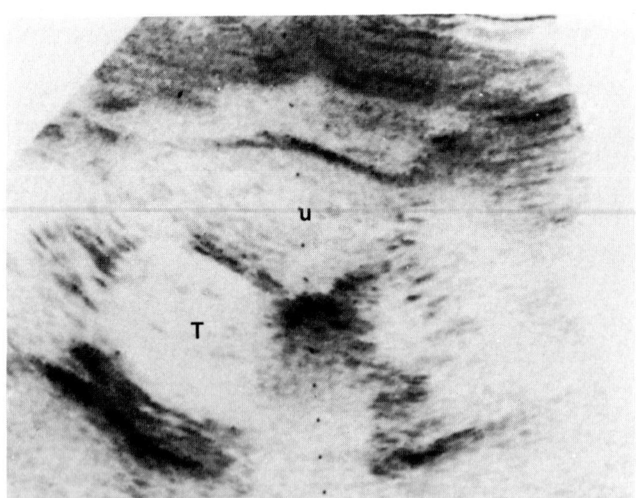

Figure 144–6. Granulosa–thecal cell tumor. A transverse section of a 6-cm complex, hypoechoic mass with fine internal echoes situated posterior to the uterus. (T = tumor; u = uterus.)

embryonic gonad or the mesenchyme of the ovary. These tumors account for only 5 per cent of all ovarian tumors.

Granulosa-Thecal-Luteal Cell Tumors

Collectively, granulosa-thecal-luteal cell tumors account for most of the ovarian stromal tumors. They may be seen at any age, but two thirds occur after menopause. These tumors are obviously a spectrum of histologic makeup in which any of three cells may predominate. In approximately 20 per cent of the cases, the granulosa cell predominates; in 20 per cent there is a mixture of granulosa and thecal cells; and in the remainder there is a pure thecal cell type; the pure luteoma is rare. These tumors are variable in size; they are usually 5 to 10 cm in diameter, but may be seen up to 20 and 30 cm. In a small number of cases these tumors may present with isosexual pseudoprecocious puberty that occurs before the age of five years. Overt feminization may occur in 85 to 90 per cent of cases. The incidence of endometrial and breast cancer has been reported to be higher in patients with estrogen-producing tumors. These tumors are usually multilocular cystic masses that may have fine internal echoes (Fig. 144–6). Predominantly solid tumors have also been reported. Thecomas have been described as tumors that, because of the dense fibrous component, cause acoustic shadowing without histologic evidence of calcification.

Sertoli-Leydig Cell Tumors

Originally called *arrhenoblastoma* and now often termed *androblastoma,* Sertoli-Leydig cell tumors often have a virilizing rather than feminizing effect. They account for less than 1 per cent of all ovarian tumors and are seen in young women with signs and symptoms of masculinization by virtue of their androgen production. Some of these tumors may, however, be associated with increased estrogen production or may have no endocrine manifestations. These tumors are indistinguishable from the granulosa-thecal-luteal cell tumors and therefore may be multilocular, predominantly solid masses with hemorrhagic and cystic degeneration or may be solid tumors in some cases (Fig. 144–7).

Fibromas

These tumors of nonspecialized mesenchymal ovarian stroma account for approximately 10 per cent of all ovarian tumors. Ten per cent are bilateral, and they usually range in size from 5 to 10 cm. They may be multiple in approximately 10 per cent of cases. They are seen most commonly in menopausal and postmenopausal women. Approximately 50 per cent of cases, in tumors greater than 6 cm, present with ascites. Meigs' syndrome, which typically includes an ovarian fibroma associated with ascites and hydrothorax, is extremely uncommon and may be present with other ovarian tumors. The sonographic description of ovarian fibromas is very incomplete; the gross morphology of the tumor suggests that these will be predominantly solid masses that may have cystic areas of necrosis and hemorrhage (Fig. 144–8).

Benign Ovarian Germ Cell Tumors

Approximately 20 per cent of all benign ovarian tumors are of germ cell origin. They usually occur at an earlier age than epithelial tumors and are seen most commonly between the ages of 10 and 30.

Benign Cystic Teratoma

Benign cystic teratoma, or dermoid cyst, accounts for the overwhelming majority of tumors of germ cell origin. The majority of these tumors are benign, although, if seen in the postmenopausal woman, they have a higher incidence of malignancy or malignant degeneration (1 per cent). There is an incidence of 10 to 20 per cent bilaterality, and familial occurrence has been reported in twins and triplets. These tumors are often discovered incidentally, although they may present with acute abdominal catastrophe from torsion and rupture. Benign cystic teratomas are usually 5 to 10 cm in size when clinically evident and are rarely very large unless malignant. There are a number of sonographic features considered characteristic which have been described. They are present, however, in only about one third of the cases. These features include (1) midline or paramidline location (Fig. 144–9), (2) unilocular or multilocular cyst with either internal echoes or a mural echogenic mass (Fig. 144–10), (3) "fat/fluid" or "hair/fluid" level (Fig. 144–11), and (4) poorly echogenic mass with either a very echogenic or echopoor center (Fig. 144–9). Probably the most characteristic and specific finding of a benign cystic teratoma is the echogenic, acoustically shadowing, inner mural component. This does not necessarily contain calcified material such as teeth (Fig. 144–12) but may rather represent matted hair and sebum. Often, this may be the only find-

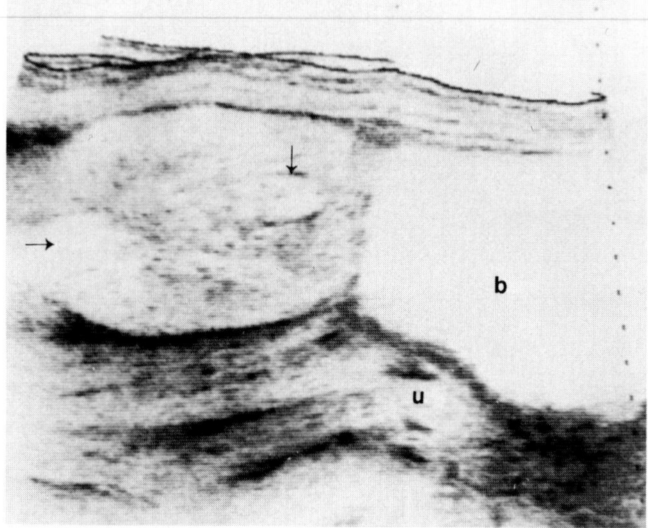

Figure 144–7. Sertoli-Leydig cell tumor. Both hypoechoic solid and small cystic components *(arrows)* give this tumor its typical sonographic features. (b = bladder; u = uterus.)

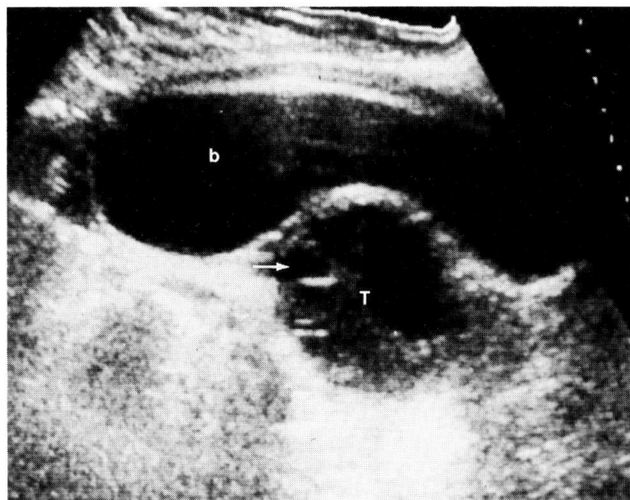

Figure 144–8. Fibroma. Although this tumor is mostly solid, there are cystic areas *(arrow)* that probably correspond to necrosis and hemorrhage. (b = bladder; T = tumor.)

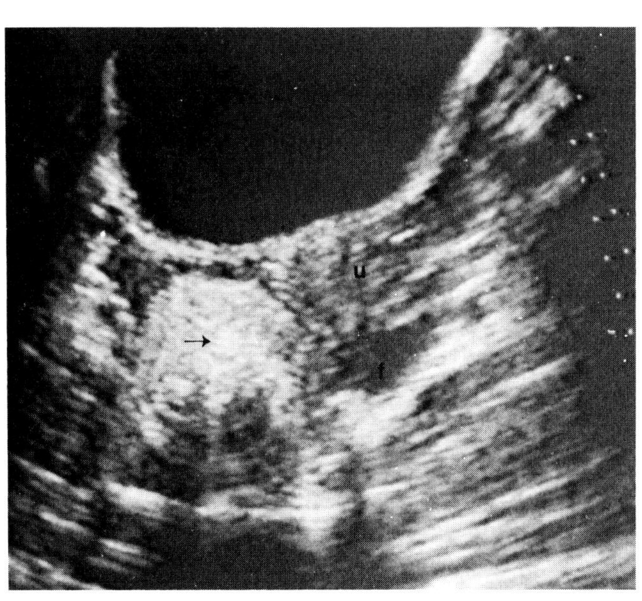

Figure 144–9. Teratoma. A transverse image of a benign teratoma situated just to the right of the uterus. Note that the very echogenic mass has some beam attenuation and a more echogenic center *(arrow)*. (u = uterus; f = fluid in cul-de-sac.)

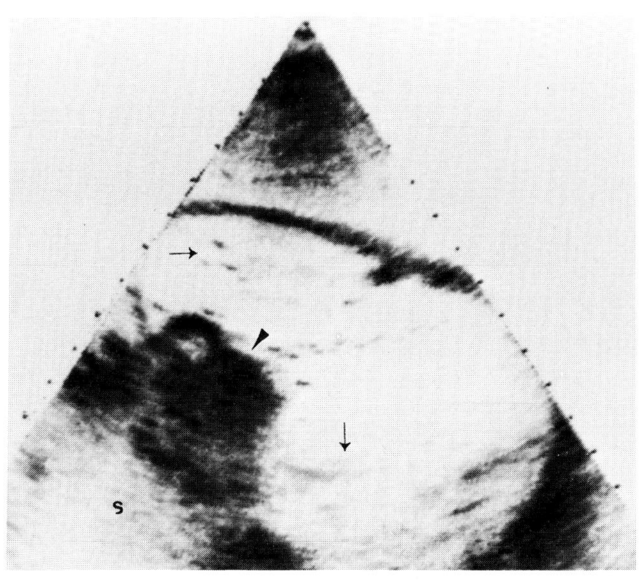

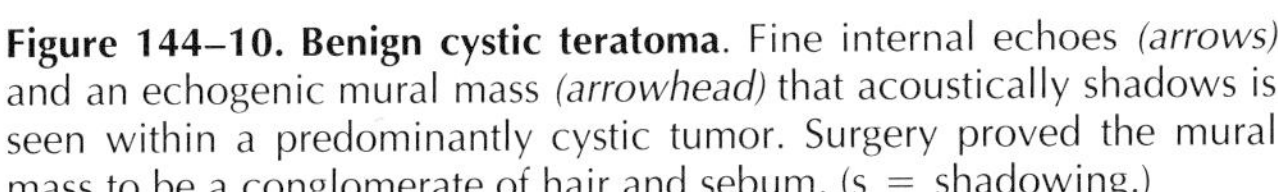

Figure 144–10. Benign cystic teratoma. Fine internal echoes *(arrows)* and an echogenic mural mass *(arrowhead)* that acoustically shadows is seen within a predominantly cystic tumor. Surgery proved the mural mass to be a conglomerate of hair and sebum. (s = shadowing.)

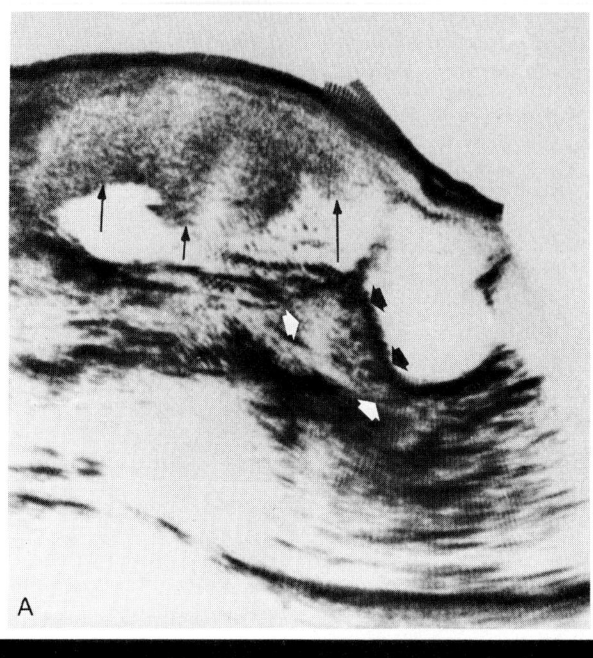

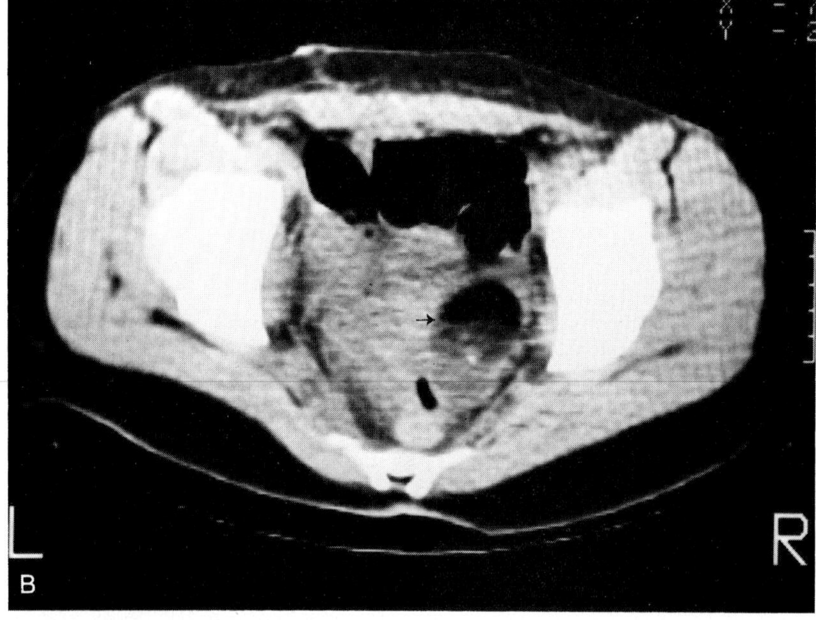

Figure 144–11. *A,* Large **benign ovarian teratoma** is seen anterior to the uterus *(arrowheads).* This mass contains an echogenic fluid layer anteriorly *(arrows).* (*A* reproduced with permission from Bowie JD: Ultrasound in gynecology. In Sabbagha RE: Diagnostic Ultrasound Applied to Obstetrics and Gynecology. New York, Harper and Row, 1980, p 286). *B,* Computed tomography of a benign cystic teratoma of the right ovary demonstrates that fat is the nondependent portion of the fat-fluid interface *(arrow).* The calcific nidus was found to be a tooth at surgery.

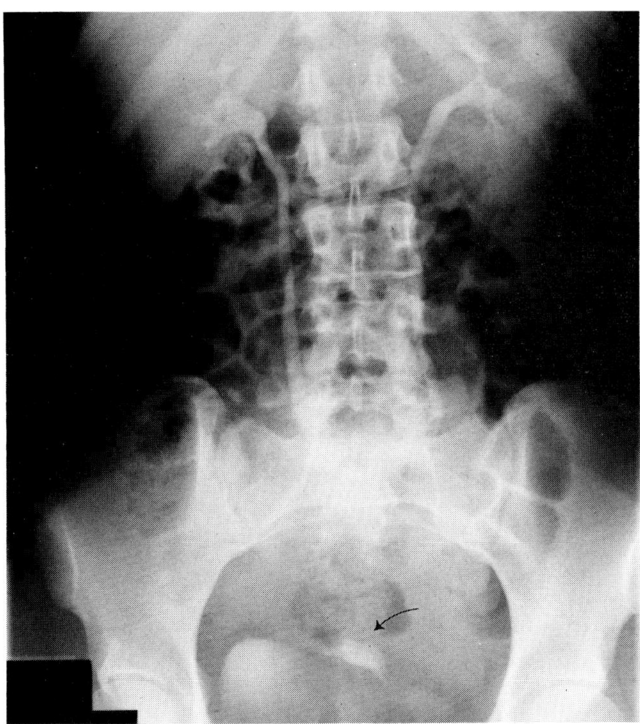

Figure 144–12. Abdominal radiograph taken during a urogram demonstrates a **left adnexal mass** with a recognizable tooth *(arrow).*

ing evident within the pelvis and it may simulate bowel gas. This confusing picture has been termed the "tip of the iceberg" (Fig. 144–13) and is probably one of the reasons why approximately 25 per cent of all benign cystic teratomas are not demonstrated on ultrasound. The CT criteria for cystic teratomas include a fat/fluid level and mural calcification, whereas an MRI may demonstrate fat intensity, chemical-shift artifact, fluid interfaces, and a "palm-tree" papillary projection within the cystic component of the mass. Rupture of a benign cystic teratoma is quite rare, occurring in less than 1 per cent of cases. Rupture may be either within the peritoneum or into adjacent organs such as the bladder, small bowel, rectum, sigmoid, or vagina. Acute rupture of a benign cystic teratoma, with acute peritonitis, has been reported to be more common with pregnancy (Fig. 144–14). Benign cystic teratomas have been found to be associated with ovarian epithelial tumors. For unknown reasons, infertility may be associated with benign cystic teratomas. Solid teratomas tend to occur in the younger, often prepubertal, age group and are often quite large. They are predominantly solid with cystic spaces, and some authorities consider these tumors malignant until proven otherwise.

TUMOR-LIKE NON-NEOPLASTIC OVARIAN CYSTS

Functional cysts are the most common cause of ovarian enlargement in young women. The practitioner of ovarian sonography needs a strong understanding of the normal hormonal and physiologic changes expressed by the ovary during the normal menstrual cycle. The normal newborn ovary usually contains at least 40,000 primordial follicles that lie dormant until after the menarche. With the menarche, the hypothalamic-pituitary-ovarian hormonal axis produces a three-phase menstrual cycle. The follicular phase, which is the phase of active follicular growth, commences the first day after menses and continues until ovulation. Multiple small ovarian cysts, usually measuring less than 15 mm in diameter, are usually seen by ultrasound (Fig. 144–15). These follicles and corpora lutea should be considered normal transient physiologic structures. A dominant follicle, usually of 17 to 25 mm in size, emerges under the influence of estrogen and follicle-stimulating hormone. With maturity, it is referred to as the *graafian follicle,* and it responds to the mid-cycle surge of luteinizing hormone from the pituitary gland. Ovulation occurs within 24 hours, with the follicle rupturing and releasing the ovum. With ovulation the remaining theca and granulosa cells enlarge, forming the corpus luteum. The corpus luteum produces progesterone, which is necessary for successful endometrial implantation. If the released ovum is fertilized, human chorionic gonadotropin prevents regression of the corpus luteum. Eventually, placental production of progesterone is established and the corpus luteum regresses. The luteal phase of the ovarian cycle may demonstrate a cystic or hemorrhage-filled cystic corpus luteum. The corpus luteum may persist for up to 10 to 12 weeks in a normal pregnancy (Fig. 144–16).

The follicular cyst, therefore, occurs during every normal ovulatory menstrual cycle, reaching a maximum size of usually 25 to 30 mm. Although the cyst usually disappears with ovulation, occasionally the follicle fails to rupture and may even continue to grow, sometimes reaching a diameter of 8 to 10 cm (Fig. 144–17). These clear follicular cysts usually contain clear serous fluid.

Corpus luteum cysts may or may not occur with each pregnancy. The corpus luteum cyst may also reach a size of 8 to 10 cm. If they are larger than 6 cm or if they persist beyond the sixteenth week of pregnancy, surgical intervention may be required because of the possibility of rupture, torsion, or hemorrhage.

Both of these functional cysts are usually incidental, and the patient is often unaware of their presence. Complications of their growth may be their reason for presentation and may necessitate medical or surgical intervention. When simple cysts are incidentally discovered, it is often suggested that they be re-examined at the end of the next menstrual period when ovarian activity is at its minimum. Sonographically, both follicular cysts and corpus luteum cysts may be smooth, thin-walled, and unilocular. Both may, however, have a complex internal architecture, septa, or fine internal echoes on examination with high-frequency transducers (see Fig. 144–17). Either may hemorrhage, producing complex adnexal

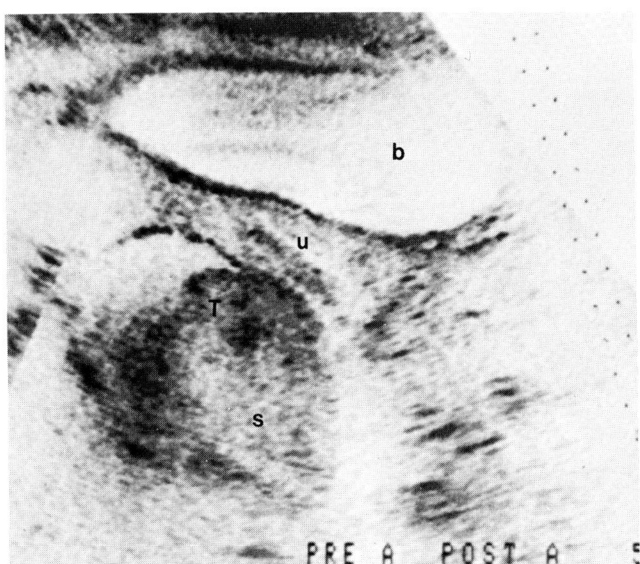

Figure 144–13. Teratoma. Solid mass behind the uterus (u) with strong acoustic interface anteriorly and shadowing posteriorly. This image might easily be misinterpreted as bowel. The bulk of the tumor (T) is difficult to visualize, thus the designation "tip of the iceberg." (b = bladder.)

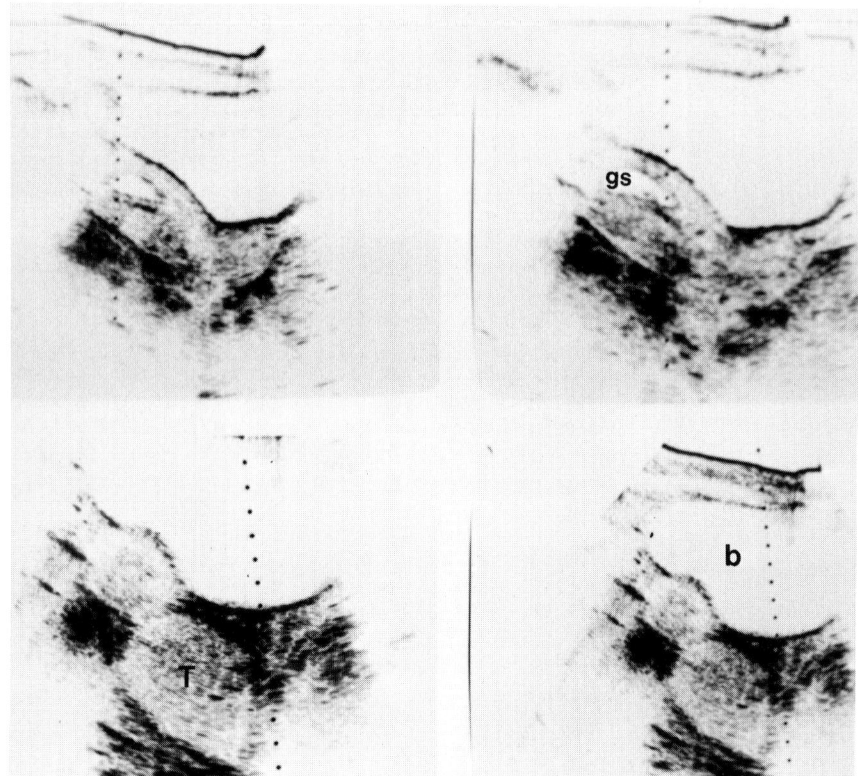

Figure 144–14. A 7-cm **benign teratoma** is seen coincident with an otherwise normal six-week gestation. (gs = gestational sac; T = teratoma; b = bladder.)

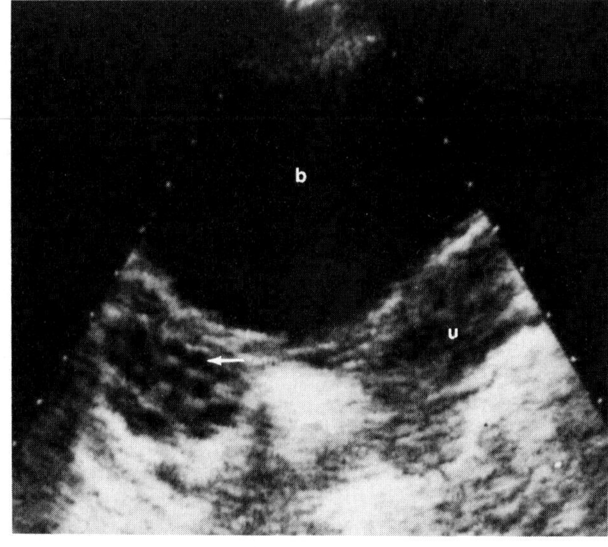

Figure 144–15. Transverse image of the right ovary demonstrates multiple 5-mm **physiologic cysts** *(arrow)* of the follicular phase of the menstrual cycle. (u = uterus; b = bladder.)

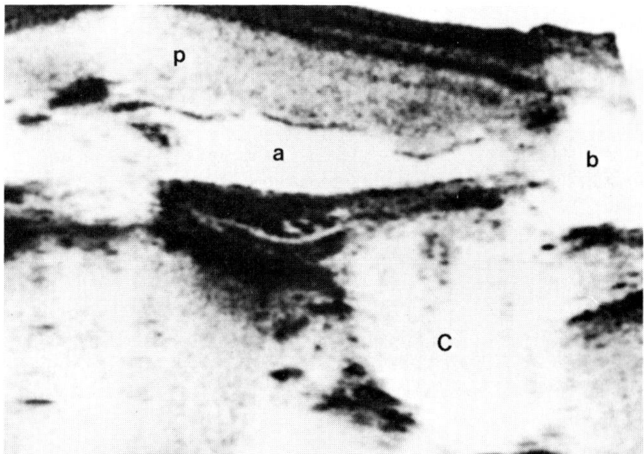

Figure 144–16. A 9-cm **corpus luteum cyst of pregnancy** seen at 20 weeks. Surgery was performed without complication. Some fine internal echoes suggested hemorrhage, which was confirmed at surgery. (C = corpus luteum; p = placenta; b = bladder; a = amniotic cavity.)

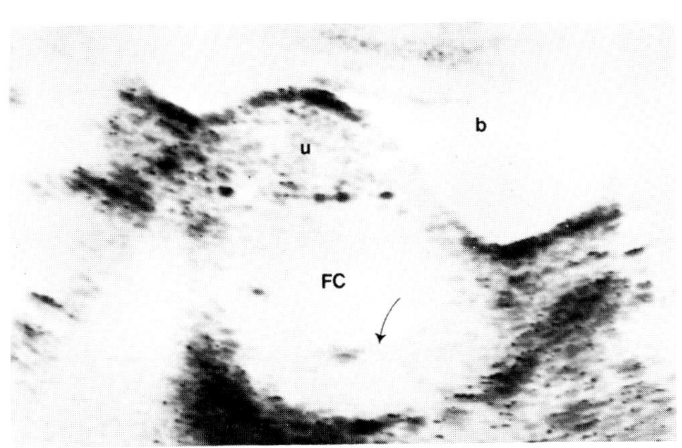

Figure 144–17. Follicular cyst. Longitudinal section reveals a cystic mass behind the uterus. There is dependent echo-producing particulate matter suggesting hemorrhage *(arrow)*. (b = bladder; u = uterus; FC = follicular cyst.)

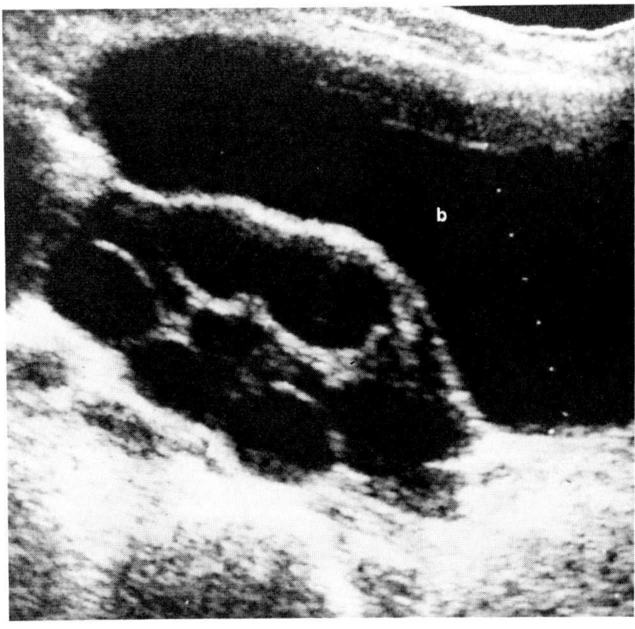

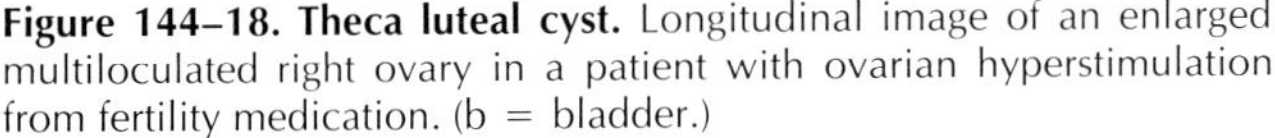
Figure 144–18. Theca luteal cyst. Longitudinal image of an enlarged multiloculated right ovary in a patient with ovarian hyperstimulation from fertility medication. (b = bladder.)

masses simulating any of a number of diseases that may cause acute pelvic pain.

Another very rare form of a functional cyst is the theca lutein cyst. Unlike the previously mentioned cysts, the theca lutein cysts are frequently bilateral and multilocular. These cysts are usually seen in association with extremely excessive levels of production of human chorionic gonadotropin, particularly encountered in patients with gestational trophoblastic disease, and in patients undergoing ovulation induction (as part of the clinical spectrum of the ovarian hyperstimulation syndrome) (Fig. 144–18). Thecal lutein cysts also may rarely be associated with multiple pregnancies or erythroblastosis fetalis. These multilocular cystic ovarian masses actually represent multiple hyperstimulated follicular cysts, which because they may reach sizes of 15 to 20 cm are extremely fragile and predisposed to hemorrhage and rupture. Involution occurs following removal of the source of gonadotropin.

Bibliography

Bowie JD: Ultrasound in gynecology. In Sabbagha RE (ed): Diagnostic Ultrasound Applied to Obstetrics and Gynecology. New York, Harper and Row, 1980, pp 259–300.

Buy JN, Ghossain MA, Sciot C, et al: Epithelial tumors of the ovary: CT findings and correlation with ultrasound. Radiology 178:881–818, 1991.

Ehren IM, Mahour GH, Isaacs H: Benign and malignant ovarian tumors in children and adolescents. Am J Surg 147:339–344, 1984.

Fleischer AC, James AE, Millis JB, Julian C: Differential diagnosis of pelvic masses by gray scale sonography. AJR 131:469–476, 1978.

Fleisher AC, Wentz AC, Jones HW, et al: Ultrasound evaluation of the ovary. In Callen P (ed): Ultrasonography in Obstetrics and Gynecology. Philadelphia, WB Saunders Company, 1983.

Ghossain MA, Buy JN, Lignére C, et al: Epithelial tumors of the ovary: Comparison of MR and CT findings. Radiology 181:863–870, 1991.

Hall DA, Hann LE, Ferruci JT, et al: Sonographic morphology of the normal menstrual cycle. Radiology 133:185–188, 1979.

Hasan A, Amr S, Issa A, Bata M: Ovarian tumors complicating pregnancy. Int J Gynecol Obstet 21:279–282, 1983.

Katsube Y, Berg JW, Silverberg SG: Epidemiologic pathology of ovarian tumors. Int Gynecol Pathol 1:3–16, 1982.

Laing FC, Volney FVD, Marks WM, et al: Dermoid cysts of the ovary: Their ultrasonographic appearances. Obstet Gynecol 57:99–104, 1981.

Lawson TL, Albarelli JN: Diagnosis of gynecologic pelvic masses by gray scale ultrasonography: Analysis of specificity and accuracy. AJR 128:1003–1006, 1979.

Moyle JW, Rochester D, Sider L, et al: Sonography of ovarian tumors: Predictability of tumor type. AJR 141:985–991, 1983.

Novak ER, Woodruff JD: Novak's Gynecologic and Obstetrical Pathology, 8th ed. Philadelphia, WB Saunders Company, 1979.

Rosenberg ER, Trought WS: The ultrasonographic evaluation of large cystic pelvic masses. Am J Obstet Gynecol 139:579–586, 1981.

Serou SF, Scully RE: Histologic typing of ovarian tumors. In International Histological Classification of Tumors No. 9. Geneva, World Health Organization, 1973.

Togashi K, Nishimura K, Itoh K, et al: Ovarian cystic teratomas: MR imaging. Radiology 162:669–673, 1987.

Williams AG, Mettler FA, Wicks JD: Cystic and solid ovarian neoplasms. Semin Ultrasound 4:166–182, 1983.

145 Malignant Ovarian Masses

Cirrelda Cooper

Ovarian cancer is an insidious disease, asymptomatic in its early stages. Over the course of a lifetime, it strikes one in 70 women. It is currently the leading cause of gynecologic cancer death. Most patients (60 to 70 per cent) are diagnosed relatively late in the course of their disease, when the prognosis is poor. Overall five-year survival is a depressing 35 per cent and has not significantly changed in recent years, despite advances in treatment.

Ovarian cancer increases in frequency with age and is therefore most common in postmenopausal women. The incidence is greatest in middle and upper class women in industrialized countries, occurring in 33 per 100,000 women in the United States each year. Other risk factors include a family history of ovarian cancer, nulliparity, and prior breast cancer.

Malignancies arising in the ovary are classified in terms of their tissues of origin. The vast majority of tumors are of epithelial origin. Stromal–sex cord tumors include granulosa-thecomas, Sertoli-Leydig cell tumors, and small cell and fibromatous masses. Germ cell lines produce malignant teratocellular carcinomas and dysgerminomas. Extraovarian primary tumors, chiefly those arising in the colon, breast, and stomach, metastasize to the ovaries, simulating both the macroscopic and microscopic features of tumors originating in the ovary.

Patients often present with abdominal distension, symptoms related to gastrointestinal or genitourinary tract compression, or nonspecific constitutional complaints. A pelvic mass may be evident on abdominal palpation or, more often, with pelvic examination. In many cases, ultrasound is initially used to confirm the presence of a mass and assess its internal characteristics.

The prognosis and management of patients with ovarian cancer are primarily based on the stage of disease, which is determined using the International Federation of Gynecology and Obstetrics (FIGO) guidelines (Table 145–1). Preoperative radiographic imag-

TABLE 145–1. STAGING OF OVARIAN CARCINOMA (FIGO) AND SURVIVAL RATES

Stage	5-Year Survival Rate
I. Tumor Confined to the Ovaries	80–90%
A. Unilateral	
B. Bilateral	
C. With positive peritoneal washings	
II. Pelvic Extension of Tumor	40–60%
A. To uterus or fallopian tubes	
B. To other pelvic tissues	
C. With malignant ascites or positive peritoneal washings	
III. Tumor Involves Abdominal Peritoneal Cavity or Retroperitoneal/Inguinal Nodes	10–15%
A. Microscopic seeding of abdominal peritoneal cavity	
B. Abdominal implants <2 cm	
C. Abdominal implants >2 cm, retroperitoneal or inguinal nodes	
IV. Distant Metastases Including Spread to Liver Parenchyma and Pleura	<5%

ing is limited because patients with ovarian carcinoma undergo detailed surgical staging at the time of their initial diagnosis. Intravenous urography may be obtained to delineate the course of the ureters and to exclude obstruction. Colonic invasion or the presence of a primary colon cancer can be evaluated by barium enema, particularly in patients over 40, those with left-sided masses, or if clinical symptoms suggest gastrointestinal involvement. On occasion, preoperative CT may be requested to delineate the extent of disease. During staging laparotomy, the surgeon resects the uterus, both ovaries, and the omentum; aspirates intraperitoneal fluid; lavages the peritoneal cavity; and samples retroperitoneal and pelvic nodes. Peritoneal surfaces are carefully inspected and biopsied. An additional goal of surgery is to remove obvious tumor because survival is improved if the remaining tumor volume can be decreased to less than 2 cm.

After adjuvant chemotherapy, patients who are asymptomatic and clinically free of disease require a second-look laparotomy to resect residual masses and assess for microscopic tumor. Overall survival depends on (a) the stage of disease at initial laparotomy, (b) the grade of the tumor, (c) the amount of residual tumor remaining after surgery, and (d) the postoperative response to chemotherapy.

MALIGNANT EPITHELIAL NEOPLASMS OF THE OVARY

Ovarian cancers of epithelial origin constitute 90 to 95 per cent of all ovarian primary cancers and are divided by histologic appearance into serous, mucinous, endometrioid, clear cell, Brenner, and undifferentiated subtypes. In terms of clinical behavior, however, the subtypes are indistinguishable. Serous and mucinous cystadenocarcinomas are most prevalent. In many tumors, histology is mixed.

Serous cystadenocarcinoma is the most common variety of malignant ovarian tumor. These tumors are more likely to be malignant and, when they are malignant, are more likely to be bilateral (up to 60 per cent in some series) than their mucinous counterparts. Current imaging techniques cannot reliably differentiate serous from mucinous tumors and often cannot distinguish malignant from benign ovarian masses. As a general rule, masses with solid components are more likely to be malignant than those that are purely cystic. Tubo-ovarian abscesses, endometriomas, complicated physiologic cysts, as well as benign ovarian neoplasms may closely resemble ovarian cancers.

Because ultrasound is used to confirm and characterize pelvic masses, it is often the initial imaging modality in patients with ovarian cancer. The sonographic appearance of epithelial malignancies is variable and nonspecific. Typically these masses are large, complex, and heterogeneous in echotexture with multiple anechoic cystic spaces, irregular thickened and nodular septations, papillary projections, and focal solid masses (Figs. 145–1 and 145–2). Internal architectural detail is better displayed by transvaginal ultrasound than transabdominal ultrasound or CT.

Recent studies indicate that Doppler and color flow imaging are useful in assessing ovarian masses. Malignant tumors characteristically have neovascularity, areas of flow in small, low-resistance vessels. Because similar findings in normal women may be seen during ovulation, pregnancy, or the luteal phase, premenopausal women should be studied during the early phase of the menstrual cycle, before day 10, and repeat studies may be useful for confirmation of abnormal findings. The periphery of the mass can be mapped using color flow as a guide to locate vessels for pulsed Doppler. The pulsatility index (PI = the difference between peak systolic and end diastolic velocities divided by mean flow velocity) and resistivity index (RI = the difference between peak systolic and end diastolic velocities divided by peak systolic velocity) are then calculated. Ovarian masses supplied by vessels with a low RI ($\leq$0.4) and low PI ($\leq$1.0) by Doppler are likely to be malignant (Fig. 145–3). Neovascularity may be seen in some benign masses as well, including dermoids and abscesses. In a large-scale study, Kurjak et al. found a positive predictive value of 98 per cent for ovarian malignancy using transvaginal Doppler with color flow, detecting several early Stage I ovarian cancers.

Although computed tomography (CT) is not needed preoperatively to stage ovarian cancer, some patients, particularly those with nonspecific symptoms, will undergo CT scanning in their initial evaluation. The CT appearance of ovarian epithelial carcinoma is a large complex unilateral or bilateral pelvic mass with cystic regions of near-water density and thick irregular walls interspersed with soft-tissue density masses (Fig. 145–4). Solid components characteristically enhance after intravenous contrast administration. Regions of high attenuation that do not enhance indicate blood or fluid with a high protein content. Calcifications, in the wall of the tumor or in soft-tissue components, and prominent enhancing tumoral vessels may also be present.

Currently magnetic resonance imaging (MRI) is neither more specific nor more sensitive than other modalities in the detection and diagnosis of ovarian cancer. With its multiplanar capabilities MRI is particularly useful in delineating complex anatomic relationships in patients with large or bilateral adnexal masses otherwise difficult to separate from the uterus or where invasion into other pelvic organs is suspected (Fig. 145–5). A combination of coronal and axial images is generally most useful.

Cystic and necrotic components of ovarian carcinomas have relatively low signal intensity on T_1-weighted images and increase in signal intensity with progressive T_2-weighting. While both T_1- and T_2-weighted images are equally likely to demonstrate an adnexal mass, T_1 images with gadolinium enhancement afford better contrast between cystic and solid components and improve delineation of internal architecture. Some malignant ovarian masses have variations in their T_1 and T_2 values as a result of areas of hemorrhage and necrosis. Mucinous tumors contain loculated fluid collections that have various T_1 and T_2 signal intensities because of their differing protein content. Tumoral vessels, particularly prominent in predominantly solid masses, are well-demonstrated with rapid-acquisition gradient echo sequences.

Ovarian epithelial malignancies spread locally to the uterus and fallopian tubes and the other ovary. Early spread to the peritoneum is particularly characteristic, but ovarian cancer also spreads via lymphatics to retroperitoneal, pelvic, and diaphragmatic nodes. In the late stage, hematogenous dissemination to the liver and other organs may also occur. Ascites and peritoneal metastases are commonly found dependently in the pelvic cul-de-sac and along the perihepatic and right diaphragmatic surfaces. They are likely found in the former region because of the local origin of the tumor and gravity and in the latter because of the flow patterns of peritoneal fluid, which drains along the paracolic gutter to the inferior aspect of the diaphragm. Transdiaphragmatic lymphatics may lead to the involvement of anterior mediastinal nodes.

Whereas ultrasound is an excellent imaging modality for evaluating ovarian masses, it is limited in assessing the presence and extent of metastatic disease. Peritoneal implants and omental metastases are difficult to detect sonographically unless detailed, directed, near-field scanning is used. MRI is also deficient in its ability to delineate small peritoneal implants because of its poor spatial resolution compared with CT. Calcified metastases that lack signal may also be missed on MRI. Serosal involvement of the bowel may be demonstrated by barium enema or small bowel studies; less commonly, calcified metastases are visible on plain abdominal films.

CT is overall the best imaging modality for assessment of intraperitoneal tumor spread. Omental metastases have a variable appearance, ranging from thick soft-tissue masses (omental "cakes") to fine linear and nodular infiltration of the omental fat. Peritoneal metastases may appear as a sheet-like soft-tissue coating of perito-

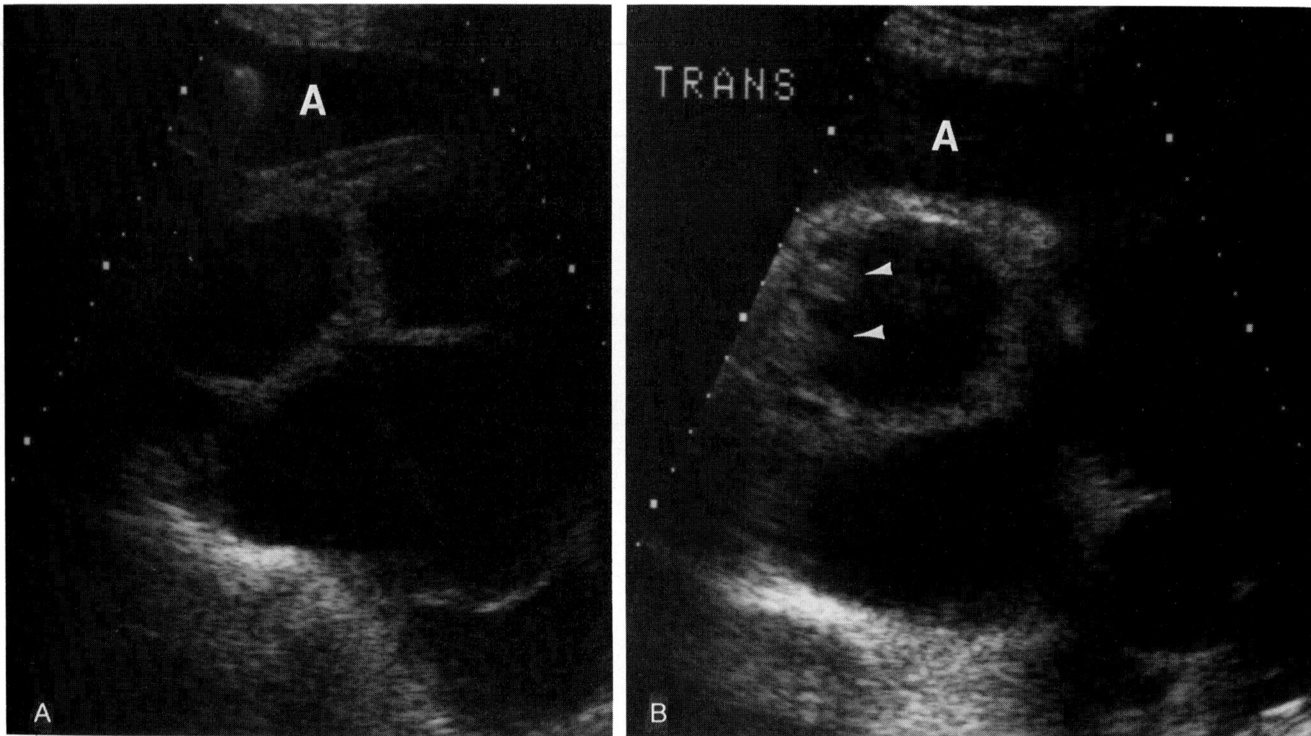

Figure 145–1. Serous cystadenocarcinoma—bilateral. *A,* Pelvic ultrasound demonstrates a large, complex, primarily cystic mass with thick, irregular septations in the right pelvis. (A = ascites.) *B,* Soft-tissue excrescences *(arrowheads)* project into cystic spaces in the left pelvic mass. Ascites is also present (A).

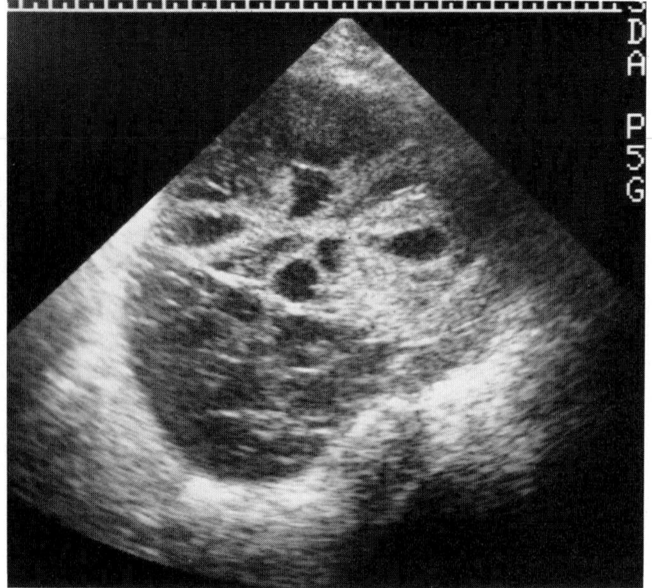

Figure 145–2. Mucinous cystadenocarcinoma—unilateral. A large multiloculated mass with heterogeneous echogenicity arises in the right ovary. The sonographic appearance is not specific for a mucinous primary and could be seen with other malignant cell types. Benign masses, including endometriomas, may have a similar appearance.

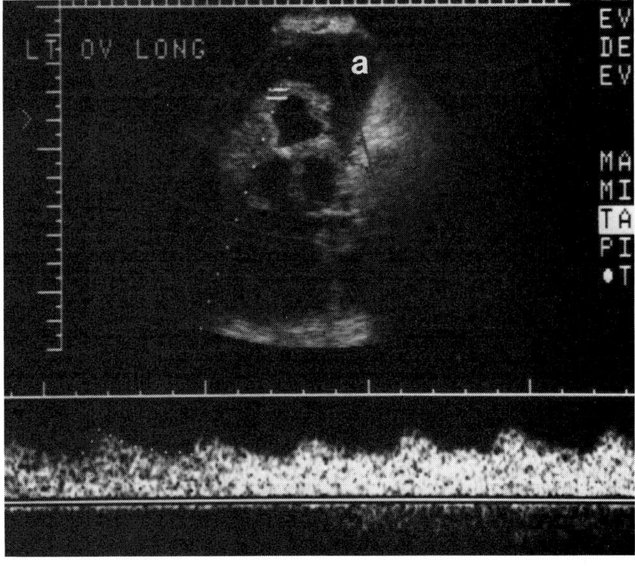

Figure 145–3. Doppler evaluation of ovarian carcinoma. High diastolic flow in low-resistance vessels (RI = 0.34; PI = 0.44) indicates neovascularity within a malignant endometrioid tumor of the ovary. Malignancy is also suggested by the thick nodular septations and focal soft-tissue components within the mass and by the presence of ascites (a).

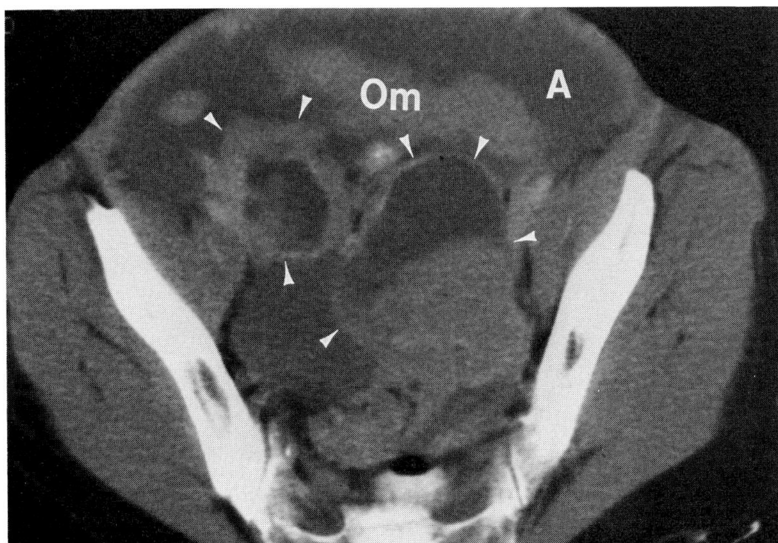

Figure 145–4. CT scan of ovarian carcinoma. Bilateral complex cystic and solid ovarian masses *(arrowheads)* are seen in the pelvis in this patient with serous cystadenocarcinoma. Ascites (A) and omental metastases (Om) are also present.

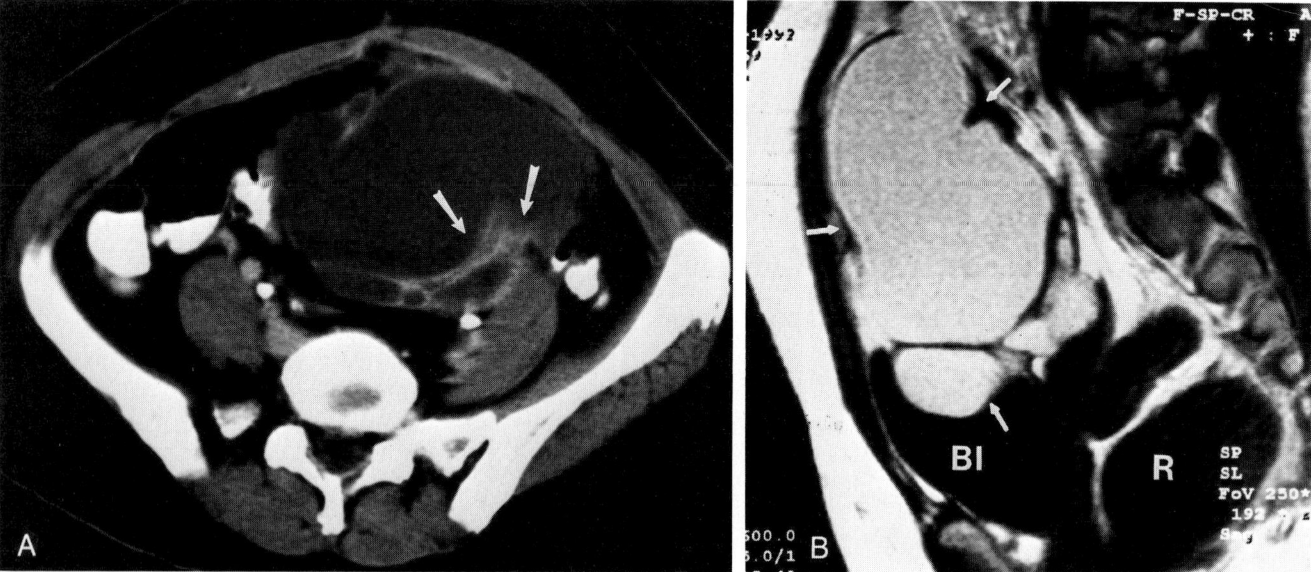

Figure 145–5. CT scan and MRI of ovarian cystadenocarcinoma. *A,* CT demonstrates a large, multiseptated cystic pelvic mass with focal areas of wall thickening and increased soft-tissue attenuation *(arrows). B,* The multiloculated cystic character of the mass *(arrows)* is well seen on a sagittal T_1-weighted MRI. The mass impresses the dome of the urinary bladder (Bl). The rectum (R) is partially fluid-filled.

neal and mesenteric surfaces or, more commonly, as small nodular masses or focal areas of thickening (Fig. 145–6). Unfortunately, CT fails to detect at least 40 per cent of peritoneal implants because masses less than 2 cm in size are not reliably seen. Factors that have been shown to influence detection of peritoneal masses include location, size, and presence of adjacent ascites. Ascites is seen in roughly half of patients with peritoneal metastases.

Pathologically, 30 per cent of serous cystadenocarcinomas contain psammomatous calcification, although only 12 per cent are visible on plain radiographs. In the case of ovarian cancer, small calcified peritoneal foci should be regarded as highly suspect for metastatic disease even if no soft-tissue component is present (Fig. 145–7). Likewise, the presence of nodal calcification, particularly in the absence of granulomatous disease, may also indicate metastatic disease.

Parenchymal liver metastases due to hematogenous spread are a late finding in ovarian cancer. Liver lesions in conjunction with a radiologic picture otherwise suggestive of primary ovarian cancer should prompt a search for an alternate primary site in the stomach or colon. Occasionally, loculated perihepatic fluid or peritoneal metastases may indent the liver contours so deeply that they simulate hematogenous intrahepatic metastases. Careful assessment of the relationship of the mass to the liver margin is necessary because peritoneal metastases will respect anatomic boundaries, such as the bare area of the liver.

Pseudomyxoma peritonei is a rare condition characterized by widespread dissemination of thick, gelatinous, mucinous material throughout the peritoneal cavity. Although it may be due to pancreatic or appendiceal tumors, malignant mucinous ovarian tumors are most often responsible. The classic CT appearance is multiple loculated intraperitoneal fluid collections, slightly above water density, which cause mass effect on adjacent organs, displacing bowel and indenting the contours of the liver and spleen (Fig. 145–8). Septations within the fluid are frequently thickened or calcified.

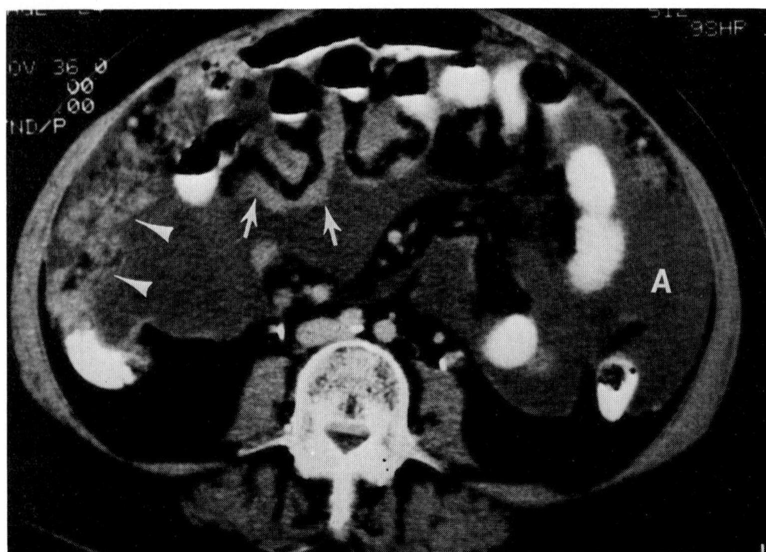

Figure 145–6. Peritoneal carcinomatosis. CT scan through the mid-abdomen demonstrates diffuse carcinomatosis secondary to ovarian carcinoma. An omental "cake" *(arrowheads),* extensive peritoneal metastases resulting in sheet-like coating of the small bowel mesentery *(arrows),* and ascites (A) are evidence of tumor spread.

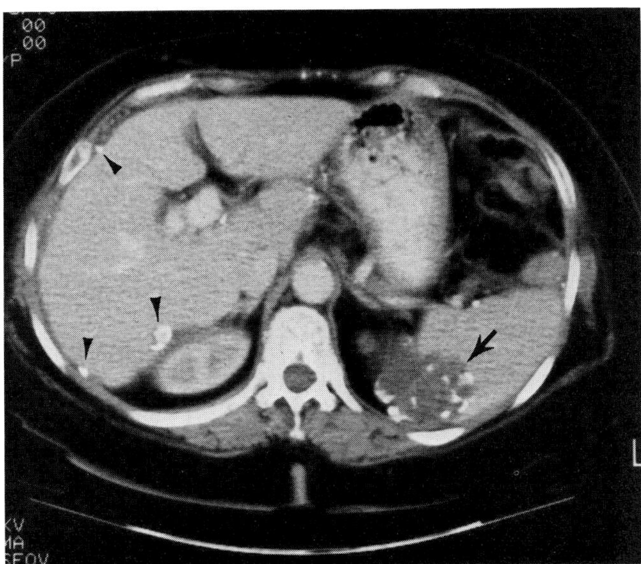

Figure 145–7. Calcified peritoneal metastases. Multiple densely calcified peritoneal implants along the liver capsule *(arrowheads)* represent metastatic spread from a serous cystadenocarcinoma of the ovary. A large soft-tissue mass with focal calcifications also invades the spleen *(arrow)*.

Loculated ascites alone is not pathognomonic for pseudomyxoma peritonei and may be seen with malignant serous tumors as well. Aspiration of mucin-containing peritoneal fluid is diagnostic.

SECOND-LOOK LAPAROTOMY IN OVARIAN CARCINOMA

After chemotherapy, patients who are clinically free of disease undergo a second-look laparotomy to assess for residual gross or microscopic tumor. If no cancer is found, the patient is spared the toxicity of further chemotherapy. In those with residual disease, therapy can be appropriately redirected.

Imaging has a role in evaluating some patients before second-look surgery because the detection of residual tumor may preclude re-exploration. Various studies of the use of CT before second-look laparotomy have shown CT to be highly specific for recurrent tumor (in the range of 80 to 100 per cent) but relatively insensitive (generally ranging from 30 to 50 per cent). Using high-resolution equipment and careful technique, Megibow et al. achieved a sensitivity of nearly 80 per cent. They noted the utility of correlating results of the patient's initial staging laparotomy with follow-up scans, because tumor most commonly recurs at sites of previously resected disease. When CT findings suggest residual tumor, percutaneous needle biopsy can be used for confirmation. A negative CT, however, cannot substitute for laparotomy because small peritoneal masses and microsopic disease are not reliably detected.

SCREENING FOR OVARIAN CANCER

In the hope that earlier detection will result in a significantly higher rate of cure than is currently possible, a number of large-scale studies have been undertaken to evaluate the role of ultrasound in screening for ovarian cancer. In more than 5000 asymptomatic pre- and postmenopausal women, Bhan et al. found that 6 per cent had persistent ovarian masses but only 0.2 per cent of the total had primary or secondary ovarian malignancies. The odds that a sonographically demonstrated mass represented an ovarian neoplasm were 1 in 2, but only 1 in 37 was malignant. In postmenopausal women, Goswamy et al. found adnexal masses in 3 per cent, with a 0.1 to 0.2 per cent rate of cancer. A more recent study by van Nagell et al. showed very similar results. The detection of benign epithelial tumors during screening is not without benefit, because an estimated 10 to 12 per cent would be expected to undergo malignant degeneration if left untreated.

The cost of widespread screening programs and their ultimate effectiveness have yet to be determined. In an individual patient with an adnexal mass, the following factors are associated with an increased likelihood of ovarian malignancy:

SIZE. Rulin et al. demonstrated in postmenopausal women that 64 per cent of masses larger than 10 cm were malignant, whereas 3 per cent of those less than 5 cm were.

ARCHITECTURE. Complex masses with increased solid components are more likely to be malignant. Thin-walled, simple-appearing cysts, particularly when smaller than 5 cm, are rarely malignant.

PERSISTENCE. Follow-up examination is useful in questionable lesions, particularly in premenopausal women in whom physiologic cysts are common.

DOPPLER STUDIES. Masses that demonstrate a low RI ($\leq$0.4), a low PI ($\leq$1.0), or evidence of neovascularity on color flow imaging are worrisome.

ELEVATED CA125 LEVELS. Increased levels of CA125, a tumor-associated antigen, should raise the level of suspicion of malignancy, particularly in postmenopausal women. Because it is not found in all women with ovarian malignancies, a normal CA125 is not reassuring.

SUGGESTION OF METASTATIC DISEASE. Ascites, lymph node, liver, or peritoneal masses point to carcinoma.

STROMAL–SEX CORD MALIGNANCIES

Neoplasms arising from sex cord or stromal cell lines comprise 3 to 6 per cent of all ovarian tumors. Because histologic appearance

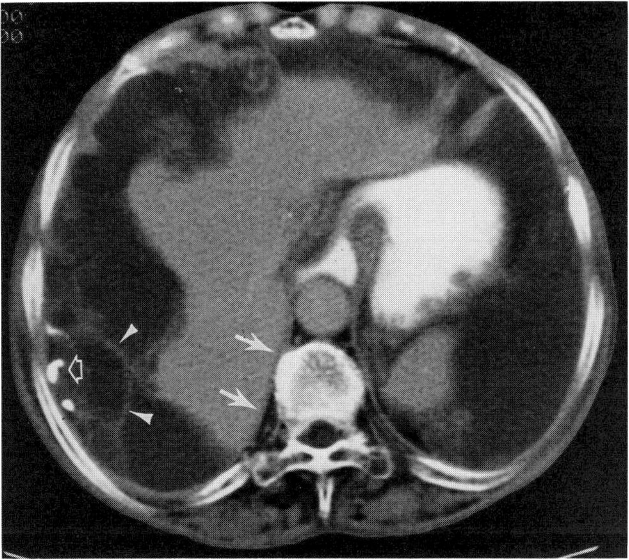

Figure 145–8. Pseudomyxoma peritonei. CT demonstrates loculated low attenuation collections that deeply indent the liver and, to a lesser extent, the spleen. Note that the "bare area" *(arrows)* of the liver is respected. Septations *(arrowheads)* and focal calcifications *(open arrow)* are also present.

does not accurately predict biologic behavior in these masses, their actual rate of malignancy is difficult to determine. Some consider all granulosa cell tumors to be malignant, while malignant thecomas and fibrosarcomas are extremely rare. The vast majority of Sertoli-Leydig cell tumors behave in a benign fashion.

Granulosa cell tumors, which account for 6 per cent of ovarian cancers, typically range between 5 and 15 cm in size and vary in appearance from homogeneously solid to multicystic masses. Unlike epithelial malignancies, granulosa cell cancers are unilateral and generally have an excellent prognosis because 90 per cent are Stage I (confined to the ovary) at diagnosis. The prognosis is worse in patients diagnosed over the age of 40, with large masses, or with extraovarian spread.

GERM CELL LINE MALIGNANCIES

Germ cell malignancies are uncommon, accounting for less than 5 per cent of all ovarian neoplasms. Subtypes include dysgerminoma; endodermal sinus tumor; embryonal tumor; malignant (immature) teratoma; and, rarely, choriocarcinoma. As is the case with testicular neoplasms, mixed histology is often present. Dysgerminoma, the most common germ cell tumor, resembles testicular seminoma in its radiosensitivity. Malignant or immature teratoma comprises tissues from all three germ cell layers, at least one of which is lacking in differentiation (Fig. 145–9). Only 2 per cent of benign teratomas undergo malignant change.

Germ cell malignancies typically affect postpubertal girls and young women. In the pediatric population, 85 per cent of malignant ovarian masses are of germ cell origin. Patients commonly present with abdominal pain (87 per cent) and/or mass (85 per cent). Ten per cent have acute symptoms related to rupture, torsion, or hemorrhage. Biologic markers such as elevated alpha-fetoprotein and human chorionic gonadotropin levels are common in some subtypes. Overall, the prognosis for Stage I tumors is good, particularly with dysgerminomas. Many of these patients can be treated with a unilateral oophorectomy to preserve fertility. However, the prognosis for patients with malignant degeneration of a previously benign teratoma is poor.

On imaging studies, these masses are typically large (averaging more than 15 cm in diameter), unilateral, and primarily solid, al-

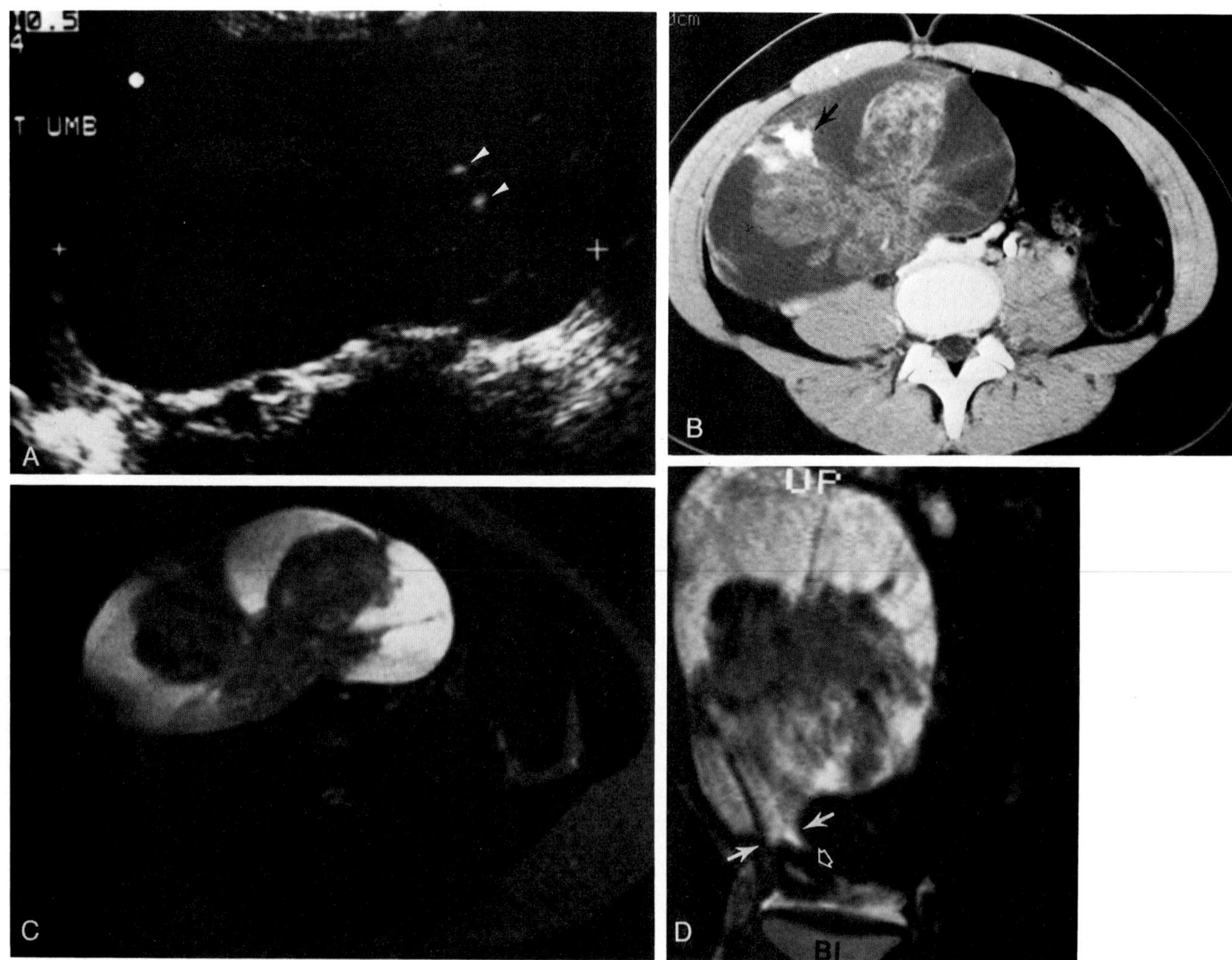

Figure 145–9. Malignant teratoma of the ovary in a 12-year-old girl. *A,* Ultrasound demonstrates a large heterogeneous left abdominal mass with cystic and solid regions as well as punctate echogenic foci due to calcification *(arrowheads). B,* CT section through the mid-abdomen shows coarse calcifications typical for malignant teratoma *(arrow)* within a well-circumscribed mass. Central solid components are surrounded by lower attenuation cystic regions. *C,* T_2-weighted axial MRI at a corresponding level demonstrates increased signal in peripheral cystic regions. The calcifications seen on CT are not apparent. Central soft-tissue components and septations are again visible. *D,* Coronal T_2-weighted MRI shows a large pedunculated mass arising in the pelvis *(arrows)* with central solid components and peripheral septated cystic regions. The uterus *(open arrow)* is identified by its high-signal endometrial stripe. (Bl = urinary bladder.)

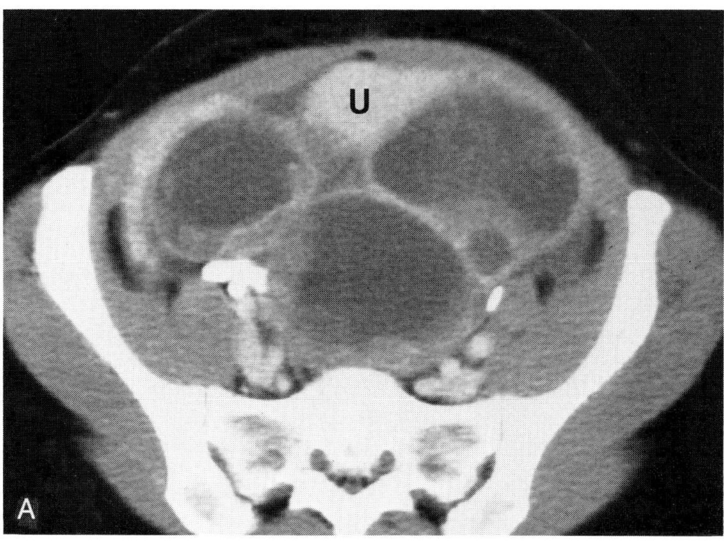

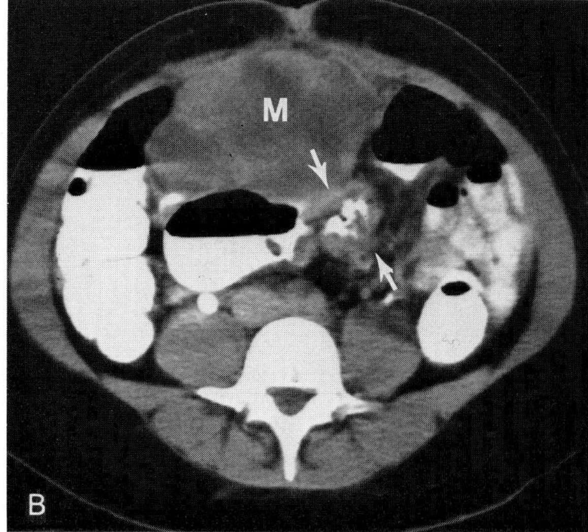

Figure 145–10. Metastatic colon carcinoma to the ovaries. *A,* CT shows shows large bilateral cystic and solid pelvic masses indistinguishable in appearance from primary ovarian cancer. (U = uterus.) *B,* At a more cephalad level, a focal area of bowel wall thickening and luminal narrowing in the sigmoid colon proved to be a primary colon carcinoma *(arrows).* Stranding densities in the adjacent fat indicate tumor spread into the mesentery. A portion of the pelvic mass is seen anteriorly (M).

though cystic, hemorrhagic, or necrotic areas are common. Bilateral primary masses are seen in 15 per cent of dysgerminomas but less frequently in other subtypes. Calcifications in dysgerminomas are typically stippled, in contrast to the coarse bone fragments seen in immature teratoma. Sixty to seventy per cent of patients have disease confined to the ovary at diagnosis. Modes of tumor spread include direct extension into adjacent organs and lymphatic and hematogenous dissemination. Lung, liver, and lymph node metastases are more common than with epithelial tumors. Ascites is found in 20 per cent, while 7 per cent will have an associated benign dermoid.

SECONDARY OVARIAN MALIGNANCIES

Fifteen per cent of malignant ovarian masses are the consequence of metastatic disease, most commonly from the breast, colon, or stomach. Less frequent primary sites include the pancreas, lung, endometrium, gallbladder, small bowel, and kidney. Melanoma, carcinoid, leukemia, and lymphoma occasionally spread to the ovaries. The term ''Krukenberg tumor'' is often used to refer to all ovarian metastases or those from gastrointestinal primaries, but it is more properly used to indicate a specific histologic pattern of mucin-containing signet cells within a sarcomatous stroma, generally from a gastric primary.

The clinical manifestations of metastatic ovarian tumors vary. Involvement of the ovary by breast cancer is frequent but often not apparent clinically or radiographically. Before current hormonal and chemotheraputic treatment, one third of breast cancer patients who underwent surgical castration were found to have unsuspected ovarian metastases. Other patients initially present with symptoms relating to the metastatic pelvic mass, rather than symptoms of their primary tumor. In fact, almost one third of patients with metastatic ovarian masses are initially suspected to have a primary ovarian carcinoma. Most of these patients will prove to have tumor originating in the gastrointestinal tract.

Secondary spread to the ovary is more common in pre- and perimenopausal women. It is a poor prognostic sign, associated with extraovarian metastases in more than 90 per cent of patients.

Ovarian metastases are often bilateral, large, and lobulated. Breast and gastric metastases may appear cystic but are usually predominantly solid. With current imaging techniques, colonic metastases are virtually indistinguishable from the mixed cystic and solid masses characteristic of primary ovarian epithelial carcinomas (Fig. 145–10). Even pathologically the distinction is often difficult.

Ascites, peritoneal nodularity, and omental metastases are common features of both primary ovarian cancers and malignancies that spread to the ovary secondarily. Hematogenous spread to the liver is relatively uncommon with ovarian primaries but is quite frequent with metastases. The stomach and colon in particular should be carefully evaluated for primary tumors if liver metastases are detected. It is prudent to consider the possiblity of ovarian metastases in any patient with an ovarian mass, particularly if there is a prior history of malignant disease or if liver lesions are present.

Bibliography

Amendola MA, Walsh JW, Amendola BE, et al: Computed tomography in the evaluation of carcinoma of the ovary. JCAT 5:179–186, 1981.

Bhan V, Amso N, Whitehead MI, et al: Characteristics of persistent ovarian masses in asymptomatic women. Br J Obstet Gynaecol 96:1384–1391, 1989.

Bourne T, Campbell S, Steer, et al: Transvaginal colour flow imaging: A possible new screening technique for ovarian cancer. Br Med J 299:1367–70, 1989.

Brenner DE, Shaff MI, Jones HW, et al: Abdominopelvic computed tomography: Evaluation in patients undergoing second-look laparotomy for ovarian carcinoma. Obstet Gynecol 65:715–719, 1985.

Buy J-N, Ghossain MA, Sciot C, et al: Epithelial tumors of the ovary: CT findings and correlation with US. Radiology 178:811–818, 1991.

Buy J-N, Moss AA, Ghossain MA, et al: Peritoneal implants from ovarian tumors: CT findings. Radiology 169:691–694, 1988.

Castro JR, Klein EW: The incidence and appearance of roentgenologically visible psammomatous calcification of papillary cystadenocarcinoma of the ovaries. AJR 88:886–891, 1962.

Cho KC, Gold BM: Computed tomography of Krukenberg tumors. AJR 145:285–288, 1985.

Clarke-Pearson DC, Brandy LC, Dudzinski M, et al: Computed tomography in evaluation of patients with ovarian carcinoma in complete clinical remission. JAMA 255:627–630, 1986.

Demopoulos R, Touger L, Dubin N: Secondary ovarian carcinoma: A clinical and pathological evaluation. Int J Gynecol Pathol 6:166–175, 1987.

Finkler NJ, Benacerraf B, Lavin PT, et al: Comparison of serum CA 125, clinical impression, and ultrasound in the preoperative evaluation of ovarian masses. Obstet Gynecol 72:659–63, 1988.

Fukuda T, Ikeuchi M, Hashimoto H, et al: Computed tomography of ovarian masses. JCAT 10:990–996, 1986.

Gerhenson DM: Malignant germ-cell tumors of the ovary. Clin Obstet Gynecol 28:824–838, 1985.

Ghossain MA, Buy J-N, Ligneres C, et al: Epithelial tumors of the ovary: Comparison of MR and CT findings. Radiology 181:863–70, 1991.

Goldhirsch A, Triller JK, Greiner R, et al: Computed tomography prior to second-look operation in advanced ovarian cancer. Obstet Gynecol 62:630–633, 1983.

Goswamy RK, Campbell S, Whitehead MI: Screening for ovarian cancer. Clin Obstet Gynaecol 10:621–642, 1983.

Hricak H: MRI of the female pelvis: A review. AJR 146:1115–1122, 1986.

Johnson RJ, Blackledge G, Eddleston B, et al: Abdomino-pelvic computed tomography in the management of ovarian carcinoma. Radiology 146:447–452, 1983.

Jolles CJ: Ovarian cancer: Histogenetic classification, histologic grading, diagnosis, staging, and epidemiology. Clin Obstet Gynecol 28:787–799, 1985.

Khan O, Cosgrove DO, Fried AM, et al: Ovarian carcinoma follow-up: US versus laparotomy. Radiology 159:111, 1986.

Kurjak A, Zalud I, Alfirevic Z: Evaluation of adnexal masses with transvaginal color ultrasound. J Ultrasound Med 10:295–297, 1991.

Mata JM, Inaraja L, Rams A, et al: CT findings in metastatie ovarian tumors from gastrointestinal tract neoplasms (Krukenberg tumors). Gastrointest Radiol 13:242–246, 1988.

Megibow AJ, Bosniak MA, Ho AG, et al: Accuracy of CT in detection of persistent or recurrent ovarian carcinoma: Correlation with second-look laparotomy. Radiology 166:341–345, 1988.

Megibow AJ, Hulnick DH, Bosniak MA, et al: Ovarian metastases: Computed tomographic appearances. Radiology 156:161–164, 1985.

Mitchell DG, Hill MC, Hill S, et al: Serous carcinoma of the ovary: CT identification of metastatic calcified implants. Radiology 158:649–652, 1986.

Moyle JW, Rochester D, Sider L, et al: Sonography of ovarian tumors: Predictability of tumor type. AJR 141:985–991, 1983.

Rulin MC, Preston AL: Adnexal masses in postmenopausal women. Obstet Gynecol 70:578–581, 1987.

Saul PB: Sex cord stromal tumors. Clin Obstet Gynecol 28:839–845, 1985.

Silverberg E, Boring CC, Squires TS: Cancer statistics 1990. CA 40:9–26, 1990.

Silverman PM, Osborne M, Dunnick NR, et al: CT prior to second-look operation in ovarian cancer. AJR 150:829–832, 1988.

Sparks JM, Varner RE: Ovarian cancer screening. Obstet Gynecol 77:787–792, 1991.

Stanhope CR, Smith JP: Germ cell tumours. Clin Obstet Gynecol 10:357–364, 1983.

Stern J, Buscema J, Rosenchien N, et al: Can computed tomography substitute for second-look operation in ovarian carcinoma? Gynecol Oncol 11:82–88, 1981.

Stevens SK, Hricak H, Stern JF: Ovarian lesions: Detection and characterization with gadolinium-enhanced MR imaging at 1.5T. Radiology 181:481–488, 1991.

van Nagell JR, DePriest PD, Puls LE, et al: Ovarian cancer screening in asymptomatic women by transvaginal sonography. Cancer 68:458–426, 1991.

Weiner Z, Thaler I, Beck D, et al: Differentiating malignant from benign ovarian tumors with transvaginal color flow imaging. Obstet Gynecol 79:159–162, 1992.

Young RH, Scully RE: Ovarian sex cord–stromal tumours: Recent advances and current status. Clin Obstet Gynecol 11:93–127, 1985.

The Breast

146 Breast Imaging Techniques

Christopher R.B. Merritt

SCREENING AND DIAGNOSIS

Diagnostic imaging plays two important roles in breast evaluation: screening and diagnosis. The most important role of breast imaging is in screening asymptomatic women for occult carcinoma. The objective of screening is early detection rather than specific characterization of an abnormality. Screening for breast cancer requires high sensitivity. Currently, mammography is the only breast imaging technique suitable for screening. By showing early changes associated with carcinoma, mammography may allow detection of cancer two years before it becomes palpable. The early detection of breast carcinoma results in a reduced likelihood of lymph node and distant metastases. This, in turn, is likely to result in improved long-term survival and provides some options for the management of primary tumor.

Because screening often does not provide a specific diagnosis, further clarification is frequently required. This is necessary to selecting patients for biopsy and avoiding procedures that add unnecessary risk or cost. Understanding the role of current and emerging breast imaging techniques requires an appreciation of the different objectives of screening and diagnosis as well as the imaging methods that complement mammography. The most important complement to mammography in breast diagnosis is ultrasonography because of its capability to differentiate solid and cystic lesions. Other diagnostic breast imaging techniques include computed tomography (CT), magnetic resonance imaging (MRI), digital image processing, and Doppler ultrasonography. In selected patients these methods have the potential of adding further specificity in the characterization of abnormalities identified by mammography and may permit the identification of abnormalities not shown by mammography. Complementary modalities overcome some of the weaknesses of mammography that are encountered in women with dense or dysplastic breast tissue or in the breasts of young, pregnant, or lactating females. These methods are useful following biopsy, augmentation mammoplasty, radiation therapy, or infection and often clarify equivocal mammographic or clinical findings, leading to a more accurate final diagnosis.

MAMMOGRAPHY

Carefully performed mammography is the single most important imaging modality for evaluation of the female breast, mainly because of its role in screening. Large studies have established the capability of mammography in the identification of preclinical (nonpalpable) carcinoma. In the Breast Cancer Detection Demonstration Project, in which mammography was performed on over 275,000 women, mammography was the only technique that detected 47 per cent of the cancers found, including 65 per cent of the cancers less than 1 cm in diameter.

Mammography is one of the most technically demanding of radiologic examinations, and diagnostic accuracy is likely to be compromised if technique is poor. The detection of microcalcifications and subtle alterations of soft-tissue architecture requires excellent spatial and contrast resolution. This can be achieved only by the use of proper equipment dedicated to the performance of mammography. The quality of mammography is also profoundly affected by the training and experience of the technologist who performs the examination and the diagnostician who supervises and interprets it. Modern mammographic technique now allows excellent image quality with minimal radiation to the breast. Even the most conservative estimates indicate the risk to the patient of carcinoma induction by the radiation used in modern mammography is negligible in relation to the benefits of early cancer detection.

Three methods have been used to perform mammography: film-screen mammography, xeromammography, and electron radiography. Today the majority of mammograms performed in the United States are done using film-screen techniques.

Film-Screen Mammography

Early mammography was performed using relatively insensitive industrial film that required large doses of radiation (often several rads) for a two-view examination. Efforts early in the 1970s led to the perfection of systems using a combination of single-emulsion film and an image-intensifying screen that permitted a significant reduction in mammographic exposure. Film-screen mammography now allows performance of a two-view examination of the breast with an average glandular dose of 0.1 to 0.2 rad.

Film-screen mammography must be performed with radiographic equipment especially designed for mammography. In order to enhance tissue contrast by taking advantage of the photoelectric effect, low–kilovolt peak (kVp) techniques are used, ranging from 25 to 28 kVp. Most x-ray tubes have molybdenum anodes, filtered with 0.3 mm molybdenum. The mammographic unit must be equipped to allow vigorous compression of the breast so that uniform penetration of the low-energy x-ray beam is achieved. Current systems also use small focal spot x-ray tubes and long tube-to-film distances to reduce geometric distortion. Microspot tubes are available with focal spot sizes of less than 300 μm, allowing magnification of suspicious areas for more precise evaluation. Moving grids to reduce scattered radiation are also available on dedicated systems, allowing more effective evaluation of dense breast tissue. With a grid, however, radiation doses may be increased up to threefold compared with nongrid film-screen mammography, unless higher speed film-screen combinations are substituted. The routine examination usually consists of craniocaudal and lateral views, although most radiologists now substitute oblique views for lateral views. Exaggerated medial and lateral craniocaudal views are sometimes necessary to supplement routine views. If a grid is available, it may be used to improve image quality in patients in whom it is not possible to compress the breast to a thickness of 4 to 5 cm.

The advantages of film-screen mammography include minimal radiation; low cost; and, unlike xeromammography, lack of dependence on complicated image processing hardware. High-quality images are possible when film-screen mammography is performed with dedicated radiographic equipment and vigorous compression.

Xeromammography

After several years of clinical trials, xeromammography was introduced in 1971 as an alternative for the high-dose film mammography then available. Unlike film-screen mammography, in which the image receptor is the film-screen combination, xeromammography uses a semiconductor plate composed of aluminum coated with selenium as the image receptor. Prior to exposure, an electric charge is placed on the plate. This charge is altered when the plate is exposed to x-rays. X-rays passing through the breast selectively discharge the plate in proportion to the density of the overlying tissue. The exposed plate contains a latent image of the breast composed of a pattern of electric charges. After exposure, the plate is sprayed with a negatively charged blue toner that is attracted to charged areas remaining on the plate after exposure. The image is then transferred to the surface of a sheet of paper, where it is fixed by heating. The resulting xerogram may then be viewed by reflected (overhead) light. An advantage of xeromammography is the property of edge enhancement, which facilitates detection of high-contrast objects, such as breast microcalcifications. Although xeromammography was popular during the 1980s, it has largely been replaced by film-screen mammography.

COMPLEMENTARY IMAGING MODALITIES

Ultrasonography

Ultrasound has been used in the diagnostic evaluation of the breast for more than 30 years and has emerged as a useful complement to mammography. The breast may be examined using either hand-held real-time scanners or dedicated automated breast scanners, many of which use a water path. High-resolution, real-time, small parts scanners operating at 5.0 to 10.0 MHz allow identification of masses as small as 1 to 2 mm within the breast (Fig. 146–1). These instruments are well suited for the characterization of palpable masses and are capable of differentiating cystic from solid masses—a distinction not possible with mammography. Ultrasound also aids in the diagnosis of nonpalpable masses seen on mammography. At the present time, sonography is used as an adjunct to mammography and physical examination. A screening role for ultrasonography has not been demonstrated. For the cystic versus solid characterization of clinically or mammographically detected masses, ultrasound is highly accurate. Solid lesions identified with ultrasound, however, cannot be characterized as benign or malignant with sufficient confidence to obviate the need for histologic confirmation of diagnosis. The role of breast ultrasound is summarized in Table 146–1.

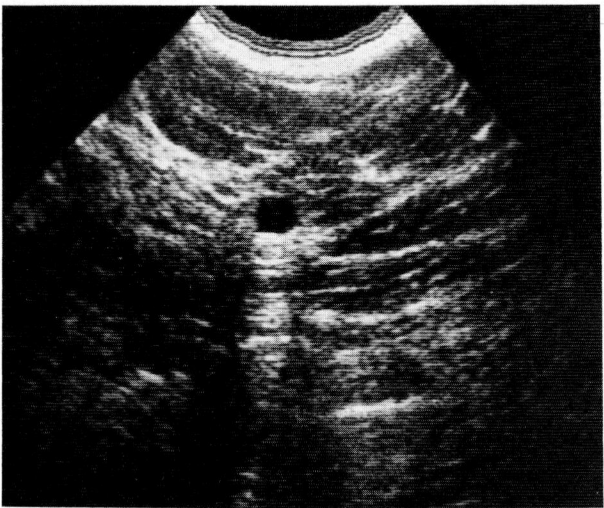

Figure 146–1. Real-time ultrasound scan obtained with a small-parts scanner operating at 10 MHz clearly shows a 3-mm cyst within the breast. Ultrasonography allows highly reliable differentiation of solid and cystic masses.

TABLE 146–1. INDICATIONS FOR ULTRASOUND MAMMOGRAPHY

1. To characterize a mass found on mammography as solid or cystic.
2. To characterize a clinically palpable mass not seen on mammography as solid or cystic.
3. To localize a mass for aspiration or biopsy.
4. To serve as the primary imaging examination of a woman younger than 30 who presents with a palpable mass.
5. To determine whether a localized abscess is present in a woman with acute mastitis.
6. To provide additional information when dense or dysplastic breast tissue renders mammographic findings indeterminate.

Advantages of sonography include the tomographic image it provides, the absence of ionizing radiation, its high accuracy in differentiating solid from cystic lesions, and its ability to provide diagnostic information in the dense or dysplastic breast. Ultrasound is not impeded by the presence of breast implants, as is mammography, and permits early identification of implant leakage. Disadvantages include problems in imaging the fatty breast; its inability to detect microcalcifications; and, of particular importance, its lack of sufficient sensitivity in detection of nonpalpable carcinoma to support its use in screening.

The use of Doppler ultrasound to identify the presence of tumor neovascularity in breast lesions is currently under investigation, and several reports have indicated promising results in differentiating benign and malignant masses. Doppler characteristics of tumor neovascularity that have been described include high flow velocity and low vascular impedance due to arteriovenous shunting.

Computed Tomography

CT has been used experimentally for breast evaluation. Studies performed after intravenous administration of iodinated contrast material have shown increased accumulation of contrast in carcinomas of the breast. Without contrast administration, it may not be possible to differentiate benign fibrocystic changes from carcinoma. The presence of CT values in excess of 25 units above baseline after contrast administration supports a diagnosis of carcinoma, although false-positive results are seen with a variety of benign diseases, including fibroadenomas, abscesses, and others. The time, expense, and radiation involved in CT of the breast render this examination of limited clinical utility at present.

Magnetic Resonance Imaging

MRI is emerging as a promising adjunct to mammography and ultrasonography in breast evaluation. MRI produces tomographic breast images in a noninvasive fashion. Optimal imaging requires the use of special coils to maximize sensitivity and spatial resolution. The value of MRI in the breast is the high tissue contrast possible and the enhancement of breast lesions with MRI contrast agents. Imaging sequences using fat suppression and gadopentetate dimeglumine infusion have been shown to permit differentiation of ductal and lobular carcinomas of the breast from benign conditions including fibrocystic condition and fat necrosis. Preliminary reports suggest that MRI may be superior to sonography in the evaluation of fatty and mildly dysplastic breasts. Gadolinium-enhanced MRI also appears to be a promising method for examination of patients with postoperative changes. With mammography, differentiation of

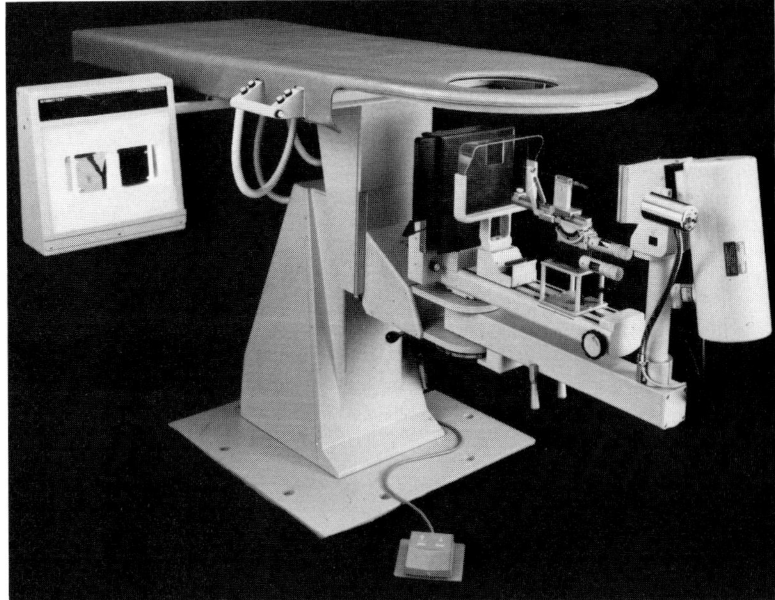

Figure 146–2. Mammography plays a key role in the localization of nonpalpable abnormalities for needle biopsy or excision. Stereotactic guidance provided by specialized mammographic units such as the one shown in this illustration permits rapid and precise biopsy of suspicious areas in the breast.

postoperative scarring from residual or recurrent cancer may be difficult. Using MRI differences in contrast enhancement often permits differentiation of these abnormalities. Good visualization of the tissue around silicon implants is another reported advantage of MRI. Although MRI provides excellent contrast resolution, spatial resolution with MRI is less than with mammography. The expense and limited throughput of current magnetic resonance scanners is a disadvantage. If MRI proves to have real potential in breast diagnosis, the development of low-cost dedicated breast units may be stimulated.

Stereotactic Localization

Although complementary methods of breast imaging improve specificity, many patients with breast lesions ultimately require histologic diagnosis. Since many abnormalities within the breast are not palpable, mammography and ultrasound are important in localizing lesions for excision, aspiration, or core needle biopsy. Stereotactic attachments for mammographic machines (Fig. 146–2) aid in precise needle placement for biopsy or localization prior to excision. These devices use a shift of position of the x-ray tube to produce exposures in which the position of the abnormality on the resulting films is used to calculate the location of the abnormality within the breast. This permits highly accurate needle localization or biopsy of the suspicious area and reduces the need for more expensive and invasive excisional biopsy procedures in many patients.

Digital Mammography

In conventional film-screen mammography, the x-ray film serves as both the image receptor and the viewing medium. Image capture requires high latitude, which conflicts with image display require-

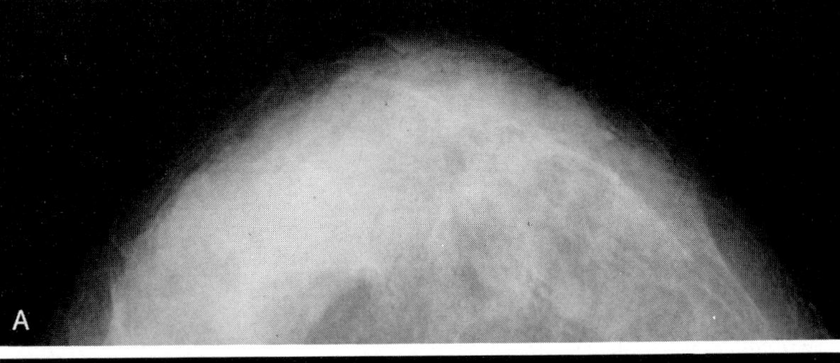

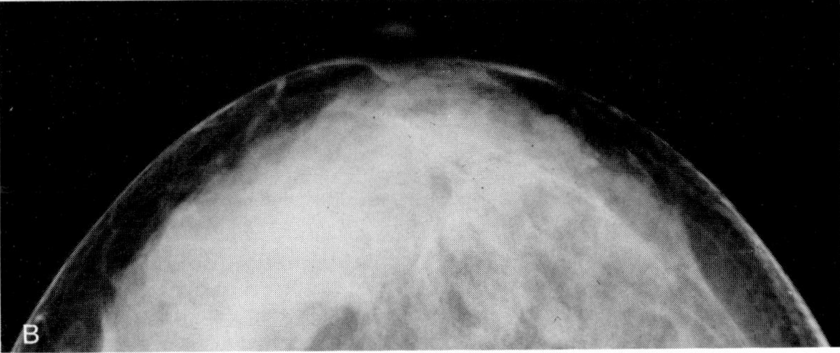

Figure 146–3. Digital mammography permits processing of breast images to improve the visibility of subtle findings. An unenhanced image is shown in *A*. After computer enhancement *(B)*, more detail is visible. Although still in development, digital methods are expected to become increasingly important in mammography.

ments for high contrast. These problems are addressed by film digitization or direct digital generation of mammographic images using laser-scanned photostimulable phosphor detectors or detector arrays. The full dynamic range of the breast may be captured using digital methods, and digital image processing may be used to display selected features (Fig. 146–3). Digital mammography at levels of spatial resolution comparable to film-screen mammography requires large amounts of digital storage, and display terminals are expensive. Despite these limitations, digital mammography and image processing are likely to play an increasingly important role in breast imaging in the future. A particularly exciting possibility is the development of automated analysis of digital mammograms using neural networks or other advanced intelligent systems.

Bibliography

Feig SA: Breast masses. Mammographic and sonographic evaluation. Radiol Clin North Am 30:67–92, 1992.

Gold RH, Sickles EA, Bassett LW, et al: Diagnostic imaging of the breast. Invest Radiology 19(Suppl):S43–S53, 1984.

Kopans DB, Meyer JE, Sadowsky N: Medical progress: Breast imaging. N Engl J Med 310:960–967, 1984.

Kopans DB: Nonmammographic breast imaging techniques. Current status and future developments. Radiol Clin North Am 25:961–971, 1987.

Moskowitz M: Mammography to screen asymptomatic women for breast cancer. AJR 143:457–459, 1984.

Pierce WB, Harms SE, Flamig DP, et al: Three-dimensional gadolinium-enhanced MR imaging of the breast: Pulse sequence with fat suppression and magnetization transfer contrast. Work in progress. Radiology 181:757–763, 1991.

147 Normal Roentgen Anatomy of the Breast

Thomas Lee Pope, Jr.

The development of a milk-producing organ during the Jurassic period 160 million years ago provided mammals with an evolutionary advantage over their predecessors. Today, however, diseases of the breast are among the leading causes of morbidity and mortality in women. One of the keys to improved survival in this malady is early diagnosis, and the mammogram is currently the imaging gold standard in this regard.

Knowledge of pathologic states, however, is difficult without an understanding of the basic normal anatomy. This chapter briefly reviews the basic normal roentgen and ultrasonographic anatomy of the breast. Histologic and gross features are included only as they pertain to the radiographic image. The important role of parenchymal patterns in the interpretation of breast images is also discussed.

ROENTGEN ANATOMY

The basic radiographic densities in the normal breast are fat, soft tissue, and calcium. The areola, nipple, skin, and breast parenchyma are all soft-tissue density. The subcutaneous and supporting fat represent the fat density. Calcifications also occur frequently in normal structures, as is discussed later. The major rationale for the low-kilovoltage technique used in mammography is to optimize the density distinction between these tissues. The basic roentgen features of each anatomic area are considered briefly below.

The Nipple and Areola

The nipple is a conical or cylindrical structure that protrudes from the center of the areola. It is covered with epidermis and has 10 to 15 lactiferous ductule openings. The technically adequate mammogram will image the nipple as a soft-tissue density in profile protruding anteriorly from the breast (Fig. 147–1). Many women have diminutive nipples or even inverted ones, and these should not necessarily be considered suspicious findings (Figs. 147–2 and 147–19). However, an inverted nipple with other roentgen abnormalities is a potentially ominous finding, as is discussed in Chapter 149. A potential pitfall in interpretation is a nipple that has not been placed in profile, as this may be misdiagnosed as a breast mass (Fig. 147–3).

The areola is a soft-tissue density situated centrally and anteriorly on the normal study and is difficult to see in most females. Some women will have prominent areolae, but these usually cause no diagnostic difficulties (Fig. 147–4).

The Skin

The combined width of the cutaneous epidermis and dermis is 0.5 to 2.0 mm histologically. Mammographically, skin is seen as a thin line of soft-tissue density surrounding the breast. Normal mammographic skin thickness varies from 0.7 to 2.7 mm, with the thickest areas being medial and inferior. Alterations in skin thickness or contour are important secondary effects of pathology. On film-screen mammography, unilateral skin thickness of more than 2.5 mm is suspicious for underlying pathology (Fig. 147–5).

Subcutaneous Fat

The normal breast contains fat of varying thickness and distribution beneath the skin, circumferentially surrounding the parenchymal elements, and interspersed between parenchymal tissue. This fat should be uniform in density throughout without distortion (Fig. 147–6).

At irregular intervals throughout the lobules of fat are soft-tissue strands 1 to 2 mm thick that take a curved course from the breast parenchyma to the skin's inferior surface. Best demonstrated by gross dissection and extending from the muscular fascia to the dermis, these septa—named Cooper's ligaments—represent a honeycomb network of fibrous tissue that completely encloses fat lobules throughout the breast and lends support to the breast paren-

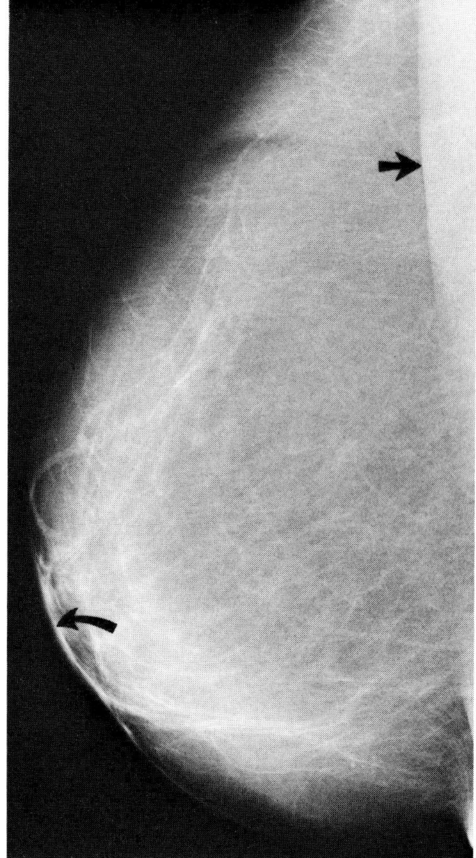

Figure 147–1. Oblique view of the left breast shows proper technique with the nipple in profile *(curved arrow)* and the pectoralis major muscle oriented parallel to the x-ray beam *(arrow)*. This muscle landmark shows that the technologist has reached very close to the chest wall.

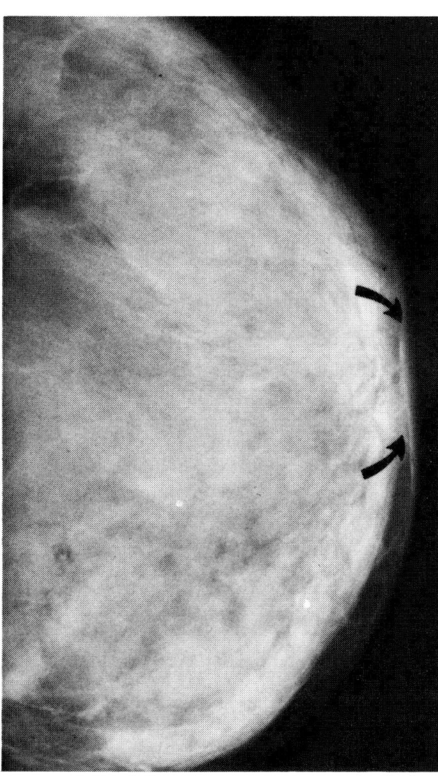

Figure 147–2. Craniocaudad (CC) view of the right breast of a woman who has had retracted nipples since childhood *(curved arrows)*. This is a common normal variant.

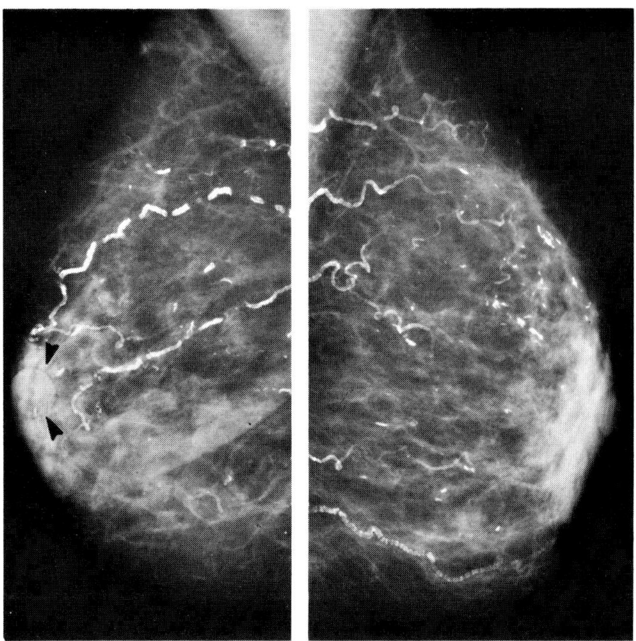

Figure 147–3. CC views of a 68-year-old woman showing a nipple that has not been placed in profile *(arrowheads)*. Note that the "pseudomass" is surrounded by air. This technical problem should not be misdiagnosed as a breast mass.

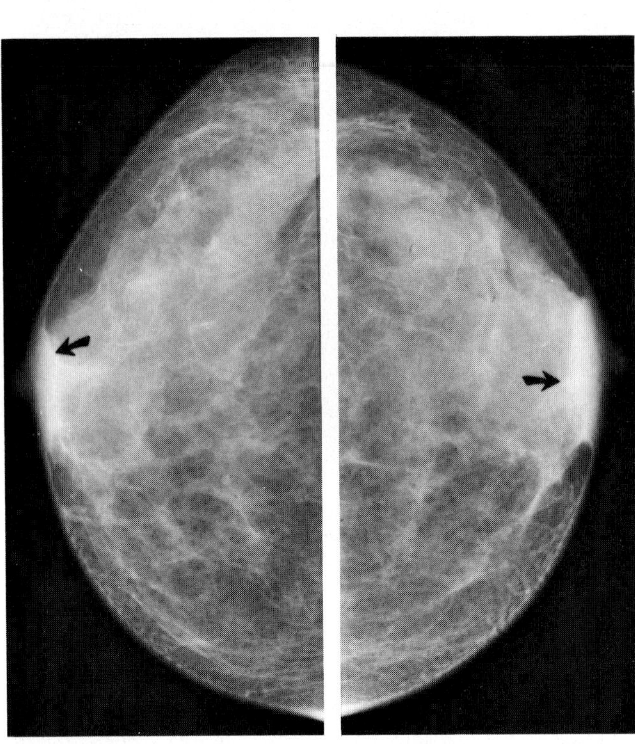

Figure 147–4. CC views of both breasts in a woman with prominent areolae *(curved arrows).* This is a normal variant and should not be mistaken for pathology.

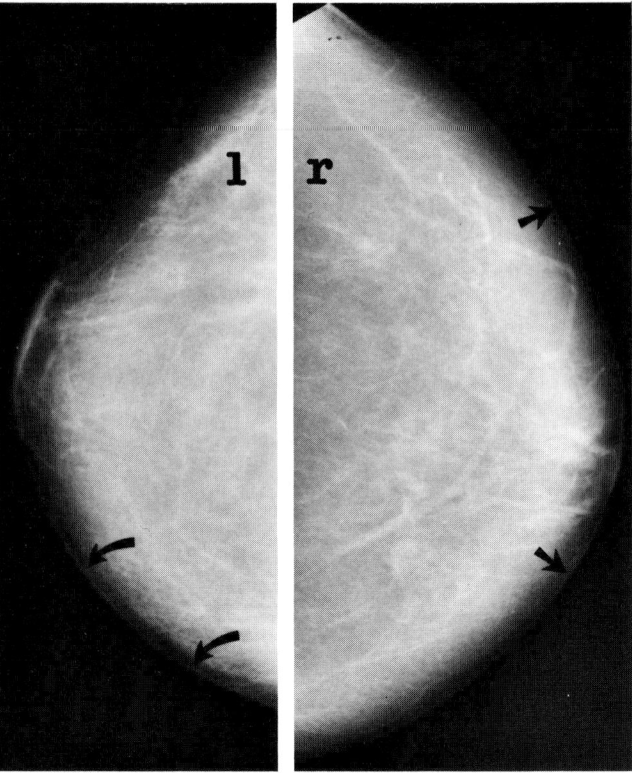

Figure 147–5. CC views of both breasts in a 58-year-old woman treated by lumpectomy and radiation therapy show skin thickening on the left of approximately 4 mm *(curved arrows).* The right breast shows a normal skin thickness of approximately 1 mm *(arrows).*

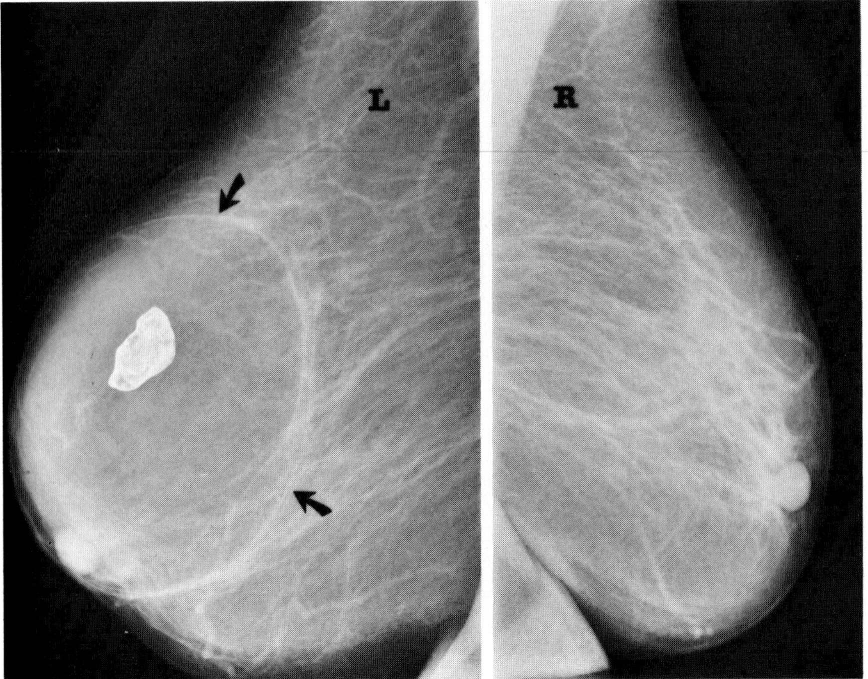

Figure 147–6. Oblique views of a 67-year-old woman with palpable mass in the left breast show a totally fatty replaced left breast and a fatty density with a large calcification representing a lipoma *(arrows).* A minimal amount of glandular tissue is present in the subareolar region on the right.

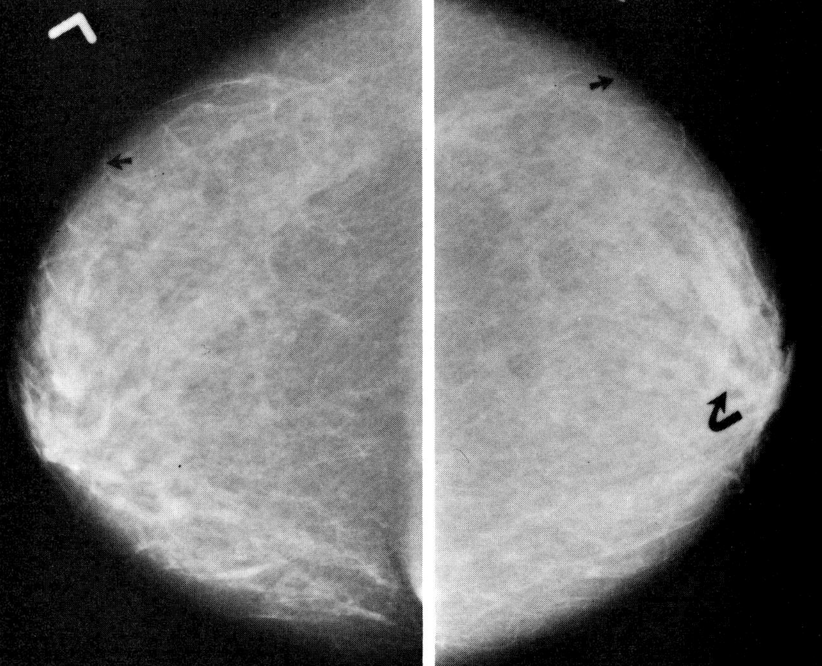

Figure 147–7. CC views of a bilateral mammogram in a 51-year-old woman show normal Cooper's ligaments *(arrows)*. These should always be curved and approximately 1 to 2 mm in thickness. Incidentally noted is ductal ectasia in the subareolar region on the right *(curved arrow)*.

chyma. Radiographically, these thin lines are best demonstrated in the subcutaneous fat and should always be slightly curved between the skin surface and the parenchyma. Straightening or thickening of Cooper's ligaments may indicate pathology in the underlying adjacent parenchyma (Figs. 147–7 and 147–8).

Breast Parenchyma and Stroma

The majority of soft-tissue density on the mammogram is composed of glandular tissue, the parenchyma and its supporting structure, the stroma. In the normal mammogram, the distribution of glandular elements may be variable, but usually they are concentrated in the subareolar and upper outer quadrant regions of the breast (Fig. 147–9). Asymmetry is common, however, and without other clinical or mammographic abnormalities should not be considered pathologic. Some women, however, may require close follow-up because of asymmetry (Fig. 147–10).

In the premenopausal nulliparous woman, glandular elements may be quite dense and occupy most of the volume of the breast (Fig. 147–11). In the lactating breast, glandular elements are also much more prominent because of the engorged milk-producing structures (Fig. 147–12). In both of these instances, soft-tissue masses may be obscured by these normal glandular elements. The other extreme in density is in the postmenopausal female after the glandular elements have involuted. Histologically, glandular structures are still present but are too small to be imaged on the mammogram. In this instance, there is total fatty replacement of the breasts. Soft-tissue densities are much more easily seen in this breast pattern (Fig. 147–13).

The variation in the volume of glandular tissue occupying the normal breast between these two extremes determines the parenchymal pattern. Some studies have shown higher rates of breast cancer with certain breast parenchymal patterns. However, most authorities today believe that the type of parenchymal pattern has little clinical or radiographic significance. Our report usually includes a comment about the amount of residual glandular tissue, but this is mainly for statistical reasons and may make us look more closely at our mammograms.

Other "Normal" Features

There are other mammographic findings that occur with such frequency that it is rational to call them "normal." Many normal women will exhibit very prominent skin pores, and these are imaged as uniformly distributed lucencies covering the breast on all projec-

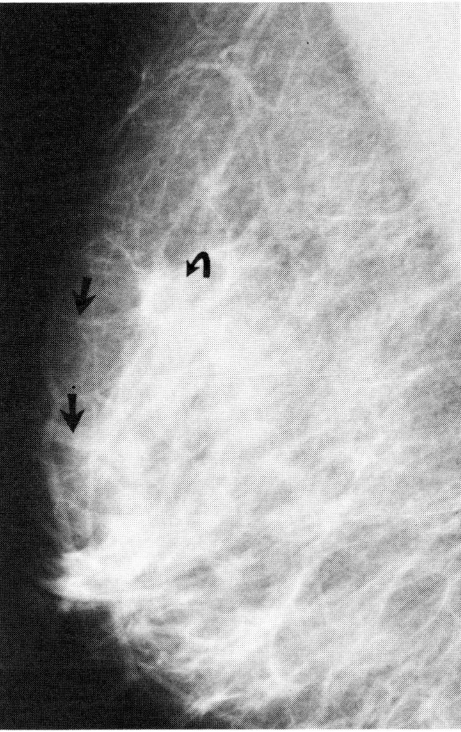

Figure 147–8. Oblique view of a 50-year-old woman with a 2-cm carcinoma in the upper half of the breast *(curved arrow)*. Thickening of the adjacent Cooper's ligaments is noted *(arrows)*.

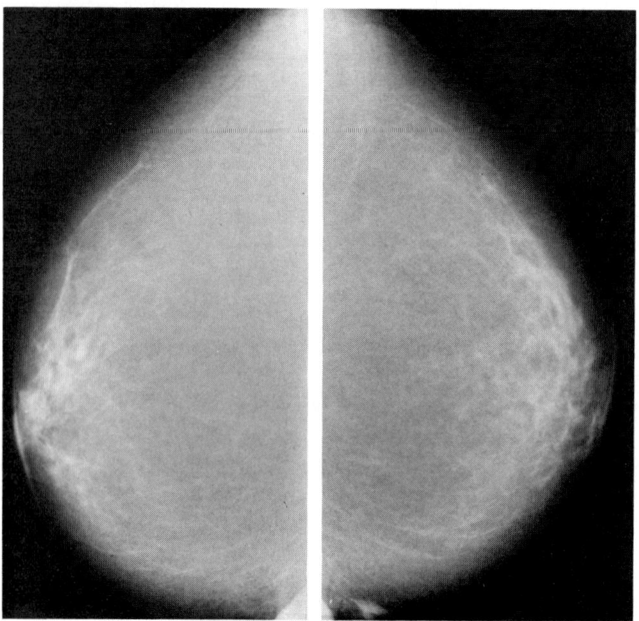

Figure 147–9. Bilateral mammogram on a woman with glandular tissue concentrated mainly in the upper outer quadrants of each breast. In the normal study, this is where most of the glandular tissue characteristically resides.

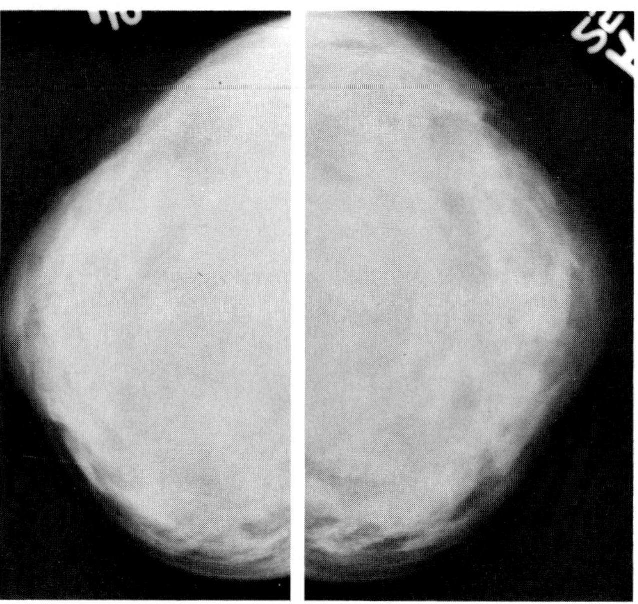

Figure 147–11. Bilateral CC views of a film-screen mammogram in a 40-year-old woman with dense residual fibroglandular tissue. Soft-tissue masses may be obscured by this degree of density in some women.

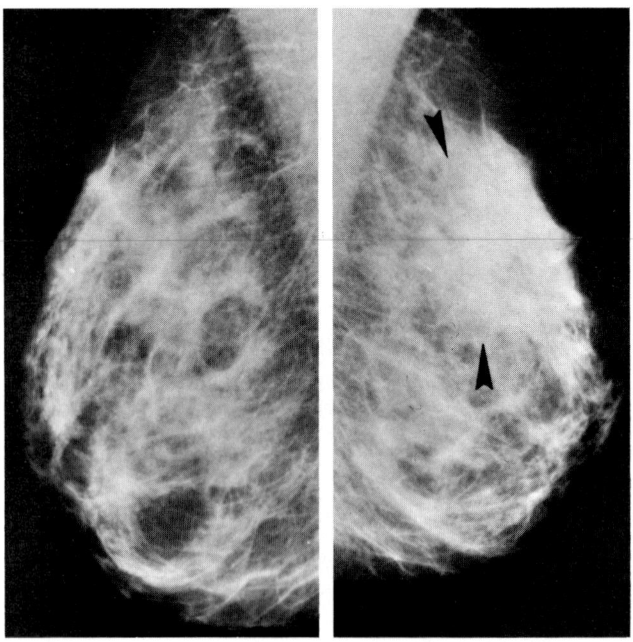

Figure 147–10. Oblique views of a 45-year-old woman showing asymmetry in the upper outer aspect of the right breast *(arrowheads)*. There were no associated clinical findings, and biopsy was not performed. Asymmetry without other clinical or mammographic findings is not a reliable sign of pathology.

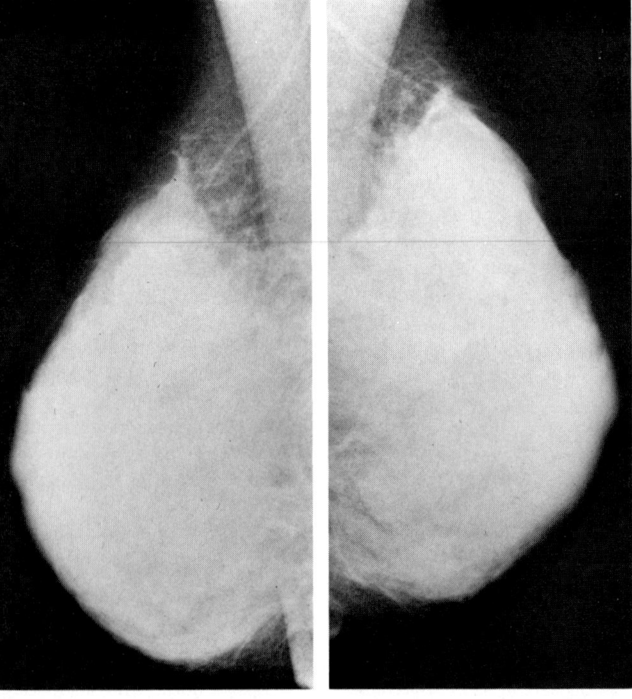

Figure 147–12. Oblique views of a film-screen mammogram of a 30-year-old woman during lactation show the concentration of dense glandular elements in this clinical situation.

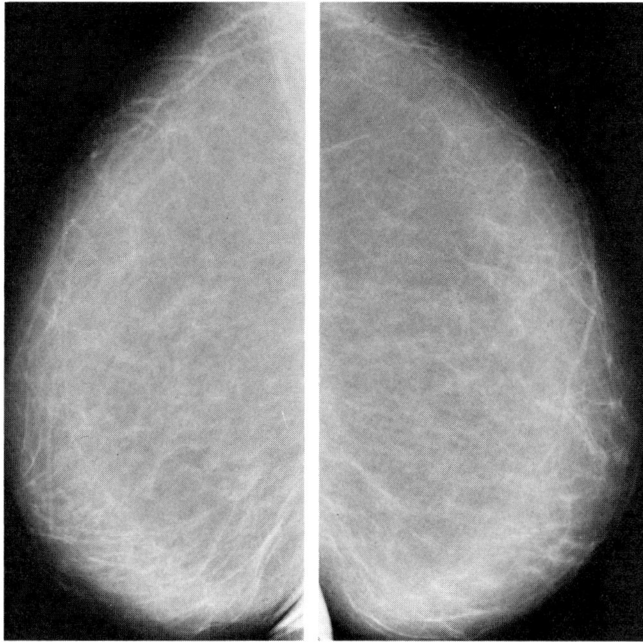

Figure 147–13. Bilateral film-screen study in a multiparous 48-year-old woman with a totally fatty replaced breast. Connective tissue strands and vessels can be seen as thin linear soft-tissue densities.

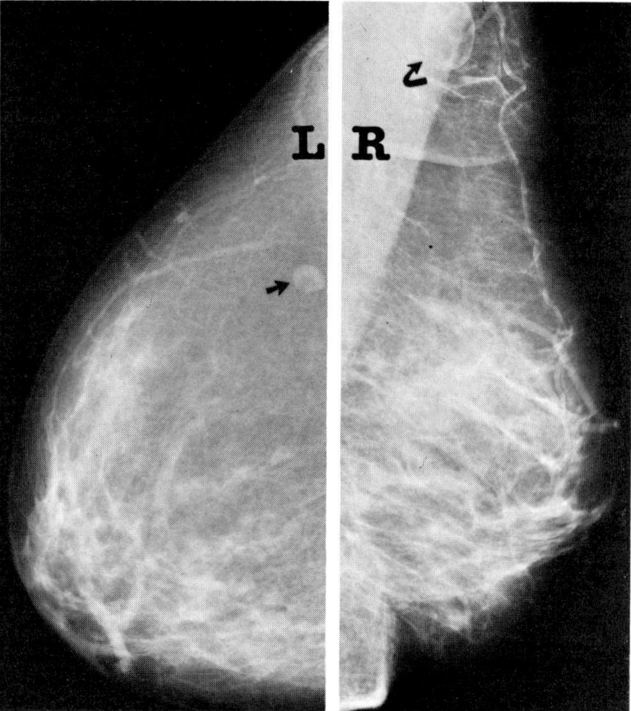

Figure 147–15. Oblique mammograms in two different patients. The left study shows a characteristic intramammary node with its fatty hilum *(arrow).* The examination on the right shows fatty replaced nodes in the axilla *(curved arrow).* An intramammary lymph node should have a central fatty hilum to be definitively called normal.

tions (Fig. 147–14). Prominent skin pores should not be confused with pathology. Another common entity is the intramammary lymph node (Fig. 147–15). These well-demarcated soft-tissue densities range in size from 2 mm to 3 cm and are generally located in the upper outer quadrants of the breast. They should show a central fatty hilum to be definitively classified as nodes, and replacement of this normal fatty hilum by soft-tissue density is better than size as a pathologic criterion (Fig. 147–16).

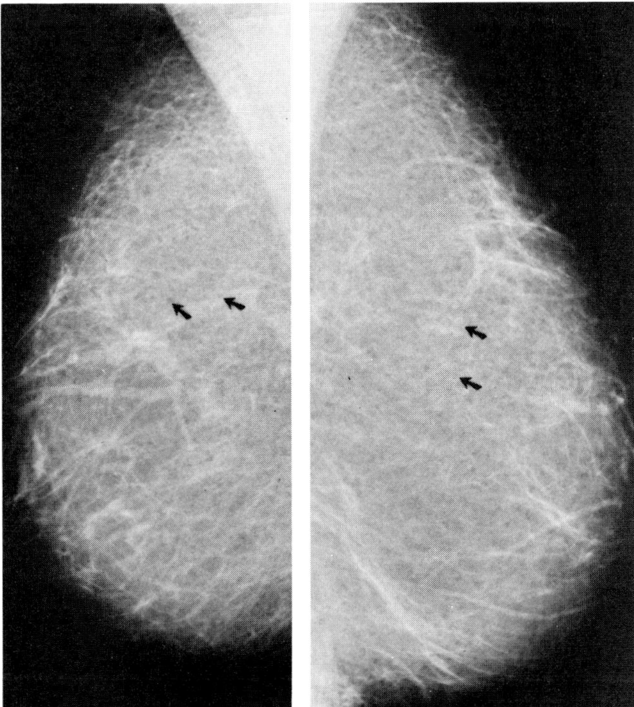

Figure 147–14. Oblique views of a 38-year-old woman show very prominent skin pores causing regularly spaced lucencies on the mammogram.

Blood vessels may be visualized in atrophic breasts as linear undulating soft-tissue densities. Veins are usually larger than arteries and do not show atherosclerotic change. Arteries are usually smaller and in older women may show typical parallel linear calcifications. There is no documented strong relationship of arterial calcification to anything other than aging (Fig. 147–17). Punctate skin calcification can also be produced by underarm deodorants. These densities are usually located in the axillae and may be confused with microcalcifications. Patients should be requested not to wear deodorant before undergoing mammography (Fig. 147–18). Calcifications on the skin mimicking microcalcifications can also be produced by zinc oxide ointment, and it is important to know if a patient is wearing this cream (Fig. 147–19).

Other unusual causes of calcifications are tattoos and keloids. However, these should be obvious and not present diagnostic difficulties. Other calcifications routinely occur in the normal breast, particularly in the lactiferous ductules, but these are discussed elsewhere.

Moles and some dermal skin growths are common on the breast and are usually easily diagnosed clinically. It is important to document their skin location with a radiopaque marker to avoid misdiagnosing them as breast masses (Fig. 147–20).

THE MALE BREAST

The male breast is histologically similar to that of the female except that it is smaller, and under normal circumstances only

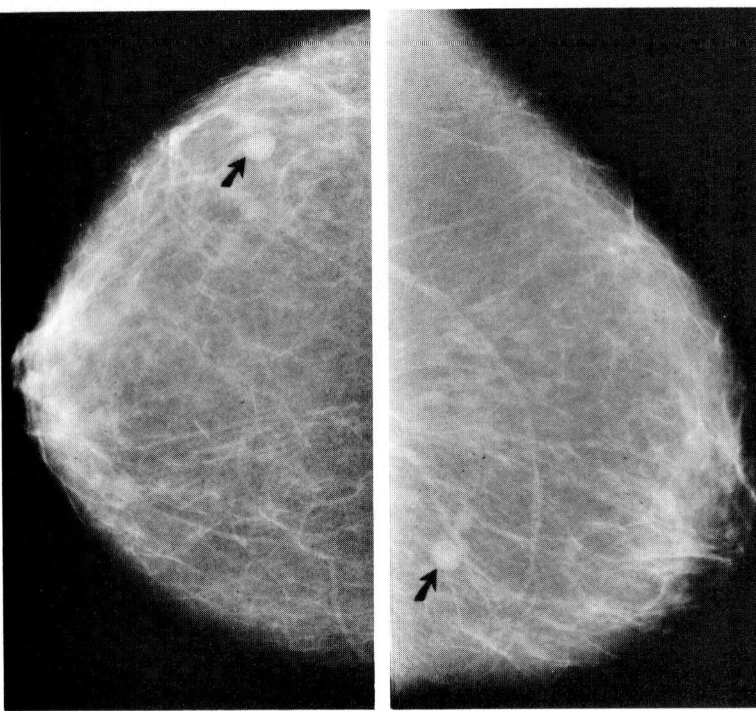

Figure 147–16. Craniocaudad *(left)* and oblique *(right)* views of the left breast in a 37-year-old woman with a history of breast carcinoma on this side treated by lumpectomy and radiation therapy. A well-demarcated 7-mm density with no fatty hilum is noted. This was surgically removed and was a benign lymph node. However, the lack of the fatty hilum and the history of carcinoma were appropriate reasons for biopsy.

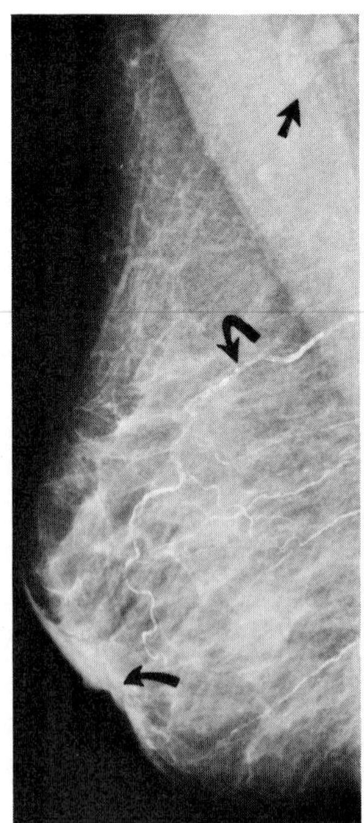

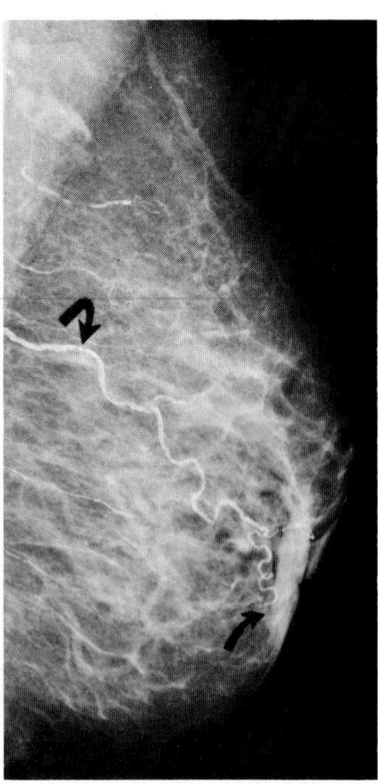

Figure 147–17. Bilateral mammogram on a 70-year-old woman showing the classic arterial calcification *(curved arrows),* fatty replaced nodes in the axillae *(straight short arrow),* and inverted nipples, which had been present since childhood *(curved arrows).*

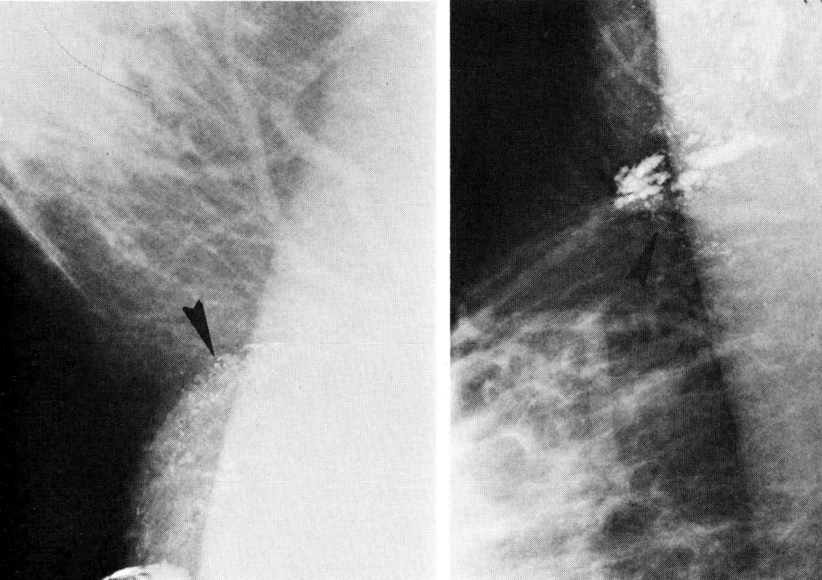

Figure 147–18. Coned-down view of oblique projections of both breasts show punctate calcific densities in the axillae caused by deodorant *(arrowheads)*. Patients should be asked not to wear deodorant prior to their examination, as it may be misinterpreted as microcalcifications.

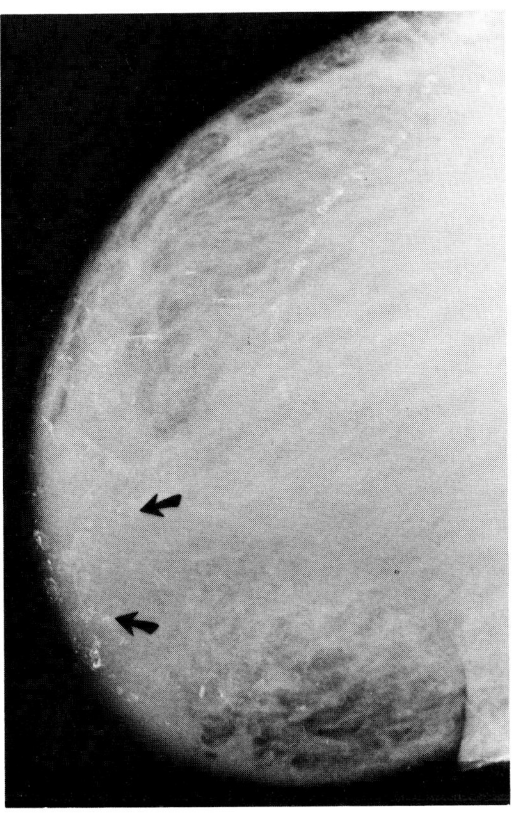

Figure 147–19. Oblique view of the left breast in a woman with clinical mastitis shows "pseudocalcifications" caused by zinc oxide cream *(arrows)*. These should not be misdiagnosed as microcalcifications.

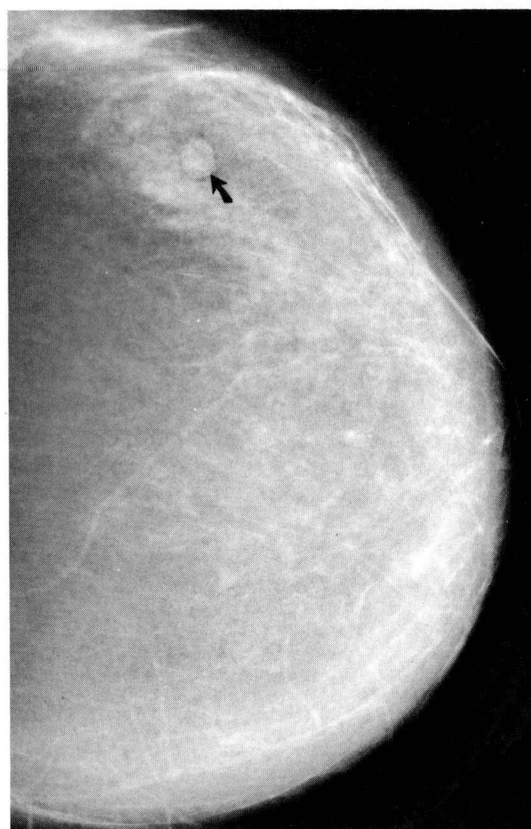

Figure 147–20. CC view of a right breast showing well-demarcated density surrounded by air in the left lateral aspect of the breast. The woman had a nevus on the skin in this exact location. It is very important to know if the skin lesions are present to avoid misdiagnosing them as masses.

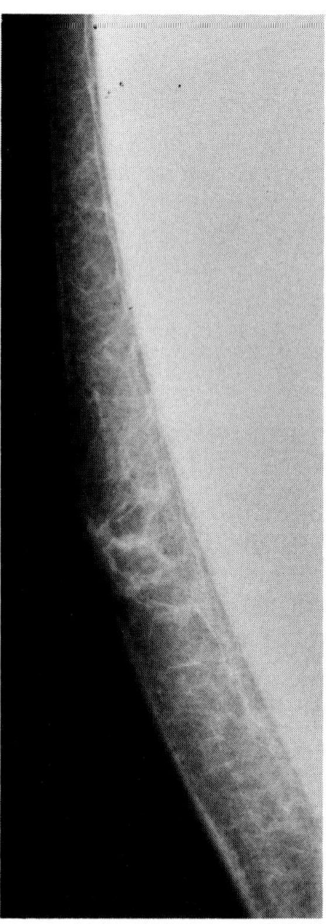

Figure 147–21. Oblique mammogram of the left breast in a male showing paucity of glandular elements. The large soft-tissue density posteriorly is the pectoralis major muscle.

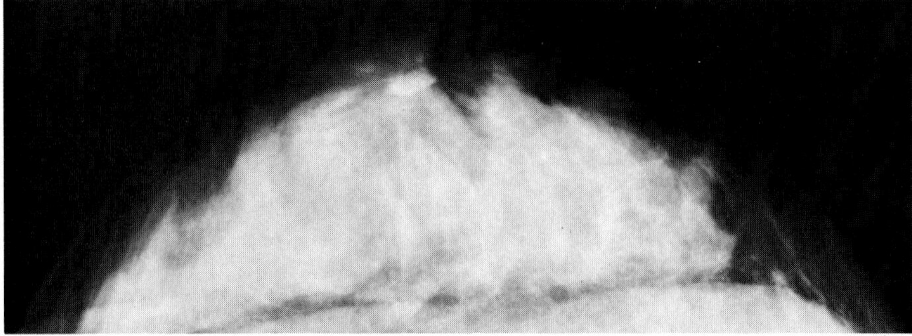

Figure 147–22. CC mammogram in a man with gynecomastia shows substantial enlargement of the breast with marked soft-tissue density throughout. No other radiographic abnormality is seen.

rudimentary ductules and a small amount of fat are present. Mammography in males shows predominantly fat with minimal soft-tissue ductular structures (Fig. 147–21). In obese and older men and in males on steroid therapy, fat may accumulate in the benign breast in varying quantities. A common clinical situation encountered in the male is gynecomastia, or a benign proliferation of glandular elements either unilaterally or bilaterally. This condition is most often idiopathic and commonly seen during puberty, but it has a number of other etiologies. The mammogram in this situation looks very much like that of a female (Fig. 147–22).

Acknowledgments

I wish to thank Angie Overby and Dese Simpson for their always excellent secretarial assistance.

Bibliography

Azzopardi JG: Problems in Breast Pathology. Philadelphia, WB Saunders Company, 1979.

Boyd NF, O'Sullivan B, Fishell E, et al: Mammographic patterns and breast cancer risk: Methodologic standards and contradictory results. JNCI 72:1253–1259, 1984.

Carlile T, Kopecky KJ, Thompson DJ, et al: Breast cancer prediction and the Wolfe classification of mammograms. JAMA 254:1050–1053, 1985.

Egan RL, Mosteller RC: Breast cancer mammographic patterns. Cancer 40:2087–2090, 1977.

Haagensen DC: Diseases of the Breast. Philadelphia, WB Saunders Company, 1986.

Kapdi C, Parekh NJ: The male breast. Radiol Clin North Am 21:137–148, 1983.

Lindfors KK, Kopans DB, McCarthy KA, et al: Breast-cancer metastasis to intramammary lymph nodes. AJR 146:133–136, 1986.

Sadowsky N, Kopans DB: Breast cancer. Radiol Clin North Am 21:51–65, 1983.

Wellings SR, Wolfe NJ: Correlative studies of the histological and radiographic appearance of the breast parenchyma. Radiology 129:299–306, 1978.

Wolfe JN: Breast patterns as an index of risk for developing breast cancer. AJR 126:1130–1139, 1976.

148 Benign Diseases of the Breast

Marc J. Homer

The term *fibrocystic disease* is used so differently by gynecologists, surgeons, radiologists, and pathologists that essentially it no longer conveys a specific meaning. Painful breasts, breasts with multiple cysts, nodular breasts, and breasts that are excessively tender during phases of the normal menstrual cycle have all been lumped together under the term *fibrocystic disease*. Forms of this disease include mastitis fibrosa cystica, chronic cystic mastitis, fibroadenomatosis, cystic mastopathy, adenosis, mazoplasia, and mammary dysplasia. Many clinicians now believe that most types of fibrocystic disease are not a disease in the usual sense of the word but rather represent a spectrum of physiologic changes. Depending on the criteria used by the pathologist, every breast contains areas of fibrocystic disease. In the opinion of many physicians knowledgeable about the breast, since fibrocystic disease no longer has a clearly defined meaning, the phrase *fibrocystic change* may be more appropriate. For this reason, the term *fibrocystic disease* is not used in this chapter.

THE ROLE OF MAMMOGRAPHY IN BENIGN BREAST DISEASE

Mammography can detect occult benign breast disease and can often demonstrate the total extent of clinical palpable benign breast disease. But since no action is taken for the presence of benign breast disease, this is really not the purpose for performing mammography in women with fibrocystic change. The real role of mammography in benign breast disease is as an additional examination of the breast for the exclusion of a malignant process. The physical examination of the painful breast or the breast with multiple masses obviously will be less sensitive than usual in detection of malignancy. Mammography serves a crucial complementary role to help exclude malignancy. It is true that with many patients having marked fibrocystic change, both breast palpation and the initial mammogram will be difficult to interpret. Yet when the patient returns for a repeat mammogram and breast palpation at a later date, it is far easier for the radiologist to compare area to area on the mammogram in search of any significant interval change than it is for the clinician to recall from his or her chart record the precise size, consistency, and location of every palpable abnormality.

Mammographic Signs of Benign Breast Disease

The cardinal mammographic signs of benign breast disease are mass, asymmetrical density, microcalcification, and an incongruity between the overall breast density and the patient's age. The first three of these signs are also primary signs of breast carcinoma and therein lies much of the difficulty in mammographic interpretation. Signs of benign breast disease may be identical to signs of malignant breast disease, and often differentiation is absolutely impossible. Ninety per cent of all masses and asymmetrical densities prove to be benign. Similarly, almost all macrocalcifications and 90 per cent of microcalcifications within the breast prove to be benign.

Mammography is an exquisitely sensitive but often nonspecific examination. Rather than trying to guess whether a specific mammographic abnormality is a manifestation of a benign or a malignant process, the radiologist instead should be deciding whether the area needs immediate biopsy or appropriate follow-up examinations. Radiologists are in error if they believe that mammography can reliably differentiate between a benign and a malignant process. This role should be left to the pathologist with his or her microscope. The remainder of this chapter illustrates some of the more prevalent forms of benign disease of the breast, including benign breast masses, inflammatory disorders and trauma, benign breast calcifications, and abnormal breast density.

BENIGN BREAST MASSES

Cysts

Breast cysts form from the enlargement and dilatation of the lactiferous ducts. While they are commonly multiple, a breast cyst may on occasion be solitary (Fig. 148–1). Cysts occur mainly in women 30 to 50 years of age and are found less frequently in younger and older women. Simple breast cysts contain clear fluid and are lined by a single layer of epithelial cells. The size and number of cysts may wax and wane during the menstrual cycle and over the course of years (Fig. 148–2). Typically cysts do not calcify, but on rare occasions they may have a thin border of calcium. Although traditional teaching relies on the sharp border of a cyst to differentiate it from a malignant mass, this sign is unreliable. Commonly, a large border of a benign cyst may appear poorly defined when overlapped by areas of normal breast stroma (Fig. 148–3). A collapsed cyst or one that has just been aspirated may also possess quite irregular margins. Conversely, some forms of breast cancer such as medullary carcinoma may have very sharp borders.

If a cyst is palpable, it can and should be easily differentiated from a solid mass by a simple needle aspiration. This is a procedure that, in effect, is both diagnostic and therapeutic. There is a controversy among clinicians about the usefulness of the cytologic examination of the aspirated fluid. Some believe that if the fluid is a clear yellow transudate, any potentially significant information gained from cytologic analysis is so minimal that the cost and time involved are not routinely justified. Other clinicians send all aspirated fluid for cytologic examination.

With the use of ultrasound, the characterization of a nonpalpable mass as solid or cystic has become straightforward. A nonpalpable, noncalcified mass should be examined by ultrasound if there is any possibility that it could represent a cyst. If it proves to be a cyst on ultrasound, then, depending on the preference of the ultrasonographer and the referring physician, it can be aspirated under ultrasound guidance or it can be followed periodically. If the mass proves to be a complex cyst or solid mass, it should be excised to rule out the possibility of a malignancy.

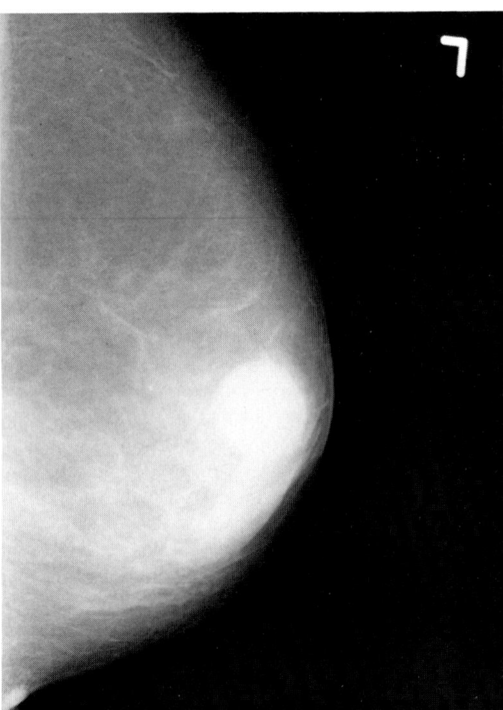

Figure 148–1. This subareolar mass has the typical features of a cyst, including sharply defined borders and no calcification. It was aspirated and totally collapsed, thereby proving its etiology.

Fibroadenoma

A fibroadenoma is a tumor that develops under the hormonal influence of estrogen. It is a firm mass composed of a proliferation of connective tissue and epithelial cells. Typically these tumors begin to appear after puberty, are commonly present up through age 30, and eventually involute, undergoing mucoid degeneration and hyalinization. During this involutionary process they may develop calcifications varying in appearance from punctate microcalcifications to popcorn macrocalcifications (Fig. 148–4). Clinically these tumors are firm, smooth, freely mobile within the breast, and lobulated.

When the fibroadenoma possesses characteristic macrocalcifications, its diagnosis is clear. However, when the mass is noncalcified or contains punctate microcalcifications, differentiation from malignancy becomes a real concern. The traditional teaching is that the smooth, sharp margins of a fibroadenoma serve as a differential point between benign and malignant. However, commonly the margins of a benign fibroadenoma may appear irregular (Fig. 148–5). In addition, margins of the benign fibroadenoma may be obscured by normal breast stroma so that evaluation of its entire border is impossible. Ultrasound examination will demonstrate a solid mass with weak internal regular homogeneous echoes. In practice, if the mass is solitary, even a "typical" ultrasonic appearance suggestive of a fibroadenoma will not stop an excisional biopsy. A fibroadenoma may sometimes grow to a very large size and the descriptive term *giant fibroadenoma* is then used. However, histologically there is no difference between it and a small fibroadenoma, and it has no higher incidence of malignancy. Although the fibroadenoma is a benign tumor, a low rate of malignant transformation has been reported. Some have advocated excision of a solitary fibroadenoma in the older woman because of this possibility.

Phylloides Tumor

Many have incorrectly used this term interchangeably with *giant fibroadenoma*. Although these two benign masses are indistinguishable mammographically, histologically these tumors are distinct from each other. A phylloides tumor (also called cystosarcoma phylloides) is characteristically a large, noncalcified mass and may be poorly marginated on some borders. It is often associated with enlarged veins (Fig. 148–6). Pathologists grade the phylloides tumor by features such as the number of mitoses per high-power field, the degree of cellular atypia present, and the appearance of the stroma. A benign phylloides tumor may be treated by simple excision, but if it is not totally excised, it may recur locally. A malignant phylloides tumor is aggressively treated by mastectomy.

Fat-Containing Masses

These are uncommon benign breast masses. As a general rule, a totally lucent, sharply marginated mass in the breast need not be biopsied, since the etiology will be either a galactocele or a lipoma. Similarly, a solitary mass containing fatty components within it often need not be excised to rule out the possibility of malignancy.

Lymph Nodes

The usual appearance of a lymph node on mammography is that of a noncalcified mass with sharp margins measuring less than 1.5 cm in size, often containing a visible cleft. When lymph nodes are

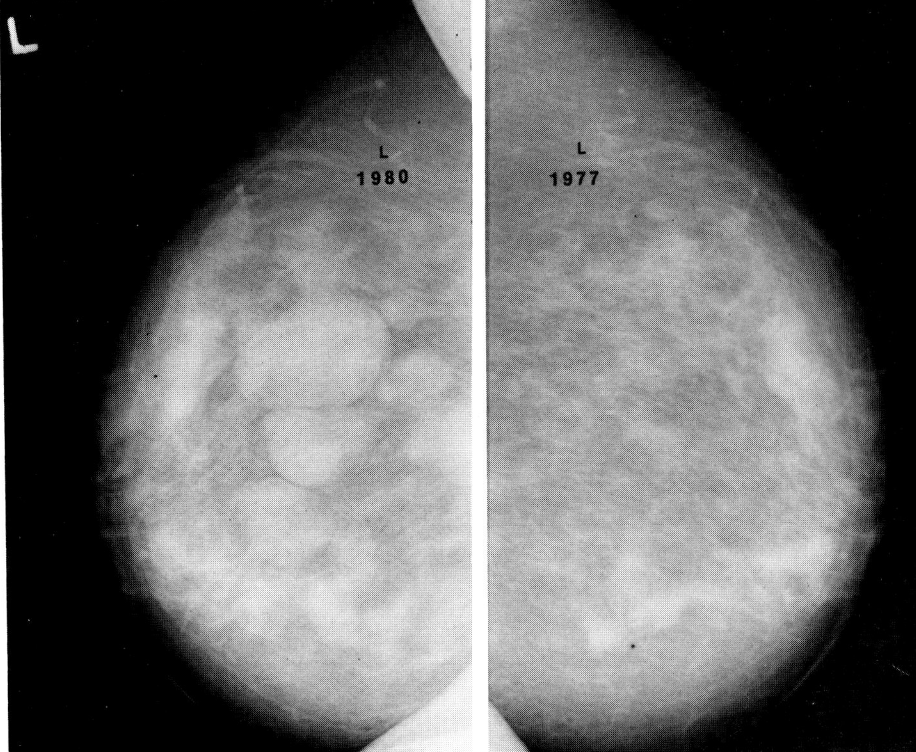

Figure 148–2. Between 1977 and 1980, **the cysts in the left breast increased in size and new ones have developed**. A similar pattern was present in the right breast.

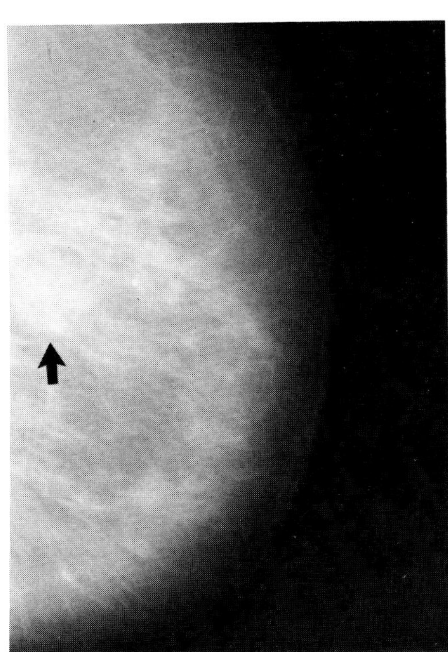

Figure 148–3. This poorly marginated, noncalcified mass with apparent angular borders *(arrow)* proved to be **a simple benign cyst** on excisional biopsy.

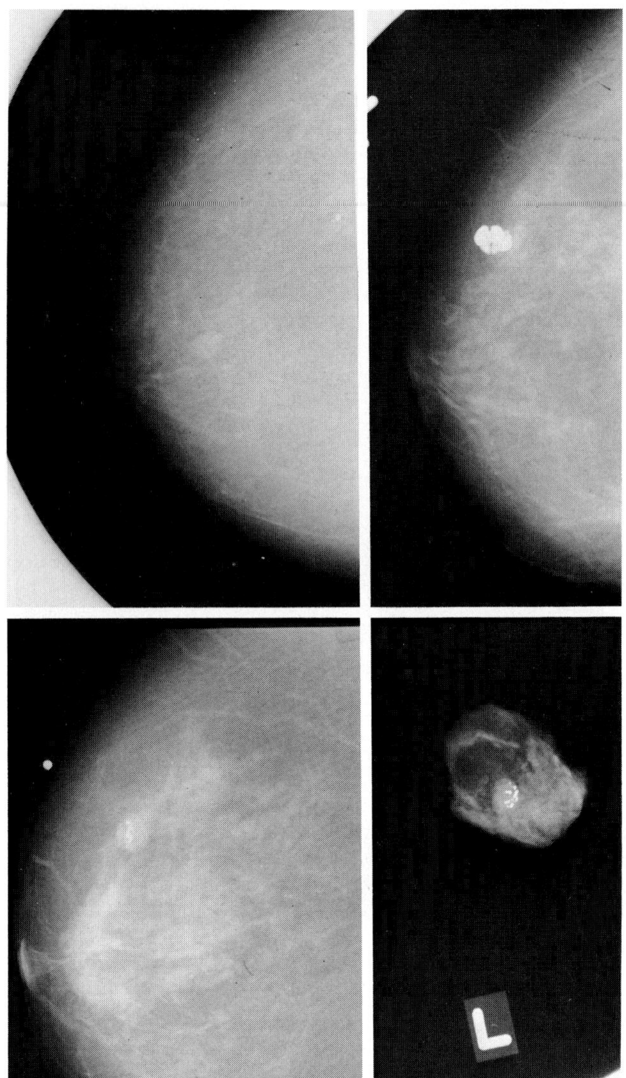

Figure 148–4. These different **fibroadenomas** range in appearance from noncalcified masses to ones containing dense macrocalcifications.

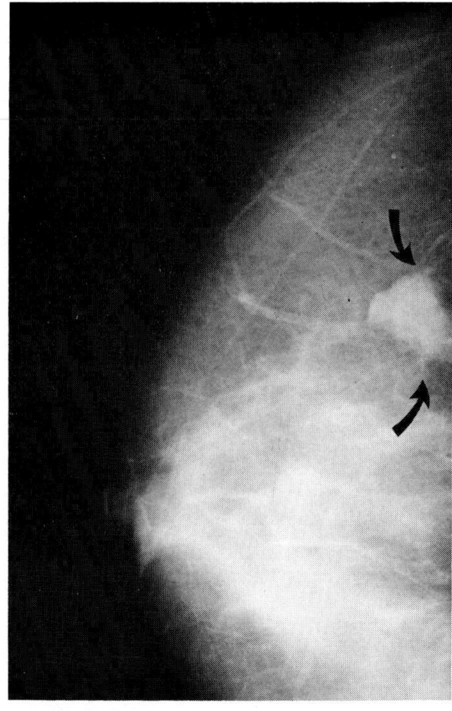

Figure 148–5. Although the margins of this mass were irregular and stellate *(arrows),* this proved to be **a benign fibroadenoma** on biopsy.

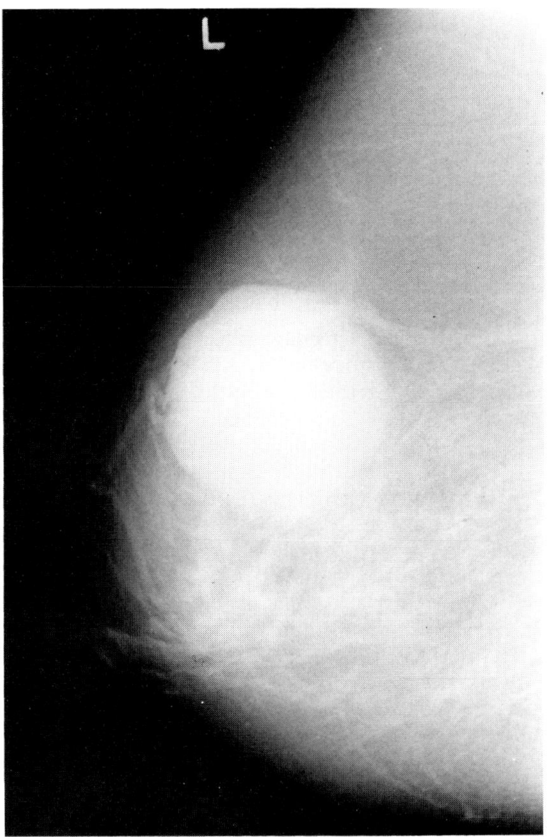

Figure 148–6. Notice the enlarged vein posterior to this large **benign cystosarcoma phylloides**.

multiple and are located in the axilla, the diagnosis is straightforward (Fig. 148–7). Often they are imaged only on the lateral view because of their axillary location. Benign lymph nodes may sometimes be larger than 1.5 cm when they are replaced by fat, and this fat can be recognized on the mammogram by its lucent appearance. Difficulties arise when the lymph node is solitary and is located in a position other than the axilla. The intramammary lymph node is a well-recognized entity and is exactly analogous to the intraparenchymal lymph node in the lung presenting as a coin lesion, for which a biopsy is usually necessary to exclude carcinoma.

Papilloma

The most common cause of a bloody nipple discharge is benign intraductal papilloma, which is composed of proliferative ductal epithelial tissue. This lesion may be multiple and is usually so small that in most instances the mammogram is entirely normal. The most frequent location of a papilloma is in the retroareolar area. On occasion it grows large enough to appear as a well-circumscribed mass that may contain microcalcification. A papilloma may obstruct the duct in which it is growing, and in this situation the pathologically enlarged duct rather than the papilloma itself may be identified by mammography.

Ductography may be done to evaluate the woman with a persistent unilateral nipple discharge (Fig. 148–8). This procedure involves identification and cannulation of the pathologically enlarged duct orifice and injection of contrast material to identify the papilloma or carcinoma that may be the underlying cause of the discharge. If the discharge is not spontaneous and is not an exudate, the chance of identifying the enlarged orifice is greatly diminished. In many hospitals ductography is not a commonly requested procedure, since in most cases the surgeon is able to identify the quadrant of the abnormal duct by noting where palpation causes the discharge to be expressed. Knowing this, the surgeon can usually identify the pathologic ductal system at surgery with direct inspection through a circumareolar incision.

INFLAMMATORY DISORDERS AND TRAUMA

Acute Mastitis

Acute mastitis is an infection that typically occurs in younger women during lactation. The involved breast is tender, swollen, and red. The patient is usually febrile and has an elevated sedimentation rate and a leukocytosis. Enlarged painful axillary lymph nodes may be palpable. Treatment consists of antibiotic therapy. The mammographic features are those of generalized skin thickening and increased stromal markings (Fig. 148–9). Although the mammographic features are indistinguishable from those of an inflammatory breast carcinoma, clinically there is usually little problem differentiating acute mastitis from inflammatory breast carcinoma. While the former is unusual in older patients and common in younger women, the reverse is true for the latter. Patients with acute mastitis are septic, while those with inflammatory carcinoma are not, although their sedimentation rate may be slightly elevated.

On occasion, an underlying abscess will be found within the breast involved with acute mastitis, and this abscess may have to be surgically drained. Rarely a breast abscess may be indolent. When this occurs in the older woman, differentiation from carcinoma is usually impossible, and an excisional biopsy is performed since clinically the abscess presents as a painless firm mass, often fixated, with poorly marginated or stellate borders. Indolent infectious agents such as tuberculosis and actinomycosis have been reported as etiologies.

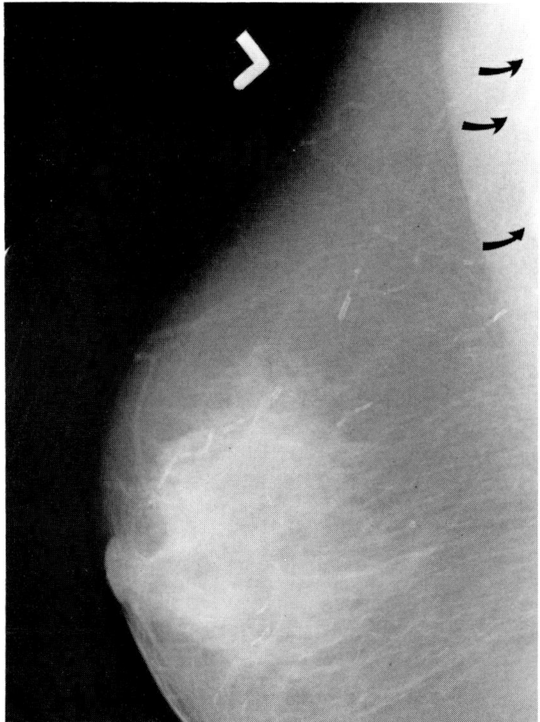

Figure 148–7. Multiple lymph nodes *(arrows)* are present in the axillary tail of the breast.

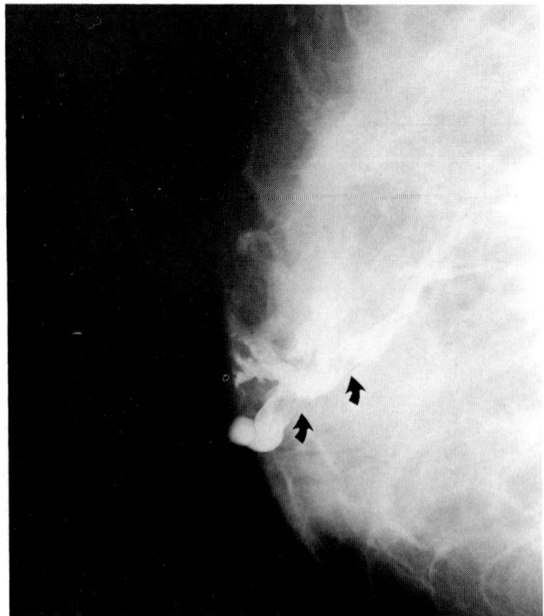

Figure 148–8. This lateral view from a ductogram revealed **two solitary papillomas** *(arrows)* in a dilated ductal system.

Chronic Mastitis

This entity is also referred to as *plasma-cell mastitis* and *fat necrosis.* Unlike acute mastitis, it is not an infection, is often occult, and is found in elderly women. No therapy is required, and biopsy is mandated only in those cases in which this entity presents as a localized abnormality so that carcinoma must be ruled out. The etiology of this process is not clear and probably is multifactorial. A history of antecedent trauma may be obtained in some cases. Fat necrosis is commonly present after surgical biopsy (iatrogenic trauma). Some believe that chronic mastitis is related to ducts losing their normal integrity as the patient ages, with resultant development of ductal ectasia. Ductal contents leak out into the breast stroma, evoking an aseptic reaction, and some have applied the term *chemical mastitis* to this sequence of events.

When one or more ductal systems are involved with chronic mastitis, this process is recognized to be benign and further evaluation is unnecessary. The large macrocalcifications with polarity toward the nipple have a characteristic appearance (Fig. 148–10). Chronic mastitis or fat necrosis may present as a localized abnormality and may appear ominous on mammography, with features including a poorly marginated or stellate mass, sometimes even containing bizarre microcalcifications (Fig. 148–11). Biopsy to exclude carcinoma is unavoidable in this circumstance.

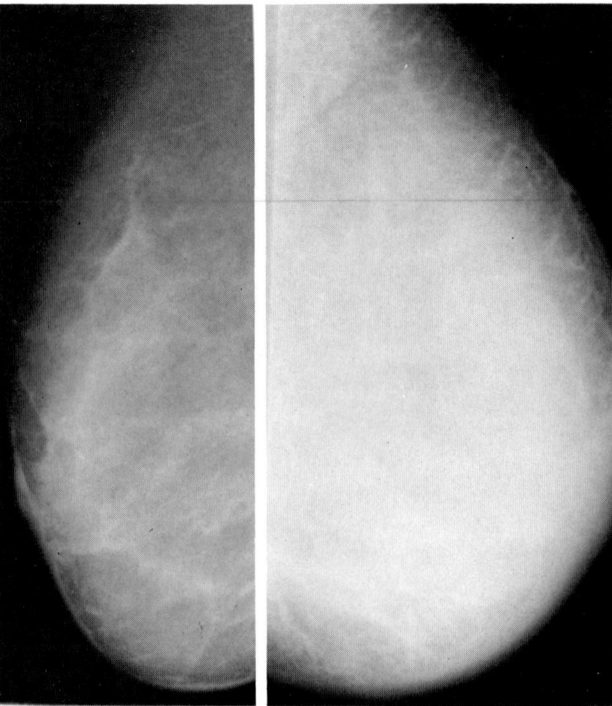

Figure 148–9. Compared with the normal left breast, **the right breast is enlarged, with increased stromal markings and generalized skin thickening**. This young lactating woman had acute mastitis on the right.

Hematoma and Contusion

Bleeding into the breast is most often the result of direct trauma (including breast biopsy) or a bleeding diathesis. Trauma may result in laceration of breast tissue and hemorrhage can accumulate into this space with formation of a hematoma. This hematoma will appear as a noncalcified, very sharply marginated mass. The appearance and natural history of a breast hematoma are similar to those of a pulmonary hematoma. The mass will decrease in size over time (Fig. 148–12). It may totally resolve or may leave residual architectural distortion. Bleeding into the breast may not form a hematoma but rather may dissect through the breast tissue. In this

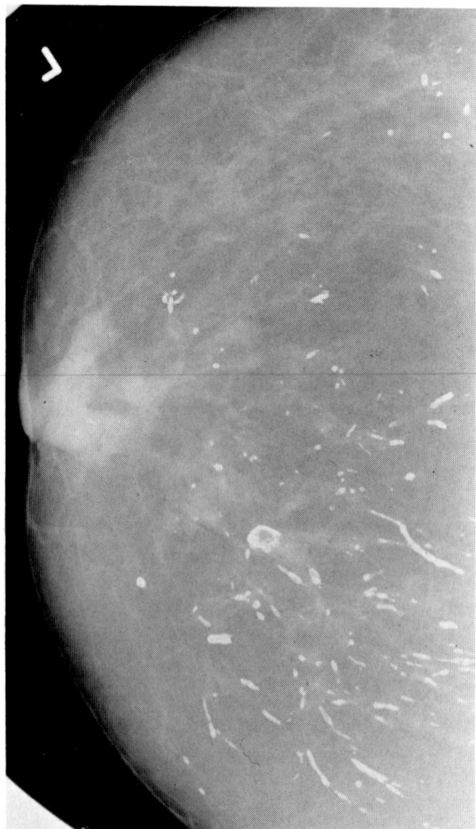

Figure 148–10. These bizarre macrocalcifications have polarity toward the nipple and are a manifestation of fat necrosis. The pathologically enlarged subareolar ducts were excised and were found to contain inspissated debris in areas of severe ductal ectasia. The contralateral breast had similar findings.

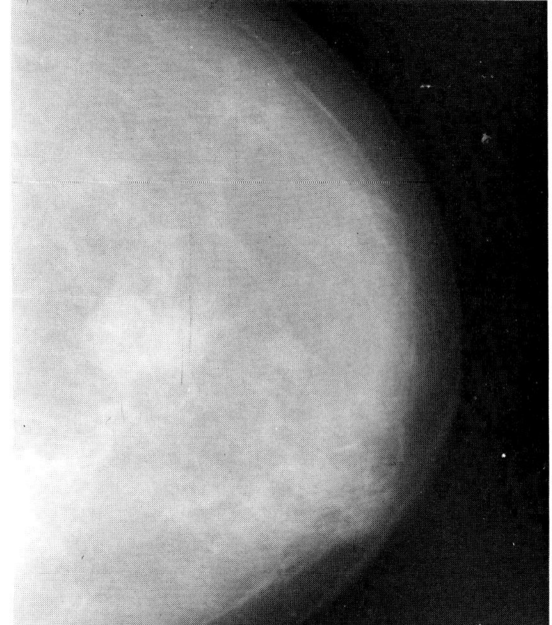

Figure 148–11. Although the large irregular mass located centrally in the breast was thought to be malignant, excisional biopsy revealed an area of **localized fat necrosis**.

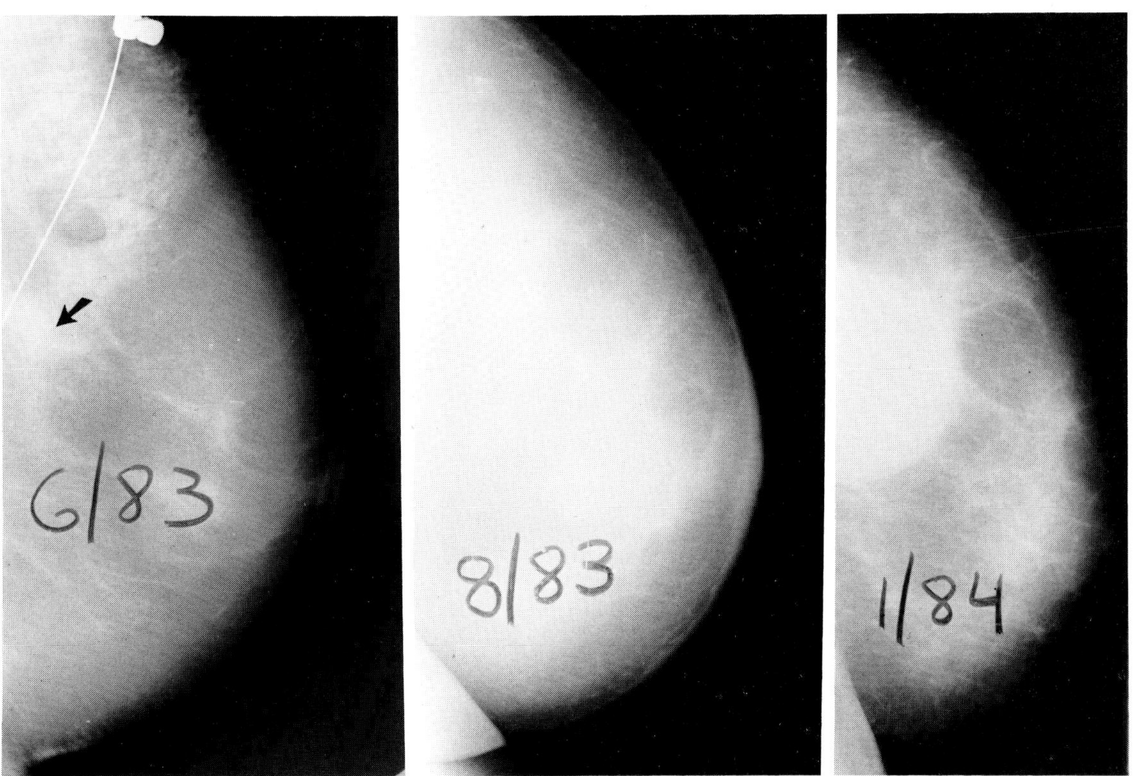

Figure 148–12. In June 1983, a percutaneous needle localization was performed for the excision of a **nonpalpable carcinoma** *(arrow)*. Two months later, **a large hematoma** is present, which is smaller in January 1984.

TABLE 148–1. ANALYSIS OF BREAST CALCIFICATIONS

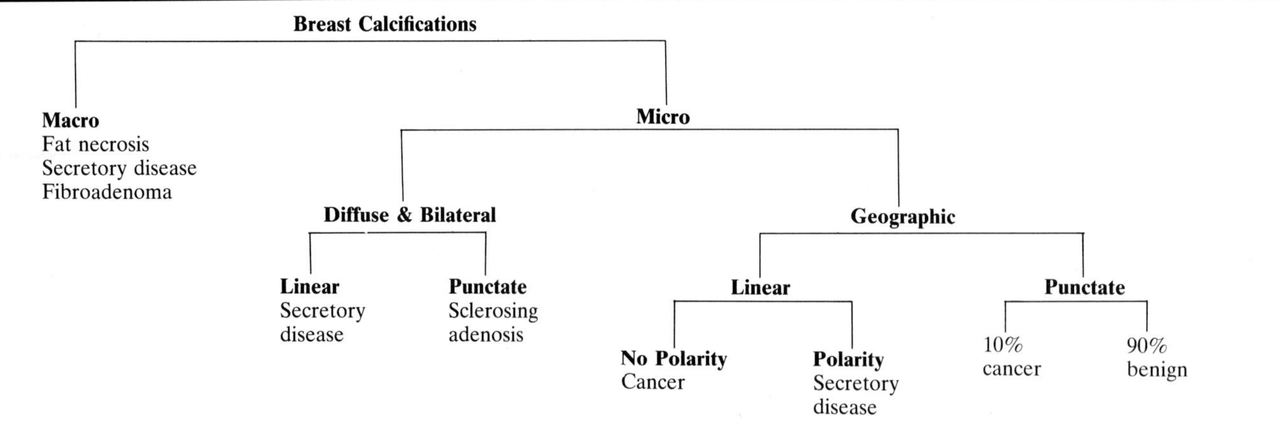

situation the mammogram will show increased stromal density in the area of hemorrhage. Over time, as the hemorrhage is resorbed, the stromal density returns to normal. Again the analogy with the lung is applicable, and the natural history of this process is similar to that of a pulmonary contusion, with progressive resolution over several days.

BENIGN BREAST CALCIFICATIONS

Developing a logical approach to the analysis of breast calcifications has been a frustrating exercise for radiologists, since numerous classifications have been proposed and none is entirely satisfactory. In analyzing calcifications within the breast, the radiologist must take into account many features, including the location of the calcifications; the volume of the breast containing the calcifications; the appearance of the surrounding breast parenchyma; and the size, shape, and orientation of the calcifications. As a general rule it is fair to say that macrocalcifications are benign, as are linear calcifications with polarity toward the nipple. Microcalcifications may be either benign or malignant. For the purposes of this review, a microcalcification will be defined as one measuring less than 0.5 mm in every diameter. Most microcalcifications prove to be related to benign breast disease. Even when the radiologist offers an educated guess as to the probability of whether a group of microcalcifications will be benign or malignant, most geographic clusters will be excised anyway. A simple schema for the analysis of breast calcifications is given in Table 148–1.

Macrocalcifications

Macrocalcifications are most often associated with benign breast disease and may be found in previously described entities such as fibroadenoma and fat necrosis (chronic mastitis). Secretory disease and ductal ectasia may also produce macrocalcifications. The calcifications usually have a linear appearance, since they are related to the orientation of the ducts and have a polarity toward the nipple (Fig. 148–13). The distribution is variable and can range from involvement of both breasts to involvement of only one ductal system.

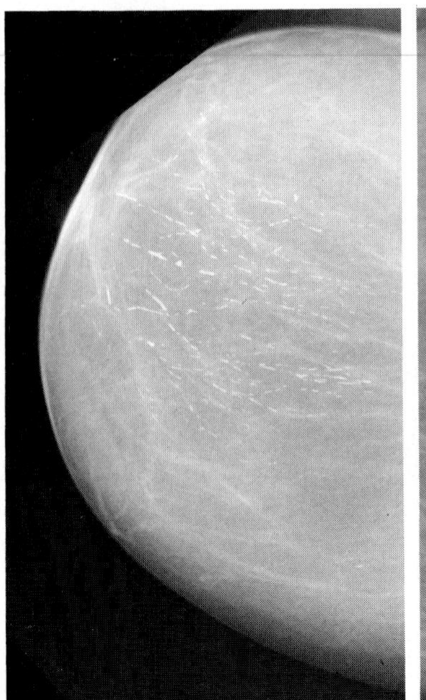

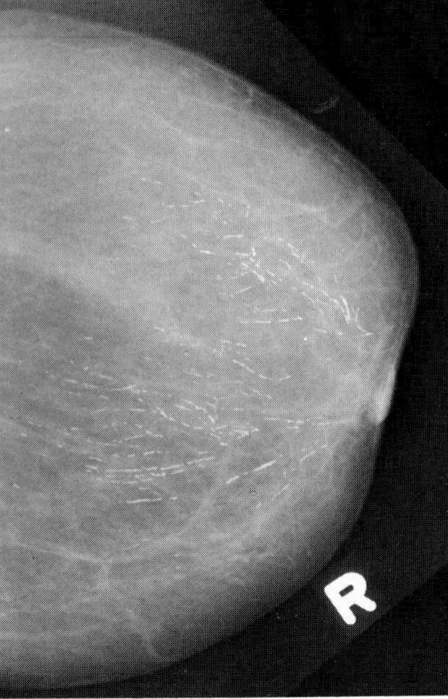

Figure 148–13. There is extensive **bilateral secretory disease and diffuse linear macrocalcifications** with polarity toward the nipple.

Diffuse Microcalcifications

Microcalcifications that are distributed diffusely through both breasts are a manifestation of benign fibrocystic change. When they are punctate, the histologic appearance is usually that of an entity called *sclerosing adenosis*. This is a good descriptive term, since the pathologist is able to identify fields of fibrosis as well as adenosis with the microcalcifications present in both of these areas. When diffuse microcalcifications are linear, they are a manifestation of secretory disease.

Geographic Microcalcifications

Geographic linear branching microcalcifications without polarity are usually a manifestation of malignancy. Geographic punctate microcalcifications are associated with malignancy in approximately 10 per cent of cases and benign disease in 90 per cent of cases. Using finely detailed mammograms, including magnification techniques, attempts are being made to reliably differentiate benign from malignant punctate microcalcification. This is an exciting area of research and if it proves reliable, needless biopsies will be avoided.

BREAST DENSITY

Over the life of the woman, the overall breast stromal pattern changes. As a female passes through adolescence the amount of breast stroma is on the increase. The total amount waxes and wanes with each pregnancy and finally as the woman approaches and passes through menopause, the breast stroma is eventually replaced by fat. A dense breast in a 35-year-old woman probably reflects a normal pattern, while in a 70-year-old woman this density is abnormal and reflects fibrocystic change. In the transitional ages between 40 and 60, difficulty exists in knowing how much density is allowable in the breast, since there is so much variation. Suffice it to say that in practice, the presence of bilateral symmetrical dense breast stroma at any age lowers the sensitivity of the mammographic examination but does not in and of itself generate a radiographic recommendation for a biopsy. A great difference of opinion exists as to whether the patient with abnormally prominent ductal tissue and dense stromal pattern has a higher risk for developing breast carcinoma. With the latest guidelines of the American Cancer Society recommending a baseline mammogram on women 35 to 40 years of age, annual mammography or mammography every other year on women 41 to 49 years of age, and annual mammography on all women over the age of 50, this controversy has become somewhat less important.

Bibliography

Greenblatt RB, Samaras C, Vasquez JM, Nezhat C: Fibrocystic disease of the breast. Clin Obstet Gynecol 25:365–371, 1982.
Hoeffken W, Lanyi M: Mammography. In Benign Diseases of the Female Breast. Philadelphia, WB Saunders Company, 1977, pp 82–155.
Paulus DD: Benign diseases of the breast. Radiol Clin North Am 21:27–50, 1983.
Schwartz GF: Benign neoplasms and inflammations of the breast. Clin Obstet Gynecol 25:373–385, 1982.

149 Radiologic Diagnosis of Breast Cancer

Norman L. Sadowsky and Elsie Levin

Mammography is the only reliable method of consistently detecting nonpalpable breast cancer. One must distinguish between the diagnostic mammogram, done to evaluate the patient with abnormal signs or symptoms, and the screening mammogram, used to detect occult cancer in the patient without signs or symptoms. This chapter is organized with this distinction in mind, although it should be realized that there is an overlap. An occult lesion can reach a seemingly palpable size and still be undetected by physical examination because of its location, size of the breast, surrounding fibrocystic nodularity, or the soft consistency of the lesion (as in medullary and colloid carcinomas). On the other hand, a tiny lesion may be palpable because of its consistency and/or peripheral location (Fig. 149–1).

SCREENING

Breast cancer is a common disease in the United States. One woman in nine (11 per cent) born in this country will develop breast cancer. It has been predicted that in 1993, 182,000 new cases of invasive breast cancer will be discovered, and 47,000 women will die of this disease. The size of the lesion at detection is related to the incidence of positive regional nodes, and the presence or absence of positive nodes is the most important factor in long-term survival. Hendriks found that cancers discovered in screening measured 1.3 cm in diameter (decreasing to 1.1 cm in the third round of screening) compared to 2.8 cm in nonscreened control group women, and that positive lymph node status was 20 per cent and 48 per cent in the screened and nonscreened groups, respectively. Theoretically, early detection should be associated with reduced mortality, a fact that has been demonstrated to be true among women in all age groups.

Symptomatic

It is important to stress that a ''negative'' mammogram must not result in delaying a biopsy in a patient with a suspicious mass in the breast. There are many reasons for a ''negative'' mammogram

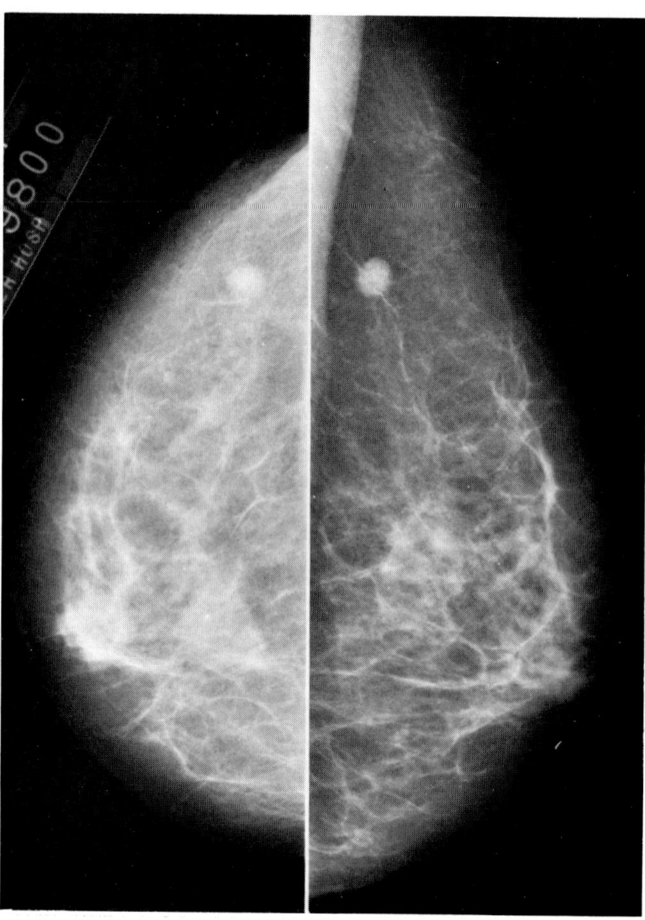

Figure 149–1. A 67-year-old woman with a 9-mm **palpable mass in the axillary tail of the left breast** discovered by the patient. Original craniocaudal view did not include the lesion, but exaggerated lateral turned craniocaudal view, guided by the radiologist's physical exam, and routine medio-lateral oblique view show a well-defined lesion with irregular borders which was an infiltrating ductal carcinoma.

in a patient with palpable breast cancer. Approximately 5 to 10 per cent of all cancers detected in screening will be found by palpation alone. A palpable cancer may be missed on mammography because of (1) observer error, (2) unusual location so that it is not included on the film, (3) a dense parenchymal pattern that hides the lesions, or (4) failure of the lesion to produce a recognizable abnormality. Therefore, it is extremely important that mammograms be interpreted with all available clinical information. The mammographic report should reflect the radiologist's knowledge of the clinical problem and should specifically state the presence or absence of radiologic findings related to that problem.

The most important element in any radiologic breast evaluation program is the leadership provided by an actively involved, interested, and well-trained radiologist. Under ideal circumstances every symptomatic patient should be examined by the radiologist to ensure that the area of concern is adequately examined. In addition to the two routine views (the craniocaudal and oblique mediolateral), special views may be necessary to ensure that the lesion is included on the film (Fig. 149–2). We often use a metallic marker on palpable abnormalities (Fig. 149–3) and fine surgical wire to mark scars (see Fig. 149–19).

Interpretation and Technique

The key to detecting abnormalities is recognizing asymmetry; all radiographically demonstrated lesions are either focal or generalized asymmetries. Therefore, we recommend that during viewing of the initial mammogram (or baseline study) films be arranged so that the right and left craniocaudal (and mediolateral oblique) projections are viewed as mirror images back to back, allowing similar areas to be compared. Breasts are usually symmetric in distribution of par-

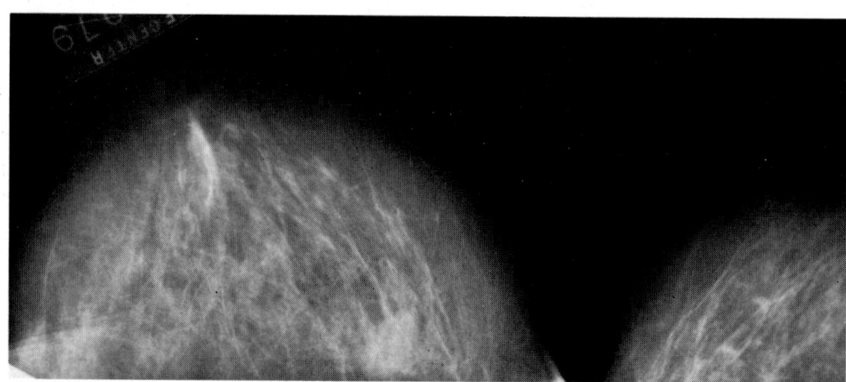

Figure 149–2. A 62-year-old woman with self-discovered **palpable mass in the upper medial right breast** not shown on routine craniocaudal view. This special exaggerated medial craniocaudal view, with the medial aspect of both breasts compressed and imaged, was done after the radiologist's physical examination.

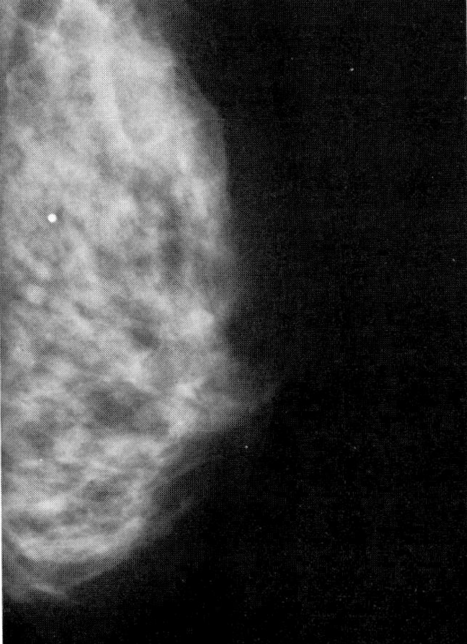

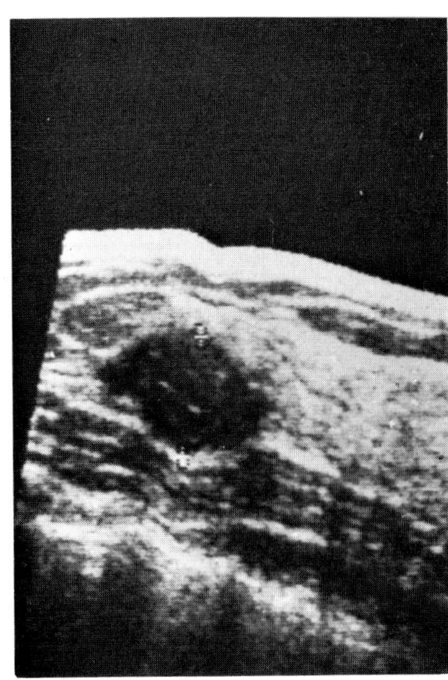

Figure 149–3. A 35-year-old woman whose mother had breast cancer at age 39 years. A metallic marker was placed over **a palpable thickening in the upper central left breast.** No lesion could be seen on mammograms (medio-lateral oblique shown) but ultrasound shows a solid mass. Biopsy was recommended, which revealed infiltrating ductal carcinoma with negative regional nodes.

enchymal densities so that by viewing them as matched pairs, they serve as their own controls, and any subtle but significant difference in density may be more readily seen (Fig. 149–4). On subsequent examinations, instead of comparing the right with the left breast, the right craniocaudal should be compared with the previous right craniocaudal, etc. When there are multiple previous examinations, it is helpful to compare a remote study rather than the most recent previous examination. This can make subtle changes in density more obvious. Comparison with previous mammograms is essential, and in the postmastectomy patient this is the only control available. We also recommend that film mammograms be placed on a view box with extraneous light blocked off; this can virtually eliminate the need to bright-light well-exposed films.

Special techniques such as magnification and compression spot films can be extremely useful in evaluating questionable findings (Fig. 149–5).

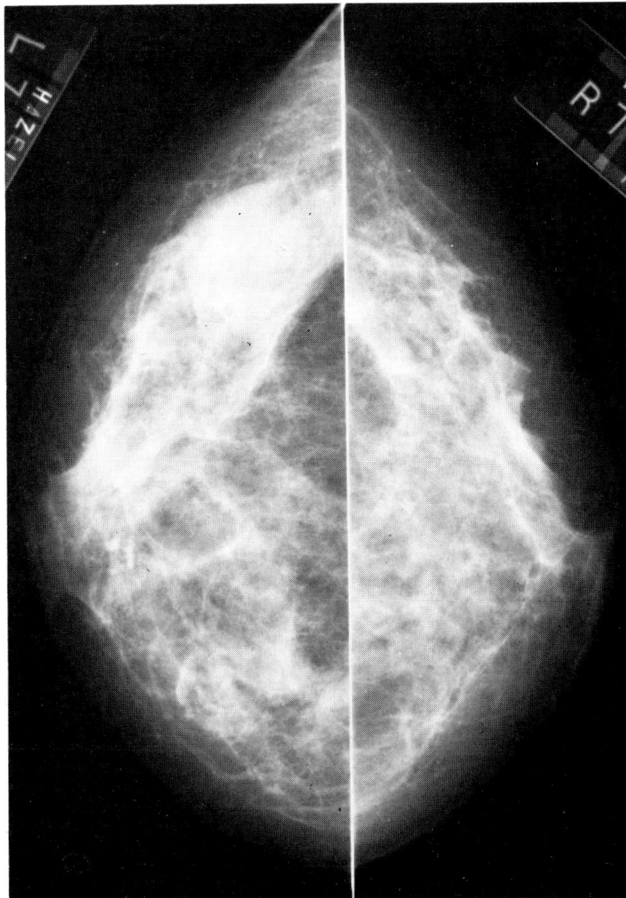

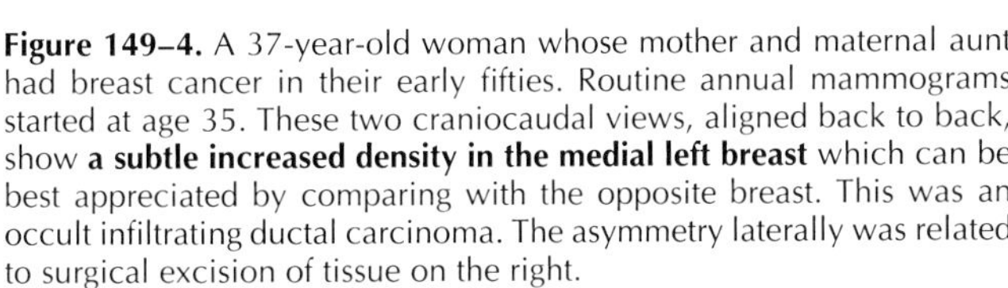

Figure 149–4. A 37-year-old woman whose mother and maternal aunt had breast cancer in their early fifties. Routine annual mammograms started at age 35. These two craniocaudal views, aligned back to back, show **a subtle increased density in the medial left breast** which can be best appreciated by comparing with the opposite breast. This was an occult infiltrating ductal carcinoma. The asymmetry laterally was related to surgical excision of tissue on the right.

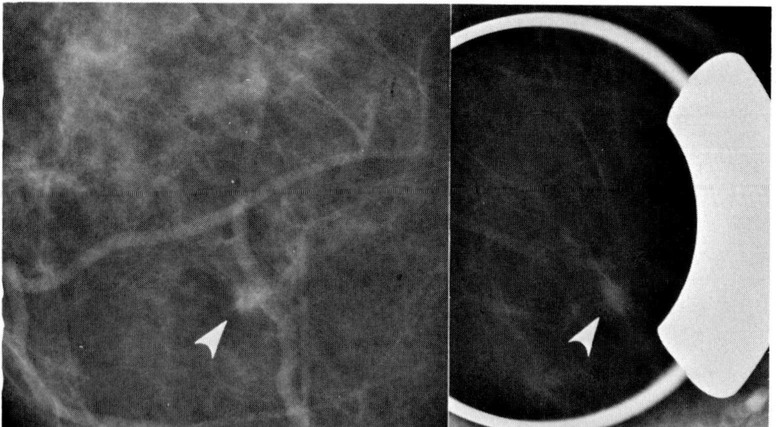

Figure 149–5. A 51-year-old woman whose mother had breast cancer at age 55 years and who has had routine screening mammograms annually for six years. Latest examination showed **a small area of increased density obscured by overlying vein** *(arrow)* seen in the craniocaudal view only. Special compression spot film that resulted in projecting the vein differently revealed the presence of a 3 × 5 mm irregular mass medially. The mass was then found in a repeat lateral view, which was a 90-degree lateromedial projection in which the lesion was seen superiorly. Biopsy showed a tiny infiltrating ductal carcinoma.

Film/screen examinations must be performed with dedicated mammography equipment specially designed to give vigorous breast compression, short exposure time, and high resolution. A moving grid affords higher contrast and resolution with a modest increase in dosage. A dedicated mammographic film processor is also a necessity to produce high-contrast films with reduced artifacts and lower dose. Establishing a quality assurance program is mandatory to maintain image quality and is one of the requirements for accreditation by the American College of Radiology.

Directed ultrasound can be helpful in evaluating a palpable mass or a nonpalpable mammographically demonstrated mass. We use hand-held ultrasound as an adjunct to mammography to determine whether a mass is solid and/or cystic. Often, a patient presents with a mass after attempted aspiration has yielded no fluid and the mammogram is inconclusive; ultrasound can tell us whether the mass is a cyst that was "missed" by the needle or is indeed solid and therefore should be biopsied. The most gratifying use for ultrasound is in the patient who presents with a palpable mass that is obscured by dense breast tissue (see Fig. 149–3). We use ultrasound as the first procedure for a mass in pregnancy or in very young women, followed by a single-view spot mammogram if indicated. Ultrasound can also be used as a guide to aspiration of palpable and nonpalpable cysts, for wire localization of a solid lesion prior to biopsy, and as a guide to fine needle aspiration and core biopsy of solid masses. Ultrasound is not effective as a stand-alone screening procedure.

RADIOLOGIC APPEARANCES OF BREAST CANCER

The primary sign of breast cancer is the presence of a dominant mass, usually with ill-defined margins. How well the mass is seen depends on its size, its location, and the density of surrounding parenchyma. With the exception of a purely radiolucent lesion such as a galactocele, lipoma, or lipid cyst of fat necrosis or a partial lucent lesion such as a hamartoma, and a heavily calcified fibroadenoma, a mass lesion cannot be definitively called benign on the basis of its mammographic appearance alone.

Secondary signs of breast cancer are (1) asymmetric density, (2) architectural distortion, (3) skin changes (thickening and/or retraction), (4) asymmetric ducts, (5) asymmetric vessels, (6) adenopathy, and (7) microcalcifications.

Primary Signs—Mass

A malignant mass can have many shapes, ranging from obvious malignancy to a virtually benign appearance.

Spiculated Mass. The classic carcinoma has a central mass surrounded by a sunburst pattern of radiating, thin spicules due to the fine extensions of tumor cells into the surrounding tissue and the desmoplastic response of the tissue to the tumor (Fig. 149–6). Clinically the mass feels significantly larger than it appears on the mammogram because the palpatory findings include not only the carcinoma but also the surrounding desmoplastic reaction. The fibrosis is responsible for the term *scirrhous* and is usually caused by an infiltrating ductal carcinoma, which constitutes 75 per cent of all invasive carcinomas. Invasive lobular carcinoma, which has a poor prognosis, can occasionally produce a similar scirrhous response (Fig. 149–7*A*).

Density with a Ragged Border. This type of lesion is often subtle and may present as an asymmetric density with vague margins. It is a variant of the spiculated mass with scirrhous elements arising in a dense dysplastic area of the breast so that at times only one margin is appreciated (Fig. 149–7*B*).

Smooth Mass. The perfectly smooth carcinoma is relatively rare but does occur. Usually, one can identify a tell-tale sign that the lesion is not just a simple benign cyst. Such signs include lobulation, a small comet tail projecting from one of the borders, a flattening of one side of the lesion, or a very slight irregularity in a seemingly smooth lesion (Fig. 149–8). These features are better appreciated on spot compression magnification views which should be done in the craniocaudal and 90-degree lateral projections.

The relatively rare intracystic carcinoma is very often completely smooth in contour, but it may have a subtle flattening on one border at the point of attachment to the cyst wall, especially if it is caught tangentially (Fig. 149–9). These carcinomas are often located close to or in the subareolar region and cannot be distinguished radiologically from an intraductal papilloma that has obstructed the duct and formed a cyst around itself. These lesions tend to be papillary within the cyst, and the prognosis is usually good. Any dominant mass in the subareolar area must be regarded with suspicion even if it appears benign. Ultrasound can be very helpful in determining the true nature of the lesion. Aspiration may yield bloody fluid, and after aspiration, the palpable mass does not disappear completely or may recur soon afterward.

The appearance of a new lesion in a postmenopausal patient, even if it is quite smooth and small, should be regarded with some suspicion, especially if the woman is being examined annually because of a history of breast cancer. In such a case, one might expect to find a very early lesion that retains its smooth appearance before it becomes infiltrating (Fig. 149–10). A detailed medication history is important because postmenopausal women on estrogen replacement therapy can and do develop cysts as well as generalized increased density, especially when estrogen replacement has been begun many years after menopause. Other medications that can cause cysts are diuretics, antihypertensive medications, cardiac drugs including calcium channel blockers, cholesterol-lowering

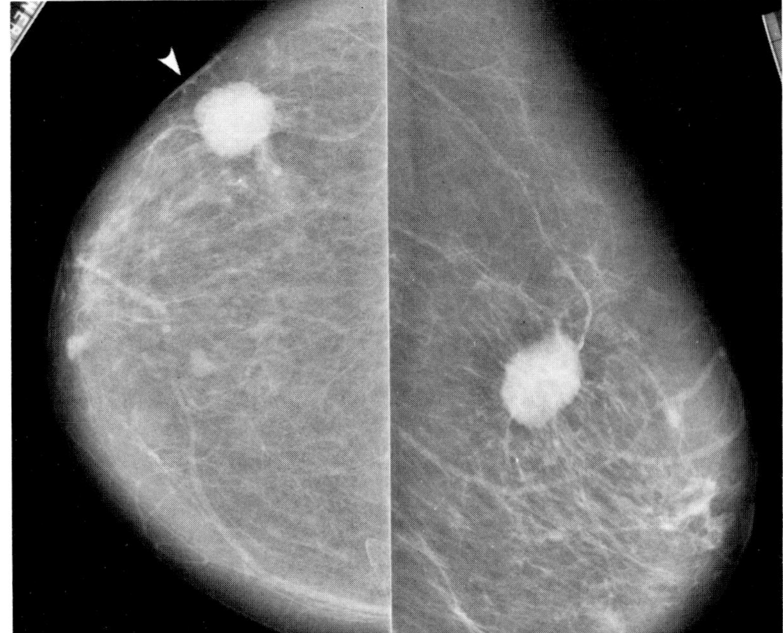

Figure 149–6. A 74-year-old woman with **a palpable mass in the left upper outer quadrant.** Craniocaudal and lateral views show typical sunburst appearance with large central mass and rays extending from the periphery. Note retraction of the skin on the craniocaudal view *(arrow)* and the extreme density of the lesion seen well against a background of fat.

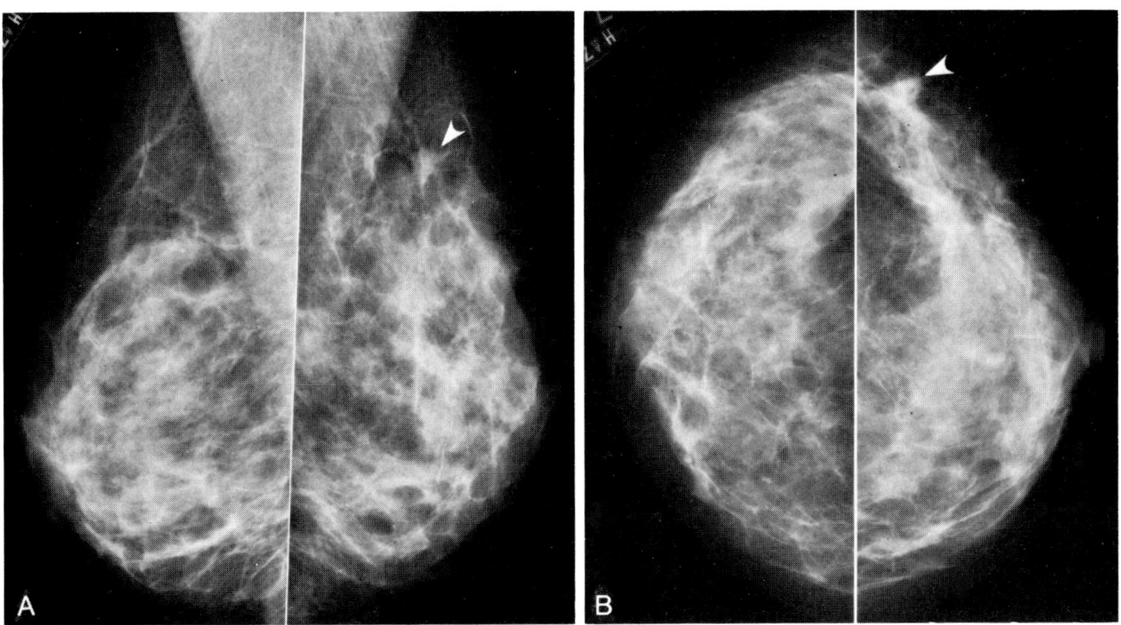

Figure 149–7. *A,* Left and right medio-lateral oblique views of a 47-year-old woman with **a palpable mass in the upper outer quadrant of the right breast.** Subtle sclerotic distortion seen superiorly in the right breast *(arrow)* is due to invasive lobular carcinoma, which has provoked a scirrhous reaction. Note asymmetry of veins superiorly, with larger veins on the normal side. *B,* Craniocaudal views of the same patient showing the carcinoma as an asymmetrical density *(arrow)* extending out from a background of fibrocystic tissue. There is very slight retraction of the overlying skin.

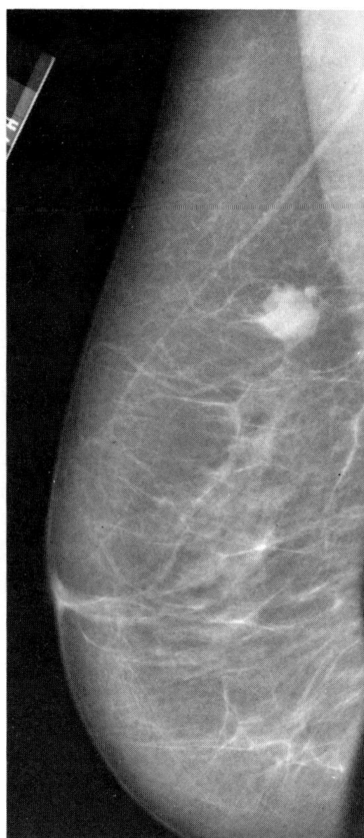

Figure 149–8. A 68-year-old woman with **a nonpalpable lesion in the upper outer quadrant of the left breast.** The lesion appears on the lateral view as a smooth mass with an irregular comet tail anteriorly and some flattening posteriorly.

agents, and levothyroxin. State-of-the-art ultrasound with a 7.5-mHz transducer can be extremely helpful in distinguishing small cysts from solid lesions. If the lesion does not meet all of the ultrasound criteria for a cyst, ultrasound-guided aspiration can be performed.

The medullary carcinoma is usually a single, dominant, well-demarcated mass that may appear smooth in its entire circumference. It is characterized pathologically as a homogeneous mass with large cells containing pleomorphic nuclei and many mitoses. A lymphocytic infiltration is usually seen throughout the tumor unaccompanied by a desmoplastic reaction. This type of tumor grows by expansion rather than by infiltration so that the contour remains smooth. The lesion is soft and, therefore, can reach a large size before becoming palpable (Fig. 149–11). Central necrosis and liquefaction of this tumor can occur, yielding an abscess-like fluid on aspiration.

The mucinous or colloid carcinoma may also appear as a smooth mass that grows by pushing rather than infiltration. This carcinoma is composed of groups of well-differentiated cells floating in or surrounded by mucin and usually occurs in older women. Like the medullary carcinoma, the mucinous carcinoma may be quite soft, and these two lesions are indistinguishable radiologically and clinically (Fig. 149–11).

LOBULATED MASS. The presence of a smooth, lobulated mass in the breast is most often due to a fibroadenoma. However, carcinomas can present in a similar way. The presence of an irregular border or other secondary signs of carcinoma must be used to differentiate these lesions. A newly appearing solid mass or one that has increased in size, unless possessing the characteristic calcifications of fibroadenoma, should have a histologic diagnosis by either surgical removal or core biopsy (Fig. 149–12).

Secondary Signs of Breast Cancer

Subtle changes may be associated with the clinical finding of a palpable mass, or the radiologic finding of a mass lesion may exist alone as the only indicator of cancer.

ASYMMETRIC DENSITY. Asymmetry in the density of the breast obviously can be appreciated only by comparing mirror image areas. When associated with a palpable asymmetric thickening or mass, asymmetry is an indication for biopsy. When seen alone, without any other findings, the asymmetric density must be regarded with suspicion; other procedures such as ultrasound and compression spot films can help in evaluating this finding (Fig. 149–13).

ASYMMETRIC DUCTS. The prominent duct pattern is usually due to periductal collagenosis and not due to dilatation of ducts. The most common place to see prominent ducts is in the subareolar region. Normally the distribution is symmetric, extending toward the base of the breast, especially into the upper outer quadrant. Asymmetry of ducts on one side, either as a discrepancy in size or number of ducts, should make one search for other signs of carcinoma. The finding of asymmetric ducts and the presence of a palpable mass should arouse suspicion of an underlying carcinoma. Compression spot films with or without magnification can be helpful in evaluating this finding, as can ultrasound. Isolated asymmetric prominent ducts in the absence of a palpable mass or abnormal findings by ultrasound or special mammographic views are not sufficient evidence to prompt biopsy.

Unilateral duct ectasia is an unusual sign of carcinoma, but when present it should alert one to the possibility of an underlying carcinoma. The carcinoma can be within the duct, causing obstruction, or it can be deep in the breast; in the latter case, the duct can often be seen extending into the parenchyma and ending in an area of subtly increased density (Fig. 149–14). Papillomatosis can give rise to dilated ducts, sometimes bilaterally, and inflammatory duct ectasia is usually bilateral.

ARCHITECTURAL DISTORTION. A cancer seen only as architectural distortion is often nonpalpable. When distortion is visible in two projections, it warrants biopsy (Fig. 149–15). The finding is due to the desmoplastic reaction around the carcinoma, which may be microscopic in size. History and physical examination are very important, since one must be sure that there is no history of previous biopsy or drained abscess in the area, common causes of distortion of the breast. Ultrasound can occasionally distinguish these entities from carcinoma. Comparison with previous examinations is also helpful.

DIFFUSE INCREASE IN DENSITY. A diffuse overall increase in density of the breast is a late finding and often represents a diffusely infiltrating carcinoma (especially infiltrating lobular carcinoma) (Fig. 149–16). Inflammatory carcinoma of the breast is characterized by the clinical appearance of inflammation (redness, skin thickening, and edema), but unlike an abscess it is usually not tender. Pathologically inflammatory carcinoma is characterized by plugging of dermal lymphatics with tumor cells that produce the marked skin thickening. The generalized edema is evident on the mammogram as a diffuse increase in density, and the lymphatic engorgement may produce Kerley's B lines running perpendicular to the skin. Skin thickening can be recognized on the mammogram before it becomes clinically apparent. Very often there is no discrete mass seen by mammography, possibly because the edema has obscured the lesion (Fig. 149–17).

SKIN CHANGES. Retraction of the skin, nipple, or areola occurs when a lesion either has spread through the ducts toward the surface or has elicited a desmoplastic reaction extending to the periphery. Some lesions causing skin retraction can be very small and arise in the periphery of the breast close to the skin (Fig. 149–18). Lesions deeper in the breast can produce an extensive network of spicules, which reach the skin and subareolar ducts, or these lesions can

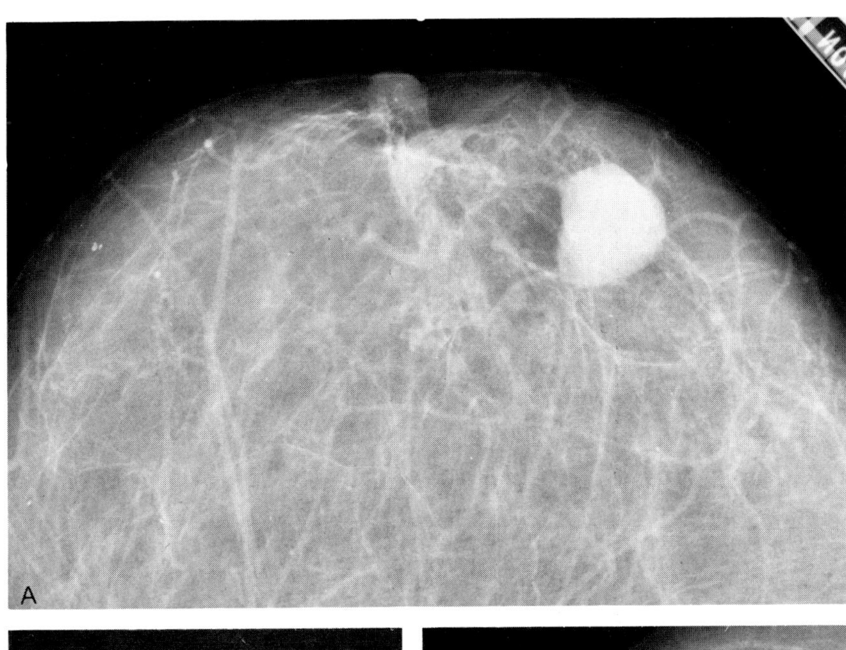

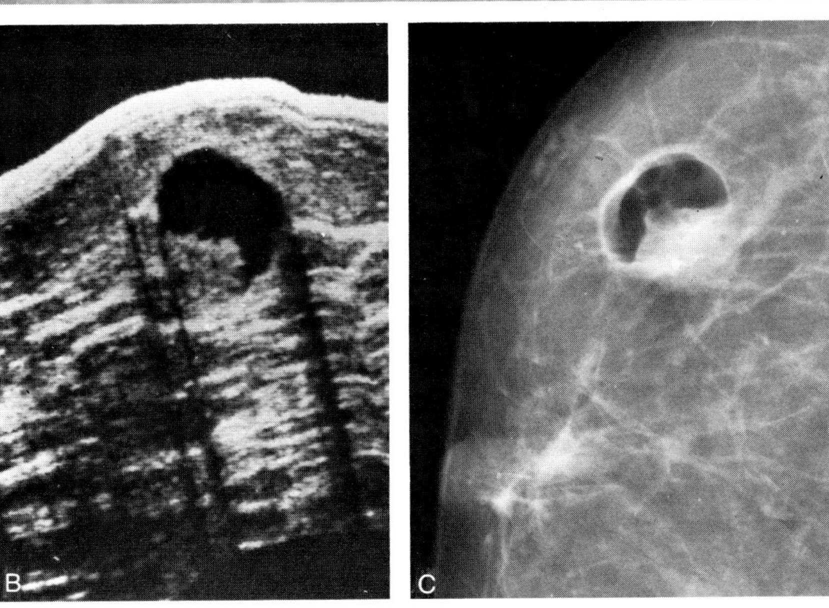

Figure 149–9. A 73-year-old woman with **a soft palpable mass lateral to the left nipple.** *A,* Craniocaudal mammogram shows a dense smooth mass with flattening and gross calcification inferiorly. *B,* Ultrasound showed that the mass was a cyst with a solid inferior component. Aspiration by the radiologist yielded clear yellow fluid. *C,* The pneumocystogram confirms the extent of the solid component. The surgical specimen was a classic intracystic papilloma, which cannot be distinguished from an intracystic carcinoma radiologically.

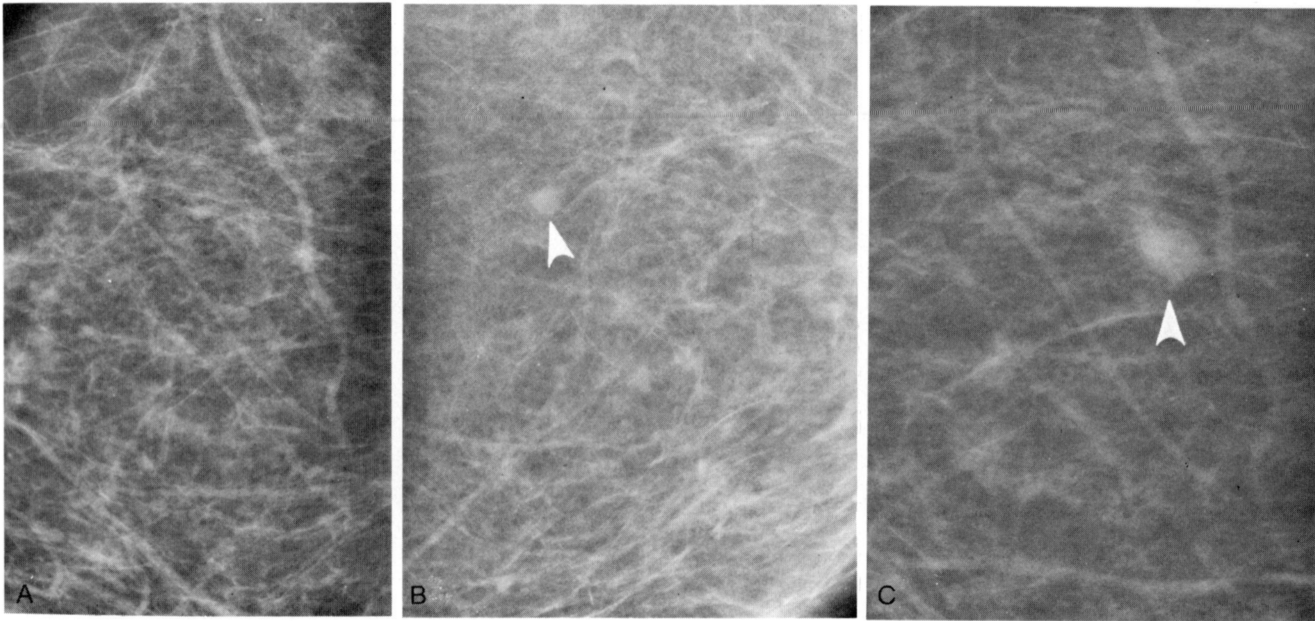

Figure 149–10. A 58-year-old woman with previous right mastectomy for carcinoma 15 years earlier. *A,* Craniocaudal view on the left was the thirteenth exam, used for comparison with the fourteenth exam *(B)* done one year later, which shows **a subtle nodule appearing centrolaterally** *(arrow).* Biopsy was advised, but surgery was not done. Fourteen months later *(C),* the lesion has increased from 5 to 7 × 10 mm. This was a medullary carcinoma, which is usually a slow-growing tumor. Note veins that appear prominent in *(A)* and *(C),* showing how variable and unreliable this sign is.

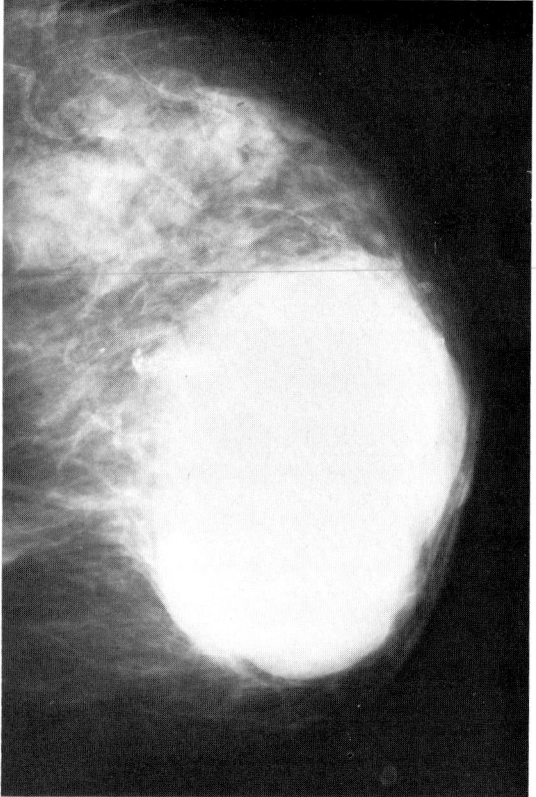

Figure 149–11. A 75-year-old woman with **a huge soft mass in the left breast.** Lateral mammogram shows a smooth-walled lobulated mass that was a colloid carcinoma, indistinguishable from a huge medullary carcinoma.

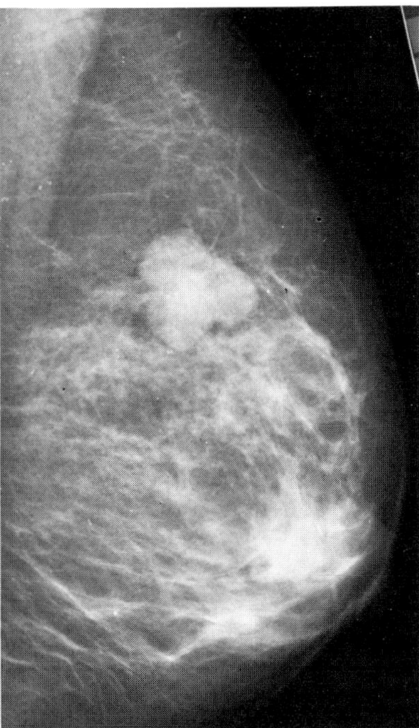

Figure 149–12. This 73-year-old woman found **a lump in her left breast superomedially.** The medio-lateral oblique mammogram shows a trilobular well-defined mass with slight comet tail irregularity superiorly. This was a ductal carcinoma with invasion.

tether the skin through Cooper's ligaments and cause retraction to occur.

Skin thickening may indicate blocked lymphatic drainage (see Fig. 149–21*B*), or it can be caused by actual tumor in the dermal lymphatics producing the peau d'orange of inflammatory carcinoma, as described previously. Metastatic spread via skin lymphatics from the opposite breast can cause thickening of the skin medially. Skin thickening, however, is not unique to breast cancer. Additional causes include acromegaly, cellulitis, abscess, diffuse fat

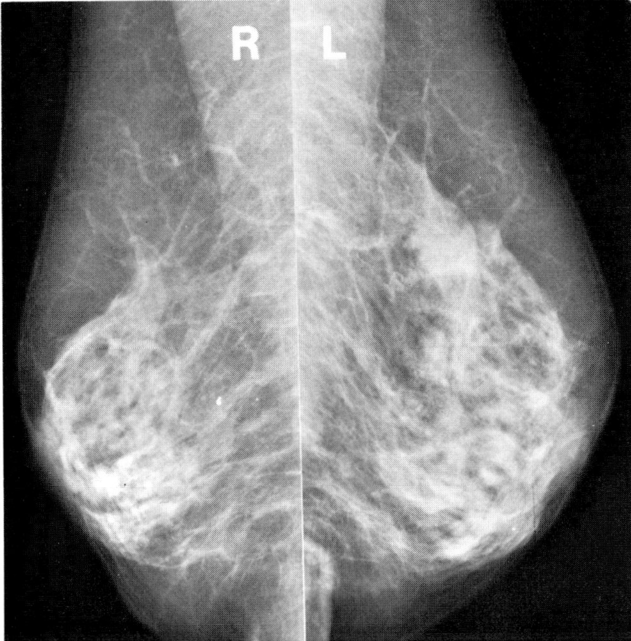

Figure 149–13. This 78-year-old woman had **a palpable mass in the left upper outer quadrant.** Aspiration yielded no fluid. Medio-lateral oblique mammograms of the right and left breast show an area of increased density in the left breast superiorly. Ultrasound demonstrated a solid mass, and excisional biopsy revealed infiltrating ductal carcinoma. The patient was treated with lumpectomy and radiation (see Fig. 149–19).

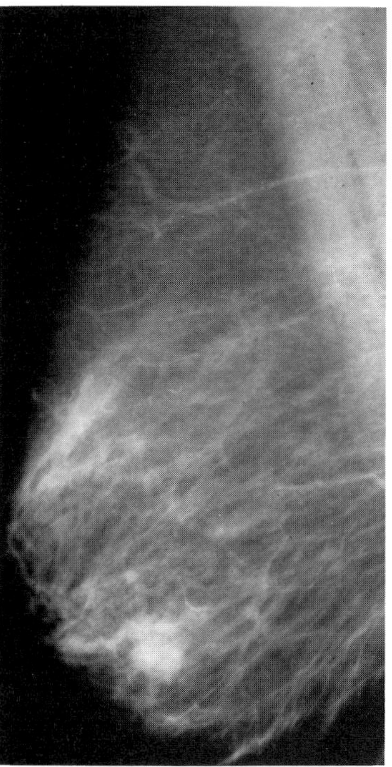

Figure 149–14. A 48-year-old woman presented with **yellow discharge from the right nipple.** Mediolateral oblique view shows a single dilated duct leading to a mass in the inferior central breast, which was infiltrating carcinoma. Note vascular calcifications.

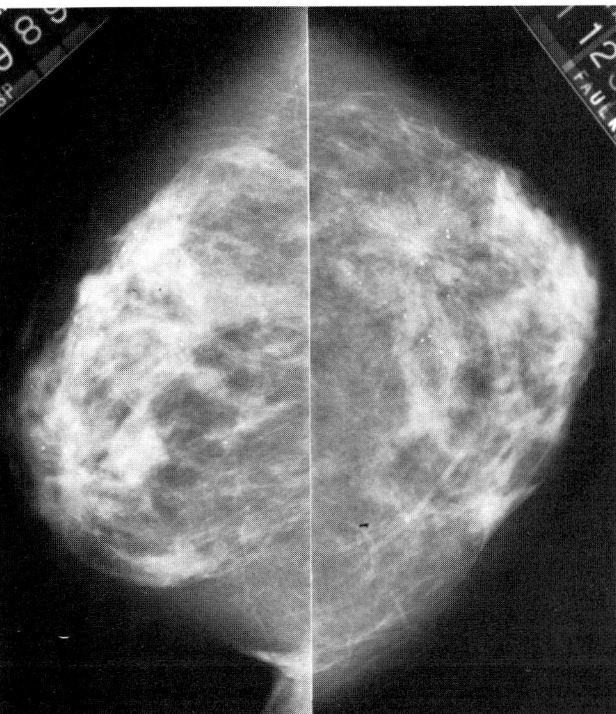

Figure 149–15. A 56-year-old woman with no palpable mass. Right lateral and craniocaudal mammograms reveal **starburst distortion with some surrounding calcifications** in the upper outer quadrant. The primary lesion was quite small, with a great deal of desmoplastic reaction giving rise to this distortion.

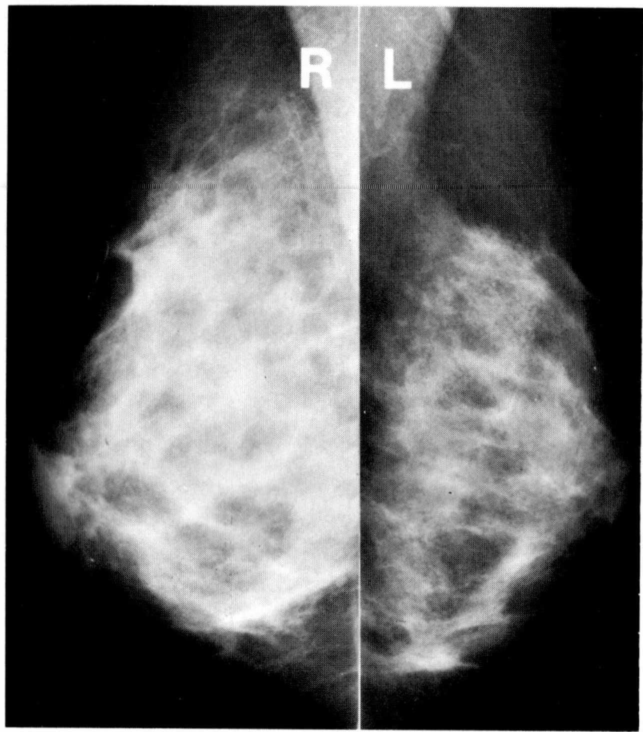

Figure 149–16. A 38-year-old woman with **a palpable mass in the superior right breast.** Comparative right and left medio-lateral oblique films shown with a wire placed on the mass. Note the generalized increased density of the right breast as well as skin thickening about the areola and extensive calcification. This proved to be an infiltrating ductal carcinoma with edema related to positive nodes but with no tumor found in dermal lymphatics.

necrosis, congestive heart failure, and dermatologic conditions. Usually these can be distinguished clinically. Irradiation of the breast following lumpectomy for carcinoma often produces skin edema that is distributed in a characteristic fashion in the periareolar region extending medially and inferiorly (Fig. 149–19).

Paget's disease is usually discovered clinically with characteristic eczematoid appearance involving the nipple and areola, which can progress to a weeping, ulcerating lesion. Radiologically, there are frequently no skin findings, but occasionally Paget's disease is seen as a thickening of the skin of the areola or the nipple, or both. This is virtually always associated with a ductal carcinoma deeper in the breast (see Fig. 149–14), and often calcification can be seen coursing through the ducts toward the nipple, even extending out onto the skin to involve the nipple and areola (Fig. 149–20).

VASCULAR ASYMMETRY. This sign is not a very important one of carcinoma, since it can be seen normally and can even vary at different times in the same patient depending on the degree or method of compression. In our experience, asymmetric vessels are most often seen with obvious carcinomas and are occasionally seen in the contralateral normal breast (see Fig. 149–7*A*). A marked asymmetry of vascularity indicates that the breasts should be examined more carefully, especially when associated with a palpable mass. Dodd has found a ratio of venous diameters of at least 1.4 to 1 in 75 per cent of patients with relatively large breast cancers.

AXILLARY NODES. Involved axillary nodes represent a failure of early detection and significantly worsen the prognosis. Unfortunately, in some women, enlarged axillary nodes may be the first sign of carcinoma. Such adenopathy is usually associated with a

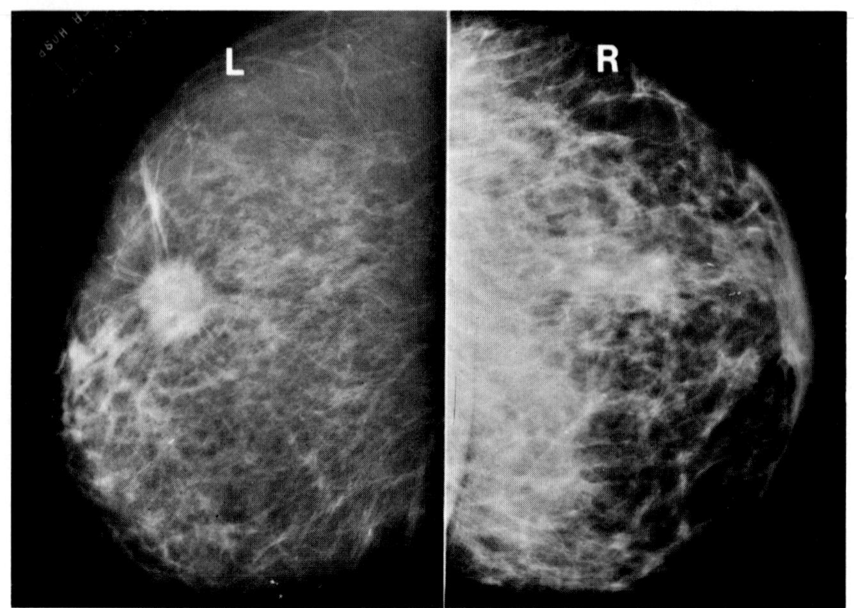

Figure 149–17. A 76-year-old woman presents with **bilateral breast cancer.** Sunburst lesion on the left (lateral view) and typical inflammatory carcinoma on the right (craniocaudal view). A mass is not seen in the right breast, but there is some ductal calcification. Skin thickening and diffuse edema on the right are obvious, especially by comparison with the left.

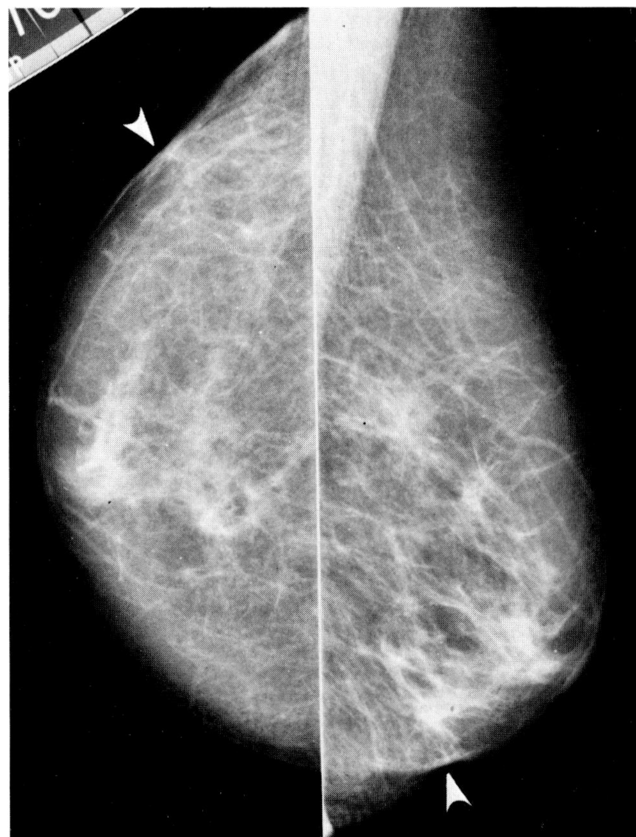

Figure 149–18. A 77-year-old woman with previous biopsy in the upper outer quadrant of the left breast. Routine craniocaudal and lateral mammograms show skin retraction laterally in the craniocaudal view of the left breast at a previous biopsy site *(arrow)*. Retraction of inferior skin seen on the lateral view *(arrow)* was not evident on the previous exam and was the only sign of **a poorly differentiated carcinoma** that extended to within 2 mm of the dermis.

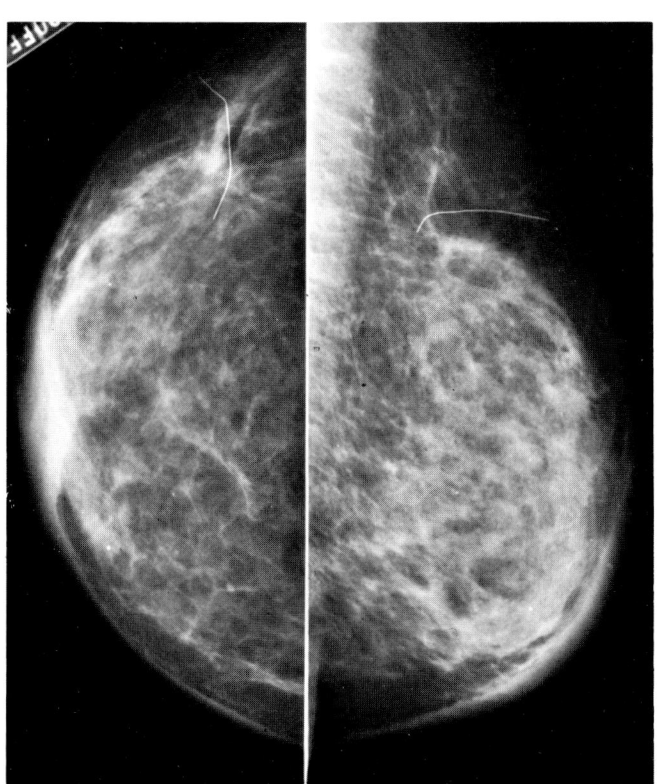

Figure 149–19. Same patient as in Figure 149–13. Craniocaudal and lateral views of the left breast showing **typical changes following lumpectomy and irradiation**. The wire is placed on the lumpectomy scar; distortion beneath the scar can be confused with that seen in carcinoma. The distribution of skin thickening following irradiation tends to be periareolar, inferior, and medial even if the lesion is in the upper outer quadrant, as it was in this case. This distribution of edema is thought to be related to dependency.

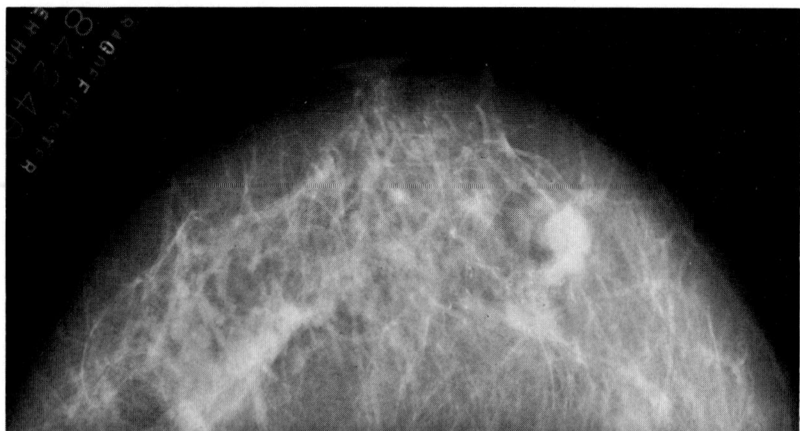

Figure 149–20. A 59-year-old woman presented with **slight thickening of the right breast and scaling of the nipple.** Craniocaudal view shows two nodular lesions in the medial breast, which were infiltrating ductal carcinomas. Note the widespread calcifications extending along ducts reaching the nipple, resulting in Paget's disease. Such intraductal involvement corresponds to the pathologic term *comedo carcinoma.*

mammographically evident lesion in the ipsilateral breast. At times, the primary tumor in the breast is microscopic and cannot be found even by pathologic sectioning of the mastectomy tissue (Fig. 149–21*B*).

Radiographically, metastatic nodes are usually dense, without fatty centers, and have lobulated or angulated borders. Individually, they tend to be large (over 2.5 cm) and may be matted together with loss of the pericapsular fat line. Metastatic nodes may be smooth and indistinguishable radiologically from reactive hyperplasia. Benign nodes, even if enlarged, can often be distinguished by their fatty centers (Fig. 149–21*A*).

CALCIFICATIONS. Clustered microcalcifications are the single most common sign of early breast carcinoma and very often occur as the only sign in such cases. Calcifications in the breast are often so obviously benign that they present no diagnostic problem, as when associated with fibroadenoma, secretory disease, arteriosclerosis, or skin deposits. A fairly common and somewhat misdiagnosed form of benign calcifications is milk-of-calcium within tiny cysts as described by Sickles and Abele (Fig. 149–22).

It is imperative to obtain craniocaudal and 90-degree lateral spot magnification views of the microcalcifications in order to make the diagnosis of benign milk-of-calcium. On the craniocaudal view, the calcifications tend to appear round and faint with blurred margins, whereas on the 90-degree lateral view, the calcifications appear more dense and assume a linear or curvilinear configuration as the calcium settles, forming a meniscus in the bottom of a tiny cyst. If an oblique magnification view is obtained instead of the recommended 90-degree lateral magnification view, this characteristic appearance may not be discernible.

Skin calcifications are usually easily distinguished because of the characteristic central lucency and distribution close to a skin surface, often in the medial and inferior aspects of the breast or in the axillary tail. In some cases it may be necessary to perform a localization procedure to place the calcifications in a tangential position to prove that they are dermal and therefore benign.

The microcalcifications found in association with 40 per cent of malignant masses also present no diagnostic problem (Fig. 149–23). When microcalcifications are the only visible abnormality, they do present difficulties. Mammography's ability to detect microcalcifications has made pathologists more aware of their presence in microscopic sections, and when special stains are used, 60 per cent of cancers may be found to contain calcifications. Radiography of the specimen may show that as many as 86 per cent of carcinomas contain calcium.

Characteristics of Tumor Calcifications. Suspicious calcifications are small, usually varying from 100 to 300 μ, but rarely they may be as large as 2 mm. Malignant calcifications tend to be pleomorphic varying in size, shape, and density. Of particular concern are the linear or branching (casting) forms and the so-called granular-type calcifications. The calcifications may be clustered (five or more calcifications within 1 cm^3 of tissue) or may be more widespread within a segment of the breast. In ductal carcinoma in situ (DCIS) of the comedo type, the calcifications may line up in the course of a duct system. The micropapillary and cribriform types of DCIS are usually more rounded and are seen in multiple clusters. The calcifications of comedo carcinoma are usually a fairly good indication of the extent of disease within the breast so that excising a 2-cm margin of tissue around the visible calcifications will result in complete excision in 86 per cent of cases. The calcification of comedo carcinoma occurs in necrotic tumor cells in the center of the ducts, creating the casting appearance. In the micropapillary or cribriform type of DCIS, the calcification is occurring in fluid secreted by the tumor cells and therefore tends to be more spotty in distribution. Because of this difference, the calcifications in comedo DCIS are a very good marker of the extent of disease, whereas the spotty nature of the calcifications in cribriform and

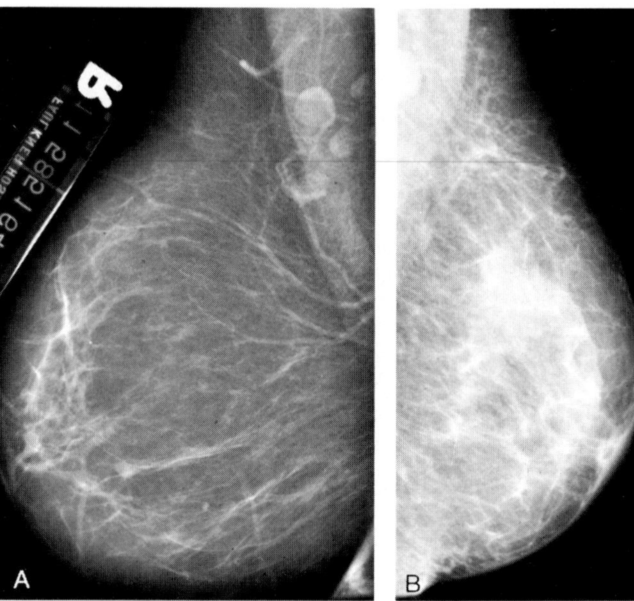

Figure 149–21. *A,* **Normal benign fatty axillary lymph nodes.** *B,* **Metastatic lymph node** in a 46-year-old woman who presented with an erythematous left breast and skin thickening. No mass was found in the breast, but axillary lymph nodes were palpable. The edema was due to lymphatic obstruction, and there were no tumor cells in dermal lymphatics, indicating that it was not inflammatory carcinoma.

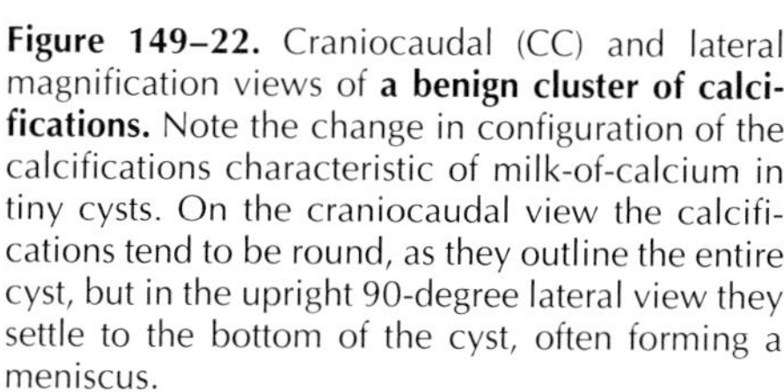

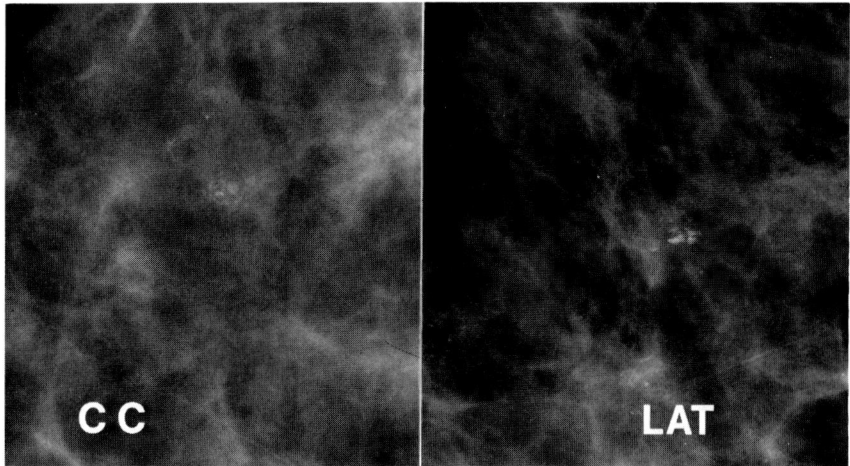

Figure 149–22. Craniocaudal (CC) and lateral magnification views of **a benign cluster of calcifications.** Note the change in configuration of the calcifications characteristic of milk-of-calcium in tiny cysts. On the craniocaudal view the calcifications tend to be round, as they outline the entire cyst, but in the upright 90-degree lateral view they settle to the bottom of the cyst, often forming a meniscus.

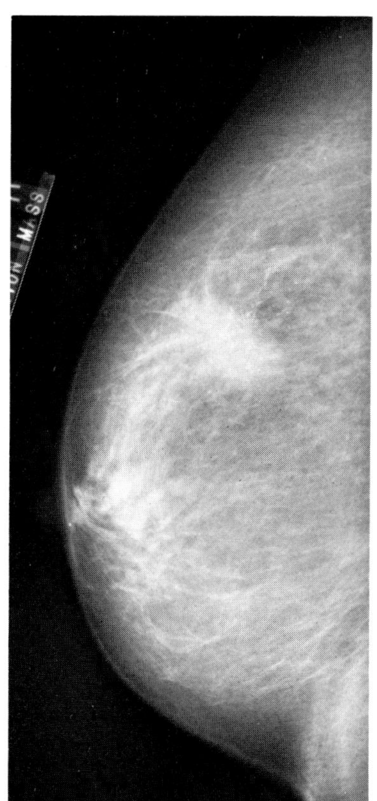

Figure 149–23. A 78-year-old woman with **palpable mass in the upper central right breast**. The lateral view shows a typical irregular carcinoma with diffuse calcifications.

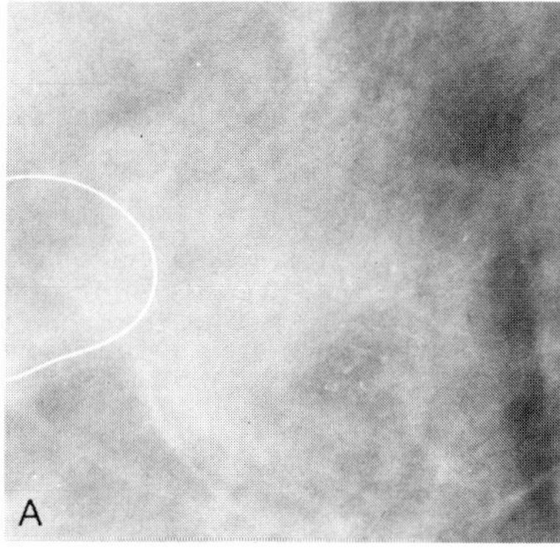

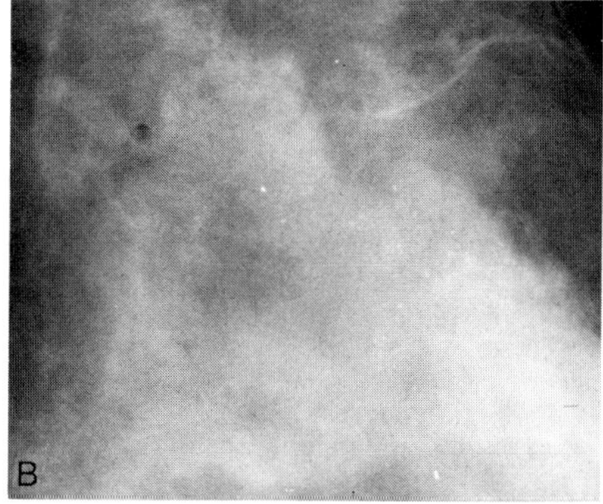

Figure 149–24. *A*, A magnification lateral view of a 39-year-old woman showing many more calcifications than could be appreciated by routine (nonmagnified) views. The pleomorphism of the calcifications could be appreciated only in the magnification view. This was **invasive ductal carcinoma**. *B*, Lateral magnification view of an asymptomatic 42-year-old woman shows many more calcifications than routine film and demonstrates lack of pleomorphism. The calcifications were believed to be benign, but we still recommended biopsy which showed proliferative changes with **ductal hyperplasia, adenosis, and papillomatosis,** but no carcinoma.

micropapillary DCIS make them not good markers for the extent of disease. A fairly tight cluster of calcifications over an area of 1 cm or less is the most suggestive finding. If the calcifications are more widespread but located in only one quadrant of the breast, biopsy is also recommended (Fig. 149–24). Carcinomatous calcifications can be quite widespread (Fig. 149–25), but generally if the calcifications are spread symmetrically throughout both breasts, they are more likely to be benign. Duct carcinoma with comedo elements can often develop widespread calcifications coursing along the duct system (see Fig. 149–20).

LOCALIZATION OF OCCULT LESIONS

Mammography guided localization must be used prior to an attempt at excision of nonpalpable suspicious lesions. Biopsy without prior localization often results in failure to remove the lesion in question or in unnecessarily wide excisions. The goal of early detection is not only to improve survival but to afford the possibility of breast preservation with good cosmesis. We use the spring hooked wire technique in which a needle is placed near (within 5 mm or less) or through the lesion in question and the wire is then passed (after loading) to the tip of the needle. The needle is then withdrawn, leaving the hooked wire in place. The depth of the lesion along the course of the wire is measured by placing a metallic marker (BB) at the skin entrance and imaging the length of wire to the lesion. We then provide a stiffening cannula of appropriate length for the surgeon to pass over the wire to the lesion.

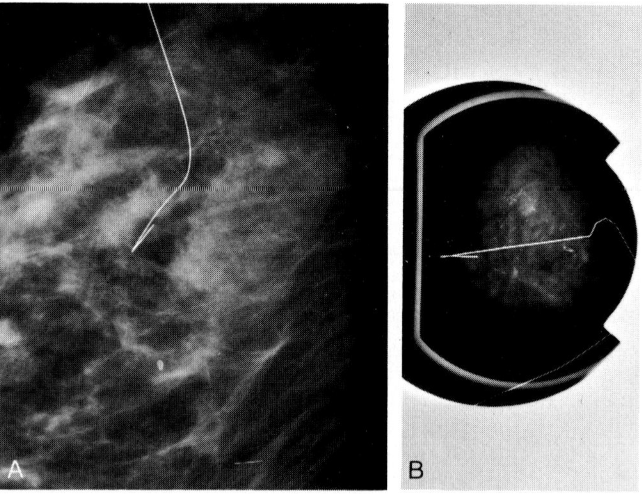

Figure 149–26. *A,* Final film of **hooked wire localization for typical malignant calcifications**. *B,* A compression specimen radiograph (different case) showing more calcifications than were seen on the preoperative mammogram. Patient had invasive ductal carcinoma.

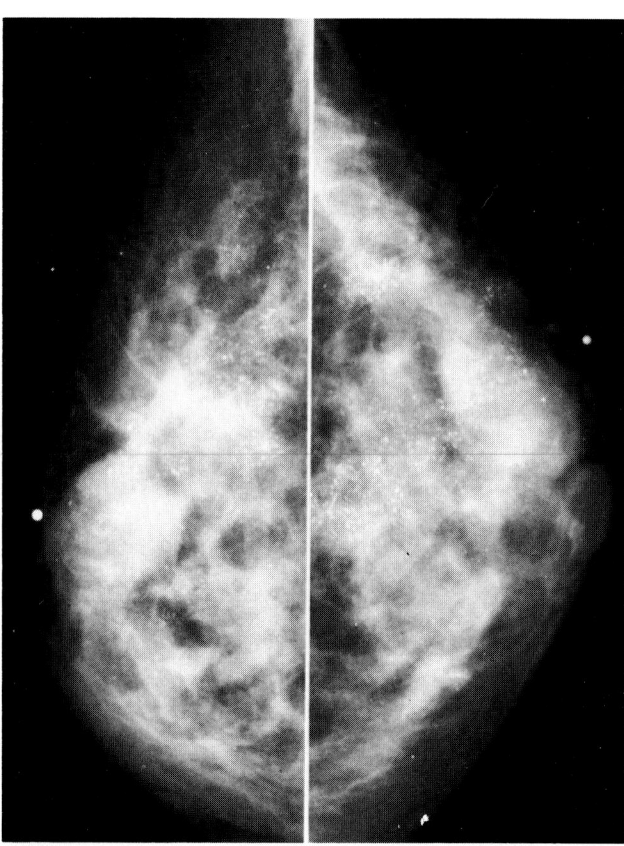

Figure 149–25. A 42-year-old woman with **a palpable mass in the right superolateral subareolar area.** The superior breast felt like "woody thickening." Right lateral and craniocaudal mammograms show a 2-cm mass lesion with a metallic marker over it. Diffuse pleomorphic calcifications spread throughout the breast. The mass was invasive ductal carcinoma, and the calcifications represent comedo (intraductal) carcinoma. Sometimes such diffuse calcifications are the only sign of malignancy with or without a palpable mass.

A specimen radiograph should be obtained in all cases whether dealing with a mass lesion or calcifications. Compression of the specimen is essential, and magnification of the specimen is recommended. The preoperative localization films should be available when reviewing the specimen radiograph to ensure that the localized lesion was removed and to aid in the evaluation of margins. The specimen radiograph is also invaluable to the pathologist in selecting areas for frozen section (Fig. 149–26).

FINE NEEDLE ASPIRATION AND CORE BIOPSY

Fine needle aspiration cytology and core biopsy using ultrasound or stereotactic mammographic guidance is playing a larger role in the diagnostic evaluation of benign and malignant disease. If the diagnosis of cancer is established, options can be discussed with the patient and a one-step surgical procedure can be performed. On the other hand, if a definitive benign diagnosis is made, such as fibroadenoma, surgery can be avoided. Positive diagnosis of a benign lesion is best made by core biopsy. As the procedure of stereotactic and ultrasound-guided fine needle aspiration and core biopsy becomes more efficacious and widely used, earlier diagnosis will be possible and the cost of screening will be reduced as the necessity for open biopsy of benign lesions decreases.

CONCLUSION

As the efficacy of mammographic screening becomes more widely appreciated, lesions at earlier stages will be more commonly detected, and the radiographic findings of palpable carcinoma will be less common. An awareness of the associated mammographic findings of occult breast carcinoma is necessary.

These findings are often not pathognomonic, but refinements of preoperative radiographically guided localization techniques permit early surgical investigation. The ability to detect and remove early breast cancer not only will result in reduced mortality, but also will offer more women the possibility of breast preservation. An understanding of this by women and their physicians will stimulate demand for breast screening.

Bibliography

Bassett LW (ed): Breast imaging-current status and future directions. Radiol Clin North Am 30(1), 1992.
Bassett LW, Kimme-Smith C: Breast sonography. AJR 156:449–455, 1991.
D'Orsi CJ, Mendelson EB: Interventional breast ultrasonography. Semin Ultrasound, CT, MR 10:132–138, 1989.
Feig SA: The importance of supplementary mammographic views to diagnostic accuracy. AJR 151:40–41, 1988.
Harris JR: Breast Diseases, 2nd ed. Philadelphia, J.B. Lippincott, 1989.
Jackson UP: The role of US in breast imaging. Radiology 177:305–311, 1990.
Kopans DB: Breast Imaging. Philadelphia, J.B. Lippincott, 1989.
Moskowitz M: Breast cancer screening: All's well that ends well, or much ado about nothing. AJR 151:659–665, 1988.
Parker SH, Lovin JD, Jobe WE, et al: Non-palpable breast lesions: Stereotactic automated large core breast biopsies. Radiology 180:403–407, 1991.
Parker SH, Jobe WE, Dennis MA, et al: US-guided automated large-core biopsy. Radiology 187:507–511, 1993.
Sickles EA: Periodic mammographic follow-up of probably benign lesions: Results in 3184 consecutive cases. Radiology 179:463–468, 1991.
Sickles EA: Breast masses: Mammographic evaluation. Radiology 173:297–303, 1989.
Sickles EA: Breast calcifications: Mammographic evaluation. Radiology 160:289–293, 1986.
Stomper PC, Connolly JH: Mammographic features predicting an extensive intraductal component in early stage infiltrating ductal carcinoma. AJR 158:269–272, 1992.
Tabar L: Control of breast cancer through screening mammography. Radiology 174:655–656, 1990.
Tabar L: Teaching Atlas of Mammography, 2nd ed. Stuttgart and New York, Thieme Stratton, 1985.

INDEX

Note: Page numbers in *italics* refer to illustrations; page numbers followed by t refer to tables.

B

C

D

E

F

G

H

I

J

K

M

N

O

P

T

U

W

X

Y

Z

ISBN 0-7216-3699-3